# SURGICAL ONCOLOGY

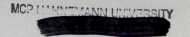
# SURGICAL ONCOLOGY

## CONTEMPORARY PRINCIPLES & PRACTICE

*Kirby I. Bland, MD*

*Professor and Chairman*
*Department of Surgery*
*University of Alabama, Birmingham*
*Deputy Director*
*Comprehensive Cancer Center*
*Surgeon-in-Chief*
*Kirklin Clinic*
*Birmingham, Alabama*


*John M. Daly, MD*

*Chairman*
*Department of Surgery*
*Lewis Atterbury Stimson Professor*
*Surgeon-in-Chief*
*The New York Hospital–Cornell Medical Center*
*New York, New York*


*Constantine P. Karakousis, MD, PhD, FACS*

*Chief*
*Surgical Oncology*
*Kaleida Health*
*Professor of Surgery*
*State University of New York, Buffalo*
*Buffalo, New York*

**McGRAW-HILL**

Medical Publishing Division

New York   St. Louis   San Francisco   Auckland   Bogotá   Caracas   Lisbon   London
Madrid   Mexico City   Milan   Montreal   New Delhi
San Juan   Singapore   Sydney   Tokyo   Toronto

**McGraw-Hill**

*A Division of The McGraw·Hill Companies*

SURGICAL ONOCOLOGY

1 2 3 4 5 6 7 8 9 0   KGPKGP   0 9 8 7 6 5 4 3 2 1 0

ISBN 0-8385-8736-4


This book was set in Minion by the PRD Group.
The editors were Michael Medina, Kathleen McCullough, Curt Berkowitz, and Scott Kurtz.
The production supervisor was Richard Ruzycka.
The cover design was by Innovative Design.
The interior designer was Joan O'Connor.
The index was prepared by Steve Shimer.
Quebecor World/Kingsport was printer and binder.

This book is printed on recycled, acid-free paper.


Library of Congress
Cataloging-in-Publication Data

Cataloging-in-Publication data is on file for this title at the Library of Congress.

# CONTENTS

List of Contributors    vii
Preface    xv
Acknowledgments    xvi

## PART I. GENERAL ASPECTS OF CANCER

CHAPTER 1. CANCER EPIDEMIOLOGY    3

A.    DEMOGRAPHICS OF THE INCIDENCE
AND GEOGRAPHIC DISTRIBUTION OF CANCER    3
*Curtis Mettlin and Margaret M. Mooney*

B.    ETIOLOGY OF CANCER    15

I. Mechanisms of Multistage Carcinogenesis    15
*Adelaide M. Carothers, Monica M. Bertagnolli,
and I. Bernard Weinstein*

II. Nutrition-Related Carcinogenesis    44
*Peter Greenwald, Susan M. Pilch, and Sharon S. McDonald*

III. Carcinogenesis by Physical Agents    78
*Joel S. Greenberger*

IV. Viral Carcinogenesis    92
*Frank J. Jenkins and Linda J. Hoffman*

CHAPTER 2. RECENT ADVANCES IN THE BIOLOGY
OF CANCER INVASION AND METASTASIS    101
*Lee M. Ellis, Robert Radinsky, and Isaiah J. Fidler*

CHAPTER 3. OVERVIEW OF CLINICAL ONCOLOGY    123

A.    PRINCIPLES OF SURGICAL ONCOLOGY    123
*John M. Daly and Kirby I. Bland*

B.    RADIATION AS A THERAPEUTIC MODALITY
IN ONCOLOGY    137
*Herman D. Suit, Bruce Borgelt, Alfred Smith,
and Ira J. Spiro*

C.    SYSTEMIC CHEMOTHERAPY OF SOLID
TUMORS    147
*Matthew R. Smith and Bruce A. Chabner*

D.    REGIONAL CHEMOTHERAPY
FOR SOLID TUMORS    159
*Maurizio Vaglini, Marcello Deraco, and Elisabetta
Pennacchioli*

E.    GENE THERAPY FOR SURGICAL
MALIGNANCIES    181
*Michael A. Morse, H. Kim Lyerly, and Bryan M. Clary*

F.    MOLECULAR BIOLOGY    191
*Alan M. Yahanda and Alfred E. Chang*

CHAPTER 4. DIAGNOSIS AND STAGING    217

A.    SURGICAL TECHNIQUES IN SOLID TUMORS    217
*Natale Cascinelli, Filiberto Belli, and Leonardo Lenisa*

B.    IMAGING TECHNIQUES IN THE DIAGNOSIS
AND FOLLOW-UP OF CANCER INTERVENTIONAL
RADIOLOGY IN ONCOLOGY    223
*Revathy B. Iyer and Chusilp Charnsangavej*

C.    NUCLEAR IMAGING IN THE DIAGNOSIS
AND FOLLOW-UP OF CANCER    235
*Tim Akhurst and Steven M. Larson*

D.    PATHOLOGY AND STAGING FOR SURGICAL
ONCOLOGY    279
*Peter M. Banks and William G. Kraybill*

CHAPTER 5. SPECIAL DIAGNOSTIC AND THERAPEUTIC
TECHNIQUES    389

A.    LAPAROSCOPY IN MALIGNANT DISEASES    389
*G. Dean Roye and Joseph F. Amaral*

B.    ENDOSCOPY IN CANCER: DIAGNOSTIC
AND THERAPEUTIC ASPECTS    411
*Rosario Vecchio and Bruce V. MacFadyen, Jr.*

C.    CRYOSURGERY FOR SOLID TUMORS    429
*Andrew A. Gage*

D.    LASERS, CAVITRON ULTRASONIC SURGICAL
ASPIRATION, AND PHOTODYNAMIC
THERAPY FOR SOLID TUMORS    457
*David Fromm, Mark Herman, and David Kessel*

CHAPTER 6. NUTRITION AND CANCER    473
*Michael H. Torosian*

## PART II. ORGAN SYSTEM CANCER

CHAPTER 7. NEOPLASMS OF THE SKIN    483

A.    PRECANCEROUS LESIONS AND CARCINOMA
IN SITU, SQUAMOUS CELL CARCINOMA
(EPIDERMOID CARCINOMA), AND BASAL
CELL CARCINOMA    483
*Charles J. McDonald, Michelle Krause, Raymond G. Dufresne,
and Leslie Robinson-Bostom*

v

B.  MALIGNANT MELANOMA   505
*Constantine P. Karakousis, Kirby I. Bland,
and Charles M. Balch*

CHAPTER 8. CANCERS OF THE HEAD AND NECK   519
*Joseph Espat, John F. Carew, and Jatin P. Shah*

CHAPTER 9. NEOPLASMS OF THE LUNG   545
*Nael Martini and Robert J. Ginsberg*

CHAPTER 10. NEOPLASMS OF THE MEDIASTINUM   571
*Christine L. Lau and R. Duane Davis, Jr.*

CHAPTER 11. CARCINOMA OF THE ESOPHAGUS   609
*Nasser K. Altorki*

CHAPTER 12. NEOPLASMS OF THE STOMACH   623
*D. Scott Lind and Stephen B. Vogel*

CHAPTER 13. EXOCRINE NEOPLASMS
OF THE PANCREAS   637
*Tara M. Breslin, Peter W. T. Pisters, Jeffrey E. Lee,
James L. Abbruzzese, and Douglas B. Evans*

CHAPTER 14. HEPATOBILIARY NEOPLASMS   659
A.  PRIMARY HEPATIC NEOPLASMS   659
*Ravi S. Chari, David P. Foley, and William C. Meyers*
B.  NEOPLASMS OF THE EXTRAHEPATIC
BILIARY TRACT   673
*Peter J. Allen and Yuman Fong*

CHAPTER 15. NEOPLASMS OF THE SMALL
INTESTINE   685
*Joshua T. Rubin*

CHAPTER 16. NEOPLASMS OF THE LARGE BOWEL   697
A.  CANCER OF THE COLON   697
*Leyo Ruo and Jose G. Guillem*
B.  CANCER OF THE RECTUM   725
*Victor E. Pricolo and Kirby I. Bland*
C.  ANAL CANCER   745
*John H. Scholefield and John MA Northover*

CHAPTER 17. UROLOGIC NEOPLASMS   753
A.  CANCER OF THE KIDNEY AND URETER   753
*Inoel Rivera and Zev Wajsman*
B.  CANCER OF THE BLADDER   769
*Sherri Machele Donat and William R. Fair*
C.  CANCER OF THE PENIS AND URETHRA   791
*David A. Corral and Curtis A. Pettaway*
D.  CANCER OF THE PROSTATE   813
*Peter N. Schlegel, Sarah K. Girardi, and E. Darracott
Vaughan, Jr.*
E.  CANCER OF THE TESTIS   839
*Steve W. Waxman and E. David Crawford*

CHAPTER 18. GYNECOLOGIC NEOPLASMS   853
A.  CANCER OF THE VULVA AND VAGINA   853
*Dennis S. Chi, Borys Mychalczak, and William J. Hoskins*
B.  CANCER OF THE CERVIX
AND UTERINE FUNDUS   883
*Thomas W. Burke and Charles Levenback*
C.  CANCER OF THE FALLOPIAN TUBE   897
*Cheung Wong and M. Steven Piver*
D.  GESTATIONAL TROPHOBLASTIC TUMORS   903
*Cheung Wong and M. Steven Piver*
E.  CANCER OF THE OVARY   911
*Elizabeth A. Poynor and William J. Hoskins*

CHAPTER 19. NEOPLASMS OF THE BREAST   951
*Maureen A. Chung and Kirby I. Bland*

CHAPTER 20. SARCOMAS   983
A.  SARCOMAS OF THE SOFT TISSUES   983
*Constantine P. Karakousis*
B.  SARCOMAS OF BONE   1015
*Patrick P. Lin and John H. Healey*

CHAPTER 21. NEOPLASMS OF THE ENDOCRINE
SYSTEM   1055
*Jeffrey A. Norton*

CHAPTER 22. BENIGN AND MALIGNANT
MESOTHELIOMA   1069
*Sunil Singhal and Larry R. Kaiser*

CHAPTER 23. SURGICAL ONCOLOGY IN THE MANAGEMENT
OF LYMPHOMAS   1103
*Omaida C. Velazquez and Linda S. Callans*

CHAPTER 24. METASTATIC CANCER   1113
A.  BRAIN METASTASES   1113
*Rajesh K. Bindal, Ajay K. Bindal, and Raymond Sawaya*
B.  PULMONARY METASTASES   1125
*Hiroshi Takita*
C.  HEPATIC METASTASES   1133
*David E. Rivadeneira and John M. Daly*
D.  MANAGEMENT OF PERITONEAL SURFACE
MALIGNANCY: APPENDIX CANCER
AND PSEUDOMYXOMA PERITONEI, COLON
CANCER, GASTRIC CANCER, ABDOMINOPELVIC
SARCOMA, AND PRIMARY PERITONEAL
MALIGNANCY   1149
*Paul H. Sugarbaker*
E.  MANAGEMENT OF MALIGNANT PLEURAL
AND PERICARDIAL EFFUSIONS
AND MALIGNANT ASCITES   1177
*Harvey I. Pass and Barbara Temeck*

*Index*   1193

*Color plates appear between pages 368 and 369.*

# LIST OF CONTRIBUTORS

**JAMES L. ABBRUZZESE, MD**
Chairman, Department of Gastrointestinal
Medicine, Oncology, and Digestive Diseases
University of Texas
M.D. Anderson Cancer Center
Houston, Texas

**TIM AKHURST, MBBS, FRACP**
Research Associate
Nuclear Medicine Service
Department of Radiology
Memorial Sloan-Kettering Cancer Center
New York, New York

**PETER J. ALLEN, MD**
Surgeon
Department of Surgery
Walter Reed Army Medical Center
Washington, DC

**NASSER ALTORKI, MD**
Professor of Surgery
Cornell University Medical College
Attending Thoracic Surgeon and
Former Chief of Thoracic Service
Memorial Sloan-Kettering Cancer Center
New York, New York

**JOSEPH F. AMARAL, MD**
President and Chief Executive Officer
Rhode Island Hospital
Director of Laparoscopic Surgery
Brown University School of Medicine
Providence, Rhode Island

**CHARLES M. BALCH, MD**
Executive Vice President and
Chief Operating Officer
American Society of Clinical Oncology
Alexandria, Virginia

**PETER M. BANKS, MD**
Clinical Professor of Pathology
Director of Hematopathology
University of North Carolina
Chapel Hill, North Carolina
Carolinas Medical Center
Charlotte, North Carolina

**FILIBERTO BELLI, MD**
Department of General Surgery
National Cancer Institute
Milan, Italy

**MONICA M. BERTAGNOLLI, MD**
Associate Professor
Department of Surgery
Weill Medical College of
Cornell University
Brigham & Women's Hospital
Boston, Massachusetts

**AJAY K. BINDAL, MD**
Staff Surgeon
Section of Neurosurgery
St. Joseph Hospital
Houston, Texas

**RAJESH K. BINDAL, MD**
Department Resident
Neurological Surgery
Indiana University School of Medicine
Indianapolis, Indiana

**KIRBY I. BLAND, MD**
Professor and Chairman
Department of Surgery
University of Alabama at Birmingham
School of Medicine
Deputy Director
UAB Comprehensive Cancer Center
Birmingham, Alabama

**BRUCE BORGELT. MD, PhD, MPH**
Assistant Professor of Radiation Oncology
Harvard Medical School
Massachusetts General Hospital
Boston, Massachusetts

**TARA M. BRESLIN, MD**
Assistant Professor of Surgery
University of Wisconsin
Clinical Science Center
Madison, Wisconsin

**THOMAS W. BURKE, MD**
Professor of Gynecologic Oncology
University of Texas
M.D. Anderson Cancer Center
Houston, Texas

**LINDA S. CALLANS, MD**
Assistant Professor
Department of Surgery
Hospital of the University of Pennsylvania
Philadelphia, Pennsylvania

**JOHN F. CAREW, MD**
Assistant Professor of Otorhinolaryngology
Weill Cornell Medical College
New York, New York

**ADELAIDE M. CAROTHERS, MD**
Assistant Professor
Department of Surgery
Weill Cornell Medical College
Senior Research Associate
Strang Cancer Prevention Center
New York, New York

**NATALE CASCINELLI, MD**
Scientific Director
National Cancer Institute
Milan, Italy

**BRUCE A. CHABNER, MD**
Professor of Medicine
Harvard Medical School
Physician, Massachusetts General Hospital
Boston, Massachusetts

**ALFRED E. CHANG, MD**
Professor of Surgery
Chief, Division of Surgical Oncology
Department of Surgery
University of Michigan
Ann Arbor, Michigan

**RAVI S. CHARI, MD**
Assistant Professor
of Surgery and Cell Biology
University of Massachusetts Medical School
Director, Gastrointestinal Surgery
University of Massachusetts
Memorial Medical Center
Worcester, Massachusetts

**CHUSLIP CHARNSANGAVEJ, MD**
Professor of Radiology and
Deputy Division Head for Research
University of Texas
M.D. Anderson Cancer Center
Houston, Texas

**DENNIS CHI, MD**
Clinical Assistant Surgeon
Gynecology Service
Department of Surgery
Memorial Sloan-Kettering Cancer Center
New York, New York

**MAUREEN A. CHUNG, MD, PhD**
Assistant Professor of Surgery
Brown University School of Medicine and
Women's and Infants' Hospital
Providence, Rhode Island

**BRYAN M. CLARY, MD**
Assistant Professor of Surgery
Duke University Medical Center
Durham, North Carolina

**DAVID A. CORRAL, MD**
Assistant Professor of Urology
Roswell Park Cancer Institute
Buffalo, New York

**E. DAVID CRAWFORD, MD**
Professor of Urologic Oncology
University of Colorado
Health Sciences Center
Denver, Colorado

**JOHN M. DALY, MD**
Lewis Atterbury Stimson Professor
Chairman, Department of Surgery
Weill Medical College of Cornell University
Surgeon-in-Chief
New York Presbyterian Hospital
of Weill Cornell Medical Center
New York, New York

**R. DUANE DAVIS, Jr., MD**
Associate Professor of Cardiothoracic Surgery
Department of Surgery
Duke University Medical Center
Durham, North Carolina

**MARCELLO DERACO, MD**
Department of Surgery
National Cancer Institute of Milan
Milan, Italy

**SHERRI MACHELE DONAT, MD**
Assistant Attending Surgeon
Memorial Sloan-Kettering Cancer Center
New York, New York

**RAYMOND G. DUFRESNE, MD**
Associate Professor of Dermatology
Director, Division of Dermatological Surgery
Brown University School of Medicine and
Rhode Island Hospital
Providence, Rhode Island

**LEE M. ELLIS, MD**
Associate Professor of Surgery and
Cancer Biology
University of Texas
M.D. Anderson Cancer Center
Houston, Texas

**NOCIF JOSEPH ESPART, MD**
Assistant Professor of Surgery
University of Illinois at Chicago
Chicago, Illinois

**DOUGLAS B. EVANS, MD**
Professor of Surgery
Department of Surgical Oncology
University of Texas
M.D. Anderson Cancer Center
Houston, Texas

**WILLIAM R. FAIR, MD**
Chairman of the Clinical Advisory Board of Health
Member Emeritus
Memorial Sloan-Kettering Cancer Center
New York, New York

**ISAIAH J. FIDLER, DVM, PhD**
R.E. "Bob" Smith Distinguished Chair in Cell Biology
Professor and Chairman
Department of Cancer Biology
University of Texas
M.D. Anderson Cancer Center
Houston, Texas

**DAVID P. FOLEY, MD**
Chief Resident in Surgery
University of Massachusetts Medical School
Worcester, Massachusetts

**YUMAN FONG, MD**
Attending Physician
Memorial Sloan-Kettering Cancer Center
New York, New York

**DAVID FROMM, MD**
Pennberthy Professor of Surgery
Department of Surgery
Wayne State University
Detroit, Michigan

**ANDREW GAGE, MD, FACS**
Professor of Surgery Emeritus
School of Medicine and
Biomedical Sciences
State University of New York
Buffalo, New York

**ROBERT J. GINSBERG, MD**
Professor of Surgery
Cornell University Medical College
Chief of Thoracic Surgery
Memorial Sloan-Kettering Cancer Center
New York, New York

**SARAH K. GIRARDI, MD**
Clinical Assistant Professor of Urology
Weill Medical College of Cornell University
Attending, North Shore University Hospital
Manhasset, New York

**JOEL S. GREENBERGER, MD**
Professor and Chairman
Department of Radiation Oncology
University of Pittsburgh
School of Medicine
Pittsburgh, Pennsylvania

**PETER GREENWALD, MD, DrPH**
Director, Division of Cancer Prevention
National Cancer Institute
National Institutes of Health
Bethesda, Maryland

**JOSE G. GUILLEM, MD, MPH**
Associate Member
Memorial Sloan-Kettering Cancer Center
Associate Professor of Surgery
Cornell University Medical College
New York, New York

**JOHN H. HEALEY, MD**
Chief, Orthopaedic Service
Department of Surgery
Memorial Sloan-Kettering Cancer Center
New York, New York

**MARK HERMAN, MD**
Chief Resident in Surgery
Wayne State University
Detroit, Michigan

**LINDA J. HOFFMAN**
Department of Infectious Diseases
and Microbiology
University of Pittsburgh
School of Medicine
Pittsburgh, Pennsylvania

**WILLIAM J. HOSKINS, MD**
Deputy Physician-in-Chief
Disease Management Teams
Chief, Gynecology Service
Memorial Sloan-Kettering Cancer Center
New York, New York

REVATHY B. IYER, MD
Radiologist and
Assistant Professor of Radiology
University of Texas
M.D. Anderson Cancer Center
Houston, Texas

FRANK JENKINS, PhD
Associate Professor of Pathology and
Infectious Diseases and Microbiology
University of Pittsburgh
School of Medicine
Pittsburgh, Pennsylvania

LARRY R. KAISER, MD
The Eldridge L. Eliason Professor of Surgery
Director of Thoracic Surgery
Hospital of the University of Pennsylvania
Philadelphia, Pennsylvania

CONSTANTINE P. KARAKOUSIS, MD, PhD
Professor of Surgery
School of Medicine and Biomedical Sciences
State University of New York at Buffalo and
Chief of Surgical Oncology
Kaleida Health
Millard Filmore Hospital
Buffalo, New York

DAVID KESSEL, PhD
Professor of Pharmacology
Wayne State University
Detroit, Michigan

MICHELLE KRAUSE, MD
Clinical Instructor
Department of Dermatology
Brown University School of Medicine
and Rhode Island Hospital
Providence, Rhode Island

WILLIAM G. KRAYBILL, MD
Associate Professor of Surgery
State University of New York at Buffalo
Chief, Soft Tissue Melanoma and
Bone Service
Surgical Oncology Division
Roswell Park Cancer
Buffalo, New York

STEVEN M. LARSON, MD
Professor of Radiology
Weill Medical College of Cornell University
Chief, Nuclear Medicine Service
Department of Radiology
Director
Laurent and Alberta Gerschel PET Center
Memorial Sloan-Kettering Cancer Center
New York, New York

CHRISTINE L. LAU, MD
Senior Resident
Department of Surgery
Duke University Medical Center
Durham, North Carolina

JEFFREY E. LEE, MD
Associate Professor of Surgery
Department of Surgical Oncology
University of Texas
M.D. Anderson Cancer Center
Houston, Texas

LEONARDO LENISA, MD
Department of General Surgery
S. Pio X Hospital
Milan, Italy

CHARLES LEVENBACK, MD
Associate Professor of Gynecologic Oncology
University of Texas
M.D. Anderson Cancer Center
Houston, Texas

PATRICK P. LIN, MD
Assistant Professor
Department of Orthopaedics
Department of Surgical Oncology
University of Texas
M.D. Anderson Cancer Center
Houston, Texas

DAVID SCOTT LIND, MD
Associate Professor of Surgery
Department of Surgery
University of Florida at Gaineville
College of Medicine
Gainesville, Florida

H. KIM LYERLY, MD
Professor of Surgery
Professor of Immunology
Associate Professor of Pathology
Duke University Medical Center
Durham, North Carolina

BRUCE V. MACFADYEN, MD
Professor of Surgery
University of Texas at Houston
Medical School
Houston, Texas

NAEL MARTINI, MD
Professor of Surgery
Cornell University Medical College
Attending Thoracic Surgeon and
Former Chief of Thoracic Service
Memorial Sloan-Kettering Cancer Center
New York, New York

**CHARLES J. McDONALD, MD**
Professor and Chairman
Department of Dermatology
Brown University School of Medicine
and Rhode Island Hospital
Providence, Rhode Island

**SHARON S. McDONALD, MS**
The Scientific Consulting Group, Inc.
Gaithersburg, Maryland

**CURTIS METTLIN, PhD**
Epidemiologist
Roswell Park Cancer Institute
Buffalo, New York

**WILLIAM C. MEYERS, MD**
Gerald Haidak Professor and Chairman
Department of Surgery
University of Massachusetts Medical School
Surgeon-in-Chief
University of Massachusetts Memorial Hospital
Worcester, Massachusetts

**MARGARET M. MOONEY, MD**
Medical Officer
American College of Surgeons Oncology Group
Chicago, Illinois

**MICHAEL A. MORSE, MD**
Assistant Professor of Medicine
Duke University Medical Center
Durham, North Carolina

**BORYS MYCHALCZAK, MD**
Clinical Associate Professor
Department of Radiation Oncology
Memorial Sloan-Kettering Cancer Center
New York, New York

**JOHN MA NORTHOVER, MD**
Consultant Surgeon
St. Mark's Hospital
Harrow, Middlesex
United Kingdom

**JEFFREY A. NORTON, MD**
Professor and Vice Chairman
Department of Surgery
Memorial Sloan-Kettering Cancer Center
New York, New York

**HARVEY I. PASS, MD**
Professor and Director
Chief, Thoracic Oncology
Wayne State University
Karmanos Cancer Institute
Chief, Thoracic Surgery
John A. Dengell Veterans Hospital
Detroit, Michigan

**ELISABETTA PENNACCHIOLI, MD**
Department of Surgery
National Cancer Institute of Milan
Milan, Italy

**CURTIS A. PETTAWAY, MD**
Associate Professor of Urology
University of Texas
M.D. Anderson Cancer Center
Houston, Texas

**SUSAN M. PILCH, PhD**
Division of Cancer Prevention
National Cancer Institute
National Institutes of Health
Bethesda, Maryland

**PETER W.T. PISTERS, MD**
Associate Professor of Surgery
Department of Surgical Oncology
University of Texas
M.D. Anderson Cancer Center
Houston, Texas

**M. STEVEN PIVER, MD**
Professor of Gynecology
State University of New York at Buffalo
Founder and Director of the Gilda Radner
Familial Ovarian Cancer Registry
Roswell Park Cancer Institute
Senior Gynecologic Oncologist
Sisters of Charity Hospital
Buffalo, New York

**ELIZABETH A. POYNOR, MD**
Clinical Assistant Attending Surgeon
Gynecology Service
Memorial Sloan-Kettering Cancer Center
New York, New York

**VICTOR E. PRICOLO, MD**
Professor of Surgery
Brown University School of Medicine
Women's and Infants' Hospital
Providence, Rhode Island

**ROBERT RADINSKY, PhD**
Associate Professor of Cancer Biology
University of Texas
M.D. Anderson Cancer Center
Houston, Texas

**DAVID E. RIVADENEIRA, MD**
Assistant Surgeon
Department of Surgery
New York Presbyterian Hospital
Weill Cornell Medical Center
New York, New York

**INOEL RIVERA, MD**
Assistant Professor of Surgery
University of Florida
Gainesville, Florida

**LESLIE ROBINSON-BOSTOM, MD**
Assistant Professor of Dermatology
Director, Division of Dermatopathology
Brown University School of Medicine and
Rhode Island Hospital
Providence, Rhode Island

**G. DEAN ROYE, MD**
Assistant Professor of Surgery
Brown University School of Medicine
Providence, Rhode Island

**JOSHUA RUBIN, MD**
Associate Professor of Surgery
Interim Chief, Division of Surgical Oncology
University of Pittsburgh School of Medicine
Division of Surgical Oncology and Biologic Therapy
Pittsburgh, Pennsylvania

**LEYO RUO, MD**
Surgical Oncology Fellow
Memorial Sloan-Kettering Cancer Center
New York, New York

**RAYMOND SAWAYA, MD**
Professor and Chairman
Department of Neurosurgery
University of Texas
M.D. Anderson Cancer Center
Houston, Texas

**PETER N. SCHLEGEL, MD**
Associate Professor and Vice Chairman
Department of Urology
Weill Medical College of Cornell University
New York Presbyterian Hospital
New York, New York

**JOHN H. SCHOLEFIELD, MD**
Professor of Surgery
Division of Gastrointestinal Surgery
University Hospital
Nottingham
United Kingdom

**JATIN P. SHAH, MD, FACS,**
Hon FRCS (Edinburgh)
Hon FDSRCS (London)
Professor of Surgery
Weill Cornell Medical College
E.W. Strong Chair in
Head and Neck Oncology
Chief, Head and Neck Service
Memorial Sloan-Kettering Cancer Center
New York, New York

**SUNIL SINGHAL, MD**
Resident-in-Surgery
Johns Hospkins University
School of Medicine
Baltimore, Maryland

**ALFRED SMITH, PhD**
Professor of Radiation Oncology
Harvard Medical School
Massachusetts General Hospital
Boston, Massachusetts

**MATTHEW R. SMITH, MD, PhD**
Instructor in Medicine
Harvard Medical School
Assistant Physician
Massachusetts General Hospital
Boston, Massachusetts

**IRA J. SPIRO, MD, PhD**
Associate Professor of Radiation Oncology
Harvard Medical School
Massachusetts General Hospital
Boston, Massachusetts

**PAUL H. SUGARBAKER, MD, FACS, FRCS**
Director, Surgical Oncology
Washington Cancer Institute
Washington, DC

**HERMAN D. SUIT, MD, DPhil**
Andres Soriano Professor of Radiation Oncology
Harvard Medical School
Massachusetts General Hospital
Boston, Massachusetts

**HIROSHI TAKITA, MD, DSc**
Associate Clinical Professor of Surgery
School of Medicine and Biomedical Sciences
State University of New York at Buffalo
Millard Fillmore Hospital
Buffalo, New York

**BARBARA TEMECK, MD**
Wayne State University
Detroit, Michigan

**MICHAEL H. TOROSIAN, MD**
Clinical Director,
Breast Surgical Research
Program Director,
Surgical Oncology Fellowship
Fox Chase Cancer Center
Philadelphia, Pennsylvania

**MAURIZIO VAGLINI, MD**
Department of Surgery
National Cancer Institute of Milan
Milan, Italy
Deceased

**E. DARRACOTT VAUGHAN, Jr., MD**
Professor and Chairman
Department of Urology
Weill Medical College of Cornell University
Urologist-in-Chief
New York Presbyterian Hospital
New York, New York

**ROSARIO VECCHIO, MD**
Fellow, Department of Surgery
University of Texas at Houston
Medical School
Houston, Texas

**OMAIDA C. VELAZQUEZ, MD**
Assistant Professor
Department of Surgery
Hospital of the University of Pennsylvania
Medical Center
Philadelphia, Pennsylvania

**STEPHEN B. VOGEL, MD**
Professor of Surgery
University of Florida at Gainesville
College of Medicine
Department of Surgery
Gainesville, Florida

**ZEV WAJSMAN, MD**
Professor of Surgery
University of Florida at Gainesville
Head, Urologic Oncology
Shands Hospital of the
University of Florida
Chief of Service
Veterans Administration Medical Center
Gainesville, Florida

**STEVE W. WAXMAN, MD**
Associated Urologists, Inc.
Indianapolis, Indiana

**I. BERNARD WEINSTEIN, MD**
Frode Jenson Professor of Medicine
Professor of Genetics and Development
Public Health Director Emeritus
Herbert Irving Comprehensive Cancer Center
Columbia-Presbyterian Medical Center
of Columbia University
New York, New York

**CHEUNG WONG, MD**
Assistant Professor of Obstetrics and
Gynecology
University of Vermont
Burlington, Vermont

**ALAN M. YAHANDA, MD**
Assistant Professor of Surgery
Division of Surgical Oncology
Department of Surgery
University of Michigan
Ann Arbor, Michigan

# PREFACE

The Editors of *Surgical Oncology: Contemporary Principles and Practice* acknowledge that solid tumors presenting to the oncologist and surgeon comprise the majority of malignant tumors that affect humans; we further acknowledge their physical, psychological, and socioeconomic impact on society. The scientific community has witnessed extraordinary advances in the therapy of neoplastic diseases of various sites over the past decade. Implicit in the management of these neoplasms is the cognitive and technical application of approaches that integrate surgery, radiation oncology, medical oncology, pathology, diagnostic radiology and imaging, genetics, pharmacology, immunology, and biostatistics among other disciplines. Each of these major disciplines contributes only a small component of the diagnostic and therapeutic approaches to clinical care; hence comprehensive planning by the general oncologic surgeon is essential to the successful management of any solid tumor.

Although there are many treatises currently available that integrate scientific rationale, clinical trials, and multidisciplinary approaches to solid tumor management, the authors have made an investment in the development of this work to provide the reader with a comprehensive text that illustrates basic cognitive principles essential to the therapy of various benign and malignant solid tumors. The explosion of scientific information is a consequence of investment and research by industrialized nations. As a result of advances in genetic and molecular biology, many hospitals and clinics are currently integrating sound, innovative principles into their screening, counseling, and therapeutic clinical projects. It is these new developments as well as the integration of advanced oncologic principles that initiated the ambitious task of organizing this volume. This work has therefore brought together many contributing authors who are renowned in their discipline for the therapy of specific neoplasms, organ systems, and the related metabolic and pathologic derangements that alter basic physiology. This text, although considered by the Editors to be comprehensive with regard to technical and operative considerations necessary to the surgical management of oncologic diseases, is not intended to replace operative atlases or standard textbooks of surgery, medicine, pathology, and physiology. Further, this book should not be considered a definitive treatise on many of the pathophysiological abnormalities that present to the general surgeon or oncologist involved in the management of tumors of various organ sites. Rather, *Surgical Oncology: Contemporary Principles and Practice* is organized to familiarize residents, fellows, and practitioners of general surgical oncology with state-of-the-art surgical principles and techniques essential to contemporary clinical management of solid tumors.

In developing this work, it was the Editors' intent, therefore, that it would coexist with and embrace other major surgical and oncologic reference texts dedicated to the treatment of individual organ system neoplasms. Hence, each chapter includes a comprehensive bibliography of carefully selected journal articles, reviews, and books that support the use of these commonly embraced surgical principles to give the reader a counterviewpoint for selection of therapy. Thus, this tome shoul be considered a distillation of seminal contributions of innumerable investigators—surgeons, internists, radiation oncologists—to the art and science of oncologic disease therapy.

*Surgical Oncology: Contemporary Principles and Practice* has been organized into 24 chapters formulated by histologic or organ system presentation and/or discipline of practice. For the majority of chapters presented, pertinent anatomy and physiology, history of presentation, technical considerations, and clinical and quality of life outcomes are extensively reviewed. This volume is not intended to represent an atlas of surgical techniques but rather one that embraces principles and management *strategies* for technical, operative, and clinical care initiatives.

Although some overlap exists among the chapters relative to organ system diseases, the chapter authors have made every effort to minimize repetition and duplication except where controversial or state-of-the-art issues are presented as opposing viewpoints. Moreover, the Editors have made every effort to ensure documentation that addresses contemporary problems that confront the general surgical oncologist. This work was therefore organized to document advanced concepts for the conduct of safe, expeditious, and anatomically planned procedures which incorporate well-recognized oncologic principles and operative approaches.

Throughout the text, the authors have sought to supplement this edition with the supportive history of the evolution and chronology of therapeutic principles. To develop and publish a comprehensive treatise on the various organ system cancers encountered by general surgical oncologists demands cooperation among the Editors and multiple contributors for each chapter, all of whom are active clinicians, researchers, and/or health-related professionals. We are therefore most appreciative of efforts of the authors and their editorial assistants who were responsible for the development of the individual chapters included in *Surgical Oncology: Contemporary Principles and Practice*.

In summary, the Editors have organized this book with the specific goal of documenting basic surgical tenets for the management of various solid neoplasms. These principles have been tested in the field of valid scientific knowledge and query and are supported as well by insights gained in multidisciplinary practice. We therefore gratefully acknowledge that the opportunity to develop *Surgical Oncology: Contemporary Principles and Practice* is the response to an immense challenge. We are hopeful that the Editors' diligence in the task has been served by achieving this goal.

*Kirby I. Bland, MD*
*John M. Daly, MD*
*Constantine P. Karakousis, MD*

# ACKNOWLEDGMENTS

The Editors are deeply indebted to the authors who contributed to *Surgical Oncology: Contemporary Principles and Practice*. We have striven to include reviews of the most pertinent clinical problems presented to practicing general surgeons and surgical oncologists. While this volume is limited specifically to oncologic diseases that present dilemmas in surgical practice, its overall purpose is to reflect on common clinical presentations managed in the perioperative and operative settings. We appreciate each contributor's efforts toward completion of this comprehensive work.

The untold hours essential to prepare this treatise represent time taken from busy clinical practices, research laboratories, and our families. Therefore, the diligent efforts of the contributors to provide insightful, state-of-the-art presentations are gratefully acknowledged. The updating of scientific knowledge by these contributors is therefore praiseworthy because of their choice of selective illustrations, tables and references to bring this text to its readable state of completeness and comprehensiveness.

Further, the Editors wish to pay tribute to the diligent work by the staff members of Appleton & Lange, who have made publication of this edition possible. Special appreciation is due to Edward Wickland, former Vice President and Publisher of the Appleton & Lange International Business and Professional Group, who provided the principal encouragement and support for initiation of this first edition of *Surgical Oncology: Contemporary Principles and Practice* and who encouraged us to bring this project to completion. Both Michael Medina, Sponsoring Editor, and Kathleen McCullough, Managing Editor of Development for the book, provided strong support for the completion of this edition: the former in the later stages and the latter through all phases of its preparation.

Editorial assistants JoAnn Ulatowski of Kaleida Health in Buffalo, Patricia A. Sullivan of Cornell Medical Center, Abby Crear of Brown University, and Caryl Johnston of the University of Alabama in Birmingham were especially helpful with oversight and facilitation of the editorial process. The Editors are deeply indebted to all of them.

The Editors also pay respect and gratitude to our residents and research fellows in surgery, medicine, radiation oncology, and other disciplines for their intellectual stimulation and encouragement to proceed with the development of this edition of the book. To the faculty and residents who have reviewed manuscripts, have offered opinions and suggestions, and have provided acknowledgment through their interest, critiques, and enlightening commentary, the Editors are also appreciative.

To our immediate families and friends who expressed interest and encouragement in the development of this text, we appreciate your indulgence for the time out of our togetherness that has allowed us to pursue the ambitious goal of preparing what we consider to be a comprehensive, readable text that embraces the general principles and practice of specific oncologic management problems faced by surgeons.

The Editors concur that the goals set forth by the editorial staff and the publisher could have only been achieved with the immense dedication to task that is evident in the contributions by the authors, the artists, and our editorial assistants.

It should also be acknowledged that Dr. Maurizio Vaglini, leading author of the chapter on regional treatments for solid tumors, passed away in August 2000. He had contributed significantly to the development of local treatment of cancer patients. He founded the Italian Society for Regional Cancer Treatment, and in March 2000, he was elected president of the International Society for Regional Cancer Treatments. He will be greatly missed.

# PART I

# GENERAL ASPECTS OF CANCER

# CHAPTER 1

# CANCER EPIDEMIOLOGY

## 1A / DEMOGRAPHICS OF THE INCIDENCE AND GEOGRAPHIC DISTRIBUTION OF CANCER

*Curtis Mettlin and Margaret M. Mooney*

### INTRODUCTION

It is nearly axiomatic in medicine that the best care is patient-oriented, with diagnosis, treatment, and follow-up made with sensitivity to the great variability of disease and response to treatment in different individuals. A sometimes less emphasized perspective holds that some aspects of disease and health can only be appreciated in groups of patients. For example, an epidemic is a well-recognized disease phenomenon that is imperceptible in an individual but can be observed when the disease experiences of multiple persons in a common time and space are documented. Similarly, physicians often evaluate patients in terms of risk factors. For this to be done, the patient must be seen as a member of a class of persons who share a trait that confers on the individual the probability of a particular outcome. Although a population perspective may seem somewhat foreign to the patient-oriented practitioner, it is one routinely applied in medical care.

The concept that important aspects of disease can be appreciated only when viewed in a group context is the essence of epidemiology. Epidemiology studies the distribution and processes of disease and health in populations. Although epidemiology is a quantitative science, it is distinguished from statistics by its underpinnings in disease, as opposed to mathematical, theory. Cancer epidemiology is the application of the general epidemiologic perspective to the class of disease defined by its underlying neoplastic pathology.

The practical uses of cancer epidemiology are several. As mentioned above, cancer epidemiology identifies risk factors for disease that can help classify persons for whom special preventive interventions may be especially appropriate. Screening for early detection of cancer in persons at high risk, counseling persons with family history of disease, chemoprevention for persons with precursor conditions, and avoidance of exposures to carcinogens in the workplace

or environment are all illustrations of applications to individuals. Because of its population-based approach, however, epidemiology may be most useful when applied at the community or societal level. Allocations of health resources can be rationalized by the epidemiologist's quantification of different levels of need in different populations, and future need can be projected from the trends in data observed across time. Measuring the potential health impact of regulation of carcinogens, determining the appropriate content of health education, assessing the effectiveness of disease screening, and monitoring the quality of care across health systems also are examples of societal applications of cancer epidemiology.

At a more fundamental level, epidemiology is a tool for understanding disease etiology. By comparative study of populations having different traits and histories of exposure, epidemiologic methods can lead to identifying causes of disease even when the biologic mechanisms are not understood. Past examples of success at this include the quantification of the effect of cigarette smoking and asbestos and radon exposure on lung cancer risk, and the importance of reproductive history in affecting breast cancer risk. Current research in this vein includes studies of diet and cancer causation, the effects of chemical carcinogens in the environment, population genetics studies, and studies of viral exposures and cancer risk to name just a few.

### HISTORICAL ASPECTS

Although the development of cancer epidemiology as a scientific discipline is relatively recent, epidemiologic insight has a rich history. Ramazzini of Padua, Italy, reported in 1713 that breast cancer occurred more frequently among nuns, a phenomenon we now account for by recognizing nulliparity as a risk factor for this disease.

Similarly, Rigoni-Stern's analyses of late eighteenth-century deaths in Verona showed breast cancer to be five times more common in nuns than among other women. In 1775, the English surgeon Percivall Pott described the common occurrence of scrotal cancer among chimney sweeps as the result of their chronic exposure to soot. Harting and Hesse investigated the high frequency of respiratory diseases among miners in the Black Forest regions. Their careful investigation and classification of causes of death clearly linked the occurrence of lung cancer with the mining environment. Ludwig Rehn observed an epidemic of bladder cancer among workers in the aniline dye industry, and his 1895 observations are looked upon as important to the development of modern industrial hygiene. These and other landmark studies have been reviewed by Holleb and Randers-Pehrson[1] and by Shimkin.[2] More modern classics of epidemiology include Wynder's[3] case control study strongly linking lung cancer to cigarette smoking and Selikoff's[4,5] multiple studies linking mesothelioma and lung cancer to occupational asbestos exposure.

Credit for progress in epidemiology also must be given to the public health officials who have developed the modern systems of cancer reporting and registration that permit monitoring of disease trends by characteristics of time, person, and place. The first large-scale cancer registry in the United States was established in Connecticut in 1935, and the National Cancer Institute undertook national surveys of the occurrence of cancer in 1937 and 1947. After the passage of the National Cancer Act in 1971, the Surveillance, Epidemiology and End Results (SEER) program of the National Cancer Institute was initiated in several geographic areas of the United States, with case ascertainment beginning with the 1973 diagnoses.[6] The National Cancer Data Base (NCDB) was established in 1989 as the first national resource dedicated to monitoring cancer care in the United States.[7] The NCDB is a joint project of the American College of Surgeons Commission on Cancer and the American Cancer Society. It is the latest in a series of cancer registration projects, which started with the first bone sarcoma registry in 1920.

## DESCRIPTIVE EPIDEMIOLOGY

Descriptive epidemiology is the quantification of disease rates and trends overall in subgroups. The subgroups that further define the descriptive epidemiology of a disease can be several, but typically include characteristics such as a person's age, sex, and race; region; and time period.

The concept of rate is essential to epidemiology. A disease rate incorporates three components: a numerator, a denominator, and a time frame. The numerator is the number of events of interest. In the case of incidence, the event is the occurrence of an instance of disease, and for mortality the event is the occurrence of death from a disease. The term *incidence* or *mortality* can be used correctly to refer to a number of cases or deaths, but an incidence rate or mortality rate must always specify a denominator and time frame. Thus, although the incidence of cancer in the United States in 1997 is estimated to be 1,257,800, the incidence rate is 410 per 100,000. Using incidence rates as opposed to numbers of cases makes it possible to compare disease patterns in different regions or at different times in a standardized manner. The number of cases of cancer tends to

increase over time simply as a function of the growth in the population and the increasing numbers of persons at risk of disease. Using rate as a measure controls for the effects of changes in the denominator and allows one to judge whether underlying incidence has changed independent of the effects of population change.

Another essential concept of descriptive epidemiology is the age specificity of rates. Most diseases, and especially cancer, exhibit different frequencies of occurrence in groups of different ages. If two populations differ in their age makeup, their characteristic disease rates will be influenced by that difference. To compare the two groups meaningfully, it is preferable to compare their age-specific rates. The comparison of the rates of each age subgroup for the comparison populations will control for the potential bias of the overall rate comparison. Age standardization is a further refinement of this principle. Age standardization statistically weights age-specific rates so that they can be combined. The combined (age-adjusted) rates for the different populations can then be compared as though the groups did not differ in age. Age standardization is particularly valuable when examining trends in rates across time. Because the population of the United States has been growing progressively older throughout this century, rates that are not age-standardized will show much greater increase across time than will age-standardized rates.

The best data on cancer incidence is from population-based cancer registries, where the complete enumeration of all occurrences of disease can be linked to a complete enumeration of the population. The United States, however, is not totally covered by registries having this degree of completeness of information. The SEER program of the National Cancer Institute bases most of its rate computations on data from nine different population registries from different parts of the country representing an estimated 13.9% of the United States' population.[6] Trends in cancer incidence, mortality, and patient survival are extrapolated to the entire country from this data bank. The SEER data base contains information on 2.0 million in situ and invasive cancers diagnosed between 1973 and 1994. Approximately 120,000 new cases are accessioned yearly. The SEER data are the principal source of information for the estimates of cancer incidence reported in the annual *Cancer Facts and Figures* reports of the American Cancer Society.[8] Another source of population-based data for the United States is the North American Association of Central Cancer Registries, which combines data from 19 registries that cover about one-third of the entire population.[9]

Hospital-based registries are important components of the cancer surveillance system. Hospital-based registries are the main sources of documentation of cancer incidence used by population-based central registries. In addition, as will be discussed later in this chapter, hospital cancer registries are the principal means of evaluating the quality of cancer patient care. However, hospital cancer registries are seldom a suitable basis for measuring disease rates. A single hospital usually has data only on some of the patients in a region and, depending on location and referral patterns, may have a patient population that overrepresents specific age, race, or socioeconomic groups. Tertiary-care facilities may tend to admit more patients with advanced disease or rarer conditions, and therefore yield an even further skewed description of a region's cancer profile at a given point in time.

Mortality data are much more completely ascertained than are incidence data. Virtually all deaths in the United States are reported by death certificate to state vital statistics bureaus and to the National Center for Health Statistics. Information on each death includes age at death, sex, geographic area of residence, and underlying and contributing causes of death. Although errors in certification do occur, all persons dying with cancer as an underlying cause are recorded as cancer deaths. These reporting practices have been in place for many years so that long-term trends for the entire United States can be observed.

The descriptive epidemiology of cancer also encompasses disease outcomes, and observed survival is the usual measure used for this purpose.[10] The observed survival rate is the proportion of cancer patients surviving for a specified length of time after diagnosis. It is typically the case that not all of the patients in a population will have been observed for the same period of time. Patients diagnosed many years prior will have been followed for long periods and patients diagnosed more recently will have been followed for short periods. In addition, the vital status of some patients will not be known because they have lost contact with the registry that was following them. Actuarial procedures adjust observed survival rates for these sources of uncertainty. An additional adjustment method used in SEER reports is the relative survival rate. The relative survival rate adjusts observed survival by expected mortality in a population. It represents the likelihood that a patient will not die from causes associated specifically with his or her cancer at some specified time after diagnosis. It is always larger than the observed survival rate for the same group of patients.

Although some error is inevitable, the sources from which most cancer statistics are derived are subject to quality control. Data are audited and tumor registrars receive continuing education to stay abreast of changes in cancer treatment and disease classification. Incidence, mortality, and survival rates, however, may be affected by many factors other than error or the underlying forces of disease. Changes in diagnostic criteria can cause a condition that would not be classified as an incident case at one time to be so classified at another time. This may be especially troublesome when the incidence of histologic subtypes of disease are being described. Changes in diagnosis and detection technology also will influence incidence rate. For example, prostate cancer incidence increased markedly following the widespread adoption of prostate-specific antigen testing in the United States. In an earlier era, breast cancer rates increased with the popularization of mammographic screening. Increased disease screening will result in earlier cancer detection and this can affect survival rates.

Earlier detection also creates a lead time, which is the interval between the time the disease is detected by screening and the time it would otherwise have been detected.[11] This adds to the overall time between diagnosis and death and, therefore, longer survival. The lead time effect, however, is a bias because it is only a lengthening of the period the person is known to have the disease rather than an extension of life by delay in death. Comparisons of the overall survival of different populations or changes in survival across time also may be biased by differences in the types of cancer diagnosed. For example, increased detection of early prostate cancer, which has a relatively good survival rate, and decreased incidence of lung cancer, which has a much poorer survival rate, will result in an improved aggregate survival rate even when the survival rates associated with each of the diseases is unchanged.

## UNITED STATES CANCER MORTALITY

Cancer is the second leading cause of death in the United States, exceeded only by heart disease. In 1900, cancer ranked much lower as a cause of death, and its rising importance as a public health problem is the result of several factors. One major factor is that the incidence of several of the diseases that formerly were leading causes of death have been reduced. Influenza, diarrheal diseases, TB, and several other acute and contagious diseases are no longer the threats they once were. Even if nothing else were to change, cancer would rise in significance only as a result of declines in other diseases. However, there also has been an actual increase in the rates for cancer partly as a consequence of the aging of the population. Cancer is a much more common condition in older populations, and lengthening life expectancy carries an increase in risk of cancer. Increased exposure to carcinogens is a third factor. Tobacco use achieved epidemic proportions in this century, and lung cancer rates swelled as a result. The effects of other factors are less easily identified but include the effects of environmental chemical contamination, increased exposure to ionizing radiation, and dietary change.

Although cancer mortality has been rising in the United States throughout this century, the trend has been more favorable in recent years.[12] Figure 1A-1 shows the age-adjusted cancer mortality rates by sex and race from the SEER reports for the 1973 to 1994 interval. Men have higher cancer death rates than women and blacks have higher mortality rates than whites for both males and females.[6] In 1990, the cancer death rate reached 321.8 per 100,000 for black men

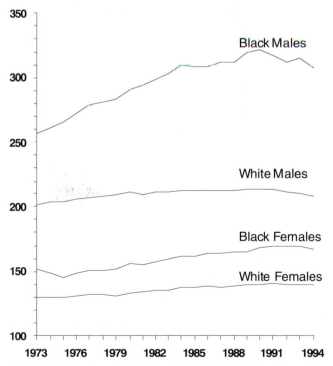

**FIGURE 1A-1.** Trends in United States age-adjusted mortality rates per 100,000 for all sites by sex and race, 1973–1994.

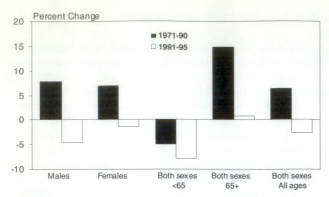

**FIGURE 1A-2.** Trends in United States age-adjusted mortality rates per 100,000 for all sites by age and sex, 1971–1990 vs. 1991–1995.

---

and 213.7 per 100,000 for white men. The highest rates for women occurred in 1991 when the rate in white women was 140.6 deaths per 100,000 and 169.7 per 100,000 for black women. The impact of the downturn in rates occurring about 1990 is further illustrated in Fig. 1A-2, where it is shown that the decline was greater in males and in persons younger than age 65.[13] Although the rates for the entire population were rising from 1971 to 1990 and only declined thereafter, a decline in cancer incidence in persons younger than 65 was evident even before 1990.

These declines are attributable to multiple factors. Lung cancer in men reached its highest incidence in the early 1980s and then began to decline. Because of the risk of death associated with lung cancer, declines in incidence rapidly affect mortality rates. A decline in United States' breast cancer mortality rates beginning about 1990 was reported in 1994. In another recent report based on SEER data, the risk of death for patients treated for prostate cancer was observed to have decreased significantly between 1973 and 1990.[14] These trends for some of the most common cancers converged with the previously established declining mortality trends for stomach cancer, testis cancer, Hodgkin's disease, uterine cancer, and a variety of childhood cancers, and resulted in the overall decline.

Continued monitoring will tell whether these trends represent a long-term change in direction in the cancer death rate. Even if the declines continue, cancer will be the second leading cause of death in virtually every community in the United States for years to come. Furthermore, the decline in mortality is in the age-adjusted rate, but as the proportion of the population living to the advanced ages when risk of cancer is greatest increases, the number of persons diagnosed with cancer and dying from it probably will continue to increase.

## UNITED STATES CANCER INCIDENCE

The association of aging and cancer risk is shown in the age-specific cancer rates of Fig. 1A-3.[6] These data also show that after age 55, men have significantly greater risk of cancer occurrence than do women. One contributor to this difference is the greater lung cancer risk in men that is associated with their historical high smoking prevalence. Another factor is that the most common cancer in men, prostate

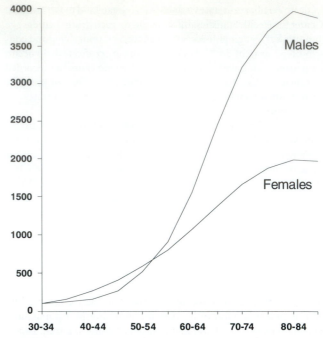

**FIGURE 1A-3.** Cancer incidence rates per 100,000 by age and sex for all sites from Surveillance Epidemiology and End Results registry regions, 1990–1994.

---

cancer, occurs late in life, whereas common cancers in women such as breast, uterine, cervical, and ovarian cancer occur more toward midlife.

Figures 1A-4 and 1A-5 show the most common cancers diagnosed in men and women during the 1990 to 1994 interval.[6] In men prostate cancer, at a rate of 160.7 per 100,000, is twice as common as the second-most-common cancer, lung cancer (79.4 per 100,000). Similarly, in women breast cancer incidence (110.2 per 100,000) far exceeds the incidence of lung cancer at 42.4 per 100,000. Colon and rectum cancer occupies an intermediate position in both men and women.

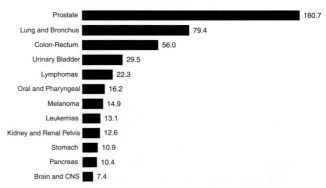

**FIGURE 1A-4.** Age-adjusted incidence rates per 100,000 for leading cancers in males from Surveillance Epidemiology and End Results registry regions, 1990–1994.

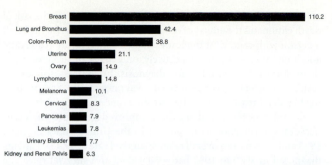

**FIGURE 1A-5.** Age-adjusted incidence rates per 100,000 for leading cancers in females from Surveillance Epidemiology and End Results registry regions, 1990–1994.

Trends in age-adjusted incidence rates for five cancers are shown in Fig. 1A-6.[6] The most striking recent trend has been the dramatic increase in prostate cancer. Between 1988 and 1992 prostate cancer rates increased 79.4%, from 106.0 per 100,000 to 190.1 per 100,000. Incidence fell during the following 2 years, reaching 144.0 per 100,000 by 1994. This rise and fall provides one of the clearest illustrations of the impact of changing diagnosis on disease rates. Prostate-specific antigen testing became widespread following published reports in 1989 of its sensitivity to the detection of prostate cancer in men not otherwise suspected of having the disease. Although this explains the dramatic increase, the reasons for the subsequent fall in rates are less clear. One factor is that the extensive screening of the population reduced the reservoir of disease that potentially could be detected. The lower rates in recent years, therefore, may represent the true baseline rate at which prostate cancer develops in the population. Another possible contributor to the decline is reduced rates of screening.

Breast cancer in women has had a long-term increase in recent decades. In 1973 breast cancer incidence in the United States was 82.5 per 100,000, and by 1994 the rate was 109.7 per 100,000. Different explanations have been suggested for this rise. Changes in reproductive variables such as delay in childbearing may increase risk. More sensitive mammographic screening is another possibility, as are environmental changes such as increased pesticide contamination.

The incidence of colon and rectum cancer is virtually unchanged in the last 20 years, but this overall pattern conceals differences in trends in colon and rectum cancer. Between 1973 and 1994 colon cancer rates were unchanged, but rectum cancer rates declined 16.1%. Overall lung cancer incidence in the United States reached a peak of 59.6 per 100,000 in 1992, and by 1994 this rate had fallen to 55.9 per 100,000. Lung cancer rates began to fall in men before they did in women due to the earlier decline in cigarette smoking rates in men.

Melanoma has the lowest incidence of those cancers shown in Fig. 1A-6, but the change in incidence for this cancer has been the greatest. The overall melanoma incidence rate doubled between 1973 and 1994, from 5.7 per 100,000 in 1973 to 12.5 per 100,000 in 1994. Melanoma incidence has been increasing 4% annually in recent years. This long-term trend is generally attributed to the greater solar damage to exposed skin that can occur in conjunction with changes in dress and leisure activity.

Cancer among children is rare, only 14.1 cases per 100,000 children.[6] Incidence is slightly higher among whites (14.4) than blacks (11.8 per 100,000). Leukemias (4.3 per 100,000) and cancer of the brain and other parts of the nervous system (3.4 per 100,000) account for more than half of the cancers among children. Even though cancer incidence has increased, cancer mortality

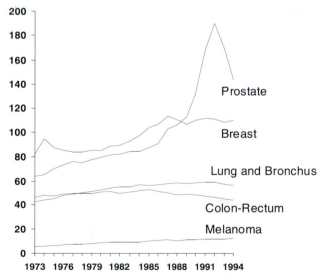

**FIGURE 1A-6.** Trends in age-adjusted incidence rates per 100,000 for selected sites from Surveillance Epidemiology and End Results registry regions, 1973–1994. Breast and prostate rates are based on sex-specific populations. Others are total population rates.

rates among children have decreased dramatically, by 42%. Cancer mortality has decreased among black as well as white children. Mortality has decreased for every cancer site; most rates have decreased by at least 50%.

## CANCER SURVIVAL

Cancer survival rates vary by stage at diagnosis, patient age, and treatment, but most importantly by the specific diagnosis. Figure 1A-7 shows 5-year relative survival rates for the most common cancers diagnosed in the 1986 to 1993 interval.[6] Because these rates are

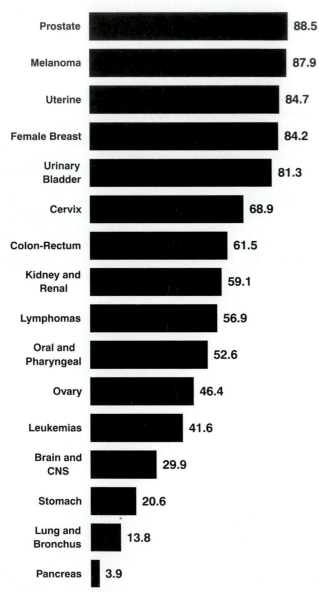

**FIGURE 1A-7.** Five-year relative survival rates for patients diagnosed 1986–1993 in Surveillance Epidemiology and End Results registry regions. Prostate, uterine, breast, cervical, and ovarian rates are sex-specific rates. Others are for both sexes combined.

adjusted for the life expectancy of the general population, the risk of death eliminates the effects of other causes of death that might befall a person with cancer. At the low extreme of survival are pancreatic and lung cancers, where, respectively, only 3.9% and 13.8% of patients survive 5 years following diagnosis. In contrast, for several common cancers, 5-year relative survival rates exceed 80%, including bladder, breast, uterine, and prostate cancers, and melanoma.

Overall cancer survival rates have improved continually in recent decades. Cancer patients diagnosed in the United States between 1973 and 1976 had an overall relative survival rate of 49.4%. Patients diagnosed in 1980 to 1982 had a 50.9% relative survival rate. The most recent data for all cancers diagnosed in the United States in 1986 to 1993 reveal an overall relative survival of 57.9%. Some of this increase is the result of improved treatment of cancer and increased probability of cure. A portion of the overall improvement in patterns of outcome is the result of the increase in the proportion of cancers with a relatively good prognosis, i.e., prostate cancer and melanoma, in the total mix of cancers.

Cancer survival rates have increased dramatically for children since the 1960s. For all sites combined, the 5-year relative survival rate has increased from less than 30% to nearly 70%. Among acute lymphocytic leukemia patients diagnosed during the early 1960s, less than 5% survived 5 years. For 1983 to 1990, three-fourths survived their disease at least 5 years past diagnosis.[6]

## INTERNATIONAL VARIATIONS IN CANCER

With cancer so serious a public health problem in the United States, it is possible to overlook the fact that from a worldwide perspective, the cancer burden of the United States is not exceptional. Many countries maintain national or regional cancer incidence registries and most collect national death data. The World Health Organization (WHO) monitors mortality trends and the International Agency for Research on Cancer (IARC) compiles incidence data from population-based registries. Incidence reports are published periodically in the *Cancer in Five Continents* series. International comparisons also are reported by the American Cancer Society in its annual statistics reviews, and it is from this source that the cancer death rates shown in Figs. 1A-8 and 1A-9 are selectively drawn.[15]

The range of cancer death rates across countries is quite large. Some extremes of rates may be the result of poorer systems of death certification that may prevail in less-developed nations. Striking differences are observed, however, even when modern industrialized countries are compared. For example, in Sweden men have only 65% the overall cancer mortality of that of men in France (128.6 per 100,000 versus 197.4 per 100,000). In women, Japan, at 75.2 per 100,000, has a cancer mortality rate that is only 68% that of the United States.

It is difficult to provide a general explanation for international variations in overall rates. Rates are age-adjusted to control for differences in life expectancy, but competing causes of death may result in the overall mortality in a region being more attributable to causes of death other than cancer. Some of the differences also are the products of different levels of medical care available in the different regions. More important, however, are differences in incidence rates and the types of cancer that are most common in the regions. Japan,

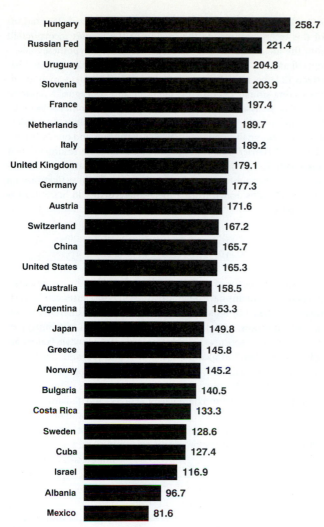

**FIGURE 1A-8.** Age-adjusted death rates per 100,000 male population for all sites of cancer in different countries.

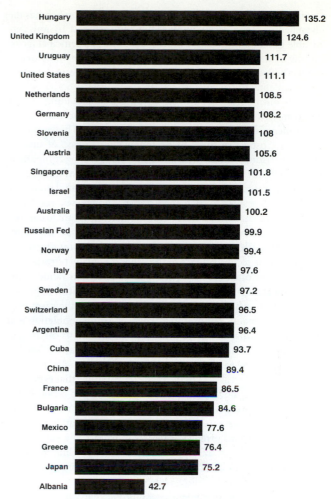

**FIGURE 1A-9.** Age-adjusted death rates per 100,000 female population for all sites of cancer in different countries.

for example, has lower cancer mortality rates in women largely because breast cancer has a much lower incidence in Japan. In men, high mortality rates tend to be associated with high rates of lung cancer. These differences often provide clues concerning the etiology of cancer. The low incidence of breast cancer in Japan has been correlated with dietary differences; the Japanese diet is lower in animal fat content than the typical diet in high-risk western nations. Lung cancer rate variations similarly further demonstrate the causal role of tobacco, with high-rate regions tending to have higher levels of cigarette consumption.

## ANALYTIC EPIDEMIOLOGY

An alternative approach to descriptive epidemiology is analytic epidemiology. Analytic epidemiology is the inference of causal relationships from comparisons of group data. The particular value of

analytic epidemiology is that it may mimic the experimental method of the laboratory scientist without the actual purposeful induction of pathology. Several different analytic epidemiology research designs that are often applied in cancer research have been described previously.[16] These include correlation, retrospective case control, prospective trials, and intervention trials. A relatively newer tool is meta-analysis, which combines multiple studies to make inferences that might not be made from the results of different studies evaluated independently.

Correlation is the epidemiologic tool best known to the general scientific community. The scattergrams that chart the association, for example, of per capita consumption of a nutrient with disease rates are familiar to most persons interested in cancer prevention research. There are logical extensions of the correlational method that also have been used. Migrant studies examine the rates of disease in migrant populations relative to rates in the host country's native population and/or rates among the nonmigrating populations of the country of origin. Similarly, changes in exposure rates across time can be correlated with changes in disease risk.

As an initial level of inquiry, the correlational approach has the advantage of being easily employed at minimal cost by any person able to plot and calculate the associations. The principal factor limiting inferences from correlational studies is the inability to distinguish between associations of etiologic significance and those that are coincidental to true disease causes.

Case-control studies have the advantage of providing greater opportunity for methodologic rigor with modest increases in the requirements for cost, time, effort, and expertise. This approach involves retrospective study of persons with a disease of interest and comparison to similar measurements made among comparable persons without the disease. Very often, in order to minimize the confounding effects of other variables, the two populations are matched with respect to such characteristics as age, sex, residence, socioeconomic status, or other factors thought important to control.

Case-control studies usually rely upon recall of past exposures by research subjects as assessed by questionnaire or interview. Although there is some evidence of the validity of many retrospective measures, they often are imprecise tools of uncertain validity. Another important limitation imposed by the case-control approach is the extent to which the technique "overmatches" the cases with comparison persons. For example, where an entire population is at uniform risk of disease due to exposure to a ubiquitous carcinogen or promoter, no comparison of cases and controls drawn from that population will reveal the presence of risk.

The principal weakness of the case-control study, that exposures be observed post hoc and reconstructed by subject recall, is addressed by the prospective or cohort research design. Prospective studies entail the measurement of exposure at one point in time and assessment of the occurrence of disease outcomes at a subsequent date. An advantage of this approach is that the baseline measurement is unlikely to be confounded by the presence of disease or faulty recall by respondents.

The highest level of epidemiologic proof, that which approximates most closely the true experiment or clinical trial, is the intervention trial. In spite of the higher level of proof provided by intervention trials, there are a number of difficulties associated with them, including such problems as noncompliance by intervention subjects and changes in habits among control subjects. Finally, the intervention trial requires greater commitment of effort, expertise, time, and funds than any other analytic epidemiology method. Because of their resource requirements and the difficulty of conducting them, intervention trials are done only infrequently. Examples of trials that have been completed include randomized controlled trials of mammography and placebo controlled trials of various possible chemopreventives such as β-carotene and synthetic vitamin A derivatives.

Meta-analysis is the application of statistical techniques to combine the results of several independent studies investigating a particular topic. It is not limited to any particular field or type of neoplasm. According to Sacks and colleagues[17] meta-analysis is primarily used with clinical trial data to increase statistical power by increasing sample size, to resolve uncertainty when studies do not agree, to provide improved estimates of effect size, and to answer additional questions not posed at the inception of the studies. Although the use of meta-analysis has increased dramatically over the past two decades since its initial description by Glass in 1977,[18,19]

its widespread application has not gone uncriticized. Limitations of this technique include the quality of the studies incorporated into the meta-analysis and heterogeneity of the hypotheses investigated and the data collected.[20] In an analysis of discrepancies between 12 large, randomized clinical trials and 19 meta-analyses investigating similar hypotheses, LeLorier and colleagues[21] reported that meta-analyses did not adequately predict outcomes 35% of the time. In no case, however, did the randomized clinical trial data and the meta-analysis give statistically significant and opposite conclusions. LeLorier and colleagues suggest that the results of their analysis indicate that the single odds ratio generated by a meta-analysis oversimplifies the complex issue under investigation and that conclusions drawn from a meta-analysis should be cautiously interpreted.

## CANCER RISK FACTORS

It is largely by means of analytic epidemiology that the major causes of cancer in humans have been identified. These causes can be variously classified, but it has become conventional to differentiate voluntary exposures, so-called life-style factors, from involuntary or environmental exposures. The most significant life-style factors are tobacco and diet, but alcohol use, sexual and reproductive behavior, and leisure activities that increase sunlight exposure also have been related to risk. Important environment causes of human cancer include exposure to chemicals, particles, and radiation in the environment. The following discussion highlights the descriptions of cancer risk factors summarized in the periodic reports of the National Cancer Institute on cancer rates and risks.[22]

### TOBACCO

Tobacco use, and particularly cigarette smoking, is the most important cause of cancer.[23] Of 538,000 cancer deaths that occurred in the United States in 1994, 164,118 (30.5%) were estimated to be attributable to cigarette smoking. The most common cancer resulting from cigarette use is lung cancer. Nearly 90% of lung cancer in men and 80% in women is attributable to a history of cigarette use. The risk of lung cancer for a long-time cigarette smoker is 2000 times that of the lifelong nonsmoker. Other cancers for which cigarette use is the primary causal factor include oral, esophageal, and laryngeal cancer, where direct exposure to the carcinogens in tobacco smoke accounts for at least 70% of deaths from these diseases. The systemic effects of cigarette use also have been linked to pancreatic, bladder, kidney, and cervical cancer.

Less commonly used forms of tobacco also are linked to cancer causation. Smokeless tobacco users have increased risk of cancers of the oral cavity. Pipe and cigar users have been shown to have increased risk of oral, pharyngeal, laryngeal, and esophageal cancer.

The life-style exposure of cigarette use also results in environmental exposure to nonsmokers. The risk associated with environmental tobacco smoke is much less than that for the smoker, but nonsmokers who live with a smoker are estimated to have a 30% to 50% increased risk of developing lung cancer. The United States Environmental Protection Agency (EPA) has calculated that 3000 to

6000 lung cancer deaths annually are attributable to environmental tobacco smoke.

## DIET

Because of the number of sites potentially related to diet and nutrition and the fact that everyone is exposed, the aggregate impact of diet has been estimated to be as great or greater than that of tobacco use.[24] For many years the international variations in cancer risk suggested the importance of diet as a factor in cancer cause and prevention. The contrasts in cancer risk between Asian and western populations generally have supported the notion that a lower-fat diet reduces the risk of breast, prostate, and colorectal cancers. It is difficult, however, to isolate the effects of specific aspects of diet from such comparisons because diet is so complex and calories, fat, fiber, and micronutrient content all are interrelated. Case-control and prospective studies have been useful in further quantifying the role of diet.

In the United States, increased intake of saturated and monounsaturated fats have been linked to risk of colon cancer but not with breast cancer. Greater intake of dietary fiber has been linked to reduced risk of colon and rectum cancer and to reduced polyp recurrence. One of the most reproducible epidemiologic effects has been the association between higher intake of β-carotene and reduced risk of lung cancer.[25] These observational findings led to controlled trials of β-carotene supplementation in men at high risk of lung cancer (e.g., cigarette smokers and asbestos workers). These studies had the surprising result of showing no protective effect for β-carotene in reducing lung cancer risk. In fact, there was some evidence of increased risk that led to early termination of the trials in some instances.

The experience with the β-carotene trials has reinforced our appreciation of the limits to inferring specific mechanisms of action from observations of dietary habits. It may be more valid to use the accrued epidemiologic data to make general dietary recommendations. One such recommendation is that the typical diet should include ample intake of fruits, vegetables, and grain products and limited meat intake. Such a diet would maximize exposure to fiber and potentially protective micronutrients such as vitamins A, C, and E; lignans; and phytoestrogens while reducing calories and fat intake that may increase risk.

## HORMONES, REPRODUCTIVE VARIABLES, AND SEXUAL BEHAVIOR

Estrogen replacement therapy at menopause has been linked to increased risk of endometrial cancer.[26] Addition of progestin to estrogen replacement therapy has been shown to mitigate this risk. The evidence that estrogen replacement therapy increases the risk of breast cancer is less conclusive, and the effects, if any, appear to be limited to long-term use. Oral contraceptive use, particularly use of the estrogen-progestin combination, has been linked to 40% to 50% reduced risk of ovarian and endometrial cancer. Although extensively studied, there is little evidence of significantly increased risk of breast cancer associated with oral contraceptive

use. Diethylstilbestrol (DES) was once prescribed during pregnancy to reduce the risk of miscarriage, but was discontinued when shown to be ineffective. In 1971 it was demonstrated that young women exposed to DES in utero had an increased risk of a rare cancer, clear-cell adenocarcinoma of the cervix. Similarly exposed male offspring experienced greater incidence of undescended testes and testicular cancer.

Nulliparity and delayed age of first childbearing are risk factors for breast cancer. Multiple sex partners and early age of first intercourse are established risk factors for cervical cancer.

## OCCUPATION

Carcinogenic agents identified in industrial and occupational settings have been catalogued by the International Agency for Research on Cancer (IARC).[27] Lung cancer is the most common tumor linked to occupational carcinogen exposures, and asbestos is the most common occupational carcinogen. Other known carcinogens in the workplace include metals, solvents, dusts, radiation, and chemicals. A broad range of tumor types is involved, including bladder, nasal cavity and sinuses, larynx, pharynx, mesothelium, skin, soft tissue, liver, and the lymphatic and hematopoietic organs.

Occupational cancer is not limited to industrial settings. Several pesticides and herbicides have been shown to be potential human carcinogens in laboratory studies, and farmers, railroad right-of-way workers, and other applicators of such materials have high exposures to these agents. DDT and its metabolites have been detected in higher levels in breast and lung cancer patients compared to controls, and increased incidence of pancreatic cancer in DDT manufacturing workers also has been observed. The evidence linking pesticide or herbicide exposure to human cancer, however, is not strong or consistent, but the possibility of an association justifies that prudence and proper protective practices be employed in the use of these chemicals. In addition to the chemical exposure related to their work, farmers may have unique viral exposures related to contact with animal herds and flocks.

## POLLUTION

Carcinogens are ubiquitous in the environment as a result of their natural presence and contamination from industrial wastes, engine exhaust, and other artificial sources.[28] Although potent at higher concentrations, the risk posed by ambient pollutants in the environment is attenuated by dilution as they spread through air, water, and soil. On the other hand, with the population so broadly exposed to pollution, its effects are difficult to distinguish from the natural background risk of disease. This may cause the magnitude of the risk of pollution to be underestimated.

Increased lung cancer incidence has been correlated with residence in urban areas with poor air quality, but it is difficult to isolate the effects of the air quality from the effects of cigarette use that is also more prevalent among urban residents. Radon exposure in homes on radon-emitting geologic formations can reach levels comparable to the uranium mining environment, which are known to be carcinogenic to the lung. The EPA has estimated that radon may account for as many as 13,000 lung cancer cases a year in the United States.

Drinking water can be contaminated with carcinogens from manufacturing; from leakage from hazardous dumpsites, as well as mining, agriculture, and forestry. Chlorination to control microbial infestations also is known to lead to the formation of chemical by-products with carcinogenic potential. Water carries asbestos particles that may affect the gastrointestinal tract. Water also carries dissolved radon, which can be released into the air when water is sprayed for washing or showering.

## MEDICINES AND MEDICAL PROCEDURES

In addition to the effects of hormones previously noted, several types of medication are associated with cancer.[29,30] Alkylating agents used for the treatment of cancer are recognized to increase subsequent risk of leukemia; Hodgkin's disease; non-Hodgkin's lymphoma; and breast, lung, ovary, brain, and gastrointestinal cancers. Immunosuppresive drugs, radiation therapy, and radioactive drugs are associated with subsequent increased cancer risk in a similarly wide range of sites. Other drugs not related to cancer treatment also appear to increase cancer risk. Phenacetin, for example, is associated with increased kidney cancer risk. On the other hand, several studies suggest that nonsteroidal anti-inflammatory drugs (NSAIDs) reduce the risk of colon cancer and the occurrence of adenomatous polyps.[31]

Diagnostic radiation is the largest single source of exposure of the general population to ionizing radiation.[32] Early practitioners of radiology suffered high cancer death rates as a result of ignorance of the risk their work posed to their health. Safety standards, equipment, and dose levels involved in radiology practice have changed considerably since those early years, and little excess risk is now seen in the physicians using or the patients exposed to diagnostic x-rays.

## SUNLIGHT

Nonmelanoma skin cancer is the most common of all cancers, and its chief cause is ultraviolet-B (UV-B) radiation from sun exposure.[33] Although less common in incidence, melanoma is a more significant cause of mortality, and risk of melanoma is also very related to sun exposure. The etiology of both types of skin cancer illustrates that the interaction between host susceptibility and exposure to risk can accentuate disease risk. Skin pigmentation is a natural defense to UV-B damage, and a light complexion is associated with increased risk of disease independent of the effect of exposure level. Thus, whites have greater rates of nonmelanoma skin cancer and melanoma than blacks or Hispanics residing in the same region. Nearly everyone, however, is exposed to sunlight and most do not experience skin cancer of any form. It appears that the human cell has mechanisms to repair UV-B–induced damage to the DNA and thereby avoid the progression to cancer. This repair capability is not present among persons with the inherited disease xeroderma pigmentosum who have hypersensitivity to sunlight and high risk of skin cancers, including melanoma.

Sunlight may have a cancer preventive role through its influence on vitamin D metabolism. Some studies have found lower levels of certain sunlight-induced vitamin metabolites in persons who experience cancer compared to controls. Prostate cancer mortality has been shown to have a geographic distribution in the United States consistent with a protective effect of sunlight. These associations between vitamin D and cancer risk, however, have not been reproducible in all studies.

## VIRUSES

The first viral cause of cancer was Rous's discovery of a virus associated with sarcomas in chickens. Although discoveries of, among others, feline and mouse leukemia viruses followed, the identification of human cancer viruses was slower in coming. Burkitt's lymphoma, a tumor found mainly in subtropical Africa, eventually was associated with the Epstein-Barr virus (EBV). Liver cancer, common in underdeveloped regions, was linked to hepatitis B virus (HBV). Viruses are believed capable of inducing cancer by their ability to integrate segments of genetic information into the human chromosome.

Modern techniques of molecular biology have made the detection of new classes of viruses possible.[34] Perhaps of greatest public health significance are retroviruses. The retrovirus HTLV (human T-cell leukemia virus) is associated with a leukemia found predominantly in Japan and the Caribbean. A related retrovirus, HIV (human immunodeficiency virus) is the means of transmission of AIDS, and, therefore, is responsible for the occurrence of the associated cancer, Kaposi's sarcoma. HPV (human papilloma virus) is yet another virus suspected of playing an important role in human cancer by its association with cervical cancer.[35]

## GENETICS

For no epidemiologic field is it more difficult to summarize the state of the art than for cancer genetics. In recent years the focus of cancer epidemiology has shifted from an emphasis on the effects of environmental and life-style factors to greater interest in genetic determinants of susceptibility. This may be in part a result of researchers' failure to account for the bulk of cancer incidence by enumeration of exposures to carcinogens. However, it must also be related to the advances that have been achieved in basic genetics research. Instead of only being able to characterize predilections to cancer crudely from racial or familial memberships, it is now possible to observe the specific genetic makeup in an individual that affects his or her risk.

The discovery of specific genes that either can be activated to induce cancer (promoter genes) or inactivated to suspend an individual's protections against cancer (suppressor genes) makes it possible to more accurately quantify an individual's risk.

Based on this known measure of genetic risk, it is more possible now that preventive interventions may be specifically targeted rather than only broadly applied. Specific genes identified for cancer include the breast and ovarian cancer gene *BRCA1*, the renal cancer gene *VHL*, the hereditary nonpolyposis colorectal cancer mismatch repair genes *MLH1* and *MSH2*, the Wilms' tumor *WT1* gene, the *RB1* retinoblastoma gene, and the *APC* gene for familial adenomatous polyposis–associated colon cancers.[36]

Although discoveries such as these represent tremendous research accomplishments, perhaps the greater challenge facing cancer epidemiology is unraveling the gene-environment interactions that possibly involve all cancers occurring in humans. To this end, epidemiologic methods are increasingly linking biomarkers of human susceptibility to observation of environmental exposure. For example, Ambrosone and colleagues [37] have observed that n-acetyltransferase-2 genetic polymorphisms interact with cigarette smoking to affect breast cancer risk, even though neither factor was associated with risk independently. Freedman and colleagues[38] similarly have reported on the interaction of dietary habits and the presence of evidence of p53 mutations in the etiology of colorectal cancer. Many other investigations of this type can be expected in the literature in the future.

## PATTERNS OF CARE RESEARCH

Although epidemiology historically has been oriented toward issues of cancer cause and prevention, in recent years epidemiologic methods have been used increasingly to study the distribution pattern of cancer care in large patient populations. The purposes of such research are several. One objective is to describe the translation of innovations in cancer treatment developed in research settings to care provided at the community level. A typical question is to assess whether a treatment demonstrated to be effective in a clinical trial or academic setting retains its effectiveness when broadly implemented in the health care system. A second purpose can be to evaluate the quality of care provided to different types of cancer patients, in different regions, and in different types of settings. For example, does it matter in terms of quality or length of life whether a particular type of cancer patient is treated in a smaller community hospital as opposed to a larger academic center?

Two different approaches to studying patterns of cancer patient care have emerged. The hospital-based approach uses the local treatment setting as the primary unit of analysis and describes regional or national patterns of care as an aggregate of these individual settings. An alternative is the population-based approach, which describes the care provided to all patients within a defined population. This latter approach relies on data collected by central population-based registries, whereas the former usually relies on data from the individual hospital registry. The advantages of the population-based approach are that it is unbiased by the patient selection factors that may affect the makeup of an individual hospital's patient population and can eliminate duplicate reports from patients treated in multiple institutions. The elimination of duplicate reports allows for more accurate determination of rates. The hospital-based strategy has the advantage of collecting data from the source closest to the delivery of care. This permits more timely data to be collected and collection of more detailed data concerning treatment than is normally available to central tumor registries. These differences between the two strategies may be more theoretical than practical, since both methods have generally yielded similar results when both are applied to the same question.[39]

The National Cancer Data Base (NCDB) is a major example of the hospital-based approach. The NCDB is a joint project of the Commission on Cancer of the American College of Surgeons and the American Cancer Society. It is a cancer management and outcomes database for health care organizations. The NCDB provides a comparative summary of patient care that can be used by communities and participating hospitals for self-assessment. The NCDB is also an integral part of the cancer program approval process of hospitals conducted by the Commission on Cancer. Hospital participation in the NCDB has increased throughout its history. In 1988, 597 hospitals reported data to the NCDB and by 1994 that number had grown to 1227. It is estimated that the NCDB data for a given year include approximately 60% of the total number of new cancers diagnosed in the United States.[7]

The National Cancer Institute SEER program has been the primary resource for population-based patterns of care research in the United States. An illustration of the application of SEER data to this field of research is the study of trends in breast cancer diagnosis and treatment by Ernster and colleagues.[40] They observe that treatment of ductal carcinoma in situ of the breast by mastectomy decreased from 71% of all cases in 1983 to 43.8% in 1992. Treatment by lumpectomy increased from 25.6% to 53.3% of all cases. They further observed that treatment patterns varied substantially by geographic region. Other SEER-based reports have focused on patterns of care for colorectal cancer and ovarian cancer. Although SEER data are often generalized to the entire United States, this may not always be appropriate because SEER data are derived predominantly from the western United States.

Patterns of cancer care in Europe are monitored by EUROCARE, a collaboration of 30 population-based registries under the auspices of the International Agency for Research on Cancer. A recent analysis of colorectal cancer patterns of care demonstrated substantial variation in the proportions of patients treated by resection.[41] Some registries reported overall resection rates as low as 58%, whereas others had rates as high as 92%. The proportions of patients receiving adjuvant or palliative chemotherapy ranged from 1% to 12% depending on region. The differences in treatment patterns were correlated to variation in colorectal cancer survival rates in the different European regions studied.

## SUMMARY

Its descriptive and analytic functions place modern cancer epidemiology at the forefront of cancer research and public health practice. Its particular strength lies in its relevance to the disease experience of human populations rather than to a laboratory model of uncertain relevance. It draws upon and is closely linked, however, to many other fields of research, including basic molecular sciences, carcinogenesis, biophysics, genetics, endocrinology, immunology, and virology. On the clinical side, epidemiology plays an important role in monitoring and measuring progress in the control of cancer. Increasingly, issues of the quality and distribution of cancer care are being seen as health care issues amenable to study by epidemiologic methods.

Given the range of areas of cancer research where epidemiology is applied, the future direction of the field is likely to be toward greater specialization. Several subspecialties already have emerged. Molecular or genetic epidemiology, pharmacoepidemiology, environmental epidemiology, clinical epidemiology, and social epidemiology are all examples of specialized fields where epidemiologic training is now offered. This trend toward specialization also leads epidemiology to greater integration with basic and clinical sciences. Hopefully, this will result in even greater research progress and contributions to public health.

## REFERENCES

1. Holleb AI, Randers-Pehrson MB (eds): *Classics in Oncology.* New York, American Cancer Society, 1987.

2. Shimkin MB: *Contrary to Nature.* Washington, DC, U.S. Department of Health, Education and Welfare Pub 76-720, 1977, pp 60–74.

3. Wynder EL, Graham EA: Tobacco smoking as possible etiologic factor in brochogenic carcinoma: Study of six-hundred and eighty-four proved cases. JAMA 143:329, 1950.

4. Selikoff IJ et al: Asbestos exposure and neoplasia. JAMA 143:329, 1964.

5. ——— et al: Relationship between exposure to asbestos and mesothelioma. N Engl J Med 272:560, 1965.

6. Ries LAG et al (eds): *SEER Cancer Statistics Review, 1973–1994.* Bethesda, MD, National Cancer Institute Pub 97-2789, 1997.

7. Menck HR et al: The growth and maturation of the National Cancer Data Base. Cancer 80:2296, 1997.

8. American Cancer Society: *Cancer Facts and Figures—1997.* Atlanta, GA, American Cancer Society, 1997.

9. Howe HL, Lehnherr M (eds): *Cancer in North America, 1989–1993, vol 1: Incidence.* Sacramento, CA, North American Association of Central Cancer Registries, 1997.

10. Flemming ID et al: *AJCC Cancer Staging Manual.* Philadelphia, Lippincott, 1997, pp 11–20.

11. Fink DJ, Mettlin CJ: Cancer detection: The cancer-related checkup guidelines. In GP Murphy et al (eds): *American Cancer Society Textbook of Clinical Oncology,* 2nd ed. Atlanta, GA, American Cancer Society, 1995, pp 178–193.

12. Cole P, Rodu B: Declining cancer mortality in the United States. Cancer 78:2045, 1996.

13. Office of Cancer Communications: Questions and answers on trends in cancer mortality. National Cancer Institute, National Institutes of Health. Press release, November 15, 1996.

14. Krongrad A et al: Mortality in prostate cancer. J Urol 156:1084, 1996.

15. Parker SL et al: Cancer statistics 1997. Ca Cancer J Clin 47:5, 1997.

16. Mettlin C: Descriptive and analytic epidemiology: Bridges to cancer control. Cancer 62:1680, 1988.

17. Sacks HS et al: Meta-analysis of randomized controlled trials. N Engl J Med 316:450, 1987.

18. Glass GV: Integrating findings: The meta-analysis of research, in *Review of Research in Education,* LS Shulman (ed): New York, Peacock, 1977, pp 351–379.

19. Altman DG: Statistics in medical journals: Developments in the 1980s. Stat Med 10:1897, 1991.

20. Eysenck HI: Systematic reviews: Meta-analysis and its problems. Br Med 309:789, 1994.

21. LeLorier J: Discrepancies between meta-analysis and subsequent large randomized controlled trials. N Engl J Med 337:536, 1997.

22. Harras A et al (eds): *Cancer Rates and Risks,* 4th ed. Washington, DC, NIH Pub 96-691, 1996.

23. Shopland DR: Cigarette smoking as a cause of cancer. In *Cancer Rates and Risks,* 4th ed, A Harras et al (eds). Washington, DC, NIH Pub 96-691, 1996, pp 67–72.

24. Clifford C et al: Diet and cancer, in *Cancer Rates and Risks,* 4th ed, A Harras et al (eds). Washington, DC, NIH Pub 96-691, 1996, pp 73–76.

25. Mettlin C: Chemoprevention of cancer: Will it work? Int J Cancer 10:18, 1997.

26. Schairer C: Hormones, in *Cancer Rates and Risks,* 4th ed, A Harras et al (eds). Washington, DC, NIH Pub 96-691, 1996, pp 83–86.

27. Blair A: Occupation, in *Cancer Rates and Risks,* 4th ed, A Harras et al (eds). Washington, DC, NIH Pub 96-691, 1996, pp 94–98.

28. Cantor KP: Air and water pollutants, in *Cancer Rates and Risks,* 4th ed, A Harras et al (eds). Washington, DC, NIH Pub 96-691, 1996, pp 56–60.

29. Tucker MA: Anticancer drugs, in *Cancer Rates and Risks,* 4th ed, A Harras et al (eds). Washington, DC, NIH Pub 96-691, 1996, pp 64–66.

30. Hoover RN: Immunosuppressives and other drugs, in *Cancer Rates and Risks,* 4th ed, A Harras et al (eds). Washington, DC, NIH Pub 96-691, 1996, pp 87–89.

31. Suh O et al: Aspirin use, cancer, and polyps of the large bowel. Cancer 72:1171, 1993.

32. Boice JD: Ionizing radiation, in *Cancer Rates and Risks,* 4th ed, A Harras et al (eds). Washington, DC, NIH Pub 96-691, 1996, pp 90–93.

33. Scotto J: Solar radiation, in *Cancer Rates and Risks,* 4th ed, A Harras et al (eds). Washington, DC, NIH Pub 96-691, 1996, pp 103–106.

34. Blattner WA: Viruses, retroviruses, and associated malignancies, in *Cancer Rates and Risks,* 4th ed, A Harras et al (eds). Washington, DC, NIH Pub 96-691, 1996, pp 107–110.

35. Hildesheim A: Herpes simplex virus type 2 and human papillomaviruses, in *Cancer Rates and Risks,* 4th ed, A Harras et al (eds). Washington, DC, NIH Pub 96-691, 1996, pp 80–82.

36. Li F, Fraser M: Familial factors, in *Cancer Rates and Risks,* 4th ed, A Harras et al (eds). Washington, DC, NIH Pub 96-691, 1996, pp 77–79.

37. Ambrosone CB et al: Cigarette smoking, n-acetyltransferase 2 genetic polymorphisms, and breast cancer risk. JAMA 276:1494, 1966.

38. Freedman AN et al: Familial and nutritional risk factors for p53 overexpression in colorectal cancer. Cancer Epidem Biom Prev 5:239, 1996.

39. Mettlin CJ et al: Comparison of breast, colorectal, lung and prostate cancers in the National Cancer Data Base to the Surveillance, Epidemiology and End Results data. Cancer 79:2052, 1997.

40. Ernster VL et al: Incidence and treatment for ductal carcinoma in situ of the breast. JAMA 275:913, 1996.

41. Gatta G et al: Substantial variation in therapy for colorectal cancer across Europe: EUROCARE analysis of cancer registry data for 1987. Eur J Cancer 32:831, 1996.

# MECHANISMS OF MULTISTAGE CARCINOGENESIS

*Adelaide M. Carothers, Monica M. Bertagnolli, and I. Bernard Weinstein*

## INTRODUCTION AND HISTORICAL PERSPECTIVE

The purpose of this chapter is to provide a conceptual basis for understanding the complex nature of carcinogenesis and to detail ways in which environmental and life-style exposures to carcinogens together with endogenous and dietary factors contribute to this multistage process. The scope of material covered will include discussions on multistage carcinogenesis, carcinogen metabolism, mutagenesis and DNA repair, signal transduction, biomarkers for cancer epidemiology, and chemoprevention. As a new millennium begins an appreciation of the long history of carcinogenesis studies and an overview of the breadth of knowledge gained in the last several decades is instructive.

Recognition that particular types of voluntary and occupational exposures were associated with specific types of cancers dates to the eighteenth century. In 1713, the Italian physician Ramazzini correlated the increased incidence of breast cancer among nuns with celibacy.[1] Today, we recognize that parity reduces the risk of breast cancer, especially in woman under 30 years of age. In 1761, Hill published a treatise warning of the hazards of tobacco snuff. He observed that this popular habit was the cause of nasal polyps. In 1775, Sir Percivall Pott described his observation that young males working as chimney sweeps risked cancer of the scrotum because of their exposure to coal tar and soot (Fig. 1B-1). The industrial development of the nineteenth century brought awareness of the role of specific occupational exposures in human cancer causation. Furthermore, the discovery of x-rays by Roentgen and of radioactivity produced by the element radon by Curie extended the categories of cancer-inducing agents.

Throughout the twentieth century enormous progress has been made in defining the pathologic cellular and molecular events in carcinogenesis, as well as elucidating mechanistically how various agents initiate and promote this process. Major technologic progress also has fueled these scientific advances. Important work in both of these areas was published in the decade between 1910 and 1920. The few historical examples noted below illustrate the large temporal gaps that have occurred between the formulation of seminal hypotheses and their scientific validations. For instance, Peyton Rous demonstrated that cell-free extracts from chickens could transmit cancer-causing factors, a finding that suggested the existence of tumor viruses. For more than half a century his work was largely ignored. It was not until 1976 when the etiologic factor was identified as the v-*src* gene carried by the acutely transforming Rous sarcoma virus, the first recognized viral oncogene, that Rous was vindicated. Similarly, in 1914, Theodor Bovari hypothesized that chromosomal alterations might cause cancer. Based on his studies of sea urchins, he postulated that tumors could be initiated by aneuploid chromosome complements arising from defects in mitoses. His descriptions of mitotic irregularities (spindle defects and multipolar mitoses) presaged notions of genomic instability and the unicellular origins of cancer. As with Rous's work, proof that carcinogenesis involves the loss of genes awaited discoveries of the 1970s when it was learned that tumorigenicity could be suppressed by fusing malignant cells with normal ones or by the transfer of specific normal chromosomes. The final cytogenetic confirmation of his hypothesis was reported in 1983 when the first tumor suppressor gene, *RB1,* was identified.

Thus, scientific discoveries in cancer research have formed bridges that link great intervals of time. Another example of these intellectual connections occurred in the first half of the twentieth century. In 1915, Yamagiwa and Ichikawa showed that skin cancer could be induced by the repeated painting of coal tar on the ears of rabbits. This result invoked earlier notions by Virchow that chronic irritation by physical or chemical means could lead to cancer. The isolation of dimethylbenzanthrene (DMBA) and other active ingredients in coal tar was reported in 1930 by two independent groups of investigators, one led by Kennaway and the other by Hieger, thus identifying the specific chemicals in coal tar that had been implicated as a human carcinogen by Percivall Pott in the eighteenth century. The structure of DMBA is shown in Fig. 1B-2*A*. These studies formed the basis for further characterizations of a series of polycyclic aromatic hydrocarbons (PAHs) as chemical initiators of carcinogenesis and stimulated epidemiologic studies of cancer in the workplace.

Although Pott was the first to record a work-related cancer in his treatise on the hazards of coal tar for chimney sweeps, in the late nineteenth century other physicians began reporting associations

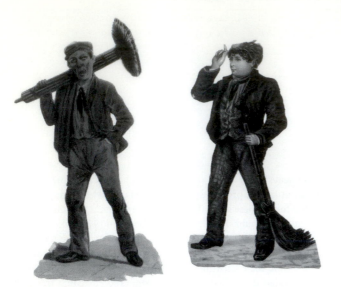

**FIGURE 1B-1.** Nineteenth-century English die-cuts depicting chimney sweeps. (See also Plate 1.)

**TABLE 1B-1.** OCCUPATIONALLY RELATED CANCERS

| OCCUPATION | CAUSATIVE AGENT | CANCER TYPE |
| --- | --- | --- |
| Fuchsin dye industry | 4-Aminobiphenyl | Bladder |
| Chemical industry | 2-Naphthylamine | Bladder |
| Chemical industry | Benzene | Myeloid leukemia |
| Plastics industry | Vinyl chloride | Hepatic angiosarcoma |
| Mining | Radon | Large cell lung |
| Mining | Cadmium | Prostate |
| Insulation industry | Asbestos | Mesothelioma |
| Furniture manufacturing | Wood dust | Nasal sinus adenocarcinoma |
| Farming/construction | Sunlight (UV-radiation) | Skin |

between specific occupations and increased cancer incidence. Beginning in the 1860s, Germany became the leading manufacturer of synthetic dyes. In 1895 a surgeon in Frankfurt, Ludwig Rehn, reported a cluster of bladder carcinomas in dye factory workmen. Epidemiologic studies implicated the arylamine, 2-naphthylamine (Fig. 1B-2*B*) as a probable carcinogen. In 1938, Heuper and coworkers confirmed this conclusion by documenting that dietary administration of this agent induced bladder tumors in dogs. Table 1B-1 lists several different types of human cancers that have

recognized occupational associations. As indicated above, by 1940 at least two chemical classes, PAHs and arylamines, were known to cause cancers in laboratory animals, and also implicated as cancer-causing agents in humans. For more detailed reviews on the history of scientific advances in carcinogenesis, the works cited in references 2 to 4 are recommended.

The last decades of the twentieth century have witnessed the emergence of modern genetics, culminating in the complete sequence analysis of several organisms (*Escherichia coli, Sacchavomyces cerevisiae, Helicobacter pylori, Caenohabditis elegans*) and imminently the entire human genome. Molecular biology and cytogenetics have provided important new concepts and tools for studying cancer causation. Research during the last several decades has validated the multistage hypothesis of the carcinogenic process and shown that the many stages reflect, at least in part, the progressive accumulation of mutations in cellular oncogenes and growth suppressor genes together with alterations in the structure of chromosomes. Within the last 20 years, the focus in cancer research has shifted to studies at the macromolecular level that have yielded profound insights into the biochemistry and molecular biology of cancer cells. A large number of cellular oncogenes and growth suppressor genes have been identified. In deciphering the roles each of these growth-regulating genes plays, the importance of the "gatekeeper" controls exerted by certain genes in different tissues (e.g., *RB1* in the retina; *APC* in the colon; *WT1* in the kidney; and *BRCA1* in the breast) has been appreciated. Derangements of various regulatory circuits that control gene expression, cell cycle progression, cell growth, differentiation, and apoptosis, have been identified in many types of cancers.[5]

The study of chemical carcinogenesis also has fostered the development of several therapeutic tools to fight cancer. During the middle decades of this century, basic research was performed to examine the biochemistry of cancer, particularly intermediary metabolism. This work, in turn, provided important insights into the deregulation of energy metabolism and biosynthetic and catabolic pathways in cancer cells. This knowledge provided a rationale for developing several very useful chemotherapeutic agents, especially antimetabolites and various cytotoxic compounds. Parallel biochemical studies in the field of chemical carcinogenesis revealed insights into

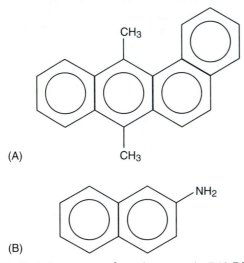

**FIGURE 1B-2.** Structures of carcinogens. *A.* 7,12-Dimethylbenz[*a*]anthracene, a polycyclic aromatic hydrocarbon (PAH). *B.* 2-Naphthylamine, an aryl amine.

carcinogen metabolism, activation, macromolecular binding, and detoxification.[6,7] Starting in 1980 when it was discovered that the *src* gene was a tyrosine kinase, biochemical studies have focused on the pathways of signal transduction and the control of gene expression in vitro and in vivo. This exploration holds great promise for the advancement of cancer research because it emphasizes the intelligence system of the cell rather than its building blocks and energy sources. Studies originating in the 1970s emphasized the use of cell culture systems, but with the recent advent of transgenic and gene disruption technologies to produce specific germ-line mutations in mice, this approach is providing powerful new model systems for understanding mechanisms of carcinogenesis. Since cells in vivo both react to and integrate signaling from neighboring cells of the same or different types, as well as from the extracellular milieu, this approach should vastly expand our knowledge of these events and thus facilitate novel strategies for cancer prevention and treatment.

Research in the area of signal transduction has illustrated parallels between the actions of tumor-promoting chemicals and naturally occurring hormones. Within the last several decades, studies on the diverse biologic effects of estrogens have been a focus because numerous epidemiologic studies demonstrate the cancer risks of estrogens in humans, and because chronic exposure of laboratory animals to various estrogens can induce tumors in target tissues. Like tumor promoters, hormones are potent inducers of cell proliferation, and they alter gene expression in treated cells. Tumor promoters will be discussed in greater detail later in this chapter. An outcome of the work on estrogens has been the development of antiestrogens (e.g., tamoxifen and raloxifene), drugs that appear to be effective in the chemoprevention of cancer. Moreover, these studies have encouraged the search for environmental chemicals that have estrogenic activity and that may act as tumor promoters. Numerous plants produce compounds of this type (e.g., phytoestrogens), and humans may be exposed to these compounds via the diet. In addition, pesticides of two classes (e.g., 2,2-bis-(*p*-chlorophenyl)-1,1,1-trichloroethane [DDT] and polychlori–nated biphenyls [PCBs]) have been found to exert estrogenic and/or tumor-promoting activity in various experimental systems. Human exposures to the latter agents occur from various sources of environmental pollution, but their carcinogenic risks to humans are not well established.

With this historical perspective as a background, this chapter will review recent findings on molecular mechanisms of chemical carcinogenesis. Many of the causes of cancer in humans are exogenous. These issues will be emphasized in order to focus the reader on the practical benefits of eliminating and/or limiting exposure to these external factors. Furthermore, the example of antiestrogens noted above suggests that modification of host responses to cancer-causing agents may be a useful strategy for preventing cancer or delaying its onset. This approach, termed *chemoprevention*, will be explored further. Certain contributors to cancer are endogenous agents; these factors will also be discussed. For many types of cancer, the precise causes are not known with certainty. Therefore, the continuation of basic research on cancer causation is an essential component of a comprehensive approach to cancer control. For instance, differences in the metabolism and detoxification of cancer-causing chemicals may affect an individual's cancer risk. Research that identifies these

differences is likely to suggest interventions for reducing risks in particular populations. The applications of these and other biomarkers to the recently developed field of molecular epidemiology will be discussed. Many promising new approaches for cancer chemoprevention using dietary and pharmaceutical agents are presently under investigation. The results of these studies should also have applications in treating and preventing the recurrence of specific cancers, thus increasing cure rates and extending patient survival. Finally, some future perspectives of cancer research will be addressed.

## MECHANISMS OF MULTISTAGE CARCINOGENESIS

### THE MULTISTAGE CANCER MODEL

The development of a fully malignant tumor involves complex interactions between both exogenous and endogenous factors. The exogenous factors include exposures to various types of environmental insults and individual life-style choices and/or circumstances; the endogenous factors may derive from genetic, hormonal, or immunologic characteristics of the individual. Infectious agents are also contributors. Examples of viruses that are implicated in cancer causation include the association of hepatitis B and C virus infections with liver cancer, of Epstein-Barr virus (EBV) with Burkitt's lymphoma, of human papillomavirus (HPV) with cervical cancer, and of human herpesvirus 8 (HHV8) with Kaposi's sarcoma. Examples of other infectious agents that play a role in causing cancer are the bacterium *H. pylori*, which is associated with stomach cancer, and the parasite *Orpisthorchis viverrini*, which is associated with cholangiocarcinoma.[8] The fact that the vast majority of cancers affect individuals over the age of 55 years suggests that carcinogenesis and aging may share some common mechanisms, and illustrates that multifactorial, multistage carcinogenesis requires a protracted *latency* period, typically decades in humans. In addition, carcinogenesis often proceeds through multiple discernible stages (Fig. 1B-3). This basic concept has been illustrated in clinical-pathologic studies in humans and in many different experimental models. A review of several of the approaches that illustrate this multistep model is instructive. From a pathologic perspective, precancerous lesions undergo stepwise changes. At the cellular level, tumors typically evolve morphologically and functionally from well-differentiated cells that resemble the normal parental type to a poorly differentiated or anaplastic unspecialized cell. Cancer cell growth also follows the multistage model since it is characterized by progressive infiltration, invasion, and destruction of the surrounding tissue, a process that ultimately leads to the development of metastasis.

In 1941, Berenblum[9,10] first stated the notion that certain chemicals that are incapable of inducing tumors alone can by cotreatment potentiate the action of a carcinogen. These agents have since been designated *tumor promoters,* a term first applied by Rous[11] in 1944. In the years that followed, studies of initiating chemical carcinogens and tumor-promoting agents have defined three critical stages in carcinogenesis: *initiation, promotion,* and *progression.* Initiation involves cellular DNA damage that results in an irreversible genetic

## 1. Initiation

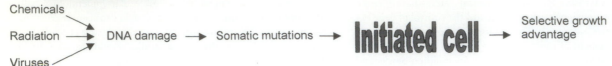

Chemicals

Radiation → DNA damage → Somatic mutations → **Initiated cell** → Selective growth advantage

Viruses

## 2. Promotion

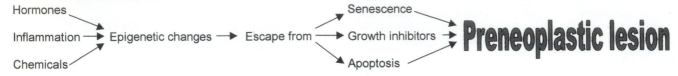

Hormones

Inflammation → Epigenetic changes → Escape from → Senescence / Growth inhibitors / Apoptosis → **Preneoplastic lesion**

Chemicals

## 3. Progression

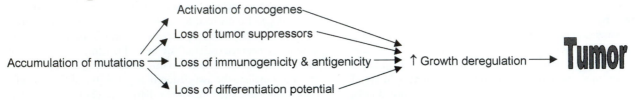

Accumulation of mutations → Activation of oncogenes / Loss of tumor suppressors / Loss of immunogenicity & antigenicity / Loss of differentiation potential → ↑ Growth deregulation → **Tumor**

## 4. Metastasis

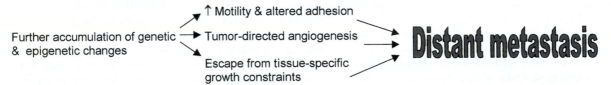

Further accumulation of genetic & epigenetic changes → ↑ Motility & altered adhesion / Tumor-directed angiogenesis / Escape from tissue-specific growth constraints → **Distant metastasis**

**FIGURE 1B-3.** Multistage carcinogenesis.

---

alteration of the target cell. The heritable change is assumed to confer upon the initiated cell a selective growth advantage or to extend its life span. The promotion phase of carcinogenesis encompasses those events needed to produce a benign lesion from the progeny of initiated cells. Regarding initiating and promotional exposures, it appears that a threshold level is required for the latter but not the former. During the progression phase, the conversion of a benign lesion to a malignant tumor is effected. Progression also includes the further evolution of a tumor that causes it to manifest increasing degrees of malignancy. The experimental models that have been devised to discriminate the effects of initiating and promoting agents are discussed below.

### THE CLONAL ORIGIN OF CANCER MODEL

The idea that carcinogenesis is a multistage process logically stems from *the clonal origin of cancer* concept. As already noted, Bovari was

the first to articulate the stemline idea. However, the concept that cancer arises from a single initiated cell has been revisited throughout the twentieth century by other investigators. For instance, in 1937, Furth and Kahn[12] demonstrated that passage of a transplantable leukemia from one mouse to another could be achieved using a single cell. Cytogeneticists have compiled convincing evidence supporting the clonal origin of cancer hypothesis as well. Although multiple karyotypic alterations in metaphase chromosomes are typical in a late-stage neoplasm, relatively few deviations from the normal banding pattern appear in certain types of leukemias. Acute promyelocytic leukemia illustrates the fact that single rather than multiple chromosomal aberrations are pathognomonic in certain leukemias; a (15;17) translocation is the only cytogenetic anomaly in 90% of cases. For this reason, leukemia and lymphoma cells were used for karyotypic comparisons with their normal counterparts. In 1960, Nowell and Hungerford[13,14] described a specific chromosomal abnormality detectable in chronic myelogenous leukemia (CML). The small acrocentric chromosome found in leukemic cells of CML

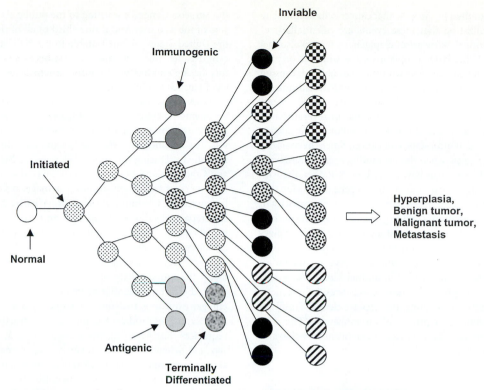

**FIGURE 1B-4.** Clonal expansion and evolution of genetically heterogeneous cells.

patients was designated the Philadelphia chromosome. This work strongly supported the clonal origin of cancer concept because consistently the same genetic alteration, a balanced translocation, was observed in all cases of a specific human cancer. Figure 1B-4 depicts the clonal evolution of neoplasia. Interestingly, cytogenetic studies of the 1970s and 1980s provided evidence that malignant cells are more genetically unstable than normal cells of the same type.[15] These observations have since coalesced with mutational mechanism and DNA repair studies by others to create another important concept in cancer biology, the idea that cancer cells display a *genomic instability* phenotype.

## GENETIC VERSUS EPIGENETIC FACTORS IN CANCER PROGRESSION

Based on the large number of mutations detectable in tumor cells and considering that the spontaneous rate of mutation in mammalian somatic cells is very low ($<10^{-9}$ per cell per generation), Loeb et al.[16,17] proposed in 1974 that cancer cells exhibit a *mutator phenotype*. The mutator concept provided a mechanism to explain how tumors can acquire their numerous different abnormal growth characteristics. The phenotypic properties of tumor cells, Loeb suggested, reflect their genotypes, which have accumulated random mutations in genes specifying regulators of cell growth and survival. His concept stated that tumor evolution is driven by genetic instabil-

ity in which clones of tumor cells are selected for increased survival ability and growth advantage. These selected cell populations, in turn, expand and are subject to further selection as their growth conditions continue to change over time.

The outcome of genomic instability eventually is *tumor cell heterogeneity*. This genetic variability arguably is the driving force for both clonal selection and tumor progression. Indeed, the genetic diversity created by mutator tumor cells may account for some or all of their phenotypic differences that include invasive and metastatic capacity, transplantability, antigenic properties, drug sensitivity or resistance, growth rates, metabolism, and morphology. Experimental evidence in colon cancer supports the mutator phenotype concept and is discussed later in this chapter with regard to DNA repair mechanisms. A recent alternative or additional explanation of the genomic instability of cancer cells is *aneuploidy* (an abnormal chromosome number).[18,19] Symmetrical segregation of chromosomes depends on the diploid complement of mitosis-regulating genes. The eventual loss of a chromosome containing one or more of these regulators in turn destabilizes the karyotype of progeny cells. This loss promotes further instability in the clonal descendants.

The tendency of neoplastic cells to randomly mutate at high frequency or to become aneuploid is likely to be only one of several mechanisms for tumor progression. The importance of epigenetic events in tumor progression is well substantiated in the literature and indicates that alterations in signal transduction pathways and gene expression are also critical. Thus, these issues are also discussed in some detail below. Implied in the view that cancer cells accumulate mutations is the realization that these events are essentially irreversible. A more optimistic view arises if epigenetic factors also fuel tumor progression. If the latter is operative, the stimulus or promotional factor theoretically may be withdrawn or ablated, causing tumor cells to revert to a more normal phenotype or to be eliminated. Evidence that epigenetic factors can play an important role, at least at early stages of carcinogenesis, is the fact that in several tissues (breast, skin, thyroid, and colon) nodules, papillomas, or adenomas precede the clinical manifestation of cancer. Since the majority of these lesions can regress when the promoting agent is removed, mutation(s) may not necessarily have caused them. Rather, these lesions may be induced by a chronic alteration of gene expression that is inappropriate for the tissue of origin.[20] Moreover, the capacity of malignant embryonic carcinoma cells to generate apparently normal mosaic mice when transferred into blastocysts indicates that epigenetic influences can markedly modify the cancer phenotype.[21–23] In this context it is noteworthy that chemopreventive agents are effective in reducing tumor formation in animal bioassays, as well as in humans, even though they appear to act through epigenetic mechanisms. Therefore, epigenetic influences are clearly significant contributors to the multistage process of carcinogenesis. This concept has shaped recent directions in cancer chemotherapy that also are addressed in this chapter.

## DNA DAMAGE AND MUTATION INDUCTION

An essential aspect of chemical carcinogenesis is DNA damage. Different types of DNA damage are induced by exogenous chemical and physical agents, as well as those generated endogenously by host factors. DNA damage is not an inevitable consequence of exposure to carcinogens because most of these compounds are subject to metabolic conversions and detoxification. Moreover, DNA lesions can be repaired (see below). Carcinogens damage DNA by forming covalent modifications of the bases, sugar moieties, or phosphate backbone. The covalent attachment of a carcinogen to DNA produces an *adduct*. Because adducts may be bulky and affect the conformation of DNA, these lesions can alter both the structure and function of the DNA template during replication and transcription. Alternatively, both small and bulky adducts may change the base-pairing ability of a modified base. The mutagenic consequences of these alterations are described later.

As previously noted, the association of certain occupations with cancers encouraged investigators to examine the precise causative agents. The first causal association between lung cancer and a life-style factor, cigarette smoking, was made in 1950 by Doll and Hill in Britain and by Wynder and Graham in the United States. Shortly thereafter it was shown that other forms of tobacco use caused cancer, and a dose-response relationship was established. Other types of neoplasia are also more common in smokers, especially cancer of the tissues of the upper aerodigestive system (lip, mouth, nasopharynx, larynx, and esophagus), as well as of the bladder and pancreas. Also, a high tar content was demonstrated to compound the damaging effects of cigarettes or cigars. Cigarette smoking combined with other exposures (asbestos, radon, or alcohol) engenders a synergistic effect on cancer risk. In 1964, the U.S. government published the Surgeon General's warning to the public about the health dangers of tobacco use. About one-third of all of the cancer deaths in the United States are attributable to cigarette smoking, and in recent decades, this epidemic has also been seen in women. Hence, this disease emphasizes the importance of the subject of chemical carcinogenesis in humans.

DNA adducts were discovered and characterized in various experimental systems in the 1960s, paving the way for in vitro and in vivo experiments on cellular transformation and mutation analysis. For instance, in 1960 the UV-induced thymidine dimer was identified.[24] During this time, Miller et al.,[25] Brookes and Lawley,[26] and Craddock and Magee[27] also discovered and characterized various types of carcinogen-induced damage to DNA. A mechanism for correcting UV-induced lesions in DNA, termed nucleotide excision repair, was discovered in 1964 and was subsequently found to be deficient in persons with the rare human inherited disease xeroderma pigmentosum.[28] In the early 1970s, McCann, Ames, and coworkers[29] devised a simple reversion assay using bacteria to rapidly assess the mutagenicity of putative carcinogens. This innovation sparked efforts to identify more environmental and life-style carcinogen exposures, to define the frequency and types of DNA adducts these exposures produced, and to characterize their mutagenic consequences. Furthermore, the recognition that an inherited DNA repair deficiency predisposed xeroderma pigmentosum patients to skin cancer implied that DNA repair competence can play a major role in determining individual susceptibility to carcinogens.

### EXOGENOUS DNA DAMAGE AND CANCER CAUSATION

International variations in incidence and the effects of migration, as well as time trends, support the view that a substantial percentage (70–80%) of cancer is due to environmental factors.[30] Consistent with this view is the fact that lung and colon cancers, which are common cancer sites associated with the highest number of annual deaths, are strongly linked with exogenous causes (cigarette smoking and diet, respectively). As indicated above, damage to the DNA of target tissues in humans stems from environmental, occupational, and individual life-style exposures to both chemical and physical agents (ionizing radiation, UV light, asbestos, etc.). Table 1B-2 summarizes general facts about chemical carcinogens and introduces topics that will be expanded on further in the following text. The primary classes of chemical carcinogens include *polycyclic aromatic hydrocarbons* (PAHs), *arylamines* and *heterocyclic amines,* and *alkylating agents*. PAHs are ubiquitous in the environment. The best-studied PAH carcinogen is benzo[*a*]pyrene (BP). PAHs are present in indoor and outdoor air pollution, industrial and automotive emissions, cigarette smoke, and in smoked and charbroiled meat and fish. The volatile emissions from frying foods with unrefined cooking oils[31] and aerosols from frying meat[32] represent newly identified forms of indoor air pollution. Along with other PAHs, BP was identified in fume samples from heated peanut oil.[33] These findings suggest that protracted exposure to the emitted fumes from cooking oils may contribute to lung cancer risk.

Among the many hundreds of carcinogens present in cigarette smoke, arylamines and heterocyclic amines in particular are correlated with causing bladder cancer. Bladder cancer is the sixth most

## TABLE 1B-2. BIOLOGICAL AND BIOCHEMICAL FACTS ABOUT CHEMICAL CARCINOGENS

1. There is a dose-dependent relationship between exposure to carcinogens and cancer incidence and an inverse relationship with respect to the latency time.
2. Carcinogenesis is a multistep process that often includes three distinct phases: initiation, promotion, and progression.
3. The latency time between exposure and tumor detection is about 5–20 years in humans.
4. Chemical carcinogens are subject to metabolic activation and detoxification.
5. The metabolic activation or detoxification of chemicals, and the repair capabilities for specific DNA lesions, can differ for different species, organs, and cell types within a tissue.
6. Activated forms of chemical carcinogens are electrophiles that covalently bind to nucleophilic residues on cellular macromolecules (DNA, RNA, and proteins).
7. The number of carcinogen-DNA adducts measured in cells often correlates with an agent's carcinogenic potency, but other factors also play a role.
8. The metabolism of chemical carcinogens also contributes to oxidant stress that can enhance the carcinogenic process.
9. Endogenous factors (ROS, deaminations, alkylations, etc.) can also cause DNA damage and lead to mutations in vivo.
10. The DNA repair capabilities of the host are important in carcinogenesis; deficient repair of carcinogen-induced DNA damage increases the probability of mutations and promotes genomic instability.
11. Individual differences in cancer susceptibility can have a genetic basis since heritable polymorphisms can alter the activities of certain drug metabolizing and detoxifying enzymes.

common malignancy in the United States, where each year there are about 50,000 new cases. Cigarette smoking increases bladder cancer risk 2- to 10-fold, and occupational exposure to arylamines (benzidine and 2-naphthylamine) increases this risk 40- to 100-fold. Three specific arylamines in cigarette smoke are implicated by epidemiologic studies to cause bladder cancer: 3- and 4-aminobiphenyl (ABP) and 2-naphthylamine. In addition, alkylating $N$-nitroso derivatives of nicotine are present in cigarette smoke. The abundant nicotine product 4-(methylnitrosamino)-1-(3-pyridyl)-1-butanone (NNK) is a highly effective inducer of lung cancer in rats and generates elevated levels of a particular type of DNA damage, $O^6$-methylguanine. The $^{32}$P-postlabeling technique has been used to identify several carcinogen-DNA adducts. It has been used to demonstrate bulky lesions from PAHs and aromatic amines, as well as methyl- and ethyl-DNA adducts. Adduct levels are higher in specimens from tissues, blood, and urine of smokers than of nonsmokers. The mutagenic consequences of these lesions are discussed below.

The consumption of carcinogens in the diet has received considerable attention over the last decade. Dietary exposure may contribute to the incidence of cancers affecting the gastrointestinal tract. In 1977, Sugimura and co-workers[34] reported that burnt and brown surfaces of cooked meat and fish were highly mutagenic in the Ames

*Salmonella* assay. Subsequently, many different types of heterocyclic amines were identified from charred meat and fish. These compounds are divided into three categories: imidazoquinolines, imidazoquinoxalines, and imidazopyridines (reviewed in reference 35). Combustion or the pyrolysis of proteins generates all of these chemicals. The most abundant heterocyclic amine formed in cooked meat is 2-amino-1-methyl-6-phenylimidazo-[4,5-$b$]pyridine (PhIP). This chemical also was found in cigarette smoke. PAHs, including BP, are also consumed in the diet. For instance, levels of BP in charcoal-broiled steak and hamburger are 9 to 50 µg/kg.[36,37] In addition to the presence of NNK in cigarette smoke, $N$-nitroso compounds are formed in the digestive tract from nitrates and nitrites in water and various amines in foods. Dietary sources of nitrosamines include cured meats, whiskey, and beer. For an extensive review of orally active carcinogens, see reference 38.

Other sources of dietary carcinogens are the contaminants produced by microorganisms such as the molds *Aspergillus flavus* and *A. parasiticus*. These organisms produce mycotins, including aflatoxin $B_1$, a chemical that can contaminate improperly stored grains and nuts. Globally, aflatoxin $B_1$ contamination contributes to the incidence of hepatocellular carcinoma, especially in regions where hepatitis B virus infection is endemic. Indeed, the two agents appear to interact synergistically in causing liver cancer in regions of southern China and sub-Saharan Africa. Aflatoxin $B_1$ exposure in the United States is 25 to 75 ng/day; in certain locations of China, the exposures were reported to be at least three times higher. Reference 39 is recommended for a detailed discussion of aflatoxin $B_1$ and carcinogenesis.

The physical agents that damage DNA that are relevant to cancer causation include UV radiation from sunlight and ionizing radiation due to the medical use of x-rays, atomic bomb and nuclear reactor disasters, or environmental exposures to the α particles of radon. UV exposure causes adjacent pyrimidines in DNA to be covalently linked forming a four-membered ring structure, the cyclobutane pyrimidine dimer. This bulky lesion produces a bend in the DNA axis and is mutagenic. Patients afflicted with xeroderma pigmentosum are unable to repair these dimers and consequently suffer a 1000-fold increased risk of developing skin cancer. Among whites in the United States, skin cancer is the most common type of cancer.[40] The incidence rate of basal cell carcinoma in the United States is 300 per 100,000 and increasing annually by about 10%. Malignant melanoma is also associated with sunlight exposure. Melanoma represents <3% of skin cancers but accounts for roughly two-thirds of total skin cancer deaths due to its metastatic nature. Moreover, increases in the incidence of melanoma have been the largest of all cancers in the United States. Melanoma incidence and mortality rates increased dramatically from 1973 to 1994 by 120.5% and 38.9%, respectively.[41] Thus, the incidence of all forms of skin cancer continues to increase in this country. For the most part, this form of cancer is avoidable, particularly if the young (<18 years) are properly protected from prolonged sun exposures.

The primary exposure to ionizing radiation in the United States is from radioactive elements in the earth that decay continuously and form additional radioactive elements in the process. One of the products generated during the decay of uranium is radon 222. The solid α-emitting daughters resulting from this radionuclide can be deposited on the mucous lining of the bronchial airways by inhalation. Certain geologic locations naturally release high levels of radon that can contaminate houses. Insulation may trap radon in basements and in ground floors. This form of pollution is particularly harmful because individuals residing in contaminated dwellings are likely to experience exposures of relatively long duration. The association of radon and cancer is supported by epidemiologic studies that have documented the marked increased risk of lung cancer in miners exposed to high doses of radon. Ionizing radiation generates ions and free radicals that can randomly collide with cellular macromolecules and break chemical bonds. Whereas x-rays and $\gamma$-rays produce sparse ionizing events along their paths, $\alpha$ particles emitted from radon produce a very dense ionization track that is potentially more damaging. The mutagenic properties of these types of physical damaging agents and of chemical carcinogens of different classes are discussed below.

## METABOLIC ACTIVATION AND DETOXIFICATION OF CHEMICAL CARCINOGENS

Chemical carcinogens are genotoxic because in vivo they bind covalently to DNA and induce mutations in somatic cells. In general, these chemicals tend to be lipophilic, a property that enables them to be transported by lipoproteins via the circulatory system and to penetrate cell membranes. As indicated above, a major source of exposure to carcinogens is via the diet or through inhalation. Both the uptake and metabolism of carcinogens is markedly affected by dietary components. This issue will be discussed later under the topic of chemoprevention. The metabolism of genotoxic carcinogens is effected in two stages. In *phase I,* a polar reactive group is added to the carcinogen molecule, converting it to a suitable form for reaction with *phase II* enzymes. Typically, phase I reactions are *oxidations,* whereas phase II reactions are *conjugations.* For chemical carcinogens, phase I reactions are generally activating, whereas phase II reactions usually result in detoxification. Examples of the oxidations carried out in phase I reactions are microsomal monooxygenations, cytosolic and mitochondrial oxidations, as well as cyclooxygenase-mediated cooxidations. Other types of phase I reactions include reductions, hydrolyses, and epoxide hydrations. Using endogenous substrates (sugars, amino acids, glutathione [GSH], etc.), phase II enzymes conjugate the reactive carcinogen intermediate to yield water-soluble products that are readily excreted. The untoward result of phase I reactions is often the conversion of a weakly reactive carcinogen to a potent electrophile. An electrophilic intermediate is capable of attacking nucleophilic constituents of macromolecules (proteins, RNA, DNA) to form covalent adducts (see reference 42 for review).

Phase I monooxygenation of genotoxic chemicals is catalyzed by either cytochrome P450 or flavin adenine dinucleotide (FAD)–containing enzymes. Both types of monooxygenases are abundantly located in microsomal fractions of cells. Heme-containing mixed-function monooxygenases constitute a large superfamily that carry out oxygenations in which one atom of molecular oxygen ($O_2$) is reduced to water in a reaction that requires NADPH. In vertebrates, the most active site for carcinogen metabolism is the liver, but it can occur in other tissues, including the skin and aerodigestive system. P450s are also expressed in steroid-producing tissues such as the adrenal gland, ovary, and testis, as well as in steroid-responsive tissues of mesodermal origin. In the liver, P450s oxidize steroid hormones and bile pigments, as well as chemicals. P450s that metabolize chemical carcinogens are mainly members of the CYP1 family. For instance, CYP1A1 and CYP1B1 metabolically activate PAHs. CYP1A1 is expressed in human lung and is readily induced by PAHs in cigarette smoke and exhaust emissions.[43] CYP1A2, which is expressed mostly in the liver, is involved in the activation of arylamines, heterocyclic amines, and aflatoxin $B_1$. On the other hand, the metabolic activation of low-molecular-weight carcinogens including benzene and alkylating $N$-nitrosamines is performed by CYP2E1. The expression levels of certain inducible P450 isoforms in vivo can be influenced by recent prior exposure to other chemicals such as therapeutic drugs, flavones from fruits and vegetables, alcohol, and insecticides. CYP1B1 is inducible in extrahepatic tissues by the aryl hydrocarbon receptor agonist 2,3,7,8-tetrachorodibenzo-*p*-dioxin and is expressed constitutively in steroidogenic tissues. The importance of certain P450s in carcinogenesis is dramatically demonstrated in the case of CYB1B1-null mice.[44] When wild-type mice were treated with DBA to induce tumors, 70% developed lymphomas, whereas only 7.5% of treated CYB1B1-null animals developed this cancer. Thus, CYB1B1-deficiency confers resistance to PAH-induced tumors in vivo.

Important reactions for the activation of PAHs are *epoxidation* and *aromatic hydroxylation.* The metabolic activation of PAHs to protein-binding intermediates was first reported by E. Miller[45] in 1951; subsequently, Gelboin[46] demonstrated the ability of P450-containing microsomes to catalyze the binding of BP to DNA in vitro. Figure 1B-5 shows the conversion of BP to its ultimate form, the 7,8-epoxide. The aromatic hydroxylation by a hydrolase then converts this epoxide to two stereochemically distinct *trans-*7,8-dihydrodiols, which then are converted by a monooxygenase to yield the 7,8-dihydrodiol-9,10-epoxide products. This ultimate epoxide product is highly reactive and binds to cellular DNA. The 7,8-diol-9,10-epoxides of BP bind primarily to the N-2 position of guanine in DNA.[47] Ultimate carcinogens have variable half-lives; the longer these species persist, the more DNA damage they can inflict. The mutagenic consequences of these carcinogen-DNA adducts is discussed below.

Another means by which BP and other carcinogens can be activated is *cooxidation* during prostaglandin biosynthesis. Via this route, arachidonic acid, a polyunsaturated lipid, undergoes two consecutive reactions with cyclooxygenase (Cox) -1 or -2. In the first oxidation reaction, prostaglandin G, a hydroperoxy endoperoxide, is formed. The additional peroxidase activity of these enzymes mediates the second reaction to generate prostaglandin $H_2$. During the latter conversion, both the hydroxylation of BP and expoxidation of BP-7,8-dihydrodiol can occur. In addition to cyclooxygenases, epoxidation of the BP *trans-*7,8-dihydrodiol can be effected by lipoxygenase, another critical enzyme in arachidonic acid metabolism.[48] It now appears likely that these reactions play a significant role in metabolically activating chemical carcinogens in extrahepatic tissues that are not replete with cytochrome P450 and FAD monooxygenase activities.[49] All tissues express the constitutive Cox-1 activity and different ones express the several lipoxygenase isoforms and/or may sustain enhanced activities of the inducible Cox-2. Thus, this

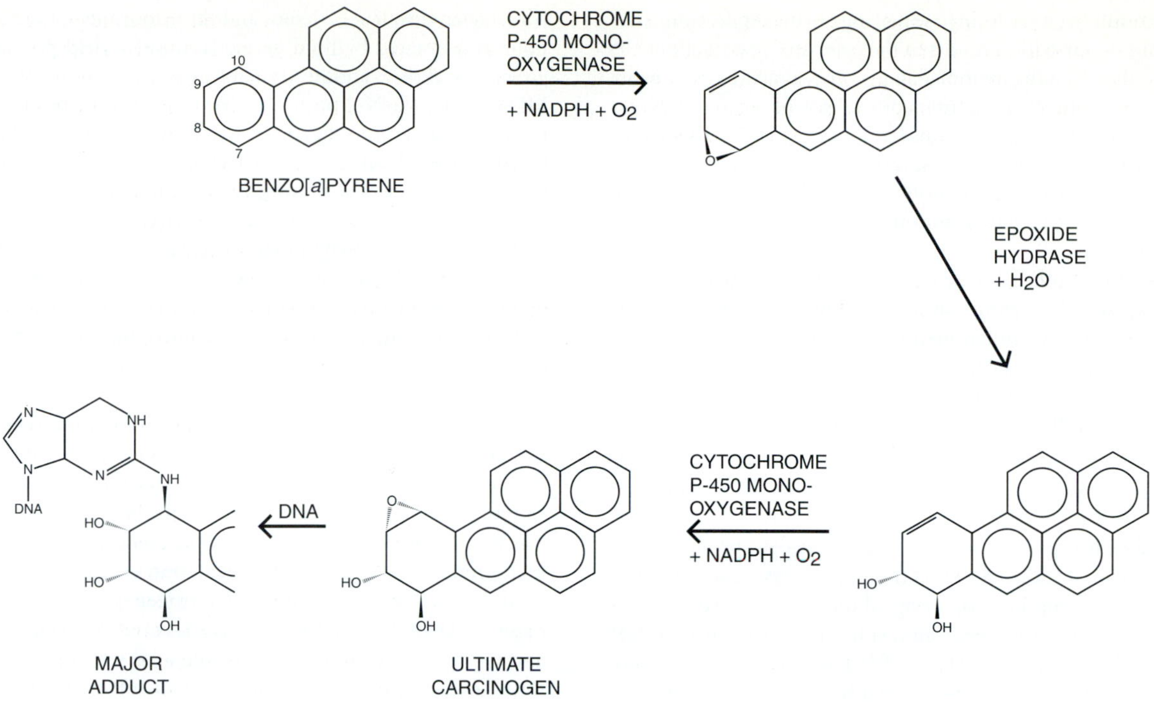

**FIGURE 1B-5.** Metabolic conversion of benzopyrene to its ultimate carcinogenic form.

situation is likely to apply in the intestinal tract. Carcinogens consumed in the diet are distributed via the enterohepatic circulation directly to the intestine. As discussed below, agents that reduce the activity of Cox-2 are chemopreventive for colon polyps and adenomas.

Phase II reactions that detoxify the metabolic intermediates of BP before they can attack DNA include conjugations of these intermediates to sulfate, glucuronide, or GSH. The enzymes that perform these reactions are sulfotransferases, uridine diphosphate (UDP) glucuronyl transferases, and glutathione transferases, respectively. In general, these conjugation products are more polar, less toxic, and more easily excreted. Lastly, the nonenzymatic hydrolysis of the dihydrodiol expoxide of BP to the 7,8,9,10-tetrahydrotetrol form blocks its ability to attack nucleophilic species.

The above discussion was limited to the metabolism of BP as an example of a PAH carcinogen. Like BP, aflatoxin $B_1$ is also metabolized by phase I enzymes to an epoxide. The reactive intermediate of aflatoxin $B_1$ is an unstable sulfate ester that is subsequently formed in a phase II reaction. This reactive species binds mainly to the N-7 position of guanine in DNA. Metabolic activation by P450s of NNK and other nitrosamines yields alkylated bases in DNA, primarily guanine (see below). For a detailed discussion of the mechanisms of nitrosamine bioactivation and carcinogenesis, see reference 50. Like aflatoxin $B_1$, arylamines and heterocyclic amines typically are activated in phase II reactions. After first undergoing a phase I hydroxylation, these compounds can either be detoxified by conjugation or converted to unstable and highly reactive sulfate esters. If the reactive intermediate is produced, it mainly binds to the C-8 position of guanine in DNA. For an extensive review of the metabolism of these and other toxicants see reference 49.

## ENDOGENOUS DNA DAMAGE

Ames and colleagues[51] have emphasized that damage to DNA from endogenous sources is a major contributor to both carcinogenesis and aging. Four categories of DNA damage can arise spontaneously from endogenous sources: *deaminations, alkylations, base losses,* and *oxidations.* The magnitude of DNA damage from endogenous sources in vivo is influenced by cell-type-specific processes, dietary factors, inflammatory responses, and environmental or life-style exposures to chemical and physical genotoxicants. Furthermore, the relative activities of drug-metabolizing phase I and II enzymes may influence the levels of endogenous DNA damage. The metabolism of carcinogens can generate oxidant stress.[52] For example, the metabolism of BP and the PCB 2,3,7,8-tetrachlorodibenzo-*p*-dioxin (TCDD), by P450 enzymes produces oxidative damage to DNA.[53,54] Cigarettes provide a potent cocktail of toxins. A single inhalation of tobacco smoke is estimated to contain about $10^{16}$ reactive (reduced) oxygen species (ROS),[55] and oxidant damage to plasma proteins is detectable following exposure to cigarette smoke.[56] Furthermore, certain isoforms of cytochrome P450s can both increase DNA-adduct levels as well as stimulate other oxidative processes.

The amount of spontaneous DNA damage of various types is extensive and occurs continuously in many types of cells. DNA bases can undergo spontaneous hydrolytic and nitrosative deaminations. Pyrimidine bases are more susceptible to spontaneous deamination than are purines. Deamination of cytosine, adenine, guanine, and 5-methylcytosine (2% to 7% of total cytosine present in the mammalian genome) yields uracil, hypoxanthine, xanthine, and thymine, respectively. If these changes fail to be corrected, single base mutations result from errors in base pairing during replication. Also, spontaneous depurination results in the estimated loss of about $10^4$ purines per day from the mammalian genome, a rate that is roughly 100 times greater than the spontaneous release of pyrimidines and 500 times greater than the deamination of cytosine.[57] This spontaneous depurination results from severing of the glycosyl bond that links the purine base to the deoxyribose sugar. As noted below, these lesions are referred to as *abasic sites* and are potentially mutagenic if they persist.

Endogenous DNA damage can arise from normal aerobic metabolism, as well as from pathophysiologic conditions such as chronic infection and inflammation. The generation of ROS is widespread in biologic materials and includes peroxyl (ROO˙) and alkoxyl (RO˙) radicals and nitric oxide (NO˙). Generation of these species occurs in cells during normal metabolism and by photosensitization. Sensitized immune effector cells release hydrogen peroxide ($H_2O_2$) and superoxide ($O_2^{˙-}$) extracellularly. $H_2O_2$ and $O_2^{˙-}$ are also formed intracellularly in response to growth factors, hormones, and tumor-promoting agents. The transient production of $H_2O_2$ in growth-stimulated cells is thought to serve a second messenger role in the amplification of signal transduction events.[58,59] A discrete phase of programmed cell death (apoptosis) also involves the intracellular production of $H_2O_2$.[60,61] The reaction of $H_2O_2$ with iron or copper chelates generates the highly damaging hydroxyl radical (HO˙). Although HO˙ is the most reactive oxidant, $H_2O_2$, which is relatively more stable, is potentially damaging because it may be converted to HO˙. Targets for the damaging effects of oxidative processes are cellular macromolecules (DNA, proteins, and membrane lipids). Although cells have elaborate defense mechanisms to combat oxidant damage, nonetheless the chronic nature of this assault is thought to contribute to various degenerative diseases, aging, and cancer.

Hydroxyl radicals produce a large variety of types of damage to DNA, including base modifications, lesions in sugar residues, single- and double-strand breaks, abasic sites, and nucleoprotein-DNA cross-links. ROS attack different positions of the bases in DNA to generate more than 30 distinct modifications. Highly sensitive detection methods such as gas chromatography/mass spectrometry and high-pressure liquid chromatography have been used to isolate and quantitate DNA oxidation products in DNA samples from mammalian cells.[62] Oxidation of guanine in DNA yields 8-oxoguanine (8-oxoG). Oxidation of cytosine can give rise to 5,6-dihydroxy-5,6-dihydrocytosine, an unstable product that is converted to 5-hydroxycytosine (5-HC), 5-hydroxyuracil (5-HU), and 5,6-dihydroxy-5,6-dihydrouracil (Ug). These modifications are both prevalent and mutagenic. Indeed, each day between $10^4$ and $10^5$ 8-oxoG residues are produced per cell in mammals.[51]

In addition to interfering with normal membrane fluidity and receptor-ligand interactions, lipid peroxidation can also lead to the formation of lesions in DNA. For example, α,β-unsaturated aldehydes such as acrolein and crotonaldehyde are widespread in the environment and both can be found in foods and cigarette smoke. These compounds also are formed by lipid peroxidation, and they can generate exocyclic etheno-dNTP adducts of DNA bases that block Watson-Crick base pairing.[63] Carbonyl compounds such as malondialdehyde (MDA) are formed nonenzymatically by lipid peroxidation and enzymatically during metabolic conversion of eicosanoids (prostaglandins, leukotrienes, and thromboxanes). Carbonyl compounds generated by lipid peroxidation can yield propanodeoxyguanosine (PdG), another type of exocyclic base adduct in DNA. MDA attacks the N-2 position of deoxyguanosine residues in DNA to produce a pyrimidopurinone derivative ($M_1G$). This $M_1G$ lesion was detected at levels of about 5000 per cell in normal human liver.[64] Oxidative processes also produce base propenals in DNA that efficiently react with MDA to yield the $M_1G$ adducts.[65] The level of $M_1G$ present in normal human pancreas is similar in magnitude to that of 8-oxoG.[66] The mutagenic consequences of these lesions are described below. Oxidation of thiol residues in proteins can alter the cellular redox balance, producing pleiotrophic effects on the physiology of cells that include changes in calcium flux and alterations in gene expression.[67]

In addition to the above types of oxidative damage, cellular DNA can also be alkylated by the addition of methyl or ethyl groups to the bases. Thus, endogenous nitrosamines formed from the reaction of secondary or tertiary amines with $N_2O_4$ can alkylate DNA. The transfer of —$CH_3$ groups in normal metabolism by *S*-adenosylmethionine also can lead to the alkylation of DNA. Alkylations can occur at any of the oxygen and nitrogen positions on the four bases in DNA (Fig. 1B-6), but are favored to occur at the N-7 and O-6 positions of guanine, as well as the N-3 position of adenine. Levels of both $O^6$-methylguanine and $O^4$-methylthymine have been measured in the DNA of liver and esophageal specimens and

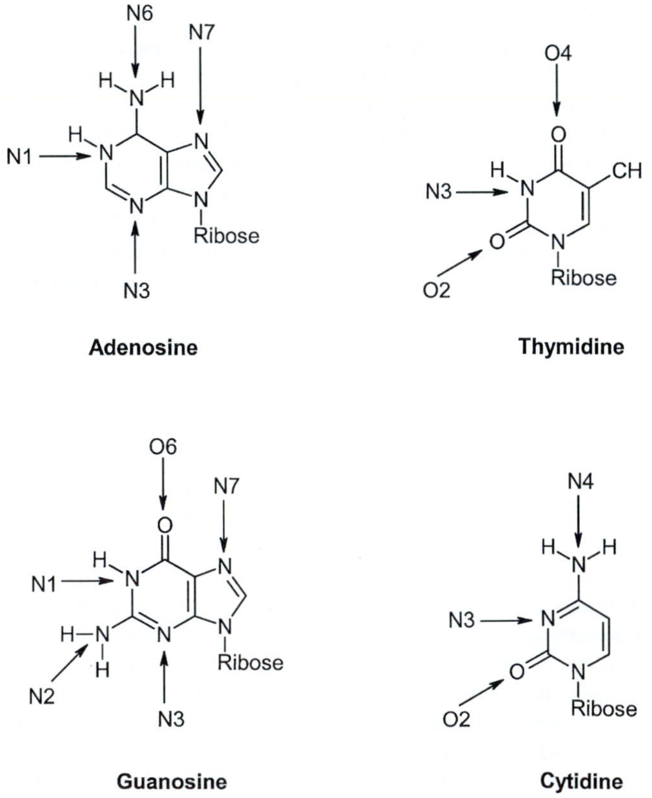

**FIGURE 1B-6.** Sites of electrophilic attack on bases in DNA.

peripheral blood leukocytes from individuals unexposed to alkylating chemicals.[68] Thus, these types of damage occur in humans.

Nitric oxide (NO·) is a biologic messenger that mediates many normal physiologic functions, including vasodilation, neurotransmission, platelet aggregation, and peroxyl radical scavenging. Furthermore, NO· is released by activated inflammatory cells (phagocytes, neutrophils, and macrophages). However, derivatives of NO· form reactive nitrogen species (RNS) that can damage DNA by nitrosation, nitration, and deamination. Autoxidation of NO· forms nitrous anhydride ($N_2O_3$) that can deaminate DNA after nitrosating the primary amine groups of the bases.[69] The deamination of dG and dA was detected at high frequency in DNA of human tracheobronchial epithelial cells following the treatment with gas-phase cigarette smoke, suggesting that some of its damaging effects may involve RNS.[70] In combination with ROS, RNS can also generate various oxidation products of DNA. For instance, reaction of NO· with $O_2^-$ forms the extremely reactive peroxynitrite (ONOO−). ONOO− and HO· are highly damaging species because they can produce potentially lethal double-strand breaks in genomic DNA. In addition, lipid peroxidation by ONOO− leads to the formation of etheno adducts in vivo.[71] Also, carbon dioxide can react with ONOO−, thus potentiating the nitrating effects of this RNS.[72] The involvement of NO· overproduction in carcinogenesis has been reviewed recently.[73,74]

## MUTATION INDUCTION DUE TO ENDOGENOUS OR EXOGENOUS DNA DAMAGE

As indicated above, different types of DNA-damaging chemicals form distinct types of lesions in DNA that, in turn, influence the mutational specificity of these agents. The relative potency of a chemical agent with respect to the induction of mutations is a function of several variables. These variables include the number of adducts or other types of lesions that are formed in the DNA of target cells and the DNA conformation at the modification site. The conformation of the DNA lesion can influence both its repair rate and its effects on base pairing and DNA replication. PAH carcinogens primarily modify the N-2 position of guanine and N-6 position of adenine. In duplex DNA, the BP adduct lies in the minor groove.[75] A preferred sequence for modification by BP is a run of guanines (5′-GGGG-3′). Adduct formation can render the modified purine residues noninstructional during DNA replication because the base-pairing functionality is occluded. Typically, this leads to insertion of adenine opposite the modified guanine, resulting in a transversion base substitution mutation (G:C→T:A) in the daughter cell. In the case of a modified adenine residue, this leads to an A:T→T:A transversion. Arylamines and heterocyclic amines, on the other hand, modify the C-8 position of guanine. The N-2 position of guanine may also be adducted to a minor extent. The adducts of arylamines and heterocyclic amines favor insertion of the carcinogen moiety into duplex DNA, displacing the affected guanine to an extrahelical position. This model is called *base displacement*.[76] Although the C-8 position of guanine is not involved in base pairing, studies have shown that the position of the carcinogen within the DNA helix can be stabilized by stacking interactions with neighboring bases and that adenine is the best-fitting pairing partner when this modified region undergoes DNA replication.[77] The most prevalent mutation induced by arylamines, therefore, is also a G:C→T:A point mutation. As mentioned above, aflatoxin $B_1$ forms adducts at the N-7 position of guanine. This DNA adduct primarily results in G:C→T:A substitutions that are induced directly by the adduct or indirectly because the liability of the modified dG yields an abasic site. In summary, bulky chemical carcinogens mainly induce single base transversion mutations. In general, PAH carcinogens are more potent mutagens than arylamines, since lower adduct levels are needed to achieve the same mutation frequency.

Alkylating chemicals are mutagenic because the two major lesions they produce in DNA, $O^6$-methyl-dG and $O^4$-methyl-dT, interfere with normal base pairing and thereby cause misinsertions during DNA replication to yield the transition mutations G:C→A:T and T:A→C:G, respectively. The ring nitrogens of bases are more nucleophilic than are the oxygen moieties. Thus, the N-7 position of guanine and the N-3 position of adenine are most reactive. However, $N^7$-alkyl-dG is not mutagenic per se because it does not interfere with normal base pairing. Both $N^3$-alkyl-dA and $N^3$-alkyl-dG block DNA replication and consequently are lethal lesions unless they are repaired. The preferred sequence target for $O^6$ modification of guanine residues in DNA by alkylating chemicals is 5′-GpG-3′. Alkylating agents can be either mono- or bifunctional. The latter class has two reactive groups and may either form adducts at adjacent bases or form DNA interstrand and intrastrand and DNA-protein cross-links. Several chemotherapeutic drugs are of this type, such as nitrogen mustards and melphalan. Cross-links formed between two complementary strands of DNA (interstrand) cause the most toxicity. These chemicals are also capable of inducing chromosomal breaks (*clastogenic* effects) due to the hydrolysis of unstable reaction products. The electrophilic attack on oxygen and phosphodiester linkages by alkylating chemicals can result in the formation of phosphotriesters. Moreover, alkylation modifications may weaken the *N*-glycosidic bond which, in turn, can cause depurination or depyrimidation and thus lead to the formation of an abasic site. For an in-depth review of chemical carcinogens with regard to the related nucleic acid chemistry, see reference 76.

Extensive characterization of the types of mutations induced by chemical carcinogens in mammalian cells cultured in vitro and in several eukaryotes (yeast, flies, and rodents) has been performed over the last three decades.[78] These studies have defined the types, locations, and frequencies of spontaneous and damage-induced mutations at different selectable loci. In addition to model systems, the study of tumors in animals has also provided a means of identifying oncogenes as potential targets for the mutagenic action of chemical carcinogens and for establishing that these mutated genes play a causative role in specific types of cancer. Important initial studies in this area examined the ability of carcinogens to induce mammary tumors in rats.[79,80] In these studies, the types of mutations present in the H-*ras* oncogene of the resulting tumors were determined and correlated with the mutational specificity of the specific chemical carcinogen used in treating the animals.

More recent studies have demonstrated that a very useful in vivo target for examining somatic mutations in humans is the tumor suppressor gene *TP53*. This gene encodes a transcriptional activator and is commonly found to be mutated in many different types of tumors, especially adult carcinomas (>50%). Missense mutations

**TABLE 1B-3.** SPECIFICITY OF MUTATIONS ENGENDERED BY ENDOGENOUS DNA DAMAGE

| TYPES OF DAMAGING AGENTS | TYPES OF BASE ALTERATIONS | CONVERSION | PRIMARY MUTATION TYPE |
|---|---|---|---|
| Nitric oxide (NO·) | Deamination | $dC \rightarrow A{:}T$ | $G{:}C \rightarrow A{:}T$ |
| | | 5-Methyl-dC $\rightarrow$ T | $G{:}C \rightarrow A{:}T$ |
| | | $dG \rightarrow$ xanthine | $G{:}C \rightarrow A{:}T$ |
| | | | $A{:}T \rightarrow G{:}C$ |
| Gylcosylase activity, ROS from oxidants, Unstable carcinogen-DNA adducts (N-7) | Depurination | $dG \rightarrow$ abasic site | $G{:}C \rightarrow T{:}A$ |
| | | $dA \rightarrow$ abasic site | $A{:}T \rightarrow T{:}A$ |
| Alkylating chemicals | $O^6$-methyl-dG | | $G{:}C \rightarrow A{:}T$ |
| Spontaneous alkylation | $O^6$-methyl-T | | $T{:}A \rightarrow C{:}G$ |
| Nitric oxide (NO) | NO· | | $C{:}G \rightarrow T{:}A$ |
| | 8-oxo-G | | $G{:}C \rightarrow T{:}A$ |
| | 5-HU | | $C{:}G \rightarrow T{:}A$ |
| ROS from oxidants or ionizing radiation | Ug | | $C{:}G \rightarrow T{:}A$ |
| | 5-HC | | $C{:}G \rightarrow T{:}A$ |
| MDA | $M_1G$ | | $G{:}C \rightarrow T{:}A$ & $G{:}C \rightarrow A{:}T$ |
| MDA | PdG | | $G{:}C \rightarrow T{:}A > G{:}C \rightarrow A{:}T$ |
| Vinyl chloride | Etheno-dC | | $C{:}G \rightarrow T{:}A$ |
| Peroxidized lipids | Etheno-dA | | $A{:}T \rightarrow G{:}C$ |

in the evolutionarily conserved DNA binding domain (exons 5–8) of the *TP53* gene produce an abnormal phenotype. Virtually all of the mutations in this coding region affect the conformation of the protein and block its transactivation ability. Two features of *TP53* make this gene useful for gaining insights into the etiology of human cancers. First, the conserved coding region is a large enough target to allow a wide diversity of mutational changes to be scored. Since chemical carcinogens tend to induce single base substitutions, this feature is important. Second, missense mutations are much more prevalent in the *TP53* gene of tumors, rather than nonsense mutations (TGA, TAA, TAG). The mutational spectrum would be biased if the latter type of mutation were the more prevalent form.

There is an international registry on human tumor *TP53* sequence data, and by 1998 data of over 8000 alleles were entered. The best correlations between the observed mutation spectra and exogenous cancer-causing exposures are for lung, liver, and skin tumors. In these cases, the types of mutations are consistent with the known specificity of putative causative agents, PAHs from tobacco smoke, aflatoxin $B_1$, and UV radiation, respectively. Also, prior studies in model systems indicated that the mutational frequency of a given DNA lesion and its relative rate of repair strongly depend on the local DNA sequence context. Therefore, the appearance of mutational *hotspots* in the *TP53* gene that are distinct for each tumor type is also a significant finding. For example, in liver tumors obtained from regions of China and Africa where aflatoxin $B_1$ contamination is common, mutations in the suppressor gene typically were G:C→T:A transversions located at codon 249. In lung cancers, G:C→T:A mutations were also detected, but the great majority of these changes were located at different sites (codons 157 and 179). In skin cancers, the characteristic mutations in *TP53* were transition mutations at dipyrimidines, which is consistent with the etiologic

agent, sunlight. In the case of skin tumors, the most affected *TP53* codon was 278. Thus, the *TP53* sequence registry appears to provide strong evidence that specific exogenous carcinogen exposures play an initiating role in human cancer causation.[81]

As noted above, various forms of oxidant stress together with chronic infection, inflammation, and/or exposures to tumor-promoting substances can generate a variety of DNA lesions in vivo. Presumably, these endogenous types of DNA damage are also a source of mutation during the carcinogenesis process. The major types of such mutations are listed in Table 1B-3, which summarizes recently published studies.[82–92] It is of interest that among the point mutations that arise spontaneously or from endogenous damage, transitions are the most prevalent. It should also be stressed that strand breaks are often intermediates in the repair of oxidized or deaminated bases or abasic sites. Therefore, although single base substitution mutations are usually induced by oxidants, the types of DNA damage produced by endogenous agents are considerably more complex. Similarly, radiation generates ionization events within cells that produce the types of DNA damage observed to occur by endogenous processes but at different yields. The prevalent mutations associated with ionization, though, are not base substitutions but rather are large deletions, insertions, or inversions resulting from double-strand breaks.

The above discussion emphasizes mainly the effects of exogenous chemical carcinogens and endogenous factors in the causation of point mutations in cellular DNA, which then drive the carcinogenic process. However, it is apparent that cancer cells, and in some cases precursor lesions, frequently bear numerous additional types of genomic damage. These include the frequent occurrence of DNA regions that display loss of heterozygosity (presumably due to recombination), gene amplification, altered patterns of DNA methylation (reflecting changes in chromatin structure and gene expression), and various chromosomal abnormalities (aneuploidy, translocations, inversions, insertions, and deletions). However, at the present time, it is not known to what extent these abnormalities are driven by damage to DNA from exogenous chemical carcinogens or endogenous agents. The underlying molecular mechanisms for these events are not yet understood with certainty. It seems likely that chemical carcinogens can play a causative role in the induction of these abnormalities since they are also seen in carcinogen-induced rodent cancers. Obviously, this subject requires more intensive research, since these diverse types of genomic abnormalities are characteristic of many types of human cancers and insights into their pathogenesis might suggest new approaches to cancer prevention. This topic is discussed in greater detail below under the heading of genomic instability.

## DNA REPAIR MECHANISMS

During evolution, organisms have evolved many DNA repair mechanisms to avoid the mutagenic consequences of various types of DNA damage. These include the proofreading capabilities of DNA polymerases, as well as the activities of numerous factors involved in DNA metabolism and the maintenance of chromosome integrity. Absent proper processing, DNA damage can be mutagenic, carcinogenic, and teratogenic. Furthermore, as illustrated by the cancer-prone autosomal inherited disease Werner's syndrome, DNA damage also contributes to aging. Table 1B-4 summarizes five evolutionarily conserved pathways for the repair of various types of DNA damage. The first two categories, *direct damage reversal* and *base excision repair*, represent the primary defenses against endogenous DNA damage,

## TABLE 1B-4. DNA REPAIR PATHWAYS

| PATHWAY | TARGETS/MECHANISMS |
|---|---|
| Direct damage reversal | Alkylated bases, principally $O^6$-methyl-dG |
| Base excision repair | Oxidized bases, *N*-alkylated purines, uracil and hypoxanthine in DNA due to deamination |
| Nucleotide excision repair | Bulky carcinogen-DNA adducts, UV photoproducts, and inter- and intrastrand lesions that distort DNA conformation |
| Mismatch repair | Replication errors, alkylated bases, and mispairs remaining after recombination |
| Double-strand break repair | Site-specific recombination and DNA double-strand end rejoining |

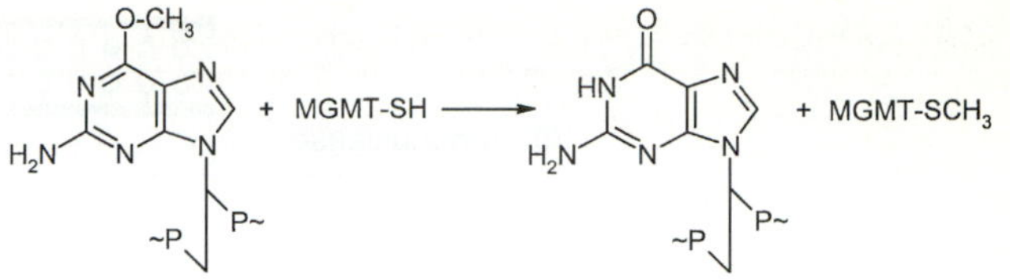

**FIGURE 1B-7.** Direct damage reversal.

as well as important defense mechanisms against certain exogenous chemical carcinogens.

## DIRECT DAMAGE REVERSAL

The *MGMT* gene located on chromosome 10q26 encodes the single human example of a protein responsible for direct damage reversal. *MGMT* encodes $O^6$-*methylguanine-DNA methyltransferase*, a monomeric protein of 21,700 kDa. As illustrated in Fig. 1B-7, this protein reacts with $O^6$-methyldG in DNA to remove the alkyl group, leaving the base intact. The reaction is stoichiometric; thus each molecule of alkyltransferase removes a single alkyl moiety, which then becomes covalently bound to a cysteine residue present on the methyltransferase protein. The alkylation of this protein, in turn, inactivates its repair function. The mammalian $O^6$-methyltransferase does not efficiently repair the mutagenic $O^4$-methylT lesion in DNA.[93,94] Compared to $O^6$-methyldG, the rate of methyl transfer to the repair protein is several hundred times slower for $O^4$-methylT. An alternative pathway for removal of $O^4$-methylT in vivo is nucleotide excision repair (NER, see below).[95] Interestingly, the human *MGMT* product inhibits $O^4$-methylT repair by binding nonproductively to the lesion and thereby blocking access to the damage site by NER factors.[96] Exactly how the efficient removal of $O^4$-methylT is regulated in normal human cells that express *MGMT* is not yet fully understood.

The possible cancer-preventing effect of this repair pathway is compromised by the fact that expression of the *MGMT* gene is not uniform in mammalian tissues. Inhibition of *MGMT* expression by epigenetic means ("gene silencing") may cause the absence of methyltransferase activity from certain tissues and consequently alkylation DNA repair deficiency. To illustrate that tissues variably express $O^6$-methyltransferase, the human liver normally contains the highest level of activity, whereas the lowest level is found in myeloid precursor cells.[95] Furthermore, treatment of animals with alkylating chemicals preferentially induced tumors in tissues that tend to express lower levels of this repair activity. *MGMT* expression in tumors and cell lines is variable as well, and is suppressed in 20% to 30% of human tumors. Human cell lines displaying this phenotype (designated Mer$^-$) characteristically are deficient in alkylation repair and show higher frequencies of mutation and sister chromatid exchange than do wild-type cells. The inhibition of this repair activity, in turn, sensitizes tissues and cells to the toxicity and clastogenicity (chromosome-damaging effects) of chemotherapeutic nitrogen mustards such as 1,3-bis(2-chloroethyl)-1-nitrosourea (BCNU).[97,98] Because expression of *MGMT* is modulated epigenetically, it is subject to change. Hence, certain human tumors may

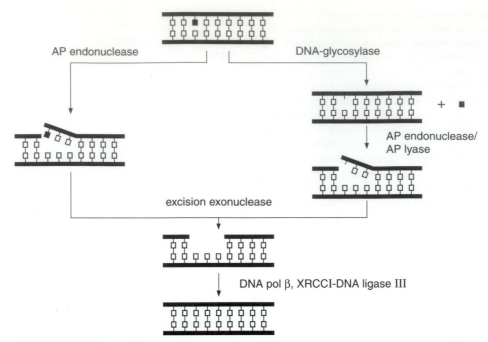

**FIGURE 1B-8.** Base excision repair.

acquire resistance to alkylating chemotherapeutic agents by increasing the expression of this gene relative to the normal surrounding tissue. In this case, the use of a selective *MGMT* inhibitor such as O[6]-benzylguanine in combination chemotherapy with alkylating agents may prove beneficial.[99] Increasing the expression of *MGMT* in normal tissue was shown to have positive consequences in vivo. For instance, transgenic mice expressing the human *MGMT* were resistant to induction of thymic lymphomas by *N*-methyl-*N*-nitrosourea.[100] In addition, mice were rescued from the myelotoxicity of exposure to BCNU by an ex vivo gene therapy technique that introduced an *MGMT* expression vector into their bone marrow stem cells.[97,98] However, mice genetically engineered to be *MGMT* null, although extremely sensitive to the toxicity of an alkylating chemical, nonetheless were not prone to developing neoplasias and had a normal life span,[101] presumably because the repair to alkylated DNA can be accomplished through alternative DNA mechanisms in vivo. The idea that different repair processes are functionally redundant in higher eukaryotes is discussed below.

## BASE EXCISION REPAIR

Typically, the various types of endogenous DNA damage are structurally subtle in comparison to those produced by some of the more bulky types of exogenous chemical carcinogens. The latter types of lesions tend to induce greater conformational distortions in the helical structure of DNA. The second repair pathway listed in Table 1B-4, base excision repair (BER), is responsible for removing most of the DNA damage that arises spontaneously as a result of endogenous agents, as well as in response to ionizing radiation (α particles and x-

and γ-rays). This repair process sequentially utilizes the activities of two classes of enzymes, *DNA-glycosylases* and *apurinic/apyrimidinic (AP) endonucleases,* and is depicted in Fig. 1B-8. To repair an AP site, a specific AP endonuclease first incises or nicks DNA immediately adjacent to the lesion. This nicking is achieved by hydrolyzing one of the phosphodiester bonds either 5′ or 3′ to the abasic sugar. Although AP sites constitute single-strand breaks, there are many chemically distinct end groups found at the termini of these breaks. In order to allow repair synthesis by DNA polymerase β, all 3′-termini must be restored to hydroxyl groups and all 5′-termini converted to phosphate groups. The filled site is then sealed by DNA ligase III in association with an accessory protein, XRCC1. An alternative means of repairing an AP site involves cleavage on the 3′ side of the lesion by an *AP lyase.* Lyase activity causes the β-elimination of the 3′ phosphate at the site of the excised damaged base. AP endonucleases and DNA-glycosylases may or may not be bifunctional and display this additional lyase activity. The ability of AP lyases to incise 3′ of a damaged base allows the diesterase activities of certain AP endonucleases to correct different 3′-blocking lesions. Examples of these lesions include 3′-phosphoglycolate esters, 3′-deoxyribose-5-phosphate esters, and 3′-phosphates. The principal human AP endonuclease is encoded by the *APE* gene residing on chromosome 14q11.2-12. Key activities of the BER pathway, including AP endonuclease, DNA polymerase β, and XRCC1-DNA ligase III, are essential since the loss of any of the corresponding genes causes embryonic lethality.[102]

AP endonuclease apparently plays a role in coordinating cellular responses to oxidative stress since a reduction of cellular AP endonuclease protein by expression of antisense *APE* mRNA in human HeLa cells resulted in hypersensitivity to the lethal effects of oxidants. *Ape*-knockout mice are inviable; therefore, the functional properties of the product are essential in development. *Saccharomyces cerevisiae* that are null for *Apn1*, the yeast homolog of *APE*, are hypersensitive to the cytotoxic effects of monofunctional alkylating chemicals and display a mutator phenotype, since their spontaneous mutation rate is 6- to 12-fold higher than that of wild-type cells.[103] The higher mutation rate characteristic of these cells is further evidence that AP sites are endogenous premutagenic lesions in eukaryotes. Increased *APE* activity may be required in solid tumors that contain hypoxic cells, since colon adenocarcinoma cells displayed increased *APE* expression in response to hypoxic stress.[104] A highly sensitive assay to quantitate the in vivo frequency and distribution of AP sites was recently reported and used to show that the number of AP sites varied in normal rat tissues.[105] This assay may be useful in human studies on the base excision repair pathway and for determining its importance in carcinogenesis.

DNA glycosylases recognize and excise various altered bases from DNA and work sequentially with AP endonucleases in the BER pathway. These enzymes are usually small in size (<30 kDa) with no metal cofactor or exogenous energy source requirements. Glycosylases hydrolyze the *N*-glycosidic bond linking the base to the deoxyribose sugar, leaving an abasic site that then is removed by an AP endonuclease with 5′ nicking and phosphodiesterase activities. All enzymes of this category strongly favor incising on double-stranded DNA and catalyze the release of single free bases as reaction products. Table 1B-5 lists the human glycosylases identified thus far and describes their repair specificities that are detailed in published reports.[106–114] Uracil-DNA glycosylases from distant species are highly conserved. All human tissues express this activity in a cell-cycle-specific manner. Expression of the *UNG1* gene is stimulated about 10-fold in late $G_1$ phase of the cell cycle and preceding a 2- to 3-fold increase in enzyme activity during S phase. Of interest is the fact that certain of these glycosylases (hOGG2 and TDG) recognize the aberrant pairing of bases with normal hydrogen bonding (8-oxo-dG:A and G:T). Also of interest are the very broad substrate specificities displayed by some of these enzymes (AAG and hNTH1).

## NUCLEOTIDE EXCISION REPAIR

Nucleotide excision repair (NER) is an evolutionarily conserved pathway for the removal of bulky, conformationally distorting DNA adducts. Over the last decade, the factors that carry out this repair have been cloned and characterized biochemically; a detailed description of the activities of NER components is reviewed in reference 115. Two subpathways operate for NER, one that performs *global genome repair* and another that carries out repair of the transcribed strand of actively expressed genes known as *transcription-coupled repair*. Global genome repair is considerably slower than transcription-coupled repair. Inherited deficiencies in NER capabilities are found in patients with xeroderma pigmentosum (XP). Individuals with XP display extreme dermal photosensitivity that leads to skin cancer. Interestingly, these individuals are prone to no other form of cancer. XP complementation studies have identified seven groups (XPA to G) reflecting mutations in seven different NER genes. Another clinical manifestation of NER deficiency is the brittle hair syndrome, trichothiodystrophy, in which XPB and XPD mutations are detected. However, individuals with this affliction are

### TABLE 1B-5. CLONED HUMAN DNA GLYCOSYLASES

| GLYCOSYLASE | GENE DESIGNATION | DAMAGED BASES EXCISED |
|---|---|---|
| Uracil DNA glycosylase | *UNG1* | Uracil and the cytosine oxidation products, isodialuric acid 5-hydroxyuracil, and alloxan |
| 8-Oxoguanine DNA glycosylase | *hOGG1* | 8-Oxo-dG paired with dC, T, or dG |
| 8-Oxoguanine DNA glycosylase | *hOGG2* | 8-Oxo-dG paired with dA after DNA synthesis has incorporated 8-OxodGTP |
| 3-Methyl-adenine DNA glycosylase | *AAG* | 3-Methyl-dA, 3-methyl-dG, 7-methyl-dG, 8-oxo-dG, hypoxanthine, etheno-dG, and etheno-dA |
| G/T mismatch-specific glycosylase | *TDG* | 5-Methyl-dC deamination product at 5′-CpG-3′ sequences |
| Human endonuclease III homolog | *hNTHI* | 17 oxidation products including thymine glycol, 5-hydroxycytosine, 5-hydroxy-6-hydrothymine, 5,6-dihydroxycytosine, and 5-hydroxyuracil |

not prone to skin cancer. Inherited loss of the transcription-coupled repair subpathway of NER falls into two complementation groups (A and B) of Cockayne's syndrome. These individuals also are not susceptible to cancer; rather this disorder is associated with developmental and neurologic abnormalities. The pleiotrophic nature of the clinical manifestations of NER deficiencies indicates that NER constituents play many distinct roles in development.

The basic molecular mechanism for NER involves six steps and is depicted in Fig. 1B-9. Rate limiting for this repair mechanism is DNA damage recognition and incision, not the actual repair synthesis. Bulky DNA adducts are first recognized by XPC in association with another protein, hHR23B.[116] Subsequently, NER components are recruited to the lesion site to effect the remaining steps of incising the DNA 5′ and 3′ of the lesion site, removing the damaged oligonucleotide and resynthesizing the complementary sequence followed by ligation to seal the 3′ nick. Both NER subpathways utilize several protein subunits of the RNA polymerase II holoenzyme transcription factor TFIIH to catalyze opening of the lesion site and to facilitate repair complex assemble. Indeed, XPB and XPD are integral components of TFIIH. Thus, following damage recognition, TFIIH, XPA, and RPA proteins are recruited to assemble the repair

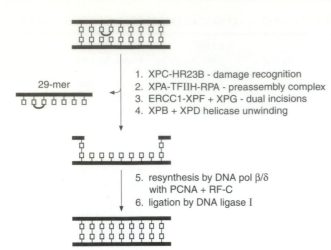

29-mer

1. XPC-HR23B - damage recognition
2. XPA-TFIIH-RPA - preassembly complex
3. ERCC1-XPF + XPG - dual incisions
4. XPB + XPD helicase unwinding

5. resynthesis by DNA pol β/δ
   with PCNA + RF-C
6. ligation by DNA ligase I

**FIGURE 1B-9.** Nucleotide excision repair.

machinery. XPA is a DNA binding protein with affinity for single-stranded damaged sites. RPA is a single-strand DNA binding protein that is thought to bind to the undamaged DNA strand to fully open and stabilize the repair complex. Interactions with RPA then allow engagement of the endonucleases ERCC1-XPF and XPG that make the dual incisions 5′ and 3′ of the lesion, respectively. The 3′ incision by XPG precedes that made by ERCC-XPF. Through interactions with other proteins, XPG serves additional roles in DNA repair. For example, its interacting with proliferating nuclear cell antigen (PCNA) stimulates repair synthesis. The XPB and XPD helicases unwind the DNA to release the approximately 30-nucleotide-long segment containing the adduct. XPB unwinds DNA in a 3′→5′ direction, whereas XPD unwinds in the opposite direction. For the NER pathway, repair synthesis is performed by both DNA polymerase β and δ. PCNA and replication factor C (RF-C) are required at this stage to promote processivity by the polymerases. Finally, DNA ligase I is thought to join the 5′ end of the newly synthesized patch to the repaired duplex sequence.

The two genes mutated in Cocayne's syndrome specify proteins that interact with the RNA polymerase II transcription apparatus. It has been described that CS-A and CS-B patients show defective repair of UV-induced photodimers, as well as oxidized bases in DNA, lesions that are corrected by two distinct repair mechanisms.[118] Interaction of XPG with hNTH1, the BER protein listed in Table 1B-5, promotes binding of the glycosylase to oxidized bases in DNA.[117] Importantly, mismatch repair-deficient cells are also deficient in the coupling of repair with transcription.[119] These findings suggest that the role of TFHII in repair should be expanded to include recognition and recruitment of the appropriate repair machinery for all types of DNA damage that stall transcription elongation. In this case, the requirement for specific changes in the configuration of components of the elongation complex are projected that would allow its displacement from the lesion site permitting the access and assembly of appropriate repair complexes. Thus, it is likely that CS-A and CS-B proteins play a structural role facilitating the access to sites of DNA damage by different repair apparatuses. Cells lacking the function of the breast and ovarian cancer susceptibility gene, *BRCA1*, also are hypersensitive to ionizing radiation and oxidant stress. By

analogy, *BRCA1* mutant cells are defective in transcription-coupled repair of oxidized bases in DNA, as well,[120] further supporting the view that factors from different pathways converge during transcription to mediate many different kinds of repair.

## MISMATCH REPAIR

Unlike NER, mismatch repair activity is lost in sporadic as well as specific types of familial cancers in humans. Hence, the gene products elaborated by this repair pathway act as tumor suppressors. Mismatch repair (MMR) corrects replication errors that have escaped the proofreading functions of DNA polymerase. The MMR pathway corrects several types of replication errors as well as G:T mismatches. Also, this repair system acts on recombination intermediates that contain mispaired bases due to partial homology. Also, MMR corrects template misalignments or slippages of a single base or as many as four nucleotides in simple repetitive sequences. This defect is expected to arise during replication of repetitive sequence tracts when the primer and template strand transiently disassociate and then re-anneal in a misaligned configuration allowing synthesis to resume. The potential consequence of such misalignments is a frame shift mutation where one or more base pairs are either added or deleted. If the unpaired base(s) arose from the primer strand, continued synthesis results in the elongation of the repeat element. However, if the unpaired base(s) was derived from the template strand, resumed synthesis results in the shortening of this element, causing a deletion. Finally, mismatches can arise if a hairpin structure forms between imperfect palindromes (e.g., inverted repeats). MMR corrects these different lesions and maintains genetic fidelity because the mechanism apparently discriminates the parental template strand from the faultily replicated daughter strand and reproduces the original sequence of the former.

Damage recognition and recruitment of an MMR complex uses primarily heterodimers of two proteins: hMSH2:hMSH6 (hMutSα). Additional human MutS homologs include hMSH3 and hMSH4. A heterodimer of hMSH2:hMSH3 (hMutSβ) binds to substrates that contain extrahelical nucleotides (2–4) such as those formed by misalignment. The hMutSα complex attaches to G:T mispairs with the highest affinity but also recognizes insertion or deletion loops of 1–2 nucleotides. MMR also relies on the binding of a heterodimer of hMLH1:hPMS2 (hMutLα); a third homolog, hPMS1, has also been identified. Unlike NER, the mechanistic details are yet to be determined for this pathway. As shown in Fig. 1B-10, a mismatch is recognized by hMutSα, which then uses a nick in either the 3′ or 5′ direction for strand discrimination. This nick can be placed as far as a thousand nucleotides away. Although the mechanism by which eukaryotic cells effect strand discrimination is still unknown, it is thought that mismatch proteins may recognize breaks in the daughter strand or may interact with proteins involved in DNA synthesis at the replication fork. After hMutSα and hMutLα binding, the DNA between the nick and the mismatch is removed by exonuclease digestion to a point beyond the mismatch site. The resulting single-strand gap is filled by DNA polymerase δ and/or ε and sealed by ligase.

The biochemistry of MMR in human cells is currently under intense study since it was discovered that this pathway is defective

G/T mismatch

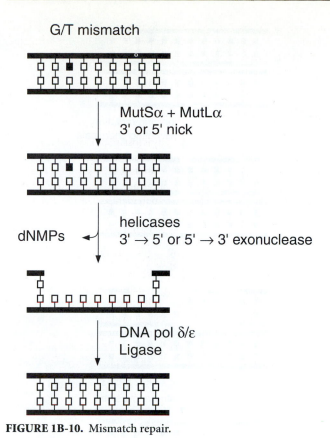

**FIGURE 1B-10.** Mismatch repair.

in a heritable form of human cancer. In 1993 Lynch described an autosomal cancer susceptibity syndrome in which affected families develop cancers mainly in the proximal colon.[121] Other affected tissues in these pedigrees include endometrium, ovary, and stomach. Lynch syndrome kindred develop cancer at an age younger than 50 years, and kindred is defined as families in which at least three relatives in two generations have colorectal cancer. The syndrome, also known as hereditary nonpolyposis colon cancer (HNPCC), is relatively common, affecting about 23,000 individuals in the United States annually and accounting for 15% to 20% of colon cancer cases in industrialized nations. Mutations in *hMSH2, hMLH1, hPMS1,* or *hPMS2* genes account for colon cancer predisposition and are detected in 92% of HNPPC patients. All four genes are thought to be classical tumor suppressors. Noninherited inactivating mutations in these genes, occurring during tumor development, are also found in some sporadic colon carcinomas (13%). Moreover, the expression of these genes in some sporadic colon tumors is silenced due to DNA methylation. The importance of the MMR genes in carcinogenesis was confirmed in mice deficient in *Mlh1, Pms1, Pms2,* and *Msh2;* with the exception of *Pms1,* all of these animals are prone to developing adenomas, lymphomas, and sarcomas by 1 year of age.[122–126]

The association of HNPCC with MMR was made when it was observed that cell lines established from patients showed marked changes in the lengths of simple repeat sequences throughout the genome. This phenotype was designated *microsatellite instability.* The human genome contains many different types of repeat elements including about $10^5$ microsatellite sequences. Elements of this type contain iterated sequences such as poly(GT)$_n$, where n is 20 or more base pairs in length.

Other characteristics of MMR-deficient cell lines established from HNPCC individuals are of interest. For example, these cells display an inappropriate response to treatment by the base analog 6-thioguanine in that they fail to undergo growth arrest in $G_2$ phase of the cell cycle. The importance of growth arrest in response to DNA damage (checkpoint control) is discussed below. Moreover, these cells have a 10- to 1000-fold higher spontaneous mutation rate, and they tend to be resistant to the cytotoxicity of alkylating chemicals. Thus, defects in MMR correlate with a tolerance of DNA damage. On the other hand, these cell lines tend to have a more normal karyotype than cell lines established from sporadic colon tumors. Recent reviews on this topic can be found in references 127 to 129.

A conundrum that has prompted much discussion is the basis of the tissue specificity of cancer types associated with different repair deficiencies. Unanswered questions include the following. Why do XP patients, in whom all tissues are deficient in NER, show only a susceptibility to skin cancer? Why are individuals deficient in MMR prone to colon cancer preferentially? In HNPCC kindred, tumors arise in the epithelium of the colon and endometrium presumably because these targets are favored either to acquire the "second hit" inactivating the remaining wild-type MMR allele, or because these tissues provide a permissive microenvironment for outgrowth (e.g., clonal selection) of preneoplastic cells, or both. Some studies of MMR knockout mice support these ideas. For instance, lymphoma-prone *Pms2*$^{-/-}$ mice showed increased numbers of intestinal adenomas when crossed with the *Min*$^{+/-}$ mouse that is heterozygous for the tumor suppressor *Apc.*[130] This result suggests that reduced *Apc* function makes the murine small bowel a permissive site for carcinognesis. The notion that colon epithelium is a favorable site to acquire a "second hit" suggests that carcinogens and dietary micronutrients may play a very important role in modulating the incidence of colon cancer in humans. (See Cancer Chemoprevention later in this chapter.) Indeed, the tumor number was increased in *Msh2*-null mice exposed to an alkylating carcinogen, ethyl methane sulfonate.[131] Also, the skin of knockout mice lacking the NER *Xpa* gene displayed a marked sensitivity to UV and PAH carcinogens.[132]

Mismatch repair also plays an editing role that limits reciprocal recombination events. This activity may be relevant to cancer because of its importance in maintaining genomic stability. Reciprocal recombination usually occurs between sequences at identical positions on homologous chromosomes, but may also occur at similar sequences at nonallelic or ectopic locations. The dispersed repetitive sequences in eukaryotic genomes can serve as substrates for ectopic recombination events since they share various degrees of homology at the DNA sequence level. Gene rearrangements (deletion, duplication, inversion, or translocation) may occur at these sites because the elements have diverged to a point of partial sequence homology. In this event, rearrangements are made by a crossing over process called *homeologous recombination.* Products of this type of recombination increase in yeast with defective MMR.

Another nonreciprocal type of recombination is called *gene conversion*. Events of this kind involve the unidirectional transfer of information from one chromosome to another. Gene conversions are nonrandomly associated with crossing over via the formation of a heteroduplex intermediate that can be resolved in either a crossover or noncrossover mode. Incomplete gene conversion is inferred to occur in yeast that are MMR-deficient because the frequency of post-meiotic segregation is increased. The precise mechanism by which MMR suppresses recombination is not known at this time. However, it is thought that steps in the process involve the interference with strand assimilation, branch migration, or resolution of recombination intermediates. Studies of cell lines derived from $Msh2^{-/-}$ mice showed promiscuity with respect to intergenomic and intragenomic recombination.[124] Therefore, it is warranted to assume that MMR defects confer a hyperrecombination phenotype in vivo, but this has not yet been established in humans.

## DOUBLE-STRAND BREAK REPAIR

The repair of double-strand breaks (DBSs) engendered by chemicals, ionizing radiation and oxidant stress, or other means is critical for cell survival. DBS repair is carried out by a recombination mechanism or by specialized recombinases. The model for the recombination mechanism (Fig. 1B-11) was proposed by Szostak and co-workers[133] in 1983. In this model, the ends of a double-strand break in DNA are first modified by exonuclease to generate single-stranded 3′ ends. These DNA ends, in turn, invade a homologous duplex and prime repair synthesis in a reaction that creates a region of double-strand gene conversion. A crossover structure called a Holliday junction arises on either side of the gene conversion, and these junctions branch-migrate to produce regions of heteroduplexed DNA that are repaired in a separate reaction. The Holliday junctions can be resolved independently in either plane, resulting in different types of crossover products. Proteins required for this form of DSB repair include those encoded by *hRAD51*, the human homolog of the bacterial recombination factor RecA, as well as RPA.[134] Evidence to support this recombination model was obtained in mammalian cells, and double-strand breaks were repeatedly shown to strongly stimulate recombination in vivo.

DSB is efficiently carried out in eukaryotic cells by end joining in a reaction that does not depend on base-pairing interactions. Variants of rodents cells that are hypersensitive to ionizing radiation led to the identification of three genes required for the end-joining mechanism, *XRCC4*, *XRCC5*, and *XRCC7*. The former encodes a protein designated Ku70, whereas the latter two encode subunits of the DNA-dependent protein kinase holoenzyme, DNA-PK, designated Ku80 and DNA$_{CS}$-PK, respectively (for a review of DNA-PK, see reference 135). Ku70 and Ku80 form a heterodimer that together have ATP-dependent helicase activity and high affinity for DNA ends. DNA$_{CS}$-PK is the 465-kDa catalytic subunit of DNA-PK and a member of the phosphatidylinositol 3-kinase family. It is thought that the Ku complex, upon binding to DNA, protects the ends from nuclease and also aids in aligning them for rejoining. DNA$_{CS}$-PK, which is inactive until bound in a ternary complex at a break site, then is engaged by the Ku heterodimer. The DNA ends are aligned prox-

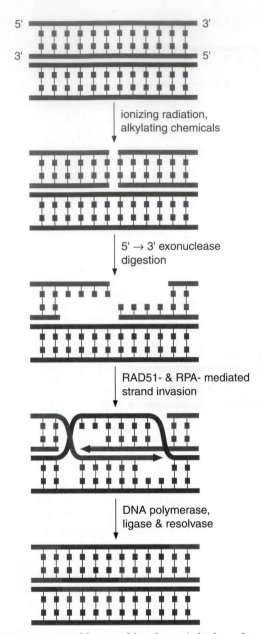

**FIGURE 1B-11.** Double-strand break repair by homologous recombination. (See also Plate 2.)

imally, and the kinase attached to one DNA end phosphorylates the catalytic subunit of the kinase attached to the opposing DNA end. This *trans* phophorylation inactivates further DNA$_{CS}$-PK activity. Subsequent repair steps are likely to include removal of 3′ blocking damage or other end modifications, followed by DNA polymerase–mediated synthesis and/or ligation by DNA ligase IV. Further details on DSB repair are provided in reference 136. Both Ku70 and Ku80 mice display a severe combined immunodeficiency (SCID) phenotype and are hypersensitive to ionizing radiation and alkylating chemicals that produce DNA strand breaks.[137–139] Moreover, DNA$_{CS}$-PK null mice develop thymic lymphomas, suggesting that *XRCC7* is a tumor suppressor gene for T cells of the cell-mediated immune system.[140]

## GENOMIC INSTABILITY AND DEREGULATED CELL CYCLE CONTROL

Upon review of the different pathways of DNA repair, it can readily be appreciated that different types of damage tend to be incurred at different stages of the cell cycle. For instance, cells in $G_0/G_1$ phase are expressing their tissue-specific functions and are quiescent. Hence, they are most vulnerable to damage by oxidative processes and carcinogens that produce DNA lesions subject to BER and NER. Actively dividing cells, though, may suffer incomplete or error-prone replication and require mismatch correction, whereas cells undergoing mitosis risk chromosomal breakage during the segregation of sister chromatids. Conserved genetic pathways exist in eukaryotes to transiently arrest progression through the cell cycle in response to DNA damage to allow the faithful completion of each phase of the cell cycle before advancing on to the next. *Checkpoint* genes encode the proteins that perform these surveillance functions. Thus, cell cycle checkpoints are regulatory mechanisms that ensure high-fidelity transmission of genetic information from one cell generation to the next.

The maintenance of checkpoint pathways preserves genomic stability under normal circumstances and especially following DNA damage. *DNA damage checkpoints* arrest cells in the $G_1$ phase of the cell cycle to prevent DNA replication of a damaged template before entry into S phase. Mediators of the DNA damage checkpoint can also slow DNA synthesis in S phase to modify replicative lesion processing (e.g., proofreading, bypass, and repair). A decreased rate of DNA synthesis in response to DNA damage can be effected by checkpoint controls over both origin initiation and replication fork progression. Finally, the DNA damage checkpoint also arrests cells in $G_2$ to prevent deletions that would result from unrepaired double-strand breaks during the compaction of chromosomes. Two other cell cycle checkpoint systems monitor M phase to prevent aneuploidy. The *spindle checkpoint* inhibits anaphase progression when chromosomes are not properly attached to the mitotic spindle. In eukaryotes, the centrosome undergoes precise duplication to generate two poles for the mitotic spindle. The *spindle pole body duplication checkpoint* prevents monopolar or polypolar mitoses that would cause ploidy changes when chromosomes are improperly segregated to a surviving daughter cell. Thus, in eukaryotes there exist DNA replication checkpoints, spindle assembly checkpoints, and cytokinesis checkpoints. The consequences of checkpoint control failure were recently reviewed in reference 141.

During carcinogenesis, the tendency for evolving tumor cells to abrogate growth constraints and to avoid apoptosis frequently leads to the loss of checkpoint controls and the acquisition of genomic instability as an early heritable trait. Indeed, cells with defective checkpoints presumably have an advantage when selection favors multiple genetic changes, and cancer cells therefore are typically missing some checkpoints, allowing for a greater rate of genomic change. As mentioned above, the multistage process of carcinogenesis is driven by the progressive acquisition of mutations in numerous genes (see Mechanisms of Multistage Carcinogenesis). It also appears that in at least some neoplasias, the evolving tumor cell acquires a mutator phenotype that further enhances tumor progression. *Mutator* cells display a higher incidence of spontaneous mutations than their normal, wild-type counterparts. However, an increased mutation rate per se does not fully explain the prevalence of mutations in tumors compared to normal cells. A selective growth advantage favors the propagation and instability of initiated cells, but not their normal counterparts in their tissue context. As discussed above, the initiated cells subsequently undergo successive rounds of clonal expansion (see Fig. 1B-4). By acquiring genomic instability, the evolving tumor cells obtain the means for both tumor progression and tumor heterogeneity. An increased mutation rate may accelerate the process, but it is not necessary or sufficient for tumorigenesis; rather selection is the driving force for tumor growth.

Tumor cells are now thought to display either of two qualitatively different types of genomic instability designated *MIN* for *microsatellite instability* and *CIN* for *chromosomal instability*.[142] As described above, the MIN phenotype is associated with HNPCC, results from the inheritance of an inactive mismatch repair gene, and is unusual in sporadic colorectal cancers. When considering all forms of colorectal, endometrial, and gastric cancers, MIN tumors represent about 13%, and for all other types of tumors, the MIN phenotype is quite rare (<2%). On the other hand, the CIN phenotype is very common in several types of human cancer and can result from mutations in numerous genes that normally regulate progression through $G_2$ and M. The precise nature of the human genes conferring CIN properties to tumors is yet to be discovered. Some of these regulators include known tumor suppressor genes such as *RB*, *TP53*, and *CDKN2A*$^{INK4A}$, conferring heritable cancer predisposition of different types. Newly identified CIN genes include *hMAD2* and *hBUB1*,[143,144] and the gene predisposing women to breast and ovarian cancer, *BRCA1*. The mutant version of this tumor suppressor causes a defective $G_2/M$ checkpoint with centrosome amplification.[145] However, studies in yeast suggest that CIN genes encode all checkpoint surveillance regulators including those specifying DNA damage responses, as well as the regulators of chromosome condensation and segregation, and kinetochore and centrosome structure and function. Given that many genes regulate these numerous processes, there are consequently many mutational targets. Therefore, CIN is by far the most prevalent type of instability in tumors. Moreover, the CIN phenotype can account for all of the usual chromosomal abnormalities evident in human tumors, including aneuploidy, loss of heterozygosity, and karyotype changes.

## SIGNAL TRANSDUCTION AND GENE EXPRESSION

As mentioned previously in this chapter, the multistage process of carcinogenesis in experimental systems can often be divided into three qualitatively different phases: initiation, promotion, and progression. A number of exogenous and endogenous agents can specifically enhance the process of tumor promotion (see Fig. 1B-4).

**TABLE 1B-6.** BIOLOGICAL AND BIOCHEMICAL FACTS ABOUT TUMOR PROMOTERS

1. Tumor promoters enhance the tumor-inducing potential of carcinogens but are not genotoxicants.
2. The activity of tumor promoters requires repeated exposures after the application of a genotoxic initiating agent.
3. Discontinuation of the promoting stimulus can reverse the tumor enhancing effect, but with prolonged treatments, tumor progression becomes irreversible.
4. Tumor promoters can both increase the number of tumors and shorten the latency period.
5. Tumor promoters stimulate cell cycle entry ($G_0 \rightarrow G_1$), activate signal transduction pathways, and alter gene expression.

The means by which these agents interact with specific cellular receptors, and the subsequent mechanism by which recognition of this event is transmitted to the nucleus to alter gene expression and thereby induce specific biological responses is known as *signal transduction*. Tumor promoters achieve their effects by causing aberrant activation of signal transduction pathways. Thus, they act through epigenetic mechanisms to affect cell proliferation and differentiation in contrast to the actions of mutagenic carcinogens that directly target DNA. Table 1B-6 lists several biologic characteristics that are typical of tumor promoters.

The first recognition that certain agents were extremely potent in promoting tumor formation came from studies on mouse skin carcinogenesis that employed croton oil (isolated from the plant *Croton tiglium*) as the tumor promoter. Subsequent studies indicated that the active compound was a phorbol ester. Figure 1B-12 illustrates the distinction between the initiation and promotion phases of carcinogenesis, and shows that a suboptimal dose of an initiating (e.g., genotoxic) carcinogen followed by repeated administrations of a tumor promoter yielded skin tumors, whereas none or very few tumors arose in the absence of the promoter. The combination of an initiating carcinogen together with tumor promoter applications increased the yield of skin tumors and shortened the latency time for their appearance. The most extensively studied experimental tumor promoter is the compound 12-*O*-tetradecanoylphorbol-13-acetate (TPA). This compound, like all tumor promoters, does not target DNA directly and is, therefore, not directly mutagenic. Instead, it enters cells and binds to and activates the function of the enzyme, *protein kinase C* (PKC). PKC constitutes a family of lipid-regulated serine and threonine protein kinases that play important roles in signal transduction pathways that control cell proliferation, differentiation, and apoptosis. PKCs also play important roles in mediating the actions of specific growth factors, cytokines, and the products of oncogenes. There are twelve distinct isoforms of this enzyme and individual isoforms differ with respect to their specific subcellular locations and cellular functions. Thus, increased expression of the epsilon isoform of PKC (PKCε) can enhance the in vitro conversion of normal cells to tumor cells, whereas the delta isoform of PKC (PKCδ) often inhibits cell growth (for review see references 146–148).

Examples of endogenous activators of signal transduction include growth factors, cytokines, hormones, eicosinoids, and neurotransmitters. The actions of several growth factors and cytokines are mediated by their binding to membrane-associated receptors that have tyrosine kinase activities. Ligand binding to these receptors often leads to the activation in the cytoplasm of the Ras protein and/or related small GTP-binding proteins. Activated Ras, in turn, initates the activation of a cascade of protein kinases, termed MAP kinases, finally resulting in the phosphorylation and activation of specific transcription factors in the nucleus. These signal transduction pathways explain how the exposure of cells to growth factors and other agonists leads to changes in gene expression, and thereby leads to alterations in specific cellular functions. Recent studies indicate that PKCα and PCKε play direct roles in enhancing the activities of these MAP kinase pathways, thus helping to

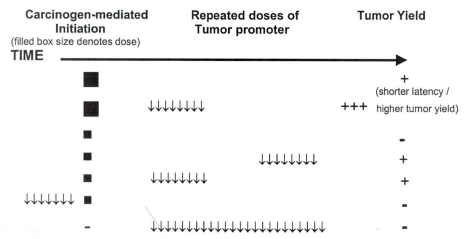

**FIGURE 1B-12.** Relationship between exposure to a genotoxic initiating carcinogen and a nongenotoxic tumor promoter in a two-stage model of carcinogenesis. (*Adapted from reference 140*).

explain the molecular mechanisms of action of TPA and related tumor promoters.[149]

There is experimental evidence that, in addition to TPA, several other types of chemicals have tumor-promoting activity in various organ systems in rodents. These include phenobarbitol, saccharine, and several halogenated organic compounds. The latter compounds include several pesticides. Although not all of these agents activate PKC, it seems likely that they act through similar pathways of signal transduction, thereby altering gene expression and enhancing carcinogenesis. Alternatively, it is possible that chronic exposures to some of these so-called nongenotoxic agents also induce mutations in DNA through indirect effects, for example, via the formation of activated forms of oxygen or through other mechanisms that eventually lead to DNA damage, as previously decribed (see DNA Damage and Mutation Induction).

The subjects of tumor promotion and alterations in gene expression are also central to the phenomenon of hormonal carcinogenesis, since hormones are not directly mutagenic, but act by binding to specific nuclear receptors that control gene transcription. These mechanisms help to explain how estrogenic compounds can enhance the development of breast and endometrial cancers and how androgens can enhance the development of prostate cancer.

Thus, the multistage process of carcinogenesis is often driven by interactions between multiple exogenous and endogenous factors, and is mediated by both genetic and epigenetic mechanisms. Furthermore, there are numerous examples in experimental systems in which initiating carcinogens, tumor promoters, or other chemical and physical agents interact synergistically with microbial agents in the carcinogenic process, both in vivo and in cell culture. It seems likely, therefore, that certain human cancers are caused by interactions between chemical agents and viruses or other infectious agents (see Mechanisms of Multistage Carcinogenesis and reference 150), that separately have weak or no carcinogenic activity. Epidemiologic studies have suggested several examples of these multifactor interactions. For instance, the high incidence of liver cancer in Africa and certain regions of Asia appears to be due to synergistic interactions between hepatitis B virus and aflatoxin $B_1$ or other carcinogens in the diet. Nasopharyngeal cancer in Asia and Burkitt's lymphoma in Africa appear to be due to an interaction between Epstein-Barr virus and nitrosamines or tumor promoters present in the diet. Cervical cancer may be due to an interaction between specific strains of human papillomavirus and carcinogens present in cigarette smoke or from other sources. Gastric cancer may be due to interactions between the bacterium *H. pylori* and dietary factors, and colorectal cancer may be due to interactions between the bacterial flora in the colon and dietary factors. Therefore, in future studies on the causation of specific human cancers, it is important to consider the likelihood of synergistic interactions between multiple types of environmental and endogenous factors.[146,147]

## CANCER CHEMOPREVENTION

The rapidly expanding field of cancer chemoprevention seeks to identify natural or synthetic compounds that will prevent or reverse the process of carcinogenesis. Because carcinogenesis is a multifactorial process that occurs over many years, it is difficult to prove a direct cancer-modulating effect of any single environmental agent. Nevertheless, insights derived from epidemiologic studies help to define both the causes of cancer and the means to achieve tumor prevention. In 1975, Armstrong and Doll[151] examined differences in cancer incidence and mortality in various parts of the world, and related these differences to nation-specific dietary practices. These data suggested that cancer incidence, particularly for colorectal and breast cancer, is highest for societies consuming the greatest amounts of meat and total fat. These researchers cautioned that diet-cancer associations also might be explained by secondary associations with environmental agents other than diet, or by economic or genetic effects. Multiple studies conducted over the subsequent 25 years provide evidence that diet does affect cancer incidence, perhaps by altering the metabolism of various carcinogens, or by enhancing the body's ability to eliminate preneoplastic cells.

In addition to harmful dietary factors such as the carcinogens in grilled meats (see DNA Damage and Mutation Induction) and the high fat in red meat, numerous dietary substances may be inhibitors of carcinogenesis. For example, many studies suggest that diets rich in fruits, vegetables, and certain grains offer protection against various cancers. As one might imagine, it is very difficult to identify the specific components of these foods that are responsible for the cancer-preventing activity. Hundreds of natural compounds have been screened in cell culture and animal cancer models to identify the most promising chemopreventive agents for use in human clinical trials.

Epidemiologic studies suggest that natural or synthetic hormones can also modulate the behavior of some epithelial cancers, such as those of the breast and prostate. Cancers sensitive to hormone treatments tend to be less advanced and better differentiated. It is reasonable to predict, therefore, that hormonal agents can also be used for primary cancer prevention. This theory is supported by the recent success of tamoxifen in preventing malignancies in a phase III randomized trial involving women at high risk for breast cancer.[152] Hormonal modulation of tumors may even occur through dietary constituents. For example, the phytoestrogens are a class of plant-derived compounds that have weak estrogenic or antiestrogenic effects, depending upon the dose and the model system studied.[153] It is possible that these agents provide protection from certain cancers when present in sufficient quantities in the diet. As shown in Table 1B-7, chemopreventive agents can be divided into several categories based on their predominant effect on target cells. These divisions are somewhat arbitrary, as most of the chemopreventive agents have multiple activities. Representative examples of agents from each category are briefly described below.

## MODIFIERS OF DETOXIFYING ENZYMES

As discussed in the section DNA Damage and Mutation Induction, phase II detoxifying enzymes are involved in the conjugation and excretion of a variety of carcinogenic chemicals, such as benzo[*a*]pyrene, found in cigarette smoke, and the food contaminant aflatoxin $B_1$. Increased activity of certain phase II enzymes, such as glutathione *S*-transferase, is associated with prevention of neoplasia in several model systems.[154] Increased expression of NAD(P)H:oxidoreductase is correlated with chemopreventive

## TABLE 1B-7. CHEMOPREVENTIVE AGENTS

| MECHANISMS | EXAMPLES OF AGENTS |
| --- | --- |
| Upregulate detoxifying enzymes | Isothiocyanates, dithiolthiones, allyl sulfides, Oltipraz |
| Prevent oxidative damage | β-Carotene; vitamins A, E, and C; selenium; plant phenolics; caffeic acid |
| Maintain DNA integrity | Folic acid |
| Promote differentiation | Vitamin A, retinoids |
| Decrease cell proliferation | DFMO, calcium, vitamin D |
| Inhibit angiogenesis | Genistein, selective Cox-2 inhibitors |
| Block cancer-associated growth factors | Tamoxifen, finasteride, phytoestrogens, aromatase inhibitors |
| Alter arachidonic acid metabolism | NSAIDs, Ω-3 fatty acids |

actions.[155] The flavonoid-related compound present in bee propolis, caffeic acid phenethyl ester (CAPE), induces NAD(P)H expression in liver cells.[156] Phase II enzyme activity can be induced by a number of different dietary agents. Several inducers of phase II detoxifying enzymes are found in fruits and vegetables, including sulforaphane, an isothiocyanate found in broccoli,[157] and various allyl sulfides present in garlic and other members of the onion family.[158] Oltipraz is a chemopreventive drug used originally for the treatment of schistosomiasis. Oltipraz induces phase II enzymes and inhibits both benzo[a]pyrene- and aflatoxin B$_1$–induced carcinogenesis.[159] Oltipraz is a potentially useful chemopreventive drug in regions of the world where aflatoxin-associated tumors are common, and interventional trials are being carried out in China.

## ANTIOXIDANTS

A significant body of evidence suggests that reactive oxygen species act as initiators and/or tumor promoters.[160] As discussed earlier in DNA Damage and Mutation Induction, oxygen radicals are produced as a result of inflammation and are capable of producing mutagenic DNA damage.[161] A wide variety of agents with chemopreventive activity are free radical scavengers, and their efficacy in tumor prevention is attributed to this antioxidant activity. Polyphenols, which constitute approximately 10% to 20% of green tea, are potent antioxidants and antitumor agents.[162] Purified polyphenols, such as (−)-epigallocatechin gallate, prevent intestinal and respiratory tumor formation in rodents treated with carcinogens.[163,164] Other promising plant-derived antioxidants that are effective in preventing intestinal tumors in animal models include curcumin, a compound derived from turmeric,[165] CAPE,[166] and (+)-catechin, which is present in grape skins.[167]

Although animal studies suggest that antioxidants are effective chemopreventive drugs, human trials with these agents have yielded mixed results. In a study from Linxian, China, a region with a high incidence of cancer of the esophagus and gastric cardia, dietary supplementation with the antioxidants, β-carotene, vitamin E, and selenium for 5 years reduced cancer mortality by 13%.[168] On the other hand, studies of skin and lung cancers in the United States and Finland failed to associate β-carotene or vitamin E use with a decrease in the incidence of these cancers.[169,170] In addition to its role as an antioxidant, β-carotene can enhance carcinogenesis by inducing cytochrome P450s.[171] Data from the southern United States, a region of relative selenium deficiency, suggest that selenium supplementation may be responsible for the favorable results observed in the Linxian trial.[172] Additional human studies of antioxidants for prevention of both cancer and cardiovascular disease are in progress.

## MAINTENANCE OF DNA INTEGRITY

An important protection against cancer is the ability to repair DNA damage and maintain normal DNA metabolism (see DNA Repair Mechanisms). DNA repair capacity can be diminished due to mutation in the genes governing DNA repair, a condition that is present in a small portion of epithelial tumors. It is likely, though, that the expression or activities of different mediators of DNA repair and metabolism may be altered in human cancers. Hypomethylation of DNA is associated with epithelial carcinogenesis, particularly for the lower intestinal tract. The loss or gain of methylation at 5′-CpG-3′ sequences in mammalian cells can epigenetically alter gene expression. Folic acid is involved in the transfer of methyl groups to DNA, and dietary supplementation of folic acid may prevent hypomethylation of DNA at CpG sites.[173] Thus, the maintenance of normal DNA metabolism can also be affected by diet. Several dietary and epidemiologic studies suggest that folic acid protects against colon cancer[174,175]; however, its efficacy as a chemopreventive agent for human colon cancer has yet to be rigorously tested.

## DIFFERENTIATION AGENTS

Retinoids are a class of drugs that function as differentiation agents for epithelial cells.[172] After binding to specific retinoid receptors, these compounds modulate epithelial proliferation, cell growth, and apoptosis. Vitamin A is a natural retinoid that is necessary for normal vision, reproduction, and growth of epithelial tissue.[176,177] Retinoids can prevent carcinogenesis in a number of animal models of epithelial cancer.[178] Human studies suggest that retinoids suppress cancers of the upper aerodigestive tract and possibly prevent respiratory cancers in smokers.[179] Unfortunately, the currently tested retinoids exhibit side effects, such as dry skin, conjunctivitis, and hypertriglyceridemia, and they are highly teratogenic. The use of retinoids to prevent cancer is therefore limited to short-duration treatments in high-risk individuals.

## DECREASE CELL PROLIFERATION

Difluoromethylornithine (DFMO) is a synthetic compound that inhibits ornithine decarboxylase, an enzyme catalyzing polyamine synthesis. The naturally occurring polyamines, putrescine, spermidine, and spermine, are essential for cell proliferation,[180] and inhibition of polyamine synthesis by DFMO reduces the proliferation of epithelial cell populations in vivo. DFMO is presently under investigation as a chemopreventive strategy for several different cancers, including skin, breast, colon, bladder, prostate, and cervical tumors.

Increased dietary calcium has been associated with a decreased incidence of cancer, particularly lower gastrointestinal malignancies. Calcium inhibits cell proliferation, possibly through effects on PKC, and is particularly effective in animal models employing a high-fat diet.[181] Calcium suppresses ornithine decarboxylase in rat colon explants, and may therefore exert its activities in a manner similar to that of DFMO.[182] A recently completed phase III trial of calcium in patients with colorectal adenomas showed a 19% decrease in adenoma recurrence in subjects taking 1.2 g of calcium per day.[183] Finally, ursodeoxycholic acid (UDCA) is a bile acid that modulates the growth and differentiation of intestinal cells through a PKC-mediated pathway. This agent also inhibits carcinogen-induced tumor formation in rodents,[184] and is currently under investigation in human phase II studies for colon cancer prevention.

## ANTIANGIOGENESIS AGENTS

In order for a single tumor cell to become a tumor mass, either locally as the primary tumor or remotely as a metastatic deposit, angiogenesis must occur. Agents capable of inhibiting the formation of new blood vessels, therefore, show promise as chemopreventive agents. Genistein, the active constituent of soy, is an isoflavonoid that prevents carcinogen-induced rodent breast and colon neoplasia.[185,186] Genistein has a number of different chemopreventive properties, including weak antiestrogenic effects,[187] protein tyrosine kinase inhibition,[185] and antioxidant activity.[188] Some of the chemopreventive effect of genistein may be due to its inhibition of blood vessel development,[189] an effect that may be mediated through transforming growth factor β (TGF-β1) signaling.[190] Although their primary activity is inhibition of prostaglandin synthesis, selective inhibitors of Cox-2 may also inhibit angiogenesis. For example, Celecoxib inhibits fibroblast growth factor–induced corneal angiogenesis in the rat, and augments apoptosis in tumor-associated endothelial cells.[191] The relative contribution of the antiangiogenic effects of these compounds to their antitumor effects is presently unknown.

## BLOCKADE OF CANCER-ASSOCIATED GROWTH FACTORS

The cellular defects associated with carcinogenesis occur at all levels of growth control, including the regulation provided through interactions of specific growth factors and hormones with their receptors. TGF-β is an example of a factor that delivers a negative growth signal to epithelial cells. TGF-β exerts an antiproliferative effect upon mammary and intestinal epithelial cells in rodents[192,193] loss of TGF-β receptor signaling is associated with intestinal tumor formation.[192] One of the chemopreventive activities of retinoids or genistein may be induction of TGF-β in target tissues such as skin, intestine, and respiratory epithelium.[190,194]

Several epithelial tissues, such as breast, prostate, endometrium, and ovary, are sensitive to regulation by steroid hormones. This fact was used successfully to develop chemotherapeutic regimens, and estrogen and androgen blockade are routinely used to treat breast and prostate cancers. Since cancers most often arise in the postreproductive era of life, it may also be possible to use hormonal modulation to prevent tumors. Success in this approach was demonstrated with the use of tamoxifen for breast cancer prevention. A recent prospective, randomized, placebo-controlled trial of tamoxifen for the prevention of breast cancer in high-risk women showed a 45% decrease in cancer incidence in women on 10 mg of tamoxifen twice daily.[152] Finasteride is an inhibitor of testosterone-5-alpha reductase that suppresses androgen production and is currently used to treat benign prostatic hypertrophy. In its early stages, prostate cancer is responsive to androgen withdrawal, and it is therefore possible that finasteride will also have an antitumor effect.[195] Furthermore, diets rich in fruits and vegetables contain phytoestrogens, compounds that bind estrogen receptors and exert weak estrogenic or antiestrogenic effects, depending upon the model studied.[153] The importance of these effects in humans has not been established.

## MODULATORS OF ARACHIDONIC ACID METABOLISM

Arachidonic acid is metabolized to tissue-specific prostaglandins through a reaction catalyzed by the enzymes Cox-1 and Cox-2. Arachidonic acid metabolism is sensitive to the composition of the lipid membrane, and can be modulated by altering the types of fatty acid substrates that are ingested. This influence may be important in the development of cancers of the breast, colon, and prostate, as several epidemiologic studies suggest that the nature of the fatty acids ingested influences cancer risk. In animal studies, polyunsaturated omega-6 fatty acids stimulate epithelial growth, whereas diets enriched in long-chain omega-3 fatty acids protect against abnormal epithelial proliferation.[196]

The most compelling evidence for an association between arachidonic acid metabolism and cancer development is provided by study of tumorigenesis in transgenic animals lacking genes for either form of the cyclooxygenase enzyme Cox-1 or Cox-2. Crossing animals prone to skin or intestinal tumors with those lacking either enzyme yielded a dramatic decrease in tumor formation.[197,198] When the knockout mice study data are taken together with the wealth of epidemiologic and animal model data showing that Cox-inhibiting NSAIDs decrease the incidence of epithelial tumors,[199] the view that these enzymes play a significant role in carcinognesis is impressive. The long-term use of aspirin or other NSAIDs is associated with a 40% to 50% decrease in the incidence of colorectal adenomas and cancers. As discussed in the section Mechanisms of Multistage Carcinogenesis, the cyclooxygenase enzymes are capable of activating chemical carcinogens. Inhibition of Cox activity by NSAIDs, therefore, may also block DNA adduct formation and the initiation phase of carcinogenesis. The NSAID sulindac mediates regression of rectal adenomas in patients with familial adenomatous polyposis, an inherited colon cancer predisposition syndrome caused by germline mutation of the *APC* gene. Several human clinical trials are under way to evaluate the efficacy of arachidonic acid metabolism inhibition in prevention of colorectal tumors. Agents under current investigation include aspirin, as well as selective inhibitors of Cox-2. Recent studies suggest that NSAIDs and their derivatives can also inhibit tumor development and growth by Cox-independent mechanisms (for review see reference 200).

## SUMMARY OF HUMAN CANCER CHEMOPREVENTION TRIALS

To be effective, chemopreventive agents must be given to generally healthy people over long periods of time, perhaps even requiring use from adolescence onward. For a chemopreventive agent to reach the stage of human clinical trials, therefore, it must have extremely low toxicity. These rigorous demands make the design and execution of human cancer chemoprevention trials difficult and costly. In many cases, modulation of a "biomarker" for cancer development can be used as an earlier or "surrogate" indicator in chemoprevention studies. A biomarker is a physiologic variable that is highly correlated with cancer development. One example of a biomarker is the presence of an adenomatous polyp in the colon. Most phase I and II and many phase III chemoprevention studies use biomarker modulation as an end point, thus reducing the time and expense of the trials.

The gold standard for chemoprevention studies remains the prospective, randomized placebo-controlled trials. Most prospective, randomized chemoprevention studies completed to date have utilized cohorts at high risk for a single disease. Examples of these studies include measurements of adenoma regression by NSAIDs in subjects with familial adenomatous polyposis,[201] or the use of tamoxifen in women over 60 years of age or with a history of lobular carcinoma in situ.[147] There have been three large prospective, randomized, placebo-controlled studies of the effect of chemopreventive agents on cancer, with multiple potential tumor sites as end points. The Physicians Health Trial randomized patients beginning in 1982 to receive β-carotene, aspirin, or placebo. Because of a significant decrease in cardiovascular mortality in the aspirin arm of the study, this arm was unblinded and analyzed in 1988. Presently, there was no significant impact of daily aspirin use on cancer mortality.[202] Results of the β-carotene arm are pending. Two additional large chemoprevention studies are in progress. In the Women's Health Study, beginning in 1992, female nurses were randomly assigned to receive β-carotene, α-tocopherol (vitamin E), aspirin, or placebo. The end points of this 8-year study include cancer of the breast, lung, and colon. Finally, the National Institutes of Health Women's Health Initiative is a study of the effect of dietary calcium and vitamin D, exercise, and smoking cessation, with multiple end points, including cancer incidence.

## MOLECULAR EPIDEMIOLOGY

The above-described advances in our understanding of the cellular and molecular mechanisms involved in multistage carcinogenesis provide new concepts and methods for elucidating the specific causes of human cancer and also for determining the cancer susceptibility of individuals or subpopulations within our society. The joining together of more traditional epidemiologic studies with specific laboratory assays on biologic fluids and tissue specimens as a source of "biomarkers," has created a new field called molecular epidemiology. Several highly sensitive and specific laboratory assays can be used as biomarkers of specific factors related to the following parameters: (1) genetic and acquired host susceptibility; (2) metabolism and tissue levels of carcinogens; (3) levels of covalent adducts formed between carcinogens and DNA or other macromolecules (e.g., hemoglobin); and (4) early cellular responses to carcinogen exposure, including sister chromatid exchange, micronuclei, DNA repair, altered gene expression, and mutations in cellular oncogenes and tumor suppressor genes. Samples that can be used for these assays include blood, urine, saliva, cytology specimens, and tissue biopsies. These methods are now applied in a broad spectrum of epidemiologic studies, and they offer great promise for expanding the scientific basis for human cancer prevention. Many of the biomarkers used in this field are also useful in dietary studies and as surrogate end points in clinical trials of chemopreventive agents. For reviews of this field see references 146, 147, 203, and 204.

## FUTURE DIRECTIONS

It is apparent from the above review that within the past few decades, exciting progress has been made in identifying some of the causes of cancer and of the cellular and molecular mechanisms involved in the multistage process of carcinogenesis. At the same time, there are still major gaps in our current knowledge. With respect to causation, these deficiencies include: (1) clarification of the specific causative factors involved for several major types of human cancer, specifically breast, prostate, and colon cancer; (2) clarification of the relative roles of environmental and/or life-style choices versus hereditary factors and their possible interactions in cancer causation; (3) identification of the specific dietary agents that either enhance or inhibit the development of specific types of cancer; and (4) further elucidation of roles of infectious agents in the etiology of cancer. With respect to remaining gaps in our knowledge of the underlying cellular and molecular mechanisms of carcinogenesis, important future areas of research include: (1) a more detailed understanding of the critical genetic mutations, as well as the epigenetic changes in gene expression that occur during multistage carcinogenesis; (2) the mechanisms responsible for genomic instability in cancer and possibly premalignant cells; and (3) a more precise understanding of the molecular mechanisms of action of tumor promoters, hormones and their agonists, and oxidative damage in carcinogenesis. Moreover, the relatively recent discoveries of new viral and bacterial causes of human cancers (e.g., Kaposi's sarcoma and gastric cancer) should encourage investigators to continue to search for new infectious agents in the future. Hopefully, advances in these areas of research will provide new biomarkers for epidemiology and clinical studies that will allow strategies for cancer prevention to be tested in humans. Eventually, the validation of prevention strategies for specific types of cancer will prove effective in reducing the cancer burden if combined with adequate public awareness and the commitment to implement these strategies. Lastly, advances in the understanding of signal transduction pathways mediating cell proliferation and checkpoint control will continue to provide new strategies for cancer therapy. Thus, the development of selective inhibitors that target tumor initiation, promotion, and progression; genomic instability; growth; survival; and metastasis should provide more effective strategies for both cancer prevention and therapy.

## REFERENCES

1. Ramazzini B: *De Morbis Artificium Diatriba* (translated by WC Wright). Chicago, University of Chicago Press, 1940.

2. Weinstein IB: From chimney sweeps to oncogenes. Mol Carcinogen 1:2, 1980.

3. Lawley PD: Historical origins of current concepts of carcinogenesis. Adv Cancer Res 65:17, 1994.

4. Witkowski JA: The inherited character of cancer—An historical survey. Cancer Cells 2:229, 1990.

5. Sgambato A et al: Abnormalities in cell cycle control in cancer and their clinical implications. Tumori 84:421, 1998.

6. Miller E: Some current perspectives on chemical carcinogenesis in humans and experimental animals. Cancer Res 38:1479, 1978.

7. Weinstein IB: The origins of human cancer: Molecular mechanism of carcinogenesis and their implications for cancer prevention and treatment. Cancer Res 48:4135, 1988.

8. Holzinger F et al: Mechanisms of biliary carcinogenesis: A pathogenetic multi-stage cascade toward cholangiocarcinoma. Ann Oncol 10:122, 1999.

9. Berenblum I: The mechanism of carcinogenesis: A study of the significance of cocarcinogenic action and related phenomena. Cancer Res 1:807, 1941.

10. Berenblum I: Carcinogenesis and tumor pathogenesis. Adv Cancer Res 2:129, 1954.

11. Friedewald WF, Rous P: The initiating and promoting elements in tumor production: An analysis of the effects of tar, benzpyrene, and methylcholanthrene on rabbit skin. J Exp Med 80:101, 1944.

12. Furth J, Kahn MC: Am J Cancer 31:276, 1937.

13. Nowell PC, Hungerford, DA: A minute chromosome in human granulocytic leukemia. Science 132:1497, 1960.

14. Nowell PC: Chromosomes and cancer: The evolution of an idea. Adv Cancer Res 62:1, 1993.

15. Nowell PC: The clonal evolution of tumor populations. Science 194:23, 1976.

16. Loeb LA et al: Errors in DNA replication as a basis of malignant changes. Cancer Res 34:2311, 1974.

17. Loeb LA: Cancer cells exhibit a mutator phenotype. Adv Cancer Res 72:25, 1998.

18. Duesberg P et al: Genetic instability of cancer cells is proportional to their degree of aneuploidy. Proc Natl Acad Sci USA 95:13,692, 1998.

19. Lengauer C et al: Genetic instability in colorectal cancers. Nature 386:623, 1997.

20. Prehn RT: Cancers beget mutations *versus* mutations beget cancers. Cancer Res 54:5296, 1994.

21. Brinster RL: Effect of cells transferred into the mouse blastocyst on subsequent development. J Exp Med 140:1049, 1974.

22. Papaioannou VE et al: Fate of teratocarcinoma cells injected into early mouse embryos. Nature 258:70, 1975.

23. Illmensee K, Minz B: Totipotency and normal differentiation of single teratocarcinoma cells cloned by injection into blastocysts. Proc Natl Acad Sci USA 73:549, 1976.

24. Beukers R, Berends W: Isolation and identification of the irradiation product of thymine. Biochim Biophys Acta 41:550, 1960.

25. Miller, EC et al: The comparative carcinogenicities of 2-acetylaminofluorene and its *N*-hydroxy metabolite in mice, hamsters, and guinea pigs. Cancer Res 24:2018, 1964.

26. Brookes P, Lawley PD: Evidence for the binding of polynuclear aromatic hydrocarbons to the nucleic acids of mouse skin: Reaction between carcinogenic power of hydrocarbons and their binding to deoxyribonucleic acid. Nature 202:781, 1964.

27. Craddock VM, Magee PN: Analysis of bases of rat-liver nucleic acids after administration of the carcinogen dimethylnitrosamine. Biochem J 100:724, 1966.

28. Cleaver JE: Defective repair replication of DNA in xeroderma pigmentosum. Nature 218:652, 1964.

29. McCann J et al: Detection of carcinogens as mutagens in the *Salmonella*/microsome test: Assay of 300 chemicals. Proc Natl Acad Sci USA 72:5135, 1973.

30. Doll R, Peto R: The causes of cancer: Quantitative estimates of avoidable risks of cancer in the United States today. J Natl Cancer Inst 66:1191, 1981.

31. Shields PG et al: Mutagens from heated Chinese and U.S. cooking oils. J Natl Cancer Inst 87:836, 1995.

32. Thiebaud HP et al: Airborne mutagens produced by frying beef, pork, and soy-based food. Food Chem Toxicol 33:821, 1995.

33. Chiang TA et al: Mutagenicity and polycyclic aromatic hydrocarbon content of fumes from heated cooking oils produced in Taiwan. Mutat Res 381:157, 1997.

34. Nagao M et al: Mutagenicity of protein pyrolysates. Cancer Lett 2:335, 1977.

35. Schut HAJ, Snyderwine EG: DNA adducts of heterocyclic amine food mutagens: Implications for mutagenesis and carcinogenesis. Carcinogenesis 20:353, 1999.

36. van Maanen JM et al: Formation of aromatic DNA adducts in white blood cells in relation to urinary excretion of 1-hydroxypyrene during consumption of grilled meat. Carcinogenesis 15:2263, 1994.

37. Lijinsky W: The formation and occurrence of polynuclear aromatic hydrocarbons associated with food. Mutat Res 259:251, 1991.

38. Scimeca JA: Naturally occurring orally active dietary carcinogens, Chap 2, in *Handbook of Human Toxicology,* J Massaro (ed). Boca Raton, FL, CRC Press, 1997, pp 409–466.

39. Dragan YP, Pitot HC: Aflatoxin carcinogenesis in the context of the multistage nature of cancer, in *The Toxicology of Aflatoxins* DL Eaton, JD Groopman (eds). San Diego, CA, Academic Press, 1994, pp 179–206.

40. Brash DE: Sunlight and the onset of skin cancer. Trends Genet 10:410, 1997.

41. Hall HI et al: Update on the incidence and mortality from melanoma in the United States. J Am Acad Dermatol 40:35, 1999.

42. Ioannides C, Parke DV: The cytochrome P4501 gene family of microsomal hemoproteins and their role in the metabolic activation of chemicals. Drug Metab Rev 22:1, 1990.

43. Gonzalez FJ, Gelboin HV: Role of human cytochromes P450 in the metabolic activation of chemical carcinogens and toxins. Drug Metab Rev 26:165, 1994.

44. BUTERS JT et al: Cytochrome P450 CYP1B1 determines susceptibility to 7,12-dimethylbenz[*a*]antracene-induced lymphomas. Proc Natl Acad Sci USA 96:1977, 1999.

45. MILLER EC: Studies on the formation of protein-bound derivatives of 3,4-benzpyrene in the epidermal fraction of mouse skin. Cancer Res 11:100, 1951.

46. GELBOIN HV: A microsome-dependent binding of benzo[*a*]pyrene. Cancer Res 29:1272, 1969.

47. JEFFREY AM et al: Structure of benzo[*a*]pyrene-nucleic acid adducts formed in human and bovine bronchial explants. Nature 269:348, 1977.

48. BYCZKOWSKI JZ, LULKARNI AP: Lipoxygenase-catalyzed epoxidation of benz[*a*]pyrene-7,8-dihydrodiol. Biochem Biophys Res Commun 159:1199, 1989.

49. HODGSON E: Metabolism of toxicants, Chap 3 in *A Textbook of Modern Toxicology*, 2d ed, E Hodgson and PE Levi (eds). Stamford, CN, Appleton & Lange, 1997, pp 51–84.

50. HECHT SS: Biochemistry, biology, and carcinogenicity of tobacco-specific *N*-nitrosamines. Chem Res Toxicol 6:559, 1998.

51. AMES B et al: Oxidants, antioxidants, and the degenerative diseases of aging. Proc Natl Acad Sci USA 90:7915, 1993.

52. GUENGERICH FP: Reactions and significance of cytochrome P-450 enzymes. J Biol Chem 266:10019, 1991.

53. LEADON SA et al: Production of oxidative DNA damage during the metabolic activation of benzo[*a*]pyrene in human mammary epithelial cells correlates with cell killing. Proc Natl Acad Sci USA 85:4365, 1988.

54. PARK JY et al: Induction of cytochrome P4501A1 by 2,3,7,8-tetrachlorodibenzo-*p*-dioxin or indolo(3,2,-*b*)carbazole is associated with oxidative DNA damage. Proc Natl Acad Sci USA 93:2322, 1996.

55. HEFFNER JE, REPINE JE: Pulmonary strategies for antioxidant defense. Am Rev Respir Dis 140:531, 1989.

56. REZNICK AZ et al: Modification of plasma proteins by cigarette smoke as measured by protein carbonyl formation. Biochem J 286:607, 1992.

57. LINDAHL T: DNA repair enzymes. Annu Rev Biochem 51:61, 1982.

58. SCHRECK R, BAEURERLE PA: A role for oxygen radicals as second messengers. Trends Cell Biol. 1:39, 1991.

59. FINKEL T: Oxygen radicals and signaling. Curr Opin Cell Biol 10:248, 1998.

60. DYPBUKT JM et al: Different prooxidant levels stimulate growth, trigger apoptosis, or produce necrosis of insulin-secreting RINm5F cells. J Biol Chem 269:30553, 1994.

61. JOHNSON TM et al: Reactive oxygen species are downstream mediators of p53-dependent apoptosis. Proc Natl Acad Sci USA 93:11,848, 1996.

62. DIZDAROGLU M: Chemical determination of oxidative DNA damage by gas chromatography-mass spectrometry. Methods Enzymol 234:3, 1994.

63. BARTSCH H et al: Formation, detection, and role in carcinogenesis of ethenobases in DNA. Drug Metab Rev 26:349, 1994.

64. CHAUDHARY AK et al: Detection of endogenous malondialdehyde-deoxyguanosine adducts in human liver. Science 265:1580, 1994.

65. DEDON PC et al: Indirect mutagenesis by oxidative DNA damage: Formation of the pyrimidopurinone adduct of deoxyguanosine by base propenal. Proc Natl Acad Sci USA 95:11,113, 1998.

66. KADLLUBAR FF et al: Comparison of DNA adduct levels associated with oxidative stress in human pancreas. Mutat Res 405:125, 1998.

67. POWIS G et al: Redox signalling and the control of cell growth and death. Pharm Ther 68:149, 1995.

68. KANG H et al: A highly sensitive and specific method for quantitation of O-alkylated DNA adducts and its application to the analysis of human tissue DNA. Environ Health Perspect 99:269, 1993.

69. WINK DA et al: DNA deaminating ability and genotoxicity of nitric oxide and its progenitors. Science 254:1001, 1991.

70. SPENCER JP et al: DNA damage in human respiratory tract epithelial cells: Damage by gas phase cigarette smoke apparently involves attack by reactive nitrogen species in addition to oxygen radicals. FEBS Lett 375:179, 1995.

71. YERMILOV V et al: Effects of carbon dioxide/bicarbonate on induction of DNA single-strand breaks and formation of 8-nitroguanine, 8-oxoguanine, and base propenal mediated by peroxynitrite. FEBS Lett 399:67, 1996.

72. NAIR J et al: Etheno adducts in spleen DNA of SJL mice stimulated to overproduce nitric oxide. Carcinogenesis 19:2081, 1998.

73. LIU RH, HOTCHKISS JH: Potential genotoxicity of chronically elevated nitric oxide: A review. Mutat Res 339:73, 1995.

74. TAMIR S, TANNENBAUM SR: The role of nitric oxide (NO˙) in the carcinogenic process. Biochim Biophys Acta 1288:F31, 1996.

75. JEFFREY AM et al: Benzo[*a*]pyrene-7,8-dihydrodiol 9,10-oxide adenosine and deoxyadenosine adducts: Structure and stereochemistry. Science 206:1309, 1979.

76. SINGER B, GRUNBERGER D: *Molecular Biology of Mutagens and Carcinogens*. New York, Plenum Press, 1983.

77. NORMAN D et al: NMR and computational characterization of the *N*-(deoxyguanosin-8-yl)aminofluorene adduct [(AF)G] opposite adenosine in DNA: (AF)G[*syn*].A[*anti*] pair formation and its pH dependence. Biochemistry 28:7462, 1989.

78. FRIEDBERG E et al: *DNA Repair and Mutagenesis*. Washington, DC, ASM Press, 1995.

79. SUKUMAR S et al: Induction of mammary carcinoma in rats by nitroso-methyl urea involves malignant activation of H-*ras-1* locus by single point mutations. Nature 306:658, 1983.

80. ZARBL H et al: Direct mutagenesis of Ha-*ras-1* oncogene by *N*-nitro-*N*-methyl urea during initiation of mammary carcinogenesis in rats. Nature 315:382, 1985.

81. HUSSAIN SP, Harris CC: Molecular epidemiology of human cancer: Contribution of mutation spectra studies of tumor suppressor genes. Cancer Res 58:4023, 1998.

82. WINK DA et al: DNA deaminating ability and genotoxicity of nitric oxide and its progenitors. Science 254:1001, 1991.

83. ROUTLEDGE MN et al: DNA sequence changes induced by two nitric oxide donor drugs in the supF assay. Chem Res Toxicol 7:628, 1994.

84. SHIBUTANI S et al: Insertion of specific bases during DNA synthesis past the oxidation-damaged base 8-oxodG. Nature 349:431, 1991.

85. PANDYA GA, Moriya M: 1,N6-ethenodeoxyadenosine, a DNA adduct highly mutagenic in mammalian cells. Biochemistry 35:11,487, 1996.

86. MORIYA M et al: Mutagenic potency of exocyclic DNA adducts: Marked differences between *Escherichia coli* and simian kidney cells. Proc Natl Acad Sci USA 91:11,899, 1994.

87. HASHIM MF, Marnett LJ: Sequence-dependent induction of base pair substitutions and frameshifts by propanodeoxyguanosine during in vitro DNA replication. J Biol Chem 271:9160, 1996.

88. HASHIM MF et al: Replication of template-primers containing propanodeoxyguanosine by DNA polymerase beta: Induction of base pair substitution and frameshift mutations by template slippage and deoxynucleoside triphosphate stabilization. J Biol Chem 272:20,205, 1997.

89. FINK SP et al: Mutagenicity in Escherichia coli of the major DNA adduct derived from the endogenous mutagen malondialdehyde. Proc Natl Acad Sci USA 94:8652, 1997.

90. BASU AK et al: Mutagenic and genotoxic effects of three vinyl chloride-induced DNA lesions: 1,N6-ethenoadenine, 3,N4-ethenocytosine, and 4-amino-5-(imidazol-2-yl)imidazole. Biochemistry 32:12,793, 1993.

91. KREUTZER DA, ESSIGMANN JM: Oxidized, deaminated cytosines are a source of C→T transitions in vivo. Proc Natl Acad Sci USA 95:3578, 1998.

92. KAMIYA H et al: Induction of mutation of a synthetic c-Ha-ras gene containing hypoxanthine. Cancer Res 52:1836, 1992.

93. SASSANTAR M et al: Relative efficiencies of the bacterial, yeast, and human DNA methyltransferases for the repair of O6-methylguanine and O4-methylthymine: Suggestive evidence for O4-methylthymine repair by eukaryotic methyltransferases. J Biol Chem 266:2767, 1991.

94. ZAK P et al: Repair of O6-methylguanine and O4-methylthymine by the human and rat O6-methylguanine-DNA methyltransferase. J Biol Chem 269:730, 1994.

95. SAMSON L, REJEWSKY MF: Alternative pathways for the in vivo repair of O6-alkylguanine and O4-alkylthymine in Escherichia coli: The adaptive response and nucleotide excision repair. EMBO J 7:2261, 1988.

96. SAMSON L et al: Mammalian DNA repair methyltransferase shield O4MeT from nucleotide excision repair. Carcinogenesis 18:919, 1997.

97. MAZE R et al: Increasing DNA repair methyltransferase levels via bone marrow stem cell transduction rescues mice from the toxic effects of 1,3-bis(2-chlorethyl)-1-nitrosourea, a chemotherapeutic alkylating agent. Proc Natl Acad Sci USA 93:206, 1996.

98. CHINNASAMY N et al: O6-benzylguanine potentiates the in vivo toxicity and clastogenicity of temozolomide and BCNU in mouse bone marrow. Blood 89:1566, 1997.

99. DOLAN ME, Pegg AE: O6-benzylguanine and its role in chemotherapy. Clin Cancer Res 3:837, 1997.

100. LIU L et al: Rapid repair of O6-methylguanine-DNA adducts protects transgenic mice from N-methylnitrosourea-induced thymic lymphomas. Cancer Res 54:4648, 1994.

101. TSUZUKI T et al: Targeted disruption of the DNA repair methyltransferase gene renders mice hypersensitive to alkylating agent. Carcinogenesis 17:1215, 1996.

102. WILSON DM, THOMPSON LH: Life without DNA repair. Proc Natl Acad Sci USA 94:12,754, 1997.

103. RAMOTAR D et al: Cellular role of yeast Apn1 apurinic endonuclease/3'-diesterase: Repair of oxidative and alkylation DNA damage and control of spontaneous mutation. Mol Cell Biol 11:4537, 1991.

104. WALKER LJ et al: A role for the human DNA repair enzyme HAP1 in cellular protection against DNA damaging agents and hypoxic stress. Nucleic Acids Res 22:4884, 1994.

105. NAKAMURA J et al: Highly sensitive apurinic/apyrimidinic site assay can detect spontaneous and chemically induced depuration under physiological conditions. Cancer Res 58:222, 1998.

106. O'CONNOR TR, LAVAL F: Isolation and structure of a cDNA expressing a mammalian 3-methyladenine-DNA glycosylase. EMBO J 9:3337, 1990.

107. SAMSON L et al: Cloning and characterization of a 3-methyladenine DNA glycosylase cDNA from human cells whose gene maps to chromosome 16. Proc Natl Acad Sci USA 88:9127, 1991.

108. CHAKRAVARTI D et al: Cloning and expression in Escherichia coli of a human cDNA encoding the DNA repair protein N-methylpurine-DNA glycosylase. J Biol Chem 266:15710, 1991.

109. NAKAMURA J et al: Highly sensitive apurininic/apyrimidinic site assay can detect spontaneous and chemically induced depuration under physiological conditions. Cancer Res 58:222, 1998.

110. NEDDERMANN P et al: Cloning and expression of human G/T mismatch-specific thymine-DNA glycosylase. J Biol Chem 271:12,767, 1996.

111. ASPINWALL R et al: Cloning and characterization of a functional human homolog of Escherichia coli endonuclease III. Proc Natl Acad Sci USA 94:109, 1997.

112. ROSENQUIST TA et al: Cloning and characterization of a mammalian 8-oxoguanine DNA glycosylase. Proc Natl Acad Sci USA 94:7429, 1997.

113. HAZRA TK et al: The presence of two distinct 8-oxoguanine repair enzymes in human cells: Their potential complementary roles in preventing mutation. Nucleic Acids Res 26:5116, 1998.

114. DIZDAROGLU M et al: Excision of products of oxidative DNA damage by human NTH1 protein. Biochemistry 38:243, 1999.

115. DE LAAT WL et al: Molecular mechanism of nucleotide excision repair. Genes Devel 13:768, 1999.

116. SUGASAWA K et al: Xeroderma pigmentosum group C protein complex is the initiator of global genome nuclear excision repair. Molec Cell 2:223, 1999.

117. KLUNGLAND A et al: Base excision repair of oxidative DNA damage activated by XPG protein. Molec Cell 3:33, 1999.

118. COOPER P et al: Defective transcription-coupled repair of oxidative base damage in Cockayne syndrome patients from XP group G. Science 275:990, 1997.

119. MELLON I et al: Transcription-coupled repair deficiency and mutations in human mismatch repair genes. Science 272:557, 1996.

120. GOWEN LC et al: BRCAI required for transcription-coupled repair of oxidative DNA damage. Science 281:1009, 1998.

121. LYNCH HT et al: Overview of natural history, pathology, molecular genetics, and management of HNPC (Lynch Syndrome). Int J Cancer 69:38, 1996.

122. BAKER SM: Male mice defective in the DNA mismatch repair gene PMS2 exhibit abnormal chromosome synapsis and meiosis. Cell 82:309, 1995.

123. BAKER SM et al: Involvement of Mlh1 in DNA mismatch repair and meiotic crossing over. Nature Genet 13:336, 1996.

124. de WIND N et al: Inactivation of the mouse Msh2 gene results in mismatch repair deficiency, methylation tolerance, hyperrecombination, and predisposition to cancer. Cell 82:321, 1995.

125. REITMAIR AH et al: Spontaneous intestinal carcinomas and skin neoplasms in MSH2-deficient mice. Cancer Res 56:3842, 1996.

126. PROLLA TA et al: Tumor susceptibility and spontaneous

mutation in mice deficient in Mlh1, Pms1, and Pms2 DNA mismatch repair. Nature Genet 18:276, 1998.

127. KOLODNER RD: Mismatch repair: Mechanism and relationship to cancer susceptibility. TIBS 20:397, 1995.

128. MODRICH P, LAHUE R: Mismatch repair in replication fidelity, genetic recombination and cancer biology. Annu Rev Biochem 65:101, 1996.

129. SCHÄR J, JIRICNY J: Eukaryotic mismatch repair, in *Nucleic Acids and Molecular Biology,* vol 12, F Eckstein, DMJ Lilley (eds). Berlin, Springer-Verlag, 1998.

130. BAKER SM et al: Enhanced intestinal adenomatous poly formation in Pms2-/-:Min mice. Cancer Res 58:1087, 1998.

131. DE WIND N et al: Mouse models for hereditary nonpolyposis colorectal cancer. Cancer Res 58:248, 1998.

132. DE VRIES A et al: Increased susceptibility to ultraviolet-B and carcinogens of mice lacking the DNA excision repair gene *XPA*. Nature 377:169, 1995.

133. SZOSTAK J et al: The double-strand break repair model for recombination. Cell 33:25, 1983.

134. SHINOHAR A et al: Cloning of human, mouse and fission yeast recombination genes homologous to *RAD51* and *resA*. Nature Genet 4:239, 1993.

135. SMITH GCM, JACKSON SP: The DNA-dependent protein kinase. Genes Devel 13:916, 1999.

136. KANAAR R et al: Molecular mechansims of DNA double-strand break repair. Trends Cell Biol 8:483, 1998.

137. ZHU C et al: Ku86-deficient mice exhibit severe combined immunodeficiency and defective processing of V(D)J recombination intermediates. Cell 86:379, 1996.

138. NUSSENZWEIG A et al: Hypersensitivity of *Ku80*-deficient cell lines and mice to DNA damage: The effects of ionizing radiation on growth, survival, and development. Proc Natl Acad Sci USA 94:13,588, 1997.

139. GU Y et al: Ku70-deficient embryonic stem cells have increased ionizing radiosensitivity, defective DNA end-binding activity, and inability to support V(D)J recombination. Proc Natl Acad Sci USA 94:8076, 1997.

140. JHAPPAN C et al: DNA-PKcs: A T-cell tumor suppressor encoded at the mouse *scid* locus. Nature Genet 17:483, 1997.

141. PAULOVICH AG et al: When checkpoints fail. Cell 88:315, 1997.

142. LANGAUER C et al: Genetic instabilities in human cancers. Nature 396:643, 1998.

143. LI Y, MCKEON F: Identification of a human mitotic checkpoint gene: hsMAD2. Science 274:246, 1996.

144. CAHILL DP et al: Mutations of mitotic checkpoint genes in human cancers. Nature 392:300, 1998.

145. XU X et al: Centrosome amplification and a defective $G_2$-M cell cycle checkpoint induce genomic instability in BRCA1 exon 11 isoform-deficient cells. Molec Cell 3:389, 1999.

146. WEINSTEIN IB et al: Molecular biology and molecular epidemiology of cancer, in *Cancer Prevention and Control,* P Greenwald et al (eds). New York, Marcell Dekker, 1995, pp 83–110.

147. WEINSTEIN IB et al: Molecular mechanisms of mutagenesis and multistage carcinogenesis, in *The Molecular Basis of Cancer,* J Mendelsohn et al (eds). Philadelphia, WB Saunders, 1995, pp 59–85.

148. CACACE A et al: PKC epsilon functions as an oncogene by activating the RAF kinase. Oncogene 13:2517, 1996.

149. SOH J-W et al: Novel roles of specific isoforms of protein kinase C in activation of the c-*fos* serum response element. Mol Cell Biol 19:1313, 1999.

150. RYSERM HJ-P: Chemical carcinogenesis. N Engl J Med 285:721, 1971.

151. ARMSTRONG B, DOLL R: Environmental factors and cancer incidence and mortality in different countries, with special reference to dietary practices. Int J Cancer 15:617, 1975.

152. WICKERHAM DL et al: The initial results from NSABP Protocol P-1: A clinical trial to determine the worth of tamoxifen for preventing breast cancer in women at increased risk. Presented at the 34th Annual Meeting, ASCO, 1998, Plenary Session.

153. STRAUSS L et al: Dietary phytoestrogens and their role in hormonally dependent disease. Toxicol Lett 1998; 102–103:349, 1998.

154. KELLOFF GJ et al: Chemopreventive drug development: Perspectives and progress. Cancer Epidemiol Biomarkers Prev 3:85, 1994.

155. BENSON AM et al: Increase of NAD(P)H:quinone reductase by dietary antioxidants: Possible role in protection against carcinogenesis and toxicity. Proc Natl Acad Sci USA 77:5216, 1997.

156. JAISWAL AK et al: Caffeic acid phenethyl ester stimulates human antioxidant response element-mediated expression of the NAD(P)H:quinone oxidoreductase (*NQO1*) gene. Cancer Res 57:440, 1997.

157. ZHANG Y et al: A major inducer of anticarcinogenic protective enzymes from broccoli: Isolation and elucidation of structure. Proc Natl Acad Sci USA 89:2399, 1992.

158. WARGOVICH MJ: Allyl sulfide, a flavor component of garlic (*Allium sativum*), inhibits dimethylhydrazine-induced colon cancer. Carcinogenesis 8:487, 1987.

159. WATTENBERG LW, BUEDING E: Inhibitory effects of 5-(2-pyrazinyl)-4 methyl-2,2-dithiol-3-dione (oltipraz) on carcinogenesis induced by benzo[*a*]pyrene, diethylnitrosamine and uracil mustard. Carcinogenesis 7:1379, 1986.

160. KENSLER TW et al: Free radicals as targets for cancer chemoprevention: Prospects and problems, in *Cellular and Molecular Targets for Chemoprevention,* VE Steele et al (eds). Boca Raton, FL, CRC Press, 1992, pp 173–191.

161. REID TM, LOWE LA: Tandem double CC-TT mutations are produced by reactive oxygen species. Proc Natl Acad Sci USA 90:3904, 1993.

162. WANG J-Y et al: Inhibition of N-nitrosodiethylamine and 4-(methylnitrosamine)-1-(3-pyridyl)-1-butanone-induced tumorigenesis in A/J mice by green tea and black tea. Cancer Res 52:1943, 1992.

163. FUJITA Y et al: Inhibitory effect of (-)-epigallocatechin gallate on carcinogenesis with N-ethyl-N-nitro-N-nitrosoguanidine in mouse duodenum. Jpn Cancer Res 80:503, 1989.

164. XU Y et al: Inhibition of tobacco-specific nitrosamine-induced lung tumorigenesis in A/J mice by green tea and its major polyphenol as antioxidants. Cancer Res 52:3875, 1992.

165. RAO CV et al: Chemoprevention of colon carcinogenesis by dietary curcumin, a naturally occurring plant phenolic compound. Cancer Res 55:259, 1995.

166. PAOLINI M et al: Co-carcinogenic effect of beta-carotene. Nature 398:760, 1999.

167. WEYANT WJ et al: (+)-catechin inhibits intestinal tumor formation and suppresses focal adhesion kinase (FAK) activation in the Min/+ mouse. Cancer Res. In press.

168. RAO CV et al: Chemoprevention of colon carcinogenesis by phenylethyl-3-methylcaffeate. Cancer Res 55:2310, 1995.

169. LI JY et al: Nutrition intervention trials in Linxian, China: Multiple vitamin/mineral supplementation, cancer incidence, and disease-specific mortality among adults with esophageal dysplasia. J Natl Cancer Inst 85:1492, 1993.

170. THE ALPHA TOCOPHEROL BETA CAROTENE STUDY GROUP. The effect of vitamin E and beta carotene on the incidence of lung cancer and other cancers in male smokers. N Engl J Med 330:1029, 1994.

171. HENNEKINS CH et al: Lack of effect of long-term supplementation with beta carotene on the incidence of malignant neoplasms and cardiovascular disease. N Engl J Med 334:1145, 1996.

172. CLARK LC et al: Effects of selenium supplementation for cancer prevention in patients with carcinoma of the skin. JAMA 276:1957, 1996.

173. CHRISTMAN JK et al: Reversibility of changes in nucleic acid methylation and gene expression induced in rat liver by severe dietary methyl deficiency. Carcinogenesis 14:551, 1993.

174. BIRD CL et al: Red cell and plasma folate, folate consumption, and the risk of colorectal adenomatous polyps. Cancer Epidemiol Biomarkers Prev 4:709, 1995.

175. GIOVANNUCCI E et al: Folate, methionine, and alcohol intake and risk of colorectal adenoma. J Natl Cancer Inst 85:875, 1993.

176. LOTAN R: Retinoic receptors and retinoid-regulated differentiation markers as intermediate endpoints in chemoprevention. Proc Am Assoc Cancer Res 35:684, 1994.

177. GOODMAN DS: Vitamin A and retinoids in health and disease. N Engl J Med 310:1023, 1984.

178. MOON RC et al: Inhibition of carcinogenesis by retinoids. Cancer Res 43:2469S, 1983.

179. LIPPMAN S et al: Retinoid chemoprevention studies in upper aerodigestive tract and lung carcinogenesis. Cancer Res 54:2025S, 1994.

180. MARTON LJ, PEGG AE: Polyamines as targets for therapeutic intervention. Annu Rev Pharmacol Toxicol 35:55, 1995.

181. XUE L et al: Influence of dietary calcium and vitamin D on diet-induced epithelial cell hyperproliferation in mice. J Natl Cancer Inst 91:176, 1999.

182. ARLOW FL et al: Attenuation of azoxymethane-induced colonic mucosal ornithine decarboxylase and tyrosine kinase activity by calcium in rats. Cancer Res 49:5884, 1989.

183. BARON JA et al: Calcium supplements for the prevention of colorectal adenomas. Calcium Polyp Prevention Study Group. N Engl J Med 340:101, 1999.

184. WALI RK et al: Mechanism of action of chemoprotective ursodeoxycholate in the azoxymethane model of rat colonic carcinogenesis: Potential roles of protein kinase C-alpha, -beta II, and -zeta. Cancer Res 55:5257, 1995.

185. BARNES S: Effect of genistein on in vitro and in vivo models of cancer. J Nutr 16:777s, 1995.

186. LAMARTINIERE CA et al: Genistein suppresses mammary cancer in rats. Carcinogenesis 16:2833, 1995.

187. MARTIN PM et al: Phytoestrogen interaction with estrogen receptors in human breast cancer cells. Endocrinology 103:1860, 1978.

188. PETERSON TG, BARNES S: Genistein inhibits both estrogen and growth factor-stimulated proliferation of human breast cancer cells. Cell Growth Diff 7:1345, 1996.

189. FOTSIS T et al: Genistein, a dietary-derived inhibitor of in vitro angiogenesis. Proc Natl Acad Sci USA 90:2690, 1993.

190. KIM H et al: Mechanisms of action of the soy isoflavone genistein: Emerging role for its effects via transforming growth factor $\beta$ signaling pathways. Am J Clin Nutr 68:1418S, 1998.

191. MASFERRER JM et al: Celecoxib: A specific cox-2 inhibitor with anti-angiogenic and anti-cancer activities. Proc Am Assoc Cancer Res 40:396, 1999.

192. ROBERTS AB, SPORN MB: Transforming growth factor $\beta$. Adv Cancer Res 51:107, 1988.

193. SIBRESTEIN GB, DANIEL CW: Reversible inhibition of mammary gland growth by transforming growth factor-$\beta$. Science 237:291, 1987.

194. GLICK AB et al: Complex regulation of TGF$\beta$ expression by retinoic acid in the vitamin A–deficient rat. Development 111:1081, 1991.

195. GROMLEY GJ et al: The effect of finasteride in men with benign prostatic hyperplasia. N Engl J Med 327:1185, 1992.

196. LIM JTE et al: Sulindac derivatives inhibit growth and induce apoptosis in human prostate cancer cell lines. Biochem Pharmacol (in press).

197. ROSE DP: Dietary fatty acids and prevention of hormone-responsive cancer. Proc Soc Exp Biol Med 216:224, 1997.

198. OSHIMA M et al: Suppression of intestinal polyposis in $Apc^{del716}$ knockout mice by inhibition of cyclooxygenase 2 (COX-2). Cell 87:803, 1996.

199. CHULADA PC et al: Cyclooxygenase-1 and -2 deficiency decrease spontaneous intestinal adenomas in the Min mouse. Proc Am Assoc Cancer Res 39:195, 1998.

200. GUPTA RA, DUBOIS RN: Aspirin, NSAIDs, and colon cancer prevention: Mechanisms? Gastroenterology 114:1095, 1998.

201. GIARDIELLO FM et al: Treatment of colonic and rectal adenomas with sulindac in familial adenomatous polyposis. N Engl J Med 328:1313, 1993.

202. GIOVANNUCCI E et al: Aspirin use and the risk for colorectal cancer and adenoma in male health professionals. An Intern Med 121:241, 1994.

203. PERERA FP: Environment and cancer: Who are susceptible? Science 278:1068, 1997.

204. PERERA FP, WEINSTEIN IB: Molecular epidemiology and carcinogen-DNA adduct detection: New approaches to studies of human cancer causation. J Chron Dis 35:581, 1982.

# NUTRITION-RELATED CARCINOGENESIS

*Peter Greenwald, Susan M. Pilch, and
Sharon S. McDonald*

## INTRODUCTION

Advances in the understanding of carcinogenesis suggest that complex interactions among both exogenous (e.g., environmental) and endogenous (e.g., genetic, hormonal) factors related to carcinogenesis may be required for the development of a malignancy, and that transitions between successive stages of cancer development can be influenced by these various factors.[1] The human diet is an exogenous factor that has been associated with risk modifications for various types of cancer, a result of the diet's diverse and complex composition.[2,3] Specific macronutrients and micronutrients, as well as naturally occurring phytochemicals, have demonstrated both beneficial and adverse effects on cancer risk, with some linked to interactions at the molecular level.[4–7] For example, folic acid currently is thought to have an influence on DNA methylation and, consequently, on proto-oncogene expression.[6] Thus, *nutrition-related carcinogenesis* is broadly defined here to include any aspects of cancer etiology and development that are related to, or influenced by, dietary constituents or dietary patterns. Such dietary influences may either inhibit or enhance cancer risk and may exert their influences through biochemical or genetic mechanisms.

Factors such as amount and type of dietary fat intake, intake of vegetables and fruits, alcohol consumption, total energy intake, level of physical activity, and obesity are all part of an intricate and inseparable interaction of lifestyle choices that can contribute to cancer risk. These factors possibly build upon individual susceptibilities derived from a complex array of polygenetic risk determinants.[8] For example, a recent cohort study of heavy smokers designed to determine the relative contributions of genetic polymorphisms—CYP1A1 (cytochrome P450 1A1 [MspI, exon 7 variant]) and glutathione *S*-transferase M1 (GSTM1)—and plasma micronutrients to levels of polycyclic aromatic hydrocarbon-DNA (PAH-DNA) adducts, reported that the presence of the exon 7 CYP1A1 variant was associated with a doubling of PAH-DNA adduct levels; also, adducts were inversely associated with plasma levels of retinol, β-carotene, and α-tocopherol. These findings indicate that a subgroup of smokers may be at increased risk of DNA damage—and possibly lung cancer—as a result of the combined effect of genetic susceptibility and low levels of plasma micronutrients.[9] In another study, a high consumption of monounsaturated fats (mostly from olive oil) was associated with a significantly decreased risk of colorectal tumors with wild-type Ki-*ras* genotype, but not of Ki-*ras* mutated tumors. Conversely, a high calcium intake was associated with a decreased risk of Ki-*ras* mutated tumors, but not of wild-type tumors.[10] Such findings suggest that the potential cancer-protective effects of dietary constituents can, in some cases, depend on the specific genotypes of the target cells.[10]

Concordance for disease in twin pairs also has provided insight into the relative contributions of environmental and genetic factors to disease occurrence. A cohort study, conducted among white male U.S. veterans, assessed the effect of inherited predisposition for cancer in 5690 monozygotic (MZ) twins and 7248 dizygotic (DZ) twins.[11] Concordance for death from cancer at all sites was higher among MZ twins than among DZ twins (overall rate ratio, 1.4), suggesting a possible role for inherited predisposition. However, approximately one-third of the MZ twins died from smoking-associated cancers, supporting the influence of environment on cancer risk. Overall, these findings are consistent with earlier studies of MZ and DZ twin pairs in the United States and northern Europe,[12–15] which suggests that inherited disposition does not explain a large proportion of all cancers or of all cancer mortality.[11] A recent report of breast and ovarian cancer development in only one of two identical twins who both have an inherited BRCA1 mutation clearly illustrates the very real possibility of differences in phenotypic expression of such mutations.[16] It is possible that genetic contributions to cancer risk may be overwhelmed by environmental influences, including lifestyle choices such as smoking and diet.[11]

Although conclusive evidence regarding the relationships between dietary factors and cancer development is not yet available, a large body of epidemiologic evidence and corroborating experimental studies strongly supports relationships between dietary constituents and the risk of specific cancers, suggesting that, in general, vegetables and fruits, dietary fiber, and certain micronutrients appear to be protective against cancer, whereas fat, excessive calories, and alcohol seem to increase cancer risk.[2,3,17] It follows that a proactive approach to cancer prevention through diet modification is a prudent lifestyle choice that may reduce cancer risk and appears to be beneficial to overall good health.

## HISTORICAL OVERVIEW

Diet and cancer research leads from epidemiologic and experimental studies are developed systematically through in vitro and in vivo preclinical research; limited human studies; and, when warranted, large-scale, randomized clinical prevention trials. Although the value of epidemiologic evidence has recently been questioned,[18] by providing initial clues that can spark scientific interest and suggest directions for future research epidemiologic studies remain essential to the hypothesis-building process. Epidemiologic studies are often the only pragmatic or ethically acceptable way to link exposures to human disease.[19] In practice, epidemiologic evidence must be judged objectively with regard to control of confounding, study design, magnitude, consistency, temporality, biologic plausibility, dose response, and coherence (i.e., no conflict of the effect with generally known information about the biology and natural history of the disease), and possibility of bias [for example, recall bias and "wish" bias (the extent to which an investigator believes a hypothesis is true)].[19,20] Critical evaluation and meaningful distillation of epidemiologic study results have played and will continue to play a key role in the identification of dietary factors related to cancer risk.

One of the earliest major contributions to our understanding of an association between tumor formation and dietary influence stemmed from the investigations of Albert Tannenbaum in the 1940s. His research efforts exploring high-fat diets, caloric restriction, and tumor formation in mice are regarded as landmark studies. Results demonstrated that increasing the fat content of the animals' basic ration enhanced the formation of spontaneous mammary and chemically induced skin tumors,[21] and that restriction of caloric intake to about 60% of the ad libitum intake inhibited both tumor formation and the average time at which tumors appeared.[22] Subsequent studies to determine whether tumor formation is dependent on diet composition as well as on the degree of caloric restriction provided evidence that a high-fat diet—implicating some direct property of fat—enhanced tumor formation independently of a general caloric effect, in terms of both incidence and average time of appearance.[23]

In the mid-1950s, investigators began to direct their research efforts toward a search for substances that could modulate cancer initiation, promotion, and progression. In the mid-1970s, this approach to cancer prevention was named *chemoprevention* by Michael B. Sporn,[24] an innovator in cancer research who recognized that the multistep nature of carcinogenesis provided numerous opportunities for pharmacologic intervention to prevent, slow, or halt the cellular progression toward malignancy. Sporn[25] pioneered chemoprevention research with laboratory studies of retinol (vitamin A) and retinoids (less toxic synthetic analogues of retinol), demonstrating their ability to inhibit both processes of malignant transformation and tumor promotion. The rationale for this approach was based on the ability of retinoids to control normal cell differentiation and proliferation in essentially all epithelia that are targets for the development of invasive carcinoma, such as lung, colon, breast, ovary, and bladder.[26,27] Over the past two decades, researchers have identified hundreds of potential chemopreventive agents that are heterogeneous and mechanistically diverse; these include micronutrients, naturally occurring nonnutritive compounds, and synthetics.

In the 1970s, many epidemiologic studies focused on indices of β-carotene (provitamin A), which is converted to vitamin A in the body as needed. In the United States, most vitamin A intake is actually in the form of β-carotene in fruits and vegetables. In 1981, Peto[28] and colleagues published a comprehensive review of the collective epidemiologic evidence that correlated blood levels of "preformed" vitamin A and either blood levels or dietary intake of carotenoids (mostly β-carotene), as estimated from vegetable and fruit intake, with cancer risk. The review concluded that the inverse association for vitamin A reported in small prospective studies needed to be confirmed and, because dietary intake has little effect on blood retinol, the factors that influenced blood retinol levels needed to be determined. With regard to carotenoids, sufficient epidemiologic evidence existed to suggest that investigating the potential anticancer effects of β-carotene, and possibly other carotenoids, was warranted.[28] The encouraging epidemiologic evidence, as well as corroborating laboratory investigations, provided a strong rationale for the conduct of randomized, controlled clinical intervention trials with β-carotene. Such trials, described more fully later in this chapter, were initiated in the early 1980s.

The government's interest in and dedication to cancer research received impetus in 1971 with the signing of the National Cancer Act. This legislation, enacted in response to a report of the National Panel of Consultants on the Conquest of Cancer, enlarged the authorities and responsibilities of the director of the National Cancer Institute

(NCI) and committed the nation to plan and develop an expanded, intensified cancer research program that included an emphasis on prevention and diet-related investigations.[29,30] Coupled with this legislative mandate for cancer research, White House conferences and congressional hearings conducted during the 1970s explored the state of knowledge concerning the status and health effects of nutrition in the United States. Issues and questions raised prompted several government-sponsored reports concerning risk factors and chronic diseases, including diet and cancer, that were published in the 1980s.

In 1981, *The Causes of Cancer: Quantitative Estimates of Avoidable Cancer in the United States Today,*[31] commissioned as a background report to the U.S. Congress, summarized the evidence relating lifestyle and other environmental factors, such as diet, tobacco, occupation, sunlight, and ionizing radiation, to cancer rates. This landmark report suggested that, in most parts of the United States in 1970, about 75% to 80% of cancer cases might have been avoidable and estimated that dietary factors were associated with approximately 35% of all cancers.

In 1982, the Committee on Diet, Nutrition, and Cancer of the National Research Council (NRC) published *Diet, Nutrition, and Cancer,*[32] a comprehensive report commissioned by the NCI. The report concluded that, based on the available evidence, cancers of most major sites are influenced by dietary patterns. The committee took an important proactive step by formulating interim dietary guidelines for the general public that were both consistent with good nutrition and likely to reduce cancer. The committee also recommended that, because future epidemiologic and experimental research was likely to provide new insights into the diet and cancer association, the NCI should establish mechanisms to review the guidelines at least every 5 years.

Maintaining the momentum of widespread national interest in health promotion, *The Surgeon General's Report on Nutrition and Health*[2] was issued by the Department of Health and Human Services (DHHS) in 1988. Although the report was developed for use by policymakers, it offered lessons that could be applied directly to the public. Acknowledging that current concerns about nutrition and health had expanded beyond the need to prevent deficiencies, the report reviewed the effects of typical American dietary patterns on chronic disease incidence, including cancer, and concluded that overconsumption of some dietary components—particularly fat—combined with low intake of dietary sources of complex carbohydrates and fiber (vegetables, fruits, and whole grains) was a major health concern for Americans. It suggested that modifying dietary practices could reduce the high rates of some cancers and other chronic diseases and supported the Dietary Guidelines for Americans that had been jointly issued in 1985 by the U.S. Department of Agriculture and DHHS.

In response to the overwhelming amount of information on diet and disease released to the public by the media, with little guidance as to how to separate fact from fallacy, the Food and Nutrition Board of the NRC established the Committee on Diet and Health in 1984. The committee was charged with undertaking a comprehensive analysis of the scientific literature on diet and major chronic diseases, including cancer, atherosclerotic cardiovascular diseases, hypertension, obesity, osteoporosis, and diabetes. Findings of the 1989 report *Diet and Health: Implications for Reducing Chronic Disease Risk*[3] were similar to those of previously published reports. The general conclusions stated that a comprehensive review of the epidemiologic, clinical, and laboratory evidence highly suggests that diet influences the risk of certain forms of cancer, especially cancers of the esophagus, stomach, large bowel, breast, lung, and prostate; and that, although not characterized or clearly identified, most chronic diseases in which nutritional factors play a role (including cancer) also have determinants such as other environmental and genetic influences. The report included proposed dietary recommendations, which were in general agreement with those provided by other expert panels in the United States.

By the early 1990s, it was generally accepted that diet is a contributing factor to the onset or progression of certain types of cancer and that a prudent selection of some foods (e.g., vegetables and fruits), as well as the avoidance or decreased consumption of others (e.g., those high in animal fat), might influence an individual's cancer risk. Improvements in the sensitivity and reliability of diet-related cancer research methodology facilitated the identification of specific dietary constituents as potential carcinogens or anticarcinogens. This knowledge, combined with public concern about the risk of cancer associated with dietary intake, a concern that resulted from media reports on the toxicity and/or carcinogenicity of specific food items and constituents, prompted the NRC to convene the Committee on Comparative Toxicity of Naturally Occurring Carcinogens in 1993. This committee was charged "to examine the occurrence, toxicologic data, mechanisms of action, and potential role of natural carcinogens in the causation of human cancer, including relative risk comparisons with synthetic carcinogens and a consideration of anticarcinogens," and to assess "the impact of these natural carcinogens on initiation, promotion, and progression of tumors."[33] The committee concluded that, because the majority of naturally occurring and synthetic dietary constituents were present below the levels at which any significant adverse biologic effect would be expected, such constituents were not likely to contribute significantly to cancer risk. Further, it determined that existing concentration and exposure data and risk assessment methods were insufficient to address definitively the respective roles of natural versus synthetic dietary compounds in cancer causation and prevention. The committee also concluded that evidence suggests that the contribution of excess macronutrients and excess calories to cancer causation in the United States outweighs that of individual food microchemicals, both natural and synthetic. Finally, the committee acknowledged the difficulty of diet-related risk assessment, given the complexity of the human diet and the multitude of unknown interactions among its components.

## CURRENT STATUS OF DIET AND CANCER RESEARCH

### DIETARY FAT, CALORIES, PHYSICAL ACTIVITY, AND BODY SIZE

A large body of international epidemiologic evidence and experimental data suggests that certain lifestyle factors, including the amount and type of dietary fat consumed, total caloric intake, phys-

ical activity, and obesity, influence the risk of cancer at several sites, most predominantly the postmenopausal breast, colon-rectum, and prostate.[2,3,34,35] Diet and cancer studies show that, in general, diets low in animal fat and red meats tend to protect against cancer, whereas diets high in fat, especially saturated fat, and total calories seem to increase cancer risk. Similarly, regular physical activity and leanness are associated with lower risk for some cancers, whereas a sedentary lifestyle, weight gain, and obesity appear to enhance cancer development.

TOTAL FAT AND CALORIC INTAKE. Correlational and immigrant studies provide a basis for hypotheses linking dietary fat, cancer incidence, and mortality in humans. Population studies that compare per capita fat consumption with cancer incidence or mortality consistently demonstrate strong, positive correlations between total dietary fat and animal intakes and cancers of the colon, breast, and prostate.[2,3] Studies of individuals who move from countries where both fat/animal intake and cancer rates are low, including many Asian countries, to countries where consumption of fat and red meat are high and cancer incidence and mortality rates are high, such as the United States, provide further evidence for a promotional role of fat in cancer development.[2,3,36,37] Many of these studies reveal progressively higher cancer rates in the children and grandchildren of the first-generation immigrants. Results of case-control and cohort studies are often less consistent, depending on the type of cancer and the population being investigated.

Confounding the hypotheses that either fat or caloric intake, or both, affect cancer risk is the very high correlation between fat and caloric intake. In general, diets high in fat are also high in calories. Thus, an effect that appears to be due to a high-calorie diet may actually be due to a diet high in fat, or vice versa. In such analyses, it is critical to adjust for one factor (either fat or calories) when attempting to determine the impact of the other on cancer risk. However, many studies fail to take this step and, because of inaccuracies in dietary ascertainment, epidemiology may not be able to reliably disentangle dietary fat from calories.

BREAST CANCER. The roles of fat and calories in the development of postmenopausal breast cancer remain controversial. Animal studies conducted more than 50 years ago supported a strong relationship between dietary fat intake and mammary tumor risk when animals were allowed to eat freely; however, the relationship was less clear when caloric intake was restricted.[22,23] A review of data from 100 experiments involving mice or rats suggested a specific, independent, tumor-enhancing effect of fat intake on mammary tumor incidence.[38] The same review indicated a more general, tumor-promoting effect of total caloric intake.

Epidemiologic studies provide conflicting results regarding the association of fat and breast cancer.[39,40] International correlations between fat intake and breast cancer incidence and mortality rates are high, averaging approximately 0.8.[34,35,39] Similarly, migrant studies support an increased risk for breast cancer as eating patterns shift from a low-fat, high-fiber diet to a high-fat, low-fiber "western" diet.[36,41] Most case-control studies suggest modest positive associations between fat intake and risk for breast cancer.[39,40] A meta-analysis of 12 case-control studies found a significant direct relationship between breast cancer risk and saturated fat intake in postmenopausal women.[42] Another meta-analysis based on fat intake in a series of case-control studies found a relative risk (RR) of 1.21 for breast cancer.[43] Interestingly, case-control studies of the recurrence of breast cancer suggest a poorer prognosis among postmenopausal women with the highest intake of fat.[44–46]

In contrast, large cohort studies generally have failed to demonstrate a link between dietary fat intake and breast cancer risk.[39,40] Two separate meta-analyses reported RRs of 1.0143 and 1.0547 for cohort studies investigating the impact of dietary fat on breast cancer development. One study of approximately 26,000 Norwegian women reported a relative risk for breast cancer of 2.44 among women who ate meat at least five times per week, compared with those who ate meat no more than twice per week.[48] However, results of the Nurses' Health Study, which followed some 89,538 women for 8 years, indicated that fat intake did not affect breast cancer incidence.[49]

Several factors may explain the inconclusive nature of these epidemiologic data, including inaccuracy in dietary assessment methods, insufficient variation in fat intake within a study population, interaction of correlated variables, differences in data collection and analysis methods, inaccuracy in dietary assessment, an insufficient follow-up period, failure to distinguish between premenopausal and postmenopausal women, and the importance of diet before adulthood.[39]

*COLORECTAL CANCER.* International correlation studies demonstrate strong, positive associations between colorectal cancer incidence and consumption of red meat and animal fats.[2,3,34,35,50] A number of case-control and cohort studies, including investigations using adenomatous polyps as markers of risk, also support the associations with red meat, with data from fat intake less convincing.[51–54] Cooking methods may contribute to the role of fat in promoting colorectal cancer. High-temperature methods of cooking meats, including grilling, frying, and broiling, produce compounds shown to possess carcinogenic activity in animals.[50]

The number of calories consumed also appears to play a role in the development of colorectal cancer. One analysis revealed a statistically significant positive association between energy intake and colorectal cancer risk in 12 of 17 case-control studies.[50] A similar result was found in a combined analysis in which data from 13 case-control studies were pooled; interestingly, this analysis found no energy-independent association between total fat intake and colorectal cancer risk.[55] Researchers postulate that high intakes of food stimulate the intestinal mucosa, which, in turn, increases the likelihood of cell division. In contrast, restricting caloric intake in animals reduces the rate of cell division and inhibits the formation of tumors of the colon. A study in which the caloric intake of obese subjects was reduced by one-third similarly produced a statistically significant drop in rectal cell proliferation, which is commonly used as a biomarker for colorectal lesions.[56]

*PROSTATE CANCER.* Numerous case-control and cohort studies suggest an inverse relationship between risk for prostate cancer and consumption of either animal fat or high-fat foods, especially red meat.[57] Polyunsaturated fats do not appear to be associated with cancer of the prostate, however.[57] In a cohort study of 52,000 male health professionals in the United States, prostate cancer risk was found to increase with consumption of red meat (RR = 2.64) but not with fat from poultry, dairy products, or fish.[58]

International and ethnic differences in prostate cancer incidence indicate that the effects of etiologic factors, including diet, may vary across populations. A study of the role of diet in the development of prostate cancer in blacks, whites, and Asians in the United States and Canada reported an overall significant, direct relationship with saturated fat; the highest risk (RR = 4.1; highest versus lowest quintiles of intake) was reported for Japanese Americans, and the lowest risk (RR = 0.91) was for whites.[37] Notably, differences in saturated fat intake accounted for only an estimated 10% of the difference in prostate cancer incidence between blacks and whites, and an estimated 15% of the difference in incidence between whites and Asians. These data support the hypothesis that other environmental factors, such as lifestyle, and/or genetics may be etiologic agents of prostate cancer.

TYPE OF FAT. Although the relationship between total fat intake and cancer risk continues to be debated, a growing body of literature suggests that the primary link between fat and risk for some cancers may be due to the type of fat consumed rather than, or in addition, to total fat intake.

*BREAST CANCER.* A recent meta-analysis of 97 animal experiments studying the effect of various types of fatty acids on mammary tumor incidence found that n-6 polyunsaturated fatty acids (PUFAs) had a strong tumor-enhancing effect, saturated fats had a weaker tumor-enhancing effect, n-3 PUFAs had a small (not significant) protective effect, and monounsaturated fats had no significant effect.[59] It has been suggested that n-6 PUFAs may enhance breast cancer invasion and metastasis via eicosanoid production, whereas n-3 PUFAs may have a suppressive effect via the same mechanism.[60] However, the specific roles of various types of fat and fatty acids in altering breast cancer risk in humans have not yet been clearly established.

International comparisons indicate that diets high in n-6 PUFAs (such as found in corn oil) are associated with increased breast cancer risk.[61–63] In contrast, consumption of oleic acid, a monounsaturated fatty acid found in olive oil, and n-3 PUFAs, which are present in certain fish and fish oils, do not increase and may even reduce the risk of breast cancer.[61–66] A recent study suggested no association between breast cancer and saturated fat intake (RR = 0.95), compared with PUFAs (RR = 0.70), oleic acid (RR = 0.81), and olive oil (RR = 0.87), each of which showed an inverse relationship with breast cancer risk.[67,68] One case-control study of primarily postmenopausal breast cancer patients found direct associations between increased breast cancer risk and the concentration of trans fatty acids (RR = 1.4, P < 0.001) and PUFAs (RR = 1.26) in gluteal adipose tissue. The most significant effect of trans fatty acids (RR = 3.65) was seen at the lowest tertile.[69] In a recent short-term dietary intervention, increases in n-3/n-6 PUFA ratios were significantly greater in breast adipose tissue than in gluteal adipose tissue, suggesting that the latter may not be a useful surrogate for changes in breast tissue.[70]

*COLORECTAL CANCER.* Data from international correlation and case-control studies consistently link animal fat and red meat to colon cancer but do not support an association with vegetable fat.[2,3,51,53] A cohort study of more than 47,000 U.S. male health professionals found a highly significantly elevated risk (RR = 1.71) between colon cancer and consumption of red meat but failed to demonstrate an association with any specific type of fat.[51] Further epidemiologic data suggest a protective effect of the consumption of fish or fish oil, calculated as a proportion of total or animal fat, on colorectal cancer risk.[64,71]

**PROSTATE CANCER.** After adjustment for energy intake, data from a large cohort study suggested that α-linolenic acid increased the risk for prostate cancer (RR = 3.43), in contrast with saturated fat (RR = 0.95), monounsaturated fat (RR = 1.58), and linoleic acid (RR = 0.64), which were not significantly associated with the disease.[58] Low plasma levels of α-linolenic acid were associated with reduced prostate cancer risk in a smaller case-control study.[72] A recent review of epidemiologic and experimental evidence suggested that n-3 PUFAs may retard prostate cancer progression.[60]

**PHYSICAL ACTIVITY AND BODY SIZE.** Numerous cohort and case-control studies have investigated the roles of physical activity (energy expenditure), weight, body size [as measured through body mass index (BMI)], and weight gain in relation to cancer risk. The strongest associations thus far have been found with breast and colon cancer.[73] Diets high in fat and/or calories, as just described, contribute to obesity, as does little or no regular physical activity. The interplay of fat, calories, physical activity, and obesity most likely work in concert to influence cancer risk.

**BREAST CANCER.** Weight, body size, and physical activity appear to influence breast cancer risk, particularly in relation to menopausal status. Yet another emerging hypothesis suggests that high caloric intake and rapid growth during youth increase breast cancer risk.[74] Epidemiologic data provide the foundation for the proposed role of body weight or, perhaps more accurately, percentage body fat or BMI, and breast cancer risk.[74–79] In such studies, obesity prior to menopause appears to protect against breast cancer, whereas postmenopausal obesity is associated with increased risk.[78,80] The relationship between adipose tissue and circulating estrogens is thought to direct this differential role of obesity. Many obese premenopausal women have irregular cycles, or fail to ovulate, thus creating an environment in which levels of circulating estrogens are relatively low. Gaining weight after age 18 and being overweight during the premenopausal years, however, appear to ultimately increase a woman's risk for breast cancer after menopause,[79–81] particularly in women who never used postmenopausal hormones.[82] Similarly, weight loss prior to, as well as after, menopause is associated with reduced risk.[80]

With the onset of menopause, estrogen derived from the conversion of androgens in adipose tissue predominates. When compared with their leaner counterparts, obese postmenopausal women may have an elevated risk for breast cancer owing to reduced levels of sex hormone-binding globulin and higher levels of circulating estrogen secondary to the increased metabolic activity in adipose tissue.[76,83]

Case-control and cohort studies consistently suggest that approximately 4 hours or 4000 kcal of physical activity or exercise per week—either on the job or during leisure time, or both—can markedly reduce the risk for breast cancer.[84–86] At least one study showed that additional exercise may lower cancer risk even further.[85]

While leading to weight loss as well as loss of body fat, sustained physical activity, helps reduce circulating levels of estrogen and progesterone, and possibly cancer risk. All women should be encouraged to exercise regularly and avoid weight gain.

**COLORECTAL CANCER.** Both leanness and regular physical activity, whether recreational or occupational, have been consistently associated with a reduced risk for colorectal cancer in men and, in many cases, women.[50,87–91] This protective effect has been observed for both adenomas and cancer and appears to be strongest for lesions of the colon.[89,92–94] Physical activity may modulate cancer risk by any one or more of several proposed mechanisms, including stimulation of immune function, bile acid metabolism, and colonic peristalsis, and reduction in intestinal transit time.[50]

Obesity, which suggests a lack of physical activity and/or excess energy intake, also is directly related to colorectal cancer risk. Data from the Nurses' Health Study indicate that women with a BMI greater than 29 kg/m$^2$, as compared with women with a BMI less than 21 kg/m$^2$, had a relative risk for colon cancer of 1.45.[90]

**PROSTATE CANCER.** Current data do not support a relationship between prostate cancer and obesity in adults.[57,95] However, a recent study of nearly 48,000 men participating in the Health Professionals Follow-up Study found that obesity during childhood (age 10 or under) had a strong inverse association with prostate cancer, whereas tallness was a strong predictor of metastatic disease (for heights >73 in. versus <69 in.). These relationships were strengthened for more aggressive disease states. The preadult hormonal milieu was cited as the underlying etiologic system driving these associations.[96] Lean body mass and high percentage muscle mass in adult men increase the risk of prostate cancer; possibly, elevated levels of circulating androgens may be responsible.[57,95]

## VEGETABLES, FRUITS, AND WHOLE GRAINS

Epidemiologic data are overwhelmingly supportive of the protective effects of vegetables, fruits, and whole grains on cancer risk. In general, the relationship between high consumption of vegetables and fruits and reduced cancer risk appears to be stronger for cancers of the alimentary and respiratory tracts (e.g., colon, lung, oral cavity) than for hormone-related cancers, such as breast cancer.[97,98] A review summarizing the results from more than 200 case-control and cohort studies found a probable protective effect for cancers of the breast, colon, endometrium, oral cavity and pharynx, pancreas, and bladder; and convincing evidence for inverse associations with cancers of the stomach, esophagus, and lung.[97] Raw vegetables had especially consistent anticarcinogenic characteristics, being protective in 85% of the studies. Vegetables from the allium family (e.g., onion, garlic), carrots, green vegetables, cruciferous vegetables (e.g., cabbage, broccoli, cauliflower), and tomatoes were highly protective in 70% or more of the studies. Total fruits, specifically citrus fruits, were protective in about 65% of the studies.

Numerous constituents found in vegetables and fruits might contribute to these anticancer effects, including dietary fiber, micronutrients (e.g., vitamins A, C, and E; folate; β-carotene; selenium; calcium), and nonnutritive phytochemicals (e.g., dithiolethiones, flavonoids, terpenes, and isothiocyanates). These dietary constituents are chemically diverse; thus, their mechanisms of action and interactive effects with regard to reducing cancer risk are likely to differ for specific cancer sites. This section includes a brief discussion of selected evidence linking some micronutrients and specific types of cancer, to illustrate the possible contributions from specific constituents of vegetables and fruits. A more comprehensive discussion of micronutrients and cancer is presented later in this chapter.

## VEGETABLES AND FRUITS

*LUNG CANCER.* The collective evidence from epidemiologic studies generally concludes that both vegetables and fruits are important in the etiology of lung cancer.[97,99,100] Protective associations have been seen for foods such as carrots, tomatoes, citrus fruits, raw vegetables, green vegetables, cruciferous vegetables, and allium vegetables, with the risk for low intakes about twice that of high intakes.[97,98,101] Several recent reviews of prospective and retrospective studies found associations between reduced risk and either vegetable and/or fruit intake or quantification of serum markers (e.g., carotenoids and vitamin C) as a measure of their consumption.[17,97,102] Data on individual constituents (e.g., β-carotene and other carotenoids, vitamins C and E, dithiolethiones, and isothiocyanates) provide abundant evidence for protective effects against lung cancer.[99,103–109] For example, an ecologic study of diet and lung cancer in the South Pacific reported an inverse association with the carotenoid lutein (but not for α- or β-carotene), which accounted for 14% of the variation in incidence in Fiji, where lung cancer rates are markedly lower than that for other islands.[106] However, stronger evidence seems to support a protective effect from vegetables and fruits as whole foods rather than from their individual vitamins, antioxidants, or nonnutritive constituents.[99,110,111]

*HEAD AND NECK CANCER.* Vegetables and fruits exhibit strong, consistent protective effects for cancers of the esophagus, oral cavity, and larynx in the majority of case-control and prospective cohort studies.[17,97,104,105,112] Consumption of carrots, citrus fruits, and green vegetables is consistently linked to prevention of cancer of the oral cavity, and green vegetables, salad, oranges, and tangerines to prevention of cancers of the larynx.[17,97] Five of six epidemiologic studies found associations between cancers of the head and neck and vitamins C and E.[105] The antioxidant action of β-carotene and vitamin E may result in regression of oral leukoplakia, a premalignant lesion for oral cancer.[113]

*COLORECTAL CANCER.* Vegetables, especially raw and green vegetables, consistently demonstrate protective effects against colorectal cancer.[97,105,114,115] Recent studies have suggested that the high consumption of vegetables and fruits may reduce total colorectal cancer incidence by half [odds ratio (OR) = 0.49].[116,117] Cruciferous vegetables, in particular, are linked closely with a decrease in rectal cancer.[50,97] Generally, fruits have demonstrated a less strong connection to cancers of the colon and rectum than vegetables.[17]

In some studies, specific micronutrients have been strongly linked to colorectal cancer. β-Carotene and vitamin C supplementation has been associated with strong to moderate decreases in ab-

normal colonic crypt cell proliferation in subjects with adenomatous polyps.[103,105,118] It is possible that the antioxidative action of either β-carotene, especially in the promotion phase of carcinogenesis,[119] or one or more of the other carotenoids present in high-carotenoid vegetables, may protect against colorectal cancer development.[115,120] Calcium has been linked to the prevention of cancers of the colon and rectum in case-control and cohort studies, but results are inconsistent.[50,54,121,122] Both modest and protective nonsignificant effects against colorectal neoplasia have been found with vitamin E.[123]

Data for a protective effect on colon cancer by vitamin C have been less consistent than that for rectal cancer (4/8 versus 4/6 studies)[104] but are supportive of a protective association.[105,118] Observational and experimental studies have linked the risk of colorectal cancer to selenium intake,[124] vitamin D,[50,54] iron,[125] and lycopene and lutein.[126] No association has been found with vitamin A.[50]

*BREAST CANCER.* A recent expert panel suggested that a diet high in vegetables and fruits ranked as the major recommendation for breast cancer prevention (along with the avoidance of alcohol).[17] Research and reviews regarding the protective effects of vegetable and fruit consumption on breast cancer are numerous[97,105,127–129]; data are generally more consistent for a protective effect of vegetables, particularly green vegetables, than for fruits.[17,130] For example, in a large, case-control study of about 13,000 women, consumption of carrots or spinach more than twice weekly was associated with almost a 50% reduction in breast cancer risk (OR = 0.56).[131] Soy products, including tofu, have been linked to protection against cancer in 63% of studies on breast cancer,[17] possibly as a result of their phytoestrogen content.[132,133]

Some case-control and follow-up studies have demonstrated the effectiveness of several microconstituents in breast cancer prevention. These include vitamin A,[134] vitamin C,[104,105,127,134] vitamin E,[105,135] β-carotene,[103,127,136,137] folic acid,[109] and selenium.[134,138] Overall, however, data are inconsistent.

*PROSTATE CANCER.* Evidence supporting the protective effects of vegetables and fruits on prostate cancer is limited and often inconsistent.[17,57,97] A comprehensive review recently determined that only 17% of case-control studies demonstrated a statistically significant protective effect of at least one vegetable or fruit on prostate cancer. Five of seven cohort studies found some protective effect; the other two reported no association.[17] For example, leafy green vegetables were significantly associated with a protective effect, as was vegetarianism.[139] In a large cohort study, tomato-based foods such as tomatoes, tomato sauce (but not tomato juice), and pizza were seen as especially protective against prostate cancer. In addition, out of 52 vegetables and fruits, this study found strawberries to be the single significantly protective fruit to show an inverse association (OR = 0.80).[140] In general, the protective effects of vegetables and fruits against prostate cancer are less well established than for cancers at other sites.[17]

In a recent study, β-carotene appeared to be protective at all stages of prostate cancer.[141] However, other studies of β-carotene have reported inconsistent results (three of five studies showed inverse associations).[103] Promising results have been seen in several vitamin E studies: one case-control study of unspecified tocopherols[141]; another case-control study in Hawaii that reported an inverse, nonsignificant association with γ-tocopherol only[142]; and a third study in which a 78% reduction (significant) was observed for α-tocopherol.[143] Protective associations also have been observed for vitamin D,[144–146] nonspecified retinoids,[142,143] and calcium and iron.[143] Data do not support a protective association with vitamin C and prostate cancer.[104,147]

*OTHER CANCERS.* Inverse relationships between the high consumption of vegetables and fruits and cancer risk have been demonstrated at several other cancer sites, including the stomach,[97,105,112,148] pancreas,[97] bladder,[97,112] and cervix.[112] Carrots and green vegetables have demonstrated particularly consistent cancer inhibitory activity against cancer of the bladder, and raw and green vegetables against stomach cancer.[97] Fruit consumption has been linked to a reduced risk of pancreatic cancer in five out of five studies[104]; also, between a twofold and threefold protective effect for stomach cancer was reported in seven of eight studies.[104,149] Individual fruits, particularly citrus fruits, have demonstrated a consistent protective effect against stomach cancer.[97] Endometrial cancer has been reported to be inversely associated with the intake of green vegetables, fruit, and whole grains.[150] After adjusting for confounding variables, one case-control study found an inverse association between ovarian cancer risk and the high intake of green vegetables and whole-grain bread or pasta.[151]

In some studies, specific constituents have been investigated. For example, selenium and folic acid reduced the risk of ovarian[152] and pancreatic[109] cancers, respectively.[109,152] Vitamin A and/or β-carotene, as well as total carotenoids, increased regression rates in cervical dysplasia as measured by cervical intraepithelial neoplasia, a commonly studied precursor of cervical cancer.[153] Further, several reviews have found a generally strong inverse relationship between stomach cancer with β-carotene,[103] vitamins C and E (12 of 13 studies),[105] and vitamin C alone (7 of 7 studies).[104]

## WHOLE GRAINS

*LUNG CANCER.* A limited number of epidemiologic studies connect lung cancer to the consumption of whole grains, and cereal products; no studies showed any relationship between the consumption of these foods and the incidences of tumors and cancers of the lung.[17] One experimental study, however, reported that cereal-fed rats developed fewer lung tumors than those fed semipurified diets.[154]

*HEAD AND NECK CANCER.* Consumption of whole grains is not strongly linked to head and neck cancer. In general, as the degree of refining for grain and cereal products increases, their cancer-protective effects decrease.[155–157] However, this generalization is based on only a few studies, because research in this area is limited.

*COLORECTAL CANCER.* Research reviews demonstrate clear correlations between an increased intake of whole grains, as well as dietary fiber from whole grains, and decreased colorectal cancer.[97,114] Fiber alone, however, probably does not account entirely for this protective association; case-control studies show that legumes, also high in dietary fiber, do not appear to protect against colorectal cancer.[97]

*BREAST CANCER.* Few data are available on an association between whole grains, per se, and breast cancer. However, as already noted, whole grains are a major source of dietary fiber. The possible relationship between dietary fiber and breast cancer is discussed in the following section on dietary fiber.

*PROSTATE CANCER.* Few studies have investigated the relationship between whole grains and prostate cancer to any appreciable degree. One Swedish study found an inverse but statistically nonsignificant association between fiber and prostate cancer in advanced cases (RR = 0.82) and at all stages (RR = 0.82).[141]

## DIETARY FIBER

The concept of a cancer-preventive role for dietary fiber was advanced in the early 1970s following Burkitt's observations that certain chronic diseases prevalent in westernized societies, such as colon cancer, diverticular disease, gallstones, and ischemic heart disease, were rarely found in African populations who consumed diets of predominately fiber-rich foods.[158] Since that time, a growing body of epidemiologic, experimental, and clinical evidence has suggested that colorectal and breast cancer risk, and possibly the risk of cancers at other sites—including the esophagus, mouth, pharynx, stomach, prostate, endometrium, and ovary—may be decreased by increasing the intake of dietary fiber and fiber-rich foods, including vegetables, fruit, and whole grains.[2,3,17,97,101]

Even though an impressive collection of data exists that generally suggests a beneficial relationship between dietary fiber and cancer, study results are somewhat inconsistent, and the exact role of total dietary fiber, as well as specific types of fiber, in cancer development remains unresolved. Because dietary fibers from different sources vary in composition, it is unlikely that all will be equally protective against cancer.[3,17,159,160] The complexities of fiber and the lack of standardized analytical methods for extracting and quantifying the fiber content of foods remain important issues.[161] Other confounding factors in the study of dietary fiber in health and disease include the different chemical and physical properties of each type of fiber (i.e., solubility, fermentability); the impact of storage, processing, and food preparation on the physical and chemical nature of fiber; the lack of specific food composition data for types of dietary fiber and total fiber; and issues related to dietary assessment, such as recall bias. Inconsistencies in results across animal studies can reflect methodologic variables, including species and strain of animal used; type, amount, and mode of administration of carcinogen; type and amount of fiber consumed; timing of fiber administration in the carcinogenic process; and study length.[162]

Because specific food composition data on fiber are limited, many epidemiologic studies have examined associations between cancer risk and dietary fiber based on food consumption patterns. As discussed in a previous section, in the majority of epidemiologic studies, the consumption of vegetables and fruits, both high-fiber food groups, is associated consistently with a reduced risk of cancer at most sites.[17,97,101] However, a major confounding factor in assessing results from such studies is that in addition to fiber, plant foods contain numerous components that may contribute to the reduced cancer risk associated with high-fiber diets. Vegetables and fruits contain many naturally occurring potential anticarcinogens, including micronutrients such as β-carotene, vitamins C and E, and selenium (discussed in the previous section, Vegetables and Fruits) and various nonnutritive phytochemicals, including phytoestrogens, carotenoids, organosulfur compounds, isothiocyanates, flavonoids, indoles, and terpenes (some of which are discussed in the following section Micronutrients). These dietary components may have both complementary and interactive mechanisms of action with each other and with dietary fiber.[4,163] The assessment of effects on cancer risk due to fiber can be further complicated by the presence of significant correlations among dietary fiber, dietary fat, and caloric intakes.

COLORECTAL CANCER. A number of extensive reviews of epidemiologic and experimental studies on dietary fiber and colorectal cancer risk have been published.[53,54,159,164–167] The hypothesis that dietary fiber is protective against colorectal cancer is generally supported by correlation studies and international comparisons. The majority of these studies show strong-to-moderate support for the protective effect of dietary fiber and fiber-rich foods; furthermore, some studies indicate that fiber may modulate the risk-enhancing effects of fat in colorectal cancer development. For example, colon cancer risk was lower in Finland, where the average fiber intake was twice that in Denmark and New York, even though all three populations had a high fat intake (34% to 37%).[168–169] A recent population-based, case-control study reported that higher intakes of dietary fiber were inversely associated with colon cancer risk in both older men (RR = 0.5) and older women (RR = 0.7) and that the protective effect was slightly stronger among those with proximal tumors.[114]

Two large, multicenter randomized controlled trials, the Polyp Prevention Trial (PPT) and the Wheat Bran Fiber Study (WBFS), reported that nutritional intervention with a high-fiber diet and a high-fiber cereal supplement, respectively, did not inhibit the recurrence of colorectal adenomas.[170–171] The PPT and WBFS studied men and women at increased risk for colorectal cancer. Trial entry criteria included having a history of colorectal adenomas, which are considered to be precursors of most colorectal cancers.

Epidemiologic observations suggest the possibility of differences in risk factors for colonic tumors at different sites. In less developed countries with a low incidence of colon cancer, most tumors are found in the proximal colon, but in affluent countries with high incidence, the majority of colonic tumors are in the distal colon.[172] If risk factors vary for different colonic sites, the effects of dietary fiber intake, as well as putative protective mechanisms, may also vary throughout the colonic lumen.[172,173] Results from one investigation of vegetable and fruit consumption and colon cancer incidence in postmenopausal women indicated that vegetable and fruit fiber may be more important in lowering the risk for distal tumors than for proximal tumors, possibly via the dilution of carcinogens through increased bulk in the distal colon.[174] In the Health Professionals Follow-up Study, a reduced risk of distal colon adenoma was observed with increased intake (highest quintile) of fruit fiber (RR = 0.81) and soluble fiber (RR = 0.69), but not for cereal or vegetable fibers, or for insoluble fiber.[175]

Fibers from different plant sources appear to vary in their protective properties for colorectal cancer; for example, data indicate

that wheat bran inhibits colon tumor development in animals more effectively than either corn bran or oat bran[176,177] and that its effects might be enhanced by certain micronutrients or phytochemicals.[178] Wheat bran fiber supplementation also has been reported to reduce rectal mucosal proliferation significantly in high-risk individuals with a family history of colorectal cancer.[179] In patients with resected colon adenomas, wheat bran fiber supplementation significantly reduced concentrations of fecal bile acids, which may act as tumor promoters,[180] but had no significant effects on proliferation rates in the rectal mucosa.[181]

Several mechanisms have been proposed for a protective effect on colorectal cancer. One direct mechanism by which dietary fiber reduces the risk of colorectal cancer may be absorption of water by insoluble dietary fiber; this increases fecal bulk, diluting the concentration of carcinogens in the feces, and also decreases transit time, thus reducing the possibility of effective interaction with colonic mucosal cells. The direct binding of carcinogens to nondegradable dietary fibers produces a similar decrease in potential carcinogenic interaction within the large bowel. Possible indirect mechanisms include stimulation of microbial growth, which increases fecal bulk and small-chain fatty acid (SCFA) production; alteration of the production of bile acids; influence on the production of cellular initiators and promoters that affect cell proliferation; and effects of SCFAs, particularly butyrate, on luminal pH.[164] Results of one study[182] indicate that the type of dietary fiber may influence the amount of diacylglycerol (DAG) produced through enhanced activity of intestinal flora; DAG activates protein kinase C, an enzyme that plays a key role in cell growth control and tumor promotion.[183] Dietary wheat bran, but not corn or oat bran, significantly decreased the levels of fecal DAG in premenopausal women,[182] an interesting result considering the superior effectiveness of wheat bran in inhibiting colon tumors in animal models.[176,177]

BREAST CANCER. Both epidemiologic and experimental data suggest that dietary fiber intake may be protective for breast cancer.[97,129,184–186] One in-depth review of available evidence summarizing the current status of breast cancer epidemiology concluded that dietary influences may, to some degree, explain the wide variations in breast cancer rates among racial, religious, and geographic groups.[187] In a review of seven case-control studies that assessed the relationship between breast cancer and fiber or fiber-rich foods, six studies indicated that diets high in fiber or cereal reduced the risk of breast cancer, and one study suggested a weak protective effect of vegetable fiber.[166] A meta-analysis of original data from 12 case-control studies, in populations with very different breast cancer risks and dietary habits, found a significant decrease in breast cancer risk among women in the highest quintile of dietary fiber intake compared with the lowest quintile, even after adjusting for total fat intake.[188] A recent case-control study reported a reduced breast cancer risk for the highest quartile of intake for total dietary fiber (RR = 0.51), grain fiber (RR = 0.65), vegetable fiber (RR = 0.56), and fruit fiber (RR = 0.77), with significant dose-response relationships for all except fruit fiber.[189] In contrast to one case-control study that found no association between fiber and breast cancer risk in Italian women,[67] findings in another Italian study suggested that cellulose reduced breast cancer risk, particularly in premenopausal women; no protective effect was observed for soluble fibers, noncellulose polysaccharides, or lignin.[190] Overall, the influence of fiber, per se, on breast cancer development, relative to the contributions of other constituents in fiber-rich foods, is not yet clear.[186,187] It is notable that in Finland, where the intake of both dietary fat and fiber is high, women have a significantly lower risk of breast cancer incidence and mortality than women in the United States, who generally consume a high-fat diet that is relatively low in fiber.[184] A modifying influence of fiber on breast cancer risk associated with high-fat intake may in part explain the lower risk of breast cancer in Finnish women.[184] Although limited, data from animal studies support the epidemiologic evidence indicating that dietary fiber may reduce breast cancer risk.[185]

It has been suggested that the risk of breast cancer, as well as other hormone-dependent cancers, may be influenced by dietary factors through alteration of hormone production, metabolism, or actions at the cellular level.[62,185,191,192] High-fiber intake is associated with low plasma levels of all major biologically active sex hormones, high levels of sex hormone binding globulin (SHBG), low percentages of free estradiol and free testosterone, and low urinary and high fecal estrogen excretion. Dietary fiber may influence estrogens, which are primarily associated with breast cancer etiology, through alteration of the microbial population and enzymes in the intestinal tract, reducing the deconjugation of estrogens and, thus, the amount available for reabsorption. Further, phytoestrogens, which have weak estrogenic activity and appear to compete with estrogens for receptor-binding sites, thus potentially reducing breast cancer risk, are produced in the intestine from fiber-related precursors.[62] Dietary phytoestrogens also increase the synthesis of SHBG in the liver,[193] thereby increasing plasma SHBG levels and, consequently, reducing the availability of sex hormones to their target organs.[186]

OTHER CANCERS. Although epidemiologic data link vegetable and fruit consumption with other cancers, including those of the lung, stomach, prostate, and endometrium, limited evidence is available linking dietary fiber per se and risk for these cancers.[57,99,194,195] Data from some studies have suggested inverse relationships between fiber intake and cancers of the esophagus, mouth, pharynx, and stomach.[112,166] Two studies reported that crude fiber[196] and vegetable fiber,[197] but not fruit or cereal fiber,[197] were associated with a decreased risk of ovarian cancer.

The association of a high-fiber, vegetarian diet with a reduced prostate cancer risk was demonstrated in a cohort study that found a significant decrease in prostate cancer risk with the frequent consumption of beans, lentils, and peas (RR = 0.53); fresh citrus fruit (RR = 0.88); nuts (RR = 0.79); tomatoes (RR = 0.60); and raisins, dates, and other dried fruit (RR = 0.62).[198] Investigation of the association between diet and sex hormone metabolism in vegetarian and nonvegetarian men demonstrated that plasma levels of testosterone and estradiol-17β were significantly lower in vegetarians than in omnivores and were significantly and inversely related to crude and dietary fiber intakes.[199] A metabolic epidemiologic study among Seventh Day Adventist men determined by in vitro assays that both percentage and amount of bound steroid hormones were directly related to levels of dietary lignin.[200] Neutral detergent fiber, hemicellulose, and cellulose did not demonstrate significant binding abilities. Such results emphasize the need to clarify the relationships between steroid-hormone metabolism, dietary fiber components, and prostate cancer risk.[199,200]

## MICRONUTRIENTS

Epidemiologic studies have demonstrated cancer-protective relationships for foods high in antioxidant micronutrients such as vitamin C, β-carotene, vitamin E, and selenium, as well as the micronutrients vitamin A, calcium, and folate.[3,17,103,105,122,201]

It is more likely that several, rather than single, micronutrients contribute to the overall protective effects seen in epidemiologic and experimental studies. For example, the beneficial effect of high vegetable and/or fruit consumption cannot be explained completely by either β-carotene or total provitamin A carotenoid intakes.[99] Microconstituents may, in fact, be markers for other dietary component(s) or a synergistic group of constituents that have preventive properties.[202] For example, a cohort study by Yong and colleagues[203] recently reported that a combination of vitamins E and C and carotenoids was more protective (RR = 0.48) than any of these individually (RRs = 0.82, 0.49, 0.55, respectively). To help ensure adequate intake of cancer-protective agents, current recommendations suggest consumption of a variety of foods rich in micronutrients, namely, vegetables, fruits, and whole grains.

The antioxidant micronutrients, including β-carotene (provitamin A), vitamins E and C, and selenium, have been of considerable interest to investigators in cancer research.[6,97,204] Reactive oxygen species such as superoxide, nitric oxide, and hydroxyl radicals, formed continuously as a result of biochemical reactions in the human body, can cause significant oxidative damage to nucleic acids, lipids, and proteins. Such damage is considered to be an important factor in carcinogenesis. Also, environmental carcinogens, including some found in food, are believed to contribute to oxidative stress. Common sources of carcinogens include tobacco smoke, industrial pollution, and food contaminants such as aflatoxins, heterocyclic aromatic amines (HAAs), and pesticide residues.[205,206]

The human body has certain defense mechanisms that repair cellular damage caused by oxidants and free radicals, for example, enzymes such as glutathione peroxidase, superoxide dismutase, and catalase. However, these defenses frequently cannot counteract all oxidative attacks. Fortunately, evolution has provided plants with numerous antioxidant constituents as protection against environmental damages resulting from oxidation; thus, consumption of plant foods may be beneficial in terms of reduced cancer risk.[119,135,207,208] Because reactive oxygen species appear to be involved at all stages of cancer development, dietary antioxidants may be effective throughout the carcinogenic process.

VITAMIN A AND β-CAROTENE. Dietary vitamin A consists of preformed vitamin A found in the fats and oils of animal products, plus vitamin A produced from some carotenoids, most notably β-carotene, in the body. Vitamin A influences cell differentiation, and a deficiency of this micronutrient leads to hyperplastic changes in epithelial tissues, such as are observed in certain precancerous conditions; thus, vitamin A is believed to be most effective in the promotion stage of carcinogenesis.[119] As early as the 1950s, researchers observed that vitamin A decreased the incidence and degree of chemically induced hyperplasia in the mouse prostate gland in vitro.[209] In the 1960s and early 1970s, vitamin A, as well as some of its less toxic analogues, were a research focus in carcinogenesis inhibition, resulting in a considerable body of somewhat inconsistent data.[3,17]

Published reviews of epidemiologic studies that focused primarily on indices of β-carotene (provitamin A) have consistently reported strong support for a significant protective effect of dietary β-carotene on lung cancer.[99,103,112] One recent review noted that associations of either high intakes of β-carotene–rich vegetables and fruits or high blood concentrations of β-carotene with reduced cancer risk were most consistent for lung and stomach cancer. Esophageal cancer showed limited but promising risk reduction.[103] Reported results for the effects of both β-carotene and vitamin A were equivocal for prostate cancer[57] and indicated a possible protective effect of β-carotene for breast cancer.[74] For colon cancer, some case-control studies reported significantly reduced risk at high intakes,[210] but overall, data suggested only a modest risk reduction.[103] In contrast, one trial with β-carotene showed no evidence of benefit for prevention of nonmelanoma skin cancer in persons previously treated for skin cancer.[211] Two trials designed to prevent colorectal polyps in high-risk individuals found no evidence of a reduction in polyp incidence, and no evidence of harm, after 4 years of intervention.[212,213]

**VITAMIN C.** More than 80% of the vitamin C in western diets comes from vegetables and fruits. Citrus fruits and berries are the best sources of vitamin C, and some vegetables are particularly good sources (e.g., green peppers, broccoli). In addition to its antioxidant effects, which also include reconstituting the active forms of vitamin E, vitamin C plays a role in the synthesis of connective tissue protein. Thus, vitamin C status may affect the integrity of intercellular membranes and have consequences with regard to inhibiting tumor spread.[61,145,202,214]

Epidemiologic evidence for a protective effect of diets high in vitamin C–containing vegetables and fruits is strong and consistent for cancers of the oral cavity, esophagus, and stomach, but moderate and less consistent for colon and lung cancers. Data do not support an association with prostate cancer and the evidence for breast cancer is conflicting.[104,105,147] A review of more than 50 case-control and cohort studies that investigated intakes of vegetables and fruits and vitamin C and E, reported that, across studies, individuals in the highest category of vegetable and fruit intake had approximately 40% less risk of gastrointestinal and respiratory tract cancers than those in the lowest intake levels.[105] Indices of vitamin C computed from vegetable and fruit intakes were also associated with lower risk in these studies. In a 30-year, prospective, follow-up study of 1900 men studied for prostate cancer risk, both vitamin C and β-carotene were positively associated with overall survival but no relationship was associated with the risk of prostate cancer.[147] To date, no large-scale human intervention studies using vitamin C alone have been reported.

**VITAMIN E.** In the United States, the primary dietary source of α-tocopherol, the most active and abundant form of vitamin E, is vegetable oils, including olive, canola, safflower, and sunflower oils. Vegetables and fruits combined provide about 20% of the intake of this fat-soluble nutrient,[97] and vitamin E is also present in whole-grain products.[135] A major antioxidant function of vitamin

E is to protect PUFAs in cell membranes from attack by free radicals, thereby interfering with lipid auto-oxidation.[135,202] Vitamin E also helps to keep selenium in the reduced state, thus facilitating the antioxidant activities of this mineral.[97]

Epidemiologic studies that have investigated associations between cancer risk and diets high in vitamin E are limited in number and show inconsistent results, possibly because estimating dietary vitamin E is difficult.[105] A review of 10 studies of vitamin E intake and 8 measuring serum vitamin E levels in relation to breast cancer risk reported an overall inconclusive relationship.[135] Another review found significant regression of premalignant lesions in the oral cavity for vitamin E alone and in combination with β-carotene.[113] One case-control study that examined the association between micronutrient intake and colorectal adenomas reported that men in the highest quartile of vitamin E intake were about one-fifth as likely to develop adenomas as men in the lowest quartile (OR = 0.22 for men; OR = 0.74 for women).[125] In the recently completed Alpha-Tocopherol, Beta-Carotene Cancer Prevention Study (ATBC Study),[215] conducted in Finland with more than 29,000 male cigarette smokers at high risk for lung cancer, 34% fewer cases of prostate cancer and 16% fewer cases of colorectal cancer were diagnosed among men who received daily vitamin E supplements. Although these results suggest a protective effect of vitamin E, prostate and colon cancers were not primary study end points. Further research targeted at these cancers is needed before conclusions can be drawn about the potential of vitamin E for their prevention. Also, a recent review suggests that the antioxidant effects of γ-tocopherol may be superior to those of α-tocopherol and that studies on the role of vitamin E in colorectal cancer should consider all tocopherols.[216]

**SELENIUM.** The trace mineral selenium is found in grains and vegetables as well as in seafood and domesticated animal meats.[50] Dietary assessment of selenium can be problematic; levels in plant foods depend on the soil in which plants grow, and levels in meats depend on the animals' feed.[97] Thus, selenium status is best determined by biochemical measures, such as blood or toenail selenium levels rather than by dietary analysis. Although not an antioxidant per se, selenium functions as a cofactor for glutathione peroxidase, an enzyme that may protect against oxidative tissue damage.[97,202] Additional protective mechanisms of selenium may include alterations in carcinogen metabolism, production of cytotoxic selenium metabolites, inhibition of protein synthesis, stimulation of apoptosis, and effects on the endocrine and immune systems.[217]

Cancer mortality international correlation studies suggest an inverse association between selenium status and cancer incidence.[218] Also, animal studies strongly support a cancer-protective effect of selenium at several sites.[219–222] Data from case-control and cohort studies, however, have not been convincing for those cancer sites investigated, including lung, breast, and stomach cancers.[74,99,195] A review of 10 cohort studies found a consistent pattern of increased cancer risk for various cancer sites associated with lower serum selenium levels.[223] More recently, data from a prospective study that examined the association of serum selenium levels and development of ovarian cancer indicated that women in the highest tertile, compared with the lowest tertile, were four times less likely to develop ovarian cancer (OR = 0.23).[152] A randomized, controlled clinical intervention showed significant reductions in total cancer mortality (RR = 0.5), total cancer incidence (RR = 0.63), and incidences of lung (RR = 0.54), colorectal (RR = 0.42), and prostate (RR = 0.37) cancer, for individuals who received selenium supplements, compared with controls.[217] These positive findings support the cancer-protective effect of selenium but must be confirmed in independent intervention trials. Determining the optimal form and dose level of selenium for use in clinical trials—effective and toxic doses are quite close—is complicated by differences in toxicity thresholds among individuals.

**CALCIUM.** Dairy products are the major source of dietary calcium; green, leafy vegetables also are good sources. Calcium acts as a functional element in cells providing structure, membrane rigidity, and permeability.[122] It is theorized that calcium could decrease the risk of colorectal cancers by binding potentially carcinogenic compounds such as secondary bile acids, as well as by slowing mucosal proliferation and increasing cell differentiation.[224–226] Numerous studies have demonstrated these effects of calcium on colonic cells both in vitro and in vivo for rodents and humans.[122] A recent study reported that shifting from a dairy product–rich to a dairy product–free diet significantly increased the cytotoxicity of human fecal water, an accepted risk marker for colon cancer, but did not affect genotoxicity, suggesting that dairy products may act at the level of tumor promotion rather than initiation.[227]

Many epidemiologic studies have suggested an association between dietary calcium and decreased carcinogenesis, primarily in colorectal cancer.[54,122] A recent review found that although several ecologic studies have demonstrated inverse associations between calcium intake and colorectal cancer mortality, many case-control and cohort studies have yielded inconsistent results.[54] Five of seven studies conducted within the past 3 years found no protective effect against colon and/or rectal carcinogenesis for either dietary calcium and/or dairy product consumption.[228–232] One positive study found a substantial inverse relationship between calcium and the risk for adenomatous polyps (OR = 0.7, P = 0.10)[233] and another found the same result in men (OR = 0.44, P = 0.57) but not in women.[125] Calcium appeared to modify the effect of total fat intake on the risk for adenomatous polyps.[233] A recent quantitative summary of 24 epidemiologic studies using stratified analyses and regression analysis found an overall lack of support for the hypothesis that calcium prevents colorectal neoplasia (cohort studies, RR = 0.9; case-control studies, RR = 0.88).[224]

**FOLATE.** Appreciable quantities of folate (folic acid), a B vitamin, are found in green vegetables, cruciferous vegetables, oranges, whole grains, wheat bran, legumes, seeds, and some organ meats.[50] One review of folic acid and carcinogenesis found strong inverse associations between intakes of folic acid and folic acid–rich foods and cancers of the colon, rectum, and breast.[109] The actions of folate and methionine, an essential amino acid, have been found to protect against both colorectal adenomas and colorectal cancers.[50,125,234,235] In a cohort of almost 48,000 male health professionals, Giovannucci and colleagues[140] found a significant positive association between colon cancer and increased alcohol consumption, with concurrent inadequate intakes of folate and methionine. In a case-control study

that evaluated possible associations between dietary folate, iron, calcium, and vitamins A, C, and E, folate was also associated with a reduced risk for colorectal adenomas (OR = 0.39, 0.08).[125] Significant protection has been observed for cancers of the colon (OR = 0.51), but not the rectum (OR = 2.12), with the risk for colon cancer almost five times higher (OR = 4.79) for men with a high-alcohol, low-folate, low-protein diet compared with a low-alcohol, high-folate, high-protein diet.[235] It has been suggested that folate may prevent hypomethylation of DNA[236]; DNA hypomethylation is an early step in colorectal carcinogenesis.[237,238] Aberrant patterns of hypomethylation may lead to changes in DNA conformation that contribute to genetic instability, which might result in oncogene expression, contributing to the development of colorectal tumorigenesis.[239,240]

## PHYTOCHEMICALS

Numerous phytochemicals, nonnutritive plant-derived compounds, are being studied for their potential cancer-preventive or cancer-enhancing effects.[87,241–244] Vegetables, fruits, whole grains, teas, soy and soy products, and other plants and plant products contain a wide variety of phytochemicals, including organosulfides, isothiocyanates, indoles, monoterpenes, dithiolethiones, polyphenols, thioethers, flavonoids, tannins, protease inhibitors, and non(vitamin A)-active carotenoids.[87,241–243] Phytochemicals and some of their sources include thioethers (garlic, onions, leeks), terpenes (citrus fruits), plant phenols (grapes, strawberries, apples), polyphenols (green tea), indoles and isothiocyanates (cruciferous vegetables such as cabbage, broccoli, cauliflower), and isoflavonoid phytoestrogens (soy, soy products).[50,87,241,242] Selected phytochemicals and their sources are listed in Table 1B-8.

The exact mechanisms by which many phytochemicals act are not yet clear. It is recognized, however, that those with cancer-preventive effects can be grouped generally as blocking agents, agents that suppress promotion, and antioxidants, and that some substances may show more than one effect.[241,245] Specific mechanisms for particular compounds are varied. Some act by scavenging reactive carcinogens, which, in turn, prevents the metabolic activation of carcinogens or tumor promoters; for example, ellagic acid, a polyphenol found in berries and nuts, inhibits DNA-carcinogen adduct formation.[246] Others may act by inducing or inhibiting phase I or phase II xenobiotic detoxification enzymes, for example, sulforaphane in broccoli[247] and brassinin in cabbage.[248] Phase I enzyme reactions result in more readily water-soluble metabolites that facilitate subsequent phase II enzyme-mediated conjugation reactions and excretion of modified xenobiotic compounds. Modulation of phase I and II activities is characteristic of blocking agents, such as flavonoids, organosulfides, indoles, and isothiocyanates.[61,145,158,249–252] Other phytochemicals, such as monoterpenes, appear to act as tumor-suppressing agents. Through the modulation of oncogene or proto-oncogene expression or function, suppressing agents interfere with the carcinogenic process in cells that would otherwise become malignant.[243,244,252,253]

A comprehensive review of the phytochemicals-cancer relationship is beyond the scope of this discussion. Thus, selected examples are presented briefly here.

**TABLE 1B-8.** SELECTED PHYTOCHEMICALS IN FRUITS AND VEGETABLES

| GROUP | PHYTOCHEMICALS | SOURCE |
|---|---|---|
| Organosulfur compounds | Allyl mercaptan | *Allium* sp. vegetables (garlic and onion) |
| | Allyl methyl disulfide | *Allium* sp. vegetables (garlic and onion) |
| | Allyl methyl trisulfide | *Allium* sp. vegetables (garlic and onion) |
| | Diallyl sulfide | *Allium* sp. vegetables (garlic and onion) |
| | Diallyl disulfide | *Allium* sp. vegetables (garlic and onion) |
| | Diallyl trisulfide | *Allium* sp. vegetables (garlic and onion) |
| Carotenoids | β-Carotene | Vegetables and fruits |
| | α-Carotene | Vegetables and fruits |
| | Lutein | Vegetables and fruits |
| | Zeaxanthin | Vegetables and fruits |
| | Cryptozanthin | Vegetables and fruits |
| | Astaxanthin | Vegetables and fruits |
| | Lycopene | Vegetables and fruits (tomatoes) |
| Cinnamic acids | Caffeic acid | Fruits, coffee beans, and soybean |
| | Ferulic acid | Fruits and soybeans |
| | Chlorogenic acid | Fruits, coffee beans, and soybean |
| Isothiocyanates | Benzyl isothiocyanate | Cruciferous vegetables |
| | Phenethyl isothiocyanate | Cruciferous vegetables |
| Flavonoids | Quercetin | Vegetables and fruits |
| | Rutin | Vegetables and fruits |
| | Tangeretin | Citrus fruits |
| | Nobiletin | Citrus fruits |
| Glucosinolates | Glucobrassicin | Cruciferous vegetables |
| | Glucotropaeolin | Cruciferous vegetables |
| | Glucoberin | Cruciferous vegetables |
| | Progoitrin | Cruciferous vegetables |
| Indoles | Indole-3-cabinol | Cruciferous vegetables |
| | Indole-3-acetonitrile | Cruciferous vegetables |
| Isoflavones | Genistein | Soybeans |
| | Daidzein | Soybeans |
| Polyphenols | Ellagic acid | Berries, nuts |
| | Curcumin | Tumeric |
| | Tea polyphenols | Green tea, black tea |
| Phytates | Inositol hexaphosphate | Cereals and legumes |
| Protease inhibitors | Leupeptin | Beans and seeds |
| | Soybean protease inhibitors | Soybeans |
| Terpenes | D-Limonene | Citrus fruit oils |
| | D-Carvone | Caraway seed oil |
| | Glycyrrhizic acid | Licorice root |
| | Glycyrrhetinic acid | Licorice root |

SOURCE: Adapted from M-T HUANG et al (eds): *Food Phytochemicals for Cancer Prevention I: Fruits and Vegetables.* Washington, D.C., American Chemical Society, 1994.

PHYTOESTROGENS. Dietary phytoestrogens, that is, isoflavonoid (e.g., genistein, daidzein) and plant lignans, are found in seeds, legumes, flaxseed, fruits, berries, and grain and vegetable fibers.[254,255] The mammalian lignans, enterlactone (Enl) and enterodiol (End), which are formed from plant lignans by the action of intestinal bacteria, and urinary concentrations of lignans correlate directly with consumption of phytoestrogen-containing plant foods.[255,256] Epidemiologic studies of Asian populations who regularly consume soybean seeds and soy-based foods from childhood through adulthood reveal markedly lower incidence rates for both breast and colon cancer, and possibly for prostate cancer, when compared with persons in western countries where soy products are rarely consumed.[132,255,257,258] Studies of vegetarians who consume soy products also suggest a decreased risk for breast and colon cancer within this population.[257,259] A recent study in Australian women reported an inverse relationship between breast cancer risk and urinary excretion of phytoestrogens (a measure of plant phytoestrogen intake).[260] A review of 26 animal studies in which dietary soy or soybean isoflavonoid was used found a cancer-protective effect, defined as a reduction in tumor incidence, latency, or number, in 65% of the studies.[258]

In vitro and animal studies suggest that phytoestrogens mimic the activity of endogenous estrogens by binding to the estrogen receptor. Although the affinity of phytoestrogens to estrogen receptors is tens to thousands times lower than that of endogenous estrogens, this activity of the plant-derived agents still allows for weak estrogenic and antiestrogenic effects.[255,258,259]

Phytoestrogens have been shown to inhibit proliferation of human breast cancer cells that depend on estrogen to replicate.[255,258] Further, by inducing production of sex hormone–binding globulin and inhibiting the enzyme aromatase, phytoestrogens indirectly reduce the amount of circulating steroid hormones, which may be associated with reduced breast cancer risk.

ORGANOSULFUR COMPOUNDS. A cancer-protective effect for members of the *Allium* family (e.g., onions, garlic, and chives), which contain numerous organosulfur compounds, has been suggested by case-control, cohort, and animal studies.[50,174,261] Diets containing *Allium* vegetables were associated with significantly reduced risk for colorectal cancer in four of five case-control studies.[50] Additional studies suggest that frequent and high consumption of *Allium* vegetables lowers the incidence of stomach cancer.[243] In animal studies, administration of diallyl sulfide (DAS) and/or its analogues, isolated from *Allium* vegetables, has been shown to inhibit carcinogen-induced tumors of the colon, esophagus, uterine cervix, liver, lung, and forestomach.[243,244]

Several mechanisms by which organosulfur compounds may act have been identified.[243,244] Some studies suggest that the primary chemopreventive mechanism of DAS may involve inhibition of the metabolism of certain carcinogens (e.g., nitrosamines) to more active intermediates by inactivation of specific cytochrome P450s. DAS also appears to act as an anticarcinogenic agent via induction of detoxification enzymes.[244,262]

CAROTENOIDS. Common green, yellow-red, and yellow-orange vegetables and fruits contain more than 40 carotenoids in addition to β-carotene that can be absorbed and metabolized by humans, including lutein, zeaxanthin, cryptoxanthin, lycopene, α-carotene, phytofluene, phytoene, astaxanthin, canthaxanthin, and crocetin.[263,264] As a class, carotenoids exhibit strong antioxidant activity, increase metabolic detoxification, increase cellular communication, and have anti-inflammatory properties.[263,265] Preliminary human metabolic studies on lutein and lycopene, the two major dietary carotenoids, and zeaxanthin, a dihydroxycarotenoid isomeric to lutein, have established that these compounds undergo oxidation in vivo, clearly demonstrating their antioxidant capabilities (Khachik et al, 1995).[264] Experimental data provide support for the cancer-preventive potential of carotenoids.[263]

Epidemiologic evidence also supports a carotenoid-cancer relationship. Using updated carotenoid data,[266,267] Ziegler and colleagues[268] reanalyzed results from a study of diet and cancer conducted during 1980 and 1981.[269,270] The reanalysis indicated that men in the lowest quartile of α-carotene intake had more than twice the risk of men in the highest quartile; corresponding risks associated with intakes of β-carotene and lutein-zeaxanthin increased only about 60%, suggesting that β-carotene is not the dominant protective factor in vegetables and fruit.[268] A case-control study of serum micronutrient levels (highest versus lowest tertiles) in Japanese-American men indicated that α-carotene (RR = 0.19), β-carotene (RR = 0.10), β-cryptoxanthin (RR = 0.25), and total carotenoids (RR = 0.22) all significantly reduced the risk of aerodigestive tract cancers; no association was observed for carotenoids and prostate cancer.[271] However, one prospective cohort study reported an inverse association between lycopene and prostate cancer risk (RR = 0.79).[140] Analysis of prostate tissue has determined that lycopene is present in biologically active concentrations, supporting the hypothesis that lycopene could have direct cancer-protective effects within the prostate.[272] Reduced risk of breast cancer has been associated with breast adipose concentrations of β-carotene (RR = 0.30), lycopene (RR = 0.32), lutein-zeaxanthin (RR = 0.68), and retinyl palmitate (RR = 0.61).[273]

GREEN TEA POLYPHENOLS. Epidemiologic studies of Japanese and Chinese tea drinkers have suggested that green tea consumption is associated with a reduced risk for cancers of the alimentary and digestive tracts.[274–277] For instance, a case-control study in Shanghai, China, recently reported an inverse association for green tea consumption (highest tertile versus lowest tertile) and cancer risk in the colon (men, RR = 0.82; women, RR = 0.67), rectum (men, RR = 0.72; women, RR = 0.57), and pancreas (men, RR = 0.63; women, RR = 0.53). The trends were statistically significant for both rectal and pancreatic cancers.[275] The major green tea polyphenols (GTPs) include (−)-epicatechin, (−)-epigallocatechin, (−)-epicatechin-3-gallate, and (−)-epigallocatechin-3-gallate (EGCG). The primary constituent of green tea, EGCG, has been shown to markedly reduce duodenal and colon tumor incidence and number in rats.[274] Oral administration of polyphenolic compounds isolated from green tea (GTP), a water extract of green tea (WEGT), or epicatechin derivatives present in green tea consistently protected against the development of cancers of the lung, forestomach, esophagus, duodenum, colon, liver, pancreas, and mammary gland in laboratory animals; topical and oral administration similarly inhibited skin tumorigenesis in mice.[276]

Experimental data suggest that GTPs are strong inhibitors of the monooxygenases that normally metabolize carcinogens to their more reactive intermediates. Some green tea constituents also can scavenge carcinogenic electrophiles, whereas others appear to modulate enzymes associated with cell proliferation, such as protein kinase C, DNA polymerase, and RNA polymerase. Studies also have found that the addition of GTP extracts to the diets of mice induced hepatic estradiol 2-hydroxylation, which has been associated with a reduced risk for breast cancer.[244,278–280]

INDOLES AND ISOTHIOCYANATES. Indoles and isothiocyanates, derived from the hydrolysis of glucosinolates, are present in cruciferous vegetables (e.g., broccoli, cauliflower, cabbage, brussels sprouts, turnips, kale).[243] Epidemiologic studies consistently demonstrate a strong, inverse relationship between consumption of diets high in cruciferous vegetables and cancer incidence,[97,101,281] a finding supported by animal studies.[282–284] Consumption or administration of cruciferous vegetables, indoles, and/or isothiocyanates increases the activity of phase I and phase II enzymes, consequently influencing the metabolism of carcinogens.[243,280] The mechanisms by which cruciferous vegetables exert their cancer-protective effects have been recently reviewed.[285]

One of the more extensively studied indoles, indole-3-carbinol (I3C), inhibits carcinogen-induced mammary tumors in rats and is effective in several other animal models,[244,280,286] but some evidence of tumor enhancement also has been reported.[286] Evidence suggests that I3C may protect against breast cancer by modulation of cytochrome P450-dependent estradiol metabolism, causing a shift from the C-16α hydroxylation pathway (which promotes estrogen activity) to the C-2 hydroxylation pathway (which decreases estrogen activity).[243,280]

When administered prior to the carcinogen, isothiocyanates have been shown to inhibit a variety of chemically induced tumors, including tumors of the lung, esophagus, colon, mammary gland, liver, and forestomach, in animals.[241,244] These compounds most likely exert their effect by blocking the metabolism of carcinogens through the inactivation of selective P450 enzymes.[244] Isothiocyanates also have been shown to increase the activity of phase II enzymes and increase tissue glutathione levels.[241,244] Two promising isothiocyanates present in cruciferous vegetables include phenethyl isothiocyanate (PEITC),[287] and sulforaphane.[247,288] A recent study reported that 3-day-old broccoli sprouts contained 10 to 100 times the amount of the glucosinolate of sulforaphane as mature plants, and that sprout extracts were highly effective in reducing the development of rat mammary tumors.[289]

## ALCOHOL

Epidemiologic data support a direct association of alcohol intake with aerodigestive cancers—cancers of the oral cavity, pharynx, esophagus, and larnyx—where alcohol acts synergistically with smoking to increase risk.[3,290–292] Increased risks for breast, colorectal, prostate, liver, and pancreatic cancers also have been linked to alcohol intake.[3,291–296] However, both the exact measure of the influence of alcohol consumption on cancer risk and the mechanism(s) by which alcohol exerts its observed effects are still unknown. Also, data across studies is not entirely consistent. Difficulties in interpretation can arise because precise figures for alcohol consumption by

individuals can be difficult to obtain. Also, increases in relative risks are small, calling into question their reliability; small changes in risk might be accounted for by bias.[297] Further, the role of confounding factors, particularly smoking, as well as the numerous chemicals other than alcohol in alcoholic beverages, may not be clear.[291] Investigations of effect modification by factors such as age, menopausal status, body size, exogenous estrogen usage, and family history have been conducted, but results are mixed; effect modifications warrant further study.[297] Differences in genetic susceptibilities of individuals and populations likely also contribute to the difficulty of establishing a clear alcohol–cancer relationship. Heritable differences for the ability to metabolize carcinogens, DNA repair capability, genomic instability, and altered expression of proto-oncogenes and tumor suppressor genes are all factors that contribute to determining the risk of carcinogenesis.[298]

AERODIGESTIVE CANCER. Along with tobacco use, micronutrient deficiencies, and consumption of pickled vegetables, salted fish, and very hot beverages, excessive consumption of alcoholic beverages is considered to be an important risk factor for aerodigestive cancers.[290] A comprehensive review concluded that the results from epidemiologic studies consistently support the carcinogenicity of alcoholic beverages at the oral cavity, pharynx, larynx, and esophagus; further, a dose-response relationship is observed in most studies.[290] For example, in a case-control study for esophageal cancer in lifelong nonsmokers, risk increased with daily consumption of four to eight drinks (RR = 2.7) and eight or more drinks (RR = 5.4), compared with consumption of fewer than four drinks (RR = 1.0).[299] Although risk associated with specific types of alcoholic beverages differs across studies, the association with total alcohol consumption has been consistent.[290] Numerous reports indicate that alcohol consumption and tobacco use have a multiplicative effect on aerodigestive cancers.[3,290,291,300] To illustrate, smoking combined with alcohol consumption increased the risk of oral cancer in Japanese men to three times that of smoking only (OR = 6.2 versus 2.2).[301]

BREAST CANCER. Results across epidemiologic studies indicate that breast cancer risk increases with total alcohol intake, regardless of whether the beverage is beer, wine, on spirits.[293] One meta-analysis of 28 case-control studies and 10 cohort studies reported an estimated 11% increase in risk for daily alcohol intake equivalent to 1 drink; results supported a dose-response relationship.[293] In the Netherlands Cohort Study, conducted in more than 62,000 postmenopausal women, elevated risk (RR = 1.72) was found among women who consumed at least 30 g (two to three drinks) of alcohol daily.[302] A case-control study in Switzerland that included both premenopausal and postmenopausal women reported a significant dose-response relationship with an OR of 2.7 for daily consumption of more than four drinks, compared with abstainers.[303] Alcohol-related risk appeared to be higher in premenopausal women (OR = 5.4, ≥ 1 drinks per day) than in postmenopausal women (OR = 1.3, ≥ 1 drinks per day), but no noticeable interaction was observed with any hormonal or reproductive factors.[303] Two population-based, case-control studies, one in postmenopausal women[304] and one in women under 45 years of age (1474 premenopausal, 171 postmenopausal),[305] investigated the timing of alcohol consumption as it relates to breast cancer risk. For postmenopausal women, no clear differences in risk associated with alcohol consumption at age 25 years, age 40 years, and in the recent past were observed. Data indicated a significant dose-response relationship for increased risk with an OR = 1.63 for daily consumption of 19 to 32 g alcohol (about 2 to 2.5 drinks), compared with abstainers.[304] For women under 45 years of age, data suggested that breast cancer risk was not influenced by alcohol consumption during the teenage years or early adulthood, but average intake during the most recent 5-year interval was associated with increased risk (RR = 1.7) for women who consumed 14 or more drinks per week.[305] Consumed at this level, alcohol had a greater effect on women with advanced regional or distant disease (RR = 2.4), suggesting that alcohol possibly acts as a tumor promotor or growth enhancer.[305]

Findings that indicate moderate alcohol intake influences estrogen metabolism support the suggestion that increased bioavailability of estrogens is a possible mechanism for a breast cancer–alcohol link.[306–309] In a long-term, randomized, crossover study investigating the effects of alcohol consumption on estrogen levels in premenopausal women, daily consumption of 30 g of alcohol was associated with increased levels of plasma estrone, plasma estradiol, and urinary estradiol in the periovulatory phase of the menstrual cycle.[309] Overall, data on the relationship between alcohol consumption and levels of female sex hormones have been inconsistent.[194] A recent investigation reported a threefold increase in circulating estradiol in postmenopausal women on estrogen replacement therapy (ERT) with moderate alcohol consumption, but no significant change in control women.[307] Data from the Iowa Women's Health Study, which classified breast cancer cases according to the presence of estrogen receptor (ER) and progesterone receptor (PR) status, showed that the combination of alcohol consumption (≥ 4 g/day) and ERT use (ever used) may be more strongly associated with ER−/PR− breast cancer (RR = 2.6) than with ER+/PR+ breast cancer (RR = 1.8) or ER+/PR− breast cancer (RR = 1.3), compared with abstainers who never used ERT.[61,62,310] Such findings suggest that interactions between alcohol and other risk factors may vary by ER/PR status and may contribute to the difficulty of defining the possibly complex etiologic role of alcohol on breast carcinogenesis.[61,62,310]

ENDOMETRIAL CANCER. It has been well established that a hyperestrogenic state is directly related to risk for endometrial cancer.[194,311] However, data linking alcohol consumption, which may influence bioavailability of estrogens, to endometrial cancer risk are not definitive. A review of six case-control studies of alcohol and endometrial cancer, as well as follow-up data from the Iowa Women's Health Study, concluded that, although inconsistent, data generally indicate either no association or a weak protective effect.[194] A more recent population-based, case-control study in Wisconsin women reported that, compared with abstainers, women consuming two or more drinks daily had a higher risk of endometrial cancer (RR = 1.27).[312] In women consuming one or more drinks daily, risks of endometrial cancer were greater for women over 55 years of age (RR = 1.07) versus women 55 years of age or less (RR = 0.58); postmenopausal women (RR = 1.05) versus premenopausal women (RR = 0.20); women in the highest tertile of body weight (RR = 1.27) versus women in the lowest tertile (RR = 0.92); and women currently using hormone replacement (RR = 1.56) versus women who had never used hormone replacement (RR = 0.70). It is possible

that inconsistent findings in previous studies may be the result, in part, of differences in study subjects in one or more of these factors, yielding subgroups at relatively higher or lower risk for endometrial cancer.[312]

PROSTATE CANCER. Although data from most studies do not support a significant link between alcohol consumption and prostate cancer,[292] several studies have reported positive results. One study in Utah reported an increased risk associated with total alcohol consumption among men 67 years of age and less (RR = 1.65) and with wine consumption among men older than 67 years (RR = 1.57); all men had aggressive tumors.[313] A case-control study in Uruguay found an increased risk of prostate cancer for men who drank more than 61 mL of beer daily (RR = 3.2), but no significant increases were observed for wine, hard liquor, or total alcohol consumption.[314] However, in a Swedish case-control study, current use of beer or wine was not associated with increased risk, whereas current drinkers of hard liquor showed increased risk (OR = 1.4).[315] Data from the Swedish study indicated a significant trend for years of alcohol use and prostate cancer risk, but not for total alcohol consumption. A recent report of the first large, population-based, case-control study in U.S. blacks and whites that focused specifically on alcohol use reported that, compared with never-users, prostate cancer risk increased with the amount of alcohol consumed (trend significant), with significantly elevated risks for men who consumed 22 to 56 drinks per week (OR = 1.4) and 57 or more drinks per week (OR = 1.9).[296] This finding was consistent for blacks and whites, for young and old subjects, and for different types of alcoholic beverages and was not affected by adjustment for possible confounders such as tobacco use, family history of prostate cancer, or other dietary factors. Mechanisms by which alcohol might influence prostate cancer risk are unclear.

COLORECTAL CANCER. Numerous epidemiologic studies have investigated a potential association between alcohol consumption and the risk of colorectal cancer.[54,294,316,317] Data have not been consistent, and the magnitude of reported associations between alcohol consumption and risk of colorectal cancer is generally small. A meta-analysis of 27 case-control and follow-up studies found a small increase in risk (RR = 1.10) for consumption of two drinks daily (approximately 24 g of alcohol) that did not vary according to gender or site within the large bowel.[317] However, results from follow-up studies (RR = 1.32) suggested a stronger relationship than those from case-control studies (RR = 1.07). A more recent qualitative review reported that of the 20 general-population studies that examined alcohol consumption and colon cancer, 12 reported a positive association. Of the 19 studies that examined alcohol consumption and rectal cancer, 12 reported a positive association; beer appeared to be directly related to rectal cancer in men more often than in women.[54] The author noted that inconsistencies in findings may be a result of several factors, including a small number of cases in some studies, as well as differences in control groups, methods of assessing consumption, and preferred beverages across countries and between men and women.[54]

Some studies suggest that the effects of alcohol on colorectal cancer risk may depend on intake levels of other nutrients. Analysis of data from the Health Professionals Followup Study showed that, overall, men who drank more than two drinks daily—about 20 to 30 g alcohol—were at higher risk of developing colon cancer (RR = 2.07) than men who drank less than one-quarter of a drink daily. However, men in the highest quintiles of methionine and folate intakes who consumed more than 20 g alcohol daily were not at increased risk (RR = 0.79, RR = 1.03, respectively). In contrast, inadequate intake of folate and methionine significantly increased alcohol-associated risk for total colon cancer (RR = 3.30), proximal colon cancer (RR = 2.70), and distal colon cancer (RR = 7.44), even after adjustment for age, history of polyps or endoscopy, smoking, level of physical activity, BMI, intakes of red meat and total energy, and multivitamin use.[318] In the ATBC study, colorectal cancer risk increased with ethanol consumption (RR = 2.7, >27.7 g ethanol daily) among men who did not receive β-carotene, whereas men who received 20 mg β-carotene daily showed no increase in risk (based on data after 3 years of follow-up). These data suggest that β-carotene supplementation may have attenuated the effects of alcohol on colorectal cancer risk in this cohort.[319]

## DIETARY CARCINOGENS

The human diet is a highly complex and variable mixture of naturally occurring and synthetic chemicals, including chemicals that have been identified as carcinogens.[33] Although synthetic chemicals such as food additives, pesticides, and other environmental contaminants have been accorded greater research and public attention, these chemicals are estimated to represent less than 1% of the carcinogens found in foods.[320,321] Most dietary carcinogens can be categorized as natural pesticides and toxins produced by plants for protection against fungi, insects, and animal predators; mycotoxins are secondary metabolites produced by molds in foods; or substances produced during food preparation, such as HAAs, PAHs, and N-nitroso compounds (NOCs).[320,322] Food sources of some selected dietary carcinogens are presented in Table 1B-9.

Evaluation of the risk posed by dietary carcinogens requires knowledge of human exposure as well as information on carcinogenic potency. The limitations of current dietary assessment methods and the lack of concentration data for many potentially carcinogenic constituents of foods make reliable exposure estimates difficult.[33] Biomarkers of exposure such as carcinogen-DNA adducts and carcinogen metabolites in blood and urine are being developed that should increase the reliability of exposure estimates.[323] One common mechanism of most carcinogens, including naturally occurring dietary carcinogens, is the formation of adducts with cellular macromolecules such as DNA. Some compounds are intrinsically reactive toward DNA, whereas others require metabolic activation.[324] DNA-carcinogen adducts have been used as measurable end points in laboratory studies to assess carcinogen exposure, carcinogen metabolism, mutagenesis, and tumorigenesis.[323,325]

Determination of potential carcinogenicity is based on information obtained from epidemiologic observations, animal models, and in vitro systems. Animal carcinogenicity data have been compiled in the Carcinogenic Potency Database, a standardized resource that includes results for 1230 chemicals tested in long-term animal experiments.[326] Approximately 50% of all chemicals tested, both synthetic and naturally occurring, have been shown

to be carcinogenic in animal tests.[327] Extrapolation from the near-toxic doses used in animal tests to risk for humans consuming low doses is difficult without understanding the carcinogenic mechanisms involved and considering the level of human exposure.[322] Mitogens likely act by increasing cell proliferation, but only at near-toxic levels; thus, a threshold level generally exists, below which cell proliferation does not occur. For such compounds, the cancer risk for humans may be lower than that indicated by animal data.[322] In contrast, mutagens can cause DNA damage at low doses; thus, the carcinogenic risk associated with mutagens in animal testing might be highly significant for humans. Current high-dose animal testing does not provide the information required to predict with a high degree of confidence the increased human risk from low-dose exposure.[33,322,328]

NATURALLY OCCURRING DIETARY CARCINOGENS. Plant foods contain thousands of phytochemicals, naturally occurring compounds that represent various chemical classes and exhibit diverse molecular structures. Very few dietary plants or their crude extracts, in which carcinogenic constituents are typically highly diluted, have been shown to be carcinogenic; in contrast, animal studies have provided evidence for the carcinogenicity of a large number of individual plant constituents fed at high doses. Only a small fraction of the potential carcinogens produced by plant foods have been tested systematically.[321] For example, cabbage contains 49 naturally occurring pesticides—including glucosinolates, indoles, isothiocyanates, cyanides, alcohols, ketones, phenols, and tannins—but only a few, such as allyl isothiocyanate, sinigrin, and caffeic acid, have been tested for carcinogenicity.[321,328] Safrole and estragole—carcinogenic alkenylbenzenes found in herbs and spices—and their metabolites, which show greater carcinogenic potency than the parents compounds, have been reported to form DNA adducts in both in vitro and in vivo studies and to exhibit genotoxic activity as measured by unscheduled DNA synthesis.[329,330] The significance of DNA adducts in the etiology of human cancer, however, is unclear.

The difficulties in assessing the risk of naturally occurring plant-derived carcinogens are well illustrated by the case of caffeic acid. It is widely distributed in plants and causes forestomach squamous cell carcinomas in male mice and in female rats, and renal tubular cell hyperplasia and adenomas in mice. As noted by the Committee on the Comparative Toxicity of Naturally Occurring Carcinogens,[33] the relevance of these positive findings to humans is uncertain because data are not available on the carcinogenicity of caffeic acid in humans, very high doses were used in the animal studies, humans do not have a forestomach, and the renal lesions were related to toxic lesions. In vitro, caffeic acid may act either as a pro-oxidant or an antioxidant, depending upon the experimental conditions employed, and it has been observed to be both protective and enhancing when administered orally in combination with known carcinogens.[33] Many of the foods in which caffeic acid is present are also high in fiber, vitamins A, E, and C, β-carotene, and numerous other protective compounds that might significantly affect the fate of caffeic acid in the body.

Reliable data for concentrations of natural pesticides in plant foods and amounts of plant foods consumed may not be available. For example, a U.S. Food and Drug Administration study estimated

**TABLE 1B-9.** DIETARY CARCINOGENS

| COMPOUND | FOOD SOURCE |
| --- | --- |
| **NATURALLY OCCURRING** | |
| Caffeic acid | Apples, pears, plums, cherries, carrots, celery, lettuce, potatoes, endive, grapes, eggplant, thyme, basil, anise, sage, dill, caraway, rosemary, tarragon, coffee beans |
| Allyl isothiocyanate | Cabbage, cauliflower, Brussels sprouts, mustard, horseradish |
| Safrole | Nutmeg, mace, pepper, cinnamon, natural root beer |
| Estragole | Basil, fennel, tarragon |
| Carvacrol | Marjoram |
| Furocoumarins | Lime, citrus oils, carrots, celery, parsley, parsnips |
| Hydrazines | Mushrooms |
| Pyrrolizidine | Herbal teas (comfrey) |
| **MYCOTOXINS** | |
| Aflatoxins | Corn, peanuts, seed nuts, peanut butter |
| Ochratoxin A | Grains, green coffee beans |
| T-2 toxin | Barley, maize, safflower seeds, cereals |
| Zearalenone | Feed grains, soybean, maize, wheat |
| Fumonisins | Corn |
| Deoxynivalenol | Wheat, maize |
| Nivalenol | Wheat, maize, barley |
| **PRODUCED DURING FOOD PREPARATION** | |
| Urethane | All fermented and yeast-leavened foods: wines, yogurt, soy sauce, sake, ale, beer, bread |
| *Heterocyclic Aromatic Amines* | |
| 2-amino-3-methylimidazo[4,5-*f*]quinoline (IQ) | Broiled beef and salmon; fried ground beef and fish |
| 2-amino-3,8-dimethylimidazo[4,5-*f*]quinoxaline(8-MeIQx) | Barbecued chicken, fish, and pork; broiled beef, chicken, mutton, and pork; fried bacon, ground beef, and fish |
| 2-amino-3,4,8-trimethylimidazo[4,5-*f*]quinoxaline (4,8-DiMeIQx) | Barbecued chicken and pork; broiled chicken and mutton; fried bacon, ground beef, and fish; smoked mackerel |
| 2-amino-1-methyl-6-phenylimidazo[4,5β]pyridine (PhIP) | Barbecued pork and fish; broiled beef, chicken, mutton, and fish; fried bacon, fish, ground beef, and ground pork |
| 2-amino-9*H*-pyrido[2,3-*b*]indole | Barbecued fish; broiled beef, chicken, and mutton |
| *Polycyclic Aromatic Hydrocarbons* | |
| Pyrene | Charcoal-broiled/grilled steak, beef patties, chicken, frankfurters, and pork; bacon; liquid smoke; smoked fish |
| Benz(α)anthracene | Charcoal-broiled/grilled steak, beef patties, chicken, frankfurters, and pork; liquid smoke; smoked fish |
| Chrysene | Charcoal-broiled/grilled steak, beef patties, chicken, frankfurters, and pork; bacon; smoked fish |
| Benz (α)pyrene | Charcoal-broiled/grilled steak, beef patties, chicken, frankfurters, and pork; bacon; liquid smoke; smoked fish |
| *N-Nitroso Compounds* | |
| N-Nitrosomethylamine | Cured meats; fried bacon; millet flour and grain products; dairy and cheese products; pickled/fermented vegetables; beer and whiskey |
| N-Nitrosoethylamine | Cured meats, salami; millet flour and grain products |
| N-Nitrosobutylamine | Cured meats; smoked chicken; dried fish |
| N-Nitrosopyrrolidine | Cured meats; fried bacon; broiled squid; pickled vegetables; mixed spices; dried chilies |
| N-Nitrosopiperidine | Cured meats; fried bacon; peppered salami; pepper; mixed spices; pickled vegetables |

Source: Derived from Scheuplein,[320] Ames and Gold,[321] Stavric,[347] Wagstaff,[331] IARC Working Group,[332] Lijinsky,[344] Tricker and Preussmann,[376] Committee on Comparative Toxicity of Naturally Occurring Carcinogens.[33]

the U.S. per capita dietary exposure to furocoumarins—several of which are carcinogenic in animals and humans, including psoralen and bergapten—to be 1.3 mg per person per day, with lime being the major dietary source.[331] However, exposure may range from 0.13 to 13 mg per person per day, considering the variance in estimates of both furocoumarin levels and consumption data.[331] Because of the uncertainties in dietary exposure and the paucity of carcinogenicity data available for specific furocoumarins, no conclusions can be drawn about the overall effects of these compounds on human health. This statement could be made fairly for most naturally occurring dietary carcinogens.

Generally, dietary exposure to natural pesticides can be controlled by selecting genetic strains of plants that produce lower concentrations and by reducing plant stress during the growing season. Particular natural pesticides that are carcinogenic in animals might be bred out of crops if research indicates they could be hazardous to humans.[328] Increasing the level of natural pesticides by breeding as an alternative to synthetic pesticides must be considered cautiously in view of their potential health effects.

**MYCOTOXINS.** Mycotoxins elicit a wide range of toxic responses in animals and humans; some are potent animal carcinogens and appear to contribute to human cancer risk.[332] Mycotoxin contamination of crops such as peanuts, cottonseed, tree nuts, corn, wheat, barley, and other cereals is common and is influenced by temperature, harvesting practices, insect infestation, and moisture levels in the field and in storage.[332] The carcinogenic risks to humans from several mycotoxins—including aflatoxins, fumonisins, ochratoxin A, zearalenone, deoxynivalenol, nivalenol, fusarenone X, and T-2 toxin—have been reviewed and evaluated by the International Agency for Research on Cancer (IARC).[332] The evaluation concluded that aflatoxin $B_1$ and naturally occurring mixtures of aflatoxins are genotoxic and carcinogenic to humans, whereas the fumonisins and ochratoxin A are possibly carcinogenic to humans.

High levels of aflatoxins, produced by *Aspergillus* species, are found in groundnuts and maize in regions of Africa, southeast Asia, and southern China, where these foods are dietary staples. Meat, milk, and eggs from animals fed contaminated feed are additional sources of exposure to aflatoxins.[33] Contamination of corn, cottonseed, and peanuts in the United States occurs at high levels in some years but generally is much lower than in less developed countries.[332] For example, aflatoxin $B_1$ exposure in southern China can be as high as 75 to 250 µg/d, compared with 25 to 75 ng/d in the United States.[333] Epidemiologic studies show a strong direct association between aflatoxin intake in Africa and China and risk for primary liver cancer.[332,334,335]

Because assessing dietary exposure to aflatoxins has been problematic, research has focused on the development and validation of aflatoxin-DNA adducts as molecular biomarkers of exposure.[336] Aflatoxin $B_1$ requires metabolic activation of its carcinogenic form, the 8,9-epoxide, which can bind to guanine and cytosine in DNA.[323,337] A review of data from animal and human studies that measured urinary excretion of aflatoxin-DNA adducts by molecular dosimetry suggested that these adducts are useful markers of exposure.[323] In a prospective study of more than 18,000 men in Shanghai, data demonstrated a significant increase in the relative risk (3.4) for liver cancer in individuals in whom urinary aflatoxin-

DNA adducts were detected.[338] Studies also indicate synergistic interactions of aflatoxin with both viral B hepatitis and alcohol consumption in humans.[338,339]

The aflatoxin 8,9-epoxide can undergo detoxification through the actions of phase II enzymes such as the glutathione S-transferases. Oltipraz, a dithiolethione that induces phase II enzymes, has been shown to reduce aflatoxin-DNA adducts in animal models.[340] Common dietary phytochemicals may protect against aflatoxins by this mechanism. Chlorophyllin, a derivative of chlorophyll, is a potent inhibitor of aflatoxin-DNA adduct formation and hepatocarcinogenesis in trout at levels found in human foods.[341]

Elimination of exposure to aflatoxins is not possible because of the ubiquitous nature of aflatoxin-producing molds. At least 50 countries have established regulatory programs for aflatoxins.[342] Such efforts should continue, especially in less developed countries, where aflatoxins present a significant risk to human health.

**PRODUCTS OF FOOD PREPARATION AND PROCESSING.** Food preparation and preservation are major sources of dietary carcinogens, including heterocyclic aromatic amines (HAAs), formed during frying, grilling, and charring high-protein foods; polycyclic aromatic hydrocarbons (PAHs), formed during broiling and smoking food; and NOCs, formed in salting and pickling foods cured with nitrate or nitrite.[320,325,332,343,344] HAAs, PAHs, and nitrosamines are genotoxic compounds that form DNA adducts after metabolic activation.[324,345] In a study of aromatic-DNA adducts in human breast tissue, the aromatic adduct level for breast cancer cases was 2.5-fold higher than for controls (6.1 versus 2.3 nucleotides per 108),[346] suggesting that aromatic compounds, such as HAAs and PAHs, may play a role in breast cancer etiology. Also, other data on adducts suggest that cooking-induced carcinogens in meat may contribute to colorectal cancer risk.[53,323]

*HETEROCYCLIC AROMATIC AMINES.* HAAs have generated considerable research interest and are the focus of several comprehensive reviews.[332,343,347,348] These compounds are potent mutagens and animal carcinogens, causing cancers of the liver, colon, mammary gland, skin, and Zymbal gland in rodent models.[343,349–351] Of greatest concern is the class of HAAs known as aminoimidazoazaarenes. An evaluation of four of these—2-amino-3-methylimidazo[4,5-$f$]quinoline (IQ); 2-amino-3,4-dimethylimidazo[4,5-$f$]quinoline (MeIQ); 2-amino-3,8-dimethylimidazo[4,5-$f$]quinoxaline (8-MeIQx); and 2-amino-1-methyl-6-phenylimidazo[4,5β]pyridine (PhIP)—concluded that IQ is probably, and MeIQ, 8-MeIQx, and PhIP are possibly, carcinogenic to humans.[332] Cooking methods such as pan frying, broiling, and grilling, which result in high food surface temperatures, are most likely to produce HAAs,[352–354] in contrast with stewing, steaming, poaching, and microwaving.[354,355] PhIP and 8-MeIQx are the most prevalent HAAs identified in cooked meats.[347,354]

Animal studies have demonstrated the formation of HAA-DNA adducts in numerous tissues, including liver, colon, mammary gland, spleen, small intestine, stomach, kidney, pancreas, heart, lung, and brain,[356–360] and the ability of PhIP and IQ to induce aberrant crypt foci in mice.[361] The metabolic activation of HAAs in humans is hypothesized to occur via N-oxidation to form N-hydroxy metabolites followed by O-acetylation to form N-acetoxy arylamines that bind to DNA. These steps are catalyzed by cytochrome P450A2 and acetyltransferase-2, respectively.[362] The polymorphism of these enzymes in humans has been investigated for potential relevance to colorectal cancer risk.[362,363] Individuals who were both rapid *N*-oxidizers and rapid acetylators had nearly three times the risk of developing colorectal cancer as individuals who were both slow *N*-oxidizers and slow acetylators. Consumption of well-done red meat also was associated with increased risk. "Rapid-rapid" individuals with a preference for well-done meat had a 6.45-fold greater risk of developing colorectal cancer than "slow-slow" individuals who preferred rare or medium meat.[362] Conflicting results have been obtained in other similar studies, however.[351]

Urinary excretion of cooking-associated HAAs and their metabolites is being investigated as a biomarker of exposure to HAAs in humans.[323] In one study, consumption of pan-fried fish, beef, or bacon resulted in a measurable excretion of MeIQx and its metabolites[364] and confirmed earlier data on the interindividual variability of urinary excretion.[365] A comparison of urinary excretion of MeIQx by black, white, and Asian men found that blacks, who excreted the most MeIQx, also consumed the greatest combined amount of bacon, pork or ham, and sausage or luncheon meats.[366]

Other dietary components might influence the bioavailability and biologic effects of HAAs. Animal studies indicate that dietary fat increases the carcinogenicity of HAAs.[367,368] Feeding PhIP resulted in more aberrant crypts in the lower intestine of male rats on a high-fat versus low-fat diet, and increased dietary calcium reduced aberrant crypt formation at both dietary fat levels.[368] Wheat bran has the potential to bind MeIQx in the large intestine and protect against mucosal damage.[369] Inhibitory effects on the initiation of hepatocarcinogenesis in rats by IQ were found for β-carotene, α-tocopherol, glutathione, vanillin, quercetin, and diallyl sulfide, all naturally occurring dietary antioxidants.[370]

The potential carcinogenic risk to humans from dietary HAAs has been estimated in several studies, with increased risk ranging from $1 \times 10^{-4}$ to $1 \times 10^{-3}$.[348,350,354,355] A recent U.S. estimate is based on a comprehensive database of reported levels of HAAs in foods, dietary intakes of foods containing HAAs from nationwide surveys, and cancer potencies derived from the results of animal bioassays.[354] The estimated upper-bound cancer risk is $1.1 \times 10^{-4}$, which corresponds to 28,000 cancers in the U.S. population, with PhIP accounting for 46% of the risk, followed by MeIQx (27%), 2-amino-3,4,8-trimethylimidazo[4,5-*f*]quinoxaline (4,8-DiMeIQx) (15%), IQ (7%), and 2-amino-9*H*-pyrido[2,3-*b*]indole (6%).[354] A recent case-control study reported an increased breast cancer risk for women in the highest quartiles of exposure for IQ (OR = 3.34), MeIQx (OR = 2.13), and PhIP (OR = 2.59).[371] In view of the possible role of HAAs in human cancer development, minimizing exposures to HAAs by prudent selection of lower-temperature cooking techniques for meat and by avoiding overcooking may be advisable.

*POLYCYCLIC AROMATIC HYDROCARBONS.* The primary source of PAHs is the incomplete combustion of fossil fuels.[345] Several PAHs found to be carcinogenic in animals when administered orally have been detected as contaminants in both animal and human foods.[344,372] PAHs also form when cooking meats over an open flame. Fat dripping onto the coals and the subsequent deposition of PAHs that rise with the smoke onto the meat contribute significantly

to PAH exposure.[344] Benzo(*a*)pyrene, the most carcinogenic PAH, has been reported at levels up to 50 μg/kg in charcoal-broiled steaks and ground beef, five times greater than benzo(*a*)pyrene levels in some less fatty pork cuts and chicken.[344]

Several studies have demonstrated a consistent association between recent consumption of charbroiled foods and increased PAH-DNA adduct concentrations in peripheral white blood cells.[323,373,374] Dietary PAHs from grilled beef may dose-dependently elevate both PAH-DNA adducts in white blood cells and excretion of 1-hydroxy-pyrene in urine, indicating substantial bioactivation of dietary PAHs.

Available exposure and carcinogenicity data are insufficient to allow a reliable estimate of the contribution of dietary PAHs to carcinogenic risk for humans.[344] However, it is prudent to reduce exposures to PAHs by modifying food preparation techniques. Oven cooking, cooking with a heat source above the meat, separation of meat from smoke while cooking, and microwaving all result in food containing minimal amounts of PAHs.[344]

*N-NITROSO COMPOUNDS.* Smoked, salted, and pickled meats and fish, as well as salted or pickled vegetables, are dietary sources of NOCs. For example, nitrates added to meats and fish to retard spoilage can combine with amines and amides to form nitrosodimethylamine.[325] NOCs also can be formed endogenously at various sites, such as the oral cavity and the stomach, from nitrites and amines present in the diet.[375]

NOCs administered orally in animals, including nonhuman primates, consistently elicit carcinogenic responses.[376,377] The genotoxicity of NOCs, coupled with the strength of animal study data, suggest that NOCs may be a significant etiologic risk factor for human cancer.[378] Epidemiologic studies have demonstrated a direct correlation between exposure to both exogenous and endogenous nitrosamines and cancers of the stomach, esophagus, nasopharynx, urinary bladder, and liver.[325,332,376] In a recent case-control study, consumption of foods high in nitrosodimethylamine was associated with a 79% increased risk of upper aerodigestive tract cancer.[325] A comprehensive review and evaluation of available evidence concluded that Chinese-style salted fish is carcinogenic to humans and may contribute to nasopharyngeal carcinoma in southern China.[332]

The formation of endogenous NOCs may be inhibited by naturally occurring compounds in foods. Such inhibition, which has been observed for ascorbic acid, tocopherols, retinoids, phenolic compounds, and sulfhydryl compounds, as well as tea, orange peel, and certain fruit and vegetable juices,[325,379–381] may contribute to the generally protective effect of vegetables and fruits on carcinogenic risk that is consistently observed in epidemiologic studies.[97,101,281]

## CHEMOPREVENTION RESEARCH

Chemoprevention research assesses the potential of specific chemical substances, many occurring naturally in foods, to prevent cancer initiation and to either slow down or reverse the progression of premalignant lesions to invasive cancer. The concept of using chemopreventive agents to reduce cancer risk is firmly based on epidemiologic and experimental evidence from the last two decades that indicates specific compounds may influence carcinogenesis at various sites, including the oral cavity, esophagus, stomach, colon/rectum, lung,

**TABLE 1B-10.** IN VITRO SCREENS

| CELL SUBSTRATE | CARCINOGEN | PROMOTER | END POINT: INHIBITION OF |
|---|---|---|---|
| Human lung tumor cells (A427) | None | None | Anchorage independent growth inhibition |
| Mouse epidermal cells (JB6) | None | TPA | Anchorage independent growth inhibition |
| Rat tracheal epithelial (RTE) cells | B(a)P | None | Transformed foci or colonies |
| Mouse mammary organ culture (MMOC) | DMBA | TPA | Hyperplastic alveolar nodules |
| Human epidermal keratinocytes | None | TPA | Metabolic cooperation enhancement |
| Primary human (foreskin) cells | Propane sultone | None | Calcium tolerance inhibition |

ABBREVIATIONS: B(a)P = benzo(a)pyrene; DMBA = 7,12-dimethylbenz(a)anthracene; TPA = 12-O-tetradecanoylphorbol-13-acetate.
SOURCE: The Chemoprevention Investigational Studies Unit, Division of Cancer Prevention, National Cancer Institute.

breast, and prostate.[382] Individuals at high risk for specific cancers, as determined by detection of genetic mutations, currently have limited options to reduce that risk. For such individuals, a chemopreventive strategy could potentially either prevent further DNA damage that might enhance carcinogenesis or suppress the appearance of the cancer phenotype.[62,63,383]

Chemoprevention research is necessarily linked to diet and cancer research and represents a logical research progression. Dietary epidemiologic studies have provided initial leads for the identification of numerous naturally occurring candidate chemopreventive agents,[97,101,204,281] and laboratory studies have identified many potential agents that suppress carcinogenesis in animal models.[384] Since the inception of the National Cancer Institute's (NCI) chemoprevention program in 1987, more than 400 agents have been entered, and of these, more than 250 have been tested in animal screens. Promising chemopreventive agents being investigated include micronutrients (e.g., vitamins A, C, and E, β-carotene, molybdenum, calcium); phytochemicals (e.g., indoles, polyphenols, isothiocyanates, flavonoids, monoterpenes, organosulfides); and synthetics (e.g., vitamin A derivatives, piroxicam, tamoxifen, 2-difluoromethylornithine [DFMO], oltipraz).[385]

### PRECLINICAL AND EARLY-PHASE CLINICAL TESTING.
Preclinical development for chemopreventive agents includes initial assessment of compound efficacy using in vitro cell screening systems (Table 1B-10). Agents with chemopreventive effect in these preliminary tests are then nominated for one or more site-specific, whole-animal in vivo assays (Table 1B-11). Based on the results, compounds are then prioritized for extended efficacy, preclinical toxicity, and clinical testing. Agents found to have high efficacy and low toxicity at this phase of development are assigned high priority for clinical evaluation.[386] Clinical development plans have been established by the NCI for a number of naturally occurring constituents in foods, including curcumin, genistein, indole-3-carbinol, 1-perillyl alcohol, PEITC, 1-selenomethionine, GTP, 18β-glycyrrhetinic acid, calcium, β-carotene and other carotenoids, vitamin A, vitamin E, and vitamin D$_3$ (and its analogues).

Phase I clinical trials, which generally use a limited number of healthy human subjects, are designed to determine the dose-related safety and toxicity of the proposed chemopreventive agent. The dose and schedule of administration are based on achieving plasma levels in humans that are likely to be safe and to show effectiveness based on the preclinical toxicology and efficacy data from animal

**TABLE 1B-11.** IN VIVO CHEMOPREVENTION SCREENING SYSTEMS (ANIMAL MODELS)

| ORGAN MODEL | SPECIES | CARCINOGEN | END POINT: INHIBITION OF |
|---|---|---|---|
| Lung | Hamster | DEN | Adenocarcinoma |
| Trachea | Hamster | MNU | Squamous cell carcinoma |
| Colon | Mouse | MAM | Adenocarcinoma |
| | Rat | AOM | Adenocarcinoma |
| | Rat | AOM | Foci of Aberrant Crypts |
| | Rat | PhIP | Adenocarcinoma |
| Mammary | Mouse (transgenic) | None | Adenocarcinoma |
| | Rat | MNU | Adenocarcinoma |
| | Rat | DMBA | Adenocarcinoma |
| Bladder | Mouse | OH-BBN | Transitional cell carcinoma |
| Skin | Mouse | DMBA/TPA | Papilloma/ carcinoma |
| Pancreas | Hamster | BOP | Adenocarcinoma, Carcinoma |
| Prostate | Rat | MNU/ Testosterone | Carcinoma |
| Lymphatic | Mouse (transgenic) | None | Lymphoma |

ABBREVIATIONS: AOM = azoxymethane; BOP = N-nitrosobis (2-oxopropyl)amine; DEN = N,N-diethylnitrosamine; DMBA = 7,12-dimethylbenz(a)anthracene; MAM = methylazoxymethanol; MNU = N-methyl-N'-nitrosourea; OH-BBN = N-butyl-N-(4-hydroxybutyl) nitrosamine; PhIP = 2-amino-1-methyl-6-phenylimidazo[4,5-f]pyridine; TPA = 12-O-tetradecanoylphorbol-13-acetate.
SOURCE: The Chemoprevention Investigational Studies Unit, Division of Cancer Prevention, National Cancer Institute.

and in vitro screening assays. Pharmacokinetics also are assessed, including parameters of absorption, distribution, metabolism, and excretion.[387]

Phase II clinical trials evaluate agent efficacy in a larger group of subjects at high risk for specific cancers. They also provide data that characterize dose, safety, and toxicity in the selected population. Two important objectives of phase II trials include identifying biochemical, genetic, cellular, or tissue biomarkers of cancer that can be used to estimate the potential for neoplastic progression; and determining whether the chemopreventive agent being tested can affect the modulation of that biomarker. Biomarkers are described in more detail below. Agents found to have high efficacy and low toxicity in Phase II clinical trials are investigated further in large-scale Phase III intervention trials conducted with a large number of subjects over an extended period. The NCI currently is sponsoring more than 80 Phase II and Phase III trials that are directed at 12 major cancer targets, including colon, prostate, breast, lung, bladder, cervix, head and neck, esophagus, skin, liver, and multiple myeloma.

## BIOMARKERS

*RISK/INTERMEDIATE BIOMARKERS.* The validation of biomarkers that can detect early, specific changes correlated significantly to carcinogenesis reversal or progression is crucial for progress in cancer prevention. Used as predictors of cancer, these biomarkers can help identify individuals at high risk for cancer who could serve as target populations for intervention trials. Such biomarkers include carcinogen exposure biomarkers (e.g., urinary mutagens, carcinogen-DNA adducts) and genetic predisposition (e.g., mutations in APC, BRCA1, BRCA2, MLH1, MLH2; Li-Fraumeni syndrome; ataxia telangiectasia; xeroderma pigmentosum; mutagen sensitivity; genetic polymorphisms in carcinogen metabolizing enzymes).[385] As surrogate end points, biomarkers that can be modulated have the potential for assessing the efficacy of preventive interventions, including both dietary and chemopreventive interventions, with a cost-effectiveness and relative speed not possible when cancer incidence is used as the end point. Besides improving trial efficiency, biomarkers are essential to applied prevention research because of their unique potential to provide insights into mechanisms of action as well as sound rationales for the design of large-scale trials.[386,388]

Despite the identification and investigation of numerous potential biomarkers, no intermediate end point has yet been validated as an accurate predictor of future cancer incidence. Several factors are considered when evaluating the potential of an intermediate biomarker to serve as an end point in clinical prevention studies. The biomarker must be expressed differently in normal and high-risk tissue, with clear evidence of progression from normal tissue to premalignant state to cancer. The intermediate biomarker should be on the causal pathway for carcinogenesis or closely associated with the pathway and, ideally, should appear early in carcinogenesis, providing a greater chance for achieving successful preventive intervention, with a consequent reduction in cancer risk. Acceptable intermediate biomarkers must be highly sensitive, specific, and reproducible, and they must be modulatable by the preventive intervention being evaluated. Further, the validation of biomarkers as end points in prevention research requires correlation of their

modulation to a decreased rate of a related cancer.[386,388] It is possible that batteries of biomarker measurements, especially those that represent the diverse pathways possible in carcinogenesis, may be more useful than single biomarkers in characterizing high-risk groups and in defining modulatable risks.[385] Examples of intermediate biomarkers include intraepithelial neoplasia, hyperproliferation, genomic instability, oncogene overexpression and tumor suppressor loss, growth factor and growth factor receptor overexpression, differentiation biomarkers (e.g., G-actin, cytokeratins), and biochemical changes (e.g., prostate-specific antigen levels).[385] NCI-sponsored phase II clinical trials are currently testing chemopreventive agents using a variety of dysplasia-based histologic biomarkers, including prostatic intraepithelial neoplasia (PIN), cervical intraepithelial neoplasia (CIN), ductal carcinoma in situ (DCIS), dysplastic oral leukoplakia, colorectal adenomas, bronchial dysplastic metaplasia, and actinic keratosis.

*BIOMARKERS OF DIETARY INTAKE.* Biomarkers that reflect specific dietary changes can be used to monitor compliance in dietary intervention studies. They also can be used to compare and/or validate various dietary assessment approaches that are used to estimate the same dietary factor. Certain dietary biomarkers have a well-defined quantitative relationship with intake. For example, 24-hour urinary nitrogen excretion represents about 80% of the total daily nitrogen ingested as protein.[389] Also, measurement of energy expenditure with the double-labeled water method is identical to total daily energy intake, assuming that individuals are in energy balance.[390] Many biomarkers of dietary intake currently in use, however, are based on blood or tissue concentrations of food constituents such as fatty acids and vitamins, and their quantitative relationship with daily intake may vary among individuals and populations.[389] Even so, biomarkers data can complement dietary intake and increase confidence in intake estimated by other dietary assessment methods. To illustrate, a study of the correlation of n-3 fatty acids in plasma phospholipids with consumption estimated by a 180-item quantitative food frequency questionnaire (FFQ) reported correlation coefficients of 0.51 and 0.49 for eicosapentaenoic acid (EPA) and docosahexaenoic acid (DHA), respectively. Also, the FFQ and plasma phospholipid concentrations classified individuals into the same quartiles in 39% of cases, with others generally classified in adjacent quartiles.[391] Another study in men with prostate cancer found correlations between fish consumption reported by FFQ and EPA composition in erythrocyte membranes and adipose tissue of 0.44 and 0.38, respectively. Results were similar for DHA.[392] The presence of prostate cancer did not significantly affect the correlations; however, correlations were lower in blacks (EPA: 0.28, 0.15) than in whites (EPA: 0.50, 0.49). Identification and evaluation of the use of biomarkers of dietary intake for both validation and interpretation of dietary assessments is an important research priority in nutrition-related carcinogenesis.

**LARGE-SCALE CLINICAL INTERVENTION TRIALS.** Randomized, large-scale phase III clinical intervention trials are considered the best means available to determine whether dietary and chemopreventive interventions reduce cancer risk; these trials are a logical conclusion in the stepwise, scientific approach to cancer prevention research. Usually involving thousands of subjects, these trials can take many years to complete; they include interventions in both high-risk populations and the general population. Although phase III trials are conducted primarily to determine the efficacy of the intervention, efforts to validate potential biomarkers as surrogate end points for cancer also can be integrated into the trial design. Selected ongoing, completed, and closed NCI-sponsored large-scale intervention trials are described briefly below.

## DIETARY MODIFICATION TRIALS

***Polyp Prevention Trial (PPT).*** The PPT was a multicenter, randomized, controlled dietary intervention trial that examined the effect of a low-fat (20% of calories from fat), high-fiber (18g/1000 cal), high-vegetable and high-fruit (five to eight daily servings, combined) dietary pattern on the recurrence of adenomatous polyps of the large bowel.[393,394] Because such polyps are precursors of most colorectal cancers, an intervention that reduces polyp occurrence has a strong probability of reducing cancer incidence. Men and women aged 35 years and older were eligible to participate in PPT if they had one or more adenomatous polyps removed within 6 months of randomization and no history of colorectal cancer, inflammatory bowel disease, or large bowel resection. Between June 1991 and January 1994, 1037 individuals were randomized to the intervention and 1042 to the control group. Participants received extensive dietary and behavioral counseling on how to meet their dietary goals. Controls were expected to continue their customary dietary intake. Results of the PPT were reported in 2000 and showed that diet did not affect the growth of precancerous colorectal polyps.[170] However, follow-up studies of participants will increase our understanding of nutritional factors that may influence critical molecular, cellular or tissue-level events in colorectal cancer formation.

***Women's Health Initiative (WHI).*** The WHI, which began in the fall of 1993, is a 10-year, multidisciplinary trial that includes both dietary and chemopreventive interventions. This trial is examining the effects of (1) a low-fat eating pattern (20% of calories from fat) that is high in vegetables, fruits, and fiber; (2) hormone replacement therapy; and (3) calcium and vitamin D supplementation on the prevention of cancer, cardiovascular disease, and osteoporosis in about 63,000 postmenopausal women of all races and socioeconomic strata. In addition to the randomized clinical trial, the WHI includes prospective surveillance of another 100,000 women for etiologic factors and predictors of future illnesses. Also, community-based intervention studies will seek effective ways to promote behaviors aimed at preventing cancer, cardiovascular disease, and osteoporosis.[395]

## CHEMOPREVENTION TRIALS

***Linxian Trials.*** The Linxian trials, conducted by the NCI in collaboration with the Chinese Institute of the Chinese Academy of Medical Sciences, were two randomized, double-blind chemoprevention trials to determine whether daily ingestion of vitamin-mineral supplements would reduce incidence and mortality rates for esophageal cancer in a high-risk population in Linxian, China, where approximately 20% of all deaths result from esophageal cancer. Begun in 1986, the general population trial randomized more

than 30,000 individuals, who received one of four combinations of supplements each day for 5 years, at doses equivalent to 1 to 2 times the U.S. Recommended Daily Allowances (RDAs). Combinations included retinol and zinc; riboflavin and niacin; vitamin C and molybdenum; and β-carotene, vitamin E, and selenium. The second study, the dysplasia trial, enrolled 3318 individuals with evidence of severe esophageal dysplasia; subjects were randomized to receive either a placebo or a daily supplement of 14 vitamins and 12 minerals, at 2 to 3 times the U.S. RDAs, for 6 years.

Results of the general population study indicated a significant benefit for those receiving the β-carotene–vitamin E–selenium combination—a 13% reduction in the cancer mortality rate, due largely to a 21% drop in stomach cancer mortality.[396] Also, this group experienced a 9% reduction in deaths from all causes, a 10% decrease in deaths from strokes, and a 4% decrease in deaths from esophageal cancer. The effects of the β-carotene–vitamin E–selenium combination began to appear within 1 to 2 years after the intervention began and continued throughout the study; the other three combinations did not affect cancer risk. A reduction in mortality from esophageal cancer was reported for the dysplasia trial.[397] Analysis of esophageal dysplasia data showed that supplementation had a significant beneficial effect; individuals receiving supplements were 1.2 times as likely to have no dysplasia after 30 and 72 months of intervention, compared with individuals receiving the placebo.[398] Postintervention follow-up is continuing. The results of these trials are encouraging but may not be directly applicable to western cultures, where populations tend to be well nourished and not deficient in multiple micronutrients, in contrast to the Linxian community.

***Women's Health Study.*** The Harvard Women's Health Study (WHS) is a chemoprevention trial that was designed to evaluate the risks and benefits of low-dose aspirin, β-carotene, and vitamin E in the primary prevention of cardiovascular disease and cancer in healthy postmenopausal women in the United States.[399,400] Begun in 1992, the WHS has enrolled approximately 40,000 female nurses, ages 45 and older, without a history of either disease. Participants are randomized to treatment or placebo groups for 2 years following a 3-month nonrandomized run-in phase. In response to the lack of benefit for β-carotene seen in closed trials, the WHS has now removed β-carotene supplementation from its intervention. The study will continue to evaluate aspirin and vitamin E.

***Closed β-Carotene Trials.*** This section summarizes briefly three large-scale, randomized β-carotene trials for which accrual has been closed and results reported. Long-term follow-up is continuing for these trials. The laboratory data and epidemiologic studies that linked high intakes of β-carotene–containing foods and high blood levels of β-carotene to a reduced risk of lung cancer provided strong hypotheses for the interventions used in these recently closed chemoprevention trials. Although the results were not as expected, these studies demonstrated the difficulty of isolating a single component of a healthful diet as the one beneficial element and exemplified the need for large-scale clinical trials to determine not only efficacy, but also safety.[401]

The Physicians' Health Study (PHS), a general population trial in 22,000 U.S. physicians that evaluated the effect of aspirin and β-carotene supplementation on the primary prevention of cardiovascular disease and cancer, began in 1982. The aspirin component of the PHS ended in 1987, because a benefit of aspirin on risk of first heart attack (44% reduction) was found. The treatment period for β-carotene continued until December 1995; data showed no significant evidence of benefit or harm from β-carotene for either cardiovascular disease or cancer.[402]

The Alpha-Tocopherol, Beta-Carotene Lung Cancer Prevention Study (ATBC Study), conducted in Finland, and the Beta-Carotene and Retinol Efficacy Trial (CARET) both were carried out in populations at high risk for lung cancer. The ATBC Study investigated the efficacy of vitamin E (α-tocopherol) alone, β-carotene alone, or a combination of the two compounds in preventing lung cancer among more than 29,000 male cigarette smokers ages 50 to 69, with an average treatment or follow-up of 6 years. Unexpectedly, this study showed a 16% higher incidence of lung cancer in the β-carotene group. However, 34% fewer cases of prostate cancer and 16% fewer cases of colorectal cancer were diagnosed among men who received vitamin E.[215,403] In the ATBC Study, the adverse effects of β-carotene were observed at the highest two quartiles of ethanol intake, indicating that alcohol consumption may enhance the actions of β-carotene.[403] CARET tested the efficacy of a combination of β-carotene and retinol (as retinyl palmitate) in male and female former heavy smokers and in men with extensive occupational asbestos exposure. This trial was terminated in January 1996 after 4 years of treatment, when data showed an overall 28% higher incidence of lung cancer in participants receiving the β-carotene–retinyl palmitate combination.[404] Excluding those exposed to asbestos, male current smokers in CARET showed a 39% higher incidence,[401] compared with the 16% higher incidence in the ATBC Study,[403] suggesting a possible adverse effect for supplemental retinol.

The results of these trials have led some to suggest that β-carotene should no longer be a candidate for inclusion in any future health interventions. However, before such an extreme position is taken, it is necessary to have a better understanding of the reasons for the unanticipated findings from the ATBC Study and CARET, especially considering that no increase in lung cancer incidence was observed in the 11% of men in the PHS who were current smokers.[402] Several possible explanations for the unanticipated outcomes of these β-carotene trials have been considered. The timing of the intervention may have been wrong.[404–407] The median follow-up of 6 years may have been too short, either to show any effect on carcinogenesis or to reverse or overcome lung cancer risk factors, particularly in active smokers. The continuing posttrial follow-up will help to clarify this issue.[404,405] Further, many heavy smokers and asbestos-exposed individuals may have already developed the initial stages of lung cancer prior to supplementation. Although evidence prior to the trials suggested that β-carotene may be more effective at later stages of carcinogenesis, this might not be the case, resulting in little benefit once initiation has occurred. Judging by the fact that the β-carotene effect appeared after only 2 years of supplementation, it is probable that the observed effect was related to the growth of cells that had already undergone malignant transformation.[405,407] It has been suggested that antioxidants such as β-carotene might prevent apoptosis of abnormal cells by scavenging the reactive oxygen species that ordinarily act as an agent of programmed cell death.[406]

However, inappropriate timing of the intervention does not fully explain the excess risk observed in the ATBC Study and CARET in individuals receiving supplements. Another consideration is that in combination with cigarette smoke and/or asbestos exposure, the high doses used (ATBC Study, 20 mg β-carotene; CARET, 30 mg β-carotene + 25,000 IU preformed vitamin A) may have had pro-oxidant effects rather than cancer-protective effects.[405–408] Direct oxidative attack of β-carotene by extremely reactive constituents of high-intensity cigarette smoke in the lungs of heavy smokers may induce the formation of β-carotene products that have pro-oxidant activity.[408] In asbestos workers, the inflammatory process in the asbestos-exposed lung—characterized by increased amounts of superoxide and hydrogen peroxide, both reactive oxygen species—may provide a favorable environment for the formation of pro-oxidant products of β-carotene.[408] Another possibility for the observed results is competitive inhibition by β-carotene of the antioxidant activity of other dietary carotenoids, such as α-carotene, lutein, and so on. α-Carotene, for example, has been reported to show higher potency than β-carotene in suppressing tumorigenesis in animal lung and skin models.[409]

It is noteworthy that participants with higher serum β-carotene concentrations at entry into the ATBC Study[403] and CARET[401] developed fewer lung cancers during the course of the trial, even among those who received β-carotene supplements. Baseline serum concentrations of β-carotene reflect total intake of vegetables and fruits, which contain numerous other antioxidants, as well as many naturally occurring potential anticarcinogens that may exert their effects through diverse mechanisms; the β-carotene serum levels may simply be a marker for the actual protective agents. Thus, this finding is in agreement with epidemiologic evidence linking β-carotene-containing foods and lung cancer and reaffirms the importance of including an abundance of plant foods in our diets.[403,408]

## TRENDS AND DIRECTIONS

Clearly, the scope of nutrition-related carcinogenesis is broad and incredibly complex. Thus, it follows that directions for future research in this very important area will also be wide-ranging and will continue to focus on clarifying the contributions to cancer risk of dietary patterns and of the specific macronutrients, micronutrients, and nonnutritive constituents found in foods. Within this context, however, certain research-related considerations warrant special attention in the design of studies and interpretation of their findings, if diet and cancer research is to play an optimally valuable role in future cancer prevention strategies. Identification of genetic susceptibility factors and gene-nutrient interactions and clarification of their significance; refinement and judicious use of statistical techniques such as meta-analysis; development of more reliable dietary assessment methodology; and validation of surrogate end point biomarkers for cancer are some of the areas that will benefit from focused research efforts.

Genetic susceptibility includes inheritable variations in carcinogen-metabolizing enzymes (polymorphisms); germline mutations in tumor-associated genes; and inherited differences in DNA adduct formation and DNA repair mechanisms.[410] Recognizing the genetic polymorphisms that affect the susceptibility of individuals to carcinogens will be important to correct interpretation of study data and subsequent development of logical and effective preventive approaches. For example, polymorphisms in the GST genes that encode glutathione-*S*-transferases—enzymes important in the detoxification of reactive electrophiles—could influence the cancer-preventive potential of those phytochemicals that either induce or inhibit these enzymes. Cancer researchers are beginning to develop innovative approaches to define the role of genetic susceptibility in epidemiologic studies. To illustrate, NAT2, which codes for *N*-acetyltransferase, an enzyme that catalyzes the formation of mutagenic products from HAAs formed in cooked meats and fish, is a gene that is known to be polymorphic and that has been studied epidemiologically for various cancer sites.[410] The NAT2 polymorphism classifies individuals into fast and slow acetylators. In contrast to earlier studies in which findings suggested that fast acetylators have a greater risk for colorectal cancer than slow acetylators,[410,411] a recent case-control study found that acetylator status alone did not increase colorectal cancer risk.[412] However, fast acetylators were at greater risk from frequent meat consumption (particularly fried), and slow acetylators appeared to be at greater risk from high alcohol consumption and smoking cigarettes.[412] This type of study, which identifies susceptible subpopulations, will allow epidemiologists to gain a better understanding of true diet-cancer associations, as well as the underlying mechanisms that affect disease development.

To maximize the amount of useful information that can be acquired from clinical studies, development of robust new statistical techniques and appropriate use of existing methodology are essential for effective diet and cancer research. For example, to help overcome the limitations resulting from data sparseness, a two-stage hierarchical model was recently developed to improve the effect estimates of gene-environment interactions.[413] Used to estimate NAT2 genotype-specific dietary effects on adenomatous polyps, the model suggested that colorectal polyp risk increased with increasing red meat consumption among slow acetylators, but not among fast acetylators,[413] the exact opposite of the results from some earlier investigations.[410,411] Such inconsistencies underscore the need for precise, reliable statistical approaches.

Meta-analysis, a statistical technique that combines the outcomes from a series of different investigations and attempts to mitigate the apparent contradictions across studies, is frequently used in diet and cancer research as an approach to handling published data from a large number of individual studies with a limited number of subjects. It is, however, a controversial statistical tool with inherent weaknesses. One limitation of meta-analysis is that most dietary studies use the same dietary assessment tool, the FFQ, which is validated by diet records. Thus, if there is a flaw in the FFQ that produces a systematic error (e.g., measurement or misclassification), meta-analysis only serves to magnify the error or solidify the belief that the error is a fact.[414] Further, meta-analysis does not account for biases present in original studies and may introduce new bias by inappropriately pooling heterogeneous studies. Keeping in mind its limitations, meta-analysis, used appropriately and carefully, can be a useful statistical tool to provide insight into the diet and cancer relationship. However, to help ensure that it will be used appropriately, techniques of meta-analysis should be included in training programs for those who may be involved in cancer research, and criteria for conducting meta-analysis should be clearly delineated.[415]

The development of validated, reliable dietary assessment techniques, along with expansion of existing databases on food com-

position, is critical to achieving valid findings in either dietary epidemiologic or dietary intervention studies. The consistently poor agreement of dietary assessment methods with one another—even under the best of conditions—and the inconsistency of results regarding nutrient-cancer relationships suggest that there may be serious limitations to the accuracy achievable using common measurement techniques.[416] The FFQ, which has been widely used in cohort studies as an instrument of dietary measure, has the advantage of being low cost and easy to administer—important factors when studying a large population.[417–419] Correlation coefficients (the correlation of intake for specific food items with intake from a diet record) in the range of 0.4 to 0.7 are most common.[417,420] Although acceptable by current standards, these coefficients are far from convincing and are not uniform from study to study. Diet records are currently considered the "gold standard" against which FFQs are evaluated. However, research suggests that people keeping a diet record may underestimate their usual intake by about 20%.[390,421] The exact reasons for such inaccuracy have not been determined, although social desirability—that is, the tendency of an individual to convey an image (dietary or other) in keeping with social norms and to avoid criticism in a testing situation—could bias self-reported dietary intake and, thus, may affect risk estimates by creating a large downward bias.[422] Also, the very act of keeping a diet record may cause individuals to alter their intake.[419] Given the inherent problems in current dietary assessment methods, the development of valid and reliable dietary biomarkers to assess and monitor dietary intake—for example, serum carotenoids as a marker of vegetable and fruit intake[423]—could be of considerable value in nutrition intervention research.

Because cancer development is a relatively infrequent event, on a population scale, both epidemiologic studies and clinical intervention trials that use cancer incidence as the end point must use a large number of subjects who are usually followed for many years, resulting in expensive and time-consuming research efforts. Short-term intervention studies are generally considered to be an attractive alternative. The success of short-term studies, however, is dependent on the availability of valid and reliable intermediate biomarkers that can substitute for a clinical cancer end point. As noted earlier, biomarkers used as surrogate end points for cancer must meet certain criteria with regard to sensitivity, specificity, reproducibility, modulation by the intervention, and correlation of the modulation to reduced cancer risk. Studies are sorely needed to critically evaluate promising intermediate biomakers with regard to their predictive value for cancer incidence. It must be recognized that the studies required to evaluate these surrogate end points thoroughly may be as large, long, and expensive as the intervention trials they were designed to replace.[424] Once validated, however, intermediate end points will provide a practical approach for testing the possible cancer-preventive effects of dietary patterns or dietary constituents.

The scope of future cancer prevention strategies could be broadened considerably by combining modifications in eating behavior with chemoprevention approaches. Such strategies might reduce cancer incidence through early intervention for individuals who are at increased risk for specific types of cancer. Developing effective methods for identifying individuals at high risk will become increasingly important. The medical community can play an important role in recognizing and promoting the merits of a preventive approach to cancer and in identifying those individuals who might benefit from preventive interventions specifically tailored for their particular risk profile, based on genetic susceptibility, lifestyle choices and other environmental exposures, history of premalignant lesions, or a combination of these factors.

## SUMMARY

Based on a convincing body of available epidemiologic, experimental, and clinical evidence, the existence of a causal link between diet and cancer is irrefutable. In general, dietary fat, excessive calories, obesity, alcohol, and some methods of food preparation such as grilling and smoking appear to increase cancer risk, whereas vegetables and fruits, dietary fiber, and certain micronutrients appear to be protective against cancer. The independent effects of specific types of fat and of individual dietary fiber components on cancer risk have yet to be determined. Also, considering the chemical diversity of dietary constituents, their mechanisms of action and possible interactive effects with regard to reducing or enhancing cancer risk might be expected to differ for specific cancer sites and likely are complex and difficult to unravel. It is unlikely that any particular plant food constituent or class of constituents will prove to be a "magic bullet" in the prevention of cancer. More likely, plant food constituents play complementary roles with regard to cancer risk, suggesting that the optimal diet should include a wide variety of vegetables, fruits, and whole grains.

Results from cancer epidemiology must be interpreted judiciously, because dietary factors that contribute to either increased or decreased cancer risk can be influenced by individual genetic susceptibility. The relative prevalence and/or distribution of polymorphisms, mutations in tumor-associated genes, and/or differences in DNA repair mechanisms and adduct formation within the populations targeted in epidemiologic studies may affect individual responses to both dietary risk factors and protective factors and thus may contribute to some of the inconsistencies observed across individual epidemiologic studies.

At present, large-scale, randomized clinical trials—even though they require a considerable investment of time and resources—remain the best approach available to evaluate the effectiveness of specific dietary or chemopreventive interventions in reducing the risk of cancer development. While diet and cancer research continues, numerous advisory groups are in agreement that, to benefit overall health and reduce cancer risk, the most prudent approach for the public is to adopt a low-fat, high-fiber diet that includes a variety of vegetables, fruits, and whole grains; to limit consumption of alcohol; and to maintain a healthy body weight.

## REFERENCES

1. WEINSTEIN IB et al: Molecular biology and epidemiology of cancer, in *Cancer Prevention and Control,* P. Greenwald et al (eds). New York, Marcel Dekker, 1995, pp 83–110.
2. U.S. DEPARTMENT OF HEALTH AND HUMAN SERVICES: *The Surgeon General's Report on Nutrition and Health.* Washington, DC, NIH Publication No. 88-50210. Public Health Service, 1988, pp 1–78.
3. NATIONAL ACADEMY OF SCIENCES, NATIONAL RESEARCH COUNCIL, COMMISSION ON LIFE SCIENCES, FOOD AND NUTRITION BOARD: *Diet and Health: Implications for Reducing Chronic Disease Risk.* Washington, DC, National Academy Press, 1989.
4. WATTENBERG LW: Chemoprevention of cancer by naturally occurring and synthetic compounds, in *Cancer Chemoprevention,* L Wattenberg et al (eds). Boca Raton, CRC Press, 1992, pp 19–39.
5. BLOCK G: Micronutrients and cancer: Time for action? J Natl Cancer Inst 85(11):846, 1993 (Editorial).
6. VAN POPPEL G, VAN DEN BERG H: Vitamins and cancer. Cancer Lett 114:195, 1997.
7. HECHT JR: Dietary fat and colon cancer. Adv Exp Med Biol 399:157, 1996.
8. GREENWALD P et al: Fat, caloric intake, and obesity: Lifestyle risk factors for breast cancer. J Am Diet Assoc 97:24, 1997.
9. MOONEY LA et al: Contribution of genetic and nutritional factors to DNA damage in heavy smokers. Carcinogenesis 18:503, 1997.
10. BAUTISTA D et al: Ki-*ras* mutation modifies the protective effect of dietary monounsaturated fat and calcium on sporadic colorectal cancer. Cancer Epidemiol Biomark Prev 6:57, 1997.
11. BRAUN MM et al: A cohort study of twins and cancer. Cancer Epidemiol Biomark Prev 4:469, 1995.
12. HRUBEC Z, NEEL JV: Contribution of familial factors to the occurrence of cancer before old age in twin veterans. Am J Hum Genet 34:658, 1982.
13. KAPRIO J et al: Cancer in adult same-sexed twins: A historical cohort study. Prog Clin Biol Res 69(C):217, 1981.
14. HOLM NV et al: Studies of cancer aetiology in a complete twin population: Breast cancer, colorectal cancer and leukaemia. Cancer Surv 1(1):17, 1982.
15. CEDERLOF R, FLODERUS-MYRHED B: Cancer mortality and morbidity among 23,000 unselected twin pairs, in *Genetic and Environmental Factors in Experimental and Human Cancer,* HV Gelboin (ed). Tokyo, Japan Sci. Soc. Press, 1980, pp 151–160.
16. DIEZ O et al: Differences in phenotypic expression of a new *BRCA1* mutation in identical twins. Lancet 350:713, 1997.
17. WORLD CANCER RESEARCH FUND: *Food, Nutrition and the Prevention of Cancer: A Global Perspective.* Washington, DC, American Institute for Cancer Research, 1997.
18. TAUBES G: Epidemiology faces its limits: The search for subtle links between diet, lifestyle, or environmental factors and disease is an unending source of fear—but often yields little certainty. Science 269:164, 1995.
19. WEED DL, KRAMER BS: Induced abortion, bias, and breast cancer: Why epidemiology hasn't reached its limit. J Natl Cancer Inst 88:1698, 1996.
20. WEED DL, GORELIC LS: The practice of causal interference in cancer epidemiology. Cancer Epidemiol Biomark Prev 5:303, 1996.
21. TANNENBAUM A: The genesis and growth of tumors. III. Effects of a high fat diet. Cancer Res 2:468, 1942.
22. TANNENBAUM A: The dependence of tumor formation on the degree of caloric restriction. Cancer Res 5:609, 1945.
23. TANNENBAUM A: The dependence of tumor formation on the composition of the calorie-restricted diet as well as on the degree of restriction. Cancer Res 5:616, 1945.
24. SPORN MB: Approaches to prevention of epithelial cancer during the preneoplastic period. Cancer Res 36:2699, 1976.
25. SPORN MB, NEWTON DL: Chemoprevention of cancer with retinoids. Fed Proc 38:2528, 1979.

26. SPORN MB: Carcinogenesis and cancer: Different perspectives on the same disease. Cancer Res 51:6215, 1991.

27. SPORN MB, ROBERTS AB: Interactions of retinoids and transforming growth factor-β in regulation of cell differentiation and proliferation. Mol Endocrinol 5:3, 1991.

28. PETO R et al: Can dietary beta-carotene materially reduce human cancer rates? Nature 290:201, 1981.

29. TISEVICH DA: Legislative history of the National Cancer Institute and the National Cancer Program. Cancer 78:2620, 1996.

30. KNIPMEYER MC: Legislative history of the National Cancer Institute. Cancer 78:2618, 1996.

31. DOLL R, PETO R: The causes of cancer: Quantitative estimates of avoidable risks of cancer in the United States today. J Natl Cancer Inst 66:1191, 1981.

32. NATIONAL ACADEMY OF SCIENCES, NATIONAL RESEARCH COUNCIL, COMMITTEE ON DIET NUTRITION AND CANCER: *Diet Nutrition and Cancer.* Washington, DC, National Academy Press, 1982.

33. COMMITTEE ON COMPARATIVE TOXICITY OF NATURALLY OCCURRING CARCINOGENS, BOARD ON ENVIRONMENTAL STUDIES AND TOXICOLOGY, COMMISSION ON LIFE SCIENCES, NATIONAL RESEARCH COUNCIL: *Carcinogens and Anticarcinogens in the Human Diet.* Washington, DC, National Academy Press, 1996.

34. ROSE DP et al: International comparisons of mortality rates for cancer of the breast, ovary, prostate, and colon and per capita food consumption. Cancer 58:2363, 1986.

35. HURSTING SD et al: Types of dietary fat and the incidence of cancer at five sites. Prev Med 19:242, 1990.

36. ZIEGLER RG et al: Migration patterns and breast cancer risk in Asian-American women. J Natl Cancer Inst 85:1819, 1993.

37. WHITTEMORE AS et al: Prostate cancer in relation to diet, physical activity, and body size in blacks, whites, and Asians in the United States and Canada. J Natl Cancer Inst 87:652, 1995.

38. FREEDMAN LS et al: Analysis of dietary fat, calories, body weight, and the development of mammary tumors in rats and mice: A review. Cancer Res 50:5710, 1990.

39. WYNDER EL et al: Breast cancer: Weighing the evidence for a promoting role of dietary fat. J Natl Cancer Inst 89:766, 1997.

40. GOLDIN BR, GORBACH SL: Hormone studies and the diet and breast cancer connection. Adv Exp Med Biol 364:35, 1994.

41. PARKIN DM: Studies of cancer in migrant populations. IARC Sci Publ 123:1, 1993.

42. HOWE GR et al: Dietary factors and risk of breast cancer: Combined analysis of 12 case-control studies. J Natl Cancer Inst 82:561, 1990.

43. BOYD NF et al: A meta-analysis of studies of dietary fat and breast cancer risk. Br J Cancer 68:627, 1993.

44. VERREAULT R et al: Dietary fat in relation to prognostic indicators in breast cancer. J Natl Cancer Inst 80:819, 1988.

45. GREGORIO DI et al: Dietary fat consumption and survival among women with breast cancer. J Natl Cancer Inst 75:37, 1985.

46. HOLM L-E et al: Treatment failure and dietary habits in women with breast cancer. J Natl Cancer Inst 85:32, 1993.

47. HUNTER DJ et al: Cohort studies of fat intake and the risk of breast cancer—A pooled analysis. N Engl J Med 334:356, 1996.

48. GAARD M et al: Dietary fat and the risk of breast cancer: A prospective study of 25,892 Norwegian women. Int J Cancer 63:13, 1995.

49. WILLETT WC et al: Dietary fat and fiber in relation to risk of breast cancer—An 8-year follow-up. JAMA 268:2037, 1992.

50. KUNE GA: Diet, in *Causes and Control of Colorectal Cancer: A Model for Cancer Prevention,* Anonymous. Boston, Kluwer Academic Publishers, 1996, pp 69–115.

51. GIOVANNUCCI E et al: Intake of fat, meat, and fiber in relation to risk of colon cancer in men. Cancer Res 54:2390, 1994.

52. GIOVANNUCCI E, WILLETT WC: Dietary factors and risk of colon cancer. Ann Med 26:443, 1994.

53. POTTER JD et al: Colon cancer: A review of the epidemiology. Epidemiol Rev 15:499, 1993.

54. POTTER JD: Nutrition and colorectal cancer. Cancer Causes Control 7:127, 1996.

55. HOWE GR et al: The relationship between dietary fat intake and risk of colorectal cancer: Evidence from the combined analysis of 13 case-control studies. Cancer Causes Control 8:215, 1997.

56. STEINBACH G et al: Effect of caloric restriction on colonic proliferation in obese persons: Implications for colon cancer prevention. Cancer Res 54:1194, 1994.

57. KOLONEL LN: Nutrition and prostate cancer. Cancer Causes Control 7:83, 1996.

58. GIOVANNUCCI E et al: A prospective study of dietary fat and risk of prostate cancer. J Natl Cancer Inst 85:1571, 1993.

59. FAY MP et al: Effect of different types and amounts of fat on the development of mammary tumors in rodents: A review. Cancer Res 57:3979, 1997.

60. ROSE DP: Dietary fatty acids and cancer. Am J Clin Nutr 66:998, 1997.

61. TAOLI H et al: Dietary habits and breast cancer: A comparative study of United States and Italian data. Nutr Cancer 16:259, 1991.

62. KAIZER L et al: Fish consumption and breast cancer risk: An ecological study. Nutr Cancer 12:61, 1989.

63. MARTIN-MORENO JM et al: Dietary fat, olive oil intake and breast cancer risk. Int J Cancer 58:774, 1994.

64. CAYGILL CPJ et al: Fat, fish, fish oil and cancer. Br J Cancer 74:159, 1996.

65. CARROLL KK: Nutrition and cancer: Fat, in *Nutrition, Toxicity, and Cancer,* IR Rowland (ed). Boca Raton, CRC Press, 1991, pp 439–453.

66. LIPWORTH L et al: Olive oil and human cancer: An assessment of the evidence. Prev Med 26:181, 1997.

67. FRANCESCHI S et al: Intake of macronutrients and risk of breast cancer. Lancet 347:1351, 1996.

68. LA VECCHIA C et al: Olive oil, other dietary fats, and the risk of breast cancer (Italy). Cancer Causes Control 6:545, 1995.

69. KOHLMEIER L et al: Adipose tissue *trans* fatty acids and breast cancer in the European Community Multicenter Study on Antioxidants, Myocardial Infarction, and Breast Cancer. Cancer Epidemiol Biomark Prev 6:705, 1997.

70. BAGGA D et al: Dietary modulation of omega-3/omega-6 polyunsaturated fatty acid ratios in patients with breast cancer. J Natl Cancer Inst 89:1123, 1997.

71. HILL MJ: Diet and cancer: A review of scientific evidence. Eur J Cancer Prev 4:3, 1995.

72. GANN PH et al: Prospective study of plasma fatty acids and risk of prostate cancer. J Natl Cancer Inst 86:281, 1994.

73. U.S. DEPARTMENT OF HEALTH AND HUMAN SERVICES: *Physical Activity and Health: A Report of the Surgeon General.* Atlanta, GA, US Department of Health and Human Services, 1996.

74. HUNTER DJ, WILLETT WC: Nutrition and breast cancer. Cancer Causes Control 7:56, 1996.

75. ALBANES D: Energy balance, body size, and cancer. Crit Rev Oncol Hematol 10:283, 1990.

76. BALLARD-BARBASH R, SWANSON CA: Body Weight: Estimation of risk for breast and endometrial cancers. Am J Clin Nutr 3:437S, 1996.

77. KULLER LH: The etiology of breast cancer—From epidemiology to prevention. Public Health Rev 23:157, 1995.

78. LA VECCHIA C et al: Body mass index and post-menopausal breast cancer: An age-specific analysis. Br J Cancer 75:441, 1997.

79. BRINTON LA, SWANSON CA: Height and weight at various ages and risk of breast cancer. Ann Epidemiol 2:597, 1992.

80. TRENTHAM-DIETZ A et al: Body size and risk of breast cancer. Am J Epidemiol 145:1011, 1997.

81. RADIMER K et al: Relation between anthropometric indicators and risk of breast cancer among Australian women. Am J Epidemiol 138(2):77, 1993.

82. HUANG Z et al: Dual effects of weight and weight gain on breast cancer risk. JAMA 278:1407, 1997.

83. POTISCHMAN N et al: Reversal of relation between body mass and endogenous estrogen concentrations with menopausal status. J Natl Cancer Inst 88:756, 1996.

84. BERNSTEIN L et al: Physical activity and reduced risk of breast cancer in young women. J Natl Cancer Inst 86:1403, 1994.

85. THUNE I et al: Physical activity and the risk of breast cancer. N Engl J Med 336:1269, 1997.

86. FREIDENREICH CM, ROHAN TE: Physical activity and risk of breast cancer. Eur J Cancer Prev 4:145, 1995.

87. SANDLER RS: Epidemiology and risk factors for colorectal cancer. Gastroent Clin N Am 25:717, 1996.

88. NEUGUT AI et al: Leisure and occupational physical activity and risk of colorectal adenomatous polyps. Int J Cancer 68:744, 1996.

89. ENGER SM et al: Recent and past physical activity and prevalence of colorectal adenomas. Br J Cancer 75:740, 1997.

90. MARTINEZ ME et al: Leisure-time physical activity, body size, and colon cancer in women. J Natl Cancer Inst 89:948, 1997.

91. COLDITZ GA et al: Physical activity and reduced risk of colon cancer: Implications for prevention. Cancer Causes Control 8:649, 1997.

92. GIOVANNUCCI E et al: Physical activity, obesity, and risk for colon cancer and adenoma in men. Ann Intern Med 122:327, 1995.

93. GIOVANNUCCI E et al: Physical activity, obesity, and risk of colorectal adenoma in women (United States). Cancer Causes Control 7:253, 1996.

94. SANDLER RS et al: Physical activity and the risk of colorectal adenomas. Epidemiology 5:602, 1995.

95. ANDERSSON S-O et al: Body size and prostate cancer: A 20-year follow-up study among 135,006 Swedish construction workers. J Natl Cancer Inst 89:385, 1997.

96. GIOVANNUCCI E et al: Height, body weight, and risk of prostate cancer. Cancer Epidemiol Biomark Prev 6:557, 1997.

97. STEINMETZ KA, POTTER JD: Vegetables, fruit, and cancer prevention: A review. J Am Diet Assoc 96:1027, 1996.

98. NEGRI E et al: Vegetable and fruit consumption and cancer risk. Int J Cancer 48:350, 1991.

99. ZIEGLER RG et al: Nutrition and lung cancer. Cancer Causes Control 7:157, 1996.

100. SCHORAH CJ: Micronutrients, antioxidants and risk of cancer. Bibl Nutr Dieta 52:92, 1995.

101. BLOCK G et al: Fruit, vegetables, and cancer prevention: A review of the epidemiological evidence Nutr Cancer 18:1, 1992.

102. DREWNOWSKI A et al: Serum β-carotene and vitamin C as biomarkers of vegetable and fruit intakes in a community-based sample of French adults. Am J Clin Nutr 65:1796, 1997.

103. VAN POPPEL G, GOLDBOHM RA: Epidemiologic evidence for β-carotene and cancer prevention. Am J Clin Nutr 62:1393S, 1995.

104. BLOCK G: Vitamin C and cancer prevention: The epidemiologic evidence. Am J Clin Nutr 53:270S, 1991.

105. BYERS T, GUERRERO N: Epidemiologic evidence for vitamin C and vitamin E in cancer prevention. Am J Clin Nutr 62:1385S, 1995.

106. LE MARCHAND L et al: An ecological study of diet and lung cancer in the South Pacific. Int J Cancer 63:18, 1995.

107. COLLINS A et al: Micronutrients and oxidative stress in the aetiology of cancer. Proc Nutr Soc 53:67, 1994.

108. OCKE MC et al: Repeated measurements of vegetables, fruits, β-carotene, and vitamins C and E in relation to lung cancer. Am J Epidemiol 145:358, 1997.

109. JENNINGS E: Folic acid as a cancer-preventing agent. Med Hypotheses 45:297, 1995.

110. DIPLOCK AT: Safety of antioxidant vitamins and β-carotene. Am J Clin Nutr 62:1510S, 1995.

111. WEBER P et al: Vitamin C and human health—A review of recent data relevant to human requirements. Int J Vitam Nutr Res 66:19, 1996.

112. ZIEGLER RG: Vegetables, fruits, and carotenoids, and the risk of cancer. Am J Clin Nutr 53:251S, 1991.

113. GAREWAL HS et al: Response of oral leukoplakia to beta-carotene. J Clin Oncol 8:1715, 1990.

114. SLATTERY ML et al: Plant foods and colon cancer: An assessment of specific foods and their related nutrients (United States). Cancer Causes Control 8:575, 1997.

115. WITTE JS et al: Relation of vegetable, fruit, and grain consumption to colorectal adenomatous polyps. Am J Epidemiol 144:1015, 1996.

116. SHANNON J et al: Relationship of food groups and water intake to colon cancer risk. Cancer Epidemiol Biomark Prev 5:495, 1996.

117. DENEO-PELLEGRINI H et al: Vegetables, fruits, and risk of colorectal cancer: A case-control study from Uruguay. Nutr Cancer 25:297, 1996.

118. CAHILL RJ et al: Effects of vitamin antioxidant supplementation on cell kinetics of patients with adenomatous polyps. Gut 34:963, 1993.

119. GERSTER H: β-carotene, vitamin E and vitamin C in different stages of experimental carcinogenesis. Eur J Clin Nutr 49:155, 1995.

120. FREEDMAN AN et al: Familial and nutritional risk factors for p53 overexpression in colorectal cancer. Cancer Epidemiol Biomark Prev 5:285, 1996.

121. KLEIBEUKER JH et al: Calcium supplementation as prophylaxis against colon cancer? Dig Dis 12:85, 1994.

122. LIPKIN M, NEWMARK H: Calcium and the prevention of colon cancer. J Cell Biochem 22(Suppl):65, 1995.

123. LONGNECKER MP et al: Serum alpha-tocopherol concentration in relation to subsequent colorectal cancer: Pooled data from five cohorts. J Natl Cancer Inst 84:430, 1992.

124. REDDY BS et al: Chemoprevention of colon cancer by organoselenium compounds and impact of high- or low-fat diets. J Natl Cancer Inst 89:506, 1997.

125. TSENG M et al: Micronutrients and the risk of colorectal adenomas. Am J Epidemiol 144:1005, 1996.

126. NARISAWA T et al: Inhibitory effects of natural carotenoids, α-carotene, β-carotene, lycopene and lutein, on colonic aberrant crypt foci formation in rats. Cancer Lett 107:137, 1996.

127. YUAN J-M et al: Diet and breast cancer in Shanghai and Tianjin, China. Br J Cancer 71(6):1353, 1995.

128. HOLMBERG L et al: Diet and breast cancer risk: Results from a

population-based, case-control study in Sweden. Arch Intern Med 154:1805, 1994.

129. NUNEZ C et al: Estudio caso-control de la relacion dieta y cancer de mama en una muestra procedente de tres problaciones hospitalarias espanolas. Repercusion del consumo de alimentos, energia y nutrientes. Rev Clin Esp 196:75, 1996.

130. HUNTER DJ et al: A prospective study of the intake of vitamins C, E, and A and the risk of breast cancer. N Engl J Med 329:234, 1993.

131. LONGNECKER MP et al: Intake of carrots, spinach, and supplements containing vitamin A in relation to risk of breast cancer. Cancer Epidemiol Biomark Prev 6:887, 1997.

132. HERMAN C et al: Soybean phytoestrogen intake and cancer risk. J Nutr 125:757, 1995.

133. MOLTENI A et al: *In vitro* hormonal effects of soybean isoflavones. J Nutr 125:751S, 1995.

134. VAN'T VEER P et al: Tissue antioxidants and postmenopausal breast cancer: The European Community Multicentre Study on Antioxidants, Myocardial Infarction, and Cancer of the Breast (EURAMIC). Cancer Epidemiol Biomark Prev 5:441, 1996.

135. KIMMICK GG et al: Vitamin E and breast cancer: A review. Nutr Cancer 27:109, 1997.

136. FREUDENHEIM JL et al: Premenopausal breast cancer risk and intake of vegetables, fruits, and related nutrients. J Natl Cancer Inst 88:340, 1996.

137. CHAJES V et al: Alpha-tocopherol and hydroperoxide content in breast adipose tissue from patients with breast tumors. Int J Cancer 67:170, 1996.

138. IP C, LISK DJ: Enrichment of selenium in allium vegetables for cancer prevention. Carcinogenesis 15(9):1881, 1994.

139. EWINGS P, BOWIE C: A case-control study of cancer of the prostate in Somerset and east Devon. Br J Cancer 74:661, 1996.

140. GIOVANNUCCI E et al: Intake of carotenoids and retinol in relation to risk of prostate cancer. J Natl Cancer Inst 87:1767, 1995.

141. ANDERSSON S-O et al: Energy, nutrient intake and prostate cancer risk: A population-based case-control study in Sweden. Int J Cancer 68:716, 1996.

142. NOMURA AMY et al: Serum micronutrients and prostate cancer in Japanese Americans in Hawaii. Cancer Epidemiol Biomark Prev 6:487, 1997.

143. VLAJINAC HD et al: Diet and prostate cancer: A case-control study. Eur J Cancer 33:101, 1997.

144. GANN PH et al: Circulating vitamin D metabolites in relation to subsequent development of prostate cancer. Cancer Epidemiol Biomark Prev 5:121, 1996.

145. ADLERCREUTZ H et al: Diet and plasma androgens in postmenopausal vegetarian and omnivorous women and postmenopausal women with breast cancer. Am J Clin Nutr 49:433, 1989.

146. GRAHAM S et al: Diet in the epidemiology of carcinoma of the prostate gland. J Natl Cancer Inst 70:687, 1983.

147. DAVIGLUS ML et al: Dietary beta-carotene, vitamin C, and risk of prostate cancer: Results from the Western Electric Study. Epidemiology 7:472, 1996.

148. HERTOG MGL et al: Fruit and vegetable consumption and cancer mortality in the Caerphilly Study. Cancer Epidemiol Biomark Prev 5:673, 1996.

149. O'TOOLE P, LOMBARD M: Vitamin C and gastric cancer: Supplements for some or fruit for all? Gut 39:345, 1996.

150. LA VECCHIA CL et al: Nutrition and diet in the etiology of endometrial cancer. Cancer 57:1248, 1986.

151. LA VECCHIA CL et al: Dietary factors and the risk of epithelial ovarian cancer. J Natl Cancer Inst 79:663, 1987.

152. HELZLSOUER KJ et al: Prospective study of serum micronutrients and ovarian cancer. J Natl Cancer Inst 88:32, 1996.

153. MANETTA A et al: β-Carotene treatment of cervical intraepithelial neoplasia: A phase II study. Cancer Epidemiol Biomark Prev 5:929, 1996.

154. CHUNG F-L et al: Inhibition of the tobacco-specific nitrosamine-induced lung tumorigenesis by compounds derived from cruciferous vegetables and green tea. Ann NY Acad Sci 686:186, 1993.

155. WINN DM et al: Diet in the etiology of oral and pharyngeal cancer among women from the southern United States. Cancer Res 44:1216, 1984.

156. MCLAUGHLIN JK et al: Dietary factors in oral and pharyngeal cancer. J Natl Cancer Inst 80:1237, 1988.

157. FRANCESCHI S et al: Risk factors for cancer of the tongue and the mouth. Cancer 70:2227, 1992.

158. BURKITT DP: Epidemiology of cancer of the colon and rectum. Cancer 28:3, 1971.

159. GREENWALD P, CLIFFORD C: Fiber and cancer: Prevention research, in *Dietary Fiber in Health and Disease,* D Kritchevsky, C Benfield (eds). St. Paul, Eagen Press, 1995, pp 159–173.

160. FAIVRE J et al: Diet and large bowel cancer, in *Advances in Nutrition and Cancer,* V Zappia et al (eds). New York, Plenum Press, 1993, pp 107–118.

161. SPILLER GA: Definition of dietary fiber, in *CRC Handbook of Dietary Fiber in Human Nutrition,* 2d ed, GA Spiller (ed). Boca Raton, CRC Press, 1993, pp 15–18.

162. BURNSTEIN MJ: Dietary factors related to colorectal neoplasms. Surg Clin North Am 73(1):13, 1993.

163. SCHATZKIN A, KELLOFF G: Chemo- and dietary prevention of colorectal cancer. Eur J Cancer 31A:1198, 1995.

164. HARRIS PJ, FERGUSON LR: Dietary fibre: Its composition and role in protection against colorectal cancer. Mutation Res 290:97, 1993.

165. TROCK B et al: Dietary fiber, vegetables, and colon cancer: Critical review and meta-analyses of the epidemiologic evidence. J Natl Cancer Inst 82:650, 1990.

166. SHANKAR S, LANZA E: Dietary fiber and cancer prevention. Hematol Oncol Clin North Am 5:25, 1991.

167. KRITCHEVSKY D: Epidemiology of fibre, resistant starch and colorectal cancer. Eur J Cancer Prev 4:345, 1995.

168. REDDY BS et al: Metabolic epidemiology of large bowel cancer: Fecal bulk and constituents in high-risk North American and low-risk Finnish populations. Cancer 42:2832, 1978.

169. JENSEN OM et al: Diet, bowel function, fecal characteristics, and large bowel cancer in Denmark and Finland. Nutr Cancer 4:5, 1982.

170. SCHATZKIN A et al: Lack of effect of a low-fat, high-fiber diet on the recurrence of colorectal adenomas. Polyp Prevention Trial Study Group. N Engl J Med 342:1149, 2000.

171. ALBERTS DS et al: Lack of effect of a high-fiber cereal supplement on the recurrence of colorectal adenomas. Phoenix Colon Cancer Prevention Physicians' Network. N Engl J Med 342:1156, 2000.

172. KLURFELD DM: Dietary fiber-mediated mechanisms in carcinogenesis. Cancer Res 52:2055S, 1992.

173. FOLINO M et al: Dietary fibers differ in their effects on large bowel epithelial proliferation and fecal fermentation-dependent events in rats. J Nutr 125:1521, 1995.

174. STEINMETZ KA et al: Vegetables, fruit, and colon cancer in the Iowa Women's Health Study. Am J Epidemiol 139(1):1, 1994.

175. PLATZ EA et al: Dietary fiber and distal colorectal adenoma in men. Cancer Epidemiol Biomark Prev 6:661, 1997.

176. KRITCHEVSKY D: *Evaluation of Publicly Available Scientific Evidence Regarding Certain Nutrient-Disease Relationships: 5. Dietary Fiber and Cancer* (prepared for *Food Safety and Applied Nutrition*, FDA, DHHS, Washington, DC). Rockville, MD, Federation of American Societies for Experimental Biology, Life Sciences Research Office, 1991, pp 1–21.

177. PILCH S: *Physiological Effects and Health Consequences of Dietary Fiber.* Bethesda, MD, Federation of American Societies for Experimental Biology, Life Sciences Research Office, 1987.

178. ALABASTER O et al: Dietary fiber and the chemopreventive modelation of colon carcinogenesis. Mutation Res 350:185, 1996.

179. ROONEY PS et al: Wheat fibre, lactulose and rectal mucosal proliferation in individuals with a family history of colorectal cancer. Br J Surg 81:1792, 1994.

180. ALBERTS DS et al: Randomized, double-blind, placebo-controlled study of effect of wheat bran fiber and calcium on fecal bile acids in patients with resected adenomatous colon polyps. J Natl Cancer Inst 88:81, 1996.

181. ALBERTS DS et al: The effect of wheat bran fiber and calcium supplementation on rectal mucosal proliferation rates in patients with resected adenomatous colorectal polyps. Cancer Epidemiol Biomark Prev 6:161, 1997.

182. REDDY BS et al: Biochemical epidemiology of colon cancer: Effect of types of dietary fiber on colonic diacylglycerols in women. Gastroenterology 106:883, 1994.

183. MOROTOMI M et al: Production of diacylglycerol, an activator of protein kinase C, by human intestinal microflora. Cancer Res 50:3595, 1990.

184. ROSE DP: Dietary fiber and breast cancer. Nutr Cancer 13:1, 1990.

185. ROSE DP: Dietary fiber, phytoestrogens, and breast cancer. Nutrition 8(1):47, 1992.

186. ROSE DP: Diet, hormones, and cancer. Annu Rev Public Health 14:1, 1993.

187. LIPWORTH L: Epidemiology of breast cancer. Eur J Cancer Prev 4:7, 1995.

188. HOWE GR et al: Dietary intake of fiber and decreased risk of cancers of the colon and rectum: Evidence from the combined analysis of 13 case-control studies. J Natl Cancer Inst 84:1887, 1992.

189. DE STEFANI E et al: Dietary fiber and risk of breast cancer: A case-control study in Uruguay. Nutr Cancer 28:14, 1997.

190. LA VECCHIA C et al: Fibers and breast cancer risk. Nutr Cancer 28:264, 1997.

191. ADLERCREUTZ H: Diet and sex hormone metabolism, in *Nutrition, Toxicity, and Cancer.* IR Rowland (ed). Boca Raton, CRC Press, 1991, pp 137–195.

192. ADLERCREUTZ H et al: Diet and breast cancer. Acta Oncol 31:175, 1992.

193. THOMPSON LU: Antioxidants and hormone-mediated health benefits of whole grains. Crit Rev Food Sci Nutr 34(5&6):473, 1994.

194. HILL HA, AUSTIN H: Nutrition and endometrial cancer. Cancer Causes Control 7:19, 1996.

195. KONO S, HIROHATA T: Nutrition and stomach cancer. Cancer Causes Control 7:41, 1996.

196. TZONOU A et al: Diet and ovarian cancer: A case-control study in Greece. Int J Cancer 55:411, 1993.

197. RISCH HA et al: Dietary fat intake and risk of epithelial ovarian cancer. J Natl Cancer Inst 86(18):1409, 1994.

198. MILLS PK et al: Cohort study of diet, lifestyle, and prostate cancer in Adventist men. Cancer 64:598, 1989.

199. HOWIE BJ, SHULTZ TD: Dietary and hormonal interrelationships among vegetarian Seventh-Day Adventists and non-vegetarian men. Am J Clin Nutr 42:127, 1985.

200. ROSS JK et al: Dietary and hormonal evaluation of men at different risks for prostate cancer: Fiber intake, excretion, and composition, with *in vitro* evidence for an association between steroid hormones and specific fiber components. Am J Clin Nutr 51:365, 1990.

201. DORGAN JF, SCHATZKIN A: Antioxidant micronutrients in cancer prevention. Hematol Oncol Clin North Am 5:43, 1991.

202. ROCK CL et al: Update on the biological characteristics of the antioxidant micronutrients: Vitamin C, vitamin E, and the carotenoids. J Am Diet Assoc 96:693, 1996.

203. YONG L-C et al: Intake of vitamins E, C, and A and risk of lung cancer. Am J Epidemiol 146:231, 1997.

204. STEINMETZ KA, POTTER JD: Vegetables, fruit, and cancer. II. Mechanisms. Cancer Causes Control 2:427, 1991.

205. LOFT S, POULSEN HE: Cancer risk and oxidative DNA damage in man. J Mol Med 74:297, 1996.

206. JACOB RA, BURRI BJ: Oxidative damage and defense. Am J Clin Nutr 63:985S, 1996.

207. DIPLOCK AT: Antioxidants and disease prevention. Food Chem Toxicol 34:1013, 1996.

208. COZZI R et al: Ascorbic acid and β-carotene as modulators of oxidative damage. Carcinogenesis 18:223, 1997.

209. LASNITZKI I: The influence of hypervitaminosis on the effect of 20-methylcholantrene on mouse prostate glands grown *in vitro.* Br J Cancer 9:434, 1955.

210. ENGER SM et al: Dietary intake of specific carotenoids and vitamins A, C, and E, and prevalence of colorectal adenomas. Cancer Epidemiol Biomark Prev 5:147, 1996.

211. GREENBERG ER et al: A clinical trial of beta carotene to prevent basal-cell and squamous cell cancers of the skin. N Engl J Med 323:789, 1990.

212. GREENBERG ER et al: A clinical trial of antioxidant vitamins to prevent colorectal adenoma. N Engl J Med 331:141, 1994.

213. MACLENNAN R et al: Randomized trial of intake of fat, fiber, and beta carotene to prevent colorectal adenomas. J Natl Cancer Inst 87:1760, 1995.

214. LA VECCHIA CL et al: Dietary factors and the risk of breast cancer. Nutr Cancer 10:205, 1987.

215. ALPHA-TOCOPHEROL BETA-CAROTENE CANCER PREVENTION STUDY GROUP, HEINONEN OP et al: The effect of vitamin E and beta carotene on the incidence of lung cancer and other cancers in male smokers. N Engl J Med 330(15):1029, 1994.

216. STONE WL, PAPAS AM: Tocopherols and the etiology of colon cancer. J Natl Cancer Inst 89:1006, 1997.

217. CLARK LC et al: Effects of selenium supplementation for cancer prevention in patients with carcinoma of the skin. JAMA 276:1957, 1996.

218. SCHRAUZER GN et al: Cancer mortality correlations studies. III: Statistical associations with dietary selenium intakes. Bioinorg Chem 7:23, 1977.

219. GOODWIN PJ, BOYD NF: Critical appraisal of the evidence that dietary fat intake is related to breast cancer risk in humans. J Natl Cancer Inst 79:473, 1987.

220. ALBERTS DS et al: Effects of dietary wheat bran fiber on rectal

epithelial cell proliferation in patients with resection for colorectal cancer. J Natl Cancer Inst 82:1280, 1990.

221. KELLOFF GJ, BOONE CW (eds): Clinical development plan: *I*-Selenomethionine. J Cell Biochem 26S(Suppl):202, 1996.

222. IP C et al: Potential of food modification in cancer prevention. Cancer Res 54:1957S, 1994.

223. COMSTOCK GW et al: Serum retinol, beta-carotene, vitamin E, and selenium as related to subsequent cancer of specific sites. Am J Epidemiol 135:115, 1992.

224. BERGSMA-KADIJK JA et al: Calcium does not protect against colorectal neoplasia. Epidemiology 7:590, 1996.

225. GOVERS MJAP et al: Calcium in milk products precipitates intestinal fatty acids and secondary bile acids and thus inhibits colonic cytotoxicity in humans. Cancer Res 56:3270, 1996.

226. BOSTICK RM: Human studies of calcium supplementation and colorectal epithelial cell proliferation. Cancer Epidemiol Biomark Prev 6:971, 1997.

227. GLINGHAMMAR B et al: Shift from a dairy product-rich to a dairy product-free diet: Influence on cytotoxicity and genotoxicity of fecal water—potential risk factors for colon cancer. Am J Clin Nutr 66:1277, 1997.

228. KAMPMAN E et al: Fermented dairy products, dietary calcium and colon cancer: A case-control study in the Netherlands. Int J Cancer 59:170, 1994.

229. PRITCHARD RS et al: Dietary calcium, vitamin D, and the risk of colorectal cancer in Stockholm, Sweden. Cancer Epidemiol Biomark Prev 5:897, 1996.

230. KEARNEY J et al: Calcium, vitamin D, and dairy foods and the occurrence of colon cancer in men. Am J Epidemiol 143:907, 1996.

231. MARTINEZ ME et al: Calcium, vitamin D, and the occurrence of colorectal cancer among women. J Natl Cancer Inst 88:1375, 1996.

232. BOUTRON M-C et al: Calcium, phosphorus, vitamin D, dairy products and colorectal carcinogenesis: A French case-control study. Br J Cancer 74:145, 1996.

233. MARTINEZ ME et al: Association of diet and colorectal adenomatous polyps: Dietary fiber, calcium, and total fat. Epidemiology 7:264, 1996.

234. BIRD CL et al: Red cell and plasma folate, folate consumption, and the risk of colorectal adenomatous polyps. Cancer Epidemiol Biomark Prev 4:709, 1995.

235. GLYNN SA et al: Colorectal cancer and folate status: A nested case-control study among male smokers. Cancer Epidemiol Biomark Prev 5:487, 1996.

236. GIOVANNUCCI E et al: Folate, methionine, and alcohol intake and risk of colorectal adenoma. J Natl Cancer Inst 85:875, 1993.

237. VOGELSTEIN B et al: Genetic alterations during colorectal-tumor development. N Engl J Med 319:525, 1988.

238. LASHNER BA et al: Effect of folate supplementation on the incidence of dysplasia and cancer in chronic ulcerative colitis. Gastroenterology 97:255, 1989.

239. EL-DIERY WS et al: High expression of the DNA methyltransferase gene characterizes human neoplastic cells and progression stages of colon cancer. Proc Natl Acad Sci USA 88:3470, 1991.

240. FEINBERG AP, VOGELSTEIN B: Hypomethylation of ras oncogenes in primary human cancers. Biochem Biophys Res Commun 111:47, 1983.

241. WATTENBERG LW: Inhibition of carcinogenesis by minor dietary constituents. Cancer Res 52:2085S, 1992.

242. STAVRIC B: Role of chemopreventers in human diet. Clin Biochem 27(5):319, 1994.

243. HUANG M-T et al: Cancer chemoprevention by phytochemicals in fruits and vegetables. An overview, in *Food Phytochemicals for Cancer Prevention I. Fruits and Vegetables,* M-T Huang et al (eds). Washington, DC, American Chemical Society, 1994, pp 2–16.

244. SMITH TJ, YANG CS: Effects of food phytochemicals on xenobiotic metabolism and tumorigenesis, in *Food Phytochemicals for Cancer Prevention I. Fruits and Vegetables,* M-T Huang et al (eds). Washington, DC, American Chemical Society, 1994, pp 17–48.

245. WATTENBERG LW: Prevention-therapy-basic science and the resolution of the cancer problem: Presidential address. *Cancer Res* 53:5890, 1993.

246. CONSTANTINOU A et al: The dietary anticancer agent ellagic acid is a potent inhibitor of DNA topoisomerases *in vitro.* Nutr Cancer 23(2):121, 1995.

247. ZHANG Y et al: Anticarcinogenic activities of sulforaphane and structurally related synthetic norbornyl isothiocyanates. Proc Natl Acad Sci USA 91:3147, 1994.

248. MEHTA RG et al: Cancer chemopreventive activity of brassinin, a phytoalexin from cabbage. Carcinogenesis 16(2):399, 1995.

249. BILLINGS PC et al: Protease inhibitor suppression of colon and anal gland carcinogenesis induced by dimethylhydrazine. Carcinogenesis 11:1083, 1990.

250. LIPPMAN JM et al: Modulation by 13-cis retinoic acid of biologic markers as indicators of intermediate endpoints in human oral carcinogenesis. Prog Clin Biol Res 339:174, 1990.

251. MANSON MM et al: Mechanism of action of dietary chemoprotective agents in rat liver: Induction of phase I and II drug metabolizing enzymes and aflatoxin $B_1$ metabolism. Carcinogenesis 18:1729, 1997.

252. WARGOVICH MJ: Experimental evidence for cancer preventive elements in food. Cancer Lett 114:11, 1997.

253. WATTENBERG LW: Chemoprevention of cancer. Prev Med 25:44, 1996.

254. ADLERCREUTZ H et al: Dietary phytoestrogens and cancer: *in vitro* and *in vivo* studies. J Steroid Biochem Mol Biol 41:331, 1992.

255. BARRETT J: Phytoestrogens. Environ Health Perspect 104:478, 1996.

256. ADLERCREUTZ H: Diet, breast cancer, and sex hormone metabolism. Ann NY Acad Sci 595:281, 1990.

257. OKUBO K et al: Soybean saponin and isoflavonoids, in *Food Phytochemicals for Cancer Prevention I. Fruits and Vegetables,* M-T Huang et al (eds). Washington, DC, American Chemical Society, 1994, pp 330–339.

258. WISEMAN H: Role of dietary phyto-oestrogens in the protection against cancer and heart disease. Biochem Soc Trans 24:795, 1996.

259. ADLERCREUTZ H: Phytoestrogens: Epidemiology and a possible role in cancer protection. Environ Health Perspect 103:103, 1995.

260. INGRAM D et al: Case-control study of phyto-oestrogens and breast cancer. Lancet 350:990, 1997.

261. WARGOVICH MJ et al: Allium vegetables: Their role in the prevention of cancer. Biochem Soc Trans 24:811, 1996.

262. HABER-MIGNARD D et al: Inhibition of aflatoxin $B_1$- and *N*-nitrosodiethylamine-induced liver preneoplastic foci in rats fed naturally occurring allyl sulfides. Nutr Cancer 25:61, 1996.

263. KELLOFF GJ, BOONE CW (eds): Clinical development plan: β-carotene and other carotenoids. J Cell Biochem 20(Suppl):110, 1994.

264. KHACHIK F et al: Lutein, lycopene, and their oxidative metabolites in chemoprevention of cancer. J Cell Biochem 22(Suppl):236, 1995.

265. STAHL W et al: Biological activities of natural and synthetic carotenoids: Induction of gap junctional communication and singlet oxygen quenching. Carcinogenesis 18:89, 1997.

266. MANGELS AR et al: Carotenoid content of fruits and vegetables: An evaluation of analytic data. J Am Diet Assoc 93:284, 1993.

267. CHUG-AHUJA JK et al: The development and application of a carotenoid database for fruits, vegetables, and selected multi-component foods. J Am Diet Assoc 93:318, 1993.

268. ZIEGLER RG et al: Importance of α-carotene, β-carotene, and other phytochemicals in the etiology of lung cancer. J Natl Cancer Inst 88:612, 1996.

269. ZIEGLER RG et al: Dietary carotene and vitamin A and risk of lung cancer among white men in New Jersey. J Natl Cancer Inst 73:1429, 1984.

270. ZIEGLER RG et al: Carotenoid intake, vegetables, and the risk of lung cancer among white men in New Jersey. Am J Epidemiol 123:1080, 1986.

271. NOMURA AMY et al: Serum micronutrients and upper aerodigestive tract cancer. Cancer Epidemiol Biomark Prev 6:407, 1997.

272. CLINTON SK et al: cis-trans Lycopene isomers, carotenoids, and retinol in the human prostate. Cancer Epidemiol Biomark Prev 5:823, 1996.

273. ZHANG S et al: Measurement of retinoids and carotenoids in breast adipose tissue and a comparison of concentrations in breast cancer cases and control subjects. Am J Clin Nutr 66:626, 1997.

274. KIM M et al: Preventive effect of green tea polyphenols on colon carcinogenesis, in Food Phytochemicals for Cancer Prevention II. Teas, Spices, and Herbs, C-T Ho et al (eds). Washington, DC, American Chemical Society, 1994, pp 51–55.

275. JI B-T et al: Green tea consumption and the risk of pancreatic and colorectal cancers. Int J Cancer 70:255, 1997.

276. KELLOFF GJ, BOONE CW (eds): Clinical development plan: Tea extracts, green tea polyphenols, epigallocatechin gallate. J Cell Biochem 26S(Suppl):236, 1996.

277. YANG CS et al: Effects of tea on carcinogenesis in animal models and humans, in Dietary Phytochemicals in Cancer Prevention and Treatment, American Institute for Cancer Research (ed). New York, Plenum Press, 1996, pp 51–61.

278. STONER GD, MUKHTAR H: Polyphenols as cancer chemopreventive agents. J Cell Biochem 22(Suppl):169, 1995.

279. ANONYMOUS: Food Phytochemicals for Cancer Prevention II. Teas, Spices, and Herbs. Washington, DC, American Chemical Society, 1994, p 51.

280. MICHNOVICZ JJ, BRADLOW HL: Dietary cytochrome P-450 modifiers in the control of estrogen metabolism, in Food Phytochemicals for Cancer Prevention I. Fruits and Vegetables, M-T Huang et al (eds). Washington, DC, American Chemical Society, 1994, pp 282–293.

281. STEINMETZ KA, POTTER JD: Vegetables, fruit, and cancer. I. Epidemiology. Cancer Causes Control 2:325, 1991.

282. FONG AT et al: Modulation of diethylnitrosamine-induced hepatocarcinogenesis and O6-ethylguanine formation in rainbow trout by indole-3-carbinol, beta-naphthoflavone, and Aroclor 1254. Toxicol Appl Pharmacol 96:93, 1988.

283. DASHWOOD RH et al: Quantitative inter-relationships between aflatoxin B1 carcinogen dose, indole-3-carbinol anti-carcinogen dose, target organ DNA adduction and final tumor response. Carcinogenesis 10:175, 1989.

284. BRESNICK E et al: Reduction in mammary tumorigenesis in the rat by cabbage and cabbage residue. Carcinogenesis 11:1159, 1990.

285. VERHOEVEN DTH et al: A review of mechanisms underlying anticarcinogenicity by brassica vegetables. Chem Biol Interact 103:79, 1997.

286. KELLOFF GJ et al: Clinical development plan: Indole-3-carbinol. J Cell Biochem 26S(Suppl):127, 1996.

287. KELLOFF GJ et al: Clinical development plan: Phenethyl isothiocyanate. J Cell Biochem 26S(Suppl):149, 1996.

288. ZHANG Y et al: A major inducer of anticarcinogenic protective enzymes from broccoli: Isolation and elucidation of structure. Proc Natl Acad Sci USA 89(6):2399, 1992.

289. FAHEY JW et al: Broccoli sprouts: An exceptionally rich source of inducers of enzymes that protect against chemical carcinogens. Proc Natl Acad Sci USA 94:10367, 1997.

290. KATO I, NOMURA AMY: Alcohol in the aetiology of upper aerodigestive tract cancer. Eur J Cancer B Oral Oncol 30B(2):75, 1994.

291. DRIVER HE, SWANN PF: Alcohol and human cancer (review). Anticancer Res 7:309, 1987.

292. LONGNECKER MP: Alcohol consumption and risk of cancer in humans: An overview. Alcohol 12:87, 1995.

293. LONGNECKER MP: Alcoholic beverage consumption in relation to risk of breast cancer: Meta-analysis and review. Cancer Causes Control 5:73, 1994.

294. KUNE GA, VITETTA L: Alcohol consumption and the etiology of colorectal cancer: A review of the scientific evidence from 1957 to 1991. Nutr Cancer 18:97, 1992.

295. HIATT RA: Alcohol consumption and breast cancer. Med Oncol Tumor Pharmacother 7:143, 1990.

296. HAYES RB et al: Alcohol use and prostate cancer risk in US blacks and whites. Am J Epidemiol 143:692, 1996.

297. SCHATZKIN A, LONGNECKER MP: Alcohol and breast cancer: Where are we now and where do we go from here? Cancer 74(3)(Suppl):1101, 1994.

298. SPITZ MR: Risk factors and genetic susceptibility. Cancer Treat Res 74:73, 1995.

299. TAVANI A et al: Risk factors for esophageal cancer in life-long nonsmokers. Cancer Epidemiol Biomark Prev 3:387, 1994.

300. BLOT WJ: Esophageal cancer trends and risk factors. Semin Oncol 21:403, 1994.

301. TAKEZAKI T et al: Tobacco, alcohol and dietary factors associated with the risk of oral cancer among Japanese. Jpn J Cancer Res 87:555, 1996.

302. VAN DEN BRANDT PA et al: Alcohol and breast cancer: Results from the Netherlands Cohort Study. Am J Epidemiol 141(10):907, 1995.

303. LEVI F et al: Alcohol and breast cancer in the Swiss Canton of Vaud. Eur J Cancer 32A:2108, 1996.

304. LONGNECKER MP et al: Lifetime alcohol consumption and breast cancer risk among postmenopausal women in Los Angeles. Cancer Epidemiol Biomark Prev 4:721, 1995.

305. SWANSON CA et al: Alcohol consumption and breast cancer risk among women under age 45 years. Epidemiology 8:231, 1997.

306. GAPSTUR SM et al: Synergistic effect between alcohol and estrogen replacement therapy on risk of breast cancer differs

by estrogen/progesterone receptor status in the Iowa Women's Health Study. Cancer Epidemiol Biomark Prev 4:313, 1995.

307. GINSBURG ES et al: Effects of alcohol ingestion on estrogens in postmenopausal women. JAMA 276:1747, 1996.

308. LONGNECKER MP: Do hormones link alcohol with breast cancer? J Natl Cancer Inst 85:692, 1993.

309. REICHMAN ME et al: Effects of alcohol consumption on plasma and urinary hormone concentrations in premenopausal women. J Natl Cancer Inst 85:722, 1993.

310. FREUDENHEIM JL et al: Risks associated with source of fiber and fiber components in cancer of the colon and rectum. Cancer Res 50:3295, 1990.

311. SWANSON CA et al: Moderate alcohol consumption and the risk of endometrial cancer. Epidemiology 4:530, 1993.

312. NEWCOMB PA et al: Alcohol consumption in relation to endometrial cancer risk. Cancer Epidemiol Biomark Prev 6:775, 1997.

313. SLATTERY ML, WEST DW: Smoking, alcohol, coffee, tea, caffeine, and theobromine: Risk of prostate cancer in Utah (United States). Cancer Causes Control 4:559, 1993.

314. DE STEFANI E et al: Tobacco, alcohol, diet and risk of prostate cancer. Tumori 81:315, 1995.

315. ANDERSSON S-O et al: Lifestyle factors and prostate cancer risk: A case-control study in Sweden. Cancer Epidemiol Biomark Prev 5:509, 1996.

316. FRANCESHI S, LA VECCHIA C: Alcohol and the risk of cancers of the stomach and colon-rectum. Dig Dis 12:276, 1994.

317. LONGNECKER MP et al: A meta-analysis of alcoholic beverage consumption in relation to risk of colorectal cancer. Cancer Causes Control 1:59, 1990.

318. GIOVANNUCCI E et al: Alcohol, low-methionine-low-folate diets, and risk of colon cancer in men. J Natl Cancer Inst 87:265, 1995.

319. GLYNN SA et al: Alcohol consumption and risk of colorectal cancer in a cohort of Finnish men. Cancer Causes Control 7:214, 1996.

320. SCHEUPLEIN RJ: Perspectives on toxicological risk—an example: Foodborne carcinogenic risk. Crit Rev Food Sci Nutr 32(2):105, 1992.

321. AMES BN, GOLD LS: Dietary carcinogens, environmental pollution, and cancer: Some misconceptions. Med Oncol Tumor Pharmacother 7(2/3):69, 1990.

322. ABBOTT PJ: Carcinogenic chemicals in food: Evaluating the health risk. Food Chem Toxicol 30(4):327, 1992.

323. STRICKLAND PT, GROOPMAN JD: Biomarkers for assessing environmental exposure to carcinogens in the diet. Am J Clin Nutr 61:710s, 1995.

324. DIPPLE A: DNA adducts of chemical carcinogens. Carcinogenesis 16(3):437, 1995.

325. BELAND FA, POIRIER MC: Significance of DNA adduct studies in animal models for cancer molecular dosimetry and risk assessment. Environ Health Perspect 99:5, 1993.

326. GOLD LS et al: The sixth plot of the Carcinogenic Potency Database: Results of animal bioassays published in the general literature 1989 to 1990 and by the National Toxicology Program 1990 to 1993. Environ Health Perspect 103:3, 1995.

327. AMES BN: Profet M. Nature's pesticides. Nat Toxins 1:2, 1992.

328. AMES BN, GOLD LS: Animal cancer tests and cancer prevention. J Natl Cancer Inst Monogr 12:125, 1992.

329. PHILLIPS DH: DNA adducts derived from safrole, estragole and related compounds, and from benzene and its metabolites, in DNA Adducts: Identification and Biological Significance, K Hemminki et al (eds). Lyon, International Agency for Research on Cancer (IARC Scientific Publications No. 125), 1994, pp 131–140.

330. HOWES AJ et al: Structure-specificity of the genotoxicity of some naturally occurring alkenylbenzenes determined by the unscheduled DNA synthesis assay in rat hepatocytes. Food Chem Toxicol 28(8):537, 1990.

331. WAGSTAFF DJ: Dietary exposure to furocoumarins. Regul Toxicol Pharmacol 14:261, 1991.

332. IARC WORKING GROUP: IARC Monographs on the Evaluation of Carcinogenic Risks to Humans, Vol 56. Lyon, International Agency for Research on Cancer, 1993.

333. GONZALEZ FJ: Genetic polymorphism and cancer susceptibility: Fourteenth Sapporo Cancer Seminar. Cancer Res 55:710, 1995.

334. GROOPMAN JD et al: Epidemiology of human aflatoxin exposures and their relationship to liver cancer. Prog Clin Biol Res 395:211, 1996.

335. WANG L-Y et al: Aflatoxin exposure and risk of hepatocellular carcinoma in Taiwan. Int J Cancer 67:620, 1996.

336. GROOPMAN JD et al: Molecular biomarkers for aflatoxins and their application to human cancer prevention. Cancer Res 54:1907S, 1994.

337. YU F-L et al: Studies on the binding and transcriptional properties of aflatoxin $B_1$-8,9-epoxide. Carcinogenesis 15(8):1737, 1994.

338. QIAN G-S et al: A follow-up study of urinary markers of aflatoxin exposure and liver cancer risk in Shanghai, People's Republic of China. Cancer Epidemiol Biomark Prev 3:3, 1994.

339. ROSS RK et al: Urinary aflatoxin biomarkers and risk of hepatocellular carcinoma. Lancet 339(8799):943, 1992.

340. KENSLER TW et al: Chemoprotection by inducers of electrophile detoxication enzymes. Basic Life Sci 61:127, 1993.

341. BREINHOLT V et al: Dietary chlorophyllin is a potent inhibitor of aflatoxin $B_1$ hepatocarcinogenesis in rainbow trout. Cancer Res 55:57, 1995.

342. VAN EGMOND HP: Rationale for regulatory programmes for mycotoxins in human foods and animal feeds. Food Additives Contam 10(1):29, 1993.

343. EISENBRAND G, TANG W: Food-borne heterocyclic amines. Chemistry, formation, occurrence and biological activities. A literature review. Toxicology 84:1, 1993.

344. LIJINSKY W: The formation and occurrence of polynuclear aromatic hydrocarbons associated with food. Mutation Res 259:251, 1991.

345. DIPPLE A et al: Chemical and mutagenic specificities of polycyclic aromatic hydrocarbon carcinogens. Adv Exp Med Biol 354:101, 1994.

346. PERERA FP et al: Carcinogen-DNA adducts in human breast tissue. Cancer Epidemiol Biomark Prev 4:233, 1995.

347. STAVRIC B: Biological significance of trace levels of mutagenic heterocyclic aromatic amines in human diet: A critical review. Food Chem Toxicol 32(10):977, 1994.

348. NAGAO M, SUGIMURA T: Carcinogenic factors in food with relevance to colon cancer development. Mutation Res 290:43, 1993.

349. GOODERHAM NJ et al: Assessing human risk to heterocyclic amines. Mutation Res 376:53, 1997.

350. ADAMSON RH et al: Extrapolation of heterocyclic amine carcinogenesis data from rodents and nonhuman primates to humans. Arch Toxicol 18(Suppl):303, 1996.

351. VINEIS P: Biomarkers, low-dose carcinogenesis and dietary exposures. Eur J Cancer Prev 6:147, 1997.

352. SKOG K et al: Effect of cooking temperature on the formation of

heterocyclic amines in fried meat products and pan residues. Carcinogenesis 16(4):861, 1995.

353. JOHANSSON MAE, JÄGERSTAD M: Occurrence of mutagenic/carcinogenic heterocyclic amines in meat and fish products, including pan residues, prepared under domestic conditions. Carcinogenesis 15(8):1511, 1994.

354. LAYTON DW et al: Cancer risk of heterocyclic amines in cooked foods: An analysis and implications for research. Carcinogenesis 16(1):39, 1995.

355. FELTON JS et al: Chemical analysis, prevention, and low-level dosimetry of heterocyclic amines from cooked food. Cancer Res 52:2103S, 1992.

356. KADERLIK KR et al: Metabolic activation pathway for the formation of DNA adducts of the carcinogen 2-amino-1-methyl-6-phenylimidazo[4,5-b]pyridine (PhIP) in rat extrahepatic tissues. Carcinogenesis 15(8):1703, 1994.

357. SNYDERWINE EG et al: DNA adduct levels of 2-amino-1-methyl-6-phenylimidazo-[4,5b]pyridine (PhIP) in tissues of cynomolgus monkeys after single or multiple dosing. Carcinogenesis 15(12):2757, 1994.

358. DAVIS CD et al: Enzymatic phase II activation of the N-hydroxylamines of IQ, MeIQx, and PhIP by various organs of monkeys and rats. Carcinogenesis 14(10):2091, 1993.

359. PFAU W et al: Pancreatic DNA adducts formed in vitro and in vivo by the food mutagens 2-amino-1-methyl-6-phenylimidazo[4,5-b]pyridine (PhIP) and 2-amino-3-methyl-9H-pyrido[2,3-b]indole (MeA″C). Mutation Res 378:13, 1997.

360. SCHUT HAJ et al: Formation and persistence of DNA adducts of 2-amino-3-methylimidazo[4,5-f]quinoline (IQ) in CDF₁ mice fed a high omega-3 fatty acid diet. Mutation Res 378:23, 1997.

361. KRISTIANSEN E et al: The ability of two cooked food mutagens to induce aberrant crypt foci in mice. Eur J Cancer Prev 6:53, 1997.

362. LANG NP et al: Rapid metabolic phenotypes for acetyltransferase and cytochrome P4501A2 and putative exposure to foodborne heterocyclic amines increase the risk for colorectal cancer or polyps. Cancer Epidemiol Biomark Prev 3:675, 1994.

363. KADLUBAR FE et al: Polymorphisms for aromatic amine metabolism in humans: Relevance for human carcinogenesis. Environ Health Perspect 98:69, 1992.

364. STILLWELL WG et al: Human urinary excretion of sulfamate and glucuronide conjugates of 2-amino-3,8-dimethylimidazo[4,5-f]quinoxaline (MeIQx). Cancer Epidemiol Biomark Prev 3:339, 1994.

365. LYNCH AM et al: Intra- and interindividual variability in systemic exposure in humans to 2-amino-3,8-dimethylimidazo[4,5-f]quinoxaline and 2-amino-1-methyl-6-phenylimidazo[4,5-b]pyridine, carcinogens present in cooked beef. Cancer Res 52:6216, 1992.

366. JI H et al: Urinary excretion of 2-amino-3,8-dimethylimidazo[4,5-f]quinoxaline in white, black, and Asian men in Los Angeles County. Cancer Epidemiol Biomark Prev 3:407, 1994.

367. GHOSHAL A et al: Induction of mammary tumors in female Sprague-Dawley rats by the food-derived carcinogen 2-amino-1-methyl-6-phenylimidazo[4,5-b]pyridine and effect of dietary fat. Carcinogenesis 15(11):2429, 1994.

368. WEISBURGER JH et al: Role of fat and calcium in cancer causation by food mutagens, heterocyclic amines. Proc Soc Exp Biol Med 205(4):347, 1994.

369. RYDEN P, ROBERTSON JA: The effect of fibre source and fermentation on the apparent hydrophobic binding properties of wheat bran preparations for the mutagen 2-amino-3,8-dimethylimidazo [4,5-f]quinoxaline (MeIQx). Carcinogenesis 16(2):209, 1995.

370. TSUDA H et al: Chemopreventive effects of β-carotene, α-tocopherol and five naturally occurring antioxidants in initiation of hepatocarcinogenesis by 2-amino-3-methylimidazo [4,5-f]quinoline in the rat. Jpn J Cancer Res 85:1214, 1994.

371. DE STEFANI E et al: Meat intake, heterocyclic amines, and risk of breast cancer: A case-control study in Uruguay. Cancer Epidemiol Biomark Prev 6:573, 1997.

372. HATTEMER-FREY HA, TRAVIS CC: Benzo-a-pyrene: Environmental partitioning and human exposure. Toxicol Ind Health 7(3):141, 1991.

373. ROTHMAN N et al: Contribution of occupation and diet to white blood cell polycyclic aromatic hydrocarbon-DNA adducts in wildland firefighters. Cancer Epidemiol Biomark Prev 2:341, 1993.

374. VAN MAANEN JMS et al: Formation of aromatic DNA adducts in white blood cells in relation to urinary excretion of 1-hydroxypyrene during consumption of grilled meat. Carcinogenesis 15(10):2263, 1994.

375. HIETANEN E, BARTSCH H: Gastrointestinal cancers: Role of nitrosamines and free radicals. Eur J Cancer Prev 1(Suppl 3):51, 1992.

376. TRICKER AR, PREUSSMANN R: Carcinogenic N-nitrosamines in the diet: Occurrence, formation, mechanisms and carcinogenic potential. Mutation Res 259:277, 1991.

377. THORGEIRSSON UP et al: Tumor incidence in a chemical carcinogenesis study of nonhuman primates. Regul Toxicol Pharmacol 19:130, 1994.

378. SHUKER DEG, BARTSCH H: DNA adducts of nitrosamines, in DNA Adducts: Identification and Biological Significance, K Hemminki et al (eds). Lyon, International Agency for Research on Cancer (IARC Scientific Publications No. 125), 1994, pp 73–89.

379. SHENOY NR, CHOUGHULEY ASU: Inhibitory effect of diet related sulphydryl compounds on the formation of carcinogenic nitrosamines. Cancer Lett 65:227, 1992.

380. HELSER MA et al: Influence of fruit and vegetable juices on the endogenous formation of N-nitrosoproline and N-nitrosothiazolidine-4-carboxylic acid in humans on controlled diets. Carcinogenesis 13(12):2277, 1992.

381. XU GP et al: Effects of fruit juices, processed vegetable juice, orange peel and green tea on endogenous formation of N-nitrosoproline in subjects from a high-risk area for gastric cancer in Moping County, China. Eur J Cancer Prev 2:327, 1993.

382. KELLOFF GJ et al: Chemopreventive drug development: Perspectives and progress. Cancer Epidemiol Biomark Prev 3:85, 1994.

383. FRIEND SH et al: Oncogenes and tumor-suppressing genes. N Engl J Med 318:618, 1988.

384. STEELE VE et al: Preclinical efficacy evaluation of potential chemopreventive agents in animal carcinogenesis models: Methods and results from the NCI chemoprevention drug development program. J Cell Biochem 20(Suppl):32, 1994.

385. KELLOFF GJ et al: Risk biomarkers and current strategies for cancer chemoprevention. J Cell Biochem 25S:1, 1996.

386. KELLOFF GJ et al: Progress in cancer chemoprevention: Perspectives on agent selection and short-term clinical intervention trials. Cancer Res 54(Suppl):2015S, 1994.

387. KELLOFF GJ et al: Approaches to the development and marketing approval of drugs that prevent cancer. Cancer Epidemiol Biomark Prev 4:1, 1995.

388. HONG WK, LIPPMAN SM: Cancer chemoprevention. J Natl Cancer Inst Monogr 17:49, 1995.

389. KAAKS RJ: Biochemical markers as additional measurements in studies of the accuracy of dietary questionnaire measurements: Conceptual issues. Am J Clin Nutr 65:1232, 1997.

390. BLACK AE et al: Measurements of total energy expenditure provide insights into the validity of dietary measurements of energy intake. J Am Diet Assoc 93:572, 1993.

391. ANDERSEN LF et al: Very-long-chain n-3 fatty acids as biomarkers for intake of fish and n-3 fatty acid concentrates. Am J Clin Nutr 64:305, 1996.

392. GODLEY PA et al: Correlation between biomarkers of omega-3 fatty acid consumption and questionnaire data in African American and Caucasian United States males with and without prostatic carcinoma. Cancer Epidemiol Biomark Prev 5:115, 1996.

393. SCHATZKIN A et al: The Polyp Prevention Trial I: Rationale, design, recruitment, and baseline participant characteristics. Cancer Epidemiol Biomark Prev 5:375, 1996.

394. LANZA E et al: The Polyp Prevention Trial II: Dietary intervention program and participant baseline dietary characteristics. Cancer Epidemiol Biomark Prev 5:385, 1996.

395. HENDERSON MM: Nutritional aspects of breast cancer. Cancer 76:2053, 1995.

396. BLOT WJ et al: Nutrition intervention trials in Linxian, China: Supplementation with specific vitamin/mineral combinations, cancer incidence, and disease-specific mortality in the general population. J Natl Cancer Inst 85:1483, 1993.

397. LI J-Y et al: Nutrition intervention trials in Linxian, China: Multiple vitamin/mineral supplementation, cancer incidence, and disease-specific mortality among adults with esophageal dysplasia. J Natl Cancer Inst 85:1492, 1993.

398. MARK SD et al: The effect of vitamin and mineral supplementation on esophageal cytology: Results from the Linxian Dysplasia Trial. Int J Cancer 57:162, 1994.

399. BURING JE, HENNEKENS CH: The Women's Health Study: Summary of the study design. J Myocardial Ischemia 4:27, 1993.

400. BURING JE, HENNEKENS CH: The Women's Health Study: Rationale and background. J Myocardial Ischemia 4:30, 1993.

401. OMENN GS et al: Risk factors for lung cancer and for intervention effects in CARET, the Beta-Carotene and Retinol Efficacy Trial. J Natl Cancer Inst 88:1550, 1996.

402. HENNEKENS CH et al: Lack of effect of long-term supplementation with beta carotene on the incidence of malignant neoplasms and cardiovascular disease. N Engl J Med 334:1145, 1996.

403. ALBANES D et al: α-Tocopherol and β-carotene supplements and lung cancer incidence in the Alpha-Tocopherol, Beta-Carotene Cancer Prevention Study: Effects of base-line characteristics and study compliance. J Natl Cancer Inst 88:1560, 1996.

404. OMENN GS et al: Effects of a combination of beta carotene and vitamin A on lung cancer and cardiovascular disease. N Engl J Med 334:1150, 1996.

405. RAUTALAHTI M et al: Beta-carotene did not work: Aftermath of the ATBC study. Cancer Lett 114:235, 1997.

406. POTTER JD: β-Carotene and the role of intervention studies. Cancer Lett 114:329, 1997.

407. ERDMAN JW et al: Beta-carotene and the carotenoids: Beyond the intervention trials. Nutr Rev 54:185, 1996.

408. MAYNE ST et al: β-Carotene and lung cancer promotion in heavy smokers—A plausible relationship? J Natl Cancer Inst 88:1513, 1996.

409. NISHINO H: Cancer chemoprevention by natural carotenoids and their related compounds. J Cell Biochem 22(Suppl):231, 1995.

410. ISHIBE N, KELSEY KT: Genetic susceptibility to environmental and occupational cancers. Cancer Causes Control 8:504, 1997.

411. ROBERTS-THOMSON IC et al: Diet, acetylator phenotype, and risk of colorectal neoplasia. Lancet 347:1372, 1996.

412. WELFARE MR et al: Relationship between acetylator status, smoking, diet and colorectal cancer risk in the north-east of England. Carcinogenesis 18:1351, 1997.

413. ARAGAKI CC et al: Hierarchical modeling of gene-environment interactions: Estimating NAT2* genotype-specific dietary effects on adenomatous polyps. Cancer Epidemiol Biomark Prev 6:307, 1997.

414. BYAR DP, FREEDMAN LS: Clinical trials in diet and cancer. Prev Med 18:203, 1989.

415. WEED DL: Meta-analysis under the microscope. J Natl Cancer Inst 89:904, 1997.

416. HEBERT JR, MILLER DR: Methodologic considerations for investigating the diet-cancer link. Am J Clin Nutr 47:1068, 1988.

417. WILLETT WC et al: The use of a self-administered questionnaire to assess diet four years in the past. Am J Epidemiol 127:188, 1988.

418. KUSHI LH: Gaps in epidemiologic research methods: Design considerations for studies that use food-frequency questionnaires. Am J Clin Nutr 59:180S, 1994.

419. JACQUES PF et al: Comparison of micronutrient intake measured by a dietary questionnaire and biochemical indicators of micronutrient status. Am J Clin Nutr 57:182, 1993.

420. FESKANICH D et al: Reproducibility and validity of food intake measurements from a semiquantitative food frequency questionnaire. J Am Diet Assoc 93:790, 1993.

421. MERTZ W et al: What are people really eating? The relation between energy intake derived from estimated diet records and intake determined to maintain body weight. Am J Clin Nutr 54:291, 1991.

422. HEBERT JR et al: Social desirability bias in dietary self-report may compromise the validity of dietary intake measures. Int J Epidemiol 24:389, 1995.

423. ROCK CL et al: Responsiveness of carotenoids to a high vegetable diet intervention designed to prevent breast cancer recurrence. Cancer Epidemiol Biomark Prev 6:617, 1997.

424. SCHATZKIN A et al: Surrogate end points in cancer research: A critique. Cancer Epidemiol Biomark Prev 5:947, 1996.

# CARCINOGENESIS BY PHYSICAL AGENTS

*Joel S. Greenberger*

## INTRODUCTION

Perhaps the best understood system of physical carcinogenesis has come from evaluation of ionizing irradiation–induced leukemias and lymphomas in experimental animals and in humans. Classic examples from the first half of the twentieth century include the development of osteogenic sarcoma of the jaw in radium watch-dial painters, the induction of acute leukemia in British patients treated with orthovoltage irradiation for ankylosing spondylitis, and leukemia development in the epillated survivors of the atomic bombings at Hiroshima and Nagasaki. These examples have emphasized the importance of understanding the risks and epidemiology of ionizing irradiation–induced tumors. However, there are numerous other reports of induction of tumors by other physical agents that are also of potential importance to the surgical oncologist. There remains a significant concern for induction of squamous cell and basal cell carcinomas of the skin and malignant melanoma by ultraviolet (UV) irradiation. There is also epidemiologic evidence for the association of an increased risk of skin carcinogenesis by UV radiation exposure in specific genotypic human populations.

In this chapter, I will review the basic science data, clinical observations, and clinical epidemiologic evidence for induction of tumors in humans and experimental animals by physical agents. There is concern over the risk of living in the vicinity of nuclear power reactors. There remains continuing concern about nuclear irradiation accidents, widespread use of radioisotopes in clinical medicine, and expanding use of linear accelerators and other radiotherapy devices in the treatment of cancer. Therefore, ionizing irradiation–induced tumors should remain the most notable focus in carcinogenesis in the sociopolitical environment of the twenty-first century. I will review data on UV-light carcinogenesis and the evidence (or lack thereof) for induction of leukemia and solid tumors by microwave irradiation, electromagnetic irradiation (EMR), and hyperthermia-associated tumors.

As is the case with many inherited or acquired forms of cancer, the involvement of physical agents in carcinogenesis occurs in an association with multiple other factors, including the genetic background of the affected population (or inbred animal strain); the presence of cocarcinogens in the environment, including dietary factors; and the past or synchronous exposure to alkylating agents or other chemotherapeutic agents in the setting of radiation therapy–associated carcinogenesis. This chapter should provide the surgical oncologist with basic background information on relevant principles of radiation biology and molecular biology of use in assessing the role of a suspect physical carcinogen in the etiology of a specific tumor. The information may be of value in determining the influence of these factors in patients presenting with other specific medical and surgical conditions.

## HISTORICAL OVERVIEW

### THERMAL CARCINOGENESIS

There has been an anecdotal association of tumor formation at the site of wound healing in thermal burn recovery. These clinical observations led to basic cell biology experiments in the role of heat alone or with ionizing irradiation in carcinogenesis.[1–4] The proliferative response of fibroblasts, endothelial cells, and other connective tissue elements in wound healing and burn recovery has been well studied.[2] Initial reports of formation of squamous cell carcinomas, desmoid tumors, or soft tissue sarcomas at the site of burn injuries have been confirmed, but the incidence is very low.[2] In the recent era of burn therapy using sulfadiazine and nitrate-based compounds, as well as other wound-healing topical treatments, concern has arisen for possible cocarcinogenic effects of these agents, systemic agents as well as steroids in organ transplant recipients, broad-spectrum antibiotics and their carrier vehicles, as well as some of the associated systemic agents that are delivered to recovering burn patients.[2]

Animal model systems have demonstrated the role of heat injury as a carcinogen or cocarcinogen.[1,3,4] Hyperthermia can be synergistic with ionizing irradiation for cell killing.[4] The effects of hyperthermia on modulation of irradiation carcinogenic effects in vitro have also been described.[4] Heat injury and ionizing irradiation are very different with respect to the mechanisms of molecular biologic damage. Although ionizing irradiation has been classically defined as a primary damaging agent for nuclear DNA, recent evidence suggests that this damage is communicated to cytoplasmic organelles, including the mitochondria, by transfer of stress-activating protein kinase (SAP-kinase) molecules to the mitochondrial membrane.[5] Transfer of other stress-induced proteins, including BAX, BAD, and p53 from nucleus to mitochondria, has been demonstrated in heat as well as UV and x-irradiation exposure.[5,6] Localization of these molecules at the mitochondria has been shown to increase mitochondrial permeability, leakage of cytochrome C, and activation of the caspase pathway, resulting in nuclear fragmentation and apoptosis.[5] Hyperthermic induction of similar forms of molecular damage has recently been demonstrated.[4] Since heat-induced malignant transformation of cells in culture has been associated with doses in the linear portion of the heat survival curve, in the sublethal or repairable dose range it has been hypothesized that repair mechanisms for heat injury may incorporate in some respects the repair mechanisms for radiation injury. The heat shock proteins (HSPs) in yeast have been demonstrated to be the most important analogs of the SAP kinases in mammalian cells.[7] Heat shock injury, eliciting a repair process in yeast, bacteria, and mammalian cells, has been associated with activation of repair mechanisms that can lead to misrepair of DNA,[7] induction of mutations,[7] and accumulation of genetic lesions that may facilitate deregulation of repressor genes, activation of oncogenes, or both in malignant transformation.[4] A common pathway for the biologic sequelae of physical agent carcinogenesis may be the alteration of mutator gene transcripts, which can result in defective repair of point mutations and defective correction of infrequently occurring genetic lesions.[8]

In the clinic, the development of tumors at burn sites has usually been in the setting of massive total body or high-percentage surface area burns in which healing has been associated with significant scar formation.[2] Scar carcinogenesis resulting from heat injury, other wound repair injury, or chemical burns has also been associated with a detectable incidence of tumor formation at the site of the scar.[2]

The etiology of heat-associated carcinogenesis must be evaluated in concert with the potential role of the cytokine "storm" that follows heat injury.[2,9] Up-regulation of transcription and protein production of tumor growth factor β (TGF-β), interleukin 1 (IL-1), tumor necrosis factor α (TNF-α), and other cytokines associated with injury[9] may play a role in facilitating growth of a clone of cells with altered genotype, allowing uncontrolled proliferation. Such progression of cell growth may lead to rapid tumor formation in the setting of wound or burn repair. The incidence of these forms of tumor is very low,[2] but may be significantly increased in frequency in the setting of specific human genotypes that predispose a person to either a defective stress response and/or an altered cytokine response to injury.

## ELECTROMAGNETIC IRRADIATION–INDUCED CANCER

There has been significant concern in the lay press over the past two decades about the possibility of an increased incidence of certain forms of tumors in residential areas close to high-tension electrical power lines.[10–13] A prominent lawsuit against the New York Power and Light Company in the early 1980s accentuated the fear and concern about this possibility.[13] Experimental evidence for induction of tumors by radiation in the electromagnetic or microwave range is available from tissue culture and animal experiments.[14] Furthermore, cocarcinogenic effects of electromagnetic radiation (EMR) and x-rays have recently been reported.[14] The biologic effects of EMR on cells have been hypothesized to relate to reorientation of molecular structures in cells aligned with the source of the magnetic radiation.[14] Cells cultured within electromagnetic fields have been reported to show either minimal or no effects of such irradiation on cell doubling, saturation density, and chromosomal stability.[11]

With the advent of medical usage of nuclear magnetic resonance imaging (MRI), now common throughout the United States and much of the world, basic science and animal research studies have focused on the effects of prolonged exposure to EMR.[15] The data show a lack of convincing evidence for either a direct carcinogenic or indirect cocarcinogenic effect of irradiation in the microwave or EMR spectrum.[10–11,16–20] Because of continued community concern about the clustered incidence of cancer in specific regions geographically associated with high-voltage power lines, further investigation in this subject will undoubtedly be forthcoming.[13] The difficulty in attributing cancer clusters to a specific etiologic agent is not restricted to the concern about electromagnetic power lines. Similar concerns arose in Sheffield, England, and in areas of western Europe during the 1980s and 1990s with proliferation of nuclear power plants.[21] A recent review of the subject of cancer and leukemia clusters near nuclear power stations in the United Kingdom and Britain was reported at the International Congress on Molecular Biology of Cancer in Hamburg, Germany, in June of 1997.[21] Consensus reports from epidemiologists and pediatric and medical oncologists reviewing the data showed no association of cancer and leukemia clusters to the proximity of nuclear power stations. Similar analysis with respect to microwave or electromagnetic irradiation has also been published[15–20] and reveals no compelling, significant geographic association at this point.

A second recent concern in the United States has been over reports of brain tumor formation in individuals who used cellular telephones, holding such devices close to the temporal bone for prolonged periods. A recent report analyzing potential effects of electromagnetic irradiation from cellular telephones, including epidemiologic and cancer cluster data, confirmed the absence of a significant effect of cellular telephone usage to the incidence of brain tumors.[22,178] Nevertheless, it appears that concern about potential carcinogenic effects of microwave ovens, cellular telephones, and even EMR from the screens of personal computers continues to stimulate epidemiologic research into these areas. At the present time, there is no convincing evidence that any of these forms of radiation is carcinogenic or acts as a cocarcinogen with other environmental or chemical agents, except in isolated tissue culture experiments using permanent cell lines that may already be primed for malignant transformation.[14] Permanent tissue culture lines often have undergone one or multiple genetic changes associated with long-term passage in culture, and such changes can prime such cell lines for a rapid response to very low or even background levels of environmental factors such as medium change, temperature change, or pH changes.[22,23]

## ULTRAVIOLET IRRADIATION CARCINOGENESIS

There is clear evidence that UV irradiation induces multiple forms of clinical skin cancers in humans and experimental animals. This evidence is based on several strong epidemiologic studies of squamous cell carcinoma, basal cell carcinoma, and malignant melanoma. In these studies, the following conclusions have been clearly confirmed and reconfirmed:

1. The incidence of malignant melanoma, as well as other forms of skin cancer, is statistically significantly increased in individuals exposed to sunlight in a direct dose-response fashion.[24–31]
2. The incidence of malignant melanoma and other forms of skin cancer is significantly increased in fair-skinned white subjects exposed to UV irradiation.[32]
3. Residence at high altitudes (Boulder, Colorado, study) is associated with a significantly increased incidence of skin cancer for relatively equivalent times of exposure to sunlight compared to matched populations residing at sea level.[32,33]

With respect to squamous cell carcinoma and basal cell carcinoma, premalignant lesions are identified in regions of relatively increased UV exposure on the human body (nose, prominent zygomatic arch of the facial bones, ears, forehead, and top of the head in individuals with thinning hair or male pattern baldness).[33] Premalignant lesions, including actinic keratosis and dysplastic lesions, are increased in exposed areas of the body, such as arms, hands, and legs in individuals working outdoors in the sunlight for prolonged periods.[24,33]

The mechanism of cell killing by UV irradiation has prompted both the application of UV light in skin cell killing as in the use of psoralens and UV-A therapy for mycosis fungoides and hairy cell leukemia,[34] as well as the use of UV irradiation–attenuating sunblock agents in sunscreen products now widely used throughout the western world.[35]

The molecular mechanism of cell killing and carcinogenesis by UV irradiation has been rigorously studied. Unlike ionizing irradiation, UV irradiation affects tissues only to the degree of penetration of the visible light spectrum, usually 2 to 3 mm from the skin or intracavitary surface.[36–46] This knowledge has been useful in developing photodynamic therapy (PDT) of some cancers and premalignant lesions of the esophagus, airway, or abdominal or thoracic cavity.[47] Patients are administered Photofrin (protoporphyrin) systemically with uptake of the compound in all tissues, and then receive locally penetrating visible light through a thoracoscopic or esophagoscopic approach to provide local tumor killing only in the area of light exposure.[47] The limitations of this technique, in fact, represent the limitations of penetration into tissue of UV light in the visible (UV) spectrum, which is approximately 2 to 3 mm.[48–49]

Cell culture studies have documented the initial events in UV damage to cellular DNA.[31–35,50–53] Cyclobutane dimers are rapidly formed,[30,42,52] and it is the process of repair or misrepair of these dimers that causes point mutation, frameshift mutation, and (in some cases) base deletion mutations that can initiate the process of carcinogenesis.[30,31,36–42,50] Common, well-known molecular biologic pathways probably follow these genetic changes, including activation of oncogenes, inhibition of suppressor genes, or alteration of mutator genes.[8,40–41,49]

The process of UV light carcinogenesis alone or with topically applied chemicals[46] has been well-documented in animal models of skin carcinogenesis. Furthermore, specific in-bred mouse strains have been shown to display a higher incidence of skin carcinogenesis relative to dosage of light calculated in energy units of joules over UV irradiation exposure in other mouse strains. The role of induction of heat shock proteins, early response genes, stress response genes, and cytokine responses to DNA damage appears to be similar in UV-irradiated cells compared to those subjected to thermal injury or, as will be described, with ionizing irradiation injury.[7,8]

Of importance to the surgical oncologist is the association of UV-induced skin cancers with areas of sun exposure and other cocarcinogens associated with skin tumors. These include genotypic propensity in patients with xeroderma pigmentosum or other conditions, chemicals in the skin, or racial or ethnic epidemiologic predisposition.[24–31,50–53] Of prime importance is the early diagnosis of malignant melanoma, which has been recently facilitated by improved teaching methods and the widespread use of the Wallace-Clark staging system for scoring skin lesions.[54–59] A prime directive in teaching surgical oncology over the last three decades has been the systematic approach toward understanding the patterns of spread of malignant melanoma, and the role of lymph node dissection in the treatment of extremity lesions. Although surgical approaches to malignant melanoma have been largely limited to wide local excision and selective clinical trials of lymph node dissection, the routine use of prophylactic lymph node removal remains controversial. It is likely that immunologic and gene therapy approaches to the treatment of malignant melanoma will be prominent in the next decade.[59]

The clear association of UV irradiation with induction of squamous cell carcinoma, basal cell carcinoma, and malignant melanoma makes this physical agent a critical factor in the diagnosis and management of patients with skin malignancies and for analysis of the role of genotype in counseling their families who may be at risk for induction of similar tumors.

## CARCINOGENESIS BY IONIZING IRRADIATION

Within years after the discovery of radium by Marie and Pierre Curie in 1895, and x-irradiation by Konrad Roentgen in 1896, radiation workers began to report sporadic events of skin and bone tumors, first on the hands and later in other parts of the body, in close proximity to radiation sources.[60,61] The first radiation biology studies demonstrating tumorigenesis as a result of ionizing irradiation came from studies in rodents, hamsters, and other small mammals.[61] It was not until the 1940s, when low-voltage (orthovoltage) irradiation became commonly used to treat benign skin conditions, including acne, tonsillitis in children, and foot deformities, that a significant incidence of thyroid nodules and bone tumors in irradiated subjects was reported.[62–83] This clinical evidence was supported by other data from watch-dial painters, who used a radium-based luminescent paint and often licked the tips of their paintbrushes to apply the paint in small quantities to the numbers on watches. These individuals suffered a significant incidence of osteogenic sarcomas of the jaw.[1,61]

The atomic bomb explosions at Hiroshima and Nagasaki, Japan, in 1945, provided the first true evidence of the induction of leukemia in humans.[84] Although the loss of life from explosive heat, concussion, and fire from these bombings far exceeded the subsequent death from leukemia or other tumors, precise evaluation of the epillated survivors revealed a clear effect of ionizing irradiation on inducing leukemia in humans.[77,84–87] Further study of the second and third generations of the survivors of the Hiroshima and Nagasaki bombings has confirmed the original reports of William C. Moloney,[84] at the Atomic Bomb Casualty Commission, that despite the true detectable increased incidence, ionizing irradiation was in fact a relatively poor leukemogen in humans. This fact has been confirmed by many more recent studies showing that patients who received curative irradiation therapy alone for Hodgkin's disease had a lower incidence of secondary leukemia compared to those receiving combination chemotherapy and irradiation, particularly alkylating agents, in the combination chemotherapy regimen.[78,88–90] The data established that alkylating agent chemotherapy was in fact a potent leukemogenic stimulus in humans.[90] Although a relatively poor leukemogen compared to alkylating agents, there is much information in molecular biologic studies, animal experiments, and human epidemiology to support a clear hazard of ionizing irradiation as a carcinogen in humans. From the Japanese atomic bomb exposure in 1945, Chernobyl reactor accident in 1986, and in other irradiation contamination accidents, thyroid cancer induction from irradiation-produced iodine 131 is a clear hazard[75,91–92] and far exceeds the incidence of leukemia incidence.[93–102]

For the surgical oncologist, there are many situations in which previous exposure to ionizing irradiation may play a role not only in the etiology of a current cancer, but may also affect the likelihood of cancer recurrence, pattern of recurrence, or even the possibility of a second tumor formation.

## CURRENT STATUS OF PHYSICAL CARCINOGENESIS

This section deals in greater detail with review of recent information regarding ionizing irradiation carcinogenesis and leukemogenesis in humans and the risks to specific clinical populations.

### MOLECULAR MECHANISM OF IONIZING IRRADIATION INDUCTION OF LATE TISSUE EFFECTS, INCLUDING TUMOR FORMATION

Stem cells are defined as those cells capable of both self-renewal and differentiation to one or more pathways. These cells exist in nearly all human tissues, including bone marrow, skin, the gastrointestinal tract, and in most glandular tissues. Stem cells have recently been identified in the adult human brain, liver, and skeletal muscle. Current evidence suggests that all adult tissues have cells that could demonstrate the capacity for self-renewal and differentiation. Elegant experiments demonstrated that irradiation induction of chromosomal abnormalities occurred in the stem cells of mice such that transplantation of these stem cells resulted in the chromosomal marker being detected in multiple differentiated hematopoietic lineages.[103–107] Irradiation killing of stem cell populations was first demonstrated by Till and McCulloch[104] using the now classic colony-forming unit spleen (CFU-S) assay. Killing of stem cells by irradiation of the gastrointestinal tract demonstrated by Withers,[105] in the germ cells,[106] and other tissues confirmed the profound and significant effect of irradiation on killing the most primitive cells in each tissue. Irradiated stem cells were shown to be capable of repair by mechanisms of either sublethal damage repair or potentially lethal irradiation damage repair.[107] The molecular mechanisms of each form of repair have now been partially elucidated and shown to involve the rapid induction of early-response genes and transcriptional activators in the nucleus of irradiated cells, followed by transport of SAP kinases from the nucleus to mitochondria.[5,6]

The earliest molecular biologic steps in induction of early-response genes and transcriptional activators in the nucleus occur within minutes of exposure and follow even more rapid x-irradiation production of hydroxyl radicals, singlet oxygen molecules, and other free radical species that bind to DNA and cause strand breaks.[107] These radiation chemistry events occur within $10^{-13}$ seconds of exposure.[107] These molecular biologic responses are an order of magnitude slower than those of radiation chemotherapy, but still rapid in a cell biology time frame. Transport from nucleus to mitochondria of other molecules, including BAX and BAD, and resultant increase over the next 30 to 60 min of mitochondrial membrane permeability, leakage of cytochrome C, and activation of caspases, poly(adenosine diphosphate-ribose) polymerase (PARP), and DNA fragmentation follow.[5,6] The earliest postirradiation events have been elucidated in hematopoietic cells and confirmed in epithelial cells in culture.[107–109]

The molecular pathways involved in irradiation damage and repair are highly complex and overlap with mechanisms of killing by withdrawal of growth factors and induction of apoptosis by tumor necrosis factor $\alpha$ (TNF-$\alpha$) or FAS binding to FAS ligand. A common pathway appears to be caspase 3.[6] Ionizing irradiation induces both apoptosis and blocks in the $G_1/S$ phase and $G_2/M$ phase of the cell cycle. These molecular biologic events have been shown to occur in vivo as well as in vitro.[6,110]

Secondary events following irradiation damage have also been shown to play a significant role in the mechanism of radiation killing and probably also in carcinogenesis. Irradiation is associated with induction of transcription of mRNA for TGF-$\beta$, TNF-$\alpha$, IL-1,[5,110] von Willebrand factor (vWf),[111] ICAM-1, and multiple other molecules involved in the tumoral and cell surface stress response to DNA-damaging agents.[110] Several of these stress response gene products can be cellular toxins themselves and contribute to cell death; for example, TNF-$\alpha$ shows a clear damaging effect in its release as a response to irradiation and adds to the damage induced by the irradiation itself.[110] Knowledge of the histopathologic correlates to the early x-ray-induced molecular biologic events include cellular swelling, cellular exudates, nuclear fragmentation, and blood vessel endothelial swelling. These findings led to studies attempting to protect normal tissues from irradiation damage through administration of corticosteroids, nonsteroidal anti-inflammatory agents, and other compounds designed to prevent the induction of free radical oxygen and hydroxyl radicals by irradiation.

The capacity of cells to repair irradiation damage appears to be both cell-type-specific and tissue-specific.[107] Spermatogonia and oogonia, as well as lymphocytes, have been shown to be most sensitive to irradiation, dying an intermitotic or interphase death.[107] Most hematopoietic and epithelial stem cells die a "mitotic" death, progressing through the $G_1/S$ phase and into $G_2$ phase, dying during mitosis.[107] It is well known that if cells are irradiated in logarithmic or growth phase and then placed into plateau phase, where cell contact is maintained and cell division is prevented, that the cells may continue to function physiologically for some time.[112] However, when these same cells are stimulated to divide, death occurs during mitosis.[112] A similar situation may occur in nondividing or nonproliferative tissues in vivo, such as those in the brain, muscle, and other connective tissues in the body. Injured, but nondying (nondividing), cells within tissues are known to up-regulate production of cellular adhesion molecules and serum amyloid A,[113] and also produce a delayed secondary burst of transcription of mRNA for genes in the cellular stress response, including TNF-$\beta$, TGF-$\alpha$, and IL-1.[110,114–115] Whether sustained production of cytokines following irradiation of injured and nondying cells and/or delayed secondary induction of production of these cytokine messages occurs as part of the carcinogenic process is not known. However, the late effects of irradiation damage are believed to be attributable to delayed effects on slowly proliferating or nonproliferating tissues.[107,110]

The late sequelae of irradiation damage usually involve migration into the irradiated field of fibroblasts and resulting scar formation. Thickening and "woodiness" of heavily irradiated areas of human skin and muscle is known to occur from 18 months to 2 years after irradiation.[118,119] The most common site of this delayed injury is in muscle tissue following 6500 to 7000 cGy irradiation over 7 weeks to the extremities for radiation therapy of soft tissue sarcomas.[116–119]

Many of the patients who are cured and survive for many years develop delayed radiation fibrosis in the heavily irradiated tissue.[107,110] With moderate doses of irradiation in the range of 4500 to 5000 cGy to the chest wall, as in primary radical radiotherapy of breast cancer, thickening of the skin over the chest where the entry point of the medial tangent occurs, and along the anterior axillary line where the lateral tangent enters, has been well documented.[117] The late irradiation effects of fibrosis in the pelvis often produce bladder fibrosis, resulting in a decrease in bladder volume seen in cervical and endometrial cancer patients who are cured by radical radiotherapy to the pelvis.[119] Similar late fibrosis occurs in the anterior rectal wall and bladder of men irradiated with external beam therapy for prostate cancer at a radiation volume usually in the upper region of the prostate radiotherapy dosage. These adult male survivors may develop clinically relevant fibrosis of the anterior rectal wall.

The late effects of radiotherapy on induction of scar formation or fibrosis are quite relevant to the understanding of radiation carcinogenesis. Several studies have documented a low but detectable increased incidence of leukemia or solid tumor formation following megavoltage irradiation for extremity lesions, intra-abdominal tumors, thoracic tumors, as well as endometrial tumors or other pelvic malignancies.[94,119–144] The incidence in each example is low, and in some cases is not statistically significant above control age-matched cohorts. In contrast, patients treated with orthovoltage irradiation (using lower-energy x-rays with a greater degree of bone resorption), particularly those receiving multiple courses of small fractions of radiotherapy over several years (as was the case in the treatment of children with histiocytosis X, and in British patients with ankylosing spondylitis), have a higher incidence of secondary leukemia.[64–90] Radiation biologists have hypothesized that the lower fractional doses occurring over multiple cycles over multiple years provide for a "mutagenic" dose to the hematopoietic microenvironment, including stromal cells and hematopoietic stem cells, rather than the lethal dose that is sustained by modern megavoltage radiotherapy, which delivers 6 to 7 weeks of higher doses per fraction using higher-energy beams with ultimately less bone resorption[107,145–167] (Fig. 1B-13C).

Although the incidence of leukemia induced by irradiation is increased by smaller fractions of orthovoltage irradiation, a reverse phenomenon appears to be true for the induction of bone tumors by radiotherapy. Ionizing irradiation has been reported to induce osteogenic sarcoma,[128] chondrosarcoma,[128] and other sarcomas[117] in patients receiving high doses of irradiation to isolated bones, usually for treatment of childhood tumors.[90,128] The incidence is quite low but is above background control levels.[78] The incidence is decreased in children who have received megavoltage irradiation therapy for treatment of malignancies of childhood compared to those patients treated in the 1940s and 1950s who received orthovoltage irradiation.[72] Since in the current era patients presenting with bone tumors who have a history of radiation therapy will have received megavoltage irradiation beams, further detectable incidence is expected to be very low.

There has been significant concern in recent years about the possible induction of breast cancer in children treated for Hodgkin's disease[138–140,168] and of lung cancer by irradiation in women treated with primary radiotherapy for breast cancer.[73,141,142] This concern is justified given the increased incidence of lung cancer in uranium miners exposed to polonium gas and radon-exposed populations[169–175] (Table 1B-12). Although the original analyses of these cancer patients failed to emphasize the significant role of the cofactor of cigarette smoking, there were detectable cases of lung cancer in miners who were nonsmokers. Reports of radon-induced lung cancer and the setting of national standards for reducing radon gas levels in the basements of houses built in areas of high radon gas leakage from the core of the earth emphasizes the continued concern over radiation induction of lung cancer.[174,175] Several studies followed large numbers of women cured of early-stage breast cancer by primary radiotherapy with a specific focus on the lung in the tangential margins of the radiation fields used to encompass the breast. A significant number of cases of lung cancer have been reported, and analysis of these patients (taking into account smoking history and family history of multiple malignancies) is in progress in several large studies.[83–141] Because of the concern for lung cancer induction by irradiation, most radiation oncologists now minimize the volume of lung in the irradiation field by using three-dimensional treatment planning techniques and setting tangential beams to avoid significant volumes of lung.[141] Furthermore, techniques of using a matched anterior field to treat the supraclavicular nodal region (and also the apex of the lung) are now being eliminated whenever possible in favor of protocols in which the nodes are not treated (the incidence of supraclavicular recurrence has been shown to be exceedingly low).[141] Protocols of combination chemotherapy with irradiation usually plan that the chemotherapy is an effective treatment for nodal micrometastases from breast cancer in supraclavicular nodes. The techniques used in the 1970s of irradiating the internal mammary nodes by en fasse techniques have been abandoned, thus eliminating the volume of lung deep to the sternum. A summary of known irradiation-induced tumors and clinical settings in which such tumors might be detected is shown in Tables 1B-13 and 1B-14.

## FUTURE TRENDS AND DIRECTIONS

With the use of more sophisticated chemotherapeutic drugs and combined modality protocols, radiation oncologists and medical oncologists have become increasingly concerned about drug and x-ray interactions at the molecular and cellular level. Studies of induction of second tumors in multimodality protocols for treatment of Hodgkin's disease, ovarian cancer, gynecologic cancer, soft tissue sarcomas, and other tumors of childhood have led to several major conclusions, which are summarized in Table 1B-13.

It is clear that the addition of alkylating agents to the treatment of patients receiving large volumes of irradiation in their treatment course increases the risk for induction of second malignancies (Table 1B-14). It is also clear that combination chemotherapy programs in which alkylating agents are eliminated or reduced can greatly decrease the chance for induction of tumors.

Although several physical agents have been associated with induction of tumors in experimental animals and in humans, concern resides in exposure to UV light and even more so to ionizing irradiation. Curative combined modality programs for the treatment of many human cancers are increasingly focusing on ways to

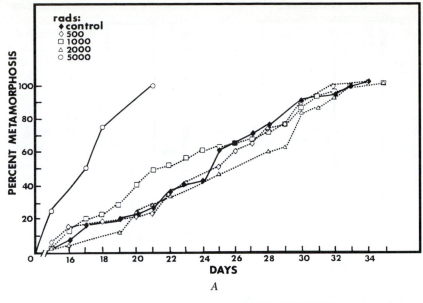

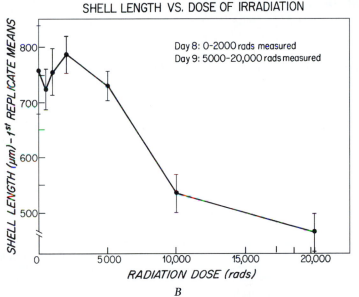

**FIGURE 1B-13.** Representative examples of ionizing irradiation–induced growth alteration at low irradiation doses, compared to cell killing at high doses. *A.* Growth rate of the snail *Crepitula fornacata* larvae irradiated to each given dose and then followed for metamorphosis or *B.* shell length. Notice increased metamorphosis and growth at low irradiation doses, compared to larval killing at higher doses. (*Reprinted with permission from Greenberger et al.*[170]) *C.* Hematopoietic cell colony production by continuous bone marrow cultures derived from leukemia-prone CBA/Ca mice irradiated to a dose known to induce leukemia at around 150 days of age, compared to long-term bone marrow cultures from 6 to 8 week, age-matched, nonirradiated mice—notice increased colonies (left hand panel) at 7 weeks by cultures from irradiated mice. (*Reprinted by permission from Greenberger et al.*[160])

reduce the irradiated volume or eliminate radiation from the therapeutic program. Due to other side effects of ionizing irradiation on developing organs, prophylactic cranial irradiation and prophylactic nodal irradiation have been eliminated from many protocols

treating pediatric leukemia, testicular cancer, and non-Hodgkin's lymphomas.[123,124] However, the continuing importance of radiotherapy in the management of patients with breast cancer, prostate cancer, cervical cancer, and endometrial cancer makes it extremely

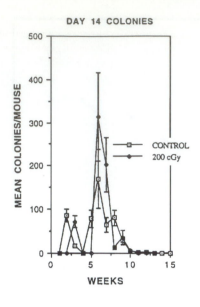
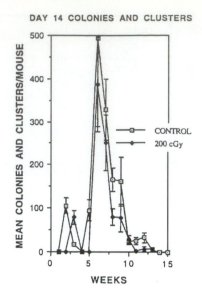

C

**FIGURE 1B-13.** (*Continued*)

critical to minimize conditions that might lead to radiation induction of bone tumors, soft tissue tumors, and leukemia in these people who are being cured of their primary cancers at high frequency.

With respect to tumor induction by microwave irradiation, electromagnetic irradiation, heat, and UV light, many precautions and public concerns have brought these areas of investigation to the forefront. Further information should be forthcoming, and until such results of carefully controlled trials are published, further concern for the role of these modalities in carcinogenesis must be placed secondary to the concern over ionizing irradiation.

Research efforts and developments in the area of physical carcinogenesis will undoubtedly follow well-established pathways of analysis of the molecular biology of cancer. These areas involve applying information gains from the human genome project to the determination of the specific gene pathways involved in the susceptibility of human tissues in specific organs to the transforming effects

**TABLE 1B-12.** MALIGNANCIES IN HUMANS IN THE SETTING OF PREVIOUS IRRADIATION EXPOSURE AND/OR RADIATION THERAPY

| CANCER | SETTING | SUSPECTED INCIDENCE REFERENCE |
|---|---|---|
| Leukemia | Multiple course orthovoltage irradiation, total lymphoid irradiation, and combination chemotherapy for Hodgkin's disease | Ankylosing spondylitis, Hodgkin's disease, multiple course irradiation of "benign" conditions[64,133,144] |
| B-cell lymphoma | Total lymphoid irradiation | Hodgkin's disease[90,122] |
| Osteogenic sarcoma Chondrosarcoma | Bone-seeking isotope accumulation, high-dose orthovoltage or megavoltage irradiation | Radium watch-dial painters, high-dose irradiation of tumors of childhood, soft tissue sarcoma[116,134] |
| Thyroid cancer | Radioisotope accumulation during nuclear fallout, thyroid irradiation (orthovoltage or megavoltage beams) | Nuclear accidents, radiation therapy for histiocytosis X, "benign" tumors of the head and neck[80] |
| Squamous cell carcinoma Basal cell carcinoma Malignant melanoma | Multiple course orthovoltage irradiation | Exposure to orthovoltage irradiation or radioisotopes[82] |

**TABLE 1B-13.** FACTORS INVOLVED IN INDUCTION OF TUMORS BY IONIZING IRRADIATION IN HUMANS

Incidence of second tumors appears to increase directly with:
- Volume of body irradiated
- Total dose
- Simultaneous exposure to alkylating agents
- Genetic predisposition to irradiation transformation (Fanconi's anemia, Cockayne syndrome, Bloom's syndrome)

Induction of tumors by ionizing irradiation in humans appears to decrease under the following conditions:
- Combined modality therapies utilize chemotherapy drugs other than alkylating agents
- Significant volume of bone marrow is non-irradiated
- Increasing age of the patient

of physical carcinogens. A major area in both basic and clinical research involves analysis of molecular mechanisms of the late effects of damage to cells and tissues by physical carcinogenic agents. The research trends and investigation should focus around several major categories.

## APPLICATION OF INFORMATION FROM THE HUMAN GENOME PROJECT TO ANALYSIS OF SUSCEPTIBILITY TO PHYSICAL CARCINOGENS

With the mapping of the human genome, it should be possible in the next decade to define specific genes in groups of genes that are involved in the early response of cells and specific tissues to ionizing irradiation damage. It is well known that some groups of patients respond to ionizing irradiation and standard fractionation with a brisk normal tissue response in the gastrointestinal tract, skin, and bone marrow. It is likely that early response to the acute effects of radiation damage may involve not only susceptibility to irradiation damage of chromosomes within specific cells, but also to a very sensitive response of associated cell populations in the immune system to the elaboration of humoral mediators and response to cytokines involved in the vascular and tissue repair process within each organ. Once the categories of genes are identified and patients can be genotyped with respect to expression of variants of the genes associated with hyper-responsiveness, it will be possible to modify radiation doses and fractionation to make patient responses more equivalent with respect to the normal tissue outcomes of radiotherapy. This has not been possible to date except with those patients who have the rare genetically determined hypersensitivity to irradiation such as Fanconi's anemia, Bloom's syndrome, or ataxia-telangiectasia. It should be possible within the next decade to present a map of the genomic expression patterns in individual patients to determine their susceptibility to both acute and late effects of ionizing irradiation. With this map in hand, clinical radiation oncologists should be able to tailor irradiation doses and field sizes to produce an equivalent tumor response in the setting of a specific hyperresponsiveness or relative resistance to that irradiation dose and fractionation scheme. These data should translate into a better understanding of physical carcinogenesis by ionizing irradiation as well. Those patients likely to suffer acute or chronic radiation side effects at lower equivalent doses would be expected to be those likely to be at higher risk for radiation carcinogenesis.

Even with analysis of data from the human genome project, it may be that there will be a disparity between acute and late side-effect induction by radiation and irradiation carcinogenesis. These trends will prove to be very important with respect to planning the integration of radiotherapy with chemotherapy and other modalities in the hope of providing long-term local control with radiotherapy and minimizing radiation carcinogenesis. The human genome project

**TABLE 1B-14.** TUMOR INDUCTION BY IONIZING IRRADIATION

| TUMOR CELL TYPE | CLINICAL EPIDEMIOLOGIC EVIDENCE | RADIATION DOSE ASSOCIATED WITH INCREASED INCIDENCE | REFERENCE |
|---|---|---|---|
| Thyroid papillary/follicular carcinoma | Total-body irradiation exposure, thyroid irradiation | 100–500 cGy | 80 |
| Acute leukemia | Orthovoltage irradiation, total-body irradiation | 100–1000 cGy (RVA factors involved) | 122, 137, 128, 144 |
| Osteogenic sarcoma | Orthovoltage irradiation, radioisotope deposition | Bone doses in the range of 10,000–20,000 cGy | 129 |
| Soft tissue sarcomas | Orthovoltage irradiation for chest wall or extremity conditions | 6000–8000 cGy | 129, 134 |
| B-cell lymphoma | Total-body irradiation with or without alkylating agent chemotherapy | 4000–6000 cGy | 90, 122 |

results should also be very important with respect to analyzing patient outcomes following nuclear accidents or nuclear radiation exposure. Individuals at higher risk for radiation carcinogenesis due to specific gene expression patterns might be those requiring intervention by delivery of tumor-suppressing gene therapy, the derivation of which should also be possible after analysis of the human genome project results. Other individuals may be candidates for more intensive surveillance with expectations of a higher incidence of tumor induction. Those individuals exposed to ionizing irradiation who are categorized to be at lower risk for radiation induction of tumors would be those subjected to a lower frequency of surveillance visits, and those who might not require intervention with a suppressive gene therapy approach. These future trends can only be outlined at the present time, since data from the human genome project is not yet available.

## ANALYSIS OF THE MOLECULAR MECHANISMS OF LATE EFFECTS OF IRRADIATION DAMAGE AND APPROPRIATE INTERVENTION

Research is well on the way toward understanding the molecular mechanisms of late radiation effects, fibrosis, neovasculature formation, and late transformation of slowly repopulating cell groups in specific organs. Once it becomes clear that specific cytokines are involved in the late expression of irradiation damage (TGF-β, IL-1α, TNF-α, and others), it may be possible to intervene with appropriate antisense gene therapy, administration of immune-modulating pharmaceutical agents at appropriate times, or other such strategies to prevent the expression of late irradiation effects. Individuals highly susceptible to induction of late effects, including those that received high radiation doses, high-volume tissue irradiation, or combination chemotherapy, might be watched more closely, and with appropriate timing of demonstration of involvement of tissues with respect to susceptibility to late effects would then have appropriate intervention. The molecular mechanism of the late effects is currently being delineated in large numbers of laboratories. By the end of the first decade of the next century, much information should be available to allow physicians and scientists to determine the molecular mechanism of late effects of radiation and to design appropriate interventions.

## UNDERSTANDING OF THE PRECISE GENES AND GENE PATTERNS INVOLVED IN RADIATION CARCINOGENESIS

The role of tumor suppressor genes, oncogenes, and mutator genes in carcinogenesis seems to be an established paradigm. However, there will be new information gained in the next decade with respect to the interaction of these genes and gene products in irradiation carcinogenesis. It appears likely that cofactors involved in gene expression and the suppression of regulatory genes in cells will also be well elaborated. Interaction between different groups of physical carcinogens, including UV light, heat, and even electromagnetic irradiation can be more specifically analyzed and reported. It would then be possible for molecular interventions to occur in very basic ways. The drug discovery programs and small molecule development programs in many pharmaceutical and biotechnology companies are paving the way for the substitution of large-molecular-weight cytokine and anticytokine therapies with small molecules that can stimulate receptors or suppress gene activation. With a complete understanding of the molecular pathways involved in radiation carcinogenesis, it may be possible in the next decade to design small-molecule pharmaceuticals that could be delivered to patients highly susceptible to radiation carcinogenesis. It is also possible that the modification of the receptors in specific organs for the effect of gene products of oncogenes can be modulated by administration of small molecules.

## GERM LINE GENE THERAPY FOR RADIOPROTECTION

As a leap into the next century, it may be premature but certainly appropriate to speculate on the long-term effects of a complete understanding of irradiation carcinogenesis. The field of germ cell gene therapy has recently been opened with the announcement by the National Institutes of Health of permission to begin experimental animal and even human embryo research. Certainly by the end of the next century it will be possible to genetically alter the human fetus at the earliest stages of development, perhaps even preimplantation of the fertilized ovum. With an understanding of the molecular biology of irradiation carcinogenesis, it may be possible to genetically modify the human embryo to resist irradiation carcinogenesis at the most basic levels. Why would one wish such a strange intervention? This might well be a question posed to officials in the National Aeronautics and Space Administration, who are interested in techniques of cryopreservation of space travelers who will be placed in cryosleep for long journeys. Certainly with the advent of technology in space vehicle design, techniques will become available to produce lightweight space vehicles that can resist ionizing irradiation from cosmic rays. However, the cryopreserved sleeping astronaut might be well served by having functional radiation-inducible oncogene suppression of all cells in the body during a continuous exposure to low-level cosmic irradiation for many years of cryosleep during journeys to faroff destinations. Ionizing irradiation has been shown to induce mutations even in frozen cells in liquid nitrogen containers, so such speculation is not irrelevant to the future of transportation.

## SUMMARY

Carcinogenesis by physical agents remains a topic of great concern to all surgical oncologists who are involved in combined modality protocols that involve radiotherapy. The routine use of megavoltage ionizing irradiation in the treatment of cancer has provided lasting benefits to thousands of patients; however, the known induction of cancer by ionizing irradiation makes this a true double-edged sword in the fight against cancer. Although the overwhelming concern rests with ionizing irradiation–induced tumors, UV light–induced skin cancer remains a second clear focus for consideration and evaluation of any patient presenting with basal cell carcinoma, squamous cell carcinoma, or malignant melanoma.

Although the most common radiation-induced cancers remain thyroid cancer and leukemia, surgical oncologists should be aware of prior irradiation exposure when analyzing the appearance of soft tissue tumors and bone tumors in patients who have been successfully treated with combined modality therapies for childhood cancer or are long-term survivors of chest wall radiotherapy for breast cancer or Hodgkin's disease. The biggest challenge for clinical and basic researchers in the next decade is to define the precise molecular mechanism of irradiation-induced cancer and to provide strategies for sound therapeutic intervention, because this population is at high risk for induction of second tumors.

## REFERENCES

### HYPERTHERMIA CARCINOGENESIS

1. BAKER DG et al: The effect of hyperthermia on radiation-induced carcinogenesis. Radiat Res 115:448, 1998.
2. HARISIADIS L et al: Oncogenic transformation and hyperthermia. Br J Radiol 53:479, 1980.
3. CLARK EP et al: Hyperthermic modulation of x-ray-induced oncogenic transformation in C3H10T1/2 cells. Radiat Res 88:619, 1981.
4. RAAPHORST GP et al: Oncogenic transformation of C3H10T1/2 mouse embryo cells by x-rays, hyperthermia, and combined treatments. Cancer Res 46:14, 1986.

### ELECTROMAGNETIC RADIATION CARCINOGENESIS

5. KHARBANDA S et al: Role for Bcl-xl as an inhibitor of cytosolic cytochrome-C accumulation in DNA damage-induced apoptosis. Proc Natl Acad Sci USA 94:6939, 1997.
6. EPPERLY MW et al: Overexpression of MnSOD in 32D cl 3 cells increases irradiation resistance by stabilization of the mitochondrial membrane and inhibition of caspase-3 and PARP activation. Proc Natl AACR Annual Meeting 40:551(#3634), 1999.
7. MIVECHI NF et al: Lower heat shock factor activation and binding and faster rate of HSP-70A messenger RNA turnover in heat sensitive human leukemias. Cancer Res 52:6815, 1992.
8. VEIGLE ML et al: Biallelic inactivation of hMLH1 by epigenetic gene silencing, a novel mechanism causing human MSI cancers. Proc Natl Acad Sci USA 95:8698, 1998.
9. MUGGENBURG BA et al: The biological effects of radium-224 injected into dogs. Radiat Res 146:171, 1996.
10. LINET MS et al: Residential exposure to magnetic fields and acute lymphoblastic leukemia in children. N Engl J Med 337:1, 1997.
11. LACY-HULBERT A et al: Biological responses to electromagnetic fields. FASEB J 12:395, 1998.
12. OLSEN JH et al: Residence near high-voltage facilities and risk of cancer in children. Br Med J 307:891, 1993.
13. KIRKPATRICK D: Can power lines give you cancer? Fortune Magazine December 31:83, 1990.
14. WALLECZEK J et al: Increase in radiation-induced HPRT gene mutation frequency after nonthermal exposure to nonionizing 60 Hz electromagnetic fields. Radiat Res 151:489, 1999.
15. POOL R: Flying blind: The making of EMF policy. Science 250:523, 1990.

16. WERTHEIMER N, LEEPER E: Electrical wiring configurations and childhood cancer. Am J Epidemiol 109:273, 1979.
17. VERKASALO PK et al: Risk of cancer in Finnish children living close to power lines. Br Med J 307:985, 1993.
18. FEYCHTING M, AHLBOM A: Magnetic fields and cancer in children residing near Swedish high voltage power lines. Am J Epidemiol 138:467, 1993.
19. SAVITZ DA et al: Case-control study of childhood cancer and exposure to 60-Hz magnetic fields. Am J Epidemiol 128:21, 1988.
20. LONDON SJ et al: Exposure to residential electric and magnetic fields and risk of childhood leukemia. Am J Epidemiol 134:923, 1991.
21. INSKIP PD et al: Leukemia following radiotherapy for uterine bleeding. Radiat Res 122:107, 1990.

### UV LIGHT CARCINOGENESIS

22. CLARK WH: Tumor progression and the nature of cancer. Br J Cancer 64:631, 1991.
23. BETTEGA D et al: Cell density dependence of transformation frequencies in C3H/10T1/2 cells exposed to x-rays. Int J Radiat Oncol Biol Phys 56:989, 1989.
24. WILLIAMS C et al: Clones of normal keratinocytes and a variety of simultaneously present epidermal neoplastic lesions contain a multitude of p53 gene mutations in a xeroderma pigmentosum patient. Cancer Res 58:2449, 1998.
25. REARDON JT et al: In vitro repair of oxidative DNA damage by human nucleotide excision repair system: Possible explanation for neurodegeneration in xeroderma pigmentosum patients. Proc Natl Acad Sci USA 94:9463, 1997.
26. SIJBERS AM et al: Xeroderma pigmentosum Group F caused by a defect in a structure-specific DNA repair endonuclease. Cell 86:811, 1996.
27. ABRAHAMS PJ et al: Inheritance of abnormal expression of SOS-like response in xeroderma pigmentosum and hereditary cancer-prone syndromes. Cancer Res 56:2621, 1996.
28. RAHA M et al: Mutagenesis by third-strand-directed psoralen adducts in repair-deficient human cells: High frequency and altered spectrum in a xeroderma pigmentosum variant. Proc Natl Acad Sci USA 93:2941, 1996.
29. GOZUKARA EM et al: The human DNA repair gene, ERCC2 (XPD), corrects UV hypersensitivity and UV hypermutability of a shuttle vector replicated in xeroderma pigmentosum Group D cells. Cancer Res 54:3837, 1994.
30. SATOH MS et al: DNA excision-repair defect of xeroderma pigmentosum prevents removal of a class of oxygen free radical-induced base lesions. Proc Natl Acad Sci USA 90:6335, 1993.
31. DUMAZ N et al: Specific UV-induced mutation spectrum in the p53 gene of skin tumors from DNA-repair-deficient xeroderma pigmentosum patients. Proc Natl Acad Sci USA 90:10529, 1993.
32. GILCHRIST BA et al: The pathogenesis of melanoma induced by ultraviolet light. N Engl J Med 340:1341, 1999.
33. KELLY JW et al: Sunlight: A major factor associated with the development of melanocytic nevi in Australian school children. J Am Acad Dermatol 30:40, 1994.
34. YOUNG AR et al: Photobiology and 5-MOP photochemoprotection from UVR-induced DNA damage in humans: The role of skin type. J Invest Dermatol 97:942, 1991.
35. NELEMANS PJ et al: Effect of intermittent exposure to sunlight on melanoma risk among indoor workers and sun-sensitive individuals. Environ Health Perspect 101:252, 1993.

36. JONASON AS et al: Frequent clones of p53-mutated keratinocytes in normal human skin. Proc Natl Acad Sci USA 93:14025, 1996.

37. REN ZP et al: Benign clonal keratinocyte patches with p53 mutations show no genetic link to synchronous squamous cell precancer or cancer in human skin. Am J Pathol 150:1791, 1997.

38. DUMAZ N et al: Can we predict solar UV radiation as the causal event in human tumors by analyzing the mutation spectra of the p53 gene? Mutat Res 307:375, 1994.

39. PONTEN F et al: UV light induces expression of p53 and p21 in human skin: effect of sunscreen and constitutive p21 expression in skin appendages. J Invest Dermatol 105:402, 1995.

40. TAKEUCHI N et al: Frequent p53 accumulation in the chronically sun-exposed epidermis and clonal expansion of p53 mutant cells in the epidermis adjacent to base cell carcinoma. J Invest Dermatol 104:928, 1995.

41. REN Z et al: Two distinct p53 immunohistochemical patterns in human squamous cell skin cancer, precursors, and normal epidermis. Int J Cancer 69:174, 1996.

42. DANDLIKER PJ et al: Oxidative thymine dimer repair in the DNA helix. Science 275:1465, 1997.

43. LABAHN J et al: Structural basis for the excision repair of alkylation-damaged DNA. Cell 86:321, 1996.

44. LU ML et al: UV irradiation-induced apoptosis leads to activation of a 36-kDa myelin basic protein kinase in HL-60 cells. Proc Natl Acad Sci USA 93:8977, 1996.

45. SVOBODA DL et al: Defective bypass replication of a leading strand cyclobutane thymine dimer in xeroderma pigmentosum variant cell extracts. Cancer Res 58:2445, 1998.

46. LINK CJ et al: Pentoxifylline inhibits gene-specific repair of UV-induced DNA damage in hamster cells. Radiat Oncol Invest 4:115, 1996.

47. STEWART F et al: What does photodynamic therapy have to offer radiation oncologists (or their cancer patients)? Radiotherapy Oncol 48:233, 1998.

48. NISHIGORI C et al: Evidence that DNA damage triggers IL-10 cytokine production in UV-irradiated murine keratinocytes. Proc Natl Acad Sci USA 93:10354, 1996.

49. CLEAVER JE et al: Overexpression of the XPA repair gene increases resistance to UV radiation in human cells by selective repair of DNA damage. Cancer Res 55:6152, 1995.

50. TAKAYAMA K et al: Defects in the DNA repair and transcription gene ERCC2 in the cancer-prone disorder xeroderma pigmentosum Group D. Cancer Res 55:5656, 1995.

51. KEENEY S et al: Correction of the DNA repair defect in xeroderma pigmentosum Group E by injection of a DNA damage-binding protein. Proc Natl Acad Sci USA 91:4053, 1994.

52. EVENO E et al: Different removal of UV photoproducts in genetically related xeroderma pigmentosum and trichothiodystrophy diseases. Cancer Res 55:4325, 1995.

53. SUNG P et al: Human xeroderma pigmentosum Group D gene encodes a DNA helicase. Nature 365:852, 1993.

## IONIZING IRRADIATION AND RADON

54. ROUSH GC et al: Inter-clinician agreement on the recognition of patients with cutaneous malignant melanoma: studies of melanocytic nevi, VI. Br J Cancer 64:373, 1990.

55. ELDER DE et al: Dysplastic nevus syndrome: A phenotypic association of sporadic melanoma. Cancer 46:1787, 1980.

56. NORDLUND JJ et al: Demographic study of clinically atypical (dysplastic) nevi in patients with melanoma and comparison subjects. Cancer 46:1005, 1986.

57. SWERDLOW AJ et al: Benign melanocytic naevi as a risk factor for malignant melanoma. Br Med J 292:1555, 1986.

58. WICK MM et al: Clinical characteristics of early cutaneous melanoma. Cancer 45:2684, 1980.

59. ELDER DE, HERLYN M: Antigens associated with tumor progression in melanocytic neoplasia. Pigment Cell Res 82:136, 1992.

60. HUTCHISON GB: Late neoplastic changes following medical irradiation. Radiology 105:645, 1972.

61. MOLE RH: Ionizing radiation as a carcinogen: Practical questions and academic pursuits. Br J Radiol 48:157, 1975.

62. KARLSSON P et al: Intracranial tumors after radium treatment for skin hemangioma during infancy: A cohort and case-control study. Radiat Res 148:161, 1997.

63. GREEN DM et al: Congenital anomalies in children of patients who received chemotherapy for cancer in childhood and adolescence. N Engl J Med 325:141, 1991.

64. HOLM L-E: Cancer occurring after radiotherapy and chemotherapy. Int J Radiat Oncol Biol Phys 19:1303, 1990.

65. GEARD CR, CHEN CY: Micronuclei and clonogenicity following low- and high-dose-rate gamma-irradiation of normal human fibroblasts. Radiat Res 124:S56, 1990.

66. ALEXANDER FE, GREAVES MF: Ionizing radiation and leukemia potential risks: Review based on the workshop held during the Tenth Symposium on Molecular Biology of Hematopoiesis and Treatment of Leukemia and Lymphomas at Hamburg, Germany, on July 5, 1997. Leukemia 12:1319, 1998.

67. SALVATI M et al: A report on radiation-induced gliomas. Cancer 67:392, 1991.

68. WALTER AW et al: Secondary brain tumors in children treated for acute lymphoblastic leukemia at St. Jude Children's Research Hospital. J Clin Oncol 16:3761, 1998.

69. OOTSUYAMA A, TANOOKA H: Threshold-like dose of local β irradiation repeated throughout the life span of mice for induction of skin and bone tumors. Radiat Res 125(1):98, 1991.

70. SHORE RE: Overview of radiation-induced skin cancer in humans. Int J Radiat Oncol Biol 57:809, 1990.

71. COGGLE JE, WILLIAMS JP: Experimental studies of radiation carcinogenesis in the skin: A review. Int J Radiat Biol 57:797, 1990.

72. BOWDEN GT et al: Biological and molecular aspects of radiation carcinogenesis. Radiat Res 121:235, 1990.

73. MATTSSON A et al: Incidence of primary malignancies other than breast cancer among women treated with radiation therapy for benign breast disease. Radiat Res 148:152, 1997.

74. DELONGCHAMP RR et al: Cancer mortality among atomic bomb survivors exposed in utero or as young children, October 1950–May 1992. Radiat Res 147:385, 1997.

75. KLUGBAUER S et al: A new form of RET rearrangement in thyroid carcinomas of children after the Chernobyl reactor accident. Oncogene 13:1099, 1996.

76. BONIVER J et al: Cellular events in radiation-induced lymphomagenesis. Int J Radiat Biol 57:693, 1990.

77. LAND CE et al: Incidence of salivary gland tumors among atomic bomb survivors, 1950–1987. Evaluation of radiation-related risk. Radiat Res 146:28, 1996.

78. CUMBERLIN RL et al: Carcinogenic effects of scattered dose associated with radiation therapy. Int J Radiat Oncol Biol Phys 17:623, 1989.

79. ELKIND MM: Repair processes in the treatment and induction of cancer with radiation. Cancer 65:2165, 1990.

80. FOGELFELD L et al: Recurrence of thyroid nodules after surgical removal in patients irradiated in childhood for benign conditions. N Engl J Med 320:835, 1989.

81. HOWE GR, MCLAUGHLIN J: Breast cancer mortality between 1950 and 1987 after exposure to fractionated moderate-dose-rate ionizing radiation in the Canadian fluoroscopy cohort study and a comparison with breast cancer mortality in the atomic bomb survivors' study. Radiat Res 145:694, 1996.

82. FRY RJM: Radiation carcinogenesis in the whole-body system. Radiat Res 126:157, 1991.

83. MILLER AB et al: Mortality from breast cancer after irradiation during fluoroscopic examinations in patients being treated for tuberculosis. N Engl J Med 321:1285, 1989.

84. LANGE RD et al: Leukemia in atomic bomb survivors. J Hematol IX:731, 1954.

85. PIERCE DA et al: Studies of the mortality of atomic bomb survivors. Report 12, Part I. Cancer 1950–1990. Radiat Res 146:1, 1996.

86. PIERCE DA et al: Analysis of time and age patterns in cancer risk for A-bomb survivors. Radiat Res 126:171, 1991.

87. NERIISHI K et al: The observed relationship between the occurrence of acute radiation effects and leukemia mortality among A-bomb survivors. Radiat Res 125:206, 1991.

88. ANDRE M et al: Treatment-related deaths and second cancer risk after autologous stem-cell transplantation for Hodgkin's disease. Blood 92:1933, 1998.

89. NYANDOTO P et al: Second cancer among long-term survivors from Hodgkin's disease. Int J Radiat Oncol Biol Phys 42:373, 1998.

90. TRAVIS LB et al: Second cancers following non-Hodgkin's lymphoma. Cancer 67:2002, 1991.

91. KLUGBAUER S et al: Detection of a novel type of RET rearrangement (PTC5) in thyroid carcinomas after Chernobyl and analysis of the involved RET-fused gene RFG51. Cancer Res 58:198, 1998.

92. INSKIP PD et al: Thyroid nodularity and cancer among Chernobyl cleanup workers from Estonia. Radiat Res 147:225, 1997.

93. BAVERSTOCK KF, THORNE MC: Radiological protection and the lymphatic system: The induction of leukemia consequent upon the internal irradiation of the tracheobronchial lymph nodes and the gastrointestinal tract wall. Int J Radiat Biol 55:129, 1989.

94. CALDWELL GG et al: Leukemia among participants in military maneuvers at a nuclear bomb test. JAMA 244:1575, 1980.

95. BAKER RJ et al: High levels of genetic change in rodents of Chernobyl. Nature 380:707, 1996.

96. DUBROVA YE et al: Human minisatellite mutation rate after the Chernobyl accident. Nature 380:683, 1996.

97. RAHU M et al: The Estonian study of Chernobyl cleanup workers: II. Incidence of cancer and mortality. Radiat Res 147:653, 1997.

98. TEKKEL M et al: The Estonian study of Chernobyl cleanup workers: I. Design and questionnaire data. Radiat Res 147:641, 1997.

99. FUGAZZOLA L et al: Molecular and biochemical analysis of RET/PTC4, a novel oncogenic rearrangement between RET and ELE1 genes, in a post-Chernobyl papillary thyroid cancer. Oncogene 13:1093, 1996.

100. KYOIZUMI S et al: Somatic cell mutations at the glycophorin A locus in erythrocytes of atomic bomb survivors: Implications for radiation carcinogenesis. Radiat Res 146:43, 1996.

101. SHIMIZU Y et al: Studies of the mortality of A-bomb survivors. 9. Mortality, 1950–1985: Part 1. Comparison of risk coefficients for site-specific cancer mortality based on the DS86 and T65DR shielded Kerma and organ doses. Radiat Res 118:502, 1989.

102. JANOWSKI M et al: The molecular biology of radiation-induced carcinogenesis: Thymic lymphoma, myeloid leukemia, and osteosarcoma. Int J Radiat Oncol Biol 57:677, 1990.

103. GREENBERGER JS: Long-term hematopoietic cultures, in *Methods In Hematology*, vol 11, D Golde (ed). New York, Churchill Livingstone, 1984, pp 203–243.

104. TILL JE, MCCULLOCH EA: A direct measurement of the radiation sensitivity of normal mouse bone marrow. Radiat Res 14:213, 1961.

105. WITHERS HR et al: Response of mouse intestine to neutrons and gamma rays in relation to dose fractionation and division cycle. Cancer 34:39, 1974.

106. WITHERS HR et al: Radiation survival and regeneration characteristics of spermatogenic stem cells of mouse testis. Radiat Res 57:88, 1974.

107. HALL EJ: *Radiobiology for the Radiologist*. Philadelphia, JB Lippincott, 1978.

108. FITZGERALD TJ et al: Increase in low-dose-rate x-irradiation resistance of factor dependent hematopoietic progenitor cells by recombinant murine GM-CSF. Int J Rad Oncol Biol Phys 17:323, 1989.

109. ——— et al: Resistance of hematopoietic stem cells to x-irradiation at clinical low-dose-rate is induced by several classes of oncogenes. Radiat Res 122:44, 1990.

110. EPPERLY MW et al: Prevention of late effects of irradiation lung damage by manganese superoxide dismutase gene therapy. Gene Ther 5:196, 1998.

111. JAHROUDI N et al: Ionizing irradiation increases transcription of the von Willebrand factor gene in endothelial cells. Blood 88:3801, 1996.

112. NAPARSTEK E et al: Persistent production of granulocyte-macrophage colony-stimulating factor (CSF-1) by cloned bone marrow stromal cell line D2XRII after x-irradiation. J Cell Physiol 126:407, 1986.

113. GOLTRY KL et al: Induction of serum amyloid A inflammatory response genes in irradiated bone marrow cells. Radiat Res 149:570, 1998.

114. GREENBERGER JS et al: Role of bone marrow stromal cells in irradiation leukemogenesis. Acta Haematol 96:1, 1996.

115. ——— et al: Stromal cell involvement in leukemogenesis and carcinogenesis. *In Vivo* 10:1, 1996.

116. WINGREN G et al: Soft tissue sarcoma and occupational exposures. Cancer 66:806, 1990.

117. GIVENS SS et al: Angiosarcoma arising in an irradiated breast. Cancer 64:2214, 1989.

118. LIPPMAN SM, HONG WK: Second malignant tumors in head and neck squamous cell carcinoma: The overshadowing threat for patients with early stage disease. Int J Radiat Oncol Biol Phys 17:691, 1989.

119. ARAI T et al: Second cancer after radiation therapy for cancer of the uterine cervix. Cancer 67:398, 1991.

120. MILLER RW, BOICE JD JR: Cancer after intrauterine exposure to the atomic bomb. Radiat Res 147:396, 1997.

121. KAWAMURA S et al: Prevalence of uterine myoma detected by ultrasound examination in the atomic bomb survivors. Radiat Res 147:753, 1997.

122. CURTIS RE et al: Solid cancers after bone marrow transplantation. N Engl J Med 336:897, 1997.

123. OLSEN JH: Risk of second cancer after cancer in childhood. Cancer 57:2250, 1986.

124. HARRIS JR, COLEMAN CN: Estimating the risk of second primary tumors following cancer treatment. J Clin Oncol 7:5, 1989.

125. CAVAZZA A et al: Post-irradiation malignant mesothelioma. Cancer 77:1379, 1996.

126. SAGMAN U et al: Second primary malignancies following diagnosis of small-cell lung cancer. J Clin Oncol 10:1525, 1992.

127. HEYNE KH et al: The incidence of second primary tumors in long-term survivors of small-cell lung cancer. J Clin Oncol 10:1519, 1992.

128. SCHWARTZ CL: Long-term survivors of childhood cancer: The late effects of therapy. Oncologist 4:45, 1999.

129. DUNST J et al: Second malignancies after treatment for Ewing's sarcoma: A report of the Cess-Studies. Int J Radiat Oncol Biol Phys 42:379, 1998.

130. KIMBALL DALTON VM et al: Second malignancies in patients treated for childhood acute lymphoblastic leukemia. J Clin Oncol 16:2848, 1998.

131. RON E et al: Tumors of the brain and nervous system after radiotherapy in childhood. N Engl J Med 319:1033, 1988.

132. KREISSMAN SG et al: Incidence of secondary acute myelogenous leukemia after treatment of childhood acute lymphoblastic leukemia. Cancer 70:2208, 1992.

133. DETOURMIGNIES L et al: Therapy-related acute promyelocytic leukemia: A report on 16 cases. J Clin Oncol 10:1430, 1992.

134. JOHNSTONE PAS et al: Tumors in dogs exposed to experimental intraoperative radiotherapy. Int J Radiat Oncol Biol Phys 34:853, 1996.

135. YAHALOM J et al: Breast cancer in patients irradiated for Hodgkin's disease: A clinical and pathologic analysis of 45 events in 37 patients. J Clin Oncol 10:1674, 1992.

136. SHAPIRO CL, MAUCH PM: Radiation-associated breast cancer after Hodgkin's disease: Risk and screening in perspective. J Clin Oncol 10:1662, 1992.

137. WITHERSPOON RP et al: Secondary cancers after bone marrow transplantation for leukemia or aplastic anemia. N Engl J Med 321:784, 1989.

138. CHUNG CT et al: Increased risk of breast cancer in splenectomized patients undergoing radiation therapy for Hodgkin's disease. Int J Radiat Oncol Biol Phys 37:405, 1997.

139. BHATIA S et al: Breast cancer and other second neoplasms after childhood Hodgkin's disease. N Engl J Med 334:745, 1996.

140. HILDRETH NG et al: The risk of breast cancer after irradiation of the thymus in infancy. N Engl J Med 321:1281, 1989.

141. LAVEY RS et al: Impact of radiation therapy and/or chemotherapy on the risk of for a second malignancy after breast cancer. Cancer 66:874, 1990.

142. CURTIS RE et al: Leukemia risk following radiotherapy for breast cancer. J Clin Oncol 7:21, 1989.

143. RON E et al: Tumors of the brain and nervous system after radiotherapy in childhood. N Engl J Med 319:1033, 1988.

144. PUI C-H et al: Secondary acute myeloid leukemia in children treated for acute lymphoid leukemia. N Engl J Med 321:136, 1989.

145. OKUMOTO M et al: Lack of evidence for the involvement of Type-C and Type-B retroviruses in radiation leukemogenesis of NFS mice. Radiat Res 121:267, 1990.

146. SILVER ARJ et al: Radiation-induced chromosome 2 rearrangement and initiation of murine acute myeloid leukemia. Radiat Res 121:233, 1990.

147. HUMBLET C et al: Further studies on the mechanism of radiation-induced thymic lymphoma prevention by bone marrow transplantation in C57BL mice. Leukemia 3:813, 1989.

148. RESNITZKY P et al: Absence of negative growth regulation in three new murine radiation-induced myeloid leukemia cell lines with deletion of chromosome 2. Leukemia 6:1288, 1992.

149. GREENBERGER JS et al: In vitro quantitation of lethal and leukemogenic effects of gamma irradiation on stromal and hematopoietic stem cells in continuous mouse bone marrow culture. Int J Rad Oncol Biol Phys 8:1155, 1982.

150. ——— et al: Effects of low dose rate irradiation on plateau phase bone marrow stromal cells in vitro: Demonstration of a new form of nonlethal physiologic alteration of support of hematopoietic stem cells. Int J Rad Oncol Biol Phys 10:1027, 1984.

151. NAPARSTEK E et al: Biologic effects of in vitro x-irradiation of murine long-term bone marrow cultures on the production of granulocyte-macrophage colony stimulating factors. Exp Hematol 13:701, 1985.

152. ——— et al: Induction of growth alterations in factor-dependent hematopoietic progenitor cell lines by cocultivation with irradiated bone marrow stromal cell lines. Blood 67:1395, 1986.

153. ——— et al: Induction of malignant transformation of co-cultivated hematopoietic stem cells by x-irradiation of murine bone marrow stromal cells in vitro. Cancer Res 46:4677, 1986.

154. ——— et al: Morphology of cell-to-cell contact between x-irradiated plateau phase bone marrow stromal cell lines and cocultivated factor-dependent cell lines leading to leukemogenesis in vitro. SEM 1:247, 1987.

155. GREENBERGER JS et al: Alteration in hematopoietic stem cell seeding and proliferation by low dose rate irradiation of bone marrow stromal cells in vitro. Int J Rad Oncol Biol Phys 14:85, 1988.

156. GREENBERGER JS et al: Hematopoietic stem cell and marrow stromal cell specific requirements for gamma-irradiation leukemogenesis in vitro. Exp Hematol 18:408, 1990.

157. SANTUCCI MA et al: Gamma-irradiation response of cocultivated bone marrow stromal cell lines of differing intrinsic radiosensitivity. Int J Rad Oncol Biol Phys 18:1083, 1990.

158. GREENBERGER JS: Toxic effects on the hematopoietic microenvironment. Exp Hematol 19:1101, 1991.

159. ROMANIK EA et al: Sequence analysis of mutational hot spots in the endogenous and transfected CSF-1 receptor in gamma-irradiation induced factor-independent subclones of clonal hematopoietic progenitor cell lines. Radiat Oncol Invest Clin Basic Res 1:94, 1993.

160. GREENBERGER JS et al: Effects of irradiation of CBA/Ca mice on hematopoietic stem cells and stromal cells in long term bone marrow cultures. Leukemia 10:514, 1996.

161. ASTIER-GIN T et al: Identification of malignant cell clones in radio-induced murine thymic lymphomas by viral and cellular probes. Leukemia 4:307, 1990.

162. MILLER RC et al: The effects of the temporal distribution of dose on oncogenic transformation by neutrons and charged particles of intermediate LET. Radiat Res 124:S62, 1990.

163. BRENNER DJ, HALL EJ: The inverse dose-rate effect for oncogenic transformation by neutrons and charged particles: A plausible interpretation consistent with published data. Int J Radiat Biol 58:745, 1990.

164. SECKER-WALKER LM et al: Secondary acute leukemia and myelodysplastic syndrome with 11q23 abnormali. Leukemia 12:840, 1998.

165. ISHII K et al: Decreased incidence of thymic lymphoma in AKR mice as a result of chronic, fractionated low-dose total body irradiation. Radiat Res 146:582, 1996.

166. ULLRICH RL: Effects of split doses of x-rays or neutrons on lung tumor formation in RFM mice. Radiat Res 83:138, 1980.

167. SILVER A, COX R: Telomere-like DNA polymorphisms associated with genetic predisposition to acute myeloid leukemia in irradiated CBA mice. Proc Natl Acad Sci USA 90:1407, 1993.

168. LEMON HM et al: Inhibition of radiogenic mammary carcinoma in rats by estriol or tamoxifen. Cancer 63:1685, 1989.

169. BOICE JD JR: Radon, your home or mine? Radiat Res 147:135, 1997.

170. GREENBERGER JS et al: X-irradiation effects on growth and metamorphosis of gastropod larvae (Crepidula fornicata): A model for environmental radiation teratogenesis. Arch Environ Contam Toxicol 15:227, 1986.

171. LUBIN JH et al: Estimating lung cancer mortality from residential radon using data for low exposures of miners. Radiat Res 147:126, 1997.

172. LUTZE LH et al: Radon-induced deletions in human cells: Role of nonhomologous strand rejoining. Cancer Res 52:5126, 1992.

173. SCHOENBERG JB et al: Case-control study of residential radon and lung cancer among New Jersey women. Cancer Res 50:6520, 1990.

174. NERO AV JR: Estimated risk of lung cancer from exposure to radon decay products in US homes: A brief review. Atmospheric Environ 22:2205, 1988.

175. SACCOMANNO G et al: Relationship of radioactive radon daughters and cigarette smoking in the genesis of lung cancer in uranium miners. Cancer 62:1402, 1988.

176. MILLER SC et al: NF-kβ or AP-1-dependent reporter gene expression is not altered in human U937 cells exposed to power-line frequency magnetic fields. Radiat Res 151:310, 1999.

177. GOSWAMI PC et al: Proto-oncogene mRNA levels and activities of multiple transcription factors in C3H10T1/2 murine embryonic fibroblasts exposed to 835.62 and 847.74 MHz cellular phone communication frequency radiation. Radiat Res 151:300, 1999.

178. MOULDER JE et al: Cell phones and cancer: What is the evidence for a connection? Radiat Res 151:513, 1999.

# VIRAL CARCINOGENESIS

*Frank J. Jenkins and Linda J. Hoffman*

## INTRODUCTION

The study of viral carcinogenesis has been and continues to be one of the most exciting areas of viral research. Early knowledge that some animal viruses could cause tumors suggested that some human cancers would fall under the description of infectious diseases and could possibly be prevented by vaccines. As discussed by Weiss,[1] approximately 15% of human cancers have now been attributed to viral infections. The research on these viruses and their role in cancer formation has resulted in some of the most important scientific discoveries over the last three to four decades. The discovery of oncogenes and their cellular counterparts (protooncogenes), as well as tumor suppressor genes, are a direct result of tumor virus research. Much of what we would now describe as basic molecular biology is also a result of this research, including mechanisms of cellular transformation, cell cycle control, messenger RNA splicing, and discovery of reverse transcriptase. Human viruses that are known, or strongly suspected, to be involved in the development of human cancers include several members of the human herpesvirus and papovavirus families, as well as human T-cell leukemia virus 1 (HTLV-1) and the hepatitis viruses B (HBV) and C (HCV). As our ability to detect previously unrecognized viral agents continues to improve, it is likely that additional viruses will be added to this list.

## HISTORICAL OVERVIEW

As long ago as the early 1900s, it was suspected that an individual agent (described as a filterable agent) was responsible for development of a leukemia[2] and later, a sarcoma, in chickens.[3] The studies on avian sarcoma led to the discovery of Rous sarcoma virus,[4] one of the most widely studied tumorigenic retroviruses. Approximately 25 years later, endogenous retroviruses were discovered, and one was reported to be responsible for creating a predisposition to breast cancer in certain strains of mice (termed mouse mammary tumor virus, MMTV).[5] These reports were followed by the discovery of the first animal DNA tumor viruses in the late 1950s and early 1960s. Realization that many different animal viruses, both RNA and DNA viruses, could cause tumor formation in different animal models led to an intensive search for homologous human viruses, a search that is continuing today. Fortunately, none of the human viruses that are involved in the formation of human cancer produce malignant tumors as a normal consequence of viral infection. Infection by these viruses therefore results in an increased risk of cancer development, and may be considered as one step in the multistep process of oncogenesis.

## CURRENT STATUS

The human viruses that have been identified as cofactors in cancer development belong to five separate families: the Flaviviridae, Hepadnaviridae, Herpesviridae, Papovaviridae, and Retroviridae (Table 1B-15). The viral mechanism(s) involved in tumorigenesis have been identified for some, but not all, of these viruses. These mechanisms, as discussed below, include interference with tumor suppressor genes, increasing cellular proliferation, and alterations of cellular gene expression.

### PAPOVAVIRIDAE

The Papovaviridae family consists of the genera *Polyomavirus* and *Papillomavirus*. The virions of this family are nonenveloped with an icosahedral capsid containing a double-stranded, covalently closed, circular DNA genome that is approximately 5 to 8 kb in length.[6,7]

**PAPILLOMAVIRUSES.** There are over 70 separate human papillomaviruses identified to date.[8] Infection with papillomavirus is generally subclinical, resulting in the formation of a benign wart in genital, upper respiratory, and digestive tracts, as well as various cutaneous sites. The majority of all papillomavirus lesions are benign and contain viral DNA in an episomal form. The viral genome consists of a long control region (LCR), and two classes of genes (early and late) that are identified by the timing of their expression during viral replication.[9] The early genes consist of E1 and E2, which function in viral replication and transcriptional control of viral genes; E4 and E5, whose functions are not well understood; and E6 and E7, which function to inhibit regulators of cell cycle control, resulting in cellular proliferation. The late genes consist of the structural proteins encoded by L1 and L2.[9,10]

Human papillomaviruses (HPVs) are associated with cervical cancer and epidermodysplasia verruciformis (EV). The association between HPV and cervical cancer is strong. Greater than 95% of cervical cancers contain HPV DNA, mostly HPV-16 or HPV-18, although several others have also been detected.[11] The presence of HPV-16 and 18 in cervical cancers appears to be related to the oncogenic potential of these HPV types. Both HPV-16 and -18 can immortalize human keratinocytes, whereas other types that are considered low risk for tumor formation (such as HPV-6 and -11) do not exhibit this function.[8] Further, although all HPV viruses can transform rodent cells, the high-risk viruses exhibit a greater efficiency of transformation compared to the low-risk viruses.

The only papillomavirus genes that are required for immortalization of human keratinocytes and the transformation of rodent cells in the laboratory are the E6 and E7 genes.[12,13] However, immortalized human keratinocytes are not transformed, since they do not exhibit anchorage independence and do not form tumors in nude mice. Thus cancer development requires more than just the presence of the virus, supporting the idea that viral infection is only one step leading toward oncogenesis. This is further supported by the observation that cervical cancer is rare compared to the incidence of HPV infection in women.[11]

**TABLE 1B-15.** HUMAN VIRUSES ASSOCIATED WITH CANCER

| HUMAN VIRUS | ASSOCIATED CANCER(S) |
| --- | --- |
| Papovaviridae: | |
|   Papillomavirus | |
|     Types 16, 18* | Cervical cancer |
|     Types 5 and 8* | Epidermodysplasia verruciformis |
|   Polyomavirus | |
|     BK virus | Cerebral Tumors |
|     JC virus | Astrocytomas |
| Hepadnaviridae: | |
|   Hepatitis B virus | Hepatocellular carcinoma |
| Flaviviridae: | |
|   Hepatitis C virus | Hepatocellular carcinoma |
| Herpesviridae | |
|   Epstein-Barr virus | Endemic Burkitt's lymphoma |
| | Nasopharyngeal carcinoma |
| | Lymphoproliferative disease |
| | Hodgkin's lymphoma |
|   Human herpesvirus 8 | Kaposi's sarcoma |
| | Body-cavity–based lymphoma |
| | Multicentric Castleman's disease |

*These are the major HPV types associated with the listed cancer.

The mechanism of HPV transformation has been linked to the function(s) of the E6 and E7 proteins. The E7 protein interacts with the cellular tumor suppressor protein RB.[14] The function of RB is to prevent cell cycle progression at the $G_1$/S boundary[15] (Fig. 1B-14). In a normal cell cycle, hypophosphorylated RB protein binds to the cellular transcription factor E2F, preventing it from triggering cell proliferation. Phosphorylation of the RB protein by a cell cycle–dependent kinase (CDK) results in the release of E2F and the progression of the cell cycle through the $G_1$/S boundary. Once in the M phase, the RB protein is dephosphorylated, allowing it to rebind to E2F. The HPV E7 protein binds to the hypophosphorylated form of RB, resulting in the release of E2F and progression of the cell cycle (Fig. 1B-14). A comparative analysis of the E7 proteins has demonstrated that the protein encoded by low-risk HPVs binds RB with a lower affinity than the protein encoded by high-risk HPVs. This lowered binding affinity correlates with the decrease in transformation efficiency of the low-risk viruses.[8,11]

The E6 protein binds a different cellular tumor suppressor protein, the p53 protein.[16] The p53 protein, unlike RB, is not constitutively produced in the cell, but instead is induced in response to DNA damage. The function of the p53 protein is to either place the cell in G1 arrest for repair of the damaged DNA or to force the cell into apoptosis in cases where the damage is extensive.[17,18] The p53 gene is the most commonly mutated gene in human cancers and is therefore recognized as a common target for tumorigenesis.[19] The binding of the E6 protein to p53 results in the inhibition of the p53's activity, and targets the protein for ubiquitin-dependent degradation. Interestingly, there is an absence of p53 somatic mutations in anogenital HPV-positive tumors, suggesting that the E6 protein functions at the protein level and does not induce genetic mutations.[20] Similar to the E7 protein, the E6 protein encoded by low-risk HPVs has been reported to bind less efficiently to p53 than the E6 protein from high-risk viruses.[21,22] Recently, the E6 protein has also been reported to induce a telomerase activity that could assist in cellular immortalization by stabilizing the lengths of the telomeres.[23]

In most HPV cancers, the viral genome is integrated into the cellular genome. This is in contrast to normally infected cells in which the viral DNA is maintained in an episomal form. Although the location of viral DNA integration in the cellular chromosome appears to be random, the integration sites within the viral genome consistently disrupt the E1 and E2 genes. The proteins encoded by these two genes serve as repressors of HPV E6 and E7 transcription, and therefore disruption of these genes results in nonregulated expression of E6 and E7, increasing the chances of cellular transformation.

In summary, although HPV-induced transformation obviously requires viral infection, infection alone is insufficient for tumor formation. Other factors felt to be involved in tumor formation include the establishment of a chronic infection, enhanced or overexpression of the E6/E7 genes and the accumulation of somatic mutations.

**POLYOMAVIRUSES.** This section includes the two human polyomaviruses, JC and BK, as well as SV40, a highly related monkey polyomavirus. SV40 has been included because most of our understanding of polyomavirus oncogenesis comes from extensive studies on this virus. In addition, SV40 was found to be a contaminant of early poliovirus vaccines and was inadvertently administered to thousands of individuals, potentially increasing their risk for developing a polyoma-induced tumor.[25] Fortunately, there has not been an association seen between SV40 and any human cancers to date.

Under normal circumstances, polyomavirus infections are generally subclinical and can persist for varying lengths of time. The BK and JC viruses can cause clinical disease following infection, but generally only in individuals who are immunosuppressed. BK-associated diseases include an acute hemorrhagic cystitis or respiratory tract disease, nephritis, and meningoencephalitis. JC virus infections are associated with development of progressive multifocal leukoencephalopathy (PML).[24] Tumor formation by human polyomaviruses is not a normal consequence of viral infection in humans. However, both human polyomaviruses have been found in rare instances in some tumors, most notably astrocytomas with JC virus and cerebral tumors with BK virus.[24] Tumor formation in the viruses' natural host is believed to be a result of an abortive infection in which the viral replicative cycle is interrupted. Consequently, progeny are not produced, but some viral genes are expressed, resulting in the development of a tumor.

The strongest evidence for polyomaviruses as tumor viruses comes from studies on the effect of viral DNA in nonpermissive cells, such as those from a species other than the virus's natural host. BK virus has been shown to induce tumors in hamsters, mice, and rats, whereas JV virus has induced tumors in hamsters and different strains of monkeys.[24] The SV40 virus can induce tumors in newborn hamsters and some strains of mice.[26]

The induction of tumors by the polyomaviruses is the result of the expression of its early genes termed T(umor) antigens. SV40 encodes two tumor antigens, large T and small t, whereas polyoma

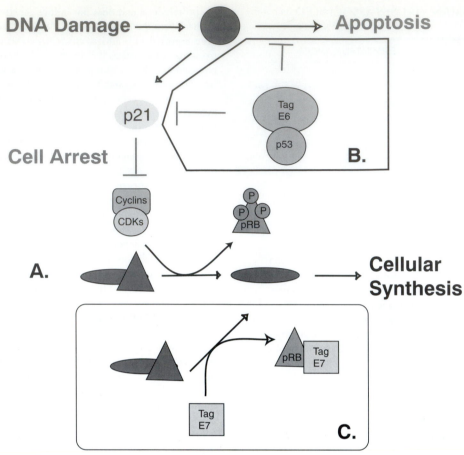

**FIGURE 1B-14. Actions of Viral Oncogenes on Cellular Tumor Suppressor Proteins.** *A.* Phosphorylation of pRB by cellular cyclins and CDKs results in the release of the cellular transcriptional factor E2F, resulting in cellular synthesis. *B.* DNA damage results in the induction of the p53 protein, which can push the cell into apoptosis or can induce p21, which causes the cell to arrest at the $G_1/S$ boundary. The SV40 T antigen (Tag) and papillomavirus E6 protein bind p53, preventing the induction of apoptosis or the p21 protein. *C.* The SV40 Tag or papillomavirus E7 protein bind to hypophosphorylated pRB, resulting in premature release of E2F and the onset of cellular synthesis. (See also Plate 3.)

encodes four tumor antigens, large T, middle T, small T, and tiny T.[27] In SV40, the large T protein can transform cells in culture, but at lowered efficiency compared to the combination of large and small T genes. The large T protein of SV40 binds to both p53 and Rb. This contrasts with the large T protein of polyomavirus, which binds Rb but not p53. Interestingly, the major transforming protein of polyomavirus is the middle T.[27]

## HEPATITIS VIRUSES

Primary hepatocellular carcinoma (HCC) is the eighth most frequent human tumor seen worldwide,[28] with an estimated 250,000 new cases developing each year.[29] The incidence of HCC in the United States and northern Europe is below 5 cases per 100,000 each year, whereas the incidence in some regions of sub-Saharan Africa, China, and Southeast Asia are much higher (>30 cases per 100,000 individuals). Two different human viruses, the hepatitis B and C viruses (HBV and HCV), have been associated with the development of HCC. Two significant risk factors for development of HCC are cirrhosis of the liver and chronic infections with either HBV or HCV. There is a considerable amount of time (20 to 30 years) between infection with either virus and the onset of cancer. In most cases, the development of HCC begins with an acute hepatitis, followed by the development of a chronic hepatitis, which leads to liver cirrhosis and finally liver cancer.

**HEPATITIS B VIRUS (HBV).** The hepatitis B virus belongs to the Hepadnaviridae family. The virus consists of an enveloped particle that is 42 nm in diameter and contains a circular, partially double-stranded DNA molecule that is approximately 3.2 kb in length.[30] The viral genome contains at least four open reading frames that encode for two core antigens (HBc and HBe), an envelope antigen (HBs), a DNA polymerase (P protein), and a protein of unknown function (gene X). HBV primarily infects hepatocytes, with viral replication occurring in the cytoplasm. Infection is mostly noncytopathogenic, and integration of the viral genome into cellular chromosomes can occur. A primary HBV infection can be subclinical or can result in acute hepatitis. Approximately 5% to 10% of adults with a primary HBV infection will go on to develop a chronic viral infection, with 10% to 25% of these individuals ultimately developing HCC.[31] Among newborns, the incidence of chronic infection increases to 60% to 80%.[28]

Harrison[29] has described three potential mechanisms for HBV-related carcinogenesis. First, that insertion of the viral genome into a cellular chromosome results in the disruption of normal cellular gene expression leading to the development of a transformed phenotype. Arguing against this mechanism is the understanding that DNA integration is not part of the HBV life-cycle and analyses of integration sites of HBV DNA in HCC tumors have failed to detect a common site. However, it has also been reported that integration of the HBV genome results in expression of the HBV X gene product, which is believed to be a transactivator of both viral and cellular genes. Whether the X protein plays a causative role in HBV-related HCC remains to be determined. A second proposed mechanism is that the virus encodes a viral oncogene. However, viral DNA has not been shown to be capable of transforming cells in culture. Furthermore, the length of time between viral infection and tumor formation (three to five decades) argues against the presence of an oncogene. The third proposed mechanism is a chronic viral infection that results in chronic hepatitis and cirrhosis, which produce a constant cellular regeneration that ultimately leads to the development of cancer in an indirect manner. As discussed below, the third mechanism has also been proposed for the hepatitis C virus.

**HEPATITIS C VIRUS (HCV).** HCV is a member of the Flaviviridae family, containing a single-stranded RNA genome that is completely unrelated to HBV.[29] HCV is the major cause of non-A–non-B hepatitis, and therefore is a significant player in chronic hepatitis and liver disease.[28] The prevalence rate of HCV in the United States is approximately 1.8%.[32] The majority of primary HCV infections are mildly symptomatic such that most infections are not diagnosed until the development of a chronic infection. Approximately 60% to 80% of all primary HCV infections develop into chronic infections.[28] There is no DNA intermediate formed during viral replication, so integration of the genome into cellular DNA does not occur. Although the precise mechanism of HCV-related liver cancer is unknown, it is hypothesized (similar to HBV) to be due to the constant cellular regeneration that occurs during a chronic infection in the presence of cirrhosis damage.[29]

## HERPESVIRUSES

Human herpesviruses have been linked to one or more human cancers since the early 1960s. Currently two members of this family have strong associations with human tumors; Epstein-Barr virus (EBV) and human herpesvirus 8 (HHV-8).

**EPSTEIN-BARR VIRUS (EBV).** EBV was the first human virus associated with a human cancer. The virus was discovered through the combined efforts of Denis Burkitt, an English surgeon, and Anthony Epstein, a pathologist. Burkitt reported on the presence of a malignant lymphoma that was endemic in children in the African malaria belt, later termed Burkitt's lymphoma (BL).[33] He speculated in 1964 that a virus might be involved in the development of this tumor, and this insight led to a collaboration with Epstein, who later discovered EBV in cancerous B cells from a BL patient.[34] EBV has been associated to varying degrees with several human cancers, including endemic BL, nasopharyngeal carcinoma, Hodgkin's lymphoma, lymphoproliferative disease, gastric carcinoma, salivary gland tumors, and, more recently, smooth muscle tumors occurring in immunocompromised individuals.

EBV infection is ubiquitous throughout the world with greater than 90% of the population seropositive for EBV antibodies.[35] A primary infection that occurs during childhood is often asymptomatic or presents as a mild upper respiratory tract infection. However, in teenagers or adults, primary infections often present as infectious mononucleosis. Transmission of EBV is predominantly through saliva. In a primary infection, EBV infects the epithelial layer of the pharyngeal mucosa, producing a lytic viral replication and subsequent infection of infiltrating B cells (Fig. 1B-15).[36] The infection of epithelial cells results in the production of a strong immune response that is believed to mediate the clearing of infected cells that are undergoing lytic viral replication and to force the virus into a latent infection in B cells.[37] The B cell is the most widely accepted site of EBV latency, which is characterized by the presence of the viral genome and the absence of virus production.[38] EBV latency has been divided into three types based on the pattern of viral gene expression (see Fig. 1B-15).[39] Interestingly, the different types of EBV latency have been shown to correlate with different types of human cancers (Table 1B-16).

*BURKITT'S LYMPHOMA (BL).* There are two types of BL, endemic BL (eBL), which occurs in equatorial regions of Africa, and sporadic BL (sBL), which occurs in low incidence throughout the world.[40] EBV is present in almost all cases of eBL (>97%) but not

## TABLE 1B-16. EBV-ASSOCIATED CANCERS

| MALIGNANCY | EBV SEROLOGY (% POSITIVE) | LATENT EBV GENE EXPRESSION |
|---|---|---|
| Endemic BL | 100 | Type I |
| Nasopharyngeal carcinoma | 100 | Type II |
| Hodgkin's disease | | Type II |
|   Mixed cellularity | 80–90 | |
|   Lymphocyte depleted | 80–90 | |
|   Nodular sclerosing | 30–40 | |
| Post-transplant | | |
| Lymphoproliferative disease (PTLD) | >90 | Type III |
| AIDS-associated | | |
|   lymphoproliferative disease | >95 | Type III |

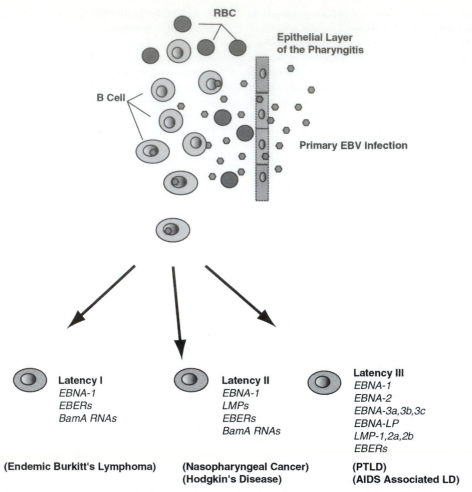

**FIGURE 1B-15.** EBV Replication and Latency. A primary EBV infection of the epithelial layer of the pharynx results in lytic viral replication that spreads to infiltrating B cells. Infected B cells serve as sites of viral latency, which is divided into three types based on viral gene expression. (See also Plate 4.)

sBL (ranging from 15% to 80%). Both forms of BL contain a translocation of the c-*myc* gene from chromosome 8 to one of the IgG regulatory domains contained on chromosomes 2, 14, or 22, with chromosome 14 representing the most common target.[39] The presence of this translocation in both EBV-positive and EBV-negative BL tissues indicates the translocation may be responsible for tumor formation, and EBV infection thus acts as a cofactor rather than a true etiologic agent. Cells from an eBL tumor express the type 1 latency pattern of gene expression (see Fig. 1B-15).

*NASOPHARYNGEAL CARCINOMA (NPC).* NPC has a high incidence rate in Hong Kong and the southern provinces of China. An intermediate incidence rate occurs in some areas of Africa, Alaska, and Greenland, whereas a low incidence rate is present in Europe and North America.[39] EBV is present consistently in NPC tumors regardless of the region or ethinicity of the patient.[41] As a result of the geographic restrictions on the presence of NPC, tumor devel-

opment is felt to be a combination of EBV infection and dietary or environmental factors. NPC cells exhibit the type 2 latency pattern of gene expression in which Epstein-Barr nuclear antigen 1 (EBNA-1), latent membrane protein 1 (LMP-1), and the EBV-encoded RNAs are produced (see Fig. 1B-15).

*HODGKIN'S DISEASE (HD).* HD has an incidence rate of 2 to 4 per 100,000 population per year in western Europe and the United States. Approximately 20% of all HD tumors contain EBV DNA, although there is some degree of variability depending on the histologic subtype (see Table 1B-16).[42] Like NPC, EBV-containing HD cells exhibit the type 2 latency pattern of gene expression (see Fig. 1B-15).

*LYMPHOPROLIFERATIVE DISEASE (LD).* LD is a B-cell lymphoma that occurs in immunocompromised individuals such as AIDS and transplant recipient patients.[43,44] The majority of the

LD tumors contain EBV DNA. In these individuals, the immune system becomes defective through immunosuppression (transplant patients) or through loss of CD4 T-cells (AIDS patients) which allows for a proliferation of EBV-immortalized B cells. EBV-containing LD cells exhibit the type 3 latency pattern of gene expression (see Fig. 1B-15) in which all the latent EBV genes are produced. Consequently, these cells are highly immunogenic, which may explain the absence of LD in immunocompetent individuals.

*X-LINKED LYMPHOPROLIFERATION (XLP).* This is an extremely rare disease in males who carry a genetic defect on the X chromosome.[45] Children who carry this defect and become infected with EBV generally die within 2 to 3 weeks from liver and/or bone marrow failure (approximately 65%). Those that survive the acute infection die several years after the initial infection from an EBV-associated lymphoma.[45]

Gastric carcinoma (GC) has also been associated with EBV. Almost all cases of undifferentiated GC contain the EBV genome, while differentiated GC cases rarely contain viral DNA.[46] More recently, smooth muscle tumors in immunosuppressed children and teenagers have been found to also contain EBV DNA.[47]

The exact mechanism(s) of EBV-induced transformation is not known. Several of the latency proteins such as EBNA-1, EBNA-2, EBNA-3, EBNA-6, and LMP-1 have been shown to be necessary for cellular immortalization.[39] The EBNA-1 protein is required for maintenance of the viral genome as an episome in latently infected B cells. The EBNA-2 protein acts as a transactivator of both viral and cellular genes. The LMP-1 protein has been shown to upregulate bcl-2 and can produce morphological transformation of a rat cell line as evidenced by a lowered growth requirement for serum, reduced anchorage dependence, and the ability of the transformed cells to produce tumors in nude mice. LMP-1 is felt to be responsible for the majority of the EBV-related growth alterations of infected B cells. As a result, some investigators have defined EBNA-2 and LMP-1 as viral oncogenes.[39] However, evidence that neither EBNA-2 nor LMP-1 are expressed in eBL cells and the fact that EBNA-2 is absent in NPC suggests that these two genes are not the only EBV-encoded oncogenes. It may be that there is more than one pathway for EBV-induced carcinogenesis. Table 1B-17 lists the different EBV latent genes along with their proposed function and latency pattern in which they are expressed.

**HUMAN HERPESVIRUS 8 (HHV-8).** HHV-8 was first reported in 1994 by Chang and colleagues as present in biopsies of Kaposi's sarcoma (KS).[48] KS is a neoplasm with a suspected endothelial origin that is seen in four distinct populations. *Classic or Mediterranean KS* affects predominantly older men (>60 years) of Mediterranean, eastern European, or Jewish background. *African or endemic KS* is found in the sub-Saharan region of Africa and represents approximately 10% of all malignancies in this region.[49] *Iatrogenic or immunosuppressive KS* is seen in organ transplant patients who have an estimated 400- to 500-fold increase in KS lesions.[50] Reduction of immunosuppression in these patients often results in a reversion of the KS lesion.[51–53] *AIDS-associated or epidemic KS* is the most common malignancy seen in AIDS patients and is now well recognized as an AIDS-defining cancer.[50,54]

In 1994, using representational difference analysis, Chang and colleagues[48] described the detection of DNA sequences in AIDS-associated KS lesions belonging to a new human herpesvirus termed Kaposi's sarcoma–associated herpesvirus (KSHV). More recently, this virus has been given the designation of human herpesvirus 8 (HHV-8). The entire HHV-8 genome has been sequenced and the predicted amino acid sequences encoded by different viral genes were found to share homology to proteins encoded by herpesvirus saimiri (HVS) and Epstein-Barr virus (EBV).[55,56] HVS and EBV both belong to the *Gammaherpesvirinae*, a subfamily of herpesviruses that are capable of immortalizing cells and persisting in lymphocytes.

HHV-8 DNA sequences have been found in over 95% of all KS tissues, including classical and iatrogenic, demonstrating that HIV infection is not required for the onset of cancer.[48,57–61] HHV-8 DNA sequences have also been found in two unusual types of lymphomas termed body-cavity–based lymphoma (BCBL) and multicentric Castleman's disease (MCD).[62–64] The HHV-8 DNA sequences in the BCBLs have been found to be present at higher levels than those seen in the KS tissues, although this may reflect the heterogeneity of the KS lesion compared to the relative homogeneity of a B-cell lymphoma. In addition, most of the HHV-8–positive

**TABLE 1B-17. EBV LATENT PROTEINS**

| EBV LATENCY PROTEIN (ALTERNATIVE NAME) | REQUIRED FOR IMMORTALIZATION | KNOWN/PROPOSED FUNCTION | LATENCY PATTERN |
|---|---|---|---|
| EBNA-1 | Yes | Maintenance of viral episome | I, II, III |
| EBNA-2 | Yes | Regulation of viral gene transcription | III |
| EBNA-3a (EBNA-3) | Yes | Regulation of viral gene transcription | III |
| EBNA-3b (EBNA-4) | No | Regulation of viral gene transcription | III |
| EBNA-3c (EBNA-6) | Yes | Regulation of viral gene transcription | III |
| EBNA-LP (EBNA-5) | No | Induction of cell cycle | III |
| LMP-1 | Yes | Induction of cell proliferation | II, III |
| LMP-2a (TP-1) | No | Regulation of viral latency | II, III |
| LMP-2b (TP-2) | No | Regulation of LMP-2a function | II, III |
| EBERs 1 and 2 | No | Small RNA | I, II, III |
| BamHI A transcripts | —— | —— | I, II, III |

lymphomas were also infected with EBV, although a few EBV-negative and HHV-8–positive lymphomas have been reported.

HHV-8 DNA has been detected in peripheral blood mononuclear cells (PBMCs) and semen of KS patients at times prior to and following the onset of KS.[55,65–68] Viral DNA has also been found in semen and saliva samples from healthy HIV-negative subjects.[69,70] The epidemiology of KS has strongly suggested that the infectious agent is transmitted by sexual intercourse. The detection of HHV-8 DNA in semen samples supports this hypothesis. Further, seroepidemiologic studies examining the seroprevalence of HHV-8 among different human cohorts have supported the concept that HHV-8 is transmitted sexually.[71–74] Sexual transmission is not the only method of viral transmission, however, as evidenced by reports of HHV-8 seropositive children and transmission of virus from mother to child.[75–78] Interestingly, HHV-8 does not appear to be spread through infected blood, even though virus has been detected in PBMCs of seropositive individuals. In one study of injecting drug users, HHV-8 seroprevalence was found to be similar to that of the general population, suggesting that HHV-8 is not readily spread through contaminated blood.[79]

The seroprevalence of HHV-8 in the general population is between 5% and 11% depending on the serologic assay. Given that KS, BCBL, or MCD is extremely rare among the general population, HHV-8 viral infection, much like the other human viruses discussed in this chapter, is not sufficient for tumor formation. However, the serology and epidemiologic studies clearly support a cofactor role for HHV-8 in the onset of these cancers. Another factor required for carcinogenesis may include immunosuppression, since it is generally shared by many patients with KS. Clearly, the AIDS-related or epidemic form of KS and the posttransplant form of KS occur in a background of immunosuppression. The classic or Mediterranean form of KS may also be viewed as related to a type of immunosuppression, since this form occurs primarily in men over the age of 60.

Although the exact mechanism of HHV-8–induced transformation is not currently known, analysis of the viral genome has revealed several proteins that share significant homology with cellular proteins. These genes include homologs for interleukin 6, cyclin D, Bcl-2, macrophage inhibitory factors, interferon regulatory factor, FLICE inhibitory protein, and a G-protein–coupled receptor. The possible roles of some of these proteins in viral oncogenesis has been recently reviewed.[80]

## HUMAN T-CELL LEUKEMIA VIRUS TYPE 1 (HTLV-1)

HTLV-1 was discovered as the first human retrovirus in 1980 from T-cell lymphoblastoid cell lines and primary PBMCs from a patient with adult T-cell leukemia (ATL).[81] HTLV-1 is now recognized as a required cofactor in the development of ATL. In Japan, where HTLV-1 is endemic, approximately 1 to 2 million people are estimated to be infected with 10 to 20 million infected individuals present worldwide.[82] The HTLV-1 virion consists of an enveloped, spherical nucleocapsid containing two copies of a 9-kb RNA genome.[83] Transmission of HTLV-1 can occur by intercourse, contaminated blood products, or vertically from mother to fetus.[84] Since HTLV-1 is a retrovirus, its replicative cycle includes the production of a DNA copy of the viral genome, which then becomes integrated into cellular DNA. Once integrated, the provirus is carried from parent to daughter cells.

ATL occurs in approximately 1 out of every 1000 to 2000 HTLV-1–infected individuals. The length of time between viral infection and ATL development is 20 to 30 years.[82] This long latency period between infection and tumor formation suggests that other cellular or molecular events must occur for development of ATL. Further, HTLV-1 infection alone is insufficient for oncogenesis, since the vast majority of HTLV-1–infected individuals will not develop ATL. A number of research studies have implicated the Tax protein of HTLV-1 in tumorigenesis. The Tax protein is a highly promiscuous transactivator, upregulating the HTLV-1 LTR as well as numerous cellular genes such as IL-2, granulocyte-macrophage colony stimulating factor (GM-CSF), transforming growth factor β (TGF-β), c-*myc*, vcam-1, c-*fos*, and c-*erg*.[85] Given that insertion of the provirus into cellular DNA is random, along with the very long incubation period between infection and tumor formation, it seems likely that HTLV-1–induced transformation is due to a prolonged transactivation of cellular genes and accumulation of other genetic defects (such as mutations in p53).

## SUMMARY

The past 10 to 15 years of research has resulted in an explosion of evidence demonstrating a role for different human viruses in the development of human cancer. Unlike many of the animal oncogenic viruses, the human viruses discussed in this chapter do not produce tumors as a consequence of their normal viral replicative cycle. Instead, they appear to serve as one additional cofactor for cancer development. Viral infection does not ensure development of cancer. Rather, viral infection under appropriate circumstances such as immunosuppression or chronic infection greatly increases the risk of cancer development. Identification of human viruses involved in the development of cancer, along with understanding the mechanisms of viral replication and viral-induced oncogenesis, will aid in the development of effective antiviral therapies that will ultimately serve to prevent viral infection and viral-induced cancer.

## REFERENCES

1. WEISS RA: Introducing viruses and cancer, in *Viruses and Human Cancer*, JR Arrand, DR Harper (eds). Oxford, England, BIOS Scientific Publishers, 1998, pp 1–16.
2. ELLERMAN V, BANG O: Experimentelle Leukamie bei Huhnern. Zentralb Bakteriol 46:595, 1908.
3. ROUS P: A transmissible avian neoplasm: sarcoma of the common fowl. J Exp Med 12:696, 1910.
4. ROUS P: Transmission of a malignant new growth by means of cell-free filtrate. JAMA 56:198, 1911.
5. BITTNER JJ: Some possible effects of nursing on the mammary gland tumor incidence in mice. Science 84:162, 1936.
6. COLE CN: Polyomavirinae: The viruses and their replication, in *Fields Virology*, BN Fields et al (eds). Philadelphia, Lippincott-Raven, 1996.

7. ORTH G: Papillomaviruses—Human, general features, in *Encyclopedia of Virology*, RG Webster, A Granoff (eds). San Diego: Academic Press, 1994, pp 1013–1021.

8. PHILLIPS AC, VOUSDEN KH: Human papillomaviruses and cancer, in *Viruses and Human Cancer*, JR Arrand, DR Harper (eds). Oxford, England, BIOS Scientific Publishers, 1998, pp 39–64.

9. LAIMINS LA: Regulation of transcription and replication by human papillomavirus, in *DNA Tumor Viruses*, DJ McCance (ed). Washington, DC: ASM Press, 1998, pp 199–222.

10. NEAD MA, McCANCE DJ: Activities of the transforming proteins of human papillomaviruses, in *DNA Tumor Viruses*, DJ McCance (ed). Washington, DC: ASM Press, 1998, pp 223–250.

11. ZUR HAUSEN H: Papillomavirus infections—A major cause of human cancers. Biochim Biophys Acta 1288:F55, 1996.

12. VOUSDEN KH et al: The E7 open reading frame of human papillomavirus type 16 encodes a transforming gene. Oncogene Res 3:167, 1988.

13. HAWLEY-NELSON P et al: HPV16 E6 and E7 proteins cooperate to immortalize human foreskin keratinocytes. EMBO J 8:3905, 1989.

14. DYSON N et al: The human papillomavirus-16 E7 oncoprotein is able to bind the retinoblastoma gene product. Science 243:934, 1989.

15. WEINBERG RA: The retinoblastoma protein and cell cycle control. Cell 81:323, 1995.

16. WERNESS BA et al: Association of human papillomavirus types 16 and 18 E6 proteins with p53. Science 248:76, 1990.

17. GOTTLIEB TM, OREN M: p53 in growth control and neoplasia. Biochim Biophys Acta 1287:77, 1996.

18. HOPPE-SEYLER F, BUTZ K: Tumor suppressor genes in molecular medicine. Clin Invest 72:619, 1994.

19. CARSON DA, LOIS A: Cancer progression and p53. Lancet 346:1009, 1995.

20. SCHEFFNER M et al: The state of the p53 and retinoblastoma genes in human cervical carcinoma cell lines. Proc Natl Acad Sci USA 88:5523, 1991.

21. CROOK T et al: Degradation of p53 can be targeted by IIPV E6 sequences distinct from those required for p53 binding and transactivation. Cell 67:547, 1991.

22. LECHNER MS, LAIMINS LA: Inhibition of p53 DNA binding by human papillomavirus E6 proteins. J Virol 68:4262, 1994.

23. KLINGELHUTZ AJ et al: Telomerase activation by the E6 gene product of human papillomavirus type 16. Nature 380:79, 1996.

24. LEDNICKY JA, BUTEL JS: Polyomaviruses and human tumors: A brief review of current concepts and interpretations. Frontiers Biosci 4:d153, 1999.

25. EDDY BE et al: Identification of the oncogenic substance in rhesus monkey kidney cell cultures as simian virus 40. Virology 17:65, 1962.

26. GIRARDI AJ et al: Development of tumors in hamsters inoculated in the neo-natal period with vacuolating virus, SV40. Proc Soc Exp Biol Med 109:649, 1962.

27. BECK GR JR et al: Introduction to tumor viruses: Adenovirus, simian virus 40, and polyomavirus, in *DNA Tumor Viruses*, DJ McCance (ed). Washington, DC, ASM Press, 1998, pp 51–86.

28. BRECHOT C: Hepatitis B and C viruses and primary liver cancer. Baillieres Clin Haematol 10:335, 1996.

29. HARRISON TJ: Viral hepatitis and primary liver cancer, in *Viruses and Human Cancer*, JR Arrand, DR Harper (eds). Oxford, England, BIOS Scientific Publishers, 1998, pp 17–38.

30. GROB PJ: Hepatitis B: Virus, pathogenesis and treatment. Vaccine 16:S11, 1998.

31. MASON WS et al: Hepatitis B virus replication, liver disease, and hepatocellular carcinoma, in *DNA Tumor Viruses*, DJ McCance (ed). Washington, DC, ASM Press, 1998, pp 251–298.

32. ALTER MJ: Epidemiology of hepatitis C. Hepatology 26:62S, 1997.

33. BURKITT DP: A sarcoma involving the jaws in African children. Br J Surg 46:218, 1958.

34. EPSTEIN MA et al: Virus particles in cultured lymphoblasts from Burkitt's lymphoma. Lancet 1:702, 1964.

35. KARIMI L, CRAWFORD DH: Epstein-Barr virus: Mechanisms of oncogenesis, in *DNA Tumor Viruses Oncogenic Mechanisms*, G Barbanti-Brodano et al (eds). New York, Plenum Press, 1995, pp 347–374.

36. SIXBEY JW et al: Epstein-Barr virus replication in oropharyngeal epithelial cells. N Engl J Med 310:1225, 1984.

37. SCHWARZMANN F et al: Epstein-Barr viral gene expression in B-lymphocytes. Leukemia Lymphoma 30:123, 1998.

38. THORLEY-LAWSON DA et al: Epstein-Barr virus and the B cell: That's all it takes. Trends Microbiol 4:204, 1996.

39. ARRAND JR: Epstein-Barr virus, in *Viruses and Human Cancer*, JR Arrand, DR Harper (eds). Oxford, England, BIOS Scientific Publishers, 1998, pp 65–92.

40. BURKITT DP: The discovery of Burkitt's lymphoma. Cancer 51:1777, 1983.

41. MILLER G: Epstein-Barr virus: Biology, pathogenesis, and medical aspects, in *Fields Virology*, BN Fields et al (eds). New York, Raven Press, 1990, pp 1921–1958.

42. DEACON EM et al: Epstein-Barr virus and Hodgkin's disease: Transcriptional analysis of virus latency in the malignant cells. J Exp Med 177:339, 1993.

43. MACMAHON EME et al: Epstein-Barr virus in AIDS-related primary central nervous system lymphoma. Lancet 338:969, 1991.

44. RANDHAWA PS et al: Expression of Epstein-Barr virus-encoded small RNA (by the EBER-1 gene) in liver specimens from transplant recipients with post-transplantation lymphoproliferative disease. N Engl J Med 327:1710, 1992.

45. PURTILO DT: Epstein-Barr virus-induced diseases in the X-linked lymphoproliferative syndrome and related disorders. Biomed Pharmacother 39:52, 1985.

46. IMAI S et al: Gastric carcinoma: Monoclonal epithelial malignant cells expressing Epstein-Barr virus latent infection protein. Proc Natl Acad Sci USA 91:9131, 1994.

47. LEE ES: The association of Epstein-Barr virus with smooth-muscle tumors occurring after organ transplantation. N Engl J Med 332:19, 1995.

48. CHANG Y: Identification of herpesvirus-like DNA sequences in AIDS-associated Kaposi's sarcoma. Science 266:1865, 1994.

49. WAHMAN A et al: The epidemiology of classic, African, and immunosuppressed Kaposi's sarcoma. Epidemiol Rev 13:178, 1991.

50. LEVINE AM: AIDS-related malignancies: The emerging epidemic. J Natl Cancer Inst 85:1382, 1993.

51. PENN I: Kaposi's sarcoma in organ transplant recipients. Transplantation 27:8, 1979.

52. PENN I: Cancers following cyclosporine therapy. Transplantation 43:32, 1987.

53. PETERMAN TA et al: The aetiology of Kaposi's sarcoma. Cancer Surv 10:23, 1991.

54. STEIN M et al: AIDS-related Kaposi's sarcoma: A review. Isr J Med Sci 30:298, 1994.

55. MOORE PS et al: Primary characterization of a herpesvirus agent associated with Kaposi's sarcoma. J Virol 70:549, 1996.

56. Russo JJ et al: Nucleotide sequence of the Kaposi sarcoma-associated herpesvirus (HHV8). Proc Natl Acad Sci USA 93:14862, 1996.

57. Su IJ et al: Herpesvirus-like DNA sequence in Kaposi's sarcoma from AIDS and non-AIDS patients in Taiwan. Lancet 345:722, 1995.

58. Huang YQ et al: Human herpesvirus-like nucleic acid in various forms of Kaposi's sarcoma. Lancet 345:759, 1995.

59. Dupin N et al: Herpesvirus-like DNA sequences in patients with Mediterranean Kaposi's sarcoma. Lancet 345:761, 1995.

60. Collandre H et al: Kaposi's sarcoma and a new herpesvirus. Lancet 345:1043, 1995.

61. Boshoff C et al: Kaposi's sarcoma–associated herpesvirus in HIV-negative Kaposi's sarcoma. Lancet 345:1043, 1995.

62. Cesarman E et al: Kaposi's sarcoma–associated herpesvirus-like DNA sequences in AIDS-related body-cavity-based lymphomas. N Engl J Med 332:1186, 1995.

63. Nador RG et al: Herpes-like DNA sequences in body-cavity-based lymphoma in HIV-negative patients. N Engl J Med 333:943, 1995.

64. Ansari MQ et al: Primary body cavity–based AIDS-related lymphomas. Am J Clin Pathol 105:221, 1996.

65. Bigoni B et al: Human herpesvirus 8 is present in the lymphoid system of healthy persons and can reactivate in the course of AIDS. J Infect Dis 173:542, 1997.

66. Lefrere JJ et al: Detection of human herpesvirus 8 DNA sequences before the appearance of Kaposi's sarcoma in human immunodeficiency virus (HIV)-positive subjects with a known date of HIV seroconversion. J Infect Dis 174:283, 1996.

67. Gupta P et al: Detection of Kaposi's sarcoma herpesvirus DNA in semen of homosexual men with Kaposi's sarcoma (Abstr). AIDS 10:1596, 1996.

68. Pastore C et al: Distribution of Kaposi's sarcoma herpesvirus sequences among lymphoid malignancies in Italy and Spain. Br J Haematol 91:918, 1995.

69. Bobroski L et al: Localization of human herpesvirus type 8 (HHV-8) in the Kaposi's sarcoma tissues and the semen specimens of HIV-1 infected and uninfected individuals by utilizing in situ polymerase chain reaction. J Reprod Immunol 41:149, 1998.

70. Calabro ML et al: Detection of human herpesvirus 8 in cervicovaginal secretions and seroprevalence in human immunodeficiency virus type 1–seropositive and –seronegative women. J Infect Dis 179:1534, 1999.

71. Kedes DH et al: The seroepidemiology of human herpesvirus 8 (Kaposi's sarcoma–associated herpesvirus): Distribution of infection in KS risk groups and evidence for sexual transmission. Nature Med 2:918, 1996.

72. Martin JN et al: Sexual-transmission and the natural history of human herpesvirus 8 infection. N Engl J Med 338:948, 1998.

73. Melbye M et al: Risk factors for Kaposi's-sarcoma-associated herpesvirus (KSHV/HHV8) seropositivity in a cohort of homosexual men, 1981–1996. Int J Cancer 77:543, 1998.

74. Verbeck W et al: Seroprevalence of HHV-8 antibodies in HIV-positive homosexual men without Kaposi's sarcoma and their clinical follow-up. Am J Clin Pathol 109:778, 1998.

75. Sitas F et al: Increasing probability of mother-to-child transmission of HHV-8 with increasing maternal antibody titer for HHV-8 [letter]. N Engl J Med 340:1923, 1999.

76. Gessain A et al: Human herpesvirus 8 primary infection occurs during childhood in Cameroon, Central Africa. Int J Cancer 81:189, 1999.

77. Andreoni M et al: High seroprevalence of antibodies to human herpesvirus-8 in Egyptian children: Evidence of nonsexual transmission. J Nat Cancer Inst 91:465, 1999.

78. Bourboulia D et al: Serologic evidence for mother-to-child transmission of Kaposi sarcoma-associated herpesvirus infection [letter]. JAMA 280:31, 1998.

79. Bernstein KT et al: Factors associated with human herpesvirus type 8 (HHV-8) infection in an injecting drug user cohort. Submitted for publication.

80. Moore PS, Chang Y: Kaposi's sarcoma–associated herpesvirus-encoded oncogenes and oncogenesis. J Natl Cancer Inst 23:65, 1998.

81. Poiesz BJ et al: Detection and isolation of type C retrovirus particles from fresh and cultured lymphocytes of a patient with cutaneous T-cell lymphoma. Proc Natl Acad Sci USA 77:7415, 1980.

82. Uchiyama T: Human T cell leukemia virus type I (HTLV-I) and human diseases. Ann Rev Immunol 15:15, 1997.

83. Coffin JM: Retroviridae: The viruses and their replication, in Fields Virology, BN Fields et al (eds). Philadelphia: Lippincott-Raven, 1996, pp 1767–1847.

84. Yao J, Wigdahl B: Human T cell lymphotrophic virus type I genomic expression and impact on intracellular signaling pathways during neurodegenerative disease and leukemia. Frontiers Biosci 5:D138, 2000.

85. Taylor GP, McClure M: Human oncoretroviruses, in Viruses and Human Cancer, JR Arrand, DR Harper (eds). Oxford, England, BIOS Scientific Publishers, 1998, pp 109–144.

# CHAPTER 2

# RECENT ADVANCES IN THE BIOLOGY OF CANCER INVASION AND METASTASIS

*Lee M. Ellis, Robert Radinsky, and Isaiah J. Fidler*

## INTRODUCTION

Metastasis is the major cause of death from cancer. The treatment of cancer poses a major problem to clinical oncologists, because, by the time many cancers are diagnosed, metastasis has in many cases already occurred. The presence of multiple metastases makes complete eradication by surgery, radiation, chemotherapy, or biotherapy nearly impossible. Exacerbating the problems of treating metastatic disease is the fact that tumor cells in different metastases, and in some instances even different regions within an individual metastatic lesion, may respond differently to treatment. Although numerous promising anticancer drugs and biotherapeutic agents have been developed, their effectiveness is still hindered by the presence of resistant cancer cells. Tumor cell resistance to current therapeutic modalities is the single most important reason for the lack of successful treatment in many types of solid neoplasms. In part, the emergence of treatment-resistant tumor cells is due to the heterogeneous nature of malignant neoplasms. Indeed, this phenotypic diversity, which permits selected variants to develop from the parent tumor, implies not only that the primary tumor and metastases can differ in their response to treatment, but also that the biology of individual metastases can differ markedly from one another.

Insight into the molecular mechanisms regulating the pathobiology of cancer metastasis as well as a better understanding of the interaction between the metastatic cell and the host environment should provide a foundation for the design of new therapeutic approaches. Furthermore, the development of in vivo and in vitro models that will allow for the isolation and characterization of cells possessing metastatic potential within both primary tumors and metastases will be invaluable in the design of more effective therapeutic modalities.

## THE PATHOGENESIS OF CANCER METASTASIS

The phenomenon of cancer metastasis is a dynamic one that, for descriptive purposes, may be divided into a series of sequential steps (Fig. 2-1). Malignant cells that eventually develop into established metastases must survive a series of potentially lethal interactions with host homeostatic and immune mechanisms, the outcome of which is influenced by both host factors and the intrinsic properties of the tumor cells (reviewed in references 1–3).

The essential steps in the formation of a metastatic lesion are summarized as follows:

1. After the initial unicellular or multicellular transforming event, survival and progressive growth of neoplastic cells is initially supported with nutrients supplied from the local microenvironment by simple diffusion.
2. Vascularization must occur next for a tumor mass to exceed approximately 2 mm in diameter. The synthesis and secretion of tumor angiogenesis factors play a key role in establishing a neo-capillary network from the surrounding host tissue.[4–8]
3. Local invasion of the surrounding host stroma by some tumor cells can occur by several mechanisms. Rapidly proliferating

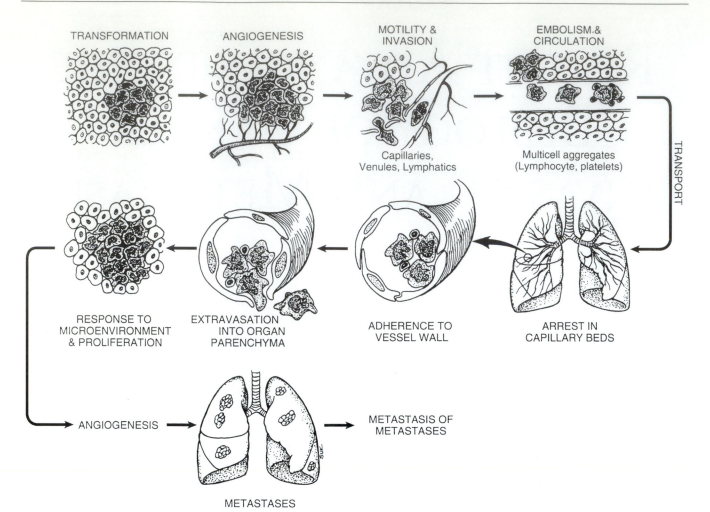

TRANSFORMATION

ANGIOGENESIS

MOTILITY & INVASION

EMBOLISM & CIRCULATION

Capillaries, Venules, Lymphatics

Multicell aggregates (Lymphocyte, platelets)

TRANSPORT

RESPONSE TO MICROENVIRONMENT & PROLIFERATION

EXTRAVASATION INTO ORGAN PARENCHYMA

ADHERENCE TO VESSEL WALL

ARREST IN CAPILLARY BEDS

ANGIOGENESIS

METASTASIS OF METASTASES

METASTASES

**FIGURE 2-1.** The pathogenesis of cancer metastasis. To produce metastases, tumor cells must detach from the primary tumor, invade the extracellular matrix and enter the circulation, survive in the circulation to arrest in the capillary bed, adhere to subendothelial basement membrane, gain entrance into the organ parenchyma, respond to paracrine growth factors, proliferate and induce angiogenesis, and evade host defenses. The pathogenesis of metastasis is therefore complex and consists of multiple sequential, selective, and interdependent steps whose outcome depends on the interaction of tumor cells with homeostatic factors. (*From Fidler.*[2] *Reproduced with permission.*)

tumors create mechanical pressure that pushes cells into areas of low resistance.[9] In contrast, tumors that grow within the major body cavities can shed cells that seed the mucosal or serosal surfaces of other organs, thereby establishing secondary growths. Such routes of tumor cell dissemination are secondary in importance to the spread of tumor cells via hematogenous or lymphatic channels. Tumor cell invasion of blood and lymphatic vessels is enhanced by the production of lytic enzymes such as lysosomal hydrolases and type IV collagenase from either tumor cells, host inflammatory cells, or host stromal cells.[10–13] A strong correlation also exists between the ability of tumor cells to adhere to basement membrane components such as fibronectin and laminin and their metastatic capabilities.[14] In fact, fragments or peptides

of laminin or fibronectin that contain the cell-surface binding sites can markedly inhibit metastasis.[14–16]

4. Once the tumor breaches the stroma of the circulatory system, detachment and embolization of small tumor cell aggregates occurs, with most tumor cells being rapidly destroyed. Radiolabeling studies have shown that for most tumors, fewer than 0.1% of tumor cells that enter the circulation survive to form metastases.[17] Thus, the presence of tumor cells in the blood does not equate with the formation of metastasis. Circulating tumor cells are unquestionably more susceptible to various host immune and nonimmune defenses, including blood turbulence and the trauma associated with arrest, transcapillary passage, and lysis by lymphocytes, monocytes, and natural killer (NK) cells.[18–22]

5. Once the tumor cells have survived the hostile environment of the circulation, they must arrest in the capillary beds of distant organs, either by adhering to capillary endothelial cells or by adhering to subendothelial basement membrane that may be exposed.[23]

6. Extravasation occurs next, probably by mechanisms similar to those that influence initial invasion.

7. Survival and growth within the organ parenchyma and the development of second-order metastases complete the metastatic cascade. To survive and grow in the organ parenchyma, the metastatic cells must develop a vascular network and evade the host immune system. These metastases, when they have attained a certain size, may then give rise to additional metastases, the so-called metastasis of metastases.

For production of clinically relevant metastases, each of the steps of the metastatic process must be completed.[1,24] Failure to complete one or more steps (e.g., inability to invade host stroma, a high degree of antigenicity, inability to grow in a distant organ's parenchyma) eliminates the cells. Because few cells survive this cascade to establish secondary foci, the development of metastases could represent the chance survival of a few tumor cells or could represent the selection from the parent tumor of a subpopulation of metastatic cells endowed with properties that enhance their survival. Data generated by our laboratory and many others strongly support the latter possibility.

The first experimental proof for metastatic heterogeneity in neoplasms was provided in 1977 by Fidler and Kripke[25] in their work with the murine B16 melanoma. Using a modification of the fluctuation assay of Luria and Delbruck,[26] they showed that different tumor cell clones, each derived from an individual cell isolated from the parent tumor, varied dramatically in their ability to produce pulmonary nodules following intravenous inoculation into syngeneic recipient mice. Control subcloning procedures demonstrated that the observed diversity was not a consequence of the cloning procedure.[25] The finding that preexisting tumor cell subpopulations proliferating in the same tumor exhibit heterogeneous metastatic potential has since been confirmed in numerous laboratories using a wide range of experimental animal tumors of different histories and histologic origins (reviewed in references 1, 3, 9, 27). In addition, studies using nude mice as models for metastasis of human neoplasms have shown that several human tumor lines and freshly isolated tumors also contain subpopulations of cells with widely differing metastatic properties.[28–33] This demonstration of heterogeneity required that the tumor cells be implanted into the correct anatomic sites.

The data demonstrating metastatic heterogeneity in neoplasms and those showing that the outcome of metastasis is also dependent on host factors support the concept that metastasis is selective and is not a random process.[1,2,34–36] Notwithstanding its implications for the value of current therapeutic strategies, the role of metastatic subpopulations of tumor cells in generating metastases offers a rational strategy for eventually combating this disease, whereas an entirely random process would be far less amenable to therapeutic manipulation. In other words, metastasis is governed by mechanisms that can be studied and ultimately understood in sufficient detail to allow the development of rational therapeutic interventions.

## ORIGIN OF BIOLOGIC DIVERSITY IN NEOPLASMS

A substantial body of evidence, gained from studies on human and experimental animal neoplasms, now indicates that most neoplasms are populated by cells with different biologic characteristics. Cells obtained from individual tumors have been shown to differ with respect to many properties, including morphology, metabolic characteristics, antigenic or immunogenic potential, growth rates, karyotypes, production of extracellular matrix proteins, sensitivity to destruction by NK or cytotoxic T lymphocytes, cell-surface receptors for lectins, hormone receptors, drug and radiation sensitivities, invasiveness, and the ability to metastasize.[1–3,27,37–41] Biologic heterogeneity is not just confined to cells in primary tumors; it is equally prominent among the cells populating metastases.

Whether neoplasms are heterogeneous and contain subpopulations of tumor cells with different metastatic propensities is no longer at issue. The more interesting problem is to understand how this extensive cellular heterogeneity originates and is maintained and controlled. For example, do metastatic variant cells arise early or late in the development of malignant neoplasms? Once metastatic cells develop in a neoplasm, do they have a growth advantage over nonmetastatic cells so that, with the passage of time, metastatic cells constitute the majority of cells in a neoplasm? How is the proportion of metastatic cells to nonmetastatic cells regulated? Answers to some of these questions are now available. They may help oncologists and surgeons make decisions critical to the timing and sequence of multimodality treatments for primary tumors and metastases.

Clinical observations of human neoplasms have suggested that spontaneous tumors tend to undergo a series of changes during the course of the disease. For example, a growth that initially appeared to be a benign tumor changes over a period of months or years into a malignant, lethal tumor. Extensive studies in murine mammary tumor systems led Foulds[42–46] to describe this phenomenon of tumor evolution as "neoplastic progression." Foulds defined tumor progression as "acquisition of permanent, irreversible qualitative changes in one or more characteristics of a neoplasm."[42] This evolution of tumors is gradual, and tumor cells proceed toward increased autonomy from their host by changes in various properties over time. The acquisition or loss of various characteristics can be independent of each other. Moreover, because tumor progression can occur over periods of months or even years, the behavioral characteristics of a neoplasm in any given individual may vary at different stages of the disease. Because tumors progress in their host, it is not surprising that tumor progression is also influenced by host homeostatic factors, which serve as selection pressures.[41,47–51] Some tumors originate from multiple transformed cells. In these tumors, the presence of diverse cellular populations may merely reflect the diverse parentages, although additional diversification is almost certainly necessary to explain the high degree of biologic heterogeneity. However, most human cancers probably result from the proliferation of a single transformed cell,[52–55] and the generation of biologic diversity in such tumors must therefore reflect a complex pattern of clonal diversification during tumor progression[42,48] (Fig. 2-2).

Tumors of unicellular origin may exhibit metastatic heterogeneity at very early stages in their development. We base this conclusion

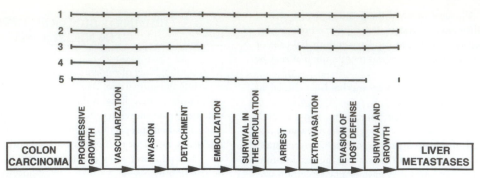

**FIGURE 2-2.** To produce metastases, tumor cells must complete every step in the process. If they fail to complete one or more steps, the cells are eliminated. For example, a cell that can induce angiogenesis but is not motile-invasive will not produce a metastasis. The prediction of metastatic potential therefore requires a multiparametric analysis. (*From Fidler.*[2] *Reproduced with permission.*)

on data generated by studies from this laboratory on the in vivo behavior of murine embryo fibroblasts transformed by an oncogenic virus.[40] Six colonies of BALB/c embryo fibroblasts, each derived from a single cell, were infected in vitro with mouse sarcoma virus and then propagated as individual cell lines. When viable cells from the clones were injected into the tail vein of BALB/c mice, the number of lung nodules produced by each clone differed markedly. Because the parent cell population was derived from a single transformed cell, these data indicate that rapid phenotypic diversification occurs. Similarly, when the clones from two colonies (one of high and one of low experimental metastatic capacity) were subcloned and evaluated in the same manner, both clones exhibited metastatic heterogeneity. Interestingly, the clone with higher metastatic capacity exhibited a greater degree of variability than the clone with lower metastatic capacity. Thus, despite originating from a single cell, by the time of the first subcloning 6 weeks after initial transformation, the so-called clones already contained subpopulations of cells with different metastatic properties. These data also demonstrate that the generation of metastatic heterogeneity in neoplasms does not require a prolonged latency period of months or even weeks, but that it can occur quite rapidly.

The cellular composition of different metastases in the same host is heterogeneous, both within a single metastasis (intralesional heterogeneity) and among different metastases (interlesional heterogeneity). This heterogeneity reflects two major processes: the selective nature of the metastatic process and the rapid evolution and phenotypic diversification of clonal tumor cell populations during progressive tumor growth (which itself results from the inherent genetic and phenotypic instability of many clonal populations of tumor cells) (Table 2-1).

Like primary neoplasms, metastases may have a unicellular or a multicellular origin.[9,56,57] To determine whether individual metastases are clonal in their origin and whether different metastases can be produced by different progenitor cells, a series of experiments were carried out utilizing the fact that x-irradiation of tumor cells induces random chromosome breaks and rearrangements that serve as "markers." Talmadge and co-workers[56] examined the metastases

that arose from subcutaneously growing tumors produced by K-1735 mouse melanoma cells that had been x-irradiated to induce chromosomal damage. They reasoned that if a metastasis were derived from a single cell, all the chromosome spreads examined within an individual metastasis would exhibit the same karyotype. In contrast, if a metastasis had been formed from more than one progenitor cell, its constituent cells would exhibit different chromosomal arrangements, assuming, of course, that the different cells involved carried distinguishable karyotypic markers.

The cellular composition of 21 individual metastases was analyzed after cultivation of cells from individual solitary metastases.

**TABLE 2-1.  POSSIBLE MECHANISMS FOR THE GENERATION OF BIOLOGICAL HETEROGENEITY WITHIN CANCER METASTASES**

A. Multicellular origin—polyclonal
B. Unicellular origin—monoclonal
  1. Genetic
    a. DNA repair alterations
    b. DNA replication infidelity
    c. DNA amplification
    d. Karyotypic alterations
      1. Rearrangements—deletion, inversion, translocation
      2. Breakage
      3. Aneuploidy
    e. Changes in transcriptional or translational regulatory control
    f. Cell fusion
  2. Epigenetic
    a. Cellular interactions and communication
      1. Tumor cell–tumor cell
      2. Tumor cell–host cell
    b. Microenvironment
      1. Hormonal influences
      2. Growth factors
      3. Inducers of differentiation or apoptosis

In 10 metastases, all the chromosomes were normal, making it impossible to establish whether they were of unicellular or multicellular origin. In the other 11 lesions, unique karyotypic patterns of abnormal marker chromosomes were found, suggesting that each metastasis originated from a single progenitor cell. This experiment, however, did not resolve whether metastases arose as a consequence of individual cells or homogeneous clumps (i.e., a multicellular embolus of cells with the same chromosome marker) surviving in the bloodstream, but it did establish that many metastases can originate from single cells. Moreover, the finding that different metastases are populated exclusively by cells with different chromosome markers indicates that different metastases can originate from different progenitor cells.

Subsequent experiments by Fidler and Talmadge[58] demonstrated that when heterogeneous clumps of two different K-1735 melanoma cell lines were injected intravenously to be arrested in the lung vasculature, the resultant metastases were all of unicellular origin. These results suggest that whether an embolus is homogeneous or heterogeneous, metastases can still originate from a single proliferating cell. Clonality of metastases has also been reported for different tumors, including mammary carcinoma, fibrosarcoma, and melanoma.[22,59–61]

Despite a clonal origin, most metastases undergo rapid diversification. We base this conclusion on experiments using B16 and K-1735 melanoma cell clones bearing identifiable biochemical or karyotypic markers. These studies demonstrated not only that the majority of metastases are of clonal origin but also that variant clones with diverse phenotypes are formed rapidly, thus generating significant cellular diversity within individual metastases.[9,62–64]

Collectively, these observations indicate that different metastases arise from different progenitor cells, a finding that can account for the well-documented differences in the behavior of individual metastases in the same patient, including differences in response to therapy. However, even within individual metastases of proven clonal origin, heterogeneity can develop rapidly to create significant intralesional heterogeneity.

## HOST AND TUMOR INTERACTIONS IN PATHOGENESIS OF METASTASIS

In humans and in experimental rodent systems, numerous examples exist in which malignant tumors metastasize to specific organs (for review, see references 34–36, 65, 66). Two arguments have been advanced previously to explain organ-specific metastasis. In 1889, Paget[67] proposed that the growth of metastases is influenced by the interaction of particular tumor cells (the "seed") with the unique organ's environment (the "soil") and that metastases resulted only when the seed and soil were compatible. Forty years later, Ewing challenged Paget's seed-and-soil theory and proposed that the pattern of metastasis is controlled by purely mechanical factors that are a result of the anatomic structure of the vascular system.[68] In a review of clinical studies on organ-specific metastasis of some tumors, Sugarbaker[69] concluded that common *regional* metastatic involvements could be attributed to anatomic or mechanical considerations such as efferent venous circulation or lymphatic drainage

to regional lymph nodes, but that *distant* organ metastases represent a unique pattern of organ specificity. Experimental[34–36,65,66] and clinical[70] confirmation of this observation suggest that the microenvironment of each organ influences the implantation, invasion, survival, and growth of particular tumor cells.

Although the ability of some tumor cells to proliferate in the parenchyma of some organs is ultimately associated with the development of organ-specific metastasis, the mechanistic basis of this interaction remains largely unknown. The successful metastatic cell, referred to two decades ago as the "decathlon champion,"[71] must today be viewed also as a cell receptive to its environment,[1,66,72] that is, during the metastatic cell's interaction with a number of host cells and systems, signals from endocrine, paracrine, or autocrine pathways, alone or in combination, could stimulate or inhibit tumor cell proliferation, with the eventual outcome dependent on the net balance of positive and negative regulators.

## ORGAN-DERIVED GROWTH FACTORS

A mechanism for site-specific tumor growth involves interactions between receptive metastatic cells and the organ environment, possibly mediated by local growth factors (GFs). Although the involvement of particular peptide GFs is speculative in organ-specific metastasis, these factors are known to mediate the growth of normal and neoplastic cells.[73] Evidence supporting organ-specific GFs for metastatic cells has been obtained, in part, from experiments on the effects of organ-conditioned medium on the growth of particular neoplastic cells. The presence of stimulatory or inhibitory factors in a particular tissue correlated with the site-specific pattern of metastasis (for reviews, see references 34–36, 65, 66). For example, lung-conditioned medium stimulated the in vitro growth of lung-colonizing K-1735 melanoma cells, and to a lesser degree, the growth of liver-colonizing M-5076 cells.[33] High lung-colonizing B16-F10 murine melanoma cells or high ovary-colonizing B16-O10 cells were growth-stimulated by lung- or ovary-conditioned medium, respectively, whereas extracts of other tissues were in each case found to be inhibitory.[34,35] To date, only a few of these organ-derived GFs have been isolated and purified to homogeneity. A potent growth-stimulatory factor was isolated from lung-conditioned medium.[65,74] This transferrinlike factor stimulated epithelial tumor cell growth better than melanoma cell growth.[74] Other investigators have shown that stromal cells in the bone produce a factor that stimulates the growth of human prostatic carcinoma cells.[75]

Conversely, a number of tissue-specific inhibitors have been isolated and purified. Transforming growth factor beta 2 (TGF-β2) was isolated and purified from kidney cell–conditioned medium. Mammastatin, a physiologic mammary growth regulator, was isolated from normal mammary cell–conditioned medium and found to selectively inhibit the growth of transformed human mammary cell lines in culture.[76] Finally, a growth inhibitory factor, amphiregulin, was isolated and found to be expressed in several normal tissues, including the placenta and ovary.[77] Together, this evidence suggests a role for organ-derived paracrine GFs in the regulation of tumor cell proliferation. Once the new factors are purified to acceptable homogeneity, more definitive analyses of organ-specific paracrine factors involved in site-specific metastasis will be possible.[78]

Different concentrations of hormones in individual organs, differentially expressed local factors, or paracrine GFs may all influence the growth of malignant cells at particular sites.[36,66] For example, specific peptide GFs are concentrated in distinct tissue environments. One example is insulinlike growth factor I (IGF-I). IGF-I is synthesized in most mammalian tissue, its highest concentration being in the liver.[79] This GF stimulates cell growth by controlling cell-cycle progression through $G_1$.[80] A recent study demonstrated that carcinoma cells metastatic to the liver were growth-stimulated by hepatocyte-derived IGF-I, correlating with IGF-I receptor density on the metastatic versus nonmetastatic tumor cells. The correlation suggests a potential mechanism of selection in the process of liver colonization.[81] Another example is TGF-β. The principal sources of this peptide are the platelets and bone, suggesting that they have roles in healing and remodeling processes.[82,83] Many transformed cells produce increased levels of TGF-β and simultaneously lose their sensitivity to its growth inhibitory effects.[82] Interestingly, moderately or highly metastatic murine fibrosarcoma cells were growth-stimulated by TGF-β1, whereas nonmetastatic and transformed cells of the identical lineage were growth-inhibited, similar to the nontransformed parental cell lines.[84] Clonal stimulation or inhibition of human colon and renal carcinoma cells by TGF-β1 has also been observed and correlated with differential expression of its receptors.[85] The importance of the inhibitory effect of TGF-β is best defined by its role in colorectal cancers with microsatellite instability. In tumors from patients with hereditary nonpolyposis colon cancer, mutations in mismatch repair genes oftentimes lead to mutations in the TGF-β receptor. This mutation in the receptor is thought to lead to loss of the growth inhibitory pathway regulated by TGF-β, and thus may contribute to colon cancer tumor progression.[86,87] The mechanisms responsible for the observed altered GF responses are currently under investigation. At the least, these results indicate that the receptive metastatic cell (as compared to its nonmetastatic counterparts) may acquire altered responses to GF signals (for reviews, see references 1, 34, 36, 66).

## TISSUE-SPECIFIC REPAIR FACTORS

Host factors (autocrine or paracrine) that control organ repair and/or regeneration may also affect the proliferation of malignant tumor cells. It is interesting to speculate that metastatic cells may therefore proliferate in secondary organs that produce compatible GFs; that is, GFs similar to those involved in the cellular regulation of the normal tissue from which the primary tumor originated. For example, human colon carcinoma (HCC) cells utilize and respond to specific GFs that regulate normal colonic epithelium.[88–90] Some of these identical factors also regulate homeostasis and tissue renewal and repair in the liver (i.e., TGF-α and hepatocyte growth factor [HGF]).[91,92] Do these same factors and receptors participate in the regulation of HCC growth at the metastatic liver-specific site? There is evidence they do. For instance, subsequent to partial hepatectomy (60%), the liver undergoes rapid cell division termed *regeneration*. Recently, transplantation experiments in our laboratory using HCC cells were performed in nude mice that had been subjected to either partial hepatectomy (60%), nephrectomy, or control abdominal surgery.[93] Colon cancer cells implanted subcutaneously

demonstrated accelerated growth in partially hepatectomized mice but not in nephrectomized or control mice. Conversely, human renal carcinoma cells established as micrometastases in the lungs of nude mice underwent significant growth acceleration following unilateral nephrectomy, but not hepatectomy.[93] As described above, the primary organ-specific site of the metastatic colon cancer is the liver, whereas the primary metastatic site of renal carcinoma is the lung. Thus, liver regeneration in the nude mouse stimulated the growth of HCC cells. Additionally, Van Dale and Galand[94] inoculated rat colon adenocarcinoma cells intraportally and showed a dramatic increase in the incidence and growth of tumor colonies in the liver of partially hepatectomized rats as compared to sham-operated controls.

Recently, TGF-α was described as a physiologic regulator of liver regeneration by means of an autocrine mechanism.[89] TGF-α production by hepatocytes might also have a paracrine role, stimulating proliferation of adjacent nonparenchymal cells.[90] Furthermore, TGF-β may be a component of the paracrine regulatory loop, controlling hepatocyte replication at the late stages of liver regeneration.[95] Therefore, when normal tissues such as liver are damaged (possibly by invading tumor cells[35,65]), GFs are released to stimulate normal organ tissue repair, and these factors may also stimulate the proliferation of receptive malignant tumor cells. Hence, tumor cells that either originate from or have affinities for growth in a particular organ can respond to physiologic signals that may produce organ-specific responses.

## ORGAN-SPECIFIC GROWTH REGULATION OF THE METASTATIC CELL

Successful metastasis depends in part on the interaction of favored tumor cells with a compatible milieu provided by a particular organ environment. Recent experimental evidence using different model systems suggests that paracrine stimulation of tumor cells by organ-derived GFs is one mechanism that determines the target organ preference of disseminated cancer cells.[36] Therefore, a modern interpretation of Paget's 1889 seed-and-soil hypothesis must take into account that organ-specific metastasis results from the proliferation of tumor cells differentially expressing GF receptors and that local GFs, organ-repair factors, or paracrine GFs stimulate the growth of malignant cells with receptors.

To distinguish the malignant potential of different Dukes' stage HCCs, our laboratory analyzed their growth in the liver parenchyma, the most common site of metastasis.[96] A reproducible bioassay of hepatic metastasis was developed whereby tumor cells from HCC surgical specimens were inoculated into the spleens of nude mice.[28,30,31,36,97] From this site, tumor cells gain access to the bloodstream and then reach the liver, where they proliferate into tumor colonies. The growth of HCC in the liver directly correlated with the metastatic potential of the cells, that is, cells from surgical specimens of primary HCCs classified as either modified Dukes' stage D or liver metastases produced significantly more colonies in the livers of nude mice than cells from a Dukes' stage B human colon primary tumor.[30,31] Radioactive distribution analyses of both Dukes' stage B and D HCC cells demonstrated that shortly after intrasplenic injection, similar numbers of tumor cells reached the liver microvasculature.[28,97] Thus, the mere presence of viable tumor cells in a particular organ does not always predict that the cells will proliferate to produce metastases.

These experiments stress that the sites of metastasis are determined not solely by the characteristics of the neoplastic cells but also by the microenvironment of the host tissue. Experimental evidence to date strongly indicates that metastases result when the seed and soil are matched.[1,72,98] Therefore, the production of HCC tumors in the livers of nude mice was determined by the ability of the HCC cells to proliferate in the liver parenchyma rather than by the ability of the cells to reach the liver.[97]

To select and isolate metastatic subpopulations of HCC cells with increasing growth potential in the liver parenchyma from heterogeneous primary HCCs, cells were derived from a surgical specimen of a Dukes' stage B2 primary HCC. These HCC cells were established in culture (KM12C) or injected into the subcutis, cecum, and spleen of nude mice.[30,31,97] Progressively growing tumors were then isolated and established in culture. Implantation of these four culture-adapted lines into the cecum or spleen of nude mice produced a few metastatic foci in the liver. HCC cells from these few liver metastases were expanded into culture and reinjected into the spleen of nude mice to provide a source for further cycles of selection. With each successive in vivo selection cycle, the metastatic ability of the isolated and propagated cells increased. Four cycles of intrasplenic selection yielded cell lines (KM12L4) with a very high metastatic efficiency as measured by the ability to proliferate in the liver parenchyma of nude mice. In analogous studies of Dukes' stage D primary HCC, highly metastatic cell lines were isolated, but successive selection cycles for growth in the liver only slightly increased their metastatic properties.[30,31] These results demonstrated that highly metastatic cells can be selected from early-stage HCC and that orthotopic implantation of HCC cells in nude mice is a valid model for determining metastatic potential.[28,30,31,97]

A mechanism that would explain the interaction between distinct HCC cells and the liver-specific environment could involve the proliferation of tumor cells differentially expressing certain GF receptors and their response to liver-specific paracrine GFs or organ-repair factors. Indeed, highly metastatic HCC cells from Dukes' stage D or surgical specimens of liver metastases respond to mitogens associated with liver regeneration induced by hepatectomy in nude mice.[1,93] Following partial hepatectomy, the liver undergoes rapid cell division. This process of liver regeneration involves quantitative changes in hepatocyte gene expression. TGF-α was recently shown to be one regulator of liver regeneration[91,95] and proliferation of normal colonic epithelial cells.[89,90] TGF-α exerts its effect through interaction with the epidermal GF receptor (EGF-R), a plasma membrane glycoprotein that contains within its cytoplasmic domain a tyrosine-specific protein tyrosine kinase (PTK) activity. The binding of TGF-α to the EGF-R stimulates a series of rapid responses, including phosphorylation of tyrosine residues within the EGF-R itself and within many other cellular proteins, hydrolysis of phosphatidyl inositol, release of $Ca^{2+}$ from intracellular stores, elevation of cytoplasmic pH, and morphological changes.[99] After 10 to 12 h in the continuous presence of EGF or TGF-α, cells are committed to synthesize DNA and to divide.[99,100]

EGF-Rs are present on many normal and tumor cells.[99–101] Increased levels and/or amplification of EGF-R has been found in many human tumors and cell lines, including breast cancer,[102] gliomas,[103]

lung cancer,[104] bladder cancer,[105] tumors of the female genital tract,[106] the A431 epidermoid carcinoma,[107] and colon carcinoma.[101] These results suggest a physiologic significance of inappropriate expression of the EGF-R tyrosine kinase in abnormal cell growth control. Whether TGF-α can also regulate the proliferation of metastatic HCC cells in the liver or lymph nodes is unclear. We recently examined the expression and function of EGF-R in a series of HCC cell lines whose liver metastatic potential differed. The results demonstrated that the expression of EGF-R at the mRNA and protein levels directly correlated with the ability of the HCC cells to grow in the liver parenchyma and hence produce hepatic metastases.[101] The EGF-Rs expressed on metastatic HCC cells were functional, based on in vitro growth stimulation assays using picogram concentrations of TGF-α, and specific, as shown by neutralization with anti-EGF-R or anti-TGF-α antibodies. Moreover, EGF-R–associated PTK activity also paralleled the observed EGF-R levels. Immunohistochemical analysis of the low-metastatic parental KM12C HCC cells demonstrated heterogeneity in the EGF-R–specific staining pattern, with <10% of the cells in the population staining intensely for EGF-R, whereas the in vivo selected highly metastatic KM12L4 and KM12SM HCC cells exhibited uniform, intense staining. Western blotting confirmed the presence of higher EGF-R protein levels in the metastatic KM12L4 and KM12SM cells than in the low-metastatic KM12C cells. Finally, isolation of the top and bottom 5% EGF-R-expressing KM12C cells by fluorescence-activated cell sorting (FACS) confirmed the association between levels of EGF-R on HCC cells and the production of liver metastases.[101]

The binding of EGF to its receptor on KM12C cells and several metastatic variants was nonlinear on a Scatchard plot, indicating there were two classes of receptors: the binding affinity of the major class was more than a magnitude less than that of the minor class. Metastatic KM12L4 cells selected in vivo after intrasplenic injection into nude mice expressed >2.5-fold the parental KM12C levels of both high- and low-affinity EGF-R. Two classes of EGF-R have been detected in human squamous carcinoma A431 cells; high-affinity EGF-Rs constitute 5% to 10% of the total EGF binding capacity.[108] High-affinity EGF binding has been shown to play an important role in EGF/TGF-α signal transduction, explaining why the $ID_{50}$ for EGF-stimulated cell proliferation (measured at 46 n$M$ for human foreskin fibroblasts) is similar to the $K_d$ for high-affinity binding but two orders of magnitude lower than the $K_d$ for low-affinity binding.[99,100] The demonstrated functionality of high-affinity-binding EGF-R is also important physiologically, since the level of EGF is extremely low, ranging from 20 to 27 μ$M$ in serum and ranging from 1 to 5 ng/g in tissue.[109] Furthermore, treatment with monoclonal antibody (Mab) 108 (which binds to the high-affinity EGF-R) inhibits the growth of human tumor cells in culture and in nude mice.[110] Collectively, these data suggest that high-affinity EGF-R binding is the primary means for in vivo stimulation of cells by TGF-α.[99,100,111]

We also observed a correlation between increased copy number of chromosome 7, EGF-R expression, and the ability of HCC to produce metastasis in the livers of nude mice. About 95% of KM12L4 cells had a chromosome 7/12 or 7/4 ratio >1.0 as compared with only 14% of KM12C cells, indicating a higher proportion of metastatic cells carried extra copies of chromosome 7. Gains of as many as 10 copies of particular chromosomes have been reported by fluorescent in situ hybridization (FISH) analyses in other solid tumors.[112,113] Dukes' stage C HCCs often exhibit additions of chromosomes 8 and 12 and a loss of chromosome 17.[112–114] The correlation between chromosome copy number and the potential of HCC cells to produce liver metastasis may be direct and specific or indirect and nonspecific. Alternatively, the observed correlation may be a reflection of genetic instability, which can lead to any of a number of gene mutations or deletions on other chromosomes, which in turn may increase tumor cell proliferation and growth in the liver.[114] Several independent reports implicated gene sequences on chromosome 7 in the process of invasion and metastasis.[115] An increased copy number of chromosome 7, shown to be associated with high expression of the EGF-R, has been detected in advanced melanoma[116] and in cancer of the breast,[102] bladder,[113] pancreas,[117] and brain.[118] These data suggest that increases in chromosome 7 copy number, and thus in EGF-R expression, may increase metastatic propensity.

The analyses described show a direct correlation between EGF-R on variant cell lines isolated from HCC and ability to produce liver metastases in nude mice. These findings are likely to be more generalized because in our recent analysis of formalin-fixed paraffin-embedded colon carcinoma surgical specimens for EGF-R transcripts using a rapid colorimetric in situ mRNA hybridization (ISH) technique,[119] we found that cell-surface hybridization with EGF-R–antisense hyperbiotinylated oligonucleotide probes in primary and metastatic colon carcinoma specimens directly correlated with immunohistochemistry and Northern blot analyses. Moreover, unlike Northern analyses, ISH showed intratumoral heterogeneity in EGF-R gene expression and identified particular cells expressing high levels of EGF-R in the tissues.[119]

Collectively, these data suggest an involvement of the EGF-R in tumor progression and dissemination and indicate a potential use of this receptor as a target for therapy (for reviews, see references 120–122). Anti-EGF-R Mabs, which block ligand binding, prevent the growth in culture of cells that are stimulated by EGF or TGF-α as well as the growth of human tumor xenografts bearing high levels of EGF-R.[121,122] Recent studies have also indicated that anti-EGF-R Mabs substantially enhance the cytotoxic effects of doxorubicin (DXR) or cis-diammine-dichloroplatinum on well-established xenografts.[123,124] Furthermore, clinical trials with squamous cell carcinoma of the lung have demonstrated the capacity of the anti-EGF-R Mabs to localize in such tumors and to achieve saturating concentrations in the blood for more than 3 days without toxicity.[121] Other therapeutic approaches targeting the EGF-R include strategies using EGF or TGF-α conjugated to toxins,[125,126] inhibitors of receptor dimerization,[127] antisense RNA, PTK inhibitors preferential for the EGF-R,[128] or receptor dominant-negative strategies.[129] These studies strongly support the premise that overexpressed EGF-Rs on malignant cells can be targeted for therapeutic intervention.

## ORGAN-SPECIFIC MODULATION OF THE INVASIVE PHENOTYPE OF METASTATIC CARCINOMA CELLS

As described thus far, the interaction of tumor cells with an organ environment can modulate the cells' tumorigenic properties and metastatic behavior.[1,36] The implantation of HCC cells into the subcutis (ectopic site) or the wall of the cecum (orthotopic site) results in locally growing tumors.[30,31] Metastasis to distant organs, however, was produced only by tumors growing in the wall of the cecum.[30,31] This difference in production of distant metastasis directly correlated with the influence of the organ environment on the production of degradative enzymes by the HCC cells.[130]

The ability of tumor cells to degrade connective tissue extracellular matrix (ECM) and basement membrane components is a prerequisite for invasion and metastasis.[11,131–133] Among the enzymes involved in degradation of the ECM are the metalloproteinases, a family of metal-dependent endopeptidases.[132] These proteinases are produced by connective tissue cells as well as many tumor cells and include enzymes with degradative activity for interstitial collagen, type IV collagen, type V collagen, gelatin, and proteoglycans. The $M_r$ 72,000 type IV collagenase is a neutral metalloproteinase capable of degrading type IV collagen within the triple helical domain, resulting in one-fourth amino terminal and three-fourths carboxyterminal fragments from the intact molecule.[134,135] The enzyme is mostly secreted into an extracellular milieu in a proenzymatic form.[132]

Increased expression of the $M_r$ 72,000 collagenase type IV has been demonstrated in HCC cells compared with that of normal mucosa cells,[136] and the metastatic capacity of HCC cells from orthotopic sites in nude mice directly correlates with the production of this enzyme activity.[30,31,130] Thus, intracecal tumors (in nude mice) of metastatic HCC cells secreted high levels of 92- and 68-kDa gelatinase activities, whereas HCC cells growing subcutaneously (not metastatic) did not produce or secrete the 68-kDa gelatinase activity.[130,137] Moreover, histologic examination of the HCC cells growing in the subcutis or cecum of nude mice revealed that mouse fibroblasts produced a thick pseudocapsule around the subcutaneous but not cecal tumors.[137] These differences suggested that the organ environment profoundly influenced the ability of metastatic cells to produce ECM-degradative enzymes.

Since recent analyses have demonstrated that the interaction of stromal fibroblasts can influence the tumorigenicity[138–140] and biologic behavior of tumor cells,[141,142] we investigated whether organ-specific fibroblasts could directly influence the invasive ability of HCC cells. Coculturing fibroblasts from skin, lung, and colon of nude mice with highly invasive and metastatic KM12SM HCC cells[137] showed that HCC cells adhered to and invaded through mouse colon and lung, but not skin fibroblasts. Moreover, nude mouse skin fibroblasts (ectopic environment), but not colon or lung fibroblasts (orthotopic environments), inhibited the production of 72-kDa type IV collagenases (gelatinases) by highly invasive and metastatic KM12SM HCC cells. This inhibition was due to a specific interaction between the HCC cells and skin fibroblasts. We based this conclusion on the data showing that nude mouse skin fibroblasts did not decrease the production of a 72-kDa type IV collagenase or the invasive capacity of the human squamous cell carcinoma A431 cells. These data, therefore, directly correlated with our studies showing that the KM12SM cells can grow in the wall of the cecum and the subcutis of nude mice, but are invasive only from the wall of the cecum.[30,31] Moreover, HCCs in the subcutis did not produce type IV collagenase.[130] The present in vitro data directly correlate with the in vivo findings and suggest that fibroblasts populating the ectopic and orthotopic organs influence the invasive phenotype of HCC cells.

Mesenchymal cells such as fibroblasts play an essential role in the differentiation and biologic behavior of both normal and neoplastic epithelial cells.[139,140,142,143] Fibroblasts can produce factors that influence tumor cell growth, invasion, and metastasis,[144] which ones depending on the stage of differentiation of the tumor cells.[139,140,145] For example, in human melanoma, skin fibroblasts inhibited the in vitro growth of cells from nevi but stimulated the in vitro growth of invasive melanoma cells.[142] Similarly, the in vitro growth of normal rat prostate cells was inhibited by fibroblasts from the prostate, whereas growth of prostate cancer cells was accelerated.[139] Although growth stimulation of human tumor cells by cultured fibroblasts has been well documented,[138] the in vitro growth of human breast and colon carcinoma cells[146] or mouse breast carcinoma cells[147,148] is enhanced by fibroblasts (or factors produced by fibroblasts) derived from the tissue of origin (orthotopic), but not by fibroblasts from ectopic tissues.

There are several mechanisms by which stromal cells and tumor cells interact and influence each other. Both in vitro and in vivo studies suggested that cell-to-cell contact is important,[149,150] and that at the epithelial cell junction, both cancer cells and fibroblasts have an altered capacity to synthesize basement membrane molecules.[151] Epithelial cells produce a variety of GFs that can influence fibroblast function, whereas fibroblasts produce ECM that can be tissue-specific.[83,152] GFs can induce and alter ECM gene expression,[83] and the ECM can, in turn, influence the type and level of GF, and even their receptor expression, in different cells.[153] Organ-specific ECM molecules have been shown to influence clonal growth of tumors,[154,155] probably by regulation of cell-cell adhesion and differentiation,[156] maintenance of cell shape controlling response to hormones and GFs,[94] and expression of tissue-specific proteins.[83,152,154]

There is now increasing evidence that fibroblasts derived from different anatomic sites in the adult display functional phenotypic heterogeneity in their morphology, interaction with steroid hormones, growth capacity, and production of cytokines.[141] One possible regulator of metalloproteinase activity is the family of tissue inhibitors of metalloproteinases (TIMPs), which can inhibit interstitial collagenase, stromelysin, and the 92-kDa type IV collagenase.[157,158] TIMP-2 can also bind specifically to 72-kDa type IV collagenase.[132,159] Furthermore, transfection of 3T3 fibroblasts with antisense DNA of TIMP resulted in the production of tumorigenic and metastatic cells.[159] In our study using anti-TIMP Mabs, we did not observe TIMP expressed differently in HCC cells in the subcutis and the cecum. As our data showed, low levels of type IV collagenolytic activity in subcutis tumors were caused by low production of the 92- and 64-kDa type IV collagenases, not by TIMP inhibition of type IV collagenase.

The organ factors that modulate type IV collagenase production in the cecal wall and subcutis were also analyzed. Various GF and cytokines have been shown to modulate the level of cell-secreted metalloproteinases and serine proteinases. Production of collagenases in normal fibroblasts can be induced by various tissue factors, for example, interleukin 1 (IL-1),[160] EGF, TGF-β, platelet-derived growth factor (PDGF),[161] and tumor-cell collagenase stimulatory factor.[162] Similarly, TGF-β induces synthesis of urokinase-type plasminogen activator in lung carcinoma cells[163] and increases production of the 72-kDa type IV collagenase in fibroblasts.[164] Welch and co-workers[165] found that TGF-β at a concentration as low as 50 μg/mL can maximally enhance the production of 92- and 72-kDa type IV collagenases and heparinase in rat 13762NF mammary adenocarcinoma MTLn3 cells. Pretreatment of MTLn3 cells with TGF-β significantly enhanced lung colonization after the cells were injected into the tail vein of a rat (Welch PNAS). In contrast, TGF-β can inhibit transcription of transin (rat stromelysin, matrix metalloproteinase 3),[166] whose expression is correlated with the progression of squamous cell carcinoma.[167] In different organs, the normal stroma surrounding primary tumors of KM12 HCC cells may contain dissimilar levels of these or other GFs, and this difference may affect the production and secretion of type IV collagenases, heparinases, and other tissue-degrading enzymes.

The exact mechanism by which nude mouse skin fibroblasts inhibit collagenase production by KM12SM cells was actively pursued by our laboratory. Since recombinant human interferon α (IFN-α) and IFN-γ have been shown to modulate the invasive capacity of human melanoma cells under in vitro conditions,[168] we examined the effects of IFN-α, -β, and -γ on the production of gelatinase activity by KM12SM HCC cells. Whereas all the r-IFNs inhibited gelatinase production (68 kDa), only inhibition by IFN-β (fibroblast IFN) was significant.[137]

We therefore investigated whether IFN-β or other IFNs could affect the production of gelatinase activity in other tumor cells or in normal cells, for example, fibroblasts. To that end, we established a cell line from a surgical specimen of human renal cell carcinoma.[169] This cell line, designated KG-2, can be transplanted into nude mice, where it is tumorigenic in the subcutis (ectopic) and kidney (orthotopic). This tumor produces spontaneous metastasis to lung tissue only from orthotopic implantation. KG-2 human renal cell carcinoma cells growing in the kidney and KG-2 lung metastases secrete higher levels of the 72-kDa gelatinase than do cells growing in the subcutis.[169,170] Under culture conditions, the gelatinase level in the culture supernatants of KG-2 cells was increased by their cultivation with mouse kidney or lung fibroblasts, whereas the cocultivation of KG-2 cells with mouse skin fibroblasts resulted in a significant reduction of gelatinase activity similar to our results with HCC cells.[137,170] Treatment with either IFN-β-serine or r-IFN-γ (but not IFN-α) decreased production of 72-kDa gelatinase and invasion through Matrigel by metastatic human renal cell carcinoma KG-2 cells.[170] The KG-2 cell invasion through Matrigel was induced by the conditioned media from human kidney fibroblast cultures.[170] Neither human IFN-α nor -β was detected by immunoassays in the media conditioned by kidney fibroblasts. Although Matrigel could contain mouse IFNs, treatment with various amounts of anti-mouse IFN-α or -β Mabs did not enhance KG-2 cell invasion through Matrigel. Thus, we concluded that the inhibition of invasion was directly caused by addition of r-IFNs.[170]

Importantly, these inhibitory effects were independent of the antiproliferative activity of r-IFNs. For example, IFN-α produced the highest levels of cytostasis but did not significantly affect gelatinase production. Moreover, the r-IFNs did not modulate production of the 72-kDa gelatinase in normal human fibroblasts, suggesting that the action of r-IFNs on gelatinase production and invasion may be specific to certain types of cells, including those of human renal cell carcinoma. Shapiro and co-workers[171] suggested that the modification of metalloproteinase production in alveolar macrophages by IFN-γ occurs at a pretranslational level. We found an approximately 70% decrease in the 72-kDa gelatinase steady-state mRNA level in

KG-2 human renal cell carcinoma cells treated with 100 U/mL of r-IFN-β-serine or r-IFN-γ, suggesting that the r-IFN–mediated inhibition of gelatinase production in KG-2 cells also occurred at a pretranslational level.[170] Improvement in the use of IFNs for treatment of any other neoplasm is dependent on a better understanding of the mechanisms by which IFNs regulate different functions of tumor cells, perhaps through the invasive phenotype.

## TUMOR ANGIOGENESIS

Angiogenesis is mediated by multiple molecules that are released by both tumor cells and host cells, including endothelial cells, epithelial cells, mesothelial cells, and leukocytes. Among these molecules are members of the fibroblast growth factor (FGF) family, vascular endothelial cell growth factor (VEGF) (or vascular permeability factor, vasculotropin), interleukin 8 (IL-8), angiogenin, angiotropin, EGF, fibrin, nicotinamide, platelet-derived endothelial cell growth factor (PD-ECGF), PDGF, TGF-α, TGF-β, and tumor necrosis factor α (TNF-α).[4,8,172–174] Angiogenesis consists of sequential processes emanating from microvascular endothelial cells.[172] To generate capillary sprouts, endothelial cells must proliferate, migrate, and penetrate host stroma, the direction of migration generally pointing toward the source of angiogenic molecules. The capillary sprout subsequently expands and undergoes morphogenesis to yield a capillary. Although most solid tumors are highly vascular, their vessels are not identical to normal vessels of normal tissue. There are differences in cellular composition, permeability, blood vessel stability, and regulation of growth.[175]

With few exceptions, benign neoplasms are sparsely vascularized and tend to grow slowly, whereas malignant neoplasms are highly vascular and fast-growing.[4,8,173] The increase in vasculature also increases the probability that tumor cells will enter the circulation and possibly give rise to metastasis.[176] Immunohistochemical staining of breast cancer sections with antibodies against factor VIII, a protein expressed only on the surface of endothelial cells, allowed Weidner and co-workers[177,178] to determine the density of microvessels. The number of microvessels in microscopic fields selected from the most vascular areas ("hot spots") of the sections correlated directly with metastasis and inversely with survival.

Most, but not all, recent studies concluded that increased microvessel density in the areas of most intense neovascularization is a significant and independent prognostic indicator in early-stage breast cancer (reviewed elsewhere in this volume).[177–187] Studies with other neoplasms such as prostate cancer, melanoma, ovarian carcinoma, gastric carcinoma, and colon carcinoma also support the conclusion that the angiogenesis index is a useful prognostic factor.[188–193] The expectation that an angiogenesis index can identify all patients with occult metastatic disease or those with probable distant metastases may be unrealistic, however.[4,5] First, human tumors are heterogeneous and consist of subpopulations of cells with different biologic properties.[1,27,38,39,72,78,194,195] Heterogeneity of angiogenic molecule expression has recently been documented in human renal carcinomas and HCCs.[196,197] Second, the process of cancer metastasis is sequential and selective and consists of a series of interlinked independent steps.[1,195,198] To produce clinically relevant metastases, tumor cells must complete all the steps in this process. Tumor cells that can induce intense angiogenesis but cannot survive in the circulation or proliferate in distant organs will not produce metastases[1,4,195,198] (Fig. 2-2). Like all other steps in the metastatic cascade, angiogenesis is necessary but not sufficient for the pathogenesis of a metastasis. Third, although not all large angiogenic tumors can produce metastasis, inhibition of angiogenesis prevents the growth of tumor cells at both the primary and secondary sites and thus can prevent the development of clinically relevant metastases.[8,199]

The role of the immune system in the regulation of angiogenesis is well established. Angiogenesis is essential to homeostasis, and its extent is influenced by leukocytes, such as mast cells, T-lymphocytes, and macrophages and their cytokines.[200–209] Cutaneous melanoma provides a clear model of these relationships. Lymphoid-mediated angiogenesis has been recognized in cutaneous melanoma. Increased vascularity at the vertical base of human melanoma is associated with poor prognosis.[210] A local inflammatory reaction consisting of T-lymphocytes and macrophages is often associated with invasive cutaneous melanoma, and an intense inflammatory reaction is often associated with increased risk of metastasis, suggesting that inflammatory-associated angiogenesis may contribute to melanoma dissemination.[211–214]

Immunologic mechanisms are involved in the physiologic angiogenesis that occurs subsequent to wound healing.[207,215,216] Systemic chemotherapy has been shown to retard wound healing, and this may be due to the decreased immune response and its contribution to wound healing; whether this is mediated by inhibition of angiogenesis is not clear.[217–219] We have investigated the role of vascularization of tumors and its effect on tumor size in immunosuppressed mice. Similar to previous studies using immunosuppressed mice (by adult thymectomy followed by whole body x-irradiation), the subcutaneous growth of the weakly immunogenic B16 melanoma was retarded in myelosuppressed mice as compared with control mice.[220] Further evidence implicating myelosuppression in the retardation of tumor growth and vascularity was obtained from doxorubicin (DXR)-pretreated animals injected with normal spleen cells one day before tumor challenge. Tumor growth in these mice was comparable to that in control mice.[221] These studies were repeated in athymic mice with very similar results, suggesting that the tumor vascularization observed in DXR-treated mice reconstituted with spleen cells was not mediated solely by T-lymphocytes. Since reconstitution with spleen cells enhanced vascularization of the B16 tumors, the results suggest that myelosuppressive chemotherapeutic drugs like DXR can inhibit host-mediated vascularization and thus inhibit tumor growth and support the concept that developing tumors can usurp homeostatic mechanisms to their advantage.[72]

In a more recent study of HCC specimens we examined the role of infiltrating cells in angiogenesis.[209] Our initial studies of HCC patients with various stages of disease demonstrated a correlation between VEGF expression, vessel count, and metastasis formation[193] (Fig. 2-3). However, we identified some patients who had a high vessel count but relatively low VEGF expression, and so hypothesized that other factors contribute to angiogenesis. In 96 HCC specimens, we found very little expression of PD-ECGF in the cancer epithelium (only 5% of patients), whereas in infiltrating cells we found that most specimens demonstrated expression of PD-ECGF

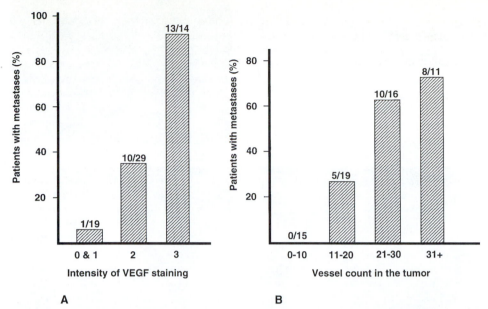

**FIGURE 2-3.** Relationship between VEGF expression and *A.* metastasis and *B.* vessel count and metastasis. The prevalence of metastatic disease increases as the intensity of VEGF expression or vessel count increases. (*From Takahashi et al.*[193] *Reproduced with permission.*)

in infiltrating cells (83%).[209] Double-staining for PD-ECGF and CD68 (specific for macrophages) or CD3 (specific for lymphocytes) demonstrated many infiltrating cells simultaneously staining for PD-ECGF and CD68. Other infiltrating cells stained positive for PD-ECGF and CD3. The intensity of staining for PD-ECGF in infiltrating cells correlated with vessel counts. Northern blot analysis revealed that colon cancer specimens and normal mucosa expressed relatively high levels of PD-ECGF mRNA, whereas transcripts were not detectable in colon cancer cell lines. These data suggest that infiltrating cells may contribute to angiogenesis in HCC and may provide a redundant mechanism for tumor neovascularization.[209]

**REGULATION OF ANGIOGENIC AND ANTIANGIO-GENIC FACTORS.** The survival of tumors and thus their metastasis is dependent upon the balance of endogenous angiogenic and antiangiogenic factors such that the outcome favors increased angiogenesis.[4] In many normal tissues, factors which inhibit angiogenesis predominate.[8] However, many neoplastic cells switch from an angiogenesis-inhibiting to an angiogenesis-stimulating phenotype upon transformation, as was observed in cultured fibroblasts from patients with Li-Fraumeni syndrome.[222] The switch to the angiogenic phenotype coincides with the loss of the wild-type (wt) allele of the p53 tumor suppressor gene and is the result of reduced production of antiangiogenic factor TSP-1. p53 may regulate other angiogenic molecules. In glioblastoma and hepatocellular carcinoma cell lines, mutant (mt) p53 has been shown to increase the promoter activity of the B-FGF gene, whereas wt p53 decreased expression of B-FGF.[223] Our lab, as well as others, has demonstrated that mt p53 (or loss of wt p53) may increase VEGF expression.[224,225]

Furthermore, reintroduction of wt p53 into HCC cells with a mt p53 gene causes a decrease in VEGF expression.[226]

Our laboratory has investigated the role of cell density in the regulation of B-FGF expression in human renal cell carcinoma cells.[227] By in situ mRNA hybridization (ISH) and Northern blot hybridization, we found an inverse correlation between increasing cell density and B-FGF expression. This finding was confirmed at the protein level as well as by immunohistochemistry and ELISA. Tumor cells harvested from dense cultures (low B-FGF expression) and plated under sparse conditions expressed high levels of B-FGF. Similar data were obtained in endothelial cells. The effect was not mediated by a soluble factor released into the culture medium.

Recent clinical observations noting an antiangiogenic effect of IFNs in tumors that express high levels of B-FGF led us to investigate whether IFNs could modulate the expression of B-FGF.[8,228,229] IFN-α and IFN-β but not IFN-γ downregulated the expression of B-FGF mRNA and protein in HRCC[230] (Fig. 2-4). This effect was independent of the antiproliferative effects of IFNs. The downregulation of B-FGF required a long exposure of cells to a low concentration of IFNs. Moreover, once IFN was withdrawn, cells resumed production of B-FGF. These observations are consistent with clinical experience indicating that IFN-α must be given for many months to induce a response.[229] The incubation of human bladder, prostate, colon, and breast carcinoma cells with noncytostatic concentrations of IFN-α or IFN-β also inhibited B-FGF production. The underlying mechanism for this modulation remains unclear, however.

Mechanisms regulating another angiogenic factor, VEGF, have also been investigated. Initial observations from human tumors examined by ISH have demonstrated that VEGF expression is

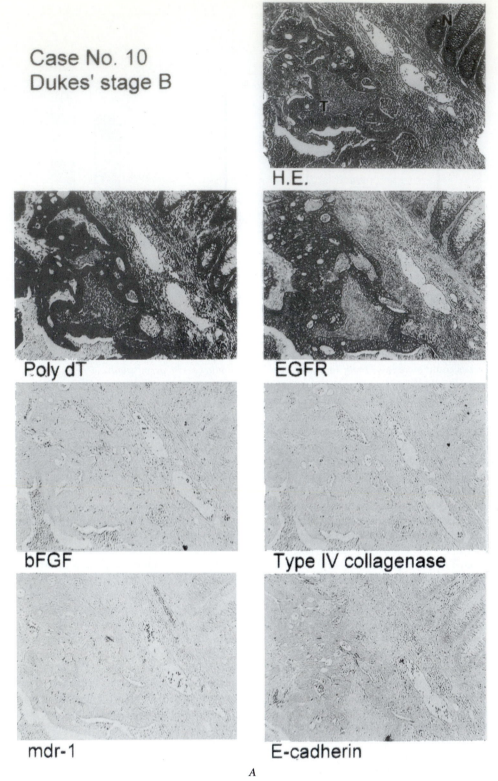

Case No. 10
Dukes' stage B

H.E.

Poly dT

EGFR

bFGF

Type IV collagenase

mdr-1

E-cadherin

*A*

**FIGURE 2-4.** In situ hybridization analyses for metastasis-related genes in tumors from patients with *A.* Dukes' stage B (*panel A*) and *B.* Dukes' stage D disease. Tumor cells from patients with Dukes' stage D disease expressed higher levels of metastasis-related genes than patients with Dukes' stage B disease. (H.E., hematoxylin and eosin, ×275.) (*From Kitadai et al.*[196] *Reproduced with permission.*) (See also Plate 5.)

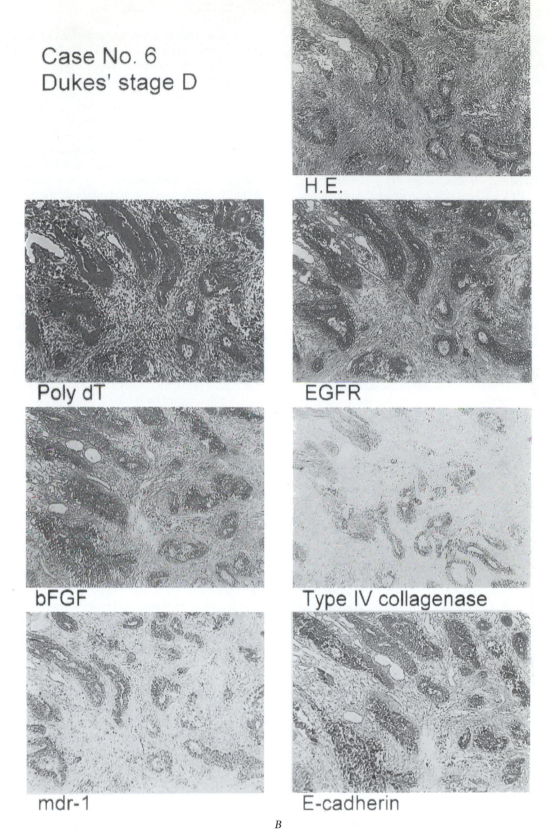

Case No. 6
Dukes' stage D

H.E.

Poly dT

EGFR

bFGF

Type IV collagenase

mdr-1

E-cadherin

B

**FIGURE 2-4.** (*Continued*)

increased in necrotic areas of tumors.[231,232] In vitro studies have confirmed that the VEGF level is increased in response to hypoxia, probably due to both increased transcription and mRNA stability.[233–236] Numerous cytokines and GFs have also been shown to increase VEGF expression. Most studies have been done in glioblastoma cell lines, a tumor system that is highly dependent upon VEGF for induction of angiogenesis. Cytokines and GFs that have been shown to upregulate VEGF expression include IL-1, IL-6, IL-8, TGF-β, PDGF, hepatocyte GF, EGF, and B-FGF.[237–244]

In contrast to the inverse correlation of cell density and B-FGF expression, we found that cell density and VEGF expression were directly related.[245] HCC cell lines were grown under sparse and confluent conditions and VEGF mRNA expression was determined. VEGF expression was increased two- to fivefold in confluent cells compared to cells grown under sparse conditions. Cells were then plated sparsely and grown for various time periods. VEGF expression increased as cell density increased. To determine if a soluble factor mediated the increase in VEGF expression in cells grown to confluence, sparsely plated cells were grown in conditioned media from confluent cells. VEGF expression was increased in these cells but not to the same level as cells grown to confluence.

VEGF expression is also regulated by certain oncogenes and tumor suppressor genes. Signal transduction pathways of *src* have been shown to be involved in hypoxia-mediated VEGF expression; this induction of VEGF was inhibited by genistein, an inhibitor of tyrosine kinases.[246] Studies done with v-*src* transfection into 293 and U87 cells demonstrated a four- to fivefold increase in VEGF promoter activity that corresponded to an increase in VEGF message. Overexpression of wt p53 suppressed VEGF expression in 293 cells, whereas mt p53 had no effect on VEGF.[247] Further experiments showed that transfection of wt p53 can inhibit the increased promoter activity of VEGF induced by v-*src*. This suggests that wt p53 is downstream of v-*src*.[247]

In rodent and human colonic epithelial cells, transformation by activated *ras* oncogenes upregulates VEGF.[247–249] As noted in other studies, transfection of the v-*src* oncogene also increased VEGF. That the human VEGF/VPF promoter contains four potential AP1 sites, which are key components of the *ras* signal pathway, suggests that mutant *ras* genes may upregulate angiogenic activity via direct transcriptional control of VEGF/VPF. Collectively, these data show that the transformation by a dominant oncogene contributes to in vivo tumorigenicity by both upregulation of GF/receptor activity and by upregulation of angiogenic molecules.[222,247–249]

Our laboratory has investigated the role of c-*src* in the regulation of VEGF in HCC using established cell lines with decreased c-*src* activity (by stable antisense transfection). These cell lines were dramatically reduced in tumorigenicity and growth in nude mice. Downregulation of c-*src* activity caused a significant decrease in the cellular mRNA expression of VEGF and secreted VEGF protein with the decrease proportional to the decrease in c-*src* activity. Under hypoxic conditions, cells with decreased *src* activity had a less than twofold increase in VEGF expression, whereas parental cells had a greater than fiftyfold increase.[250]

ORGAN MICROENVIRONMENT REGULATION OF METASTASIS/ANGIOGENESIS-RELATED GENES. Our laboratory has demonstrated that expression of certain angiogenic factors is dependent upon the site of implantation of tumor cells. When human renal cell carcinoma was implanted in different organ microenvironments in nude mice, the expression of B-FGF was 10 to 20 times higher in those tumors implanted in the kidney than in those implanted in the subcutaneous tissues.[197] The kidney tumors were more highly vascularized than tumors implanted in the subcutis. In sharp contrast, the expression of IFN-β was high in and around the subcutaneous tumors, whereas no IFN-β was found in the human renal cell carcinomas growing in the kidney. This study also demonstrated that B-FGF expression differed between the parental cell line and metastatic clone. The alteration in B-FGF level by the site of implantation was due to adaptation to the organ microenvironment inasmuch as cells reestablished in culture returned to the levels found in vitro after 4 weeks in culture.[197]

The organ-specific expression of IL-8 (an angiogenic GF associated with metastatic potential of melanoma cells) was examined in two human melanoma cell lines.[251] The A375P (parental) and A375SM (metastatic clone) lines were implanted into the subcutis, spleen (producing liver metastasis), and tail vein (producing lung metastasis). By Northern blot and immunohistochemical analyses, subcutaneous tumors expressed the greatest amount of IL-8, followed by lung lesions, and lastly liver lesions. The expression of IL-8 in the metastatic clone was higher in tissue culture than the parental line, but relative levels of IL-8 in the other organs were similar to the parental line. This effect was not due to the size, density, or subpopulation of cells. Cells cocultured with keratinocytes or well-differentiated human hepatoma cells produced similar relative amounts of IL-8 as found in in vivo tumor extracts. Stimulation with cytokines indigenous to those particular organs again produced similar results to the in vivo studies.

To determine the role of site of tumor implantation on VEGF expression, tumor angiogenesis, tumor cell proliferation, and metastasis formation, we implanted a gastric cancer cell line (KKLS) in orthotopic (stomach) and ectopic (subcutaneous) locations in nude mice.[252] Tumors in the stomach demonstrated greater vascularization, higher levels of VEGF expression, and greater proliferation than tumors in the subcutaneous tissues. In addition, 70% (7/10) of the tumors implanted in the stomach produced metastasis, but no metastases were evident in mice whose tumors were implanted subcutaneously. These data suggest that the expression of VEGF, vascularization, metastasis, and proliferation of human gastric cancer cells are regulated, in part, by the organ microenvironment.

Ongoing studies are examining the mechanism by which genes are regulated at specific sites. The possibilities include cell-to-cell contact and changes in the cytoskeleton of tumor cells regulating gene expression. Alternatively, a paracrine mechanism may be responsible for activation or inactivation of certain genes through receptor binding and signal transduction pathways. Understanding the mechanisms that regulate site-specific expression of invasion and metastasis and angiogenesis-related genes should allow more rational development of site-specific therapies for metastasis to individual organs.

## MULTIPARAMETRIC STUDIES EXAMINING METASTASIS-RELATED GENES

Since multiple steps must be successfully completed in order for a tumor cell to form a metastasis, it follows that multiple factors must be expressed at levels that allow the tumor cell to transgress each step of the metastatic cascade.[1] Most studies, however, focus on the expression of individual factors and their role in metastasis formation. These studies ultimately lead to the conclusion that expression of these genes is necessary but not sufficient to induce the metastatic potential of these tumors. Because discrete steps in the pathogenesis of metastasis are regulated by independent genes, the identification of cells capable of metastasis formation requires multiparametric analysis. Examining tumor tissues for concurrent expression of several genes that regulate different steps in metastasis should permit identification and quantitation of cells with metastatic potential among those comprising an individual patient's tumor.

In order to determine the feasibility of the use of multiparametric analysis in predicting the metastatic behavior of tumors, we used a rapid ISH technique developed in our laboratory[119] to examine expression of EGFR (growth), bFGF and IL-8 (angiogenesis), type IV collagenase (invasion), E-cadherin and CEA (adhesion) and mdr-1 (drug resistance) in metastatic and nonmetastatic HCC cells.[253] This initial study showed that the mRNA levels of specific genes differed between metastatic and nonmetastatic cells.

We then investigated the expression of several metastasis-related genes in HCC specimens of various stages of disease.[254] We found differential expression of metastasis-related genes between metastatic and nonmetastatic tumors (see Fig. 2-5). In addition, patients with Dukes' stages C and D tumors had more uniform staining of these genes, in contrast to a more heterogeneous staining pattern in nonmetastatic tumors. More recently, we examined expression of metastasis related genes in archival surgical specimens of primary HCCs (minimum 5-year follow-up) to determine whether ISH analysis of metastasis-related genes could be used to predict metastatic potential. Specimens from patients with Dukes' stage D tumors were also analyzed. These tumors served as a type of internal control in that we hypothesized that patients who initially presented with a Dukes' stage B tumor, but developed a metachronous recurrence, had expression of metastasis-related genes similar to tumors from patients with Dukes' stage D disease. This study revealed intertumoral and intratumoral heterogeneity for expression of metastasis-related genes. The expression of bFGF, collagenase type IV, EGF-R, and mdr-1 mRNA was higher in Dukes' stage D than in Dukes' stage B tumors. All patients with Dukes' stage B tumors who developed metachronous recurrence had high expression of EGFR, bFGF, and collagenase type IV. Multivariate analysis revealed that high levels of expression of collagenase type IV and low levels of expression of E-cadherin were independent factors associated with recurrent disease. We have observed similar findings in studies on specimens from patients with prostate and pancreatic cancers. It is important to note that in these patients, altered expression of specific factors predicted metastatic potential, but this observation should not lead to the conclusion that these factors alone were sufficient to produce metastasis. It is more likely that the other factors necessary for metastasis were already present in sufficient amounts to allow transgression through that specific step in the metastatic cascade. It is only when *all* of the factors necessary to complete the metastatic cascade are expressed at the requisite level can a tumor cell metastasize. In the above studies, it is possible that all of the tumors possessed the necessary machinery to produce metastasis with the exception of high levels of collagenase type IV and decreased levels of E-cadherin. Only those tumors with the latter characteristics developed metastasis, however.

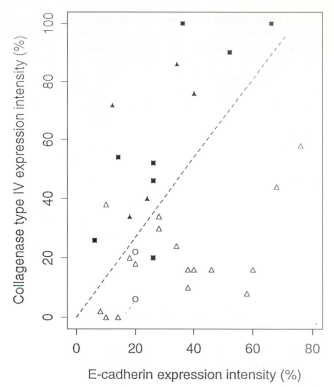

**FIGURE 2-5.** Ratio of E-cadherin to collagenase type IV mRNA expression in HCC specimens from patients with various stages of disease. Those patients who presented with metastasis or who developed metastasis had higher collagenase type IV to E-cadherin ratios than those with early-stage disease. Open circle = Dukes' stage A specimens; open triangle = Node-negative tumors with no evidence of disease at 5 years; solid triangle = Node-negative tumors with metachronous recurrence; solid square = Dukes' stage D specimens. (*From Kitadai et al.*[196] *Reproduced with permission.*)

## CONCLUSIONS

A primary goal of cancer research is an increased understanding of the molecular mechanisms mediating the process of cancer metastasis. Analyses of cancer cells (the seeds) and the microenvironment (the soil) have increased our understanding of the biologic mechanisms mediating organ-specific metastasis. Insight into the molecular mechanisms regulating the pathobiology of cancer metastasis as well as a better understanding of the interaction between the metastatic cell and the host environment should produce a foundation for new therapeutic approaches. In this chapter, we summarized new experimental findings demonstrating that the host organ's microenvironment can profoundly influence the biologic behavior of metastatic tumor cells, including resistance to chemotherapy, the production of degradative enzymes, angiogenesis, and proliferation at the metastatic site. Each of these studies indicates that the production of clinically relevant metastases depends, in part, on the interaction of particular tumor cells with specific organ environments. Therefore, the successful metastatic cell whose complex phenotype helps make it the decathlon champion[71] must be viewed today as a cell receptive to its environment. The analyses presented herein add important evidence to support the concept that cancer metastasis is not a random process; it is a highly regulated process that can now be studied on the molecular level. This new knowledge should eventually lead to the design and implementation of more effective therapies for this disease, ones that will refine the use of all treatment modalities, including surgery, chemotherapy, radiotherapy, and biotherapy.

## Acknowledgments

*The authors thank Walter Pagel for editorial assistance. This work was supported in part by American Cancer Society Career Development Award #94-21 (L.M.E.), and by Cancer Center Support Core Grant CA 16672 and grant R35-CA42107 from the National Cancer Institute, National Institutes of Health and ROI-CA74821 (L.M.E.).*

## REFERENCES

1. FIDLER IJ: Critical factors in the biology of human cancer metastasis: Twenty-eighth G.H.A. Clowes Memorial Award Lecture. Cancer Res 50:6130, 1990.

2. FIDLER IJ: Molecular biology of cancer: invasion and metastasis, in *Cancer: Principles and Practice of Oncology,* VT Devita Jr et al (eds). Philadelphia: Lippincott-Raven, 1997, pp 135–152.

3. FIDLER IJ, BALCH CM: The biology of cancer metastasis and implications for therapy. Curr Probl Surg. 24:137, 1987.

4. FIDLER IJ, ELLIS LM: The implications of angiogenesis to the biology and therapy of cancer metastasis. Cell 79:185, 1994.

5. ELLIS LM, FIDLER IJ: Angiogenesis and breast cancer metastasis. Lancet 346:388, 1995.

6. FOLKMAN J, TYLER K: Tumor angiogenesis: Its possible role in metastasis and invasion, in *Cancer Invasion and Metastasis: Biologic Mechanisms and Therapy*, SB Day et al (eds). New York: Raven Press, 1997, pp 95–103.

7. FOLKMAN J: What is the evidence that tumours are angiogenesis dependent? J Natl Cancer Inst 82:4, 1990.

8. FOLKMAN J: Angiogenesis in cancer, vascular, rhuematoid and other disease. Nature Med 1:27, 1995.

9. POSTE G et al: Evolution of tumor cell heterogeneity during progressive growth of individual lung metastases. Proc Natl Acad Sci USA 79:6574, 1982.

10. LIOTTA LA: Tumor invasion and metastases—Role of the extracellular matrix: Rhoads Memorial Award Lecture. Cancer Res 46:1, 1986.

11. LIOTTA LA et al: Role of collagenases in tumor cell invasion. Cancer Metastasis Rev 1:277, 1982.

12. MATRISIAN LM: The matrix-degrading metalloproteinases. Bioessays 14:455, 1992.

13. STETLER-STEVENSON WG et al: The activation of human type IV collagenase proenzyme. J Biol Chem 264:1353, 1989.

14. ALBINI A et al: The in vitro invasiveness and interaction with laminin of K-1735 melanoma cells. Evidence for different laminin-binding affinities in high and low metastatic variants. Clin Exp Metastasis 7:437, 1989.

15. HUMPHRIES MJ et al: A synthetic peptide from fibronectin inhibits experimental metastasis of murine melanoma cells. Science 223:467, 1986.

16. IWAMOTO Y et al: A synthetic laminin pentapeptide, inhibits experimental metastasis formation. Science 238:1131, 1987.

17. FIDLER IJ: Metastasis: quantitative analysis of distribution and fate of tumor emboli labeled with 125-I-5-iodo2-deoxuridine. J Natl Cancer Inst 45:773, 1970.

18. FIDLER IJ et al: Characterization in vivo and in vitro of tumor cells selected for resistance to syngeneic lymphocyte-mediated cytotoxicity. Cancer Res 36:3160, 1976.

19. DAVEY GC et al: Immunity as the predominant factor determining metastasis by murine lymphomas. Br J Cancer 40:590, 1979.

20. HANNA N, FIDLER IJ: The role of natural killer cells in the destruction of circulating tumor emboli. J Natl Cancer Inst 65:801, 1980.

21. MANTOVANI A et al: Cytolytic activity of circulating human monocytes on transformed and ultraformed human fibroblast. Int J Cancer 23:28, 1979.

22. TALMADGE JE, ZBAR B: Clonality of pulmonary metastases from the bladder 6 subline of the B16 melanoma studied by Southern hybridization. J Natl Cancer Inst 78:315, 1987.

23. KRAMER RH et al: Metastatic tumor cells adhere preferentially to the extracellular matrix underlying vascular endothelial cells. Int J Cancer 26:639, 1980.

24. ELLIS LM, FIDLER IJ: Angiogenesis and metastasis. Eur J Cancer 32A:2451, 1996.

25. FIDLER IJ, KRIPKE ML: Metastasis results from preexisting variant cells within a malignant tumor. Science 197:893, 1977.

26. LURIA SE, DELBRUCK M: Mutations of bacteria from virus sensitivity to virus resistance. Genetics 28:491, 1943.

27. HEPPNER G: Tumor heterogeneity. Cancer Res 44:2259, 1984.

28. GIAVAZZI R et al: Metastatic behavior of tumor cells from primary and metastatic human colorectal carcinomas implanted into different sites in nude mice. Cancer Res 46:1928, 1986.

29. KOZLOWSKI JM et al: Metastatic behavior of human tumor cell lines grown in the nude mouse. Cancer Res 44:3522, 1984.

30. MORIKAWA K et al: In vivo selection of highly metastatic cells from surgical specimens of different primary human colon carcinomas implanted into nude mice. Cancer Res 48:1943, 1988.

31. MORIKAWA K et al: Influence of organ environment on the growth, selection, and metastasis of human colon carcinoma cells in nude mice. Cancer Res 48:6863, 1988.

32. NAITO S et al: Growth and metastasis of tumor cells isolated from a human renal cell carcinoma implanted into different organs of nude mice. Cancer Res 46:4109, 1986.

33. NAITO S et al: Different growth pattern and biologic behavior of human renal cell carcinoma implanted into different organs of nude mice. J Natl Cancer Inst 78:377, 1987.

34. HART IR: "Seed and soil" revisited: Mechanisms of site-specific metastasis. Cancer Metastasis Rev 1:5, 1982.

35. NICOLSON GL: Cancer metastasis: Tumor cell and host organ properties important in metastasis to specific secondary sites. Biochim Biophys Acta 948:175, 1988.

36. RADINSKY R: Growth factors and their receptors in metastasis. Cancer Biol 2:169, 1991.

37. CROUCH EC et al: Heterogeneity in the production of collagens and fibronectin by morphologically distinct clones of a human tumor cell line: Evidence for intratumoral diversity in matrix protein biosynthesis. Cancer Res 47:6086, 1987.

38. FIDLER IJ: Tumor heterogeneity and the biology of cancer invasion and metastasis. Cancer Res 38:2651, 1978.

39. FIDLER IJ, HART IR: Biological diversity in metastatic neoplasms: Origins and implications. Science 217:998, 1982.

40. FIDLER IJ, POSTE G: The cellular heterogeneity of malignant neoplasms: Implications for adjuvant chemotherapy. Semin Oncol 12:207, 1985.

41. NICOLSON GL: Generation of phenotypic diversity and progression in metastatic tumor cells. Cancer Met Rev 3:25, 1984.

42. FOULDS L: The experimental study of tumor progression. A review. Cancer Res 14:327, 1954.

43. FOULDS L: The histologic analysis of mammary tumors of mice. I. Scope of investigations and general principles of analysis. J Natl Cancer Inst 17:701, 1956.

44. FOULDS L: The histologic analysis of mammary tumors of mice. II. The histology of responsiveness and progression. The origins of tumors. J Natl Cancer Inst 17:713, 1956.

45. FOULDS L: The histologic analysis of mammary tumors of mice. III. Organoid tumors. J Natl Cancer Inst 17:755, 1956.

46. FOULDS L: The histologic analysis of mammary tumors of mice. IV. Secretion. J Natl Cancer Inst 17:783, 1956.

47. KLEIN G, KLEIN E: Immune surveillance against virus-induced tumors and non-rejectability of spontaneous tumors: Contrasting consequences of host-versus-tumor evolution. Proc Natl Acad Sci USA 74:2121, 1977.

48. NOWELL PC: The clonal evolution of tumor cell populations: Acquired genetic lability permits stepwise selection of variant sublines and underlies tumor progression. Science 194:23, 1976.

49. NOWELL PC: Mechanisms of tumor progression. Cancer Res 46:2203, 1986.

50. NOWELL PC: Chromosomal and molecular clues to tumor progression. Semin Oncol 16:116, 1989.

51. PREHN RT: Tumor progression and homeostasis. Adv Cancer Res 23:203, 1976.

52. FEARON ER et al: Clonal analysis of human colorectal tumors. Science 238:193, 1987.

53. FRIEDMAN E et al: Clonality of parathyroid tumors in familial multiple endocrine neoplasia type I. N Engl J Med 321:213, 1989.

54. MULERIS M et al: Chromosomal study demonstrating the clonal evolution and metastatic origin of a metachronous colorectal carcinoma. Int J Cancer 38:167, 1986.

55. VOGELSTEIN B et al: Allelotype of colorectal carcinomas. Science 244:207, 1989.

56. TALMADGE JE et al: Evidence for the clonal origin of spontaneous metastases. Science 217:361, 1982.

57. KERBEL RS: Growth dominance of metastatic cancer cell: Cellular and molecular aspects. Adv Cancer Res 55:87, 1990.

58. FIDLER IJ, TALMADGE JE: *The Origin and Progression of Cancer Metastases.* New York, Alan R. Liss, 1984.

59. OOTSUYAMA A et al: Evidence by cellular mosaicism for monoclonal metastasis of spontaneous mouse mammary tumors. J Natl Cancer Inst 78:1223, 1987.

60. KORCZAK B et al: Genetic tagging of tumor cells with retrovirus vectors: Clonal analysis of tumor growth and metastasis in vivo. Mol Cell Biol 8:3143, 1988.

61. HU F et al: Clonal origin of metastasis in B16 murine melanoma: A cytogenetic study. J Natl Cancer Inst 78:155, 1987.

62. NICOLSON GL: Generation of phenotype diversity and progression in metastatic tumors. Cancer Metastasis Rev 3:25, 1984.

63. OLSSON L: Phenotypic diversity of malignant cell populations: Molecular mechanisms and biological significance. Cancer Res 3:91, 1986.

64. TALMADGE JE et al: The development of biological diversity and susceptibility to chemotherapy in cancer metastases. Cancer Res 44:3801, 1984.

65. NICOLSON GL: Cancer progression and growth: Relationship of paracrine and autocrine growth mechanisms to organ preference of metastasis. Exp Cell Res 204:171, 1993.

66. RADINSKY R: Paracrine growth regulation of human colon carcinoma organ-specific metastases. Cancer Metastasis Rev 12:345, 1993.

67. PAGET S: The distribution of secondary growths in cancer of the breast. Lancet 1:571, 1889.

68. EWING J: *Neoplastic Diseases.* Philadelphia, WB Saunders, 1928.

69. SUGARBAKER EV: Patterns of metastasis in human malignancies. Cancer Biol Rev 2:235, 1981.

70. TARIN D et al: Mechanisms of human tumor metastasis studied in patients with peritoneovenous shunts. Cancer Res 44:3584, 1984.

71. FIDLER IJ: Tumor heterogeneity and the biology of cancer invasion and metastasis. Cancer Res 38:2651, 1978.

72. FIDLER IJ: Modulation of the organ microenvironment for treatment of cancer metastasis. J Natl Cancer Inst 87:1588, 1995.

73. DEUEL TF: Polypeptide growth factors: Roles in normal and abnormal cell growth. Annu Rev Cell Biol 3:443, 1987.

74. CAVANAUGH PG, NICOLSON GL: Purification and some properties of a lung-derived growth factor that differentially stimulates the growth of tumor cells metastatic to the lung. Cancer Res 49:3928, 1989.

75. CHACKAL-ROY M et al: Stimulation of human prostatic carcinoma cell growth by factors present in human bone marrow. J Clin Invest 84:43, 1989.

76. ERVIN PR et al: Production of mammastatin, a tissue-specific growth inhibitor, by normal human mammary cells. Science 244:1585, 1989.

77. PLOWMAN GD et al: The amphiregulin gene encodes a novel epidermal growth factor-related protein with tumor-inhibitory activity. Mol Cell Biol 10:1969, 1981.

78. HART IR et al: Molecular aspects of the metastatic cascade. Biochim Biophys Acta 989:65, 1989.

79. ZARRILLI R et al: Multiple levels of control of insulin-like growth factor gene expression. Mol Cell Endocrinol 101:R1, 1994.

80. STILES CD et al: Dual control of cell growth by somatomedins and platelet-derived growth factor. Proc Natl Acad Sci USA 76:1279, 1979.

81. LONG L et al: A regulatory mechanism for carcinoma cells metastatic to the liver. Cancer Res 54:3732, 1994.

82. ROBERTS AB et al: Transforming growth factor β: Possible roles in carcinogenesis. Br J Cancer 57:594, 1988.

83. ROBERTS AB et al: Transforming growth factor type beta: Rapid induction of fibrosis and angiogenesis in vivo and stimulation of collagen formation in vitro. Proc Natl Acad Sci USA 83:4167, 1986.

84. SCHWARZ LC et al: Loss of growth factor dependence and conversion of transforming growth factor-β1 inhibition to stimulation in metastatic H-ras-transformed murine fibroblasts. Cancer Res 48:6999, 1988.

85. FAN D et al: Clonal stimulation or inhibition of human colon carcinomas and human renal carcinoma mediated by transforming growth factor-β1. Cancer Commun 1:117, 1989.

86. MARKOWITZ SD, ROBERTS AB: Tumor suppressor activity of the TGF-beta pathway in human cancers. Cytokine Growth Factor Rev 7:93, 1996.

87. PARSONS R et al: Microsatellite instability and mutations of the transforming growth factor beta type II receptor gene in colorectal cancer. Cancer Res 55:5548, 1995.

88. GOODLAND R et al: Intravenous but not intragastric urogastrone-EGF is trophic to the intestine of parenterally fed rats. Gut 28:573, 1987.

89. MALDEN L et al: Expression of transforming growth factor alpha messenger RNA in normal and neoplastic gastrointestinal tract. Int J Cancer 43:380, 1989.

90. MARKOWITZ SD et al: Growth stimulation by coexpression of transforming growth factor-alpha and epidermal growth factor receptor in normal and adenomatous human colon epithelium. J Clin Invest 86:356, 1990.

91. MEAD JE, FAUSTO N: Transforming growth factor may be a physiological regulator of liver regeneration by means of an autocrine mechanism. Proc Natl Acad Sci USA 86:1558, 1989.

92. MICHALOPOULOS GK: Liver regeneration: Molecular mechanisms of growth control. FASEB J 4:176, 1990.

93. GUTMAN M et al: Accelerated growth of human colon cancer cells in nude mice undergoing liver regeneration. Invasion Metastasis 14:362, 1994.

94. vanDALE P, GALAND P: Effect of partial hepatectomy on experimental liver invasion by intraportally injected colon carcinoma cells in rats. Invasion Metastasis 8:217, 1988.

95. GRUPPOSO PA et al: Transforming growth factor receptors in liver regeneration following partial hepatectomy in the rat. Cancer Res 50:1464, 1990.

96. RUSSELL AH et al: Adenocarcinoma of the proximal colon: Sites of initial dissemination and patterns of recurrence following surgery alone. Cancer 53:360, 1984.

97. GIAVAZZI R et al: Experimental nude mouse model of human colorectal cancer liver metastases. J Natl Cancer Inst 77:1303, 1986.

98. RADINSKY R, FIDLER IJ: Regulation of tumor cell growth at organ-specific metastases. In Vivo 6:325, 1992.

99. vanderGEER P et al: Receptor protein-tyrosine kinases and their signal transduction pathways. Annu Rev Cell Biol 10:251, 1994.

100. SCHLESSINGER J: Allosteric regulation of the epidermal growth factor receptor kinase. J Cell Biol 103:2067, 1986.

101. RADINSKY R et al: Level and function of epidermal growth factor receptor predict the metastatic potential of human colon carcinoma cells. Clin Cancer Res 1:19, 1995.

102. SAINSBURY JRC et al: Epidermal growth factor receptors and oestrogen receptors in human breast cancer. Lancet i:364, 1986.

103. BIGNER SH et al: Characterization of the epidermal growth factor receptor in human glioma cell lines and xenografts. Cancer Res 50:8017, 1990.

104. HARRIS AL, NEAL DE: *Epidermal Growth Factor and Its Receptor in Human Cancer.* Chichester, England, Ellis Horwood, 1987.

105. BERGER MS et al: Evaluation of epidermal growth factor receptors in bladder tumours. Br J Cancer 56:533, 1987.

106. GULLICK WJ et al: Expression of epidermal growth factor receptors on human cervical, ovarian, and vulvar carcinomas. Cancer Res 46:285, 1986.

107. ULLRICH AL et al: Human epidermal growth factor receptor cDNA sequence and aberrant expression of the amplified gene in A431 epidermoid carcinoma cells. Nature 309:418, 1984.

108. KAWAMOTO T et al: Growth stimulation of A431 cells by epidermal growth factor: Identification of high-affinity receptors for epidermal growth factor by an anti-receptor antibody. Proc Natl Acad Sci USA 80:1337, 1983.

109. HIRATA Y et al: Plasma concentration of immunoreactive human epidermal growth factor (urogastrone in man). J Clin Endocrinol Metab 40:440, 1980.

110. BELLOT F et al: High-affinity epidermal growth factor binding is specifically reduced by a monoclonal antibody, and appears necessary for early responses. J Cell Biol 110:491, 1990.

111. DEFIZE LHK et al: Signal transduction by epidermal growth factor occurs through the subclass of high affinity receptors. J Cell Biol 109:2495, 1990.

112. STEINER MG et al: Chromosomes 8, 12, and 17 copy number in Astler-Coller stage C colon cancer in relation to proliferative activity and DNA ploidy. Cancer Res 53:681, 1993.

113. WALDMAN FM et al: Centromeric copy number of chromosome 7 is strongly correlated with tumor grade and labeling index in human bladder cancer. Cancer Res 51:3807, 1991.

114. KERN SE et al: Allelic loss in colorectal carcinoma. JAMA 261:3099, 1989.

115. COLLARD JG et al: Genetic analysis of invasion and metastasis. Cancer Surv 7:691, 1988.

116. KOPROWSKI H et al: Expression of the receptor for epidermal growth factor correlates with increased dosage of chromosome 7 in malignant melanoma. Somatic Cell Molec Genet 11:297, 1985.

117. KORC M et al: Enhanced expression of epidermal growth factor receptor correlates with alterations of chromosome 7 in human pancreatic cancer. Proc Natl Acad Sci USA 83:5141, 1986.

118. HENN W et al: Polysomy of chromosome 7 is correlated with overexpression of the erbB oncogene in human glioblastoma cell lines. Hum Genet 74:104, 1986.

119. RADINSKY R et al: A rapid colorimetric in situ mRNA hybridization technique for analysis of epidermal growth factor receptor in paraffin-embedded surgical specimens of human colon carcinomas. Cancer Res 53:937, 1993.

120. KHAZAIE K et al: EGF receptor in neoplasia and metastasis. Cancer Metastasis Rev 12:255, 1993.

121. MENDELSOHN J: The epidermal growth factor receptor as a target for therapy with antireceptor monoclonal antibodies. Semin Cancer Biol 1:339, 1990.

122. MODJTAHEDI H, DEAN C: The receptor for EGF and its ligands: Expression, prognostic value and target for therapy in cancer (review). Int J Oncol 4:277, 1994.

123. BASELGA J et al: Antitumor effects of doxorubicin in combination with anti-epidermal growth factor receptor monoclonal antibodies. J Natl Cancer Inst 85:1327, 1993.

124. FAN Z et al: Blockade of epidermal growth factor receptor function by bivalent and monovalent fragments of 225 anti-epidermal growth factor receptor monoclonal antibodies. Cancer Res 53:4322, 1993.

125. PHILLIPS PC et al: Transforming growth factor—*Pseudomonas* exotoxin fusion protein (TGF–PE38) treatment of subcutaneous and intracranial human glioma and medulloblastoma xenografts in athymic mice. Cancer Res 54:1008, 1994.

126. SIEGALL CB et al: Selective killing of tumor cells using EGF or TCG-Pseudomonas exotoxin chimeric molecules. Semin Cancer Biol 1:345, 1990.

127. LOFTS FJ et al: Specific short transmembrane sequences can inhibit transformation by the mutant neu growth factor receptor in vitro and in vivo. Oncogene 8:2813, 1993.

128. BUCHDUNGER E et al: A protein-tyrosine kinase inhibitor with selectivity for the epidermal growth factor receptor signal transduction pathway and potent in vivo antitumor activity. Proc Natl Acad Sci USA 91:2334, 1994.

129. KASHLES O et al: A dominant negative mutation suppresses the function of normal epidermal growth factor receptors by heterodimerization. Mol Cell Biol 11:1454, 1991.

130. NAKAJIMA M et al: Influence of organ environment on extracellular matrix degradative activity and metastasis of human colon carcinoma cells. J Natl Cancer Inst 82:1890, 1990.

131. TESTA JE, QUIGLEY JP: Reversal of misfortune: TIMP-2 inhibits tumor cell invasion. J Natl Cancer Inst 83:740, 1991.

132. STETLER-STEVENSON WG: Type IV collagenases in tumor invasion and metastasis. Cancer Metastasis Rev 9:289, 1990.

133. McDONNELL S, MATRISIAN LM: Stromelysin in tumor progression and metastasis. Cancer Metastasis Rev 9:305, 1990.

134. FESSLER L et al: Identification of the procollagen IV cleavage products produced by specific tumor collagenase. J Biol Chem 259:9783, 1984.

135. LIOTTA LA et al: Metastatic potential correlates with enzymatic degradation of basement membrane collagen. Nature 284:67, 1980.

136. LEVY A et al: Increased expression of the 72 kDa type IV collagenase in human colonic adenocarcinoma. Cancer Res 51:439, 1991.

137. FABRA A et al: Modulation of the invasive phenotype of human colon carcinoma cells by organ specific fibroblasts of nude mice. Differentiation 52:101, 1992.

138. BRATTAIN MG et al: Enhancement of growth of human colon tumor cell lines by feeder layers of murine fibroblasts. J Natl Cancer Inst 69:767, 1982.

139. CHUNG LWK: Fibroblasts are critical determinants in prostatic cancer growth and dissemination. Cancer Metastasis Rev 10:263, 1991.

140. CAMPS JL et al: Fibroblast-mediated acceleration of human epithelial tumor growth in vivo. Proc Natl Acad Sci USA 87:75, 1990.

141. BENATHAN M et al: Modulatory growth effects of 3T3 fibroblasts on cocultivated human melanoma cells. Anticancer Res 11:491, 1991.

142. CORNIL I et al: Fibroblast cell interaction with human melanoma cells affecting tumor cell growth are a function of tumor progression. Proc Natl Acad Sci USA 88:6028, 1991.

143. CUNHA GR, CHUNG LWK: Stromal-epithelial interaction: I. Induction of prostatic phenotype in urothelium of testicular feminized (TFm/y) mice. J Steroid Biochem 14:1317, 1981.

144. BASSET P et al: A novel metalloproteinase gene specifically expressed in stromal cells of breast carcinomas. Nature 348:699, 1990.

145. TANAKA H et al: Enhancement of metastatic capacity of fibroblast-tumor cell interaction in mice. Cancer Res 48:1456, 1988.

146. MUKAIDA H et al: Significance of freshly cultured fibroblasts from different tissues in promoting cancer cell growth. Int J Cancer 48:423, 1991.

147. MILLER FR et al: Growth regulation of mammary tumor cells in collagen gel cultures by diffusible factors produced by normal mammary gland epithelium and stromal fibroblasts. Cancer Res 49:6091, 1989.

148. ENAMI J et al: Growth of normal and neoplastic mouse mammary epithelial cells in primary culture: Stimulation by conditioned medium from mouse mammary fibroblasts. Jpn J Cancer Res 74:845, 1983.

149. KEDINGER M et al: Importance of a fibroblastic support for in vitro differentiation of intestinal endodermal cells and for their response to glucocorticoids. Cell Differentiation 20:171, 1987.

150. KEDINGER M et al: Intestinal tissue and cell cultures. Cell Differentiation 36:71, 1986.

151. BOUZIGES F et al: Altered deposition of basement-membrane molecules in co-cultures of colonic cancer cells and fibroblasts. Int J Cancer 48:101, 1991.

152. REID LM: *Extracellular Matrix and Hormonal Regulation of Synthesis and Abundance of Messenger RNAs in Cultured Liver Cells.* New York, Raven Press, 1988.

153. GORDON PB et al: Extracellular matrix heparan sulfate proteoglycans modulate the mitogenic capacity of acidic fibroblast growth factor. J Cell Physiol 140:584, 1988.

154. DOERR R et al: Clonal growth of tumors on tissue-specific biomatrices and correlation with organ site specificity of metastases. Cancer Res 49:384, 1989.

155. ZVIBEL I et al: Heparin and hormonal regulation of mRNA synthesis and abundance of autocrine growth factors: Relevance to clonal growth of tumors. Mol Cell Biol 11:108, 1991.

156. HAY ED: *Cell-Matrix Interaction in the Embryo: Cell Shape, Cell Surface, and Their Role in Differentiation.* New York, Alan Liss, 1984.

157. KHOKA R et al: Antisense RNA-induced reduction in muting TIMP levels confers oncogenicity on Swiss 3T3 cells. Science 243:947, 1989.

158. WILHELM SM et al: SV40-transformed human lung fibroblasts secrete a 92-kDa type IV collagenase which is identical to that secreted by normal human macrophages. J Biol Chem 264:17213, 1989.

159. GOLDBERG GI et al: Human 72-kilodalton type IV collagenase forms a complex with a tissue inhibitor of metalloproteinases designated TIMP-2. Proc Natl Acad Sci USA 86:8207, 1989.

160. POSTLETHWAITE AE et al: Interleukin 1 stimulation of collagenase production by cultured fibroblasts. J Exp Med 157:801, 1983.

161. CHUA CC et al: Induction of collagenase secretion in human fibroblast cultures by growth promoting factors. J Biol Chem 260:5213, 1986.

162. ELLIS SM et al: Monoclonal antibody preparation and purification of a tumor cell collagenase-stimulatory factor. Cancer Res 49:3385, 1989.

163. KESKI-OJA J et al: Regulation of the synthesis and activity of urokinase plasminogen activator in A549 human lung carcinoma cells by transforming growth factor-beta. J Cell Biol 106:451, 1988.

164. OVERALL CM et al: Independent regulation of collagenase, 72-kDa progelatinase, and metalloendoproteinase inhibitor expression in human fibroblasts by transforming growth factor-beta. J Biol Chem 25:1860, 1989.

165. WELCH DR et al: Transforming growth factor-beta stimulates mammary adenocarcinoma cell invasion and metastatic potential. Proc Natl Acad Sci USA 87:7678, 1990.

166. KERR LD et al: Transforming growth factor beta 1 and cAMP inhibit transcription of epidermal growth factor and induced transin RNA. J Biol Chem 263:16999, 1988.

167. OSTROWSKI LE et al: Expression pattern of a gene for a secreted metalloproteinase during late stage of tumor progression. Mol Carcinogen 1:13, 1988.

168. Hujanen ES, Turpeenniemi-Hujanen T: Recombinant interferon alpha and gamma modulate the invasive potential of human melanoma in vitro. Int J Cancer 47:576, 1991.

169. Gohji K et al: The importance of orthotopic implantation to the isolation and biological characterization of a metastatic human clear cell renal carcinoma in nude mice. Int J Oncol 2:23, 1993.

170. ——— et al: Human recombinant interferons beta and gamma decrease gelatinase production and invasion by human KG-2 renal carcinoma cells. Int J Cancer 58:380, 1994.

171. Shapiro SD et al: Immune modulation of metalloproteinase production in human macrophages: Selective suppression of interstitial collagenase and stromelysin biosynthesis by interferon-gamma. J Clin Invest 86:1204, 1990.

172. Folkman J: How is blood vessel growth regulated in normal and neoplastic tissue?—G.H.A. Clowes Memorial Award Lecture. Cancer Res 46:467, 1986.

173. Auerbach W, Auerbach R: Angiogenesis inhibition: a review. Pharmacol Ther 63:265, 1994.

174. Folkman J, Klagsburn M: Angiogenic factors (review). Science 235:442, 1987.

175. Folkman J, Cotran R: Relation of vascular proliferation to tumor growth. Int Rev Exp Pathol 16:207, 1976.

176. Liotta LA et al: Quantitative relationships of intravascular tumor cells, tumor vessels, and pulmonary metastases following tumor implantation. Cancer Res 34:997, 1974.

177. Weidner N et al: Tumor angiogenesis and metastasis-correlation in invasive breast cancer. N Engl J Med 324:1, 1991.

178. ——— et al: Tumor angiogenesis: a new significant and independent prognostic indicator in early-stage breast carcinoma. J Natl Cancer Inst 84:1875, 1992.

179. Gasparini G et al: Intratumoral microvessel density and p53 protein: correlation with metastasis in head-and-neck squamous-cell carcinoma. Int J Cancer 55:739, 1993.

180. Obermair A et al: Tumoral vascular density in breast tumors and their effect on recurrence-free survival. Chirurgery 65:611, 1994.

181. Toi M et al: Tumor angiogenesis is an independent prognostic indicator in primary breast carcinoma. Int J Cancer 55:371, 1993.

182. Visscher DW et al: Prognostic significance of image morphometric microvessel enumeration in breast carcinoma. Anal Quant Cytol Histol 15:88, 1993.

183. Horak ER et al: Angiogenesis, assessed by platelet/endothelial cell adhesion molecule antibodies, as an indicator of node metastases and survival in breast cancer. Lancet 340:1120, 1992.

184. Bosari S et al: Microvessel quantitation and prognosis in invasive breast carcinoma. Hum Pathol 23:755, 1992.

185. Hall N et al: Is the relationship between angiogenesis and metastasis in breast cancer real? Surg Oncol 1:223, 1992.

186. Van Hoef ME et al: Assessment of tumour vascularity as a prognostic factor in lymph node negative invasive breast cancer. Eur J Cancer 29A:1141, 1993.

187. Axelsson K et al: Tumor angiogenesis as a prognostic assay for invasive ductal breast carcinoma. J Natl Cancer Inst 87:997, 1995.

188. Weidner N et al: Tumor angiogenesis correlates with metastasis in invasive prostate carcinoma. Am J Pathol 143:401, 1993.

189. Graham CH et al: Extent of vascularization as a prognostic indicator in thin (<0.76 mm) malignant melanomas. Am J Pathol 145:510, 1994.

190. Hollingsworth HC et al: Tumor angiogenesis in advanced stage ovarian carcinoma. Am J Pathol 147:33, 1995.

191. Maeda K et al: Tumour angiogenesis and tumour cell proliferation as prognostic indicators in gastric carcinoma. Br J Cancer 72:319, 1995.

192. Takahashi Y et al: Significance of vessel count and vascular endothelial growth factor and its receptor (KDR) in intestinal-type gastric cancer. Clin Cancer Res 2:1679, 1996.

193. Takahashi Y et al: Expression of vascular endothelial growth factor and its receptor, KDR, correlates with vascularity, metastasis, and proliferation of human colon cancer. Cancer Res 55:3964, 1995.

194. Liotta LA, Stetler-Stevenson WG: Tumor invasion and metastasis: An imbalance of positive and negative regulation (review). Cancer Res 51:5054s, 1991.

195. Poste G, Fidler IJ: The pathogenesis of cancer metastasis. Nature 283:139, 1979.

196. Kitadai Y et al: Multiparametric in situ mRNA hybridization analysis to detect metastasis-related genes in surgical specimens of human colon carcinomas. Clin Cancer Res 1:1095, 1995.

197. Singh RK et al: Organ site-dependent expression of basic fibroblast growth factor in human renal cell carcinoma cells. Am J Pathol 145:365, 1994.

198. Fidler IJ et al: The biology of cancer invasion and metastasis. Adv Cancer Res 28:149, 1978.

199. O'Reilly MS et al: Angiostatin: A novel angiogenesis inhibitor that mediates the suppression of metastases by a Lewis lung carcinoma. Cell 79:315, 1994.

200. Sidky YA, Auerbach R: Lymphocyte-induced angiogenesis in tumor-bearing mice. Science 192:1237, 1976.

201. Meininger CJ, Zetter BR: Mast cells and angiogenesis. Semin Cancer Biol 3:73, 1992.

202. Fidler IJ: Lymphocytes are not only immunocytes (guest editorial). Biomedicine 32:1, 1980.

203. Fidler IJ et al: Influence of immune status on the metastasis of three murine fibrosarcomas of different immunogenicities. Cancer Res 39:3816, 1979.

204. Miguez M et al: Lymphocyte-induced angiogenesis: correlation with the metastatic incidence of two murine mammary adenocarcinomas. Invasion Metastasis 6:313, 1986.

205. Freeman MR et al: Peripheral blood T lymphocytes and lymphocytes infiltrating human cancers express vascular endothelial growth factor: A potential role for T cells in angiogenesis. Cancer Res 55:4140, 1995.

206. Polverini P et al: Activated macrophages induce vascular proliferation. Nature 269:804, 1977.

207. Sunderkötter C et al: Macrophages and angiogenesis. J Leukocyte Biol 55:410, 1994.

208. Leek RD et al: Cytokine networks in solid human tumors: Regulation of angiogenesis. J Leukocyte Biology 56:423, 1994.

209. Takahashi Y et al: Platelet derived endothelial cell growth factor in human colon cancer angiogenesis: Role of infiltrating cells. J Natl Cancer Inst 88:1146, 1996.

210. Srivastava A et al: The prognostic significance of tumor vascularity in intermediate thickness (.76–4.0 mm thick) skin melanoma: A quantitative histologic study. Am J Pathol 133:419, 1988.

211. Smolle J et al: Vascular architecture of melanocytic skin tumors. Pathol Res Practice 185:740, 1989.

212. Ruiter DJ et al: Major histocompatibility antigens and the mononuclear inflammatory infiltrate in benign nevomelanocytic proliferation and malignant melanoma. J Immunol 129:2808, 1982.

213. Klausner JM et al: Unknown primary melanoma. J Surg Oncol 24:129, 1983.

214. BROCKER EG et al: Macrophages in melanocytic naevi. Arch Dermatol Res 284:127, 1992.

215. DIPIETRO LA, POLVERINI PJ: Angiogenic macrophages produce the angiogenic inhibitor thrombospondin 1. Am J Pathol 143:678, 1993.

216. RAPPOLEE DA et al: Wound macrophages express TGF-α and other growth factors in vivo: Analysis by mRNA phenotyping. Science 241:708, 1988.

217. FUMAGALLI U et al: Effects of intraperitoneal chemotherapy on anastomotic healing in the rat. J Surg Res 50:82, 1991.

218. NOH R et al: The effect of doxorubicin and mitoxantrone on wound healing. Cancer Chemother Pharmacol 29:141, 1991.

219. HENDRICKS T et al: Inhibition of basal and TGF-β-induced fibroblast collagen synthesis by antineoplastic agents: Implications for wound healing. Br J Cancer 67:545, 1993.

220. FIDLER IJ, GERSTEN DM: Effect of syngeneic lymphocytes on the vascularity, growth, and induced metastasis of the B16 melanoma, in Neoplasm Immunity: Experimental and Clinical, R Crispen (ed). New York, Elsevier, 1980, pp 3–15.

221. GUTMAN M et al: Leukocyte-induced angiogenesis and subcutaneous growth of B16 melanoma. Cancer Biother 9:163, 1994.

222. DAMERON KM et al: Control of angiogenesis in fibroblasts by p53 regulation of thrombospondin-1. Science 265:1502, 1994.

223. UEBA T et al: Transcriptional regulation of basic fibroblast growth factor gene by p53 in human glioblastoma and hepatocellular carcinoma cells. Proc Natl Acad Sci USA 91:9009, 1994.

224. KIESER A et al: Mutant p53 potentiates protein kinase C induction of vascular endothelial growth factor. Oncogene 9:963, 1994.

225. KOURA AN et al: Regulation of genes associated with angiogenesis, growth, and metastasis by specific p53 mutations in a murine melanoma cell line. Oncol Rep 4:475, 1997.

226. BOUVET M et al: Adenovirally mediated wild-type p53 gene therapy downregulates vascular endothelial growth factor expression in human colon cancer. Surg Forum 48:806, 1997.

227. SINGH RK et al: Cell density-dependent modulation of basic FGF by interferon-beta (abstract). Proc Am Assoc Cancer Res 36:87, 1995.

228. TAKAHASHI K et al: Cellular markers that distinguish the phases of hemangioma during infancy and childhood. J Clin Invest 93:2357, 1994.

229. EZEKOWITZ RAB et al: Interferon alfa-2a therapy for life-threatening hemangiomas of infancy. N Engl J Med 326:1456, 1992.

230. SINGH R et al: Interferons alpha and beta down-regulate the expression of basic fibroblast growth factor in human carcinomas. Proc Natl Acad Sci USA 39:231, 1994.

231. BROWN LF et al: Expression of vascular permeability factor (vascular endothelial growth factor) and its receptors in adenocarcinomas of the gastrointestinal tract. Cancer Res 53:4727, 1993.

232. BROWN LF et al: Increased expression of vascular permeability factor (vascular endothelial growth factor) and its receptors in kidney and bladder carcinomas. Am J Pathol 143:1255, 1993.

233. SHWEIKI D et al: Vascular endothelial growth factor induced by hypoxia may mediate hypoxia-initiated angiogenesis. Nature 359:843, 1992.

234. SHIMA DT et al: Hypoxic induction of vascular endothelial growth factor (VEGF) in human epithelial cells is mediated by increases in mRNA stability. Febs Lett 370:203, 1995.

235. IKEDA E et al: Hypoxia-induced transcriptional activation and increased mRNA stability of vascular endothelial growth factor in C6 glioma cells. J Biol Chem 34:19761, 1995.

236. LEVY AP et al: Transcriptional regulation of the rat vascular endothelial growth factor gene by hypoxia. J Biol Chem 270:13333, 1995.

237. KOOCHEKPOUR S et al: Vascular endothelial growth factor production is stimulated in response to growth factors in human glioma cells. Oncol Rep 2:1059, 1995.

238. STAVRI GT et al: Hypoxia and platelet-derived growth factor-BB synergistically upregulate the expression of vascular endothelial growth factor in vascular smooth muscle cells. Febs Lett 358:311, 1995.

239. TSAI JC et al: Vascular endothelial growth factor in human glioma cell lines: Induced secretion by EGF, PDGF-BB, and bFGF. J Neurosurg 82:864, 1995.

240. SILVAGNO F et al: In vivo activation of met tyrosine kinase by heterodimeric hepatocyte growth molecule promotes angiogenesis. Arterioscler Thromb Vasc Biol 15:1857, 1995.

241. DETMAR M et al: Keratinocyte-derived vascular permeability factor (vascular endothelial growth factor) is a potent mitogen for dermal microvascular endothelial cells. J Invest Dermatol 105:44, 1995.

242. COHEN T et al: Interleukin 6 induces the expression of vascular endothelial growth factor. J Biol Chem 271:736, 1996.

243. LI J et al: Induction of vascular endothelial growth factor gene expression by Interleukin-1β in rat aortic smooth muscle cells. J Biol Chem 270:308, 1995.

244. PERTOVAARA L et al: Vascular endothelial growth factor is induced in response to transforming growth factor-β in fibroblastic and epithelial cells. J Biol Chem 269:6271, 1994.

245. KOURA AN et al: Regulation of vascular endothelial growth factor expression in human colon carcinoma cells by cell density. Cancer Res 56:3891, 1996.

246. MUKHOPADHYAY D et al: Hypoxic induction of human vascular endothelial growth factor expression through c-src activation. Nature 375:577, 1995.

247. MUKHOPADHYAY D et al: Wild-type p53 and v-src exert opposing influences on human vascular endothelial growth factor gene expression. Cancer Res 55:6161, 1995.

248. RAK J et al: Mutant ras oncogenes upregulate VEGF/VPF expression: Implications for induction and inhibition of tumor angiogenesis. Cancer Res (Adv in Brief) 55:4575, 1995.

249. RAK J et al: Oncogenes as inducers of tumor angiogenesis. Cancer Met Rev 14:263, 1995.

250. ELLIS LM et al: Down-regulation of vascular endothelial growth factor in a human colon carcinoma cell line transfected with an antisense expression vector specific for c-src. J Biol Chem (in press).

251. GUTMAN M et al: Regulation of interleukin-8 expression in human melanoma cells by the organ environment. Cancer Res 55:2470, 1995.

252. TAKAHASHI Y et al: Site-dependent expression of, human vascular endothelial growth factor, angiogenesis and proliferation in human gastric carcinoma. Int J Oncol 8:701, 1996.

253. KITADAI Y et al: In situ hybridization technique for analysis of metastasis-related genes in human colon carcinoma cells. Am J Pathol 147:1238, 1995.

254. KITADAI Y et al: Multiparametric in situ mRNA hybridization analysis to predict disease recurrence in patients with colon carcinoma. Am J Pathol 149:1541, 1996.

# CHAPTER 3

# OVERVIEW OF CLINICAL ONCOLOGY

## 3A / PRINCIPLES OF SURGICAL ONCOLOGY

*John M. Daly and Kirby I. Bland*

The surgical oncologist occupies a unique position in the management of the patient with cancer. Most cancer patients undergo some form of operative therapy for the diagnosis, primary treatment, or management of complications during the course of treatment for their neoplastic disease. Survival statistics of patients with cancer treated surgically have plateaued; earlier detection through selective screening and multimodal therapy should further improve cure rates. Inclusion of radiation therapy or chemotherapy into treatment programs often preserve comparable overall survival rates while permitting less extensive operations compared with surgical resection alone, thus enhancing cosmesis and function. The surgical oncologist is responsible for the initial diagnosis and management of many types of cancer. Knowledge of tumor staging and the natural history of the disease should be integrated into a multimodal approach to treatment in concert with the medical oncologist and the radiation therapist. The guiding principles of the surgical oncologist should be the accurate diagnosis and staging of the cancer with adequate operative removal of locoregional disease (Fig. 3A-1).

The surgical oncologist's role varies with the type of cancer. For example, curative operations may be performed on patients with primary breast, head and neck, gastrointestinal, gynecologic, lung, skin, and urinary tract malignancies. In other forms of cancer, such as lymphoma, the surgeon may provide diagnostic and staging information. In patients with hematologic malignancies, the surgeon may provide vascular access or manage complications related to chemotherapy or radiation therapy.

### PREOPERATIVE ASSESSMENT: CLINICAL DIAGNOSIS AND STAGING

On the first examination of the patient with cancer, a complete history and physical examination are indispensable before further judgments can be made regarding laboratory testing and treatment. Common symptoms range from anorexia, nausea, vomiting, hematemesis, abdominal pain, melena, and hematochezia in patients with gastrointestinal cancer to anorexia, productive cough, and hemoptysis in lung cancer, to an enlarging mass in breast and soft tissue tumors. Symptoms generally correspond to the sites involved, but nonspecific symptoms such as night sweats and weight loss may be the initial manifestations of an underlying neoplastic tumor. The duration of symptoms may indicate the aggressiveness of the cancer. The degree of impairment should be noted, as this will influence treatment decisions regarding palliation.

The patient's past medical history often provides clues to the diagnosis. The medical history also reveals environmental factors such as smoking, alcohol ingestion, or exposure to asbestos or aniline dyes that can be related to organ-specific sites of tumor development. Finally, a thorough medical history provides an important index of operative risk for the patient.

Physical examination should begin with a general assessment, proceed through a systemic examination, and then focus on the specific sites suggested by the medical history. Simple screening examinations, such as a complete pelvic examination with uterine cervical Pap smear and fecal occult blood testing, should be performed.

In addition to routine laboratory tests such as complete blood count, coagulation profile, multichannel serum biochemistry profile, and chest roentgenography, other studies are useful in determining the primary tumor site and extent of disease. The oncologist frequently requires assays for tumor markers in the blood or urine as well as radiologic studies.

Serum tumor markers have been most useful in following the patient's response to therapy (Table 3A-1). Serum markers such as carcinoembryonic antigen, β-human chorionic gonadotropin, TA-90, thyroglobulin and α-fetoprotein are useful in the management of patients with specific tumors.[1–3]

**TABLE 3A-1.** SERUM TUMOR MARKERS APPLICABLE IN SURGICAL ONCOLOGY

| TUMOR SITE | APPROVED AND UNAPPROVED TUMOR BIOMARKER | ANTIGEN SOURCE | APPLICATION SCORE* |
|---|---|---|---|
| Alimentary tract (stomach, pancreas, colorectum | CEA† | Oncofetal epithelium | 2,3,4 |
| | CA 19-9 | Mucin-type glycoprotein | 2,3,4 |
| | CA 50, CA 195, CA 72-4, TAG 72 | Mucin-type glycoprotein | 4 |
| Prostate | PSA† | Prostate glycoprotein, serine protease | 1,2,3,4 |
| | PAP† | Prostate cellular protein | 3,4 |
| Liver (hepatocellular adenocarcinoma | AFP† | Carrier protein liver cell | 1,2,3,4 |
| | CEA† | Hepatocellular oncofetal epithelium | (?3),4 |
| Ovary | CA 125† | Glycoprotein, surface protein of ovarian cell | (?2),3,4 |
| | PLAP (Regan isoenzyme) | Heat-stable acid phosphatase of placental origin | (?2),4 |
| | Beta-HCG (embryonal teratoblastoma) | Urinary HCG peptide | 2,4 |
| Breast | CEA† | Oncofetal epithelium of neoplasm | 4 |
| | CA 15-3 | Similar antigen from milk fat globules and membranes of breast cancer metastasis | 3,(?4) |
| | CAM26, M29, CA27.29, MCA | Antigenic high-molecular-weight glycoprotein (mucin) | Unknown |
| Testicle (germ cell origin) | AFP† | Serum carrier protein testicular cell (malignant teratoblastoma) | 2,3,4 |
| | Beta-HCG (embryonal teratoblastoma) | Malignant teratoblastoma carrier protein | 2,3,4 |
| | LDH† and PLAP† (seminoma) | Heat-stable phosphatase and dehydrogenase, seminoma origin | 3,4 |
| Thyroid | Thyroglobulin† | Thyroid hormone inversely correlates with TSH | 1,(?3),4 |
| | Calcitonin† (medullary cancer) | Parafollicular C cell of thyroid | 1–4 |
| | NSE (medullary cancer) | Glycolytic isoenzyme specific to parafollicular C cell | 4 |
| Lung | NSE (SCCL) | Isoenzyme with specific antigenicity to SCCL | 4 |
| | CK-BB (SCCL) | Creatine kinase brain isoenzyme | ?2 |
| Neuroendocrine: | | | |
|   Carcinoid | 5-HIAA† | Peptide urinary metabolite of indole acetic acid | 2,(?3,?4) |
|   Neuroblastoma | NSE | Isoenzyme with antigenicity to neuroendocrine neural blastogenic cells | 4 |
|   Pancreas | Insulin | Nonbeta islet cell of the pancreas | 1,2,4 |
|   Stomach | Gastrin | G cell gastric antrum | 1,2,3,4 |
|   Pituitary | ACTH | Anterior pituitary hormone | 1,2,3,4 |
| Bone | Alkaline phosphatase | Heat-stable phosphatase with bone fraction specificity | 2,3,4 |
| Head and neck | SCC | Squamous cell antigenicity | 3,4 |
| Trophoblastic | HCG (hydatidiform mole, invasive mole, and choriocarcinoma) | Urinary and serum marker of gestational trophoblasts | 2,3,4 |
| Myeloma | Bence Jones immunoglobulins† | Urinary light chain immunoglobulin G protein | 2,3 |

*Application score: 1 = screening; 2 = diagnosis; 3 = prognosis; 4 = monitoring course and therapeutic responses.
† Denotes approval by the Food and Drug Administration.
ABBREVIATIONS: CEA = carcinoembryonic antigen; AFP = alpha-fetoprotein; SCC = squamous cell carcinoma; PAP = prostatic acid phosphatase; LDH = lactic dehydrogenase; 5-HIAA = 5-hydroxyindole acetic acid; ACTH = adrenocorticotropic hormone; PSA = prostate-specific antigen; beta-HCG = beta-human chorionic gonadotrophic hormone; PLAP = placental alkaline phosphatase; TSH = thyroid-stimulating hormone; NSE = neuron-specific enolase; SCCL = small cell carcinoma of the lung.

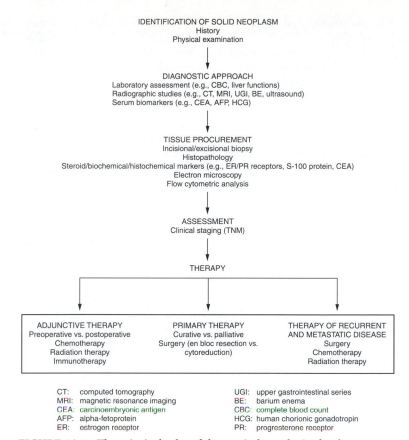

IDENTIFICATION OF SOLID NEOPLASM
History
Physical examination

DIAGNOSTIC APPROACH
Laboratory assessment (e.g., CBC, liver functions)
Radiographic studies (e.g., CT, MRI, UGI, BE, ultrasound)
Serum biomarkers (e.g., CEA, AFP, HCG)

TISSUE PROCUREMENT
Incisional/excisional biopsy
Histopathology
Steroid/biochemical/histochemical markers (e.g., ER/PR receptors, S-100 protein, CEA)
Electron microscopy
Flow cytometric analysis

ASSESSMENT
Clinical staging (TNM)

THERAPY

| ADJUNCTIVE THERAPY | PRIMARY THERAPY | THERAPY OF RECURRENT AND METASTATIC DISEASE |
|---|---|---|
| Preoperative vs. postoperative Chemotherapy Radiation therapy Immunotherapy | Curative vs. palliative Surgery (en bloc resection vs. cytoreduction) | Surgery Chemotherapy Radiation therapy |

CT:   computed tomography
MRI:  magnetic resonance imaging
CEA:  carcinoembryonic antigen
AFP:  alpha-fetoprotein
ER:   estrogen receptor

UGI:  upper gastrointestinal series
BE:   barium enema
CBC:  complete blood count
HCG:  human chorionic gonadotropin
PR:   progesterone receptor

**FIGURE 3A-1.** The principal roles of the surgical oncologist for the management of solid tumors.

The surgical oncologist relies heavily on preoperative imaging for diagnosis, staging, and planning the operation. Most commonly, a dynamic helical computed tomography (CT) scan is the first and only radiologic test required to assess an intraabdominal process. Magnetic resonance imaging (MRI) is helpful for extremity sarcomas, retroperitoneal tumors, and the assessment of bowel-wall penetration of rectal tumors.[4] Endoscopic ultrasound has a major role in the preoperative assessment of esophageal, gastric, pancreatic, and rectal tumors. Ultrasound is user-dependent, but in experienced centers is a superb modality for evaluating tumors involving the hepatobiliary system. The use of preoperative angiography has been drastically reduced with the advent of Duplex ultrasound, MRI angiography, and contrast-enhanced helical CT scanning. However, preoperative arteriography can be useful in patients under consideration for hepatic artery infusional therapy. Mammography is useful for detecting occult breast masses and areas of suspicious microcalcifications, for stereotactic needle biopsies, and for providing needle localization of occult mammographic abnormalities for excisional biopsy. Radionuclide scans are useful for evaluating the presence of bone metastases in patients with symptomatic musculoskeletal complaints. Radiolabeled octreotide, cholesterol, and carcinoembryonic antigen (CEA) scans have utility in staging patients with carcinoid, adrenal, and colorectal tumors, respectively.[5,6] Positron emission tomography (PET) scanning complements other diagnostic modalities for lung, melanoma, and gastrointestinal cancers and may prove ultimately to be more cost effective. Diagnostic sensitivity, specificity, and accuracy are 85% to 90% or better when assessing for primaries, metastases, or recurrence. Utilizing PET scanning altered patient management in 15% to 44% of patients with recurrent colorectal cancer, lung cancer, lymphoma, and melanoma (Table 3A-2).

## PATHOLOGIC DIAGNOSIS AND STAGING

The importance of accurate pathologic diagnosis in the proper surgical treatment of cancer patients cannot be overstated. The

**TABLE 3A-2.** ALTERED PATIENT MANAGEMENT WITH PET SCANNING

| DISEASE | NO. OF PATIENTS | CHANGE IN TREATMENT |
|---|---|---|
| Recurrent colorectal cancer | 93 | 38% |
| Lung cancer | 159 | 41% |
| Lymphoma | 74 | 15% |
| Melanoma | 50 | 44% |

SOURCE: From Conti PS et al:[6] Reproduced with permission.

determinations of histologic grade, primary site, and surgical resection margins provide critical information.

Diagnosis can frequently be made by the use of fine-needle aspiration (FNA). Diagnosis using FNA (22- to 25-gauge needle) techniques concurs with the surgical pathologic diagnosis in 97% of tested lymph nodes in patients with metastatic solid tumors and 77% of primary breast tumors examined. This technique is rapid, minimally traumatic, and highly accurate for diagnosis of a clearly palpable mass or a radiographically visible lesion. False-positive results are rare; false-negative results may occur because of the small sample size and the site of the lesion. With the use of FNA techniques in combination with helical CT scans and ultrasound, deep nonpalpable lesions have become amenable to diagnosis with minimal morbidity. Tumor cell implantation of the aspiration site is rare. FNA cytology is particularly useful in diagnosing palpable masses in the breast or thyroid or palpable suspected nodes in the neck, axilla, or groin. However, aspiration cytology cannot be relied on for grading solid tumors, for subdividing types of lymphoma, or for making an accurate diagnosis after radiation treatment, but a positive diagnosis of malignancy greatly facilitates diagnostic and treatment planning.

When an accurate diagnosis of tumor type and grade is necessary and cannot be accomplished by FNA, an incisional or excisional biopsy is required. Care should be taken in the planning of a surgical biopsy so as not to jeopardize later surgical extirpation or the use of skin flaps. In general, large soft tissue lesions (5 to 7 cm) that are deeper than the superficial fascia are best sampled by incisional biopsy to provide a diagnosis and allow planning for a definitive procedure. Small (<2 cm) superficial lesions should be managed by excisional biopsy with a view toward further treatment depending on tumor type, grade, and depth of invasion. Frozen-section diagnosis should not be relied on to provide accurate histologic grade and information about invasion depth. Surgical margins of resection should be evaluated by frozen-section or permanent section examination of a properly marked and oriented specimen.

The surgical staging of intraabdominal tumors with a concomitant decrease in morbidity has improved with minimal access surgery. Utilizing small incisions and ports with one-way valves, surgical instruments and cameras can be introduced into the $CO_2$ gas–distended abdomen for exploration, direct organ ultrasound, tissue biopsy, peritoneal cytology, and sometimes curative resection. Many surgical oncologists utilize laparoscopic techniques to rule out carcinomatosis prior to laparotomy for pancreatic, gastric, and hepatic malignancies. Limiting laparotomy only to patients who may benefit from resection reduces patient morbidity, time to definitive therapy, duration of hospitalization, and cost.

## SURGICAL THERAPY

### PRIMARY (DEFINITIVE) SURGICAL THERAPY

The surgeon should convey to the patient and the family a reasonable expectation that a definitive (primary) procedure can be completed following the diagnosis and staging of a cutaneous or visceral malignancy. Although the following section deals with the assessment

of operative risk, knowledge of the general medical condition of the patient is a requisite to the performance of a safe operation with low morbidity and mortality rates. Thus, in terms of planning the primary operation, the surgeon must integrate the following parameters: the physiologic status of the patient, the stage and location of the tumor, the expectations for curability or palliation of the malignancy, and the histopathologic features of the neoplasm.[7] The cardinal principle for primary curative surgery includes the total removal of gross and microscopic neoplastic tissues. When total extirpation of the neoplasm is possible, an accurate assessment of the specimen and margins allows pathologic staging with exacting tissue data in regard to gross and microscopic disease that is confined to the locoregional anatomic site of the primary. In many cancers, simple extirpation of the tumor with a "free" tissue margin (microscopic) is curative for the majority of lesions (e.g., cutaneous melanoma cured in 80% to 90% with local excision). By contrast, despite free surgical margins and negative nodes histologically in aggressive, small (T1) cancers of certain individuals (e.g., breast cancer in young patients with a high S-phase and high nuclear grade), distant metastases may be expected on an exponential basis with time. These patients may require adjuvant therapies despite pathologically free margins with definitive surgical treatment. The integration of tumor biology with the stage of disease is an additional requirement in the responsibilities of the oncologic surgeon, as required by these distinctly different clinical scenarios.

## PRIMARY SURGICAL THERAPY IN THE ERA OF COMBINATION MODALITIES

Surgery, similar to other therapeutic modalities, has its own inherent risks and side effects, some of which may be permanent in terms of the effect on cosmesis, form, and function. The past 20 years have witnessed a progressive reduction in the radicality of operative procedures for various operative sites, the primary paradigm being that of breast cancer.[8–11] The trend toward conservation-type surgery has been attributed to a change in the pathophysiologic perceptions by the oncologic surgeon of the methods by which tumor dissemination occurs. Contemporary tumor biology suggests that tumor progression is not always orderly or stereotypic through the regional nodes, but rather it may directly involve distant sites following hematogenous dissemination. The biologic observation that distant dissemination may occur with a bypass of the regional lymphatic channels mitigates the need or rationale for radical en bloc resection of the primary site and the regional nodes. However, the major factor for change of the scope and extent of oncologic surgical procedures has been the development of alternative (adjunctive) effective modalities, namely, radiation and chemotherapy. The melding of these adjuvant approaches with surgery resulted from a rising consciousness by surgeons of the limits and goals of operative therapy (Table 3A-3). With adjunctive modalities, the extent of the surgical procedure and its undesirable complications can be restricted while achieving results that are equivalent to those following radical surgery (e.g., segmental mastectomy plus irradiation versus modified radical mastectomy). When similar results can be achieved with conservative approaches, the choice would obviously favor a combination modality that preserves organ function and cosmesis.

**TABLE 3A-3.** LUMPECTOMY VERSUS LUMPECTOMY AND IRRADIATION VERSUS MASTECTOMY FOR EARLY-STAGE BREAST CANCER

| SURVIVAL CATEGORY AND TREATMENT GROUP | JUNE 1984 | | DECEMBER 1987 | |
| --- | --- | --- | --- | --- |
| | PATIENTS AT RISK (NO.) | SURVIVAL (%) | PATIENTS AT RISK (NO.) | SURVIVAL (%) |
| Disease-free survival: | | | | |
| Total mastectomy | 67 | 66 | 281 | 67 |
| Lumpectomy | 78 | 63 | 278 | 64 |
| Lumpectomy and irradiation | 88 | 72 | 307 | 71 |
| Distant disease-free survival: | | | | |
| Total mastectomy | 67 | 72 | 297 | 74 |
| Lumpectomy | 83 | 70 | 302 | 71 |
| Lumpectomy and irradiation | 88 | 76 | 313 | 74 |
| Overall survival: | | | | |
| Total mastectomy | 81 | 76 | 345 | 82 |
| Lumpectomy | 100 | 85 | 363 | 83 |
| Lumpectomy and irradiation | 98 | 85 | 359 | 84 |

Trends similar to those depicted earlier for breast cancer have been observed for other anatomic sites. Abdominoperineal resections (APR) are done less frequently than are low anterior resections for rectal cancer.[12] The trend in conservation-type approaches for this organ site requires adjuvant therapies (chemotherapy and radiation therapy) to achieve locoregional control equivalent to APR. In past decades, amputation for extremity sarcomas was the primary modality of treatment for 40% to 50% of patients treated in cancer centers throughout North America. Presently, the application of combination modalities has reduced the amputation rate for this malignancy to 5% to 10%. Although contemporary oncology demands an appreciation of the utility of adjuvant therapies, surgical treatment as a primary modality remains indispensable and maintains a primary role in the management of malignancies, as in the past. The surgeon must have a clear perspective of the objectives of the operative procedure, i.e., to produce maximum cytoreductive or ablative effect on the tumor with minimal disturbance of cosmesis and organ function. These potential objectives of the procedure are at least partly contradictory. The challenge for the oncologic surgeon is the application of the optimal meld of the objectives for each tumor and, indeed, for each case. Obviously, the "blend" of these objectives for each histologic type depends on the availability of effective adjuvant modalities. If the latter are available and efficacious, the surgeon can perform a more conservative operation; in the absence of tumor responsiveness to adjuvant modalities, a more radical approach may be essential. In the context of present knowledge of tumor biology, axillary dissection should be more thorough and radical for melanoma (e.g., Patey dissection of levels I to III) than for breast cancer (e.g., sampling level I and low-level II). These tenets are essential because local recurrence near the primary site or in the nodal drainage area for melanoma has dire prognostic implications; this clinical presentation does not portend the same ominous consequences for breast cancer.

With conservative or radical primary therapy of the neoplasm, the conduct of the procedure is essential to the outcome. The availability of effective adjuvant modalities and a plan to implement these therapies does not condone less precise technical aspects of the surgical procedure. The surgeon must obtain and ensure the maximum effect on the tumor within the surgical constraints consciously chosen. The application of technically precise approaches exercised by surgeons in various cancer centers has allowed the selective application of combination modalities to emerge as state-of-the-art conservation-type approaches (e.g., segmental mastectomy plus radiation therapy for breast cancer or preoperative radiation and local excision for rectal carcinoma). For example, the rate of amputation to treat extremity sarcomas has remained stable at 5% to 6%, since limb salvage approaches became standardized. Preliminary results from Roswell Park Cancer Institute suggest that the rate of local recurrence was 24% in the period 1977 to 1982, 15% in the period 1983 to 1987, and 10% in the years 1988 to 1991. Because therapeutic strategies and the application of adjuvant modalities have remained static since the late 1970s, the progressive decline in local recurrence with limb salvage over these years perhaps reflects the increasing familiarity by the staff with operative technique, patient selection, and staging to ensure more commonly that a successful limb salvage procedure can be achieved.[13-16] The latter procedure necessitates that wide (or radical) tissue margins be procured about the tumor in three dimensions when tissue with little functional or cosmetic importance is available; these margins are deliberately reduced (compromised) in the vicinity of functionally significant structures such as vital organs, arteries, and nerves. A structure to be preserved with limb salvage is exposed both proximally and distally and thereafter is approached from its aspect away from the tumor, so that extrication of this structure may be achieved while the sheath originally encircling the structure is left attached to the tumor.

Although the semantics of wide (radical) resection versus conservative-type (local) excision need to be preserved for purposes of scientific (technical) communication and for a determination of the need for other adjuvant modalities, the type of procedure that is actually completed defies an easy classification and may be intermediate with features of both radical and conservative approaches. As an example, a sarcoma in the region of the groin may require exposure of the iliac vessels proximally (by use of many of the technical steps of radical groin dissection or abdominoinguinal incision) and the superficial femoral vessels distally. These technical events are followed by resection of involved portions of the lower abdominal wall, the anterior and/or medial compartments of the thigh, with infrequent removal of the femoral nerve. Following circumferential freeing of the entire specimen, the iliofemoral vessels are resected, and vascular continuity is reestablished with prosthetic grafts. In the resected specimen, pathologists may identify margins varying from 3 to 15 cm in the majority of areas about the tumor; however, the margins may be as narrow as 0.5 cm in small areas in which the tumor was adjacent to the femur or femoral nerve. Despite attempts for the differentiation of conservative versus radical procedures that are well entrenched in clinical parlance, it is obvious that the minimal margin of 0.5 cm is the determinant for the classification of the procedure and provides a major pathologic discriminant for the necessity of adjuvant modalities of local control (i.e., chemotherapy or radiation). The accepted minimal margin required for an operation to be adequate can usually be determined from the surgical literature; however, the extent of the minimal margin and the tissues composing this compromised area of resection assume great importance when predicting recurrence.[17] An operation in which the circumferential margins in three dimensions about the tumor are uniformly less than 1 cm is associated with a much higher potential for locoregional recurrence than an operation in which the minimal margin of 1 cm is restricted to a small surface area of the specimen. Furthermore, a 0.5-cm margin around an intramuscular sarcoma that is superficially composed of a strong fascial layer (the dissection having been completed outside the compartment) may be considered adequate; similar margins composed only of muscle within a muscular compartment are grossly inadequate.

In the context of applications of multimodal approaches, surgery becomes highly discriminating. This discipline procures wide margins three dimensionally around the tumor mass for tissues that are not functionally (or cosmetically) essential, while diminishing marginal excisions along functionally essential structures.[12] As observed earlier, this procedure would be termed neither radical nor conservative. Despite a paucity of nomenclature to classify the procedure technically, this approach in itself may achieve local control by a reduction of potential microscopic residual sites that may be effectively destroyed (controlled) by other adjuvant modalities. Thus, this primary definitive approach may be the maximal therapeutic modality that can be offered to the patient within the constraints chosen and on the basis of the availability and efficacy of other modalities or technical considerations imposed by the local or regional anatomy. The necessity of reducing the depth of margins near anatomic structures that are functionally essential should not dampen the resolve to achieve wide margins in other portions of the tumor when this is technically feasible.

In the era of combination therapeutic modalities to treat solid tumors, the dichotomy for the differentiation of radical and conservative operative procedures loses its crucial significance. The practice of contemporary surgical oncology demands comprehensive and adequate surgical extirpation when possible. This practice can be very conservative in the presence of adjuvant modalities that provide effective local control; the design of the procedure should be radical when the size of the tumor is significant, when it has an adverse impact on function (neuromuscular or vascular), and when the available adjuvant modalities are ineffectual.

## GENERAL PRINCIPLES OF PRIMARY TUMOR RESECTION

An en bloc resection of the primary tumor is a requisite of tumor control, and ablation should be done when technically possible. This axiom implies that all (and potentially microscopic) disease is eradicated operatively when contiguous tissue planes and/or organs are included in the operative specimen. The en bloc technique further dictates that the neoplasm be resected intact with the incorporation of the biopsy incision and structures involved by or near the tumor without violation of tissue planes contiguous to the tumor or of tissues interposed between the structures to be resected.[12] It is the responsibility of the surgeon to be fully cognizant of the optimal application of surgical instrumentation that will be required for the procedure. In general, scalpel dissection with tissues being divided under tension can proceed in fractions of millimeters and, therefore, is safe and efficacious for dissection of nontransparent tissues. This technique also has great value in the development of viable tissue flaps, in which the maintenance of the vascular supply is essential to the integrity and viability of the skin. Metzenbaum scissors or electrocautery dissection may be preferable for the division of transparent tissues, such as adhesions, particularly within recesses when the scalpel cannot be easily manipulated. A regard for the safety and conduct of the procedure and the demand of tumor ablation are principal concerns of the responsible surgeon. Typically, during dissection about a large tumor, the surgeon must constantly orient himself or herself with the perspective of dissection in a three-dimensional spatial configuration, remaining cognizant of the demands for exposure and safety near vital structures. In general, the surgeon must follow the planes of least resistance about the tumor as long as the planes are grossly and microscopically free of disease. When the dissection necessitates a compromise of wide margins near vital structures, frozen-section pathologic analyses are recommended, with an operative description and orientation of the margins of the specimen forwarded to the pathology laboratory. With exercise of the aforementioned tenets, dissection in sites that are easiest to mobilize first will allow mobilization of the specimen and adequate, safe dissection of previously difficult areas.

Intraoperative palpation of the neoplasm alone is often an insufficient criterion to determine its resectability. For example, a sarcoma or carcinoma that presents at the base of the mesentery should not be termed unresectable merely on the basis of its anatomic location; the exposure and dissection of superior mesenteric vessels is essential to determine its resectability and may be accomplished with wide mesenteric margins that allow the salvage of mesenteric vasculature and, hence, a preservation of the blood supply to the midgut. Thus, the term *nonresectable* or *unresectable* should be reserved for an anatomic demonstration of the involvement of vital structures in which a resection would be likely to result in the patient's death (e.g., hepatic trisegmentectomy in nutritionally compromised and elderly patients) or incompatibility with a meaningful quality of life (e.g., hemicorporectomy for advanced sarcoma of the pelvis). In addition, fixation is not a reliable criterion of unresectability. Frequently, normal structures, such as the iliacus and psoas, appear "fixed" on palpation. However, sarcomas that originate in this area generally are resectable. Furthermore, solid tumors (e.g., sarcoma) that involve the pubic bone may also appear fixed; however, such lesions are easily resectable with free margins because normal contiguous structures can be resected en bloc with the primary lesion.

Finally, the surgeon must be cognizant of the purpose of the procedure and its expected benefit (Table 3A-4). A risk versus benefit ratio for the potential of the operation to be curative or palliative must be considered when the risk of operative morbidity and mortality are significant. Although the operative risk should be minimized for all patients, the exercise of prudent judgment and experience are primary and may determine that a minimally invasive or nonoperative approach is in the best interests of the patient when an operation has mainly palliative value.

## CONSIDERATIONS OF LOCAL VERSUS SYSTEMIC PRESENTATION OF CANCER

Primary surgical therapy is concerned initially with eradication of the tumor mass in its earliest locoregional stage. This primary therapeutic approach will allow accurate pathologic staging of the cancer. The expected 5- and 10-year survival rates will depend on the

**TABLE 3A-4.** MULTIPLE SURGICAL STRATEGIES USED IN THE MANAGEMENT OF SOLID TUMORS

| TYPE OF SURGERY | RATIONALE | EXAMPLES |
| --- | --- | --- |
| Primary (Definitive) | Definitive therapy of primary tumor and regional site(s) of disease<br><br>Organization of therapeutic strategies with other oncology and medical disciplines | Segmental mastectomy<br>Colon resection<br>Radiation oncology<br>Medical oncology<br>Pediatric oncology<br>Endocrinology consultation |
| Cytoreductive | Reduction of tumor volume of primary, regional, or metastatic foci to enhance responsiveness to adjuvant modalities | Ovarian carcinoma<br>Lymphoma (Burkitt's) |
| Palliative | Enhance organ function<br>Relieve symptoms of progressive disease<br>Enhance quality of life<br>Diminish immediate mortality | Bypass/resection of colon cancer obstruction<br>"Toilet" mastectomy<br>Gastrectomy for hemorrhage from carcinoma<br>Brain metastasis from melanoma with neurologic symptoms |
| Metastatic disease | Curative intent<br>    Staging determines solitary focus of metastasis<br>Noncurative intent<br>    Operative cure unlikely<br>    Palliation achieved only with resection of metastases | Colorectal hepatic metastasis<br>Soft tissue/bone sarcoma metastatic to lung<br>Regional lymph node dissection for skin/vascular fixation of melanoma or squamous carcinoma |
| Emergency | Immediate operative intervention essential to avoid death | Viscus perforation: stomach, small bowel, or colon<br>Major gastrointestinal hemorrhage<br>Intraabdominal abscess with sepsis |
| Rehabilitation reconstruction | Enhance quality of life<br>Enhance form, function, and cosmesis | Free-tissue transfer to neck for reconstruction following esophageal-laryngeal resection<br>Transabdominal myocutaneous flap for radical/modified-radical mastectomy |
| Vascular access | Provide venous access for administration of chemotherapeutic agents, antibiotics, and blood components<br>Essential when peripheral venous routes are lost for blood drawing or administration purposes<br>Administration of local parenteral nutrition following loss of enteral route for transient or permanent intervals | Implantable subcutaneous venous ports<br>Hickman catheters<br>Central venous catheters |

stage of the primary tumor and the specific prognostic parameters evident for each histologic type and organ site. Substantial rates of long-term survival and cure may be achieved with surgical therapy alone, if the primary tumor is determined to be localized clinically and pathologically. The long-term survival rates and cure of malignant melanomas currently approach 80% to 90% because of earlier diagnosis and treatment owing to improved public awareness. Previous studies from the surgical era in which an operation was the sole modality for therapy of breast and colorectal carcinoma have documented substantial 10-year survival rates. By contrast, cancers of the pancreas and lung have had much shorter long-term survival times. The latter tumors are typical of those in which the tumor's biology (e.g., aggressive morphologic features with high metastatic frequency) is the predominant determinant of survival, especially when diagnosis and therapy are delayed. Experimental evidence confirms that dormant (occult) metastatic cells may be present in the early stages of growth of the primary tumor and gives rise to the concept that cancer is often a "systemic disease" from its inception.

An additional cardinal principle of curative definitive surgery recognizes the therapy of regional disease.[18] With the possible exception of regional infusion or isolation perfusion for in-transit metastasis from cutaneous melanoma, surgical therapy remains the most effective modality for the management of locoregional disease in the majority of solid tumors. Locoregional disease should thus be viewed as a potentially curable state. As observed earlier, the majority of patients with an extension of the primary tumor to regional sites will have distant occult disease and sustain an expected frequency of relapse during follow-up. The proportion who do not have distant metastasis at the time of definitive operative therapy may have prolonged survival beyond 10 years following surgical therapy. Locoregional recurrence and survival are dependent on a number of discriminant factors, i.e., clinical nodal status, number of nodes, prior disease-free interval, and tumor biology (e.g., high versus low nuclear grade, diploid versus aneuploid, and percent S-phase). Increasingly, evidence of adverse tumor biology of the primary lesion has provided objective determinants for the therapy of occult systemic disease to provide enhancement of the disease-free survival time.

## CYTOREDUCTIVE SURGICAL THERAPY

The rationale for cytoreductive surgery has been an evolutionary process for the recognition of the benefits of removal of residual gross disease. The objective of this therapeutic approach is the reduction of the volume of the primary and regional or metastatic foci to provide enhancement of the tumor's responsiveness to effective adjuvant modalities. Thus, in the selective advanced cancers (e.g., ovarian carcinoma or Burkitt's lymphoma), the resection of bulky disease may provide improvement in organ function and, thus, quality of life. The surgeon must be cognizant of all therapeutic modalities of value for selective histopathologic types because cytoreductive surgery may be injurious to the host in whom adjuvant radiation and/or chemotherapy are ineffectual. The classic example of the latter is a "frozen" pelvis secondary to adenocarcinoma of the rectum, for which pelvic exenteration is not only ineffectual palliation but is highly likely to provide significant morbidity and mortality without

a salutary benefit for short-term recovery or the enhancement of quality of life.

## PALLIATIVE SURGICAL THERAPY

This category of surgical intervention shares common features with attempts to complete primary (definitive) resection of solid tumors. Palliation implies the therapeutic attempt to provide patient benefit (improved survival or quality of life) in the absence of cure. Although the initial intent of the procedure may be curative, intraoperative staging and the assessment of tumor characteristics may convert the elective curative procedure to one that is purely palliative. Examples of the latter include procedures initiated to extirpate solid tumors that threaten or impede vital function (e.g., pulmonary carcinoma obstructing a bronchus or a carcinoma obstructing the colon), to provide relief of pain or intolerable symptoms (e.g., "toilet" mastectomy for ulcerated breast carcinoma), or to abrogate impending symptoms and the morbidity of advanced disease (e.g., gastrectomy performed for hemorrhage related to advanced gastric carcinoma with metastasis).

## SURGICAL THERAPY OF METASTATIC DISEASE

Although much data are available with regard to the mechanistic concepts for tumor dissemination by lymphatic and hematogenous routes, little is understood of the tumor biology that initiates or inhibits the pathophysiologic event of metastasis. A malignant tumor may disseminate by four routes, i.e., direct infiltration of contiguous tissues, lymphatic channels, vascular invasion, or exfoliation and implantation in serous cavities. In addition, many histopathologic variants of cancer may disseminate by more than one route; thus, orderly spread of the neoplasm is not predictable. Examples may include patients with melanoma or breast, lung, or colorectal carcinomas who may be determined with staging to have distant disease in multiple metastatic sites (e.g., lung, liver, bone, or brain) without evidence of regional lymphatic metastases. The patterns and frequencies of metastatic dissemination for various human tumors are summarized in Table 3A-5.

When approaching metastatic disease, the oncologic surgeon must differentiate a procedure performed with curative intent from an operation in which the likelihood of rendering the patient free of disease is remote. Three tenets must be satisfied in consideration of the resection of metastatic disease:

1. A limited volume of metastatic disease within a single organ site (i.e., the absence of metastatic disease in other organs)
2. Evidence that the anatomic site can be resected with gross and microscopic free margins without interference or impairment in the vital function of the organ
3. Acceptable morbidity and mortality rates following resection

Examples include selected patients with solitary or limited foci of hepatic metastases from colorectal carcinomas; 5-year survival rates have exceeded 30% for selected patients. Furthermore, similar 5-year survival rates following pulmonary resections can be expected for metastases of soft tissue or bone sarcomas and colorectal carcinoma.

**TABLE 3A-5. ESTIMATED FREQUENCY FOR PATTERNS OF NEOPLASTIC SPREAD FOR SOME COMMON HUMAN CANCERS**

| NEOPLASM | HEMATOGENOUS | LYMPHATIC | LOCAL INFILTRATION[†] |
|---|---|---|---|
| Adenocarcinoma: | | | |
| Breast | 4* | 3 | 2 |
| Endometrium | 1 | 2 | 1 |
| Ovary | 2 | 3 | 4 |
| Stomach | 4 | 4 | 3 |
| Pancreas | 4 | 4 | 3 |
| Colon | 3 | 3 | 1 |
| Kidney | 2 | 2 | 2 |
| Prostate | 3 | 3 | 3 |
| Liver | 1 | 1 | 4 |
| | | | |
| Epidermoid carcinoma: | | | |
| Lung | 4 | 3 | 2 |
| Oropharynx | 1 | 3 | 3 |
| Larynx | 1 | 3 | 2 |
| Cervix | 1 | 4 | 3 |
| | | | |
| Transitional cell carcinoma: | | | |
| Bladder | 2 | 3 | 4 |
| | | | |
| Cutaneous neoplasm: | | | |
| Squamous cell carcinoma | 1 | 2 | 1 |
| Melanomas | 3 | 3 | 2 |
| Basal cell carcinomas | 0 | 0 | 1 |
| | | | |
| Sarcomas: | | | |
| Bones | 4 | 1 | 1 |
| Soft tissue | 4 | 1 | 3 |
| Brain neoplasms | 0 | 0 | 4 |

*0 = Does not occur; 1 = 1% to 15%; 2 = 15% to 30%; 3 > 30%; 4 > 50%.
[†] Expressed as local recurrence.
SOURCE: Modified from Morton DL: *Cancer Medicine*. Philadelphia, Lea & Febiger, 1993, p. 530.

As effective systemic therapy continues to evolve for the treatment of these organ sites, the cure rates of metastasectomy may increase. In contradistinction, the majority of cutaneous melanomas and adenocarcinomas of pancreatic, gastrointestinal, and hepatic primary sites are only rarely amenable to curative pulmonary resection. However, should a solitary metastasis to the lung be determined by CT in the absence of recurrent or residual disease in other anatomic sites, surgical resection is warranted. Similarly, a solitary metastasis to the brain from lesions of various histologic types (i.e., melanoma,

adenocarcinoma, carcinoma, or renal cell carcinoma) should be considered for resection when extracranial residual disease has been excluded. In addition, the neurologic sequelae of a major intracranial resection must be considered because function may be influenced profoundly when critical neurologic tracts or lobes are removed. Adjuvant whole-brain irradiation and high-dose corticosteroid therapy may be an option in lieu of operative intervention when major neurologic impairment is expected following surgical resection. With the planning of the surgical therapy of metastatic disease one must consider additional factors that influence the risk-benefit ratio of operative intervention relative to the tumor's histologic type and staging.

## ONCOLOGIC SURGERY OF THE FUTURE

### SURGICAL INTERVENTION FOR SMALL TUMOR VOLUME

The great majority of the solid neoplasms of humans have undergone a minimal 30 exponential cellular replications (divisions) prior to obtaining the size of 1 cm$^3$. Mathematically, this 1-cm$^3$ nodule consists of approximately 1 billion neoplastic cells following division. Thus, between 36 and 40 divisions on this exponential scale represent a state of the host with rapid demise. If we assume that, biologically, a cancer has its origin from a single cell, it is highly probable that the majority of neoplasms have resided within the body for a minimum of 2 years, and many as long as 10 years, prior to their detection by physical, radiographic, biochemical, or immunologic methods. Should the science and art of early detection evolve in the next decade to apply more sophisticated, specific, and sensitive methods, it is theoretically conceivable that common solid organ neoplasms of the breast, colorectum, prostate, and lung may be curable if diagnosed in Tis or T1 stages. It is with this volume of tumor that the surgeon would have the greatest biologic impact and produce predictable therapeutic responses; these early stages imply the absence of regional disease but may still have established (occult) clones of metastatic foci. In addition, currently established traditional diagnostic techniques with radiographic, biochemical, and immunohistochemical methods may be enhanced (or complemented) with evolving diagnostic measures (e.g., radiolabeled monoclonal antibody markers that can be identified radiographically or by hand-held radiodetection probes). Predictably, the impact of early diagnosis will be translated into enhanced disease-free and overall survival rates.

### RADIOIMMUNOGUIDED SURGERY AND IMMUNOSCINTIGRAPHY IN CANCER DIAGNOSIS AND THERAPY

Major advances of the past two decades for the treatment of cancer include the introduction of adjuvant therapies (chemotherapy and radiation therapy) for various solid neoplasms. Despite these additive measures for tumor control, adjuvant nonsurgical therapies have not significantly altered the outcome of cancer-related deaths and, in many circumstances, have escalated treatment complications (major and minor) associated with the administration of these therapies. Until adjuvant approaches provide a risk-benefit ratio which enhances the tumoricidal effect, contemporary technology may allow therapists to use in vivo diagnostic agents which improve preoperative staging of smaller tumor volumes and, thus, provide early surgical intervention for curative or cytoreductive purposes. Furthermore, these in vivo imaging agents may be of value to monitor the locoregional and distant extent of metachronous disease.

Following the identification of tumor-associated globulin (TAG) by the antibody, an agent (linker) that targets a gamma-emitting radioisotope to the complex may result in the latter's destruction. Polyclonal antibodies and monoclonal antibodies have been used in this technology to enhance tumor specificity and targeting sensitivity. Monoclonal antibodies are derived by cell-fusion techniques from long-lived tissue culture lines of cells; thus, single antibodies are purified to homogeneity. By contrast, polyclonal antibodies are derived from the sera of an immunized animal (i.e., goat or rabbit). Monoclonal antibodies are usually derived from immunized mice. By contrast, with tumor-specific antigens, tumor-associated antigens are identified on tumor membrane surfaces, the cytoplasm, and restricted sites of cells in developing embryos. Because these sites are highly restricted in their distribution, they may be useful in identifying tumors for diagnostic or therapeutic purposes. Approximately 90% of studies in radiopharmaceutical chemistry have used the radioisotopes $^{131}$In and $^{99m}$Tc for these purposes. The majority of studies for radioimaging incorporates either $^{111}$In or $^{99m}$Tc. Indium has a half-life of 2.8 days; technetium has a half-life of 6 hours.

## DIAGNOSTIC LAPAROSCOPY AS AN ADJUNCT IN MANAGEMENT OF MALIGNANCY

The advantages of laparoscopy over laparotomy are well documented. The two procedures are equivalent in revealing metastatic and nodal disease, but laparoscopy requires a shorter hospital stay, causes less pain, allows an earlier return to normal activities, produces less adhesion formation, and reduces the psychological debilitation attending the aforementioned factors. Given these benefits, it is reasonable to apply laparoscopy whenever possible in the evaluation of oncology patients.

Laparoscopy is an effective method for determining the resectability of intraabdominal malignancies with expected low cure rates. This advantage is especially important for disease considered to be unresectable following negative or equivocal noninvasive diagnostic measures. As many as 40% of patients with cancer of the stomach, esophagus, pancreas, and liver benefit from laparoscopy with the avoidance of nontherapeutic laparotomy. In large part, this benefit is related to the diagnostic capability of laparoscopy to detect small (1- to 2-mm) hepatic and peritoneal metastases that are not discernible by CT scanning or other contemporary imaging modalities.

Nodal status is an important determinant of treatment alternatives for various malignancies. Patients with cancer of the cervix, cancer of the prostate, or lymphoma may undergo laparoscopic staging, which allows a shorter hospital stay and causes less morbidity; nodal yield and visceral assessment are the same as in traditional (open) staging laparotomy. Laparoscopy is also useful to monitor the effectiveness of treatment. It is ideally suited for "second-look" procedures because it is an outpatient procedure, is more accurate than noninvasive imaging modalities, and is associated with a reduced incidence of de novo adhesion formation when compared to conventional laparotomy. Further, this technique is beneficial for evaluating the objective responsiveness of certain neoplasms to chemotherapy [e.g., ovarian carcinoma, especially with evidence of elevation of specific biomarkers for this neoplasm (CA-125)]. It should be noted, however, that laparoscopy does not rule out the presence of occult disease; rather, it serves to document the presence of gross visible disease unappreciated radiographically with state-of-the-art imaging methods.

Laparoscopic staging is currently being used more commonly in oncology clinics to provide supportive measures for patients with various malignancies, such as directed placement of intraabdominal infusion port devices in patients with ovarian cancer or gastrostomy in patients with advanced head and neck malignancy. Moreover, increasingly complex palliative procedures (such as cholecystojejunostomy and gastrojejunostomy) and primary surgical management of malignant disease (such as colorectal resection for carcinoma) are being performed more frequently. Long-term results, especially with regard to the efficacy of these modalities to treat solid tumors, remain undetermined.

## CARDIAC RISK ASSESSMENT

The patient's pertinent history of prior cardiac events should be recorded, including valvular disease, hypertension, ischemic heart disease, congestive heart failure, and angina. Chest pain is graded on a scale of 1 to 4 according to physical tolerance to exercise.

Furthermore, the surgeon and anesthesiologist must be aware of pertinent cardiac medications and noncardiac drugs that affect myocardial performance (e.g., digitalis, nitroglycerin, or diuretics). Congestive heart failure may be determined on the basis of paroxysmal nocturnal dyspnea, orthopnea, tachycardia, or lower-extremity edema. In addition, congestive heart failure may be determined solely by cardiac auscultation or estimations of performance and radiographic criteria (e.g., cardiac enlargement with changes of prominent pulmonary vasculature). Before initiating a major oncologic operation on the patient who is 65 years of age or older with a known cardiac history, it is advisable to place a Swan-Ganz catheter preoperatively to ensure an intraoperative estimation of myocardial performance. This method was used to allow the identification of patients with prohibitive cardiac risk and is valuable in directing therapies that enhance cardiac performance prior to the operation. Based on hemodynamic data (e.g., pulse rate, stroke index, cardiac index, left ventricular stroke work, and oxygen transport measurement), patients may be stratified into one of the following classes.

*Stage I*: Individuals with no abnormalities.
*Stage II*: Individuals with mild functional deficits who require aggressive intraoperative and postoperative monitoring parameters.
*Stage III*: Individuals with mild-to-moderate deficits who require preoperative hemodynamic and pulmonary intervention (e.g., inotropic therapy, respiratory toilet, volume replacement, or blood replacement).

*Stage IV*: Individuals with profound uncorrectable deficits of function that make them unsuitable for the proposed operative procedure.

The anesthesiologist may wish to obtain a multiple-gated acquisition (MUGA) scan to evaluate the kinetics of myocardial function; MUGA scans provide information for ventricular functional assessment that correlates well with myocardial performance (e.g., ventricular ejection fraction). An evaluation of the coronary circulation to determine important hemodynamic alterations is provided by both the dipyridamole–thallium 201 scintigram and coronary angiography. Based on the findings of these two studies, preoperative coronary bypass and monitoring with Swan-Ganz catheters may be essential to optimize cardiac function for patients with Stages II and III disease prior to the proposed oncologic procedure.

The incidence of cardiovascular disease had increased to 18% for women and more than twice that (37%) for men. Therefore, cardiac complications represent a leading cause of death in the elderly patient undergoing operative management. In elderly patients undergoing general surgical procedures, postoperative cardiac complications were evident in 12% and cardiac-related death in 2% representing 20% of potentially preventable deaths.

Early reviews and studies suggested a risk of reinfarction of approximately 30% when nonelective surgery occurred within 3 months of myocardial infarction; this risk decreased to 15% between 3 and 6 months and was 5% when the operation was performed more than 6 months following the infarction. These reports suggested that the mortality rate associated with an acute myocardial infarction ranges from 54% to 70%. More contemporary reports of reinfarction frequency following invasive monitoring and technologic advances suggest an improvement in cardiac-related mortality rates. A reinfarction rate of 6% within 3 months of a recent myocardial infarction has been observed. This rate decreased to 2% for the 3 to 6 months following infarction. Other investigators also observed an improvement through perioperative invasive monitoring and anesthetic approaches to diminish cardiac morbidity and mortality rates.

Advancing age represents a profound risk for a subsequent cardiac event. In patients older than 70 years of age, the risk of perioperative cardiac death increases by tenfold. In addition, elderly patients are more subject to emergency operations and this increases the cardiac complication rate fourfold. Cardiac risk index (CRI) was applied in the 1970s as the state-of-the-art risk assessment parameter. As previously noted, this index was the first prospective tool to provide a multivariant analysis for the assessment of cardiac risk. A patient's preoperative Dripps-ASA classification had strong univariate correlation with the cardiac outcome. However, with discriminant analysis, it did not add a statistically significant increment in classification power to the multifactorial index.

## TECHNIQUES FOR CARDIAC RISK ASSESSMENT

*Step 1.* The results of the history and physical examination should preempt any nonivasive or invasive diagnostic technical procedure in the assessment of cardiac risk. The review of systems with the identification of comorbid events (e.g., recent or past myocardial infarction, syncope, angina, pulmonary edema, valvular disease, peripheral vascular disease, or hepatic and renal failure) is requisite to the testing. The physical examination should document peripheral pulses, cardiac rate and rhythm, evidence of murmurs, cardiomegaly, peripheral edema, and associated hepatic disease. The laboratory tests must be comprehensive and include a complete blood count, electrolyte levels, blood urea nitrogen concentration, serum creatinine and serum glutamic oxalic transaminase levels, and arterial blood gas measurements. The basic assessment of any adult patient being prepared for major oncologic procedures should include an electrocardiogram that provides an evaluation of the cardiac rhythm and rate, evidence of previous infarction, ischemia, and ventricular hypertrophy.

*Step 2.* The Goldman CRI or Detsky MMI may be calculated to assist in the cardiac risk analysis. Despite the numeric considerations as an advantage to identify risk, these noninvasive tools are far from precise. An evaluation of all parameters with clinical judgment is advisable. The Detsky MMI equates the score with probability ratios and calculates the posttest probability of a serious cardiac event that is dependent on the type of procedure planned. The acquisition of one-third of such complications indicates death. MMI scores exceeding 15 are considered high risk; Goldman CRI classes III and IV are high risk.

*Step 3.* For major oncologic procedures in which the predicted indices for elderly patients are few (Goldman CRI less than 14 or Detsky MMI less than 16), many recommend the bicycle exercise test to provide a further prediction of risk. Those individuals who cannot perform for 2 min (raising pulse more than 99) are considered high risk.

*Step 4.* When the anticipated risk of the oncologic procedure is unequivocally lower than the projected benefit (e.g., palliation, enhanced survival, and improved quality of life), the operation should be performed. Should the risk significantly exceed that of the "average" patient, additional measures to complete the preoperative evaluation are advisable to assess the risk further. However, no invasive test or mathematics formula will substitute for sound clinical judgment and experience in the management of high-risk patients. When extensive cardiac or peripheral vascular disease is evident and an urgent or emergency operation is indicated, it is advisable to consider additional evaluations (e.g., echocardiography, coronary angiography, stress electrocardiography, or nuclear medicine testing).

By consensus, hemodynamic monitoring during the perioperative period is essential for the high-risk cardiac patient. Arterial lines and pulmonary artery catheters are valuable to assess and monitor hemodynamic variations in high-risk surgical patients (mean age, 68 years) who had previously been "cleared" by internists on the basis of clinical assessment alone. Operative mortality rate can be reduced substantially with a correction of deficits, optimization of perioperative fluid management with volume resuscitation and restriction, diuretics, afterload reduction, and inotropic drugs. Such invasive hemodynamic monitoring should continue for at least 48 hours because this is the period of risk in which fluid is rapidly mobilized into the intravascular compartment. Postoperative heart failure has a biphasic peak, often occurring immediately postoperatively or within the subsequent 24 to 48 hours. Most myocardial infarctions result within 72 hours of surgery; subsequent myocardial infarctions occur between the fourth and sixth postoperative days. In addition, up to one-half of patients with significant coronary artery disease do not have angina; thus, continual monitoring for arrhythmias, malperfusion, blood pressure, or mental status alterations is essential.

## PULMONARY RISK ASSESSMENT

Dyspnea is the primary symptom that provides an assessment of respiratory function and is graded from I to IV relative to physical tolerance to graded levels of physical activities.

*Grade I*: Dyspnea initiated by moderate exercise (e.g., running or climbing stairs).
*Grade II*: Dyspnea related to mild exercise (e.g., walking).
*Grade III*: Dyspnea initiated with minor activity (e.g., dressing or bathing).
*Grade IV*: Dyspnea at rest.

The recognition and recording of bronchopulmonary diseases that may be exacerbated with changes in activity, temperature, or medication should be noted. Chronic bronchitis with the attendant signs and symptoms of sputum production, cough, and dyspnea also should be noted. Chronic use of tobacco (whether cigarettes, pipes, or cigars) should alert the physician to potentially coexisting chronic obstructive pulmonary disease (COPD) and the possible necessity for long-term intubation postoperatively.

## ENDOCRINE DISORDERS

Juvenile or adult-onset diabetes mellitus with insulin or oral hypoglycemic medication requirements signals the necessity of control and perioperative monitoring of the serum glucose level. As a consequence of the stress of a major operation, diabetes mellitus may initiate an exaggerated gluconeogenic response manifested as hyperglycemia. With this augmented gluconeogenic response, sugar (glucose) recycling and refractory responses to the action of insulin in organ and muscle tissues are identified as a result of these increased metabolic demands. Prompt intensive monitoring of electrolyte derangements and alterations of the plasma glucose level are essential to avoid hyperosmolar dehydration. Identifiable stress in the diabetic patient is a reason to limit the glucose intake to 150 g/day and to monitor plasma and urine glucose values as a guide to appropriate doses of insulin. A lack of attention to these monitoring parameters will initiate osmotic diuresis, glucosuria, and the potential for hyperosmolar coma if they are left uncorrected. It is the surgeon's charge to avoid both hypoglycemia and hyperglycemia. Furthermore, the hyperglycemic state may initiate glycosylation of circulatory pro-

teins with important alteration of their immune function. Thus, immune proteins may be subject to adverse alterations that confer a loss of immunocompetence to the patient. The continuous intravenous infusion of glucose is the preferred method for correcting and controlling fluctuations of the plasma glucose level in the critically ill diabetic patient undergoing preparation for or being subjected to an operation.

Patients with established thyroid disorders require a careful preoperative evaluation to establish the presence of the hyperthyroid or hypothyroid state. These common disorders may be recognized among critically ill intensive care patients and are easily diagnosed by laboratory screening parameters. An identification of the hypothyroid state requires an immediate intravenous infusion of levothyroxine (synthroid). Thyrotoxic crisis requires immediate medical intervention with beta-blocker administration. Blocking the synthesis of thyroid hormone with propylthiouracil may be essential in the hyperthyroid state.

Any patient who has had a previous operation for adrenal disease should be queried by history and physical examination for the potential coexistence of adrenocortical insufficiency. Adrenocortical insufficiency in the critically ill patient occurs most commonly secondary to previous or current corticosteroid therapy and is identified as an inadequate response to stress. Individuals who have identifiable hormonal insufficiency following partial or total adrenal-ectomy require perioperative replacement of steroids with hydrocortisone (100 mg every 8 h); weaning from these higher maintenance doses over 3 to 5 days postoperatively is possible when the unstressed, noncatabolic state is evident.

## SECOND INTERVAL OF RISK (3 TO 30 DAYS POSTOPERATIVELY)

Invasive sepsis is a major cause of morbidity and death during the second interval of risk period (days 3 to 30).[19] A risk assessment of this prolonged interval incorporates an evaluation of the patient's immunologic and physiologic functional abilities to abrogate potential complications (e.g., sepsis) that may occur following major surgical intervention. Invasive sepsis of major proportions is defined as a culture-proven focus of infection that exists in a major body cavity, an identifiable culture-proven bacterium derived from blood culture, ascending cholangitis, or confirmed (culture and sensitivity) pneumonia. Risk assessments of infectious risks during this interval suggest that age is an independent risk predictor, as are other associated major medical diagnoses (e.g., cancer, previous therapy with irradiation and/or chemotherapy, depletion of fat stores, muscle cachexia, ascites, and vitamin deficiencies) (Table 3A-6).

Surgical infection is defined as the postoperative toxic state that ensues following systemic dissemination of bacteria or their toxins from a defined focus within body cavities or tissues. By definition, major bacterial sepsis is a culture-proven focus of infection that involves any organ site or soft tissues (e.g., hepatobiliary tree, upper and lower gastrointestinal tract, and pulmonary and renal systems). Because major oncologic procedures commonly require resections of major viscera and organs, adverse technical events or

**TABLE 3A-6.  OPERATIVE SITES: INCIDENCE OF POSTOPERATIVE INFECTIONS AT THE OPERATIVE AREAS**

| OPERATION | INCIDENCE (%) | TYPE OF INFECTION | MAJOR PATHOGENS |
|---|---|---|---|
| Intradural craniotomy | 4–8 | Wound | Staphylococcus aureus |
| | 0.5–1 | Meningitis/abscess | Gram-negative |
| Head and neck | 15–40 | Wound | S. aureus gram-negative anaerobes |
| Pulmonary | 0.5–6 | Wound | S. aureus, gram-negative aerobes |
| | 1–2 | Empyema | |
| Laparotomy | 2–4 | Wound | Anaerobes, gram-negative |
| Gastric resection | 5–10 | Wound | Streptococcus, anaerobes |
| Biliary tract | 3–10 | Wound | Gram-negative enterococci, Clostridia |
| Colon resection | 8–40 | Wound | Anaerobes |
| | 2–10 | Abdominal abscess | Gram-negative aerobes |
| Mastectomy | 1–3 | Wound | S. aureus, gram-negative aerobes |

SOURCE: Bartlett JG: Choosing and using antibiotics, in *Surgical Care*, RE Condon, JJ DeCosse (eds). Philadelphia, Lea & Febiger, 1980.

errors may result in bacterial contamination and subsequent invasive sepsis. Patient survival is dependent on immediate recognition of the infectious focus and its eradication by abscess drainage or resection of the contaminated focus. In addition, immunocompetence is a major determinant of the metabolic and immunologic events that will transpire and predict the patient's response to the catabolic septic insult. Various techniques have been proposed to assess the probability of an infection within this risk interval of 3 to 30 days postoperatively. Risk assessments have been described for organ system–related events (cardiac versus pulmonary) and for specific operative conditions (e.g., peritonitis or hepatobiliary infection). Each analysis has indicated that age is an independent risk factor for morbidity and death. In addition, the patient with cancer has an increased risk for major morbidity that is related to the specific medical diagnosis, the extent (stage) of the neoplasm, metabolic status (e.g., weight loss, catabolism, total fat stores, ascites, edema, or vitamin deficiency), and previous treatment with irradiation or chemotherapy. Catabolic states in individuals with profound body wasting with loss of fat and protein stores impart an increased risk for minor and major complications; preoperative enteral or parenteral nutritional repletion may be advisable in severely malnourished states.[20]

## OPERATIVE RISK IN THE ELDERLY PATIENT

Life spans in western societies are becoming longer; thus, surgical illness in the elderly patient will have increasing ramifications for the future. With growth of the elderly population, this population may account for 50% of all surgical emergencies and comprise 75% of postoperative deaths. Unmistakably, the increasing morbidity and mortality rates of elderly patients are attributed primarily to the expected decrease in physiologic reserve with concurrent comorbid states. The operative risk thus increases exponentially with age; the mortality rate increases principally from the failure of cardiac and pulmonary reserves. A consistent increase in mortality rates for elective surgery occurs with age; at least a threefold increase in the mortality rate was projected when emergency surgery is performed. Of interest, mortality rates for both elective and emergency surgery appear to be declining, and this is based primarily on improvements in perioperative anesthesia, invasive monitoring, and advanced surgical (technical) expertise. For patients 90 years of age and older, the postoperative mortality rate was approximately 2% for elective surgery, 16% for urgent cases, and 45% for emergency procedures. Of interest, the long-term prognosis following surgery in the elderly patient is generally excellent.

As described previously, the prevalence of disease states that enhance the surgical risk (e.g., ischemic heart disease and COPD) will increase proportionately as the population ages. Thus, pneumonia and cardiac failure are considered the principal causes of postoperative complications and deaths in surgical patients older than age 65 years. Although improvements have been made in their recognition and treatment, thromboembolism, pulmonary embolism, and acute postoperative confusion still remain common clinical events noted in elderly patients. The management of major oncologic procedures performed on elderly patients thus requires a high level of awareness for the magnitude and frequency of adverse events expected in this group.

Thus, the surgical oncologist should recognize the relevance of tumor biology and the patient's clinical condition in determining an overall treatment plan.

## SELECTED REFERENCES

1. MARTIN EW JR et al: CEA-directed second look surgery in the asymptomatic patient after primary resection of colorectal carcinoma. Ann Surg 202:310, 1985.
2. MOERTEL CG et al: An evaluation of the carcinoembryonic antigen (CEA) test for monitoring colon cancer. JAMA 270:943, 1993.
3. SCHWARTZ MK: Tumor markers in diagnosis and screening, in *Human Tumor Markers*, SW Ting et al (eds). Amsterdam, Elsevier Science, 1987.
4. BOTET JF et al: Preoperative staging of gastric cancer: Comparison of endoscopic ultrasonography and dynamic CT. Radiology 181:426, 1991.
5. KVOLS LK et al: Evaluation of a radiolabeled somatostatin analog (1-123 octreotide) in the detection and localization of carcinoid and islet cell tumors. Radiology 187:129, 1993.

6. Conti PS et al: PET and 18F-FDG in oncology: A clinical update. Nucl Med Biol 23:717, 1996.

7. Duke JH, Miller TA: Salt and water: Fluid and electrolyte problems, in *Surgical Care*. R Condon, J DeCosse (eds). Philadephia, Lea & Febiger, 1980.

8. Fisher B: Lumpectomy (segmented mastectomy) and axillary dissection, in *The Breast: Comprehensive Management of Benign and Malignant Diseases*. KI Bland, EM Copeland (eds). Philadelphia, WB Saunders, 1991, pp 634–652.

9. Fisher B et al: Five-year results of a randomized clinical trial comparing total mastectomy and segmental mastectomy with or without radiation in the treatment of breast cancer. N Engl J Med 312:665, 1985.

10. Fisher B et al: Trauma and the localization of tumor cells. Cancer 20:23, 1967.

11. Fisher B et al: Eight-year results of a randomized clinical trial comparing total mastectomy and lumpectomy with or without irradiation in the treatment of breast cancer. N Engl J Med 320:822, 1989.

12. Enker WE et al: En bloc pelvic lymphadenectomy and sphincter preservation in the surgical management of rectal cancer. Ann Surg 203:426, 1986.

13. Karakousis CP et al: Limb salvage in soft tissue sarcomas with selective combination of modalities. Eur J Surg Oncol 7:71, 1991.

14. Karakousis CP et al: Feasibility of limb salvage and survival in soft tissue sarcomas. Cancer 57:484, 1986.

15. Shiu MH et al: Surgical treatment of 297 soft tissue sarcomas of the lower extremity. Ann Surg 182:597, 1975.

16. Abbas JH et al: The surgical treatment and outcome of soft-tissue sarcoma. Arch Surg 116:765, 1981.

17. Karakousis CP et al: Changes in survival with clinical stage I malignant melanoma. J Surg Oncol 34:155, 1987.

18. Bilchik AJ et al: Universal application of intraoperative lymphatic mapping and sentinel lymphadenectomy in solid neoplasms. Cancer J Sci Am 4:351, 1998.

19. Bartlett JG: Choosing and using antibiotics, in *Surgical Care*. RE Condon, JJ DeCosse (eds). Philadephia, Lea & Febiger, 1980.

20. Redmond HP, Daly JM: Preoperative nutritional therapy in cancer patients is benefical, in *Debates in Clinical Surgery*. R Simmons (ed). Chicago, Mosby Year Book, 1991.

# 3B / RADIATION AS A THERAPEUTIC MODALITY IN ONCOLOGY

*Herman D. Suit, Bruce Borgelt, Alfred Smith, and Ira J. Spiro*

## CURRENT CLINICAL RESULTS

The goal in the management of the cancer patient is to achieve eradication of all local, regional and distant disease and to have no treatment-related morbidity. This is being achieved in a growing proportion of patients, and radiation is playing an increasingly important role in realization of that goal.

Radiation has been employed in oncology for about 100 years. Over that time it has been under continuous development and refinement. It is important to note that clinical experience has demonstrated radiation to be a highly effective therapeutic modality in treating selected tumors with reference to pathologic types, anatomic sites, and stages of disease. Radiation is a particularly elegant modality for treating patients with small to modest sized tumors at several sites. This is due to the potential of achieving a high degree of tumor control and doing so with the preservation of near-normal anatomy, function, and cosmesis. For locally advanced lesions, the outcome is less satisfactory due to the larger number of tumor clonogens* and the extent to which tumor growth has damaged normal tissue. In many of the latter patients, results have been improved substantially by combining relatively conservative surgery with moderate radiation dose levels. Further, the combination of radiation with chemotherapeutic agents has often achieved gains in both local and distant control. In addition, the remarkable advances in imaging techniques, namely CT, MRI, and ultrasound (US), have made the implementation of ultraprecise radiation treatment methods achievable in the clinic. Magnetic resonance spectroscopy and positron emission tomography (PET) are showing potential to assess the physiologic state of the neoplasm. This information should be of value in predicting tumor response and, thus, of major value in designing treatment for the individual patient. Fortunately, future prospects are rich with potential for continued advances in patient treatment as the present modalities are further improved and combined with qualitative new approaches, such as genetic, immunologic, antiangiogenic and other methods.

Here we discuss the therapeutic applications of ionizing radiation. Table 3B-1 provides a simple review of the success rate cur-rently being achieved by radiation in the treatment of cancer patients. Shown are outcomes by radiation treatment alone or combined with other modalities for a variety of anatomic sites, clinical stages, and pathologic tumor types. These data from many cancer centers document that radiation alone or combined with other modalities can be employed so as to achieve clinically valuable rates of long-term disease-free survival for patients with a broad spectrum of tumor types and sites.

## CLINICAL RADIATION BIOLOGY

Ionizing radiations cause cell death, principally by the production of ionizations in DNA, either directly or indirectly through radiation-produced free radicals. Some of these events result in biochemical changes that cannot be repaired or that are repaired in a defective manner. Damaging such sites in the DNA often results in cell death. The observed differences in cell sensitivity to radiation arise from the cell's ability to repair radiation damage and to do so correctly. The genetic determinants of this repair ability are under intensive investigation.[1-4] The expectation is that as these critical repair genes are identified, the molecular biologist will be able to determine those tumors that are likely to be especially radiation sensitive or resistant, thereby permitting the clinician to plan the radiation dose schedule most appropriate for the particular patient.

At this point, we present a brief review of a few rather straightforward aspects of clinically relevant radiation biology. First, mammalian cells are very sensitive to the killing action of ionizing radiation. Figure 3B-1 shows a survival curve for the human squamous cell carcinoma cell line, HeLa.[†] A surviving cell is one with the capacity to produce a continuously expanding progeny; the experimental endpoint is colony formation. Thus, a cell that loses this reproductive integrity may retain essentially normal metabolic function but would be judged to be dead in this radiobiologic context. An important but not always appreciated fact is that radiation-killed cells may display active proliferation for several postradiation generations before the progeny undergo pyknosis and lyse. This is illustrated in Fig. 3B-2, which shows the progeny of a radiation-killed

---

*Tumor clonogens are cells with the capacity to proliferate and produce a continuously expanding progeny. That is, one surviving clonogen would, by this definition, proliferate and result in a regrowth of the tumor.

[†]This was the first experiment performed using mammalian cells and colony formation as the endpoint.

**TABLE 3B-1.** FIVE-YEAR ACTUARIAL RESULTS OBTAINED BY RADIATION ALONE OR COMBINED WITH SURGERY OR CHEMOTHERAPY IN THE TREATMENT OF CANCER PATIENTS

| ANATOMIC SITE | STAGE | LOCAL CONTROL (%) | REFERENCE | NOTES |
|---|---|---|---|---|
| **RADIATION ALONE** | | | | |
| Glottis | T1 | 93 | 14 | |
| Tongue, oral | T1 | 86 | 15 | |
| Tongue, base | T1 | 89 | 16 | |
| Tonsil | T1 | 81 | 17 | |
| Hodgkin's disease | I–IIA | 75 | 18 | 20-yr freedom from any relapse |
| Uterine cervix | IB (<5 cm) | 97*, 99** | 19 | *Pelvic tumor control, **central tumor control |
| | IB (5–7.9 cm) | 84*, 93** | 19 | *Pelvic tumor control, **central tumor control |
| Prostate | A2,B | 85–87 | 20 | 10-yr lymph node dissection negative, external beam |
| | T1,T2 | 83–100 | 21 | 18–37 mo median follow-up, transperoneal implant |
| Uveal melanoma | Local | 97 | 12 | Proton treatment |
| **RADIATION AND SURGERY WITH OR WITHOUT CHEMOTHERAPY** | | | | |
| Breast | I | 87 | 22 | Local excision, 10 yr follow-up |
| Chondrosarcoma, skull base | M0 | 92 | 13 | 10-yr follow-up, proton treatment |
| Soft tissue sarcoma | M0 | 86 | 23 | Either pre- or postoperative with total gross excision |
| Rectum | T1*,T2 | 90–96 | 24,25 | *Unfavorable |
| Medulloblastoma | T2,T3,T4 | 82* | 26 | *In posterior fossa |
| Parotid gland | T1,T2 | 93 | 27 | |
| **RADIATION AND CHEMOTHERAPY** | | | | |
| Anus | I–III | 88 | 28 | |
| Esophagus | M0 | 55 | 29 | |
| Ewing's sarcoma | Localized | 86 | 30 | |
| Non-Hodgkin's lymphoma, bone | IE | 90 | 31 | ≥2 yr follow-up |

L59 cell.[6] Several postradiation division cycles occurred prior to the metabolic death of the entire progeny. For a postradiation cell population to result in a colony, there must be at least 50 cells. "Colonies" of fewer than 50 cells are classed as abortive and are not counted.

The survival curve presented in Fig. 3B-1 is a plot of log survival fraction (SF) against dose. The curve shape shown in Fig. 3B-1 is typical of virtually all reported survival curves for x-irradiated mammalian cells: an initial shoulder and then a straight line, where cell death increases exponentially with dose. There is no shoulder on the curve for many lymphoid and germinal cell lines. In radiation oncology, the most commonly used descriptor of radiation sensitivity is the $SF_2$, or the fraction of cells that survive a dose of 2 Gy, with 2 Gy selected as the endpoint since the great bulk of clinical radiation oncology uses dose fractions of 1.8 to 2 Gy. The $SF_2$ is ≈0.3 to 0.5 for epithelial and mesenchymal tumor cells grow-

ing in vitro under "optimal" metabolic conditions. The $SF_2$'s for lymphoid cell lines are much lower at ≈0.1 to 0.3, while glioblastoma multiforme cell lines are higher at ≈0.5 to 0.6. Were these values to obtain for tumor cells irradiated in vivo, the standard daily dose of 2 Gy, would be expected to kill some 60% of tumor cells. For tumor and normal tissue cells studied in vitro and in vivo, the $SF_2$ appears to be relatively constant for multiple doses. Thus, were the $SF_2$ to be 0.4 in vivo and to be constant after each of a series of equal doses, the fraction of cells surviving 30 treatments of 2 Gy would be extremely small, for example, $10^{-12}$. The implication of these calculations for the response of a model tumor system is that the difference between success and failure to eradicate the tumor could be attributed to an extremely small absolute number of surviving cells. Actually, essentially all local failures would be expected to regrow from <10 cells that had survived the radiation treatment.[7]

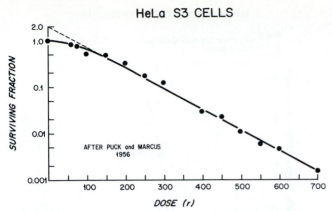

**FIGURE 3B-1.** The relationship between radiation dose and fraction of HeLa cells surviving a single radiation dose. (*From Puck and Marcus.*[5])

surviving clonogens during each intertreatment interval. The effect would be to increase the net number of tumor clonogens that must be inactivated by the radiation dose to achieve a specified tumor control probability (TCP).

Fourth, the radiation sensitivity of a cell varies with its position in the cell replication cycle. Actually, the most sensitive cycle phases are M and the $G_1S$ interface, while the most resistant phase is S. Thus, the probability of inactivation of a tumor is a function of (1) the number of tumor clonogens; (2) the radiation sensitivity of the clonogens; (3) the proliferation rate of clonogens that are surviving at the start of each intertreatment interval; and (4) the distribution of the clonogens among the cell cycle phases at the instant of each radiation treatment.

Fifth, metabolite concentration in the microenvironment affects cellular radiation sensitivity. The $pO_2$ at irradiation is thoroughly documented to be a very powerful determinant of the cell's radiation sensitivity. Namely, sensitivity varies by a factor of 3 for irradiation at $pO_2 \leq 1$ mmHg (resistant) to that at $\geq 20$ mmHg (near maximum sensitivity). A low sulfhydryl concentration confers an increased sensitivity of cells.

An important question is: what is the difference in sensitivity between the cells of the tumor and normal tissue? There is a small difference in sensitivity that favors the normal epithelial and mesenchymal cell; this is judged to be due to a slightly greater repair capacity or a higher frequency of accurate repair. Even a small difference may be extremely important if that difference were exponentiated over a series of 30 to 35 fractions.

Second, the probability of killing all of the clonogens of a tumor for a defined radiation dose is, of course, a function of the number of clonogens. The dose to inactivate all of the clonogens in a population of cells at a specified probability increases linearly with log number of clonogens.

Third, the number of tumor clonogens may increase during the course of fractionated dose irradiation due to proliferation of the

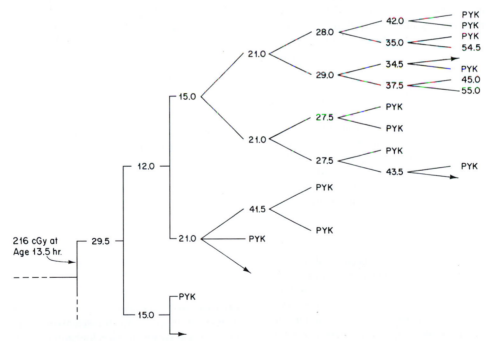

**FIGURE 3B-2.** The cell division record of the progeny of a single L59 cell.[6] The numbers on the lines between the branching points refer to the interdivision time in hours. PYK indicates that the cell became pyknotic.

For tumors, there are factors that affect tumor control probability beyond radiation dose, number of clonogens, and so forth. These include the presence of an immune rejection reaction by the host against the tumor. One potential avenue for enhancing the efficacy of radiation is augmentation of the immune rejection reaction. For epithelial-mesenchymal tumors, efforts in this direction have not, as yet, achieved important successes. For tumors of the body surface or epithelial lining of hollow organs, there is some loss of tumor clonogens by exfoliation. The consequence is a lesser net or effective number of tumor clonogens. Clinical experience indicates that there is a higher probability of tumor control following radiation alone against exophytic tumors than for tumors of the same volume that are infiltrative.

In all experimental animal studies of spontaneous tumors as autochthonous tumors or as early generation transplants growing in syngeneic animals, tumor control frequency increases in an orderly manner with dose. For obvious reasons, this relationship between dose and response over the full range in TCP cannot be demonstrated for human tumors. Tumor control increases with radiation dose as shown in Fig. 3B-3A for a spontaneous mouse mammary carcinoma growing as third-generation transplants in syngeneic mice.[8] When plotted on a linear grid, the curve approximates a sigmoid shape. When plotted on a Logit TCP-log dose grid, the dose-response curve is almost a straight line (Fig. 3B-3B). The dose to inactivate a tumor at a given probability, say the $TCD_{50}$ (dose to achieve control in half of the irradiated tumors), increases with tumor volume (number of tumor clonogens), as has been shown in a series of mouse mammary carcinoma tumors.[9]

For clinical data from a particular trial, there may well be no evidence of a dependence of local control on dose. This is due to several factors: (1) a narrow range of doses employed; (2) a limited number of dose levels; (3) modest numbers of patients at each dose level; and (4) substantial heterogeneity among the population of tumors in any clinical study. Of course, heterogeneity can be diminished by performing the study on a more narrow strata of patients, that is, by limiting accession to the study to a defined histologic type, range in volume, anatomic site, exophytic or infiltrative presentation, hemoglobin, gender (for certain tumors), and so on. Any heterogeneity makes the dose-response curve less steep; hence, detecting the impact of a modest dose differential on TCP would be difficult in most clinical studies because of the heterogeneity with reference to the above-mentioned response determinants. Heterogeneity is greater between tumors than between normal tissues. This is reflected in the steeper slopes of dose-response curves for normal tissues than for tumor control. This is illustrated by Fig. 3B-4, which presents dose-response curves for local control of squamous cell carcinoma and necrosis of the normal tissues of the oral cavity[10] in a prospective randomized dose escalation study on canine patients. This set of data constitutes the basis for the only complete dose-response curves for subjects other than rodents. The relationship between dose and tumor control in an individual patient would be quite steep. The flatness of the observed dose-response relationships in clinical data is primarily due to intertumoral heterogeneity. Intratumoral heterogeneity affects slope to a minimal degree.[11] This means that there is strong justification for efforts to utilize advanced technology to

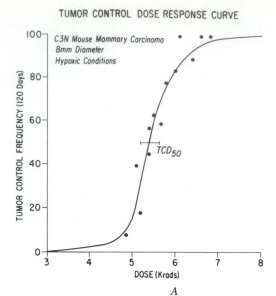

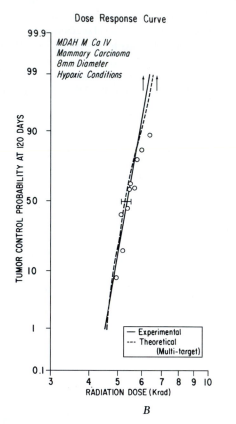

**FIGURE 3B-3.** The plot of the dose-response curve of 8-mm-diameter third-generation transplants of a spontaneous mammary carcinoma in syngeneic mice. Radiation was by a single dose given under locally hypoxic conditions. The data are plotted on a linear-linear grid. (*From Suit.*[8]) B. The data in part A plotted on a logit-log dose grid.

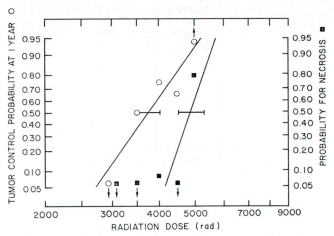

**FIGURE 3B-4.** A plot of tumor control of squamous cell carcinoma of the oral cavity and of normal tissue damage in canines randomly assigned to different dose levels and treated in 10 equal doses. (*From Gillette et al.*[10])

improve the dose distribution and, hence, the option of administering a higher dose. Any dose increment will result in a higher TCP.

The relationship between the dose-response curves for tumor control and normal tissue damage and for uncomplicated tumor control is presented in Fig. 3B-5. The point of clinical interest is the curve for the frequency of uncomplicated local control. This desired outcome increases to a maximum and then, with further dose increments, declines steeply to a point where there are virtually no subjects with tumor control who are also free of complications.

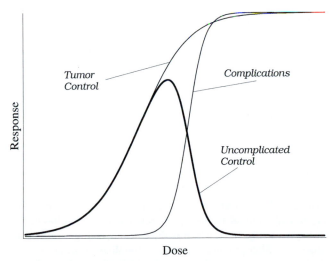

**FIGURE 3B-5.** The relationship in a model system between the dose-response curves for tumor control and normal tissue damage and the consequent curve for uncomplicated local control.

This means that the clinician is, in every treatment plan, balancing the expected tumor control probability versus the probability of symptomatic damage to the normal tissues. The clinical efficacy of a radiation treatment will accordingly be a function of the separation between these two dose response curves (tumor control versus damage to normal tissues).

## RADIATION TREATMENT METHODS

There are two major strategies for increasing the frequency of achieving eradication of tumor and having no treatment-related morbidity. These are (1) to develop radiation techniques that yield superior dose distributions (smaller treatment volumes); and (2) to enhance the differential biologic effectiveness of the radiation on the tumor and the normal tissues (for example, dose fractionation, radiation sensitizers, immunomodulators, radiation protectors, certain of the chemotherapeutic agents, and so forth).

The first approach has been used regularly over the history of radiation oncology with repeated success. These include the following: (1) increases in the energy of x-ray beams, for example, 110 kV → 180 kV → 250 kV → $^{60}$Co → 4–35 MeV linear accelerators; (2) use of radium and radon and, more recently, $^{192}$Ir, $^{125}$I and other isotopes in brachytherapy (this now includes stereotactic and CT-controlled brachytherapy); (3) introduction of electron beams; (4) portal films and on-line portal imaging systems, simulators; (5) computer-based treatment planning; (6) intraoperative electron beam therapy; (6) particle beam techniques (proton, helium ion beams); (7) three-dimensional treatment planning with intensity modulation; and (8) biomathematical modeling of the biologic effect on each structure being irradiated, for example, probabilities of tumor control and damage to normal structure. This allows the clinician to go beyond relying exclusively on the physical dose distribution and to assess the likely biologic effect. In the coming decade, treatment technique development will be substantially enhanced with the implementation of intensity modulation strategies for x-ray and proton beams.

The only disadvantage to the patient is the irradiation of tissues and structures that are uninvolved by tumor. Hence, there is sustained pressure to improve the quality of our treatment plans and the ability to execute them. One may question the yield of further efforts to reduce treatment volume. Will we not lose more than might be gained due to underestimates of the extent of the tumor? If this were true, the result would be failures at the edge of the smaller treatment volumes, that is, marginal misses. Fortunately, the answer is no. The use of CT, MRI, US, PET, and other imaging systems by the radiation oncologist permits the secure identification of most of the critical nontarget tissues and structures and the ability to exclude them from the treatment volume. Essentially all of the treatment-related morbidity arises in tissues not judged to be invaded by tumor. For example, in treatment of carcinoma of the urinary bladder, there is no risk in the exclusion of the small and large bowel, sacral plexus, and bony pelvis from the treatment volume. For many treatment situations, there is an extremely low probability of involvement of the eye, spinal cord, liver, kidney, heart, and so on. With current treatment methods, these structures are irradiated only because of technical limitations or lack of effort by the radiation oncologist. Current radiation techniques employ large treatment volumes relative to the treatment volumes of surgery at many anatomic sites. This difference between the two treatment volumes is potentially an important source of solid information upon which studies of reductions of treatment volume may be based.

In present clinical radiation oncology, ≥90% of treatments are administered by external beam techniques. Figure 3B-6A presents the depth dose profile along the central axis of a 10-MeV x-ray beam. For many treatment situations, a beam modifier is employed to achieve a dose distribution that more closely conforms to the target. These are wedge and compensator filters; the beams may be modified dynamically in complex patterns by using sophisticated multi-leaf collimator systems. To illustrate this process, in Fig. 3B-6B we show the "coronal" view of a standard 10-MeV x-ray beam and of a 10-MeV beam that has passed through a wedge filter to produce a 45° slope to the isodose curves being presented. The dose distribution obtained by using a pair of such beams at 90° is presented in Fig. 3B-7. There is a good confinement of dose to the target region.

A treatment method that has achieved substantial popularity is ultrasound-directed $^{125}$I brachytherapy for early-stage carcinoma of the prostate. This technique requires the depositing of an array of $^{125}$I seeds in a planned geometric distribution. From the patient's viewpoint, this procedure has the advantage of requiring only 1 day for the treatment. Dose levels are 140 to 160 Gy, when calculated for total decay of the isotope. Further, the results at 5 years are quite comparable to those obtained by radical surgery or by external beam radiation therapy.

Proton beam therapy has the powerful attraction of delivering a uniform dose across the target with zero dose just deep to the target for each beam path. To compare the depth dose curves of the 10-MeV x-ray beam with that of a beam of protons of a single energy, for example, 160 MV, and for a 160-MV proton beam that has been energy-modulated to achieve a 7-cm spread-out Bragg peak (sobp), study Fig. 3B-8. This physical advantage means a superior dose distribution for many treatment situations, that is, a lesser dose beyond the defined target. The ultimate technical development of external beam radiation therapy is intensity modulation, namely, dynamic beam modulation during the irradiation of each beam path. This can be achieved with x-rays and protons. To demonstrate the gain in dose confinement, examine Fig. 3B-9, which shows the dose distribution using intensity-modulated proton and x-ray beams for treating a patient with carcinoma of the nasopharynx. These sophisticated methods are just now being introduced into special cancer centers and should be widely available by 2010.

We make mention here of two impressive outcome results derived from using proton beams. First, the actuarial 5-year local control and survival of 1005 patients treated by protons for their uveal melanoma are 96% and 80%, respectively.[11] These results are fully comparable to those achieved by enucleation. The dose was 70 Gy, given in five fractions of 14 Gy, that is, an exceptionally aggressive dose. Useful vision has been retained in 90% of patients. Loss of visual function was observed to be dependent on lesion size and location; patients

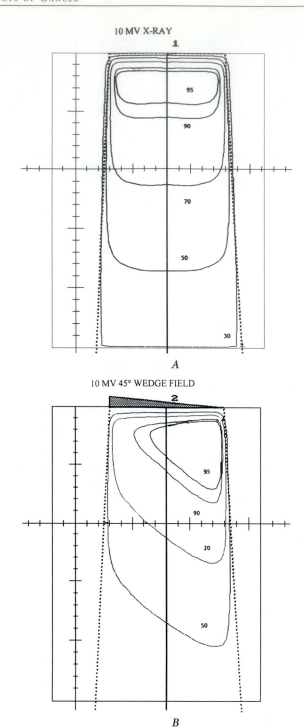

**FIGURE 3B-6A AND B.** These graphs present the depth dose profiles of a normal 10-MeV x-ray beam and one that has passed through a wedge filter, which is thick at one end and thin at the other. This filter produces a change in the slope of the dose across the beam from horizontal to an angle of 45°. The marks on the line that crosses the beam and the line to the left of the beam profile are centimeter markers.

## 10 MeV 45° WEDGE PAIR

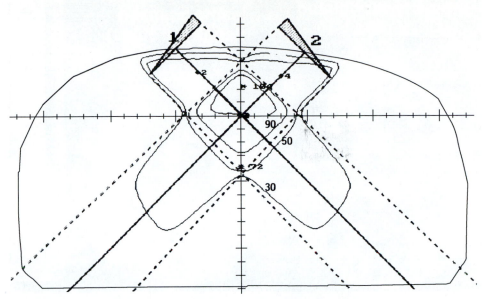

**FIGURE 3B-7.** The combination of two 45° wedged fields at 90° to each other can achieve a good dose distribution. Note that there is dose beyond the intended target.

whose tumors were close to the fovea or disc were less likely to retain useful vision. Second, the experience at Massachusetts General Hospital with 180 patients with chondrosarcoma of the skull base is a 10-year local control rate of 92%.[12] Because distant metastases were infrequent, local control was almost synonymous with survival.

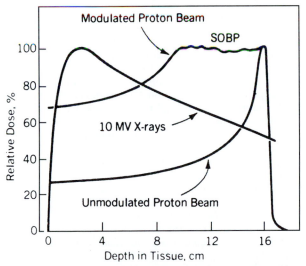

**FIGURE 3B-8.** The depth dose profiles of a 10-MeV x-ray, a proton beam of protons of a single energy, such as 160 MV, and a 160-MV beam that has been modulated to provide a spread-out Bragg peak of ≈7 cm.

## COMBINED MODALITY THERAPY

The rationale for combining radiation and conservative surgery is simple and straightforward. Namely, the efficacy of radiation alone to eradicate a tumor mass at a very high probability decreases with tumor volume or the number of tumor clonogens. Hence, radiation in moderate dose levels can be expected to inactivate the subclinical disease foci that have extended beyond the gross mass, that is, the surgical resection specimen. Thus, the patient need not be exposed to the morbidities associated with radical surgery or radical radiation dose levels. This approach has been proved to be of great efficacy for tumors at several anatomic sites. Namely, consider the success of conservative surgery and moderate-dose radiation in the management of patients with early-stage carcinoma of the breast, soft tissue sarcoma, tumors in the low anterior section of the rectum, and tumors at several sites in the head and neck region (see Table 3B-1).

By combining radiation and chemotherapeutic agents, a decrease in the local failure rate and also in the rate of distant metastasis in multiple instances has been observed. Consider the treatment outcomes for patients with Ewing's sarcoma (primitive neuroectodermal tumor; PNET); carcinomas of the anus, colorectum, urinary bladder, esophagus, and nasopharynx; small cell carcinoma of lung, and so on (see Table 3B-1).

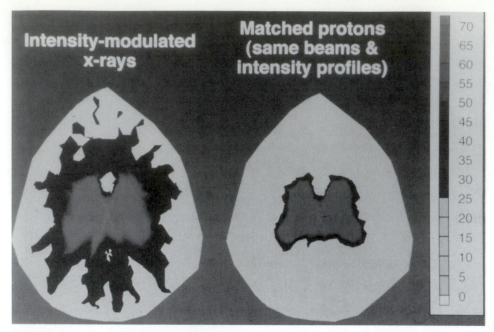

**FIGURE 3B-9.** Dose distributions achieved by intensity modulation techniques for x-ray and for proton beam irradiation of cancer of the nasopharynx. (*This figure was generously provided by Dr. T. Lomax, Paul Sherrer Institute, 1997.*)

A particularly interesting potential is the prospect of physiologic and genetic characterizations of the tumor and the normal tissues in the individual patient with reference to those properties that determine response. To the extent that this is accomplished, the clinician would have the capability to design the best feasible treatment for the particular patient.

## REFERENCES

1. YARNOLD JR: Molecular aspects of cellular responses to radiotherapy. Radiotherapy Oncol 44:1, 1997.
2. BRISTOW RG et al: The p53 gene as a modifier of intrinsic radiosensitivity: Implications for radiotherapy. Radiotherapy Oncol 40:197, 1996.
3. GORDON AT, MCMILLAN TJ: Molecular basis of radiation sensitivity, in *Molecular Biology for Oncologists,* JR Yarnold et al (eds). London, Chapman and Hall, 1996, pp 166–175.
4. POWELL SN et al: How do cells repair DNA damage caused by ionising radiation? In *Molecular Biology for Oncologists,* JR Yarnold et al (eds). London, Chapman and Hall 1996, pp 176–184.
5. PUCK TT, MARCUS PI: Action of x-rays on mammalian cells. J Exp Med 103:653, 1956.
6. THOMPSON LH, SUIT HD: Proliferation kinetics of X-irradiated mouse L cells studied with time-lapse photography. Int J Radiat Oncol Biol Phys 13:391, 1967.
7. SUIT HD et al: Time distribution of recurrences of an immunogenic and non-immunogenic tumor following local irradiation. Radiat Res 73:251, 1978.
8. SUIT HD: Radiation biology: A basis for radiotherapy, in *Textbook of Radiation Therapy,* GH Fletcher (ed). Philadelphia, Lea and Febiger, 1966, pp 65–97.
9. SUIT HD et al: Radiation response of C3H mouse mammary carcinoma evaluated in terms of cellular radiation sensitivity, in *Cellular Radiation Biology,* RP Shalak (ed). Baltimore, Williams & Wilkins, 1965, pp 514–530.
10. GILLETTE EL et al: Response of canine oral carcinomas to heat and radiation. Int J Radiat Oncol Biol Phys 13:1861, 1987.
11. SUIT H et al: Clinical implications of heterogeneity of tumor response to radiation therapy. Radiotherapy Oncol 25:251, 1992.
12. GRAGOUDAS ES et al: Intraocular recurrence of uveal melanoma after proton beam irradiation. Ophthalmology 99:760, 1992.
13. MUNZENRIDER JE et al: Skull-based tumors: Treatment with 3-d planning and fractionated x-ray and proton radiotherapy, in *Textbook of Radiotherapy,* S Leibel, T Phillips (eds). Philadelphia, Saunders, 1998.
14. PEREZ CA, BRADY LW: *Principles and Practice of Radiation Therapy.* Philadelphia, Lippincott, 1992.
15. WANG CC: *Radiation Therapy for Head and Neck Neoplasms.* New York, Wiley-Liss, 1997, p 131.
16. WANG CC: *Radiation Therapy for Head and Neck Neoplasms.* New York, Wiley Liss, 1997, p 200.
17. WANG CC: *Radiation Therapy for Head and Neck Neoplasms.* New York, Wiley Liss, 1997, p 195.
18. HOPPE RT: Radiation therapy in the management of Hodgkin's disease. Semin Oncol 17:704, 1990.
19. EIFEL PJ et al: The influence of tumor size and morphology on the outcome of patients with FIGO stage IB squamous cell carcinoma of the uterine cervix. Int J Radiat Oncol Biol Phys 29:9, 1994.

20. Cox J: *Radiation Oncology: Rationale, Technique, Results.* St Louis, Mosby, 1994, p 597.
21. Blasko JC et al: Should brachytherapy be considered a therapeutic option in localized prostate cancer? Urologic Clin NA 23:633, 1996.
22. Cox JD: Moss' *Radiation Oncology: Rationale, Technique, Results.* St Louis, Mosby, 1994, p 372.
23. Suit HD et al: Treatment of the patient with stage $M_O$ sarcoma of soft tissue. J Clin Oncol 6:854, 1988.
24. Ng AK et al: Sphincter preservation therapy for distal rectal carcinoma: A review. Cancer 79:671, 1997.
25. Chakravarti A et al: Long-term follow-up of patients with rectal cancer managed by local excision with and without adjuvant therapy. Ann Surg 230:49, 1999.
26. Tarbell NJ et al: The change in patterns of relapse in medulloblastoma. Cancer 68:1600, 1991.
27. Spiro IJ et al: Carcinoma of the parotid gland: Analysis of treatment results and patterns of failure after combined surgery and radiation therapy. Cancer 71:2699, 1993.
28. Cox JD: Moss' *Radiation Oncology: Rationale, Technique, Results.* St Louis, Mosby, 1994, p 493.
29. Coia IR: Chemoradiation: A superior alternative for primary management of esophageal carcinoma. Semin Radiat Oncol 4:157, 1994.
30. Dunst J et al: Radiation therapy in Ewing's sarcoma: An update of the CESS 86 trial. Int J Radiat Oncol Biol Phys 32:919, 1995.
31. Fairbanks R et al: Treatment of stage IE primary lymphoma of bone. Int J Radiat Oncol Biol Phys 28:363, 1994.

# 3C / SYSTEMIC CHEMOTHERAPY OF SOLID TUMORS

*Matthew R. Smith and Bruce A. Chabner*

## INTRODUCTION

Chemotherapy is now an integral part of the treatment of most patients with cancer. Historically, anticancer drugs have been primarily used to treat unresectable or metastatic tumors. However, chemotherapy has become increasingly important in the management of clinically localized and surgically resectable malignancies. In these situations, drugs used in combination with surgery and/or radiation therapy decrease the chance of postoperative recurrence and allow for a more limited and potentially function-sparing surgery. As our knowledge of effective combined modality therapy continues to evolve, the role of chemotherapy may further expand to improve the survival and quality of life of patients with a variety of solid tumors.

## BRIEF HISTORY OF CHEMOTHERAPY

In most cases, cancer is a systemic disease at the time of diagnosis. Surgical resection of the primary tumor mass provides effective local control but does not address the problem of distant microscopic metastases. For more than a century, thoughtful investigators have sought effective systemic therapy for human malignancies. The first suggestion for systemic therapy arose from the toxicity of sulfur mustard gas, a biologic warfare agent used during World War I. Based on the myelosuppression and lymphoid aplasia associated with mustard gas, nitrogen mustard was used to treat patients with lymphoid malignancies. In 1943, physicians at Yale University noted the regression of a mediastinal mass in a patient with Hodgkin's disease following treatment with nitrogen mustard, the first demonstration of an effective systemic treatment for a human malignancy.[1] The conceptual basis for the activity of mustard gas was not defined until more than a decade later when deoxyribonucleic acid was identified as the target for this alkylating agent.

The early experience with alkylating agents led investigators to design analogues of compounds involved in metabolic pathways required for cell growth. Vitamins and nucleic acid bases proved to be the most vulnerable metabolic targets. In the late 1940s, scientists from American Cyanamid synthesized analogues of folic acid, including aminopterin and methotrexate.[2] Sidney Farber later demonstrated that treatment with these antifolates resulted in marked but transient responses in children with acute lymphoblastic leukemia. Prospects for the treatment of cancer with drugs dramatically es-

calated in the following decade. In 1951, Hitchings, Elion, and colleagues at Burroughs-Wellcome evaluated a series of purine analogues and demonstrated antitumor effects in animals, leading to the successful development of 6-thioguanine and 6-mercaptopurine.[3] Corticosteroids were subsequently shown to have cytotoxic activity in childhood leukemia and lymphoma.[3]

Natural products are the source of a variety of novel anticancer agents. During their evaluation of natural products for the treatment of diabetes in the 1950s, scientists at Eli Lilly discovered the antimitotic and cytotoxic activity of the vinca alkaloids.[4] In the 1960s, natural product research resulted in the discovery of mitomycin C (a novel alkylating agent), bleomycin (a DNA cleaving peptide), the anthracyclines (topoisomerase II inhibitors), the taxanes (inhibitors of microtubule function), and the camptothecins (topoisomerase I inhibitors).[5]

## THE BIOLOGY OF CANCER CHEMOTHERAPY

The essential properties of cancer cells that distinguish them from their normal counterparts include excess cellular proliferation, invasive capacity, metastatic potential, ability to induce new blood vessel formation, and ability to escape immune surveillance. While each of these malignant properties is the starting point for new drug development efforts, most current chemotherapy agents act primarily by inhibiting cellular proliferation.

The cell cycle involves a series of regulated steps that result in cellular reproduction. The central events of the cell cycle are synthesis of DNA (S phase) and cell division (M phase). The uncontrolled cellular proliferation of most cancer cells results from acquired mutations in the genes that regulate the cell cycle.[6] The activity of most chemotherapy agents is restricted to a specific phase of the cell cycle. The S phase–specific agents interfere with DNA synthesis by a variety of mechanisms including depletion of nucleotide biosynthetic pools, covalent modification of DNA, cleavage of DNA, and inhibition of enzymes involved in DNA topology. Most M phase–specific agents arrest cells in mitosis by interfering with normal microtubule function.

Apoptosis or programmed cell death is the common pathway of cellular demise following chemotherapy-induced growth arrest.[7] Apoptosis involves an orderly series of biochemical events that result in condensation of chromatin, disintegration of the nucleus, and fragmentation of DNA. The apoptotic cell is rapidly phagocytosed by macrophages and epithelial cells. Mutation of the genes that regulate programmed cell death (including the p53 tumor suppressor gene) are an important mechanism of resistance to chemotherapy agents.

## MODELS FOR CHEMOTHERAPY

The first major conceptual model of tumor growth and response to chemotherapy was the log-kill model developed by Skipper and Schabel at the Southern Research Institute.[8] This model is based on quantitative chemotherapy studies in murine leukemia. The basic principles of the Skipper-Schabel model are as follows:

1. *Fractional cell kill.* Each dose of chemotherapy kills a constant fraction of the cell population. Cell kill is a function of the drug dose and the schedule of administration. For most agents, cell kill correlates with the area under the drug concentration time curve (CT, or AUC).
2. *Importance of dose intensity.* During the time period between cycles of treatment, tumor cells resume proliferation. Therefore, the highest drug doses and shortest periods between treatment cycles result in the highest rates of cell kill.
3. *Drug resistance.* Exposure of tumors to single-agent chemotherapy rapidly results in an outgrowth of drug-resistant cells. Therefore, combinations of drugs are more effective than single agents because drug combinations may prevent the outgrowth of resistant cells.
4. *Cell cycle dependency of cell kill.* Most anticancer drugs have their greatest effect on actively proliferating cells. The rate of cell proliferation slows, and the number of nonproliferating cells increases with expansion of the tumor mass. Thus, chemotherapy is most effective when the tumor burden is lowest and cell proliferation is most active.

The Skipper-Schabel model established a fundamental understanding of the kinetics of cell kill and the mechanisms of drug resistance. In addition, the Skipper-Schabel model provided the rational basis for design of combination chemotherapy regimens.

In the 1970s, Norton and Simons extended the Skipper-Schabel model using a Gompertzian model of cell growth and regression.[9] In exponential growth, the rates of tumor growth and regression in response to treatment are constant. In the Gompertzian model, the rates of tumor growth and regression decrease with increasing tumor size. According to the Norton-Simons hypothesis, the fractional cell kill of larger slow-growing tumors is smaller than the fractional cell kill of smaller tumors. For example, chemotherapy that results in a 2-log kill of a tumor containing $10^{11}$ cells may result in a 5-log kill in a tumor containing $10^9$ cells. The hypothesis predicts that the greater fractional cell kill in smaller tumors is balanced by the faster regrowth of residual tumor. This observation may explain why earlier standard chemotherapy for patients with advanced and metastatic solid tumors typically has a modest impact on survival. In addition, this observation may explain why standard adjuvant treatment of most solid tumors has a greater impact on disease-free survival than on overall survival. The Norton-Simons hypothesis established the theoretical basis for the use of more intensive chemotherapy against very small tumors in the adjuvant or minimal-disease setting.

## MODELS OF DRUG RESISTANCE

In 1943, Luria and Delbruck[10] determined that bacteria developed resistance to bacteriophage infection at random times during culture and often before exposure to the bacteriophage. Based on these observations, they developed a mathematical model to estimate the probability of identifying a given property in a bacterial culture based on the size of the bacterial population, a surrogate for the number of generations represented in the culture.

In 1979, Goldie and Coldman[11] applied the Delbruck-Luria model to the problem of drug resistance in human cancers. Using reasonable estimates of cell mutation rates, their analyses suggest that the probability of drug resistance dramatically increases over an approximately 2-log increase in tumor cell number. Assuming a mutation rate of 10-6, the Goldie-Coldman model predicts a <10% probability of drug resistance in a tumor containing 105 cells compared to a >99% probability of drug resistance in a tumor containing 107 cells. These kinetic observations were influential in developing both the concept of combination chemotherapy and the rational basis for adjuvant chemotherapy. However, predictions of the Goldie-Coldman hypothesis may be inaccurate based on the higher than expected rate of mutation in cancer cells (especially cells with mutations in the p53 tumor-suppressor gene), the possibility of single genetic events resulting in resistance to several classes of agents, and the potential that treatment itself may increase the mutation rate.

## PHARMACOKINETICS OF CHEMOTHERAPY

Pharmacokinetics is the study of drug absorption, distribution, metabolism, and excretion. The safe administration of cancer chemotherapy requires an understanding of pharmacokinetics since most chemotherapy agents have narrow therapeutic indices. The information presented in this section is derived from several sources.[12,13]

For orally administered drugs, absorption refers to transport across the gastrointestinal mucosa. The degree of drug absorption is often expressed as bioavailability or the ratio of the AUC after oral administration and the AUC after intravenous administration. Bioavailability is reduced by poor oral absorption and high first-pass metabolism in the liver.

Following administration, drugs distribute from the plasma or central compartment into peripheral tissue compartments. Pharmacokinetic compartments are mathematical constructs that may not correspond to physiologically defined spaces. Drug distribution to various compartments is determined by drug solubility, mechanisms of transport, and degree of protein binding. Drugs that distribute to peripheral compartments have the potential to reenter the plasma compartment. The pharmacokinetics of drugs that are extensively distributed are usually characterized by a long terminal half-life that depends on the rate of redistribution. Drug distribution may dramatically influence the activity and toxicity of schedule-dependent drugs. For example, methotrexate readily distributes into third spaces, including ascites and pleural effusions. Slow redistribution of methotrexate from these third space "reservoirs" may cause prolonged and severe drug toxicity, including myelosuppression and mucositis. Accordingly, methotrexate is contraindicated for patients with large-volume ascites or pleural effusions.

Metabolism is the most critical and complex determinant of the pharmacokinetics for many agents. Drug metabolism may involve specific metabolic pathways, general detoxification pathways in the liver, metabolism in peripheral tissues, spontaneous decomposition, or formation of adducts with biological macromolecules. Chemotherapy agents that resemble physiologic substances are often metabolized by the corresponding specific metabolic pathway. For example, nucleoside analogues are prodrugs that require activation by conversion to nucleoside triphosphates by purine and pyrimidine salvage pathways. Similarly, some antifolates are polyglutamated by the same mechanisms used to metabolize natural folates. Chemotherapy agents that do not resemble physiologic substances are usually metabolized by detoxification pathways in the liver. The most important of these hepatic metabolic pathways is oxidation or conjugation by the cytochrome P-450 class of enzymes. Some drugs are not metabolized but rather cleared by excretion of the parent compound.

Excretion of most cytotoxic drugs and their metabolites is accomplished by either the liver or kidneys. Both renal and biliary excretion are complex processes. Chemotherapy agents may undergo renal filtration, secretion, and reabsorption. Measured or estimated creatinine clearance is often used as a surrogate for the glomerular filtration rate (GFR). However, estimates of GFR may be inaccurate and do not provide information about the potential contribution of renal secretion and reabsorption to renal excretion. Biliary excretion involves several known transport systems including P-glycoprotein and the multifunctional organic anion transporter. Following biliary excretion, some drugs or metabolites are reabsorbed in the small intestine, leading to enterohepatic circulation. Bilirubin is commonly used as a marker of impaired biliary excretion. Both renal and biliary excretion can be modulated by disease or concurrent medications.

The fundamental concept of pharmacokinetics is drug clearance or elimination from the body. After single-dose administration, drug clearance is typically calculated as:

$$AUC = dose/clearance$$

where AUC (area under the concentration time curve) represents the total drug exposure integrated over time. For a given drug dose, the AUC increases with decreasing drug clearance.

Clearance is a function of drug distribution and elimination. In the simplest pharmacokinetic model,

$$Clearance = VK$$

where V is the volume of distribution and K is the elimination constant. The larger the volume of the distribution, the smaller the initial plasma concentration. The elimination constant is inversely proportional to the drug half-life. With a short drug half-life, the elimination constant is high and drug concentrations decline rapidly.

The pharmacokinetics of a drug may vary from one patient to another. Interpatient pharmacokinetic variability may result from differences in absorption, distribution, metabolism, and excretion (Table 3C-1). Interpatient pharmacokinetic variability may account for the differences in toxicity between patients treated with same drug dose and schedule.

**TABLE 3C-1. POTENTIAL SOURCES OF INTERPATIENT PHARMACOKINETIC VARIABILITY**

Differences in absorption
Nausea or vomiting
Diarrhea
Altered gastrointestinal motility
Patient compliance
Concurrent medications
Differences in distribution
Differences in body composition
Pleural effusions
Ascites
Differences in metabolism
Inherited differences in enzyme activity
Liver disease
Concurrent medications
Differences in excretion
Hepatic dysfunction
Renal dysfunction
Concurrent medications

## TOXICITY OF CHEMOTHERAPY

The safe administration of chemotherapy requires an understanding of the potential acute and delayed side effects of treatment. The factors that determine the adverse effects of treatment include the drug, the condition of the target tissues, and the patient's ability to eliminate the drug.

Dose-limiting toxicity is defined as the adverse effect that limits dose escalation. In some cases, the dose-limiting toxicity may be ameliorated by another drug or intervention. For example, treatment with hematopoietic growth factors may permit dose escalation of drugs associated with myelosuppression.[14]

The adverse effects of chemotherapy may be acute and/or delayed. For example, the acute dose-limiting toxicity of the nucleoside analogue fludarabine monophosphate is reversible myelosuppression. However, high-dose fludarabine monophosphate may cause severe delayed neurologic toxicity with cortical blindness and coma 4 to 6 weeks after treatment. Delayed toxicity may be difficult to distinguish from the toxicity that results from repetitive drug administration. For example, doxorubicin is associated with cardiac toxicity, and this toxicity is related to both the peak plasma drug concentration and cumulative dose. Schedules of doxorubicin administration that reduce the peak plasma drug concentration diminish but do not prevent cumulative dose-related cardiac toxicity.

The toxicity of treatment may vary between patients. This variation may result from differences in the condition of target tissues related to the extent of disease or prior treatment. For example, treatment-related myelosuppresion may be more severe for patients with bone marrow involvement or decreased bone marrow reserve due to previous radiation therapy or chemotherapy. Differences in toxicity may also result from interpatient variation in drug-metabolism. For example, patients with liver disease may have increased toxicity from vincristine or paclitaxel due to decreased hepatic metabolism and biliary excretion. Interpatient variation in drug metabolism may also result from genetic differences. For example, the major route of 5-fluorouracil elimination is metabolic conversion to dihydrofluorouracil by the enzyme dihydropyrimidine dehydrogenase. Rare individuals with inherited deficiency of this enzyme have markedly increased toxicity from standard doses of 5-fluorouracil.

## MECHANISMS OF DRUG RESISTANCE

Clinical drug resistance may occur by a variety of mechanisms (Table 3C-2).[15] Resistance to a single drug may occur by several different mechanisms, and a single mechanism may result in resistance to multiple, structurally distinct compounds. Most mechanisms of drug resistance have been defined in experimental systems. There is limited information about the role of specific mechanisms of resistance in clinical treatment failures.

The general cellular mechanisms of drug resistance include decreased drug accumulation, altered drug metabolism, altered drug targets, and increased repair of drug targets. These cellular mechanisms of drug resistance may result from mutation, gene amplification or deletion, or altered transcriptional regulation of the drug target.

Some mechanisms of resistance are specific to particular classes of drugs. For example, a common mechanism of resistance to methotrexate is increased expression of its cellular target, dihydrofolate reductase. Other mechanisms of resistance involve more general regulatory or metabolic pathways and confer resistance to several classes of drugs. For example, mechanisms of resistance involving DNA repair or cell death pathways result in resistance to multiple classes of chemotherapy agents.

The classic mechanism of de novo and acquired resistance to multiple drugs is expression of P-glycoprotein, a family of membrane proteins that function as drug efflux pumps.[16,17] P-Glycoprotein–associated multiple drug resistance (MDR) is characterized by cross-resistance to a broad array of natural products, including the anthracyclines, antitumor antibiotics, vinca alkaloids, and epipodophyllotoxins. P-Glycoprotein expression is associated with a poor outcome in a variety of human malignancies, including leukemia, breast cancer, ovarian cancer, and renal cell carcinoma.

Similar phenotypes of resistance to multiple drugs have been associated with expression of other membrane proteins. For example, MRP is a membrane protein involved in energy-dependent transport of glutathione-conjugated compounds.[18] MRP expression results in cross-resistance to a variety of natural products, and this MDR phenotype is similar to that associated with P-glycoprotein expression.

## CHEMOTHERAPY STRATEGIES

### COMBINATION CHEMOTHERAPY

With few exceptions, the use of multiple drug treatment regimens or combination chemotherapy is more effective than single-agent chemotherapy. De novo resistance to a single agent is common, even in clinically responsive tumors. In addition, initially sensitive tumors may rapidly acquire resistance to a single chemotherapy agent by either outgrowth of a resistant clone or selection of somatic mutations that confer drug resistance. Combination chemotherapy may overcome both of these resistance phenomena.

The principles for the development of new combination chemotherapy regimens include the use of drugs with single-agent activity in the target disease, different mechanisms of action, nonoverlapping toxicities to allow the use of each drug in full dose, and nonoverlapping mechanisms of resistance (Table 3C-3). These principles are not absolute, and the combination of drugs based on their single-agent activity may override other considerations. For example, the CHOP (cyclophosphamide, adriamycin, vincristine, and prednisone) regimen for treatment of lymphoma includes agents with overlapping toxicities and common mechanisms of resistance.

### PRIMARY CHEMOTHERAPY

Several human malignancies are curable by treatment with chemotherapy alone (Table 3C-4). These include gestational trophoblastic tumors, testicular germ cell tumors, Hodgkin's disease, some subtypes of non-Hodgkin's lymphoma, acute myeloid and lymphoid leukemias, and hairy cell leukemia. The recognition of the potential curative role of primary chemotherapy is important. In many of these diseases, debulking surgery is unnecessary and may reduce the probability of long-term remission by delaying primary systemic treatment.

### MULTIMODALITY THERAPY

The management of many solid tumors involves a combination of surgery, radiation therapy, and chemotherapy. In multimodality treatment, chemotherapy may be used to downstage the primary

---

**TABLE 3C-2.** MECHANISMS OF DRUG RESISTANCE

Decreased drug accumulation
Decreased drug activation
Increased drug inactivation
Increased repair of drug-induced damage
Alteration in drug target
Alteration in normal cell death pathways

---

**TABLE 3C-3.** PRINCIPLES OF COMBINATION CHEMOTHERAPY

Single-agent activity in the target disease
Different mechanisms of action
Nonoverlapping toxicities to allow for the use of each drug in full dose
Nonoverlapping mechanisms of resistance

## TABLE 3C-4. MALIGNANCIES OFTEN CURED BY PRIMARY CHEMOTHERAPY

Gestational trophoblastic tumors

Germ cell tumors

Hodgkin's disease

Non-Hodgkin's lymphoma (some subtypes)

Acute myeloid leukemia

Acute lymphoid leukemia

Hairy cell leukemia

---

tumor, increase the efficacy of local radiation therapy, or treat microscopic metastatic disease. The purpose and timing of chemotherapy may vary with the tumor type and stage of disease (Table 3C-5). Several examples are provided here.

Women with high-risk node-positive and node-negative breast cancer are typically treated with breast-conserving surgery, adjuvant chemotherapy, and local radiation therapy.[19] In contrast, women with inflammatory breast cancer are routinely treated with chemotherapy followed by local treatment.[20,21] Neoadjuvant chemotherapy improves the local-regional control and disease-free survival rates in women with inflammatory breast cancer, and their outcome is correlated with primary tumor response.

Approximately one-half of patients who undergo radical cystectomy for invasive transitional cell carcinoma will develop metastatic disease.[22] Because of the high distant failure rate and significant morbidity of radical cystectomy, combined modality treatment with transurethral resection followed by concurrent chemotherapy and radiation therapy has been evaluated as an alternative approach to management of muscle invasive bladder cancer. Prospective trials of multimodality "bladder-sparing" therapy for selected patients with invasive bladder cancer have reported excellent long-term disease-free and overall survival rates.[23,24] Randomized prospective trials will be required to determine the equivalence of bladder-sparing multimodality therapy and radical cystectomy.

Most patients with clinically localized esophageal cancer treated with surgery alone will develop local or distant disease recurrence. The addition of radiation and/or chemotherapy prior to surgical resection has been evaluated as a method for improving local control and distant control rates.[25,26] Prospective randomized trials of surgery alone versus neoadjuvant chemoradiation followed by surgery suggest that multimodality therapy is superior to surgery alone. Additional randomized trials to evaluate the value of multimodality therapy for patients with clinically localized esophageal cancer are ongoing.

## ADJUVANT CHEMOTHERAPY

Adjuvant chemotherapy is administered to patients without clinically detectable disease following local treatment with surgical resection and/or radiation therapy. By treating microscopic metastatic disease, adjuvant chemotherapy is designed to improve the survival of patients at high risk of disease relapse. The theoretical advantages of adjuvant chemotherapy compared to treatment of clinically apparent metastatic disease are compelling. By treating patients with very small tumor burden, most of the obstacles associated with treatment of solid tumors are mitigated, including the problems of drug delivery to a poorly vascularized tumor, de novo drug resistance, low growth fraction, and tumor heterogeneity.

Adjuvant chemotherapy improves the outcome of patients with breast cancer, colorectal cancer, laryngeal cancer, osteosarcoma, and Wilms' tumor. Adjuvant chemotherapy has not improved the outcome of many other malignancies associated with high relapse rates. This absence of benefit in these other diseases may reflect the limited

## TABLE 3C-5. MULTIMODALITY TREATMENT OF SOLID TUMORS

| TREATMENT APPROACH | DISEASE | RESULTS | REFERENCES |
|---|---|---|---|
| Surgery followed by chemotherapy and radiation therapy | Stage II–III rectal cancer | Improved local control and survival | GITSG 1985[39] GITSG 1986[40] Krook et al 1991[41] |
| | Stage I–II breast cancer | Improved local control and survival | Overgaard et al 1997[42] Ragaz et al 1997[43] |
| Chemotherapy and radiation therapy followed by surgery | Stage II–III esophageal cancer | Improved survival | Al-Sarraf et al 1996[44] Walsh et al 1997[45] |
| | Stage III non-small-cell lung cancer | Improved survival | Dillman et al 1993[46] |
| | Stage III breast cancer | Improved local control and survival; organ conservation | Perloff et al 1988[47] Hortobagyi 1990[48] |
| Chemotherapy and radiation therapy without surgery | Stage II–III anal cancer | Improved survival compared to surgery; organ preservation in most patients | UKCCCR 1991[49] Bartelink et al 1997[50] |
| | Stage III–IVB laryngeal cancer Stage II–III hypopharyngeal cancer | Organ preservation in most patients; decreased distant relapse rate | VA 1991[51] Lefebvre et al 1996[52] |

ABBREVIATIONS: GITSG = Gastrointestinal Tumor Study Group; UKCCCR = United Kingdom Coordinating Committee on Cancer Research; VA = Veterans affairs.

activity of current chemotherapy regimens or the absence of adequate randomized clinical trials. In some cases, the major limitation appears to be the absence of adequate trials. For example, cisplatin-based chemotherapy for metastatic bladder cancer is associated with complete and partial response rates that exceed the chemotherapy response rates for metastatic breast cancer or colorectal cancer.[27] While most randomized trials of adjuvant chemotherapy for high-risk bladder cancer have demonstrated no benefit, these trials were underpowered to detect an improved outcome of a magnitude similar to that associated with adjuvant chemotherapy for breast and colorectal cancers.[28]

## NEOADJUVANT CHEMOTHERAPY

The use of chemotherapy prior to definitive local treatment of the primary tumor is termed *neoadjuvant chemotherapy*. Neoadjuvant chemotherapy has several potential advantages compared to adjuvant chemotherapy, including early treatment of microscopic metastatic disease, the ability to directly assess tumor response to chemotherapy, and the potential ability to downstage the primary tumor. The disadvantages of neoadjuvant chemotherapy include the loss of the precision associated with initial surgical staging, the potential delay in definitive local treatment, and increased operative risk following chemotherapy and radiation therapy.

Several solid tumors are effectively treated with neoadjuvant chemotherapy, including osteosarcoma, anal tract cancers, bladder cancer, laryngeal cancer, lung cancer, esophageal cancer, and inflammatory or locally advanced breast cancer. For example, the primary treatment of most squamous and cloacogenic cancers of the anal canal is chemotherapy combined with radiation therapy.[29] Combined chemoradiation for anal cancers is associated with excellent organ-preservation and disease-free survival rates. Abdominoperitoneal resection is recommended when combined chemoradiation therapy does not result in a complete response.

## HIGH-DOSE CHEMOTHERAPY

Autologous bone marrow or stem cell transplantation involves the intravenous administration of hematopoietic progenitor cells to reconstitute marrow function for patients following treatment with high-dose chemotherapy.[30] The hematopoietic progenitor cells can be derived from either the patient's bone marrow or peripheral blood prior to treatment. This approach allows for the administration of myelosuppressive drugs in doses that exceed the usual maximum-tolerated dose. Since most cytotoxic drugs are administered in doses that correspond to the linear range of the dose-response curve, the administration of high-dose chemotherapy followed by stem cell rescue has the potential to improve response rates and survival.

The role of high-dose chemotherapy in the treatment of most solid tumors is undefined. High-dose chemotherapy has resulted in "salvage" or long-term remissions in selected patients not expected to benefit from standard chemotherapy. Favorable results have been reported in breast cancer, neuroblastoma, and testicular cancer.[31–33] Randomized trials are required to evaluate the role of high-dose chemotherapy in the management of these diseases.

## CHEMOTHERAPY AGENTS

This section and Table 3C-6 provide a brief overview of chemotherapy agents commonly used for the treatment of solid tumors. This information is derived from several sources, and the reader is referred to these sources for a more comprehensive discussion of individual chemotherapy agents.[34,35] Current information should be obtained from the manufacturer prior to initiating therapy.

## ALKYLATING AGENTS

The alkylating agents are a class of compounds that covalently modify biologic macromolecules, including RNA, DNA, and proteins. The cytotoxic effects of alkylating agents are due to covalent modifications of DNA that result in either interstrand DNA crosslinks or base modifications leading to depurination and single-strand DNA breaks.

Cyclophosphamide is the most commonly used alkylating agent. Cyclophosphamide is a prodrug that is converted to several active compounds by hepatic microsomal metabolism. Cyclophosphamide has less hematologic and gastrointestinal toxicity than other alkylating agents because of rapid inactivation of active cyclphosphamide metabolites in hematopoietic stem cells and gastrointestinal mucosa. Cyclophosphamide and cyclophosphamide metabolities are cleared by renal excretion. Resistance to cyclophosphamide results from decreased cellular entry–increased cellular export, increased intracellular inactivation, and increased DNA repair.

Cyclophosphamide and other alkylating agents are commonly used to treat solid tumors and hematologic malignancies, including breast cancer, non-Hodgkin's lymphoma, and multiple myeloma. The major toxicities of cyclophosphamide include myelosuppression, nausea, vomiting, and gonadal failure. Hemorrhagic cystitis may result from the accumulation of toxic metabolites in the urine. Cyclophosphamide increases the risk of transitional cell carcinoma of the bladder.

## ANTHRACYCLINES AND DNA INTERCALATORS

The DNA intercalators share a common chemical structure and mechanism of action. DNA intercalators have a planar aromatic ring structure that allows them to bind between adjacent base pairs of DNA. This binding alters DNA supercoiling and causes inactivation of topoisomerase II and other enzymes that regulate DNA topology. The DNA intercalators appear to kill cells by promoting topoisomerase-mediated DNA damage.

The DNA intercalators are one of the most important classes of antineoplastic agents. The DNA intercalators in clinical use include the anthracyclines (doxorubicin, daunorubicin, epirubicin, idarubicin), mitoxantrone, dactinomycin, and amsacrine. The

**TABLE 3C-6.** SUMMARY OF COMMON CHEMOTHERAPY AGENTS FOR SOLID TUMORS

| AGENT | CLASS | INDICATIONS | CLEARANCE | SIDE EFFECTS |
|---|---|---|---|---|
| Aminoglutethimide | Aromatase inhibitor | Breast cancer | Renal excretion | Drowsiness, nausea, rash |
| Bicalutamide | Antiandrogen | Prostate cancer | Metabolism | Hepatotoxicity |
| Bleomycin | Antitumor antibiotic | Testis cancer, lymphoma, squamous cell carcinoma | Renal excretion | Allergic reactions, mucositis, pulmonary fibrosis, Raynaud's phenomenon |
| Carboplatin | Platinum compound | Head and neck cancer, lung cancer, lymphoma, ovarian cancer | Renal excretion | Nausea/vomiting, myelosuppression |
| Cisplatin | Platinum compound | Bladder cancer, lung cancer, ovarian cancer, testis cancer | Renal excretion | Myelosuppression, nausea/vomiting, neuropathy, ototoxicity, renal toxicity |
| Cyclophosphamide | Alkylating agent | Breast cancer, lymphoma, sarcoma, Wilms' tumor | Hepatic metabolism, renal excretion | Hemorrhagic cystitis, myelosuppression, nausea/vomiting, SIADH |
| Dacarbazine | Alkylating agent | Hodgkin's disease, melanoma, sarcoma | Hepatic metabolism, renal excretion | Flulike syndrome, myelosuppression, nausea/vomiting |
| Docetaxel | Taxane | Breast cancer, lung cancer, ovarian cancer | Hepatic metabolism | Cardiac toxicity, hypersensitivity reaction, myelosuppression, nausea/vomiting, neuropathy |
| Doxorubicin | Anthracycline | Bladder cancer, breast cancer, lymphoma, sarcoma | Hepatic metabolism | Cardiac toxicity, mucositis, myelosuppression, nausea/vomiting |
| Estramustine | Antimicrotubule agent | Prostate cancer | Hepatic metabolism | Estrogenic effects, fluid retention, nausea |
| Etoposide | Topoisomerase II inhibitor | Small cell lung cancer, sarcoma, testis cancer | Hepatic metabolism, renal excretion | Allergic reactions, CNS toxicity, hepatotoxicity, hypotension, nausea/vomiting, second malignancies |
| Fluorouracil | Antimetabolite | Breast cancer, gastrointestinal cancers, head and neck cancers | Hepatic metabolism | Cerebellar ataxia, diarrhea, myocardial ischemia |
| Flutamide | Antiandrogen | Prostate cancer | Metabolism, renal excretion of metabolities | Diarrhea, hepatotoxicity |
| Gemcitabine | Pyrimidine analogue | Pancreatic cancer, lung cancer, bladder cancer | Metabolism | Myelosuppression |
| Goserelin | LHRH agonist | Breast cancer, prostate cancer | Metabolism | Hot flashes, loss of libido, osteoporosis, weight gain |
| Interferon-$\alpha$ | Cytokine | Kaposi's sarcoma, lymphoma, melanoma, renal cell carcinoma | Renal excretion | Cardiovascular toxicity, CNS toxicity, fever, flulike syndrome |
| Interleukin-2 | Cytokine | Melanoma, renal cell carcinoma | Renal excretion | Capillary leak syndrome, cardiovascular toxicity, CNS toxicity, fever, flulike syndrome |
| Ifosfamide | Alkylating agent | Lymphoma, sarcoma, testis cancer | Hepatic metabolism, renal excretion | CNS toxicity, hemorrhagic cystitis, myelosuppression, nausea/vomiting, SIADH |
| Irinotecan | Topoisomerase I inhibitor | Colorectal cancer | Hepatic metabolism | Diarrhea, myelosuppression |

(continues)

**TABLE 3C-6.** (*Continued*)

| AGENT | CLASS | INDICATIONS | CLEARANCE | SIDE EFFECTS |
|---|---|---|---|---|
| Leuprolide | LHRH agonist | Breast cancer, prostate cancer | Hepatic metabolism | Hot flashes, loss of libido, osteoporosis, weight gain |
| Megestrol acetate | Progestational agent | Breast cancer, endometrial cancer | Renal excretion | Weight gain, thromboembolic events |
| Methotrexate | Folate antagonist | Bladder cancer, breast cancer, choriocarcinoma, head and neck cancer, lymphoma | Renal excretion | Hepatotoxicity, myelosuppression, nausea/vomiting, pulmonary toxicity, renal toxicity |
| Mitomycin | Antitumor antibiotic | Gastrointestinal cancers | Hepatic metabolism, renal excretion | Hepatotoxicity, myelosuppression, pulmonary toxicity, renal toxicity |
| Mitoxantrone | Anthroquinone | Breast cancer, lymphoma, prostate cancer | Hepatic metabolism, biliary excretion | Cardiac toxicity, myelosuppression, nausea/vomiting |
| Nilutamide | Antiandrogen | Prostate cancer | Metabolism, renal excretion of metabolites | Impaired dark adaptation |
| Paclitaxel | Taxane | Breast cancer, lung cancer, ovarian cancer | Hepatic metabolism | Cardiac toxicity, hypersensitivity reaction, myelosuppression, nausea/vomiting, neuropathy |
| Prednisone | Corticosteroid | Lymphoma, prostate cancer | Renal excretion of metabolites | Fluid retention, hyperglycemia, muscle weakness, osteoporosis |
| Tamoxifen | Antiestrogen | Breast cancer | Hepatic metabolism | Hot flashes, nausea, hepatotoxicity, endometrial carcinoma |
| Thiotepa | Alkylating agent | Bladder cancer, breast cancer, ovarian cancer | Renal excretion | Myelosuppression, nausea/vomiting |
| Topotecan | Topoisomerase I inhibitor | Breast cancer | Renal excretion | Fever, myelosuppression, rash |
| Vinblastine | Vinca alkaloid | Bladder cancer, lymphoma, testis cancer, prostate cancer | Hepatic metabolism | Myelosuppression |
| Vincristine | Vinca alkaloid | Lymphoma, sarcoma | Hepatic metabolism | Neurotoxicity |
| Vinorelbine | Vinca alkaloid | Breast cancer, lung cancer, prostate cancer | Hepatic metabolism | Myelosuppression, neurotoxicity |

ABBREVIATIONS:  SIADH = syndrome of inappropriate secretion of antidiuretic hormone; LHRH = luteinizing hormone-releasing hormone.

anthracyclines have a broad spectrum of clinical activity, including breast cancer, sarcoma, Hodgkin's and non-Hodgkin's lymphoma, multiple myeloma, and acute lymphoid and myeloid leukemias. Mitoxantrone is used to treat breast cancer, prostate cancer, lymphoma, and leukemia. Dactinomycin is used to treat several pediatric malignancies. The major clinical use of amsacrine is in the treatment of myeloid leukemias.

The major toxicities of the anthracyclines include myelosuppression, mucositis, alopecia, and cardiac toxicity. The anthracyclines are vesicants and must be administered through a freely flowing and newly placed intravenous catheter. Extravasation into subcutaneous tissues can result in severe local injury.

## ENDOCRINE THERAPY

The growth and differentiation of the breast, endometrium, and prostate are regulated by gonadal steroids. Malignancies that arise from these sites are often dependent on hormones for growth. Endocrine or hormonal therapies that decrease circulating gonadal steroid levels or interfere with hormone-receptor interactions represent effective therapies for malignancies of the breast, endometrium, and prostate.

Antiestrogens are commonly used for the adjuvant treatment of primary breast cancer in postmenopausal women and for the treatment of metastatic disease in patients with tumors that express the estrogen receptor. The standard adjuvant treatment for primary breast cancer in premenopausal women is cytotoxic chemotherapy. However, oophorectomy and suppression of ovarian estrogen production with luteinizing hormone–releasing hormone (LHRH) agonists are effective adjuvant therapies for premenopausal women with tumors that express the estrogen receptor. In addition, part of the effectiveness of cytotoxic chemotherapy in premenopausal women appears to result from the treatment-related ovarian suppression.

Treatment of recurrent or advanced endometrial carcinoma is associated with a 10% to 30% response rate and a median response duration of 10 to 20 months. Patients with tumors that are well differentiated and express high levels of the progesterone receptor have the greatest probability of response. There is no evidence to support the use of adjuvant progestational agents following hysterectomy for endometrial carcinoma.

The standard management of metastatic prostate cancer is androgen deprivation by either orchiectomy or suppression of testicular androgen production with LHRH agonists. Androgen deprivation has a >90% response rate in metastatic prostate cancer and a median duration of response of 18 to 24 months. In men with locally advanced prostate cancer (clinical stage T3 tumors), treatment with the combination of external beam radiation therapy and adjuvant androgen deprivation results in superior disease-free and overall survival rates than external beam radiation therapy alone.

## FOLATE ANTAGONISTS

Folate antagonists act by inhibiting one or more biosynthetic steps involving folate coenzymes. Methotrexate and all other clinically important folate antagonists act predominantly by inhibiting the enzyme dihydrofolate reductase, resulting in decreased synthesis of tetrahydrofolate. The formation of thymidine, a key step in purine biosynthesis, is the only folate coenzyme-mediated one-carbon transfer reaction resulting in the conversion of tetrahydrofolate to dihydrofolate. Dihydrofolate reductase regenerates tetrahydrofolate from dihydrofolate. In rapidly dividing cells, inhibition of dihydrofolate reductase results in decreased thymidine triphosphate pools, decreased DNA synthesis, and eventual cell death.

Methotrexate is extensively distributed after intravenous administration. Patients with pleural effusions or ascites are at increased risk of methotrexate toxicity due to accumulation of methotrexate in these third spaces, followed by slow redistribution with sustained concentrations in the serum.

The primary metabolite of methotrexate is 7-hydroxy methotrexate. Methotrexate and methotrexate metabolites are converted to active polyglutamates within the cell. Methotrexate is cleared predominantly by renal excretion. There are several known mechanisms of methotrexate resistance, including increased expression of dihydrofolate reductase, decreased transport, and decreased polyglutamate formation.

The major toxicities of methotrexate include neutropenia, mucositis, hepatotoxicity, renal toxicity, and pulmonary toxicity. Leucovorin (D,L-$N$5-formyltetrahydrofolate) is commonly administered to rescue patients from toxicity when methotrexate is administered in high doses. Methotrexate is used for the treatment

of a variety of malignancies including acute leukemia, lymphoma, choriocarcinoma, breast cancer, and transitional cell carcinoma.

## PLATINUM COMPOUNDS

The platinum compounds are metal complexes that form covalent bonds with proteins and nucleic acids. The cytotoxic effects of the platinum compounds appears to involve formation of interstrand and intrastrand DNA cross-links, resulting in DNA breaks.

There are two platinum compounds in clinical use: cisplatin and carboplatin. These agents have a broad spectrum of clinical activity and are commonly used to treat testis cancer, urothelial malignancies, ovarian cancer, small cell lung cancer, non-small cell lung cancer, head and neck cancers, and lymphomas. Cisplatin and carboplatin appear to have similar but not identical patterns of clinical activity. Randomized trials of combination chemotherapy suggest that cisplatin is superior to carboplatin for the treatment of testicular germ cell tumors.[36]

Carboplatin is cleared by renal excretion. Cisplatin is cleared by renal excretion and formation of covalent adducts with proteins and nucleic acids. The toxicities of cisplatin include myelosuppression, renal toxicity, ototoxicity, and neurotoxicity. The dose-limiting toxicity of carboplatin is myelosuppression. In contrast to cisplatin, the nonhematologic side effects of carboplatin are mild.

## PURINE AND PYRIMIDINE ANTIMETABOLITES

Nucleotide antimetabolites are a class of antineoplastic agents that mimic purines or pyrimidines. Most purine and pyrimidine analogues are prodrugs that are active only following conversion to the nucleotide form. Nucleotide antimetabolites mediate their antitumor effects by a variety of mechanisms, including inhibition of nucleic acid biosynthesis and incorporation into nascent RNA or DNA.

The pyrimidine analogue 5-fluorouracil (5-FU) is one of the most commonly used cancer chemotherapy agents. Following entry into the cell by carrier-mediated transport, 5-FU is converted to several nucleotide metabolites, including 5′-fluorouridine triphosphate (FUTP), 5′-fluorodeoxyuridine monophosphate (FdUMP), and 5′-fluorodeoxyuridine triphosphate (FdUTP). The biologic action of 5-FU is mediated by the incorporation of FUTP into RNA, incorporation of the FdUTP into DNA, and inhibition of DNA synthesis by covalent inaction of thymidylate synthetase by FdUMP. Covalent inactivation of thymidylate synthetase by 5-FU requires formation of a ternary complex between FdUMP, thymidylate synthetase, and folate coenzymes. Leucovorin increases the biologic activity of 5-FU by stabilizing formation of this ternary complex.

5-FU is used to treat a variety of malignancies, including colon, breast, and head and neck cancers. The major toxicities of 5-FU are stomatitis, diarrhea, and myelosuppression.

## TAXANES

The taxanes, paclitaxel and docetaxel, have a novel mechanism of action and a broad spectrum of clinical activity. Paclitaxel was isolated from the bark of the western yew tree, *Taxus brevifolia*. Docetaxel was isolated from the leaves of the European yew tree. Both of these taxanes are now produced by synthetic methods.

Paclitaxel and docetaxel inhibit normal disassembly of microtubules by reversible high-affinity binding to polymerized microtubules. This disruption of normal microtubule function results in biologic effects similar to those associated with the vinca alkaloids, including inhibition of cellular movement, secretion, and mitosis. Resistance to the taxanes results from altered expression or mutation of tubulin subunits and increased expression of *P*-glycoprotein.

The taxanes have a broad spectrum of clinical activity, including cancers of the breast, ovary, head and neck, lung, and prostate. The major side effects of the taxanes include severe allergic reactions, myelosuppression, alopecia, sensory neuropathy, myalgias, arthralgias, and bradycardia. Premedication with dexamethasone, cimetidine, and diphenhydramine are required to reduce the risk of severe allergic reactions during drug adminstration.

## TOPOISOMERASE I INHIBITORS

Camptothecin was isolated from the stem wood of the Chinese tree *Camptotheca accuminata*. Semisynthetic derivatives of camptothecin, including 9-amino-20(*S*)-camptothecin (9-AC), topotecan, and irinotecan (CPT-11), are an important new class of chemotherapeutic agents. The camptothecins inhibit topoisomerase I, an enzyme that functions in transcription and DNA replication by relaxing supercoiled DNA. Inhibition of topoisomerase I results in single-strand DNA breaks and cell death. Resistance to the camptothecins appears to involve altered expression or mutation of topoisomerase I.

The camptothecins have activity in several solid tumors, including colorectal cancer, gastric cancer, small cell lung cancer, and non-small cell lung cancers. The campothecins have similar toxicities. The major toxicities of topotecan include myelosuppression, alopecia, rash, and fever. Treatment with irinotecan is associated with myelosuppression and diarrhea. The major toxicities of 9-aminocamptothecin include myelosuppression, diarrhea, nausea, vomiting, and hemmorrhagic cystitis.

## TOPOISOMERASE II INHIBITORS

Etoposide (VP-16) and teniposide (VM-26) are semisynthetic derivatives of podophyllotoxin, a medicinal product from the May apple or American mandrake plant. The cytotoxicity of these agents results from inhibition of topoisomerase II, leading to double-stranded DNA breaks.

Etoposide has a wide range of clinical activity, including small cell lung cancer, testis cancer, sarcoma, neuroblastoma, Wilms' tumor, Hodgkin's and non-Hodgkin's lymphoma, and acute leukemia. Teniposide also appears to have a broad spectrum of activity, although its major use involves pediatric malignancies.

The major toxicities of etoposide and teniposide are myelosuppression, nausea, vomiting, alopecia, peripheral neuropathy, and secondary malignancies.

## VINCA ALKALOIDS

There are three vinca alkaloids approved for use in the United States: vincristine, vinblastine, and vinorelbine. Vincristine and vinblastine are derived from the periwinkle plant, *Vinca rosea* or *Catharanthus roseus*. Vinorelbine is a semisynthetic vinca alkaloid with distinctive lipophilic properties.

The vinca alkaloids reversibly bind to tubulin and disrupt microtubule-dependent processes, including cytoskeletal function, membrane trafficking, cell motility, and mitosis. Although the primary mechanism of action appears to involve inhibition of mitosis, the diverse biologic effects of microtubule disruption may explain the cytotoxic effects of the vinca alkaloids in both dividing and nondividing cells. Resistance to the vinca alkaloids may result from overexpression of *P*-glycoprotein (MDR1 gene) or mutation of the $\alpha$ or $\beta$ subunits of tubulin, leading to decreased vinca alkaloid binding.

Despite similar chemical structures and a common mechanism of action, the clinical activity and toxicity of the vinca alkaloids vary considerably. Vincristine is used as a component in combination chemotherapy for Hodgkin's disease, non-Hodgkin's lymphoma, rhabdomyosarcoma of childhood, Wilms' tumor, and neuroblastoma. The dose-limiting toxicity of vincristine is peripheral neuropathy. Vinblastine has activity in Hodgkin's and non-Hodgkin's lymphoma, testis cancer, prostate cancer, and histiocytosis X. The dose-limiting toxicity of vinblastine is myelosuppression. Vinorelbine has activity in non-small cell lung cancer, breast cancer, and prostate cancer. The major side effects of vinorelbine are myelosuppression and neurotoxicity. The neurotoxicity of vinorelbine is less than that associated with vincristine.

## BIOLOGIC RESPONSE MODIFIERS

Biologic response modifiers are macromolecules that produce antitumor effects, primarily by augmentation of natural host defense mechanisms. The most commonly used biologic response modifiers are interleukin-2 and interferon-$\alpha$.

Interleukin-2 is a protein produced by activated T-lymphocytes. Interleukin-2 has a variety of biologic effects and plays a central role in normal immune regulation. Interleukin-2 is used clinically to treat metastatic renal cell carcinoma and melanoma. Interleukin-2 has no direct cytotoxic activity and appears to mediate disease responses by nonspecific immune activation. Treatment with interleukin-2 is associated with capillary leak syndrome, cardiovascular toxicity, central nervous system toxicity, fever, and a flulike syndrome.

The interferons are a family of proteins produced by cells in response to viral infection or mitogenic stimulation. The interferons have a variety of immunomodulatory and antiproliferative effects. Interferon-$\alpha$ is produced by macrophages and lymphocytes. Interferon-$\alpha$ is used clinically to treat a variety of malignancies, including renal cell carcinoma, melanoma, low-grade lymphoma, and chronic myelogenous leukemia. Treatment with interferon-$\alpha$ is associated with cardiovascular toxicity, central nervous system toxicity, fever, and a flulike syndrome. The toxicity of interleukin-2 and interferon-$\alpha$ are dose- and schedule-dependent.

## NEW DRUG EVALUATION

New drug development has only recently focused on the identification of agents with activity against epithelial malignancies. Accordingly, there are few drugs with activity against the most common human malignancies, including cancers of the lung, colon, breast, and prostate. Improved strategies of identifying agents with activity against these malignancies will improve the systemic treatment of common solid tumors.

The traditional approach to new drug discovery involves screening libraries of synthetic compounds and natural products for cytotoxic activity. Prior to 1985, the National Cancer Institute screened new compounds for anticancer activity using murine models of leukemia. That strategy identified agents with activity in leukemia but relatively few agents that were effective against common solid tumors. In 1985, the Developmental Therapeutics Program of the NCI established a primary in vitro screen in which new agents are evaluated for their ability to inhibit the growth of 60 different human cancer cell lines.[37] This disease-oriented strategy is based on the hypothesis that the in vitro activity against human cancer cell lines predicts selective activity in the corresponding human malignancy.

In addition to identifying potential therapeutic applications of new chemotherapeutic agents, the NCI 60 cell-line screen provides a method for characterizing new agents. Patterns of activity are analyzed using the COMPARE algorithm.[38] A similar pattern of activity may indicate related molecular structures, modes of action, and mechanisms of resistance. The COMPARE algorithm has been applied productively to many classes of chemotherapy agents, including topoisomerase II inhibitors, pyrimidine biosynthesis inhibitors, and tubulin-active agents. The NCI 60 cell-line screen and COMPARE algorithm have been used to select several compounds for entry into clinical trials, including KRN 5500, flavopiridol, UCN-01, a depsipeptide, and a quinocarmycin analog.

In recent decades, the dramatic expansion of knowledge about the molecular pathways that cause cancer has provided new avenues for cancer treatment. As a result of these basic research efforts, there are now several hundred compounds at various stages of development for the treatment of human malignancies. Many of these drugs have novel cellular targets and mechanisms of action. This exciting era of rational drug discovery holds the promise of new agents with greater efficacy and less toxicity.

## REFERENCES

1. GOODMAN LS et al: Nitrogen mustard therapy. J Am Med Assoc 251:2255, 1984.
2. BERTINO JR: Karnofsky memorial lecture. Ode to methotrexate. J Clin Oncol 11:5, 1993.
3. ZUBROD CG: Historic milestones in curative chemotherapy. Semin Oncol 6:490, 1979.
4. NOBLE RL: The discovery of the vinca alkaloids—Chemotherapeutic agents against cancer. Biochem Cell Biol 68:1344, 1990.
5. KENNEDY BJ: Evolution of chemotherapy. CA 41:261, 1991.
6. SHERR CJ: Cancer cell cycles. Science 274(5293):1672, 1996.
7. FISHER DE: Apoptosis in cancer therapy: Crossing the threshold. Cell 78:539, 1994.
8. SKIPPER HE: Laboratory models: Some historical perspective. Cancer Treat Rep 70:3, 1986.
9. NORTON L, SIMON R: The Norton-Simon hypothesis revisited. Cancer Treat Rep 70:163, 1986.
10. LURIA SE, DELBRUCK M: Mutations of bacteria from virus sensitivity to virus resistance. Genetics 28:491, 1943.
11. GOLDIE JH, COLDMAN AJ: A mathematical model for relating the drug sensitivity of tumors to their spontaneous mutation rate. Cancer Treat Rep 63(14):1727, 1979.
12. RATAIN MJ, SCHILSKY RL: Principles of pharmacology and pharmacokinetics, in The Chemotherapy Sourcebook, MC Perry (ed). Baltimore, Williams & Wilkins, 1992, pp 22–35.
13. RATAIN MJ, PLUNKETT W: Pharmacology, in Cancer Medicine, 4th ed, JF Holland et al (eds). Baltimore, Williams & Wilkins, 1997; Chap 58, pp 875–889.
14. ANONYMOUS: American Society of Clinical Oncology. Recommendations for the use of hematopoietic colony-stimulating factors: evidence-based clinical practice guidelines. J Clin Oncol 12:2471, 1994.
15. RINGBORG U, PLATZ A: Chemotherapy resistance mechanisms. Acta Oncologica 35(Suppl)5:76, 1996.
16. NOOTER K, STOTER G: Molecular mechanisms of multidrug resistance in cancer chemotherapy. Pathology, Res Prac 192:768, 1996.
17. LING V: Multidrug resistance: Molecular mechanisms and clinical relevance. Cancer Chemother Pharmacol 40(Suppl):S3, 1997.
18. LAUTIER D et al: Multidrug resistance mediated by the multidrug resistance protein (MRP) gene. Biochem Pharm 52(7):967, 1996.
19. OVERMOYER BA: Chemotherapy in the management of breast cancer. Cleveland Clin J Med 62(1):36, 1995.
20. PEREZ EA et al: Management of locally advanced breast cancer. Oncology 11(9 Suppl 9):9, 1997.
21. SINGLETARY SE et al: New strategies in locally advanced breast cancer. Cancer Treat Res 90:253, 1997.
22. MCCAFFREY JA et al: Combined modality therapy for bladder cancer. Oncology 11(Suppl 9):18, 1997.
23. DOUGLAS RM et al: Conservative surgery, patient selection, and chemoradiation as organ-preserving treatment for muscle-invading bladder cancer. Semin Oncol 23:614, 1996.
24. KACHNIC LA et al: Bladder preservation by combined modality therapy for invasive bladder cancer. J Clin Oncol 5(3):1022, 1997.
25. AJANI JA: Current status of new drugs and multidisciplinary approaches in patients with carcinoma of the esophagus. Chest 113(Suppl 1):112S, 1998.
26. FORASTIERE AA et al: Multimodality therapy for esophageal cancer. Chest 112(Suppl 4):195S, 1997.
27. SMITH MR, KANTOFF PW: Neoadjuvant and adjuvant chemotherapy for invasive bladder cancer. Semin Oncol 22:625, 1995.
28. DIMOPOULOS MA, MOULOPOULOS LA: Role of adjuvant chemotherapy in the treatment of invasive carcinoma of the urinary bladder. J Clin Oncol 16:1601, 1998.
29. STAFFORD SL, MARTENSON JA: Combined radiation and chemotherapy for carcinoma of the anal canal. Oncology 12(3):373, 381; discussion 382, 384, 38, 1998.
30. APPELBAUM FR: The use of bone marrow and peripheral blood stem cell transplantation in the treatment of cancer. CA 46(3):142, 1996.

31. GRADISHAR WJ et al: High-dose chemotherapy for breast cancer. Ann Int Med 125(7):599, 1996.

32. KLETZEL M, KIM AR: Autologous bone marrow transplantation in pediatric solid tumors. Cancer Treat Res 77:333, 1997.

33. BOKEMEYER C et al: The use of dose-intensified chemotherapy in the treatment of metastatic nonseminomatous testicular germ cell tumors. German Testicular Cancer Study Group. Semin Oncol 25(2 Suppl 4):24, discussion 45, 199, 1998.

34. Chemotherapeutic drugs, in *The Chemotherapy Sourcebook,* Sec 2, MC Perry (ed). Baltimore, Williams & Wilkins, 1992, pp 286–497.

35. RATAIN M: Pharmacology of Cancer Chemotherapy, in *Cancer Principles and Practice of Oncology,* 5th ed, VT Devita et al (eds). Philadelphia, Lippincott-Raven, 1997, pp 375–512.

36. HORWICH A et al: Randomized trial of bleomycin, etoposide, and cisplatin compared with bleomycin, etoposide, and carboplatin in good-prognosis metastatic nonseminomatous germ cell cancer: A Multi-institutional Medical Research Council/European Organization for Research and Treatment of Cancer Trial. J Clin Oncol 15(5):1844, 1997.

37. GREVER MR et al: The National Cancer Institute: Cancer drug discovery and development program. Semin Oncol 19:622, 1992.

38. WEINSTEIN JN et al: An information-intensive approach to the molecular pharmacology of cancer. Science 275(5298):343, 1997.

39. GASTROINTESTINAL TUMOR STUDY GROUP: Prolongation of disease-free interval in surgically treated rectal carcinoma. N Engl J Med 312:1465, 1985.

40. ———: Survival after postoperative combination treatment of rectal cancer. N Engl J Med 315:1295, 1986.

41. KROOK JE et al: Effective surgical adjuvant therapy for high-risk rectal carcinoma. N Engl J Med 324:709, 1991.

42. OVERGAARD M et al: Postoperative radiotherapy in high risk premenopausal women with breast cancer who receive adjuvant chemotherapy. Danish Breast Cancer Cooperative Group 82b Trial. N Engl J Med 337:949, 1997.

43. RAGAZ J et al: Adjuvant radiotherapy and chemotherapy in node-positive premenopausal women with breast cancer. N Engl J Med 337:956, 1997.

44. AL-SARRAF M et al: Progress report of combined chemoradiotherapy versus radiotherapy alone in patients with esophageal cancer: An intergroup study. J Clin Oncol 15:277, 1997.

45. WALSH TN et al: A comparison of multimodality therapy and surgery for esophageal adenocarcinoma. N Engl J Med 335:509, 1996; 336:374, 376, 1997.

46. DILLMAN RO et al: Randomized trial of induction chemotherapy plus radiation therapy versus radiation alone in stage III non-small cell lung cancer (NSCLC): Five year followup of CALGB84-33 (abstract). Proc Am Soc Clin Oncol 12:329, 1993.

47. PERLOFF M et al: Combination chemotherapy with mastectomy or radiatiotherapy for stage III breast carcinoma: A cancer and leukemia group B study. J Clin Oncol 6:261, 1988.

48. HORTOBAGYI GN: Comprehensive management of locally advanced breast cancer. Cancer 66:1387, 1990.

49. UKCCCR ANAL CANCER TRIAL WORKING PARTY: Epidermoid anal cancer: Results from the UKCCCR randomized trial of radiotherapy alone versus radiotherapy, 5-fluorouracil, and mitomycin. Lancet 348:1049, 1996.

50. BARTELINK H et al: Concomitant radiotherapy and chemotherapy is superior to radiotherapy alone in treatment of locally advanced anal cancer: Results of a phase III randomized trial of the European Organization for the Research and Treatment of Cancer Radiotherapy and Gastrointestinal Cooperative Groups. J Clin Oncol 15:2040, 1997.

51. THE DEPARTMENT OF VETERANS AFFAIRS LARYNGEAL CANCER STUDY GROUP: Induction chemotherapy plus radiation compared with surgery plus radiation in patients with advanced laryngeal cancer. N Engl J Med 324:1685, 1991.

52. LEFEBVRE JL et al: Larynx preservation in pyriform sinus cancer: Preliminary results of a European Organization for Research and Treatment of Cancer phase III trial. EORTC Head and Neck Cancer Cooperative Group. J Natl Cancer Inst 88:890, 1996.

# 3D / REGIONAL CHEMOTHERAPY FOR SOLID TUMORS

*Maurizio Vaglini, Marcello Deraco, and Elisabetta Pennacchioli*

## INTRODUCTION

Restricted until recently to treatment of "off-limits" tumors, regional chemotherapies are currently used as neoadjuvant therapies for reducing to a level of conservative operability tumors that would otherwise be in need of major disfiguring or amputative surgery, or as adjuvant therapies in cancers at high risk of local recurrence or dissemination, particularly in the abdominal cavity.

At present, thanks to important studies in basic research and to the scientific rigor of physicians and scientific societies strictly devoted to locoregional therapies, these treatment modalities are more and more frequently employed. There are many prospective randomized clinical trials in this field that provide clear answers to more specific questions.

The theory supporting the use of regional chemotherapy is based on two assumptions. First, locoregionally delivered chemotherapeutic agents generate a higher drug concentration within the tumor-bearing area and thus should improve the overall response over that of systemic chemotherapy. Second, if the infused target region binds most of the agent, thus limiting systemic toxicity, the drug dose can be significantly escalated. There is evidence in the literature (von Essen et al.[1] in 1968; Koyama et al.[2] in 1975; Auersperg[3] in 1978; Mavligit et al.[4] in 1981; Stephens[5] in 1981) that in treating aggressive or large localized, malignant tumors, the best results may be achieved by first reducing the size, extent, and viability of the tumors with cytoreductive chemotherapy and then eradicating the residual disease by surgery or radiotherapy.[5] Cytoreductive chemotherapy can also be used in selected patients who may already have, or are at significant risk for developing, systemic spread. In this situation, it is appropriate to use both cytoreductive chemotherapy by locoregional approach before definitive local treatment and adjuvant systemic chemotherapy following definitive local treatment. Three criteria[6] that must be fullfilled for the regional chemotherapy to succeed are as follows:

- The disease to be treated should be confined to a given region of the body.
- In order to offer some advantage over systemic therapy, the treatment should exploit the anatomic and physiologic properties of that region.
- The therapy must be safe and effective.

## HISTORICAL REVIEW

In 1946, Gilman and Philips[7] reported that experimental animal tumors regressed after the systemic administration of a war-gas product, the nitrogen mustard ($HN_2$) compound.

In 1946, Jacobsen[8] and in 1947, Rhoads[9] demonstrated that bone marrow toxicity occurred at drug levels too low to effect more than transient tumor responses. This means that the susceptibility of normal vital organs to less than cytotoxic cancer levels continues to be the limiting factor in systemic cancer chemotherapy.

In 1950, Klopp et al.[10] and Bierman et al.[11] and, in 1953, Sullivan et al.[12] found that $HN_2$ administered interarterially had an increased tumoricidal effect with lower hematologic side effects, although the drug levels were too low to obtain prolonged, significant tumor regression.

In 1958, Creech et al.[13] and Krementz et al.[14] introduced regional perfusion to the treatment of human cancer. The technique was applied to regionally confined but extensive cancer, including carcinoma, melanoma, sarcoma, and glioblastoma. The use of an extracorporeal, oxygenated circuit was adapted to maintain and deliver chemotherapeutic agents to the isolated tumor-bearing area, obtaining high-dose tumor exposure with minimal systemic effects. Drug dosage was limited only by the local tissue tolerance. The technique was applied to a variety of tumor types, but the greatest responses were seen in the melanomas of the extremities. The operative method of regional chemotherapy opened a new field of research. The main clinical research was carried out in New Orleans by Krementz et al.[14], but, as with many techniques requiring expertise, some groups utilized the method on a casual basis and the results were unsatisfactory.

In recent years, a rebirth of interest in the method has occurred, including Koops and Oldhoff[15] in 1983, Bulman and Jamieson[16] in 1980, and Aigner et al.[17] in 1983. In 1967, Cavaliere et al.[18] reported the synergism of hyperthermia and high-dose chemotherapy in vitro. The potential role of hyperthermia has been known from antiquity. In 1866, Busch,[19] who noted the regression of a sarcoma after high fever, was the first to find heat useful in cancer treatment. In 1893, Coley[20] deliberately injected patients with bacterial toxins in order to cause fever. In the early 1900s, there were many reports on the use of applied hyperthermia in cancer, but it has been in the last two decades, that there has been an enormous increase in interest in this method.

In 1975, Stehlin and associates[21] reported the enhanced effects of chemotherapy in the presence of increased temperatures in humans. From this knowledge, hyperthermia has been introduced into most locoregional treatments. Contemporaneously, a possible role for the locoregional approach has been considered to treat neoplasms showing peritoneal dissemination. In 1955, Weissberger and associates[22] reported the results of intraperitoneal $HN_2$ treatment for seven patients with ovarian cancer. Impressive control of malignant ascites was observed. In 1980, Spratt and associates[23] reported that the clinical delivery system of intraperitoneal chemotherapy in hyperthermic conditions is an effective treatment for patients with pseudomyxoma peritonei; thus this technique has been considered safe for intracavitary treatment. Koga et al.,[24] Fujimura et al.,[25] and Fujimoto et al.[26] introduced continuous hyperthermic peritoneal perfusion (CHPP) combined with mitomycin C (MMC) as a prophylactic treatment for peritoneal recurrence after surgery for gastric cancer. Yomaguchi and associates[27] reported that CHPP is an effective treatment for colon cancer associated with peritoneal dissemination. In 1996, Deraco and associates[28] reported that dose-intensive treatments combining cytoreductive surgery and CHPP have resulted in long-term survival and that the technique is well tolerated by patients. The role of extensive surgery (peritonectomy) associated with intraperitoneal chemotherapy was emphasized by Sugarbaker[29] to treat appendiceal adenocarcinoma and pseudomyxoma peritonei.

## REGIONAL CHEMOTHERAPY AND PHARMACOKINETICS

In 1974, Eckman and associates[30] developed a mathematical model detailing the potential drug concentration advantage derived from an intraarterial infusion versus intravenous administration.[31] This model describes the advantage intraarterial drug delivery has over systemic therapy as an integral equation of concentration ($C$) multiplied by time ($T$) ($C \times T$). The regional advantage also depends on the rate of drug delivery, regional blood flow, and rate of total-body clearance. The regional drug advantage is determined by three factors: (1) regional drug extraction or metabolism, (2) regional blood flow, and (3) the total-body clearance of the drug. The efficacy of regional drug extraction, metabolism, and clearance in this model defines the advantage of regional drug delivery. There is minimal regional advantage if the infused drug is cleared more rapidly systemically than regionally. This lack of advantage is particularly true for extrahepatic intraarterial infusion. Collins[31] characterizes the therapeutic index as "the ratio of drug concentration in the tumor ($AUC_T$) [AUC = area under curve] to drug concentration in the systemic circulation ($AUC_S$). The therapeutic advantage for drug delivery, $R_d$, can be expressed as the ratio ($R$) of the therapeutic index ($d$) for intra-arterial versus the therapeutic index for intravenous (IV) administration[31] (pp 23–24)":

$$R_d = \frac{(AUC_T/AUC_S)IA}{(AUC_T/AUC_S)IV} \qquad \text{(ref. 31, pp 23–24)}$$

For that region or organ that metabolizes and clears the infused drug, the therapeutic advantage is increased proportionally to the regional drug clearance. The $R_d$ also depends on the fraction of drug $E$ removed during a single pass through the target tissue:

$$R_d = \frac{Cl_{TB}}{Q(1 - E)} + 1$$

For a region not metabolizing or clearing the infused agent, the $R_d$ is a function of the regional blood flow ($Q_i$) and total-body clearance ($Cl_{TB}$):

$$R_d = \frac{Cl_{TB}}{Q_i} + 1$$

Chemotherapeutic agents rapidly cleared systemically, such as 5-fluorouracil (5-FU), may allow some regional benefit when the drug is delivered as a continuous regional infusion.

## REGIONAL DRUG SCHEDULING, DOSE, AND DRUGS

Most chemotherapeutic agents have essentially the same antineoplastic activity, whether they are administered as a single bolus dose once a month, a weekly dose, or a prolonged infusion. However, it is important to remember that their antineoplastic activity and acute toxicity correspond to the integral equation of concentration-time product ($C \times T$) or the area under the curve (AUC) rather than the peak plasma concentration $C_{max}$ achieved following bolus administration.[32,33] Both the antitumor effect and the toxicity are directly proportional to the AUC. However, the antitumor effect is determined more by the $C_{max}$ and by the time this concentration is maintained above a certain tumor cytotoxic threshold. Also, increasing the delivered drug dose does not significantly produce an increase in the peak dose $C_{max}$, but usually increases only the half-life of the terminal phase.[34] It is the AUC of the terminal phase that contributes most to the toxicity of a particular chemotherapeutic agent.

The alkylating agents nitrogen mustard, melphalan, and the nitrosoureas, plus the antitumor antibiotics MMC, dacarbazine, and cisplatin, have commonly been used in most regional chemotherapy systems.[35,36] These drugs interact rapidly with the DNA, tend not to be cell cycle dependent, and are primarily *concentration dependent* for their cytotoxic effect. On the other hand, antimetabolites such as floxuridine (FUDR), 5-FU, and methotrexate are *time dependent* and require a prolonged exposure time for their antitumor effect. Theoretically, tumor cytotoxicity can be better facilitated by significantly increasing the regional drug peak concentration rather than by increasing the time exposure of a tumor-bearing region to a chemotherapeutic agent.[37] The anthracyclines and anthracenes are primarily concentration-dependent cytocidal drugs having some time dependence.[37]

Therefore, the appropriate agents and schedule to use in regional chemotherapy would be alkylating agents or antitumor antibiotics in a high-dose, short-term infusion of approximately 1 to 2 hours. Thus, this type of scheduling generates within the regional capillary network a maximal plasma level or $C_{max}$ of drug capable of producing the appropriate intratumor drug levels.

The following are the main procedures for delivering regional chemotherapy:

- Continuous infusion of drugs intraarterially in a selected region.
- Locoregional perfusion with extracorporeal circulation.

The purpose of intraarterial chemotherapy is to achieve a clinico-pathologic improvement of the primary lesion, therefore permitting a more conservative surgical approach. The systemic drug circulation derived from the nonextracted drug is expected to control or prevent possible distant micrometastases.

The rationale behind locoregional perfusion with extracorporeal circulation (ECC) is to attempt to cure a tumor without the need to use salvage surgery. The low potential of systemic activity is related to the low leakage rate.

## INTRAARTERIAL CHEMOTHERAPY

In 1950, the first reports of intraarterial chemotherapy using nitrogen mustard were published simultaneously by Klopp and associates[10] and by Bierman and associates.[11] The theoretical basis of regional chemotherapy has remained essentially unchanged since then. The hypotheses are as follows: (1) that this technique can deliver a high concentration of the antitumor agent to localized cancers and hence produce a higher response rate than with systemic administration; and (2) that a significant amount of the drug will be removed after the first pass through the capillary bed of the target region and thus reduce the systemic drug availability and toxicity generated.

Data from in vitro tissue culture assays show that gastrointestinal tract malignancies are usually resistant to the systemic dosages of most chemotherapeutic agents.[38] Also, selection of those tumors with minimal sensitivity to systemic chemotherapy might benefit from an incremental increase in a locally delivered drug dose. This is particularly true since most chemotherapeutic agents have a very steep dose-response curve.

The advantage in delivering drugs regionally by intraarterial infusion depends on the size of the artery infused; the rate of excretion of the agents used; the amount of the agent entering the tissues, especially from the first circulation; and the amount of the agent entering the tissues that is biologically active against tumor cells. If the drug or the combination of drugs[5] is infused through an artery supplying a small area of tissues, the initial concentration of drug in the region will be higher than if a large artery supplying a large area of tissues is infused. The lower the blood flow through the artery infused, the greater will be the initial concentration of drug in the regional tissues. In clinical practice, the smallest appropriate regional artery is selected for infusion. The more rapidly the agents are excreted after they have entered the systemic circulation, the greater will be the relative effect of the initial pass through the arterial bed of the tumor.

Another important factor is the amount of drug infused that enters the tumor and reenters the venous and lymphatic circulation unchanged. It seems that this does not affect the end result, other than by allowing more time for the drug to act chemically on susceptible cells.

### LIMITATIONS OF INTRAARTERIAL CHEMOTHERAPY

Since total-body clearance $Cl_{TB}$ is inversely proportional to AUC and principally to the toxicity of a chemotherapeutic agent, the rapidity of the clearance determines the usefulness of regional drug infusion:

$$Cl_{TB} = \text{drug dose}/\text{AUC}$$

The antimetabolite FUDR used in treating hepatic metastases from colon cancer is the only situation where a chemotherapeutic agent has a truly worthwhile regional advantage. This agent has a hepatic extraction ratio of approximately 92%; therefore, the hepatic tumor drug exposure can be increased 100- to 400-fold.[39] However, 5-FU, doxorubicin, MMC, the nitrosoureas, and cisplatin are not as effectively cleared by the liver. In addition, because of the high regional blood flow (~1450 mL/min) within the liver, the tumor uptake of these agents is modest and their effectiveness on tumor response is minimal.[40] The regional pharmacokinetics of MMC, doxorubicin, and 5-FU show that during a hepatic artery infusion, the extraction ratios were only 23% to 50%. At best, the hepatic exposure is increased only 5- to 10-fold.[39,41–43] Thus, most chemotherapeutic agents do not have a realistic regional therapeutic advantage, even in treating hepatic colorectal metastases or, for that matter, pancreatic cancer.

Another problem is evident after analyzing the pharmacokinetics of intraarterial doxorubicin. Studies with intraarterial doxorubicin show that the hepatic clearance or detoxifying mechanism becomes saturated at higher drug levels.[44] Thus, using higher doxorubicin doses, the hepatic extraction fraction decreased from 0.33 to 0.22 in a rat isolation perfusion model.[45] Also, in patients with liver metastases, there can be a tremendous variation in hepatic doxorubicin clearance, and in one study the hepatic extraction ratio ranged from a low of 0.05 to 0.5, a more normal extraction fraction.[42] The therapeutic advantage of regional drug delivery for extrahepatic sites is not well defined. Thus, for the pancreas, the major portion of the infused drug dose will be cleared systemically. Systemic toxicity then remains the main dose-limiting factor. However, the venous effluent following a pancreatic, celiac infusion passes mainly through the portal system of the liver. The total-body clearance of the drugs used—5-FU, MMC, cisplatin, doxorubicin, and mitoxantrone—will be only partly dependent on the first pass, hepatic extraction, and metabolism. However, the hepatic extraction will never be enough to create a regional therapeutic advantage.

The question of the actual concentration of drug delivered to a target area represents another notable problem with regional chemotherapy. The regional drug dose is increased by intraarterial delivery only by 1 to $1\frac{1}{2}$ times that of systemic drug delivery. The initial experience in treating pancreatic cancer with regional chemotherapy produced no difference in survival over that of systemic chemotherapy.[46,47] Even though tumor response to the small increment in delivered dose is significantly better, the survival advantage for patients with pancreatic or gastrointestinal tract malignancies remains minimal.[45–48] In fact, tissue culture data show that significant improvement in response for most gastrointestinal malignancies comes only after increasing the drug dose 5 to 10 times above the systemic peak plasma concentration of the drug.[49,50]

With current techniques, regional chemotherapy increases the regional drug delivery at most by two to three times that following systemic administration.[43,51] Thus, the regional advantage does not increase drug delivery significantly enough to overcome the tumor cell resistance stemming from the P-170 drug efflux enzyme system. To be effective, 5-FU should be escalated more than 10 times the normal systemic peak plasma concentration. MMC, doxorubicin, mitoxantrone, and cisplatin only produce increased response rates of gastrointestinal tract malignancies in vitro when the plasma dose is increased from 1 mg/mL to 10 mg/mL.[49,52] Likewise, gemcitabine demonstrates only a modest in vitro activity against sensitive, human tumor cell lines after increasing the dosage from 1 mg/mL to 10 mg/mL, but resistant cell lines require that the drug dose be escalated up to 100 mg/mL.[53]

## INTRAARTERIAL INFUSION CHEMOTHERAPY FOR SOFT TISSUE SARCOMAS

Intraarterial infusion chemotherapy combines two procedures, each effective by itself: intraarterial administration and slow continuous infusion. It was in the early 1980s when some experiences suggested that preoperative intraarterial chemotherapy could improve the management of soft tissue sarcomas.[54,55,56,57] Despite the hopeful intent of neoadjuvant treatment and some encouraging reports, results are still controversial. Azzarelli and co-workers[58] employed higher doses of chemotherapy (Adriamycin (or doxorubicin) 100 mg/m$^2$ per cycle) for a longer time (200 hr) compared to previous reports (Eilber and co-workers[59] in 1988). The clinical parameter of response was highly predictive of survival: 63% versus 36% survival in the group of responders and nonresponders, respectively, whereas the pathologic parameter of response was not so predictive (Table 3D-1, Fig. 3D-1).

*TECHNIQUE.* Intraarterial infusion is performed through a catheter placed in the artery that supplies the area of the tumor.[60] The catheter is usually placed at the time of diagnostic angiography. The drug delivered intraarterially should have the following: (1) specific tropism to the tumor under treatment; (2) direct activity without the necessity of metabolic transformation; (3) easy clearance toward the interstitial space, even at low plasma concentration; (4) early catabolism or excretion by liver or kidney; and (5) good stability. In the management of soft tissue sarcomas, doxorubicin is the drug of choice. Clinical and experimental studies

**TABLE 3D-1.** INTRA-ARTERIAL INDUCTION CHEMOTHERAPY FOR SOFT TISSUE SARCOMAS: CLINICAL RESPONSE BY HISTOLOGY

| HISTOTYPE | CLINICAL RESPONSE | NO. CASES: RESPONDERS/TOTAL |
|---|---|---|
| Malignant fibrous histiocytoma | 26% | 6/23 |
| High-grade liposarcoma | 69% | 9/13 |
| Synovial sarcoma | 40% | 4/10 |
| Malignant schwannoma | 44% | 4/9 |
| Low-grade liposarcoma | 62% | 5/8 |
| Leiomyosarcoma | 29% | 2/7 |
| Unclassified sarcoma | 71% | 5/7 |
| Clear cell sarcoma | 100% | 4/4 |
| Others | 27% | 3/11 |
| Total | 46% | 42/92 |

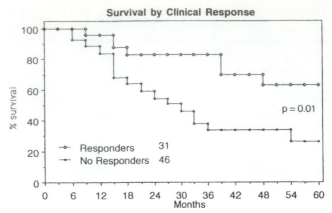

**FIGURE 3D-1.** Intraarterial induction chemotherapy for soft tissue sarcomas.

have confirmed its enhanced tissue concentration, tumor uptake, and improved effect by intraarterial administration.[60] Moreover, it improves tumor cell sensitivity to radiation therapy. The drug is administered as slow, continuous infusion, the infusional flow being controlled by an external electric pump. Infusional therapy can be repeated many times, at the classic interval of 3 to 4 weeks.

## LOCOREGIONAL PERFUSION WITH EXTRACORPOREAL CIRCULATION (ECC)

With regional intraarterial chemotherapy, the maximum regional drug escalation is only onefold to twofold over that of systemic chemotherapy. For most solid tumors, the predicted improvement in response and survival has not materialized.

Locoregional perfusion employs a system in which the tumor-bearing region is isolated and connected to a heart-lung perfusion pump (Fig. 3D-2).[35] With this regional chemotherapy system, regional drug delivery can be escalated 6 to 10 times that of a systemic dose. Regional perfusion effectively controls locoregional metastatic malignant melanoma, which is normally resistant to the entire spectrum of systemic chemotherapeutic agents.[35,61] In combination with surgery, in terms of resectability, local control rates, and aesthetic-functional results, it is also considered the most active treatment for advanced limb sarcomas.

By using ECC, physicians have learned that first the locoregional drug dose needs to be increased to approximately 5 to 10 times that of the systemic dose in order to induce a complete response (CR) or a significant partial response (PR). Second, to improve the long-term survival of patients with an advanced cancer, the tumor and tumor-bearing tissues should be surgically resected following regional chemotherapy. An important point to consider is that locoregional perfusion allows the option of exposing the tumor to hypoxia or hyperoxia and to hyperthermia. The resulting advantages[35] of regional perfusion can be summarized as follows:

1. Depending on the perfusion site, drug concentration in the isolated area is calculated to be increased 6 to 10 times that attained by systemic administration.

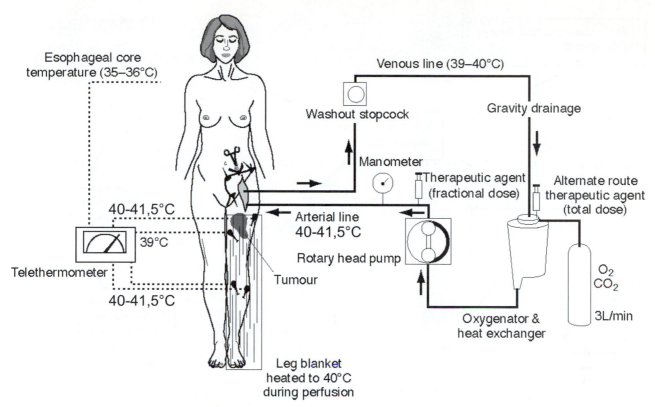

**FIGURE 3D-2.** Scheme of isolated limb perfusion.

2. Perfusion of the regional tissues is thorough and complete.
3. The use of a bubble oxygenator causes an increased $Po_2$ value, which, in effect, creates a hyperbaric chamber in the perfused area. Elevating $Po_2$ potentiates the action of alkylating agents and produces a direct tumoricidal effect by increasing the $Po_2$ level on tumor tissue. On the other hand, hypoxia increases the tumoricidal effects of such drugs as MMC and doxorubicin.
4. Heat increases the chemical activity of the alkylating agents; however, at temperatures higher than 42°C, the chemotherapeutic agents are rapidly hydrolyzed and tissue toxicity is increased. Higher temperatures increase cell metabolism and the absorption and activity of the drug as well.
5. Heparin has an antimetastatic effect, inhibiting the adhesion of tumor cells to vessel walls and their penetration into tissues to establish growth.
6. Isolation of the treated area decreases systemic toxicity and protects host immune resistance to tumor cells.
7. Wash-out of the unbound agent and toxic end products decreases systemic toxicity and regional postoperative complications.
8. Clinical observations suggest that the destruction of cancer cells in vivo initiates an autoimmunization process.
9. Patients who receive perfusion respond satisfactorily to a more conservative surgical procedure than is required when surgery is the only treatment used.

If we consider melanoma, the clinical evaluation of local recurrences and of in-transit or lymph node metastasis fails to detect regional microscopic disease, which is frequently present.[62] This explains the relative ineffectiveness of surgery in the control of locoregional disease. In clinical practice, it has been confirmed that, in these situations, perfusion is the treatment of choice for the following reasons:

• Perfusion involves the entire tumor-bearing area.
• Isolating the target area from systemic circulation allows the administration of higher dosages of antineoplastic drugs without serious side effects.
• The continuous recirculation of drugs for the duration of perfusion provides greater drug uptake by the tumor.
• High doses of drugs require lower activation energy (41.5 to 41.8°C for 90 to 120 min) to obtain an isoeffect.

## ENHANCEMENT OF LOCOREGIONAL CHEMOTHERAPY ACTIVITY IN ECC

**ENHANCEMENT BY HYPERTHERMIA.** Malignant cells appear to be selectively sensitive to thermal injury. The precise mechanism of cell death after heat exposure has not been established, but the phenomenon has been demonstrated by both in vitro and in vivo techniques. In 1989, Storm[63] reported that hyperthermia may be the most potent chemotherapeutic drug sensitizer. He showed that heat interacts synergistically with a variety of antineoplastic agents, which means that a combination of heat and antineoplastic

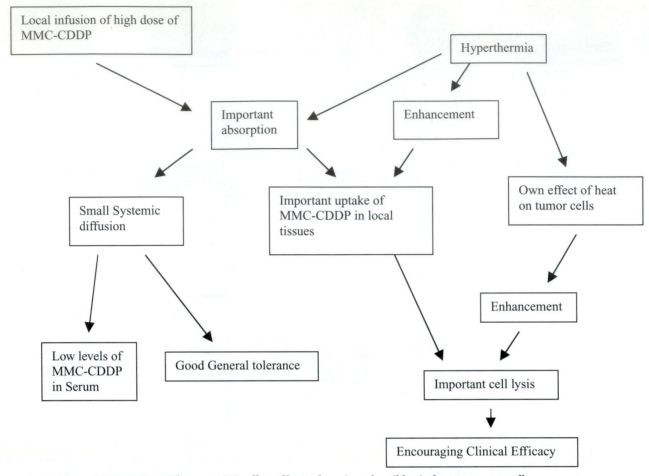

**FIGURE 3D-3.** The synergistic effect of hyperthermia and antiblastic drugs on tumor cells.

drugs frequently results in increased cytotoxicity over that predicted for an additive effect (Fig. 3D-3). However, each drug may be affected differently.[63] Hyperthermia may also overcome certain forms of drug resistance by several mechanisms, such as by the increase of cell uptake (membrane permeability), the inhibition of repair mechanisms (DNA-polymerase injury), and the temperature-dependent increases in drug action. The advantages[64] of hyperthermia are as follows: (1) synergy with chemotherapeutic drugs and ionizing radiation, (2) low host toxicity, (3) ease of control, and (4) low resistance. At temperatures from 39 to 43°C, the rate of cell inactivation is nearly linear with thiotepa, the nitrosoureas, and cisplatin. Other drugs do not follow this rule. Doxorubicin, for example, requires temperatures of 42 to 43°C before significant synergism occurs. Moreover, the drugs of choice at physiologic temperatures may not be the drugs of choice at elevated temperatures, and the drug concentration in the target tissues must be high for sufficient thermal enhancement.

Upon heating,[65] the intratumor environment becomes acidic, hypoxic, and nutritionally deprived due to vascular damage. Such a suboptimal environment in the heated tumors potentiates the response of tumor cells to hyperthermia, inhibits the repair of ther-

mal damage, and also interferes with the development of thermal tolerance. The acidic environment also potentiates the response of tumor cells to certain drugs at elevated temperatures. Clinical trials of thermochemotherapy have employed various heating methods, including local heating, hyperthermic locoregional perfusion, and whole-body hyperthermia.

**ENHANCEMENT BY HYPOXIA.** Solid tumors always present areas that are hypoperfused. Hypoxia produces some alterations in cells, that is, a reduced capacity for repair of metabolic changes. A hypoxic cell is unable to maintain a stable pH; this increases the permeability of cell membrane so that antineoplastic agents can easily move through the membrane, improving the global concentration of the drug both inside and outside the cell. Based on experimental studies that evaluated the responsiveness of tumor cells under aerobic and hypoxic conditions, Teicher and co-workers[66] classified chemotherapeutic agents in three groups:

1. Preferentially toxic in aerobic conditions (bleomycin, procarbazine, streptonigril, actinomycin D, vincristine, and melphalan).

2. Preferentially toxic under hypoxic conditions (MMC and adriamycin).
3. No major preferential toxicity to oxygenation (*cis*-diamine dichloroplatinum, 5-FU, and methotrexate).

The hypoxic condition can be created during locoregional perfusion, achieving improved efficacy for drugs potentiated by low oxygen concentration. This condition, which occurs through hypoxic infusion or perfusion with stop-flow technique, is an area of growing interest, that is, the combination of hypoxia and hyperthermia in the classic isolated limb perfusion (ILP).

## ISOLATED LIMB PERFUSION

Isolated limb perfusion (ILP) was introduced for the treatment of patients with melanoma by Creech and co-workers[13] in 1957. ILP[67] with high-dose melphalan currently produces complete responses in approximately 55% of patients with locoregional recurrent disease. The toxicity of the procedure is primarily regional and consists of edema, skin erythema, and blistering, as well as rare neuropathies or vascular complications, and is generally classified by the Wieberling method.[68] Systemic toxicity is limited, consisting of immediate postoperative nausea and vomiting and sometimes transient bone marrow depression, often caused by a high leakage rate. The addition of tumor necrosis factor α (TNFα), at doses up to 10 times the MDT, with or without interferon γ (IFNγ), allows high response rates (>80%) for locally advanced soft tissue sarcomas (Fig. 3D-4).

*TECHNIQUE.* Depending on the location of the tumor, ILP can be carried out at several different levels. The options for the upper limb are the subclavian, axillary, and brachial arteries, while in the lower limb, the external iliac, common femoral, and popliteal arteries are used (Fig. 3D-5). The perfusion level is chosen to achieve the smallest perfusion volume around the tumor, since this is related to lower morbidity. Other factors to consider when choosing the perfusion level are the size and grade of the tumor and whether it is primary or recurrent. An important point in performing the perfusion is to minimize leakage of the chemotherapeutic agents into the systemic circulation. This requires ligation or occlusion of collateral vessels, as well as the application of a tourniquet at the root of the limb. In order to prevent external heat loss, the limb is wrapped in a sterile-water-circulation thermal blanket. During the procedure, the limb temperature is monitored by thermistors inserted through the skin into the subcutaneous tissues and muscles. Once the vessels are prepared and the bandages and limb root tourniquet are in place, the limb can be connected to the extracorporeal limb perfusion circuit using appropriate catheters (Fig. 3D-6). The flow is adjusted to a rate of 35 to 40 mL/L of limb volume per minute. At low flow, it is important to ensure that the fluid level in the oxygenator reservoir remains stable and that the oxygen saturation remains above 60%. The perfusion pressure should not be more than 15 mmHg below mean systemic arterial pressure. Good flow rates are important for several reasons, including better tissue perfusion, lower drug toxicity, and better tissue temperature regulation.

During perfusion, several parameters are continuously monitored in the extracorporeal circuit. These are line pressure, arterial and venous oxygen saturation, level of the oxygenator reservoir, arterial and venous blood temperature, and subcutaneous and intramuscular temperature. Optimal parameters to be considered are the tumor oxygen concentration (partial tissue $O_2$) and the tumor blood flow.

The perfusion technique requires a bubble oxygenator along with a blood-heat exchanger, a heart-lung pump, and a circuit. The perfusion catheter is chosen according to the diameter of the vessels (range, 14 to 24 F). Priming consists of 500 mL of a saline solution (Normosol R, pH 7.4) plus 250 mL of Emagel. Perfusate flow is maintained as high and as stable as possible (range, 150 to 750 mL/min). The temperature within the tumor is maintained between 38 and 41.5°C. The drug injection depends on the treatment schedule. At the National Cancer Institute NCI of Milan, melphalan (range, 50 to 100 mg) in true hyperthermic condition (41.5°C) is used for stage III melanoma patients. The drug is injected at 41°C, and the perfusion is carried out for 60 min. With regard to sarcoma patients, TNFα is infused when the temperature at the arterial level is 38.5°C. Melphalan (50 to 100 mg) or doxorubicin (0.7 to 1.4 mg/m²) is infused in the circuit 30 min later. Perfusion lasts 90 min from the time of infusion of TNF and the temperature is maintained at 40 to 41°C. At the end of ILP, the limb is washed with aprotinin and 3.000 to 5.000 mL of saline solution for 5 to 7 min. Finally, the vessels are sutured. Blood gas values, priming, and hematochemical control are evaluated by means of serial measurements of blood samples taken at fixed intervals from the two compartments (circuit and systemic). Hemodynamic values can be measured by means of an inserted Swan-Ganz catheter. Blood pressure, ECG, urine output,

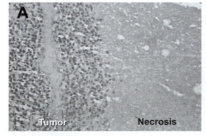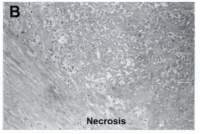

**FIGURE 3D-4.** *A.* Limb sarcoma: partial response. *B.* Limb sarcoma: complete response after isolated limb perfusion. (See also Plate 6.)

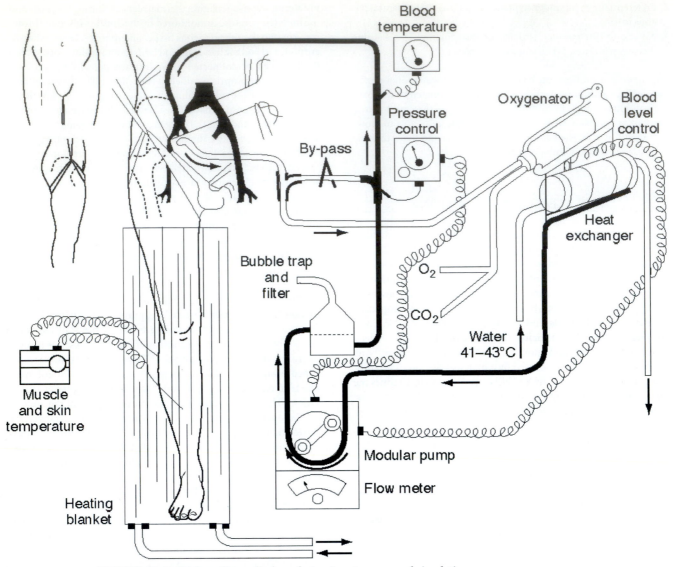

**FIGURE 3D-5.** Design of lower limb perfusion in extracorporeal circulation.

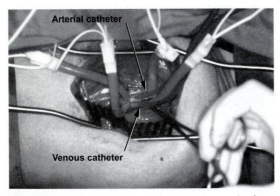

**FIGURE 3D-6.** Isolated limb perfusion: approach from the femoral vessels. (See also Plate 7.)

venous and pulmonary pressure, as well as arterial wedge pressure, can be checked at standard intervals during the procedure and for at least 2 days after ILP. Continuous leakage monitoring is carried out in patients receiving TNFα by a nuclear medicine procedure.

The therapeutic efficacy of ILP for the treatment of locally recurrent melanoma and in-transit metastasis is well established, as well for nonresectable limb sarcoma. ILP has undoubtedly led to improved survival and better results (Fig. 3D-7) than those achieved with chemotherapy (however administered: systemic, intraarterial infusion, normothermic antineoplastic perfusion), radiotherapy, and immunotherapy.

Table 3D-2 summarizes results from literature obtained in melanoma patients treated by ILP. The different characteristics of the patients (number of lesions, node involvement, and relapse status) and the treatment employed (level of tumor temperature and drug

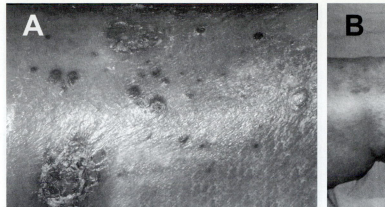
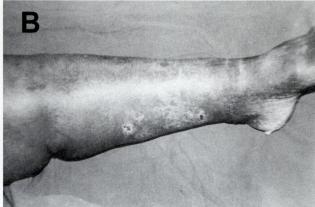

**FIGURE 3D-7.** Stage III melanoma: *A.* before isolated limb perfusion; *B.* after isolated limb perfusion. (See also Plate 8.)

dosage) provide a plausible explanation for the heterogeneous results obtained.

With regard to sarcoma patients, despite the multidisciplinary approach to the primary tumor, the incidence of local recurrence is very high. In fact, 24% to 60% of patients who undergo surgery for primary sarcomas of the limbs develop local recurrence. If this event is not associated with distant metastases, radical surgery, such as amputation or disarticulation, is the treatment advocated by

**TABLE 3D-2.** LIMB SARCOMA TREATED BY ISOLATED LIMB PERFUSION: RESULTS FROM LITERATURE

| AUTHORS | NO. OF PATIENTS | DRUG | TEMPERATURE | PR* (%) | CR* (%) | NC* (%) | PD* (%) | LIMB SALVAGE AT 2 YR(%) | MEDIAN DISEASE-FREE SURVIVAL | MEDIAN OVERALL SURVIVAL |
|---|---|---|---|---|---|---|---|---|---|---|
| Santinami (Dec. 96) | 10 | TNF (2–4 mg) Melphalan (50–100 mg) | 40–40.5°C | 2/10 | 7/10 | | | | | |
| Di Filippo (Sept. 99) | 18 | TNF (>1 mg)+ Doxorubicin | 41°C | | | | | | | |
| | | Doxorubicin (0.2–0.7 mg/kg, upper limb) | 40.5°C | 63.1 | 27.7 | 9.2 | — | | | |
| Rossi, Vaglini, & Di Filippo | 67 | Doxorubicin (0.5–1.4 mg/kg, lower limb) | 40.5–42°C | | | | | | 16.03 mo. | |
| | | TNF 0.5–3.3 mg + Doxorubicin 0.7–1.4 mg/kg | 40.5–41.8°C | | | | | | | 36.3 mo. |
| Eggermont ('96) | 186 | TNF + melphalan | 39–40°C | 57 | 18 | 22 | 3% | 82 | | |
| Olieman | 34 | TNF + IFN + melphalan | | | | | | 85 | | |
| Eggermont '96 (*J. Clin Oncology*) | | IFN + TNF + melphalan | | 64 | 18 | 10 | — | 84 | | |

*PR = partial response; CR = complete response; NC = no change; PD = progression of disease

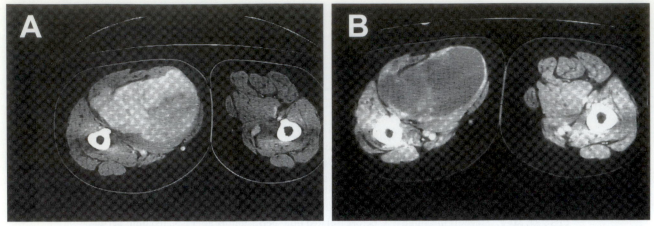

**FIGURE 3D-8.** *A.* Sarcoma of the limb; *B.* complete response after isolated limb perfusion with TNFα and adriamycin.

many authors. It is clear from the literature that patients who develop a local recurrence of high-grade sarcoma have an extremely poor survival rate due to evident or microscopic distant metastases. Consequently, it is questionable whether an extensive surgery such as amputation or disarticulation is indicated in patients at high risk of distant metastases and a poor survival, while a locoregional approach can provide an optimal local control (Fig. 3D-8).

Table 3D-3 summarizes the literature on results obtained in patients with nonresectable limb sarcoma treated by ILP.

## ISOLATED PELVIC PERFUSION

Intraarterial infusion has been used for palliation of pelvic tumors, achieving one to two times the local drug concentration attainable with intravenous dosing and resulting in a 20% to 75% palliation rate and a 20% to 31% objective response rate.[69] Isolated

pelvic perfusion has a potential therapeutic advantage over intraarterial infusion through a much higher drug concentration in the regional tissues achieved in an isolated system. This technique was first described by Creech and co-workers[13] in 1959. Based on the experience with regional perfusion of the extremities, Guadagni[79] applied antineoplastic hyperthermic pelvic perfusion for advanced rectal cancer. The drugs used in the isolated pelvic perfusion derived from protocols known to be effective in recurrent malignant neoplasms. 5-FU is an ideal agent in this incomplete vascular isolation, because it is the most effective agent against adenocarcinomas and squamous cell carcinoma of the gastrointestinal tract and is capable of rapid systemic metabolism. MMC is a potent cytotoxic agent against many malignant neoplasms and is increasingly cytotoxic in a hypoxic environment, attributes which are advantageous for this perfusion system. The technique has achieved local control of advanced and recurrent rectal cancer and has improved the quality of life. Dacarbazine and cisplatin are two of the most active agents in the treatment of metastatic melanoma,

**TABLE 3D-3.** MELANOMA OF LIMB TREATED BY ISOLATED LIMB PERFUSION: RESULTS FROM LITERATURE

| AUTHORS | YEAR | NO. OF PATIENTS | DRUG | OVERALL RESPONSE (%) | 5-YR SURVIVAL (%) | | | 10-YR SURVIVAL (%) | | |
|---|---|---|---|---|---|---|---|---|---|---|
| | | | | | II* | IIIA | IIIAB | II* | IIIA | IIIAB |
| Krementz | 1985 | 182 | Melphalan | | 64 | 35 | 31 | 58 | 28 | 28 |
| Shiu | 1986 | 18 | Nitrogen mustard | | — | 50 | 38 | — | — | — |
| Cavaliere | 1987 | 65 | Melphalan | | 80 | 56 | 33 | — | — | — |
| Hartley & Fletcher | 1988 | 39 | Melphalan | | 58 | | 29 | 44 | | 29 |
| Stehlin | 1988 | 117 | Melphalan | | 75 | 70 | 36 | — | 50 | 23 |
| Hoekstra | 1989 | 110 | Melphalan | | 74 | 67 | 40 | 63 | 45 | 34 |
| Cavaliere | 1994 | 287 | Melphalan | 84.2 | — | 53.7 | 2.07 | — | 53.7 | 20.7 |
| Vaglini | 1994 | 100 | Melphalan | 88.9 | — | 45.7 | 32.9 | — | 26.1 | 18.8 |
| Fletcher | 1994 | 21 | Cisplatin | — | | 47 | | — | | |
| Liénart & Lejeune | 1994 | 53 | TNFα + melphalan + IFNγ | 100 | | | | — | | |
| Vaglini | 1994 | 22 | TNFα + melphalan + IFNγ | 77 | | | | — | | |

* II, IIIA, and IIIAB refer to cancer stages.

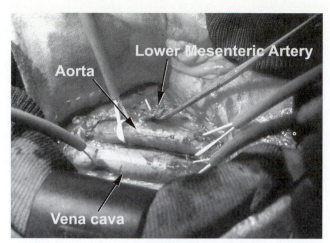

**FIGURE 3D-9.** The aorta, anterior mesenteric artery, and vena cava are dissected before cannulation. (See also Plate 9.)

and their use in hyperthermic isolated perfusion has been well documented.

*TECHNIQUE.* After anesthesia, a three-way catheter is positioned in the bladder to cool the bladder surface during hyperthermic perfusion. An inflatable sleeve is placed on each thigh to occlude the femoral vessels and is inflated to a pressure of about 200 to 300 mgHg at the beginning of hyperthermic perfusion. The vena cava and aorta are isolated by a 6- to 8-cm midline, subumbilical abdominal incision (Fig. 3D-9) above the bifurcation; all collateral branches of these vessels are isolated and dissected. The two vessels are clamped just above the inferior mesenteric artery. Two 41-cm-long catheters are inserted into the vena cava and aorta through a small incision. Catheter diameter (14 to 24 F) is selected according to vessel caliber. The venous catheter is placed in the vena cava. The end of the arterial catheter is positioned to allow perfusion of the tumor, also taking into consideration the anatomy of the vascular supply to the pelvis (aorta, iliac, and hypogastric). One catheter is connected to the venous line and the other to the arterial line of the extracorporeal circuit (Fig. 3D-10). The circuit consists of polyvinyl chloride tubes with an inner diameter of 0.95 cm for the venous line and 0.64 cm for the arterial line. The circuit includes a bubble oxygenator, a rotating pump, and a water-heat exchanger. The circuit is filled with a constant volume (750 to 1000 mL) of a liquid, which includes saline solution (500 to 700 mL) and 250 mL of plasma expander (Emagel). Heparin, at a total dose of 5000 U/L, is routinely added. The flow rate in the perfusion circuit, measured by a transducer placed in the arterial line, is kept at 250 to 400 mL/min. Local temperature is maintained at 39.5 to 40.5°C and is monitored by thermistor needles placed at different points of the pelvis (uterus, parametrium, presacral space, tumor). Drugs are added to the circuit when a tumor temperature of 39.5°C is reached. Real perfusion time from drug injection in the circuit is 90 min. Blood oxygenation during extracorporeal circulation is obtained

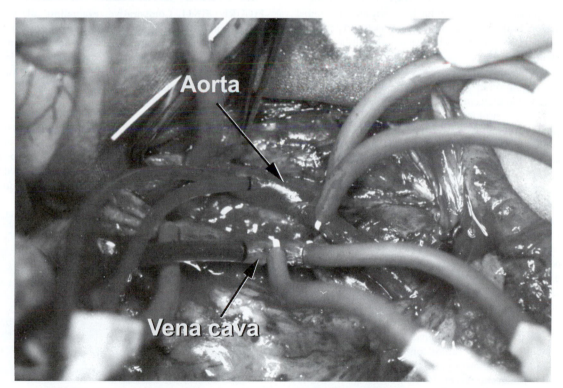

**FIGURE 3D-10.** Pelvic perfusion in extracorporeal circulation: The aorta and vena cava are cannulated.

with an $O^2$–$CO_2$ (97% and 3%, respectively) mixture. At the end of perfusion, the pelvic circuit is washed with 5 L of physiologic solution in addition to 2,000,000 IU of aprotinin to remove as much drug as possible and to antagonize bradykinin release by cell lysis. The catheters are removed and vasotomies repaired with Prolene 5-0. In selected patients, a continuous infusional pump is placed following perfusion by means of a catheter inserted in the aorta through the inferior mesenteric artery (see Fig. 3D-9). The pump used for continuous infusion is made of inert material (titanium) and weighs 250 g. Filled with a heparinized solution, the system is checked every 15 days, calibrated by radiotelemetry, and controlled by an external computer. The infusional treatment is started about 2 weeks after surgery to allow patients full recovery of their general condition and normalization of hematochemical parameters.

## LOCOREGIONAL INFUSION AND PERFUSION WITH STOP-FLOW TECHNIQUE

In 1963, Lathrop and associates[71] described a technique suitable for abdominal and pelvic perfusion using femoral cannulation and exposure of the aorta and the inferior vena cava. In a 1987 study of hyperthermic pelvic perfusion (HPP) with 5-FU, Wile and Smolin[72] reported the occlusion of the great vessels by means of balloon occlusion catheters in 11 of 27 patients with refractory pelvic cancer. In 1993, a similar technique was reported by Turk and co-workers[73] in six patients with recurrent unresectable rectal cancer who underwent perfusion with 5-FU, cisplatin, and MMC. In 1993, Aigner[74] proposed a simplified surgical technique for pelvic and abdominal hypoxic perfusion. Both occlusion of the great vessels and perfusion were done with only two catheters, which were surgically introduced through the femoral vessels.

A similar technique, using a percutaneous catheter, was later performed by Thompson et al.[75,76] in seven patients with recurrent rectal cancer who underwent perfusion with MMC and 5-FU or cisplatin. The pharmacokinetics of MMC in peripheral, portal, and aortic blood were studied by Averbach et al.[77,78] in 18 mongrel dogs under different types of major vessel occlusion. For the type of abdominal stop-flow corresponding to the methodology used in humans by Aigner,[74] the area under the curve ratios for portal blood versus systemic circulation was 2.9:1.

Recently, in a pilot study of patients with recurrent, unresectable rectal cancer, Guadagni and co-workers[79] (Fig. 3D-11) reported that pelvic perfusion performed by Aigner's technique yielded a ratio of pelvic to systemic area under the curve of MMC of 11.7:1 and a maximum pelvic MMC peak of 60 μg/mL. Evaluation of the clinical results is very difficult because of different indications, techniques of perfusion, and drug schedules used in different series. Only phase I and II clinical studies are available. The main indication for pelvic perfusion is recurrent rectal cancer.[72,73,80,81] In patients amenable to resection, 50% to 80% of the responses were reported with increased resectability, improved tumor control, and long survival[70] (Figs. 3D-12 and 13). The main indication for abdominal perfusion is advanced pancreatic cancer.[82,83] In UICC stage III and IV pancreatic carcinoma, after abdominal hypoxic perfusion, approximately 50% of patients had a measurable response, with a median survival of 10 months and a quality of life significantly improved.

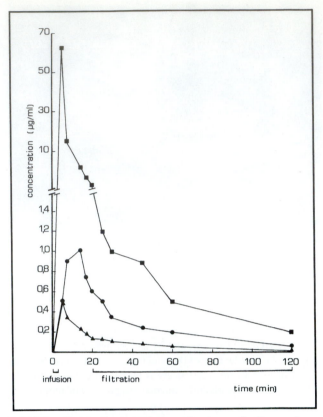

**FIGURE 3D-11.** Comparative evaluation of three plasma concentration-time profiles (caval vein blood) after three different infusions of 40 mg of MMC in an individual patient. Symbols: ■ = Intraaortic infusion with aortic and inferior caval vein stop-flow (hypoxic pelvic perfusion); ● = intraaortic infusion; ▲ = intravenous infusion.

In order to reach high regional cytostatic drug concentrations in the thoracic region, isolated thoracic perfusion has been proposed. Isolation of the chest was achieved with a coaxial stop-flow balloon catheter and a vena cava stop-flow catheter, both placed beneath the diaphragm. Both upper arms were blocked with pneumatic cuffs.[84]

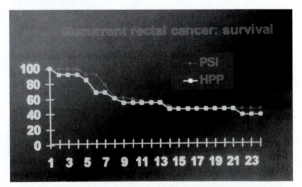

**FIGURE 3D-12.** Hypoxic pelvic perfusion (HPP): Pelvic stop-flow infusion. *(From Aigner and Keevel.[80])*

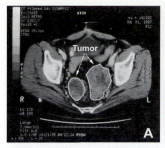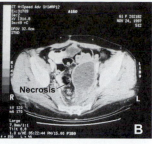

**FIGURE 3D-13.** *A.* Pelvic recurrence of ovarian cancer; *B.* complete response after hypoxic pelvic perfusion with stop-flow technique.

Pilot studies on isolated thoracic perfusion for the treatment of non-small cell lung cancer (stages IIIb and IV), lung metastases from breast cancer, and malignant lymphoma have been presented.[84–86] Preliminary results are very encouraging, and further investigations involving more patients should be carried out in the future.

*STOP-FLOW TECHNIQUE.* Hypoxic regional infusion-perfusion with stop-flow technique is carried out by both surgical and percutaneous approaches. In the surgical approach, the femoral artery and vein are exposed through a short, longitudinal incision in the groin. After systemic heparinization, stop-flow balloon catheters are introduced and positioned under radiologic control in the aorta and cava (Fig. 3D-14). The level depends on the target area. Both balloons are blocked. For isolation in the pelvis and abdominal stop-flow, pneumatic cuffs are placed on the thighs and inflated; for thoracic stop-flow, the pneumatic cuffs are positioned at the arm roots (Fig. 3D-15). For HPP, the infusion channels of the arterial and venous stop-flow catheters are connected to a saline-primed hypoxic perfusion set on a roller pump. The extracorporeal circuit also included both a hemofiltration system and a heater-cooler unit. The hypoxic perfusion circuit is maintained over 20 min (mean $22 \pm 4$ min). The temperature of the perfusate is 38.5°C. For PSI plus HPP, after occlusion of the great vessels, the drug solution is infused in the aortic catheter and left in the pelvis for 10 min. The hypoxic perfusion circuit is activated over the next 10 min to achieve a more diffuse drug distribution. Af-

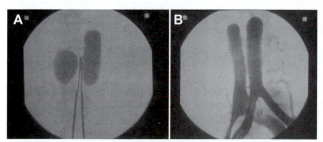

**FIGURE 3D-14.** *A.* Stop-flow balloon catheters are positioned below the renal vessels and above the aortic and vena cava bifurcation. Both balloons are inflated. *B.* Angiography of the aorta and vena cava.

ter HPP or PSI plus HPP, both catheter balloons and pneumatic cuffs are deflated and the circulation restored. The extracorporeal circuit is also used in the hemofiltration section over $80 \pm 20$ min. A polyamide hemofilter with a surface area of 2 m² is used. Thereafter, the catheters are withdrawn and the vessels are repaired.

## REGIONAL CHEMOTHERAPY PLUS HEMOFILTRATION

Hemofiltration is a technique of extracorporeal drug clearance, related in part to that of both hemodialysis and hemoperfusion. Thus, extracoporeal hemofiltration acts to artificially increase the total-body clearance through a filtration process. Used in conjunction with regional chemotherapy, this method permits the escalation of the total regional drug dose. For recapturing the peak plasma concentrations of an antineoplastic agent, hemofiltration is most effective when a steep drug gradient exists across the semipermeable membrane of the filter. Thus, through filtration, hemofiltration rapidly lowers the peak drug concentration, but it then becomes inefficient as the concentration on both sides of the filter equilibrates. Since filtration clears only the peak concentration, this technique only recaptures effectively 20% to 25% of the total drug dose.[87] With hemofiltration, the regional advantage $R_d$ is then related to $E_r$, the fraction of drug eliminated on the first pass through the tumor-bearing region; second, $E_l$, the fraction cleared by the liver, plus primarily $E_{hf}$, the fraction of drug cleared through the hemofiltration system[74]:

$$R_d = \frac{Cl_{TB}}{Q[1 - (E_r + E_l + E_{hf})]} + 1$$

## INTRAPERITONEAL CHEMOTHERAPY

In 1955, Weissberger and co-workers[22] reported the results of intraperitoneal nitrogen mustard treatment of seven patients with ovarian cancer. Impressive control of malignant ascites was observed. Unfortunately, this and other early clinical studies were unable to demonstrate any impact of intraperitoneal drug administration on response and survival in patients with intraabdominal tumor masses. Furthermore, the toxicity of the treatment was substantial. Based on these disappointing early experiences, the technique was rarely employed. In the late 1970s, Dedrick and co-workers[88] described a model based on physiologic and anatomic characteristics of the peritoneal cavity, as well as on previously reported pharmacokinetic data for some chemotherapeutic drugs, which suggested that the peritoneal cavity would be exposed to significantly more drug than the systemic circulation following direct intraperitoneal administration of the agent. In this model the tumor in the peritoneal cavity might come in contact with much higher concentrations of drug than could be achieved with systemic delivery of the same agent.

Because intraperitoneal administration of drugs relies on free-surface diffusion of the drug into tumor cells, it is critical that the drug reach the tumor within the peritoneal cavity.[89] Both experimental and clinical observations demonstrated that large treatment volumes must be employed to obtain this goal. The volumes of fluid administered should be fixed on the possibility of a multiple-day treatment program, a situation in which it is possible to develop

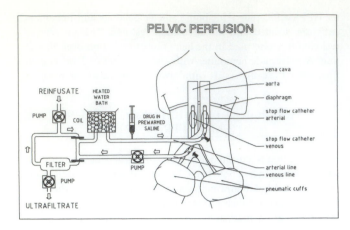

A   Scheme of hypoxic pelvic perfusion.

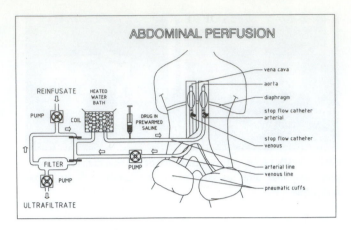

B   Scheme of hypoxic abdominal perfusion and extracorporeal circuit incorporating both hemofiltration system and heater-cooler unit.

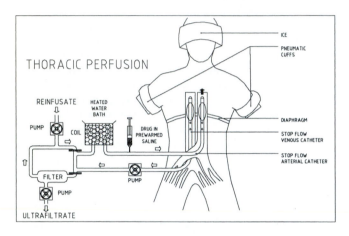

C   Scheme of isolated thoracic perfusion.

**FIGURE 3D-15.**  Scheme of locoregional perfusion with stop-flow technique.

"one-way valves" that do not permit the accidental egress of the fluid present in the cavity.

Probably the major factor determining the limitations of intraperitoneal therapy is the depth of penetration of cytotoxic agents into the tumor. This has been studied both in vitro and in vivo in experimental systems employing multiple antineoplastic agents. The conclusion has been that the direct penetration of the drugs into tissue is extremely limited, ranging from several cell layers to 1 to 3 mm from the tumor surface.[90,91] Even more important than the absolute depth of penetration of the drug into the tumor is the relative advantage for drug delivery to the tumor after intraperitoneal instillation, compared to that achieved by systemic drug administration.[89] In one experimental model with cisplatin in ovarian cancer, the relative advantage of intraperitoneal drug administration was found to be limited to 0.1 to 1 mm from the peritoneal surface. This means that the superiority of intraperitoneal cisplatin administration over intravenous delivery for ovarian cancer will be limited to those patients with very small tumor volumes when intraperitoneal treatment is initiated.

Another factor to consider is the dose-limiting toxicities of either systemic or local intraperitoneal drug administration.[89] Intraperitoneal administration of cisplatin or carboplatin results in minimal local toxicity, with systemic side effects being the limiting factor. On the other hand, intraperitoneal administration of doxorubicin or mitomycin results in minimal systemic exposure due to the dose-limiting local toxic effects of these drugs.

The major cause of the limited effectiveness of cancer chemotherapy may be the development of resistant cells. One strategy for minimizing this mechanism of treatment failure involves instituting dose-intensive regimens administered to patients with a minimum tumor burden. To reduce tumor burden, cytoreductive surgery is indicated.

In an attempt to design a treatment that would eliminate local tumor spread as a mechanism of gastrointestinal cancer recurrence, Sugarbaker and co-workers[92] performed pharmacologic studies with intraperitoneal chemotherapy early in the postoperative period. It is well known that the chemotherapeutic agents used to treat gastrointestinal cancer by an intravenous route of drug administration have response rates of 20% or less.[93] We know, however, that these

**TABLE 3D-4.** SITES OF RECURRENCE OF ABDOMINAL TUMORS

| HISTOLOGY | RESECTION SITE | PERITONEAL SITE | LIVER METASTASES | DISTANT METASTASES |
|---|---|---|---|---|
| Gastric cancer | 90 | 50 | 30 | 30 |
| Colon cancer | 60 | 50 | 50 | 20 |
| Rectal cancer | 50 | 20 | 30 | 20 |
| Sarcoma | 70 | 20 | 10 | 20 |
| Pancreatic cancer | 100 | 70 | 70 | 50 |
| Biliary tract | 70 | 50 | 50 | 20 |

drugs can be more effective if tumor cells are exposed to higher drug concentration for longer periods. The rationale is as follows:

- The resection site and abraded peritoneal surfaces are at high risk for tumor cell implantation in the postoperative period.
- If the surgeon has been careful to separate all adherent structures and if these treatments are instituted prior to the formation of new adhesions, then all intraabdominal surfaces are fully exposed to intraperitoneal chemotherapy.
- In the postoperative period the surgical techniques required for intraperitoneal drug delivery are very simple.
- Regional chemotherapy may result in increased local responses without compromising systemic effects.

*TECHNIQUE.* After surgery, using large volumes of a peritoneal dialysis solution, the abdomen is lavaged clear of blood, blood products, and tissue debris.[94] One or two liters of fluid is instilled via a Tenckhoff catheter into the peritoneal cavity. Chemotherapy instillations are then performed on postoperative days 1 and 5 or 1 and 6.

## INTRAPERITONEAL HYPERTHERMIC PERFUSION

Peritoneal carcinomatosis is the most common event in the natural history of gastrointestinal and ovarian cancer, representing the terminal stage of the disease (Table 3D-4). For a long time, it has been considered a lethal clinical entity. Recently, dose-intensive treatments combining cytoreductive surgery and intraperitoneal hyperthermic perfusion (IPHP) have resulted in long-term survival and good results. Cytoreductive surgery (CRS) means complete removal of all macroscopic tumor in the peritoneal cavity. This could require peritonectomy procedures,[95] often associated with intestinal and/or organ resections (Figs. 3D-16 and 3D-17). The present knowledge

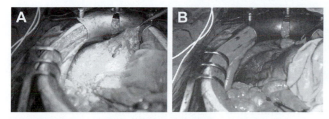

**FIGURE 3D-16.** Peritonectomy procedure: *A.* Upper right quadrant peritoneal stripping; *B.* after procedure. (See also Plate 10.)

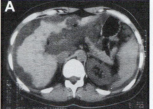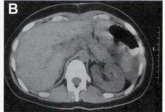

**FIGURE 3D-17.** CT scan of a patient with pseudomyxoma peritonei: *A.* Typical complete redistribution phenomenon; *B.* after complete peritonectomy.

of cell-kill kinetics with cytotoxic drugs indicates that, due to a larger proportion of cell growth fraction, micrometastases are more chemosensitive than macroscopic ones.[96,97] Even as a result of an extensive CRS or peritonectomy, free cancer cells in the peritoneal cavity could represent an ideal target for a locoregional treatment that consists of a high-dose administration of cytotoxic drugs in hyperthermic condition.

IPHP represents the natural evolution of the intraperitoneal chemotherapy that gradually developed during the last 3 decades. It has been employed by some investigators (Yonemura et al.[98], in 1991; Gilly et al.[99], in 1990; Sugarbaker et al.[100], in 1996; Deraco et al.[101], in 1996) for the treatment of peritoneal carcinomatosis. It is based on a strong scientific rationale and actually represents a fascinating area of research. The theory concerning the peritoneal plasma barrier is based on different studies[102] confirming the existing gradient between peritoneum and plasma. The barrier, represented by the submesothelial tissue and the capillary basement membrane, limits the resorption of high-molecular-weight and hydrophilic drugs, such as MMC and CDDP. The result is a longer presence of drugs in the peritoneal cavity. The hyperthermic effects on drug activity are known to be related to the following: (1) an increase in drug concentration; (2) the drug activation process; (3) intracellular alkylating index; and (4) the inhibition of the DNA repairing process. The clearance of intraperitoneal drugs is lower than of those in the plasma, which is in fact a conventional and important characteristic of a locoregional treatment. IPHP overcomes some of the common limitations of intraperitoneal chemotherapy, such as low drug penetration into tissue (no more than 1 to 3 mm in normothermic conditions) and the limited diffusion caused by postoperative adhesions and the relative local toxicity.

IPHP is an intraoperative approach that represents the synthesis of three different characteristics: the added efficacy of hyperthermia (more penetration into the tumor), the fluid dynamics of the system (better diffusion into the peritoneal cavity), and finally the mechanical filtration process (elimination of microscopic cancer residual by filter). Current indications for cytoreductive surgery and intraperitoneal chemotherapy are as follows[103]:

- Gastrointestinal cancer associated with peritoneal carcinomatosis or positive peritoneal cytology
- Perforated gastrointestinal cancer
- Peritoneal sarcomatosis
- Peritoneal mesothelioma
- Pseudomyxoma peritonei
- Peritoneal carcinomatosis from ovarian cancer
- Palliation in patients with malignant ascites

A peritoneal cancer index[103] is used to estimate the likelihood of complete cytoreduction. In the current approach to peritoneal carcinomatosis and sarcomatosis, implant size and extent of tumor distribution are the fundamental criteria for the selection of patients to treat with intraperitoneal chemotherapy.

*TECHNIQUE.* The IPHP can be performed by open abdomen technique and closed abdomen technique.

*OPEN ABDOMEN TECHNIQUE.* A self-retaining Thompson retractor is positioned, and using a running suture from the retractor's frame, the skin edges of the abdominal wound are suspended (Fig. 3D-18). Inflow line is introduced through the abdominal wound and positioned in the resection bed. Three drains are placed through separate stab wounds in the flanks and positioned between the liver and undersurface of the right hemidiaphragm, behind the spleen, and in the pelvis. These drains are secured to the skin with a purse-string suture and left in place in the postoperative period until the drainage from the peritoneal cavity subsides. The drains are connected with the extracorporeal circuit. One of two temperature probes is secured near the tip of the inflow catheter and the second in the pelvis. The wound is covered with a plastic sheet sutured to skin edges.

*CLOSED ABDOMEN TECHNIQUE.* Before closing the abdominal wall after cytoreductive surgery, four silicone catheters are placed in the abdominal cavity through the abdominal wall. Two inflow catheters are placed respectively in the right subphrenic cavity and at the deep pelvic level. Two outflow catheters are placed in the left subphrenic cavity and the superficial pelvic site (Fig. 3D-19). A continuous peritoneal monitoring of temperatures during IPHP is obtained by thermocouples placed in the abdominal cavity and subperitoneal site. After closure of the abdominal skin, the catheters are connected with the extracorporeal circuit. Once the catheters are connected with the extracorporeal circuit, using a heart-lung pump at a mean flow of 600 mL/min, a preheated solution is infused into the peritoneal cavity. The perfusate consists of Normosol R, pH 7.4 (2/3) plus Emagel (1/3). Normally, 3 to 4 L of perfusate is used for open abdomen technique and 5 to 6 L for closed abdomen technique. After achieving the true hyperthermic phase (42.5°C), the drugs are injected into the circuit inflow line. The drug regimen is chosen according to the tumor histotype and the schedule of treatment. Following perfusion, the perfusate is quickly drained and, after careful intraperitoneal observation, the abdomen closed.

POSTOPERATIVE TREATMENT. Based on reported results[24-26] that show significant changes in protein level caused by hemodilution induced by the perfusion, all patients receive preventive treatment with 10 to 20 g/day of albumin (D0 → D7) and 250 mL of fresh plasma (D0 → D3). (D0 = the day of surgery, D3 = third day after surgery, etc.) In order to prevent possible renal

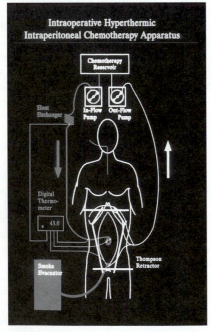

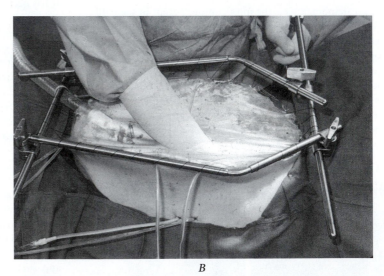

*B*

*A*

**FIGURE 3D-18.** Intraperitoneal hyperthermic perfusion: *A.* Scheme of intraperitoneal hyperthermic perfusion. *B.* Open abdomen technique (intraoperative view). (*From Sugarbaker.*[100]) (See also Plate 11.)

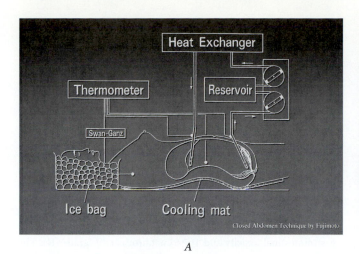
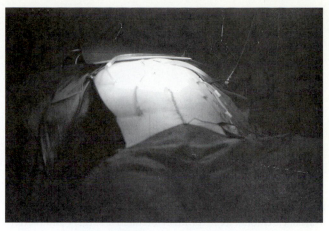

*A*                                              *B*

**FIGURE 3D-19.** Intraperitoneal hyperthermic perfusion: *A.* Scheme of intraperitoneal hyperthermic perfusion. *B.* Closed abdomen technique (intraoperative view). (*From Fujimoto.*[105]) (See also Plate 12.)

failure brought on by the high-dose administration of CDDP and MMC, all patients are treated with dopamine (3 μg/kg/min) for 72 h postoperatively and almost 3500 mL/day of IV fluids (D0 → D7).

**RESULTS OF IPHP.** Continuous hyperthermic peritoneal perfusion using CDDP and MMC combined with cytoreductive surgery was performed in 41 patients with peritoneal dissemination of gastric cancer following resection of the primary lesion.[104] According to the Japanese classification of peritoneal carcinomatosis, 25 patients had peritoneal dissemination limited to the adjacent peritoneum above the transverse colon including the greater omentum (P1) or a few to several scattered metastases in the distant peritoneum below the transverse colon (P2); 16 patients had numerous metastases to the distant peritoneum (P3). In addition to the peritoneal dissemination, 15 of the 41 patients had metastases to group 3 or 4 lymph nodes (N3,4), and 10 patients had invasion of contiguous structures (S3), such as pancreas and liver. In 7 of the 25 patients with P1 or P2 metastases, all peritoneal dissemination and lymph node metastases were removed by cytoreductive surgery in combination with gastrectomy, and all macroscopic tumor was removed (complete resection). The remaining 34 patients underwent incomplete resection. The median overall survival was 14.6 months; the 3-year survival was 28.5%. Of 14 patients who underwent a second-look operation, 7 showed a remarkable decrease in the degree of peritoneal dissemination.

In 1997, Fujimoto and co-workers[105] published the impressive results of their nonrandomized study on 48 patients submitted to aggressive surgery and IPHP using MMC alone. The 3-year and 5-year survival rates in P1, P2, and P3 patients were 41.5% and 31%, respectively (as compared to a survival rate of 0 in 18 controls submitted to surgery alone), and there was good control of the peritoneal carcinomatosis in 73% of the patients (Fig. 3D-20).

With regard to ovarian cancer, the salvage therapy has not been clearly established. The second-line chemotherapy response rate is low (22% to 37%) with a short median survival rate (43 to 61

weeks). At the NCI of Milan, for this subset of patients, it was proposed to investigate the effect of an aggressive approach consisting of surgery followed by intraperitoneal drug(s) delivery and local hyperthermia.[106] In a phase II clinical study, 27 patients with advanced and recurrent ovarian carcinoma were treated by cytoreductive surgery and intraperitoneal hyperthermic perfusion (Fig. 3D-21). Mean follow-up was 17.4 months. Patients had been surgically staged and heavily pretreated with cisplatin-based, taxol-based, or taxol/platinum–containing regimens. Complete salvage cytoreduction was achieved in 15(55%) patients, and 4 (15%) patients had residual disease < 2.5 mm. The IPHP was performed with the closed

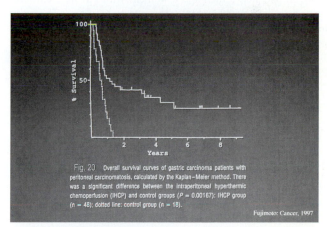

Fig. 20   Overall survival curves of gastric carcinoma patients with peritoneal carcinomatosis, calculated by the Kaplan–Meier method. There was a significant difference between the intraperitoneal hyperthermic chemoperfusion (IHCP) and control groups (P = 0.00167): IHCP group (n = 48); dotted line: control group (n = 18).

**FIGURE 3D-20.** Overall survival curves for gastric carcinoma patients with peritoneal carcinomatosis, calculated by the Kaplan-Meier method. There was a significant difference between the intraperitoneal hyperthermic chemoperfusion (IHCP) and control groups (*P* = 0.00167): IHCP group (*n* = 48), dotted line; control group (*n* = 18), continuous or solid line. (*From Fujimoto.*[105])

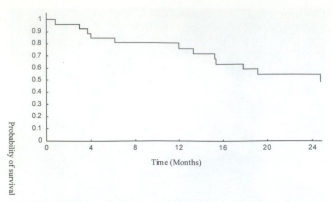

**FIGURE 3D-21.** Overall survival in 27 patients with recurrent ovarian carcinoma treated with cytoreductive surgery and IPHP.

abdomen technique, using a preheated saline perfusate containing cisplatin (25 mg/m$^2$/L) and MMC (3.3 mg/m$^2$/L) through a heart-lung pump at a mean flow of 700 mL/min for 60 min in the hyperthermic phase (42.5°C). The 2-year overall survival rate, median time to progression, and median time to local progression were 55%, 21.8 months, and 16 months, respectively. Variables that affected the overall survival rate or time to progression were residual disease, carcinomatosis extension, patient's age, and lag-time between diagnoses and treatment with CRS and IPHP. Treatment-related morbidity, mortality, and toxicity rates were 11%, 4%, and 27%, respectively.

Another area of interest for application of CRS and IPHP is the primitive peritoneal neoplasm. Peritoneal mesothelioma (PM) is a rare disease, with a poor prognosis (median survival, 4 to 12 months). At the NCI of Milan, a trial was conducted to evaluate the feasibility, morbidity, and impact on survival of patients with PM treated with CRS and IPHP (unpublished data) (Fig. 3D-22). Thirteen patients (5 men and 8 women) with PM were enrolled. The mean age was 48.5 years (range, 24 to 66 years). The mean follow-up was 12.9 months (range, 2.1 to 29.1 months). All patients had intraperitoneally disseminated disease. One (8%), 2(15%), and 10(77%) patients had benign, borderline, and malignant histotype of PM, respectively. Seven (54%) patients had previously been treated

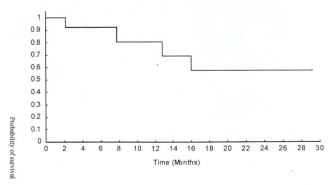

**FIGURE 3D-22.** Overall survival in 13 patients with peritoneal mesothelioma treated with cytoreductive surgery and IPHP.

with systemic chemotherapy. Five (36%), 5(36%), and 4(27%) cases, respectively, had no residual, minimal residual, and bulky residual disease after cytoreductive surgery. Due to a locoregional progression, one patient was submitted to a second procedure 1 year after the first procedure. Using a preheated saline perfusate containing cisplatin (25 mg/m$^2$/L) plus MMC (3.3 mg/m$^2$/L) or cisplatin (25 mg/m$^2$/L) plus adriamycin (7 mg/m$^2$/L) through a heart-lung pump at a mean flow rate of 600 mL/min for 60 or 90 min during the hyperthermic phase (42.5°C), the closed abdomen technique was carried out for IPHP. The two-year overall survival rate was 58%; the median progression-free survival rate was 16 months. Four patients died of disease progression, and three patients survived more than 2 years after the treatment (two with no evidence of disease (NED) and one alive with disease (AWD)). The operative morbidity rate was 20% without operative mortality. Only 3(23%) patients presented gastrointestinal toxicity and 1(7%) nephrotoxicity (grade III). The therapeutic strategy is a well-tolerated, feasible, and promising alternative in the management of selected patients with PM, which has, up to now, been considered a terminal condition without any definitive treatment.

An aggressive treatment strategy including CRS and IPHP has been advocated to treat peritoneal carcinomatosis from colon and rectal cancer.[106,107] In patients with peritoneal carcinomatosis from adenocarcinoma of the colon or appendix, the treatment is associated with a 35% morbidity rate and 5% mortality rate.[108] Extensive surgery and high intraabdominal temperature represent the major risk factors for postoperative morbidity and mortality of patients treated with this new therapeutic approach. Against the therapeutic potential, one should consider the extent of cytoreductive surgery followed by intraperitoneal hyperthermic perfusion, overall a complex procedure that requires at least a 12-hr engagement of a trained team and the support of an intensive care unit.

## REFERENCES

1. VON ESSEN CF et al: Sequential chemotherapy and radiation therapy of buccal mucosa carcinoma in South India. AJR 102:530, 1968.
2. KOYAMA H et al: Intra-arterial infusion chemotherapy of a preoperative treatment of locally advanced breast cancer. Cancer 36:1603, 1975.
3. AUERSPERG N: Intra-arterial chemotherapy and radiotherapy in locally advanced cancer of the oral cavity and oropharynx. Int J Radioat Oncol Biol Phys 4:273, 1978.
4. MAVLIGIT GM et al: Intraarterial cis-platinum for patients with inoperable skeletal tumors. Cancer 48:1, 1981.
5. STEPHENS FO: Pharmacokinetics of intra-arterial chemotherapy. Recent Results Cancer Res 86:1, 1983.
6. COIT DG: Hyperthermic isolation limb perfusion for malignant melanoma: A review. Cancer Invest 10(4):277, 1992.
7. GILMAN A, Philips FS: Biological actions and therapeutic application of β-chloroethyl amines and sulfides. Science 103:409, 1946.
8. JACOBSON LO et al: Nitrogen mustard therapy: Studies on the effect of methyl-bis (beta-chloroethyl) amine hydrochloride on neoplastic disease and allied disorders of hemopoietic system. JAMA 132:263, 1946.

9. Rhoads CP: Report on a cooperative study of nitrogen mustard (HN$_2$) therapy of neoplastic disease. Trans Assoc Am Phys 60:110, 1947.

10. Klopp CT et al: Fractional intra-arterial cancer chemotherapy with methyl-bis-amine hydrochloride. Ann Surg 132:811, 1950.

11. Bierman HR et al: The effects of intra-arterial administration of nitrogen mustard. Fifth International Cancer Congress. Paris, 1950, pp 187–188.

12. Sullivan RD et al: The treatment of human cancer with intraarterial nitrogen mustard (methyl bis (2-chloroethyl) amine hydrocloride) utilizing a simplified catheter technique. Cancer 6:121, 1953.

13. Creech O Jr et al: Chemotherapy of cancer: Regional perfusion utilizing an extracorporeal circuit. Ann Surg 148:616, 1958.

14. Krementz ET et al: Treatment of malignant tumors of the extremities by perfusion with chemotherapeutic agents. J Bone Joint Surg 41:977, 1959.

15. Koops HS, Oldhoff J: Hyperthermic regional perfusion in high-risk stage I malignant melanomas of the extremities. Recent Results Cancer Res 86:223, 1983.

16. Bulman AS, Jamieson CW: Isolated limb perfusion with melphalan in the treatment of malignant melanoma. Br J Surg 67:660, 1980.

17. Aigner K et al: Regional perfusion with cisplatinum and dacarbazine. Recent Results Cancer Res 86:239, 1983.

18. Cavaliere R et al: Selective heat sensitivity of cancer cells: Biochemical and clinical studies. Cancer 20:1351, 1967.

19. Busch. 1866. No information available.

20. Coley WB: The treatment of malignant tumors by repeated inoculations of erysipelas. A report of ten original cases. 1893. Clin Orthop 262:3, 1991.

21. Stelin JS Jr et al: Results of hyperthermic perfusion for melanoma of the extremities. Surg Gynecol Obstet 140(3):339, 1975.

22. Weissberger AS et al: Use of nitrogen mustard in treatment of serous effusions of neoplastic origin. JAMA 159:1704, 1955.

23. Spratt JS et al: Clinical delivery system for intraperitoneal hyperthermic chemotherapy. Cancer Res 40:256, 1980.

24. Koga S et al: Prophylactic therapy for peritoneal recurrence of gastric cancer by continuous hyperthethermic peritoneal perfusion. Cancer 61:232, 1988.

25. Fujimura T et al: Continuous hyperthermic peritoneal perfusion for the treatment of peritoneal dissemination in gastric cancer and subsequent second-look operation. Cancer 65:65, 1990.

26. Fujimoto S et al: Clinical outcome of combined therapy of intraoperative hyperthermochemotherapy and surgery for patients with peritoneal recurrence from gastric cancer. Reg Cancer Treat 3:181, 1990.

27. Yomaguchi A et al: Intraperitoneal hyperthermic treatment for peritoneal dissemination of colorectal cancer. Dis Colon Rectum 35(10):964, 1992.

28. Deraco M et al: Intraperitoneal hyperthermic perfusion (IPHI): Analisys of morbidity and toxicity. Oncology Reports 3:1103, 1996.

29. Sugarbaker PH: Cancer of the appendix and pseudomyxoma, in Current Therapy in colon and rectal surgery, VW Fazio (ed). Philadelphia, Decker, 1989, pp 295–301.

30. Eckman WM et al: A critical evaluation of principles governing the advantages of intraarterial infusions. J Pharmacokinet Biopharm 2:257, 1974.

31. Collins JM: Pharmacokinetics and clinical monitoring, in Cancer Chemotherapy: Principles and Practice, BA Chabner, JM Collins (eds). Philadelphia, Lippincott, 1990, pp 16–31.

32. Chan KK et al: Prediction of adriamycin disposition in cancer patients using physiologic, pharmacokinetic model. Cancer Treat Rep 62:1161, 1978.

33. Ertmann R et al: Pharmacokinetics of doxorubicin in man: Dose and schedule dependence. J Cancer Res Clin Oncol 114:509, 1998.

34. Matsushima Y et al: Time-schedule dependency of the inhibiting activity of various anticancer drugs in the clogenic assay. Cancer Chemother Pharmacol 14:104, 1985.

35. Krementz ET: Regional perfusion. Current sophistication, What Next? Cancer 57:416, 1986.

36. Muchmore JH et al: Regional perfusion for malignant melanoma and soft tissue sarcoma. A review. Cancer Invest 3:129, 1985.

37. Mitchell RB et al: Experimental rationale for continuous infusion chemotherapy, in Cancer Chemotherapy by Infusion, 2d ed, JJ Lokich (ed). Chicago, Precept Press, 1990, pp 3–34.

38. Schroy PC III et al: New chemotherapeutic drug sensitivity assay for colon carcinomas in monolayer culture. Cancer Res 48:3236, 1988.

39. Ensminger WD, Gyves JW: Regional cancer chemotherapy. Cancer Treat Rep 68:101, 1984.

40. Curt GA, Collins JM: Clinical pharmacology and infusional chemotherapy, in Cancer Chemotherapy by Infusion, 2d ed, JJ Lokich (ed). Chicago, Precept Press, 1990, pp 35–41.

41. Ensminger WD, Gyes JW: Clinical pharmacology of hepatic arterial chemotherapy. Semin Oncol 10:176, 1983.

42. Garnick MB et al: A clinical-pharmacological evaluation of hepatic arterial infusion of adriamycin. Cancer Res 39:4105, 1979.

43. Hu E, Howell SB: Pharmacokinetics of intraarterial mitomycin C in humans. Cancer Res 43:4474, 1983.

44. Chen H-SG, Gross JF: Intraarterial infusion of anticancer drugs: Theoretic aspects of drug delivery and review of responses. Cancer Treat Rep 64:31, 1980.

45. Ballet F et al: Hepatic extraction, metabolism and biliary excretion of doxorubicin in the isolated perfused rat liver. Cancer Chemother Pharmacol 19:240, 1987.

46. Theodors A et al: Intermittent regional infusion of chemotherapy for pancreatic adenocareinoma. Am J Clin Oncol 5:555, 1982.

47. Bengmark S, Andren-Sandberg A: Infusion chemotherapy in inoperable pancreatic carcinoma. Rec Res Cancer Res 86:13, 1983.

48. Aigner KR et al: Intraarterial chemotherapy with MMC, CDDP and 5-FU for non-resectable pancreatic cancer: A phase II study. Reg Cancer Treat 3:1, 1990.

49. Link KH et al: Prospective correlative chemosensitivity testing in high-dose intra-arterial chemotherapy for liver metastases. Cancer Res 46:4837, 1986.

50. Park J et al: Chemosensitivity testing of human colorectal carcinoma cell lines using tetrazolium-based colorimetric assay. Cancer Res 47:5875, 1987.

51. Dedrick RL: Arterial drug infusion: Pharmacokinetic problems and pitfalls. JNCI 80:84, 1988.

52. Link KH: Basic concepts for the application of mitomycin C in regional cancer treatment, in Mitomycin C in Cancer Chemotherapy, T Taguchi, KR Aigner (eds). Tokyo, Excerpta Medica, 1991, pp 62–71.

53. BOLD R, MCCONKEY D: Gemcitabine-induced apoptotic cell death of human pancreatic carcinoma is determined by bcl-2 content (abstr). 51st Annual Cancer Symposium. Arlington Heights, IL, Society of Surgical Oncology, 1998, p 57.

54. EILBER FR et al: Is amputation necessary for sarcomas? A seven-year experience with limb salvage. Ann Surg 192:431, 1980.

55. ———— Limb salvage for skeletal and soft tissue sarcomas: Multidisciplinary preoperative therapy. Cancer 53:2579, 1984.

56. KARAKOUSIS CP et al: Intraarterial adriamycin in the treatment of soft tissue sarcomas. J Surg Oncol 13:21, 1980.

57. KARAKOUSIS CP et al: Limb salvage in soft tissue sarcomas with selective combination of modalities. Eur J Surg Oncol 17:71, 1991.

58. AZZARELLI A et al: Intraarterial induction chemotherapy for soft tissue sarcomas. Annuals of Oncology 3 (Suppl 2):567, 1992.

59. EILBER FR et al: A randomized prospective trial using preoperative adjuvant chemotherapy (Adriamycin) in high grade extremity soft tissue sarcomas. Am J Clin Oncol 11:39, 1988.

60. AZZARELLI A et al: Intra-arterial infusion and perfusion chemotherapy for soft tissue sarcomas of the extremities, in *Clinical Management of Soft Tissue Sarcomas,* HM Pinedo, J Verweij (eds). Boston, Martinus Nijhoff Publishers, 1986, pp 103–129.

61. MUCHMORE JH et al: Regional perfusion for malignant melanoma and soft tissue sarcomas: A review. Cancer Invest 3:129, 1985.

62. CAVALIERE R et al: Hyperthermic antiblastic perfusion in the treatment of local recurrence a "in transit" metastases of limb melanoma. Semin Surg Oncol 8:374, 1992.

63. STORM FK: Clinical Hyperthermia and Chemotherapy. Radiol Clin North Am 27(3):621, 1989.

64. KOWAL CD, BERTINO JR: Possible benefits of hyperthermia to chemotherapy. Cancer Res 39:2285, 1979.

65. SONG CW: Effect of local hyperthermia on blood flow and microenvironment: A review. Cancer Res 44 (Suppl):4721s, 1984.

66. TEICHER BA et al: Classification of antineoplastic agents by their selective toxicities toward oxygenated and hypoxic tumor cells. Cancer Res 41:73, 1981.

67. VROUENRAETS BC et al: Absence of severe systemic toxicity after leakage-controlled isolated limb perfusion with tumor necrosis factor-α and melphalan. Ann Surg Oncol 6(4):405, 1999.

68. WIEBERDINK J et al: Dosimetry in isolation perfusion of the limbs by assessment of perfused tissue volume and grading of toxic tissue reactions. Eur J Cancer Clin Oncol 18:905, 1982.

69. TURK PS et al: Isolated pelvic perfusion for unresectable cancer using a balloon occlusion technique. Arch Surg 128:533, 538, 1993.

70. AIGNER KR, KEEVEL K: Hipoxic pelvic perfusion (HPP): Pelvic stop-flow infusion. Reg Cancer Treat 1:6, 1994.

71. LATHROP JC et al: Perfusion chemotherapy for gynecological malignancy. Trans N Engl Obstet Gynecol Soc 17:47, 1963.

72. WILE A, Smolin M: Hypertemic pelvic isolation-perfusion in the treatment of refractory pelvic cancer. Arch Surg 122:1321, 1987.

73. TURK PS et al: Isolated pelvic perfusion for unrectable cancer using a balloon occlusion techniques. Arch Surg 128:533, 1993.

74. AIGNER KR: Aortic stopfow infusion and hypoxic abdominal perfusion for disseminated bulky peritoneal carcinomatosis. Rationale and technique (abstr). Reg Cancer Treat 6(Suppl 1): 3, 1993.

75. THOMPSON JF et al: Stop-flow cytotoxic infusion: A simplified technique using percutaneous catheter (abstr). Reg Cancer Treat 6 (Suppl 1):51, 1993.

76. THOMPSON JF et al: A percutaneous aortic "stop-flow" infusion technique for regional cytotoxic therapy of the abdomen and pelvis. Reg Cancer Treat 7:202, 1994.

77. AVERBACH AM et al: Intraaortic stop-flow infusion: Pharmacokinetic feasibility study of regional chemotherapy for unresectable gastrointestinal cancers. Ann Surg Oncol 2:325, 1995.

78. AVERBACH AM et al: Pharmacokinetic studies of intraaortic stop-flow infusion with 14C-labeled mitomycin C. J Surg Res 59:415, 1995.

79. GUADAGNI S et al: Pharmacokinetic of mitomycin C in pelvic stopflow infusion and hypoxic pelvic perfusion with and without hemofiltration: A pilot study of patients with recurrent unresectable rectal cancer. J Clin Pharmacol 38:100, 1998.

80. AIGNER KR, KEEVEL K: Pelvic stopflow infusion (PSI) and hypoxic pelvic perfusion (HPP) with mitomycin and melphalan for recurrent rectal cancer. Reg Cancer Treat 7:6, 1994.

81. WANEBO HJ et al: Preoperative therapy for advanced pelvic malignancy by isolated pelvic perfusion with balloon-occlusion technique. Ann Surg Oncol 3:295, 1996.

82. AIGNER KR: Intraarterial infusion: Overview and novel approaches. Semin Surg Oncol 14:248, 1998.

83. FIORENTINI G et al: Intra-aortic stop-flow infusion with hypoxic abdominal perfusion in UICC stage III/IV pancreatic carcinoma: Report of a phase II study. Reg Cancer Treat 9:88, 1996.

84. AIGNER KR, SELAK E: Isolated thoracic perfusion for lung metastases from breast cancer (abstr). Reg Cancer Treat 10 (Suppl 1): 76, 1997.

85. GUADAGNI S et al: Pilot study on isolated thoracic perfusion for the treatment of non-small cell lung cancer stage IIIb and IV (abstr). Proceedings of International Cancer Conference, Perugia, Italy 1998.

86. RUSSO F et al: Thoracic perfusion with cisplatin-based regimen is very active in malignant lymphoma failing salvage high dose chemotherapy and autologous peripheral stem cell rescue (abstr). Proceedings of ASCO, Los Angeles. J Clin Oncol 17:6, 1988.

87. MUCHMORE JH: Treatment of advanced pancreatic cancer with regional chemotherapy plus hemofiltration. Semin Surg Oncol 11:154, 1995.

88. DEDRICK RL et al: Pharmacokinetic rationale for peritoneal drug administration in the treatment of ovarian cancer. Cancer Treat Rep 62:1, 1978.

89. MARKMAN M: Intraperitoneal chemotherapy. Semin Oncol 18(3):248, 1991.

90. OZALS RF et al: Pharmacokinetics of adriamycin and tissue penetration in murine ovarian cancer. Cancer Res 39:3209, 1999.

91. LOS G et al: Direct diffusion of cis-diamminedichloroplatinum (II) in intraperitoneal chemotherapy: A comparison with systemic chemotherapy. Cancer Res 49:3380, 1989.

92. SUGARBAKER PH et al: Early postoperative intraperitoneal chemotherapy as an adjuvant therapy to surgery for peritoneal carcinomatosis from gastrointestinal cancer: Pharmacological studies. Cancer Res 50:5790, 1990.

93. SUGARBAKER PH et al: Rationale for postoperative intraperitoneal chemotherapy as a surgical adjuvant for gastrointestinal malignancy. Reg Cancer Treat 1:66, 1988.

94. SUGARBAKER PH et al: Curative treatment of peritoneal carcinomatosis from grade 1 mucinous adenocarcinoma. Surg Rounds 11:45, 1988.

95. SUGARBAKER PH et al: Peritonectomy procedures. Ann of Surg 221 (1):29, 1995.

96. SCHABEL FM Jr: Concepts for systemic treatment of micrometastases. Cancer 35:15, 1975.

97. SKIPPER HE et al: Experimental evaluation of potential anticancer agents. XIII. On the criteria and kinetics associated with curability of experimental leukemia. Cancer Chemother Rep 35:1, 1964.

98. YONEMURA Y et al: Hyperthermochemotherapy combined with cytoreductive surgery for the treatment of gastric cancer with peritoneal dissemination. World J Surg 15:530, 1991.

99. GILLY FN et al: Traitment des carcinoses peritoneales par chimio-hyperthermie intra-peritoneale avec Mitomycin C. Première experience. Annal Chirurgie 44, 1990.

100. SUGARBAKER PH et al: A simplified approach to hyperthermic intraoaperative intraperitoneal chemotherapy (HIIC) using a self retaining retractor. Cancer Treat Res 82:415, 1996.

101. DERACO M et al: Intrapertioneal hyperthermic perfusion (IPHP): Analysis of morbidity and toxicity. Oncol Reports 3:1103, 1996.

102. JACQUET P, SUGARBAKER Ph: Peritoneal-plasma barrier, in Peritoneal Carcinomatosis: Principles of Management, Ph Sugarbaker (ed). Boston, Kluwer Academic Publishers, 1966, pp 53–63.

103. SUGARBAKER PH: Management of Peritoneal Surface Malignancy Using Intraperitoneal Chemotherapy and Cytoreductive Surgery: A Manual. The Ludann Company, Grand Rapids, MI, november 1998.

104. YONEMURA Y et al: Hyperthermochemotherapy combined with cytoreductive surgery for the treatment of gastric cancer with peritoneal dissemination. World J Surg 15:530, 1991.

105. FUJIMOTO S et al: Improved mortality rate of gastric carcinoma patients with peritoneal carcinomatosis treated with intraperitoneal hyperthermic chemoperfusion combined with surgery. Cancer 79(5):884, 1997.

106. DERACO M et al: Could advanced ovarian cancer be responsive to cytoreductive surgery and intraperitoneal hyperthermic perfusion? Proceedings of UICC 17th International Cancer Congress. Rio de Janeiro, August 23–28, 1998.

107. PORTILLA AG et al: Clinical pathway for peritoneal carcinomatosis from colon and rectal cancer: Guidelines for current practice. Tumori 83:725, 1997.

108. JACQUET P et al: Analysis of morbidity and mortality in 60 patients with peritoneal carcinomatosis treated by cytoreductive surgery and heated intraoperative intraperitoneal chemotherapy. Cancer 77(12):2622, 1996.

# 3E / GENE THERAPY FOR SURGICAL MALIGNANCIES

*Michael A. Morse, H. Kim Lyerly, and Bryan M. Clary*

## INTRODUCTION

Because the prognosis of advanced malignancies after the failure of surgical resection is minimally altered by standard chemotherapy and radiation, novel approaches such as gene therapy have generated considerable interest. The term *gene therapy* describes approaches that involve the introduction of genetic material that alters the phenotype of the target tissue with therapeutic implications. The initial gene therapy studies were designed to correct monogenic inherited diseases such as hemoglobinopathies. In the first human gene therapy trial, performed in patients with thalassemia in 1980, the human β-globin gene was transferred into bone marrow stem cells ex vivo prior to their reinfusion.[1] The chemical methods used for gene transfer were inefficient,[2] but retroviral vectors with greater efficiency of transfer were developed in the early 1980s. The first trial utilizing this approach was initiated in 1990; it involved the transfer of a normal adenosine deaminase (ADA) gene into the peripheral lymphocytes of patients with severe combined immunodeficiency due to ADA deficiency.[3] Over a short period of time, there has been a rapid expansion in the development of more efficient vectors and genes that can be transferred. This section reviews the current strategies for delivering and utilizing therapeutic genes, and the present and future applications of these strategies to the treatment of malignancies.

## STRATEGIES FOR ANTICANCER GENE THERAPY

Because genetic mutations result in the malignant phenotype, it is appropriate that gene transfer be used to correct gene defects (e.g., correct a tumor-promoting mutation by replacement of a tumor-suppressor gene). In contrast to the treatment of monogenic inherited defects, though, the treatment of malignancies has permitted a greater diversity of approaches using recombinant DNA technology (Table 3E-1). For example, gene transfer may confer increased sensitivity of the tumor to chemical agents ("suicide genes") or decreased sensitivity of normal tissues to chemotherapy. Transfer of cytokine, a major histocompatibility antigen, and costimulatory molecule genes may be utilized to increase the immunogenicity of a tumor. The tumor itself need not always be the target of the gene transfer. Insertion of a gene that is a dominant negative for an angiogenesis factor receptor may interfere with neovascularization. The rationale for these approaches will be discussed below.

## CORRECTION OF TUMOR SUPPRESSOR GENE DEFECTS AND INACTIVATION OF ONCOGENES

Defective tumor suppressor genes [such as p53 and Rb1-activated[4] oncogenes (such as *ras*)] are frequent causes of tumor development and represent possible targets for intervention. Defects in both alleles of tumor suppressor genes are usually required for tumorigenesis, and often consist of a combination of mutation and deletion that results in nonfunctional protein. Alterations in p53, which causes a reversible arrest in the $G_1$ phase of the cell cycle or the irreversible induction of apoptosis, is found in almost half of all malignancies. In vitro, apoptosis occurs after transfer of wild-type (wt) p53 to p53-deficient cells.[5,6] In vivo models of lung, head and neck, and colon cancers established in immunodeficient mice have revealed a reduction of tumorigenicity following introduction of wt-p53.[7–11] Transfer of p53 into tumors also renders them more sensitive to chemotherapy-induced apoptosis.[12,13] For example, when cisplatin was administered systemically following intratumoral injection of an adenoviral vector encoding wt-p53, there was a significant increase in apoptosis and tumor cell death.[14] Whether p53 must be delivered to each tumor cell harboring the defect is unclear. One study showed a reduction in tumor growth when retroviral wt-p53–transduced tumor cells were mixed with nontransduced tumor cells.[15] Because apoptotic bodies can be taken up by antigen-presenting cells and used to prime naive T cells,[16] this may occur by an immunologic mechanism. Models of ovarian[17] and breast cancer,[18] hepatoma,[19] and glioblastoma[20] have demonstrated gene delivery to the target tissue and tumor regression. Phase I studies of p53 gene therapy are now under way in unresectable hepatic metastases of colorectal cancer, primary hepatocellular carcinoma, and lung cancer using either adenoviral constructs in which the human p53 gene is expressed under the control of the cytomegalovirus promoter or naked wt-p53 plasmid DNA. At the recent 3rd European Conference on Gene Therapy of Cancer, preliminary human studies of p53 gene therapy reported regressions of hepatocellular carcinomas and evidence of necrosis and apoptosis of head and neck tumors.[21]

The inhibition of oncogene function has been attempted by a number of different strategies, including (1) antisense oligonucleotides, (2) antisense RNA, (3) ribozymes, and (4) single-chain intracellular antibodies.[22–28] Antisense oligonucleotides (ODNs), short sequences of deoxy nucleotides designed to bind in a complementary fashion to desired sequences of DNA or RNA, inhibit gene expression by interfering with transcription (hybridizing with DNA), RNA transport or splicing, or translation (binding to

**TABLE 3E-1.** GENE THERAPY STRATEGIES FOR TREATING CANCER

Correction of gene defects
   p53 gene transfer
   Oncogene antisense oligonucleotides

Immunotherapy
   Cytokine gene-transduced autologous or allogeneic tumor
   Costimulatory molecule-transduced autologous or allogeneic tumor
   HLA molecule-transduced autologous tumor
   Intramuscular injection of tumor antigen encoding genes

Prodrug-converting enzymes

Protection of normal tissues
   mdr transfer to hematopoietic progenitors

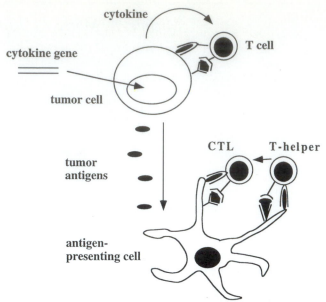

**FIGURE 3E-1.** Possible mechanisms of activity of cytokine gene transfer strategies. Autologous (or allogene) tumor cells are transfected with the cytokine (e.g., IL-2, GM-CSF, IL-4, and others) gene and subsequently secrete cytokine. It was originally postulated that this altered the cytokine milieu of the tumor cell such that naive T cells that could recognize tumor antigens would be stimulated to proliferate and ultimately migrate and kill untransfected tumor. There are increasing data that the cytokines released by the tumor cell lead to an inflammatory reaction during which antigen-presenting cells such as dendritic cells are recruited. The dendritic cells take up antigen released from the tumor cell and present it to naive T cells resulting in a potent antigen-specific immune response.

ribosomal RNA or mRNA). Although ODNs have been demonstrated to inhibit numerous oncogenes in vivo including c-*abl*, c-*fos*, c-*fes*, c-*fms*, c-*kit*, c-*myb*, c-*myc*, c-*raf*, c-*src*, and *ras*,[28] their instability, preferential accumulation in the liver and kidneys, and inefficient uptake by cells have limited their clinical applicability. One solution has been to transfer sequences that serve as templates for antisense RNA in the form of plasmids or viral vectors. This approach has been demonstrated to inhibit expression of c-*myc*, and K-*ras*[29–31] and is being tested in clinical trials of non–small cell lung cancer (K-*ras*), central nervous system (CNS) tumors (insulin-like growth factor, IGF-1), metastatic breast cancer (c-*fos*, c-*myc*), prostate cancer (c-*myc*), and Her2/neu (+) tumors. Ribozymes are RNA molecules that are able to cleave mRNA and replace a section containing a genetic defect with a normal segment.[32] Studies have demonstrated a reduction in the ability of Ha-*ras*–expressing cells to form tumors following the introduction of Ha-*ras*–targeted ribozyme.[33] As with other RNA molecules, exogenous ribozymes suffer from a lack of in vivo targeting mechanisms and rapid degradation by nucleases, although modifications to increase stability have been introduced.[34]

In summary, the replacement of defective tumor suppressor genes or the inhibition of the expression of oncogenes has been demonstrated to be efficacious in preventing tumorigenicity in preclinical models. Interestingly, despite the fact that tumors often have multiple genetic defects, correcting a single lesion may be therapeutically successful. Because of the difficulties in targeting tumor tissues after systemic administration, local administration is being employed in current clinical trials. Preliminary results from phase I studies are now being reported at international meetings.

**IMMUNOTHERAPY BY GENE TRANSFER.** Gene transfer into tumors for the purpose of increasing their immunogenicity was developed based on the hypothesis that immune responses against poorly immunogenic tumors could be induced by altering their cytokine milieu or their expression of MHC (major histocompatibility complex) class I or costimulatory molecules (Fig. 3E-1). A number of animal models have demonstrated that tumor cells, genetically engineered to secrete various cytokines [interleukin 2

(IL-2), IL-4, interferon-gamma (IFN-γ), granulocyte-macrophage colony stimulating factor (GM-CSF), tumor necrosis factor α (TNF-α), IL-6, and IL-7] induce systemic immunity capable of rejecting established tumors and subsequent tumor challenge.[35–45] Human studies with either allogeneic[46] or autologous tumor[47] transduced with cytokine genes have been initiated in patients with melanoma[48] and renal cell carcinoma.[49] Delayed-type hypersensitivity reactions at the injection sites, inflammatory infiltrates at distant metastases, and minor clinical responses have been reported. Nonetheless, difficulty in obtaining an adequate amount of autologous tumor and in efficiently transducing the genes of interest into cells that are often only slowly dividing have encumbered clinical trials of these vaccines. Although more efficient gene delivery systems have been evaluated,[50–52] two alternative approaches to delivery of cytokine genes have been proposed: vaccinations with mixtures of tumor and autologous, cytokine gene–transduced fibroblasts;[53–55] and intratumoral injection of viral vectors or plasmids encoding cytokine genes,[56] MHC, or costimulatory molecules. Clinical trials of intratumoral injections of plasmids encoding the allogeneic MHC molecule (often HLA-B7) have begun and have thus far demonstrated a few regressions at local and distant sites of patients with advanced malignancies.[57,58]

Enthusiasm for approaches designed to augment the immunogenicity of the tumor by gene transfer has dampened with the discovery that the gene-modified tumors may not themselves induce an immune response, but rather incite inflammation that results in destruction of the injected tumor cells and the release of antigens that are then processed by antigen-presenting cells (such as dendritic cells) and presented to T cells.[59] If this is the case, it may be more efficient to deliver defined tumor antigens to antigen-presenting cells in a less cumbersome fashion. Intramuscular injection of naked DNA and RNA preparations encoding known tumor antigens including carcinoembryonic antigen (CEA),[60–62] Her-2-neu, MART-1, MAGE-1, tyrosinase, gp100, MUC-1, and p21 *ras* have been demonstrated to induce antigen-specific immune responses. Although it is likely that myocytes take up the plasmid DNA, express the gene for at least 7 to 10 days,[63,64] and present epitopes of the encoded protein to T cells, antigen transfer to professional antigen-presenting cells is also possible.[65] Alternatives to the injection of naked genetic material include viral vectors such as the pox viruses (vaccinia, fowlpox, ALVAC) as vectors to introduce genes encoding prostate-specific antigen (PSA), CEA,[66] gp100, and MART-1 in patients with prostate cancer, advanced CEA-expressing gastrointestinal (GI) malignancies, and melanoma, respectively. (See later in this chapter for a more detailed discussion of these methods of gene transfer.)

Another method of utilizing gene transfer in an immunotherapy strategy is to transduce lymphocytes to make them more cytotoxic[67,68] or to make them more specific for the tumor.[69] Other cells of the immune system can be transduced with genes for an anticancer therapeutic effect. Dendritic cells, which are the most potent antigen-presenting cells and are capable of stimulating antigen-specific T-cell responses in vitro and in vivo, are being used in a number of immunotherapy strategies now. Gene modification of dendritic cells with either cytokine genes or with genes encoding tumor antigens is now under evaluation. For example, a retroviral construct encoding the tumor antigen epithelial mucin (MUC1) gene has been used for stable transfection of dendritic cells (generated from CD34+ cord blood progenitor cells). Expression of mucin was demonstrated on the cell surface, and these transfected dendritic cells were found to be potent stimulators of allogeneic CD4+ T cells.[70] More recently, Nair and colleagues have demonstrated that dendritic cells can take up mRNA-encoding CEA and induce CEA-specific T cells in vitro.

One final area of immunotherapy utilizing gene transfer technology that requires further study is the possible contribution of noncoding genetic material to the immune response. It has been demonstrated that bacterial DNA contains immunostimulatory sequence motifs that when included in plasmid vectors may influence the immune response to the protein encoded by the accompanying transferred gene.[72] Thus, it will be important to consider the benefits of these sequences (as adjuvants) as well as their possible ability to confound the interpretation of immunologic results from gene therapy studies.

## DRUG-SENSITIVITY GENES

Prodrug-converting gene therapy (also called suicide gene therapy) involves delivery of a gene whose product converts a nontoxic prodrug to a toxic metabolite, thus attempting to limit toxicity to the tumor microenvironment[73–79] (Fig. 3E-2). The most widely utilized prodrug-converting gene is the herpes simplex virus thymidine kinase (HSV-TK) gene, the enzyme product of which is

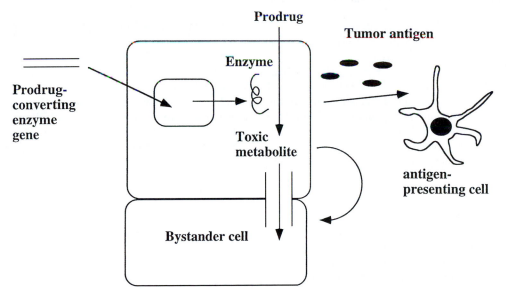

**FIGURE 3E-2.** Prodrug gene therapy strategy. Once the prodrug-converting enzyme gene is expressed, the enzyme product is capable of converting a systemically administered prodrug into a metabolite toxic to the transduced cell and bystanders via gap junctions or local release. In some models, it is also likely that immune mechanisms are involved when tumor antigen released from the transfected tumor cell as it dies is taken up by antigen-presenting cells and used to stimulate T-cell responses.

1000 times more efficient at initiating the phosphorylation of the prodrug ganciclovir (GCV) than human TK. Following the completion of triphosphorylation, the toxic metabolite is incorporated into DNA during cell proliferation, causing chain termination and cell death by apoptosis. Tumor cells transduced in vitro with HSV-TK–expressing vectors exhibit sensitivity to GCV at concentrations achievable systemically,[80] but which are below the level of significant normal tissue cytotoxicity. Other prodrug-converting gene systems under development include *Escherichia coli* cytosine deaminase, which converts 5-flucytosine into the toxic metabolite 5-fluorouracil;[81–85] the varicella-zoster virus TK, which phosphorylates 6-methoxypurine arabinonucleoside (araM);[86] the *E. coli* XGPRT, which monophosphorylates 6-thioxanthine;[87,88] DeoD, which generates the toxic 6-methylpurine;[89] and the cytochrome P450 gene, which activates cyclophosphamide.[90] A novel approach is the radiosensitization of tumors after inserting HSV-TK[91] or cytosine deaminase[92] and administering prodrugs that are converted into radiosensitizing molecules. One appealing aspect of prodrug-converting gene therapy is the "bystander effect," in which significant tumor regression occurs when only a fraction of the cells express the suicide gene.[93] This is hypothesized to result from release or transfer of a toxic metabolite from the transfected cells to the surrounding cells through gap junctions, damage to the vasculature, and/or immunologic mechanisms.[75,93–95] The presence of a bystander effect has also permitted the intratumoral or intracavitary injection of fibroblasts transfected with prodrug-converting genes instead of requiring gene transfer to the tumor. Animal models of gliomas[76,96] and meningeal disease[97] have demonstrated tumor regressions with this method. Numerous other animal models of the transfer of prodrug-converting enzymes to tumors[98–102] have similarly demonstrated regression of tumors after administration of the prodrug, but complete tumor elimination or long-term animal survival has not always been observed.

The ongoing human trials of suicide gene therapy are all in phase I and have been predominantly directed toward brain tumors, but at least one study is targeting metastatic colon cancer and another ovarian cancer. All but the colon cancer study use the HSV-TK gene. Brain tumors are well suited for this type of study because normal brain is mitotically inactive compared with tumors, permitting the targeting of retroviruses to tumor cells. Stereotactic injection of the vector into the tumor is possible, and cavities at the surgical site will accept the injection of the necessary volumes of viral supernatant. Although final results have not been published yet in manuscript form, preliminary reports suggest responses occur in some patients.[74]

## DRUG-RESISTANCE GENES

Instead of targeting a therapeutic gene to a tumor, it is also possible to deliver genes that can prevent toxicity to normal tissue while the tumor is exposed to systemically administered chemotherapy. The most extensively studied has been the multidrug resistance gene 1 (*MDR1*) that encodes p-glycoprotein, a transmembrane efflux pump[103] that is capable of extruding cytotoxic agents. Since hematopoietic toxicity is dose-limiting for many agents, it would be possible to protect bone marrow progenitors by transfer of the *MDR1* gene to just a few progenitors, and then allow for repopulation of the bone marrow with these modified cells. Indeed, amounts of *MDR1*–transduced murine hematopoietic progenitors are markedly increased after treatment with methotrexate or paclitaxel.[104] Other potential resistance genes include those encoding dihydrofolate reductase, methylguanine methyltransferase, aldehyde dehydrogenase, superoxide dismutase, and the nucleotide excision repair gene (ERCC-1). In the first reported human trial,[105] CD34+ cells selected from bone marrow or blood were transduced with a retroviral vector containing the cDNA for *MDR1* and were reinfused along with unmanipulated bone marrow into patients with various malignancies following high-dose chemotherapy. High levels of transduction of BFU-E and CFU-GM (30–70%) were observed after transduction, but only two out of five evaluable patients had MDR-transduced marrow cells detected by PCR following transplantation. Whether this method of gene therapy will have a routine role is unclear because there are several theoretical difficulties. First, current protocols utilize retroviral vectors that require cell division in order for stable integration of the gene of interest to occur.[106] Unfortunately, this may lead to differentiation of the hematopoietic progenitors and loss of the quiescent, self-renewing cells required to maintain long-term hematopoiesis.[107] Nonetheless, retrovirally transduced human hematopoietic cells have been shown in gene-marking trials to survive for extended periods of time.[108] Second, nonhematologic toxicities become dose-limiting, often only after a small increase above the hematologically limiting dose. Third, there are concerns about transducing tumor cells with the drug-resistance gene. The latter can hopefully be avoided with careful separation techniques and the incorporation of suicide genes into the vector, which would allow for the selective destruction of transduced cells in the event that a drug-resistance phenotype was conferred upon the tumor.

## DELIVERY SYSTEMS IN GENE THERAPEUTICS

The major obstacle to the gene therapy approaches described above has been the efficiency of gene delivery. Of course, different anticancer therapeutic strategies may have different gene delivery requirements, including the duration and level of expression as well as targeted expression within specific cell types (i.e., nonneoplastic vs. neoplastic). The most widely utilized class of gene-delivery vectors is based upon mutated viruses, but physiochemical methods of delivery, including liposome-DNA complexes, electroporation, and gold particle bombardment ("gene gun") have also been developed.

## VIRAL VECTORS

### RETROVIRUS

Retroviral vectors, rendered replication-incompetent by replacing their *gag, pol,* and *env* regions with the coding sequences of the gene of interest (as well as genes for selection and marker enzymes), are the best characterized and the most frequently used gene-delivery vehicle in the current clinical trials. The vectors infect the target cell and the RNA is reverse-transcribed into DNA, which then integrates into the host genome DNA, permitting stable, high-level gene expression. Because they are replication-incompetent, they must be produced in packaging cell lines that supply the structural proteins in trans. Retroviral vectors most commonly in use in gene transfer studies are derived from the Moloney murine leukemia virus (MoMuL V). Amphotropic variants of this virus are available that readily infect human cells. They are most commonly used in those trials where long-term expression is necessary and cell growth and division are possible.

Retroviral vectors have several limitations. First, they require cell proliferation for integration, and even in rapidly dividing tumors, the fraction of cells undergoing cell division at any one time is low. Second, the expression of the transduced gene may vary depending on the state of activity of the transduced cell. For example, there is low expression from the MoMuL V LTR in quiescent cells.[109] Third, appropriate viral receptors must be present on the target cell, but the receptors for some retroviruses are unknown, and thus it may not be possible to predict whether a tumor will be susceptible to transduction. Fourth, retroviral vector titers rarely exceed $10^6$ infectious units per milliliter, and thus large volumes of packaging cell supernatants are required. Fifth, retroviruses are labile at body temperature. Finally, integration that disrupts a tumor suppressor gene or activates an oncogene could increase the virulence of a tumor, although this has never been reported.[110] In order to improve delivery into tumor cells, direct injection into the tumor or tumor vasculature has been suggested for localized disease.[98,111] Furthermore, lentivirus-derived vectors have now been developed that can transduce some quiescent cells.[112] Table 3E-2 lists methods of gene transfer.

## ADENOVIRUS

Adenoviral vectors, made replication-incompetent by the deletion of the E1 gene, are large complex DNA viruses capable of transducing most quiescent and dividing cells. The adenoviral genome does not integrate into the cellular genome, but remains as an episome in the nucleus that can be lost with cellular division. In addition to transcription of the intended foreign gene, the viral genes encoded by

the adenoviral genome are also transcribed, resulting in the production of immunogenic viral proteins. Packaging cell lines have been engineered to express the E1 region in order to generate adenoviral vectors for gene therapy. The advantages of adenoviral vectors include: (1) stability and easy production of high titers of recombinant adenoviruses ($10^{12}$ pfu/mL), (2) transduction of a wide range of cell types, (3) little to no integration of the adenoviral genome in the host cell genome, (4) accommodation of large gene constructs (7.5 kb in adenovectors possessing the E1 deletion), and (5) the ability to transduce nondividing cells.[113] The major drawbacks have been the lack of specificity of cell transduction, the toxicity of adenovirus to some tissues such as the liver, and the immune host response against the recombinant adenoviral vector or vector-transduced cells. This immune response, both humoral and cell-mediated, limits the duration of transgene expression and precludes efficient secondary administration. Attempts to address the immune response include deletions of other regions of the genome that are considered immunogenic, using immunosuppressive drugs such as cyclosporin to mediate a transient attenuation of the immune response in patients previously exposed to adenovirus, switching to one of the many (>47) different adenoviral serotypes, or using vectors that lack all adenoviral gene products.[114]

## ADENOASSOCIATED VIRUS

Adenoassociated viral (AAV) vectors, single-stranded DNA parvovirus, integrate into the host genome but have not been associated with any diseases in humans. In order to produce AAV vectors for clinical trials, the replication-defective virus requires defined "helper" functions provided by coinfection with adenoviruses or herpesviruses.[115] The potential advantages of recombinant AAV vectors include the ability to transduce nondividing cells, stable integration as multicopy tandem repeats, lack of transcribed viral proteins (and thus lack of immunogenicity), and selective integration into chromosome 19 (i.e., lack of random integration.) One of the main disadvantages of utilizing recombinant AAV vectors is the arduous processing necessary to produce high-titer and wild-type free, helper-virus free viruses for use in clinical trials.

## OTHER VIRUSES

Vaccinia virus, a DNA poxvirus, does not integrate into the host genome. Its advantages are the ability to transfer large genes (up to 25-kb pairs) and the wide tissue tropism.[56] The disadvantages are the lysis of transduced cells within 2 days and the significant immune response against the vector itself, limiting attempts to repeat delivery of the target gene. Vaccinia has been most useful as a method for vaccination against tumor antigens[61] as opposed to a method to deliver genes to tumors. Poxviruses related to vaccinia, such as fowlpox and canarypox, are unable to replicate in mammalian cells and may be alternatives to vaccinia. Herpes simplex virus displays neurologic tissue tropism and thus may be useful for CNS tumors. Finally, polio-, Sindbis-, and baculovirus-based gene transfer techniques are under development.

## TABLE 3E-2.  METHODS OF GENE TRANSFER

Viral vectors
  Retrovirus
  Adenovirus
  Adeno-associated virus
  Herpes simplex
  Vaccinia, fowlpox, canarypox
  Small RNA viruses (polio, Sindbis)

Nonviral methods
  "Gene gun"
  Receptor targeted-protein and DNA complexes
  Electroporation
  Liposomes
  Naked DNA

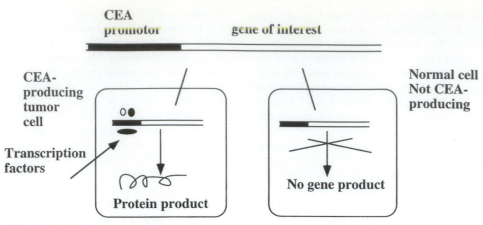

**FIGURE 3E-3.** Transcriptional control. Genes of interest are combined with a promoter that is known to be active in the tumor cell. Following gene transfection, only tumor cells with the transcription factors required for the activity of the promoter will express the gene.

## NONVIRAL METHODS OF GENE DELIVERY

### LIPOSOME-MEDIATED TRANSFECTION

Liposomes, consisting of mixtures of plasmid DNA and polycationic lipids (such as dioleoylphosphatidylethanolamine [DOPE]) with DOTMA, DOSPA, DDAB, DOTAP, DMRIE, and DC-cholesterol[116] likely fuse with the target cell membrane to achieve gene delivery. Because of their ease of preparation, stability, safety, lack of immunogenicity,[117,118] and ability to deliver genes to a wide variety of tissues,[119] DNA-liposome complexes have been studied for use both in vitro[50,51] and in vivo (by direct intratumoral injection, via bronchoscopy, and intravenously).

### OTHER NONVIRAL METHODS

Naked DNA-encoding genes of interest may be injected intramuscularly or as a coating on metallic particles administered via the high-velocity "gene gun."[120] Preclinical models using particle-mediated gene transfer into subcutaneous tumor explants have shown improved survival of tumor-bearing mice using a variety of cytokine genes, including IL-2, IL-6, and IFN-$\gamma$.[121] Some investigators have attempted to achieve targeted gene delivery through the use of synthetic complexes of DNA linked with proteins or polycationic molecules that can bind specific cellular receptors.[122] The advantages of this approach include specificity and the ability to transfer large DNA sequences. Unfortunately, the need for an endosomal lysis agent and short duration of gene expression have limited the in vivo use. If the transduction efficiency and cell-type specificity can be improved, nonviral approaches to gene transfer may become the preferred methods.

## CONTROL OF GENE EXPRESSION

Critical to the successful implementation of a gene therapy strategy is the expression of the transferred gene in the desired cell, at the appro-

priate time, in the appropriate quantity. Control over the ultimate protein production begins with regulation of gene transcription and is maintained by regulation of many other points, including the transport of the mRNA from the nucleus, the stability of the mRNA transcript, the relative affinity of the ribosomal complexes for the mRNA transcript, the stability of the newly synthesized protein, and further posttranslational modifications. Sequences within, flanking, and even at a distance from the gene of interest (such as promoters and enhancers) provide the information needed to exert these controls (Fig. 3E-3). Therefore, for the most effective gene therapy strategies, consideration must be given not only to the type of gene and transfer methodology, but also the choice of associated regulatory sequences.

## CELL TYPE-SPECIFIC REGULATORY ELEMENTS

Because it may not be possible to precisely target only tumor tissue with a gene, it is reasonable to attempt to limit expression of the gene to neoplastic cells. This has been accomplished by including regulatory elements within the delivered gene construct that control the expression of proteins produced specifically in tumor cells (e.g., CEA, $\alpha$-fetoprotein [AFP], PSA). The more widely studied targeted expression systems have been for melanoma, CEA-expressing malignancies, prostate cancer hepatomas, and c-*erb*B-2–expressing malignancies.

Because melanin production in melanocytes requires the presence of tyrosinase protein, it has been speculated that tissuespecificity of gene expression in melanoma could be achieved by use of the enhancer and promoter regions of the tyrosinase and tyrosinase-related protein (TRP). Indeed, these promoter regions have been found to have a high level of activity in 12 of 14 human and murine melanoma cell lines tested, but showed only basal levels of activity in 12 nonmelanoma cell types.[123] To extend these observations to a murine model of melanoma (B16), recombinant retroviral constructs encoding the tyrosinase promoter and HSV-TK gene were injected intratumorally into established B16 melanomas. Following treatment with the prodrug GCV, smaller tumors were observed than in saline-injected controls.

Because higher-than-baseline expression of CEA is present in most gastrointestinal malignancies and medullary thyroid, metastatic breast, and gynecologic cancers, sections of the CEA promoter have been evaluated for their ability to target tissue expression of therapeutic genes.[124,125] Introduction of the CEA promoter into retroviral vectors 5′ to coding regions for HSV-TK leads to selective sensitivity to the prodrug GCV in CEA-expressing lung and pancreatic cells.[75,126] The authors have demonstrated that intratumoral injection of murine fibroblasts producing retroviral virions encoding HSV-TK under the control of the CEA promoter leads to regression of CEA-producing pancreatic tumors in immunodeficient mice when these animals are administered systemic GCV.[75,100]

Other promoters, identified to be active exclusively in malignancies, which have been combined with therapeutic genes include AFP (hepatoma), PSA (prostate cancer), and c-erbB-2 (breast and others). In two studies in which suicide genes were placed under the control of the AFP promoter and introduced into hepatoma cell lines, there was increased cell killing of AFP-expressing tumor cell lines when compared to AFP-negative cells.[86,127] Similarly, attachment of the proximal c-erbB-2 promoter to the cytosine deaminase gene in retroviral vector constructs led to selective sensitivity to the prodrug 5-fluorocytosine (5FC) in c-erbB-2 overexpressing breast and pancreatic tumor cell lines. Tumor cell lines with low-level c-erbB-2 expression were not affected by the 5-FC.[128] The secretory leukoprotease inhibitor (SLPI) promoter, expressed in lung, breast, bladder, ovarian, endometrial, and colorectal carcinomas, has been linked to the HSV-TK gene, leading to selective sensitivity to GCV in SLPI-expressing lung and ovarian cancer cell lines.[129] Finally, a fragment from the PSA promoter has been demonstrated to actively drive gene expression in a PSA-producing prostate tumor cell line, whereas no promoter activity was detected in non-PSA-producing prostate, renal, or breast cancer cell lines.[130] In addition to utilizing promoters that regulate tumor-associated antigens, targeted expression in neoplastic cells may be achieved through the use of inducible promoters that are active predominantly in neoplastic cells. These include the multidrug resistance gene (MDR1), x-irradiation–induced tissue-type plasminogen activator, human heat shock protein (HHSP70), glucose-regulated protein (GRP78), and the early growth response gene (Egr1). Because routine treatment modalities such as chemotherapy, radiation, and hyperthermia may induce these genes, it is hoped that the expression of therapeutic genes regulated from their promoters may act synergistically with these standard forms of therapy.

## PRESENT STATUS AND FUTURE DIRECTIONS FOR CLINICAL TRIALS OF GENE THERAPY FOR MALIGNANCIES

At the present time, there are more than 100 gene therapy studies in the United States and 40 in Europe that are related to the treatment of malignancies, with most being phase I toxicity analyses. The type of tumor being targeted has varied with the therapeutic modality. For example, most cytokine gene transfer studies have been designed for melanoma and renal cell carcinoma. Suicide gene therapy has primarily been applied to brain or ovarian tumors. Tumor suppressor genes are being applied to hepatic cancers. It has been difficult to reproduce the achievements of gene transfection and ef-

ficacy demonstrated on a small scale when translated to larger-scale human studies. Nonetheless, there have been occasional reports of clinical responses. It is not clear whether gene therapy will have a role in the routine care of cancer patients in the future. If so, it will likely be in the setting of minimal residual disease after surgical resection or following chemotherapy–induced remissions. Animal models have demonstrated greatest efficacy in the setting of minimal tumor burden.

## REFERENCES

1. WOLFF J, LEDERBERG J: A history of gene transfer and therapy, in *Gene Therapeutics: Methods and Applications of Direct Gene Transfer*, J Wolff (ed). Boston, Birkhausen, 1994.
2. TZENG E et al: Gene therapy. Cur Prob Surg 33:961, 1996.
3. BLAESE R et al: T lymphocyte-directed gene therapy for ADA-SCID: Initial trial results after 4 years. Science 270:475, 1995.
4. SKUSE G, LUDLOW J: Tumor suppressor genes in disease and therapy. Lancet 345:902, 1995.
5. GOYETTE M et al: Progression of colorectal cancer is associated with multiple tumor suppressor gene defects but inhibition of tumorigenicity is accomplished by correction of any single defect via chromosome transfer. Mol Cell Biol 12:1387, 1992.
6. TAKAHASHI T et al: Wild-type but not mutant p53 suppresses the growth of human lung cancer cells bearing multiple genetic lesions. Cancer Res 52:2340, 1992.
7. DRAZEN K et al: In vivo adenoviral-mediated human p53 tumor suppressor gene transfer and expression in rat liver after resection. Surgery 116:197, 1994.
8. BADIE B et al: Adenovirus-mediated p53 gene delivery inhibits 9L glioma growth in rats. Neurol Res 17:209, 1995.
9. CLAYMAN G et al: In vivo molecular therapy with p53 adenovirus for microscopic residual head and neck squamous carcinoma. Cancer Res 55:1, 1995.
10. LIU T et al: Growth suppression of human head and neck cancer cells by the introduction of a wild-type p53 gene via a recombinant adenovirus. Cancer Res 54:3662, 1994.
11. WERTHMAN P et al: Adenoviral-p53 gene transfer to orthotopic and peritoneal murine bladder cancer. J Urol 155:753, 1996.
12. RUSCH V et al: Aberrant p53 expression predicts clinical resistance to cisplatin-based chemotherapy in locally advanced non-small cell lung cancer. Cancer Res 55:5038, 1995.
13. LOWE S et al: p53-dependent apoptosis modulates the cytotoxicity of anticancer agents. Cell 74:957, 1993.
14. FUJIWARA T et al: Induction of chemosensitivity in human lung cancer cells in vivo by adenoviral-mediated transfer of the wild-type p53 gene. Cancer Res 54:2287, 1994.
15. CAI D et al: Stable expression of the wild-type p53 gene in human lung cancer cells after retrovirus-mediated gene transfer. Hum Gene Ther 4:617, 1993.
16. ALBERT M et al: Dendritic cells acquire antigen from apoptotic cells and induce class-I restricted CTLs. Nature 392:86, 1998.
17. MUJOO K et al: Adenoviral-mediated p53 tumor suppressor gene therapy of human ovarian carcinoma. Oncogene 12:1617, 1996.
18. NIELSEN L et al: Efficacy of p53 adenovirus-mediated gene therapy against human breast cancer xenografts. Cancer Gene Ther 4:129, 1997.
19. NIELSEN L, MANEVAL D: P53 tumor suppressor gene therapy for cancer. Cancer Gene Ther 5:52, 1998.

20. KOCK H et al: Adenovirus-mediated p53 gene transfer suppresses growth of human glioblastoma cells in vitro and in vivo. Int J Cancer 67:808, 1996.

21. FARZANEH F et al: Gene therapy of cancer. Immunol Today 19:294, 1998.

22. RICHARDSON J, MARASCO W: Intracellular antibodies; development and therapeutic potential. Trends Biotech 13:306, 1995.

23. ZHANG Y et al: Retroviral vector-mediated transduction of K-ras antisense RNA into human lung cancer cells inhibits expression of the malignant phenotype. Hum Gene Ther 4:451, 1993.

24. KASHANI-SABET M et al: Suppression of the neoplastic phenotype in vivo by an anti-ras ribozyme. Cancer Res 54:900, 1994.

25. FENG M et al: Neoplastic reversion accomplished by high efficiency adenoviral-mediated delivery of an anti-ras ribozyme. Cancer Res 55:2024, 1995.

26. CALABRETTA B: Inhibition of protooncogene expression by antisense oligodeoxynucleotides: Biological and therapeutic implications. Cancer Res 51:4505, 1991.

27. AKHTAR S, IVINSON A: Therapies that make sense. Nature Gen 4:215, 1993.

28. ZHANG W: Antisense oncogene and tumor suppressor gene therapy of cancer. J Mol Med 74:191, 1996.

29. SKLAR M et al: Depletion of c-myc with specific antisense sequences reverses the transformed phenotype in ras oncogene-transformed NIH 3T3 cells. Mol Cell Biol 11:3699, 1991.

30. MUKHOPADHYAY T et al: Specific inhibition of K-ras expression and tumorigenicity of lung cancer cells by antisense RNA. Cancer Res 51:1744, 1991.

31. LEDWITH B et al: Antisense-fos RNA causes partial reversion of the transformation phenotypes induced by the c-Ha-ras oncogene. Mol Cell Biol 10:1545, 1990.

32. SULLENGER B: Gene therapy's next wave: messenger RNA repair. J Natl Inst Health Res 9:37, 1997.

33. CHANG M et al: A ribozyme specifically suppresses transformation and tumorigenicity of Ha-ras-oncogene-transformed NIH/3T3 cell lines. J Cancer Res Clin Oncol 123:91, 1997.

34. SCHERR M et al: Specific hammerhead ribozyme-mediated cleavage of mutant N-ras mRNA in vitro and ex vivo. Oligonucleotides as therapeutic agents. J Biol Chem 272:14304, 1997.

35. AOKI T et al: Expression of murine interleukin 7 in a murine glioma cell line results in reduced tumorigenicity in vivo. Proc Natl Acad Sci USA 89:3850, 1992.

36. CONNOR J et al: Regression of bladder tumors in mice treated with interleukin-2 gene-modified tumor cells. J Exp Med 177:1127, 1993.

37. FEARON E et al: Interleukin-2 production by tumor cells bypasses T helper function in the generation of an anti-tumor response. Cell 60:397, 1990.

38. DRANOFF G et al: Vaccination with irradiated tumor cells engineered to secrete murine granulocyte-macrophage colony-stimulating factor stimulates potent, specific, and long-lasting anti-tumor immunity. Proc Natl Acad Sci USA 90:3539, 1993.

39. GANSBACHER B et al: Interleukin-2 gene transfer into tumor cells abrogates tumorigenicity and induces protective immunity. J Exp Med 172:1217, 1990.

40. GANSBACHER et al: Retroviral vector-mediated gamma-interferon gene transfer into tumor cells generates potent and long lasting anti-tumor immunity. Cancer Res 50:7820, 1990.

41. GOLUMBEK P et al: Treatment of established renal cancer by tumor cells engineered to secrete interleukin-4. Science 254:713, 1991.

42. PORGADOR A et al: Interleukin 6 gene transfection into Lewis lung carcinoma tumor cells suppresses the malignant phenotype and confers immunotherapeutic competence against parental metastatic cells. Cancer Res 52:3679, 1992.

43. PORGADOR et al: Immunotherapy via gene therapy: Comparison of the effects of tumor cells transduced with the interleukin-2, interleukin-6, or interferon-γ genes. J Immunother 14:191, 1993.

44. SAITO S et al: Immunotherapy of bladder cancer with cytokine gene-modified tumor vaccines. Cancer Res 54:3516, 1994.

45. VIEWEG J et al: Immunotherapy of prostate cancer in the Dunning rat model: Use of cytokine gene modified tumor vaccines. Cancer Res 54:3516, 1994.

46. BELLI F et al: Active immunization of metastatic melanoma patients with interleukin-2-transduced allogeneic melanoma cells: Evaluation of efficacy and tolerability. Cancer Immunol Immunother 44:197, 1997.

47. ABDEL-WAHAB Z et al: A phase I clinical trial of immunotherapy with interferon-γ gene-modified autologous melanoma cells. Cancer 80:401, 1997.

48. ELLEM K et al: A case report: Immune responses and clinical course of the first human use of granulocyte-macrophage colony-stimulating-factor-transduced autologous melanoma cells for immunotherapy. Cancer Immunol Immunother 44:10, 1997.

49. SIMONS J et al: Bioactivity of autologous irradiated renal cell carcinoma vaccines generated by ex vivo granulocyte-macrophage colony-stimulating factor gene transfer. J Immunol Cancer Res 57:1537, 1997.

50. CLARY B et al: Active immunization with tumor cells transduced by a novel AAV plasmid-based gene delivery system. J Immunother 20:26, 1997.

51. PHILIP R et al: Gene modification of primary tumor cells for active immunotherapy of human breast and ovarian cancer. Clin Cancer Res 2:59, 1996.

52. JAFFEE E et al: High efficiency gene transfer into primary human tumor explants without cell selection. Cancer Res 53:2221, 1993.

53. TAHARA H et al: Clinical protocol: IL-12 gene therapy using direct injection of tumors with genetically engineered autologous fibroblasts. Hum Gene Ther 6:1607, 1995.

54. TAHARA H et al: Fibroblasts genetically engineered to secrete interleukin-12 can suppress tumor growth and induce anti-tumor immunity to a murine melanoma in vivo. Cancer Res 54:182, 1994.

55. LOTZE M, RUBIN J: Gene therapy of cancer: a pilot study of IL-4 gene modified fibroblasts admixed with autologous tumor to elicit an immune response. Hum Gene Ther 5:41, 1994.

56. LATTIME E et al: In situ cytokine gene transfection using vaccinia virus vectors. Semin Oncol 23:88, 1996.

57. NABEL G et al: Immune response in human melanoma after transfer of an allogeneic class I major histocompatibility complex gene with DNA-liposome complexes. Proc Natl Acad Sci USA 93:15388, 1996.

58. HUI K et al: Phase I study of immunotherapy of cutaneous metastases of human carcinoma using allogeneic and xenogeneic MHC DNA-liposome complexes. Gene Ther 4:783, 1997.

59. HUANG A et al: Role of bone marrow-derived cells in presenting MHC class I-restricted tumor antigens. Science 264:961, 1994.

60. CONRY R et al: Polynucleotide-mediated immunization therapy of cancer. Semin Oncol 23:135, 1996.

61. HAMILTON J et al: Phase I study of recombinant vaccinia virus (rV) that expresses human carcinoembryonic antigen (CEA) in adult patients with adenocarcinoma. Proc Am Soc Clin Oncol 961 (abstract), 1994.

62. MCANENY D et al: Results of a phase I trial of a recombinant vaccinia virus that expresses carcinoembryonic antigen in patients with advanced colorectal cancer. Ann Surg Oncol 3:495, 1996.

63. WOLFF J et al: Long-term persistence of plasmid DNA and foreign gene expression in mouse muscle. Hum Molec Gen 1:363, 1992.

64. DANKO I, WOLFF J: Direct gene transfer into muscle. Vaccine 12:1499, 1994.

65. DOE B et al: Induction of cytotoxic T lymphocytes by intramuscular immunization with plasmid DNA is facilitated by bone marrow derived cells. Proc Natl Acad Sci USA 93:8578, 1996.

66. TSANG K et al: Generation of human cytotoxic T cells specific for human carcinoembryonic antigen epitopes from patients immunized with recombinant vaccinia-CEA vaccine. J Natl Cancer Inst 87:982, 1995.

67. HWU P et al: Functional and molecular characterization of TIL transduced with the TNF-$\alpha$ cDNA for the gene therapy of cancer in man. J Immunol 150:1404, 1993.

68. CHEN S et al: Potent antitumor activity of a new class of tumour-specific killer cells. Nature 385:78, 1997.

69. ALTENSCHMIDT U et al: Specific cytotoxic T lymphocytes in gene therapy. J Mol Med 75:259, 1997.

70. HENDERSON R et al: Human dendritic cells genetically engineered to express high levels of the human epithelial tumor antigen mucin (MUC-1). Cancer Res 56:3763, 1996.

71. NAIR S et al: Induction of primary carcinoembryonic antigen (CEA)-specific cytotoxic T lymphocytes in vitro using human dendritic cells transfected with RNA. Nature Biotech 16:1, 1998.

72. SATO Y et al: Immunostimulatory DNA sequences necessary for effective intradermal gene immunization. Science 273:352, 1996.

73. MOOLTEN F: Drug sensitivity ("suicide") genes for selective cancer chemotherapy. Cancer Gene Ther 4:279, 1994.

74. FREEMAN S et al: In situ use of suicide genes for cancer therapy. Semin Oncol 23:31, 1996.

75. DIMAIO J et al: Directed enzyme pro-drug gene therapy for pancreatic cancer in vivo. Surgery 116:205, 1994.

76. CULVER K et al: In vivo gene transfer with retroviral vector-producer cells for treatment of experimental brain tumors. Science 256:1550, 1992.

77. BORRELLI E et al: Targeting of an inducible toxic phenotype in animal cells. Proc Natl Acad Sci USA 85:7572, 1988.

78. EZZEDDINE Z et al: Selective killing of glioma cells in culture and in vivo by retrovirus transfer of the herpes simplex virus thymidine kinase gene. New Biologist 3:608, 1991.

79. RAM Z et al: In situ retroviral-mediated gene transfer for the treatment of brain tumors in rats. Cancer Res 53:83, 1993.

80. MOOLTEN F: Tumor chemosensitivity conferred by inserted herpes thymidine kinase genes: Paradigm for a prospective cancer control strategy. Cancer Res 46:5276, 1986.

81. AUSTIN E, HUBER B: A first step in the development of gene therapy for colorectal carcinoma: cloning, sequencing, and expression of Escherichia coli cytosine deaminase. Mol Pharmacol 43:380, 1993.

82. CONSALVO M et al: 5-fluorocytosine induced eradication of murine adenocarcinomas engineered to express the cytosine deaminase suicide gene requires host immune competence and leaves an efficient memory. J Immunol 154:5302, 1995.

83. HUBER B et al: Metabolism of 5-fluorocytosine to 5-fluorouracil in human colorectal tumor cells transduced with the cytosine deaminase gene: Significant antitumor effects when only a small percentage of tumor cells express cytosine deaminase. Proc Natl Acad Sci USA 91:8302, 1994.

84. MULLEN C et al: Tumors expressing the cytosine deaminase gene can be eliminated in vivo with 5-fluorocytosine and induce protective immunity to wild type tumor. Cancer Res 54:1503, 1994.

85. HIRSCHOWITZ E et al: In vivo adenovirus-mediated gene transfer of the Escherichia coli cytosine deaminase gene to human colon carcinoma-derived tumors induces chemosensitivity to 5-fluorocytosine. Hum Gene Ther 6:1055, 1995.

86. HUBER B et al: Retroviral-mediated gene therapy for the treatment of hepatocellular carcinoma: an innovative approach for cancer therapy. Hum Gene Ther 88:8039, 1991.

87. BESNARD C et al: Selection against expression of the Escherichia coli hene in hprt+ mouse teratocarcinoma and hybrid cells. Mol Cell Biol 7:4139, 1987.

88. MROZ P, MOOLTEN F: Retrovirally transduced Escherichia coli hgpt genes combine selectability with chemosensitivity capable of mediating tumor eradication. Hum Gene Ther 4:589, 1993.

89. DEONARAIN M, EPENETOS A: Targeting enzymes for cancer therapy: Old enzymes in new roles. Br J Cancer 5:786, 1994.

90. WEI M et al: Experimental tumor therapy in mice using cyclophosphamide-activating cytochrome P450 2B1 gene. Hum Gene Ther 5:969, 1994.

91. KIM J et al: Selective enhancement by an antiviral agent of the radiation-induced cell killing of human glioma cells transduced with HSV-tk gene. Cancer Res 54:6053, 1994.

92. KHIL M et al: Radiosensitization by 5-fluorocytosine human colorectal carcinoma cells in culture transduced with cytosine-deaminase gene: retrovirus vector-mediated gene transfer, prodrug activation and irradiation for improved tumor therapy. Clin Cancer Res 2:53, 1996.

93. FREEMAN S et al: The "bystander effect": tumor regression when a fraction of the tumor mass is genetically modified. Cancer Res 53:5274, 1993.

94. VILE R et al: Systemic gene therapy of murine melanoma using tissue specific expression of the HSVTK gene involves an immune component. Cancer Res 54:6228, 1994.

95. BI W et al: In vitro evidence that metabolic cooperation is responsible for the bystander effect observed with HSVTK retroviral gene therapy. Hum Gene Ther 4:725, 1993.

96. BARBA D et al: Development of anti-tumor immunity following thymidine kinase-mediated killing of experimental brain tumors. Proc Natl Acad Sci USA 91:4348, 1994.

97. RAM Z et al: Intrathecal gene therapy for malignant leptomeningeal neoplasia. Cancer Res 54:2141, 1994.

98. CARUSO M et al: Regression of established macroscopic liver metastases after in situ transduction of a suicide gene. Proc Natl Acad Sci USA 90:7024, 1993.

99. BLOCK A et al: Adenoviral-mediated herpes simplex virus thymidine kinase gene transfer: regression of hepatic metastasis of pancreatic tumors. Pancreas 15:25, 1997.

100. CLARY B et al: In vivo directed enzyme pro-drug gene therapy for human pancreatic cancer. Surg Forum 46:520, 1995.

101. SMYTHE W et al: Treatment of experimental human mesothelioma using adenovirus transfer of the herpes simplex thymidine kinase gene. Ann Surg 222:78, 1995.

102. YOSHIDA K et al: Retrovirally transmitted gene therapy for gastric carcinoma using herpes simplex virus thymidine kinase gene. Cancer 75:1467, 1995.

103. GOTTESMAN M, PASTAN I: Biochemistry of multidrug resistance mediated by the multidrug transporter. Ann Rev Biochem 62:385, 1993.

104. SORRENTINO B et al: Selection of drug-resistant bone marrow cells in vivo after retroviral transfer of human MDR-1. Science 257:99, 1992.

105. HESDORFFER C et al: Phase I trial of retroviral-mediated transfer of the human MDR1 gene as marrow chemoprotection in patients undergoing high-dose chemotherapy and autologous stem-cell transplantation. J Clin Oncol 16:165, 1998.

106. MILLER D et al: Gene transfer by retrovirus vectors occurs only in cells that are actively replicating at the time of infection. Mol Cell Biol 10:4239, 1990.

107. KOC O et al: Transfer of drug resistance genes into hematopoietic progenitors to improve chemotherapy tolerance. Semin Oncol 23:46, 1996.

108. BRENNER M et al: Gene-marking to trace origin of relapse after autologous bone marrow transplantation. Lancet 341:85, 1993.

109. RUHL E et al: T cell activation status modulates retrovirus-mediated gene expression. Blood 90(Suppl):417b, 1997.

110. CORNETTA K et al: No retroviremia or pathology in long term follow-up of monkeys exposed to a murine amphotropic retrovirus. Hum Gene Ther 2:215, 1991.

111. FERRY N et al: Retroviral-mediated gene transfer into hepatocytes in vivo. Proc Natl Acad Sci USA 88:8377, 1991.

112. NALDINI L et al: In vitro gene delivery and stable transduction of nondividing cells by a lentiviral vector. Science 272:263, 1996.

113. DESCAMPS V et al: Strategies for cancer gene therapy using adenoviral vectors. J Molec Med 74:183, 1996.

114. KOCHANEK S et al: A new adenoviral vector-replacement of all viral coding sequences with 28kb of DNA independently expressing both full-length dystrophin and beta-galactosidase. Proc Natl Acad Sci USA 93:5731, 1996.

115. BERNS K, BOHENZKY R: Adeno-associated viruses: An update. Adv Virus Res 32:243, 1987.

116. FELGNER P et al: Synthetic recombinant DNA delivery for cancer therapeutics. Cancer Gene Ther 2:61, 1995.

117. NABEL E et al: Gene transfer in vivo with DNA-liposome complexes: Lack of autoimmunity and gonadal localization. Human Gene Ther 3:649, 1992.

118. STEWART M et al: Gene transfer in vivo with DNA-liposome complexes: Safety and acute toxicity in mice. Hum Gene Ther 3:267, 1992.

119. ZHU N et al: Systemic gene expression after intravenous DNA delivery into adult mice. Science 261:209, 1993.

120. YANG N et al: Developing particle-mediated gene-transfer technology for research into gene therapy of cancer. Mol Med Today 2:476, 1996.

121. SUN W et al: In vivo cytokine gene transfer by gene gun reduces tumor growth in mice. Proc Natl Acad Sci USA 92:2889, 1995.

122. WU G et al: Receptor-mediated gene delivery in vivo. Partial correction of genetic analbuminemia in Nagase rats. J Biol Chem 266:14338, 1991.

123. VILE R, HART I: In vitro and in vivo targeting of gene expression to melanoma cells. Cancer Res 53:962, 1993.

124. SCHREWE H et al: Cloning of the complete gene for carcinoembryonic antigen: analysis of its promoter indicates a region conveying cell type-specific expression. Mol Cell Biol 10:2738, 1990.

125. RICHARDS C et al: Transcriptional regulatory sequences of carcinoembryonic antigen: identification and use with cytosine deaminase for tumor-specific gene therapy. Hum Gene Ther 6:881, 1995.

126. OSAKI T et al: Gene therapy for carcinoembryonic antigen-producing human lung cancer cells by cell type-specific expression of herpes simplex virus thymidine kinase gene. Cancer Res 54:5258, 1994.

127. IDO A et al: Gene therapy for hepatoma cells using a retrovirus vector carrying herpes simplex virus thymidine kinase gene under the control of human α-fetoprotein promoter. Cancer Res 55:3105, 1995.

128. HARRIS J et al: Gene therapy for cancer using tumor-specific prodrug activation. Gene Ther 1:170, 1994.

129. GARVER R et al: Strategy for achieving selective killing of carcinomas. Gene Ther 1:46, 1994.

130. PANG S et al: Prostate tissue specificity of the prostate-specific antigen promoter isolated from a patient with prostate cancer. Hum Gene Ther 6:1417, 1995.

# 3F / MOLECULAR BIOLOGY

*Alan M. Yahanda and Alfred E. Chang*

## INTRODUCTION

Our understanding of the molecular origins of disease has expanded remarkably over the past two decades. New disease genes are being found at an unprecedented rate, and it is likely that the sequence of the entire human genome will be known within the next several years. Our current pace of discovery is unparalleled by any other period in history, and we stand at the brink of a revolution in which molecular diagnosis and treatment will become an integral part of the practice of medicine and oncology.

The integration of molecular biology into the everyday clinical practice of oncology has, in fact, already begun. It is therefore essential for the practicing physician to have a basic understanding of molecular biology, its terminology, and its techniques. The scope of this section will not permit a detailed review of molecular biology or genetics. Instead, it will focus on some fundamentals of molecular biology and molecular biologic techniques and their application in the evaluation and treatment of cancer patients. In addition, some basics of cancer genetics and familial cancer syndromes will be discussed.

## AN OVERVIEW OF MOLECULAR BIOLOGY

The information necessary for the development, functioning, and propagation of an organism is contained within its DNA and is encoded by the sequence of four nucleotides, adenine (A), guanine (G), cytosine (C), and thymidine (T). Each strand of DNA is paired to a complementary strand of DNA, resulting in the double helical structure. This pairing is specified through the interactions of the four nucleotides: an A on one strand is always paired with a T on the complementary strand, and a G on one strand is always paired with a C on the other. Consequently, the genetic information in DNA is actually redundant, being present in both strands of the pair (Fig. 3F-1).

According to the central doctrine of molecular biology, genetic information is perpetuated by replication of DNA and is expressed in the form of proteins (Fig. 3F-2). Replication of DNA occurs when the double strands of DNA separate, and each strand serves as a template for the creation of another, identical complementary strand. Within these strands of DNA are individual units called genes, which contain the information necessary for the synthesis of a specific protein. The conversion of the genetic information contained in the DNA to its corresponding protein occurs in a two-stage process. Initially, one strand of the DNA, the antisense strand, is used as a template for the synthesis of messenger RNA (mRNA) in a process termed transcription. Consequently, the nucleotide sequence of the mRNA is identical to that of the opposite strand of DNA, the sense strand. A protein is then synthesized from the mRNA by the process of translation, in which each amino acid in the protein is specified by a triplet of nucleotides in the mRNA called a codon. Any alteration of the sequence of the DNA, therefore, may have significant impact on the sequence of amino acids in the encoded protein.

Virtually every combination of three nucleotides in the DNA codes for a specific amino acid. Of the 64 possible arrangements of 4 nucleotides in a triplet sequence, 61 code for amino acids, whereas 3, called stop codons, cause termination of translation. Given that there are 20 amino acids used to synthesize proteins, almost all amino acids are represented by more than one codon. Most commonly, the last nucleotide in a triplet sequence is the most degenerate, as codons differing in the last base often code for the same amino acid. Thus, alterations in DNA sequence may not necessarily cause change in a corresponding protein. Such variations in sequence, although termed mutations, cause no functional change in protein sequence or structure. These alterations may be more appropriately termed polymorphisms or allelic variations. This degeneracy of the genetic code may, in fact, serve to ameliorate many spontaneous, sporadic mutations that may occur.

Alternative forms of a gene are termed alleles, and their existence may be normal, allowing for diversity within a population. For example, in the pioneering genetic studies of the garden pea by Gregor Mendel, he found that flower color could be either purple or white, and that these characteristics were determined by different alleles of the same gene. When an organism has two identical alleles of a gene, it is homozygous for that allele. If the organism carries two different alleles of a gene, it is heterozygous. Although allelic variation within a population is quite normal, we are most familiar with cases in which one allele is normal and another is decidedly abnormal and pathogenic. A classic example of this is the disease sickle cell anemia, in which affected individuals inherit two mutant alleles of the hemoglobin gene that code for an altered form of the protein hemoglobin S. Red blood cells containing hemoglobin S change morphology to become sickle-shaped under conditions of low oxygen tension. This example also demonstrates the concept that the appearance or functioning of an individual (the phenotype) results from the interaction of the environment and his or her genetic makeup (the genotype).

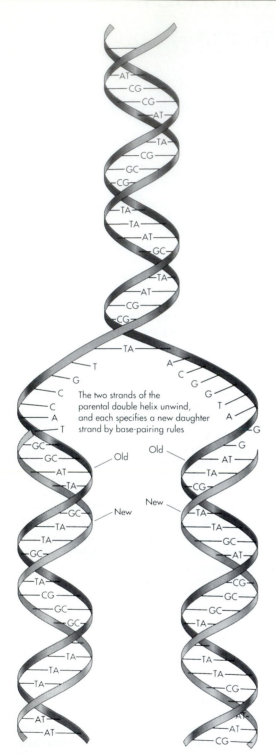

**FIGURE 3F-1.** DNA consists of two polynucleotide chains that form a double helix. The two chains are associated by a series of hydrogen bonds between nucleotides. Note the complementary pairing of bases between strands: a guanine (G) can hydrogen bond specifically with a cytosine (C) and an adenosine (A) with a thymine (T). The two strands are said to be complementary. (*Reprinted with permission from Watson.*[140])

Within figure: The two strands of the parental double helix unwind, and each specifies a new daughter strand by base-pairing rules. Old / Old / New / New

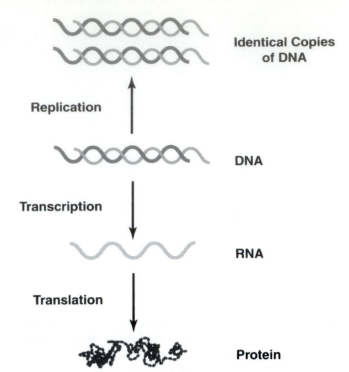

**FIGURE 3F-2.** The central doctrine of molecular biology states that the information contained in DNA is perpetuated by replication and expressed in the form of protein.

Within figure: Identical Copies of DNA / Replication / DNA / Transcription / RNA / Translation / Protein

The genetic code is remarkably conserved among all living organisms. In fact, the same codon–amino acid assignments exist in bacteria, yeast, and humans. This similarity is central to many common techniques in molecular biology and biotechnology, making possible the expression of human genes in animal or bacterial cells and the production of recombinant human proteins. Furthermore, it has made possible the identification of human gene homologues in lower animals, allowing for more facile elucidation of functional and biochemical pathways.

The length of most mRNA transcripts is significantly smaller than the sequence length of the coding genomic DNA. The reason for this discrepancy is that most genes have interruptions in their coding sequences, segments of DNA that are not represented in the mRNA, called introns. The sequence destined to be retained in the mature mRNA is transcribed from segments of the gene termed exons. The intronic sequence is removed from the primary mRNA by the process of mRNA splicing. Sites at which splicing takes place are encoded in segments of sequence that designate both splice donor and acceptor sites. This same process of splicing can actually allow one DNA sequence (i.e., gene) to code for more than one protein through alternative splicing of the mRNA transcript. By splicing out different exons, in addition to the introns, the resultant proteins may still be relatively similar in form and function, or they may be completely different with no sequence or functional homology. An example of the latter is the p16-p19$^{ARF}$ locus from which two distinct proteins are produced (Fig. 3F-3).[1]

It is estimated that there may be as many as 125,000 genes in the human genome, but only a fraction of these are expressed in a given

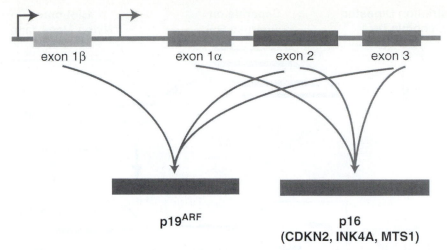

**FIGURE 3F-3.** The p16-p19[ARF] gene illustrates the process of RNA splicing. Two completely distinct products arise out of a single locus through RNA splicing and the use of different reading frames. p16 is derived from exons 1a, 2, and 3, with a promoter region depicted by the green arrow. The p19[ARF] transcript, on the other hand, is derived from exons 1b, 2 and 3, with the promoter shown in magenta. Although both transcripts share exons 2 and 3, they have different reading frames, and thus, have no amino acid sequence similarity. (See also Plate 13.)

cell at any given time. If one assumes that the number of unique mRNA transcripts isolated from a cell represents the number of expressed genes, then the average human cell expresses approximately 10,000 to 20,000 different genes.[2] Gene expression is turned on and off by a molecular switch termed a promoter, which is a sequence of nucleotides that precedes the coding portion of the gene. The promoter sequence is recognized by and binds specific proteins that are responsible for initiating transcription, the best known being an RNA polymerase that synthesizes RNA by reading the DNA as a template. Binding of RNA polymerase alone directly to the promoter may be seen in genes that are constitutively expressed in all cell types. There are, however, many cells in which genes are expressed in a more tissue- or temporal-specific manner. In these cells there are additional, specific promoter-binding proteins, or transcription factors, that permit certain genes to be expressed only in certain cells or at certain times in development. For example, a muscle cell would have the necessary transcription factors to activate the myosin gene, whereas a myeloid cell would not. Further affecting the expression of specific genes are enhancers, which are sequences of DNA that are located before the promoter. It is thought that enhancer elements also serve to bind transcription factors that influence the rate at which a gene is transcribed. Mutations in the promoter or enhancer sequences may result in an alteration in the level of gene expression by either increasing or decreasing the ability of transcription factors to bind.

## ISOLATION AND ANALYSIS OF GENES

Genomic DNA necessary for experimental or diagnostic assays can be easily isolated from both fresh and archival tissues and cells.[3] The analysis of DNA usually involves: (1) confirmation of the presence or absence of a specific gene or DNA sequence within a sample, (2) amplification and isolation of specific genes or sequences, (3) identification of variation or mutation within DNA sequences, and (4) mapping the location of a gene within the genome. Some of the techniques to analyze DNA used on a routine basis in clinical and research laboratories will be discussed in this section.

## SOUTHERN BLOTTING

Identification of a specific gene or DNA sequence within a sample of DNA that may contain thousands of genes is accomplished using the technique of Southern blotting, developed by E. M. Southern in 1975.[4] Using this technique, the DNA sequence of interest, called the probe, is radiolabeled and added to the sample of DNA (Fig. 3F-4). If a sequence complementary to that of the probe is present in the sample DNA, it hybridizes with the probe and thus can be detected. When large segments of DNA are used, such as genomic DNA, the initial step is to first cut it into smaller, more easily managed pieces using restriction endonucleases, enzymes that cleave DNA at unique and specific sequences of nucleotides. These fragments are next separated by size using electrophoresis, with smaller fragments migrating more rapidly within a gel than larger ones. At this point, if genomic DNA was used, the gel contains a continuous smear of different-sized DNA fragments without distinct bands. Because the gel is a poor medium in which to perform the subsequent hybridization steps, the fractionated DNA must be transferred and immobilized to a solid support, such as a nitrocellulose filter or nylon membrane. The radiolabeled probe, specific for the DNA sequence of interest, is then added and allowed to hybridize to the DNA immobilized on

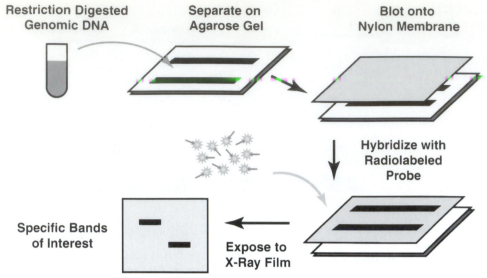

**Restriction Digested Genomic DNA**

**Separate on Agarose Gel**

**Blot onto Nylon Membrane**

**Hybridize with Radiolabeled Probe**

**Specific Bands of Interest**

**Expose to X-Ray Film**

**FIGURE 3F-4.** Southern blotting is a technique to detect DNA. The sample of DNA is separated by size in an agarose gel using electrophoresis. The separated DNA is transferred to a solid support (such as a nylon membrane) and incubated with a specific DNA probe that is radiolabeled. The probe will hybridize to its complementary DNA on the membrane. The presence and size of the DNA of interest can be detected by autoradiography.

the membrane. The probe will hybridize only to DNA fragments that contain complementary sequence. When placed on x-ray film, each complementary sequence yields a distinct band at a position determined by the size of the DNA fragment.

## LOSS OF HETEROZYGOSITY AND MICROSATELLITE INSTABILITY

A common genetic mechanism underlying many cancers is the loss of a specific gene, such as one responsible for growth regulation, or more often, loss of a larger segment of DNA in which that gene is located. In such cases, the normal tissues retain two normal copies of the gene, whereas the tumor tissue has either one or no copies of the gene. In order to document such a loss, investigators exploit naturally occurring repeated nucleotide sequences in the genome called microsatellites. These repeated sequences of 2, 3, or 4 nucleotides are of variable length (typically between 5 and 30 repeats) and are usually polymorphic. Consequently, an individual may be heterozygous at a given microsatellite locus, with a paternal allele of one length and a maternal allele of another length.[5] In such cases, the loss of one of the microsatellite alleles at a particular locus is termed loss of heterozygosity (LOH). In individuals who are homozygous for a microsatellite allele, loss of one of the alleles would not be detected and, therefore, the particular locus would be declared uninformative.

Many of these microsatellites and their flanking DNA sequences have been identified throughout the genome, and it is estimated that a microsatellite tract may be present every 30,000 to 60,000 bases. In order to determine if there has been LOH, normal and tumor DNA are amplified by the polymerase chain reaction (see later for description) using radiolabeled primers flanking the microsatellite of interest. The amplified products from normal and tumor DNA are loaded in adjacent lanes on a polyacrylamide gel and are separated by size using electrophoresis. The gel is then placed on x-ray film, and the products are visualized. Absence in tumor tissue of a microsatellite band that is present in normal tissue constitutes a loss of heterozygosity (Fig. 3F-5A). LOH studies have largely supplanted cytogenetic analysis as a means of identifying regions of DNA loss in tumor cells. This strategy has been used widely in virtually all tumor types to define areas of loss that may harbor important cancer-related genes. For example, the short arm of chromosome 17 (17q) was found to be lost in 73% of sporadic colon cancers. Using a panel of polymorphic markers spaced along 17q, the common region of loss was found to be centered around 17p13.1, the location of the p53 tumor suppressor gene.[6,7]

Microsatellite markers have also been used extensively in identifying cells that are deficient in DNA mismatch repair. Such cells lack the ability to excise and repair nucleotide mismatches that occur during DNA replication (see DNA Mismatch Repair Genes below). Microsatellites, with long tracts of repeated nucleotides, are particularly prone to mismatching, and cells with a deficient repair mechanism will manifest this by either expansion or contraction of the length of the repeats and are considered to have microsatellite instability. In assaying for microsatellite instability, paired normal and tumor DNA are processed in a manner similar to LOH. When visualized on an autoradiograph, however, the length of the microsatellite tracts from a tumor deficient in mismatch repair will differ from those of normal tissue (Fig. 3F-5B). Microsatellite instability is the hallmark of tumors resected from patients with hereditary nonpolyposis colorectal cancer in whom mutations in any of several DNA

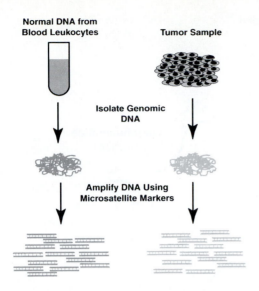

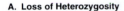

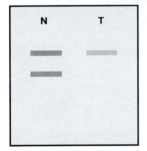
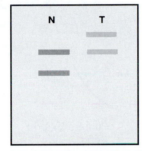

**FIGURE 3F-5.** Normal DNA is isolated from either peripheral blood lymphocytes or from normal tissue samples, and tumor DNA is obtained from tumor tissue. The DNA is amplified through the polymerase chain reaction using primers around the particular microsatellite. Paired tumor and normal DNA are run in parallel on a gel. *A.* The absence of a microsatellite band in the tumor sample demonstrates loss of heterozygosity at this locus. *B.* Expansion (shown here) or contraction of the size of a microsatellite tract in tumor tissue indicates microsatellite instability. (N = normal sample; T = tumor sample).

mismatch repair enzymes have been implicated in tumorigenesis.[8,9] Similarly, microsatellite instability has been found in many sporadic cancers, as well as in cells isolated from the urine, sputum, stool, and surgical margins of patients with corresponding primary tumors.[10,11]

## POLYMERASE CHAIN REACTION

One of the most significant advances in molecular biology has been the development of the polymerase chain reaction (PCR). This incredibly powerful technique allows a single copy of a specific DNA sequence to be amplified to yield millions or even billions of copies.

Its impact on the way that molecular biology is now practiced has been staggering. Whereas before, milligram quantities of cells or tissues were needed in order to isolate sufficient DNA for study, PCR allows the study of microscopic amounts of tissue or even single cells. The PCR machine has become a standard and indispensable piece of equipment in every molecular biology laboratory, and is now gaining wider use in clinical laboratories as well. An increasing number of diagnoses in human disease are being made at the molecular level using PCR methods (see Molecular Pathology below). The importance of PCR was recognized in 1993 when the Nobel Prize in Chemistry was awarded to Kary Mullis for his contributions to the invention and development of the technique.[12,13]

The concept of PCR is illustrated in Fig. 3F-6. A double-stranded piece of DNA containing the sequence of interest serves as the template. Two oligonucleotides (approximately 15 to 25 nucleotides in length), called primers, are designed to have sequence complementary to the sequence flanking the segment of DNA to be amplified. The template DNA and primers are heated in order to separate the double-stranded DNA into single strands (denaturation step). The mixture is then cooled to allow annealing of the primers to their complementary sequence on the template (annealing step). A DNA polymerase enzyme then uses the template strand to add complementary bases to the primer (extension step). In this manner, each double-stranded piece of DNA yields two complementary copies of the sequence of interest. These three steps are repeated multiple times, resulting in a doubling of the DNA with each cycle. If 30 cycles are used, a single DNA sequence can be amplified to $2^{30}$ (>1 billion) identical copies!

## DETECTION OF MUTATIONS

Direct sequencing of a gene is the only way to verify the presence or absence of a mutation. The most widely used method for DNA sequencing is the chain termination technique developed by Sanger and colleagues[14] in the 1970s. Central to the method are dideoxynucleotides (ddNTP), which are nucleotides that can be incorporated by DNA polymerase into an elongating DNA strand but are unable to form a phosphodiester bond with the next downstream nucleotide. Thus, incorporation of a ddNTP results in termination of the forming DNA chain. When normal deoxynucleotides (dNTPs) are mixed with a lower concentration of a specific ddNTP, the DNA polymerase will randomly incorporate both into the synthesized DNA. What results is a series of DNA chains with variable lengths that are determined during synthesis when the ddNTP was incorporated. Four separate reactions are run, one for each ddNTP, and the products of the reaction are separated on a polyacrylamide gel. A ladder of DNA bands results, with each depicting where in the sequence a particular nucleotide exists. In this manner, the nucleotide sequence of a segment of DNA can be deduced. This technique is used routinely in most molecular biology laboratories, and the process has been automated for high-output operations.

Despite its accuracy, direct DNA sequencing can be very cumbersome, especially if long segments require analysis. At best, manual or automated reactions can sequence 200 to 500 bases at a time. If a particular gene is large and a mutation cluster region has not been identified, sequencing can be costly in both time and money.

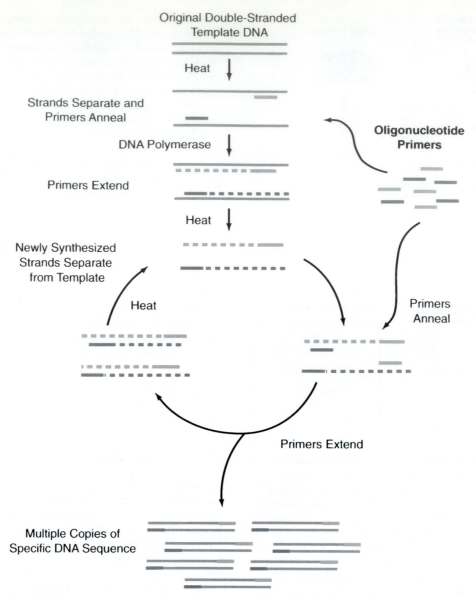

**FIGURE 3F-6.** The polymerase chain reaction is a powerful technique that allows the amplification of minute quantities of DNA.

There are a number of techniques that have been developed to more efficiently screen for mutations, particularly when multiple samples require evaluation. One such method is single-strand conformational polymorphism (SSCP) analysis, which is based on changes in the mobility of single-stranded DNA species caused by alterations in their primary sequence.[15] Single-stranded DNA has a folded, secondary structure that is dictated by the sequence of nucleotides in the strand. Differences in one nucleotide between two otherwise identical strands of DNA can be identified by alterations in the mobility of those strands through a nondenaturing electrophoretic gel. For example, a tumor that is wild-type for a gene of interest will show two bands, one corresponding to the sense strand and the other to the antisense strand. A tumor that harbors a heterozygous mutation in the gene of interest will be characterized by four bands, two corresponding to the wild-type strand and two corresponding to the mutant strands. Finally, a tumor that is homozygous for a mutation will show two bands that have a migration pattern different than that seen for the wild-type strand. The aberrantly migrating bands are then excised, and the contained DNA is isolated and sequenced to confirm the presence of an actual mutation. The increased efficiency of SSCP in screening for mutations, however, comes at the price of decreased sensitivity. At best, SSCP can detect about 80% of single base-pair mutations.[15,16] Similarly, a number of other techniques have been developed to help facilitate screening for mutations in a large number of samples. All of them, such as denaturing gradient-gel electrophoresis (DGGE) or heteroduplex analysis suffer from the same decreased sensitivity experienced with SSCP.[17,18]

As mentioned previously, the detection of a sequence variation in the DNA does not necessarily represent a pathogenic mutation. Many of these, due to the redundancy of the genetic code, may cause no change in the amino acid sequence of the resultant protein. Conversely, even those nucleotide sequence variations that result in amino acid changes may not be pathologic. For example, a mutation at codon 72 of the p53 gene that causes proline to be inserted rather than the normal arginine was identified in a group of patients with colon cancer. When a normal control population was screened, a similar frequency of this mutation was identified.[19] Thus, in order for a mutation to be considered a pathogenic one, it must be documented that its frequency is higher in the study population than in a control population, that it results in a functionally altered protein product, and ultimately that this results in a pathologic phenotype in the individual.

## ANALYSIS OF GENE EXPRESSION: mRNA

The majority of genes in a given cell are not transcribed into RNA. Therefore, a mutation may remain silent if a gene is not expressed in a particular cell type. This may explain, for example, why a germline mutation in a cancer predisposition gene may appear as a tumor in only one tissue type, even though all cells of the body contain the mutation. In order to document that a gene is expressed, one must first demonstrate that it is transcribed into mRNA and, ultimately, that this is translated into a protein.

Total cellular RNA can be isolated from cells by a variety of protocols.[3] The RNA thus isolated is an admixture of several RNA species, including ribosomal RNA (rRNA); transfer RNA (tRNA); mRNA; and unprocessed, transcribed RNA. Consequently, only a small fraction of this RNA will ever serve as templates for the synthesis of proteins. In order to narrow down the pool to those RNAs that are destined to be translated, it is necessary to isolate just the mRNA. Most eukaryotic mRNAs have long runs of adenines at one of their ends [poly(A) tail] that are added posttranscriptionally. The function of the poly(A) tail is unknown, but it can be exploited as a means of isolating mRNA for analysis. If the total RNA is exposed to a poly(T) oligonucleotide that has been immobilized to a solid support, such as cellulose or plastic beads, the poly(A) tail will bind to the complementary sequence. The other unwanted RNA species can then be washed away, leaving only the mature mRNA behind. The mRNA can then be eluted off of the poly(T) tract and recovered for study.

## NORTHERN BLOTTING

Documenting the expression of a gene and quantitating the level of that expression can be accomplished by northern blotting, a technique wittily named because of its similarity to Southern blotting. With northern blotting, RNA (total or messenger) is separated by size on a denaturing agarose gel by electrophoresis. As with Southern blotting, the RNA is transferred to nitrocellulose or a nylon mem-

brane and detected using a specific, labeled probe that hybridizes to the mRNA sequence of interest. A number of different probes can be used to detect RNA, including DNA, synthetic oligonucleotides, or RNA synthesized in vitro with DNA-dependent RNA polymerases.[3] Following hybridization, the RNA band of interest is visualized using autoradiography. Northern blotting is quantitative in that the intensity of the band is directly proportional to the amount of target RNA in the sample. Thus, differences in gene expression between samples, for example, tumor and normal tissue or stimulated and unstimulated cells, can be measured.

## REVERSE TRANSCRIPTASE PCR

When working with small amounts of sample or with rare mRNA transcripts, northern blot analysis is not feasible because it requires a significant amount of RNA to be loaded on the gel and it is limited in its ability to detect small amounts of transcript. To overcome these limitations, PCR technology has been applied to RNA in order to amplify rare messages and to facilitate their detection (Fig. 3F-7).

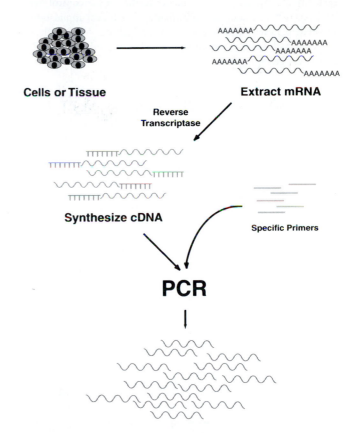

**FIGURE 3F-7.** Reverse transcriptase PCR (RT-PCR) is a sensitive method for detecting the expression of genes. The mRNA must first be converted to cDNA using the enzyme reverse transcriptase and primers that will anneal to the poly(A) tail of the mature mRNA. The resultant cDNA can then be amplified by using PCR.

The DNA polymerases used in PCR, however, are unable to utilize RNA as a template. Consequently, the RNA must first be converted to DNA for use in a PCR reaction. This conversion, however, runs counter to the direction defined by the central dogma of molecular biology, that is, DNA is transcribed into RNA, and not the reverse. This problem can be overcome by using a retroviral DNA polymerase called reverse transcriptase (RT), which uses RNA as a template for the synthesis of a complementary strand of DNA (complementary DNA or cDNA). This cDNA can then serve as the template in a standard PCR reaction. In this manner, a very small quantity of RNA can be amplified to yield millions of copies for subsequent study. The ability to quantitate gene expression by RT-PCR is controversial. Alterations in RT or PCR conditions, primer design, or template sequence and secondary structure can influence the efficiency of either the RT or PCR reactions, potentially resulting in nonlinear amplification. A number of methods have been developed to better enable RT-PCR to be used in a quantitative manner. These have included the simultaneous amplification of a control RNA sequence, which is usually from a gene with ubiquitous expression such as β-actin or glyceraldehyde 3-phosphate dehydrogenase. By normalizing the quantity of amplified target sequence to that of the control, comparisons between samples can be made.[20,21] Clinical application of RT-PCR is now routine, being used for such purposes as detecting viral pathogens or occult tumor cells in blood or tissues (see Molecular Pathology).

## ANALYSIS OF GENE EXPRESSION: PROTEIN

Proteins are synthesized by translation of the information encoded in mRNA and represent the end product of gene expression. Detection of proteins can be accomplished either by assays looking for a particular biologic function or by assays that are independent of such activity. Functional assays, however, may not be practical due to their lack of sensitivity when a protein is present in low quantity, or due to the complexity of many protein-protein interactions.[3] Furthermore, for many novel proteins, their function is unknown, making such assays impossible. Consequently, a number of techniques have been developed to detect proteins independent of their function, including western blotting, immunoprecipitation, and immunohistochemistry. All of these methods rely on antibodies that specifically bind to the protein of interest as the means of detection. A discussion of immunohistochemistry is presented in the Molecular Pathology section of this chapter.

## WESTERN BLOTTING

Proteins, and the amino acids that comprise them, are more heterogeneous than nucleic acids, making size fractionation by electrophoresis more difficult. Whereas nucleic acids represent a fairly homogeneous group of anionic molecules, there are 20 amino acids, some with positive, negative, or neutral charges. In addition, further complexity is added by the relative hydrophilic or hydrophobic nature of many amino acids and the addition of posttranslational modifications such as the addition of carbohydrate or phosphate moieties. Electrophoresis through a standard gel results in erratic migration of protein species. In order to overcome this problem, protein electrophoresis is performed in the presence of a detergent, sodium dodecyl sulfate (SDS), which binds to proteins and imparts a more uniform anionic charge. The migration of a protein through a gel to which SDS has been added is more uniform and will proceed based on the size of the protein.

Western blot analysis represents a means of detecting proteins that have been size-fractionated on an SDS-containing electrophoretic gel. Similar to the technique of Southern or northern blotting, the proteins are transferred from the gel to a solid support, such as nitrocellulose or nylon membrane. The protein blot is then incubated in a solution containing an antibody specific for the protein of interest. It is essential that a reliable, sensitive, and specific antibody be used for the best results. The antibody will bind to the protein, and its location on the blot can be visualized by a variety of detection systems. Regardless of the means of detection, the intensity of signal should correspond to the amount of protein present. Thus, western blot is used routinely for the quantification of proteins.

## CANCER IS A GENETIC DISEASE

The genetic or familial association of cancer has been recognized for centuries, but only recently has there been evidence that cancer is, in fact, a genetic disease. Malignant transformation and progression result from alterations in the genetic information within the cell (the DNA) that allow a selective growth advantage over surrounding normal cells. A current belief is that cancers arise from a multistep process of genetic alterations that result in the clonal expansion of progressively more abnormal and autonomous cells (Fig. 3F-8). The actual genes involved and the order in which they become altered may not always follow the same pattern in a given type of cancer. Instead, such models of tumor progression should

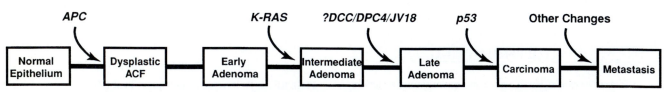

**FIGURE 3F-8.** The progression of normal colonic mucosa to cancer is thought to occur in a multistep fashion through the sequential accumulation of genetic alterations. Similar multistep models have been proposed for other tumor sites. (ACF = aberrant crypt focus) (*From Kinzler and Vogelstein,*[67] *with permission.*)

serve only as frameworks to enable us to better conceptualize the process of multistep carcinogenesis.

Genetic mutations that cause cancer can be inherited or can occur spontaneously. Those mutations that are passed from generation to generation are referred to as germline mutations. In these cases, the mutation is present in the DNA of every cell of the body and is passed on to subsequent generations through the germ cells. Cancers that arise sporadically, in the absence of any germline mutation, are called somatic mutations. In these cases only the tumor cells will harbor the mutation and their normal counterparts will not. The vast majority of cancers arise from presumed somatic mutations. There are three classes of genes that may be mutated in both inherited and sporadic cases of cancer: oncogenes, tumor suppressor genes, and DNA mismatch repair genes. Each of these gene classes will be discussed briefly and specific examples will be cited. The scope of this chapter precludes a more extensive treatment.

## ONCOGENES AND PROTOONCOGENES

Oncogenes were initially identified as genes carried by viruses that were capable of transforming infected cells. When mutated, oncogenes confer a positive or dominant growth advantage to a cell, resulting in transformation and tumorigenesis. Thus, oncogenic alleles are considered gain-of-function mutations. Oncogenes have normal cellular counterparts, known as protooncogenes, which serve important roles in the regulation of many aspects of normal cell growth and development. Protooncogenes can be grouped into several major classes based on their normal cellular function, and include growth factors or growth factor receptors, components of signal transduction pathways, and nuclear proteins or transcription factors that control gene expression. Normally, the expression of protooncogenes is tightly regulated, and consequently, normal cells do not become malignant. Homologues of protooncogenes have been identified in all multicellular organisms and their active domains are highly conserved, suggesting that their proteins serve important and integral roles in cellular function. When protooncogenes become mutated or overexpressed, however, they may contribute to cellular transformation and oncogenesis.

Transforming mutations of a protooncogene are generally those that disrupt the normal function of the protein to render it constitutively active. Mutations of the *RAS* gene family serve as an illustrative example. The *RAS* gene family comprises three similar genes: H-*RAS*, K-*RAS*, and N-*RAS*. Each of these genes encodes a guanine nucleotide-binding protein. Mutations in *RAS* genes have been identified in 10% to 15% of human cancers.[22] The K-*RAS* gene appears to be the most frequently mutated, with mutations found in approximately 50% of colon cancers, 70% to 90% of pancreatic cancers, and about 30% of lung cancers.[23–27] Most commonly, K-*RAS* mutations are found in codons 12 and 13, and to a lesser degree in codon 61. Such mutations alter the ability of the *RAS* protein to hydrolyze guanosine triphosphate (GTP) to guanosine diphosphate (GDP). GTP-bound *RAS* recruits *RAF*, another component of the *RAS* signaling pathway, and initiates a cascade of events that ultimately results in activation of growth-promoting genes.[28] The inability of mutant *RAS* to hydrolyze GTP to GDP results in constitutive activation of the *RAS* signal transduction pathway, overexpression of *RAS*-dependent growth factors, and consequent tumorigenesis.

Chromosomal translocations, a cytogenetic hallmark of many hematologic malignancies, can also result in oncogene activation and transformation. One mechanism by which this occurs is when the translocation juxtaposes a protooncogene to the enhancer or promoter element from a gene that is active in a particular cell type. In many hematologic malignancies, the translocation frequently involves either the immunoglobulin (Ig) or T-cell receptor (TCR) loci whose enhancer or promoter elements are active in leukocytes. In Burkitt's lymphoma, the translocation most commonly occurs between chromosomes 8 and 14, fusing sequence of the *MYC* protooncogene with sequence of the Ig heavy chain. A smaller number of cases of Burkitt's lymphoma (~10%) result from activation of the *MYC* gene by fusion with Ig light chain sequences on either chromosome 2 (κ locus) or chromosome 22 (λ locus). Interestingly, a different phenotype is seen when the *MYC* gene becomes fused to the TCR locus. When this translocation occurs, acute T-cell lymphocytic leukemia (T-ALL) develops. The same phenotype results when the TCR locus is juxtaposed to other oncogenes, including *LYL*-1, *TAL*-1, *TAL*-2, *TAN*-1, and *HOX*-11.[29–31]

Creation of chimeric protein products by the fusion of the gene sequence from one side of a translocation breakpoint to that of the other side of the breakpoint is another mechanism by which chromosomal translocations can produce oncogenic alleles. The classic example of such a translocation is the Philadelphia (Ph) chromosome in chronic myeloid leukemia (CML) and in some forms of acute lymphoblastic leukemias. The Ph chromosome fuses sequence of the *BCR* gene on chromosome 22 to sequence of the *ABL* gene on chromosome 9 (Fig. 3F-9). The *ABL* protooncogene is the cellular homologue of the Abelson murine leukemia virus oncogene, v-*abL*. The resultant chimeric protein is a tyrosine-specific kinase that has increased activity over that of the normal protein.[32]

A number of tumors have been identified that have multiple copies of a protooncogene (Table 3F-1). The number of amplified copies of a particular protooncogene is variable and can range from a just a few to several hundred. The amplified unit, termed an amplicon, usually contains repeated copies of a single gene; however, some may contain two or more genes. In those cases in which several genes are represented in the amplicon, it becomes difficult to determine whether one or a combination of the genes is the putative protooncogene. For example, a region of chromosome 11q13 containing several candidate protooncogenes, including *CCND1* (cyclin D1), *FGF4*, *FGF3*/int, and *EMS1*, is amplified in breast cancer and other tumors.[33,34] The presence of multiple copies of protooncogenes and overexpression of the protein has been correlated with a poor prognosis in many tumor types. In breast cancer, amplification of the protooncogene *ERBB2* (*HER2*) is associated with a worse prognosis, as is amplification of *MYC* family members in small cell cancer of the lung.[35–37]

## TUMOR SUPPRESSOR GENES

In contrast to the detection of oncogenes, in which protein overexpression is the common finding, the detection and discovery of tumor suppressor genes has been more difficult. Tumor suppressor genes are those genes whose normal function is to control

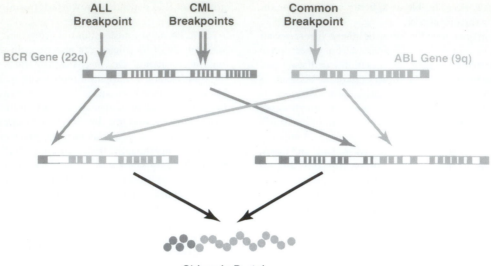

**FIGURE 3F-9.** Translocation between chromosome 22 and chromosome 9 yields the Philadelphia chromosome. The type of leukemia that results from such translocations is determined by the location of the breakpoint in the *BCR* gene. A breakpoint in the 5′ end of the *BCR* gene results in acute lymphoblastic leukemia (ALL). Those that occur in the 3′ end of the *BCR* gene result in chronic myeloid leukemia (CML). Both translocations produce a chimeric protein.

cellular growth or to promote cellular differentiation. The existence of such genes was postulated by Boveri[38] in 1914 when he hypothesized the presence of "chromosomes which inhibit division," and that "tumors with unlimited growth would arise if those inhibiting chromosomes were eliminated." Mutations in tumor suppressor genes were thought to be recessive and that the tumor phenotype required alteration of both copies of the normal gene. Accordingly, where oncogene mutations constitute a gain of function, alterations of tumor suppressor genes represent a loss of function.

The initial experimental evidence suggesting the existence of tumor suppressor genes, whose loss or mutation could lead to unconstrained cell growth, came from cell fusion studies in which hybrids made between tumor cells and normal cells resulted in inhibition of tumor cell proliferation.[39,40] It was also observed that loss of specific chromosomes from these cell hybrids could result in their reversion to an oncogenic phenotype. Subsequently, it was found that the introduction of a single normal chromosome into a tumor cell could inhibit tumor growth. In two landmark studies, a single chromosome 11, when introduced into the HeLa cervical carcinoma cell line or a Wilms' tumor cell line, would suppress growth.[41,42] These observations suggested that single chromosomes or even single genes, rather than the entire normal genome, might be sufficient to suppress tumorigenicity.

Coincident with the cell fusion experiments were the studies of Alfred Knudson[43] on sporadic and familial cases of retinoblastoma. He proposed that patients with the inherited form of retinoblastoma received a mutant copy of the disease gene from a parent through the germline, and as such the mutation was present in all cells of the body. In the presence of a normal copy of the gene, however, the retinoblastoma phenotype was masked. A mutation to the normal allele, a second "hit," would be necessary for tumor progression. On the other hand, patients with the sporadic form of retinoblastoma had two normal copies of the disease gene. Tumor development in these patients would require two separate somatic mutational events (Fig. 3F-10). This hypothesis, which has come to be known as Knudson's two-hit hypothesis, has become central to our understanding of the mechanism by which tumor suppressor genes function and the patterns of inheritance of many familial cancer syndromes. Furthermore, it served to substantiate and explain cell fusion studies that hypothesized the existence of recessive tumor genes.

It was not until 16 years following the publication of Knudson's work that the actual retinoblastoma disease gene (*RB1*) was cloned and characterized.[44,45] Since that time, retinoblastoma has served as a paradigm of a disease resulting from alterations in a tumor suppressor gene. The *RB1* gene is located on chromosome 13q14, and codes for a nuclear phosphoprotein that is expressed almost ubiquitously in tissues. The functional role of the *RB1* protein is presumably to control the progression of the cell cycle, particularly the entrance of the cell into the DNA synthesis (S) and $G_2$ phases.[46–48] Mutations in the gene result in abrogation of these cell cycle checkpoints and the unrestricted growth of cells.

Thus far, over a dozen tumor suppressor genes have been confirmed, and several more candidate tumor suppressors have been proposed. Verification that a candidate gene is, in fact, a tumor suppressor gene can be difficult. The most compelling evidence is the identification of inactivating germline mutations in the putative suppressor gene in a hereditary cancer syndrome and the loss or mutation of the remaining wild-type allele in the tumors that arise in affected family members. In the absence of an associated hereditary cancer syndrome, proof that a gene functions as a tumor suppressor must come from the identification of somatic, inactivating mutations in both alleles in sporadic cases of cancer. Even with

**TABLE 3F-1.** ONCOGENE AMPLIFICATION IN HUMAN CANCERS

| TUMOR TYPE | GENE AMPLIFIED | FREQUENCY, % |
|---|---|---|
| Neuroblastoma | MYCN | 20–25 |
| Small cell lung cancer | MYC | 15–20 |
| Glioblastoma | ERB B1 (EGFR) | 33–50 |
| Breast cancer | MYC | 20 |
| | ERB B2 (EGFR2) | ~20 |
| | FGFR1 | 12 |
| | FGFR2 | 12 |
| | CCND1 (cyclin D1) | 15–20 |
| Esophageal cancer | MYC | 38 |
| | CCND1 (cyclin D1) | 25 |
| Gastric cancer | K-RAS | 10 |
| | CCNE (cyclin E) | 15 |
| Hepatocellular cancer | CCND1 (cyclin D1) | 13 |
| Sarcoma | MDM2 | 10–30 |
| | CDK4 | 11 |
| Cervical cancer | MYC | 25–50 |
| Ovarian cancer | MYC | 20–30 |
| | ERB B2 (EGFR2) | 15–30 |
| | AKT2 | 12 |
| Head and neck cancer | MYC | 7–10 |
| | ERB B1 (EGFR) | 10 |
| | CCND1 (cyclin D1) | ~50 |
| Colorectal cancer | MYB | 15–20 |
| | H-RAS | 29 |
| | K-RAS | 22 |

SOURCE: Reproduced from Fearon,[66] with permission.

such evidence, however, the role of a gene as a tumor suppressor cannot be conclusively proven because of the difficulties in elucidating the role that the altered gene has in tumor initiation and growth, and the temporal relationship of its alteration to other genetic alterations in the tumor cell.[49]

## DNA MISMATCH REPAIR GENES

Maintaining the fidelity of the genome during DNA replication and cell division is of paramount importance for the normal growth and development of an organism. Ordinarily, cells have numerous mechanisms that constantly survey the DNA for damage or replication errors and, if present, repair them. In this manner, the integrity of the genome is assured, and the accumulation and propagation of mutations is minimized. One can imagine that if these survey and repair mechanisms were defective, genetic instability and accelerated rates of mutation would follow. If such mutations resulted in the activation of oncogenes or the inactivation of tumor suppressor genes, the affected cells would gain a malignant potential.

In the early 1990s, several investigators observed that a subset of colorectal tumors had widespread instability in microsatellite repeats in tumor DNA[50,51] and that such instability was present in the tumors of many patients affected by hereditary nonpolyposis colorectal cancer (HNPCC).[8] Simultaneously, bacterial and yeast geneticists described a set of DNA repair enzymes, termed DNA mismatch repair enzymes, that functioned to excise and repair nucleotide base mismatches that occurred during DNA replication. There were two major classes of these enzymes, mutS and mutL, and it was noted that organisms deficient in any one of these enzymes developed instability in simple repeat DNA sequences similar to those observed in HNPCC tumors. The connection between DNA mismatch repair enzymes and HNPCC was solidified when it was found that tumor cells from HNPCC patients lacked DNA mismatch repair activity in vitro.[9] Subsequently, two groups cloned and characterized the first human homologue of mutS, hMSH2, and found that it was mutated in many patients with HNPCC.[52,53] Soon thereafter, the human homologue of a mutL mismatch repair enzyme, hMLH1, was cloned and demonstrated to be altered in a subset of HNPCC patients who had normal hMSH2.[54,55]

It is now thought that DNA mismatch repair in the eukaryotic cells requires the participation of at least four other enzymes in addition to hMSH2 and hMLH1. These additional enzymes include two mutL homologues, hPMS1 and hPMS2, and two mutS homologues, hMSH6 (formerly called GTBP) and hMSH3.[56–59] Together, these enzymes complex to perform various aspects of the DNA mismatch repair process (Fig. 3F-11). The strongest mutator phenotypes, as measured by microsatellite instability, are observed with mutations in either hMSH2 and hMLH1, suggesting that the other enzymes play a less significant role in the process or that there may be some redundancy in their function. This, in fact, is the case with hMSH3 and hMSH6, where functional overlap between the two may attenuate the mutator phenotype resulting from a mutation in one or the other.[60,61]

Defects in DNA repair mechanisms have also been linked to other familial cancer predisposition syndromes, including ataxia-telangiectasia, xeroderma pigmentosum (XP), Bloom syndrome, and Cockayne syndrome. Patients with these disorders all share features of increased genetic instability, as characterized by chromosomal alterations and accelerated mutagenesis. In XP, patients have severe photosensitivity and a markedly accelerated rate of skin cancer. The underlying defects responsible for XP are deficiencies in the nucleotide excision repair pathway, which is a pathway broadly responsible for the repair of DNA damage, such as that resulting from UV radiation.[62]

## FAMILIAL CANCER SYNDROMES

Those cases of cancer in which there is a clear pattern of inheritance in a family represent only 1% of all cancers. Yet despite their rarity, insights gained from their study have proven to be invaluable

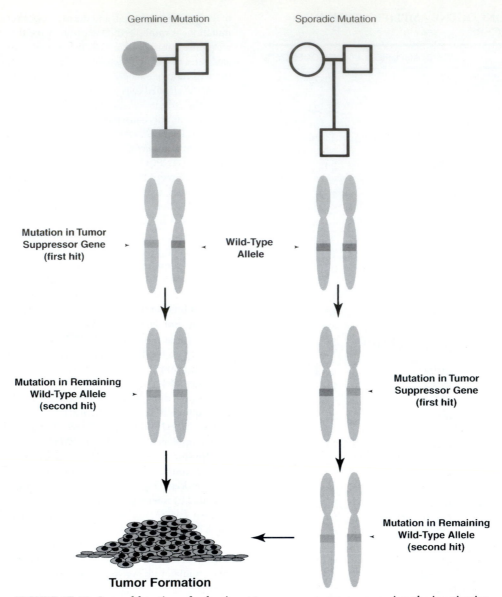

**FIGURE 3F-10.** Loss of function of a dominant tumor suppressor gene requires the inactivation of both normal copies of the gene ("two hits"). Individuals inheriting a germline mutation already have the first hit. As such, they require only one subsequent somatic inactivating event for tumor formation.

in our understanding of the pathogenesis of cancer. The presence of a germline mutation in a cancer gene affords one of the purest means of elucidating complex signaling pathways and of assessing the interaction of other cellular or environmental factors on the ultimate phenotype. Such determinations are more difficult in sporadic tumors in which the temporal relationship between gene defect and tumor progression is not as easily determined.

The majority of inherited cancer syndromes arise from the inactivation of tumor suppressor genes and follow an autosomal dominant pattern of inheritance. Accordingly, studies of cancer families were instrumental for the physical mapping and cloning of most tumor suppressor genes. As noted in the preceding section, defects in DNA excision and repair genes are also responsible for a number of inherited cancer syndromes. Included in this group may be the familial breast cancer genes *BRCA1* and *BRCA2,* which have been shown to associate with Rad51, a protein known to mediate DNA strand exchange functions necessary for normal recombination.[63–65] In contrast, there are only three inherited cancer syndromes attributed to activating germline mutations in oncogenes (*RET, MET,* and *CDK4*). A detailed review of each hereditary cancer syndrome is

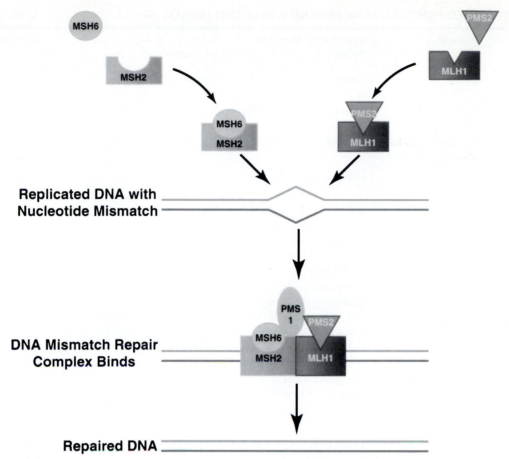

**FIGURE 3F-11.** DNA mismatch repair requires the participation of a number of repair enzymes. Mismatched bases are recognized and the complex of enzymes binds to them. The bases are then excised, the correct bases are inserted, and the strands are ligated.

beyond the scope of this chapter. A brief summary of some of the more common syndromes, however, is given in Table 3F-2. The reader may refer to reviews by Fearon,[66] Kinzler,[67] and Lindor[68] for more details.

It is clear that in the future more and more patients with cancer will be determined to have a responsible hereditary defect in either a specific tumor gene or in a modifying gene that imparts a cancer predisposition. Obtaining a thorough family history is now a necessity in the workup of any patient with cancer, especially those with a young age of onset or those with multiple tumors. The easy availability of genetic testing by many commercial laboratories has been problematic, as most physicians are not prepared to interpret the results nor to counsel the patient regarding his or her cancer risk and treatment. In a study of patients undergoing genetic testing for familial polyposis by a commercial company, it was found that only 19% of patients received genetic counseling before the test, and in 32% of cases, the physician ordering the test misinterpreted the results.[69]

Although most problems with misinterpretation are encountered with negative results, the interpretation of a positive result also can be difficult. It must be emphasized that a negative result can provide reassurance only if the predisposing mutation in the family is already known. Otherwise, a negative result may mean that the mutation was missed, that it occurred in promoter or intronic sequences not evaluated, or that a cancer predisposition may still exist due to a mutation in another known or unknown disease gene.[70] In the case of a positive result, one must be sure that the mutation, in fact, confers a cancer risk and is not merely a benign polymorphism. Therefore, when identified, patients suspected of having an inherited cancer syndrome should be offered counseling by a cancer geneticist or experienced genetic counselor both before the test is ordered and after the results are known.

## MOLECULAR PATHOLOGY

The standard approach to the diagnosis of cancer has relied upon the morphological features of cells and the surrounding stromal elements as assessed by light microscopy. At the subcellular level, electron microscopy has been employed in selected instances to help

**TABLE 3F-2.** SELECTED FAMILIAL CANCER SYNDROMES AND DISEASE GENES

| SYNDROME | PRIMARY TUMOR | ASSOCIATED CANCERS OR TRAITS | CHROMOSOME | GENE | PUTATIVE FUNCTION OF GENE |
|---|---|---|---|---|---|
| Familial retinoblastoma | Retinoblastoma | Osteosarcoma | 13q14.3 | RB1 | Cell cycle and transcription regulation E2F binding |
| Neurofibromatosis type 1 (NF1) | Neurofibromas | Neurofibrosarcoma, AML, brain tumors | 17q11.2 | NF1 | GAP for p21 ras proteins; microtubule binding? |
| Neurofibromatosis type 2 (NF2) | Acoustic neuromas, meningiomas | Gliomas, ependymomas | 22q12.2 | NF2 | Links membrane proteins to cytoskeleton? |
| Li-Fraumeni syndrome | Sarcomas, breast cancer | Leukemias, brain tumors | 17p13.1 | p53 | Apoptosis, cell cycle control, transcription factor |
| Familial adenomatous polyposis (FAP) | Colorectal cancer | Colorectal adenomatosis, gastric and duodenal polyps, desmoids, CHRPE, medulloblastoma (Turcot syndrome) | 5q21 | APC | b-catenin binding and degradation, microtubule binding, apoptosis |
| Hereditary nonpolyposis colorectal cancer (HNPCC) | Colorectal cancer | Endometrial, ovarian, gastric, hepatobiliary, and urinary tract cancers, glioblastoma (Turcot syndrome) | 2p16 3p21 2q32 7p22 2p15-16 | hMSH2 hMLH1 PMS1 PMS2 hMSH6 | DNA mismatch repair |
| Wilms' tumor | Wilms' tumor | WAGR (Wilms', aniridia, GU abnormalities, mental retardation) | 11p13 | WT1 | Transcriptional repressor |
| Familial breast cancer 1 | Breast cancer | Ovarian cancer | 17q21 | BRCA1 | Interacts with RAD51 protein, DNA repair |
| Familial breast cancer 2 | Breast cancer | Male breast cancer, pancreatic cancer, ? others | 13q12 | BRCA2 | Interacts with RAD51 protein, DNA repair |
| von Hippel-Lindau (VHL) disease | Renal cancer (clear cell) | Pheochromocytomas, retinal angiomas, hemangioblastomas | 3p25 | VHL | ?Regulates transcriptional elongation by RNA polymerase II |
| Familial melanoma | Melanoma | Pancreatic cancer, dysplastic nevi, atypical moles | 9q21 | p16 (CDKN2) | Inhibitor of CDK4 and CDK6 cyclin-dependent kinases |
| | | | 12q13 | CDK4 | Cyclin-dependent kinase |
| Cowden's disease | Breast cancer, thyroid cancer | Intestinal hamartomas, skin and oral mucosal lesions, fibrocystic change of breasts | 10q23 | PTEN (MMAC 1) | Dual-specificity phosphatase |
| Multiple endocrine neoplasia type 1 (MEN 1) | Pancreatic islet cell tumors | Parathyroid hyperplasia, pituitary adenomas | 11q13 | MEN1 | Unknown |
| Multiple endocrine neoplasia type 2 (MEN 2) | Medullary thyroid cancer | Pheochromocytoma, parathyroid hyperplasia, mucosal hamartoma | 10q11.2 | RET | Transmembrane receptor tyrosine kinase for GDNF |

ABBREVIATIONS: AML, acute myelogenous leukemia; GAP, GTPase-activating protein; CHRPE, congenital hypertrophy of the retinal pigment epithelium.
SOURCE: Reproduced from Fearon,[56] with permission.

subcategorize certain tumors (i.e., sarcomas) based upon ultrastructural features. More recently, techniques that can identify structures at the molecular level have become increasingly utilized as an adjunct to light microscopy to characterize cancers for diagnosis, prognosis, and prediction of therapeutic responsiveness. These techniques include cytogenetics, immunohistochemistry, analysis of DNA or RNA, and molecular genetics. This technology has defined a new field known as molecular pathology, which provides diagnostic information through the detection or analysis of specific molecules rather than relying on cellular anatomy.

The molecular-based methods can be applied for different purposes in evaluating tissues or fluid samples from cancer patients. The most important purpose is to establish the diagnosis of malignancy versus a benign process. Another purpose is to ascertain certain differentiation markers that may be able to indicate the tissue of origin of the malignancy or subtyping of tumor, which can have a direct bearing on subsequent therapy. Molecular tools have been utilized to stage tumors in an attempt to look for "micrometastases" in the blood, bone marrow, or regional drain lymph nodes (i.e., sentinel lymph node). Besides establishing the diagnosis of malignancy, molecular techniques have been recently utilized to test for inherited predispositions to the development of certain cancers as reviewed earlier in this chapter.

## IMMUNOHISTOCHEMISTRY

Immunohistochemistry has become a valuable molecular pathology technique to identify specific proteins (a.k.a. antigens) on the surface of tumor cells. The technique involves the binding of an antibody that is specific for a particular antigen or protein. The antibody is tagged with a marker for easy identification such as a fluorescent molecule or an enzyme (i.e., peroxidase or alkaline phosphatase) that can convert an added substrate to a colored product detectable by light microscopy. The ever-increasing number of commercially available antisera to defined antigenic determinants has made immunohistochemical techniques a required methodology in clinical pathology laboratories. The availability of automated devices for staining slides has further standardized this methodology for diagnostic purposes. Antigens recognized by available antibodies include molecules such as surface receptors, constituents of intercellular matrix, hormones or secreted products, proteins controlling cellular differentiation, and proteins controlling proliferation (Table 3F-3). Detection of the sites to which the antibody has bound can be assessed by a variety of methods, most relying on colorimetric changes that will allow easy visualization under light microscopy. The intensity of the staining in the tissue can serve as a means of measuring the levels of protein expression. Actual quantification, however, is difficult and is often dependent on the subjective interpretation of the investigator viewing the slide. Furthermore, the amount of antibody bound to its target protein may be affected by a variety of factors, including the availability of the target protein if it is already bound to or complexed by another cellular protein, the ability of the antibody to access the target protein if it is intracellular or intranuclear, and the affinity of the antibody for the protein.

A broad overview of the application of immunohistochemistry to clinical oncology is outlined in Table 3F-4. Immunohistochemistry is applied more often to the classification of tumors as opposed

## TABLE 3F-3. EXAMPLES OF COMMONLY USED ANTIGENS FOR IMMUNOHISTOCHEMICAL ANALYSIS OF TUMORS

| ANTIGENS | TISSUE EXPRESSION |
| --- | --- |
| Membrane receptors: | |
| Estrogen, progesterone | Breast carcinoma |
| Integrins | Expressed in tumors according to cell lineage |
| Her2/neu | Breast carcinoma |
| Hormones/secreted products: | |
| α-Fetoprotein | Liver, hepatocellular carcinoma, yolk sac tumors |
| CA 125 | Ovarian, cervix, endometrial, gastrointestinal, and breast carcinomas |
| Prostate-specific antigen | Hyperplastic and neoplastic prostate |
| CEA | Gastrointestinal, pancreatic, breast, and lung carcinomas |
| Intercellular matrix: | |
| Cytokeratins | Epithelial tumors |
| Desmin | Striated and parenchymal smooth muscle |
| Actin | Smooth muscle and myofibroblasts |
| Vimentin | Mesenchymal tumors; high-grade epithelial tumors |
| Cell differentiation: | |
| CD antigens for B and T cell lineages | Hematologic malignancies |
| S-100 | Melanocytic, glial, dendritic cells, sarcomas, salivary gland cancers |
| HMB-45 | Melanocytic cells |
| Cell proliferation: | |
| Ki-67 | Proliferation antigen in all cells |
| p53 | Prolonged half-life in many tumors |

## TABLE 3F-4. COMMON APPLICATIONS OF IMMUNOHISTOCHEMISTRY IN CLINICAL ONCOLOGY

- Subtyping different categories of lymphomas
- Separating undifferentiated malignancies into carcinomas, lymphomas, melanomas, and sarcomas
- Assessing prognostic markers
- Assessing therapeutic markers
- Staging for micrometastases

to the primary diagnosis of malignancy. This is best illustrated with the classification of lymphomas. The clonality of these diseases can be determined by specific common leukocyte determinants (CD antigens) present on malignant B or T cells. For solid malignancies, immunohistochemical techniques are useful to classify undifferentiated tumors into the major groupings of carcinomas, lymphomas, sarcomas, and melanomas that can direct the clinician into deciding appropriate therapeutic options. For undifferentiated carcinomas where the primary tissue of origin is unknown, immunohistochemistry can sometimes be helpful. Staining the tissue for different antigens prevalent on breast, ovarian, gastrointestinal, or prostatic tumors may help define the primary site of origin. Characterizations of tumor cells for surface receptors or proteins implicated in the cell cycle are being utilized as prognostic markers as well as indicators of how tumors may respond to specific therapies. These features of tumors will be reviewed in more detail later in this chapter.

An application for which immunochemistry has been useful is the detection of micrometastatic disease in regional or distant sites where malignant cells are too sparse to be detected by conventional stained sections. Hainsworth et al[71] reported that detection of occult micrometastases using immunohistochemical stains for mucin in node-negative breast cancer patients identified a subset of patients with decreased relapse-free and overall survival. Approximately 12% of patients with node-negative breast disease assessed by routine staining technique were found to have microscopic foci of nodal disease by immunohistochemistry. The decreased survival rate of this subgroup of patients when compared with node-negative patients is illustrated in Fig. 3F-12. Other applications where immunohistochemistry has been useful in detecting micrometastases has been the evaluation of bone marrow samples in breast cancer patients. Studies with only short-term follow-up suggest that breast cancer

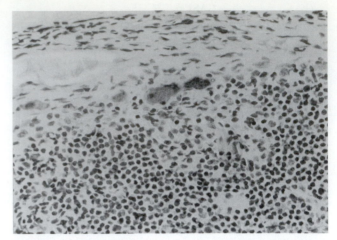

**FIGURE 3F-13.** Photomicrograph of sentinel lymph node removed from a melanoma patient. Routine hematoxylin and eosin (H&E) staining failed to reveal evidence of melanoma. Immunohistochemical staining with S-100 antibody revealed melanoma tumor cells (brown stain). (*Courtesy of Dr. Lori Lowe, Department of Pathology, University of Michigan.*) (See also Plate 14.)

patients with stage I and II resected disease identified to have a few metastatic cells in the bone marrow by immunohistochemistry have a higher risk of relapse.[72] Longer-term analysis of this type of staging is required to validate biologic significance of micrometastatic disease in the marrow of breast cancer patients.

In melanoma patients, it has become common practice to identify and remove the first draining lymph node (a.k.a. sentinel node) of a cutaneous primary lesion in order to determine if metastatic disease is present in the regional nodal basin.[73,74] Approximately 20% of the time, metastatic tumor cells will be identified in these node(s) in the absence of any clinical abnormality, and has significant prognostic and therapeutic implications for the patients. In order to reduce false-negative interpretations of the status of these nodes, it has become important to perform serial sectioning of these nodes in order not to miss a small-focus tumor. If serial sectioning is unrevealing, then immunohistochemical staining for S-100 and HMB-45 (see Table 3F-4) should be performed in order to detect microfoci of tumor (Fig. 3F-13). This type of protocol will reduce the false negative rate by 80%.[75] Routine histologic examination by light microscopy has been shown to identify one melanoma cell in a background of $10^4$ lymphoid cells. Immunohistochemistry has been able to increase the sensitivity of the examination by allowing detection of one melanoma cell in a background of $10^5$ lymphoid cells.

The use of sentinel node mapping is currently being investigated for staging the axillae in breast cancer.[76] The technique appears to be very accurate in identifying the presence of occult nodal metastatic disease. As with melanoma, it will be important to examine sentinel lymph nodes in breast cancer patients with immunohistochemical stains against tumor markers such as cytokeratins or mucins in situations where serial sectioning and standard stains are unrevealing.

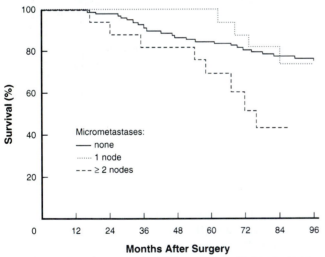

**FIGURE 3F-12.** Survival rate of patients with breast cancer after surgery. All patients had negative nodes on routine hematoxylin and eosin (H&E) staining. Immunohistochemical staining revealed micrometastatic disease in a subgroup of patients with one or two or more nodes (*Adapted from Hainsworth et al,[141] with permission.*)

**TABLE 3F-5. DNA-BASED TECHNIQUES OF MOLECULAR PATHOLOGY**

| TECHNIQUE | INFORMATION OBTAINED |
|---|---|
| DNA content | Ploidy (chromosome number); S-phase fraction |
| Southern blot | Can detect rearrangements of DNA, large deletions and amplifications |
| Polymerase chain reaction (PCR) or reverse transcriptase PCR (RT-PCR) | Can detect a small defined sequence of DNA (PCR) or messenger RNA (RT-PCR) from tissue samples |
| Fluorescence in situ hybridization (FISH) | Detection of chromosomal abnormalities in cells |
| In situ hybridization | Detection of specific RNA sequences within cells to assess gene expression |
| Single-strand conformational polymorphism (SSCP) | Detection of point mutations (substitution of single base pair) in DNA |
| Denaturing gradient gel electrophoresis (DGGE) | Detection of point mutations in DNA |

## DNA-BASED TECHNIQUES

There are several DNA-based techniques that have been adopted by pathologists to evaluate cells from tissues derived from cancer patients. A brief overview (Table 3F-5) of these methodologies and examples of their application will be reviewed in this section.

One of the earliest DNA-based techniques used was the analysis of DNA content. This involved either the measurement of chromosome number (i.e., ploidy), or the measurement of S-phase fraction. These measurements can be performed by flow cytometry image analysis microscopy. The measurement of ploidy assumes that normal cells have a diploid number of chromosomes and that malignant cells are polyploid or aneuploid in nature. The frequency of abnormal chromosome numbers generally increases with higher-grade tumors. The measurement of S-phase fraction reflects the proportion of cells that have doubled their DNA content in preparation for mitosis and reflects the rate of cellular division within a tumor. Although there are many studies correlating prognosis or certain tumor types with aneuploid status or increased S-phase fraction, these analyses are not consistent with all tumors. Furthermore, the clinical utility of these analyses has not been realized with respect to defining treatment options.

Analysis of nucleotide sequences to examine for genetic alterations from tissue specimens has been expanding over the last 15 years as we gain more knowledge regarding the genetic events giving rise to specific tumor types. This has led to the development of diagnostic molecular genetics as a tool available to the clinician. Table 3F-5 summarizes many of the available techniques that can be employed to analyze nucleotide sequences. Many of these techniques are described in more detail in the beginning of this chapter. Specific

nucleotide sequences in DNA and RNA can serve as markers for the molecular genetic diagnosis of cancers. These markers may be related to the development of the cancer (i.e., mutation in an oncogene or tumor suppressor gene) or acquired during the progression of the tumor. In either event, the fundamental principle underlying the development of cancers is that they represent the clonal expansion of genetically aberrant cells that can be identified by the specific mutations. Once acquired, the alterations in DNA tend to be irreversible and stable making them useful markers for diagnosis. Examples of certain malignancies and the genetic markers used to diagnose them are listed in Table 3F-6.

A large class of molecular genetic markers involves chromosomal rearrangements resulting from some type of recombination between DNA sequences. These rearrangements include duplication, deletions, amplifications, translocations, and inversions. Identification of these chromosomal rearrangements have been used predominantly with hematologic malignancies. Genetic testing has helped improve primary diagnosis of these hematologic malignancies as

**TABLE 3F-6. EXAMPLES OF GENETIC MARKERS USED IN THE DIAGNOSIS OF CANCERS**

| CANCERS | GENETIC MARKERS |
|---|---|
| HEMATOLOGIC MALIGNANCIES | |
| CML | Translocation of *BCR* and *ABL* genes to form chimeric *BCR-ABL* (a.k.a. Philadelphia chromosome) |
| Non-Hodgkin lymphomas, ALL, CLL | Rearrangements of antigen receptor genes |
| EBV-induced lymphomas | EBV DNA |
| Adult T-cell leukemia/lymphoma | HTLV1 DNA |
| SOLID TUMORS | |
| Ewing's sarcoma | Translocation t(11;22) (q24;q12) |
| Breast cancer | Her2/neu amplification, cytokeratin |
| Prostate cancer | PSA, PSMA, mRNA |
| Melanoma | Tyrosinase, Mage-3, mRNA |
| Colorectal cancer | DCC mutations |
| Cervical cancer | HPV-16, HPV-18 DNA |
| FAMILIAL CANCERS | |
| Breast | *BRCA1, BRCA2* mutations |
| Colorectal | *APC, MSH2, MLH1, PMS1, PMS2* mutations |
| Retinoblastoma | RB mutation |
| Li-Fraumeni syndrome | p53 mutation |
| MEN 1 and 2 | *RET* mutation |
| Kidney cancer | *VHL* mutation |
| Neurofibrosarcomas | *NF1, NF2* mutations |

well as subclassifying them. Another important application of molecular genetic techniques for the hematologic disease is the testing for low levels of residual disease after therapy, the detection of early relapse, and the detection of contamination of bone marrow used for autotransplantation.

The use of genetic molecular markers in the diagnosis and staging of solid tumors is becoming more prevalent. The first report of a molecular genetic assessment for identifying tumor cells in the circulation from a solid malignancy was in 1991.[77] This report utilized RT-PCR to detect mRNA for tyrosinase in melanoma cells within the peripheral blood. With PCR-based techniques it is now possible to detect a tumor cell among one million normal cells by identifying tumor-associated genetic markers. There is a large array of genetic markers that can detect different malignancies, some of which are listed in Table 3F-6. These markers may be specific to the tissues from which a cancer arises, such as prostate-specific antigen (PSA), or fairly nonspecific, such as cytokeratin 19, which will be common to many epithelial-derived cancers. The utility of PCR-based assays for tumor cell detection will be with the assessment of tissue samples where the genetic marker would not normally be expressed. Hence, the examination of peripheral blood, lymph nodes, bone marrow, and various body fluids (i.e., urine, sputum, stool, ascites) are sites where PCR-based assays have been investigated. Tumor types where these assays have been examined the most include melanoma and prostate cancer.

PCR-based tests for melanoma have been initially utilized to evaluate peripheral blood. Genetic markers for tyrosinase, cytokeratin 20, Mage-3, p97, muc-18, and β-HCG have been reported.[82] Tyrosinase has been the most extensively examined. In the normal, general population, tyrosinase is not detectable in the peripheral blood. Therefore, a PCR-based test to identify tyrosinase-containing melanoma cells would be highly specific. However, several studies examining for tyrosinase expression in the peripheral blood of patients with stage IV melanoma has varied from 0% to 100%, making the test very insensitive.[77–80] A major technical problem is standardizing the PCR-based test among institutions performing the assay. Because of the insensitivity of the test in peripheral blood, the prognosis of a patient with a positive RT-PCR assay for tyrosinase is unknown. Another application of PCR-based assays of genetic markers is with the examination of draining lymph nodes. The technique of identifying the "sentinel" draining lymph node in melanoma patients with clinically negative nodal examinations has become a routine clinical practice. Besides serial sectioning and immunostaining for HMB-45 and S-100, there have been reports evaluating the utility of RT-PCR to identify melanoma-involved nodes. Genetic markers such as tyrosinase and Mage-3 are being examined. Reintgen and co-workers[81] reported that melanoma patients with histologically negative sentinel nodes that were positive for tyrosine mRNA by RT-PCR had a significantly worse survival rate compared to patients with histologically negative and RT-PCR–negative sentinel nodes. Immunohistochemistry was not used in this study. Although the follow-up was only 28 months, there appears to be some utility in applying RT-PCR techniques for the evaluation of nodal disease. Caution is advised in the technical conduct of these assays as already alluded to. In addition, false-positive results can occur if benign nevus cells are present in the node. This has been observed to occur in approximately 5% of nodes examined.[81] The presence of these cells can give rise to positive RT-PCR assays that could be misinterpreted as representing melanoma micrometastasis.

The assessment of hematogenous micrometastases for prostate carcinoma has been evaluated extensively due to the specificity of PSA as a genetic marker for prostate-derived cells. Another specific marker for prostate-derived tumor cells is prostate-specific membrane antigen (PMSA). Clinical studies have shown that RT-PCR can detect circulating PSA- and PMSA-expressing cells in patients with disseminated disease and in a subgroup of patients with localized disease.[82] The reported sensitivities of detection of PSA- and PMSA-expressing cells is highly variable, and, as with melanoma, are due to the vagaries of how the assays are performed in different laboratories. The prognosis of a patient with clinically localized disease and a positive RT-PCR assay is currently not known. The use of RT-PCR for detecting PSA-expressing cells in draining lymph nodes is also in evolution. RT-PCR is more reliable than immunohistochemistry in detecting prostatic tissue in lymph nodes.[83] However, the added prognostic significance of RT-PCR–positive lymph nodes compared to standard pathologic staging still needs to be determined.

To date, the molecular genetic tests that are currently available have been most useful for their application in diagnosis. This is most apparent for the hematologic malignancies where subclassification of lymphomas and leukemias can be performed. For staging patients with solid malignancies, either in the peripheral blood or lymph nodes, the jury is still out. PCR-based technology is clearly a powerful tool that can detect a mere 1000 tumor cells in the peripheral circulation. However, it is unknown what the significance of this microscopic tumor burden is in the subsequent dissemination of disease. It is possible that such a tumor burden is too small to result in the successful metastatic spread of cancer and that immunologic surveillance is capable of destroying these microfoci of tumor cells. Further correlative survival studies need to be performed to identify the prognostic significance of PCR-based positive tests in the blood or lymph nodes of patients with clinically localized disease. In addition, optimizing and standardizing the protocols to perform these PCR-based tests will be important to establish reliable assays for clinical use.

## MOLECULAR PROGNOSTIC INDICATORS

As reviewed above, molecular-based assays have been used with increasing frequency to identify micrometastases in various sites that may have clinical relevance to staging patients. In this section, we will concentrate on molecular markers evaluated in the primary tumor that may have prognostic significance. This subject pertains much more to solid malignancies, which are very heterogeneous with respect to histologic factors and their natural history. The standard histologic analyses of primary solid malignancies include a determination of size, histologic grade, angiolymphatic invasion or perineural invasion, as well as other cellular features depending upon the tumor type. Molecular characterization of tumors is undergoing intense scrutiny and may complement standard histologic prognostic features of tumors. The types of molecular factors can be categorized

**TABLE 3F-7.** EXAMPLES OF MOLECULAR MARKERS ASSOCIATED WITH PROGNOSIS

| CATEGORY | MOLECULAR MARKER |
| --- | --- |
| Carcinogenesis | p53, K-*RAS*, *RB1*, p21, *MYC*, *DCC* |
| Cell growth | S-phase fraction, ploidy, HER-2/neu, EGFR, PCNA, Ki-67 |
| Cell death | BCL2, telomerase |
| Metastasis | Angiogenic factors (i.e., fibroblast growth factor), nm23, invasion-associated enzymes (i.e., cathepsin D, metalloproteinases, collagenases, strome-lysine), CD44E |
| Immunologic | HLA expression, cytokine production, CD40 |

into those involved with carcinogenesis, cell growth, cell death, and metastasis. Examples of selected molecular markers in these different categories are shown in Table 3F-7. A review of our current understanding of molecular markers will be reviewed for specific tumors.

## BREAST CANCER

One of the more standard DNA-based tests that have been employed with breast cancer evaluation has been ploidy and S-phase fraction. There are many review articles devoted to analyzing the utility of these tests.[84,85] On a univariate level, increased S-phase fraction is associated with decreased overall survival. Ploidy is not strongly associated with prognosis, especially when a multivariate analysis that includes the more traditional prognostic factors is performed. When such an analysis is applied with S-phase fraction, it becomes a less important prognostic indicator when histologic grading is included.[84]

Several newer molecular markers have been examined in the context of breast cancer. Among the more intensively evaluated markers are mutations of the tumor suppressor gene p53, which gives rise to overexpression of intracellular p53. Overaccumulation of p53 in breast tumor cells has been correlated with shortened survival in patients.[86,87] However, there are just as many negative studies as there are positive reports demonstrating the prognostic significance of p53.[88] The length of follow-up seems to be important since those with shorter follow-up (i.e., 60 months) had positive correlations with p53 expression compared with longer follow-up (i.e., 100 months), which demonstrated negative correlations.[88]

Another molecular marker that has been intensely studied in breast cancer is HER-2/neu. This is a marker that is expressed on the cell surface of tumor cells and has significant homology to epidermal growth factor receptor (EGFR). It is reported to be overexpressed in 10% to 30% of breast carcinomas and is associated with aggressive breast carcinomas.[89–92] It appears to be more common in ductal carcinoma in situ (DCIS) (overexpressed in 60%), especially in the high-grade variants, and has been postulated to be involved in the

evolution of these noninvasive lesions into invasive cancers. As will be reviewed later, the overexpression of HER-2/neu may predict for increased susceptibility to chemotherapeutic agents. It has also been used as a target molecule for monoclonal therapy.[93,94]

Various molecular mechanisms involved in the metastatic cascade have been evaluated for their prognostic significance. One of these mechanisms involves the elaboration of "invasion-associated" enzymes. An example of this is cathepsin D. This has been reported to be associated with more aggressive breast cancers.[95] However, the methodologies to measure cathepsin D are not standardized and are technically difficult. To date, it has not become a useful prognostic indicator. Another metastatic mechanism that has been examined is tumor angiogenesis. The ability of tumor cells to make microvessels is felt to be requisite for their ability to grow within the vasculature of a distant organ. Numerous studies have shown that measuring intratumor microvessel density predicts tumor aggressiveness in breast cancer as well as other solid malignancies.[96,97] The technique for assessing microvessel density requires immunohistochemistry, which utilizes monoclonal antibodies to stain for markers on endothelial cells (i.e., anti-CD31, anti-CD34, antifactor VIII).

There are many other molecular markers that have been examined for breast cancer. We have highlighted only a few better-known studies. The standard employment of these markers as prognostic tools is still in evolution and they should still be considered experimental. The validation of their use will require multiparametric studies that also contain the results of traditional prognostic indicators (i.e., nodal status, tumor size, grade, ER-PR content) in patients with sufficiently long follow-up. In addition, these studies need to be reproduced at different centers with separate patient databases.

## COLORECTAL CANCER

There are several studies that have evaluated DNA content (i.e., ploidy and S-phase fraction) of colorectal tumors as prognostic factors, but few have employed multiparametric analyses. One problem associated with DNA content analysis is the heterogeneity of tumors, making sampling error a potential problem, and the lack of standardized protocols to perform the assays. Nevertheless, there are a few studies to indicate that DNA content may have significant prognostic value. In these studies, patients with Duke's B and C colorectal primaries were evaluated in multivariate studies that included standard pathologic prognostic factors and demonstrated ploidy and S-phase fraction to be independent prognostic factors.[98,99]

There have been more recent studies evaluating various molecular genetic markers. The presence of mutated p53, just as in breast cancer, is controversial as to whether it correlates with a more aggressive tumor. Another gene that has been reported to be a candidate metastatic suppressor gene, nm23, is thought to dispose tumor cells to metastasize when its expression is reduced. Allelic deletions of nm23 have been associated with aneuploidy in colorectal cancers and decreased survival rates.[100] The deleted-in-colon-cancer (*DCC*) gene located on the long arm of chromosome 18 encodes for a protein that is structurally related to a class of cell adhesion molecules. It has been implicated in tumorigenesis, although its role is controversial.[101] Of interest is the observation that allelic loss of chromosome 18q21, which contains *DCC*, is associated with a poorer prognosis in patients with node-negative stage II colon cancer.[102,103] Patients with this genetic marker abnormality have survival rates similar to patients with node-positive stage III disease, and it has been proposed that this subgroup of stage II patients may benefit from adjuvant chemotherapy. These observations remain controversial, since another study was unable to confirm these results.[104] Another marker of interest relates to CD44, a cell surface glycoprotein in cell-cell interactions and cell migration. Various isoforms exist and can be detected by immunohistochemistry. The CD44H isoform is present on normal colonic epithelium and is increasingly reduced in expression in adenomas, carcinomas, and metastatic lesions, respectively.[105] Hence, loss of expression of CD44H correlates with increased aggressiveness of a tumor. On the other hand, studies involving RT-PCR–based assays indicate that increased expression of CD44E may be associated with tumor invasion and mechanisms of metastatic spread.[106]

Tumor angiogenesis has also been reported to be a prognostic factor for colorectal tumors. At least two separate studies have documented microvessel density assessed by immunohistochemistry to be associated with a poorer prognosis.[107,108] In one of these studies, a multivariate analysis that included standard histologic factors such as tumor size, grade, lymphatic and venous invasion, and Duke's stage, microvessel count proved to be an independent prognostic indicator.[108]

## MELANOMA

Cytogenetic abnormalities in melanoma patients have been studied, and correlations between stage and prognosis observed. Regional nodal metastases in patients with stage III disease show fewer total structural chromosomal abnormalities compared with tumor samples from patients with disseminated stage IV disease.[109] The most common chromosomal abnormalities occurred in regions 1p, 1q, 6q, and 11q. These observations may be important in identifying potential candidate genes involved in the pathogenesis of melanoma. In a study involving patients with stage IV disease, structural abnormalities in chromosome 7 or 11 were associated with significantly shorter survival in patients with melanoma compared to those without such abnormalities.[110] In a group of patients with localized primary melanoma, allelic losses of 6q, 9p, and 10q were associated with a decreased disease-free survival that was independent of tumor thickness.[111]

One mechanism involved in the metastatic process implicates the interaction of tumor cells with endothelial cells. An important component of this interaction is the binding of cellular adhesion molecules, known as integrins, to appropriate ligands. Endothelial cells can express important ligands known as E- and P-selectins, which bind to different integrins expressed on circulating cells. In a recent study, melanoma tumors stained for E- or P-selectins revealed that the degree of their expression in intratumoral vessels significantly correlated with the development of metastases.[111] In this same study, VLA-4, an integrin that is overexpressed in metastatic melanoma cells, was found to correlate with survival. Melanomas demonstrating positive staining in more than 50% of tumor cells

were associated with a poor outcome (50% vs. 20% mortality at 24 months).

## IMMUNOLOGIC MARKERS

Besides the markers identified in the previous sections which relate to various growth and metastatic characteristics of tumor cells, there is increasing evidence that there exist immunologic mechanisms that can modulate tumor growth. The expression of major histocompatibility (MHC) molecules is felt to be an important requisite for immune recognition of tumor cells. The ability of antigen-specific CD8[+] cytotoxic T cells to recognize and kill tumor cells requires a matching of MHC class I molecules between the T cell and tumor cells, and is known as an MHC class I–restricted response. Similarly, for immune CD4[+] T cells to engage with tumor cells, MHC class II identification between the two cells is required. It is well known that several tumor types have reduced expression of these MHC molecules, which are also subclassified as histocompatibility antigens (HLAs).[113,114] It is the reduced expression of these molecules by tumor cells that has been postulated to be a mechanism by which tumor cells escape recognition. Lee et al[115] identified an interesting association between the expression on an HLA class II phenotype, HLA-DQB1*0301, and disease recurrence in patients with stage I or II melanoma. Patients with this HLA phenotype and localized melanoma were more likely to develop recurrent disease, and this was an independent prognostic factor compared to tumor thickness, ulceration, anatomic location, and sex. Based upon what has been described of the HLA class II DQ locus, it was postulated that expression of HLA-DQB1*0301 may induce a relative state of immune tolerance in patients.

The presence of immunosuppression in a cancer patient has been attributed to the elaboration of soluble factors by the tumor. The induction of such an immunosuppressed state would theoretically result in enhanced tumor growth and metastasis. Several immunosuppressive cytokines have been reported to be secreted by certain tumors. These cytokines have adverse effects on the host in eradicating tumor, and in certain clinical reports, appear to be associated with more advanced disease and a poor prognosis. The most consistently reported cytokines in this regard are transforming growth factor β (TGF-β) and IL-10.

TGF-β is produced in five different isoforms and belongs to a superfamily of homodimeric polypeptide growth factors regulating cell growth and differentiation.[116] Animal studies suggest that the major activity of this cytokine in vivo is promotion of invasion and metastasis. The most likely mechanism by which TGF-β induces progression of carcinomas is through suppression of the immune response. In a clinical study, TGF-β was detected in 45 of 88 patients with resected lung adenocarcinomas and was associated with a poor survival.[117] The 5-year survival rate was 56% for the TGF-β–negative group, and 16% for the TGF-β–positive group. In another report, patients undergoing curative resections of colorectal cancers underwent immunohistochemical staining for TGF-β.[118] Patients with high TGF-β1 expression were 18 times more likely to have recurrence of disease compared to patients with low-expressing tumors, and this was independent of nodal status or degree of differentiation of the primary cancer. In pancreatic carcinoma, the absence of

TGF-β expression in tumors was associated with a longer postoperative survival.[119]

IL-10 is known as an immune suppressive cytokine that negatively regulates costimulatory signals involved in antigen-induced lymphocyte proliferation. Binding of IL-10 onto tumor cells can inhibit programmed cell death and promote proliferation.[116] This cytokine is known to be secreted by helper T cells, activated monocytes, and neoplastic B cells. However, it is also known to be secreted in certain tumors. The elaboration of IL-10 within basal cell carcinomas has been shown to result in an inhibition of the immune function of tumor-infiltrating dendritic cells.[120] Dendritic cells are highly potent antigen-presenting cells that are believed to be the initial cells required to trigger an immune response against tumor-associated antigens. Expression of mRNA for IL-10 has been reported in glial tumors, non–small cell lung cancers, melanoma, head and neck cancers, and renal cell cancers. The expression of IL-10 mRNA was correlated with high-grade and recurrence in glial tumors.[121]

## MOLECULAR DETERMINANTS OF SENSITIVITY TO ANTITUMOR AGENTS

Currently available therapeutic anticancer agents can be quite effective at treating a limited spectrum of tumor cell types while remaining ineffective against a larger group of carcinomas. The lack of adequate understanding of the molecular and cellular determinants of sensitivity or resistance to various antitumor reagents remains a barrier to improving existing cancer therapies. The next generation of breakthrough cancer therapies will likely be based upon the clarification of the molecular differences between normal and tumor cells, and the ability to develop antitumor reagents that can target these differences. The area of molecular markers that will predict sensitivity to antitumor antibodies will be a by-product of this effort (see Table 3F-7).

Early work in the field of cytotoxic drugs focused on the growth fraction of tumors as a predictor for responsiveness. However, it became evident that the growth rate of heterogeneous human tumors was not linear, nor was growth kinetics a predictor for drug sensitivity. Investigators began to examine other biochemical and cellular mechanisms that would confer resistance or sensitivity to specific cytotoxic drugs (Table 3F-8). One of the best understood mechanisms of drug resistance involves the expression of P-glycoprotein (P-gp), a transmembrane energy-dependent drug efflux pump that reduces drug accumulation within a cell. P-gp is encoded by the multidrug resistance (MDR1) gene, which belongs to a multigene family designated MDR. Gene transfection experiments have clearly demonstrated that the introduction and expression of MDR1 gene is sufficient to confer multidrug resistance to previously susceptible cells. Clinical trials are under way to confer this MDR phenotype to stem cells for use in bone marrow transplantation during intensive chemotherapy. The overexpression of P-gp has been reported to be an adverse prognostic factor in patients undergoing chemotherapy for acute myeloid leukemia;[123] pediatric tumors;[122,125] sarcoma; and breast, ovarian, and lung cancers.[124,126,127]

Knowing the biochemical target or receptor of a therapeutic agent can identify substrates that could act as molecular determinants of sensitivity. A well-established model of this is the determination of ER status in breast cancer patients to identify patients most likely to benefit from hormonal manipulation. An example of a marker for a cytotoxic agent is thymidylate synthase (TS), an essential enzyme in DNA synthesis that is the target for fluoropyrimidines. The presence of the TS gene and the expression of the enzyme in human colorectal and gastric tumor tissue were found to be a significant predictor as to whether patients responded to 5-fluorouracil chemotherapy.[128] In a different study of node-positive women with breast cancer who were randomized to receive six cycles of cyclophosphamide, methotrexate, and 5-fluorouracil (CMF) versus one cycle of perioperative CMF, patients with high TS levels demonstrated the most significant improvement in disease-free and overall survival.[129]

Besides efflux of drugs from a cell or identifying biochemical substrates of cytotoxic agents, other mechanisms by which cells may be resistant or sensitive to certain agents exist. Molecular tools have led to a new understanding of how chemotherapeutic agents induce cell death. Genetic mechanisms controlling a cell's pathway to repair treatment-related DNA damage, or to proceed into apoptotic death, determines whether or not tumors grow after exposure to a cytotoxic agent. Tumor suppressor gene products, such as p53, are important regulators of this process, as well as influencing expression of genes important to drug resistance. For example, wild-type p53 suppresses the promoter for the MDR1 gene, whereas the mutant form of this protein can actually stimulate the promoter, thereby enhancing multidrug resistance.[130]

Genetic markers in tumors have recently been identified to correlate with chemotherapeutic responsiveness. In glioma patients, the loss of heterozygosity of alleles on chromosomes 1p and 19q were significantly associated with chemosensitivity to combination procarbazine, lomustine, vincristine, and predicted longer disease-free survival after chemotherapy.[131] The mechanism for this association is currently unknown; however, the allelic loss suggests that a tumor suppressor gene(s) yet unidentified may be involved. In breast cancer, the expression of ERB2 (a.k.a. HER-2/neu) has been found to be a marker for responsiveness to doxorubicin. In the B-11 trial conducted by the National Surgical Adjuvant Breast and Bowel Project, patients with node-positive, ER-negative tumors were randomly assigned to receive L-phenylalanine mustard plus 5-fluorouracil (PF) or a combination of PF and doxorubicin (PAF).[132] In the group of patients who were HER-2/neu–positive, there was improved survival with PAF treatment compared to PF with a median follow-up of 13.5 years. There was no difference in survival between the two groups among the HER-2/neu–negative patients. In a confirmatory study reported by the Cancer and Leukemia Group B (CALGB),[133] there

**TABLE 3F-8.** EXAMPLES OF MOLECULAR MARKERS OF SENSITIVITY TO ANTI-TUMOR AGENTS

| | |
|---|---|
| Resistance: | MDR1 |
| | ?BCL2 |
| | |
| Sensitivity: | ER (breast) |
| | p53 (breast) |
| | HER-2/neu (breast, endometrial cancers) |
| | LOH of chromosome 1p and 19q (gliomas) |
| | Thymidine synthase (gastric, colorectal, breast cancers) |

was a strong interaction between HER-2/neu positivity and dose intensity of cyclophosphamide, doxorubicin and 5-fluorouracil (CAF) on overall survival in patients with node-positive breast cancer.[133] In this study, p53 expression was also found to be an independent prognostic marker. p53 expression also interacted with CAF dose to predict treatment outcome in multivariate analyses, although the effect was less pronounced than HER-2/neu. Similar interactions with HER-2/neu and doxorubicin have been reported for endometrial cancer.[134]

Programmed cell death, or apoptosis, is an important determinant of the response to chemotherapy. Among the genes involved in the apoptotic pathway is *BCL2*, which encodes a protein that can prevent programmed cell death induced by most chemotherapeutic drugs in in vitro models.[135–137] However, its role in determining in vivo chemoresistance has been sparsely investigated. Currently there are conflicting reports regarding the predictive value of *BCL2* expression in tumors to their responsiveness to chemotherapeutic regimens.[138,139]

In summary, the role of molecular markers in predicting responses to antitumor agents is a rapidly evolving field. It is being employed to predict therapeutic efficacy of specific chemotherapeutic regimens in the advanced disease state as well as in the adjuvant setting of micrometastatic disease.

# REFERENCES

1. HABER DA: Splicing into senescence: The curious case of p16 and p19^{ARF}. Cell 91:555, 1997.
2. LEWIN B: *Genes VI*. New York, Oxford University Press, 1997.
3. SAMBROOK J et al: *Molecular Cloning: A Laboratory Manual*, 2d ed. New York, Cold Spring Harbor Press, 1989.
4. SOUTHERN EM: Detection of specific sequences among DNA fragments separated by gel electrophoresis. J Mol Biol 98:505, 1974.
5. WEBER JL, MAY PE: Abundant class of human DNA polymorphisms which can be typed using the polymerase chain reaction. Am J Hum Genet 44:388, 1989.
6. VOGELSTEIN B et al: Allelotype of colorectal carcinomas. Science 244:207, 1989.
7. BAKER SJ et al: Chromosome 17 deletions and p53 gene mutations in colorectal carcinomas. Science 244:217, 1989.
8. AALTONEN LA et al: Clues to the pathogenesis of familial colorectal cancer. Science 260:812, 1993.
9. PARSONS R et al: Hypermutability and mismatch repair deficiency in RER+ tumor cells. Cell 75:1227, 1993.
10. JIRICNY J: Mismatch repair in cancer. Cancer Surv 28:47, 1996.
11. MAO L et al: Microsatellite alterations as clonal markers for the detection of human cancer. Proc Natl Acad Sci USA 91:9871, 1994.
12. MULLIS KB, FALOONA FA: Specific synthesis of DNA in vitro via a polymerase-catalyzed chain reaction: Meth Enzymol 155:335, 1987.
13. SAIKI RK et al: Primer-directed enzymatic amplification of DNA with a thermostable DNA polymerase. Science 239:487, 1988.
14. SANGER F et al: A new method for sequencing DNA. Proc Natl Acad Sci USA 74:560, 1977.
15. ORITA M et al: Detection of polymorphisms of human DNA by gel electrophoresis as single-strand conformation polymorphisms. Proc Natl Acad Sci USA 86:2766, 1989.
16. COTTON RG: Current methods of mutation detection. Mut Res 285:125, 1993.
17. FODDE R, LOSEKOOT M: Mutation detection by denaturing gradient gel electrophoresis. Hum Mut 3:83, 1994.
18. WHITE MB et al: Detecting single base substitutions as heteroduplex polymorphisms. Genomics 12:301, 1992.
19. OLSCHWANG S et al: Characterization of a frequent polymorphism in the coding sequence of the Tp53 gene in colonic cancer patients and a control population. Hum Genet 86:369, 1991.
20. RIEDY MC et al: Quantitative RT-PCR for measuring gene expression. Bio Techniques 18:70, 1995.
21. FILLE M et al: Quantitative RT-PCR using a PCR-generated competitive internal standard. Bio Techniques 23:34, 1997.
22. BARBACID M: ras genes. Annu Rev Biochem 56:779, 1987.
23. ALMOGUERA C et al: Most human carcinomas of the exocrine pancreas contain mutant c-K-ras genes. Cell 53:549, 1988.
24. HRUBAN RH et al: K-ras oncogene activation in adenocarcinoma of the human pancreas. Am J Pathol 143:545, 1993.
25. BOS JL: ras oncogenes in human cancer: A review. Cancer Res 49:4682, 1989.
26. FORRESTER K et al: Detection of high incidence of K-ras oncogenes during human colon tumorigenesis. Nature 327:298, 1987.
27. BOS JL et al: Prevalence of ras gene mutations in human colorectal cancers. Nature 327:293, 1987.
28. HILL CS, TREISMAN R: Transcriptional regulation by extracellular signals: Mechanisms and specificity. Cell 80:199, 1995.
29. LEDER P et al: Translocations among antibody genes in human cancer. Science 222:765, 1983.
30. SOLOMON E et al: Chromosome aberrations and cancer. Science 254:1153, 1991.
31. RABBITTS TH: Chromosomal translocations in human cancer. Nature 372:143, 1994.
32. HEISTERKAMP N et al: Localization of the c-abl oncogene adjacent to a translocation breakpoint in chronic myelocytic leukaemia. Nature 306:239, 1983.
33. KARLSEDER J et al: Patterns of DNA amplification at band q13 of chromosome 11 in human breast cancer. Genes Chrom Cancer 9:42, 1994.
34. SCHURRING E: The involvement of the chromosome 11q13 region in human malignancies: cyclin D1 and EMS1 are two new candidate oncogenes—A review. Gene 159:83, 1995.
35. ZHOU D et al: Association of multiple copies of the c-erbB-2 oncogene with spread of breast cancer. Cancer Res 47:6123, 1987.
36. SLAMON DJ et al: Human breast cancer: Correlation of relapse and survival with amplification of the HER-2/neu oncogene. Science 235:177, 1987.
37. HYNES NE: Amplification and overexpression of the erbB-2 gene in human tumors: Its involvement in tumor development, significance as a prognostic factor, and potential as a target for cancer therapy. Semin Cancer Biol 4:19, 1993.
38. BOVERI T: *The Origins of Malignant Tumors*. Baltimore, Williams & Wilkins, 1929, pp 26–27.
39. HARRIS H: The analysis of malignancy by cell fusion: the position in 1988. Cancer Res 48:3302, 1988.
40. STANBRIDGE EJ et al: Human cell hybrids: Analysis of transformation and tumorigenicity. Science 215:252, 1982.
41. SAXON PJ et al: Introduction of human chromosome 11 via

microcell transfer controls tumorigenic expression of HeLa cells. EMBO J 5:3461, 1986.

42. WEISSMAN BE et al: Introduction of a normal human chromosome 11 into a Wilms' tumor cell line controls its tumorigenic expression. Science 236:175, 1987.

43. KNUDSON AG: Mutation and cancer: Statistical study of retinoblastoma. Proc Natl Acad Sci USA 68:820, 1971.

44. FRIEND SH et al: A human DNA segment with properties of the gene that predisposes to retinoblastoma and osteosarcoma. Nature 323:643, 1986.

45. LEE W-H et al: Human retinoblastoma susceptibility gene: cloning, identification, and sequence. Science 235:1394, 1987.

46. NEVINS JR: E2F: A link between the Rb tumor suppressor protein and viral oncogenes. Science 258:424, 1992.

47. HELIN K et al: A cDNA encoding a pRB-binding protein with properties of the transcription factor E2F. Cell 70:337, 1992.

48. KAELIN WG JR et al: Expression cloning of a cDNA encoding a retinoblastoma-binding protein with E2F-like properties. Cell 70:351, 1992.

49. FEARON ER: Tumor suppressor genes, in *The Genetic Basis of Human Cancer*, B Vogelstein, KW Kinzler (eds). New York, McGraw-Hill, 1998, pp 229–236.

50. THIBODEAU SN et al: Microsatellite instability in cancer of the proximal colon. Science 260:816, 1993.

51. IONOV Y et al: Ubiquitous somatic mutations in simple repeated sequences reveal a new mechanism for colonic carcinogenesis. Nature 363:558, 1993.

52. LEACH FS et al: Mutations of a mutS homolog in hereditary nonpolyposis colorectal cancer. Cell 75:1215, 1993.

53. FISHEL R et al: The human mutator gene homolog MSH2 and its association with hereditary nonpolyposis colon cancer. Cell 75:1027, 1993.

54. PAPADOPOULOS N et al: Mutation of a mutL homolog in hereditary colon cancer. Science 263:1625, 1994.

55. BRONNER CE et al: Mutation in the DNA mismatch repair gene homologue hMLH1 is associated with hereditary nonpolyposis colon cancer. Nature 368:258, 1994.

56. KOLODNER R: Biochemistry and genetics of eukaryotic mismatch repair. Genes Dev 10:1433, 1996.

57. DRUMMOND JT et al: Isolation of an hMSH2-p160 heterodimer that restores DNA mismatch repair to tumor cells. Science 268:1909, 1995.

58. PALOMBO F et al: GTBP, a 160-kilodalton protein essential for mismatch-binding activity in human cells. Science 268:1912, 1995.

59. PAPADOPOULOS N et al: Mutations of GTBP in genetically unstable cells. Science 268:1915, 1995.

60. MARSISCHKY GT et al: Redundancy of Saccharomyces cerevisiae MSH3 and MSH6 in MSH2-dependent mismatch repair. Genes Dev 10:407, 1996.

61. UMAR A et al: Functional overlap in mismatch repair by human MSH3 and MSH6. Genetics 148:1637, 1998.

62. BOOTSMA D et al: Nucleotide excision repair syndromes: Xeroderma pigmentosum, Cockayne syndrome, and trichothiodystrophy, in *The Genetic Basis of Human Cancer*, B Vogelstein, KW Kinzler (eds). New York, McGraw-Hill, 1988, pp 245–274.

63. SCULLY R et al: Association of BRCA1 with Rad51 in mitotic and meiotic cells. Cell 88:265, 1997.

64. SHARAN SK et al: Embryonic lethality and radiation hypersensitivity mediated by Rad51 in mice lacking BRCA2. Nature 386:804, 1997.

65. BERTWISTLE D, ASHWORTH A: Functions of the BRCA1 and BRCA2 genes. Curr Opinion Genet Dev 8:14, 1998.

66. FEARON ER: Human cancer syndromes: Clues to the origin and nature of cancer. Science 278:1043, 1997.

67. KINZLER KW, VOGELSTEIN B: Lessons from hereditary colorectal cancer. Cell 87:159, 1996.

68. LINDOR NM, GREENE MH: The concise handbook of family cancer syndromes. J Natl Cancer Inst 90:1039, 1998.

69. GIARDIELLO FM et al: The use and interpretation of commercial APC gene testing for familial adenomatous polyposis. N Engl J Med 336:823, 1997.

70. PONDER B: Genetic testing for cancer risk. Science 278:1050, 1997.

71. HAINSWORTH PJ et al: Detection and significance of occult metastases in node-negative breast cancer. Br J Surg 80:459, 1993.

72. COTE RJ et al: Prediction of early relapse in patients with operable breast cancer by detection of occult bone marrow micrometastases. J Clin Onc 9:1749, 1991.

73. MORTON DL et al: Technical details of intraoperative lymphatic mapping for early stage melanoma. Arch Surg 127:393, 1992.

74. REINTGEN D: More rational and conservative surgical strategies for malignant melanoma using lymphatic mapping and sentinel node biopsy techniques. Curr Opin Oncol 8:152, 1996.

75. GERSHENWALD JE et al: Patterns of recurrence following a negative sentinel lymph node biopsy in 243 patients with stage I or II melanoma. J Clin Oncol 16:2253, 1998.

76. KRAG D et al: The sentinel node in breast cancer. N Engl J Med 339:941, 1998.

77. SMITH B et al: Detection of melanoma cells in peripheral blood by means of reverse transcriptase and polymerase chain reaction. Lancet 338:1227, 1991.

78. JUNG FA et al: Evaluation of tyrosinase mRNA as a tumor marker in the blood of melanoma patients. J Clin Oncol 15:2826, 1997.

79. CURRY BJ et al: Polymerase chain reaction detection of melanoma cells in circulation: Relation to clinical stage, surgical treatment, and recurrence from melanoma. J Clin Oncol 16:1760, 1998.

80. GLASER R et al: Detection of circulating melanoma cells by specific amplification of tyrosinase complementary DNA is not a reliable tumor marker in melanoma patients: A clinical two-center study. J Clin Oncol 15:2818, 1997.

81. SHIVERS SC et al: Molecular staging of malignant melanoma. JAMA 280:1410, 1998.

82. GANESH VR et al: Utilization of polymerase chain reaction technology in the detection of solid tumors. Cancer 82:1419, 1998.

83. DEGUCHI T et al: Detection of micrometastatic prostate cancer cells in lymph nodes by reverse transcriptase-polymerase chain reaction. Cancer Res 53:5350, 1993.

84. HEDLEY DW et al: Consensus review of the clinical utility of DNA cytometry in carcinoma of the breast. Cytometry 14:482, 1993.

85. O'REILLY SM, RICHARDS MA: Is DNA flow cytometry a useful investigation in breast cancer? Eur J Cancer 28:504, 1992.

86. THOR AD et al: Accumulation of p53 tumor suppressor gene protein: An independent marker of prognosis in breast cancers. J Natl Cancer Inst 84:845, 1992.

87. DAVIDOFF AM et al: Relation between p53 overexpression and established prognostic factors in breast cancer. Surgery 110:259, 191.

88. BARBARESCHI M: Prognostic value of the immunohistochemical expression of p53 in breast carcinomas correlates with reduced patient survival. Am J Pathol 139:245, 1991.

89. SJOGREN S et al: Prognostic and predictive value of c-erbB-2 overexpression in primary breast cancer, alone and in combination with other prognostic markers. J Clin Oncol 16:462, 1998.

90. VALERON PF et al: Quantitative analysis of p185(HER-2/neu) protein in breast cancer and its association with other prognostic factors. Intl J Cancer 74:175, 1997.

91. ALLRED DC et al: Her-2/neu in node-negative breast cancer: Prognostic significance of overexpression influenced by the presence of in situ carcinoma. J Clin Oncol 10:599, 1992.

92. IGLEHART JD et al: Increased erbB-2 gene copies and expression in multiple stages of breast cancer. Cancer Res 50:6701, 1990.

93. COBLEIGH MA et al: Efficacy and safety of Herceptin (humanized anti-Her2 antibody) as a single agent in 222 women with Her2 overexpression who relapsed following chemotherapy for metastatic breast cancer. Am Soc Clin Oncol 17:376, 1998.

94. SLAMON D et al: Am Soc Clin Oncol 17:377, 1998.

95. ISOLA J et al: Cathepsin D expression detected by immunohistochemistry has independent prognostic value in axillary node-negative breast cancer. J Clin Oncol 11:36, 1993.

96. WEIDNER N et al: Tumor angiogenesis and metastasis: Correlation in invasive breast carcinoma. N Engl J Med 324:1, 1991.

97. WEIDNER N et al: Tumor angiogenesis: A new significant and independent prognostic indicator in early-stage breast carcinoma. J Natl Cancer Inst 84:1875, 1992.

98. WITZIG TE et al: DNA ploidy and cell kinetic measurements as predictors of recurrence and survival in stages B2 and C colorectal adenocarcinoma. Cancer 68:879, 1991.

99. TAKANISKI DM JR et al: Ploidy as a prognostic feature in colonic adenocarcinoma. Arch Surg 131:587, 1996.

100. CAMPO E et al: Prognostic significance of the loss of heterozygosity of Nm23-H1 and p 53 genes in human colorectal carcinomas. Cancer 73:2913, 1994.

101. KERN SE et al: Clinical and pathological associations with allelic loss in colorectal cancer. JAMA 261:3099, 1989.

102. JEN J et al: Allelic loss of chromosome 18q and prognosis in colorectal cancer. N Engl J Med 331:213, 1994.

103. SHIBATA D et al: The DCC protein and prognosis in colorectal cancer. N Engl J Med 335:1727, 1996.

104. CARETHERS JM et al: Prognostic significance of allelic loss at chromosome 18q21 for stage II colorectal cancer. Gastroenterology 114:1188, 1998.

105. JACKSON PA et al: Relationship between stage, grade, proliferation, and expression of CD44 in adenomas and carcinomas of the colorectum. J Clin Pathol 48:1098, 1995.

106. TANABE KK et al: Expression of CD44R1 adhesion molecule in colon carcinomas and metastases. Lancet 341:725, 1993.

107. FRANK RE et al: Tumor angiogenesis as a predictor of recurrence and survival in patients with node-negative colon cancer. Ann Surg 222:695, 1995.

108. TAKEBAYASHI Y et al: Angiogenesis as an unfavorable prognostic factor in colorectal carcinoma. Cancer 78:226, 1996.

109. THOMPSON FH et al: Cytogenetics in 158 patients with regional or disseminated melanoma-subset analysis of near diploid and simple karotypes. Cancer Genet Cytogenet 83:93, 1995.

110. TRENT JM et al: Relation of cytogenetic abnormalities and clinical outcome in metastatic melanoma. N Engl J Med 322:1508, 1990.

111. HEALY E et al: Prognostic significance of allelic losses in primary melanoma. Oncogene 16:2213, 1998.

112. SCHADENDORF D et al: Association with clinical outcome of expression of VLA-4 in primary cutaneous malignant melanoma as well as P-selectin and E-selectin on intratumoral vessels. J Natl Cancer Inst 87:366, 1995.

113. VAN DUINEN SG et al: Level of HLA antigens in locoregional metastases and clinical course of the disease in patients with melanoma. Cancer Res 48:1019, 1988.

114. McDOUGALL CJ et al: Reduced expression of HLA class I and II antigens in colon cancer. Cancer Res 50:8023, 1990.

115. LEE JE et al: Malignant melanoma: Relationship of the human leukocyte antigen class II gene DQB1*0301 to disease recurrence in American joint committee on cancer stage I or II. Cancer 78:758, 1996.

116. WOJTOWICZ-PRAGA S: Reversal of tumor-induced immunosuppression: A new approach to cancer therapy. J Immunother 20:165, 1997.

117. TAKANAMI I et al: Transforming growth factor $\beta_1$ as a prognostic factor in pulmonary adenocarcinoma. J Clin Pathol 47:1098, 1994.

118. FRIEDMAN E et al: High levels of transforming growth factor beta 1 correlate with disease progression in human colon cancer. Cancer Epidemiol Biomarkers Prev 4:549, 1994.

119. FRIESS H et al: Enhanced expression of transforming growth factor beta isoforms in pancreatic cancer correlates with decreased survival. Gastroenterology 105:1846, 1993.

120. NESTLE FO et al: Human sunlight-induced basal-cell-carcinoma-associated dendritic cells are deficient in T cell costimulatory molecules and are impaired as antigen-presenting cells. Am J Pathol 150:641, 1997.

121. HUETTNER C et al: Messenger RNA expression of the immunosuppressive cytokine IL-10 in human gliomas. Am J Pathol 146:317, 1995.

122. NOOTER K, SONNEVELD P: Clinical relevance of P-glycoprotein expression in haematological malignancies. Leukemia Res 18:233, 1994.

123. HOLMES JA, WEST RR: The effect of MDR-1 gene expression on outcome in acute myeloblastic leukaemia. Br J Cancer 69:382, 1994.

124. CHAN HS et al: Immunohistochemical detection of P-glycoprotein: Prognostic correlation in soft tissue sarcoma of childhood. J Clin Oncol 8:689, 1990.

125. CHAN H et al: P-glycoprotein expression as a predictor of the outcome of therapy of neuroblastoma. N Engl J Med 325:1608, 1991.

126. HOLTZMAYER TA et al: Clinical correlates of MDR1 (P-glycoprotein) gene expression in ovarian and small cell lung carcinomas. J Natl Cancer Inst 84:232, 1993.

127. VERRELLE P et al: Clinical relevance of immunohistochemical detection of multidrug resistant p-glycoprotein in breast cancer. J Natl Cancer Inst 83:111, 1991.

128. JOHNSTON PG et al: Thymidylate synthase gene and protein expression correlate and are associated with response to 5-fluorouracil in human colorectal and gastric tumors. Cancer Res 55:1407, 1995.

129. PESTALOZZI BC et al: Prognostic importance of thymidylate synthase expression in early breast cancer. J Clin Oncol 15:1923, 1997.

130. MURREN JR, DE VITA VT JR: Another look at multidrug resistance. Principles Pract Oncol 9:1, 1995.

131. CAIRNCROSS JG et al: Specific genetic predictors of chemotherapeutic response and survival in patients with anaplastic oligodendrogliomas. J Natl Cancer Inst 90:1473, 1998.

132. PAIK S et al: erbB-2 and response to doxorubicin in patients with axillary lymph node-positive, hormone receptor-negative breast cancer. J Natl Cancer Inst 90:1361, 1998.

133. THOR AD et al: ErbB-2, p53, and efficacy of adjuvant therapy in lymph node-positive breast cancer. J Natl Cancer Inst 90:1346, 1998.

134. SAFFARI B et al: Amplification and overexpression of HER-2/neu (c-erbB2) in endometrial cancers: Correlation with overall survival. Cancer Res 55:5693, 1995.

135. WALTON MI et al: Constitutive expression of human Bcl-2 modulates nitrogen mustard and campothecin-induced apoptosis. Cancer Res 53:1853, 1993.

136. MIYASHITA T, REED JC: Bcl-2 oncoprotein blocks chemotherapy-induced apoptosis in a human leukemia cell line. Blood 81:151, 1993.

137. LASORELLA A et al: Differentiation of neuroblastoma enhances Bcl-2 expression and induces alterations of apoptosis and drug resistance. Cancer Res 55:4711, 1995.

138. BONETTI A et al: bcl-2 but not p53 expression is associated with resistance to chemotherapy in advanced breast cancer. Clin Cancer Res 4:2331, 1998.

139. VAN SLOOTEN HJ et al: Expression of bcl-2 in node-negative breast cancer is associated with various prognostic factors, but does not predict response to one course of perioperative chemotherapy. Br J Cancer 74:78, 1996.

140. WATSON JD et al (eds): Recombinant DNA. New York, Scientific American Books, 1992, p 22.

141. HAINSWORTH PJ et al: Detection and significance of occult metastases in node-negative breast cancer. Br J Surg 80:459, 1993.

142. BRODEUR GM, HOGARTY MD: Gene amplification in human cancers: Biological and clinical significance, in The Genetic Basis of Human Cancer, B Vogelstein, KW Kinzler (eds). New York, McGraw-Hill, 1998, p 162.

# CHAPTER 4

# DIAGNOSIS AND STAGING

## 4A / SURGICAL TECHNIQUES IN SOLID TUMORS

*Natale Cascinelli, Filiberto Belli, and Leonardo Lenisa*

### THE ROLE OF SURGICAL ONCOLOGY

Surgery commonly represents the first treatment option in patients with solid tumors, so the surgeon has a primary and critical role in the approach and management of cancer patients. It has been estimated that approximately 90% of cancer patients are submitted to surgical procedures for diagnosis, primary treatment, or management of complications during the course of their neoplastic disease.

Although it is commonly assumed that current management of most solid tumors should include an interdisciplinary approach among the surgeon, the medical oncologist, the radiotherapist, and the pathologist, the surgeon frequently bears the responsibility of initial diagnosis and appropriate setting of the diagnostic and therapeutic goals.

The role of the surgeon may vary according to various factors, such as the type and site of neoplasm, the stage of disease at time of diagnosis, the patient's general condition, and the emergence of disease-related complications. Generally the different roles of surgery (Fig. 4A-1) in oncology may be summarized as follows:

- Surgery may represent the appropriate initial and often definitive treatment for many solid tumors. This is the case in the curative resection of most gastrointestinal carcinomas, gynecological cancers (breast, ovary, cervix, vulvovaginal), lung cancer, melanoma, and others.
- In other cases, surgery is needed for the appropriate diagnosis (excision of an atypical mole, lymph node biopsy) and thorough staging of disease (laparotomy, laparoscopy, liver biopsy, mediastinoscopy). Sentinel node biopsy for melanoma, breast cancer, and other carcinomas may be included in this section because it is a minimally invasive surgical procedure for accurate staging of disease. Recent advances in the knowledge of genetics and gene therapy[1] are now opening a new perspective in cancer treatment, as is the case of adoptive immunotherapy and vaccine therapy.

Because fresh cancer tissue may be required in this setting, the surgeon may be needed for cancer tissue retrieval through minimally invasive procedures.

- Surgical access may be needed for administration of antineoplastic agents. The use of implantable intravascular ports (e.g., Port-a-Cath) has currently been adopted to deliver drugs in major veins, providing easy percutaneous access. Implantable pumps are used for regional high-dose drug administration, as in the case of intraarterial drug delivery in the treatment of hepatic metastases. Vascular access is required also in the treatment of patients with regionally advanced melanomas or sarcomas of limbs by means of extracorporeal perfusion or stop flow technique. The perfused substances may be drugs such as melphalan or mitomycin or cytokines [tumor necrosis factor (TNF), interleukins] and the antineoplastic effect may be potentiated by hyperthermia. Vascular access is surgically obtained at the root of the affected limb (iliac-femoral axis for lower limbs, brachial axis for upper limbs). Cannulation is followed by the perfusion through an extracorporeal pump of the solution containing the antineoplastic agents, for a period ranging from 45 to 90 min. Extracorporeal limb perfusion currently represents the treatment of choice for stage III A (M.D. Anderson classification) patients with melanoma of the limbs.[2,3] Moreover, this procedure can decrease the amputation rate in patients with sarcomas of the limbs by reducing the size of the tumor, thus permitting a conservative but radical operation.[4]
- Palliative procedures are a common feature in the management of cancer patients. Surgery may be required for the treatment of complications related to cancer, that is, bleeding (gastrointestinal haemorrhage, vascular erosion, etc.), perforation (advanced gastric or pancreatic cancer, ileal metastases from melanoma, etc.), obstructive ileus (any abdominal mass), jaundice (biliary tree and pancreatic malignancies), or asphyxia (endoluminal masses of the airway). Some patients affected by metastatic dissemination of cancer may benefit from debulking procedures aimed at preventing potential complications, reducing the tumor burden, and

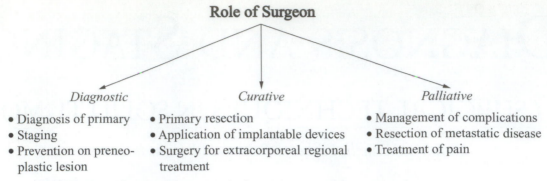

**FIGURE 4A-1.** The role of the surgeon in the management of the cancer patient.

potentiating the effects of chemotherapy, as in ovarian cancer. In strictly selected cases, resection of solitary metastases may prove beneficial in melanoma patients.[5] Hepatic resections for metastatic colorectal cancer may prolong patient survival.[6]

• Surgery may represent a useful tool in secondary prevention of cancer. There are a number of lesions currently recognized as preneoplastic that can be removed with minimal excision or resection. Such an example is the case of leukoplakia in relation with oral cancer or the genital CIN III (cervical intraepithelial neoplasia), VIN III (vaginal), VUIN III (vulvar) and PIN III (penile). The ablation of these lesions with minimal margins and little or no functional damage may prevent the onset of invasive cancer.

## HISTORY AND PHYSICAL EXAMINATION

The guiding principles for the surgical oncologist should be the accurate diagnosis and staging of the cancer in order to plan appropriate treatment correctly. In the approach to a potential cancer patient, a complete history and physical examination is the first step before further judgments can be made regarding laboratory testing and treatment. The patient's past medical history often provides clues to the diagnosis. The medical history may reveal environmental factors or habits such as smoking, alcohol ingestion, exposure to known carcinogenic agents such as asbestos or aniline dyes, which can be related to organ-specific malignancies. Inquiry into family history may reveal findings that support an initial diagnosis, suggest additional associated lesions, or influence the extent of surgical treatment. Further, a thorough medical history may provide important clues on possible operative risks for the patient. The physical examination of the patient should begin with an overall assessment, should proceed through a systematic examination, and then it should focus on the specific sites suggested by the medical history.

The main goals of a correct preoperative clinical evaluation are:

1. Establishment of the diagnosis.
2. Determination of extent of disease.
3. Planning of the best appropriate therapy to optimize the chance of cure for the patient.
4. Assessment of general or specific tumor-related conditions that

could affect negatively the operative risk and/or postoperative recovery (anemia, nutritional status, reduced cardio-respiratory performance, immunodepression, infections, metabolic impairment).
5. Determination of the need for psychological support or assistance.

The definitive diagnosis of cancer can be expressed only by a competent pathologist after appropriate retrieval of tumor samples, such as by tissue biopsy or surgical specimen. The diagnosis of cancer and determination of the type of cancer cannot be established without a biopsy. There may be clinical presentations that make the diagnosis of cancer virtually certain to the clinician, even as to the specific site of origin or histologic type, but despite these insights it is mandatory that an adequate biopsy be obtained. Details on the technique of biopsy are reported in a following paragraph.

The appropriate determination of the extent of the neoplasm, or staging of the disease, is the next requirement for the surgeon before the design and initiation of a treatment program takes place. Knowledge of the usual sites of metastasis, their recognition, and documentation by the best available diagnostic methods including efficient use of radiology, nuclear medicine, and appropriate medical oncology consultations are among the important skills of the surgical oncologist.

The presence of metastases in critical sites, which may influence therapeutic policy, should be determined with accuracy. In many situations, biopsy confirmation of metastatic disease is required, even if major surgical procedures such as laparotomy and thoracotomy are necessary, because of the impact such information has on the prognosis and therapeutic planning.

The concurrent presence of conditions reducing the performance status of the patient must carefully be assessed as it may reduce the chance of success of curative surgery even in the presence of technically resectable disease. The threatening behavior of cancer may induce the acceptance as surgical candidates of patients with an increased operative risk, but this decision must carefully take into account the potential negative effects on immediate outcome and assess the risk versus benefit ratio.

After consideration of all these aspects, the surgeon must determine the potential for cure for the patient in accordance with the principles outlined in the next paragraph.

## PRINCIPLES OF CURATIVE SURGERY

Curative operation is commonly considered the procedure capable of removing all recognizable tumor tissue with the appropriate margin around it aiming at removing microscopic tumor extensions. The concept of radicality is continuously evolving according to advances in the fields of biology, anatomy, physiology, and surgical pathology. For this reason an approach with curative intent must consider the following items.

### ANATOMIC LOCATION AND EXTENT OF TUMOR SPREAD

The surgeon must preoperatively assess the stage of disease according to current classifications. The local extent of disease must be considered in relation to tissue layers, the limits of the involved organ, and the possibility of infiltration of adjacent tissues or organs. The presence of multifocality, tumor satellitosis, or other synchronous primaries must be thoroughly investigated. These concepts are the basis of the success of more conservative treatments that maintain the same oncologic potential of cure thanks also to the development of other adjuvant therapeutic options. A paradigmatic example is given by the evolution in the treatment of invasive breast cancer. The curative approach, which started from the superradical Halsted's mastectomy evolved through modified Patey's radical mastectomy to the current adoption of quadrantectomy or lumpectomy for lesions 2 cm in diameter or less. This was also made possible by the adoption of postoperative radiotherapy on the remaining breast tissue. Lymphatic spread of disease often already exists at the time of diagnosis and is commonly underestimated by the physical examination or standard preoperative workup. This concept supports the inclusion of lymphadenectomy to primary tumor excision. The extent of lymphadenectomy (perivisceral vs. extended or superextended), the intent of lymphadenectomy (staging vs. therapeutic), or the need of en bloc dissection around the primary tumor are a matter of continuous debate among surgical oncologists in each specific field. The presence of distant metastatic sites must be evaluated in designing the appropriate operation. The appearance of distant metastases usually represents a dismal event in the prognosis of cancer patients but does not necessarily preclude a radical approach. The evaluation must consider the characteristics of the primary tumor as well as the site and number of metastases. One to three metastases from colorectal cancer in the same hepatic lobe are amenable to "radical" major hepatic resection with improved patient outcome.

### BIOLOGIC CHARACTERISTICS OF THE TUMOR

The continuous progress in the knowledge of cancer biology has led to the identification of some features that are common to all types of tumors and that may have an impact on prognosis. The recognition of these features may in some cases induce a modification in the therapeutic strategy. The prognosis and clinical behavior may depend on the specific site of origin of a given neoplasm (e.g., uveal or mucosal melanoma may differ in clinical behavior from cutaneous melanoma). The surgeon must then be aware of the tumor behavior according to site of origin and pattern of metastatic spread in order to plan an adequate strategy for the surgical approach.

### CONCEPT OF RADICALITY

Radicality can be defined as the ability of the surgeon to leave no residual disease in the surgical field. In this view, no local relapse should be observed after a "radical" resection, but every surgeon knows that this is not always feasible. The null recurrence rate is the aim of every surgical oncologist, and all surgical strategies are designed with the goal of reducing relapses of disease. Failures are mainly attributable to the lack of understanding of all anatomic and pathophysiologic aspects of cancer biology. A paradigmatic advance is represented by the evolution of the treatment of cancer of the rectum. For many years the interest of surgeons was concentrated on the distal clearance margin, which was considered safe when no less than 5 cm in length, otherwise an abdominoperineal resection was required. Nevertheless, the local recurrence rate ranged from 20% to 40%. The subsequent strategy to combine surgery with other postoperative adjuvant treatments such as radiotherapy and chemotherapy resulted in a slight decrease in pelvic recurrence rate to the level of 15% to 25%. Further improvements in our understanding of the surgical anatomy of the pelvis led to the recognition of the anatomical-functional structure called mesorectum; moreover, the advances in surgical pathology demonstrated that the lateral clearance margin was as or more important than the distal margin on the bowel wall. An appropriate operation was expressly designed including total rectum resection, mesorectum excision, and pelvic lymphadenectomy with preservation of anal sphincter and, when feasible, of the sacral nervous plexus.[7] This kind of operation has been able to reduce the pelvic recurrence rate to 4% to 8% when performed by dedicated colorectal surgeons.

Macroscopic radicality is assumed by the surgeon when all the appreciable neoplastic tissue is removed. Microscopic radicality is determined by the pathologist after analysis of the margins of the surgical specimen. Oncologic radicality is a rather complex concept combining surgical pathology findings together with cancer biology concepts. This synthesis changes continuously according to the evolution of knowledge and represents the basis for decision making in the surgical approach to the cancer patient.

## THE BIOPSY

The surgical pathologist plays a key role in the management of the cancer patient, because any suspicious lesion requires pathologic confirmation before treatment. A close collaboration is needed among surgeons and pathologists in order to obtain as much information as possible with the least invasive and traumatic approach. In this view the role of biopsy is crucial, and a skillful surgeon will obtain the best results. Prior communication with the pathologist should assess the need for special procedures in specimen retrieval, slide preparation, and fixation and staining, so as not to waste valuable material.

The technique of biopsy varies according to site and characteristics of neoplastic target considered, and can be summarized as follows.

## BIOPSY OF SUPERFICIAL TISSUES

Cutaneous lesions commonly are referred to the surgeon by the patients themselves, because they are easily noted and identified. The preferable approach to potential skin cancer is the excisional biopsy with clear margins unless otherwise required in consideration of the extent or site of disease. Shave biopsies are absolutely contraindicated, especially in pigmented lesions, as they jeopardize the correct evaluation of thickness of primary lesions in the case of melanoma. Incisional biopsies are also to be avoided in melanoma, but they may be necessary in the approach to giant congenital nevi with areas of degeneration, or in some special sites such as the eyelid, nose, ear, mouth, nipple, or genital area, where a surgical approach that may potentially interfere with cosmesis is not acceptable in the absence of a clear pathologic evidence of disease.

In special conditions, such as in ulcerated and exfoliating neoplasms, diagnostic material may be collected by direct application of the slide onto the lesion. Mucosal lesions should be managed with the same criteria outlined for cutaneous ones.

## ENDOSCOPIC SAMPLING

In the last two decades the extraordinary development of endoscopic procedures has drastically modified the approach to intracavitary and intraluminal lesions.

The routine application of endoscopy in the workup of respiratory, urinary, esophagogastroduodenal, and colonic lesions constituted clear progress in the diagnosis of these malignancies. The adoption of optic fiber flexible endoscopes permits a thorough exploration and accurate pathologic diagnosis of lesions that are difficult to access, even with open surgery. Endoscopic biopsy is accurate because the magnification of the image of the lesion and the sampling are made easy by the continuous development of more sophisticated instrumentation. The risk of bleeding or perforation of hollow viscera is well known, but is lowered by appropriate training of the operator. The methods of sampling of the lesion are established according to current knowledge about the biology of the specific tumor (single or multiple biopsies of the lesion, sampling of adjacent healthy tissue, etc.). When the lesion is suspected but is not clearly seen to be biopsied or removed, special methods of sampling are used such as brushing, washing, random sampling in presence of submucosal lesions, and aspiration.

Laparoscopy and thoracoscopy today are commonly included in the workup for staging of major malignancies such as lung cancer, lymphoma, and gastric and pancreatic carcinomas.[8] Nevertheless, after an initial period of enthusiasm, the current trend is toward a strict definition of the role of endoscopic procedures; in fact, a potential role of these procedures in causing distant intracavitary and port-site implantation has been reported.

## PERCUTANEOUS BIOPSY

This procedure is widely adopted for the sampling of lesions of subcutaneous organs, such as the breast, as well as for deep-located organs with the complementary guide of ultrasound or CT scan (thyroid, lung, liver, kidney, etc.). The samples may be collected both for cytologic analysis with a fine-needle aspiration biopsy (FNAB)[9,10] and for histologic evaluation using a thicker tissue-cutting needle (e.g., Tru-Cut or Menghini) for musculoskeletal, liver, kidney, or bone marrow biopsy.[11] One of the latest developments in the documentation of breast cancer has been the ABBI System,[12] which is a stereotactic guided device allowing a minimally invasive excision under local anesthesia and in an outpatient setting of breast lumps up to 2 cm in diameter in order to obtain a large quantity of material to be processed by the pathologist. The clear advantage is accurate identification by means of stereotactic guidance.

The potential risk of contamination through the use of percutaneous biopsy techniques through spilling of neoplastic cells in the injected field is under continuous evaluation and is still controversial. Nevertheless, the use of a fine needle and the introduction of the needle through a cutaneous access that will be subsequently excised in the case of neoplastic finding may reduce the risk of spillage in breast cancer, melanoma, and lymph node metastases. Fine-needle biopsies are mainly used to demonstrate cytologic changes of malignancy (presence or absence of malignant neoplastic cells). The precise definition of histotype is not achievable with this technique.

Diagnosis by means of needle biopsy is recommended for:

- Adequate surgical planning for melanoma and breast, thyroid, salivary gland, and other superficial neoplasms.
- Diagnosis of visceral neoplasms (liver, kidney, pancreas, lung, etc.) with the guidance of ultrasound (US) or CT scans.
- Minimally invasive diagnosis of neoplastic lesions beyond surgical resectability in order to plan an appropriate radiochemotherapeutic approach.

## INTRAOPERATIVE BIOPSY

Biopsy of neoplastic material may be required in some instances during open surgery. Commonly the tissue retrieved is processed by frozen section technique for a prompt intraoperative diagnosis.[13] The retrieval procedures can either be incision, excision, or needle core biopsy, according to anatomic and surgical pathology conditions.

Frozen sections may be required by the surgeons for:

- Diagnosis of primary lesion, if not obtainable preoperatively
- Diagnosis of previously unknown secondary lesions discovered intraoperatively
- Confirmation of radicality on surgical margins of resection or on the residual surgical field
- Diagnosis of accidental bulky lesions during routine or emergency procedures

## NODE BIOPSY

This is required for diagnosis of clinical adenopathy, both in patients with a known primary cancer and in those in whom the nodal enlargement is the first presentation of disease. In the differential diagnosis of lymphoproliferative disease, it is generally required by the pathologist that the whole lymph node be sent fresh, not in fixative liquid, to allow correct definition of histotype, and paraffin-embedded sections are commonly indicated for this purpose. On the other hand, frozen sections are very helpful in definition of nodal metastases from epithelial or melanocytic cancers. In these cases accurate intraoperative diagnosis translates into en bloc nodal dissection, the procedure of choice for the treatment of nodal metastases from carcinoma and melanoma.

Biopsy confirmation is of special importance if the interval between treatment completion and apparent recurrence is long, if the site of recurrence is atypical, if the clinical findings are equivocal, and if the morbidity of the biopsy procedure is acceptable. As in the case of the original diagnosis, tumor relapse has a profound prognostic importance and usually necessitates a radical change in therapeutic strategy.

Particular mention should be made of a new minimally invasive staging technique commonly called sentinel node biopsy, which was first introduced by Morton and co-workers[14,15] in the 1990s for the diagnosis of occult nodal metastases in melanoma patients. Its use has now been extended to breast, vulvar, penile, and other invasive carcinomas.

## REFERENCES

1. PARMIANI G, COLOMBO MP: Somatic gene therapy of human melanoma: Preclinical studies and early clinical trials. Melanoma Res 5:295, 1995.
2. STEHLIN JS, et al: Results of eleven years experience with heated perfusion for melanoma of the extremities. Cancer Res 39:2255, 1979.
3. LIENARD D et al: High dose of rTNF-a in combination with IFN-gamma and melphalan in isolated perfusion of the limbs for melanoma and sarcoma. J Clin Oncol 122:52, 1991.
4. EGGERMONT AMM et al: Limb salvage by isolated limb perfusion (ILP) with TNF and melphalan in patients with locally soft tissue sarcomas: Outcome of 270 ILPs in 246 patients. Melanoma and Sarcoma Proceedings of ASCO Meeting, Atlanta, GA, May 15–18, 1999; 18:535a.
5. WONG JH et al: The role of surgery in the treatment of nonregionally recurrent melanoma. Surgery 113:389, 1993.
6. CADY B et al: Surgical margin in hepatic resection for colorectal metastasis. Ann Surg 227:566, 1998.
7. LEO E et al: Total rectal resection, mesorectum excision and coloendoanal anastomosis: A therapeutic option for the treatment of low rectal cancer. Ann Surg Oncol 3:336, 1996.
8. GREENE FL, DORSAY D: Laparoscopic staging and investigation of intra-abdominal malignancy, in *Current Techniques in Laparoscopy*, DC Brooks, vol 11 in *Current Medicine*, Philadelphia, 1994, pp 11.1–11.9.
9. GIOVANNINI M et al: Fine-needle aspiration cytology guided by endoscopic ultrasonography: results in 141 patients. Endoscopy 27:171, 1995.
10. VALMANN P et al: Endoscopic ultrasonography-guided fine-needle aspiration biopsy of lesions in the upper gastrointestinal tract. Gastrointest Endoscop 41:230, 1995.
11. STOKER DJ et al: Needle biopsy of musculoskeletal lesion. A review of 208 procedures. J Bone Joint Surg 73B:498, 1991.
12. FERZLI GS, HURWITS JB: Initial experience with breast biopsy utilizing the advanced breast biopsy instrumentation (ABBI). Surg Endoscop 11:393, 1997.
13. FERREIRO JA et al: Accuracy of frozen section diagnosis in surgical pathology: A review of a 1-year experience with 24,880 cases at Mayo Clinic Rochester. Mayo Clinic Proc 70:1137, 1995.
14. MORTON DL et al: Technical details of intraoperative lymphatic mapping for early stage melanoma. Arch Surg 127:392, 1992.
15. REINTGEN DS et al: Lymphatic mapping and sentinel lymphadenectomy, in *Cutaneous Melanoma*, CM Balch et al (eds). St Louis, Quality Medical, 1998, p 227.

# 4B / IMAGING TECHNIQUES IN THE DIAGNOSIS AND FOLLOW-UP OF CANCER INTERVENTIONAL RADIOLOGY IN ONCOLOGY

*Revathy B. Iyer and Chusilp Charnsangavej*

## INTRODUCTION

Advances in imaging technology over the past two decades have improved the ability of diagnostic radiologists to detect, diagnose, and stage malignant tumors of various organs in the body. Significant technical development has occurred in several areas, including image data acquisition and image-processing techniques. Rapid data acquisition and better spatial resolution of new imaging technology improves the understanding of morphological, physiologic, and hemodynamic changes of tumors, and provides excellent anatomic information on tumor spread. Improved methodology for processing imaging data after data acquisition allows more precise anatomic demonstration with three-dimensional and multiplanar image reconstruction, which are essential for treatment planning. Quantification of tumor volume and monitoring internal characteristic changes in the tumor provide valuable information for treatment response evaluation. In modern oncologic practice, these imaging techniques, which include ultrasound (US), computed tomography (CT), and magnetic resonance imaging (MRI), have emerged as important and necessary modalities in the diagnosis, treatment planning, and follow-up of various tumors in the body.

Similar progress in interventional radiology has provided new options for the management of various tumors in patients who are not candidates for curative resection but whose tumors remain confined to certain anatomic regions. These discoveries have led to development of alternative treatment strategies for patients with these malignant tumors that, in general, have a very poor prognosis. The model for technical development in interventional radiology that has made most significant progress during the past two decades is in the treatment of liver cancer. The techniques have developed from the concept of occlusion of blood supply to the tumor with various occluding agents as in *embolization*, and mixing chemotherapeutic agents with occluding agents as in *chemoembolization*. Refinement in catheterization techniques allows superselective catheterization for subsegmental chemoembolization that can accomplish results similar to those achieved with subsegmental liver resection but with lower morbidity. Progress in imaging technology and needle localization has allowed image-guided percutaneous tumor ablation techniques to develop. Percutaneous tumor ablation has advanced from us-

ing various chemicals such as absolute ethanol to produce physical damage to the tumor to using temperature-controlled stimuli via a probe to create coagulation necrosis of the tumor as in cryoablation, microwave coagulation, laser-induced thermal therapy, and radiofrequency tumor ablation. With proper patient selection, these techniques offer alternative treatments for patients with malignant tumors of the liver.

This section discusses the use of modern imaging techniques in the diagnosis and staging of malignant tumors that are commonly treated by interventional radiologic procedures and how these techniques can be used for monitoring treatment and follow-up. The discussion will focus on development of related interventional radiologic techniques and the results of the treatment. Because radiologic treatment of liver tumors is a well-established intervention, our discussion will largely focus on this subject.

## HISTORICAL PERSPECTIVES AND CURRENT STATUS

### IMAGING TECHNIQUES

**ULTRASOUND (US).** US is widely available in most clinical practice settings and can be used in most parts of the body. US is well suited to imaging because it is relatively inexpensive, produces no ionizing radiation, is noninvasive, and is both fast and portable. Wide ranges of transducers are available for examination of various parts of the body depending on the needed depth of sound penetration and the tissue to be penetrated, the field of view, and the image resolution. For example, in most transabdominal examinations, 3- and 5-MHz transducers are used, whereas a 7.5-MHz transducer is preferable for examination of small parts and superficial tissues such as the breast and the thyroid gland because of its improved image resolution. The major disadvantages of US are that it is operator-dependent, it lacks tissue specificity, and it is limited by body habitus, particularly for examinations of several abdominal organs or tissues that require sound penetration through air, bone, or fat. Because of this limitation, US is more frequently used as a primary screening modality for lesion detection in general practice, or in a screening program, such as in hepatocellular carcinoma (HCC) screening in high-risk patients. However, with experienced sonographers, the technique has been successfully used for diagnosis and staging of breast cancer, particularly when combined with aspiration biopsy.

New US techniques allow real-time scanning, which produces fewer artifacts than static scanning, and improve image resolution, signal detection, and image display.[1] Vascular imaging using duplex or color Doppler flow imaging and new intravenous contrast agents such as microbubbles provide the opportunity to assess and quantify small vessels in the tumors.[2–4] Progress in transducer technology over the past decade has allowed the development of small transducer probes that can be inserted via an endoscope or a laparoscope port. Tumors in many organs, such as the esophagus, stomach, duodenum, pancreas, colon, and liver, can be diagnosed and staged for the depth of tumor invasion with high accuracy.[5–7] This technology requires the expertise of an endoscopist, but it can produce significant impact in the diagnosis and staging of various gastrointestinal malignancies, particularly when combined with aspiration biopsy.[8]

COMPUTED TOMOGRAPHY (CT). Over the past two decades, CT has been commonly used for the diagnosis and staging of various tumors in the body because it can display anatomy with excellent image resolution, and the study can be repeated on a consistent basis. CT detection and diagnosis of a lesion usually requires the use of intravenous (IV) contrast enhancement because the differences in tissue attenuation between the normal organs and pathologic processes on an unenhanced CT are frequently imperceptible. Evolution in CT technology over the past decade has made scanning faster, allowing extended anatomic coverage over a shorter time, and improved image resolution. The importance of shorter scans is not only to limit involuntary motion artifacts associated with a long scan time and to improve the image quality of early-generation scanners, but also to accommodate IV delivery of contrast material from a drip infusion technique to delivery by an automatic injector at a rate of 2 to 5 mL/s. The recent development of helical, or spiral, scanning offers an additional advantage to conventional scanning by improving scan speed so that imaging of a certain anatomic region can be done in a shorter time than with the most advanced conventional scanner during delivery of a bolus of IV contrast medium.[9–12]

In helical scanning, the x-ray tube continuously turns and rotates around the gantry, and scan data are acquired as the table transports the patient through the scanning gantry at a constant speed. Since the scan data are acquired in a continuous fashion, the extent of anatomic coverage along the axis of table advancement increases when compared to a conventional scanner. The resolution of the scan depends upon the slice thickness, the speed of table advancement, and the exposure time. With helical scanning, it is now possible to scan through the liver and the pancreas within 20 to 30 s. This scan time is even further reduced by a new generation of helical CT scanners using multiple rows of detectors. This scanning technique reduces the time needed to scan upper abdominal organs to below 10 s while maintaining the image resolution.

Faster scan time using helical CT has proven to be advantageous by allowing organs to be scanned at the proper phase of IV contrast enhancement for improved lesion detection and lesion characterization.[12–14] Volume data acquisition improves the ability to display imaging in multiple planes or in a three-dimensional format.[13,15,16]

MAGNETIC RESONANCE IMAGING (MRI). The major advantage of MRI over other imaging modalities is its ability to display inherent tissue contrast. MRI relies on the differing hydrogen atom content and T1 and T2 relaxation times of differing tissues to provide contrast between such tissues. Radiologists select imaging techniques on MRI to combine these three components variably and thereby alter image contrast to answer specific clinical questions.

MRI offers distinct advantages over CT in that it does not produce ionizing radiation and does not rely on the use of contrast agents in detecting lesions. Patients with iodine allergy or renal insufficiency are not excluded from MRI scans and may be imaged without complications related to administration of iodinated contrast agents. Although MRI does not rely on contrast agents for lesion detection, MR contrast agents can be used to gain additional information about the enhancement characteristics of the lesions and to improve lesion detection.[17] For example, the use of intravenous gadolinium (Gd) as an ionic or nonionic chelate with fast imaging sequences is important in the specific characterization of lesions such as hemangioma, focal nodular hyperplasia, and HCC. Other MR contrast agents such as manganese and superparamagnetic iron oxide particles are available for lesion detection and characterization.

Apart from its ability to display inherent tissue contrast, MRI possesses another additional advantage that may be important for treatment planning. It permits multiplanar imaging to display images in coronal and sagittal planes that further facilitate treatment planning.

Despite its many advantages, MRI is not without its drawbacks. Some patients are excluded from MRI scans, including patients with pacemakers and certain types of metallic implants that are in danger of being deflected within the confines of the strong magnetic fields. Claustrophobia is a potential problem in many individuals, although this problem could be alleviated by the increasing availability of open magnets with high field strength. Other problems include the relatively long scan time of MR, which results in motion artifacts as compared to helical CT, and the limited availability of the state-of-the-art technology, which continues to change at a rapid pace.

## CURRENT STATUS OF LIVER TUMOR IMAGING

Imaging studies for the evaluation of liver tumors have been focused on their ability to detect the lesions; to diagnose the lesions, and to distinguish benign hepatic lesions such as hemangioma, focal nodular hyperplasia, and cysts from malignant lesions such as HCC and various types of metastatic disease. Although the gold standard for the diagnosis of liver tumors remains the pathologic diagnosis, various benign tumors such as cavernous hemangioma and focal nodular hyperplasia have specific imaging characteristics and can be accurately diagnosed without using invasive procedures. Current knowledge of the imaging characteristics of liver tumors and HCC can be attributed to the progress of imaging technology, screening programs, and the aggressive treatment of small HCCs in Japan as well as the aggressive treatment of hepatic metastasis in the United States and in Europe.

**IMAGING OF HCCs.** The imaging findings of HCC are based largely on its morphology, histology, and its tumor vascularity.[18–21] Edmunson[19] classified the morphology of HCC into three types: nodular, massive, and diffuse. This classification has been accepted worldwide with minor modifications in various regions. The prevalence of each morphological type varies depending upon the stage of the disease at the time of diagnosis, the presence or absence of cirrhosis, and etiologic factors. The basic morphologic changes of the nodular type of HCC include the presence of a capsule, intratumoral architecture forming a mosaic pattern, and the presence of fat and/or areas of hemorrhage and necrosis. Most tumor nodules in the nodular type of HCC (80% to 88%) are hypervascular on angiography. In advanced cases, vascular invasion into the hepatic veins and portal vein is common and can be considered characteristic.

*US FINDINGS.* The typical appearance of a nodular HCC includes a well-circumscribed hypoechoic rim corresponding to the capsule with tumor nodules of varying echogenicity and fibrous septa in the lesion producing a mosaic pattern.[22–24] The tumors tend to produce posterior echo enhancement because the relatively soft tumor produces good through transmission against the surrounding fibrotic, cirrhotic liver. Frequently, small HCCs tend to be hypoechoic, but they can be hyperechoic because of fatty metamorphosis and clear cell histologic type.

Because the majority of nodular HCCs are hypervascular and they receive blood supply from the hepatic artery, several investigators use color Doppler US, power color Doppler US, and US angiography to enhance the visualization of HCC and distinguish it from other tumors. On color Doppler US, pulsatile waveform of the artery entering from the periphery of the lesion can be observed. Lesion enhancement following injection of carbon dioxide microbubbles into the hepatic artery makes detection of small lesions easier.[2,24]

*CT FINDINGS.* Unenhanced CT alone is not sensitive enough to detect small HCCs because the density of the tumor nodules may be uniform and indistinguishable from the surrounding hepatic parenchyma. The tumor nodule can be seen when the fibrous capsule is present or when the tumor nodule becomes inhomogeneous because of fatty metamorphosis, areas of hemorrhage or necrosis, and presence of intranodular septa. The fibrous capsule and fibrous septa can be seen as hypodense rim surrounding the tumor nodule or hypodense intratumoral linear band. The inhomogeneous pattern of intratumoral architecture is better recognized after IV contrast enhancement and will be further described.

Visualization of tumor nodules of HCC on CT requires IV contrast enhancement to distinguish the nodules from the surrounding parenchyma. The evolution of CT from conventional to helical scanning and the techniques of IV contrast have improved our understanding of the dynamics of tumor enhancement.[20,21,25–32] This knowledge has improved the diagnosis and detection of small tumors by CT. In the 1980s and the early 1990s when conventional scanning techniques following IV contrast enhancement were commonly used, the tumor nodules of HCC varied in enhancement characteristics from hypodense, to isodense, to hyperdense, and the success of small lesion detection was quite variable, from 46% to 84%.[18] Because most tumor nodules in HCC are hypervascular and the hepatic artery supplies the majority of the tumors, scanning the liver rapidly during the early phase, when peak arterial enhancement occurs, after a large-bolus IV contrast infusion results in better enhancement of the tumor nodules (Fig. 4B-1). These tumor nodules may become isodense or hypodense to the hepatic parenchyma during the portal phase, and later, when the enhanced portal vein blood increases the density of the surrounding hepatic parenchyma, enhancement of the tumor nodules becomes stable or starts to decrease. The dynamic changes of tumor enhancement and hepatic parenchymal enhancement 2 to 3 min after IV contrast enhancement can only be recognized with the rapid scanning technique of helical CT,[25,32] and could further improve with the newer generations of helical CT.

Morphologically, the fibrous capsule of the tumor, the mosaic pattern of the internal architecture, and the presence of areas of necrosis or hemorrhage can also be recognized on CT. The fibrous capsule is hypodense during the early phase but could become hyperdense during the later phase because the fibrous tissue is relatively hypovascular, but leakage of contrast material into the interstitium of the fibrous tissue increases its density during the later phase. The mosaic pattern of the tumor is a result of tumor nodules separated by fibrous septa and areas of tumor necrosis that can be identified as areas of unenhanced low-density tissue. The appearance of hemorrhage is variable; fresh blood is relatively hyperdense, whereas old blood is hypodense.

In advanced HCCs, the patterns of tumor growth are quite characteristic, resulting in the spread of tumors beyond the capsule, intrahepatic spread via the portal vein producing multiple satellite nodules in the liver, and growth of tumors in the portal and hepatic veins.

*MR FINDINGS.* The characteristics of HCC on unenhanced MR also rely on the morphological appearance of the tumor, including the fibrous capsule, the mosaic patterns, and tumor inhomogeneity due to hemorrhage and necrosis.[33–38] The capsule of the tumor has a low signal intensity on both T1- and T2-weighted images, and it is better seen on T1-weighted images. The septum and nodules-in-nodule appearance, as well as areas of tumor necrosis and hemorrhage, are frequently seen on both T1- and T2-weighted images, but they are better seen on T2-weighted images and particularly in lesions larger than 3 cm (Fig. 4B-2). Fatty metamorphosis, which is a common pathologic feature, can be seen as areas of high signal intensity on T1-weighted images.[38]

Similar to contrast-enhanced CT, dynamic fast-scanning MR technique following rapid IV contrast administration is the preferred method to detect tumor nodules.[39–42] The concept of IV Gd-based tumor enhancement is similar to that of IV-iodinated contrast-enhanced CT. The tumor nodules are better seen during the early phase of IV contrast enhancement. Lesion detection has been shown to be better in dynamic, fast scanning techniques than MR studies with iron-based contrast enhancement.[43,44] In those studies, iron-based contrast material is picked up by the Kupffer cells and the signal intensity of the normal parenchyma is reduced.

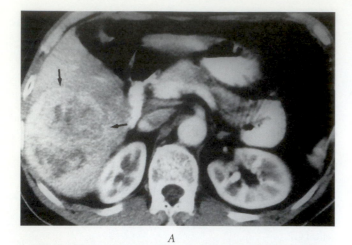

*A*

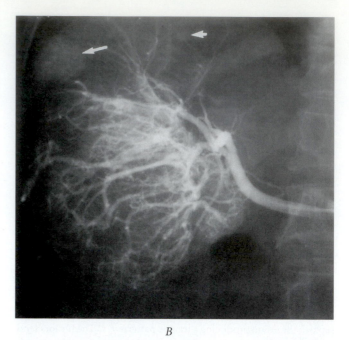

*B*

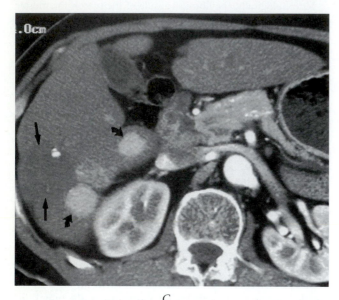

*C*

**FIGURE 4B-1.** CT of hepatocellular carcinoma before and after treatment with chemoembolization. *A.* CT scan shows a large tumor (arrows) in segment VI. Note the heterogeneous enhancement of the tumor. *B.* Right hepatic arteriogram shows hypervascular tumor. Note small foci of daughter nodules (arrows). *C.* CT scan 14 months after chemoembolization. The treated tumor (arrows) becomes hypodense, but multiple small foci (curved arrow) that show hyperdense enhancement during arterial-phase CT develop and continue to grow.

## IMAGING STRATEGIES FOR DIAGNOSIS AND STAGING

The most important goals in imaging for the diagnosis and staging of HCCs before treatment planning are to make the correct diagnosis and to identify patients who are candidates for surgery. The imaging studies should be designed to answer the following questions:

1. Is the tumor confined to a single lobe or region that makes it resectable?
2. Does the tumor invade the portal vein or hepatic veins?
3. Are there smaller lesions in other lobes or segments?
4. Is there evidence of liver cirrhosis and portal hypertension?
5. Are there any lymph node metastases?
6. Are there any other metastases?

    The current approach in the diagnosis of HCC using CT or MR is quite specific, particularly when proper techniques are used. The combination of morphological and dynamic changes in tumor enhancement after IV contrast enhancement using multiphase helical CT or dynamic MR increases the specificity of the diagnosis of HCC to 85% to 95%. The sensitivity of detecting tumor nodules for staging varies from 50% to 65% when using conventional CT but increases to 70% to 75% when multiphase helical CT or dynamic MR is used.[45,46]

    Several investigators in Japan advocate the technique of CT hepatic arteriography for the diagnosis and staging of HCC. The approach is based on hepatic arterial blood supply to the tumor nodule. With the catheter placed in the hepatic artery and CT performed while injecting the contrast material into the hepatic artery, the tumor nodule can be seen as a hyperdense enhancing lesion.[47] This technique can be performed as a single-level cine-CT for lesion diagnosis or scanning through the liver for lesion detection and staging. Others have used CT performed after lipiodol injection into the hepatic artery and CT arterial portography for staging evaluation.[48] These CT techniques have improved the sensitivity

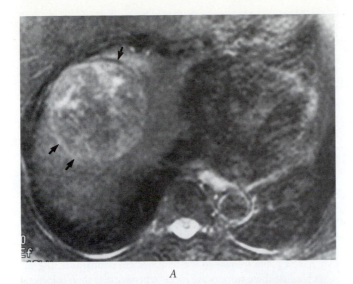

*A*

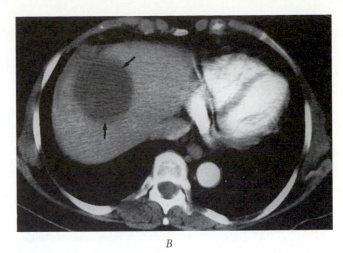

*B*

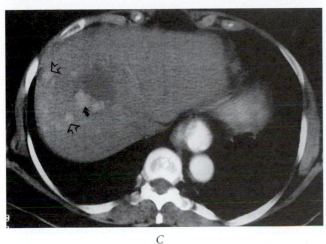

*C*

**FIGURE 4B-2.** MRI of hepatocellular carcinoma and CT after radiofrequency ablation. *A*. T2-weighted image shows large tumor in segment VIII. Note the heterogeneous intensity in the lesion and well defined capsule (arrows). *B* and *C*. CT during arterial phase of IV contrast enhancement 3 months later shows homogeneous low density of necrotic tumor (arrows). However, hyperdense enhanced nodules (curved arrow) at the caudal margin of the lesion in *C* is consistent with locally recurrent disease. Also note small satellite nodules (open arrows).

of lesion detection to 80% to 90%. However, these techniques are more invasive than IV contrast-enhanced CT or MR and have not been widely accepted for staging evaluation because of the invasiveness of the techniques. Recent advances in CT and MR technology with rapid scanning techniques and IV contrast enhancement could improve the sensitivity of lesion detection and make CT arteriography unnecessary as a routine staging procedure.[27,30,31,42,45,46]

## INTERVENTIONAL RADIOLOGY AND TREATMENT OF HCC AND LIVER METASTASIS

Surgery is the treatment option that offers the best potential for cure for HCC, particularly in properly selected patients. Data derived from liver transplantation programs and from surgery in highly selected patients suggest that patients with stage I TNM classification[49] HCC can expect a 5-year survival of 70% to 75%.[50,51] The 5-year survival rates for stage II, III, and IVA disease decrease to 60%, 40%, and

10%, respectively.[50,51] These data suggest that small tumors confined to one lobe or segment and small tumors without portal vein or hepatic vein invasion have the best chance for cure. Patients with larger tumors may also be technically resectable, provided that the hepatic functional reserves are adequate and there is no portal vein or hepatic vein invasion. However, only 10% to 30% of patients are candidates for surgery. Similarly, surgery remains the best treatment option for patients with hepatic metastasis, particularly when it is confined to the liver and limited to a certain lobe or segment. Survival rates at 5 years of 25% to 40% and a 5-year disease-free survival rate of approximately 25% have been reported in properly selected patients.[52]

When surgery is not possible in patients with cirrhosis or poor liver function reserve, chemoembolization and percutaneous tumor ablation by various techniques provide excellent options, particularly when tumors are smaller than 3 cm.

**CHEMOEMBOLIZATION OF THE LIVER.** Over the past two decades, embolization of liver tumors has been used as an alternative treatment for unresectable tumors.[53–60] The technique has progressed from mechanical occlusion of the hepatic artery to chemoembolization that requires mixing chemotherapeutic agents with embolic agents to occlude the hepatic artery. Technical refinement and experiences with various embolic agents in Japan over the past two decades suggest that chemoembolization is effective for treating HCCs smaller than 3 cm, and prolonged survival rates have been reported in this group of patients. The best results can be accomplished when segmental and subsegmental chemoembolization are used, as shown by Matsui and co-workers[57] and Uchida and associates.[56] This is probably due to an increased effectiveness of embolization of the daughter nodules and tumor invasion beyond the capsules. Recurrence rates, as reported by Matsui and co-workers[57] were 18% at 1 year, 30% at 2 years, and 33% at 3 and 4 years after treatment. The 3-year survival rates were 55% to 78% and the 4-year survival rate was 67%.

Despite the evidence from these nonrandomized single-institution studies suggesting that the treatment was most effective when iodized oil was used as a carrier of chemotherapeutic agents followed by gelatin sponge embolization, the efficacy of specific embolic agents has been subjected to debate. A randomized study reported by Hatanaka and associates[60] comparing chemoembolization using gelatin sponge and anticancer agents to chemoembolization using gelatin sponge, iodized oil, and anticancer agents showed no difference in the 1- and 5-year survival rates between the two groups, but the results were better than using iodized oil and anticancer agents without gelatin sponge. The 5-year survival in this study ranged from 18% to 28%. In multivariate analysis, extrahepatic metastasis, presence of ascites, and of tumor involving more than one lobe were important adverse prognostic indicators, whereas the type of embolic agent (iodized oil or no iodized oil) was not an important prognostic indicator.

The results of chemoembolization for HCC in Europe and in the United States were not as good as the results from Japan.[61–65] The median survival rates were between 7 and 11 months in most reports. Van Beers and colleagues,[61] in a retrospective analysis of chemoembolization of 54 patients with HCC, found that the patients who had oil retention in the tumor of greater than 50% of the tumor size lived significantly longer than the patients who had oil retention of less than 50% (1-year and 2-year survival rates of 82% and 65% vs. 27% and 0%). In addition, they also observed that the tumors in those patients who had poor oil retention were infiltrative, hypovascular, and more advanced, whereas the lesions that had oil retention of more than 50% were nodular and hypervascular. Other reasons that may contribute to the poor results of chemoembolization, particularly for tumors larger than 5 cm, are the development of collateral blood supply to the tumors, which could derive from extrahepatic collaterals such as the inferior phrenic and intercostal arteries, and intrahepatic collaterals from the interlobar peribiliary plexus.

A randomized study by a multi-institution French group[65] for the treatment of HCC comparing lipiodol chemoembolization against conservative symptomatic treatment without chemoembolization has shown that there was no survival benefit from chemoembolization (1-year survival rate of 62% vs. 43.5%). Even though chemoembolization may slow down the rate of tumor growth, the incidence of hepatic failure was higher in the chemoembolization group. It should be noted that the criteria for patient selection and the size of the tumors treated in this study were different than those treated in Japan.

The difference in the results of phase 2 single-institution clinical studies from Japan and phase 3 multi-institution trials in Europe can be interpreted to mean that in properly selected patients (tumors smaller than 3 cm, Child A classification) treated by experienced angiographers, chemoembolization can accomplish results similar to surgery, but the results cannot be repeated in multi-institutional trials performed by angiographers with different levels of expertise.

Chemoembolization of hepatic metastasis has more variable results, particularly for treatment of metastases from colorectal cancer.[52] This is probably because metastatic tumors from colorectal cancer are less vascular than HCC, and many of the tumors contain areas of fibrosis, necrosis, and mucin production. The median survival rates of patients treated with chemoembolization vary from 7 to 11 months. These results are similar to or shorter than those after systemic or intraarterial chemotherapy alone. Chemoembolization may have a palliative role in the treatment of neuroendocrine tumors because these tumors are more hypervascular than colorectal metastases.

**PERCUTANEOUS ETHANOL INJECTION (PEI).** PEI has become widely applicable for treatment of small HCCs because of the simplicity of the technique. The procedure includes placement of a 20- to 22-gauge needle under imaging guidance, most frequently US or CT, followed by an injection of dehydrated ethanol at a volume predetermined by the diameter of the tumor. Absolute ethanol causes tumor necrosis by protein denaturation. The procedure can be easily repeated to destroy the tumor completely. The effectiveness of the treatment has been shown in histopathologic studies from specimens in patients who had surgical resection after absolute ethanol injection and in clinical results.[66–69] Shiina and co-workers[68] reported complete tumor necrosis in up to 70% of their selected cases, and the remaining cases showed 70% to 90% tumor necrosis. Long-term survival rates were reported ranging from 39% to 79% at 5 years.[67–69] The results of treatment were better in patients with Child A classification and a single lesion smaller than 5 cm. Recurrence in the treated lesion was 17% according to Livraghi and colleagues,[69] but new lesions in other regions of the liver were seen in up to 83% at 5 years.

A randomized study reported by Bartolozzi and associates[70] comparing chemoembolization with the combination of chemoembolization and PEI in treating HCCs between 3 and 8 cm, showed that combination treatment produced a better response rate and lower recurrence rate, but the survival rates were not statistically significant. However, new lesions in untreated areas occurred with a similar frequency.

PEI is less effective in treating hepatic metastasis from colorectal cancer.[52] Several factors are thought to be responsible. First, the tumors are less vascular than HCC and the lack of tumor vascularity does not allow good distribution of absolute alcohol in the tumor. Second, they may contain areas of fibrosis that limit the ability for absolute ethanol to diffuse uniformly throughout the tumors. Third, the surrounding hepatic parenchyma in metastatic disease is normal, whereas the hepatic parenchyma in HCC is fibrotic. The fibrotic parenchyma associated with HCC may help contain absolute ethanol within the tumor better.

**PERCUTANEOUS TUMOR ABLATION.** The poor results achieved in treating hepatic metastasis or tumors larger than 5 cm with PEI are believed to be due to poor distribution of absolute alcohol in the tumor and limitation of the amount of absolute alcohol that can be used in each treatment session. This has led to the development over the past decade of new techniques using image guidance that can produce physical damage to the tumor.[71] Among these new techniques are cryoablation,[72] microwave tissue coagulation,[73] laser-induced thermal ablation,[74] radiofrequency tissue ablation,[75–79] and focused US thermal ablation.[80] Focused US is still under technical development and in the early phase of clinical trials. Radiofrequency ablation and cryoablation have made significant progress in their technical development and are under phase II and phase III clinical trials, whereas laser-induced thermal therapy and microwave tissue coagulation have had limited clinical trials so far. However, most of these techniques have not yet been established as standard treatments for liver tumors.

Cryoablation is tissue destruction by means of freezing to produce tissue necrosis. The technique has been applied to the treatment of prostate cancers and liver cancers by using a probe (3 to 8 mm in diameter) placed into the tumor under imaging guidance and rapidly lowering the temperature of the probe to below −100°C. The majority of the procedures are done in the operating room following laparotomy. The surgeon and the radiologist collaborate because the cryoprobe is too large to be safely manipulated percutaneously. The treatment seems to be more effective in treating tumors smaller than 5 cm, and in properly selected patients the results are similar to those achieved with hepatic resection.

Radiofrequency-induced or laser-induced thermal therapy through electrodes or a probe under imaging guidance is another attempt to create coagulative necrosis of the tumor. The heat that can be generated raises the temperature up to 90°C in the tissue 2 to 3 cm surrounding the tip of the probe or electrodes. This results in coagulative necrosis of the treated tissue. It provides an alternative method to hepatic resection for local control of metastatic tumor. Most phase I and phase II clinical trials have shown that the technique is possible and can create tumor necrosis with only minor complications. The treatment is more effective for tumors smaller than 3 cm. Complete necrosis or local control of a metastatic lesion can be achieved in approximately 44% to 66% of patients in 1 year.[75–78] Long-term results and prolonged survival rates are still to be determined.

## IMAGING AFTER INTERVENTIONAL RADIOLOGIC PROCEDURES

The goals of imaging studies after treatment by various interventional radiologic procedures include: (1) Detection of complications of the treatment, (2) determination if the entire lesion has been adequately treated, (3) detection of local recurrent disease at the treated lesion, and (4) detection of new lesions at other sites. Imaging studies are usually performed at various intervals varying from immediately following the procedure to within 1 month post treatment period, intermediate follow-up between 3 and 6 months after treatment, and long-term follow-up at 6-month intervals thereafter.

**IMAGING AFTER CHEMOEMBOLIZATION.** The radiologic appearance of treated tumors after chemoembolization depends upon the embolic materials used. When the tumors are embolized without using iodized oil, necrotic tumors are readily seen on CT as areas of uniform low density without enhancement after IV contrast medium administration. After chemoembolization with agents containing iodized oil, uniform accumulation of iodized oil within the tumor produces high-density changes[55,57] (Fig. 4B-3). The more uniform the staining throughout the tumor, the better the results.[61,62] Iodized oil becomes resorbed and eventually disappears over time, and the residual low-density necrotic tumor becomes smaller. During the immediate period after chemoembolization, gas bubbles can be seen in necrotic tumors in up to 60% of patients, and these bubbles are generally resorbed in 2 to 3 weeks. This should not be mistaken for abscess formation except in highly suspicious cases. In such cases aspiration biopsy may be needed to distinguish necrotic tumors from an abscess. Residual tumor or incomplete embolization can be seen as a soft tissue nodule that may enhance after a rapid bolus IV contrast medium infusion. The presence of a soft tissue nodule in the necrotic tumor or a tumor that is well-stained with iodized oil on immediate or long-term follow-up should suggest the possibility of residual or recurrent disease.

The changes of signal intensity on unenhanced MRI after chemoembolization are quite variable.[81,82] The signal intensity of the tumors could increase or decrease on unenhanced T1- or T2-weighted images because coagulation necrosis and hemorrhagic necrosis produce variable signal intensity changes. The necrotic tumor, however, should not enhance after IV infusion of contrast medium.

On long-term follow-up imaging, detection of locally recurrent disease and new disease can be accomplished by helical CT or fast MR scanning technique following a bolus of IV contrast medium. For hypervascular tumors such as HCC and metastatic neuroendocrine tumors, scanning during the arterial phase yields the best results in the detection of small tumor nodules (see Figs. 4B-1 and 4B-2), whereas scanning during the portal phase is preferable for hepatic metastasis from colorectal cancer. Locally recurrent disease is frequently seen at the periphery of the lesion as a nodule with soft-tissue density on CT and high signal intensity on T2-weighted MRI. Locally recurrent disease after chemoembolization frequently occurs at the hepatic surface in contact with the diaphragm or rib where it derives collateral blood supply from extrahepatic circulation such as the inferior phrenic artery, internal mammary artery, and intercostal artery (see Fig. 4B-3).

**IMAGING AFTER TUMOR ABLATION.** The appearance of the tumors after ablation are similar whether absolute ethanol, cryoablation, or thermal therapy is used.[76,82–85] These changes occur in the tumors that fully or incompletely respond to the treatment, and they reflect pathologic changes that are largely due to coagulative and hemorrhagic necrosis. The appearances on imaging studies also reflect the type of treatment. For example, PEI is frequently associated with wedge-shaped hypodensity changes of the surrounding hepatic parenchyma and hyperdense enhancement of that area after IV contrast medium treatment because of associated reflux of ethanol into the portal vein.[86,87] Perihepatic fluid collection and subcapsular hematoma are more frequent (29% to 43%) with cryoablation because larger probes are used in this method.[85]

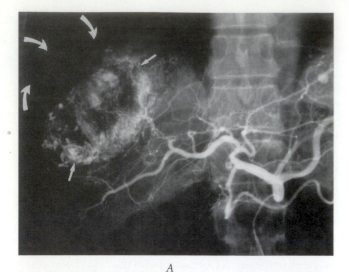

*A*

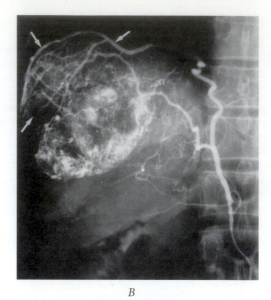

*B*

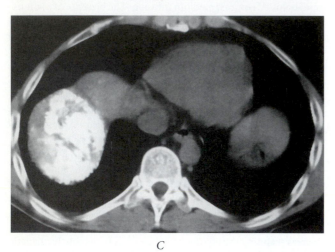

*C*

**FIGURE 4B-3.** Angiograms and CT of recurrent hepatocellular carcinoma after chemoembolization with iodized oil and gelatin sponge. *A.* Celiac angiogram shows minimal blood supply to the treated tumor. Note iodized oil staining (arrows) and the lack of staining (curved arrows) under the right diaphragm. *B.* Right inferior phrenic arteriogram shows the artery providing collateral supply to the tumor (arrows) in the areas under the diaphragm. *C.* CT after iodized oil chemoembolization shows good staining of the tumor.

When US is used to monitor the treatment, the tumors become hyperechoic and produce posterior acoustic shadowing.[72] Although this change accurately defines the site of the treated lesion, mismatch echogenicity with the surrounding tissue, particularly at the posterior wall, makes it difficult to determine if the entire lesion has been adequately treated. On immediate and long-term follow-up, the echogenicity of the treated tumors becomes heterogeneous, making it unreliable for the detection of local recurrence.

The necrotic tumors after PEI, cryoablation, and radiofrequency ablation appear hypodense on unenhanced CT and hypointense on T2-weighted images, and there is no enhancement after IV contrast medium administration[76,82,84,85] (Figs. 4B-4 and 4B-5). The well-demarcated area of low density on CT or low intensity on T2-weighted images makes it easy to recognize viable residual tumors. In most cases, a hyperdense enhancing halo can be observed at the periphery of the mass, corresponding to granulation tissue on pathologic examination.

On intermediate and long-term follow-up, the treated tumors become smaller or remain stable, but the density of the lesions re-

mains uniform. After radiofrequency ablation, locally recurrent disease frequently shows a centrifugal growth pattern from the periphery of the tumor[76,77] (Fig. 4B-6). The tumor will be hyperintense on T2-weighted images and enhances after IV contrast medium administration. Local recurrence rates were 5% to 34%, whereas new disease outside the treated lesion was reported at 22% to 36%.[75–77,79]

After cryoablation, the lesion becomes hypodense, extending to the surface of the liver. Because of pathologic changes in cryoablation associated with rupture of small vessels, high-density areas within the tumor consistent with hemorrhage are more often seen (93%) during the first few weeks of treatment.[72,85]

## FUTURE TRENDS

The clinical experiences and evidence of the past two decades suggest that minimally invasive therapy, including chemoembolization

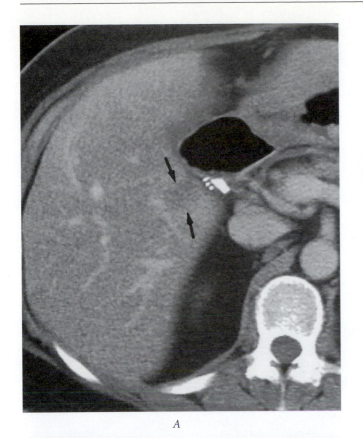

*A*

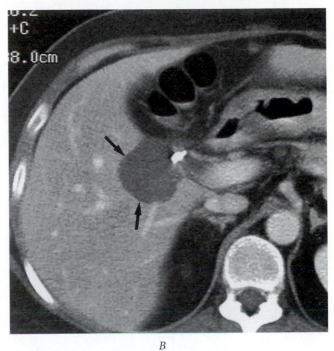

*B*

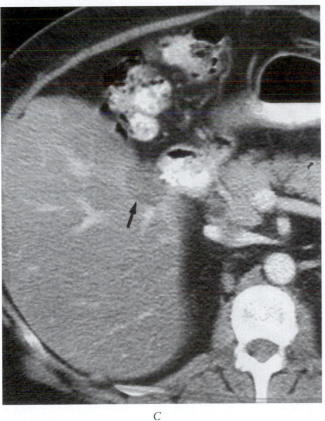

*C*

**FIGURE 4B-4.** CT before and after adequate radiofrequency ablation of metastatic colon carcinoma in segment V. *A.* CT shows 2-cm tumor (arrows) in segment V. *B.* CT 3 months after ablation. The treated tumor (arrows) becomes uniformly hypodense and well demarcated. *C.* CT 15 months after treatment shows no evidence of recurrence. The treated tumor (arrow) remains well defined and is smaller.

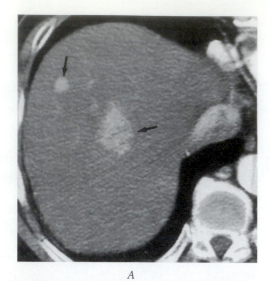

*A*

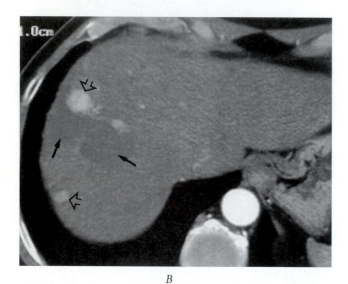

*B*

**FIGURE 4B-5.** CT of multifocal hepatocellular carcinoma before and after treatment with absolute ethanol injection. *A*. Arterial phase CT shows hyperdense enhancing tumors (arrows) in segment VII. *B*. Two months after absolute ethanol injection, the treated lesion (arrow) becomes hypodense but new lesions (open arrows) develop.

and percutaneous tumor ablation, is effective in local control of the tumor, providing that the treatment is properly and adequately targeted to the tumor. Adequate treatment in properly selected patients should yield results similar to surgery, but with lower morbidity and cost. However, there are many challenges to overcome in developing a system that guarantees precise treatment delivery to the tumor with minimal or no injury to the normal tissue and a system that can inform the operator that maximum treatment effect has been achieved. However, despite all the advances of the past two decades, one must realize that these methods of treatment are only

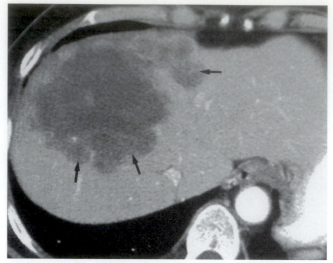

**FIGURE 4B-6.** Recurrent tumor after radiofrequency ablation shown on CT. Note the irregular nodules (arrows) at the periphery of the lesion. The center of the lesion remains necrotic.

a local treatment applied to the treated lesion. The overall biology of the tumor is not changed and tumor cells that may have been undetected and untreated will eventually grow.

## REFERENCES

1. KREMKAU FW et al: Future directions in diagnostic US. Radiology 209:305, 1998.
2. KUDO M et al: Small hepatocellular carcinoma: diagnosis with US angiography with intraarterial $CO_2$ microbubbles. Radiology 182:155, 1992.
3. NOMURA Y et al: Hepatocellular carcinoma in adenomatous hyperplasia: detection with contrast enhanced US with carbon dioxide microbubbles. Radiology 187:353, 1993.
4. NUMATA K et al: Flow characteristics of hepatic tumors at color Doppler sonography: correlation with arteriographic findings. Am J Radiol 160:515, 1993.
5. ROUEIN LD et al: Endoscopic sonography in staging rectal cancer. Am J Gastroenterol 85:1391, 1990.
6. TIO TL et al: Colorectal carcinoma: preoperative TNM classification with endosonography. Radiology 179:165, 1991.
7. DITTLER HJ, SIEWERT JR: Role of endoscopic sonography in gastric carcinoma. Endoscopy 25:162, 1993.
8. CHANG KJ et al: Endoscopic ultrasound-guided fine-needle aspiration. Gastrointest Endosc 40:694, 1994.
9. KALENDER WA et al: Spiral volumetric CT with single-breath-hold technique, continuous transport, and continuous scanner rotation. Radiology 176:181, 1990.
10. ZEMAN RK et al: Helical (spiral) CT of the abdomen. Am J Radiol 160:719, 1993.
11. HEIKEN JP et al: Spiral (helical) CT. Radiology 189:647, 1993.
12. BRINK JA et al: Spiral CT: decreased spatial resolution in vivo due to broadening of section-sensitivity profile. Radiology 185:469, 1992.

13. FISHMAN EK et al: Spiral CT of the pancreas with multiplanar display. Am J Radiol 159:1209, 1992.

14. BLUEMKE DA, FISHMAN EK: Spiral CT of the liver. Am J Radiol 160:787, 1993.

15. ZEMAN RK et al: Three-dimensional models of the abdominal vasculature based on helical CT: usefulness in patients with pancreatic neoplasms. Am J Radiol 162:1425, 1994.

16. SOYER P et al: Surgical segmental anatomy of the liver: Demonstration with spiral CT during arterial portography and multi-planar reconstruction. Am J Radiol 163:99, 1994.

17. SIEGELMAN ES, OUTWATER EK: Magnetic resonance imaging of focal and diffuse hepatic disease. Semin Ultrasound CT MRI 19:2, 1998.

18. CHOI BI et al: Small hepatocellular carcinomas and associated nodular lesions of the liver: pathology, pathogenesis, and imaging findings. Am J Radiol 160:1177, 1993.

19. KOJIRO M: Pathology of hepatocellular carcinoma, in Liver Cancer, K Okuda, E Tabor (eds). London, Churchill Livingstone, 1997, pp 165–187.

20. HONDA H et al: Hepatocellular carcinoma: correlation of CT, angiographic, and histopathologic findings. Radiology 189:857, 1993.

21. OHASHI I et al: Small hepatocellular carcinomas: Two-phase dynamic incremental CT in detection and evaluation. Radiology 189:851, 1993.

22. SHEU JC et al: Ultrasonography of small hepatic tumors using high-resolution linear-array real-time instruments. Radiology 150:797, 1984.

23. SHINAGAWA T et al: Diagnosis and clinical features of small hepatocellular carcinoma with emphasis on the utility of real-time ultrasonography. A study in 51 patients. Gastroenterology 86:495, 1984.

24. KUDO M: Ultrasound, in Liver Cancer, K Okuda, E Tabor (eds). London, Churchill Livingstone, 1997, pp 331–346.

25. BARON RL et al: Hepatocellular carcinoma: evaluation with biphasic, contrast-enhanced, helical CT. Radiology 199:505, 1996.

26. VAN LEEUWEN MS et al: Focal liver lesions: Characterization with triphasic spiral CT. Radiology 201:327, 1996.

27. OLIVER JH III et al: Detecting hepatocellular carcinoma: value of unenhanced or arterial phase CT imaging or both used in conjunction with conventional portal venous phase contrast-enhanced CT imaging. Am J Radiol 167:71, 1996.

28. VAN HOE L et al: Dual-phase helical CT of the liver: value of an early-phase acquisition in the differential diagnosis of noncystic focal lesions. Am J Radiol 168:1185, 1997.

29. LEE HM et al: Hepatic lesion characterization in cirrhosis: Significance of arterial hypervascularity on dual-phase helical CT. Am J Radiol 169:125, 1997.

30. HWANG GJ et al: Nodular hepatocellular carcinomas: detection with arterial-, portal-, and delayed-phase images at spiral CT. Radiology 202:383, 1997.

31. KANEMATSU M et al: Hepatocellular carcinoma: the role of helical biphasic contrast-enhanced CT versus CT during arterial portography. Radiology 205:75, 1997.

32. LOYER EM et al: Hepatocellular carcinoma and intrahepatic peripheral cholangiocarcinoma: enhancement patterns with quadruple phase helical CT—a comparative study. Radiology 212:866, 1999.

33. EBARA M et al: Diagnosis of small hepatocellular carcinoma: Correlation of MR imaging and tumor histologic studies. Radiology 159:371, 1986.

34. ITOH K et al: Hepatocellular carcinoma: MR imaging. Radiology 164:21, 1987.

35. KADOYA M et al: Hepatocellular carcinoma: correlation of MR imaging and histopathologic findings. Radiology 183:819, 1992.

36. RUMMENY E et al. Primary liver tumors: diagnosis by MR imaging Am J Radiol 152:63. 1989.

37. RUMMENY E et al: Central scars in primary liver tumors: MR features, specificity, and pathologic correlation. Radiology 171:323, 1989.

38. MARTIN J et al: Fatty metamorphosis of hepatocellular carcinoma: detection with chemical shift gradient-echo MR imaging. Radiology 195:125, 1995.

39. VOGL TJ et al: Hepatocellular carcinoma: evaluation with dynamic and static gadobentate dimeglumine-enhanced MR imaging and histopathologic correlation. Radiology 205:721, 1997.

40. ITO K et al: Biphasic contrast-enhanced multisection dynamic MR imaging of the liver: potential pitfalls. Radiographics 17:693, 1997.

41. FUJITA T et al: High-resolution dynamic MR imaging of hepatocellular carcinoma with a phased-array body coil. Radiographics 17:315, 1997.

42. YU JS et al: Contrast enhancement of small hepatocellular carcinoma: usefulness of three successive early image acquisitions during multiphase dynamic MR imaging. Am J Radiol 173:597, 1999.

43. YAMAMOTO H et al: Hepatocellular carcinoma in cirrhotic livers: detection with unenhanced and iron oxide-enhanced MR imaging. Radiology 195:106, 1995.

44. TANG Y et al: Detection of hepatocellular carcinoma arising in cirrhotic livers: comparison of gadolinium- and ferumoxides-enhanced MR imaging. Am J Radiol 172:1547, 1999.

45. LARSON RE et al: Hypervascular malignant liver lesions: comparison of various MR imaging pulse sequences and dynamic CT. Radiology 192:393, 1994.

46. YAMASHITA Y et al: Small hepatocellular carcinoma in patients with chronic liver damage: prospective comparison of detection with dynamic MR imaging and helical CT of the whole liver. Radiology 200:79, 1996.

47. UEDA K et al: Hypervascular hepatocellular carcinoma: evaluation of hemodynamics with dynamic CT during hepatic arteriography. Radiology 206:161, 1998.

48. TAOUREL PG et al: Small hepatocellular carcinoma in patients undergoing liver transplantation: Detection with CT after injection of iodized oil. Radiology 197:377, 1995.

49. SOBIN LH, WITTEKIND CH (eds): TNM Classification of Malignant Tumours, 5th ed. Wiley-Liss, New York, 1997.

50. FLICKINGER JC et al: Cancer of the liver, in Cancer: Principles and Practice of Oncology, 5th ed, vol I, VT Devita Jr et al. (eds). Philadelphia, Lippincott-Raven 1997, pp 1087–1114.

51. ENGSTROM PF et al: Primary neoplasms of the liver, in Cancer Medicine, 4th ed, vol II, JF Holland et al (eds). Baltimore, Williams & Wilkins, 1997, pp 1923–1938.

52. KEMENY N, FONG Y: Treatment of liver metastases, in Cancer Medicine, 4th ed, vol II. JF Holland et al (eds). Baltimore, Williams & Wilkins, 1997, pp 1939–1953.

53. YAMADA R et al: Transcatheter arterial embolization in unresectable hepatocellular carcinoma. Cardiovasc Intervent Radiol 13:135, 1990.

54. TAKAYASU K et al: Hepatic arterial embolization for hepatocellular carcinoma. Radiology 150:661, 1984.

55. OHISHI H et al: Hepatocellular carcinoma detected by iodized oil. Radiology 154:25, 1985.

56. UCHIDA H et al: Transcatheter hepatic segmental arterial embolization using lipiodol mixed with an anticancer drug and gelfoam particles for hepatocellular carcinoma. Cardiovasc Intervent Radiol 13:140, 1990.

57. MATSUI O et al: Small hepatocellular carcinoma: treatment with subsegmental transcatheter arterial embolization. Radiology 188:79, 1993.

58. NAKAMURA H et al: Treatment of hepatocellular carcinoma by segmental hepatic artery injection of adriamycin-in-oil emulsion with overflow to segmental portal veins. Acta Radiol 31:347, 1990.

59. CHUNG JW et al: Hepatic tumors: predisposing factors for complications of transcatheter oily chemoembolization. Radiology 198:33, 1996.

60. HATANAKA Y et al: Unresectable hepatocellular carcinoma: analysis of prognostic factors in transcatheter management. Radiology 195:747, 1995.

61. VETTER D et al: Transcatheter oily chemo-embolization in the management of advanced hepatocellular carcinoma in cirrhosis; results of a western comparative study in 60 patients. Hepatology 13:427, 1990.

62. VAN BEERS B et al: Transcatheter arterial chemotherapy using doxorubicin, iodized oil and gelfoam embolization in hepatocellular carcinoma. Acta Radol 30:415, 1989.

63. VENOOK AP et al: Chemoembolization for hepatocellular carcinoma. J Clin Oncol 8:1108, 1990.

64. PELLETIER G et al: A randomized trial of hepatic arterial chemoembolization in patients with unresectable hepatocellular carcinoma. J Hepatol 11:181, 1990.

65. GROUP D'ETUDE ET DE TRAITEMENT DU CARCINOME HÉPATOCELLULAIRE: A comparison of lipiodol chemoembolization and conservative treatment for unresectable hepatocellular carcinoma. N Engl J Med 332:1256, 1995.

66. EBARA M et al: Percutaneous ethanol injection for the treatment of small hepatocellular carcinoma: Study of 95 patients. J Gastroenterol Hepatol 5:616, 1990.

67. TANAKA K et al: Hepatocellular carcinoma: treatment with percutaneous ethanol injection and transcatheter arterial embolization. Radiology 185:457, 1992.

68. SHIINA S et al: Percutaneous ethanol injection therapy for hepatocellular carcinoma: results in 146 patients. Am J Radiol 160:1023, 1993.

69. LIVRAGHI T et al: Hepatocellular carcinoma and cirrhosis in 746 patients: long-term results of percutaneous ethanol injection. Radiology 197:101, 1995.

70. BARTOLOZZI C et al: Treatment of large HCC: Transcatheter arterial chemoembolization combined with percutaneous ethanol injection versus repeated transcatheter arterial chemoembolization. Radiology 197:812, 1995.

71. D'AGOSTINO HB, SOLINAS A: Percutaneous ablation therapy for hepatocellular carcinomas. Am J Radiol 164:1165, 1995.

72. LEE FT JR et al: Hepatic cryosurgery with intraoperative US guidance. Radiology 202:624, 1997.

73. MURAKAMI R et al: Treatment of hepatocellular carcinoma: value of percutaneous microwave coagulation. Am J Radiol 164:1159, 1995.

74. VOGL TJ et al: Malignant liver tumors treated with MR imaging-guided laser-induced thermotherapy: Technique and prospective results. Radiology 196:257, 1995.

75. ROSSI S et al: Percutaneous RF interstitial thermal ablation in the treatment of hepatic cancer. Am J Radiol 167:759, 1996.

76. SOLBIATI L et al: Percutaneous US-guided radio-frequency tissue ablation of liver metastases: treatment and follow-up in 16 patients. Radiology 202:195, 1997.

77. SOLBIATI L et al: Hepatic metastases: percutaneous radio-frequency ablation with cooled-tip electrodes. Radiology 205:367, 1997.

78. LIVRAGHI T et al: Saline-enhanced radio-frequency tissue ablation in the treatment of liver metastases. Radiology 202:205, 1997.

79. LIVRAGHI T et al: Small hepatocellular carcinoma: treatment with radio-frequency ablation versus ethanol injection. Radiology 210:655, 1999.

80. CLINE HE et al: Focused US system for MR imaging-guided tumor ablation. Radiology 194:731, 1995.

81. YOSHIOKA H et al: MR imaging of the liver before and after transcatheter hepatic chemo-embolization for hepatocellular carcinoma. Acta Radiol 31:63, 1990.

82. BARTOLOZZI C et al: Hepatocellular carcinoma: CT and MR features after transcatheter arterial embolization and percutaneous ethanol injection. Radiology 191:123, 1994.

83. LENCIONI R et al: Hepatocellular carcinoma: use of color Doppler US to evaluate response to treatment with percutaneous ethanol injection. Radiology 194:113, 1995.

84. SIRONI S et al: Small hepatocellular carcinoma treated with percutaneous ethanol injection: unenhanced and gadolinium-enhanced MR imaging follow-up. Radiology 192:407, 1994.

85. KUSZYK BS et al: Hepatic tumors treated by cryosurgery: Normal CT appearance. Am J Radiol 166:363, 1996.

86. YOSHIKAWA J et al: Hepatocellular carcinoma: CT appearance of parenchymal changes after percutaneous ethanol injection therapy. Radiology 194:107, 1995.

87. ITO K et al: Enhanced MR imaging of the liver after ethanol treatment of hepatocellular carcinoma: evaluation of areas of hyperperfusion adjacent to the tumor. Am J Radiol 164:1413, 1995.

# 4C / NUCLEAR IMAGING IN THE DIAGNOSIS AND FOLLOW-UP OF CANCER

*Tim Akhurst and Steven M. Larson*

## INTRODUCTION

The fundamental role of medical imaging in surgical oncology is to define where cancer is, predict how it may behave, and determine how it is responding to therapy. In almost all cases, radiologic and nuclear data need to be used in concert to provide optimum information to the referring clinician. The technologies underlying both radiologic and nuclear imaging are constantly evolving, leading to an ever-improving utility of the information given to surgical oncologists. This chapter introduces the reader to nuclear medicine methodologies, as well as outlining approaches that exist or are planned to assist surgical oncologists.

The science of nuclear medicine is constantly evolving, both in terms of mechanisms of photon detection as well as new tracer development. The fundamental principle of nuclear medicine imaging is the external detection of photon emission from radioactive tracers administered to the patient. This is in contrast to other radiographic techniques in which some form of external energy provided by a machine interacts with the mass of the patient's body. The "tracer principle" underlies nuclear medicine's imaging power, in that tracers and machines can be devised to image almost any physiologic process ranging from left ventricular ejection fraction to gene expression. Many of the radionuclides in clinical use have complex radioactive decay schemes, allowing both diagnosis and therapy to be performed with the emitted radiation.

## NUCLEAR IMAGING METHODOLOGIES

### BASIC SCIENCES (TABLES 4C-1 TO 4C-3)

**MOLECULAR IMAGING.** Nuclear medicine is a science based on the use of radiotracer methods to monitor biochemical and physiologic processes in health and disease. The principle of the tracer approach is that the administered radioactive drug (radiopharmaceutical) has no pharmacologic or physiologic effect on the biologic system that it is investigating, but that the labeled drug will be handled in the same manner as the unlabeled molecule, and in this way serve as a radiotracer. The chemical amounts of the radionuclides used in nuclear medicine are extremely small, orders of magnitude less than the contrast agents used in both CT and MRI. Specificity in nuclear medicine is achieved by the development of pharmaceuticals that are tracers of pathophysiologic processes. The simplest example of this is orally ingested radioactive iodine that is used to assess thyroid function. The biologic handling of iodine 131 ($^{131}I$) is determined by the number of protons in the nucleus and the electron shell configuration of the element, rather than the number of neutrons in the nucleus. Therefore, the biodistribution and pharmacokinetics of radioactive iodine are exactly the same as the stable isotope iodine 127. In order to model most other physiologic processes, the generation of biologic analogues that are handled in a similar fashion to the native molecule is necessary. These drugs are then labeled with radioactive elements with radioactive emissions that are suitable for detection by nuclear medicine instrumentation, such as technetium 99m ($^{99m}Tc$) and fluorine-18 ($^{18}F$).

Technetium 99m has been used to label many drugs, including bone-seeking agents, hepatobiliary agents, and renal agents (Table 4C-3). In general, good agents to label with radioactivity are those that have a high degree of affinity for their target tissue and low affinity for nontarget tissue. A washout approach is often used in nuclear medicine; the best-known example is that of bone agents that require an uptake period of 1 to 4 hr after injection. During this time, there is continuing incorporation of the tracer into the bone, as well as continued clearance of the drug from nonosseous sites by the kidneys (Fig. 4C-1). Those physiologic processes that are slower to occur, such as antibody clearance from the plasma, are often imaged with longer-lived isotopes such as $^{131}I$ rather than $^{99m}Tc$ that would have decayed by the time the targeting of the physiologic process has occurred. Therefore, part of the skill of the developmental radiochemist is in the matching of an isotope to the physiologic process that they are trying to target. A wide variety of radiotracers are in clinical use, and a number of these are listed in Table 4C-3.

**NUCLEAR MEDICINE THERAPY.** The process of radioactive decay occurs because the nucleus of the radioactive element is unstable and breaks down with the release of energy in the form of radioactive emissions in order to reach a more stable nuclear configuration. The nuclear emissions take many forms, and the most medically important are β minus, β plus (positron), x-rays, γ rays, and α particles. A general term for these emissions is *ionizing radiation*, because as the radioactive emission passes through matter, the chemicals in the path of the radiation become ionized, and in

## TABLE 4C-1. RADIOISOTOPES IN CLINICAL NUCLEAR MEDICINE DIAGNOSIS

|   |   | HALF-LIFE | RELEVANT EMISSION |
|---|---|---|---|
| * | Technetium 99m | 6.02 hr | Gamma |
|   | Iodine 123 | 13.27 hr | Gamma |
|   | Iodine 131 | 8.02 days | Gamma |
|   | Indium 111 | 2.81 days | Gamma |
|   | Gallium 67 | 3.26 days | Gamma |
|   | Thallium 201 | 72.91 hr | Gamma |
| **PET TRACERS** |   |   |   |
| * | Fluorine 18 | 110 min | Positron |
|   | Carbon 11 | 20 min | Positron |
|   | Oxygen 15 | 2 min | Positron |
|   | Gallium 66 | 9.49 hr | Positron |
|   | Yttrium 86 | 14.74 hr | Positron |
|   | Iodine 124 | 4.2 days | Positron |
| **RADIOISOTOPES IN NUCLEAR MEDICINE THERAPY** |   |   |   |
| * | Iodine 131 | 8.02 days | Beta particle |
|   | Iodine 125 | 59.41 days | Auger electron |
|   | Bismuth 213 | 45.59 min | Alpha particle |
|   | Yttrium 90 | 64 hr | Beta particle |
|   | Phosphorus 32 | 14.26 days | Beta particle |
|   | Astatine 211 | 7.21 hr | Alpha particle |
|   | Strontium 89 | 50.53 days | Beta particle |
|   | Rhenium 186 | 3.72 days | Beta particle |
|   | Samarium 153 | 46.28 hr | Beta particle |
|   | Stannum 117m | 13.6 days | Auger electron |

* Dominant tracer in category.

## TABLE 4C-2. INSTRUMENTS USED IN NUCLEAR MEDICINE

| INSTRUMENT | ROLE |
|---|---|
| • Gamma probe | Intraoperative radio (immuno) detection |
| • Whole-body counter | Dosimetry |
| • Gamma camera | Whole-body/dynamic/SPECT imaging |
| • Solid-state digital detectors | Whole-body/dynamic/SPECT imaging; possible role as intraoperative imaging devices |
| • Dual-detector gamma camera with coincidence detection | As for gamma camera with positron emission detection, inferior lesion detection compared with machines below |
| • Sodium iodide–based ring-detector PET systems | Medium-cost PET |
| • BGO-based ring-detector PET systems | High-cost, high-resolution PET |
| • Fusion devices: CT/SPECT machines | Anatomic or functional imaging device |
| • Fusion devices: CT/PET | Prototype anatomic or functional imaging device |

The use of dosimetry scanning makes it possible to tailor therapeutic doses for a particular patient that are safe and effective. For example, we use this approach to compute optimal therapeutic doses of $^{131}$I in thyroid cancer and $^{131}$I-radiolabeled antibody in non-Hodgkin's lymphoma. When a therapeutic dose of radioactivity is given, we can follow this with a posttreatment scan to assess the efficacy of dose delivery and, because of the higher count statistics, search for microscopic deposits of disease.

NUCLEAR MEDICINE DETECTOR SYSTEMS (TABLE 4C-3). The nuclear medicine device that surgical oncologists are becoming increasingly familiar with is the gamma probe. These hand-held radiation detectors are capable of focused detection of radiation and are being increasingly used intraoperatively in sentinel node detection in breast cancer and malanoma. Newer applications of this technology will include positron detection intraoperatively as well as radioimmunodetection with radiolabeled antibodies.

The stalwart of nuclear medicine has long been the gamma camera. This system can have single or multiple detectors, although the most common configuration is with two detectors. The gamma camera is capable of static planar images, whole-body planar images, as well as tomographic [single photon emission computed tomography (SPECT)] imaging, in addition to dynamic scans. These devices are optimized for detection of technetium 99m, which has a 140-keV photon emission. Newer modifications of the gamma camera include the introduction of devices with thicker sodium iodide crystals that have more photon absorption "stopping power," therefore improving the camera's capability to accurately detect more

this way energy is transferred from the radioactive emission to the tissues. In general, x-ray or γ emissions have the smallest chance of causing cell death because they do not deposit much of their energy in the body as they pass through. β particles have a much higher likelihood of causing cell death; α particles have an even higher probability of causing cell death because they deposit large amounts of energy in the tissues that they pass through. An evolving understanding of radiobiology has led to the development of therapeutic radionuclides.

The unique properties of the radionuclides used in nuclear medicine allow nuclear physicians to predict with reasonable certainty the likelihood of successful therapy as well as the toxicity of a particular radionuclide therapy. When $^{131}$I undergoes decay, it emits both γ photons as well as β particles. In thyroid cancer, the complex decay scheme of radioactive isotopes of iodine allows us to plan therapy with $^{123}$I (no β emission) or low-dose $^{131}$I (β and γ emission). Based on imaging examination with the gamma camera and blood clearance data, the total absorbed radiation dose can be estimated for normal and abnormal tissues. Several dosimetry methods have evolved for calculating the radiation doses delivered to patients. The most commonly used is called MIRD (medical internal radiation dosimetry), a system that is continually being updated and is available in booklet form from the Society of Nuclear Medicine.

**TABLE 4C-3.** COMMONLY USED RADIOPHARMACEUTICALS

| | MOST COMMONLY USED AGENT | ORGAN SYSTEM | MECHANISM OF UPTAKE |
|---|---|---|---|
| **GAMMA CAMERA** | | | |
| Technetium 99m based: | | | |
| Pertechnetate | | Thyroid | Anionic uptake |
| Phosphates | MDP | Bone | Osteoblastic activity |
| Iminodiacetic acid derivatives | HIDA | Biliary system | Bile acid formation |
| | DPTA | Renal | Glomerular function |
| | MAG3 | Renal | Glomerular function and tubular excretion |
| | DMSA | Parathyroid localization Renal parenchymal imaging | Tubular function |
| | methoxyisobutyl isonitrile | Parathyroid imaging Myocardial perfusion | |
| | | Breast scintimammography | |
| Stannous chloride | | Red cell labeling | Hemoglobin binding |
| Particulates | Sulfur colloids | Lymphoscintigraphy Liver and spleen studies | Phagocytosis |
| | Macroaggregated albumin | Lung Hepatic pump studies | Capillary occlusion |
| **IODINE:** | | | |
| $^{123}$I | I | Thyroid imaging | Iodine symporter |
| $^{131}$I | I | Thyroid imaging and therapy | Iodine symporter |
| | MIBG | Adrenal | Adrenergic pathway |
| | Antibodies | Radioimmunodetection and therapy | Target specific |
| Thallium 201 | Chloride | Heart | Potassium analogue |
| | | General tumor-seeking agent | |
| Gallium 67 | Citrate | Tumor or infection | Transferrin receptor |
| Indium 111 | Oxine | White cell labeling | |
| | Octreotide | Neuroendocrine imaging | somatostatin receptor binders |
| **PET CAMERA** | | | |
| Fluorine 18 | FDG | Glucose metabolism | Hexokinase and glucose transporters |
| | FLT | DNA turnover | Thymidine analogue |
| | FMT | Protein metabolism | Tyrosine analogue |
| | 5-FU | Kinetics of antimetabolite | 5-FU analogue |
| Carbon 11 | Various amino acids | Amino acid metabolism | Amino acid transporters |
| Yttrium 86 | Antibodies | Radioimmunodetection and dosimetry of radioimmunotherapy | Target specific |
| Gallium 66 | Antibodies | Radioimmunodetection and dosimetry of radioimmunotherapy | Target specific |
| $^{124}$I | I | Thyroid cancer imaging | Symporter |
| $^{124}$I | Antibodies | As above | Target specific |
| $^{124}$I | FIAU | Viral TK probe | Monitoring gene therapy |
| Oxygen 15 | Water | Perfusion | |

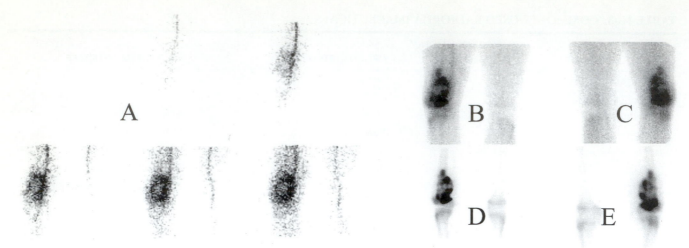

**FIGURE 4C-1.** Triple phase bone scan, soft tissue versus bone pathology. Nuclear medicine cameras are capable of rapid frame acquisitions. In this series of images labeled *A*, the initial perfusion phase of the bone scan of a patient with osteosarcoma of the distal femur is shown. The anterior images are sequential 2-s frames; they demonstrate that there is increased flow to the right leg as a whole as well as the sarcoma itself. The images labeled *B* and *C* are anterior and posterior images of the knees, taken for 5 min immediately after the early vascular phase, and constitute the blood pool component of the study. The images *D* and *E* are the anterior and posterior delayed static bone phase of the sequence, respectively. The concordance of the three phases of the scan suggests that the increased vascularity of the knee be primarily due to the bone itself rather than the soft tissues. If only the first two phases of the scan were positive then a more likely diagnosis would be overlying cellulitis.

energetic photons from $^{131}$I (single 364-keV photon) and $^{18}$F (two 511-keV photons). In addition, coincidence circuitry has been added to these devices so that they are capable of localizing positron decay from radionuclides like $^{18}$F 2-fluoro-2-deoxy-D-glucose (FDG). In spite of the higher energy associated with positron decay, there is a significant degree of attenuation of these photons, particularly in those that originate from the center of the body. In order to overcome this, transmission sources have also been added to these devices to provide attenuation correction and, therefore, more correct images.

A different approach to the detection of positron emission has been to abandon the use of a dual detector system in favor of a ring detector system. These devices are much more efficient in terms of the number of "counts" they detect for a given amount of radioactivity injected into a patient because they are collecting data in 360°. A gamma camera typically has to rotate in "32 steps" to collect the same amount of data.

Dedicated positron emission tomography (PET) devices use a different type of detector crystal, bismuth germanium oxide (BGO). The elements used to create these crystals have higher molecular weight and, therefore, more "stopping power" and thus are efficient at detecting positron emission. These machines also have either partial- or full-ring designs. In general, the dedicated BGO systems are more expensive but outperform sodium iodide crystal–based systems. Most users of these systems use attenuation correction (Fig. 4C-2).

The newest innovations in camera design incorporate x-ray CT machines to provide the attenuation maps necessary for attenuation correction. These machines will also provide functional anatomic imaging where there is fusion of the anatomic detail provided by the CT with the pathophysiologic information inherent in the nuclear medicine data. The first generation of these machines has been released and shows great promise.

Other potential innovations include "solid-state detectors" that have a lower profile and, therefore, will be potentially more flexible in terms of detector design. Hand-held cameras have been designed that will allow intraoperative imaging and therefore image-guided surgery.

The two most common scans performed in nuclear oncology at Memorial Sloan-Kettering Cancer Center (MSKCC) are $^{99m}$Tc methylene diphosphonate (MDP) bone scans and $^{18}$F FDG PET scans. The $^{99m}$Tc bone scan involves an injection of 900 to 1000 MBq of the radiotracer that targets the hydroxyapatite crystal of the bone. The most commonly used tracer is a phosphonate labeled with technetium 99m such as methylene diphosphonate of MDP. The injection of the tracer can be performed with the patient on the gamma camera, allowing the acquisition of dynamic data. The dynamic phase examines the vascularity of a body part, the immediate blood pool images providing an impression of tissue perfusion to the area, or in those cases where this is warranted, whole-body blood pool images can also be performed. The delayed whole-body images are then acquired between 3 and 6 hr after injection (see Figs. 4C-1 and 4C-3). The quality of images depends on the total number of counts acquired by the camera. This depends in part on the administered dose as well as the time taken to acquire an image over a

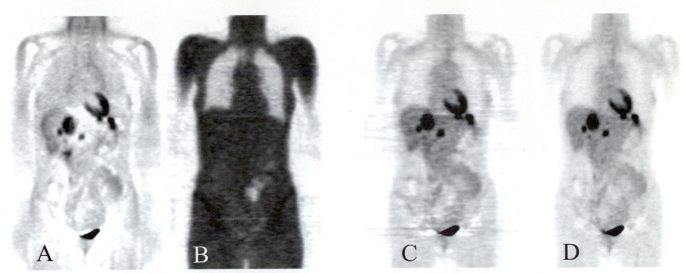

**FIGURE 4C-2.** The effect of attenuation correction on nuclear medicine images. This figure is a series of coronal images from a patient with colorectal cancer metastatic to the liver, with some normal activity within the myocardium. Note the lack of activity in the marrow of the humerii, normal uptake in the bowel and mediastinum, with normal excretion of the tracer into the urinary bladder. Image *A* represents a nonattenuation-corrected emission scan; note the paucity of counts from the center of the patient. Also note the apparent equivalent number of counts from the liver and lungs. Image *B* represents the attenuation-correction scan; this image is like a crude CT scan and represents an attenuation map of the patient. Note in *B* the trachea appearing as white in the upper mediastinum; note also the low-attenuation lungs and intestinal gas. Note also the lack of soft tissue detail, with the pelvis only just discernable from the surrounding soft tissues due to the high energy of the 511-keV photons emitted from the attenuation rod sources. Image *C* represents a filtered back-projection reconstruction of the attenuation-corrected emission images. Note how there is now a correction of the erroneous overrepresentation of the activity in the lungs as well as the underrepresentation of the activity in the center of the abdomen (segments 1, 2, 3, and 4 of the liver). Note also how the attenuation correction has introduced "noise" into the image and the appearance of streak artifacts related to the method of reconstruction. Image *D* represents an iteratively reconstructed image; this computationally intensive reconstruction algorithm reconstructs the image on a pixel by pixel basis, and therefore converges the reconstruction solution to "dots" rather than streaks. Note the absence of streak artifacts and the homogeneity of activity within the lung fields.

particular body part. In the case of bone scans, the quality of bone images also depends on the clearance of the MDP from the blood pool, and this is largely related to the renal function and hydration status of the patient. Scanning protocols can be modified to the particular needs of a particular clinical situation. For instance, 24-hr images are often needed to differentiate between soft tissue infection and osteomyelitis in the diabetic foot.

An FDG PET scan at our institution involves the injection of between 370 and 550 MBq of $^{18}$F FDG. FDG is a marker of glucose metabolism; therefore, any patient-specific process that may lead to focally increased glucose metabolism needs to be understood and avoided. For this reason, we ask our patients to rest quietly after their injection prior to scanning so that skeletal muscle uptake is not increased. In addition, the patient's overall glucose metabolism needs to be understood. If a patient's body is prompted to store glucose by a recent meal, insulin secretion is increased, and there is a shift in overall glucose handling to replenish body stores, especially

to cardiac and skeletal muscle. For this reason we always ask our patients to fast for at least 6 hr prior to the injection of FDG to limit skeletal muscle uptake. The amount of FDG the scanner detects in tissues is related to the duration of time after injection that the scan is performed. Therefore, we attempt to image all of our patients at the same time after FDG injection. All of our patients undergo both emission and transmission scans to allow for more accurate quantification of tissue activity concentrations (see Fig 4C-2). The typical FDG scan of the torso takes about 60 min.

## IMAGING OF SPECIFIC TUMOR TYPES

### NEOPLASMS OF THE SKIN

There are two main roles of nuclear medicine in skin malignancies, staging the primary tumor with lymphoscintigraphy and sentinel

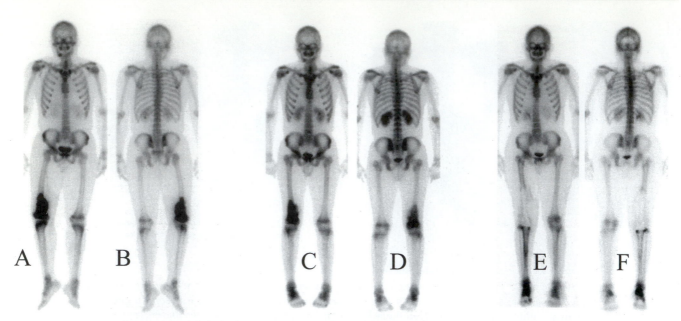

**FIGURE 4C-3.** Whole-body bone scan: Primary bone tumor. This patient with an osteosarcoma of the distal right femur underwent a whole-body bone scan as part of his initial investigation to exclude occult metastatic disease. Images *A* and *B* are anterior and posterior whole-body images, respectively. Images *C* and *D* are performed after a course of chemotherapy. Note that the scan is still markedly abnormal although there is some reduction in the intensity of uptake (compare to Fig. 4C-22, a thallium 201 scan performed at the same time). The initial prosthesis had to be removed due to infection, and a replacement prosthesis was inserted. Six months after the prosthesis was reinserted, the patient underwent a repeat bone scan. The femoral component of the prosthesis is uncomplicated, the tibial component of which appears to have some low-grade bone reaction, perhaps related to low-grade infection. Note also the increased bone turnover in the ankle due to altered mechanical action of the foot and ankle.

lymph node biopsy and the detection of metastases with a variety of tracers.

**LYMPHOSCINTIGRAPHY.** The rationale behind lymphoscintigraphy is that a particulate tracer administered into the skin will be transported by the lymphatics to draining lymph nodes. Drainage is generally along the path of least resistance from the high-pressure injection site to low-pressure sites in the tissues. Therefore, tracer injected around a skin tumor will drain into the low-pressure subdermal lymphatic plexus and from there to the draining lymph nodes. The particle size of the radiopharmaceutical agent is very important. If the particles are too large, there will be inadequate clearance from the injection site. If the particles are too small, the tracer will behave like saline and pass through, rather than be retained in, the lymph nodes. The development of a lymphoscintigraphic program involves a dialogue among surgeons, nuclear physicians, and the radiochemist to ensure the particle size is applicable to the time after injection that the surgeon wishes to operate. Dynamic gamma camera images are important in the assessment of the first lymph node draining a site because lymph drainage from the skin occurs rapidly and nodes are often seen in the first minute following injection. In general, the first node seen is usually the hottest node on delayed imaging, and by implication has the greatest lymph flow from a site and, therefore, the highest probability of containing metastatic disease. In-transit nodes are seen and may contain tumor. Drainage of truncal tumors may pass to unexpected, contralateral lymph node basins so that a large-field-of-view gamma camera image is required to image both axillae and both groins simultaneously so that a surgeon does not ignore a clinically significant lymph node basin.

Sentinel lymph node (SLN) biopsy involves the use of blue dye injected intraoperatively with or without a gamma probe to detect nodes that drain a site involved with tumor. A variety of criteria have been devised to help a surgeon decide what is a significant lymph node and when sufficient nodes have been resected to adequately stage a lymph node basin, including a fourfold reduction in counts arising from the lymph node basin. The inverse square law of physics states that the count rate detected by a gamma probe varies with square of the distance of the source from the probe (doubling the distance leads to a fourfold drop in counts). If a drop in counts is to be used as the criterion of a successful SLN biopsy, the surgeon needs to be very careful to keep the probe at the same distance from any potential source of radiation to avoid errors related to the inverse square law. The combination of a visual cue from the blue dye with the gamma probe information is more powerful than either

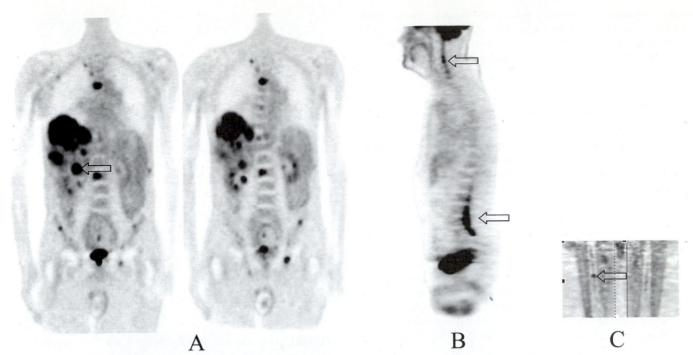

**FIGURE 4C-4.** FDG PET imaging of melanoma. Panel *A* is a series of coronal slices from a male patient who 6 months previously underwent resection of what was thought to be a solitary metastasis to his liver. The current FDG PET study is grossly abnormal with multiple recurrences in liver, spine, right adrenal (arrow), and pelvis. Panel *B*, image of a different patient, reveals increased uptake in leptomeningeal disease in the cervical and lumbar spine (arrows). A distinct advantage of FDG PET over bone scanning in melanoma is its ability to document disease in the marrow that is not evident on bone scan, as demonstrated in the last patient of this series (see panel *C*, arrow).

technique alone in the detection of sentinel nodes in melanoma patients.[1] Lymphoscintigraphy and biopsy of the sentinel node have become increasingly important in the approach to patients with Merkel cell skin tumors and melanoma in whom a regional lymph node dissection is planned.

Both Merkel cell cancers and melanomas have a propensity to disseminate widely. The role of metastasectomy is unclear, but some long-term survivors have been reported.[2] In those patients with high-risk primary cancers, careful preoperative staging is necessary to rule out widespread metastatic disease before local therapy of metastatic disease is undertaken. Both tumors can be targeted with a wide variety of tracers. Merkel cell cancer can be followed with tracers targeting its neuroendocrine phylogeny [[123]I metaiodobenzylguanidine (MIBG)], somatostatin receptors ([111]In octreotide), as well as its overexpression of glucose transporters and hexokinase ([18]F FDG PET). All three tracers have been used to document disease, and altered patterns of uptake have been associated with therapy response. Melanoma has been successfully imaged with a number of SPECT and PET tracers, including monoclonal antibodies. The increased photon flux ("counts") associated with FDG imaging have led to impressive results in terms of lesion detectability with FDG PET such that FDG PET will rapidly become the initial investigation for follow-up of patients with melanoma in those with access

to this technique (Fig. 4C-4). In an initial retrospective series at MSKCC, over one-third of patients studied had a change in their management on the basis of FDG PET performed after conventional imaging.[3] In a subsequent prospective blinded study, similar figures have also been found and the findings confirmed by several other authors.[4,5] In those patients without access to FDG PET, other tracers, including gallium 67, pentavalent [99m]Tc dimercaptosuccinic acid (DMSA), thallium 201, [99m]Tc methoxyisobutylisonitrile (MIBI) have also proved successful in imaging melanoma. If potentially resectable localized disease is found with FDG PET, then the anatomic detail of the recurrence should be investigated with either CT or MRI. A fine-cut CT of the chest and MRI of the brain should be performed as a final screen because CT and MRI are more sensitive than FDG PET in these areas, respectively.

Success rates of treatment of localized limb recurrence of many tumor types, including Merkel cell and melanoma, with regional chemotherapy administration by isolated limb perfusion can be improved by nuclear medicine. Before intensive locoregional chemotherapy is administered with the intention of potential cure, a preoperative scan with FDG PET would seem reasonable to exclude occult metastatic disease. Before the actual locoregional treatment is administered into a closed-loop system, a known amount of tracer, usually [99m]Tc labeled red blood cells, is added to the closed loop. A gamma probe positioned over the heart is used to detect a rise in counts, indicating leak of the tracer, and by inference, the chemotherapy into the systemic circulation. Following locoregional therapy, FDG PET has been used to assess response.[6]

## CANCERS OF THE HEAD AND NECK

Nuclear medicine has much to contribute to the treatment of patients with cancers of the head and neck. Lymphoscintigraphy and sentinel node biopsy techniques have been applied to patients with head and neck cancer, predominantly those with cancers of the skin. An initial report on the use of sentinel node biopsy for patients with oral cancer was disappointing. However, this was a limited study and probably should be repeated in a larger cohort.[7] Local assessment of direct invasion of advanced head and neck cancer is probably best accomplished by MRI. The decision to involve imaging in local nodal staging depends upon the wishes of the patient and the surgeon. If a neck dissection is to be performed as a therapeutic maneuver for the purposes of local control, then there is little role for imaging. If the dissection is to be performed with the intention of cure, there is a need to exclude synchronous tobacco-related cancers of the lung, and, to a lesser extent, esophagus and stomach that occur with a high incidence in patients with head and neck cancers.[8] A single helical CT of the chest will always detect more pulmonary nodules than nuclear techniques, but is less specific in terms of the diagnosis of malignancy. Because PET can characterize both regional lymph nodes that are clinically impalpable as well as detect other occult primary lesions, some groups use FDG PET and other PET tracers such as [11]C methionine (an amino acid tracer) in the preoperative workup of patients with head and neck cancer. In a small series, it appears that both [11]C methionine and FDG PET have a role in the preoperative detection of clinically N0 nodes that are moderately involved with tumor, although microscopic disease cannot be seen with any current imaging modality.[9,10] Other groups have used FDG PET successfully to localize an occult primary cancer in the group of patients who present with palpable lymph node metastases. About 30% of patients with an isolated malignant lymph node in the neck will have the primary site found with FDG PET after a complete search for the primary. The success rates of FDG PET in this setting will vary from group to group,[10–16] in part due to differing rigor of the preceding clinical examination (operative and nonoperative).

There is a shift from initial laryngectomy to radiotherapy with or without chemotherapy in the treatment of laryngeal cancer. In terms of follow-up of patients following radiotherapy, there is very promising evidence that FDG PET is a useful modality in the detection of persistent or recurrent disease.[17–19] Because FDG PET does not rely on the normal tissue planes to determine if recurrence is present, remote treatment does not impact on the detection of recurrent disease, giving PET considerable advantage over conventional imaging modalities, particularly in the postradiotherapy setting.[20] New agents showing some promise are hypoxic tumor tracers (derivatives of misonidazole) that may predict response to radiotherapy. In those centers without access to FDG PET, thallium 201 appears to perform well in the detection of recurrence.[21]

**THYROID CANCER.** The thyroid was the mainstay of nuclear medicine practice in its infancy and remains a significant part of

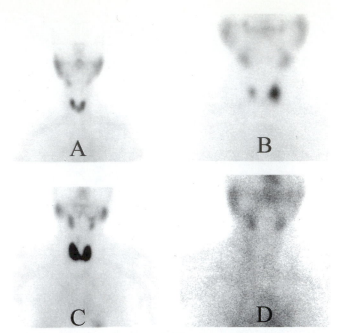

**FIGURE 4C-5.** Thyroid imaging. Image *A* is a [99m]Tc thyroid scan revealing normal uptake. Image *B* is a [99m]Tc thyroid scan revealing irregular uptake in the thyroid, consistent with a multinodular goiter, with two dominant nodules. Image *C* is a [99m]Tc thyroid scan revealing diffusely increased uptake in the thyroid gland due to Graves' disease. Image *D* is a [99m]Tc thyroid scan revealing absence of thyroid tissue due to past successful thyroidectomy and ablation with [131]I.

nuclear medicine practice both in terms of diagnosis (Fig. 4C-5), therapy, and follow-up. Ultrasound and fine-needle aspiration have added further accuracy to the diagnosis of thyroid masses characterized by nuclear imaging. The characteristic findings of a thyroid cancer on both [99m]Tc scans as well as [123]I or [131]I scans are that of a cold nodule. The diagnostic approach to a thyroid nodule will depend on local expertise. If the particular clinic is blessed with a skilled ultrasonographer and cytopathologist, then an ultrasound-guided fine-needle aspiration biopsy is a reasonable first step in the workup of a thyroid nodule. The index of suspicion for a thyroid cancer increases in a cold nodule; however, such findings are also commonly seen in adenoma and adenomatous hyperplasia and colloid cysts. Warm nodules are usually due to an adenoma with autonomous function, and rarely due to thyroid cancer. It is reasonable to follow warm or hot nodules. A number of investigators have included MIBI in the assessment of cold nodules. The role of a MIBI scan is to rule out the presence of degenerative nodules, which appear cold with MIBI, as opposed to adenoma and carcinoma, which appear warm to hot on MIBI scans.[22]

There are a number of adverse clinical and pathologic features that affect the prognosis in thyroid cancer. These include age over 45, the presence of lymphovascular invasion, extrathyroid extension, primary lesion larger than 2 cm in diameter, the presence of distant metastases, and male sex. Radioiodine ablation is recommended in these high-risk patients following total thyroidectomy. The objective

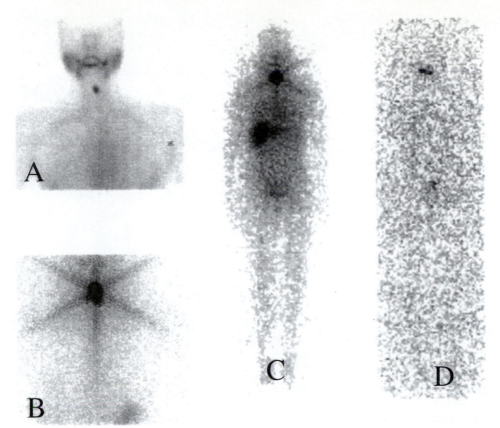

**FIGURE 4C-6.**  Thyroid remnant ablation. Figure *A* is a $^{99m}$Tc thyroid scan demonstrating residual thyroid activity in the neck of a patient with papillary thyroid cancer. Figure *B* is the $^{131}$I scan demonstrating concordant $^{99m}$Tc and $^{131}$I findings suggestive of residual thyroid tissue in the neck. Figure *C* is the postablation whole-body scan demonstrating increased uptake in the thyroid bed with no evidence of distant disease. The uptake seen in the liver is due to hepatic breakdown of the thyroglobulin made by the residual functional thyroid tissue. Figure *D* is the follow-up $^{131}$I whole-body scan revealing no pathologic foci of residual disease. Because the patient's TSH-stimulated thyroglobulin level is low, this patient was not given a further dose of therapeutic radioactive iodine.

of an ablative dose of radioactive iodine is to destroy any remaining viable normal thyroid tissue following surgery. The amount of iodine required to achieve ablation varies from patient to patient, and the doses administered in outpatient treatment vary from 1125 to 2625 MBq (30 to 70 mCi), and in some cases are limited by local governmental radiation safety regulations.

After ablation, an additional whole-body iodine scan is performed to look for occult metastatic disease (Fig. 4C-6). There are now two ways to perform these studies. The traditional way is to withdraw thyroid hormone (T-4) supplements for a sufficient time (about 6 weeks; about 4 weeks for T-3) to cause an elevated thyroid-stimulating hormone (TSH) level in response to thyroxin withdrawl (TSH >60 μIU/mL is desirable). Recombinant TSH to administer by injection is now available, although it is very expensive. The initial experience of this approach, which spares the patient a period of hypothyroidism, has been very promising. If occult disease is seen, a higher therapeutic dose of $^{131}$I is given in an attempt to destroy any metastatic tumor (Fig. 4C-7). Whole-body radioiodine scans are recommended yearly for follow-up purposes. Once two consec-

utive whole-body scans are negative, the patient can be placed on a maintenance observation schedule. The follow-up of patients with thyroid cancer is evolving, with an increasing dependence on serum thyroglobulin to detect evidence of recurrence, with whole-body iodine scans increasingly reserved for those with an elevated thyroglobulin. Iodine 131 therapy remains the key therapy for patients who develop metastatic disease. Some institutions give empirical doses of radioactive iodine; others, including our own, use a pretreatment dosimetry scan to determine the maximum permissible dose. The dose-limiting organs are the lung (in those patients with diffuse lung metastases) and the red marrow. Another side effect that although not life-threatening often limits dose is salivary gland dysfunction. Early trials of investigational agents aimed at limiting salivary gland toxicity have now been completed and appear promising.[23] Some groups have substituted MIBI for $^{131}$I or $^{123}$I in the scintigraphic detection of thyroid cancer, and detection rates appear similar.[24] The attraction of MIBI scans is that the administered scanning doses of MIBI can be a lot higher [740 to 1100 MBq (20 to 30 mCi)] compared with 74 to 370 MBq (2 to 10 mCi) for iodine,

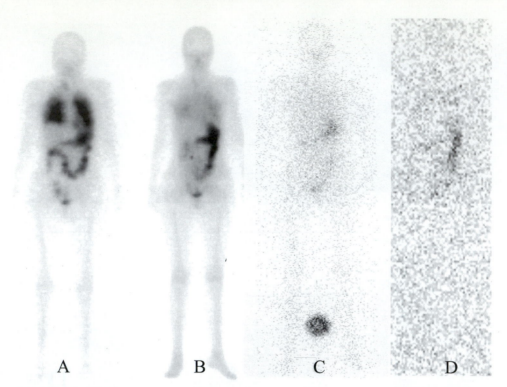

A          B          C          D

**FIGURE 4C-7.**  [131]I therapy. *A* series of images of a 24-year-old female patient with follicular variant of papillary thyroid cancer metastatic to neck and lungs are shown. This patient had previously received 982 mCi (36,334 MBq) of [131]I over a 6-year period for neck, mediastinal, and lung disease. Image *A* is a posttherapy scan performed in May 1997, 7 days after administration of 300 mCi (11,100 Mbq) of [131]I. Image *B* is a posttherapy scan performed in January 1998 showing a reduction in uptake in the lungs. Images *C* (8/98) and *D* (12/99) are follow-up scans documenting successful ablation of the lung and neck disease.

---

enabling better scan quality. The disadvantage of the MIBI approach is that there is no dosimetric information to guide the subsequent therapeutic administration of [131]I. In the search for non-iodine-avid disease that may be surgically resectable, initial studies report that FDG PET seems to outperform SPECT tracers, including MIBI.[25]

In a number of neoplasms, there appears to be an inverse relationship between the uptake of FDG and a more "specific" tracer. This appears to hold true for thyroid cancer. A number of reports have been published describing an inverse relationship between the degree of FDG uptake and the degree of [131]I uptake. It seems that there is loss of effective function of the sodium-iodine symporter as the activity of glucose transporters and hexokinase increases. This observation is important because it will allow investigators a noninvasive endpoint with which to examine the efficacy of differentiating agents in thyroid cancer, as well as possibly selecting patients in whom trials of novel therapeutic agents in thyroid cancer would be appropriate.

Medullary carcinoma of the thyroid is an interesting tumor and accumulates thallium 201, pentavalent DMSA, MIBI, as well as analogues of somatostatin. The implications of this are being explored with radioguided surgery being performed with [111]In octreotide,[26]

and early trials of yttrium-labeled somatostatin analogues are being performed for the treatment of advanced somatostatin receptor–positive disease.[27]

Initial trials with murine monoclonal antibodies in treating head and neck cancer have not lived up to their conceptual promise. One of the major impediments to effective monoclonal therapy is the development of human antimouse antibodies (HAMAs) that have precluded repeated administrations due to the rapidity of the clearance of the antibody with subsequent administrations. The observation that monoclonal antibodies can induce an immune response has lead to additional avenues of research, generating humanized monoclonal antibodies in addition to bispecific antibodies that bind either effector molecules or reporter systems.[28]

**PARATHYROID TUMORS.**  Imaging the parathyroid is a challenge to nuclear medicine clinicians; a variety of approaches have been used, including dual tracer subtraction imaging and anti-CEA antibody imaging. Subtraction imaging involves the administration of an agent (thallium 201) that localizes in the parathyroid as well as the thyroid after administering an agent that is only accumulated in the thyroid tissue ([99m]Tc pertechnetate or [123]I or [131]I). By subtracting

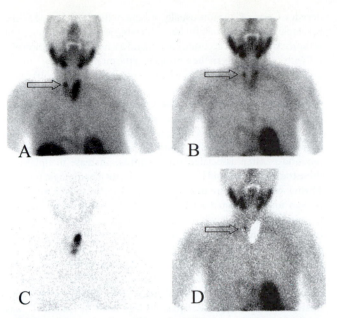

**FIGURE 4C-8.** Parathyroid imaging. This 81-year-old woman presented with recurrent hyperparathyroidism, having previously had a right hemithyroidectomy and parathyroid resection. Images *A* and *B* are early and late sestamibi studies revealing differential retention of the tracer in the region of the bed of the upper pole of the right thyroid lobe, compared to the left thyroid lobe. These images by themselves are suggestive of a parathyroid adenoma. Confirmation was obtained by the use of an [123]I scan performed on the same day, *C*, and a subtraction image *D* where the activity arising in the thyroid seen in image *C* is subtracted from the sestamibi image *B* highlighting the parathyroid adenoma (open arrows). The patient subsequently underwent resection of an enlarged parathyroid gland (0.45 g) with normalization of her serum calcium level.

the [99m]Tc activity arising in the thyroid from the [201]Th activity arising from both the parathyroid and the thyroid, activity due to the parathyroid is demonstrated. Because the two acquisitions are temporally separated, motion artifacts can produce false positives and false negatives. An alternate approach is to use [99m]Tc sestamibi that is initially taken up in both thyroid tissue and the parathyroids. Uptake of the tracer appears independent of *p*-glycoprotein expression.[29] There is selective washout from the thyroid leading to clear demonstration of the parathyroids on delayed imaging (performed 120 min later) (Fig. 4C-8). It appears that sestamibi imaging is the most accurate method of determining the site of parathyroid adenomas, outperforming ultrasound, CT, and MRI.[30] Surgery, with the assistance of sestamibi imaging, has a high likelihood of normalizing the serum calcium level.[31]

## LUNG NEOPLASMS

*EVALUATION OF THE SOLITARY PULMONARY NODULE.* In a carefully selected population, screening CT of the chest has been shown to be quite effective at detecting small malignancies in

the lung.[32] An inevitable consequence of the reporting of the utility of CT in the detection of small lung cancers in these high-risk groups will be the performance of a large number of CTs in patients who do not meet the strict criteria of the formal studies. A further consequence will be the detection of a large number of solitary pulmonary nodules. Characterizing these lesions with radiotracers should help direct patients at higher risk for cancer and in whom a more aggressive workup is needed. FDG PET is a powerful tool in the evaluation of solitary pulmonary nodules, with pathologic FDG uptake almost always being due to tumor,[33] especially in those groups at high risk of the disease.[34] The use of FDG PET as an initial investigation in evaluating such lesions is cost-effective in some models.[34] In patient populations with a high prevalence of granulomatous parenchymal inflammation, the specificity of FDG PET imaging will be much lower than the initial optimistic reports mentioned above.

*PREOPERATIVE STAGING OF LUNG CANCER.* There is a relatively high incidence of bone metastases at the time of diagnosis of the primary cancer, especially when the primary tumor is greater than 3 cm. Many groups include a preoperative bone scan in the diagnostic workup of patients with T2 lung cancers. When positive, this should be accompanied by an MRI of the head because brain and bone metastases often go hand in hand in patients with lung cancer. Lung cancer often progresses rapidly. The bone scan is imaging the bone's response to the presence of tumor, rather than the tumor itself. For this reason, bone scan lesions may be photopenic (reduced focal uptake) in rapidly progressive lung cancer.

Preoperative differential lung function studies using a combination of a ventilation agent ([99m]Tc Technegas, [99m]Tc pertechnetate, [99m]Tc DPTA aerosol, and xenon 133) as well as the perfusion agent, [99m]Tc-labeled macroaggregated albumin (MAA), can give good estimates of the differential perfusion and ventilation of the lungs. This is a useful test in those patients with borderline respiratory function in whom pneumonectomy is contemplated because it accurately predicts the postoperative respiratory function.[35] As a rule of thumb, the forced expiratory volume (FEV1) will be reduced in the postoperative setting, proportionate to the percent of perfused functioning lung removed on the perfusion agent imaging.

The appropriate staging of lung cancer for an individual patient depends on the expertise of the local surgeon and cytopathologist. At this stage, the relative merits of mediastinoscopy and FDG PET imaging are unproven, but a large multicenter trial is under way to answer this question. Mediastinoscopy and pathologic examination are both subject to sampling errors and are by necessity invasive. No imaging modality can detect very small volume disease, and a significant number of patients will be understaged by any imaging technique when compared to a subsequent thorough mediastinal lymph node dissection and pathologic examination. FDG PET is more successful at differentiating benign from malignant nodes when compared to CT.[36] A PET-directed mediastinoscopy is likely to have a higher yield of positive nodes than a CT-directed procedure. The presence of contralateral FDG-positive nodes is an ominous sign in terms of resectability. Many patients are undergoing a PET scan prior to a surgical procedure. This seems a reasonable approach because easily accessible nodes (in the supraclavicular fossa for instance) are often found with FDG PET that obviate the need for mediastinal node sampling.

Certain types of lung neoplasms are not particularly FDG avid. This is true of bronchoalveolar carcinoma and well-differentiated carcinoid tumors (adenocarcinoma with bronchoalveolar features and poorly differentiated carcinoid tumors are often FDG avid). Patients with suspected carcinoid tumors should be investigated with a specific somatostatin analogue tracer such as octreotide. When there is a clinical history of recurrent mucinous bronchoalveolar carcinoma, FDG PET has little role to play in patient management.

MEDIASTINAL TUMORS. The diagnosis of mediastinal masses can be streamlined with the aid of a clinical history, the sites of involvement, and the demographics of the patient. Thymoma is the most common mediastinal mass in adults, outranking lymphoma, endocrine masses (predominantly thyroid), and germ cell tumors. Thymoma appears in the fifth or sixth decade, usually (80%) is present in the anterior mediastinum, and about 50% of patients have associated myasthenia. Lymphoma usually presents in the third decade of life, with a second peak in the seventh and eighth

decades. Germ cell tumors usually present in the third decade of life. Serologic markers are helpful in establishing a diagnosis of germ cell tumors. Although an accurate history and a careful examination of a CT with contrast govern the approach to the management of a mediastinal mass, in those patients who potentially have a goitrous mass, an [123]I scan performed prior to the administration of intravenous contrast will rapidly give the correct diagnosis.

The normal thymus gland can often be seen on gallium scans, FDG scans, as well as in posttreatment radioiodine scans. The mechanism of uptake is not well established, but the syndrome of thymic rebound is often associated with a diffuse increase in uptake of these tracers, and should not be confused with a pathologic process. Thymic carcinomas are often FDG avid, and the degree of uptake is likely to be associated with the tumor's aggressiveness.[37] Because thymic cancers recur within the pleural space (Fig. 4C-9) if not removed in toto, the planned surgical margin could be increased if a thymic mass is FDG avid.

A common outcome of chemotherapy and or radiotherapy for lymphoma is the presence of a residual mass. The single best noninvasive test to evaluate residual masses is comparison of a pretreatment and posttreatment nuclear medicine scan. Gallium 67 was the diagnostic medium of choice in this situation. However, these scans often take 3 days to complete, leading to delays in diagnosis

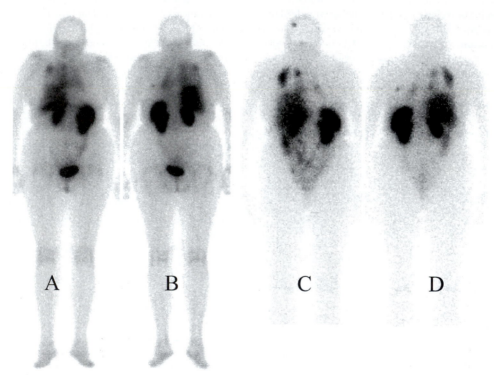

**FIGURE 4C-9.** Thymic cancer with octreotide affinity. This patient presented with a thymic mass that was resected and was found to be a poorly differentiated thymic carcinoma. This patient underwent an octreotide scan that demonstrated bilateral pleural involvement; 14 months later, in spite of chemotherapy, the patient had developed a cerebral metastasis and progressive pleural disease. The avidity of the tumor for octreotide indicates that some response could be expected with cold somatostatin, and when available yttrium 90–labeled octreotide as therapy.

and for the patient, a significant amount of time spent away from work. FDG PET appears to be a major advance in this regard because it provides the same or better information as a gallium 67 scan in 1 day.[38]

Germ cell tumors have a bimodal presentation, typically presenting in childhood in the form of mature teratoma (that are not FDG avid) and in the thirties as seminoma and nonseminomatous germ cell tumors (usually FDG avid). Unfortunately, seminoma and non-seminomatous germ cell tumors can harbor small pockets of mature teratoma. A more specialized form of FDG PET imaging requiring additional scanning time has been shown to be able to differentiate mature teratoma from scar on the basis of uptake and retention (phosphorylation) rates of FDG.[39] However, this study needs to be repeated in a larger patient group.

**ESOPHAGEAL CANCER.** When imaging the esophagus with FDG PET, one has to be cognizant of the fact that areas of inflammation are hypermetabolic and will therefore exhibit increased FDG uptake. This is particularly true of the lower esophagus, which is often mildly hypermetabolic, presumably due to low-grade esophagitis. For this reason, early-stage esophageal cancer will not be reliably detected with FDG PET. In addition, the depth of tumor invasion will also not be able to be reliably assessed.[40] The role of PET in this disease is in the detection of regional and distant malignant lymphadenopathy. The performance of FDG PET in this regard is similar to that seen in lung cancer, where disease is seen in normal-sized lymph nodes, leading to the demonstration of significant amounts of local and distant spread not seen with CT.[41] In addition, FDG PET has been used to monitor patients medically unfit for surgery that have had a course of combined chemotherapy and radiotherapy. Given the current state of our knowledge of use of FDG PET in this disease, it is probably inappropriate not to operate on patients who are otherwise fit for surgery purely on the basis of a negative posttreatment FDG PET scan. The converse is true, however, in that a lack of fall of FDG uptake and persistent uptake in an area of tumor is very likely to represent residual cancer.[42]

## CANCER OF THE STOMACH

Large primary gastric tumors can be seen with FDG PET. However, low-grade diffuse uptake is often seen, making the diagnosis of early lesions with FDG PET difficult. Due in part to gastric peristalsis, and also partial volume averaging from the primary tumor, the detection of peritumoral nodes as discrete foci of tumor is difficult with FDG PET. Regional adenopathy in the celiac axis can often be seen, however. In terms of the detection of peritoneal disease, a staging laparoscopy is a powerful diagnostic tool and is rapidly being accepted as a cost-effective procedure.[43] The role of FDG PET in addition to laparoscopy has yet to be established, as has the relative accuracy of FDG PET and CT (one small study has shown some additional benefit with PET).[44]

The efficacy of delivery of a chemotherapeutic drug to the entire peritoneum can be assessed by simply instilling a [99m]Tc-labeled particulate such as sulfur colloid or MAA and imaging the patient with a gamma camera. Many gastric cancers express CEA and, therefore, radiolabeled anti-CEA antibodies and constructs could be used to image and potentially target gastric cancers. Research into the use of monoclonal antibodies in gastric cancer is limited but ongoing in terms of antigen expression[45,46] and radioimmunoguided surgery.[47–50] Gastric motility can be assessed with radiolabeled solids and liquids, thus examining both the solid and liquid phases of gastric emptying.

## EXOCRINE PANCREATIC TUMORS

In those patients with no history of pancreatitis, the initial diagnostic test performed is helical CT with contrast.[51] Newer approaches include the use of MRI, the actual sequences and contrast agents of which are in evolution. Receiver operator characteristic (ROC) analyses of MRI and CT have varied results, possibly because of differing imaging sequences.[52,53] Pancreatic cancer and chronic pancreatitis may be indistinguishable at the bedside, and the ultrastructural characteristics of both can mimic each other on CT.[54] Many MRI/CT papers include only patients who are suspected of having pancreatic cancer, so there is an element of recruitment bias in the ROC analyses, and such high success rates may not be reproducible in the general population. FDG PET has been used to detect pancreatic cancer, and indeed pancreatic cancers are hypermetabolic.[55] Semiquantitative analysis of lesion uptake values can differentiate chronic pancreatitis from pancreatic cancer,[56] although visual interpretation appears equally successful in the diagnosis of malignancy with ROC areas of about 97%.[57] In a separate study, CT and PET were compared directly, and it appears that FDG PET performs at least as well as CT in the diagnosis of malignancy.[58] Endocrine pancreatic failure secondary to chronic pancreatitis results in hyperglycemia that has been shown to reduce the sensitivity of FDG PET.[59,60] The role for PET in diagnosis of pancreatic cancer therefore appears to be in the assessment of equivocal lesions seen in patients with or without chronic pancreatitis. CT and PET are likely to be complementary because PET is not able to define local tumor extent.

Resection of tumors of the pancreatic head often involves resection of the duodenum and biliary ampulla. These procedures are associated with persistent gastrointestinal symptoms that can be followed with nuclear medicine. Gastric emptying studies have long been used to assess gastric motility, and hepatobiliary studies are accurate in the perioperative assessment of bile leak and later in the course of recovery biliary stricture. These studies will be dealt with in more detail in subsequent paragraphs on hepatobiliary tumors.

## ENDOCRINE PANCREATIC TUMORS

Most tumors arising from the amine precursor uptake and decarboxylation (APUD) system are readily assessed with somatostatin analogues (see Figs. 4C-9, 4C-10, and 4C-11). The FDA-approved somatostatin receptor scintigraphic study (SRS) agent is [111]In octreotide. Iodine 131 and 123 MIBG have also been used to detect APUD tumors, although they do not seem to be as accurate as SRS.[61] Octreotide has a high affinity for somatostatin receptor types 2 and 5 and, to a lesser extent, type 3, with little to no affinity for receptor types 1 and 4.[62] The reported detection rates of primary APUD

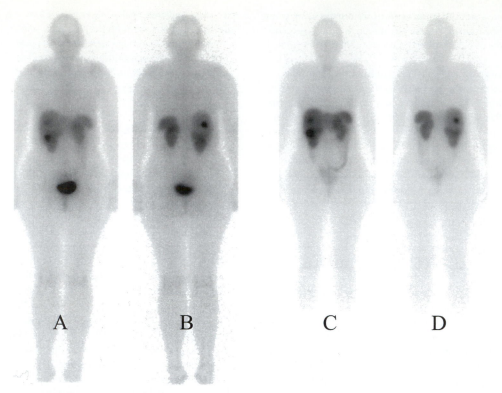

**FIGURE 4C-10.** Neuroendocrine cancers. This patient presented with a liver metastasis due to a well-differentiated neuroendocrine tumor; note the very avid lesion seen in segment 4 of the liver, with a second lesion seen more posteriorly in the liver. The remainder of the uptake seen is within physiologic limits. Images *A* and *B* were performed in March; images *C* and *D* were performed in November of the same year and show no change, indicating a stable tumor.

pancreatic tumors are 79% for gastrinomas, 100% for glucagonomas, 84% for other pancreatic APUDomas, with the exception of insulinomas, which have a detection rate of 47%.[63] An SRS study performed as the initial imaging study in patients with pancreatic endocrine tumors will not only identify the primary tumor in the majority of cases, but also any metastases within the liver with higher accuracy than CT.[61,64] The presence of SRS-positive disease suggests a patient will respond to therapeutic doses of nonlabeled octreotide by reducing hormone hypersecretion from islet cell and carcinoid tumors (see Fig. 4C-11). An additional advantage of SRS is in the assessment of patients for possible radioimmunotherapy with [111]In octreotide or [90]Y octreotide (trials of [90]Y are currently open).[27]

Carcinoid tumors may arise in the pancreas but also in the duodenal wall and lung. They will, however, be dealt with here. SRS is again very successful in imaging carcinoid tumors with detection rates of 83% to 87% of the primary tumor and 100% of the associated liver metastases when imaged with [111]In octreotide.[65,66] Atypical carcinoid is also a significant medical problem and comprises about 10% of all carcinoid tumors in the lung and is associated with a poorer prognosis than typical carcinoid. Atypical carcinoid also appears to be octreotide avid,[67] but experience with octreotide scintigraphy in atypical carcinoid is very limited.

## EXTRAHEPATIC BILIARY NEOPLASMS

### GALLBLADDER CANCER

*CHOLANGIOCARCINOMA.* The cardinal symptom of cholangiocarcinoma is painless jaundice, less frequently pruritus, abdominal pain, and weight loss are the presenting symptoms. Unless biliary manipulation has occurred, cholangitis is uncommon. The standard imaging workup of painless jaundice includes a transabdominal ultrasound or CT aimed at excluding hepatic metastases, or pancreatic cancer, that are a more common cause of painless jaundice. The finding of a mass within proximal duct dilatation is a clue to the diagnosis of cholangiocarcinoma, the level of duct dilatation providing a clue as to the site of the tumor. Functional assessment of bile flow can be achieved with hydroxy iminodiacetic acid (HIDA) derivatives labeled with [99m]Tc. Functional assessment of the biliary tree (bile flow rates) is not currently possible with radiologic techniques, although a noninvasive assessment of biliary anatomy can be performed with MRI. It is likely that the staging of bile duct malignancies by noninvasive imaging will soon be dominated by MRI, because this methodology can image both biliary anatomy as well as detect metastases.[68] Preliminary results indicate that cholangiocarcinoma is FDG avid.[69,70] FDG PET may therefore

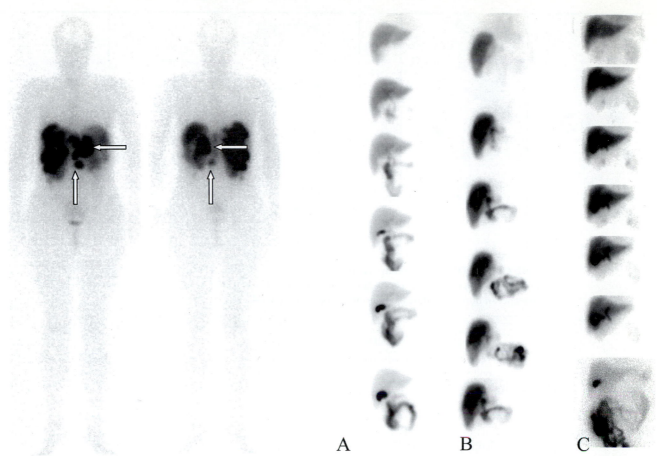

**FIGURE 4C-11.** This 52-year-old patient was referred for characterization of her known liver metastases; she was found to have a distal pancreatic lesion (horizontal arrows) as well as a retroperitoneal lymph node (vertical arrow). Subsequent biopsy revealed islet cell carcinoma. Two years after this scan she remains well and symptom-free on cold octreotide therapy, indicating that strongly positive octreotide scans can predict responsiveness to cold octreotide therapy.

**FIGURE 4C-12.** HIDA scanning. This is a series of HIDA scans demonstrating a variety of clinical situations. The images are arranged vertically, 5 min apart during the study. The images in column *A* are of a 66-year-old man with prostate cancer who developed acute abdominal pain, possibly due to acute cholecystitis. The scan is normal, excluding cholecystitis. Notice the prompt uptake of the tracer into the liver, excretion into the bile ducts and gallbladder, with emptying of the biliary system into the gut. The images in column *B* are of a patient with a prior left hepatectomy and Whipple's procedure without evidence of obstruction of biliary drainage. The images in column *C* are of a patient with upper abdominal pain who demonstrates, on scanning, a failure of drainage into the gut, due to sphincter of Oddi dysfunction. The last panel in column 3 is 3 hr after injection and demonstrates the absence of complete biliary obstruction.

be a sensitive method to detect early cholangiocarcinomas, but the specificity of low to intermediate grades of FDG uptake in the setting of sclerosing cholangitis is not yet established, because activated inflammatory cells are also FDG avid. In those patients who have undergone resection, HIDA studies are very useful in documenting bile flow (Fig. 4C-12). HIDA scans are the most accurate test in the detection of cystic duct obstruction.

**SMALL INTESTINAL NEOPLASMS.** Radiolabeled red cell studies are a powerful test in determining the site of GI bleeding that may be the presenting symptom of small bowel malignancies and are able to detect rates of bleeding that are lower than those able to be seen with conventional angiography. In these studies, a sequential series of images is acquired to provide the reader with a cine-loop to follow the passage of blood through the gut.

Neuroendocrine tumors of the proximal bowel have been discussed in the paragraphs dealing with pancreatic neoplasms. In brief, both diagnostic and therapeutic analogues of octreotide are now available, and as octreotide receptors are not highly expressed on normal bowel, the use of this class of drugs provides high tumor to background ratios, leading to highly sensitive and specific imaging.

The literature reporting the nuclear medicine imaging of leiomyomas is sparse; there are isolated reports of increased FDG uptake

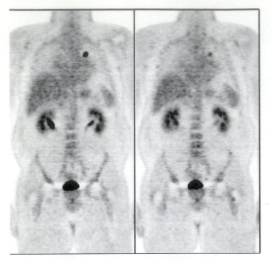
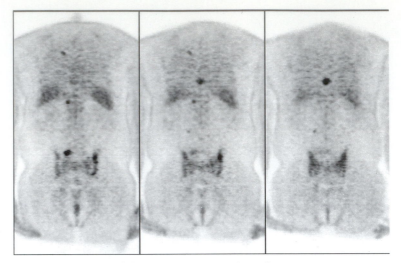

**FIGURE 4C-13.** FDG PET in leiomyosarcoma. This patient underwent FDG PET to evaluate the resectability of a right lung metastasis from a leiomyosarcoma. The FDG PET scan clearly demonstrated the presence of bone metastases, rendering the patient inoperable.

in a retroperitoneal leiomyoma,[71] and metastatic leiomyosarcoma has also been reported to be FDG avid.[72,73] It appears that FDG PET may have a role in the follow-up of patients with leiomyosarcoma (Fig. 4C-13).

Small intestinal adenocarcinoma is uncommon and no large series of patients have been reported in the nuclear medicine literature. The utility of FDG PET in the detection of recurrent disease is likely to be similar to that seen with large bowel adenocarcinoma (see the following).

**LARGE BOWEL NEOPLASMS (SEE ALSO "HEPATIC METASTASES").** Lymphoscintigraphy of the anorectal canal has been performed with injections given endoscopically.[74,75] However, sentinel node biospy guided by a gamma probe was not done in these cases. Sentinel node biopsy may be an important advance in patient management given the potential for lymph drainage outside the operative/radiotherapy field to the groin, but it has yet to be reported.

FDG PET has been recognized as a powerful tool in the detection of locoregional disease from colorectal cancer. The staging of primary colorectal cancer is currently the province of the radiologist and the endoscopist. Recent advances in the methodology of reconstruction of FDG PET scans is enabling nuclear medicine physicians to detect lymph nodes adjacent to metabolically active primary tumors (that are almost universally hypermetabolic).[76] In those patients with a large primary tumor, an FDG PET scan may be an economically effective way to determine the presence or absence of distant metastases.

In those patients with advanced colorectal cancer, FDG PET consistently is able to detect more lesions and, therefore, alter patient management in a large proportion (about 30%) of patients in whom it is performed. This is partly due to presence of tumor in normal-sized lymph nodes. The visual cue presented to a radiologist from

a malignant lesion is much stronger with PET than it is with CT, where the signal from the malignant tissue is "buried" in a large amount of anatomic information leading to higher sensitivity with PET than CT. On retrospective review, the vast majority of lesions seen with FDG PET can be seen on CT (Fig. 4C-14).

### RISING CEA LEVEL AND A NEGATIVE CT SCAN

Intraperitoneal recurrences of colorectal cancer can often not be recognized with CT. FDG PET is able to detect such cases that may present as an "isolated" rising CEA, as the signal-to-noise ratio of malignant deposits is very high with FDG PET. In the postradiotherapy setting, FDG PET appears to be more successful than MRI or CT in detecting pelvic or presacral recurrences following radiotherapy (Fig. 4C-15). A CT of the chest performed with contrast and a narrow slice thickness will detect more lesions than an FDG PET scan, but the specificity of an abnormal finding on a single CT is low. New findings on CT chest in a patient with cancer are more likely to represent metastatic disease. As outlined in the section above dealing with lung cancer, FDG PET efficiently characterizes solitary pulmonary nodules. Those pulmonary lesions appearing hypermetabolic on FDG scan, particularly in the setting of known cancer are very likely to be malignant.

**MONITORING RESPONSE TO THERAPY.** The response of primary rectal cancer to radiotherapy in 20 patients was reported by Scheipers et al.[77] They found a clear difference in the glucose metabolic rate of the primary tumor before and after radiotherapy (215 nmol/mL per minute to 77 nmol/mL per minute). At MSKCC, a group of 15 patients with T3 or N1 tumors was studied. We found that there was a good correlation between the degree of response as assessed by PET and by the pathologist and that PET outperformed

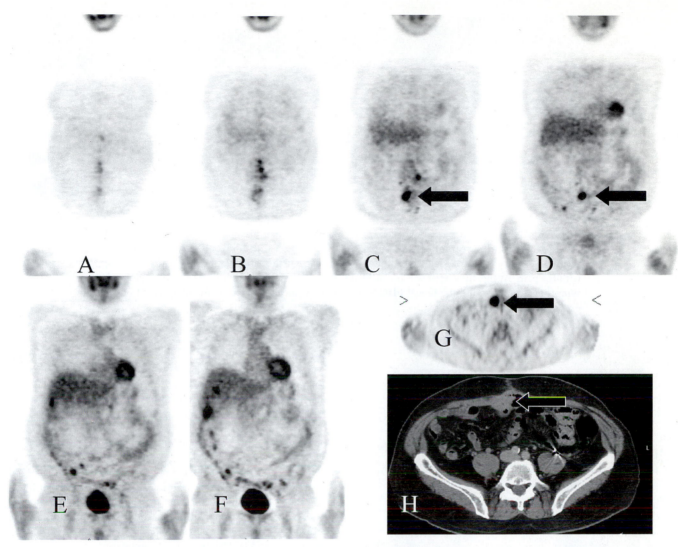

**FIGURE 4C-14.** Peritoneal recurrence of colorectal cancer. This series of coronal FDG PET images is of a man referred for possible resection of hepatic metastases. He presented with a transverse colon adenocarcinoma that was resected 7 months previously. A CT performed immediately prior to the FDG PET scan was read as no evidence of recurrent colorectal cancer outside the liver. The FDG PET was performed as a part of the post-CT workup of the patient prior to hepatic resection. The coronal images of the FDG scan (images *A* to *F*) showed a number of focal hypermetabolic deposits lining the large bowel, the inner aspect of the surgical incision, in addition to a mass (arrows) next to the anterior abdominal wall (see transaxial image *G*) that was recognized only in retrospect on CT (see image *H*). This case illustrates the difficulty radiologists have in detecting lesions from distorted anatomy after surgery, in direct contrast to the high contrast from tumor to background seen in the FDG PET scan.

CT in this regard. The best PET assessment of response was the visual assessment, which had a 60% complete concordance with the pathology response score, compared with 33% for standardized uptake value (SUV) measures and 22% for CT (Fig. 4C-16). In addition, the three patients with synchronous liver metastases were also correctly staged with FDG PET.[78]

## CANCERS OF THE KIDNEY AND URETER

Cancers of the kidney often present late, with 30% of patients having metastatic disease at diagnosis. Ultrasound is a sensitive test in the detection of renal space-occupying lesions. However, the vast majority of space-occupying lesions detected on routine ultrasound

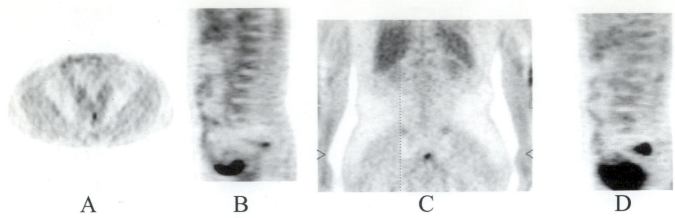

A          B          C          D

**FIGURE 4C-15.** Rectal cancer recurrence. This 62-year-old man presented with a shooting pain into the right testicle 3 years after resection of a low rectal cancer with adjuvant chemoradiotherapy. Figure *A*, *B*, and *C* are transaxial, sagittal, and coronal images of the patient at the time of presentation with his pain. At this time MRI was inconclusive. In spite of additional radiotherapy, the patient's symptoms worsened and the repeat FDG PET scan performed, *D*, revealed an enlargement of the presacral mass.

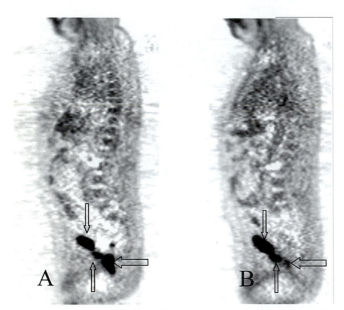

A          B

**FIGURE 4C-16.** Assessment of treatment response FDG PET. This patient with a T3 rectal cancer received induction chemoradiotherapy and was studied with FDG PET before and after therapy. The image labeled *A* is a sagittal view of the patient prior to therapy, image *B* is the posttreatment sagittal view. Notice the marked reduction in FDG in the primary tumor (horizontal arrow), urinary activity in the bladder (down arrow) and the postprostatectomy fossa (up arrow). The patient elected to not have surgery and has been followed for 2 years without endoscopic or imaging evidence of local or distant recurrence of disease. The normal marrow of the sacrum demonstrates a reduction in metabolism after radiotherapy.

are benign cysts. Thin-section CT with bolus IV contrast medium is more specific than ultrasound because it can detect enhancement and nodularity of a cystic mass as well as providing a vascular road map of the kidney. At this time no nuclear medicine test is as successful as CT in the initial workup of a renal mass.

Preoperative renal function testing and differential renal function assessment can be performed in patients prior to nephrectomy. Chromium 51–labeled ethylene diamine tetraacetic acid (EDTA) is a long-lived, glomerular-filtered renal agent that with serial blood sampling is capable of very accurate measures of glomerular filtration rate (GFR). Modifications of this approach with the shorter-lived $^{99m}$Tc DTPA have also been used and are also capable of accurate measures of GFR. Many clinics prefer to $^{99m}$Tc diethylenetriamine pentaacetic acid (DTPA) because it can be combined with gamma camera imaging to estimate differential renal function. $^{99m}$Tc mercapto acetyl glycine glycine glycine (MAG3), filtered by the glomerulus and secreted by the renal tubules, has also been used for differential renal function assessment.

Metastatic renal cell cancer is FDG avid and this should be a useful technique to apply to the monitoring of patients with metastatic cancer who are undergoing therapy. Bone scans are a sensitive modality in the detection of bone metastases. Renal metastases to bone are often osteolytic and therefore manifest themselves by cold lesions on the bone scan. Ongoing protocols involving radioimmunotherapy are under way for those patients with advanced renal cell cancer.[79]

Nuclear medicine scans are a useful method of demonstrating leaks and obstruction. $^{99m}$Tc DTPA scans are specific in demonstrating acute tubular necrosis (ATN) in the postoperative setting.

## CARCINOMA OF THE BLADDER

Most nuclear medicine tracers have some renal clearance, making it difficult to delineate tumor from luminal activity. Follow-up DTPA

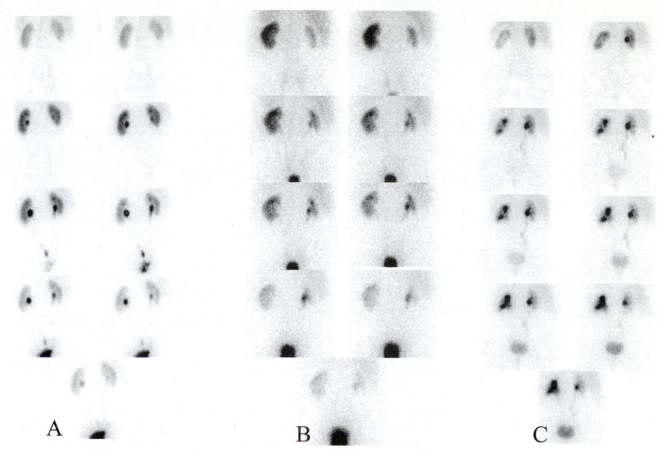

**FIGURE 4C-17.** Renal scanning. This figure comprises three panels *A, B,* and *C,* each of which is two columns wide. The images in panel *A* are of a 74-year-old male patient after cystoprostatectomy for bladder cancer who had a neobladder reconstructed. These images are 3 min apart, taken from behind the patient. The patient has mild renal parenchymal dysfunction, leading to slow uptake of the tracer, but the study reveals normal clearance of the tracer into the neobladder without evidence of leak or obstruction. The images in panel *B* are of a patient with poor renal function and a dilated left renal pelvis. The scan demonstrates a small right kidney that appears unobstructed, as well as a normally draining left kidney. The scan's findings have excluded reversible renal impairment and are consistent with a prior renal insult (probably in infancy) to the right kidney, leading to the formation of a hypoplastic right kidney. The images in panel *C* are of an obstructed left kidney: notice the continued accumulation of the tracer in a dilated right renal collecting system, the absence of a hydroureter making a pelvic-ureteric junction (PUJ) obstruction the most likely diagnosis. The right kidney is normal.

or MAG3 renal scans are useful in the detection of anastomotic stenoses leading to upper tract obstruction (Fig. 4C-17). In those patients with equivocal changes on CT following radiotherapy or with documented recurrence, FDG PET should provide useful clinical information.[80]

## CARCINOMA OF THE PENIS

The proof of principle of lymphoscintigraphic studies and sentinel node biopsy was made in a group of patients with carcinoma of the penis.[81] There has been some controversy regarding this procedure since the initial report.[82–85] The inconsistencies in the results reported may reflect a selection bias, with patients with clinically involved nodes being inappropriately subjected to the procedure. It is known that nodes completely replaced with tumor will not accumulate particulate lymphatic tracers (if the lymphatics are occluded with tumor, the tracer cannot travel along them). Penile cancer could be restudied, applying the knowledge we have learned with breast and melanoma lymphoscintigraphy (if other imaging does not reveal distant disease) to those patients with immunohistochemically positive nodes undergoing formal lymph node dissection.

## CARCINOMA OF THE PROSTATE

**STAGING.** MRI is currently the imaging modality of choice to determine the presence of capsular invasion. Interpretation of these images is difficult, and an endorectal coil is required, making this modality a tool of specialized clinics. CT and MRI both rely on the size of regional nodes to determine the presence or absence of malignant involvement. Scintigraphic approaches to the preoperative detection of involved nodes include monoclonal antibodies, including [111]In-capromab pendetide and a radiolabeled murine monoclonal antibody CYT-356, directed against prostatic-specific membrane antigen (Prostascint). Early studies with this agent are promising, appearing to be superior to CT, MRI, and ultrasound (US) in a high-risk patient group in both primary and extraprostatic disease. Capromab has accuracy rates of 92% and 81% versus a combined accuracy rate for CT, MRI, and US of 51% and 48%, respectively.[86] One of the entry criteria to the study was patients with equivocal CT findings, leading perhaps to some ascertainment bias. As the capromab technique becomes more refined, specifically in regard to imaging delayed to 120 hr after injection, results should improve further.[87] The longer half-life of indium should allow gamma probe–guided surgery.

**BONE SCANNING.** Bone scans are a very sensitive, inexpensive method of detecting skeletal metastases. The methodology of detection relies on osteoblastic activity leading to a "hot" lesion or, less commonly in prostate cancer, osteolytic lesions leading to a "cold" lesion. Not all hot lesions on a bone scan are metastatic because the mechanism of localization is not cancer specific. Bone scans can be reported qualitatively or semiquantitatively. One such semiquantitative measure, the bone scan index (BSI), has demonstrated that there is a gompertzian growth of prostate cancer.[88] The bone scan, however, is slow to respond to therapy, with responding lesions often becoming more metabolically active before resolving, leading to the so-called flare phenomenon initially described in breast cancer by Rossleigh et al.[89] and later in prostate cancer.[90] Those patients with progressive prostate cancer who have extensive skeletal metastases are difficult to assess with serial bone scans because of the gompertzian nature of the cancer's growth. The difficulties in assessing prostate cancer with the bone scan have led to the development of newer imaging techniques in nuclear medicine.

**PET IMAGING OF PROSTATE CANCER.** There have been a number of radiopharmaceutical approaches to the PET imaging of prostate cancer in animals including, [11]C choline, [18]F FDG, [18]F fluoropropyl putrescine and, more recently, [18]F 5α-dihydrotestosterone. The referring clinician needs to be aware of the patterns of uptake of FDG in prostate cancer. The initial unselected prostate cancer series reported by the MSKCC group demonstrated that not all lesions seen on bone scan were FDG avid. This was not altogether unexpected because bone scans are imaging the response of bone to the presence of tumor, rather than the cellular mass of the tumor itself. In many of the lesions, the tumor was quiescent and not FDG avid because of partially successful therapy (it is known that lytic lesions in breast cancer are more likely to be FDG avid than osteoblastic lesions[91]). In a later series of patients with hormonally refractory progressive prostate cancer we have found that FDG PET was successful in imaging a far greater number of metastatic deposits. In addition, we found that there is a reduction in FDG uptake that correlates with other measures of response both in animal[92] and in human studies.[93] The key to prostate imaging with FDG PET appears, therefore, to be patient selection, with those patients with a high Gleason score more likely to be successfully imaged.[94] Those patients with progressive hormonally refractive prostate cancer are also much more likely to be successfully imaged. It is therefore probable that poor patient selection was the underlying reason for the discouraging initial reports from a number of groups, including our own.[95–97] Malignant prostatic tissue in pelvic lymph nodes has been detected with FDG PET,[98] although these initial findings need to be confirmed in a larger series that compares FDG to standard imaging modalities.

[11]C choline research is closely associated with magnetic resonance spectroscopy research that has demonstrated increased choline content in prostatic malignancy. In a small series, [11]C choline uptake was greater than that seen with FDG,[99] suggesting that this agent may be a sensitive method of disease detection. If the degree of [11]C choline uptake correlates with the grade of malignancy, then it may be a useful agent for guiding patient management.

**PALLIATIVE NUCLEAR MEDICINE THERAPIES IN PROSTATE CANCER.** The major method of radiation-induced cell injury and death is due to double-strand DNA breaks that lead to mitotic cell death. Apoptotic cell death may be induced by other methods. The most radiosensitive part of the cell cycle is mitosis closely followed by G2M. The amount of damage caused by radiation in tissue is related to the linear energy transfer (LET) factor that describes the amount of energy lost by the incident energetic particle over the particle's path length. The higher the LET, the greater the amount of energy deposited and the more tissue damage done. β particles, such as those emitted by [32]P and [89]Sr, are considered to be relatively high LET particles.

One of the earliest reports of palliative administrations of unsealed radionuclides for bone metastases dates back to the 1940s when Pecher[100] reported on the use of strontium in the treatment of bone metastases. The recognition that both [89]Sr and [32]P lead to myelosupression led to a waning of interest in this approach to bone pain palliation. There has been a recent resurgence in interest in this type of therapy because it is very effective at reducing the pain of bone metastases with a duration of response of up to 3 months. There is, however, no evidence of prolongation of survival with radionuclide therapy of bone metastases, even though over 80% of patients will respond to the therapy.[101] Multiple doses of 148 MBq (4 mCi) of [89]Sr may be given to patients with progressive bone metastases. Repeat doses should not be given unless the patient's marrow has recovered. Marrow toxicity is common but usually spontaneously reverses, with only one reported death related to marrow toxicity. A flare reaction is seen in about 10% of patients.

*MECHANISM OF ACTION.* [89]Sr uptake is greatest in lesions that have become osteoblastic because the mechanism of uptake is related to calcium deposition. The close correlation between [89]Sr and [99m]Tc MDP uptake[102] has led to the use of MDP bone scans to estimate the likely efficacy of [89]Sr therapy.[103] [32]P is also incorporated into osteoblastic areas due to the incorporation of phosphate into the bone matrix. In addition, osteolytic bone lesions can be treated with $^{32}$P[104] because cancer cells exhibit accelerated phosphorus metabolism.[105] The use of $^{32}$P for palliation of breast cancer skeletal metastases will be dealt with in the section on breast cancer (below). Firusian and Schmidt.[106] reported the use of $^{89}$Sr in the treatment of prostate cancer. $^{89}$Sr therapy takes longer to have a therapeutic effect but is as effective as external beam radiotherapy in terms of the duration of control of painful bony metastases.[107] When used together with external beam, $^{89}$Sr potentiates the efficacy of external beam radiotherapy for the treatment of painful osseous metastases, increasing the time to retreatment and reducing the number of new painful sites of disease.[108,109]

Newer agents include rhenium 186 hydroxyethylidene diphosphate (HEDP), a radionuclide that combines the properties of a bisphosphonate[110] with the therapeutic efficacy of a β emitter. Response rates of around 80% have also been reported with this agent.[111] On-site generators of rhenium 188 are now available, making the radionuclide much less expensive, and $^{188}$Re HEDP appears to be as efficacious as $^{186}$Re HEDP with response rates of 80% reported.[112] Samarium 153 ethylene diamine tetramethylene phosphonate (EDTMP) has also been studied and has similar efficacy, toxicities, and duration of response.[113,114] Tin 117m DTPA has also been tested for the treatment of bone metastases, and response rates are similar to other agents.[115]

## CANCER OF THE TESTIS

Germ cell tumors of the testis have proved to be an elusive target for nuclear medicine imaging, particularly in the postchemotherapy setting. Gallium 67 citrate has been studied, and the study was able to determine response rates, but was unable to detect the difference between major response and complete response in seminoma patients treated with chemotherapy.[116] The role of PET in the posttreatment setting has also been studied. FDG PET, like gallium, is good at demonstrating a response, but when performed in wholebody scanning mode, is unable to detect microscopic amounts of residual tumor that may remain after chemotherapy. Fossa et al.[117] reported a group of 78 patients with nonseminomatous germ cell cancer who were left with masses smaller than 2 cm in diameter following chemotherapy. Of these 78, 51 were found to have necrosis, 22 were found to have mature teratoma, and 5 had residual germ cell tumor (2 of 5 with elevated serum marker level). In those patients with a residual mass post-chemotherapy, if the FDG uptake is high, then this suggests there is residual germ cell carcinoma present. If the FDG uptake is low, then PET cannot differentiate between necrosis and teratoma.[118] In a retrospective report of 104 patients with advanced seminoma after chemotherapy, the MSKCC group found that a residual mass of greater than 3 cm was more likely to contain viable tumor than a mass less than 3 cm (27% versus 3%).[119,120] If the approach to the patient with residual masses following chemotherapy is the same as recommended at MSKCC, where any mass remaining after chemotherapy is resected if it is greater than 3 cm in diameter, then noninvasive imaging is unlikely to affect clinical management. Where the CT of the lesion is poorly defined (a lack of fat planes), there was a greater risk of an R1 resection. Currently there is a lack of data to support the routine use of FDG PET in the evaluation of masses of greater than 3 cm in patients with seminoma. If a screening CT performed to investigate rising markers were negative, and a surgical procedure was anticipated, this would be an indication for FDG PET scanning.

## VULVAL AND VAGINAL NEOPLASMS

The major role of nuclear medicine in these cancers is to identify sentinel lymph nodes in a similar manner to that of breast cancer.[121] Renal studies can be performed to exclude obstruction, either related to the disease itself or complications of therapy. Assessment of the bony pelvis can be adequately accomplished with CT. There has been little experience with FDG PET in vulval and vaginal cancers.

## CANCER OF THE CERVIX, ENDOMETRIUM, AND UTERINE SARCOMAS

Advanced disease in all of these tumor types is FDG avid, and where there is a clinical risk of disease beyond what is surgically resectable, an FDG PET scan would be a reasonable test to rule out extensive disease (Fig. 4C-18). Rose et al.[122] in a study of 32 patients with stage IIB, IIIB, and IVA cervical cancer concluded that FDG PET accurately predicts both the presence and absence of pelvic and paraaortic nodal metastatic disease. The major advantage of FDG will be its ability to detect disease in normal-sized lymph nodes, activity within the ureters not withstanding.[123] Response assessment with FDG PET is also possible. As FDG PET becomes more widely available, the avidity of these tumors for thallium and sestamibi will be clinically less important.

## GESTATIONAL TROPHOBLASTIC DISEASE

The diagnosis of gestational trophoblastic disease remains the province of ultrasound. MRI has proved useful in the assessment of depth of involvement in uterine tumors, and is considered the gold standard in the detection of brain metastases. Radiolabeling of anti-β HCG has been performed,[124] but has not reached widespread clinical application. Gestational trophoblastic disease is FDG avid.

## CANCER OF THE OVARY

This is an interesting tumor because nuclear medicine can play a role in staging as well as a direct role in therapy with radiolabeled antibodies. The lack of FDG uptake in low-grade ovarian cancers, as well as mucinous cystadenocarcinoma, as well as the avidity for FDG of inflammatory conditions of the adnexa[125–127] makes FDG PET unreliable as a single test in the assessment of adnexal masses. Hubner[128] has reported that metastatic ovarian carcinoma is FDG avid. Standard chemotherapy regimens achieve a 75% to 80% complete clinical response after an initial optimal surgical cytoreduction. However, only 50% of these patients are visually free of disease at second-look surgery. Of those patients considered free of disease after second-look surgery, a further 50% relapse.[129] Therefore, 60% to 70% of patients with ovarian carcinoma will have recurrence after a

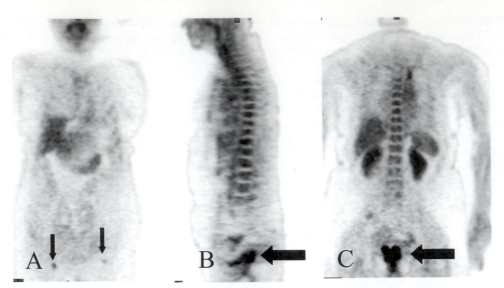

**FIGURE 4C-18.** Radiotherapy and FDG PET. There is a prolonged alteration in normal tissue metabolism of $^{18}$F FDG in response to radiotherapy. This is a case of recurrent cervical cancer imaged with FDG PET. Image *A,* an anterior coronal image of the patient demonstrates increased uptake of FDG in inguinal lymph nodes (down arrows). Image *B,* a sagittal image, reveals increased uptake in the recurrent tumor (arrow), as well as reduced activity in the normal bone marrow of the sacrum, due to the prior radiotherapy (compare with Fig. 4C-28 *J* ). Image *C,* a posterior coronal slice, reveals increased activity in the recurrent pelvic tumor. This patient has increased uptake of FDG in the remainder of her bone marrow due to prior chemotherapy.

course of chemotherapy. A careful study aimed at demonstrating a survival advantage of second-look laparotomy failed to do so.[130] It appears that patients with small-volume or microscopic disease may have a favorable prognosis compared to those patients with macroscopic disease.[131,132] Hubner's work indicates that there may be a role for FDG PET–guided exploratory laparotomy on laparoscopy to search for resectable recurrent ovarian carcinoma. Reasonable hypotheses to test at this point in time are

1. Is there a particular pattern of FDG uptake that reliably predicts surgically unresectable recurrence?
2. Does FDG-avid disease suggest the need for a debulking laparotomy?
3. Is there an additive benefit of a second-look laparotomy in the face of FDG-avid disease?

Additional research efforts with new PET tracers should attempt to increase our ability to detect microscopic deposits of disease in the hope of identifying those 25% of patients who are cured with their initial surgery and chemotherapy.

## RADIOLABELED ANTIBODIES

The high rate of local failure following chemotherapy has led to the exploration of a number of local therapies, including intraperitoneal chemotherapy and intraperitoneal radioimmunotherapy. The ini-

tial crop of radiolabeled antibodies were all murine-based, and a significant problem soon encountered was the recognition of the development of human antimouse antibodies (HAMA). If HAMA develops, a second dose of the radiolabeled antibody is rendered less effective because the murine antibody is rapidly cleared from the body. The dose-limiting organ for yttrium 90 intraperitoneal radioimmunotherapy is the bone marrow, and attempts at reducing toxicity to the marrow with EDTA have shown some promise.[133] Most initial trials also used $^{131}$I as the therapeutic isotope, and have shown some partial responses.[134] It was also found that the size of the residual mass predicted the response. The initial experience with radiolabeled antibodies lead to the substitution of $^{90}$Y for the $^{131}$I with improved results in 5-year survival demonstrated with intraperitoneal radioimmunotherapy following chemotherapy (80%) versus chemotherapy alone (80% vs. 55%, $p = 0.0035$).[135] Stratifying patients by FDG PET positivity or negativity (minimal residual disease) prior to radioimmunotherapy may lead to greater success with radioimmunotherapy.

## BREAST CANCER

Nuclear medicine has a role to play in most aspects of the care of breast cancer patients. $^{99m}$Tc sestamibi is selectively incorporated into cancer cells, a property it shares with $^{201}$Th and $^{99m}$Tc tetrofosmin. The observation that breast cancers accumulate radiotracers has led many to investigate the use of sestamibi in the workup

**TABLE 4C-4.** DEPENDENCE OF SENSITIVITY AND SPECIFICITY OF SCINTIMAMMOGRAPHY ON TUMOR SIZE AND PALPABILITY

| TOTAL NO. OF PATIENTS | NO. OF CANCERS | SENSITIVITY <1 CM OR IMPALPABLE | SPECIFICITY <1 CM OR IMPALPABLE | SENSITIVITY >1 CM OR PALPABLE | SPECIFICITY <1 CM OR PALPABLE | REFERENCE |
|---|---|---|---|---|---|---|
| 77 | | 35% | 100% | 97% | 84% | 289 |
| 246 | | | | | | 137 |
| 140 | | 54% | 93% | 95% | 75% | 290 |
| 388 | 247 | 75% | 81% | 94% | 61% | 291 |
| 70 | | | | 56% | 87% | 292 |
| | | | | 63% | 87% | 293 |
| 85 | | 97% | 90% | 50% | 90% | 294 |
| 53 | | 96.9% | | 50% | | 295 |
| 77 | | | | | | 296 |
| 420 | 355 | 98% | 89% | 62% | 91% | 136 |
| 56 | | 91% | 62% | 60% | 75% | 297 |

of women with suspected breast cancer. It appears that prone sestamibi imaging is very successful in those women with palpable breast masses and breast cancers over 1 cm in diameter. The sensitivity of scintimammography is consistently significantly lower for lesions that are either classified as impalpable or under 1 cm in size (Table 4C-4). These smaller studies have been confirmed in two large cooperative studies conducted in Europe.[136,137] Scopinaro et al.[136] reported on a group of 420 patients in whom there were 355 cancers. In those patients with cancers less than 1 cm in size, the sensitivity of the test was 44%, and for those patients with tumors less than 0.5 cm, the sensitivity dropped to 26%. They also found that for larger tumors situated close to the chest wall that sensitivity was less than expected, possibly due to scatter from the underlying muscle and motion artifacts. Palmedo et al[137] reported on the use of sestamibi scintimammography in 246 patients in whom there were 253 lesions, of which 165 were later proven malignant. Taking the patient's history and performing palpation led to an improvement in sensitivity, as illustrated by those 38 women with impalpable tumors where the sensitivity of blind scintimammogram reads was only 29%, whereas for in-house (unblinded) reads the sensitivity was 69%. False-positive results in scintimammography do occur and are primarily due to benign proliferative breast conditions such as fibrocystic disease and hypercellular fibroadenoma.[138] Small reductions in sensitivity and specificity can have a major impact on the cost effectiveness of a new imaging modality. The cost effectiveness of scintimammographic screening has been modeled. It has been found to be a very expensive method of screening and not cost-effective unless the expected incidence of cancer in the population is greater than 3%.[139] Screening scintimammography would therefore seem unsuitable for patients with palpable nodules, where the incidence of false negatives is unacceptably high (9% in the European study[137]), but it would be suited to those patients with mammographically unassessable (dense, scarred) breasts and a strong pretest likelihood of cancer (*BRCA1* or *BRCA2*-positive patients or patients with a strong family history).

$^{99m}$Tc sestamibi is a lipophilic molecule that is positively charged and has been found to be concentrated into the mitochondria of the cell.[140] It was recognized that sestamibi was not fixed in cancer cells, and interestingly, that the multidrug resistance P-glycoprotein complex expression correlated with the efflux of rates of sestamibi, suggesting that sestamibi was a substrate for that complex.[141] This observation has led to the as yet unproven hypothesis that steady-state levels of sestamibi in tumors may be a noninvasive method of assessing the expression of P-glycoprotein, although sestamibi uptake appears to be markedly reduced by chemotherapy in a nonspecific manner.[142] A relationship between the degree of sestamibi uptake and markers of aggressiveness of the tumors has been described.[143,144] However, these papers have not used a multivariate analysis to control for size and, therefore, determine that sestamibi uptake is an independent prognostic factor.

LYMPHOSCINTIGRAPHY AND SENTINEL NODE DETECTION. The concept of using radiopharmaceuticals to outline the lymphatic drainage of tumors is not a new one. The initial lymphoscintigraphic hypothesis provides a salutary lesson to those practicing lymphoscintigraphy and sentinel node biopsy today. The original approach was designed to assist planning for internal mammary lymph node resection as part of the "extended radial" mastectomy as advocated by Urban.[145] The technique involved an injection of the tracer into the rectus abdominis fascia, and a positive result was defined by the absence of uptake in one of the nodes of the internal mammary nodal chain. The hypothesis was that a node whose afferent or efferent lymphatics are occluded by tumor will not appear as a hot spot on either a lymphoscintigraphic image or be detectable with a gamma probe. This proved correct. Nevertheless, the current approach of using a radioactive particulate to help define which lymph nodes to remove for staging purposes is revolutionizing the care of the increasing numbers of women who present with early T-stage breast cancer in whom complete axillary lymphadenectomy is likely to be unnecessarily aggressive (Figs. 4C-19 and 4C-20).

The pathophysiologic hypothesis underlying sentinel node biopsy is that tumor cells will be passively carried along by the flow of lymph that surrounds a tumor. The lymph node that drains the most lymph from the area around a tumor will therefore be the node that most likely will contain tumor cells within it, given the caveat above. The addition of immunohistochemical analysis of sentinel

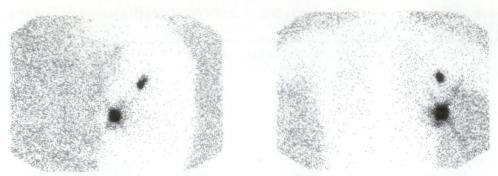

**FIGURE 4C-19.** Breast lymphoscintigraphy. This patient with a left breast cancer was referred for preoperative lymphatic mapping. Following the intradermal injection of 3.7 mBq of unfiltered $^{99m}$Tc sulfur colloid, a cobalt 57 transmission source was placed behind the patient to give the patient silhouette, and an anterior and lateral static acquisition was made. Note the lower area of activity, the injection site in the breast, with what appears to be a single node in the axilla on the anterior view. However, a second node is seen on the lateral projection; two hot nodes were found at surgery.

nodes has led to an improvement in the sensitivity of the sentinel node biopsy procedure in the detection of axillary nodal metastases.

There are many variations on the theme of lymphoscintigraphy, including 1-day[146] versus 2-day[147] protocols, blue dye[148] versus isotope alone versus combination blue dye and isotope,[149] intradermal[150] versus intramammary injection,[151] sulfur colloid[146] versus rhenium sulfur colloid[152] versus antimony colloid,[153] filtered[149] versus unfiltered sulfur colloid[154] and gamma probe only versus lymphoscintigraphy and gamma probe in combination. Each of these variations has its proponent. However, the success rate in terms of the detection of a hot sentinel node at operation of most

techniques is remarkably similar and is almost universally of the order of 94%. These techniques have such similar success rates because the lymphatic drainage of the breast appears functionally to be quite simple. The reason that intradermal administration of the tracer has been as successful as intramammary peritumoral injection of tracer is that most lymphatic channels from the breast lead to the axilla[155] and to the same sentinel nodes as the overlying skin in the majority of patients. It appears that the peritumoral lymphatic channels are the same as those draining the overlying skin, perhaps due to the embryologic derivation of the breast. SLN biopsy has a high success rate in the detection of lymph node metastases to the

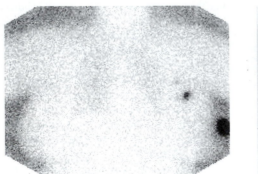

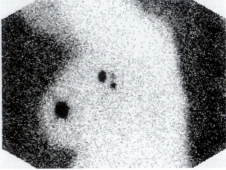

**FIGURE 4C-20.** Breast lymphoscintigraphy. This patient with a 1.6-cm left breast cancer was referred for lymphatic mapping. Following the intradermal injection of 3.7 mBq of unfiltered $^{99m}$Tc sulfur colloid, a cobalt 57 transmission source was placed behind the patient to give the patient silhouette, and an anterior and lateral static acquisition was made. Note the injection site in the lower lateral quadrant of the left breast, with three sentinel nodes demonstrated. At surgery four sentinel nodes were resected, one of which contained a 2-mm focus of metastatic cancer. Subsequent axillary resection removed an additional 15 lymph nodes, all of which contained no tumor. The case elegantly illustrates the principle of lymphatic mapping, where the images in and of themselves do not predict malignant involvement (compare with Fig. 4C-19), but serve as an accurate guide to the surgeon, who can resect the nodes predicted to be most likely to contain metastatic disease.

axilla because the pathologist is presented with only 1 to 3 nodes rather than 20 nodes harvested from an axillary dissection. The pathologist is able to section the lymph nodes more times, and to perform a more detailed examination, including immunohisto-chemistry. If the sentinel node procedure misses the node draining the most lymph from the tumor, but rather demonstrates the node accepting the second- or third-highest amount of lymph, immuno-histochemical analysis may still be positive because even if only a single cancer cell is present, it will be detected.

The Ludwig group[156] has shown that the presence of micrometa-static deposits in lymph nodes is an adverse prognostic factor. At MSKCC we have found that the combination of blue dye and in-tradermal injection of tracer is associated with the highest success rates of node detection. In addition, we have found that the in-tradermal technique is associated with a higher success rate than the intramammary approach with rapid transit to the node and is, therefore, suitable for a 1-day protocol.[157] At our hospital, in order to accommodate the early commencement of surgery, the first two or three operative patients of the morning are injected the day prior to surgery, thus mimicking the approach of the Milan oncology group. We experimented with filtering the colloidal preparation through a 0.22-$\mu$m filter. However, in spite of leading to an increase in suc-cess with the lymphoscintigram, there was a lower surgical success rate.[154] This was largely due to the presence of a diffusely hot axilla, presumably because of the ability of small colloidal particles to pass through the sentinel node and onto secondary draining nodes. If a filtered preparation is to be used, it is probably better to delay surgery to the next day, thereby allowing the smallest colloidal particles to wash out of the secondary nodes.

Positive pathology of the internal mammary node is an adverse prognostic sign. Internal mammary nodal dissection is by no means universal. Each clinic has to determine its approach to the internal mammary nodes. Demonstration of sentinel nodes in the internal mammary chain is much less common with the intradermal tech-nique than the intramammary technique. If the surgeon and patient are prepared to undertake internal mammary nodal dissection, and the primary tumor is medially situated, then an intramammary in-jection may be more likely to demonstrate a positive internal mam-mary node.

It should be noted that some researchers have expressed concerns regarding the widespread introduction of the sentinel node proce-dure into clinical practice, pointing out that randomized trials have not been performed.[158] However, there is an enormous weight of evidence supporting the sentinel node procedure, and randomized trials comparing sentinel node biopsy plus chemotherapy to com-pletion axillary lymphadenectomy plus chemotherapy are currently under way.

Bone scans have long been an essential part of the follow-up of patients with breast cancer. Bone scans are easily performed and readily available. They have the advantage of being very sensitive but the disadvantage of being relatively nonspecific. Certain sites have higher probability of being involved with disease. For instance, a solitary abnormal site in the sternum is likely to be due to a metas-tasis.

The incidence of abnormal bone scans in patients with low T-stage tumors is so low as to make routine preoperative bone scanning not cost effective.[159] The incidence of abnormalities rises up to 16%

in T3,[160] with higher numbers expected in T4 patients and, therefore, warranted to document the extent of disease. In terms of follow-up of patients treated with chemotherapy, bone scans have also been found to be useful, with increasing probability of metastases being present as the number of new lesions increases from a baseline scan.[161] Clin-icians need to be aware of the flare phenomenon that describes a transient worsening of the appearance of a bone scan related to the commencement of a successful course of chemotherapy.[90]

Gated cardiac blood pool scans (GBPS), also known as radionu-cleotide ventriculograms (RNVG) and multigated radionuclide angiograms (MUGA), have been used to monitor left ventricu-lar function in patients undergoing cardiotoxic chemotherapy. The GBPS is a reliable measure of left ventricular function because it di-rectly measures the volume of the ventricle rather than subjective bi-dimensional measures that are reported by echocardiography. The reproducibility of left ventricular ejection fractions (LVEF) mea-sured by RNVG has led to the ability to detect drops in left ventricular function before they become symptomatic, with increased sensitiv-ity shown by the exercise RNVG technique.[162,163] The risk of LVEF dysfunction increases in an almost linear fashion once a cumulative dose of 550 mg/m$^2$ of doxorubicin is reached.[164] The RNVG remains the accepted standard for assessment of LVEF for the purposes of new drug evaluation.

A variety of PET tracers have been investigated in breast cancer research, including a number of fluorinated estrogens (predomi-nantly the group led by Welsh and Katzenellenbogen)[165] as well as FDG. Minn et al.,[166] using a specially collimated gamma cam-era, demonstrated FDG uptake in metastatic breast cancers and that increasing FDG uptake in the face of chemotherapy was an adverse prognostic sign. This has been confirmed using dedicated PET scanners.[167] A number of authors have investigated the use of FDG to image primary breast cancer[167,168] and sensitivity rates are quite high.[169] Avril et al.[169,170] have cautioned that FDG PET should not be used to stage the axilla, because the sensitivity of FDG PET falls rapidly as lesion sizes fall below 1 cm in diameter.[169,170] When compared to bone scans, FDG PET may not detect as many long-standing metastases because it is recognized that lytic metastases are more metabolically active than sclerotic lesions.[166] This mirrors our experience in prostate cancer.

FDG PET has a significant role to play in the treatment of pa-tients with breast cancer, because it appears to be able to predict those patients who will respond to chemotherapy, perhaps as early as 8 days after the commencement of chemotherapy treatment, as initially suggested by Wahl et al.[171] These initial observations have been consistently confirmed by other groups.[172–176] Caution may need to be applied immediately after commencement of hormonal therapy because of the possible occurrence of a metabolic "flare" with tamoxifen therapy.[177] By rapidly assessing the response to therapy, it may be possible to accelerate a patient through the chemotherapeu-tic regimes, instituting experimental therapies earlier in a patient's course while their performance status remains good. Before a PET-based approach to chemotherapy becomes widely accepted, much larger trials need to be performed than the ones reported at this time. Fluorinated estrogens have been used successfully to image the es-trogen receptors on breast cancers, with close correlation between the in vivo image data and subsequent estrogen receptor assays.[178] It appears that the degree of uptake of estrogen-based tracers should predict responses to hormonally based therapies, and that a fall in these tracers' uptake will be correlated with response, as was shown in an initial small series by Dehdashti et al.[177]

**PALLIATIVE THERAPIES WITH RADIONUCLIDES IN BREAST CANCER TREATMENT.** Response rates of the order of 80% have been reported following the use of [89]Sr as a palliative therapy in bone pain from metastases in patients with breast cancer. [89]Sr treatment may take 7 to 10 days to provide relief. In 10% of patients, there may be a flare response, and response duration is of the order of 12 to 17 weeks (see the section on palliative therapies with radionuclides in prostate cancer above). [32]P has been used to help palliate bone metastases in patients with breast cancer. This approach was initially tried in the 1940s and 1950s with 10 responses reported by Friedell et al.[104] in a group of 12 women with breast cancer. In a series of studies performed between 1950 and 1986 reviewed by Silberstein et al.,[179] a consistent response rate of the order of 80% was seen in over 800 patients treated with a variety of regimens, most of which included androgens as [32]P response modulators. A preliminary report of a multicenter trial found no difference in the response rates of patients treated with [32]P and [89]Sr.[180] The final results of this trial in over 400 patients conducted by the International Atomic Energy Agency under the aegis of Dr. Ajit Padhy have not yet been published. The increased efficacy seen with the addition of androgens may be due to the increased incorporation of [32]P into bone induced by androgens. McEwan[181] has stressed the need for carefully designed trials to reevaluate the efficacy of [32]P in patients with bone metastases.

## SOFT TISSUE SARCOMAS

Conventional imaging modalities such as CT and MRI are the cornerstone of the initial assessment of soft tissue sarcomas. In terms of local staging, nuclear medicine does not have sufficient soft tissue resolution to compete with these modalities. Osseous involvement has been assessed with [18]F, a bone tracer, as well as [99m]Tc MDP. Sarcomas have been successfully imaged with gallium 67,[182] thallium 201,[183] [99m]Tc pryophosphate,[184] [99m]Tc sestamibi,[185] [111]In octreotide,[186] [123]I-labeled iodophenyl-9-methyl pentadecanoic acid ([123]I-BMIPP) and a tracer of fatty acid metabolism has also been used to image liposarcomas.[187] Nuclear medicine procedures can be used to grade tumors, with early reports of grades of FDG uptake being related to histologic grade,[188] subsequently confirmed.[189] There is a low negative predictive value of FDG PET in low-grade sarcomas.

**ASSESSMENT OF THERAPY RESPONSE.** Thallium scans performed in the middle of a course of chemotherapy have been shown to be predictive of final outcome of treatment.[190] FDG PET appears to be capable at assessing response, but may underestimate the degree of response due to the presence of treatment-related inflammation and capsule formation, both of which are associated with persistent FDG uptake.[191,192] Further investigation of FDG uptake patterns in relation to chemotherapy is warranted because there may be a time point after chemotherapy that most accurately predicts the ultimate response to therapy. An interesting use of nuclear medicine imaging was described by Garcia et al.,[185] who found that tumors that were negative on [99m]Tc sestamibi imaging but positive on FDG imaging were high-grade sarcomas and did not respond to chemotherapy, perhaps due to the expression of *MDR* gene by the tumor. (*MDR* is associated with rapid washout of sestamibi and therefore these lesions may be negative on sestamibi imaging.[141] This is an elegant demonstration of the potential of noninvasively characterizing a tumor and determining the correct therapeutic approach.

Isolated limb perfusion has been discussed in the section above that dealt with melanoma. Similarly, the section on breast cancer dealt with the assessment of anthracycline chemotherapy–associated cardiotoxicity with GBPS.

## BONE SARCOMAS

The initial reports of nuclear medicine imaging of bone sarcomas involved the use of the positron emitter [18]F as a fluoride ion and [85]Sr, a gamma-emitting radioisotope of strontium.[193–195] The labeling of diphosphonates with [99m]Tc rapidly supplanted these techniques. Metastatic osteosarcoma calcifies, making a [99m]Tc MDP bone scan an efficient, inexpensive way of characterizing lesions in the lung. The prolonged time course of resolution of changes in MDP uptake after therapy has led to the abandonment of this technique as an early measure of response (see Figs. 4C-1 and 4C-3; Fig. 4C-21). Alternate tracers have been assessed as measures of response and appear to correlate well with pathologic measures of response. Thallium 201 is a potassium analogue whose uptake and retention in cells is dependent on the integrity of the Na, K-ATPase pump. It is, therefore, only taken up into viable cells, and slowly diffuses out of cells. In part, the degree of uptake is proportional to perfusion of the tissue, a finding that has led to the widespread application of the tracer as a marker of myocardial perfusion and viability. Thallium was directly compared to both gallium and [99m]Tc MDP and was found to be superior to both tracers in terms of assessment of therapy response.[196] [99m]Tc sestamibi uptake is related to perfusion, and in the myocardium the tracer does not diffuse out of cells, making it an ideal tracer for myocardial imaging. It was soon recognized that sestamibi "washed out" of tumors, and it was subsequently recognized that this phenomenon was strongly associated with overexpression of the *MDR* receptor gene.[141] The implications of this are that sestamibi is a suitable tracer prior to treatment and should be thoroughly investigated to assess correlation between sestamibi washout kinetics and responsiveness to chemotherapy. Sestamibi is an inappropriate tracer to assess response, because a reduction in uptake may be due to cell death or induction of MDR.

[18]F as fluoride was the initial radionuclide used in nuclear medicine to image bone. It's use may undergo a resurgence because current detector systems, particularly the circular detector NaI systems, which offer the potential of whole-body tomographic imaging in a similar time to a standard whole-body bone scan. The increased certainty of spatial localization of areas of increased uptake with tomographic imaging should increase the specificity of bone scan reports in patients with only a few bone lesions, because planar bone scans are often incapable of distinguishing between joint-based (arthritis) and marrow or cortical lesions (malignant). FDG imaging has the potential to accurately predict response because it is imaging the

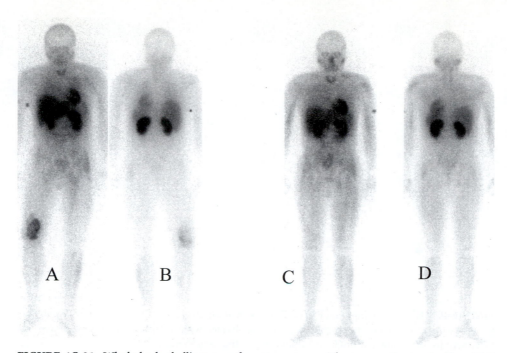

**FIGURE 4C-21.** Whole-body thallium scan for osteosarcoma. The same patient as in Figs. 4C-2 and 4C-3 was also studied with thallium 201. The images are anterior and posterior whole-body images performed before (*A* and *B*) and after (*C* and *D*) chemotherapy, respectively. Thallium 201 is a potassium analogue that is taken up in tumor due to overactivity of the Na, K-ATPase pump. The uptake in the myocardium is normal, as is the uptake in kidney, liver, spleen, and thyroid. This patient was injected through a Broviac IV line, and this explains the small focus of activity seen near the right arm in images *A* and *B* and the left arm in images *C* and *D*. The tumor is clearly demonstrated in the right knee on the pretreatment images, with a reduction in uptake on the posttreatment images. The resected femur was reported as totally necrotic. This case illustrates the utility of thallium in predicting response to therapy and the insensitivity of an early bone scan (see Fig. 4C-3) to detect postchemotherapy response.

metabolic activity of the tumor, as does thallium, with improved spatial resolution. No large trial has yet been published that compares thallium and FDG uptake in terms of response assessment. In an initial series comparing FDG and sestamibi, a potential problem with PET imaging was noted, whereby tissue healing related to treatment (Fig. 4C-22) was associated with residual FDG uptake.[191] Statistical analysis can be used to assess and determine the correct threshold of change in FDG uptake that constitutes a reproducible, clinically relevant response parameter.

## ENDOCRINE NEOPLASMS

Thyroid cancer diagnosis, therapy, and follow-up have been dealt with in the section on head and neck cancers above. Neuroendocrine tumors are thought to derive from cells originating in the neural crest. Many of these tumors express surface receptors for somatostatin; others of adrenergic lineage exhibit increased catecholamine metabolism. These characteristics have led to the development of tracers that utilize these biochemical and molecular signatures to image tumors. The two radionuclides that dominate in this area are indium 111 octreotide, marketed as Octreoscan, which targets somatostatin receptors, and metaiodobenzylguanidine (MIBG) (labeled with both [131]I and [123]I), which images "adrenergic" tumors. Somatostatin receptor scintigraphy has been discussed in the paragraphs dealing with endocrine pancreatic cancers (above). MIBG, a guanethidine derivative structurally analogous to noradrenaline, is a metabolically stable molecule in vivo. Normal MIBG uptake is seen in the heart, salivary glands, spleen, and lacrimal glands. The small amount of free iodide present is cleared under the cover of stable iodide that blocks uptake of MIBG into the thyroid. The degree of uptake in any tissue on MIBG imaging is a balance of type 1 uptake[197] into neuroendocrine tissues (often followed by incorporation into membrane bound storage granules) and depolarization-mediated efflux from the storage granules. Due to favorable dosimetry, higher doses of [123]I MIBG can be administered and normal adrenals can be seen with this radionuclide. The tracer is predominantly cleared by the kidneys with minimal excretion in the feces. Therefore, the kidneys, bladder, and bowel can be visualized on images acquired close to the time of administration. For this reason, the typical MIBG

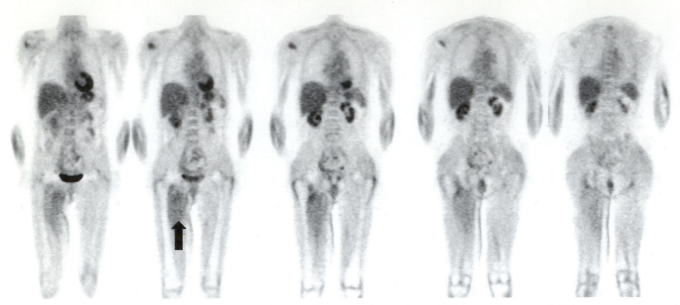

**FIGURE 4C-22.** Radiotherapy and FDG PET. A series of coronal FDG PET images is presented. This patient, with a sarcoma of the thigh, was previously treated with radiotherapy. Note the increased FDG activity in the medial thigh corresponding to the radiotherapy field (arrow). Note also the increased physiologic uptake of the tracer seen in the right latissimus dorsi muscle, due to muscle spasm, and the normal left ventricular myocardium, as well as physiologic excretion via the kidneys and bladder.

study is acquired over a number of days to exclude false positives due to bowel clearance. Shulkin et al.[198] suggest that FDG should not be considered a substitute for MIBG imaging because it not more sensitive and is potentially less specific than MIBG imaging. In centers where MIBG is not readily available, and in those patients with an incidental adrenal mass, it is probably reasonable to perform an FDG study to triage those patients with an FDG-avid mass toward a more aggressive treatment pathway.

MIBG IN PHEOCHROMOCYTOMA. MIBG is a highly sensitive and specific method of localizing pheochromocytoma tissue. Sensitivity ranges from 80% to 90%, with specificity ranges from 95% to 100%. Size has been shown to be the major determinant of the sensitivity rate with [131]I MIBG.[199] The same is likely to be true with the [123]I preparation, which in and of itself is more sensitive than [131]I MIBG.[200] Malignant forms of pheochromocytoma are rare but are difficult to treat.

[131]I MIBG therapy has been investigated and partial responses have been reported,[201,202] with anecdotal reports of durable responses.[203] In general, complete responses are rare. Concomitant chemotherapy regimes have also been tried with limited success.[204] Figure 4C-23 demonstrates increased [131]I MIBG uptake in the metastatic disease of malignant pheochromocytoma.

NEUROBLASTOMA. This tumor can be imaged by a variety of nuclear medicine techniques, including MIBG, somatostatin receptor scintigraphy (SRS) (Fig. 4C-24), [99m]Tc MDP, FDG, and [131]I-labeled 3F8, an anti-GD2 monoclonal antibody. This antibody is

more sensitive and specific than MIBG and [99m]Tc MDP, but has limited availability.[205] [99m]Tc MDP imaging is quite sensitive but nonspecific. The most specific test remains MIBG. FDG imaging compares favorably with MIBG in the setting of the untreated patient, in part due to the improved sensitivity of the camera used to detect the tumor. In the patient group who have previously received chemotherapy, it is a much more significant challenge to differentiate between regenerating marrow and residual viable tumor using FDG PET.

[131]I MIBG has been given to patients with neuroblastoma as therapy and the experience of a number of groups in a total of 255 patients has been summarized by Troncone and Ruffini.[203] Complete responses were seen in 5%, partial responses in 24%, stable disease in 29%, with 13% of patients inevaluable. Most clinicians combine MIBG therapy with chemotherapy. The preferred method of delivering radioactivity to neuroblastoma in our hospital has been using [131]I 3F8, a murine anti-GD2 monoclonal antibody. The administration of [131]I 3F8 following intensive chemotherapy for stage 4 neuroblastoma patients with minimal residual disease has led to significant improvements in the outcome of this tumor over historical controls, with long-term progression-free probabilities of 38% seen in a group at high risk of recurrence.[206] Because this trial was not randomized, the absolute effects of the chemotherapy and the 3F8 administration were not determined, but the results remain encouraging.

ADRENAL MASSES. The assessment of adrenal masses is rapidly changing. Fine-cut noncontrast CT, by detecting the high lipid content of adrenal adenomas reflected in the Hounsfield units,

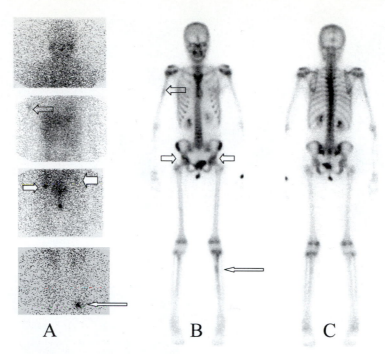

A          B          C

**FIGURE 4C-23.** This 17-year-old girl has a 3-year history of pheochromocytoma metastatic to bone. She was followed with MIBG (image *A*) and bone scans (images *B* and *C*). Note the concordant findings in the right humerus, left tibia, and the acetabulum bilaterally. Urinary contamination is seen in both studies.

is very successful at differentiating secondary deposits in the adrenal gland from adrenal adenomas.[207] Characteristic MRI findings have also been described that involve analysis of the opposed-phase MRI image in comparison to the in-phase MRI image and calculating the adrenal-spleen ratio (ASR). Lesions with an ASR of less than 70 are likely to be benign; lesions with an ASR greater than 80 are likely to be malignant.[208] In the face of a PET-positive primary lesion, it is unlikely that an adrenal secondary will not also be hypermetabolic, given a minimum size of the adrenal lesion. In a study of adrenal lesions in patients with lung cancer, FDG PET was able to correctly stratify lesions as benign or malignant on the basis of the SUV.[209]

Adrenal cortical lesions have been characterized in the past using radiolabeled cholesterol analogues, [131]I 6β-iodomethyl-19-norcholesterol (NP-59) (Figs. 4C-25 and 4C-26), [75]Seselenocholesterol, as well as gallium 67.[210–213] These scans are useful in those patients in whom there are bilateral adenomas and therefore a surgeon is having difficulty in determining on which side to operate.[214] Early published experience with FDG suggests that adrenal cortical carcinomas are hypermetabolic.[215] This is confirmed by our own experience (Fig. 4C-27).

## MESOTHELIOMA

One of the challenges in thoracic surgery is the determination of the malignant potential of incidentally demonstrated pleural plaques.

An additional challenge appears to be in the presurgical staging, because there is a very large range of survivals reported, and prognostic factors have not been fully elucidated. It was recognized that tumors exhibit increased uptake of gallium in comparison to normal tissues. This led to some preliminary studies investigating the utility of gallium in the characterization of pleural masses. The earliest descriptions of the use of gallium 67 citrate imaging suggested that gallium may be of only limited benefit in the characterization of pleurally based masses.[216,217] The main difficulties in gallium imaging are the low photon flux of the tracer due to the relatively low doses of the tracer administered, the poor spatial resolution of the cameras used to image gallium, as well as the nonspecific uptake of gallium. In the febrile patient, gallium cannot distinguish between uptake due to tumor and uptake due to infection. FDG PET is currently being actively explored as a methodology to characterize pleural plaques.[218–220] FDG is an improvement over gallium imaging in terms of rapidity of the scanning procedure as well as the achievable spatial resolution. FDG shares the problem of lack of specificity with gallium, however, in that infectious processes will be FDG avid. In addition, FDG imaging with current machines cannot distinguish between involvement of the mediastinal lymph nodes and the overlying pleura, although an isolated nodule in the mediastinum may prompt a mediastinoscopy as an early staging procedure rather than a thoracoscopy. When hybrid PET/CT machines become available, it is likely that mediastinal staging will be more accurate even in the presence of overlying pleural disease.

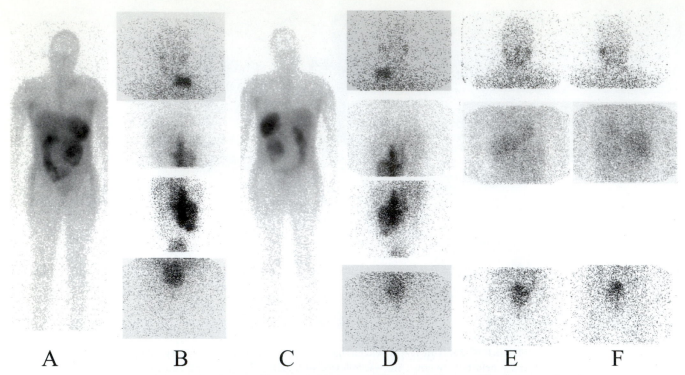

**FIGURE 4C-24.** MIBG in neuroblastoma. This 17-year-old patient with neuroblastoma was referred for MIBG, octreotide, and FDG studies to characterize her tumor. Images *A* and *C* are whole-body octreotide images demonstrating increased somatostatin receptor density in the left supraclavicular region as well as the left upper abdomen. The images in column *B* are a series of partially overlapping static MIBG studies in the anterior projection. Note the increased uptake in the left supraclavicular region, and in the left paraaortic nodes. *D* is a series of posterior static MIBG images. *E* and *F* are posttreatment MIBG static images demonstrating resolution of the pathologic uptake seen on the pretreatment scans (*B* and *D*). The amount of administered activity of MIBG is much less than that of octreotide, leading to a reduction in overall image quality, but the specificity of the tracer makes the overall utility of the MIBG images better.

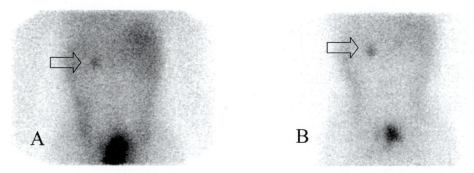

**FIGURE 4C-25.** NP59 in adrenal adenoma. This 35-year-old woman with hypertension was found on a screening CT to have a left adrenal mass; the NP59 scan reveals a functional left adrenal adenoma (open arrow) seen on the 72-(*A*) and 120-hr (*B*) postinjection images. There was resolution of hypertension with resection of the left adrenal mass.

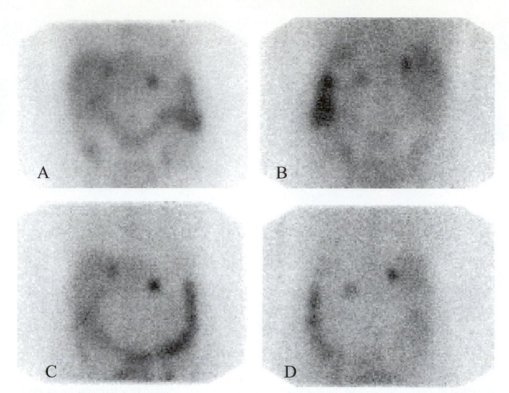

**FIGURE 4C-26.** Bilateral adrenal adenomas. This 55-year-old diabetic female with a high cortisol level was found to have enlargement of both adrenal glands on CT scan, suspicious for adrenal hyperplasia or adenoma, referred for iodine 131, NP59 scan to evaluate the possibility of adrenal adenoma. These images were acquired 72-(*A* and *B*) and 120 hr (*C* and *D*) after injection of 1.1 mCi of NP59. Patient preparation includes SSKI drops to block free iodine uptake by the stomach and thyroid and dexamethasone to suppress normal adrenal tissue. These images demonstrate physiologic excretion into the colon that alters in pattern with time, as well as bilateral adrenal uptake. Note also the influence of count statistics on image quality, with the earlier, higher count images *A* and *B* looking better than images *C* and *D*, although target to background ratio has improved with time. This patient has bilateral adrenal hyperplasia.

Semiquantitative analysis of FDG PET images appears to stratify patients into good and poor prognostic groups. Whether this is an independent prognostic factor cannot be determined because the number of patients reported was too small. Higher SUV values appeared ($p = 0.0094$) to be recorded in the sarcomatoid variety[221] as well as higher T-stage tumors.[220] Depth of chest wall invasion may be a component of the correlation between SUV values and prognosis due to partial volume averaging.[220,222] FDG PET is unable to distinguish between low-grade mesothelioma and local pleural infection. FDG PET–based treatment algorithms may be a treatment approach in the future, but a lot more work needs to be done in the interim, and hybrid machines are likely to be an essential part of this approach.

Intrapleural $^{32}$P therapy has been used as a treatment adjunct and appears to effectively reduce concomitant pleural effusions.[223] A randomized control comparing the efficacy of this approach versus other pleural-based therapies such as intrapleural chemotherapy or photodynamic therapy has not been performed. Planning for intracavitary therapies can be assisted by the use of $^{99m}$Tc tracers for distribution studies.

## LYMPHOMA

Gallium 67 citrate has been shown to be very valuable in the treatment of patients with lymphoma. Gallium uptake is normally seen in the liver, bone, spleen, salivary and lacrimal glands, nasal mucosa, thymus, and breasts. There is renal and gut clearance of the tracer leading to normal uptake early in kidneys and bladder, later in the gut. Delayed imaging is beneficial because it allows clearance of the tracer from the blood, as well as demonstrating passage of the tracer through the gut. Increased uptake is seen in benign nodes in smokers. Gallium scans need to be performed with care, with correct collimators, dosage of tracer, and including SPECT imaging. The sensitivity results of the early cooperative groups reported in 1977 and 1978 have been consistently outperformed by later studies

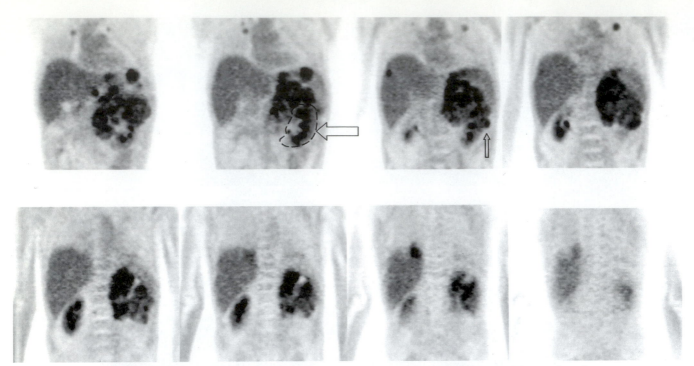

**FIGURE 4C-27.** FDG PET in adrenal cancer. This 50-year-old male initially underwent adrenal resection in 1994, and has had further rises in his cortisol level, leading to a reoperation in 1995. However, due to the presence of extensive disease, no resection was performed. The images were performed after chemotherapy. Notice the multiple metastases in liver, lung, and peritoneum. Some of the difficulties with FDG PET are demonstrated in this case; notice how the left kidney (outlined) looks similar to the peritoneal recurrences, with a lesion (up arrow) overlying the mid outer pole of the left kidney unable to be separated from the renal parenchyma.

using higher dose of tracer (low-dose sensitivity for non-Hodgkin's disease 76%[224] high-dose sensitivity 97%[225]; Hodgkin's disease low-dose sensitivity 88%,[226] high-dose 92%[225]). The sensitivity of gallium scans is slightly higher in Hodgkin's disease (HD) than non-Hodgkin's lymphoma (NHL).[227] If there is a plan to use gallium as a response marker, it is critical to perform the initial gallium scan prior to any therapy. A valid baseline scan that demonstrates gallium-avid lymphoma provides an internal control against which all subsequent scans can be compared.

### ASSESSMENT OF RESIDUAL DISEASE AFTER TREATMENT.

The earliest report of gallium scanning in lymphoma also noted the absence of gallium uptake in a lymphoma patient recently treated with vinblastine.[228] These earliest findings have held up consistently.[224,226] A recent report suggesting the appearances of the repeat gallium study performed after two cycles of chemotherapy strongly predicts final outcome in patients with aggressive NHL.[229] Similar results with HD after a single cycle have also been reported.[230] Gallium positivity in a residual mass after chemotherapy strongly predicts residual viable lymphoma.

FDG PET is currently being investigated in lymphoma. The attraction of FDG imaging is that the scan can potentially give the same result in a few hours as a gallium scan can over a number of days. There are no large cooperative studies comparing FDG PET

and gallium in the management of patients with lymphoma. Most studies of FDG PET in lymphoma report FDG alone or in comparison to conventional imaging modalities. FDG PET again appears to outperform conventional imaging in response assessment. The small series reported thus far tend to support the hypothesis that FDG PET is as good at detecting lymphomatous masses as gallium 67 imaging (Fig. 4C-28). The improved detection of lymphoma with FDG PET is due to the much greater sensitivity of the dedicated PET devices, with the improved spatial resolution that allows clearer delineation of the abnormal sites.[231]

At this institution, the majority of patients with lymphoma are treated with chemotherapy rather than surgery and/or radiotherapy, with the exception of patients with mucosa-associated lymphoid tissue (MALT)-associated lymphoma and low-grade follicular lymphoma. This systemic approach to therapy has implications for imaging, because it becomes less important to demonstrate small-volume disease on the opposite side of the diaphragm to the indicator lesion. The most important clinical indication for gallium scanning at this center is therefore response assessment. If FDG PET can independently distinguish patients at high risk of recurrence and/or those with residual viable disease, then adoption of FDG PET imaging would seem appropriate.

Nonspecific gastric uptake of gallium and FDG make the use of these tracers problematic in the assessment of gastric lymphoma.

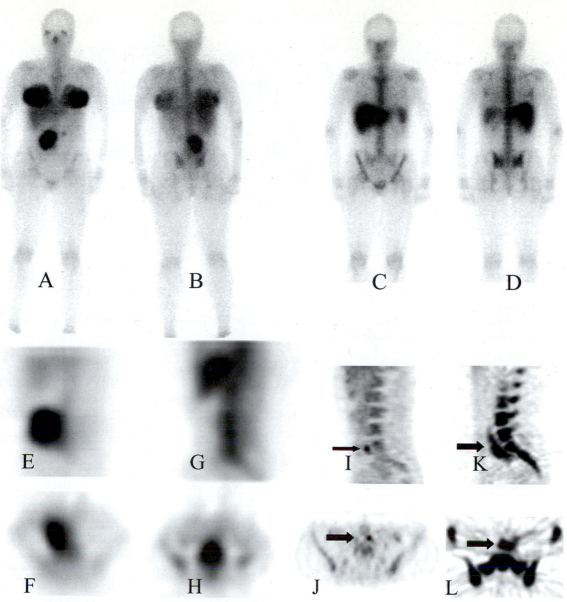

**FIGURE 4C-28.** A comparison of $^{18}$F FDG and gallium 67 imaging of lymphoma. This patient presented with a high-grade lymphoma and underwent a pretreatment $^{67}$Ga scanning for evaluation of extent of disease. Note the high degree of uptake in the right midabdomen seen in images *A* (anterior whole body) and *B* (posterior whole body). Note also in images *A* and *B* the physiologically increased uptake in the premenopausal breast tissue, normal uptake in the liver, nose, lacrimal glands, bone marrow, and to a lesser extent renal and bowel excretion. The posttreatment gallium scan revealed resolution of uptake in the abdominal mass, with increased uptake in the marrow, liver, and spleen (images *C* and *D*). Single photon emission computed tomography (SPECT) images revealed increased gallium uptake in the paraaortic nodes seen in the sagittal slice image *E* and transaxial image *F*, which completely resolved with treatment, leaving physiologic activity in the reactive marrow, images *G* (sagittal) and *H* (transaxial). An FDG PET scan performed soon after the gallium scan revealed a recurrence in a lower left paraaortic node anterior to the body of the sacrum [see images I (coronal) and *J* (sagittal)]. The patient subsequently underwent a bone marrow transplant, but had progressive disease (see images *K* and *L*). Note the intense uptake in the regenerating marrow as well as the uptake in the enlarging presacral mass. There are a number of reasons why the FDG images look so much better than the gallium images; the first is that the gamma camera cannot compete with the dedicated PET camera in terms of resolution and count statistics, and that the total number of photons coming from the patient at the time of imaging is higher with FDG than gallium because of decay.

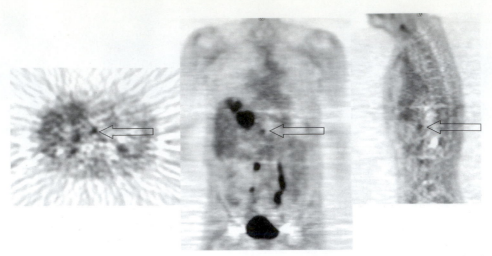

**FIGURE 4C-29.** FDG PET in malignant lymphadenopathy. This patient with potentially localized disease to the liver, thereby potentially curable with aggressive local therapy, was found to have malignant involvement in a lymph node on FDG PET (arrows). This was confirmed surgically; the patient is continuing on with chemotherapy.

There is a report of reduced sensitivity of FDG PET in MALT lymphoma.[232] There was a comprehensive examination of the utility of FDG PET as a measure of treatment response in NHL treated with chemotherapy [cyclophosphamide, doxorubicin (Adriamycin), vincristine, prednisone (CHOP) or cyclophosphamide, doxorubicin (Adriamycin), vincristine (etoposide), prednisone (CHOEP)]. Eleven patients were studied 7 and 42 days after the initiation of chemotherapy. This study found that dynamic PET data performed at 7 days after chemotherapy initiation was sufficiently sensitive to predict disease status at 16 months. Semiquantitative analysis (SUV) measures performed 42 days after onset of chemotherapy were able to differentiate those patients at high risk of recurrence.[233] This well-designed trial has proved strong evidence of the efficacy of FDG PET in determining response early in treatment.

## METASTATIC CANCER

**BRAIN METASTASES.** Nuclear medicine imaging of brain tumors has been mainly focused on the imaging of primary brain tumors. Many of the principles elucidated in these works can be applied to metastatic cancers and are therefore reported here. The most sensitive imaging modality for the detection of brain lesions is MRI. MRI and CT have some difficulty in characterizing tumors, and nuclear medicine procedures can often assist in characterizing tumors. Prior to the availability of adequate cross-sectional imaging, nuclear physicians investigated brain lesions with agents that worked predominantly by imaging the vascularity of the tumor.[234,235] The earliest PET studies of the brain were reported in 1976.[236] Once thallium 201 was recognized to be a tumor-seeking agent, it was then applied to imaging brain tumors, both primary and secondary,[237,238] and was found to be a better agent than [67]Ga- or [99m]Tc-based perfusion agents. Thallium imaging, in spite of the poor spatial resolution, is a very good method of estimating the amount of viable tumor tissue left after therapy, predicting tumor volume 2 months earlier than cross-sectional imaging.[239] Thallium accumulation is an active process requiring the presence of Na, K-ATPase, an enzyme involved in the maintenance of the transmembrane potential. There was some early concern that [201]Th accumulation only occurred in areas of the brain with a disrupted blood-brain barrier. Thallium uptake is independent of steroid administration.[240] Ratios of normal brain to tumor were shown to be prognostically significant, as was the degree of uptake of thallium, with increased accumulation seen in the higher-grade primary tumors.[241–243] The concern that thallium uptake is increased in areas of the brain with contrast enhancement has in part proved true. Those patients without enhancement and positive on thallium imaging are very likely to have malignant tumors. Thallium retention rates have proved important in the differential diagnosis of cerebral lesions. Those lesions that are malignant are likely to have prolonged retention of thallium.[244] [99m]Tc sestamibi has also been used to investigate brain lesions. It has the advantage of higher photon flux due to the higher doses administered, but a major disadvantage is the presence of MIBI uptake by the normal choroid plexus.

Amino acid tracers for SPECT and PET imaging have been used successfully to image brain tumors. The advantage of amino acid tracers is that they rapidly reach equilibrium and have very little uptake in normal brain matter. The disadvantage of amino acid tracers is that the degree of uptake is not related to the degree of aggressiveness of the tumor. FDG PET is also commonly used to assess brain lesions. The advantage of FDG PET is that the degree of uptake is related to the aggressiveness of the tumor,[245] making FDG PET a useful tool in the assessment of the aggressiveness of tumors and, therefore, in treatment planning. The major disadvantage of FDG PET is that the normal brain is very FDG avid. In order to interpret FDG PET scans, coregistration of FDG PET and CT or MRI images is often required. Maisey's group[246] has proposed a reliable method of investigating brain tumors, localizing the tumor with [11]C-labeled methionine and then characterizing the aggressiveness of the tumor with FDG PET. At MSKCC we do not currently advocate a routine FDG brain scan in patients with non-CNS tumors, because we believe that we will miss small tumors that could be detected with CT or MRI. A cooperative study currently under way is examining the relative accuracy of FDG PET and CT compared to surgical staging of the mediastinum in patients with lung cancer. A component of this study is the evaluation of the CNS and should confirm or refute our current clinical impression.

**STAGING PATIENTS WITH LIVER METASTASES.** This topic will be addressed with particular reference to colorectal cancer. The incidence of hepatic metastases in patients with end-stage colorectal cancer is as high as 70%.[247] Liver resection has the potential to produce long disease-free intervals, with a 30% 5-year survival rate.[248] The current literature reporting the relative values of FDG PET and conventional imaging modalities is marred by selection biases, differences in scanning sequences, and machines used to acquire the data. This makes a metaanalysis of the current trials very difficult to perform. When trying to characterize liver lesions, CT portography is the most sensitive modality but the least specific. FDG PET appears at least as sensitive but more specific than CT.[249–251] FDG PET appears more capable of detecting nodal metastatic disease than CT due primarily to the detection of tumor in normal-sized lymph nodes (Fig. 4C-29). FDG PET also appears to outperform CT in the detection of peritoneal disease,[249,252–255] as the signal-to-noise ratio (tumor to normal anatomy) is much higher with FDG PET than with CT (Fig. 4C-14). In those patients with rectal cancer who have a suspicious presacral mass following primary therapy, FDG PET outperforms CT and MRI,[256,257] in part because the tissue responses to radiotherapy are time-dependent and the sequence varies from patient to patient.[258–261] These are general statements based on community standard imaging practices that constantly need to be revised as the technologies used to perform the studies improve. The sensitivity of FDG PET will vary according to the time after injection that the patient is scanned, the duration of time spent scanning the liver, how close to a course of chemotherapy the scan occurs, and the type of camera used. The accuracy of CT will vary depending on slice thickness, the presence of absence of IV contrast, the use of delayed scans, and so on. In unselected patients presenting for hepatic resection, FDG PET appears to change the stage of patients previously investigated in about 30% of patients.[252,253,262]

It is not yet known, but there will probably be certain clinical situations in which a particular scanning technique should be used first. For instance, it appears FDG PET consistently outperforms CT in the detection of peritoneal deposits of disease. Therefore, those patients who at primary surgery are at high risk of peritoneal recurrence[263] would perhaps benefit from an FDG PET scan prior to a CT. Those patients with low risk of intraabdominal recurrence but high risk of liver metastasis perhaps should have a CT first to define vascular resectability, then an FDG PET scan to rule out occult disease. These important clinical questions can only be answered when much larger series are reported, examining carefully for known risk factors, and scanning with state-of-the-art equipment.

**HEPATIC ARTERIAL CHEMOTHERAPY.** Patients with hepatic metastases to the liver that are unresectable are often offered an hepatic artery pump for local chemotherapy. The literature regarding this therapeutic approach is maturing. A recent article has

demonstrated a clear improvement in hepatic disease-free status at 2 years in patients treated with a combination of pump therapy and systemic chemotherapy after resection of hepatic metastases.[264] The success of intrahepatic chemotherapy depends on the degree of success with which the therapeutic agent can target the hepatic metastasis. Using $^{99m}$Tc MAA injected into the hepatic artery via the pump, and comparing the uptake of the trace to a $^{99m}$Tc sulfur colloid study, it is possible to assess the delivery of these drugs to the liver. If the tumor is hypervascular, then the hepatic arterial therapy is likely to be successful in delivering adequate doses to the tumor. The actual response of the tumor to chemotherapy is multifactorial and, no doubt, also reflects 5-fluorouracil (5-Fu) resistance[265] as well as the dose delivered.[266,267] Likely side effects of the chemotherapy can be predicted on the basis of systemic shunting, as well as the presence of perfusion of the stomach or pancreas (Fig. 4C-30).[268]

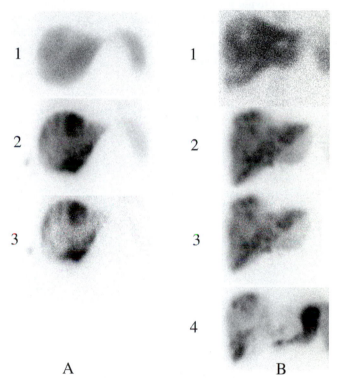

**A**                                   **B**

**FIGURE 4C-30.** Hepatic pump study. The anterior images in column A are: (1) The initial sulfur colloid study demonstrating a number of photopenic areas; (2) the pump MAA injection and sulfur colloid activity; (3) the net image created by subtracting the sulfur colloid image from the pump image. Notice the increased perfusion of the metastases by the hepatic artery, compared to the rest of the liver, and the lack of perfusion of the extrahepatic tissues. The images in column B follow the same schema, with the sulfur colloid study in the top panel, the MAA/colloid study in the middle panel, and the net image in the second to lowest panel. The lowest panel in column B is a MAA pump injection performed 9 months later, demonstrating migration of the catheter and subsequent perfusion of the stomach and spleen.

$^{68}$F-labeled 5-FU has been synthesized, and retention rates of the drug have been correlated with response rates.[269]

### NONRESECTABLE METASTATIC DISEASE TO THE LIVER.

In those patients with unresectable disease, if the results reported by Kemeny et al.[264] can be extrapolated, one would expect modest improvements in survival, given that a "hepatic death" would be the most likely clinical outcome without successful hepatic-directed therapy. Debulking procedures have a theoretical role in the treatment of hepatic metastases, in that the fewer cells present, the less likely a group of cells will be able to become resistant to a given therapy. Cryotherapy and radiofrequency (RF) ablation are methods used to treat hepatic metastases. Both suffer from potential inadequacies of therapy to lesions close to or involving major intrahepatic vessels that effectively insulate local tissues from thermal injury. Both cryotherapy and RF lead to prolonged perturbations in normal tissue architecture, making evaluation of residual or recurrent tumor problematic,[270,271] although the CT finding of a lesion following RF ablation that is larger than the pretreatment lesion may be associated with successful treatment.[272] Our initial experience with FDG PET has been positive (Fig. 4C-31), with asymmetries in residual FDG activity being associated with local recurrence.[273]

Therapeutic approaches to the treatment of hepatic metastases have included the injection of $^{90}$Y-labeled microspheres,[274] lipiodol[275] $^{131}$I labeled antibodies,[276] and epirubicin lipiodol.[277]

### PERITONEAL METASTATIC DISEASE.

Nuclear medicine techniques have been used to demonstrate the volume of peritoneal dialysate needed to ensure adequate distribution of intraperitoneal (IP) drugs.[278–281] Peritoneal scintigraphy with $^{99m}$Tc-labeled tracers is simple to perform and can reliably document the distribution of IP drugs and can triage the (re-)placement of catheters. Radiolabeled monoclonal antibodies and FDG can detect peritoneal disease, although microscopic disease cannot be as reliably detected as direct visualization. In challenging cases where access is difficult and normal tissue planes are disrupted by therapy, nuclear medicine techniques offer an alternate method of determining if recurrent disease is present. Some attempts at therapy of peritoneal carcinomatosis using therapeutic radionuclides such as $^{32}$P have been made, but have not become widespread in their application[282–284] due to a lack of specificity in their approach. More targeted therapy such as reported by Crippa et al.[285] using radiolabeled antibodies should improve the therapeutic index of these approaches.[286,287]

### PLEURAL EFFUSIONS.

These have been discussed in the section above dealing with lung cancer.

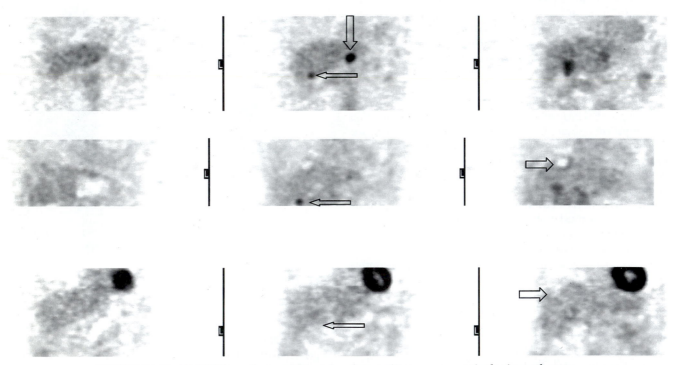

**FIGURE 4C-31.** FDG PET cryotherapy. This series of coronal images was acquired prior to therapy in January 1998 (upper panel), after cryotherapy in February 1998 (middle panel), and after an initial course of hepatic pump chemotherapy (lower panel) in April 1998. The lesion in segment 3 was resected. Notice the effect of cryotherapy in the middle panel that is resolving in the lower panel. The small lesion in the region of segment 5 was not treated with cryotherapy but was successfully treated with chemotherapy.

## CARDIAC RISK FACTOR ASSESSMENT

Many of the risk factors for solid tumors are similar to the risk factors for coronary artery disease. Preoperative cardiac risk factor assessment has been carefully evaluated in those patients undergoing vascular surgery. Myocardial scintigraphy has been shown to predict accurately the cardiac event rates in those patients undergoing major surgery. The best patients in whom to use myocardial scintigraphy are those with an intermediate risk of coronary disease.[288]

## FUTURE AVENUES OF NUCLEAR MEDICINE RESEARCH IN SURGICAL ONCOLOGY

**GENE IMAGING.** Preclinical studies have demonstrated the feasibility of imaging gene transfer in animal models. This area of research is expanding rapidly in part due to funding by the NIH. If gene expression can be reliably reported noninvasively, then medical and surgical oncologists will have powerful tools with which to tailor therapies for individual patients.

Radiolabeled antibody diagnosis and therapy is being continually evaluated, and advances in the basic science of antibody development are improving the specificity and utility of antibody-based therapies.

## REFERENCES

1. Morton DL et al: Validation of the accuracy of intraoperative lymphatic mapping and sentinel lymphadenectomy for early-stage melanoma: A multicenter trial. Multicenter Selective Lymphadenectomy Trial Group. Ann Surg 230:453, 1999; discussion, 463.
2. Coit DG: Role of surgery for metastatic malignant melanoma: A review. Semin Surg Oncol 9:239, 1993.
3. Nguyen A et al: PET scanning with [18F] 2-fluoro-2-deoxy-D-glucose (FDG) in patients with melanoma: Benefits and limitations. Clin Positron Imaging 2:93, 1999.
4. Damian DL et al: Positron emission tomography in the detection and management of metastatic melanoma. Melanoma Res 6:325, 1996.
5. Eigtved A et al: Use of fluorine-18 fluorodeoxyglucose positron emission tomography in the detection of silent metastases from malignant melanoma (In Process Citation). Eur J Nucl Med 27:70, 2000 (MEDLINE record in process).
6. Lampreave JL et al: PET evaluation of therapeutic limb perfusion in Merkel's cell carcinoma. J Nucl Med 39:2087, 1998.
7. Koch WM et al: Gamma probe-directed biopsy of the sentinel node in oral squamous cell carcinoma. Archi Otolaryngol Head Neck Surg 124:455, 1998.
8. Di Nicola V, Fiorella R: Multiple primary tumors in patients with laryngeal carcinoma: Incidence and prognostic factors. Acta Otorhinolaryngol Ital 15(6 Suppl 51):1, 1995.
9. Paulus P et al: 18FDG-PET for the assessment of primary head and neck tumors: Clinical, computed tomography, and histopathological correlation in 38 patients. Laryngoscope 108:1578, 1998.
10. Hanasono MM et al: Uses and limitations of FDG positron emission tomography in patients with head and neck cancer. Laryngoscope 109:880, 1999.
11. Bohuslavizki KH et al: F-18 FDG PET for detection of occult primary tumor in patients with lymphatic metastases of the neck region. Laryngorhinootologie 78:445, 1999.
12. Safa AA et al: The role of positron emission tomography in occult primary head and neck cancers [see comments]. Cancer J Sci Am 5:214, 1999.
13. Os AA et al: Metastatic head and neck cancer: Role and usefulness of FDG PET in locating occult primary tumors. Radiology 210:177, 1999.
14. Jungehulsing M et al: Detection of unknown primary cancer with fluor-deoxy-glucose positron emission tomography. Ann Otol Rhinol Laryngol 108:623, 1999.
15. Greven KM et al: Occult primary tumors of the head and neck: Lack of benefit from positron emission tomography imaging with 2-[F-18]fluoro-2-deoxy-D-glucose. Cancer 86:114, 1999.
16. Braams JW et al: Detection of unknown primary head and neck tumors by positron emission tomography. Int J Oral Maxillofac Surg 26:112, 1997.
17. Farber LA et al: Detection of recurrent head and neck squamous cell carcinomas after radiation therapy with 2-18F-fluoro-2-deoxy-D-glucose positron emission tomography. Laryngoscope 109:970, 1999.
18. Lowe VJ et al: Primary and recurrent early stage laryngeal cancer: Preliminary results of 2-[fluorine 18]fluoro-2-deoxy-D-glucose PET imaging. Radiology 212:799, 1999.
19. Kim HJ et al: F-18 FDG PET scan after radiotherapy for early-stage larynx cancer. Clin Nucl Med 23:750, 1998.
20. McGuirt WF et al: PET scanning in head and neck oncology: A review. Head Neck 20:208, 1998.
21. Mukherji SK et al: Thallium-201 single-photon emission CT versus CT for the detection of recurrent squamous cell carcinoma of the head and neck [see comments]. Am J Neuroradiol 20:1215, 1999.
22. Mezosi E et al: The role of technetium-99m methoxy-isobutylisonitrile scintigraphy in the differential diagnosis of cold thyroid nodules [see comments]. Eur J Nucl Med 26:798, 1999.
23. Bohuslavizki KH et al: Salivary gland protection by amifostine in high-dose radioiodine treatment: Results of a double-blind placebo-controlled study. J Clin Oncol 16:3542, 1998.
24. Sundram FX et al: Role of technetium-99m sestamibi in localisation of thyroid cancer metastases. Ann Acad Med (Singapore) 22:557, 1993.
25. Grünwald F et al: Comparison of 18FDG-PET with 131iodine and 99m Tc-sestamibi scintigraphy in differentiated thyroid cancer. Thyroid 7:327, 1997.
26. Adams S et al: Intraoperative gamma probe detection of neuroendocrine tumors. J Nucl Med 39:1155, 1998.
27. Krenning EP et al: The role of radioactive somatostatin and its analogues in the control of tumor growth. Recent Results Cancer Res 153:1, 2000.
28. Curnow RT: Clinical experience with CD64-directed immunotherapy. An overview. Cancer Immunol Immunother 45:210, 1997.
29. Bhatnagar A et al: Technetium-99m-sestamibi parathyroid scintigraphy: Effect of P-glycoprotein, histology and tumor size on detectability. J Nucl Med 39:1617, 1998.
30. Caixàs A et al: Utility of 99m Tc-sestamibi scintigraphy as a first-line imaging procedure in the preoperative evaluation of hyperparathyroidism [see comments]. Clin Endocrinol 43:525, 1995.

31. Caixàs et al: Efficacy of preoperative diagnostic imaging localization of technetium 99m-sestamibi scintigraphy in hyperparathyroidism. Surgery 121:535, 1997.

32. Henschke CI et al: Early Lung Cancer Action Project: Overall design and findings from baseline screening [see comments]. Lancet 354:99, 1999.

33. Dewan NA et al: Likelihood of malignancy in a solitary pulmonary nodule: Comparison of Bayesian analysis and results of FDG-PET scan. Chest 112:416, 1997.

34. Gambhir SS et al: Analytical decision model for the cost-effective management of solitary pulmonary nodules. J Clin Oncol 16:2113, 1998.

35. Hosokawa N et al: Prediction of postoperative pulmonary function using 99mTc-MAA perfusion lung SPECT. Nippon Igaku Hoshasen Gakkai Zasshi 55:414, 1995.

36. Saunders CA et al: Evaluation of fluorine-18-fluorodeoxyglucose whole body positron emission tomography imaging in the staging of lung cancer. Ann Thorac Surg 67:790, 1999.

37. Kubota K et al: PET imaging of primary mediastinal tumours. Br J Cancer 73:882, 1996.

38. Hoh CK et al: Whole-body FDG-PET imaging for staging of Hodgkin's disease and lymphoma. Nucl Med 38:343, 1997.

39. Sugawara Y et al: Germ cell tumor: Differentiation of viable tumor, mature teratoma, and necrotic tissue with FDG PET and kinetic modeling. Radiology 211:249, 1999.

40. Kole AC et al: Positron emission tomography for staging of oesophageal and gastroesophageal malignancy. Br J Cancer 78:521, 1998.

41. Block MI et al: Improvement in staging of esophageal cancer with the addition of positron emission tomography. Ann Thorac Surg 64:770, 1997; discussion 776.

42. Couper GW et al: Detection of response to chemotherapy using positron emission tomography in patients with oesophageal and gastric cancer. Br J Surg 85:1403, 1998.

43. Burke EC et al: Laparoscopy in the management of gastric adenocarcinoma. Ann Surg 225:262, 1997.

44. Rankin SC et al: Computed tomography and positron emission tomography in the pre-operative staging of oesophageal carcinoma. Clin Radiol 53:659, 1998.

45. Yuan M: Characterization and detection of cancer-associated antigens in patients with gastric cancer. Chung-Hua I Hsueh Tsa Chih (Chinese Med J) 73:457, 1993.

46. Ohyanagi H et al: A monoclonal antibody, KM10 reactive with human gastrointestinal cancer and its application for immunotherapy. Japan J Cancer Res 79:1349, 1988.

47. Xu G et al: Radioimmunoguided surgery in gastric cancer using 131-I labeled monoclonal antibody 3H11. Semin Surg Oncol 10:88, 1994.

48. Martin EWJ et al: Radioimmunoguided surgery using monoclonal antibody. Am J Surg 156:386, 1988.

49. Lucisano E, Bertoglio S: Role of radioimmunoguided surgery using iodine-125-labeled B72.3 monoclonal antibody in gastric cancer surgery. Semin Surg Oncol 15:212, 1998.

50. Liu BG et al: A clinical trial of radioimmunoguided surgery for gastric cancer. Chung-Hua Chung Liu Tsa Chih (Chinese J Oncol) 16:284, 1994.

51. Megibow AJ et al: Pancreatic adenocarcinoma: CT versus MR imaging in the evaluation of resectability—Report of the Radiology Diagnostic Oncology Group. Radiology 195:327, 1995.

52. Nishiharu T et al: Local extension of pancreatic carcinoma: Assessment with thin-section helical CT versus with breath-hold fast MR imaging—ROC analysis. Radiology 212:445, 1999.

53. Sheridan MB et al: Dynamic contrast-enhanced MR imaging and dualphase helical CT in the preoperative assessment of suspected pancreatic cancer: A comparative study with receiver operating characteristic analysis. AJR 173:583, 1999.

54. van Gulik TM et al: Differential diagnosis of focal pancreatitis and pancreatic cancer. Ann Oncol 10(Suppl 4):85, 1999.

55. Reske SN et al: Overexpression of glucose transporter 1 and increased FDG uptake in pancreatic carcinoma. J Nucl Med 38:1344, 1997.

56. Imdahl A et al: Evaluation of positron emission tomography with 2-[18F]fluoro-2-deoxy-D-glucose for the differentiation of chronic pancreatitis and pancreatic cancer. Br J Surg 86:194, 1999.

57. Stollfuss JC et al: 2-(fluorine-18)-fluoro-2-deoxy-D-glucose PET in detection of pancreatic cancer: Value of quantitative image interpretation [see comments]. Radiology 195:339, 1995.

58. Inokuma T et al: Evaluation of pancreatic tumors with positron emission tomography and F-18 fluorodeoxyglucose: Comparison with CT and US. Radiology 195:345, 1995.

59. Zimny M et al: Fluorine-18 fluorodeoxyglucose positron emission tomography in the differential diagnosis of pancreatic carcinoma: A report of 106 cases. Eur J Nucl Med 24:678, 1997.

60. Zimny M, Buell U: 18FDG-positron emission tomography in pancreatic cancer. Ann Oncol 10(Suppl 4):28, 1999.

61. Dresel S et al: 111IN-octreotide and 123I-MIBG scintigraphy in the diagnosis of small intestinal carcinoid tumors—results of a comparative investigation. Nuklearmedizin 35:53, 1996.

62. van Eijck CH et al: Somatostatin receptor imaging and therapy of pancreatic endocrine tumors. Ann Oncol 10(Suppl 4):177, 1999.

63. Valkema R et al: The diagnostic utility of somatostatin receptor scintigraphy in oncology. J Cancer Res Clin Oncol 122:513, 1996.

64. Termanini B et al: Distinguishing small hepatic hemangiomas from vascular liver metastases in gastrinoma: Use of a somatostatin-receptor scintigraphic agent. Radiology 202:151, 1997.

65. Kwekkeboom DJ et al: Somatostatin analogue scintigraphy in carcinoid tumours. Eur J Nucl Med 20:283, 1993.

66. Kwekkeboom DJ, Krenning EP: Somatostatin receptor scintigraphy in patients with carcinoid tumors. World J Surg 20:157, 1996.

67. Anthony LB et al: Somatostatin receptor imaging: Predictive and prognostic considerations. Digestion 57(Suppl 1):50, 1996.

68. Pavone P et al: MR cholangiopancreatography: Technique, indications and clinical results. Radiologia Medica 94:632, 1997.

69. Keiding S et al: Detection of cholangiocarcinoma in primary sclerosing cholangitis by positron emission tomography. Hepatology 28:700, 1998.

70. Berr F et al: Detection of cholangiocarcinoma in primary sclerosing cholangitis by positron emission tomography [letter]. Hepatology 29:611, 1999.

71. Okazumi S et al: Evaluation of the cases of benign disease with high accumulation on the examination of 18F-fluorodeoxyglucose PET. Kaku Igaku 30:1439, 1993.

72. Collins BT et al: Correlation of CT-guided fine-needle aspiration biopsy of the liver with fluoride-18 fluorodeoxyglucose positron emission tomography in the assessment of metastatic hepatic abnormalities. Diagn Cytopathol 21:39, 1999.

73. JADVAR H: Evaluation of rare tumors with [F-18] flurodeoxyglucose positron emission tomography. Clin Pos Imag 2:153, 1999.

74. HONG SS et al: Clinical usefulness of lymphoscintigraphy by rectal submucosal injection of radioactive colloid. Radioisotopes 32:546, 1983.

75. MISCUSI G et al: Endoscopic lymphoscintigraphy. A new tool for target surgery of rectal cancer. Surg Endosc 1:113, 1987.

76. AKHURST T et al: A comparison of reconstruction algorithms with FDG PET. Iterative reconstruction segmented attenuation correction (IRSAC) allows greater detectability than filtered back projection (FBP) (abstract). Eur J Nucl Med 26:1027, 1999.

77. SCHIEPERS C et al: The effect of preoperative radiation therapy on glucose utilization and cell kinetics in patients with primary rectal carcinoma. Cancer 85:803, 1999.

78. LARSON S et al: Tumor treatment response based on Visual and Quantitative Changes in Global tumor Glycolysis using FDG PET Imaging: The Visual response Score (VRS), and the change in total Lesion Glycolysis (dTLG). Clinical Positron Imaging 2:159, 1999.

79. DIVGI CR et al: Phase I/II radioimmunotherapy trial with iodine-131-labeled monoclonal antibody G250 in metastatic renal cell carcinoma. Clin Cancer Res 4:2729, 1998.

80. HARNEY JV et al: Uptake of 2-deoxy, 2-(18F) fluoro-D-glucose in bladder cancer: Animal localization and initial patient positron emission tomography. J Urol 145:279, 1991.

81. CABANAS RM: An approach for the treatment of penile carcinoma. Cancer 39:456, 1977.

82. GRABSTALD H: Controversies concerning lymph node dissection for cancer of the penis. Urol Clin North Am 7:793, 1980.

83. CATALONA WJ: Role of lymphadenectomy in carcinoma of the penis. Urol Clin North Am 7:785, 1980.

84. PERINETTI E et al: Unreliability of sentinel lymph node biopsy for staging penile carcinoma. J Urol 124:734, 1980.

85. PETTAWAY CA et al: Sentinel lymph node dissection for penile carcinoma: The M.D. Anderson Cancer Center experience. J Urol 154:1999, 1995.

86. HINKLE GH et al: Multicenter radioimmunoscintigraphic evaluation of patients with prostate carcinoma using indium-111 capromab pendetide. Cancer 83:739, 1998.

87. HASEMAN MK: Capromab pendetide imaging of occult lymph node metastases (editorial; comment). J Nucl Med 39:653, 1998.

88. IMBRIACO M et al: A new parameter for measuring metastatic bone involvement by prostate cancer: The Bone Scan Index. Clin Cancer Res 4:1765, 1998.

89. ROSSLEIGH MA et al: Serial bone scans in the assessment of response to therapy in advanced breast carcinoma. Clini Nucl Med 7:397, 1982.

90. POLLEN JJ et al: The flare phenomenon on radionuclide bone scan in metastatic prostate cancer. AJR 142:773, 1984.

91. COOK GJ et al: Detection of bone metastases in breast cancer by 18FDG PET: Differing metabolic activity in osteoblastic and osteolytic lesions. J Clin Oncol 16:3375, 1998.

92. AGUS DB et al: Positron emission tomography of a human prostate cancer xenograft: Association of changes in deoxyglucose accumulation with other measures of outcome following androgen withdrawal. Cancer Res 58:3009, 1998.

93. OSMAN I et al: 18-Fluorinated deoxy glucose (FDG) positron emission tomography (PET) in metastatic prostate cancer patients treated with systemic therapy. ASCO 17:1379, 1999.

94. OYAMA N et al: Fluorodeoxyglucose positron emission tomography in diagnosis of untreated prostate cancer. Nippon Rinsho. Japanese J Clini Med 56:2052, 1998.

95. SHREVE PD et al: Metastatic Prostate cancer: Initial findings of PET with 2-deoxy-2-[F-18]fluoro-D-glucose. Radiology 199:751, 1996.

96. YEH SD et al: Detection of bony metastases of androgen-independent prostate cancer by PET-FDG. Nucl Med Biol 23:693, 1996.

97. HOFER C et al: Fluorine-18-fluorodeoxyglucose positron emission tomography is useless for the detection of local recurrence after radical prostatectomy. Eur Urol 36:31, 1999.

98. HEICAPPELL R et al: Staging of pelvic lymph nodes in neoplasms of the bladder and prostate by positron emission tomography with 2-[(18)F]-2-deoxy-D-glucose. Eur Urol 36:582, 1999.

99. HARA T et al: PET imaging of prostate cancer using carbon-11-choline. J Nucl Med 39:990, 1998.

100. PECHER C: Biological Investigations with radioactive calcium and strontium: Preliminary report on the use of radioactive strontium in the treatment of metastatic bone cancer. U Cal Pub Pharmacol 11:117, 1942.

101. ROBINSON RG et al: Treatment of metastatic bone pain with strontium-89. Int J Rad Appl Instrum B 14:219, 1987.

102. BLAKE GM et al: Sr-89 therapy: Strontium kinetics in disseminated carcinoma of the prostate. Eur J Nucl Med 12:447, 1986.

103. MANETOU A, LIMOURLS GS: Prediction of tumor absorbed dose by Tc-99m-MDP scintigraphy prior to treatment with Sr-89. Anticancer Res 17:1845, 1997.

104. FREIDELL H, STORAASLI J: The use of radioactive phosphorous in the treatment of carcinoma of the breast with widespread metastases to bone. AJR 64:559, 1950.

105. MARSHAK A: Uptake of radioactive phosphorous by nuclei of liver an tumors. Science 92:460, 1940.

106. FIRUSIAN N, SCHMIDT CG: Radioactive strontium for treating incurable pain in skeletal neoplasms (author's transl). Dtsch Med Wochenschr 98:2347, 1973.

107. QUILTY PM et al: A comparison of the palliative effects of strontium-89 and external beam radiotherapy in metastatic prostate cancer. Radiother Oncol 31:33, 1994.

108. PORTER AT, McEWAN AJ: Strontium-89 as an adjuvant to external beam radiation improves pain relief and delays disease progression in advanced prostate cancer: Results of a randomized controlled trial. Semin Oncol 20(Suppl 2):38, 1993.

109. PORTER AT et al: Results of a randomized phase-III trial to evaluate the efficacy of strontium-89 adjuvant to local field external beam irradiation in the management of endocrine resistant metastatic prostate cancer. Int J Radiat Oncol Biol Phys 25:805, 1993.

110. HILLNER BE et al: American Society of Clinical Oncology guideline on the role of bisphosphonates in breast cancer. American Society of Clinical Oncology Bisphosphonates Expert Panel. J Clin Oncol 18:1378, 2000.

111. MAXON HR et al: Rhenium-186(Sn)HEDP for treatment of painful osseous metastases: Results of a double-blind crossover comparison with placebo. J Nucl Med 32:1877, 1991.

112. MAXON HR et al: Rhenium-188(Sn)HEDP for treatment of osseous metastases. J Nucl Med 39:659, 1998.

113. SERAFINI AN et al: Palliation of pain associated with metastatic bone cancer using samarium-153 lexidronam: A double-blind placebo-controlled clinical trial. J Clin Onco 16:1574, 1998.

114. TIAN JH et al: Multicentre trial on the efficacy and toxicity of single-dose samarium-153-ethylene diamine tetramethylene

phosphonate as a palliative treatment for painful skeletal metastases in China. Eur J Nucl Medi 26:2, 1999.

115. SRIVASTAVA SC et al: Treatment of metastatic bone pain with tin-117m stannic diethylenetriaminepentaacetic acid: A phase I/II clinical study. Clin Cancer Res 4:61, 1998.

116. WARREN GP, EINHORN LH: Gallium scans in the evaluation of residual masses after chemotherapy for seminoma. J Clin Oncol 13:2784, 1995.

117. FOSSA SD et al: Is postchemotherapy retroperitoneal surgery necessary in patients with nonseminomatous testicular cancer and minimal residual tumor masses? J Clin Oncol 10:569, 1992.

118. STEPHENS AW et al: Positron emission tomography evaluation of residual radiographic abnormalities in postchemotherapy germ cell tumor patients. J Clin Oncol 14:1637, 1996.

119. HERR HW et al: Surgery for a post-chemotherapy residual mass in seminoma. J Urol 157:860, 1997.

120. PUC HS et al: Management of residual mass in advanced seminoma: Results and recommendations from the Memorial Sloan-Kettering Cancer Center (see comments). J Clin Oncol 14:454, 1996.

121. DE HULLU JA et al: Sentinel lymph node procedure is highly accurate in squamous cell carcinoma of the vulva. J Clin Oncol 18(15):2811, 2000.

122. ROSE PG et al: Positron emission tomography for evaluating para-aortic nodal metastasis in locally advanced cervical cancer before surgical staging: A surgicopathologic study. J Clin Oncol 17:41, 1999.

123. SUGAWARA Y et al: Evaluation of FDG PET in patients with cervical cancer. J Nucl Med 40:1125, 1999.

124. MORAIS J et al: Anti-beta HCG abdominopelvic immunoscintigraphy in patients with resistant gestational trophoblastic disease. Nucl Med Commun 13:464, 1992.

125. ROMER W et al: Metabolic characterization of ovarian tumors with positron-emission tomography and F-18 fluorodeoxyglucose. Rofo Fortschr Geb Rontgenstr Neuen Bildgeb Verfahr 166:62, 1997.

126. ZIMMY M et al: 18F-Fluorodeoxyglucose PET in ovarian carcinoma: Methodology and preliminary results. Nuklearmedizin 36:228, 1997.

127. FENCHEL S et al: Preoperative assessment of asymptomatic adnexal tumors by positron emission tomography and F 18 fluorodeoxyglucose. Nuklearmedizin 38:101, 1999.

128. HUBNER KF et al: Assessment of primary and metastatic ovarian cancer by positron emission tomography (PET) using 2-[18F]deoxyglucose (2-[18F]FDG). Gynecol Oncol 51:197, 1993.

129. CAIN JM et al: A review of second-look laparotomy for ovarian cancer. Gynecol Oncol 23:14, 1986.

130. NICOLETTO MO et al: Surgical second look in ovarian cancer: A randomized study in patients with laparoscopic complete remission—A Northeastern Oncology Cooperative Group–Ovarian Cancer Cooperative Group Study. J Clin Oncol 15:994, 1997.

131. BARAKAT RR et al: A phase II trial of intraperitoneal cisplatin and etoposide as consolidation therapy in patients with stage II-IV epithelial ovarian cancer following negative surgical assessment. Gynecol Oncol 69:17, 1998.

132. MARKMAN M et al: Impact on survival of surgically defined favorable responses to salvage intraperitoneal chemotherapy in small-volume residual ovarian cancer. J Clin Oncol 10:1479, 1992.

133. HIRD V et al: Intraperitoneally administered 90Y-labelled monoclonal antibodies as a third line of treatment in ovarian cancer. A phase 1-2 trial: Problems encountered and possible solutions. Br J Cancer Suppl 10:48, 1990.

134. STEWART JS et al: Intraperitoneal radioimmunotherapy for ovarian cancer: Pharmacokinetics, toxicity, and efficacy of I-131 labeled monoclonal antibodies. Int J Radiat Oncol Biol Phys 16:405, 1989.

135. NICHOLSON S et al: Radioimmunotherapy after chemotherapy compared to chemotherapy alone in the treatment of advanced ovarian cancer: A matched analysis. Oncol Rep 5:223, 1998.

136. SCOPINARO F et al: A three center study on the diagnostic accuracy of 99m Tc-MIBI scintimammography. Anticancer Res 17:1631, 1997.

137. PALMEDO H et al: Scintimammography with technetium-99m methoxyisobutylisonitrile: Results of a prospective European multicentre trial. Eur J Nucl Med 25:375, 1998.

138. FENLON HM et al: Tc-99m tetrofosmin scintigraphy as an adjunct to plain-film mammography in palpable breast lesions. Clini Radiol 53:17, 1998.

139. ALLEN MW et al: A study on the cost effectiveness of sestamibi scintimammography for screening women with dense breasts for breast cancer. Breast Cancer Res Treat 55:243, 1999.

140. CARVALHO PA et al: Subcellular distribution and analysis of technetium-99m-MIBI in isolated perfused rat hearts. J Nucl Med 33:1516, 1992.

141. PIWNICA WORMS D et al: Functional imaging of multidrug-resistant P-glycoprotein with an organotechnetium complex. Cancer Res 53:977, 1993.

142. CWIKLA JB et al: The effect of chemotherapy on the uptake of technetium-99m sestamibi in breast cancer. Eur J Nucl Med 24:1175, 1997.

143. CWIKLA JB et al: Correlation between uptake of Tc-99m sestaMIBI and prognostic factors of breast cancer. Anticancer Res 19:2299, 1999.

144. OMAR WS et al: Role of thallium-201 chloride and Tc-99m methoxy-isobutyl-isonitrite (sestaMIBI) in evaluation of breast masses: Correlation with the immunohistochemical characteristic parameters (Ki-67, PCNA, Bcl, and angiogenesis) in malignant lesions. Anticancer Res 17:1639, 1997.

145. URBAN JA, CASTRO EB: Selecting variations in extent of surgical procedure for breast cancer. Cancer 28:1615, 1971.

146. HILL AD et al: Lessons learned from 500 cases of lymphatic mapping for breast cancer (see comments). Ann Surg 229:528, 1999.

147. VERONESI U et al: Sentinel-node biopsy to avoid axillary dissection in breast cancer with clinically negative lymph-nodes (see comments). Lancet 349:1864, 1997.

148. GIULIANO AE et al: Lymphatic mapping and sentinel lymphadenectomy for breast cancer (see comments). Ann Surg 220:391; discussion 398, 1994.

149. ALBERTINI JJ et al: Lymphatic mapping and sentinel node biopsy in the patient with breast cancer (see comments). JAMA 276:1818, 1996.

150. PAGANELLI G et al: Optimized sentinel node scintigraphy in breast cancer. Q J Nucl Med 42:49, 1998.

151. VERONESI U et al: Sentinel lymph node biopsy and axillary dissection in breast cancer: Results in a large series (see comments). J Natl Cancer Inst 91:368, 1999.

152. SCHNEEBAUM S et al: Gamma probe-guided sentinel node biopsy: Optimal timing for injection. Eur J Surg Oncol 24:515, 1998.

153. UREN RF et al: Mammary lymphoscintigraphy in breast cancer (see comments). J Nucl Med 36:1775, 1995.

154. LINEHAN DC et al: Sentinel lymph node biopsy in breast cancer: Unfiltered radioisotope is superior to filtered. J Am Coll Surg 188:377, 1999.

155. ROUMEN RM et al: In search of the true sentinel node by different injection techniques in breast cancer patients. Eur J Surg Oncol 25:347, 1999.

156. International (Ludwig) Breast Cancer Study Group (see comments). Prognostic importance of occult axillary lymph node micrometastases from breast cancers. Lancet 335:1565, 1990.

157. LINEHAN DC et al: Intradermal radiocolloid and intraparenchymal blue dye injection optimize sentinel node identification in breast cancer patients (see comments). Ann Surg Oncol 6:450, 1999.

158. DIXON M: Sentinel node biopsy in breast cancer: A promising technique, but it should not be introduced without proper trials (editorial). BMJ 317:295, 1998.

159. COLEMAN RE et al: Selection of patients with breast cancer for routine follow-up bone scans. Clin Oncol 2:328, 1990.

160. COX MR et al: An evaluation of radionuclide bone scanning and liver ultrasonography for staging breast cancer. Aus N Z J Surg 62:550, 1992.

161. JACOBSON AF et al: Association between number and sites of new bone scan abnormalities and presence of skeletal metastases in patients with breast cancer. J Nucl Med 31:387, 1990.

162. ALCAN KE et al: Early detection of anthracycline-induced cardiotoxicity by stress radionuclide cineangiography in conjunction with Fourier amplitude and phase analysis. Clin Nucl Med 10:160, 1985.

163. PENG NJ et al: Clinical decision making based on radionuclide determined ejection fraction in oncology patients. J Nucl Med 38:702, 1997.

164. VON HOFF DD et al: Risk factors for doxorubicin-induced congestive heart failure. Ann Int Med 91:710, 1979.

165. MINTUN MA et al: Breast cancer: PET imaging of estrogen receptors. Radiology 169:45, 1988.

166. MINN H, SOINI I: [18F]Fluorodeoxyglucose scintigraphy in diagnosis and follow up of treatment in advanced breast cancer. Eur J Nucl Med 15:61, 1989.

167. WAHL RL et al: Primary and metastatic breast carcinoma: Initial clinical evaluation with PET with the radiolabeled glucose analogue 2-[F-18]-fluoro-2-deoxy-D-glucose. Radiology 179:765, 1991.

168. KUBOTA K et al: Imaging of breast cancer with [18F]fluorodeoxyglucose and positron emission tomography. J Comput Assist Tomogr 13:1097, 1989.

169. AVRIL N et al: Metabolic characterization of breast tumors with positron emission tomography using F-18 fluorodeoxyglucose. J Clin Oncol 14:1848, 1996.

170. AVRIL N et al: Assessment of axillary lymph node involvement in breast cancer patients with positron emission tomography using radiolabeled 2-(fluorine-18)-fluoro-2-deoxy-D-glucose. J Natl Cancer Instit 88:1204, 1996.

171. WAHL RL et al: Metabolic monitoring of breast cancer chemohormonotherapy using positron emission tomography: Initial evaluation. J Clin Oncol 11:2101, 1993.

172. BRUCE DM et al: Positron emission tomography: 2-deoxy-2-[18F]-fluoro-D-glucose uptake in locally advanced breast cancers. Eur J Surg Oncol 21:280, 1995.

173. JANSSON T et al: Positron emission tomography studies in patients with locally advanced and/or metastatic breast cancer: A method for early therapy evaluation? J Clin Oncol 13:1470, 1995.

174. BASSA P et al: Evaluation of preoperative chemotherapy using PET with fluorine-18-fluorodeoxyglucose in breast cancer. J Nucl Med 37:931, 1996.

175. SMITH IC et al: Positron emission tomography using [(18)F]-fluorodeoxy-D-glucose to predict the pathologic response of breast cancer to primary chemotherapy. J Clin Oncol 18:1676, 2000 (record as supplied by publisher).

176. SCHELLING M et al: Positron emission tomography using [(18)F]fluorodeoxyglucose for monitoring primary chemotherapy in breast cancer. J Clin Oncol 18:1689, 2000 (record as supplied by publisher).

177. DEHDASHTI F et al: Positron emission tomographic assessment of metabolic flare to predict response of metastatic breast cancer to antiestrogen therapy. Eur J Nucl Med 26:51, 1999.

178. DEHDASHTI F et al: Positron tomographic assessment of estrogen receptors in breast cancer: Comparison with FDG-PET and in vitro receptor assays. J Nucl Med 36:1766, 1995.

179. SILBERSTEIN EB et al: Phosphorus-32 radiopharmaceuticals for the treatment of painful osseous metastases. Semin Nucl Med 22:17, 1992.

180. NAIR N: Relative efficacy of 32P and 89Sr in palliation in skeletal metastases. J Nucl Med 40:256, 1999.

181. MCEWAN AJ: Unsealed source therapy of painful bone metastases: An update. Sem Nucl Med 27:165, 1997.

182. PALERMO F, PATRESE P: Detection of neoplastic lesions with radiogallium (67 Ga citrate): Clinical-statistical report on 125 cases. Radiol Clin Biol 43:509, 1974.

183. COX PH et al: Thallium 201 chloride uptake in tumours: A possible complication in heart scintigraphy. Br J Radiol 49:767, 1976.

184. BLATT CJ et al: Soft-tissue sarcoma: Imaged with technetium-99m pyrophosphate. NY State J Med 77:2118, 1977.

185. GARCIA R et al: Comparison of fluorine-18-FDG PET and technetium-99m-MIBI SPECT in evaluation of musculoskeletal sarcomas. J Nucl Med 37:1476, 1996.

186. FRIEDBERG JW et al: Uptake of radiolabeled somatostatin analog is detectable in patients with metastatic foci of sarcoma. Cancer 86:1621, 1999.

187. YAMAMOTO Y et al: Iodine-123 BMIPP and Ga-67 scintigraphy in liposarcoma. Clin Nucl Med 23:609, 1998.

188. KERN KA et al: Metabolic imaging of human extremity musculoskeletal tumors by PET. J Nucl Med 29:181, 1988.

189. SCHWARZBACH MH et al: Clinical value of [18-F] fluorodeoxyglucose positron emission tomography imaging in soft tissue sarcomas. Ann Surg 231:380, 2000.

190. SUMIYA H et al: Midcourse thallium-201 scintigraphy to predict tumor response in bone and soft-tissue tumors. J Nucl Med 39:1600, 1998.

191. JONES DN et al: Monitoring of neoadjuvant therapy response of soft-tissue and musculoskeletal sarcoma using fluorine-18-FDG PET. J Nucl Med 37:1438, 1996.

192. VAN GINKEL RJ et al: FDG-PET to evaluate response to hyperthermic isolated limb perfusion for locally advanced soft-tissue sarcoma. J Nucl Med 37:984, 1996.

193. DWORKIN HJ, FILMANOWICZ EV: Radiofluoride photoscanning of bone for reticulum cell sarcoma. Early detection of bone involvement. JAMA 198:985, 1966.

194. FREY KW et al: Bone scintigraphy using strontium 85 and its clinical significance. Med Klin 62:978, 1967.

195. HOLSTI LR, PATOMAKI LK: 18F scanning of primary and

metastatic bone tumours. Ann Med Intern Fenn 56(3): 1967; 56:131,1967.

196. RAMANNA L et al: Thallium-201 scintigraphy in bone sarcoma: Comparison with gallium-67 and technetium-MDP in the evaluation of chemotherapeutic response. J Nucl Med 31:567, 1990.

197. TOBES MC et al: Effect of uptake-one inhibitors on the uptake of norepinephrine and metaiodobenzylguanidine. J Nucl Med 26:897, 1985.

198. SHULKIN BL et al: Pheochromocytomas: Imaging with 2-[fluorine-18]fluoro-2-deoxy-D-glucose PET. Radiology 212: 35, 1999.

199. NGUYEN HH et al: Tumour size: The only predictive factor for 131I MIBG uptake in pheochromocytoma and paraganglioma. Aust N Z J Surg 69:350, 1999.

200. LYNN MD et al: Pheochromocytoma and the normal adrenal medulla: Improved visualization with I-123 MIBG scintigraphy. Radiology 155:789, 1985.

201. SHAPIRO B et al: Radiopharmaceutical therapy of malignant pheochromocytoma with [131I]metaiodobenzylguanidine: Results from ten years of experience. J Nucl Biol Med 35:269, 1991.

202. SCHLUMBERGER M et al: Malignant pheochromocytoma: Clinical, biological, histologic and therapeutic data in a series of 20 patients with distant metastases. J Endocrinol Invest 15:631, 1992.

203. TRONCONE L, RUFFINI V: Nuclear medicine therapy of pheochromocytoma and paraganglioma. Q J Nucl Med 43:344, 1999.

204. SISSON JC et al: Treatment of malignant pheochromocytomas with 131-I metaiodobenzylguanidine and chemotherapy. Am J Clin Oncol 22:364, 1999.

205. YEH SD et al: Radioimmunodetection of neuroblastoma with iodine-131-3F8: Correlation with biopsy, iodine-131-metaiodobenzylguanidine and standard diagnostic modalities. J Nucl Med 32:769, 1991.

206. CHEUNG NK et al: Anti-G(D2) antibody treatment of minimal residual stage 4 neuroblastoma diagnosed at more than 1 year of age. J Clin Oncol 16:3053, 1998.

207. SZOLAR DH et al: Computed tomography evaluation of adrenal masses. Curr Opin Urol 9:143, 1999.

208. McNICHOLAS MM et al: An imaging algorithm for the differential diagnosis of adrenal adenomas and metastases. AJR 165:1453, 1995.

209. ERASMUS JJ et al: Evaluation of adrenal masses in patients with bronchogenic carcinoma using 18F-fluorodeoxyglucose positron emission tomography (see comments). AJR 168:1357, 1997.

210. PARTHASARATHY KL et al: Localization of metastatic adrenal carcinoma utilizing 67Ga-citrate. Clin Nucl Med 3:24, 1978.

211. GROSS MD et al: The relationship of I-131 6 beta-iodomethyl-19-norcholesterol (NP-59) adrenal cortical uptake to indices of androgen secretion in women with hyperandrogenism. Clin Nucl Med 9:264, 1984.

212. HOWMAN-GILES R et al: Ga-67 scintigraphy in a child with adrenocortical carcinoma. Clin Nucl Med 18:642, 1993.

213. KAO CH et al: I-131 NP-59 adrenal cortical scintigraphy in suspected primary aldosteronism. Kao-Hsiung I Hsueh Ko Hsueh Tsa Chih (Kaohsiung Journal Of Medical Sciences) 8:213, 1992.

214. GREGIANIN M et al: Nuclear medicine methods for the diagnosis of adrenal tumors. Minerva Endocrinol 20:27, 1995.

215. SCHUMACHER T et al: Imaging of an adrenal cortex carcinoma and its metastasis with FDG-PET. Nuklearmedizin 38:124, 1999.

216. WENTZ KU et al: Malignant pleural mesothelioma: Value of 67Ga scintigraphy compared to computerized tomography. ROFO Fortschr Geb Rontgenstr Nuklearmed 145:61, 1986.

217. GUERIN RA et al: Diagnosis of intrathoracic malignant tumors by means of gallium 67 isotope scanning; Limitations of the method. Nouv Presse Med 2:981, 1973.

218. CARRETTA A et al: 18-FDG positron emission tomography in the evaluation of malignant pleural diseases: A pilot study. Eur J Cardiothorac Surg 17:377, 2000.

219. BUCHMANN I et al: F-18-FDG PET for primary diagnosis differential diagnosis of pleural processes. Nuklearmedizin 38:319, 1999.

220. BENARD F et al: Prognostic value of FDG PET imaging in malignant pleural mesothelioma. J Nucl Med 40:1241, 1999.

221. BENARD F et al: Metabolic imaging of malignant pleural mesothelioma with fluorodeoxyglucose positron emission tomography (see comments) Chest 114:713, 1998.

222. KEYES JWJ: SUV: Standard uptake or silly useless value? J Nucl Med 36:1836, 1995.

223. BRADY LW: Mesothelioma: The role for radiation therapy. Semin Oncol 8:329, 1981.

224. ANDREWS GA et al: Ga-67 citrate imaging in malignant lymphoma: Final report of cooperative group. J Nucl Med 19:1013, 1978.

225. KAPLAN W et al: High dose gallium in the evaluation of lymphoma. J Nucl Med 25:P50, 1983.

226. JOHNSTON GS et al: Gallium-67 citrate imaging in Hodgkin's disease: Final report of cooperative group. J Nucl Med 18:692, 1977.

227. ANDERSON KC et al: High-dose gallium imaging in lymphoma. Am J Med 75:327, 1983.

228. EDWARDS CL, HAYES RL: Tumor scanning with 67Ga citrate. J Nucl Med 10:103, 1969.

229. JANICEK M et al: Early restaging gallium scans predict outcome in poor-prognosis patients with aggressive non-Hodgkin's lymphoma treated with high-dose CHOP chemotherapy. J Clin Oncol 15:1631, 1997.

230. FRONT D et al: Hodgkin disease: Prediction of outcome with 67Ga scintigraphy after one cycle of chemotherapy. Radiology 210:487, 1999.

231. WILLKOMM P et al: Functional imaging of Hodgkin's disease with FDG-PET and gallium-67. Nuklearmedizin 37:251, 1998.

232. HOFFMANN M et al: Positron emission tomography with fluorine-18-2-fluoro-2-deoxy-D-glucose (F18-FDG) does not visualize extranodal B-cell lymphoma of the mucosa-associated lymphoid tissue (MALT)-type. Ann Oncol 10:1185, 1999.

233. RÖMER W et al: Positron emission tomography in non-Hodgkin's lymphoma: Assessment of chemotherapy with fluorodeoxyglucose. Blood 91:4464, 1998.

234. QUINN JD Analysis of 96 abnormal brain scans using technetium 99m (pertechnetate form). JAMA 194:157, 1965.

235. HOSAIN F et al: Ytterbium-169 diethylenetriaminepentaacetic acid complex: A new radiopharmaceutical for brain scanning. Radiology 91:1294, 1968.

236. HOOP B et al: Techniques for positron scintigraphy of the brain. J Nucl Med 17:473, 1976.

237. ANCRI D, BASSET JY: Diagnosis of cerebral metastases by thallium 201. Br J Radiol 53:443, 1980.

238. ANCRI D et al: Diagnosis of cerebral lesions by thallium 201. Radiology 128:417, 1978.

239. TOMURA N et al: Thallium-201 single photon emission computed tomography in the evaluation of therapeutic response for brain tumors. Kaku Igaku 31:951, 1994.

240. KAPLAN WD et al: Thallium-201 brain tumor imaging: A comparative study with pathologic correlation. J Nucl Med 28:47, 1987.

241. BLACK KL et al: Use of thallium-201 SPECT to quantitate malignancy grade of gliomas. J Neurosurg 71:342, 1989.

242. KIM KT et al: Thallium-201 SPECT imaging of brain tumors: Methods and results (see comments). J Nucl Med 31:965, 1990.

243. ORIUCHI N et al: Clinical evaluation of thallium-201 SPECT in supratentorial gliomas: Relationship to histologic grade, prognosis and proliferative activities (see comments). J Nucl Med 34:2085, 1993.

244. TAKI S et al: 201 TI SPECT in the differential diagnosis of brain tumours. Nucl Med Commun 20:637, 1999.

245. DI CHIRO G: Positron emission tomography using [18F] fluorodeoxyglucose in brain tumors: A powerful diagnostic and prognostic tool. Invest Radio 22:360, 1987.

246. COOK GJ et al: Normal variants, artefacts and interpretative pitfalls in PET imaging with 18-fluoro-2-deoxyglucose and carbon-11 methionine. Eur J Nucl Med 26:1363, 1999.

247. TAYLOR I: Liver metastases from colorectal cancer: lessons from past and present clinical studies. Br J Surg 83:456, 1996.

248. D'ANGELICA M et al: Ninety-six five-year survivors after liver resection for metastatic colorectal cancer. J Am Coll Surg 185:554, 1997.

249. DELBEKE D et al: Staging recurrent metastatic colorectal carcinoma with PET. J Nucl Med 38:1196, 1997.

250. SOYER P et al: False-positive CT portography: Correlation with pathologic findings. AJR 160:285, 1993.

251. SOYER P et al: Hepatic metastases from colorectal cancer: Detection and false-positive findings with helical CT during arterial portography. Radiology 193:71, 1994.

252. LAI DT et al: The role of whole-body positron emission tomography with [18F] fluorodeoxyglucose in identifying operable colorectal cancer metastases to the liver. Arch Surg 131:703, 1996.

253. SCHIEPERS C et al: Contribution of PET in the diagnosis of recurrent colorectal cancer: Comparison with conventional imaging. Eur J Surg Oncol 21:517, 1995.

254. VALK PE et al: Whole-body PET imaging with [18F] fluorodeoxyglucose in management of recurrent colorectal cancer. Arch Surg 134:503; discussion 511, 1999.

255. FLAMEN P et al: Additional value of whole-body positron emission tomography with fluorine-18:2-Fluoro-2-deoxy-D-glucose in recurrent colorectal cancer. J Clin Oncol 17:894, 1999.

256. ITO K et al: Recurrent rectal cancer and scar: Differentiation with PET and MR imaging. Radiology 182:549, 1992.

257. LEHNER B et al: The value of positron emission tomography in diagnosis of recurrent rectal cancer. Zentralbl Chir 115:813, 1990.

258. COLAGRANDE S et al: Role of CT and RM in postoperative evaluation of the patient after rectal carcinoma surgery: Postoperative anatomy and nonneoplastic sequelae. Radiol Med (Torino) 89:250, 1995.

259. SOVIK E et al: Postirradiation changes in the pelvic wall: Findings on MR. Acta Radiol 34:573, 1993.

260. GUALDI GF et al: MR in rectal cancer recurrences. Radiol Med (Torino) 79:479, 1990.

261. KRESTIN GP: Diagnosis of recurrent rectal cancer: Comparison of CT and MR. ROFO Fortschr Geb Rontgenstr Nuklearmed 148:28, 1988.

262. FONG Y et al: Utility of 18F-FDG positron emission tomography scanning on selection of patients for resection of hepatic colorectal metastases. Am J Surg 178:282, 1999.

263. SHEPHERD NA et al: The prognostic importance of peritoneal involvement in colonic cancer: A prospective evaluation (see comments). Gastroenterology 112:1096, 1997.

264. KEMENY N et al: Hepatic arterial infusion of chemotherapy after resection of hepatic metastases from colorectal cancer. N Engl J Med 341:2039, 1999.

265. GORLICK R, BERTINO JR: Drug resistance in colon cancer. Semin Oncol 26:606, 1999.

266. BORZUTZKY CA, TURBINER EH: The predictive value of hepatic artery perfusion scintigraphy. J Nucl Med 26:1153, 1985.

267. LEHNER B et al: Results of liver angiography and perfusion scintigraphy do not correlate with response to hepatic artery infusion chemotherapy. J Surg Oncol 39:73, 1988.

268. KATAYAMA M et al: Hepatic arterial perfusion scintigraphy with 99mTc-MAA for assessment of the hepatic distribution of drugs given by intrahepatic arterial infusion. Kaku Igaku 33:233, 1996.

269. KISSEL J et al: Pharmacokinetic analysis of 5-[18F]fluorouracil tissue concentrations measured with positron emission tomography in patients with liver metastases from colorectal adenocarcinoma. Cancer Res 57:3415, 1997.

270. MCLOUGHLIN RF et al: CT of the liver after cryotherapy of hepatic metastases: Imaging findings. AJR 165:329, 1995.

271. KUSZYK BS et al: Hepatic tumors treated by cryosurgery: Normal CT appearance. AJR 166:363, 1996.

272. SIPERSTEIN A et al: Local recurrence after laparoscopic radiofrequency thermal ablation of hepatic tumors (see comments) Ann Surg Oncol 7:106, 2000.

273. AKHURST T et al: Flurodeoxyglucose(FDG) positron emission tomography(PET) immediately post hepatic cryotherapy predicts recurrence of tumour in the liver. Proc Ann Meeting ASCO 18:625a, 1999.

274. STRIBLEY KV et al: Internal radiotherapy for hepatic metastases II: The blood supply to hepatic metastases. J Surg Res 34:25, 1983.

275. WANG SJ et al: Hepatic artery injection of yttrium-90-lipiodol: biodistribution in rats with hepatoma. J Nucl Med 37:332, 1996.

276. YCHOU M et al: Potential contribution of 131I-labelled monoclonal anti-CEA antibodies in the treatment of liver metastases from colorectal carcinomas: Pretherapeutic study with dose recovery in resected tissues. Eur J Cancer 29A:1105, 1993.

277. BHATTACHARYA S et al: Epirubicin-lipiodol chemotherapy versus 131 iodine: lipiodol radiotherapy in the treatment of unresectable hepatocellular carcinoma. Cancer 76:2202, 1995.

278. TULCHINSKY M, EGGLI DF: Intraperitoneal distribution imaging prior to chromic phosphate (P-32) therapy in ovarian cancer patients. Clin Nucl Med 19:43, 1994.

279. DE FOMI M et al: Anatomic changes in the abdominal cavity during intraperitoneal chemotherapy: Prospective study using scintigraphic peritoneography. Bull Cancer 80:345, 1993.

280. ARNSTEIN NB et al: Adenocarcinoma of the alimentary tract: Peritoneal distribution scintigraphy. Radiology 162:439, 1987.

281. SULLIVAN DC et al: Observations on the intraperitoneal

distribution of chromic phosphate (32P) suspension for intraperitoneal therapy. Radiology 146:539, 1983.

282. OTT RJ et al: The measurement of radiation doses from P32 chromic phosphate therapy of the peritoneum using SPECT. Eur J Nucl Med 11:305, 1985.

283. McGOWAN L: Adjuvant intraperitoneal chromic phosphate therapy in a woman with early ovarian carcinoma and pelvic infection with resulting catastrophic complications. Clin Nucl Med 19:696, 1994.

284. PETERS WA et al: Intraperitoneal P-32 is not an effective consolidation therapy after a negative second-look laparotomy for epithelial carcinoma of the ovary. Gynecol Oncol 47:146, 1992.

285. CRIPPA F et al: Single-dose intraperitoneal radioimmunotherapy with the murine monoclonal antibody I-131 MOv18: Clinical results in patients with minimal residual disease of ovarian cancer. Eur J Cancer 31A:686, 1995.

286. ROSENBLUM MG et al: Clinical pharmacology, metabolism, and tissue distribution of 90Y-labeled monoclonal antibody B72.3 after intraperitoneal administration (see comments). J Natl Cancer Inst 83:1629, 1991.

287. STEWART JS et al: Intraperitoneal 131 I- and 90Y-labelled monoclonal antibodies for ovarian cancer: Pharmocokinetics and normal tissue dosimetry. Int J Cancer Suppl 3:71, 1988.

288. EAGLE KA et al: Combining clinical and thallium data optimizes preoperative assessment of cardiac risk before major vascular surgery. Ann Intern Med 110:859, 1989.

289. ARSLAN N et al: 99Tcm-MIBI scintimammography in the evaluation of breast lesions and axillary involvement: A comparison with mammography and histopathological diagnosis. Nucl Med Commun 20:317, 1999.

290. MEKHMANDAROV S et al: Technetium-99m-MIBI scintimammography in palpable and nonpalpable breast lesions. J Nucl Med 39:86, 1998.

291. PRATS E et al: A Spanish multicenter scintigraphic study of the breast using Tc 99m MIBI: Report of results. Rev Esp Med Nucl 17:338, 1998.

292. TOLMOS J et al: Scintimammographic analysis of nonpalpable breast lesions previously identified by conventional mammography. J Natl Cancer Instit 90:846, 1998.

293. TILING R et al: Limited value of scintimammography and contrast-enhanced MRI in the evaluation of microcalcification detected by mammography. Nucl Med Commun 19:55, 1998.

294. SCOPINARO F et al: 99mTc-MIBI prone scintimammography in patients with high and intermediate risk mammography. Anticancer Res 17:1635, 1997.

295. SCOPINARO F et al: 99mTc MIBI prone scintimammography in patients with suspicious breast cancer: Relationship with mammography and tumor size. Int J Oncol 12:661, 1998.

296. BECHERER A et al: The diagnostic value of planar and SPECT scintimammography in different age groups. Nucl Commun 18:710, 1997.

297. PALMEDO H et al: Scintimammography with technetium-99m methoxyisobutylisonitrile: Comparison with mammography and magnetic resonance imaging. Eur J Nucl Med 23:940, 1996.

# 4D / PATHOLOGY AND STAGING FOR SURGICAL ONCOLOGY

*Peter M. Banks and William G. Kraybill*

## THE SURGEON AND THE PATHOLOGIST

This chapter seeks to assist the surgeon in exploring pathology as a resource for patient management. Recent decades have seen an explosion of the knowledge base of both surgery and pathology. The development of sophisticated operative techniques has engendered increasing subspecialization in surgical training, accompanied by a decline in surgeons' training and participation in pathology. Thirty years ago a typical trainee spent 6 months or more in pathology and developed familiarity with pathologists and proficiency in pathology. Today, a pathology rotation is no longer required for surgical board eligibility. Surgery is not alone in its march toward subspecialization. In academic pathology programs, the demand for scholarly productivity and research requires skills in sophisticated study methods such as immunology and molecular biology. Only a small percentage of pathology trainees and pathologists are familiar with the complexities of modern surgical oncology. In many academic programs and large private pathology groups, patients are immediately routed to one or another subspecialist. This trend toward tunnel vision undermines the clinical practice setting. As surgeons and pathologists have lost their common educational moorings, so too have they lost their ability to communicate and to support one another's role in patient care. This chapter seeks to provide the reader with an outline of the means by which surgical pathologists and surgical oncologists, working together, can improve patient care.[1]

## CASE EXAMPLES

Lessons can be learned from individual case examples. Three representative cases illustrating successes and problems in the interactions of surgeons and pathologists will be discussed. The importance of communication between the surgeon and surgical pathologist is demonstrated in these examples.

### CASE 1. METASTATIC RENAL ADENOCARCINOMA SIMULATING INFLAMMATORY PSEUDOTUMOR OF LUNG

**HISTORY.** Two years previously, a 44-year-old woman underwent radical nephrectomy for renal cortical adenocarcinoma. She had been without evidence of relapse until vague pleuritic symptoms occasioned chest x-rays showing a solitary peripheral density about 4 cm in greatest dimension in the left lateral lung field. Thorough medical evaluation revealed no evidence of disease elsewhere, and she was scheduled for thoracotomy.

**SURGEON'S ACTIONS.** At thoracotomy, a firm subpleural, sharply defined mass was identified in the lateral aspect of the left upper lobe. The pleura was not puckered by this, nor was there any roughening of the overlying pleural surface. A segmental resection was performed and the specimen was sent to the pathology laboratory with a requisition slip stating "lung tumor, left upper lobe."

**PATHOLOGIST'S ACTIONS.** Evaluation of the specimen revealed a tumor 4 × 3 × 3 cm that was mottled yellow and gray and sharply demarcated. Scrape-smear cytology preparations and frozen sections were produced. Microscopically, the frozen section showed pulmonary parenchyma replaced by a spindling proliferation with areas of plump foam cells (Fig. 4D-1*A*). These appearances suggested an inflammatory process featuring fibroblasts and histiocytes, i.e., so-called inflammatory pseudotumor or plasma cell granuloma of the lung. The pathologist communicated this impression to the surgeon over the intercom.

**SURGEON'S ACTIONS.** The surgeon asked the pathologist if this was not consistent with metastasis from the renal carcinoma, diagnosed 2 years earlier.

**PATHOLOGIST'S ACTIONS.** The pathologist expressed surprise at this suggestion, not having been previously informed of the history, and told the surgeon that a review of the findings was in order with this in mind. The frozen section was studied again with the same observations. However, review of the cytology preparation allowed recognition of definite nuclear atypia among some of the plump foamy cells, as distinct from associated benign macrophages (Fig. 4D-1*B*). The pathologist reviewed the chart and in it found the pathology report from 2 years previously. This described the renal tumor as mixed low- and high-grade composition, with areas featuring a sarcomatoid spindling growth pattern. Based on this past description, the pathologist's impression changed to metastatic carcinoma consistent with renal cortical origin. This impression was

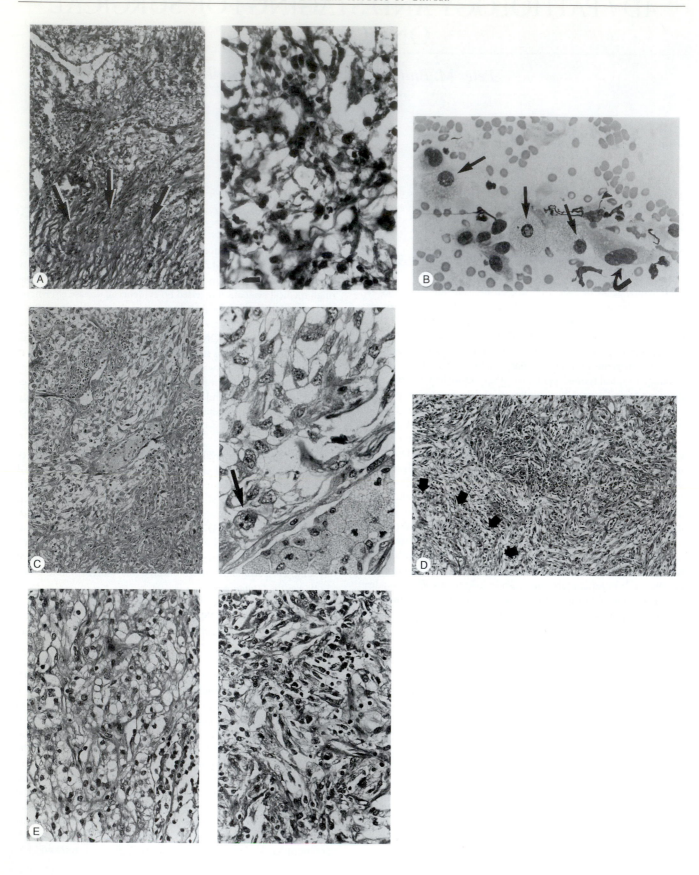

conveyed verbally to the surgeon over the intercom and documented in an intraoperative pathology report placed in the patient's chart.

**SURGEON'S ACTIONS.** Careful examination of the left lung revealed one additional small, suspicious subpleural nodule in the left middle lobe. This was removed in its entirety in another segmental resection.

**PATHOLOGIST'S ACTIONS.** The following day, permanent sections of both resected pulmonary nodules showed an overtly malignant process with a mixture of plump clear-cell epithelial features and malignant spindle cells (Fig. 4D-1C). Comparison with the original renal tumor showed similar features (Fig. 4D-1D and 4D-1E).

**OUTCOME.** The patient was told that a second small nodule of tumor had been found in the left lung but that the likelihood of further problems with tumor spread was uncertain. After 10 months without evidence of disease, there was progression of localized headaches, and a large cerebral metastasis was resected. The patient remains alive without further evidence of disease progression 4 months later.

**COMMENTS.** The pathologist's first erroneous interpretation would have been avoided if the operating room listing or pathology requisition slip had alluded to the past history of a renal carcinoma. Well-differentiated clear-cell adenocarcinomas can mimic benign foamy macrophages microscopically, so that the unwary surgeon, operating without benefit of clinical history, may accept an intraoperative diagnosis of "lipid pneumonia" or "inflammatory pseudotumor." In this case the spindling growth pattern of the sarcomatoid elements of the tumor, together with the inflammatory response in surrounding pulmonary parenchyma, gave the false impression of an inflammatory tumefactive process; i.e., so-called inflammatory pseudotumor. Because the surgeon communicated well with the pathologist from the operating room, the correct diagnosis was established intraoperatively, permitting identification of a second, radiologically inapparent metastasis. Had the pulmonary process actually been an inflammatory one, there would have been no indication for searching for additional tumors.

Renal cortical adenocarinoma is capricious in behavior. Although in this case there was subsequent metastatic disease in other organs, there are many documented cases with long sustained disease-free intervals after resection of one or even several metastases.

## CASE 2. EARLY, WELL-DIFFERENTIATED CARCINOMA OF THE BREAST IDENTIFIED BY AVOIDANCE OF INTRAOPERATIVE FROZEN SECTION

**HISTORY.** Two years previously, a 53-year-old woman underwent modified radical mastectomy for carcinoma of the right breast. Follow-up examination revealed no evidence of recurrent carcinoma; however, a subtle, ill-defined nodularity was palpable in the left (contralateral) breast, and mammography was interpreted as suspicious for malignancy.

**SURGEON'S ACTIONS.** A large, open biopsy of the suspicious quadrant was carried out. Intraoperative pathology consultation was requested.

**PATHOLOGIST'S ACTIONS.** The specimen measured 6.5 × 3.5 × 2.0 cm, and careful palpation revealed numerous small

**FIGURE 4D-1.** *A.* Frozen sections from pulmonary nodule exhibit microscopic features initially interpreted as benign inflammatory pseudotumor. Low magnification (left) shows zone of hypocellular fibrosis (arrows); high magnification (right) reveals a mixture of spindle cells, thought to be fibroblasts, and plump cells, taken to be histiocytes. *B.* Air-dried scrape-smear cytology preparation from the nodule was rapidly stained with Diff-Quik method and studied carefully after the surgeon mentioned a history of renal cortical carcinoma. In this preparation nuclei of benign foamy histiocytes appear small (straight arrows) in comparison to large, atypical nucleus of spindle cell (curved arrow). On the basis of this finding and history, the intraoperative diagnosis was changed to metastatic carcinoma, consistent with renal origin. *C.* Permanent sections the following day confirmed the intraoperative interpretation. Low magnification (left) shows whorls of spindling clear cells. At high magnification (right), there are anaplastic cellular features indicative of malignancy, including large vesicular nuclei with prominent nucleoli (arrow). Such cellular features of malignancy stand in striking contrast to those of the benign foamy histiocytes along the inferior margin of this field. *D.* Review of sections from the renal tumor 2 years previously showed microscopic features similar to those of the metastasis. In this low-magnification field, a spindling cellular growth pattern is manifest in most areas; however, in the lower left there is a zone of plump epithelial tumor cells (arrows). *E.* Higher magnification allows comparison of variation in cellular appearances within this renal cortical adenocarcinoma. An epithelioid area (left) consists of plump, foamy, clear tumor cells typical of hypernephroma. An area of spindle tumor cells (right) produces a sarcomatoid appearance. Metastases with such features can be mistaken for primary or secondary sarcomas, or intraoperatively as in this case, for benign fibroblastic processes. (*With permission, from Banks PM, Kraybill WG:* Pathology for the Surgeon. *Philadelphia, WB Saunders, 1996.*)

nodules 0.5 cm in maximum dimension. Specimen radiographs showed corresponding zones of soft tissue density. India ink was blotted over the external surface of the specimen to indicate resection planes. Sectioning of the specimen at 0.5-cm intervals revealed no single lesion that was grossly suspicious for carcinoma. The surgeon was informed that frozen section was contraindicated because of the absence of a grossly definable lesion; that margins appeared adequate, with fatty tissue enclosing all firm nodular tissue; and that microscopy would be deferred to permanent sections.

**SURGEON'S ACTIONS.** Convinced that the entire tissue region considered suspicious for malignancy had been removed, the surgeon closed the wound and told the patient that preliminary findings were all favorable, but a careful examination would take several days. The patient was scheduled for a clinic visit 5 days later.

**PATHOLOGIST'S ACTIONS.** After fixation, the pathologist sampled all firm areas and submitted 12 tissue blocks. The following day, permanent sections revealed widespread proliferative breast disease with several foci of atypical ductal hyperplasia. A single 0.3-cm focus of well-differentiated tubular carcinoma was identified (Figs. 4D-2*A* and *B*); this process did not encroach upon the inked resection surfaces. The surgeon was contacted by phone with the diagnosis.

**SURGEON'S ACTIONS.** The patient was advised that a small focus of malignancy had been successfully removed, but that there were changes of premalignancy throughout the quadrant, which carried a significant risk of subsequent malignancy. In anticipation of continued freedom from recurrence from the earlier right-sided cancer, subcutaneous mastectomy was advised and carried out. Pathologic examination revealed proliferative disease with atypical ductal hyperplasia.

**COMMENTS.** Because small, well-differentiated tubular carcinomas are difficult to distinguish from benign sclerosing lesions, the final diagnosis would have been jeopardized by freezing artifact if the pathologist had done intraoperative frozen sections. When no grossly recognizable tumor greater than 1.0 cm in diameter is present, frozen sections should be avoided.[2]

## CASE 3. PRIMARY MALIGNANT LYMPHOMA OF BONE SIMULATING SARCOMA

**HISTORY.** After 6 months of progressive discomfort while walking, a 32-year-old male prison inmate was seen in an outpatient clinic. His complaints were initially dismissed as spurious, being seen as an attempt to avoid physical labor. However, radiographs showed a large area of medullary and cortical bone destruction in the distal right femur (Fig. 4D-3*A*), and magnetic resonance imaging (MRI) studies revealed soft tissue extension. The patient was afebrile, denied fever or night sweats, and laboratory studies did not suggest an infectious process. Further evaluation, including skeletal survey and body CT, was negative for additional tumor foci. There was, however, palpable enlargement of the right (ipsilateral) inguinal lymph nodes, to about 3 cm in greatest dimension.

**SURGEON'S ACTIONS.** Using general anesthesia and a lateral approach to avoid the posterior neurovascular compartment, about 2 cm² of soft tumor tissue was curetted from the bone and surrounding soft tissues and submitted for intraoperative pathology consultation. A portion of the tissue was retained in a sterile container for potential microbial cultures.

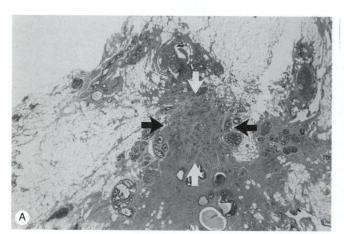
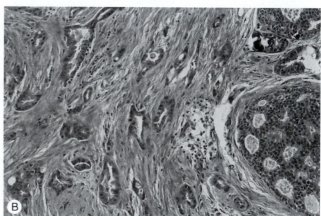

**FIGURE 4D-2.** *A*. Low magnification shows a small focus of well-differentiated tubular carcinoma (arrows) arising in the setting of profuse ductal hyperplasia and fibrosis. *B*. Intermediate magnification reveals atypical tubules of well-differentiated carcinoma within proliferative fibrosis. Such a subtle lesion could not have been diagnosed if freezing artifact had been introduced with intraoperative frozen-section preparation. In the right portion of the field are ducts showing atypical hyperplasia. (*With permission, from Banks PM, Kraybill WG: Pathology for the Surgeon. Philadelphia, WB Saunders, 1996.*)

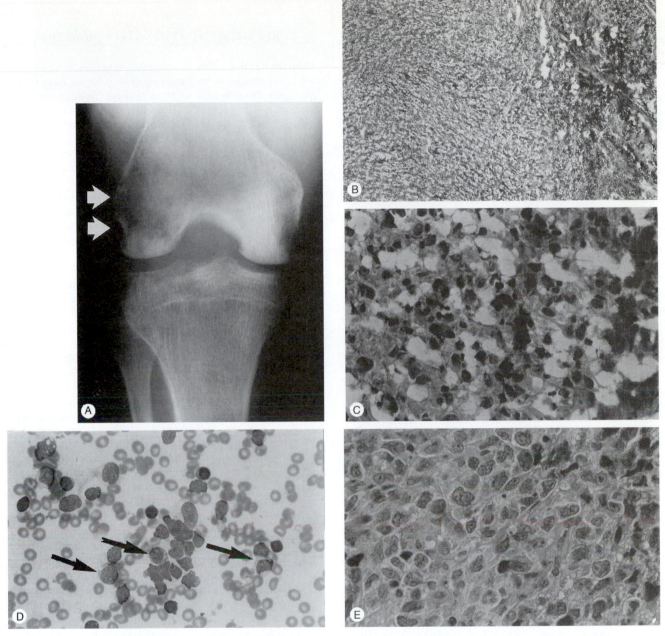

**FIGURE 4D-3.** *A*. Radiograph of right knee shows a large, irregular, poorly defined zone of bony destruction in the lateral distal femur (arrows). There is cortical destruction, and magnetic resonance imaging demonstrated extension of the process into adjacent soft tissue. *B, C*. Frozen section at low magnification reveals a cellular tumor with a diffuse growth pattern devoid of any matrix such as osteoid or chondroid substance. High magnification shows pleomorphic tumor nuclei; no neutrophils or plasma cells are present to suggest osteomyelitis. *D*. Diff-Quik–stained, air-dried imprint preparation used for intraoperative interpretation shows delicate tumor cell chromatin and scant cytoplasm (arrows). This was not consistent with osteosarcoma, chondrosarcoma, or fibrosarcoma. Therefore, intraoperative diagnosis of sarcoma was withheld (high magnification). *E*. Permanent paraffin section at high magnification shows features typical for large cell lymphoma: irregular, complex vesicular nuclei and scant, pale-staining cytoplasm. Although granulocytic or monocytic sarcomas (i.e., solid manifestations of myeloid leukemia) can simulate lymphoma morphologically, in this case both the microscopic finding of early lymph nodal involvement and immunostains showing a B-cell lymphoid phenotype ruled out such a possibility. (*With permission, from Banks PM, Kraybill WG:* Pathology for the Surgeon. *Philadelphia, WB Saunders, 1996.*)

PATHOLOGIST'S ACTIONS. Two of the six curettings were processed for immediate frozen-section study. Tissue imprints were stained with rapid Romanowsky-type method—Diff-Quik stain. Frozen sections revealed a uniform cellular neoplasm without matrix (osteoid or cartilage) production (Fig. 4D-3B and C). Tumor nuclei were moderately pleomorphic. Imprint cytology preparations showed tumor nuclei to be delicate and complexly irregular, with scant cytoplasm (Fig. 4D-3D). The surgeon was told that there was no evidence of infection and that this was a malignancy of uncertain nature. Sampling was adequate to allow definitive diagnosis with permanent sections. Portions of fresh, intact tumor were snap-frozen for storage at −70°C and the remaining tissue was processed routinely.

SURGEON'S ACTIONS. The surgeon wisely anticipated that examination of the ipsilateral inguinal lymph nodes might be crucial for tumor staging. Several nodes were excised and submitted to pathology in formalin, as was the remaining bony sampling, which had initially been kept in a sealed sterile container for the option of microbial cultures.

PATHOLOGIST'S ACTIONS. Permanent sections were available the following afternoon. These confirmed the frozen-section impression of a poorly differentiated tumor with a diffuse growth pattern (Fig. 4D-3E). Features were most consistent with a large-cell malignant lymphoma—an impression confirmed by focal involvement of germinal center regions in the sampled inguinal lymph nodes. Paraffin immunostains of the tumor showed reactivity for B-cell lymphoid antigens.

The surgeon was called, given the diagnosis, and congratulated on the forethought demonstrated in the sampling of the lymph nodes.

OUTCOME. Hematology-oncology consultants performed bilateral iliac crest bone marrow biopsies that were negative for lymphoma. The lymphoma was considered stage IIE. Six months later, after he had completed six cycles of polychemotherapy, the patient's femur showed moderate bony repair in the original distribution of the lesion and the patient's gait had improved markedly. There was no evidence of disease elsewhere.

COMMENTS. Whenever the clinical presentation and radiologic findings are atypical for a primary sarcoma of bone, intraoperative diagnosis for definitive resection is ill advised. In this case, the pathologist diagnosed the process as malignancy, not infection, and concluded that the features did not suggest common types of primary bone sarcoma. Because lymphomas are treated with radiation and/or chemotherapy, limb-sparing resection or amputation would have been inappropriate. The surgeon was wise to excise the regional lymph nodes within the single anesthetic period. If the pathologist had verbally considered lymphoma during the intraoperative discussion, the surgeon could have included the iliac crest biopsy in the same anesthetic procedure as well. The pathologist's use of imprint preparations provided cytologic detail better than that in frozen sections, achieving optimal intraoperative interpretation.

## RECOMMENDATIONS FOR PRACTICE

Although it is impossible to anticipate every clinical situation that will be encountered by the surgeon-pathologist team, there are some guidelines that will help to avoid mishaps. Nothing can replace the importance of complete knowledge of the patient's clinical history, physical exam, and radiologic and laboratory information. An understanding of the pathophysiology of each anatomic and functional system will allow the surgeon to provide appropriate diagnostic evaluation and care. By developing a differential diagnosis, the surgeon avoids an incomplete evaluation. For those patients likely to have special problems, the surgeon should alert the pathologist. Slides of previous samplings should always be reviewed prior to surgery. By discussing cases with the pathologist preoperatively, the surgeon assures informed involvement intraoperatively and post-operatively.

Intraoperative decision making requires a clear line of communication between the surgeon and the pathologist and may affect the overall success of the surgical procedure. Communication with and consultation from the pathologist should be maximized during a complex case. If unexpected appearances of tissues or organs are described to the pathologist (over the telephone or intercom), this may elicit some useful differential diagnostic insights. Likewise, careful descriptions of operative findings and individual labeling of numerous operative specimens safeguard pathologic interpretation of each. On the other hand, requesting a specimen interpretation (diagnosis) intraoperatively is justified only when there is potential impact on operative decision making or when appropriate tissue allocation needs to be secured by such means. If the pathologist has questions concerning the biopsy site, use of cautery, past medical history, or the plan of surgery, these and any other issues should be communicated to the surgeon before proceeding with issuing a report.

Postoperative communication is also important. Unexpected intraoperative findings should be communicated to the pathologist. If the pathologist has questions concerning orientation of the specimen, these should be addressed to the surgeon. If there are unexpected histologic findings, the pathologist should communicate this to the surgeon. If the pathologic examination will be prolonged, the surgeon should be notified. Occasionally, extramural consultations from subspecialty experts are required to resolve a case. Referral of cases to such specialists does not imply incompetence on the part of the pathologist. Even renowned experts at the most prestigious medical centers encounter cases that are diagnostically problematic, requiring the opinions of other renowned experts. It is far better to raise question about a diagnosis than to withhold comment and risk persisting error.

## PRINCIPLES OF PATHOLOGY FOR SURGICAL ONCOLOGY

Just as the surgical oncologist's methods for practice continue to expand with new instrumentation and techniques, so too are new diagnostic modalities broadening the pathologist's horizon. The methods most effective for definitively diagnosing a particular patient depend on the individual patient's findings. Pathology is a critical resource for the surgical oncologist. Case examples in the preceding section show both its power and some of the potential pitfalls that can lead to incorrect diagnosis and suboptimal patient management. The key to successful practice is clear communication between surgeon and pathologist, preoperatively, intraoperatively, and postoperatively. In the ensuing sections, samples are shown of appropriate recruitment of diverse methods in pathology in different specialty areas in surgical oncology. First, however, a review of the methods themselves is in order.

## GROSS EXAMINATION

The value of the gross evaluation should not be underestimated.[3] At the least, it is used to guide the selection of microscopic sampling of large resected specimens. Just to orient and assess intelligently a gross specimen such as an excisional breast biopsy requires of the pathologist considerable training and experience (Fig. 4D-4). Without proper orientation and analysis of the gross specimen, microscopy is reduced to an unreliable method and accurate pathologic staging cannot be carried out. At the most, gross evaluation can itself be the final and definitive method. For example, when breast or cutaneous neoplasms are resected, the presence of visibly intact, palpably soft fatty tissue margins is reliable (see Fig. 4D-4). In fact, intraprocedural frozen sections are not possible in such situations because adipose tissue will not freeze hard enough to allow sections for microscopic evaluation. Likewise, the pathologist's identification of a polyp within a segmental bowel resection in the operating room requires no microscopy or other methods, only a skilled eye.

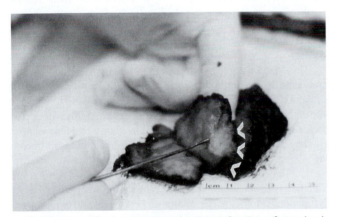

**FIGURE 4D-4.** The importance of gross evaluation of margins is exemplified by this excisional breast biopsy. After initially inking the entire specimen surface, the pathologist has sectioned the specimen in a plane to gauge the closest margin (white arrows). The tumor appears pale and opaque against the darker translucent surrounding fat (probe points to tumor). This cannot be evaluated by frozen section because the fatty tissue will not freeze hard to permit use of the method.

## CONVENTIONAL MICROSCOPY

When the pathologist poses for a photograph in the work setting, the microscope always fits into the picture. For more than 100 years, conventional hematoxylin and eosin–stained paraffin-embedded tissue sections have been used with ever-improving accuracy, as the mainstay of surgical pathology. It is truly amazing how powerful this method continues to be. Skilled, highly seasoned surgical pathologists can learn to associate subtle microscopic features with powerful markers of other modalities such as electron microscopy, immunostaining, and even molecular probes. By this means such updated, highly refined conventional microscopy becomes a practical, efficient, rapid means to diagnose previously unrecognized tumor types. Many surgeons today have not trained in pathology themselves and so do not appreciate the pathologist's need for uniformly high-quality sections on which to base their diagnoses. It is an irony that today, with so many technologic advances in medicine, such as computer-guided stereotactic surgery and laser ablation techniques, there is often a shortage of qualified histotechnologists to produce high-quality microscopic sections. The process remains highly labor intensive, demanding the same standards of time and effort required a century ago. When sectioning is substandard, subtle microscopic observations cannot be made (Fig. 4D-5). In extreme situations, tissue blocks are incorrectly oriented or worse still, negligently cut through, resulting in total loss of small biopsy specimens! Other potentials for disaster in the laboratory relate to errors in labeling tissue blocks or the glass slides, leading to diagnoses being exchanged among patients. Suffice it to say that the operation of the histology laboratory requires meticulous quality-controlled procedures to assure uninterrupted reliable services for pathologist, surgeon, and patient.

## INTRAOPERATIVE (INTRAPROCEDURAL) METHODS

Faced with the need to provide the surgeon with intraoperative findings on which further actions are predicated, the pathologist's judgment and resourcefulness are put to the test. In large part the question in the pathologist's mind can be reduced to this simple formulation: Am I certain enough about these findings to render a definite useful diagnosis? More experienced, more confident pathologists rely more heavily on clinical (and radiologic) information and gross specimen examination than do less experienced pathologists. Greater experience usually endows pathologists with more incisive intraoperative decision-making ability. For example, being asked to evaluate a wide reexcision for fibromatosis (desmoid tumor), a less experienced pathologist is likely to set about producing frozen sections for margins while inwardly struggling with doubts as to the feasibility of the effort, whereas the more seasoned pathologist will carefully evaluate the specimen with the naked eye and with palpation and then forthrightly explain to the surgeon that frozen-section microscopy is unlikely to assist further in distinguishing scar tissue secondary to the initial biopsy from residual tumor.

Since their initiation at the Johns Hopkins Hospital in 1895[4] and their establishment as a method for confirming clinical impressions

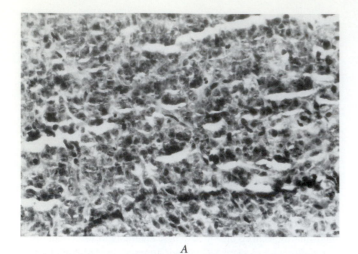

*A*

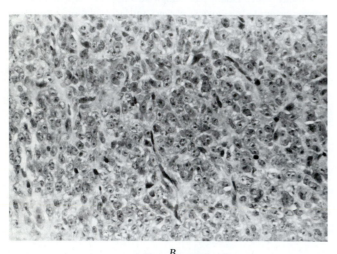

*B*

**FIGURE 4D-5.** Dependence of the pathologist upon high-quality permanent paraffin sections for accurate diagnosis is illustrated with this comparison *A.* of initial poor quality slide with *B.* Subsequently obtained high quality slide produced from the same paraffin block. Sectioning technique is poor in *A,* resulting in too thick (dark) a preparation with tearing, obscuring cellular detail. In *B* the tumor nuclei can be recognized as delicate and vesicular, supporting the correct diagnosis of malignant lymphoma. High-quality slides are necessary for accurate diagnosis, but require constant laboratory quality control efforts and well-trained, enthusiastic histotechnologists. (Hematoxylin and eosin stain, ×400.)

before commitment to resective surgery at Mayo Clinic in the 1910s,[5] frozen sections have been considered synonymous with intraoperative pathology. Although conventional paraffin-embedded sections require roughly a day to produce, with sequential tissue block fixation, dehydration, clearing, and hot wax infiltration prior to sectioning, frozen sections can be produced within minutes by rendering the tissues hard enough to section by freezing and then sectioning the frozen block with a microtome housed within a frozen space, the so-called cryotome or cryostat. The frozen sections are

then rapidly fixed (because of their extreme thinness), stained, and mounted under a coverslip for microscopic evaluation. Unfortunately, the quality of frozen sections is never as good as permanent sections. In conventional hematoxylin-eosin–stained sections, the freezing introduces a smudgy obscuration of nuclear detail (Fig. 4D-6). A method for avoiding some of the shortcomings of conventional hematoxylin-eosin–stained frozen sections is to use a supravital dye, such as methylene blue or toluidine blue on unfixed frozen sections. This provides finer nuclear detail, since most of the obscurity of nuclear features derives from fixation of the previously frozen cells (see Fig. 4D-6). Such supravitally stained preparations are coverslipped with water mounts, so that they are not permanent preparations. Ideally, both types of slides can be prepared; however, this is somewhat time consuming.

Another important means for evaluating specimens intraoperatively is through cytology preparations. Advantages include speed, the conservation of small tissue samples free of freezing artifact, suitability of bony tissues, and very high quality preparations for evaluating cellular detail. The main disadvantage is lack of tissue architecture for interpretation, but additionally there is a risk of introducing crush artifact into small tissue biopsies through imprinting or scraping such samples. Imprint preparations are produced by direct application and withdrawal of the glass slide to the fresh-cut tissue surface (Fig. 4D-7). Scrape-smear preparations are produced by scraping the edge of one end of a slide across the fresh-cut tissue surface followed by immediate smear of the accumulated cellular cluster over the surface of a different slide (see Fig. 4D-7). Imprints provide variably thick layers of intact cells, but are unreliable with fibrotic or bony tissues. Scrape-smear preparations can be produced even from bony and fibrotic tissues but larger, more delicate cells are prone to rupture. Cytology preparations can be wet-fixed in alcohol or formalin immediately before drying and stained with hematoxylin-eosin or the Papanicolau stain method to allow optimal nuclear detail (Fig. 4D-8). Preparations allowed to air-dry can be stained with modified Romanowsky methods, such as Diff-Quik stain, providing superior cytoplasmic detail (see Fig. 4D-8).

The skilled pathologist utilizes these different methods for intraoperative interpretation in accordance with the needs of the case at hand. For example, in a situation where there is high suspicion of tumor, e.g., an excisional breast biopsy for margins with a classic stellate tumor or an initial mediastinal lymph node biopsy with discrete firm gray tumor tissue apart from surrounding anthracotic nodal elements, a cytology scrape-smear preparation is a quick, convenient way to establish the diagnosis of malignancy. Likewise, in a situation with small samples, such as mediastinoscopic biopsies for lymphoma, cytology preparations can be used instead of frozen sections as a means to conserve tissue free of freeze-thaw artifact.

Supravital staining of frozen sections can be usefully added on to hematoxylin-eosin–stained preparations in cases in which superior nuclear detail is critical (e.g., bile duct biopsies for the diagnosis of malignancy) or in which the preservation of lipid material within the section is desirable (e.g., for recognition of cytoplasmic lipid granules within inactive normal parathyroid glandular cellularity vs. the absence of such granules in hyperplastic or adenomatous glands).

Intraoperative pathologic interpretations are useful in ways beyond the surgeon's decision making. By narrowing down the

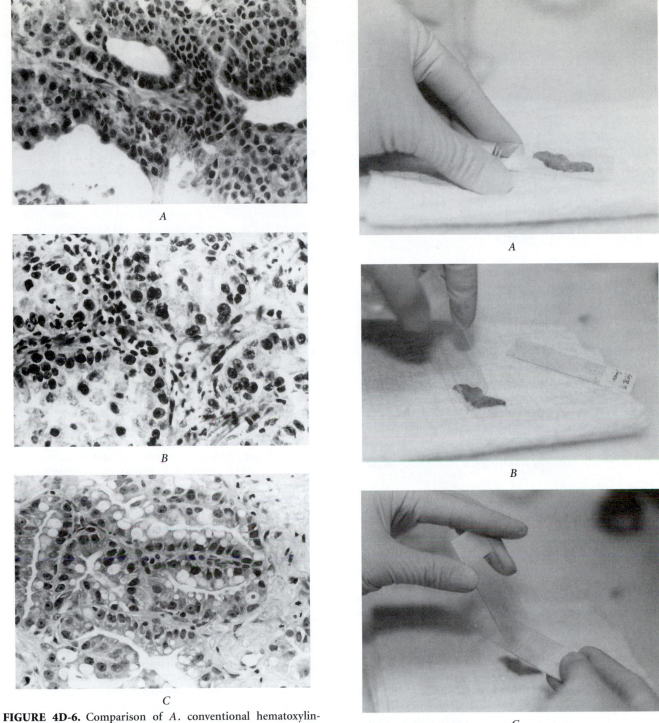

**FIGURE 4D-6.** Comparison of *A.* conventional hematoxylin-eosin–stained frozen section versus *B.* supravital polychrome methylene blue stained frozen section versus *C.* hemotoxylin-eosin–stained permanent paraffin section (all photos ×400). Note the dark smudgy nuclear appearance of the conventional frozen section (*A*) in comparison with the clearer nuclear detail but with pale cytoplasmic staining in *B*. Optimal microscopic detail is attained in the permanent paraffin section (*C*). The case is a pulmonary adenocarcinoma. When cellular details are critical for intraoperative diagnosis the pathologist can use both techniques (*A* & *B*) to complement one another.

**FIGURE 4D-7.** Comparison of methods for producing cellular monolayer slide preparations for intraoperative interpretation. *A.* Imprinting a slide against a fresh-cut surface of tumor tissue. *B.* Scraping the fresh-cut surface to extract cells onto the slide edge. *C.* Smearing the scrape preparation to produce a uniform distribution of cells on another slide. Imprinting is satisfactory for soft, cellular tumors, but the scrape-smear method is needed for successful cellular preparations when fibrosis, bone, or other matrix materials retain cells.

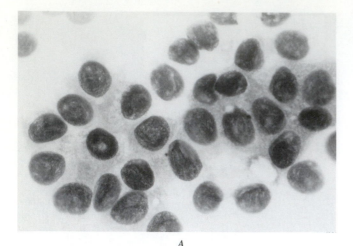

*A*

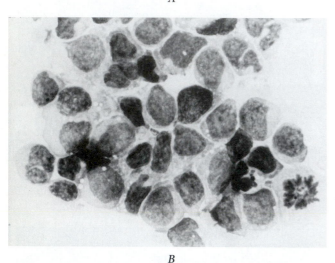

*B*

**FIGURE 4D-8.** Comparison of *A*. wet-fixed hematoxylin-eosin–stained cytology preparation to *B*. air-dried Diff-Quik–stained preparation (adenocarcinoma of lung; same case as in Fig. 4D-6, both photos ×1000). With method *A* nuclear features similar to those of stained sections are attained (compare to Fig. 4D-6), whereas with method *B* there is better cytoplasmic detail (note clear lipid vacuoles).

differential diagnosis with such immediate means of analysis, the pathologist can allocate the sampled tissues most effectively. A pulmonary lobectomy specimen need not be arduously sampled for margins and regional nodal status if a frozen-section approach has demonstrated the suspicious mass to be a hamartoma or fibrotic granuloma. If cytology preparations suggest the possibility of a histiocytic nature to a bony biopsy, tissue can be fixed for electron microscopy to demonstrate definitively the Langerhans cell's Birbeck granules specific to eosinophilic granuloma (see Fig. 4D-20).

The need for intraoperative decision making based on pathologic findings can be both stressful and rewarding for the surgeon-

pathologist team, testing the wisdom, ingenuity, and communication skills at both ends of the intercom.

## AUTOPSIES

Although "surgical pathology" is generally considered the application of pathologic interpretation to surgical specimens, autopsy findings continue to be informative, sometimes critically so, in relation to the practice of surgical oncology. Despite advances in radiologic imaging and in laparoscopic and endoscopic biopsy techniques, comparison of recent to past autopsy studies has shown little change in the percentage of major unexpected findings.[6] In many instances, the success or failure of attempts at surgical resection can be judged only by autopsy findings. Indeed, autopsy findings are used in the American Joint Committee on Cancer (AJCC) staging system for a separately designated tumor classification designated TNM.

## CYTOLOGY

A specialized area of diagnostic pathology is cytology, emphasizing cellular detail in the absence of tissue section patterns. This discipline has proved highly efficient as a cancer screening method for cervical-vaginal preparations, using time-honored Pap smear preparations or more recently introduced cytobrush or Thin-prep preparations. Other important applications of exfoliative cytology for evaluation of malignancy include body fluids (e.g., cerebrospinal, thoracentesis, or ascites fluids), intraoperative fluid washings (e.g., pelvic or bronchoalveolar), and brushing preparations from endoscopic or bronchoscopic procedures. Because pathologic interpretation depends on cellular findings alone, clinical information and experience on the pathologist's part are even more critical than in tissue section interpretation for an accurate diagnosis. Pathologists who specialize in diagnostic cytology require in-depth active experience in tissue section practice in corresponding specialty practice in order to maintain their skills, in gynecologic surgical pathology for cervical-vaginal smear interpretation, head and neck surgical pathology for cervical lymph node or thyroid aspiration biopsy interpretations, etc.

Fine-needle aspiration biopsy is a simple, quick, and inexpensive method to biopsy discrete mass lesions. It has gained widespread usage in North America after its initial development in Scandinavia.[8] The technique utilizes thin or "fine" needles (22 gauge or higher), carries with it little risk of patient discomfort, and can be used with direct palpation guidance for superficial lesions (Fig. 4D-9) or with radiologic guidance for deep masses in almost any site. Surgeons and radiologists performing this biopsy procedure need to dedicate significant time and effort, not only in perfecting their sampling approach but also in following the samples through preparation and interpretation by the pathologist (Figs. 4D-10 and 4D-11), so that they can perceive directly which approaches yield the most informative cellular harvests. Again, the team approach for surgeon and pathologist is essential for success. Just a few examples of ways in which this technique can be utilized in surgical oncology include the aspiration biopsy of lymph nodes to confirm

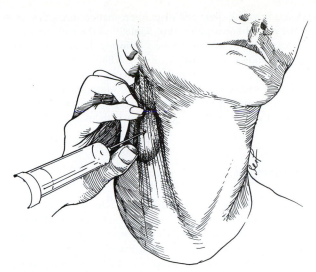

**FIGURE 4D-9.** Aspiration of a cervical lymph node. Approach in this case is behind the posterior border of the sternocleidomastoid muscle. The approach to an enlarged cervical lymph node should avoid the sternocleidomastoid or any large muscle mass. (*With permission, from Banks PM, Kraybill WG:* Pathology for the Surgeon. *Philadelphia, WB Saunders, 1996.*)

metastatic malignancy (Fig. 4D-12) vs. intercurrent events such as inflammatory lymphadenitis or malignant lymphoma (Fig. 4D-13), of thyroid nodules to detect papillary type carcinoma vs. colloid nodule (Fig. 4D-14), of pancreatic masses to establish the diagnosis of malignancy and of breast lesions to distinguish reducible cysts from carcinoma.

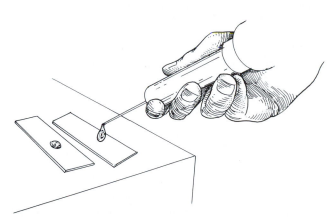

**FIGURE 4D-10.** Aspirate is expressed as a 2- to 4-mm drop on the center of a plain glass slide. When expressing the drop, place the needle, bevel side down, on the surface of the glass slide to avoid splattering the drop, with resultant excessive air-drying before the smears can be prepared. (*With permission, from Banks PM, Kraybill WG:* Pathology for the Surgeon. *Philadelphia, WB Saunders, 1996.*)

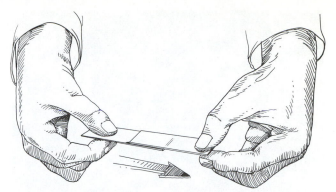

**FIGURE 4D-11.** Smear prepared by pulling the slides apart horizontally as the drop of aspirate begins to spread. The weight of the glass slide is sufficient pressure on the aspirate to make an even smear. Alternatively, the slides may be pulled apart vertically as the drop of aspirate begins to spread, creating a relatively compact circular smear. (*With permission, from Banks PM, Kraybill WG:* Pathology for the Surgeon. *Philadelphia, WB Saunders, 1996.*)

## CONVENTIONAL SPECIAL STAINS

Which stains constitute "standard" and which "special" depends on the practice of a particular laboratory. In general, pathology laboratories turn out hematoxylin-eosin–stained paraffin sections as standard fare, although some stains may be routinely carried out for certain designated types of case, for example, Giemsa stain for all gastric biopsies for the detection of *Helicobacter pylori* or acid-fast

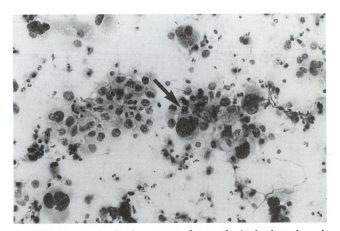

**FIGURE 4D-12.** Aspiration smear of supraclavicular lymph node from patient with lung mass, with irregular sheets of malignant tumor cells containing large, bizarre, and sometimes multinucleated tumor giant cells. Note phagocytosis of polymorphonuclear leukocytes within tumor cells (arrow), a feature of giant cell carcinoma of the lung. (Diff-Quik stain, ×250.) (*With permission, from Banks PM, Kraybill WG:* Pathology for the Surgeon. *Philadelphia, WB Saunders, 1996.*)

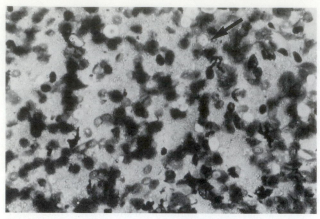

**FIGURE 4D-13.** Clear round-to-oval structures with a slightly gray center can be found scattered throughout this smear, otherwise composed of lymphocytes and red blood cells from an HIV-positive patient. Some of these structures appear to be budding (arrow). They represent *Cryptococcus neoformans*, in this case a disseminated infection in the setting of immunodeficiency. (Diff-Quik stain, ×600.) (*With permission, from Banks PM, Kraybill WG: Pathology for the Surgeon. Philadelphia, WB Saunders, 1996.*)

stain for all bronchoscopic biopsies for the detection of mycobacteria. Because of today's emphasis on immunostains (see below), many pathologists overlook the diagnostic utility of time-honored, quick, inexpensive special stains, such as periodic-acid Schiff (PAS)

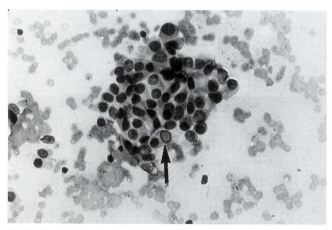

**FIGURE 4D-14.** Clusters of cells with nuclear overlap from a cellular aspiration of a thyroid mass from a 32-year-old patient. Within this cluster of thyroid cells, there are nuclei with sharply defined intranuclear inclusions (arrow) and also examples of nuclei with linear grooves. These are two of several features that support the diagnosis of papillary carcinoma of the thyroid. (Diff-Quik stain, ×400.) (*With permission, from Banks PM, Kraybill WG: Pathology for the Surgeon. Philadelphia, WB Saunders, 1996.*)

stain, mucicarmine stain, and silver impregnation methods such as argentaffin and argyrophil stains. Sometimes the pathologist can show resourcefulness by achieving a definitive diagnosis with such simple techniques, for example, distinguishing a poorly differentiated gastric carcinoma from lymphoma by demonstrating focal cytoplasmic vacuoles positive for PAS (or mucicarmine) or showing an endoscopically biopsied tumor to be a neuroendocrine type (carcinoid) with cytoplasmic granularity with an argentaffin silver stain.

## IMMUNOSTAINS

Over the past 20 years, surgical pathology has been virtually revolutionized by the development of immunostaining, a method allowing the demonstration of immunologically detected markers in conventional paraffin sections. This method has allowed the pathologist combined resolution of microscopically defined appearances with the biochemical specificity of antigens, resolved by animal, usually murine, antibodies. With this technology, enormous strides have been made in further understanding original concepts of tumor histogenesis, and indeed entire new concepts have been developed. Many early theories regarding embryonic differentiation of various mature tissues have been revised or abandoned, as immunostaining markers for basic tissue types, such as cytokeratin cytoskeletal proteins for epithelial elements, vimentin cytoskeletal proteins for mesenchymal elements, and endocrine secretory granule components such as synaptophysin or chromogranin for neuroendocrine elements, have been shown to be inducible in neoplasms from pluripotent stem cells present even in the adult organism.

Immunostains are now the favored method for classifying poorly differentiated high-grade neoplasms because they are practical, i.e., can be applied to conventional formalin-fixed paraffin sections, and because abundant published data are now present as a guide to interpreting such data. For example, when an anaplastic tumor is identified in the axillary lymph node of a woman without history or current evidence of breast carcinoma, an initial battery of immunostains narrows down the possibilities. The combination of cytokeratin and epithelial membrane antigen is a sensitive detector of carcinoma; S100 protein is sensitive for malignant melanoma (Figs. 4D-15 and 4D-16), whereas leukocyte common antigen CD45RB is sensitive for malignant lymphoma. In some cases, immunostaining can assist in pinpointing the origin of metastatic malignancy, such as with demonstration of prostate-specific antigen (Figs. 4D-17 and 4D-18).

Effective and efficient use of immunostaining requires experience and understanding on the part of the pathologist. Rather than blindly using all the potential markers available, the skilled pathologist orders only those appropriate to the differential diagnosis, often in a sequence, with the succeeding markers ordered on the basis of the outcome of the earlier ordered markers. In this manner algorithms of differential diagnosis can be developed, according to several conventional microscopic groupings.[9] Figure 4D-19 shows a schematic algorithm for the use of immunostaining markers to achieve a final, definitive diagnosis for poorly differentiated spindle cell tumors, which includes such final diagnoses as malignant melanoma, malignant peripheral nerve sheath tumor,

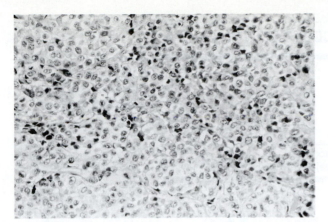

**FIGURE 4D-15.** Malignant large cell neoplasm in an excised axillary lymph node in a 67-year-old woman with no other abnormalities. The tumor is morphologically indeterminate by conventional staining with hematoxylin and eosin; it could be interpreted as a carcinoma, a lymphoma, or a melanoma. (*With permission, from Banks PM, Kraybill WG:* Pathology for the Surgeon. *Philadelphia, WB Saunders, 1996.*)

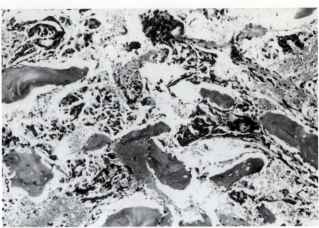

**FIGURE 4D-17.** Closed-needle biopsy of a blastic lesion of the left sixth rib in a patient with elevated level of serum prostate-specific antigen. Between the irregular geographic shapes of bony trabecula are distorted clusters of foreign polygonal cells, representing a metastatic, poorly differentiated nonhematopoietic neoplasm. (*With permission, from Banks PM, Kraybill WG:* Pathology for the Surgeon. *Philadelphia, WB Saunders, 1996.*)

angiosarcoma, malignant fibrous histiocytoma, leiomyosarcoma, and sarcomatoid variant squamous cell carcinoma.

## AUTOMATED FLOW CYTOMETRY

Cell suspensions can be analyzed at great speed and with extreme accuracy by automated flow cytometers. This method has proved useful in precise immunophenotyping of leukemias and lymphomas by establishing a neoplasm's "fingerprint" of reactivity from within a large panel of antibodies directed against lymphoid or myeloid markers.[10] Fresh, viable cells in suspension are required.

A different application of flow cytometry is the study of a cell suspension for nuclear DNA content. This can be performed on nuclei extracted from especially thick paraffin sections cut from conventional formalin-fixed paraffin-embedded tissue blocks. Two

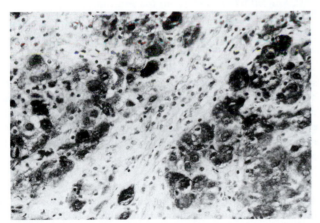

**FIGURE 4D-16.** Immunostaining of the tumor in Fig. 4D-15 for S100 protein shows combined nuclear and cytoplasmic reactivity, as demonstrated in this photograph. Other stains for keratin and CD45 were negative. This constellation of findings establishes the diagnosis of metastatic malignant melanoma, which was further substantiated by the results of other immunohistochemical studies (see text). (*With permission, from Banks PM, Kraybill WG:* Pathology for the Surgeon. *Philadelphia, WB Saunders, 1996.*)

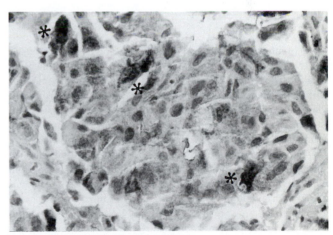

**FIGURE 4D-18.** Multifocal immunoreactivity for prostate-specific antigen (asterisks) is evident in the specimen shown in Fig. 4D-17, confirming a diagnosis of metastatic prostatic adenocarcinoma. (*With permission, from Banks PM, Kraybill WG:* Pathology for the Surgeon. *Philadelphia, WB Saunders, 1996.*)

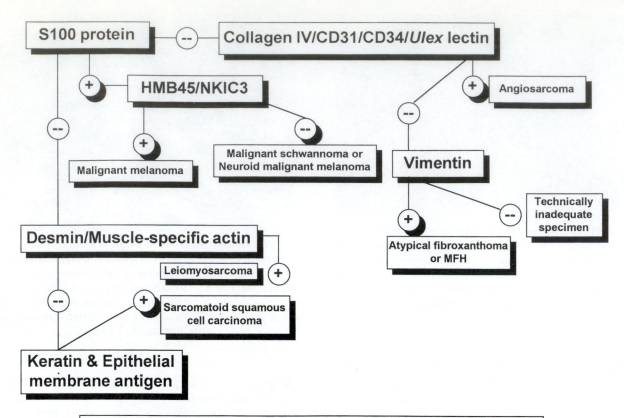

IMMUNOHISTOCHEMICAL DIAGNOSIS OF MALIGNANT PLEOMORPHIC TUMORS

**FIGURE 4D-19.** Algorithm for immunohistochemical diagnosis of pleomorphic spindle cell undifferentiated neoplasms. (*With permission, from Banks PM, Kraybill WG:* Pathology for the Surgeon. *Philadelphia, WB Saunders, 1996.*)

types of information can be obtained. First, the presence of an aneuploid peak of DNA molecular weight can be used to infer that a malignant neoplasm is present. This same determination can be of prognostic value in some tumor types. For example, paradoxically in some malignancies such as childhood neuroblastoma, the *absence* of an aneuploid peak is actually *less favorable* than if such a peak is present.[9] Second, the proportion of sampled nuclei with DNA content between diploid and tetraploid can be used to calculate the growth fraction, i.e., the percentage of cells in active DNA synthesis (S phase). In many tumors, such as breast carcinoma, the growth fraction is a predictor, if not an independent one, of prognosis.[11]

## ELECTRON MICROSCOPY

Ultrastructure is used in tumor pathology to classify poorly differentiated neoplasms and to confirm the identity of a relatively small number of tumor types with specific subcellular elements. The presence of well-developed intercellular junctions is generally a feature of epithelial rather than hematolymphoid differentiation. Electron-dense secretory granules are present in neuroendocrine but not other types of carcinoma. Organelles that are neoplasm-specific include melanosomes (melanoma), keratohyaline granules (squamous cell carcinoma), Weibel-Palade bodies (endothelial cells), and Birbeck granules (Langerhans' cells) (Fig. 4D-20). Ideally, tissue for electron microscopic study should be cut into a very thin block (less than 1 mm in thickness) and primarily fixed in glutaraldehyde. However, for diagnostic purposes, particularly when the questions to be addressed are straightforward and deal with larger, more resilient organelles such as desmosomes or intermediate filaments, tissue shaved off the fastest fixed surface of a specimen in formalin is suitable. Occasionally, tissue run back from a paraffin block is informative; however, pathologists experienced with diagnostic ultrastructure are seldom enthusiastic about such efforts.

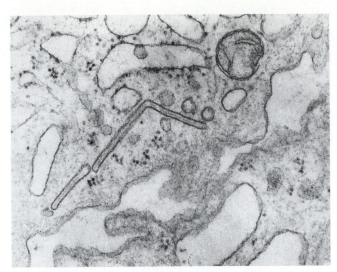

**FIGURE 4D-20.** This electron micrograph of the tissue discloses the presence of diagnostic Birbeck granules (center of fig). These are linear or curvilinear membranous inclusions that secure a diagnosis of a Langerhans' cell disease. (*With permission, from Banks PM, Kraybill WG:* Pathology for the Surgeon. *Philadelphia, WB Saunders, 1996.*)

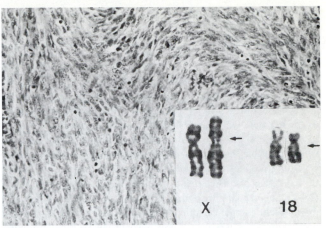

**FIGURE 4D-21.** Malignant spindle cell neoplasm of the foot in a 25-year-old man, which is histologically indeterminate. Synovial sarcoma, leiomyosarcoma, fibrosarcoma, and malignant peripheral nerve sheath tumor are all diagnostic possibilities based on conventional morphological study. Chromosomal analysis of fresh tissue (inset) from the tumor shown in the larger portion of this figure. This evaluation showed the characteristic X;18 translocation of synovial sarcoma. (*Reprinted with permission from Fletcher JA:* Cytogenetic aberrations in malignant soft tissue tumors. Adv Pathol Lab Med *4:235–246, 1991.*)

## CYTOGENETICS

Although metaphase chromosome analysis has been established as a critical diagnostic method for most forms of leukemia and for some types of lymphoma, its role in diagnosis and management of other tumors remains less clear. Although tumor type–specific chromosomal abnormalities have been identified, in most cases their presence does not add to diagnostic resolution or management considerations. An evolving exception is in the area of soft tissue classification, where recognition of certain tumors such as liposarcoma[12] or synovial sarcoma can be improved with such means (Fig. 4D-21). Unfortunately, allocating tissue for cytogenetics analysis is very fastidious, requiring fresh, preferably sterile tissue from which dividing cells can be successfully promulgated.

## MOLECULAR PROBES

The most rapidly advancing modality in scientific investigation of tumors is in the area of molecular probes, chiefly using two different methods—polymerase chain reaction (PCR) and in situ hybridization techniques. Both techniques require probes or primers consisting of nucleic acid templates that derive from chromosomal regions, such as oncogene translocations, of particular importance and ultimately deriving from observations in classical cytogenetic (chromosomal) methods. Certain translocations seem to be associated more often with particular malignancies, e.g., K-*ras* translocation with pancreatic carcinoma. As yet, such findings are not used in patient management. However, in select situations molecular probe information may be of use in differential diagnosis, such as the presence of the 11;22 translocation among blastic childhood malignancies to indicate that the tumor is of the Ewing's-primitive neuroectodermal grouping with its associated therapeutic implications.[13] Because of the extreme sensitivity of the PCR method, it can be used to detect marker sequences in archival paraffin-embedded tissue. With such practicality to recommend it, this technique is likely to become an important part of the pathologist's diagnostic armamentarium in the near future.

## CANCER STAGING

The importance of standardized systems for the staging of various malignancies cannot be exaggerated. These systems, which have been developed by the American Joint Committee on Cancer (AJCC), are based on cumulative published experience from the world literature on each individual organ (or tumor) system, have great predictive value, and allow risk stratification of patients into meaningful groupings for evaluation of new therapeutic studies.[7] Each staging system is based on accurate histopathologic diagnosis and in many instances, grading of the tumor.

Clinical staging is based on physical and radiologic findings suggesting the extent of tumor spread. Whenever practical, more definitive pathologic staging should be carried out to confirm the clinical staging findings. For example, a radiologically demonstrated tumor in the liver will be the basis for clinically assigned high stage of disease. However, biopsy may reveal a benign, unrelated process, such as focal nodular hyperplasia of the liver (see Fig. 4D-66), resulting in radically downstaging the patient by pathologic criteria. Accurate pathologic staging requires skill and effort on the pathologist's part. Both gross and microscopic findings are used in assessing tumor (T) stage. In dealing with breast specimens, initial gross measurement of maximal tumor diameter must sometimes be modified in accordance with microscopic observations, as for example when nonpalpable infiltrative lobular carcinoma insidiously extends into soft surrounding tissues, or by contrast, when a palpable "tumor" corresponds microscopically to a comedo-type duct carcinoma in situ, resulting in downstaging the tumor to Tis status. The assessment of lymph nodes for accurate nodal (N) staging may require highly sensitive immunostaining to avoid missing subtle single-cell micrometastases (see Fig. 4D-29). Detecting distant metastases, particularly in small-needle-biopsy samples, demands expertise in cytology (see Fig. 4D-12). In practice, the pathologist is most often directly involved in establishing tumor (T) and nodal (N) stage, whereas clinical findings are relied upon for metastatic (M) stage. At the completion of diagnostic evaluation, in deciding on appropriate therapy, patients with most types of malignancy should have filed in their charts a completed AJCC staging form.[7] Staging systems vary according to tumor type and organ system. The AJCC TNM system is particularly well suited for tumors such as breast carcinoma, which demonstrate a continuous range of survival in relation to T, N, and M stage (see "The Breast" and Table 4D-3). In the case of cutaneous malignant melanoma, great emphasis is placed on microstaging the primary tumor because precise measurement of maximal tumor thickness, even to one-hundreth of a millimeter, together with level of dermal tissue compartment of invasion is a highly predictive determinant of survival (see "Skin" and Table 4D-1). In some systems anatomic complexities require precise evaluation regarding local extension of the tumor for T staging. An example is laryngeal carcinoma, which has separate T-staging systems for supraglottic, glottic, and subglottic tumors (see "The Head and Neck" and Table 4D-4). For ovarian tumors, special considerations for local transperitoneal spread, rather than just lymph nodal involvement, are incorporated into a specialized T-staging gradation, in agreement with the Federation Internationale de Gynecologie et d'Obstetrique (FIGO) staging system (see "The Obstetric and Gynecologic System," Table 4D-15). The staging of lymphomas requires an entirely separate system, without a T stage at all, emphasizing distribution of involved nodal or other tissues rather than size of a primary tumor (see "The Hematolymphoid System" and Table 4D-18).

The staging system for testicular germ cell tumors is unique in that it incorporates an S component, in addition to TNM, representing serum levels of certain tumor-related substances that are of established prognostic value (see "The Male Reproductive System" and Table 4D-12). In the future, similar additions are likely to be added to staging systems for other tumors, as biochemical and molecular genetic markers are identified as predictors of survival and response to specific therapies.

In a few organ systems, staging has proved of less value. In the central nervous system, with its critical microanatomy, tumor type, grade, and location dictate therapy and prognosis. In the soft tissues accurate classification and, in some types of tumor, grading, are critical. In most cases, the predictor of survival is the presence or absence of distant hematogenous metastases (see "Soft Tissue Tumors"). Tumors of childhood are especially diverse, some exhibiting unique distributional characteristics, e.g., neuroblastoma and Wilms' tumor (see "Special Considerations of the Pediatric Patient"). Therefore, no system for these tumors has been developed by the AJCC.[7]

## SKIN

### THE SURGICAL APPROACH TO SKIN LESIONS

The skin presents the surgeon with special challenges and opportunities. As the easily visualized organ system, it may serve as a "window" on underlying maladies, e.g., pyoderma gangrenosum in patients with primary inflammatory bowel disease. Early detection of primary cutaneous neoplasms and their accurate classification and staging with microscopy are critical for effective, often curative surgical management. The surgical approach to cutaneous lesions is predicated upon the clinical differential diagnosis. Small solitary lesions can be readily excised, whereas larger, less-defined lesions, or those in anatomically "tight" locations, can be sampled with wedge or punch biopsies. Shave biopsies are useful only for very superficial lesions of epidermis and should be avoided for deep or high-profile lesions, or whenever malignant melanoma is a consideration. Surgeons are commonly brought in on a case to obtain a sample for pathologic interpretation. Usually submission of the specimen in fixative for standard turnaround time with permanent section evaluation is appropriate. Only when intraprocedural decision making is required, e.g., to decide whether margins are adequate, for example, in the resection of large carcinomas, or those in critical areas of cosmesis, are frozen sections indicated. Because of the relatively wide margins required for malignant melanoma resection, these lesions are usually first excised for precise pathologic evaluation, and then subsequently the tumor bed is widely resected. Careful orientation of any resection specimen of skin is critical for useful interpretation regarding adequacy of margins by the pathologist. Simple drawings to explain the specimen's critical margins are often effective. When one margin is of particular concern, this should be "flagged" by a diagram, sutures, or clips on the specimen, or even separate submission of the area in question. Unthinking sampling by the pathologist of all circumferential and deep planes of resection from a large specimen is rarely necessary. Visual and palpation evaluation of large resection specimens usually allows selection of a small sampling of the closest margins.

### MOHS MICROGRAPHIC SURGERY

This highly specialized technique entails conservative excision of relatively localized carcinomas, most commonly basal cell type, with detailed intraprocedural mapping of margins that are systematically evaluated by frozen section. Specially trained dermatologists apply this method to tumors with visually indistinct borders, such as morpheaform variants of basal cell carcinoma.[14]

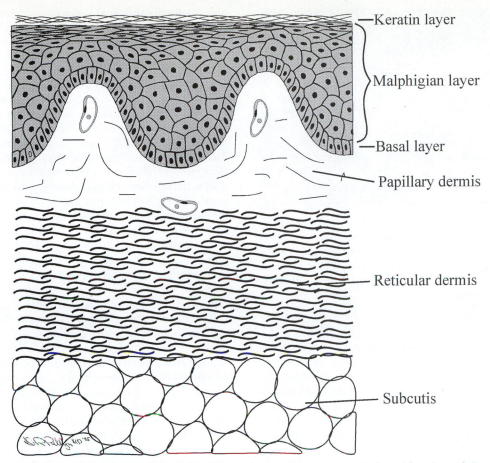

—Keratin layer

Malphigian layer

—Basal layer

—Papillary dermis

—Reticular dermis

Subcutis

**FIGURE 4D-22.** Basic histology of the skin. At the top, the gray zone is the epidermis, with its three layers indicated. (*With permission, from Banks PM, Kraybill WG:* Pathology for the Surgeon. *Philadelphia, WB Saunders, 1996.*)

## CUTANEOUS TUMORS

Neoplasms of the skin are very common and range from benign nodules such as seborrheic keratoses to potentially lethal malignancies such as malignant melanoma. Surgical management is guided by the histologic diagnosis. The most common neoplasms, both benign and malignant, derive from epithelium of the surface (epidermis) or from the associated melanocytic pigment-producing elements. Less common tumors derive from stromal elements of the dermis (e.g., vascular or fibroblastic) or epithelium of the adnexal structures such as sweat glands and hair-producing elements (Fig. 4D-22).

Sharply circumscribed elevated lesions of long duration usually correspond to seborrheic keratoses, common warts, skin tags, or papillary intradermal nevi and can simply be excised. Flat or ulcerated lesions of recent onset or with reported growth require a more cautious approach, with initial punch or wedge biopsy to guide definitive methods for removal.

Because of the visibility of cutaneous lesions, premalignant dysplastic processes are well described and generally accurately recognizable with a combination of gross inspection and the history, as observed by the patient and/or patient's spouse. Actinic keratoses are irregular, slowly growing lesions in sun-exposed areas, usually with associated dermal atrophy and telangiectasias. There are areas of rough hyperkeratosis that correspond to proliferative dysplastic epidermis microscopically. Keratoacanthomas are regular, centrally puckered, rapidly growing lesions that mimic squamous cell carcinoma, both clinically and microscopically. Lentigo maligna, or Hutchinson's freckle, is a premalignant dysplastic proliferation of melanocytes within epidermis, usually on the cheek or other sun-exposed region of older individuals. These lesions are flat, with highly variable pigmentation and irregular outline, usually of long duration. Microscopically, there are clusters ("theques") of atypical melanocytes within the epidermis but without invasion into dermis.

## SURGICAL MANAGEMENT OF CUTANEOUS MALIGNANCIES

Rare epithelial primary cutaneous malignancies include adnexal (sweat gland) carcinomas and neuroendocrine (Merkel cell)

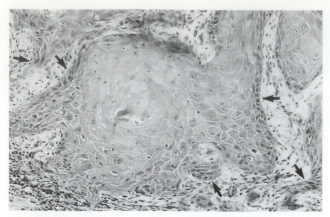

**FIGURE 4D-23.** Keratoacanthoma. The lesion consists of pale-staining keratinocytes with abundant eosinophilic cytoplasm. There is only mild cytologic atypia, which is most prominent along the advancing margins of the lesion (arrows). (*With permission, from Banks PM, Kraybill WG:* Pathology for the Surgeon. *Philadelphia, WB Saunders, 1996.*)

carcinomas. Mesenchymal malignancies arising from the dermal connective tissues include lower-grade tumors such as dermatofibrosarcoma protuberans, atypical fibroxanthoma, and Kaposi's sarcoma unrelated to immunodeficiences; higher-grade tumors include malignant lymphoma, malignant peripheral nerve sheath tumor, angiosarcoma, and Kaposi's sarcoma in immunodeficiency. These diverse neoplasms require surgical and other modes of therapy individually tailored to the specific disease process and the patient's presentation and tumor stage.

The vast majority of cutaneous malignancies are sun exposure–related carcinomas of the epidermis, basal cell or squamous type carcinomas. Although both types derive from epidermal epithe-

lium, basal cell carcinomas are so named because they retain the appearance of the basal layer epidermal cells, often with palisading arrangement of cells along the interface with dermal stroma (Fig. 4D-23). By contrast, squamous cell carcinomas are less orderly in their configuration, and usually show some (abortive) maturation into keratin-containing dying cellularity mimicking the superficial corneal layer of normal epidermis (Fig. 4D-24). As subtle as this microscopic distinction between the two types may seem, it has great predictive power regarding clinical behavior. Basal cell carcinomas are potentially locally aggressive, but almost never metastasize. Even when margins of excision are focally positive microscopically, these tumors will often not recur. Squamous cell carcinomas related to sun exposure only infrequently metastasize (less than 1% of cases), whereas those arising in other settings (burn scars, chronic ulcers, immunosuppression) have greater potential for distant spread. Both carcinoma types appear as elevated irregular nodules, centrally ulcerated in larger tumors (Fig. 4D-25). Basal cell carcinomas often appear as pearly plaques or nodules with "rolled" borders, and the most subtle and aggressive type, microscopically the sclerosing morpheaform variant, tends to insidiously infiltrate surrounding connective tissues, penetrating suture lines of the skull or other underlying neurovascular planes. Intraoperative frozen-section pathologic evaluation of resection margins is necessary for large, irregular tumors or those situated in anatomically "tight" regions such as face and neck. There is extensive experience managing patients with very small tumor burdens with ablation (cryosurgery and electrosurgery). Such methods are more often applied for basal cell tumors and should be applied to squamous cell carcinomas only selectively in favorable situations (early-stage, low-grade sun exposure lesions). In most cases of squamous cell carcinoma margins of 3 to 5 mm should be attained for smaller tumors, and margins of at least 1 cm for larger, more aggressive neoplasms, even if reconstruction will be required. In patients with large tumors at risk for regional nodal metastasis, consideration should be given to sentinel node biopsy.

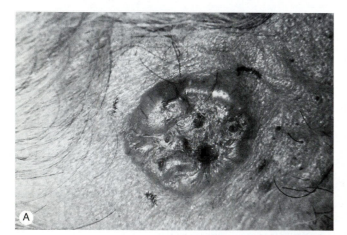

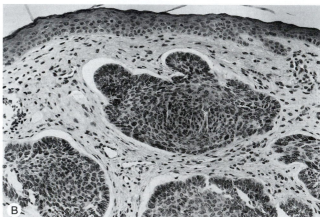

**FIGURE 4D-24.** Basal cell carcinoma. *A.* Clinically, the lesions occur on sun-exposed areas and manifest as pearly plaques or nodules, with "rolled" borders and a central zone of ulceration. *B.* Microscopically the lesions consist of nests of basophilic tumor cells with "palisading" of nuclei at the periphery; the cleftlike space surrounding the nests contains extracellular mucin. (*With permission, from Banks PM, Kraybill WG:* Pathology for the Surgeon. *Philadelphia, WB Saunders, 1996.*)

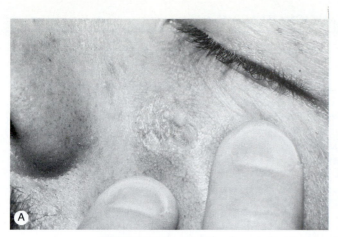
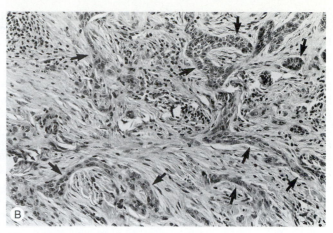

**FIGURE 4D-25.** Morpheaform (sclerosing) basal cell carcinoma. *A*. Clinically, the lesions present as ill-defined zones of cutaneous atrophy. *B*. Histologically, the lesions consist of slender nests and cords of tumor cells (arrows) in a cellular, fibrotic matrix. (*With permission, from Banks PM, Kraybill WG: Pathology for the Surgeon. Philadelphia, WB Saunders, 1996.*)

Malignant melanoma is one of the most aggressive and capricious human neoplasms. Lesions as small as 5 mm in diameter and 1 mm thick can metastasize with rapid fatality. Most cutaneous melanomas proceed sequentially through a less aggressive radial growth phase, with intraepidermal "lateral" proliferation, eventually attaining a more aggressive "vertical" growth into dermal and even subcutaneous tissues with high risk of lymphatic and hematogenous metastases.[15,16] They are composed of variably atypical melanocytes, sometimes attaining extremely anaplastic cellular features, often losing their production of pigment as evidence of "dedifferentiation" (Fig. 4D-26). Indeed, metastatic melanoma is respected by pathologists as "the great masquerader," capable of microscopically mimicking other high-grade tumors. Complete excision

of melanomas for initial pathologic microstaging is critical for prognostic and management purposes. Both depth of invasion and maximal lesional thickness are important determinants. So predictive are the microstaging findings for cutaneous melanomas that they have been incorporated as the essential criteria for tumor staging within the AJCC pathologic staging system (Table 4D-1). Width of adequate surgical resection is heavily microstage dependent. Randomized prospective trials have demonstrated that adequate margins for primary tumors measuring up to 1 mm in thickness can be as little as 1 cm.[17] Tumors greater than 1 mm in thickness require 2-cm margins. Intraoperative frozen section is almost never indicated in the resection of malignant melanoma. Historically, the role of lymph node dissection in patients without clinical evidence of

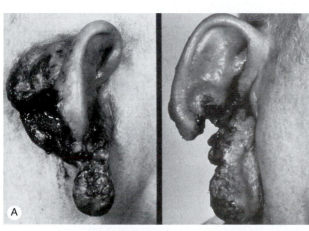
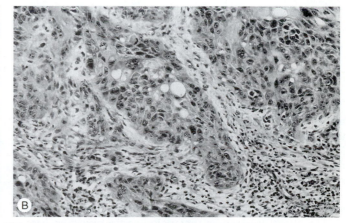

**FIGURE 4D-26.** Squamous cell carcinoma. *A*. This large, fungating lesion has partially destroyed the pinna of the ear. *B*. Histologically, the lesion consists of nests of markedly atypical keratinocytes that invade the surrounding dermis. (*With permission, from Banks PM, Kraybill WG: Pathology for the Surgeon. Philadelphia, WB Saunders, 1996.*)

**TABLE 4D-1.** AJCC STAGING SYSTEM FOR CUTANEOUS MALIGNANT MELANOMA

Primary tumor (pT):

| | |
|---|---|
| pTX | Primary tumor cannot be assessed. |
| pT0 | No evidence of primary tumor. |
| pTis | Melanoma in situ (atypical melanocytic hyperplasia, severe melanocytic dysplasia), not an invasive malignant lesion (Clark's level I). |
| pT1 | Tumor 0.75 mm or less in thickness and invades the papillary dermis (Clark's level II). |
| pT2 | Tumor more than 0.75 mm but not more than 1.5 mm in thickness and/or invades to papillary-reticular dermal interface (Clark's level III). |
| pT3 | Tumor more than 1.5 mm but not more than 4 mm in thickness and/or invades the reticular dermis (Clark's level IV). |
| pT3a | Tumor more than 1.5 mm but not more than 3 mm in thickness. |
| pT3b | Tumor more than 3 mm but not more than 4 mm in thickness. |
| pT4 | Tumor more than 4 mm in thickness and/or invades the subcutaneous tissue (Clark's level V) and/or satellite(s) within 2 cm of the primary tumor. |
| pT4a | Tumor more than 4 mm in thickness and/or invades the subcutaneous tissue. |
| pT4b | Satellite(s) within 2 cm of the primary tumor. |

Regional lymph nodes (N):

| | |
|---|---|
| NX | Regional lymph nodes cannot be assessed. |
| N0 | No regional lymph node metastasis. |
| N1 | Metastasis 3 cm or less in greatest dimension in any regional lymph node(s). |
| N2 | Metastasis more than 3 cm in greatest dimension in any regional lymph node(s) and/or in-transit metastasis. |
| N2a | Metastasis more than 3 cm in greatest dimension in any regional lymph node(s). |
| N2b | In-transit metastasis. |
| N2c | Both (N2a and N2b). |

Distant metastasis (M):

| | |
|---|---|
| MX | Distant metastasis cannot be assessed. |
| M0 | No distant metastasis. |
| M1 | Distant metastasis. |
| M1a | Metastasis in skin or subcutaneous tissue or lymph node(s) beyond the regional lymph nodes. |
| M1b | Visceral metastasis. |

Stage grouping:

| | | | |
|---|---|---|---|
| Stage 0 | pTis | N0 | M0 |
| Stage I | pT1 | N0 | M0 |
| | pT2 | N0 | M0 |
| Stage II | pT3 | N0 | M0 |
| Stage III | pT4 | N0 | M0 |
| | Any pT | N1 | M0 |
| | Any pT | N2 | M0 |
| Stage IV | Any pT | Any N | M1 |

SOURCE: With permission from the American Joint Committee on Cancer: *AJCC Cancer Staging Manual*, 5th ed. JD Fleming et al (eds). Philadelphia, Lippincott-Raven, 1997.

metastases has been highly controversial. Development of selective sentinel lymph node biopsy has allowed accurate evaluation for the presence of metastatic disease without performing complete nodal dissection. Thorough evaluation of such sentinel lymph node specimens by the pathologist with multilevel sectioning and, when needed, ancillary immunohistochemical techniques for sensitive detection of micrometastases, is critical to the successful institution of this highly specialized surgical strategy. Prospective evaluations have demonstrated a false-positive rate of 1%. Gamma probe–guided nodal localization, in combination with the use of blue dye, further enhances efficacy of the technique and accelerates the learning curve.

# THE BREAST

The common goal for surgeon and pathologist is accurate diagnosis for successful management of neoplastic breast disease. Today's attempts at ever earlier detection of breast cancer represent new challenges, as smaller, subtler lesions are the subject of study. Critical to success are open lines of communication among radiologist, pathologist, and surgeon. Regular case conferences are an effective means for maintaining high quality practice in the setting of constantly expanding knowledge and changing methodologies.

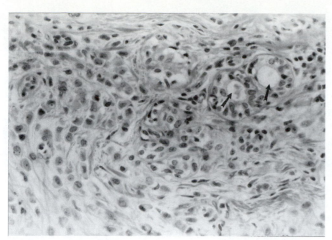

**FIGURE 4D-27.** Infiltrative adenocarcinoma of breast with mixed ductal and lobular features, a not uncommon observation. Ductal differentiation is seen in right upper field (arrows), whereas dispersed lobular pattern is most conspicuous in lower left portion of field. (Hematoxylin and eosin, ×400.)

Familiarity with the standard inventory of prototypic pathologic lesions, malignant and premalignant, and staging and other predictive markers can be acquired through use of updated templates applied by the pathologist to each biopsy or resection case. The experienced surgeon specializing in the management of breast disease comes to understand that not all lesions can be adequately described in terms of these disease prototypes. For example, while most cancers, both invasive and in situ, can be characterized as either ductal or lobular, occasional cases show overlapping microscopic features (Fig. 4D-27).

## DIAGNOSTIC SAMPLING

Fine-needle aspiration cytology samples are a rapid and convenient means to establish the malignant nature of highly suspicious lesions, e.g., large, palpable fixed tumors or suspected recurrence. Interpretations by experienced pathologists can often go further, including possibilities such as spindle cell stromal proliferations, inflammatory processes, etc.[18] However, this type of sample is not adequate for classification or grading of carcinomas. Needle-core biopsies can often be used to accurately classify carcinomas as to invasive vs. in situ and to suggest certain specific types of benign proliferations such as fibroadenoma, sclerosing adenosis, etc. The presence of calcification can also be assessed, for radiologic correlation, in needle-core sections. Accurate grading and staging of carcinomas and risk management evaluation of proliferative breast disease require larger excisional specimens.

## PATHOLOGIC EVALUATION OF LARGE SPECIMENS

Accurate orientation and careful gross evaluation of excised or resected breast specimens are critical to the pathologist's final report. Intraoperative frozen sections should not be requested unless imme-

diate decision making is to be based on the outcome, e.g., extension of margins or proceeding to axillary nodal dissection. Small lesions (less than 1 cm) should not be subjected to frozen-section interpretation because freezing artifact jeopardizes final diagnostic accuracy.[2] If margins consist of soft adipose tissue, frozen sections cannot be produced (see Fig. 4D-4). Insistence on intraoperative pathologic interpretation of such specimens by means other than careful gross examination is unreasonable and serves no purpose.

Careful orientation of excisional specimens should be indicated by the surgeon with sutures or other markings on the specimen, or by direct demonstration to the pathologist. When intraoperative pathologic evaluation is requested, adequate time should be allowed the pathologist for careful orientation and color-keyed inking of the specimen surfaces (see Fig. 4D-4). No sections should be made prior to inking of margin surfaces and a gross dictation, since these essential elements of evaluation cannot be re-created from a specimen once it has been sectioned. Even grossly benign, fatty excisional specimens should be thoroughly sampled microscopically if an earlier needle or mammotome biopsy showed malignancy, since such extensive "blind" sampling increases the likelihood of detecting foci of residual carcinoma.[19]

For particularly soft fatty specimens, an extra day of turn-around time should be allotted for the final pathology report, reflecting initial fixation of the entire intact specimen preparatory to sectioning. Sectioning a soft, unfixed fatty specimen invariably introduces distortion of tissue planes and the interrelationships between tumor and margins. Axillary dissection contents submitted separately should have a suture or other marking to indicate the highest level of lymph nodes.

Correlation of pathology with radiologic findings is often essential to address the question as to what a specific focal abnormality corresponds. Wire loop localization excision specimens should be radiographed prior to arrival in the laboratory. The pathologist, through comparison of the radiograph to the specimen, can usually isolate the suspicious lesion within a few carefully selected tissue blocks. Alternatively, when excised specimens are relatively small (less than 100 mL), the entire tissue sampling can be reduced into spatially sequenced tissue blocks, spaced over an x-ray film, and selected for processing on the basis of the presence of radiologic abnormalities, such as microcalcifications or soft tissue densities. When microscopic sections fail to demonstrate expected calcifications, radiographs can be made of the remaining paraffin-embedded blocks to ascertain whether sectioning deeper into these blocks may yet disclose the calcified lesion(s).

## SPECIAL TISSUE ALLOCATIONS

The requirements for fresh tissue allocation for biochemical assay of estrogen and progesterone receptors have been superseded in recent years by the development of highly accurate paraffin section immunostains for these same markers. Likewise, immunostaining for *erb*-B2 overexpression has recently been developed.[20] These immunostaining methods are actually superior to the direct assay, because they allow the pathologist to visualize the cells being stained by direct microscopy, assuring that it is cancer cells and not associated benign ductal elements that are being assessed. Other studies requiring fresh or fresh-frozen sections, such as ploidy analysis or cathepsin-D activity are not currently established as independent predictors of clinical outcome or as indicators for alternative management strategies. Therefore, at present the pathologist can carry out conventional fixation, which also assures optimal conventional microscopic evaluation, without compromising any special study requirements.

## CONVENTIONAL MICROSCOPIC EVALUATION

Meticulous microscopic scrutiny is required in evaluation of all breast samples because of the highly variable and sometimes focal nature of many entities. It is not unusual to encounter a single focus of lobular carcinoma in situ, occupying an area only 2 mm in maximum dimension, within a sampling of many microscopic slides totaling dozens of square centimeters in area (Fig. 4D-28). Even in straightforward cases of invasive carcinoma, subtle features such as vascular or lymphatic invasion, mitotic activity, and associated in situ carcinomatous elements demand rigorous study to detect or quantitate. Special requirements are associated with evaluation of sentinel lymph nodes, including sections at interval levels and, when no evidence of metastasis is found by conventional microscopy, immunostaining for sensitive markers such as cytokeratins or epithelial membrane antigen, in order to avoid missing subtle micrometastases[21] (Fig. 4D-29).

## REPORTING BREAST CARCINOMAS

Because options for management of breast cancer patients have created a complex multifactorial decision-making process (see

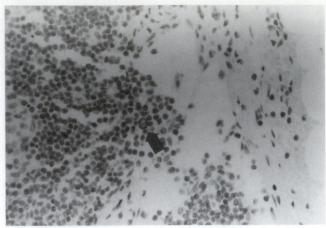

**FIGURE 4D-29.** Single cell of metastatic breast carcinoma in axillary, sentinel lymph node, detected by immunostaining (arrow). Pale capsular fibrous tissues to right side of field. Immunoperoxidase method for cytokeratin was used to detect tumor cells so rare and scattered as to be unrecognizable in conventional sections. (Ethylcarbazole color reagent, hematoxylin counterstain, ×400.)

Chapter 19, "Neoplasms of the Breast"), complete and detailed reporting of pathologic findings, both gross and microscopic, is mandatory. Most pathologists find the use of a template a practical and convenient means to assure that all requisite information has been obtained and reported in conventional terms. For the surgeon, inclusion of such standardized informational format is useful, since it allows uniform, predictable presentation of critical elements of staging and grading tumors[22] (Table 4D-2). Such template

**TABLE 4D-2. TEMPLATE FOR BREAST CARCINOMA PATHOLOGY REPORTING**

**Tumor type:** (e.g., infiltrative ductal, no special type versus other)

**Tumor size:** (Single maximum dimension)

**Focality:** (Unifocal versus multifocal—usually meaning in more than one quadrant)

**Margins:** (Single closest measurement)

**Skin or chest wall invasion:** (Present?)

**Lymphatic or vascular invasion:** (Present?)

**Tumor grade:** Multifactorial Scarff, Bloom, and Richardson, as modified by Elston, combining nuclear grade, degree of tubular growth pattern and mitotic rate for a total score ranging from 1–9[24]

**Associated duct carcinoma in situ:** Estimated percentage of tumor that is in situ versus infiltrative.

**Calcifications:** Present in tumor or in benign elements?

**Receptor status:** Strong, modest, mild, or no staining for ER and PR in immunohistochemical slide preparations.

**TNM stage:** (Current AJCC criteria)

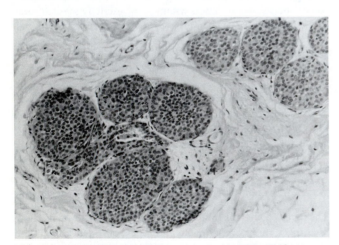

**FIGURE 4D-28.** Lobular carcinoma in situ (LCIS). Uniform neoplastic cells fill and distend this lobular unit. This high-risk lesion may be found either in isolation or in association with infiltrative carcinoma of lobular or ductal type. (*With permission, from Banks PM, Kraybill WG: Pathology for the Surgeon. Philadelphia, WB Saunders, 1996.*)

reporting does not replace conventional gross and microscopic descriptions that are specific to each individual patient and that allow for variable features that cannot be anticipated by simplified forms. Although most breast cancers can be adequately characterized in such templates, there are occasional cases that elude description in such a stock format. Examples include mucinous and adenoid-cystic variants of ductal carcinoma and certain variants of lobular-type carcinoma.

The AJCC pathologic staging system is well suited to risk stratification for breast carcinoma, with 5-year relative survival rates corresponding to stage I being 98%, stage IIIA being 55%, and stage IV being 16%. Therefore, meticulous detail on the part of pathologist is required for accurate gross and microscopic evaluation of excisional and resection specimens (Table 4D-3).

## RISK ASSESSMENT OF PROLIFERATIVE LESIONS

Due to the focal distribution and small size of some high-risk proliferative lesions, smaller biopsy samples or blocks deriving from radiologically suspicious areas in larger specimens need particularly painstaking examination, often involving the study of sections at multiple levels within the tissue block. Similarly, microscopic identification of a worrisome or atypical area, such as atypical terminal duct proliferation, justifies the evaluation of additional sections in the same block (Fig. 4D-30).

Long-term risk assessment based on excisional biopsies is predicated on thorough microscopic examination. With long-term longitudinal clinical studies, ever greater precision in recognition of subtly different lesions is required.[23] For example, fibroadenoma has a roughly twofold relative risk implication if proliferative changes are present in the epithelium of surrounding elements, but when such

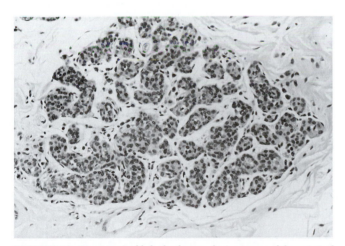

**FIGURE 4D-30.** Atypical lobular hyperplasia. Some of the acini of this lobular unit contain the same cells found in LCIS; however, none is completely filled and there is no distention, hence the diagnosis of atypical lobular hyperplasia. Compare to Fig. 4D-28. (*With permission, from Banks PM, Kraybill WG: Pathology for the Surgeon. Philadelphia, WB Saunders, 1996.*)

associated changes are not present, there appears to be no increased relative risk.

## THE HEAD AND NECK

### INTRODUCTION

The anatomy and pathology of the head and neck are uniquely complex. First, biopsies from this area are frequently small or crushed. Second, there is a wide spectrum of complex neoplasms in this area, such as the numerous subtypes of salivary gland tumors. The anatomy, with its bewildering arrangement of cavities, sinuses, and spaces, is very complex. Finally, because human interchange is directed to and through this anatomic region, patient sensitivities to any surgical-cosmetic defects are often extreme. As emphasized elsewhere in this chapter, the key to effective patient care is close communication between surgeon and pathologist. Relevant patient history, such as the source of the biopsy, the clinical impression, and past treatment with surgery, radiation, and chemotherapy, are all important to the pathologist.

### MARGINS OF RESECTION

Traditionally, the pathologist evaluates margins of resection at the time of gross evaluation of the excised tumor; however, some surgeons prefer to remove the tumor and then separately sample designated margins. Either approach is acceptable. For larger complex specimens, such as maxillectomies and cranial base resections, the surgeon may call the pathologist to the operating room to orient the specimen and point out margins of concern. Adequacy of margins varies according to anatomic location and tumor type. For squamous cell carcinoma arising in the larynx, 2 mm is sufficient, whereas for tumors of the oral cavity and hypopharynx-cervical esophagus (where submucosal spread is common), margins of at least 5 and 10 mm, respectively, are desirable. In adenoid cystic tumors, neural margins are of particular importance.

### FROZEN SECTIONS

In the head and neck region, intraoperative frozen sections are used primarily to evaluate salivary gland tumors, lymph nodes, neck masses, disorders of thyroid and parathyroid glands, and the adequacy of resection margins. Although the procedure is 95% to 98% accurate, errors do occur. The indications for frozen section are to determine diagnosis, to evaluate margins, to assure that tissue removed will be diagnostic, and to identify certain microorganisms such *Aspergillus* expeditiously. Errors can be limited by good communication between the pathologist and the surgeon.

### PREMALIGNANT LESIONS

Premalignant lesions of the mucous membranes of the head and neck usually appear as patches that are white (leukoplakia), red

**TABLE 4D-3.** AJCC SYSTEM FOR STAGING BREAST CARCINOMA

Primary tumor (T):

| | |
|---|---|
| TX | Primary tumor cannot be assessed. |
| T0 | No evidence of primary tumor. |
| Tis | Carcinoma in situ: Intraductal carcinoma, lobular carcinoma in situ, or Paget's disease* of the nipple with no tumor. |
| T1 | Tumor 2 cm or less in greatest dimension. |
| T1mic | Microinvasion 0.1 cm or less in greatest dimension. |
| T1a | Tumor more than 0.1 but not more than 0.5 cm in greatest dimension. |
| T1b | Tumor more than 0.5 cm but not more than 1 cm in greatest dimension. |
| T1c | Tumor more than 1 cm but not more than 2 cm in greatest dimension. |
| T2 | Tumor more than 2 cm but not more than 5 cm in greatest dimension. |
| T3 | Tumor more than 5 cm in greatest dimension. |
| T4 | Tumor of any size with direct extension to (a) chest wall or (b) skin, only as described below. |
| T4a | Extension to chest wall. |
| T4b | Edema (including peau d'orange) or ulceration of the skin of the breast or satellite skin nodules confined to the same breast. |
| T4c | Both (T4a and T4b). |
| T4d | Inflammatory carcinoma. |

Regional lymph nodes (N):

| | |
|---|---|
| NX | Regional lymph nodes cannot be assessed (e.g., previously removed). |
| N0 | No regional lymph node metastasis. |
| N1 | Metastasis to movable ipsilateral axillary lymph node(s). |
| N2 | Metastasis to ipsilateral axillary lymph node(s) fixed to one another or to other structures. |
| N3 | Metastasis to ipsilateral internal mammary lymph node(s). |

Pathologic classification (pN):

| | |
|---|---|
| pNX | Regional lymph nodes cannot be assessed (e.g., previously removed, or not removed for pathologic study). |
| pN0 | No regional lymph node metastasis. |
| pN1 | Metastasis to movable ipsilateral axillary lymph node(s). |
| pN1a | Only micrometastasis (none larger than 0.2 cm). |
| pN1b | Metastasis to lymph node(s), any larger than 0.2 cm. |
| pN1bi | Metastasis in 1 to 3 lymph nodes, any more than 0.2 cm and all less than 2 cm in greatest dimension. |
| pN1bii | Metastasis to 4 or more lymph nodes, any more than 0.2 cm and all less than 2 cm in greatest dimension. |
| pN1biii | Extension of tumor beyond the capsule of a lymph node metastasis less than 2 cm in greatest dimension. |
| pN1biv | Metastasis to a lymph node 2 cm or more in greatest dimension. |
| pN2 | Metastasis to ipsilateral axillary lymph nodes that are fixed to one another or to other structures. |
| pN3 | Metastasis to ipsilateral internal mammary lymph node(s). |

Distant metastasis (M):

| | |
|---|---|
| MX | Distant metastasis cannot be assessed. |
| M0 | No distant metastasis. |
| M1 | Distant metastasis (includes metastasis to ipsilateral supraclavicular lymph node[s]). |

Stage grouping:

| Stage | T | N | M |
|---|---|---|---|
| Stage 0 | Tis | N0 | M0 |
| Stage I | T1 | N0 | M0 |
| Stage IIA | T0 | N1 | M0 |
| | T1 | N1 | M0 |
| | T2 | N0 | M0 |
| Stage IIB | T2 | N1 | M0 |
| | T3 | N0 | M0 |
| Stage IIIA | T0 | N2 | M0 |
| | T1 | N2 | M0 |
| | T2 | N2 | M0 |
| | T3 | N1 | M0 |
| | T3 | N2 | M0 |
| Stage IIIB | T4 | Any N | M0 |
| | Any T | N3 | M0 |
| Stage IV | Any T | Any N | M1 |

* Paget's disease associated with a tumor is classified according to the size of the tumor.
SOURCE: With permission from the American Joint Committee on Cancer: *AJCC Cancer Staging Manual,* 5th ed. JD Fleming et al (eds). Philadelphia, Lippincott-Raven, 1997.

(erythroplasia, erythroplakia), or mixed white-red (speckled leuko-plakia). Of the three, erythroplasia is the most ominous, since these lesions frequently correspond microscopically to severe dysplasia, carcinoma in situ, or superficially invasive squamous cell carcinoma. Erythroplasias characteristically have poorly defined margins. They occur commonly in the oral cavity or oropharynx and infrequently in the larynx. In contrast, leukoplakias exhibit a broad spectrum of histologic findings. Some show only surface keratinization without significant epithelial changes, whereas others demonstrate invasive keratinizing squamous cell carcinoma. Those with dysplasia are important because they are premalignant and portend the patient's increased risk for developing malignancy.

## ORAL CAVITY

**ANATOMY.** The oral cavity extends from the skin-vermilion junction of the lips to the junction of the hard-soft palate above and the line of circumvallate papillae below. It is divided into seven major divisions: lips, anterior two-thirds of the tongue (oral, mobile tongue), floor of mouth, buccal mucosa, upper and lower alveolar ridges, hard palate, and retromolar gingiva (retromolar trigone).[24]

**BENIGN DISEASES.** Common benign conditions of the oral cavity include cystic lesions of the jaws, mucoceles, ranulas, irritation fibromas, granular-cell tumors, and ameloblastomas.

Cysts and cystlike lesions of the jaws can be divided into true cysts (those with an epithelial lining) versus pseudocysts (those without an epithelial lining) and odontogenic versus nonodontogenic cysts.

Odontogenic cysts arise from or are associated with the tooth apparatus (Fig. 4D-31). Since the subtypes share a similar histologic feature, namely, a squamous epithelial lining, accurate classification

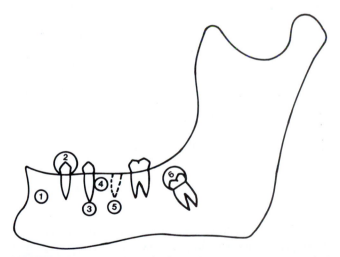

**FIGURE 4D-31.** Location of odontogenic cysts. 1 = primordial cyst, 2 = eruption cyst, 3 = radicular cyst, 4 = lateral periodontal cyst, 5 = residual cyst, and 6 = dentigerous cyst. (*With permission from Banks PM, Kraybill WG: Pathology for the Surgeon. Philadelphia, WB Saunders, 1996.*)

depends upon clinical-radiographic findings and the result of dental vitality testing. On roentgenographic exam they appear as well-circumscribed unilocular, sometimes multilocular, radiolucencies. Unless neglected, most odontogenic cysts are relatively harmless and are rarely the site of malignant change. The exception is the odontogenic keratocyst, especially the parakeratotic type. This cyst is locally aggressive, tends to recur, may be multiple, and is sometimes associated with the nevoid basal cell carcinoma syndrome.

Mucoceles arise from traumatic disruption of the ducts of minor salivary glands. As a result, mucus escapes into the soft tissue and elicits an inflammatory response. A mucocele typically presents as a solitary, 0.5 cm or less, blue, dome-shaped elevation on the lower lip and is especially common in "lip biters." Ranulas represent another type of mucus-retention phenomenon that presents in the floor of the mouth on either side of the midline. They are larger than mucoceles and result from disruption of the excretory duct of the sublingual gland and, rarely, of the submandibular gland or as a result of blockage of the excretory duct with cystic accumulation of mucus distal to the obstruction.

Irritation fibromas represent a localized fibrous tissue response to chronic trauma of the oral mucosa. They are usually seen on the lateral border of the tongue, the buccal mucosa, or the lower lip and rarely exceed 1 cm.

Granular-cell tumors are uncommon neoplasms of presumed neural origin that in the past have been inappropriately referred to as "granular-cell myoblastomas." They occur primarily on the tongue and rarely exceed 2 to 3 cm. Their smooth, firm, submucosal appearance contrasts with squamous cell carcinoma of the tongue, which is usually ulcerated. They consist of delicate pink granular cells that may elude notice microscopically and often induce pseudo-epitheliomatous hyperplasia of the overlying squamous mucosa that in superficial biopsies can be mistaken by the pathologist for a squamous cell carcinoma. To avoid this mishap, any lesion suspected of being a granular cell tumor should be adequately biopsied.

The ameloblastoma is a histologically benign, sometimes locally aggressive, odontogenic tumor that occurs primarily in the mandible (80% to 85% of all patients) and less commonly in the maxilla. It is seen in all age groups, with a peak occurrence in adults averaging 35 to 45 years of age. On radiographic exam, it presents as a unilocular or multilocular radiolucency with well-defined, often sclerotic borders. The tumor is nonencapsulated and grows as large islands or anastomosing cords of cells, with prominent nuclear palisading of the peripheral cells. Since curettage is associated with a 50% to 100% rate of recurrence, wide excision with a margin of 1 to 1.5 cm is advisable. Most ameloblastomas are radioresistant.

## MALIGNANT DISEASES

Squamous cell carcinoma is the most common malignant tumor of the oral cavity. The most frequent sites of origin are the lips, tongue, and the floor of mouth.

Some 88% to 98% of all labial squamous cell carcinomas occur on the lower lip, where they typically arise on the exposed vermilion border approximately halfway between the oral commissure and the midline. Most are well differentiated and, when small, are sometimes difficult to distinguish both clinically and microscopically from actinic keratoses. The majority of patients are men, usually between 50 and 80 years of age. Fewer than 10% of patients have cervical node metastasis at diagnosis. The average 5-year determinant survival is 82%.[25] Poor prognostic features include:

1. Tumors larger than 2.0 cm
2. Occurrence on the upper lip or oral commissure
3. Perineural invasion
4. Greater than 6 mm depth of invasion
5. Mandibular involvement
6. Cervical lymph node metastases, especially if there is extranodal spread.[25,26]

Approximately 75% of all carcinomas of the oral tongue present as painless ulcers on the lateral border. At the time of diagnosis, 30% of patients will have clinically positive cervical lymph nodes and, if the tumor crosses the midline, the incidence of contralateral or bilateral nodal metastases increases. The overall 5-year determinant survival for squamous cell carcinoma of the oral tongue is 45% to 50%.[25] Because tumors of the base of the tongue are not amenable to inspection, they tend to be more advanced at presentation. Some 50% to 75% of patients will have cervical lymph node metastasis at diagnosis, and 20% to 30% will either have or develop contralateral and/or bilateral nodal metastases during the course of their disease. The overall 5-year determinant survival rate is 25% to 30%.[25]

Squamous cell carcinomas of the floor of the mouth typically arise laterally rather than in the midline. In 50% to 75% of patients, the tumor has extended beyond the floor of the mouth to involve the tongue, gingiva, anterior tonsillar pillar, or mandible. Some 30% to 60% of patients either have or will develop cervical lymph node metastases. Of floor of mouth tumors, 15% to 30% invade the mandible. If the tumor invades the mandible, the tumor may propagate along the intraosseus inferior alveolar nerve and compromise an otherwise adequate margin of resection. The overall 5-year determinant survival rate for squamous cell carcinoma of the floor of the mouth is 35% to 50%.

Verrucous carcinoma is an exceedingly well-differentiated nonmetastasizing but locally aggressive variant of squamous cell carcinoma which, on small biopsies, is often histologically indistinguishable from a squamous papilloma or nonspecific epithelial hyperplasia. As a result, close communication between the surgeon and pathologist is necessary to establish the correct diagnosis. The tumor is rarely seen in patients below the age of 50 years and, in the oral cavity, originates primarily from the lower alveolar ridge or buccal mucosa (Fig. 4D-32). Risk factors include the use of tobacco, poor oral hygiene, and possibly the human papillomavirus. Medina et al.[27] have described variants of verrucous carcinoma that contain foci of conventional squamous cell carcinoma, so-called hybrid tumors. In their review of 104 verrucous carcinomas of the oral cavity, 19.2% were regarded as hybrid tumors. The incidence of local recurrence following treatment was higher in the hybrid group (30%) compared with that of pure verrucous carcinoma (18.2%). Their study underscores the importance of thorough microscopic sampling of verrucous carcinomas for foci of conventional squamous cell carcinoma.

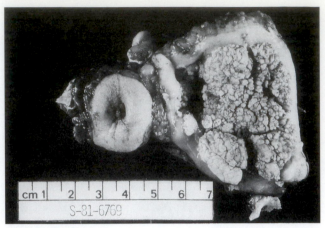

**FIGURE 4D-32.** Large verrucous carcinoma of the buccal mucosa with involvement of overlying skin (note circular portion of skin on the left with central "dimple"). (*With permission, from Banks PM, Kraybill WG:* Pathology for the Surgeon. *Philadelphia, WB Saunders, 1996.*)

## OROPHARYNX

**ANATOMY.** The oropharynx extends from the plane of the hard palate superiorly to the plane of the hyoid bone inferiorly and is continuous with the oral cavity through an opening termed the faucial isthmus. The oropharynx contains the soft palate, uvula, anterior and posterior tonsillar pillars, palatine tonsils, base of the tongue, vallecula, and posterior and lateral oropharyngeal walls.

**BENIGN DISEASES.** Although not as popular now as in the past, tonsillectomy is still the most common operation done in the oropharynx. Pathologic evaluation of tonsils for recurrent tonsillitis generally shows only lymphoid hyperplasia with or without fibrosis or, at most, foci of superficial ulceration with residual acute inflammation of the surface or within the crypts. Granules of *Actinomyces* are commonly found in the tonsillar crypts and should not be confused with the disease actinomycosis, in which the organism invades the tissue and elicits an inflammatory response.

**MALIGNANT DISEASES.** Squamous cell carcinoma and malignant lymphoma are the most common malignancies of the tonsils, accounting for 70% to 85% and 15% of all tonsillar malignancies, respectively. Because of their delicate lymphoid cellular composition, biopsies of the tonsils are more fragile and subject to crush artifact than tissue from most other sites in the head and neck. Some tonsillar carcinomas, especially those that arise from the base of the tonsillar crypts, are notorious for producing cystic cervical lymph node metastases that masquerade as a branchial cleft cyst or as a tumor of unknown origin, often without clinical abnormality on physical examination. As a result, diagnostic tonsillectomy is superior to biopsy for establishing the diagnosis. Although lymphomas of the tonsil arise in the submucosa, they can involve the overlying mucosa and thereby result in ulceration. Squamous cell carcinoma of the tonsil occurs in patients over the age of 50 years and manifests as a sore throat or a neck mass. At the time of diagnosis, 50% to 75% will have clinically enlarged cervical lymph nodes. The overall 5-year determinant survival is about 40%.[25]

## NASOPHARYNX

**ANATOMY.** The roof of the nasopharynx is the base of the skull, which slopes downward to become the posterior pharyngeal wall. The inferior limit is the plane of the hard palate. The anterior boundary is the choana, through which it is continuous with the nasal cavity. The lateral wall is composed of the torus tubarius, the eustachian tube orifice, and that portion of the mucosa of the fossa of Rosenmuller that extends to its apex and junction with the roof.[24]

**BENIGN DISEASES.** Symptomatic enlargement of the adenoids and angiofibromas are the most common benign conditions of the nasopharynx that require surgical intervention. Enlarged adenoids should be removed when they obstruct the nasopharyngeal orifice of the eustachian tube with repeated bouts of otitis media or when they occlude the nasal passages and cause labored breathing.

Angiofibroma, sometimes referred to as nasopharyngeal angiofibroma, arises from a fibrovascular nidus in the posterolateral wall of the nasal cavity but, following the lines of least resistance, secondarily involves the nasopharynx. Though histologically benign, this tumor can be locally destructive if neglected and may even extend intracranially in 5% to 20% of patients. If incompletely excised, it may recur. Histologically, the tumor is highly vascular and densely fibrous (Fig. 4D-33). The blood vessels are usually but not invariably devoid of smooth muscle and therefore incapable of vasoconstriction. As a result, biopsies of angiofibromas may lead to profuse hemorrhage.

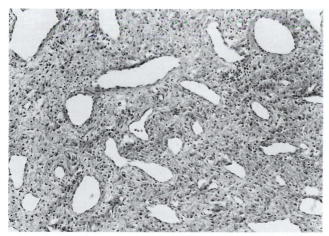

**FIGURE 4D-33.** Angiofibroma. Note the fibrous stroma and the numerous blood vessels which lack smooth muscle in their walls. (Hematoxylin and eosin, ×100.) (*With permission, from Banks PM, Kraybill WG:* Pathology for the Surgeon. *Philadelphia, WB Saunders, 1996.*)

Although malignant change in angiofibromas has been recorded, in most cases this has followed unusually high doses of irradiation.

**MALIGNANT DISEASES.** Malignant lymphoma and nasopharyngeal carcinoma are the most common malignant tumors of the nasopharynx, and both are treated primarily by radiotherapy. Nasopharyngeal carcinoma is one of the most common cancers in China and Southeast Asia but is relatively uncommon in the United States. The World Health Organization (WHO) divides nasopharyngeal carcinomas into three types: squamous cell carcinoma (WHO I), nonkeratinizing carcinoma (WHO II), and undifferentiated carcinoma (WHO III). Prognosis depends partly on histologic type. Those carcinomas that show keratinization tend to have a poorer prognosis than do those that lack keratinization. These latter types are also more responsive to irradiation therapy and are more closely associated with the Epstein-Barr virus than is squamous cell carcinoma.

## HYPOPHARYNX

**ANATOMY.** The hypopharynx extends from the plane of the hyoid bone superiorly to the lower border of the cricoid cartilage inferiorly. It consists of three regions: the pyriform sinuses, posterior pharyngeal wall, and postcricoid area.

**MALIGNANT DISEASES.** Benign disease in this area is rare. Squamous cell carcinomas of the hypopharynx are about one-third as common as those of the larynx. Approximately 65% to 85% arise in the pyriform sinus, 10% to 20% on the posterior pharyngeal wall, and 5% to 15% in the postcricoid area.[24] Since the hypopharynx is not amenable to self-inspection, patients often present with advanced tumors. Hypopharyngeal carcinomas are notorious for growing beneath intact mucosa and often extend well beyond their apparent clinical margins. Pyriform sinus tumors that extend to the apex of the sinus occasionally involve, either by direct extension or embolic spread, the ipsilateral lobe of the thyroid. Some 65% to 75% of hypopharyngeal carcinomas are associated with cervical lymph node metastases. Other nodal groups can be metastatically involved as well: retropharyngeal nodes with posterior pharyngeal wall tumors and paratracheal nodes with postcricoid tumors. The 5-year determinant survival is 20% to 40%.[25]

## LARYNX

**ANATOMY.** The superolateral border of the larynx is delineated by the tip of the epiglottis and the aryepiglottic folds, while the inferior rim of the cricoid cartilage defines the lower extent. The larynx is divided into three regions: supraglottis, glottis, and subglottis.[24]

**BENIGN DISEASES.** Common benign conditions of the larynx are vocal cord nodules, squamous papillomas, and the "keratoses." Vocal cord nodules are not true neoplasms but a stromal reaction to vocal abuse. They characteristically occur on the anterior half of the true vocal cord. Squamous papillomas of the larynx are divided into nonkeratinized and keratinized types. Nonkeratinizing papillomas occur predominantly in children, are often multiple, and are associated with the human papillomavirus (HPV) types 6 and 11. Although they often recur following excision, they have little if any malignant potential (unless irradiated). They present as pink, often confluent growths. In contrast, keratinized papilloma occurs predominantly in adults and is usually a solitary white growth. They generally are not related to HPV, but despite the fact that they show less tendency to recur, they may occasionally become malignant. The mucous membrane of the larynx, if irritated, may keratinize focally and form "leukoplakia" or keratoses. These may be innocuous, premalignant, or malignant, and consequently require biopsy.

MALIGNANT DISEASES. Squamous cell carcinoma accounts for 95% of all malignant tumors of the larynx and, based on location, is divided into three major categories: glottic, supraglottic, and subglottic. Glottic carcinomas arise from the true vocal cords or the anterior and posterior commissures. They represent 60% to 65% of all laryngeal carcinomas seen in the United States.[25] They typically arise from the anterior half of the true vocal cord. Because of their early association with hoarseness they are usually identified early. Prognosis varies according to stage. Because they are usually identified early, collectively they are associated with an 80% to 85% 5-year survival rate. More extensive glottic tumors that involve either the supraglottis or subglottis are termed transglottic tumors. These are more extensive tumors with a correspondingly worse prognosis. Supraglottic carcinomas arise from the epiglottis, false vocal cords, ventricles, aryepiglottic folds, and/or arytenoids and represent 30% to 35% of all laryngeal carcinomas. They tend to be bulky tumors and cause dysphagia, change in quality of the voice, otalgia sensation of a foreign body in the throat, or a neck mass. Supraglottic carcinomas have cervical lymph node metastases in 40% of patients and carry a 5-year survival rate of 65% to 75%. Subglottic carcinomas are the least common, representing no more than 5% of all laryngeal carcinomas. The subglottis is defined as the region from 1 cm below the apex of the ventricles to the lower border of the cricoid cartilage. Subglottic carcinomas present with airway obstruction and often require tracheotomy. Although they have cervical lymph node metastases in only 15% to 20% of patients, the primary drainage is to the paratracheal lymph nodes and thyroid gland. This site may also drain to mediastinal lymph nodes. The 5-year survival rate is 40%.

Although tumor staging for most head and neck carcinoma in the AJCC system is based on maximum tumor size, in the case of laryngeal carcinoma an intricate system has been developed reflecting progressively less favorable extension through the specialized anatomy of this region (Table 4D-4).

## NOSE AND PARANASAL SINUSES

ANATOMY. The nose and paired maxillary, ethmoid, frontal, and sphenoid sinuses form a functional unit referred to as the sinonasal tract. The nasal septum divides the nose internally into the right and left nasal cavities, each of which, in turn, communicates with the nasopharynx through openings called choanae. The

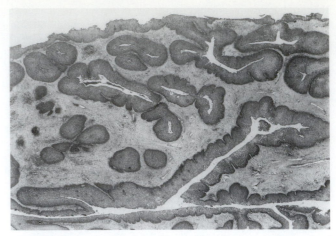

FIGURE 4D-34. Inverted papilloma. Note the inverted growth of sharply demarcated islands of epithelium. (Hematoxylin and eosin, ×100.) (*With permission, from Banks PM, Kraybill WG:* Pathology for the Surgeon. *Philadelphia, WB Saunders, 1996.*)

maxillary sinuses are usually symmetric and located in the body of each maxilla and connect to the other sinuses.

BENIGN DISEASES. Sinonasal polyps (allergic polyps, inflammatory polyps, simple polyps) are nonneoplastic inflammatory swellings of the mucosa of the nose and paranasal sinuses. Etiologically, they may be related to allergies, vasomotor rhinitis, infections, and cystic fibrosis. Some sinonasal polyps may contain reactive histiocytes and fibroblasts that have been mistaken microscopically for rhabdomyosarcoma. Inverted papillomas are histologically benign but locally aggressive head and neck tumors that, if neglected, may erode into the cranial cavity. They characteristically arise unilaterally in the nasal cavity in the region of the middle turbinate-ethmoid sinus. Microscopically, they are composed of hyperplastic ribbons of basement membrane–enclosed epithelium that grows into the underlying stroma (Fig. 4D-34). The epithelium may be squamous, respiratory, or transitional. Thorough microscopic examination is critical because 5% to 15% of inverted papillomas are associated with squamous cell carcinomas.

MALIGNANT DISEASES. Numerous "small round cell tumors" originate in the sinonasal tract. Such tumors are characterized by cells with prominent round nuclei and scant cytoplasm with or without mitoses and necrosis. This histologically similar but prognostically variable group of neoplasms includes malignant lymphoma, extramedullary plasmacytoma, olfactory neuroblastoma, primitive neuroectodermal tumor, Ewing's sarcoma, embryonal rhabdomyosarcoma, malignant melanoma, anaplastic carcinoma, and invasive pituitary adenoma. These tumors are often indistinguishable by routine hematoxylin and eosin microscopic evaluation and frequently require additional, time-consuming, specialized procedures, such as immunostaining and electron microscopy for

**TABLE 4D-4.** AJCC STAGING SYSTEM FOR LARYNGEAL TUMORS

Primary tumor (T):
TX   Primary tumor cannot be assessed.
T0   No evidence of primary tumor.
Tis   Carcinoma in situ.

Supraglottis:
T1   Tumor limited to one subsite of supraglottis with normal vocal cord mobility.
T2   Tumor invades mucosa of more than one adjacent subsite of supraglottis or glottis or region outside the supraglottis (e.g., mucosa of base of tongue, vallecula, medial wall of pyriform sinus) without fixation of the larynx.
T3   Tumor limited to larynx with vocal cord fixation and/or invades any of the following: postcricoid area, pre-epiglottic tissues.
T4   Tumor invades through the thyroid cartilage, and/or extends into soft tissues of the neck, thyroid, and/or esophagus.

Glottis:
T1   Tumor limited to the vocal cord(s) (may involve anterior or posterior commisure) with normal mobility.
    T1a   Tumor limited to one vocal cord.
    T1b   Tumor involves both vocal cords.
T2   Tumor extends to supraglottis and/or subglottis, and/or with impaired vocal cord mobility.
T3   Tumor limited to the larynx with vocal cord fixation.
T4   Tumor invades through the thyroid cartilage and/or to other tissues beyond the larynx (e.g., trachea, soft tissues of neck, including thyroid, pharynx).

Subglottis:
T1   Tumor limited to the subglottis.
T2   Tumor extends to vocal cord(s) with normal or impaired mobility.
T3   Tumor limited to larynx with vocal cord fixation.
T4   Tumor invades through cricoid or thyroid cartilage and/or extends to other tissues beyond the larynx (e.g., trachea, soft tissues of neck, including thyroid, esophagus).

Regional lymph nodes (N):
NX   Regional lymph nodes cannot be assessed.
N0   No regional lymph node metastasis.
N1   Metastasis in a single ipsilateral lymph node, 3 cm or less in greatest dimension.
N2   Metastasis in a single ipsilateral lymph node, more than 3 cm but not more than 6 cm in greatest dimension, or in multiple ipsilateral lymph nodes, none more than 6 cm in greatest dimension, or in bilateral or contralateral lymph nodes, none more than 6 cm in greatest dimension.
    N2a   Metastasis in a single ipsilateral lymph node more than 3 cm but not more than 6 cm in greatest dimension.
    N2b   Metastasis in multiple ipsilateral lymph nodes, none more than 6 cm in greatest dimension.
    N2c   Metastasis in bilateral or contralateral lymph nodes, none more than 6 cm in greatest dimension.
N3   Metastasis in a lymph node more than 6 cm in greatest dimension.

Distant metastasis (M):
MX   Distant metastasis cannot be assessed.
M0   No distant metastasis.
M1   Distant metastasis.

Stage grouping:

| Stage | T | N | M |
|---|---|---|---|
| Stage 0 | Tis | N0 | M0 |
| Stage I | T1 | N0 | M0 |
| Stage II | T2 | N0 | M0 |
| Stage III | T3 | N0 | M0 |
| | T1 | N1 | M0 |
| | T2 | N1 | M0 |
| | T3 | N1 | M0 |
| Stage IVA | T4 | N0 | M0 |
| | T4 | N1 | M0 |
| | Any T | N2 | M0 |
| Stage IVB | Any T | N3 | M0 |
| Stage IVC | Any T | Any N | M1 |

SOURCE: With permission from the American Joint Committee on Cancer: *AJCC Cancer Staging Manual*, 5th ed. JD Fleming et al (eds). Philadelphia, Lippincott-Raven, 1997.

definitive diagnosis. The olfactory neuroblastoma is the prototypical small round cell tumor of the sinonasal tract. It occurs in all age groups and typically arises as a polypoid intranasal mass attached high in the nasal cavity to the cribriform plate. Unilateral nasal obstruction and intermittent epistaxis with or without anosmia are the most common symptoms. The tumor may spread locally to involve the adjacent paranasal sinuses, orbit, or cranial cavity, or it may metastasize to cervical nodes or to more distant sites. The overall 5-year survival rate is 50% to 60%. Squamous cell carcinoma involving the maxillary sinus is the most common sinonasal malignancy. Signs and symptoms depend upon direction of tumor growth and are grouped accordingly: nasal, oral, ocular, facial, and neurologic. The 5-year survival rate ranges from 20% to 25%.

## EAR—TEMPORAL BONE

**ANATOMY.** The ear is divided into three compartments: external, middle, and inner. The external consists of the "ear," its canal and the surface of the tympanic membrane. The middle ear is composed of the bones of the middle ear and the inner surface of the tympanic membrane. The inner ear consists of the membranous and osseous labyrinths and the vestibular apparatus.

**BENIGN DISEASES.** Inflammatory diseases include otitis media, a common pediatric disease, and cholesteatoma, which results from neglected chronic inflammation of the middle ear. The surgical oncologist is seldom faced with the management of these inflammatory diseases.

Paraganglioma (glomus tumor, chemodectoma) is the commonest tumor of the middle ear and the second most common tumor of the temporal bone, acoustic neuroma being the most common. It arises from collections of paraganglion cells normally found in the adventitia of the jugular bulb, along the course of the nerve of Jacobson or nerve of Arnold. In practice, it may be impossible to determine the precise site of origin. In these instances, the all-inclusive term *jugulotympanic paraganglioma* is used. These tumors are three to six times more common in females, occur primarily in middle age, and present clinically with pulsatile tinnitus and conductive hearing loss. They are slow-growing neoplasms, but, if neglected, may extend intracranially. The diagnosis may be made angiographically. Surgical intervention requires caution (Fig. 4D-35), and if biopsies prove necessary, they should be obtained intraoperatively (with frozen-section evaluation).

Located within the dermis of the outer cartilaginous portion of the external auditory canal are a group of modified apocrine glands known as ceruminous glands. These glands can give rise to five distinct types of tumors: ceruminous adenoma, ceruminous adenocarcinoma, pleomorphic adenoma, adenoid cystic carcinoma, and mucoepidermoid carcinoma.

**MALIGNANT DISEASES.** Embryonal rhabdomyosarcoma and squamous cell carcinoma are the most common malignant tumors of the middle ear. Rhabdomyosarcoma occurs primarily in children under 5 years of age and presents as a polypoid lesion that is often mistaken, both clinically and pathologically, for an aural polyp. Close attention to cytologic details, augmented with

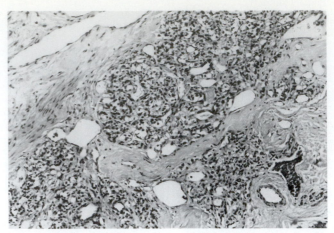

**FIGURE 4D-35.** Jugulotympanic paraganglioma. The tumor cells grow in small clusters (referred to as *Zellballen*) that are sometimes difficult to appreciate on small, crushed biopsies. Note the prominent vascularity. (Hematoxylin and eosin, ×200.) (*With permission, from Banks PM, Kraybill WG:* Pathology for the Surgeon. *Philadelphia, WB Saunders, 1996.*)

immunostains for muscle markers (myoglobin, desmin), allows distinction. Because of close proximity to the central nervous system, tumor seeding of the meninges with neurologic signs and symptoms is not uncommon. The overall 3-year relapse-free survival rate for rhabdomyosarcoma of the middle ear and mastoid is about 45%.

Squamous cell carcinoma of the middle ear and mastoid is symptomatically similar to cholesteatoma, often accounting for delay in diagnosis. Any biopsies from this area that show dysplasia should be regarded as suspicious for carcinoma, since cholesteatomas rarely if ever show this feature. About 15% will have cervical lymph node metastases and 10% will develop systemic metastases. The overall 5-year survival is about 25% to 30%.

## SALIVARY GLANDS

**ANATOMY.** The major salivary glands are paired and symmetrical. The parotid gland, the largest salivary gland, lies in front of the ear and extends from the zygomatic arch superiorly to just below the angle of the mandible inferiorly. In contrast to other salivary glands, the parotid contains a large number of intraglandular lymph nodes that may (1) show nonspecific hyperplasia and clinically masquerade as a tumor, (2) give rise to primary lymphomas, or (3) harbor metastases from tumors arising in other sites. The submandibular gland lies in the posterior floor of the mouth between the tongue, mandible, and hyoid bone. The sublingual gland, the smallest of the three major glands, rests upon the mylohyoid muscle, near the mandibular symphysis, just beneath the mucosa of the floor of the mouth.

**BENIGN AND MALIGNANT DISEASES.** Neoplasms of the salivary gland may be indistinguishable clinically from chronic

**TABLE 4D-5.  ABRIDGED CLASSIFICATION OF SALIVARY GLAND TUMORS**

| BENIGN | MALIGNANT |
|---|---|
| | *Low grade:* |
| Pleomorphic adenoma | Mucoepidermoid carcinoma |
| Basal cell adenoma | Acinic cell carcinoma |
| Warthin tumor | Adenoid cystic carcinoma |
| Oncocytoma | Basal cell carcinoma |
| Myoepithelioma | Epithelial myoepithelial carcinoma |
| Sebaceous adenoma | Myoepithelial carcinoma |
| Canalicular adenoma | Polymorphous low-grade |
| Papillary cystadenoma | adenocarcinoma |
| | Carcinoma ex pleomorphic |
| | adenoma (some) |
| | Papillary cystadenocarcinoma |
| | *High grade:* |
| | Mucoepidermoid carcinoma |
| | Carcinoma ex pleomorphic |
| | adenoma (some) |
| | Salivary duct carcinoma |
| | Undifferentiated carcinoma |
| | Squamous cell carcinoma |

SOURCE:  With permission, from Banks PM, Kraybill WG: *Pathology for the Surgeon*. Philadelphia, WB Saunders, 1996.

inflammatory diseases. Patients with chronic sialadenitis with stone formation often present with a history of recurring infection and swelling with eating. Radiographic confirmation of calculus improves diagnostic accuracy; however, 20% of submandibular and 80% of parotid calculi do not contain calcium and are therefore not radiodense. In one series, over 85% of patients who were operated upon for removal of a submandibular mass were found to have chronic inflammatory disease with sialadenitis and sialolithiasis. In contrast, over 75% of patients who present with a discrete mass in parotid gland will have a neoplasm. In general, 15% to 25% of all parotid, 40% to 60% of all submandibular, and 80% to 90% of all subligual gland neoplasms are malignant.

The heterogeneity of tumor types encountered in the salivary glands is a challenge even to the experienced pathologist (Table 4D-5). Because radical resections of neoplasms of the parotid gland may result in significant disfigurement and morbidity, the decision to perform such a procedure should not be based on frozen section or fine-needle aspiration biopsy (FNAB). Instead the pathologist establishes a definite diagnosis on permanent histologic sections. If indicated, the patient is then returned to the operating room for a definitive procedure following thorough evaluation and informed consent.

## THE NERVOUS SYSTEM

Considerations of the nervous system are not the exclusive province of the neurosurgeon.[28] Peripheral nerves and their disorders extend to every organ system and tissue. Indeed, plastic or general surgeons most often perform skeletal muscle and nerve biopsies. Even the central nervous system, with its surrounding structures giving rise to various soft tissue and osseous lesions, may be encountered by specialists in head-and-neck, orthopedic, plastic, oncologic, or dermatologic surgery. Malformations and disease processes of this system sometimes lead to encounters that are unexpected and unintentional. This section will emphasize oncologic pathology of the nervous system.

### ANATOMIC DESCRIPTION OF CENTRAL NERVOUS SYSTEM

The central nervous system (CNS) is protected by the skull and vertebral column and by the multilayered meninges. The latter are of mesenchymal derivation and consist of three layers: (1) the dura, the most superficial layer formed of dense collagenous tissue; (2) the arachnoid, a thin membrane composed largely of meningothelial cells, which serves to contain and direct the flow of cerebrospinal fluid; and (3) the pia, a delicate layer closely applied to the brain and spinal cord. Accordingly, the meninges delimit three potential spaces between the skull and brain: the epidural, subdural, and subarachnoidal. Within the skull, the dura adheres to the inner table of the calvarum. Its folds form basic anatomic landmarks that separate the compartments of the CNS. These include the falx, a midline fold separating the left and right cerebral hemispheres, and the tentorium, which separates the middle from the posterior fossa. Additionally, the dural layers envelop the major venous sinuses, including the superior and inferior sagittal, the transverse and sigmoid sinuses, and in the parasellar region the cavernous sinus. The intracranial contents thus lie within two compartments, the supratentorial and infratentorial spaces. Supratentorial structures include the cerebral hemispheres and the deep gray nuclei (the basal ganglia, thalamus, and hypothalamus). The cerebellum and the brainstem are infratentorial in location.

In the spinal canal the meninges also form three anatomic compartments: the extradural space (between the dura and the spine, there being no adhesion to the bone), the intradural-extramedullary space (within the dura but outside the substance of the spinal cord), and the intramedullary region (consisting of the spinal cord proper). Several anatomic sites surrounding the CNS represent important surgical and pathologic landmarks in that lesions arise specific to these locations, and their involvement engenders specific differential diagnoses. These sites include the sellar and suprasellar regions, the cavernous sinus, the cerebellopontine angle, the pineal region, and the base of the skull.

### PRIMARY CNS TUMORS—INTRAOPERATIVE DIAGNOSIS

Optimal surgical management of CNS tumors requires intraoperative pathology consultation to facilitate decision making. In most instances, this process includes microscopic confirmation of the presence of a neoplasm, determining whether it is primary or secondary, benign or malignant, and, if primary, of a morphological type that may lend itself to complete excision. Improved sensitivity of neuroimaging, coupled with the increased use of stereotactic biopsy, has expanded the pathologist's role to include assessment of whether the biopsy findings are consistent with the imaging abnormality. The diminutive nature of many biopsy specimens, particularly those obtained by needle and fine forceps, emphasizes the importance of combining the cytological smear method with conventional frozen-section interpretation.

Both the pathologist and the neurosurgeon must understand that the process of intraoperative diagnosis is only the first step in specimen assessment and that it has limitations. A final diagnosis, one correlating cytologic and histologic features, tumor growth pattern relative to underlying parenchyma, and clinical data with imaging characteristics, awaits review of permanent sections. The development of a differential diagnosis depends upon factors such as patient age, clinical presentation, duration of symptoms, and gross operative findings. Patient age and tumor location, in particular, become major factors in elaborating a differential diagnosis for CNS tumors (Table 4D-6). Clear communication and a collegial relationship between pathologist and neurosurgeon greatly facilitate the diagnostic effort and reduce the likelihood of "beginner's errors."

Although frozen sections provide a good working if not always precise diagnosis, several centers have recommended the cytologic smear technique for intraoperative evaluation of CNS biopsies.[29] The smear method also provides useful information regarding the cellular composition of either reactive or neoplastic processes. Smear interpretations are reported to concur with final diagnoses made on permanent sections in 90% to 95% of patients.[29] The great advantage of the smear method resides in its suitability for the study of minute fragments of tissue, allowing retention of much of the specimen for optimal processing. Imprint preparations, although produced less often than smears, are better suited for the examination of specimens firm or fibrous in nature, e.g., metastatic carcinomas in dural tissue.[30]

**APPROACH TO THE SPECIMEN.** Intraoperative tissue review should be regarded as a preliminary step, one providing information useful in operative decision making. Care must be taken to conserve tissue needed for permanent sections and, in some cases, for special procedures. Indiscriminate freezing of entire specimens should be avoided. Cauterized tissue and samples from suction bottles are usually inadequate because such specimens show distortion and obscuration of cellular and architectural features.

In the case of brain tumors in particular, material should be set aside for routine histology, special histochemical stains, and for immunostaining. Because of the tissue-sparing nature of smear or imprint preparations, even small specimens may suffice for special analyses such as ultrastructural study. The latter requires only a 1- to 2-mm fragment and, in difficult cases, may be pivotal for diagnosis. In patients where there is suspicion of hematopoietic disorders, fresh tissue should be submitted for flow cytometric studies and for the assessment of tumor clonality. Chromosomal abnormalities in brain tumors, some of diagnostic importance, can be identified using viable, fresh tissue submitted for cytogenetic analysis. Immediate freezing of specimens (with liquid nitrogen or similar methods) preserves their potential for molecular diagnosis. In cases of a possible infectious nature, a specimen should be allocated for microbial culture.

## TOPOGRAPHIC CLASSIFICATION

Topographic and histologic features are relevant not only to the diagnosis of CNS neoplasms but also play a role in determining prognosis and treatment. Location within the CNS is a major factor in narrowing down the differential diagnosis of tumors occurring in both adult and pediatric populations. Approximately 70% of tumors appearing in childhood arise in the infratentorial compartment, whereas the great majority of tumors in adults are supratentorial. A topographic distribution of tumors in relation to patient age is provided in Table 4D-6.

## HISTOLOGIC CLASSIFICATION OF BRAIN TUMORS

Tumors of the CNS account for a small but significant portion of all human tumors. Their spectrum, as evidenced by the new World Health Organization (WHO) classification (Table 4D-7) is very broad.[31] In children, the CNS is the second most common site of primary tumors. The distribution and categories of neoplasms that arise in CNS of children and adults reflect their distinctive histogenesis. The following is a brief discussion of the more important CNS tumors. Table 4D-4 provides a concise summary of common lesions. For a more detailed description of CNS tumors, the reader is referred to more complete neuropathology texts.[28,31,32]

## STAGING

In contrast to most other organ systems, staging of brain tumors does not assume importance in predicting survival or in selecting appropriate therapy. Instead, tumor classification and evidence of circumscribed versus diffusely infiltrative growth pattern assume critical importance.

## NEUROEPITHELIAL TUMORS WITH GLIAL DIFFERENTIATION

Regardless of patient age, gliomas are the most common CNS tumors. Collectively they represent nearly 50% of tumors in both the adult and pediatric population. Gliomas are classified according to predominant cell type, a feature presumably reflecting their histogenesis (see Table 4D-7).

**ASTROCYTIC TUMORS.** Astrocytomas are proliferations of neoplastic astrocytes. Such tumors vary greatly, both in morphology and biologic behavior. Astrocytomas are divided into two major groups according to their tendency to infiltrate surrounding brain parenchyma: diffusely infiltrating astrocytomas versus circumscribed astrocytomas.

**TABLE 4D-6.** TOPOGRAPHIC DISTRIBUTION OF TUMORS OF THE CENTRAL NERVOUS SYSTEM BY PATIENT AGE

| LOCATION | CHILDREN/ADOLESCENTS | ADULTS |
|---|---|---|
| *Supratentorium:* | | |
| Cerebral hemispheres | Astrocytoma | Astrocytoma |
| | Anaplastic astrocytoma | Anaplastic astrocytoma |
| | Pleomorphic xanthoastrocytoma | Glioblastoma multiforme |
| | Pilocytic astrocytoma | Metastatic carcinoma |
| | Ependymoma | Oligodendroglioma |
| | Oligodendroglioma | Ependymoma |
| | Ganglioglioma | PNET |
| | Desmoplastic infantile ganglioglioma, astrocytoma | Meningioma |
| | PNET | |
| Corpus callosum | Astrocytoma | Astrocytoma |
| | Anaplastic astrocytoma | Anaplastic astrocytoma |
| | Oligodendroglioma | Glioblastoma multiforme |
| Lateral ventricle | Ependymoma | Ependymoma |
| | Choroid plexus papilloma (>carcinoma) | Subependymoma |
| | Central neurocytoma | Choroid plexus papilloma |
| | Subependymal giant cell astrocytoma | Central neurocytoma |
| | | Meningioma |
| Third ventricle | Ependymoma | Colloid cyst |
| | Choroid plexus papilloma (>carcinoma) | Ependymoma |
| Region of third ventricle | Pilocytic astrocytoma | Astrocytoma, anaplastic astrocytoma, glioblastoma |
| | Oligodendroglioma | Oligodendroglioma |
| | Ependymoma | Ependymoma |
| Optic nerve and chiasm | Pilocytic astrocytoma | Meningioma |
| | | Pilocytic astrocytoma |
| Pineal region | Germ cell tumors | Germ cell tumors |
| | Pineoblastoma | Pineocytoma |
| | | Pineoblastoma |
| Pituitary-sellar region | Craniopharyngioma | Pituitary adenoma |
| | Germ cell tumor | Meningioma |
| | | Germ cell tumor |
| | | Metastasis |
| | | Chordoma/chondroma |
| *Infratentorium:* | | |
| Cerebellum | Medulloblastoma | Hemangioblastoma |
| | Pilocytic astrocytoma | Metastatic carcinoma |
| | Dermoid cyst | Astrocytoma (diffuse or pilocytic) |
| | | Medulloblastoma |
| Fourth ventricle | Ependymoma | Ependymoma |
| | Choroid plexus papilloma (>carcinoma) | Choroid plexus papilloma |
| | | Subependymoma |
| Cerebellopontine angle | Ependymoma | Schwannoma |
| | Choroid plexus papilloma | Meningioma |
| | | Epidermoid cyst |
| | | Choroid plexus papilloma |
| | | Glomus jugulare tumor |
| Brainstem | Astrocytoma (diffuse or pilocytic) | Astrocytoma |
| | Anaplastic astrocytoma | Anaplastic astrocytoma |
| | Glioblastoma multiforme | Glioblastoma multiforme |
| Spinal region | Ependymoma | Ependymoma |
| | Astrocytoma (diffuse or pilocytic) | Astrocytoma (diffuse or pilocytic) |
| | Meningioma | Hemangioblastoma |
| | | Meningioma |
| | | Schwannoma |
| | | Neurofibroma |
| | | Paraganglioma |

SOURCE: Modified from Scheithauer BW: Central nervous system and pituitary, in *Intraoperative Pathologic Diagnosis*, EG Silva, BB Kramer (eds). Baltimore, Williams & Wilkins, 1987.

**TABLE 4D-7.** TUMORS OF NEUROEPITHELIAL TISSUE WHO CLASSIFICATION (1993)

**Astrocytic tumor:**
Astrocytoma: variants: fibrillary, protoplasmic, gemistocytic
Anaplastic (malignant) astrocytoma
Glioblastomas: variants: giant cell glioblastoma, gliosarcoma
Pilocytic astrocytoma
Pleomorphic xanthoastrocytoma
Subependymal giant cell astrocytoma (usually in association with tuberous sclerosis)

**Oligodendroglial tumors:**
Oligodendroglioma
Anaplastic (malignant oligodendroglioma)

**Ependymal tumors:**
Ependymoma: variants: cellular, papillary, clear cell
Anaplastic (malignant) ependymoma
Myxopapillary ependymoma
Subependymoma

**Mixed gliomas:**
Oligoastrocytoma
Anaplastic (malignant) oligoastrocytoma
Others

**Choroid plexus tumors:**
Choroid plexus papilloma
Choroid plexus carcinoma

**Neuroepithelial tumors of uncertain origin:**
Astroblastoma
Polar spongioblastoma
Gliomatosis cerebri

**Neuronal and mixed neuronal-glial tumors:**
Gangliocytoma
Dysplastic gangliocytoma of cerebellum (Lhermitte-Duclos)
Desmoplastic infantile ganglioglioma
Dysembryoplastic neuroepithelial tumor
Ganglioglioma
Anaplastic (malignant) ganglioglioma
Central neurocytoma
Paraganglioma of the filum terminate

Olfactory neuroblastoma (esthesioneuroblastoma); variant: olfactory neuroepithelioma

**Pineal parenchymal tumors:**
Pineocytoma
Pineoblastoma
Mixed pineoblastoma/pineocytoma

**Embryonal tumors:**
Medulloepithelioma
Neuroblastoma: variant: ganglioneuroblastoma
Ependymoblastoma
Retinoblastoma
Primitive neuroectodermal tumors (PNETs)
Medulloblastoma: variants: desmoplastic medulloblastoma, medullomyoblastoma, melanotic medulloblastoma

Cerebral or spinal PNETs

SOURCE: From Kleihues P et al: *Histological Typing of Tumours of the Central Nervous System*, 2d ed. New York, Springer-Verlag, 1993.

Diffusely infiltrating astrocytomas with unfavorable prognosis comprise nearly 75% of all astrocytic neoplasms and form a spectrum of lesions that vary in differentiation and degree of malignancy[32] (Fig. 4D-36). Even the relatively low-grade forms are prognostically unfavorable, the 10-year survival being 20%. Criteria used for grading astrocytic tumors include degree of nuclear atypia, mitotic activity, the presence of necrosis, endothelial proliferation, etc.[28] (Fig. 4D-37). Diffusely infiltrating astrocytomas are characterized by remarkable intratumoral heterogeneity, both morphologic and genetic. This is particularly the case as they undergo progressive anaplastic transformation. The frequency of this shift to higher grade is the basis for a poor prognosis with this grouping of astrocytic neoplasms.

Relatively circumscribed astrocytomas with favorable prognosis include tumors that, in terms of their radiographic and gross appearance, are relatively circumscribed neoplasms when compared with diffuse astrocytomas previously discussed (Fig. 4D-38). This category includes pilocytic astrocytoma, pleomorphic xanthoastrocytoma, and subependymal giant cell astrocytoma. Collectively,

these tumors all exhibit distinctive clinicopathologic features, tend to be slow growing, and have a much more favorable prognosis. This is due not only to their relative circumscription but to the fact that they occur in younger patients and show less tendency to undergo anaplastic transformation. With surgical resection the majority of patients do well.

**OLIGODENDROGLIOMAS.** Estimates put the frequency of oligodendrogliomas at approximately 5% to 15% of intracranial gliomas. Although the majority occurs in adults, with a peak incidence in the fourth and fifth decades, oligodendrogliomas make up about 5% of gliomas in childhood and adolescence. Clinically, most oligodendrogliomas progress very slowly and are often associated with a long history of seizures. They may occur at any level of the neuraxis, most frequently the cerebral hemisphere, particularly the frontotemporal region. Although the majority of oligodendrogliomas are well differentiated and slow growing, a minority behaves more aggressively. As with other gliomas, oligodendrogliomas exhibit a spectrum of histologic differentiation, one

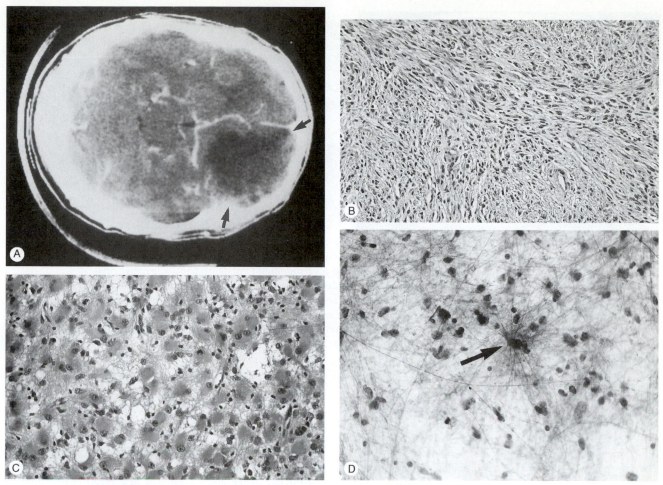

**FIGURE 4D-36.** Diffusely infiltrative low-grade glioma (fibillary astrocytoma). *A.* Contrast-enhanced CT scan. Such infiltrative gliomas (arrows) exhibit relatively low to moderate cellularity and are unassociated with a significant increase in vascularity; they lack contrast enhancement. *B.* Microscopic features of grade 2 fibrillary astrocytoma; note spindling cellular pattern. *C.* Microscopic features of grade 2 gemistocytic astrocytoma; note large, round, granular cells. *D.* This smear preparation from grade 2 astrocytoma of fibrillary type demonstrates scattered neoplastic cells with nuclear pleomorphism and variable hyperchromasia. Note their apparent lack of cytoplasm, a feature typical of isolated infiltrating cells. At the center is a stellate reactive astrocyte (arrow) with its symmetrically radiating processes. Sharply delineated, long processes crossing the field represent residual axons within the parenchyma. (Hemalum-phloxine stain.) (*With permission, from Banks PM, Kraybill WG:* Pathology for the Surgeon. *Philadelphia, WB Saunders, 1996.*)

without prognostic implication. Common to all are cellular uniformity, round nuclei, scant processes, "geometric" acutely branching capillaries, and scattered microcalcifications.

**EPENDYMOMAS.** Ependymomas represent approximately 5% of intracranial gliomas.[31] Children and adolescents are affected more often than adults. Pediatric ependymomas usually arise in the fourth ventricle, whereas those of adults are located primarily in the spinal cord. Ependymomas are reported to represent as many as 60% of spinal cord gliomas. Unlike other gliomas and regard-

less of location, ependymomas are grossly and microscopically well-demarcated tumors with "pushing borders" (Fig. 4D-39). Tumors with intraventricular components may spread through the ventricular system via foramina. A characteristic histologic feature of ependymomas is radial orientation of the processes of tumor cells around blood vessels, resulting in pseudorosette formation (see Fig. 4D-39). The WHO classification recognizes three histologic forms of ependymoma: cellular, papillary, and clear cell. Anaplastic ependymomas may occur at any site but are relatively infrequent in the spinal cord. A clinically reliable grading scheme for

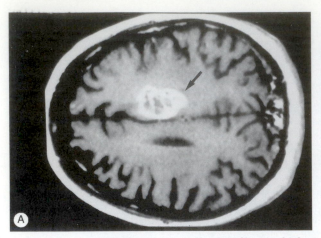
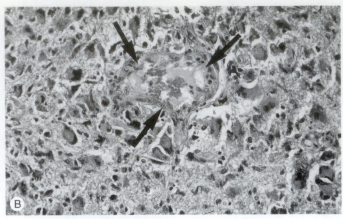

**FIGURE 4D-37.** Diffusely infiltrative high-grade astrocytoma. *A*. This grade 4 lesion (glioblastoma multiforme) shows ring enhancement corresponding to a highly cellular and vascular element, central hypodensity that equates with necrosis, and a surrounding hypodense zone of parenchymal infiltration by isolated tumor cells, as well as of edema (arrow). *B*. Microscopic appearance of grade 4 astrocytoma (glioblastoma multiforme). Key features distinguishing this common tumor from the closely related grade 3 (anaplastic) astrocytoma are endothelial proliferation (arrows) and necrosis. (*With permission, from Banks PM, Kraybill WG:* Pathology for the Surgeon. *Philadelphia, WB Saunders, 1996.*)

ependymomas has not yet been devised. Histologic criteria alone have limited significance; however, histologic grade in conjunction with such factors as patient age and DNA ploidy analysis permits distinction of low-from high-grade tumors.

Myxopapillary ependymoma is a morphologically distinct variant of ependymoma that, with few exceptions, is restricted to the cauda equina. Most occur in adults during the third or fourth decades. Presenting symptoms include pain, asymmetric sensorimotor deficits, and sphincter dysfunction. Grossly, the tumors appear either as delicately encapsulated discrete, sausage-shaped masses arising from the filum terminale or as disrupted tumors associated with local tumor seeding. Extradural lesions arising in either the postsacral or presacral regions are far less common and presumably arise from ependymal rests. Myxopapillary ependymomas show varying proportions of elongated, fibrillary, glial-appearing cells together with epithelial-like cells arranged around perivascular accumulations of mucin. These tumors should be removed intact. Their rupture forfeits the chance for surgical cure.

Subependymomas are well-circumscribed tumors that arise in the walls of the fourth ventricle. Most are asymptomatic. Symptomatic tumors, which are very uncommon, may involve any level of the ventricular system, including the septum pellucidum, foramen of Monro, and on rare occasions the center of the spinal cord. Symptoms are generally related to hydrocephalus, the result of obstruction of cerebrospinal fluid (CSF) flow or to intratumoral hemorrhage. Subependymomas consist of cells exhibiting ependymal and astrocytic differentiation. Clinical behavior is even more favorable than that of pure ependymomas; even subtotal removal results in long-term improvement. Tumor locations and successful resection appear to be the most important prognostic factors.

## EMBRYONAL TUMORS (MEDULLOBLASTOMA)

As the most common malignant CNS tumors of childhood, medulloblastomas make up approximately one-quarter of all intracranial tumors in the pediatric age group.[33] Their peak incidence is at the end of the first decade. The new WHO classification (see Table 4D-7) applies the generic designation of "primitive neuroectodermal tumor" (PNET) to small cell embryonal tumors that appear to be composed of primitive neuroepithelial progenitor cells expressing divergent glioneuronal differentiation. Most medulloblastomas arise in the roof of the fourth ventricle and commonly fill the fourth ventricle, producing symptoms of increased intracranial pressure. Less often, particularly in adults, they are situated laterally in the cerebellar hemisphere (Fig. 4D-40). Grossly, ordinary medulloblastomas are soft and clearly demarcated from surrounding brain. Seeding by CSF may be apparent either early or late in the disease course. Medulloblastomas are markedly cellular neoplasms typically composed of small cells with scant cytoplasm, variably hyperchromatic nuclei, and ill-defined cell borders (see Fig. 4D-40). Although poorly differentiated by routine light microscopy, a significant proportion show neuroblastic differentiation in the form of neuroblastic rosettes. Top surgical priorities are removal or debulking of tumor and clearing obstruction of CSF pathways, particularly at the fourth ventricle.

## MENINGOTHELIAL TUMORS

Meningiomas are dural tumors derived from arachnoidal cells. They account for about 15% of intracranial tumors and about 25% of

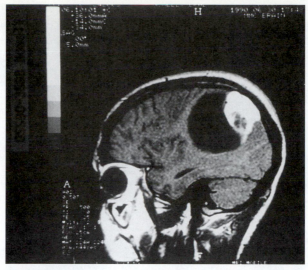

*A*

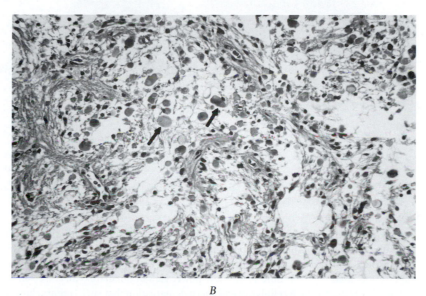

*B*

**FIGURE 4D-38.** Circumscribed, favorable astrocytoma, pilocytic type. *A*. MRI with contrast. This classic supratentorial example consists of a mural nodule of solid tumor within a cyst. Contrast enhancement is typical of pilocytic astrocytomas and, in contrast to diffuse astrocytic tumors, is not indicative of high-grade malignancy. *B*. Microscopic features of pilocytic astrocytoma. This, the most common of astrocytomas with favorable prognosis, shows considerable histologic variation, ranging from bipolar spindle cells (left) to less fibrillary cells engaged in microcyst formation. The latter pattern predominates in this example and is associated with granular body formation (arrows). (*With permission, from Banks PM, Kraybill WG:* Pathology for the Surgeon. *Philadelphia, WB Saunders, 1996.*)

intraspinal tumors. Most meningiomas become clinically apparent in midlife but they are occasionally seen in childhood. In adults there is a marked female predominance (3:1); in childhood and in the elderly there is no sex predilection. Meningimoas are multiple in nearly 8% of cases and large numbers of lesions are associated with central neurofibromatosis (NF-2). Meningiomas may arise at any level of the neuraxis, but there are sites of predilection. In neuroimaging studies strong contrast enhancement is the rule; in addition,

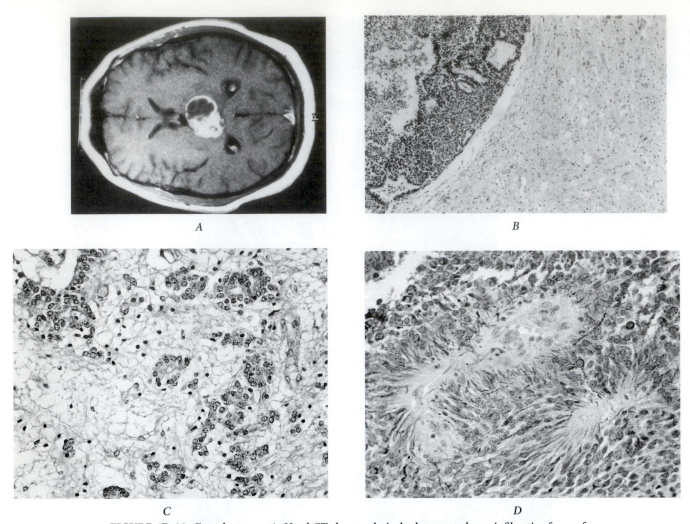

**FIGURE 4D-39.** Ependymoma. *A.* Head CT shows relatively demarcated, noninfiltrative form of glioma typically situated adjacent to the ependyma and contrast enhancing. As in the case of pilocytic astrocytoma, contrast enhancement is a typical feature and is not indicative of high-grade malignancy. Cyst formation is common. *B.* This low-power view of a hematoxylin and eosin (H&E)–stained section illustrates the high cellularity and sharp demarcation that such tumors show relative to surrounding brain parenchyma. A characteristic histologic feature is the formation of *C.* perivascular pseudorosettes and true rosettes with lumens (*D*). The latter are uncommonly seen. *C.* Glial fibrillary acidic protein (GFAP) immunostain; *D.* H&E stain. (*With permission, from Banks PM, Kraybill WG:* Pathology for the Surgeon. *Philadelphia, WB Saunders, 1996.*)

the periphery of the lesion may exhibit a "dural tail" (Fig. 4D-41). Supratentorially, they most frequently arise along the falx (see Fig. 4D-41), over the cerebral convexity, on the tuberculum sellae, in the parasellar region, in the olfactory grooves, and along the sphenoidal ridge. The posterior fossa, the cerebellopontine angle or, more anteriorly, the petroclival junction are commonly affected sites. Spinal canal meningiomas most often affect the thoracic and cervical regions. They are typically slow-growing tumors. Histo-

logically, meningiomas are divided into four general catergories that roughly reflect aggressiveness and malignant potential: meningioma, atypical meningioma, papillary meningioma, and anaplastic (malignant) meningioma. These patterns are itemized in the new WHO classification.[31] The range is broad and includes epithelial, mesenchymal, and mixed phenotypes (see Fig. 4D-41). Atypical meningiomas, papillary meningiomas, and anaplastic meningiomas are progressively more malignant.

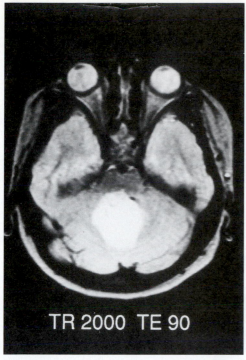

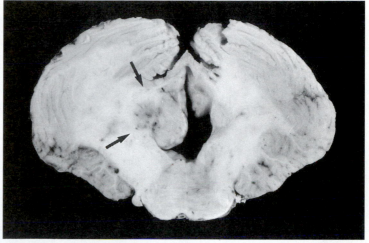

A

B

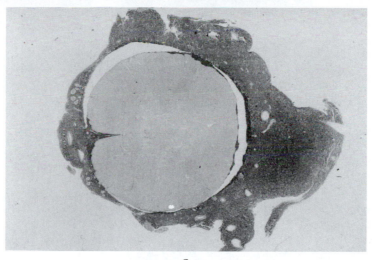

C

**FIGURE 4D-40.** Medulloblastoma. *A*. MRI with contrast. This form of primitive neuroectodermal tumor arises within the cerebellum, more often in the vermis than the hemispheres. Many extend into the fourth ventricle. Medulloblastomas are typically solid, relatively demarcated, and contrast enhancing on CT and MRI scans. *B*. This horizontal section of the cerebellum shows the tumor (arrows) to arise within the vermis and to compromise the fourth ventricle. Cerebrospinal seeding has led to the formation of a cerebellopontine angle mass and widespread leptomeningeal involvement. *C*. This transverse whole-mount section of the spinal cord shows extensive leptomeningeal dissemination as well as tumoral encasement of the otherwise unremarkable cord. *D*. This pediatric tumor of the cerebellum is a distinctive form of PNET, one often associated with loss of chromosome 17p and a relatively good response to therapy. The majority are composed of hyperchromatic, carrot-shaped cells. *E*. Homer-Wright rosettes are commonly seen and are indicative of neuroblastic differentiation. (*With permission, from Banks PM, Kraybill WG:* Pathology for the Surgeon. *Philadelphia, WB Saunders, 1996.*)

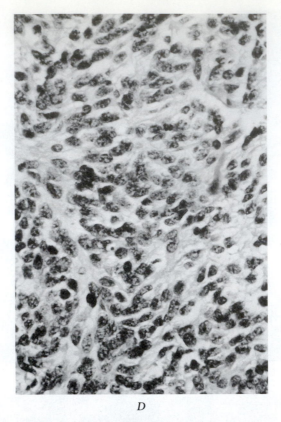

*D*

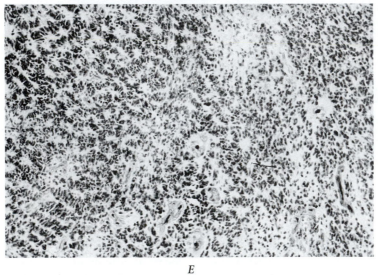

*E*

**FIGURE 4D-40.** (*Continued*)

## METASTATIC NEOPLASIA

Metastatic neoplasms can involve the brain or meninges. In the latter situation they resemble meningiomas (Fig. 4D-42). In either location they are characterized by circumscription and may be multifocal. In most instances the diagnosis is straightforward, with known prior extracranial malignancy. Metastatic carcinomas and melanomas far outnumber sarcomas. Any of these may mimic glioblastoma. Pathologic features of metastases that aid in their recognition include abrupt tumor margins, relative lack of microvascular proliferation, and absence of elongated cells with multipolar processes.

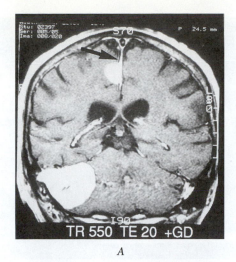

*A*

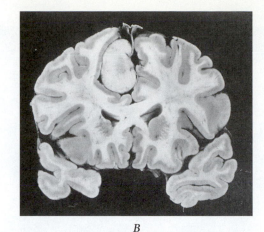

*B*

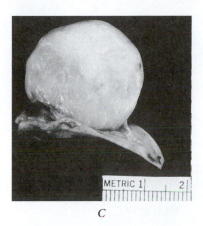

*C*

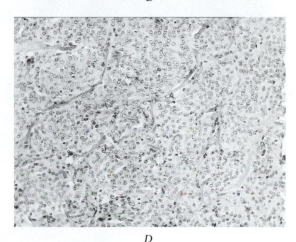

*D*

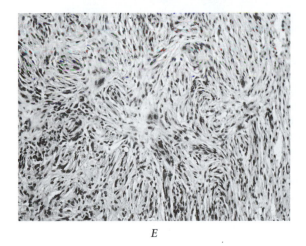

*E*

**FIGURE 4D-41.** Meningioma. *A*. MRI with contrast enhancement. This example of multiple meningiomas shows their dural attachment, marked contrast enhancement, and displacement of brain. Note a tapering dural tail (arrow) in the smaller lesion. *B*. Whole brain section. This example involves the falx from which tumor grows in a globular fashion to displace the underlying brain in a manner typical of extraaxial meningiomas. *C*. Excised specimen. The tumor is clearly dura based. Its peripheral tapered extension along the dural surface is the basis of the dural tail sign, as seen with neuroimaging in *A*. *D*. No other tumors of the central nervous system are capable of the morphologic diversity of meningiomas. Common patterns range from meningothelial tumors with *D*. A decidedly epithelial pattern to *E*. the fibrous variant composed of spindle cells associated with collagen production. (*With permission, from Banks PM, Kraybill WG: Pathology for the Surgeon. Philadelphia, WB Saunders, 1996.*)

## PITUITARY GLAND

Pituitary adenomas make up more than 75% of surgical specimens from the sellar region. Correlation of clinical and biochemical data is of particular diagnostic importance because of the broad spectrum of endocrinologic manifestations produced by pituitary adenomas.

Clinically, adenomas may appear as "functioning" tumors, i.e., associated with a clinical syndrome resulting from tumoral hormone production (hyperprolactinemia, acromegaly/gigantism, Cushing's disease), or as nonfunctioning tumors. In the latter situation, patients present with symptoms resulting from compression of adjacent neural structures, usually visual-field defects related to optic

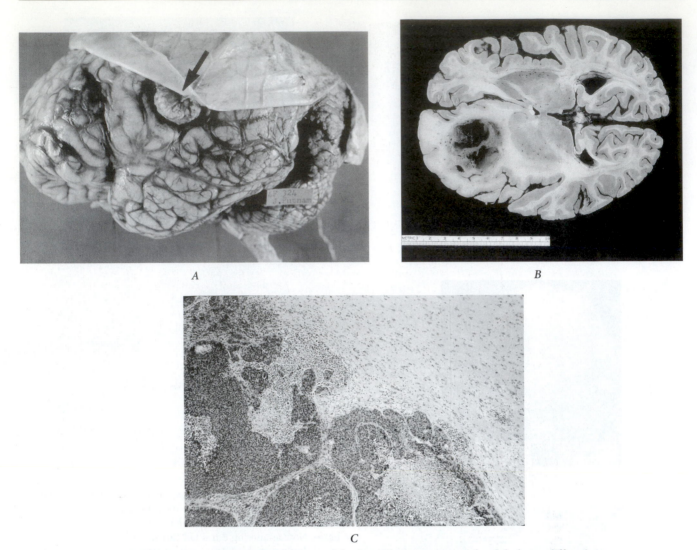

*A*

*B*

*C*

**FIGURE 4D-42.** *A*. Metastatic carcinoma of the dura. Such tumors may be globular or diffuse in their pattern of growth. Globular lesions such as this breast carcinoma (arrow) displace underlying brain and may mimic meningioma. *B*. Metastatic carcinoma in brain. Parenchymal metastases are characterized by circumscription and accompanying edema. Multiplicity is common. When the deposits are small, they tend to center upon the junction of gray and white matter. This example of metastatic oat cell carcinoma of lung in a 62-year-old man involves a frontal lobe, is well demarcated, and produces considerable mass effect. *C*. Microscopic features of metastatic carcinoma. Unlike the vast majority of gliomas, metastatic carcinomas typically form sharply demarcated deposits, ones often associated with necrosis. The surrounding brain shows edema and gliosis. (*With permission, from Banks PM, Kraybill WG:* Pathology for the Surgeon. *Philadelphia, WB Saunders, 1996.*)

chiasm compression or signs of hypopituitarism. Meaningful classification of pituitary adenomas requires not only conventional paraffin sections, but special methods, particularly immunostaining and sometimes electron microscopy.[32] These methods identify tumoral production of certain hormones.

Intraoperative diagnosis of pituitary lesions may be problematic when specimens are small. This is particularly the case in adenomas of Cushing's disease and in prolactinomas occurring in reproductive-age females. In such instances, indiscriminate frozen section is to be avoided. Instead, smears or touch preparations are preferable; they permit the identification of adenomas, minimize tissue loss for permanent sections, and represent a useful permanent record of the pathology.

## PERIPHERAL NERVOUS SYSTEM

Cranial and spinal nerve roots supply the functionally defined voluntary (sensorimotor) and autonomic systems with nerves that ramify

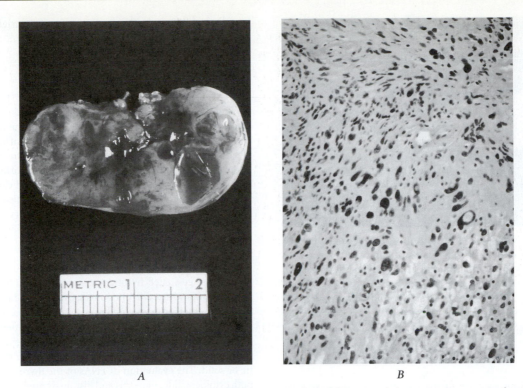

A          B

**FIGURE 4D-43.** Schwannoma. *A*. Gross appearance. Typical of this tumor is its eccentric manner of growth relative to the parent nerve (not shown), patchy yellow discoloration, and tendency to undergo cystic degeneration. *B*. Microscopic features of "ancient schwannoma." Despite their benign nature, schwannomas of long standing may show a degree of degenerative nuclear atypia readily mistaken for malignancy. Unlike sarcomas of peripheral nerves, such tumors typically lack mitotic activity. (*With permission, from Banks PM, Kraybill WG:* Pathology for the Surgeon. *Philadelphia, WB Saunders, 1996.*)

in every organ and tissue. Whether intracranial or distal within the extremities, these nerves are prone to similar diseases, both neoplastic and nonneoplastic.

## NERVE SHEATH TUMORS

This category includes tumors derived from supportive or stromal cells of peripheral nerves including Schwann cells and perineurial cells as well as fibroblasts. Although traumatic neuromas produce painful masses, these are not neoplasms but reparative proliferations of interwined nerve processes and nerve sheath elements. Variants include amputation neuroma and Morton's (intermetatarsal) neuroma. The majority of nerve sheath neoplasms are schwannomas (neurilemomas) and neurofibromas. Schwannomas consist exclusively of Schwann cells. In contrast, neurofibromas consist of Schwann cells together with perineurial cells, fibroblasts, and transitional cells. Schwannomas tend to be solitary and arise more frequently from cranial and spinal nerve roots than from peripheral nerves. Grossly, their pattern of growth is as a solid encapsulated mass, one eccentric to the parent nerve, which remains intact along-

side the tumor. Degenerative changes including lipid accumulation and cystic change are common (Fig. 4D-43), and "degenerative nuclear atypia" should not be misinterpreted as evidence of malignancy (see Fig. 4D-43). Neurofibromas are commonly multiple and usually involve major peripheral nerves or their branches. The majority of cutaneous nerve sheath tumors are neurofibromas. Unlike schwannomas, neurofibromas symmetrically enlarge the parent nerve in a fusiform fashion; they grow within the nerve substance and lack their own capsule (Fig. 4D-44).

Schwannomas and neurofibromas occur either sporadically or in the setting of neurofibromatosis (NF). Multiple neurofibromas arise in NF-1 (von Recklinghausen's disease or peripheral neurofibromatosis), whereas multiple schwannomas are associated with NF-2 (central neurofibromatosis) or with a little-known condition termed schwannomatosis. Neurofibromas are the principal lesions of NF-1, being far more common than schwannomas. Plexiform neurofibromas are diagnostic of NF-1, whereas bilateral acoustic schwannomas are pathognomonic of NF-2. Important surgical considerations surround the resection of nerve sheath tumors. Short of diffuse cutaneous tumors, the removal of neurofibroma necessarily involves resection of the parent nerve with resultant loss of its function. By contrast, with careful dissection, schwannomas can

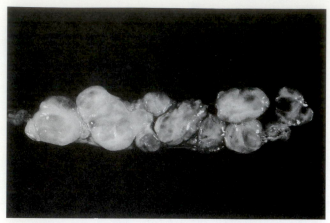

**FIGURE 4D-44.** Plexiform neurofibroma. Such tumors involve multiple nerve fascicles, are typically mucoid in texture, and often defy gross total removal. Their finding is virtually pathognomonic of von Recklinghausen's disease (NF-1). Careful tissue sampling is of importance in that 5% of such tumors undergo sarcomatous transformation. (*With permission, from Banks PM, Kraybill WG: Pathology for the Surgeon. Philadelphia, WB Saunders, 1996.*)

be removed without sacrifice of the parent nerve, preserving its function. Unlike neurofibromas, schwannomas almost never become malignant.

Malignant peripheral nerve sheath tumors (MPNSTs) are often large, partially necrotic tumors that spread within the parent nerve. Anaplastic transformation of schwannomas is an extremely rare event and most MPNSTs are derived from neurofibromas. Their overall incidence in the general population is very low (approximately 0.001%), but it is much higher among patients with NF-1 (4.6%). Because MPNSTs often arise in neurofibromas, sampling is of importance, particularly in large tumors. The majority of MPNSTs are high-grade tumors featuring necrosis and hemorrhage. Their microscopic appearance varies considerably, ranging from conventional spindle cell lesions to epithelioid variants that mimic carcinoma. Rare MPNSTs show differentiation toward skeletal muscle ("Triton tumors"), bone, cartilage, or even bona fide epithelium: mucin-producing, squamous, or neuroendocrine. Such variants are more often observed in NF-1, but also occur in sporadic tumors. These tumors are extremely aggressive and have a poor prognosis. The prognosis of MPNST relates not only to resectability but also to tumor size, location, and to association with NF-1; more centrally situated tumors, those greater than 5 cm in greatest dimension, and those occurring in the setting of NF-1 have a particularly poor prognosis. Histologic grade is not a powerful prognostic indicator. These tumors are frequently considered in relation to soft tissue tumors.

## ENDOCRINE PATHOLOGY

This section addresses the cytologic, frozen section, and final pathologic analyses of thyroid, parathyroid, and adrenal neoplasms. The

purpose is to strengthen the oncologic surgeon's insight into pathology in order to facilitate surgical decision making.[34]

## THYROID PATHOLOGY

**THYROID NODULE.** Three issues addressed during the evaluation of a patient with a thyroid nodule are the likelihood that the nodule is malignant, the microscopic type of neoplasm, and whether there is microscopic spread. About 5% to 10% of thyroid nodules are malignant. The clinical history is important in assessing risk factors. Patients at increased risk for thyroid cancer are those with a history of radiation treatment or a family history of multiple endocrine neoplasia. Such relevant clinical history and significant physical findings should be shared with the pathologist.

**FINE-NEEDLE ASPIRATION BIOPSY.** Although thyroid nodules are evaluated by other techniques, including ultrasound, thyroid scan, and thyroid function tests, fine-needle aspiration (FNA) biopsy has emerged as a favored primary diagnostic modality for thyroid nodules.[35] This method is used to screen patients with suspicious clinical findings preoperatively. All cellular aspiration material should be evaluated by a cytopathologist, whether the lesion is cystic or solid. The evaluation of FNAs of the thyroid should include both cytologic slides (smears) and histologic preparations (cell block sections). The diagnostic accuracy of FNA is excellent for papillary, anaplastic, and medullary carcinomas (Figs. 4D-45 and 4D-46). Because the diagnosis of follicular carcinoma is based on noncytologic

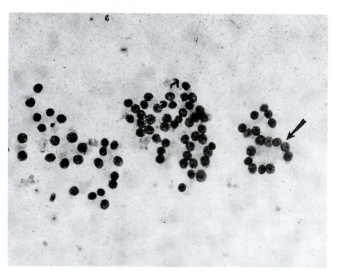

**FIGURE 4D-45.** Cytology of a follicular neoplasm of the thyroid. As is typical for follicular neoplasms, the cells in this follicular adenoma form a small follicle (arrow). The nuclei do not overlap and contain uniform chromatin. Distinction from well-differentiated follicular carcinoma is not possible on the basis of such preparations. (*With permission, from Banks PM, Kraybill WG: Pathology for the Surgeon. Philadelphia, WB Saunders, 1996.*)

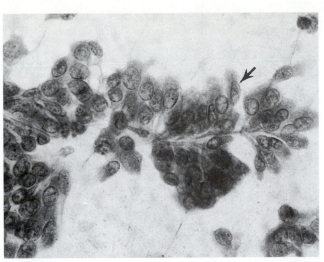

**FIGURE 4D-46.** Cytology of a papillary carcinoma of the thyroid. Note the papillary architecture of the tissue fragment, the overlapping nuclei, and the nuclear grooves (arrow) in this Papanicolaou-stained preparation. (*With permission, from Banks PM, Kraybill WG: Pathology for the Surgeon. Philadelphia, WB Saunders, 1996.*)

criteria (capsular invasion and vascular invasion), FNAs of follicular lesions are unreliable predictors of malignancy (Fig. 4D-47). In patients with cytology suspicious for lymphoma or anaplastic thyroid cancer, an incisional thyroid biopsy is required to establish the diagnosis.

The results of FNA for thyroid nodules are divided into four categories: (1) benign or negative, including colloid nodule, cyst, or thyroiditis; (2) suspicious or indeterminate, including Hurthle cell, follicular neoplasm, or findings suggestive of malignancy; (3) malignant or positive, including papillary, medullary, or anaplastic thyroid cancer, metastatic carcinoma, or lymphoma; and, finally, (4) unsatisfactory for cytopathologic evaluation. A collective review of more than 18,000 FNA specimens showed an average rate of 69% benign aspiration results, 3.5% malignant, 10% suspicious, and 17% nondiagnostic.[35] The false-negative rate was 1% to 11%; the false-positive rate, 1% to 8%. Of those patients submitted to surgical resection (i.e., those with either malignant or suspicious cytopathology), 32% later proved to have a thyroid malignancy. Of greater concern, however, is the possibility of missing a thyroid malignancy because of a false-negative FNA. In a study by Grant et al.[36] of 439 patients with benign cytopathology, only 0.7% developed thyroid cancer after an average follow-up of 6.1 years.[36]

Papillary carcinomas of the thyroid have distinct cytologic features that are easily recognized on FNA (see Figs. 4D-14, 4D-46 and 4D-47). These include papillary fronds, psammoma bodies, and characteristic nuclear features. The nuclei of papillary carcinomas are clear, with finely dispersed chromatin; they tend to overlap and often contain nuclear grooves or intranuclear cytoplasmic inclusions. In contrast, the cytologic features of medullary carcinoma are variable. Aspirates from medullary carcinomas often show single cells or small groups of spindle-shaped cells. The nuclei may be uniform or show marked pleomorphism. Clumps of extracellular amyloid, when present, support the diagnosis of medullary carcinoma. Because of its variable appearance on FNA, immunohistochemical staining for calcitonin is often necessary to establish the diagnosis of a medullary carcinoma (Figs. 4D-48 and 4D-49). Interpretation of follicular neoplasms by FNA is more problematic. Because the diagnosis of follicular carcinoma rests on transcapsular and vascular

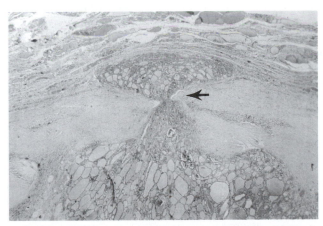

**FIGURE 4D-47.** Transcapsular penetration (arrow) in a follicular carcinoma of the thyroid. The presence of transcapsular penetration in a follicular neoplasm of a carcinoma. (*With permission, from Banks PM, Kraybill WG: Pathology for the Surgeon. Philadelphia, WB Saunders, 1996.*)

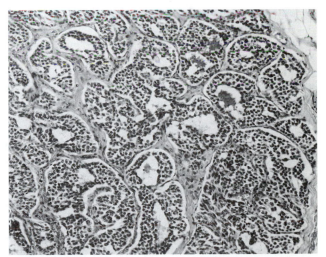

**FIGURE 4D-48.** Medullary carcinoma of the thyroid. The neoplastic cells form prominent nests in this case. Most of the cells are rather uniform, but focal spindling is present. (*With permission, from Banks PM, Kraybill WG: Pathology for the Surgeon. Philadelphia, WB Saunders, 1996.*)

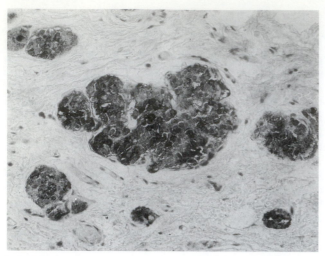

**FIGURE 4D-49.** Immunohistochemical stain for calcitonin in a primary medullary carcinoma. Note the intense cytoplasmic staining, indicating the expression of calcitonin by the neoplastic cells. (*With permission, from Banks PM, Kraybill WG:* Pathology for the Surgeon. *Philadelphia, WB Saunders, 1996.*)

invasion, FNA biopsy from the center of a follicular neoplasm is not sensitive for diagnosing follicular carcinoma; however, useful information can be gleaned. Follicular carcinomas often have a solid, microfollicular, or trabecular growth pattern and, if seen on FNA, these architectural patterns should raise concerns. Only occasionally do higher-grade follicular carcinomas manifest cytologic atypia and abundant mitotic figures allowing recognition of malignancy. FNA evaluation of follicular lesions rarely distinguishes between a benign and a malignant neoplasm; surgery is usually required for definitive diagnosis (see Figs. 4D-45 and 4D-47).

Intraoperative frozen section of thyroid nodules also has its limitations. If the surgeon recognizes the limitations of utilizing a frozen-section diagnosis, it can be a useful technique. Its two main limitations are distinguishing follicular adenoma from follicular carcinoma (see Fig. 4D-47) and distinguishing a follicular neoplasm from the follicular variant of papillary carcinoma. Follicular carcinomas are distinguished from follicular adenomas by the presence of transcapsular penetration and vascular invasion. A follicular carcinoma cannot be ruled out until the entire capsule is examined microscopically. It is neither practical nor reliable to examine an entire lesion microscopically at the time of frozen section; the probability of a false-negative frozen section interpretation cannot be eliminated. Similarly, the follicular variant of papillary carcinoma can be difficult to recognize on frozen section.[37] This neoplasm has a predominantly follicular architecture and can closely mimic follicular carcinomas in frozen section; however, cellular features disclose its true nature: optically clear nuclei with intranuclear inclusions and nuclear grooves. These nuclear features are dependent on artifacts of fixation and are not present in frozen sections. Intraoperative imprint or scrape-smear cytology may aid in recognizing a follicular-variant papillary neoplasm. By combining the findings on FNA and/or smear cytology with frozen section, the diagnosis may

be made. A lesion with follicular architecture on frozen section and papillary nuclei on FNA is most likely a follicular variant of papillary carcinoma.

As with other situations described in this chapter, optimal management of surgical specimens is dependent on good communication between the surgeon and pathologist. The thyroid and any lymph nodes should be properly oriented. Areas of special interest such as close margins should be marked. As discussed above, the capsule of the thyroid must be carefully examined grossly and microscopically to identify evidence of capsular penetration. Although perhaps imperfect, the TNM staging system does provide important prognostic information for patients with malignancies of the thyroid.

## PARATHYROID PATHOLOGY

Patients undergo surgery for primary, secondary, or tertiary hyperparathyroidism and, rarely, for parathyroid carcinoma. Patients with primary hyperparathyroidism have elevated parathyroid hormone (PTH) levels in the face of hypercalcemia. Approximately 80% of patients with primary hyperparathyroidism harbor a parathyroid adenoma, 20% have parathyroid hyperplasia, and less than 1% have a parathyroid carcinoma.[38] Multiple parathyroid adenomas are rare. Hyperparathyroidism in patients with chronic renal failure is usually due to secondary hyperparathyroidism, whereas patients with functioning kidney transplants and hyperparathyroidism usually have so-called tertiary hyperparathyroidism.[38] This represents parathyroid hyperfunction originally induced by renal failure that has subsequently become autonomous. Patients who have marked hypercalcemia, palpable neck mass, symptoms secondary to hypercalcemia, and no evidence of metastatic disease should be suspected of having parathyroid carcinoma.

Good communication between the surgeon and the pathologist is critical to the successful surgical management and diagnosis of patients with parathyroid adenomas and hyperplasia. The pathologist must be able to accurately discern that biopsied tissue is parathyroid tissue. It is the role of the surgeon to determine whether the patient has evidence of hyperplasia, with all four glands appearing abnormally enlarged, or whether the patient harbors one or more adenomas. Parathyroid adenomas are clonal neoplasms that result in single gland enlargement.[39] For the pathologist, the distinction between adenoma and hyperplasia is frequently very difficult to make. Ideally, adenomas are well encapsulated and are composed of chief or oxyphil cells arranged in sheets or nests, devoid of fat (Fig. 4D-50). They range from 300 mg to several grams. Another helpful clue for diagnosis of adenoma is the presence of a thin rim of residual normal, fatty parathyroid tissue. In contrast, parathyroid hyperplasia shows enlargement of all four glands. Hyperplastic glands usually lack the capsules of adenomas and typically retain more fat than do adenomas. Nonetheless, it is often extremely difficult to distinguish parathyroid hyperplasia from parathyroid adenoma purely by microscopic criteria. It is helpful if the surgeon submits one normal-appearing gland with any apparent adenomas.[40]

Parathyroid carcinoma usually presents in the fourth decade and is associated with hyperparathyroidism.[41] It is a rare condition

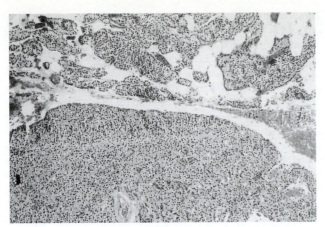

**FIGURE 4D-50.** Parathyroid adenoma. The absence of fat in the adenoma (bottom half) separates it from the residual normal parathyroid (top half). (*With permission, from Banks PM, Kraybill WG: Pathology for the Surgeon. Philadelphia, WB Saunders, 1996.*)

accounting for fewer than 1% of all patients with hyperparathyroidism. Patients may recur late after successful treatment of presumed parathyroid adenomas.[42] The initial operation should be a wide en bloc resection. Parathyroid carcinomas can be difficult to distinguish from adenomas on microscopic grounds. Parathyroid carcinomas are aggressive neoplasms that infiltrate adjacent connective tissues and other structures. These findings at the time of surgery may be useful in determining the diagnosis. Microscopically, parathyroid carcinomas are recognized by their trabecular (ribbon-like) architecture, with fibrous bands, vascular invasion, and mitotic figures.

## ADRENAL PATHOLOGY

The advent of high-resolution radiologic imaging has vastly increased detection of clinically unsuspected adrenal tumors, or so-called incidentalomas. If serum and urinary corticosteroids and catecholamine levels are normal and the tumor is less than 4 to 5 cm in size, the patient may safely be followed by serial computed tomography (CT) scans. If based upon the patient's history one suspects metastatic disease, one may then obtain a CT-guided needle aspiration for confirmation. Any tumor that is larger than 4 to 5 cm or is hormone-secreting warrants surgical resection.

## ADRENAL ADENOMA VERSUS HYPERPLASIA VERSUS CARCINOMA

Because the management is different, the differentiation of hormone-producing unilateral adenoma from bilateral hyperplasia is important. This is particularly difficult because nonfunctioning adenomas may accompany bilateral hyperplasia. The differentiation between adenoma ("aldosteronoma") and bilateral adrenocortical hyperplasia is best made by postural response studies.[43] A CT scan

will identify the adenoma, and surgery should be directed to the side with the adenoma. Adrenal vein sampling for aldosterone may also help localize aldosteronomas.[44] The differential diagnosis for primary adrenal causes of Cushing's syndrome includes glucocorticoid-producing adrenal adenoma and bilateral adrenocortical hyperplasia. If biochemical studies show elevated 24-hr urinary free cortisol levels, low plasma adrenocorticotropic hormone (ACTH) levels, and failure to suppress cortisol levels with high-dose dexamethasone, a CT scan is used to differentiate between an adenoma and primary bilateral adrenocortical hyperplasia. Surgical resection follows appropriate diagnostic evaluation. Primary adrenal neoplasms originate in cortex (adenoma, carcinoma) or in medulla (pheochromocytoma, neuroblastoma). Adrenal cortical adenomas may be either functional or nonfunctional. They are usually solitary and encapsulated and they tend to compress surrounding adrenal tissue, with resulting atrophy.[34] By contrast, hyperplastic adrenal cortical nodules are poorly defined, unencapsulated, and often multiple. The majority of adenomas are yellow and weigh less than 100 g. They are composed of either clear lipid-containing cells (Cushing's syndrome, hyperaldosteronism) or eosinophilic cells (feminizing or virilizing syndromes). Even though they are benign, adenomas may exhibit bizarre-appearing cells microscopically with large pleomorphic nuclei. Unfortunately, no single feature can be used to separate adrenal adenomas from adrenocortical carcinomas. Cumulative experience associates malignancy with weight greater than 100 g, mitotic counts greater than 60 per 50 high-power fields, bizarre mitoses, and vascular invasion.[45] Cytogenetic analysis of primary adrenocortical carcinoma reveals clonal rearrangements of several autosomes and sex chromosomes.[46] Multiple-parameter scoring systems are therefore useful for predicting outcome. Although in some instances there may be difficulty differentiating cortical adenoma from carcinoma, some carcinomas are advanced at presentation. They may weigh between 100 and 5000 g. Areas of necrosis and hemorrhage are common and are consistent with malignancy. Invasion and metastases are common. Microscopically, the presence of cells with big nuclei, hyperchromatism, and enlarged nucleoli are consistent with malignancy.[46]

## MALIGNANT VERSUS BENIGN PHEOCHROMOCYTOMA

Pheochromocytomas are adrenal medullary neoplasms that are capable of synthesizing and secreting catecholamines. These mediators are responsible for the patient's presenting symptoms: hypertension, palpitations, sweating, headaches, and paroxysmal attacks. Extraadrenal pheochromocytomas, or paragangliomas, are found anywhere from the base of the skull to the lower genitourinary tract, including the aortic bifurcation (organ of Zuckerkandl), bladder, mediastinum, and heart as well as carotid and glomus jugulare bodies. The preoperative evaluation of the patient includes an assessment for secreted catecholamines. MRI and/or CT scans may be used to attempt to localize the tumor.

Pheochromocytoma can be multifocal. Therefore, unless the pheochromocytoma is metastatic or is locally invasive, differentiating between malignant and benign conditions is a challenge. Final pathologic differentiation is often determined by the patient's postoperative course. Pathologically, pheochromocytomas are neoplasms of the adrenal medulla and are related embryologically to paragangliomas. Grossly, pheochromocytomas are well-circumscribed, large (3 to 5 cm), and gray to dark red on fresh cut section. Pheochromocytomas can show a variety of microscopic growth patterns, including trabecular, nesting, and diffuse patterns. As is the case with adrenal cortical neoplasms, it can be difficult to recognize malignancy in a pheochromocytoma. Features favoring malignancy include large size (greater than 700 g), extraadrenal location, extensive necrosis, numerous mitoses (greater than 1 per 10 high-power fields), and vascular invasion.

## IMMUNOHISTOCHEMICAL STAINS FOR ENDOCRINE TUMORS

On occasion, a patient will present to the surgeon with a metastatic endocrine tumor of unknown primary or with a tumor suspected to be a metastasis from a known site of endocrine tumor origin (Fig. 4D-51). Identification of the lesion's origin can often be achieved by immunocytochemical staining. The development of monoclonal antibodies for immunohistochemical staining has had a major impact on the practice of endocrine pathology. The three main uses for immunohistochemistry in endocrine pathology are

1. To demonstrate neuroendocrine differentiation in a poorly differentiated neoplasm that is otherwise hard to classify
2. To determine the specific tissue type of origin of a neuroendocrine tumor,
3. To provide prognostic information.

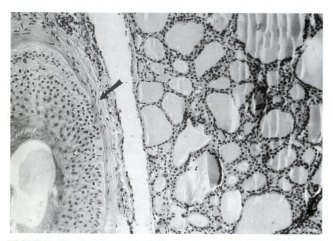

**FIGURE 4D-51.** Metastatic follicular carcinoma of the thyroid. This follicular carcinoma metastasized to the scalp. A hair follicle is present on the left (arrow) and the follicular cancer is on the right. Even in this metastasis, the microscopic characteristics of the follicles are not overtly malignant. (*With permission, from Banks PM, Kraybill WG:* Pathology for the Surgeon. *Philadelphia, WB Saunders, 1996.*)

Three immunohistochemical stains are commonly employed: chromogranins, synaptophysin, and neuron-specific enolase (NSE). The chromogranins are a family of acidic polypeptides that probably function as carrier proteins in neurosecretory granules. For this reason, they are very sensitive markers for neuroendocrine differentiation and are expressed in a diversity of neoplasms, including islet cell tumors, pheochromocytomas, pituitary adenomas, parathyroid adenomas, and carcinoid tumors. Similarly, the expression of synaptophysin, an acidic transmembrane glycoprotein, is also a relatively sensitive and specific marker of neuroendocrine differentiation. NSE is an enzyme expressed in a variety of endocrine neoplasms, but unfortunately, most commercially available antibodies to NSE lack the sensitivity and specificity necessary for them to be useful.

A wide variety of immunohistochemical stains is currently available for demonstration of the cell of origin of neuroendocrine neoplasms. Thyroglobulin is expressed by normal follicular cells of the thyroid and by most neoplasms derived from follicular cells. Although not all follicular carcinomas express this marker, its presence in a metastatic carcinoma strongly suggests origin from follicular cells of the thyroid. Similarly, the expression of calcitonin can demonstrate C-cell origin of a neoplasm (see Fig. 4D-49). Although a detailed discussion of this topic is beyond the scope of this section, immunohistochemical staining is an integral part of the pathologist's armamentarium.

## THE MEDIASTINUM

### WHAT IS THE MEDIASTINUM?

The word *mediastinum* means "median septum." In current medical usage, it is defined as the anatomic compartment bounded superiorly by the plane of the thoracic inlet (outlined by the manubrium and first ribs), inferiorly by the diaphragm, and laterally by the mediastinal parietal pleura of the left and right thoracic cavities.

Its location in the midline of the chest renders access to the mediastinum difficult, and the associated presence of large vessels and airways makes exploration hazardous. In addition, the tissues of the mediastinum, like the retroperitoneum, have a propensity for fibrosis in response to diverse pathologic processes. This combination of factors often leads to difficulty in histopathologic interpretation of biopsy specimens from the mediastinum, since they are likely to be small, fibrotic, and crushed. Mass lesions of the mediastinum are often lymphoid and may be either neoplastic or infectious, requiring special techniques such as microbial cultures, immunophenotyping, or electron microscopy for diagnosis. The role of the surgeon in diseases of the mediastinum ranges from providing diagnostic tissue so that other physicians can proceed with definitive treatment (as, for example, in lymphoma) to providing definitive surgical treatment (as in thymoma and mediastinal cysts). Both the surgeon and the pathologist must have a clear idea of the preoperative differential diagnosis and the goals of the operative procedure so that the specimen may be handled appropriately, since therapeutic considerations are so predicated on precise pathologic classification of the neoplastic process at hand.[47]

**TABLE 4D-8.** MEDIASTINAL COMPARTMENTS, CONTENTS, AND PATHOLOGIC CONDITIONS

| COMPARTMENT | DEFINITION | CONTENTS | PATHOLOGY | %* |
|---|---|---|---|---|
| Anterosuperior | Anterior and superior to pericardial sac | Trachea, esophagus, great vessels, thymus lymph nodes, nerves (vagus, phrenic), fat, connective tissue | *Primary tumors/cysts:* Thymoma (30%)* Lymphoma (25%) Germ cell tumor (20%) Cysts (5%): Thymic Bronchogenic Mesenchymal (4%) Carcinoid (thymic) Primary carcinoma *Other conditions:* Metastatic carcinoma Castleman's disease Sarcoidosis Histoplasmosis | 56% |
| Middle | Visceral compartment, between anterior and posterior compartments | Heart, great vessels, phrenic nerves, carina and bronchi, lymph nodes, connective tissue | *Primary tumors/cysts:* Cysts (60%): Pericardial Bronchogenic Lymphoma (20%) Mesenchymal (10%) Paraganglioma *Other conditions:* (as for anterior) | 19% |
| Posterovertebral | Posterior to pericardial sac | Esophagus, descending aorta, azygos vein, thoracic duct, nerves (vagus, sympathetic, intercostal), lymph nodes, fat, connective tissue | *Primary tumors/cysts:* Neurogenic (50%) Cysts (30%): Bronchogenic Enteric Mesenchymal (10%) *Other conditions:* Meningioma Extramedullary hematopoiesis | 26% |

* Frequency of primary tumors and cysts in Duke University Medical Center series of 441 cases, from Davis and Sabiston.[1]
SOURCE: With permission, from Banks PM, Kraybill WG: *Pathology for the Surgeon.* Philadelphia, WB Saunders, 1996.

## ANATOMIC DISTRIBUTION OF PRIMARY MEDIASTINAL TUMORS AND CYSTS

Different tumor types have different incidence in the various compartments, and there is strong association with age as well. The anterior-superior mediastinum is the site of the majority of primary mediastinal tumors, accounting for over half of all tumors (Table 4D-8). The posterior mediastinum is next, being the site of just over one-quarter of all tumors, and the middle is the least-frequent site. In adults, thymoma, lymphoma (usually Hodgkin's lymphoma or large cell lymphoma), and neurogenic tumors (usually neurilemoma or neurofibroma) are the most common (15% to 20% each), followed by germ cell tumors (10%) (Table 4D-9). Mesenchymal tumors, carcinomas of unknown origin, and other rare

conditions make up the rest. In children, neurogenic tumors (usually ganglioneuroma or neuroblastoma) are most common (35%), followed by lymphoma, usually lymphoblastic (25%), and germ-cell tumors, usually mature teratoma (10%). Mesenchymal tumors, often vascular, and other rare tumors account for the remainder. Cysts (pericardial, bronchogenic, or enteric) account for about 20% of primary mediastinal masses in adults and children.

## WHAT TYPE OF BIOPSY SHOULD BE DONE?

Once the decision has been made that a biopsy is necessary, what type of biopsy should be done? In the differential diagnosis of primary anterosuperior mediastinal tumors, FNA biopsy has limited

**TABLE 4D-9.** SUMMARY OF PRIMARY MEDIASTINAL TUMORS AND CYSTS

| TUMOR | ADULTS, % | CHILDREN, % |
|---|---|---|
| Neurogenic tumors | 21 | 35 |
| Thymoma | 19 | |
| Lymphoma | 13 | 25 |
| Germ cell tumor | 10 | 10 |
| Cysts | 18 | 16 |
| Mesenchymal tumors | 6 | 10 |
| Endocrine tumors | 6 | |
| Carcinomas of unknown primary | 5 | 2 |
| Other | 3 | 2 |

SOURCE: With permission, from Banks PM, Kraybill WG: *Pathology for the Surgeon.* Philadelphia, WB Saunders, 1996.

utility. The epithelial cells of thymoma or of germ cell tumor and the large cells of lymphoma all resemble one another in conventional microscopic appearance. The lymphocytes of a cortical thymoma may resemble those of a lymphoblastic lymphoma or the background lymphocytes of Hodgkin's lymphoma. Similar problems will be encountered with cutting needle biopsies. Immunostaining techniques can be performed on these types of specimens, but they are often suboptimal and inconclusive with small specimens, only delaying the definitive diagnosis. For the diagnosis of these tumors, a piece of tissue at least 1 to 2 cm in diameter is usually required to demonstrate the typical cytologic and architectural features that distinguish one tumor from another. Unless there is a compelling clinical reason to avoid anesthesia, it may be more efficient and cost-effective to proceed directly to an open biopsy procedure with intraoperative pathology monitoring to assure an adequate sampling.

## HANDLING OF THE BIOPSY SPECIMEN AND THE ROLE OF INTRAOPERATIVE FROZEN SECTION

Biopsy specimens from mediastinal masses should always be sent fresh (the entire specimen) to the pathologist for intraoperative determination of specimen adequacy and for preparation of tissue for special diagnostic techniques. Intraoperative diagnosis as a basis for immediate resection of antero-superior mediastinal masses should be carried out only when there is strong preoperative evidence of thymoma or germ cell tumor where the tumor is clearly resectable. Even in this circumstance due consideration should be given to resection without biopsy, depending upon the clinical circumstances. In contrast, the nature of cystic lesions, neurogenic tumors, and metastatic carcinoma can often be established with reasonable certainty on intraoperative frozen section. Frozen sections can also be used with the surgeon's guidance to evaluate the status of margins during definitive resection of a tumor; the surgeon must guide the pathologist to areas of particular suspicion or submit selected samples of concern separately since complete intraoperative evaluation of all margins is impractical.

## CLINICOPATHOLOGIC FEATURES OF PRIMARY MEDIASTINAL TUMORS

### THYMOMA

*CLINICAL FEATURES.* About 40% of thymomas occur in adults, associated with myasthenia gravis in older patients.[48] On radiologic studies, thymomas are solid or partially cystic masses, usually well circumscribed, in the anterosuperior mediastinum. Lymph node enlargement is so uncommon that its presence alone speaks strongly against the diagnosis of thymoma. Thymomas behave as either benign or low-grade malignant tumors with a propensity for local invasion and recurrence and a miniscule rate of true metastasis.

*GROSS APPEARANCE.* Thymomas, even when invasive, generally appear as more or less well-circumscribed masses, often with a bosselated or lobulated surface. They may occur anywhere within the thymus but are most commonly found at the base, or isthmus, where the right and left lobes join. The consistency ranges from fleshy to firm, and there are often areas of cystic degeneration (Fig. 4D-52).

*HISTOPATHOLOGY.* Thymoma is a tumor of thymic epithelial cells and is thus the only true thymic neoplasm. Carcinoid tumors, germ cell tumors, and lymphomas may all arise in the thymus, but these are tumors of cells that can be found elsewhere in the body and are thus not uniquely thymic neoplasms.

Thymomas closely resemble the normal thymus. All thymomas contain neoplastic thymic epithelial cells, and most contain nonneoplastic lymphocytes of the types normally found in the thymus. Although some classifications subdivide thymomas according to the relative proportions of lymphocytes and epithelial cells, these tumors can more usefully be classified according to the morphology of the epithelial cells. The Mueller-Hermelink classification has five categories of thymoma and has predictive value both for invasiveness and risk of relapse and death.[48,49] Medullary thymomas are composed of bland oval or spindle cells resembling those of the thymic medullas with few lymphocytes. They do not recur or metastasize. Mixed thymomas have areas of medullary thymoma admixed with areas of organoid thymoma. These tumors also do not recur even when invasive. Organoid thymomas contain areas resembling both normal thymic cortex and medulla, usually have a lobular architecture, and very closely resemble the normal thymus. They have a small but definite risk of late relapse. Cortical thymomas have large, pale epithelial cells identical to those of the normal thymic cortex with preservation of a lobular architecture. They have a risk of invasiveness and relapse. Well-differentiated thymic carcinoma is composed predominantly of epithelial cells that resemble those of cortical thymoma but with a moderate degree of cytologic atypia and occasional mitotic figures. They are almost always invasive and carry a significant risk of early relapse, even with minimal invasion. This type accounted for all the relapses and deaths from thymoma occurring within 10 years in a large series of patients from Massachusetts General Hospital.[49]

Unlike the tumors that resemble normal thymic epithelium and are considered thymomas, there are rare, poorly differentiated carcinomas that resemble carcinomas of other sites and appear to have arisen in the thymus.

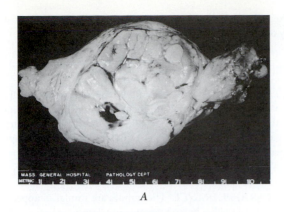

*A*

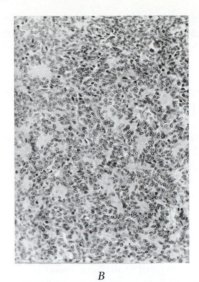

*B*

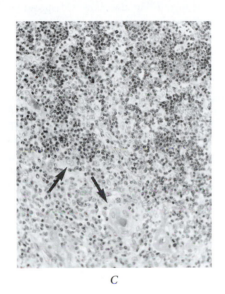

*C*

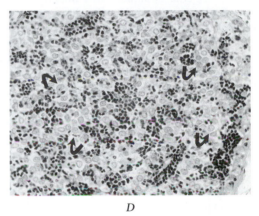

*D*

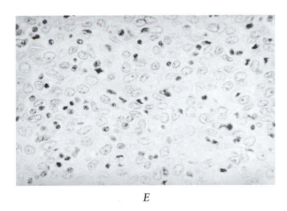

*E*

**FIGURE 4D-52.** Thymoma. *A*. Gross photograph, showing large, encapsulated tumor. *B–E*. Microscopic sections illustrating histologic subtypes of thymoma according to the Müller-Hermelink classification. *B*. Medullary thymoma, with small, oval-to-spindle cells. *C*. Organoid thymoma, with zones featuring numerous lymphocytes and other areas of epithelial cells (arrows), closely resembling normal thymus. *D*. Cortical thymoma, with large, pale epithelial cells (arrows) and many lymphocytes. *E*. Well-differentiated thymic carcinoma; the epithelial cells are smaller than those of cortical thymoma, with nuclear irregularity, moderate mitotic activity, and relatively few lymphocytes. This tumor may be confused with (large cell) lymphoma in small biopsy specimens or with intraoperative frozen section. (*With permission, from Banks PM, Kraybill WG:* Pathology for the Surgeon. *Philadelphia, WB Saunders, 1996.*)

*PERIOPERATIVE AND POSTOPERATIVE COMMUNICATION WITH THE PATHOLOGIST.* Staging is a cooperative endeavor requiring input from both the surgeon and the pathologist. The surgeon must carefully examine the thorax at the time of thymectomy. Findings of tumor extension or metastases should be communicated to the pathologist. If the tumor is invasive but resectable, areas of involved pericardium or lung should also be removed. These areas should be identified for the pathologist and the specimen should be oriented to allow effective evaluation and study. The specimen should be delivered promptly to the pathologist so that proper fixation can be achieved. Particularly if a preoperative histologic diagnosis of thymoma has not been made, tissue should be prepared for immunohistologic and electron microscopic study, in anticipation that other tumors will enter into the differential diagnosis.

## LYMPHOMAS: HODGKIN'S LYMPHOMA, LARGE CELL AND LYMPHOBLASTIC TYPES

In the mediastinum, lymphomas most often involve anterosuperior mediastinal lymph nodes and/or thymus, but they can also involve the peribronchial lymph nodes of the middle mediastinum. Different types of lymphoma call for different types of therapy. The surgeon's role in the care of the patient with mediastinal lymphoma is to provide sufficient tissue to the pathologist in a condition that will permit optimal fixation and special diagnostic studies, and, of course, to avoid unnecessary radical surgery on the basis of a misdiagnosis (clinical and/or frozen section) of thymoma or germ cell tumor. If the type of mediastinal tumor is uncertain by clinical and radiologic criteria, intraoperative frozen section and cytology are often equivocal in making this distinction as well, and definitive surgery should be deferred until permanent histologic sections are available for accurate diagnosis. When submitting tissue for intraoperative interpretation, the surgeon should inform the pathologist if the sample is from the vicinity of the thymus. This may avoid erroneous diagnosis of thymoma, based on residual thymic elements within lymphoma or some other type of neoplasm.

### HODGKIN'S LYMPHOMA

*CLINICAL FEATURES.* Hodgkin's lymphoma (HL) can occur at any age, peaking in incidence in the second through fourth decades. The majority of patients with mediastinal HL also have disease outside the mediastinum—usually cervical or occasionally axillary lymphadenopathy.

*GROSS APPEARANCE.* The tumor is virtually always invasive, involving multiple lymph nodes. As in thymoma, the presence of sclerosis in HL makes the involved nodes firm, and they are often densely adherent to one another and to pericardium or pleura. The dense sclerosis may complicate biopsy; superficial specimens are often nondiagnostic.

*HISTOPATHOLOGY.* The diagnosis requires identification of Reed-Sternberg cells in the appropriate benign cellular background. Because of the lymphocytic background and the lobular architecture, as well as the presence of proliferating thymic epithelium in some cases, HL may be difficult to distinguish from thymoma in small biopsy specimens, particularly on frozen section. For this and other reasons, adequate specimens are critical.

*STAGING AND OUTCOME.* Patients who present with mediastinal HL in the absence of cervical or axillary nodal involvement are rarely found to have disease below the diaphragm and usually receive only radiation therapy. Patients with large (more than one-third of thoracic width) masses do poorly with radiation alone and

are treated with chemotherapy as well. Survival depends almost entirely on the stage of disease at the time of diagnosis.[50]

### DIFFUSE LARGE B-CELL LYMPHOMA

*CLINICAL FEATURES.* Patients with primary large B-cell lymphoma of the mediastinum are most commonly young adults in their third and fourth decades; females predominate.[51] They are virtually all symptomatic because of a rapidly enlarging anterosuperior mediastinal mass with cough, dyspnea, and often superior vena cava (SVC) syndrome.

*GROSS APPEARANCE.* The tumors are similar in appearance to HL; they may either be firm, because of sclerosis, or soft and fleshy. Most involve the thymus but also show widespread local invasion at the time of diagnosis; a few tumors have been completely confined to the thymus, suggesting that they may indeed originate there (Fig. 4D-53).

*HISTOLOGY.* The tumors have a diffuse growth pattern and show variable amounts of fine or dense sclerosis, which does not form nodules, as in HL, but rather divides the tumor cells into small nests, mimicking carcinoma. The tumor cells are similar in size to those of well-differentiated thymic carcinoma or seminoma and, like these tumors, have abundant pale or clear cytoplasm. The nuclei vary from oval to irregular or "cleaved," with one or more prominent nucleoli; there is often a brisk mitotic rate (see Fig. 4D-53). Areas of normal thymus may be found in large biopsy specimens or in resected tumors. Immunostaining has shown that the majority of primary mediastinal large cell lymphomas are of B-cell origin.[52]

*STAGING AND OUTCOME.* There is no indication for staging laparotomy because all patients receive chemotherapy. The prognosis is not as favorable as that of HL, but it is not significantly worse than that for large cell lymphoma in general; 5-year median survivals are 40% to 60% in most series.[51]

### LYMPHOBLASTIC LYMPHOMA

*CLINICAL FEATURES.* Lymphoblastic lymphoma (LBL) is most common in children and young adults, with a sharp peak in incidence in the second and third decades and a striking male predominance.[53] In contrast to HL and mediastinal large cell lymphoma, LBL is usually a systemic disease, with early involvement of the bone marrow and other hematolymphoid organs. Mediastinal LBL is one end of a spectrum of lymphoblastic neoplasia, with T-cell acute lymphoblastic leukemia at the other end.

*GROSS APPEARANCE.* The involved thymus and lymph nodes are generally soft and fleshy, resembling other small round cell tumors and lacking the fibrotic quality of HL and large cell lymphoma. The infiltrate often extends diffusely into perithymic and perinodal fat, which gives the fat an indurated quality.

*HISTOPATHOLOGY.* The neoplastic lymphoblasts are smaller and more delicate than those of large cell lymphoma or thymoma.

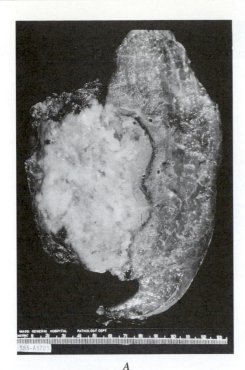

*A*

*B*

**FIGURE 4D-53.** Primary mediastinal large B-cell lymphoma *A*. Gross photograph, showing a large tumor invading the lung. *B*. Photomicrograph showing large lymphoid cells with fine, compartmentalizing sclerosis, mimicking a nonlymphoid tumor such as seminoma or well-differentiated thymic carcinoma. (*With permission, from Banks PM, Kraybill WG: Pathology for the Surgeon. Philadelphia, WB Saunders, 1996.*)

They have dispersed primitive-appearing chromatin, scant cytoplasm, inconspicuous nucleoli, and a high mitotic rate. Most patients have the immumnophenotype of immature T cells, often similar to those normally found in the thymus. The differential diagnosis includes lymphoctye-rich thymomas, small round cell tumors of childhood, such as neuroblastoma, as well as small cell carcinoma, granulocytic sarcoma, and large cell lymphoma.

***SPECIAL PATHOLOGIC STUDIES.*** Automated-flow immunophenotyping study of fresh cell suspensions is useful for the diagnosis and subclassification of LBL or leukemia; however, immunostaining of paraffin sections usually allows diagnosis, albeit in a less definitive manner.

***STAGING AND TREATMENT.*** Bone marrow aspiration and cerebrospinal fluid (CSF) examination are important for accurate staging. Treatment is with aggressive combination chemotherapy with CNS prophylaxis. Children have a relatively high likelihood of cure, but the prognosis in adults is less favorable.[53]

## GERM CELL TUMORS

***CLINICAL FEATURES.*** Mediastinal germ cell tumors occur in the same age group as testicular germ cell tumors, and may be any of the same histologic types: teratoma, seminoma (dysgerminoma), embryonal carcinoma, yolk sac (endodermal sinus) tumor, and choriocarcinoma, or a mixture of these. Patients are always symptomatic from a large anterosuperior mediastinal mass and may have SVC syndrome (20%). The majority of nonseminomatous types have elevation of serum human chorionic gonadotropin (HCG) or α-fetoprotein (AFP) levels, and these tests should be done on all males of this age group with an anterosuperior mediastinal mass.

***GROSS APPEARANCE.*** Mature teratomas are often cystic ("dermoid cysts") and may contain hair, sebaceous material, and teeth. The gross features of the other germ-cell tumors are not distinctively different from those of other malignant tumors: they are lobulated, often invasive solid masses that may have areas of necrosis (Fig. 4D-54).

***HISTOPATHOLOGY.*** The histopathology of mediastinal germ cell tumors is identical to that of gonadal tumors.[54] Mixtures of the various types are common in germ cell tumors. For this reason, these tumors must be thoroughly sampled for microscopic examination. Small biopsy specimens of germ cell tumors containing only undifferentiated malignant cells may be indistinguishable from lymphoma or thymoma (see Fig. 4D-54).

***SPECIAL PATHOLOGIC TECHNIQUES.*** Electron microscopy may be useful in characterizing seminoma. A battery of immunohistologic stains on paraffin sections can be useful in distinguishing malignant germ cell tumors from lymphoma and thymoma; useful marker antigens include placental alkaline phosphatase, cytokeratin, AFP, HCG, and leukocyte-associated antigens.

***STAGING AND OUTCOME.*** For nonseminomatous tumors, the serum AFP or HCG is an important marker for evaluation of remission status. Treatment involves resection, if possible, followed by radiation or adjuvant therapy. The prognosis varies among the different types, with mature teratoma usually being benign, seminoma being potentially aggressive but responsive to radiation and

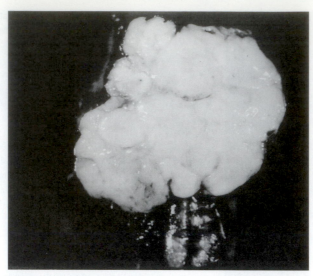

**FIGURE 4D-54.** Mediastinal seminoma. Gross photograph showing a large, encapsulated tumor. The abundant pale cytoplasm and cohesive growth are useful in distinguishing thymona from lymphoma, but the differential diagnosis can be difficult on small biopsy specimens or on a frozen section. (*With permission, from Banks PM, Kraybill WG:* Pathology for the Surgeon. *Philadelphia, WB Saunders, 1996.*)

chemotherapy, and nonseminomatous types being highly aggressive, often disseminated, and only varyingly responsive to treatment.

## NEUROGENIC TUMORS

*CLINICAL FEATURES.* Neurogenic tumors are about equal in overall frequency to thymoma and lymphoma and are by far the most common tumor in the posterior mediastinum (Table 4D-6).[47] Neurilemoma (schwannoma), neurofibroma, and ganglioneuroma are often asymptomatic and discovered by chance on chest x-ray (Fig. 4D-55). Neural tumors may be associated with back pain, dyspnea, or neurologic symptoms related to brachial or cervical plexus involvement or cord compression. The latter is seen in cases that extend into the spinal canal ("dumbbell tumors").

*GROSS APPEARANCE.* Neurilemomas (schwannomas) are well-circumscribed, firm, yellow-white nodules extending from an intercostal nerve. Neurofibromas appear as less-well-circumscribed fusiform expansions of the nerve. Ganglioneuromas are also encapsulated and firm and may have areas of cystic degeneration. Ganglioneuroblastomas and neuroblastomas have a softer, more fleshy appearance and are often poorly circumscribed and invasive. Paragangliomas are usually small and well circumscribed but tend to be very vascular.

*HISTOPATHOLOGY.* The microscopic appearance of neurogenic tumors is diverse but distinctly different from that of the above-mentioned tumor types, and in combination with strong clin-

ical lines of preoperative evidence, usually allows definitive intraoperative diagnosis. Neurilemomas (schwannomas) are composed of bland spindle cells, which focally display a characteristic palisading pattern alternating with looser, edematous areas. Neurofibromas consist of more randomly oriented oval to spindle cells that infiltrate between nerve fibers. Only rarely do these undergo malignant transformation. Ganglioneuromas are composed of mature ganglion cells and neural tissue. The ganglion cells are very large cells with round nuclei, prominent nucleoli, and characteristic abundant eosinophilic cytoplasm (see Fig. 4D-55). Ganglioneuroblastomas contain a mixture of the aforementioned features with primitive neuroblasts, which are small, round cells with a high nuclear-cytoplasmic ratio and a high mitotic rate. Neuroblastoma is composed entirely of such blastic cells, often forming characteristic Homer Wright rosettes around masses of nerve filaments. The differential diagnosis includes other small round cell tumors of childhood (in the chest, principally Ewing's sarcoma) and LBL. Paragangliomas are composed of medium-sized polygonal cells with pale cytoplasm that form characteristic nests, closely resembling normal paraganglia. Numerous small blood vessels are present in the intervening fibrous septa.

*SPECIAL TECHNIQUES.* Electron microscopy is important in the differential diagnosis of small round cell tumors of childhood. Immunostains for neurofilament protein or neuron-specific enolase may be useful.

*STAGING AND OUTCOME.* Ganglioneuroblastoma and neuroblastoma are staged according to the extent of disease. Treatment

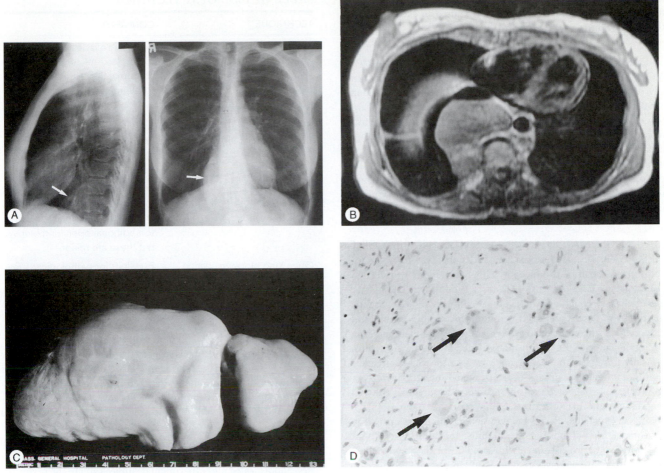

**FIGURE 4D-55.** Ganglioneuroma of the posterior mediastinum. *A*. Chest x-rays, showing a right posterior/paravertebral mediastinal mass. *B*. CT showing paravertebral location of the mass. *C*. Gross photograph, showing lobulated, smooth-surfaced masses of firm, white tissue. *D*. Photomicrograph, showing mature ganglion cells (arrows) in a background of neural tissue. (*With permission, from Banks PM, Kraybill WG:* Pathology for the Surgeon. *Philadelphia, WB Saunders, 1996.*)

is by excision for localized tumors, excision followed by radiation for invasive tumors, and chemotherapy with or without subsequent resection for widely metastatic blastic tumors.

**CYSTS.** Diverse benign cysts occur in the mediastinum, and at clinical presentation often simulate neoplasms. Radiologic imaging is critical for recognition of their cystic nature, although certain neoplasms can acquire cystic degeneration. Age and anatomic compartmental distribution aid in anticipating the correct diagnosis. Bronchogenic cysts are the most common mediastinal cysts. These are located most commonly in the middle or posterior mediastinum and are composed of all layers of the bronchial tree—smooth muscle, cartilage, and mucous glands—and are lined by respiratory epithelium. To confirm the cystic nature of the lesion and exclude the presence of malignant cells by cytopathologic examination, FNA may be useful. Although these lesions are benign and nonprogres-

sive, complete excision is advised to relieve symptoms and provide a definitive diagnosis as well as to prevent complicating infection within the cyst.

Pericardial cysts are usually discovered on routine chest x-ray in asymptomatic adults. The most common location is the right cardiophrenic angle. They are composed of a thick fibrous wall with a mesothelial lining. Needle aspiration with total drainage may be sufficient treatment. If aspiration is unsuccessful, surgical excision may be indicated to exclude malignancy.

Enteric cysts are more common in children and arise from primitive foregut. The diagnosis is usually suspected on clinical and radiologic grounds, and preoperative biopsy is not usually necessary.

Thymic cysts are uncommon but occur more frequently in patients with a history of mediastinal tumors such as HL. They are lined with either squamous or respiratory epithelium. Occasional thymomas and even thymic HL may be predominantly cystic; therefore, extensive histologic sectioning is required to exclude foci of thymoma within the wall of the cyst.

### CASTLEMAN'S DISEASE (ANGIOFOLLICULAR LYMPH NODE HYPERPLASIA).

Mediastinal Castleman's disease is usually discovered on routine chest x-ray in an asymptomatic adult. Small biopsies are usually nonspecific. The lesion consists of a large lymph node with an abundance of peculiar small follicles (involuted, "onionskin," or regressively transformed) surrounded by a broad mantle zone and penetrated by a small blood vessel. Grossly it may resemble a normal spleen. Although clinically benign and nonprogressive, excision is usually required to rule out more ominous conditions. The pathologist can usually diagnose this process intraoperatively if clinical information is provided.

### GRANULOMATOUS LYMPHADENITIS AND FIBROSING MEDIASTINITIS.

Mediastinal lymphadenopathy, usually paratracheal or hilar, can be produced by either sarcoidosis or infectious granulomas, particularly histoplasmosis. Patients with either disorder often have cough and may have pulmonary disease. The mediastinal soft tissues are infiltrated and replaced by dense fibrous tissue, which surrounds major vessels and airways and mimics invasive malignancy of the anterosuperior mediastinum.[54] Sarcoidosis typically produces nonnecrotizing granulomas; conversely, infectious granulomas are usually necrotizing and often caseous. There is sufficient overlap in clinical and histologic features that culture is mandatory if the intraoperative frozen section shows granulomas. In about half of patients there is granulomatous inflammation, and approximately 50% of those are due to fungal infection, usually histoplasmosis; some are associated with sarcoidosis; and the remainder are of unknown etiology. Sarcoidosis of lymph nodes is therefore a diagnosis of exclusion, after infections and neoplasms have been ruled out.

## THE LUNG AND THE PLEURA

### TUMORS OF THE LUNGS AND AIRWAYS

**BIOPSY TECHNIQUES.** There are many ways to obtain lung cells and tissue for diagnostic purposes: each of these has different applications, depending on the clinical situation (Table 4D-10).

Cytologic specimens provide single cells or groups of cells for microscopic evaluation. These techniques are particularly useful for diagnosis of infectious and neoplastic processes, but since only material shed into the airway is examined, they are most reliable for proximal lesions.

Bronchial and transbronchial biopsies are often too small to evaluate pulmonary architecture, but, like cytology, they may be useful for diagnosis of neoplasms and infection. In conjunction with bronchoalveolar lavage, these biopsy techniques can be more useful. If, however, pattern recognition is important for diagnosis, thoracoscopic or open lung biopsies may be required. An example of this is lymphangioleiomyomatosis, in which the distribution and spatial relationship of cells within the lung are diagnostically important.

### TABLE 4D-10. BIOPSY TECHNIQUES

| TECHNIQUE | COMMENT |
| --- | --- |
| Cytologic: Sputum, bronchial washing, bronchoalveolar lavage, fine-needle aspiration biopsy. | Small size of specimen; cannot discern architectural abnormalities; especially useful for tumors and infection. |
| Bronchial wall biopsy. | Small size of specimen; cannot discern architecture. |
| Transbronchial biopsy. | Small size of specimen; cannot discern architecture. |
| Thoracoscopic lung biopsy. | Some problems with sampling (tissue cannot be fully palpated); traumatic distortion of specimen and sometimes small size relative to traditional open lung biopsy; but these are minor. |
| Open lung biopsy/resection specimen. | Excellent for pathologic evaluation. |

SOURCE: With permission, from Banks PM, Kraybill WG: *Pathology for the Surgeon*. Philadelphia, WB Saunders, 1996.

If a pulmonary infection is suspected, microbial cultures are necessary. Depending on the routine in a particular institution, the surgeon may handle this in the operating room or send sterile tissue to the laboratory for the pathologist to allocate.

In addition to usual histologic procedures, a number of special stains for organisms, mucin, iron, and other substances, as well as immunohistochemical stains can be performed on biopsy material. These procedures can be performed by most pathology laboratories. Sophisticated and experimental studies can also be performed on lung tissue if provisions are made prior to obtaining the tissue by consulting with the pathologist and the interested investigative laboratory.

### LUNG MASSES

A mass in the lung is the most common problem presenting to the surgeon.[55] Carcinoma of the lung is usually the first concern, although a metastasis or nonmalignant lesion can present in this fashion. Although carcinoma of the lung is extremely common, the most common malignancies in the lung are metastases.

### CARCINOMA OF THE LUNG

Carcinoma of the lung is common and carries a poor prognosis; only a minority of patients qualifies for surgical resection, effectively the only chance for cure. Adult smokers are most commonly affected.[56] Location, clinical behavior, and management are related to the histologic types: squamous cell carcinoma, adenocarcinoma (including the subset called bronchioloalveolar carcinoma), small cell carcinoma, and large cell carcinoma. These histologic types are compared in Table 4D-8 and illustrated in Fig. 4D-56.

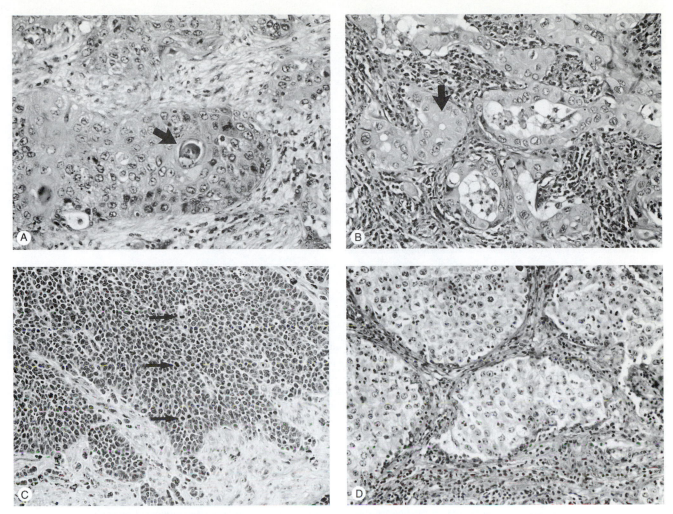

**FIGURE 4D-56.** Microscopic appearances of the major histologic types of carcinoma of the lung. *A*. Squamous cell carcinoma. There is a nest of malignant cells well demarcated from the surrounding fibrous stroma, which shows an inflammatory cell infiltrate. The cells become larger and have more abundant cytoplasm centrally, and there is keratin pearl formation (arrow). *B*. Adenocarcinoma. Tumor cells form glands (arrow), nests, and cords of cells with surrounding stroma showing an inflammatory cell infiltrate. *C*. Small cell carcinoma. Sheets of carcinoma cells are present, with numerous mitotic figures (arrows). The cells show some palisading at the border with the stroma, which is hypocellular fibrous tissue. *D*. Large cell carcinoma. Large carcinoma cells with some cytoplasmic clearing are present, but no glandular or squamous differentiation is seen. The stroma shows a moderate inflammatory cell infiltrate. All figures are taken at the same magnification. (Hematoxylin and eosin, ×200.) (*With permission, from Banks PM, Kraybill WG: Pathology for the Surgeon. Philadelphia, WB Saunders, 1996.*)

Squamous cell carcinomas are generally proximal bronchial tumors that show differentiation toward squamous epithelium in the form of intercellular bridges or keratin production. Adenocarcinomas tend to be parenchymal (peripheral) tumors that form tubules, glands, or papillae (mimicking glandular epithelium) or that secretes mucin identifiable with histochemical stains such as mucicarmine or digested periodic acid-Schiff (PAS) reagents. The latter are called solid adenocarcinomas with mucin production. Bronchioloalveolar carcinoma is a special term for well-differentiated adenocarcinoma that shows growth of tumor cells along alveolar walls with preservation of architecture (Fig. 4D-57). Small cell carcinomas lack squamous or glandular differentiation and are composed of small cells with very little cytoplasm, a high mitotic rate, and extensive necrosis. They tend to be large central rapidly growing tumors and have

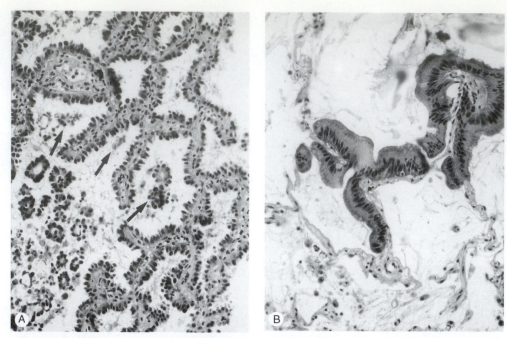

**FIGURE 4D-57.** Bronchioloalveolar subtype of adenocarcinoma. *A*. The nonmucinous variant of bronchioloalveolar carcinoma is associated with a proliferation of atypical cells along alveolar walls. The cells have a somewhat hobnail appearance as they protrude from the alveolar walls. Some papillary groups have detached themselves and are present in alveolar spaces (arrows). *B*. Mucinous bronchioloalveolar carcinoma is seen as well-differentiated mucinous epithelium growing along alveolar walls (center). The surrounding alveoli show abundant strands of mucus in their lumens. (Hematoxylin and eosin, ×200.) (*With permission, from Banks PM, Kraybill WG:* Pathology for the Surgeon. *Philadelphia, WB Saunders, 1996.*)

been associated with hormone production and paraneoplastic syndromes. Large cell carcinomas are composed of intermediate to large polygonal cells with relatively abundant cytoplasm and nuclei that usually have prominent nucleoli. Glandular and squamous differentiation are lacking.

The most important separation among these four types is the separation of small cell carcinoma from the three other types; for this purpose, these three are often collectively termed *non–small cell carcinomas*.

Frozen-section evaluation of tissues taken at the time of surgical staging (either at mediastinoscopy or thoracotomy) is useful in most cases to identify involved lymph node groups and thereby to determine operability. In resection specimens frozen sections need to be performed on bronchial margins only when gross evaluation leaves any concern or doubt as to margin adequacy.

## CARCINOID TUMOR

Carcinoid tumors are low-grade neuroendocrine malignancies. Dense-core neurosecretory granules can be demonstrated in the cytoplasm of the cells, and there is occasionally corresponding clinical evidence of hormone production.[57] Such granules may be identified by electron microscopy or with special histochemical or immunohistochemical stains. They usually occur in adults and have no relationship to cigarette smoking. Carcinoid tumors are more commonly central than peripheral and may be endobronchial, covered by intact mucosa (Fig. 4D-58). Grossly, on fresh sectioning, they are yellow or tan. Microscopically, they are made up of uniform nests or ribbons of cells with prominent, delicate vascularity. The cells are polygonal or somewhat fusiform, with central nuclei with a stippled "salt-and-pepper" chromatin and with eosinophilic or slightly basophilic cytoplasm (Fig. 4D-59). Immunohistochemical stains for neurosecretory granules (e.g., chromogranin, synaptophysin) are usually positive. The prognosis with surgical resection is excellent, even in the presence of regional lymph node metastases (5-year overall survival 90%). Atypical carcinoid tumors show neuroendocrine differentiation similar to carcinoid tumors but have increased mitotic activity, cytologic atypia, necrosis, and loss of architecture. The prognosis is less favorable than that for carcinoid tumors, with 5-year survival slightly better than 60%.[57]

Other low-grade malignant endobronchial tumors often grouped with carcinoid tumors are mucoepidermoid carcinomas and adenoid cystic carcinomas. Both are probably derived from salivary gland–type tissue that makes up the bronchial submucosal glands. In the past these low-grade carcinomas were inappropriately termed "bronchial adenomas."

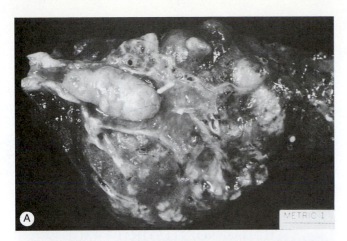

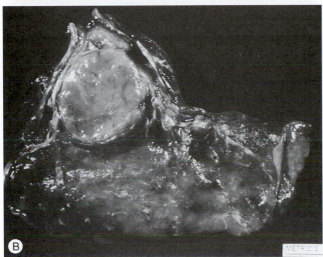

**FIGURE 4D-58.** Carcinoid tumor (gross appearance). Carcinoid tumors may be *A.* endobronchial polypoid masses or *B.* well-circumscribed nodules that compress bronchi. (*With permission, from Banks PM, Kraybill WG:* Pathology for the Surgeon. *Philadelphia, WB Saunders, 1996.*)

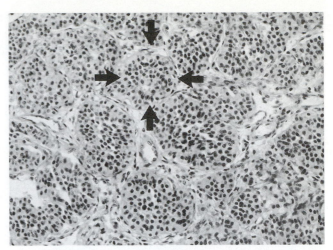

**FIGURE 4D-59.** Carcinoid tumor (microscopic appearance). Typical carcinoid tumors are composed of nests of uniform cells with centrally placed nucleoli that have a salt-and-pepper chromatin pattern. The stroma shows prominent, delicate vascularity and surrounds the tumor cells, producing a "cell ball" appearance (arrows). (Hematoxylin and eosin, ×220.) (*With permission, from Banks PM, Kraybill WG:* Pathology for the Surgeon. *Philadelphia, WB Saunders, 1996.*)

immunohistochemistry may be helpful in distinguishing a new primary from a metastasis. Anatomic patterns of metastatic carcinoma are diverse and include a single nodule, multiple nodules, localized infiltrates, diffuse lymphangitic involvement, intraarteriolar tumor emboli and endobronchial lesions. Metastatic carcinoma (and rarely sarcoma) from an occult primary site can produce a solitary mass that mimics primary neoplasm of the lung.

## PLEURAE

Whether localized or diffuse, pleural diseases manifest similar signs and symptoms: chest pain, often pleuritic, and effusion with or without associated dyspnea.

### PLEURAL BIOPSY TECHNIQUES.

*CYTOLOGIC EVALUATION.* Malignant cells in pleural fluid generally grow as three-dimensional clusters of cells with a high nuclear-to-cytoplasmic ratio and hyperchromatic nuclei, sometimes with prominent nucleoli. Reactive mesothelial cells may appear very atypical and simulate malignancy microscopically.

*CLOSED NEEDLE BIOPSY.* These samples tend to be small and sometimes include portions of the chest wall, but in selected cases they may be diagnostic.

*THORACOSCOPIC BIOPSY.* Direct visualization through the thoracoscope permits directed sampling of lesions. Sampling problems may still occur.

## BENIGN TUMORS OF THE LUNG

Benign tumors are important because of their differential diagnosis with malignant pulmonary disease. They are rare; a number have been described, including benign fibrous histiocytomas, lipomas, neurofibromas, schwannomas, hemangiomas, and others.

## METASTATIC NEOPLASMS

Tumor metastasis to the lung is extremely common; in most cases the histology of the metastasis recapitulates that of the primary site (see Fig. 4D-1). In patients with a prior history of malignant disease, an effort should be made to obtain the prior slides to allow the pathologist comparison of the features of earlier disease with those of the current lung tumor (see Fig. 4D-1). Special stains and

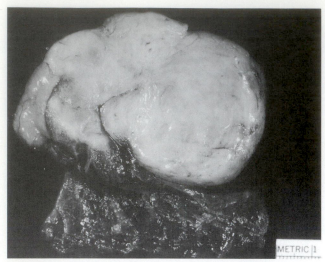

**FIGURE 4D-60.** Solitary fibrous tumor of the pleura. There is a somewhat lobulated and whorled fibrous tumor broadly attached to the visceral pleura. Histologically, these tumors are composed of paucicellular fibrous tissue that has a benign appearance. When resected with a margin of normal tissue, as in this case, such tumors do not recur. (*With permission, from Banks PM, Kraybill WG: Pathology for the Surgeon. Philadelphia, WB Saunders, 1996.*)

---

*OPEN PLEURAL BIOPSY.* The best tissue samples are obtained by this method; however, it carries with it considerable morbidity.

## LOCALIZED PLEURAL TUMORS

### SOLITARY FIBROUS TUMOR (LOCALIZED OR BENIGN FIBROUS MESOTHELIOMA).

This mesenchymal neoplasm is probably a proliferation of submesothelial fibroblasts rather than mesothelial lining cells and so, in the strictest sense, is not truly a mesothelioma. It is not related to asbestos exposure. The majority of these lesions occur as localized nodules attached to the visceral pleura; they are cured by resection (Fig. 4D-60). Microscopically, they are composed of bland-appearing fibroblasts in dense, collagenous matrix. Even the rare sarcomatous solitary fibrous tumors, presumed to represent malignant progressions, are sometimes cured with complete resection.

### PLEURAL METASTASES.

The pleura is a relatively frequent site of metastasis. In general, metastases recapitulate the microscopic features seen in the primary tumor. It is often useful to retrieve the original slides for the pathologist's comparison with the current preparations (see Fig. 4D-1).

### DIFFUSE MALIGNANCY OF THE PLEURA.

Diffuse pleural malignancies are usually metastatic carcinomas, and most patients have a prior history of carcinoma. Metastases usually resemble the primary tumor microscopically. Diffuse malignant mesotheliomas

are uncommon (Fig. 4D-61). The majority of cases are associated with a history of prior asbestos exposure often decades prior to presentation. Many, but not all, patients will have positive pleural fluid cytology, but the distinction from adenocarcinoma is difficult. Mesotheliomas are classified as epithelial, mixed epithelial and sarcomatous, and sarcomatous. One variant of sarcomatous mesothelioma is the desmoplastic mesothelioma; this is paucicellular as to closely mimic benign fibrous tissue. On the other hand, epithelial variants of mesothelioma may so closely resemble carcinoma as to require special studies. Carcinomas often but not invariably show mucin production and immunohistochemical reactivity for carcinoembryonic antigen, B72.3, and Leu-M1.[58]

## THE GASTROINTESTINAL TRACT

Through modern endoscopy the gastrointestinal (GI) tract has become accessible to visualization and biopsy. As a result, processes previously recognized at only an advanced stage can be diagnosed much earlier in their evolution. As the body's most proliferative cell population the gut mucosa is susceptible to neoplastic transformation, both benign and malignant.[59] The incidence of such neoplasms varies according to site, patient age, and population risk factors that probably relate principally to dietary and genetic contributions.[60]

Critical to the pathologist for accurate microscopic interpretation are representative and adequately large biopsy samples. Superficial inflammatory and pedunculated neoplastic processes can be recognized in small forceps biopsies, whereas deeply infiltrative submucosal lesions require larger ("jumbo") forceps biopsies. Precise identification as to location of each biopsy should be included on each specimen label and also on the requisition slip in order to leave no room for error; each biopsied site should be submitted in a separate container and placed in the container immediately after procurement. When segments of GI tract are submitted as resection specimens, they should be opened and examined by the pathologist soon after removal. This allows their recorded gross description in a state of fresh anatomic integrity and affords the pathologist the opportunity to pin out thin-walled viscera for fixation and subsequent ideal sectioning. Segmental bowel specimens, and their respective margins in proportion, shrink about 50% in length when not pinned out during fixation.[61] When circumstances require submission of stapled, closed viscera, the surgeon should disrupt the wall with a single, straight longitudinal incision as distant from the tumor as possible. Submission of such an opened specimen in a large container with formalin solution assures adequate fixation of the critical mucosal (and in most cases tumorous) surfaces.

Adequacy of surgical margins can be assessed intraoperatively by the pathologist. Although in some cases, e.g., distal rectosigmoid colonic or esophageal resections, frozen-section microscopic evaluation may be critical, in most cases gross evaluation of the opened specimen is the most accurate means to judge margins (Fig. 4D-62). Microscopic evaluation of margins is not appropriate for certain tumors, such as lymphomas and stromal tumors. Evaluation of stalk margins in cases of pedunculated polyps containing malignancy can

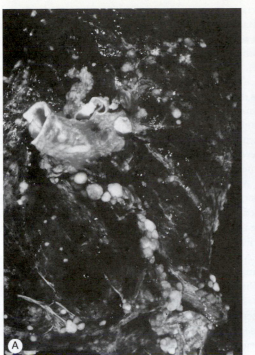
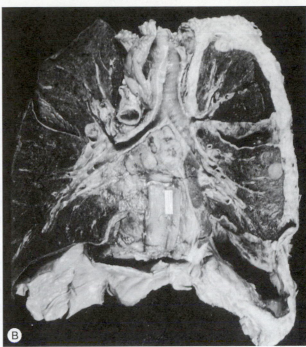

**FIGURE 4D-61.** Diffuse malignant mesothelioma. Early in their course, diffuse malignant mesotheliomas may be seen as *A*. nodules studding the visceral pleural surface, whereas late in their course, they form *B*. the classic rind surrounding the lung, sometimes extending into fissures. (*With permission, from Banks PM, Kraybill WG:* Pathology for the Surgeon. *Philadelphia, WB Saunders, 1996.*)

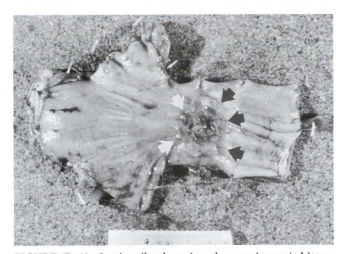

**FIGURE 4D-62.** Semisessile, ulcerating adenocarcinoma (white arrows) of the esophagus. Resection specimen including the proximal stomach shows the neoplasm arising at the superior aspect of a short segment of Barrett's esophagus (black arrows). (*With permission, from Banks PM, Kraybill WG:* Pathology for the Surgeon. *Philadelphia, WB Saunders, 1996.*)

be enhanced by sequential longitudinal sectioning of the specimen, but remains at best imprecise.

The single most important predictive factor for most GI malignancies, i.e., carcinomas and lymphomas, is the stage of a patient's disease. Regional lymph nodes should be sampled, either in continuity with the resected tumor or separately excised. Suspicious lesions in omentum or liver should likewise be selectively sampled. Staging using the AJCC system is highly predictive; however, especially in areas such as the cecum in which bowel wall is relatively thin, precise assessment of early stages of invasion requires meticulous coordinated gross and microscopic pathologic evaluation (Table 4D-11).

Neoplasms of the GI tract vary in incidence and type according to site. Most neoplasms, both benign and malignant, derive from mucosal epithelial elements and are diagnosable with endoscopic biopsy. Benign ulcers can mimic carcinomas endoscopically and microscopically, with "tumor" being simulated by edema and granulation tissue formation, and with cellular atypia and invasive growth pattern being imitated by inflammatory glandular regeneration. Biopsies should derive not only from ulcer base but also from the edge and adjacent intact mucosa.

Carcinomas of the GI tract are predominantly adenocarcinomas, with malignant gland formation, except in the esophagus and anus and anorectal junction regions where squamous cell carcinomas predominate. In North America the most common site for

**TABLE 4D-11.** AJCC STAGING SYSTEM FOR COLORECTAL TUMORS

Primary tumor (T):

TX   Primary tumor cannot be assessed.

T0   No evidence of primary tumor.

Tis   Carcinoma in situ: Intraepithelial or invasion of lamina propria.[1]

T1   Tumor invades submucosa.

T2   Tumor invades muscularis propria.

T3   Tumor invades through the muscularis propria into the subserosa, or into nonperitonealized pericolic or perirectal tissues.

T4   Tumor directly invades other organs or structures, and/or perforates visceral peritoneum.[2]

Regional lymph nodes (N):

NX   Regional lymph nodes cannot be assessed.

N0   No regional lymph node metastasis.

N1   Metastasis in 1 to 3 regional lymph nodes.

N2   Metastasis in 4 or more regional lymph nodes.

Distant metastasis (M):

MX   Distant metastasis cannot be assessed.

M0   No distant metastasis.

M1   Distant metastasis.

*Stage Grouping:*

| AJCC/UICC | | | | DUKES[3] |
|---|---|---|---|---|
| Stage 0 | Tis | N0 | M0 | — |
| Stage I | T1 | N0 | M0 | A |
| | T2 | N0 | M0 | — |
| Stage II | T3 | N0 | M0 | B |
| | T4 | N0 | M0 | — |
| Stage III | Any T | N1 | M0 | C |
| | Any T | N2 | M0 | — |
| Stage IV | Any T | Any N | M1 | — |

[1]NOTE: Tis includes cancer cells confined within the glandular basement membrane (intraepithelial) or lamina propria (intramucosal) with no extension through the muscularis mucosae into the submucosa.

[2]NOTE: Direct invasion in T4 includes invasion of other segments of the colorectum by way of the serosa; for example, invasion of the sigmoid colon by a carcinoma of the cecum.

[3]NOTE: Dukes B is a composite of better (T3, N0, M0) and worse (T4, N0, M0) prognostic groups, as is Dukes C (any T, N1, M0 and any T, N2, M0).

SOURCE: With permission from the American Joint Committee on Cancer: *AJCC Cancer Staging Manual*, 5th ed, JD Fleming et al (eds). Philadelphia, Lippincott-Raven, 1997.

adenocarcinoma is in the large bowel, followed by stomach and esophagus. Benign adenomas, either sessile or pedunculated, are limited mainly to the large bowel and may undergo malignant transformation (Fig. 4D-63). Detailed microscopic evaluation of early carcinomas arising within polyps can allow risk assessment for nodal metastasis and aid in the decision for or against segmental resection.[62] Detailed pathologic staging of resected adenocarcinomas is critical for prognosis and in planning the desirability of adjunctive therapy. Both the earlier Dukes' and the current AJCC systems include tumor size, anatomic layer of deepest tumorous infiltration, and the presence of lymph nodal metastases. The AJCC system also addresses the distribution of any positive lymph nodes (adjacent to tumor vs. root of mesentery). The pathologist's evaluation of tumor stage demands careful, time-consuming efforts at effectively sectioning rigid fixed specimens and at lymph node dissection. Thin-walled viscera present more challenging structures for estimation of deepest layer of penetration (e.g., esophagus, cecum).

An uncommon form of epithelial neoplasm of the gut is endocrine carcinoma ("carcinoid tumor"). Clinical behavior is correlated with site. Appendiceal tumors are highly favorable; those arising in small bowel often metastasize early to regional lymph nodes or liver.[63,64]

Malignant lymphomas can arise at any site in the gut, but are most common in the stomach where they are associated with chronic *Helicobacter* gastritis (Fig. 4D-64).[65] Lymphoma incidence in the intestine is increased in patients with chronic inflammatory diseases such as ulcerative colitis, Crohn's disease, and celiac disease. Resection of GI tract lymphomas is highly controversial, since this tumor type is typically very sensitive to both radiation therapy and chemotherapy. Careful surgical staging, as for carcinoma, is critical for proper patient management, and while classifying and grading lymphomas is important, staging is even more critical.[66] In addition to a large (full-thickness) biopsy of the primary tumor, sampling of regional lymph nodes and wedge and needle biopsies of liver are indicated; splenectomy is not routinely necessary for staging purposes.

Gastrointestinal stromal tumors (GIST) are most commonly encountered in the stomach and small intestine. These tumors were considered leiomyomas or leiomyosarcomas in earlier literature; however, with the advent of powerful immunostaining methods, it became clear that some showed peripheral nerve differentiation, whereas many were not demonstrably differentiated in either respect.[67] A combination of gross and microscopic findings is used by the pathologist to predict benign vs. malignant behavior. Large (greater than 3 cm), ulcerated, hemorrhagic tumors and those with microscopic evidence of proliferative activity are more likely to metastasize (Fig. 4D-65). However, cut-points in distinguishing benign from malignant are somewhat site-dependent.[68] Stromal tumors exhibit a spindle cell microscopic appearance that may resemble smooth muscle or peripheral nerve sheath differentiation. In this regard immunohistochemical stains often show differentiation that is incongruous with microscopic appearances, but there seems to be little clinical correlation with apparent histogenesis. These tumors are usually sharply circumscribed, allowing ready assessment of resection margins. Malignant GISTs tend to distantly metastasize rather than locally recur or spread to regional lymph nodes.

## THE LIVER, BILIARY TRACT, AND PANCREAS

Diseases involving the distal biliary-pancreatic ducts may profoundly affect both the liver and the pancreas. Moreover, the evaluation of

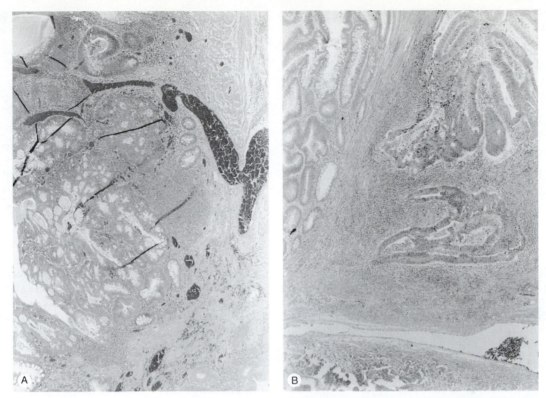

**FIGURE 4D-63.** Examples of early carcinomatous progression within large intestinal adenomas. *A.* There is only intramucosal carcinoma, consisting of abnormally dark, solid glandular elements without evidence of stromal invasion (arrows). Such early carcinoma has no access to lymphatics and so poses little risk of metastasis. *B.* There is superficial stromal infiltration, recognizable by the inflammatory cell reaction (arrows). Such early invasive carcinomas have a low, but real risk for metastasis. (*With permission, from Banks PM, Kraybill WG:* Pathology of the Surgeon. *Philadelphia, WB Saunders, 1996.*)

neoplastic diseases involving the terminal portions of the biliary and pancreatic ducts requires similar diagnostic and therapeutic tools. For these reasons, surgeons and pathologists consider these organs as a single system. The reported number of hepatic and pancreatic tumors is increasing, due in part to a true increased incidence and in part to improved detection methods. This is a group of tumors of increasing importance to the surgical oncologist.[69]

Five types of liver biopsies are used to evaluate liver diseases: percutaneous core needle biopsy, percutaneous FNA biopsy, laparoscopic needle biopsy, and open incisional or excisional biopsy. Needle core techniques utilize a cutting needle to obtain a core of tissue. Such specimens are appropriate for diagnosing diffuse diseases of the liver, such as chronic active hepatitis or cirrhosis. In contrast, the FNA is best for space-occupying lesions, especially primary and metastatic neoplasms and hepatic abscesses. Computed tomography (CT) or ultrasonography is the best method for guiding aspiration biopsy of hepatic lesions. The sensitivity of this procedure varies from 80% to 90%, with few false positives.

Intraoperative frozen-section diagnosis of an unsuspected liver mass may be essential for definitive surgical treatment. Such is the case when one or several hepatic nodules are found during resection of a GI carcinoma. Another clear indication for frozen-section diagnosis is the examination of surgical margins in hepatic resections for primary malignant hepatic neoplasms or solitary metastatic lesions. Frozen-section diagnosis of liver lesions is usually straightforward; however, three benign tumors can cause problems for the unwary pathologist: liver cell adenoma, bile duct adenoma, and angiomyolipoma. Large hepatic adenomas with cytological atypia can be virtually impossible to distinguish from well-differentiated hepatocellular carcinomas. Bile duct adenomas are asymptomatic, small, solitary or multiple nodules composed of tubular structures resembling bile ducts, which can be confused with glands of metastatic carcinoma. Angiomyolipomas may cause confusion with angiosarcoma, malignant fibrous histiocytoma, or hepatocellular carcinoma.

## BENIGN HEPATIC TUMORS

Focal nodular hyperplasia (FNH) is a well-demarcated multinodular hepatic mass in an otherwise normal liver. It is often an incidental finding at autopsy or during a CT scan or a laparotomy for

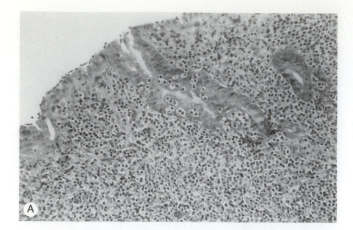

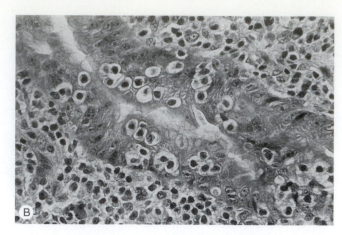

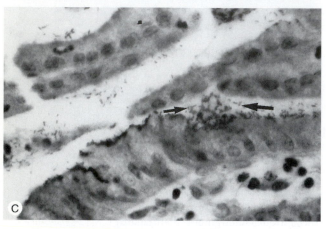

**FIGURE 4D-64.** Photomicrograph of low-grade B-cell lymphoma of mucosa-associated lymphoid tissue (MALT). *A.* Low-magnification view of gastric mucosa reveals a monomorphic lymphoid infiltrate that displaces and infiltrates mucosal epithelium. (Hematoxylin and eosin, ×10) *B.* Higher magnification shows a lymphoepithelial lesion specific for this type of lymphoma. Numerous neoplastic lymphocytes are present within glandular epithelium; ×40. *C.* Adjacent gastric mucosa with *Helicobacter pylori* organisms (arrows) in the overlying mucus. (Warthin-Starry, ×100). (See also Fig. 4D-97). (*With permission, from Banks PM, Kraybill WG:* Pathology for the Surgeon. *Philadelphia, WB Saunders, 1996*).

unrelated diseases. Dynamic CT or magnetic resonance imaging (MRI) can also raise consideration of this diagnosis. FNH is most common in females between 25 and 50 years of age. About one-third of patients report mild abdominal pain or a palpable mass. Improved imaging methods now allow better detection and earlier resection of FNH. A core needle biopsy is usually diagnostic, whereas FNA is inconclusive. Usually measuring less than 6 cm in diameter on cross section they are multinodular, yellow-brown, with a central or eccentric depressed scar that radiates toward the periphery and divides the lesion into nodules (Fig. 4D-66). Microscopically, FNA consists of nodules of normal-appearing hepatocytes. The nodules are separated by fibrous septa containing bile ducts, inflammatory cells, and abnormal arteries and veins.

Hepatocellular adenomas occur most commonly in women during their reproductive years, usually those with a history of oral contraceptive use. The most common clinical presentation is a palpable mass associated with right upper-quadrant discomfort or pain. Rupture of the adenoma leads to intraperitoneal hemorrhage. The tumors are usually single, well demarcated, and even partially encapsulated. Although there may be central necrosis, in contrast to FNH, there is no central scar. They may vary in size from 2 to 26 cm. Conventional hepatic adenomas cannot be differentiated from FNH by cytology. Malignant transformation has been reported to occur only rarely. Adenomas associated with the use of androgenic an-

abolic steroids predominate in males; they are usually multiple and small. Because of cytologic atypia these adenomas are often mistaken for hepatocellular carcinoma by FNA.

Vascular tumors are an important group of neoplasms of the liver. Cavernous hemangioma is the most common primary hepatic tumor. It can be differentiated from other mass lesions by isotope scanning or MRI.[70] Due to the risk of hemorrhage, FNA is contraindicated if hemangioma is suspected. The majority of these vascular neoplasms are incidental findings at autopsy. Only large or giant cavernous hemangiomas (10 cm or larger) require surgical treatment either because they compress adjacent structures or to avoid the risk of catastrophic hemorrhage. Infantile hemangioendotheliomas are usually asymptomatic, but they may rupture, producing congestive heart failure or thrombocytopenia. Malignant transformation has rarely been reported. Epithelioid hemangioendothelioma is a distinctive, low-grade, malignant vascular tumor that is often multicentric and usually involves both lobes.[71] It is most commonly seen in women. Patients often survive many years after diagnosis regardless of therapy. The neoplastic endothelial cells are large and epithelioid, have vacuolated cytoplasm, and lie in dense fibrous stroma. These tumors are easily mistaken microscopically for carcinomas. Angiosarcoma is a highly malignant mesenchymal tumor of the liver that can be induced by thorium dioxide or vinyl chloride exposure or by arsenical ingestion. Because it usually appears as a

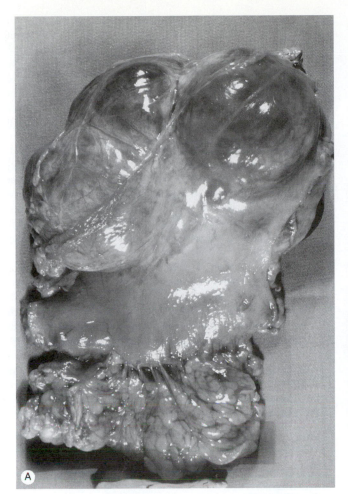

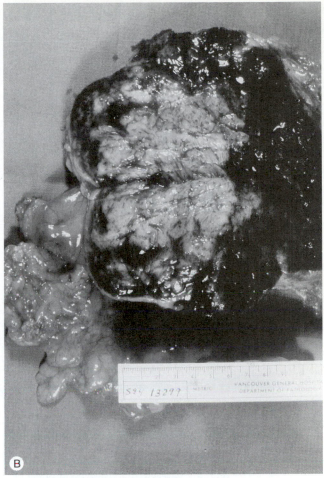

**FIGURE 4D-65.** Malignant gastric stromal tumor. *A.* Multinodular tumor arises along the lesser curvature. *B.* The cut surface shows a whorled gray appearance with extensive hemorrhage. Both large size and hemorrhage suggest malignancy, confirmed by microscopy. (*With permission, from Banks PM, Kraybill WG:* Pathology for the Surgeon. *Philadelphia, WB Saunders, 1996.*)

multinodular mass involving both hepatic lobes, angiosarcoma is rarely resectable.

Bile duct adenoma is a small (less than 1 cm), subcapsular nodule that simulates metastatic disease both grossly and microscopically. The likelihood of such misdiagnosis is increased when these nodules are multiple, found during resection of gastrointestinal adenocarcinomas, or diagnosed with intraoperative frozen sections. These benign tumors are composed of tubular structures resembling normal bile ducts.

## MALIGNANT TUMORS OF THE HEPATIC PARENCHYMA

Hepatocellular carcinoma is one of the most prevalent and most lethal cancers in the world.[72] The incidence is increasing in many parts of the world, including the United States. Hepatitis B and C viruses have both been associated with hepatocellular carcinoma.[73]

Other potential etiologies include hemochromatosis, alcoholic cirrhosis, and glycogen storage disease. The most common symptoms are weakness, malaise, abdominal pain, hepatic mass, weight loss, jaundice, anorexia, and fever. In high-risk patients, the combination of periodic serum AFP measurements, ultrasonography, CT, and FNA have allowed the detection of small tumors (less than 4 cm in diameter). Consequently, the rate of resection has increased.[74] FNA cytology allows differentiation of well to moderately differentiated hepatocellular carcinoma from metastatic disease. However, poorly differentiated hepatocellular carcinomas are difficult to distinguish from metastatic carcinoma by FNA, and core needle biopsy or open biopsy may be required for definitive diagnosis. Likewise, hepatocellular adenomas with atypia cannot be distinguished from well-differentiated hepatocellular carcinoma by FNA. These tumors may be single and small or large and multinodular (Fig. 4D-67).

Microscopically, hepatocellular carcinomas are composed of cells that resemble normal hepatocytes. The most common pattern is

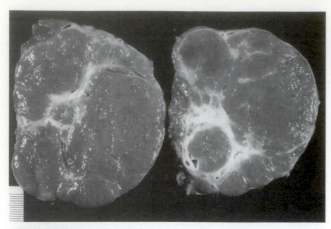

**FIGURE 4D-66.** Focal nodular hyperplasia. The central scar divides the hepatic tissue into nodules of different sizes. (*With permission, from Banks PM, Kraybill WG: Pathology for the Surgeon. Philadelphia, WB Saunders, 1996.*)

trabecular; however, sheetlike and acinar growth patterns are also relatively common. Although most hepatocellular carcinomas are well to moderately differentiated, poorly differentiated forms exist. These tumors are composed of spindle or giant cells and have a poorer prognosis. The fibrolamellar variant occurs in adolescents or young adults and has a better prognosis than the conventional hepatocellular carcinoma. It usually arises in noncirrhotic liver. FNA cytology does not distinguish this unusual variant from the conventional type of hepatocellular carcinoma. However, the distinction can be made on core needle biopsy or with intraoperative frozen sections. Microscopically, it is characterized by deeply eosinophilic cells separated into cords and trabecula by lamellar fibrous bands (Fig. 4D-68).

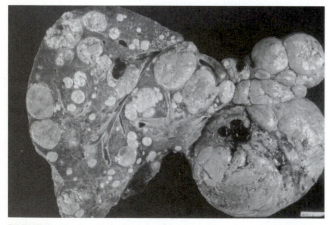

**FIGURE 4D-67.** Multinodular hepatocellular carcinoma involving both hepatic lobes and resembling metastatic carcinoma. (*With permission, from Banks PM, Kraybill WG: Pathology for the Surgeon. Philadelphia, WB Saunders, 1996.*)

Hepatoblastoma is the most common primary hepatic tumor in childhood and is associated with a high mortality rate. Over 60% of hepatoblastomas are diagnosed in children under 2 years of age.[75] Hypoglycemia, thrombocytosis, sexual precocity, and hemihypertrophy are associated with these tumors. They are usually composed of fetal hepatocytes, although frequently a mesenchymal component is present.

Cholangiocarcinoma is a malignant tumor composed of ductal structures similar to intrahepatic bile ducts. It is less common than hepatocellular carcinoma and usually arises in noncirrhotic liver. Elevated serum carcinoembryonic antigen (CEA) and CA 19-9 levels are reported in over half of patients. Ultrasonography is the best radiographic method for the detection of cholangiocarcinoma. Core needle or incisional biopsy may be necessary for definitive diagnosis, since aspiration cytology does not distinguish cholangiocarcinoma from metastatic adenocarcinoma. Cholangiocarcinomas may be multifocal or may present as a single large mass (Fig. 4D-69).

Metastatic tumors are the most common malignant neoplasms of the liver and are the prime consideration when multiple umbilicated nodules are discovered in the liver of patients over 50 years of age. Although any malignant neoplasms can disseminate and reach the liver through the bloodstream, the most common are lung carcinoma, adenocarcinoma of the gastrointestinal tract, breast carcinoma, prostatic adenocarcinoma, genitourinary carcinoma, and malignant melanoma. Frequently, it is not possible to determine the site of origin of hepatic metastasis by microscopic examination of biopsy specimens alone. Even with the aid of immunohistochemistry and electron microscopy it may be impossible to determine with certainty the origin of a metastatic tumor.[76]

## INFLAMMATORY PROCESSES OF THE GALLBLADDER AND BILIARY TREE

Early in the evaluation of a patient with biliary disease the major challenge is the distinction of inflammation versus neoplasm. Although rare compared to chronic cholecystitis, cancer of the gallbladder may occur in the setting of right upper quadrant symptoms or clinical findings initially consistent with inflammation of the gallbladder. Diffuse calcification of the gallbladder gives rise to the "porcelain gallbladder," which carries a 10% to 20% risk for malignant transformation.[77] For this reason, prophylactic cholecystectomy is recommended for patients with porcelain gallbladder. Cholangitis in western countries is most commonly caused by stones, tumors, or scarring from previous surgery. In chronic obstructive cholangitis, fibrosis of the wall of the bile ducts ensues. Entrapment of glandlike structures may microscopically simulate carcinoma. However, nonneoplastic glands are arranged in a lobular pattern that is lacking in carcinoma. Primary sclerosing cholangitis is a rare inflammatory disorder of the intrahepatic and extrahepatic bile ducts.[78] It is characterized by fatigue, pruritus, jaundice, and slow progression to cirrhosis. Approximately 50% to 70% of cases are associated with inflammatory bowel disease, mainly ulcerative colitis. Extensive fibrosis of the wall with entrapment of glandlike structures may simulate adenocarcinoma microscopically. Primary sclerosing cholangitis is a risk factor for the development of cholangiocarcinoma, particularly when associated with ulcerative colitis.

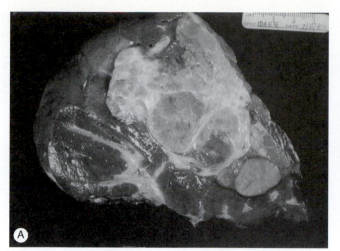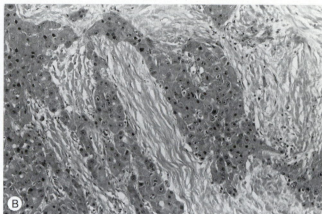

**FIGURE 4D-68.** *A.* Multinodular fibrolamellar carcinoma that arose in noncirrhotic liver. A scar reminiscent of focal nodular hyperplasia is seen. *B.* Fibrolamellar carcinoma. Cords of neoplastic, deeply eosinophilic cells with prominent nucleoli are separated by dense fibrous bands. (*With permission, from Banks PM, Kraybill WG:* Pathology for the Surgeon. *Philadelphia, WB Saunders, 1996.*)

## NEOPLASMS OF THE GALLBLADDER AND EXTRAHEPATIC BILE DUCTS

Adenomas of the gallbladder are more common in women than men and are found in 0.3% to 0.5% of gallbladders removed for cholelithiasis. They are small, usually single, and often found incidentally in cholecystectomy specimens.[79] Rarely, they occur in association with

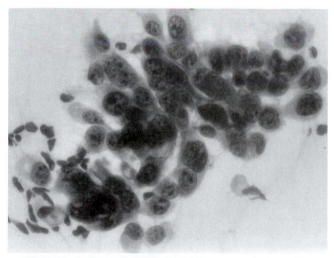

**FIGURE 4D-69.** Fine-needle aspirate from pancreas, obtained intraoperatively, contains clusters of malignant ductal epithelial cells. (Pap stain × 1000.) (*With permission, from Banks PM, Kraybill WG:* Pathology for the Surgeon. *Philadelphia, WB Saunders, 1996.*)

Gardner's syndrome or with Peutz-Jeghers syndrome. Their malignant potential is low. Although adenomas of the extrahepatic bile ducts are much less common than those that arise in the gallbladder, they mimic malignant tumors clinically because of resulting biliary obstruction. Granular cell tumors and carcinoid tumors may rarely occur in the gallbladder or extrahepatic bile duct.

Although carcinomas of the gallbladder and extrahepatic bile ducts are histologically similar, they differ in their epidemiology, clinical presentation, risk factors, and etiology. The incidence of carcinoma of the gallbladder correlates with the incidence of cholelithiasis. The initial signs and symptoms of gallbladder cancer are those of cholelithiasis. The dominant sign of extrahepatic biliary cancer is jaundice in 90% of patients. Approximately 10% to 15% of invasive gallbladder carcinomas are inconspicuous on gross examination. The macroscopic features in these cases are similar to those of chronic cholecystitis. Surgeons should request frozen sections of gallbladders removed for cholelithiasis but found to have a very thickened wall. According to their gross features, carcinomas of the extrahepatic bile ducts are classified as nodular, polypoid, or diffusely infiltrating. Both surgeons and pathologists can easily overlook the latter type of carcinoma. It has been reported that carcinoma of the bile ducts is missed in up to 20% of patients at the time of initial surgical exploration for obstructive jaundice. This is a problem area for both surgeon and pathologist. Obtaining intraoperative biopsies of high proximal carcinomas may be extremely difficult. Retrograde cholangiography with brush biopsy can sometimes successfully identify proximal extrahepatic bile duct carcinoma preoperatively. Pathologic interpretation is difficult due to the mimicry of malignancy achieved by benign, glandlike structures in the walls of bile ducts. The two most important prognostic factors are pathologic stage and histologic grade of the tumor.

## PANCREATIC NEOPLASMS

Because carcinoma of the pancreas can be difficult to distinguish from chronic pancreatitis, and because both diseases often co-exist in the same pancreas, biopsy is imperative to establish the correct diagnosis. Moreover, a great variety of neoplams with varying prognoses originate in the pancreas and must be differentiated from the rapidly lethal carcinomas. Cytologic examination of pancreatic secretions and brushings obtained during endoscopic retrograde cholangiopancreatography after secretion stimulation has produced limited diagnostic success. Because of its high sensitivity and specificity, CT- or ultrasound-guided FNA is now the preoperative method of choice for the diagnosis of pancreatic cancer.[80] Percutaneous transabdominal aspiration provides adequate material in 60% to 90% of patients, depending upon the skill of the operator. If the tumor appears resectable, FNA during laparotomy may also be done (Fig. 4D-69). Assessment of peritoneal, lymph nodal, and hepatic metastasis is done by intraoperative frozen sections if visibly suspect lesions are identified, prior to embarking on a Whipple procedure or a total pancreatectomy. The presence of hepatic, serosal, or distant nodal metastases indicates an unresectable tumor. The role of laparoscopic evaluation of these patients prior to laparotomy is being investigated and appears promising. At present, wedge or needle core biopsies are used only infrequently for the intraoperative diagnosis of pancreatic cancer. Such biopsy methods are associated with significant morbidity, and multiple samples are often necessary to obtain a definite diagnosis. Common pitfalls with frozen sections include misdiagnosis of malignancy due either to benign proliferating duct radicals in dense fibrous stroma or to perineural endocrine cell proliferation as seen in chronic pancreatitis. Both of these features closely simulate carcinoma microscopically.

In the United States, ductal carcinoma of the exocrine pancreas is the ninth most common malignancy and the second most common gastrointestinal cancer, being surpassed only by colorectal cancer. Ductal carcinoma is highly lethal.[81] Approximately 95% of patients die within 2 years of diagnosis. Although modern imaging techniques have improved our ability to identify pancreatic masses 2 cm in size or larger, differentiating carcinoma from chronic pancreatitis remains a diagnostic problem. Grossly these tumors are firm, gray-white masses with poorly defined borders. Extensive necrosis and cystic degeneration are uncommon features of conventional ductal carcinomas, but may be seen in giant cell variant carcinomas and in some endocrine carcinomas. Ductal carcinomas occur most commonly in the head of the pancreas. Mutations of the K-*ras* oncogene are found in about 90% of patients.[82] Accounting for 90% of malignant tumors of the pancreas, ductal adenocarcinoma is often deceptively well differentiated appearing microscopically (Fig. 4D-70). Of importance to the surgeon is the rare intraductal mucin-producing papillary carcinoma. Such tumors remain confined to the major pancreatic duct for several years and can therefore be cured by the Whipple procedure or total pancreatectomy.[83]

Cystic neoplasms of the pancreas are divided into three types according to their microscopic features and biologic behavior: mucinous, microcystic adenoma, and papillary and cystic tumors.[84] Mucinous cystic neoplasms of the pancreas are usually large, multiloculated, and more common in middle-aged females. About 65% of the tumors arise in the tail of the pancreas. Cystadenomas tend

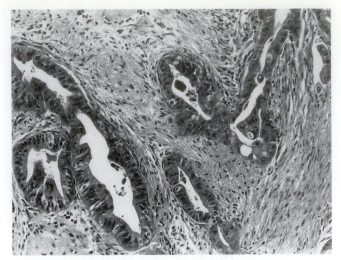

**FIGURE 4D-70.** Photomicrograph of ductal carcinoma of the pancreas, the most common form of pancreatic cancer. Abnormal ducts featuring dark, atypical epithelium are surrounded by cellular fibrous stroma. (*With permission, from Banks PM, Kraybill WG:* Pathology for the Surgeon. *Philadelphia, WB Saunders, 1996.*)

to be smaller than cystadenocarcinomas and borderline tumors. Glycogen-rich microcystic adenomas are almost invariably benign and are more common in the head of the pancreas. They are most commonly seen in females and vary in size from 2 to 20 cm. They are composed of cuboidal clear PAS-positive cells that line small cystic spaces. Mucinous cystic neoplasms are subdivided into cystadenomas, which follow a benign clinical course; borderline tumors (tumors of low malignant potential), of which only a small proportion recur or metastasize; and cystadenocarcinomas, which recur or metastasize in about 40% to 50% of patients. Some believe that CT findings are sufficiently distinctive to allow radiologic distinction of mucinous cystic tumors from pseudocysts and microcystic adenomas. However, mucinous cystic neoplasms are still confused with pseudocysts, despite claims to the contrary. FNA allows distinction of mucinous tumors from glycogen-rich microcystic adenomas. The aspirates of the former tumor usually contain abundant mucin and high concentration of CEA, whereas the aspirates of glycogen-rich microcystic adenomas show clear fluid that does not contain CEA. FNA biopsy of cystadenoma shows clusters of sheets of benign epithelial cells with vacuolated cytoplasm. In borderline mucinous tumors and cystadenocarcinomas, at least some of the epithelial cells show large, hyperchromatic nuclei and vacuolated cytoplasm. Aspirates of microcystic adenomas contain few cuboidal cells with clear cytoplasm and a small, centrally placed round nucleus. The cytology of papillary and cystic tumors consists of papillary fronds lined by one or more layers of cuboidal cells with round eccentric nuclei having finely granular chromatin. Small nucleoli may be present. Histologically, mucinous cystadenomas are lined by a benign mucinous epithelium. In borderline tumors the lining epithelium shows focal areas of carcinoma in situ alternating with benign-appearing mucinous epithelium. Cystadenocarcinomas are malignant gland-forming tumors that infiltrate the stroma. Extensive sampling is recommended in cystadenocarcinomas and borderline tumors so as to exclude foci of invasive carcinoma. Papillary cystic tumors occur almost exclusively in adolescent girls or young females. The majority of these tumors are benign and more often affect the body or tail than the head of the pancreas. They may reach a large size (average 10 cm) and may be asymptomatic. Pancreatoblastoma is a rare malignant pancreatic tumor of childhood that may produce an elevation of serum AFP levels.

Clinicopathologic correlation and immunohistochemical assessment are essential to understand the pathobiology of endocrine tumors of the pancreas that are an integral component of multiple endocrine neoplasia type I (MEN I).[85] Malignancy is difficult to evaluate on histologic grounds alone. Extension beyond the pancreas, blood vessel invasion, and metastases are the best indicators of malignant behavior. Functioning endocrine tumors account for 60% to 80% of all pancreatic endocrine neoplasms. β-cell tumors (insulinomas) are the most common functioning tumors of the pancreas (Fig. 4D-71). They produce hyperinsulinemia and hypoglycemia. The great majority (90%) of β-cell tumors are benign, small (usually less than 2 cm), and solitary. Some 1% to 3% are multiple and associated with MEN I. In contrast to β-cell tumors (insulinomas), α-cell tumors (glucagonomas) are usually malignant and produce elevated serum glucagon levels. This syndrome consists of necrolytic migratory erythema, diabetes, glossitis, normocytic anemia and a tendency to develop vein thrombosis. G-cell tumors (gastrinomas) are associated with gastric acid hypersecretion, peptic ulcers in the stomach or small bowel, diarrhea, and elevated serum gastrin levels. The majority of pancreatic gastrinomas are malignant. Somatostatin-producing tumors (D-cell tumors) are very rare. They give rise to a clinical syndrome (somatostatinoma) characterized by diabetes

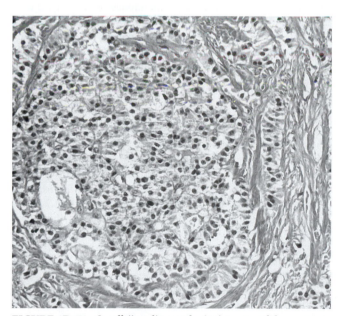

**FIGURE 4D-71.** β-cell (insulin-producing) tumor of the pancreas showing a nodule of neoplastic cells, reminiscent of a pancreatic islet. (*With permission, from Banks PM, Kraybill WG: Pathology for the Surgeon. Philadelphia, WB Saunders, 1996.*)

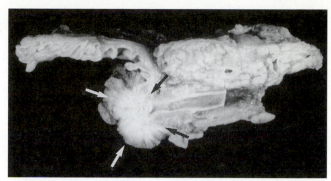

**FIGURE 4D-72.** Adenocarcinoma of the ampulla of Vater. The tumor (arrows) arose in the duodenal mucosa and extended into the common channel. (*With permission, from Banks PM, Kraybill WG: Pathology for the Surgeon. Philadelphia, WB Saunders, 1996.*)

mellitus, steatorrhea, diarrhea, cholelithiasis, and elevated serum somatostatin levels. These are malignant tumors. Tumors that produce excessive amounts of vasoactive intestinal peptide (VIP) give rise to a syndrome characterized by watery diarrhea, hypokalemia, and achlorhydria.

## AMPULLARY TUMORS

Ampullary tumors may arise from the duodenal mucosa, the common channel, the most distal portion of the common bile duct, or the pancreatic duct (Fig. 4D-72). Tubular and villous adenomas usually arise from the duodenal mucosa and may extend into the common channel. They may be either sporadic or represent a component of familial polyposis or Gardner's syndrome. Since adenocarcinomas frequently arise at the base of the adenoma, small endoscopic biopsies often miss the malignant component. The most common malignant tumors are well to moderately differentiated adenocarcinomas. Because of small glands occurring in this area, interpretation of frozen section is notoriously difficult and requires a thorough understanding of the microscopic anatomy peculiar to this site.

## EXAMINATION OF THE WHIPPLE SPECIMEN

The pathologist should dissect along the common bile duct and the main pancreatic duct and determine whether the latter joins with the distal portion of the common bile duct or empties directly into the duodenum. Sections for histologic examination should include the tumor, duodenal mucosa, common channel, common bile duct, main pancreatic duct, pancreas, and stomach. All peripancreatic and retroduodenal lymph nodes should be examined histologically. The most important margins are usually the proximal common bile duct and the plane of pancreatic transection. The gastric and duodenal margins are nearly always free of tumor in standard Whipple resections. However, these margins are of great importance in pylorus-preserving pancreaticoduodenectomy specimens.

## THE UROLOGIC SYSTEM

### RENAL MASSES

Increased use of abdominal and pelvic imaging studies such as ultrasound, CT, and MRI has improved the accuracy and rate of detection of renal masses. Many renal tumors are now diagnosed at an early stage.[86,87] Sonographically, cystic masses that are simple or are composed of adipose tissue usually require no further workup. In contrast, hyperdense or complex cysts should be investigated, often with cyst aspiration. Solid masses usually require surgery, although fine-needle aspiration (FNA) is often employed preoperatively to determine the nature of the tumor.

Percutaneous FNA is safe and reasonably accurate and allows evaluation of tumor recurrence in the renal fossa after nephrectomy, as well as distinction between renal cysts and neoplasms. Simple nephrectomy is performed in patients with end-stage kidney diseases, calculus disease, obstruction, and trauma, whereas radical nephrectomy is performed in patients with renal adenocarcinoma and other malignancies. Regardless of the condition, the pathologist weights, measures, and slices the specimen carefully at 3-mm intervals to determine multicentricity, anatomic location, and extent of the process. Pathologic staging of renal neoplasms requires evaluation of Gerota's fascia, renal vein and artery, and medulla and pelvis. Multiple sections are obtained representing both the neoplasm and the adjacent uninvolved kidney for histologic evaluation. Partial nephrectomy is useful for removal of a variety of benign lesions in the kidney and is employed in select cases with malignant tumors in which preservation of renal function is desired. In such cases it is important to document the portion of kidney removed. Intraoperative frozen sections are usually employed to assure adequacy of surgical margins.

### BENIGN TUMORS OF THE KIDNEY

Angiomyolipoma is a hamartoma composed of blood vessels, smooth muscle, and fat, and is common in patients with tuberous sclerosis. This syndrome should be looked for in all cases, particularly in patients with bilateral angiomyolipoma. Oncocytoma is a common benign epithelial tumor of adulthood with large eosinophilic cells containing numerous mitochondria; it may be difficult to distinguish from renal cell carcinoma (Fig. 4D-73). It is large, solitary, encapsulated, and mahogany-brown, with a central stellate scar. Juxtaglomerular cell tumor is a rare tumor that causes hypertension in young patients. Fibroma is a small gray-white nodule within the pyramids composed of fibroblasts and collagen, usually identified incidentally at autopsy.

### MALIGNANT TUMORS OF THE KIDNEY

Renal cell carcinoma usually occurs in patients over 60 years of age and is more common in men than women.[86,87] It usually appears as a large, solitary, circumscribed mass but multifocality is frequently observed in serially sectioned kidneys, a finding that challenges the feasibility of nephron-sparing (partial) nephrectomy. As

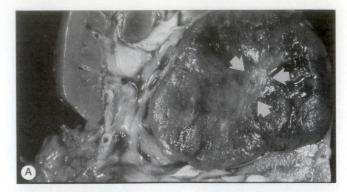

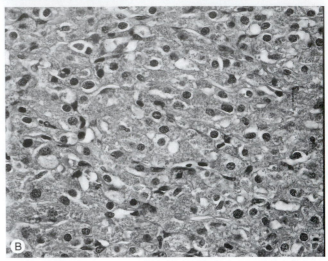

FIGURE 4D-73. Oncocytoma of the kidney. *A*. Grossly, the tumor is solitary, large, and mahogany-brown, with a characteristic central stellate scar (arrows). *B*. Microscopically, the cells are uniform with abundant eosinophilic cytoplasm. (*With permission, from Banks PM, Kraybill WG:* Pathology for the Surgeon. *Philadelphia, WB Saunders, 1996.*)

one of the great mimickers in medicine, renal cell carcinoma can first appear in other sites prior to detection of a primary renal tumor. It may produce paraneoplastic syndromes such as polycythemia (due to erythropoietin production), hypercalcemia, hypertension (due to renin production), Cushing's syndrome (due to ACTH production), feminization, masculinization, amyloidosis, and others. The most common histologic pattern is clear cell carcinoma (Fig. 4D-74). Two histologic patterns—sarcomatoid and papillary—are associated with the poorest outcomes (see Fig. 4D-1). Patients with von Hippel-Lindau syndrome, an autosomal dominant disease, often have renal cell carcinoma, and this syndrome should always be considered in patients with bilateral renal tumors.

The most important prognostic variables in renal cell carcinoma are tumor size, stage, grade, and histologic pattern. Separation of adenoma from carcinoma was originally based on a size threshold of 3 cm, but reports of metastases with smaller tumors have led most investigators to abandon the simple size criterion. A reasonable approach is to refer to small tumors as renal cortical neoplasms without

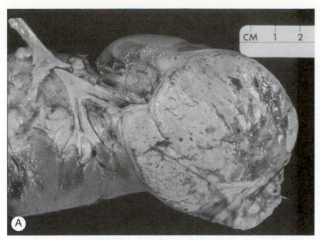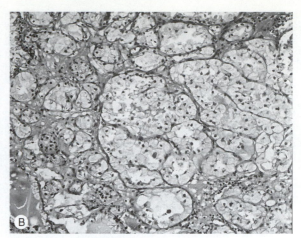

**FIGURE 4D-74.** Renal cell carcinoma, clear cell type. *A.* Grossly, the tumor is large and solitary. *B.* Microscopically, the tumor cells are uniform with abundant clear to pale cytoplasm. (*With permission, from Banks PM, Kraybill WG:* Pathology for the Surgeon. *Philadelphia, WB Saunders, 1996.*)

separating them into benign or malignant categories. Grading of renal cell carcinoma is prognostically valuable, and many pathologists use the Fuhrmann classification scheme.[86,87] DNA ploidy may also provide prognostic information.

Wilms' tumor is an unusual tumor that usually occurs in infancy and childhood, occurring as a large round tumor dwarfing the kidney. Microscopically, Wilms' tumor is composed of a mixture of primitive renal epithelial and stromal elements. Cytogenetic deletion of the short arm of chromsosome 3 is characteristic. The histologic appearance and grading of urothelial carcinoma of the renal pelvis and ureters are the same as for those corresponding neoplasms arising in the bladder (see page 350).

Nonneoplastic processes should be included in the differential diagnosis. Cysts are frequent incidental findings in the kidney and may be confused with tumors.[86] They are often associated with certain forms of chronic renal failure and with cysts in other organs. Childhood polycystic kidney disease is a rare autosomal recessive condition associated with liver and bile duct cysts and congenital hepatic fibrosis. Adult polycystic kidney disease is a common autosomal dominant condition associated with liver cysts (40%) and berry aneurysms in the circle of Willis (10% to 30%). Other cystic diseases include benign simple cysts, cystic renal dysplasia, cystic disease of the renal medulla, and dialysis associated cystic disease.

## UROTHELIAL TUMORS

In the patient presenting with signs and symptoms relating to lower urinary tract infection, cystitis and urothelial tumors are important differential diagnoses. The clinical evaluation of these patients includes physical examination, microscopic evaluation of the urine with culture, and cystoscopy. All suspect cystoscopically visible lesions should be sampled to exclude a urothelial tumor. Transurethral resection of the bladder is subject to the same artifacts seen in prostatic curettage, including cautery artifact and tissue shrinkage. Cystoscopic biopsy often shows denudation of the mucosa because of

the tenuous adherence of the urothelium to the stroma, particularly in inflamed areas. Intraoperative frozen section generally only compounds the problem of interpretation posed by small specimens and is rarely indicated in this clinical setting. Exfoliative urine cytology is an effective method for detecting urothelial carcinoma and for monitoring treatment. For carcinoma of the bladder, cytology has a sensitivity of 50% to 60% for a single specimen and 80% to 90% for multiple specimens, with a specificity of almost 100%. The sensitivity is lower for urothelial neoplasms of the upper urinary tract and for low-grade tumors such as urothelial papilloma. False-negative results can occur with advanced neoplasms. Sequential cytology samples at 3- to 6-month intervals are useful for following patients with incipient urothelial carcinoma.

There are two morphologic patterns of noninvasive (in situ) urothelial neoplasia that differ clinically and pathologically.[88] The first, noninvasive papillary urothelial carcinoma, is common and usually low grade and tends to recur multiple times prior to any stromal invasion (Fig. 4D-75). The local recurrence rate is 40% to 70%, usually within 2 years, with progression to higher grade in about 30%. The second form of urothelial neoplasia, flat carcinoma in situ, is uncommon, is usually high grade, and tends to progress to invasive carcinoma rapidly (Fig. 4D-76). Both forms of noninvasive urothelial neoplasia are initially treated by intravesicular therapy such as bacille Calmette-Guérin (BCG); however, resective surgery is often necessary in cases that progress to invasion.

Urothelial carcinoma (transitional cell carcinoma) accounts for about 90% of bladder cancers in the United States.[88] It is rare before 40 years of age and much more common in men than women. The tumors are grossly papillary, sessile, nodular, or infiltrating. Although most common in the bladder, this tumor can arise anywhere in the urinary tract. Microscopically, three grades are recognized: grade 1 consists of an orderly but thickened growth of urothelial cells with mild nuclear abnormalities such as enlargement, hyperchromasia, and variation in shape; grade 2 is similar to grade 1 except that there is greater architectural distortion with loss of cellular maturation and orderliness as well as moderate to marked nuclear abnormality; and

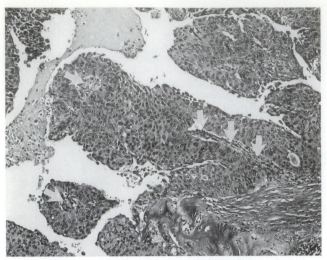

**FIGURE 4D-75.** Grade 1 noninvasive papillary urothelial carcinoma of the bladder. Papillary projections of well-differentiated epithelium contain stromal cores (arrows); stroma without tumor invasion is present in the lower right corner. (*With permission, from Banks PM, Kraybill WG:* Pathology for the Surgeon. *Philadelphia, WB Saunders, 1996.*)

grade 3 consists of urothelial cells with marked nuclear abnormalities that lack maturation and polarity. Surgery and radiation therapy are commonly utilized for invasive bladder cancer regardless of histologic features. Prognostic factors of importance include histologic type, grade, growth pattern, stage, lymphatic invasion, nuclear DNA content (ploidy), and blood group antigen expression.

Squamous cell carcinoma is the most common form of bladder cancer in countries such as Egypt, where *Schistosoma haematobium* is endemic. It may also occur in other clinical situations. Squamous cell carcinoma tends to be clinically aggressive, manifesting at a high stage. Keratinizing squamous metaplasia is considered to be a precursor lesion in some cases. Adenocarcinoma is a rare and aggressive form of bladder cancer that often arises in the urachus, in extrophic bladders, and in those infected with schistosomiasis. The tumors can be papillary, glandular, mucin-producing, of the signet ring cell type, or clear cell variants. Other rare forms of urothelial carcinoma include small cell undifferentiated carcinoma and sarcomatoid carcinoma. Benign soft tissue tumors and tumorlike conditions that occur in the bladder include inflammatory pseudotumor, postoperative spindle cell nodule, leiomyoma, pheochromocytoma, amyloidosis, and endometriosis. Malignant soft tissue tumors are rare and include sarcoma botryoides (embryonal rhabdomyosarcoma) in infants and leiomyosarcoma in adults. The bladder is rarely involved by metastatic malignancy.

## THE MALE REPRODUCTIVE SYSTEM

### PROSTATE AND SEMINAL VESICLES

There are a number of acute and chronic inflammatory conditions of the prostate. They may be important in that more chronic conditions may present with findings suspicious for carcinoma of the prostate. Granulomatous prostatitis includes morphologically distinct forms of chronic prostatitis caused by a variety of inciting agents including infection and biopsy instrumentation.[89] The majority of patients have a history of urinary tract infection. The prostate is often hard, fixed, and nodular, and cancer is often suspected clinically. Urinalysis shows pyuria and hematuria, but biopsy is required for definitive diagnosis (Fig. 4D-77). The common pathogenetic mechanism of

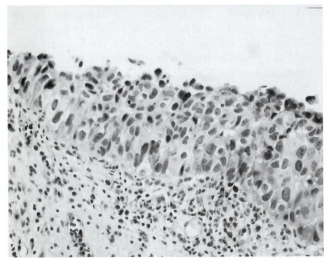

**FIGURE 4D-76.** Carcinoma in situ (flat pattern) of the bladder. Highly atypical, dark, irregular epithelial nuclei remain within the mucosal surface. (*With permission, from Banks PM, Kraybill WG:* Pathology for the Surgeon. *Philadelphia, WB Saunders, 1996.*)

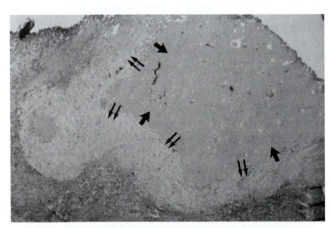

**FIGURE 4D-77.** Granulomatous prostatitis following transurethral resection. Note the central gray zone of coagulative necrosis (single arrows), surrounded by a granulomatous giant-cell reaction (double arrows). (*With permission, from Banks PM, Kraybill WG:* Pathology for the Surgeon. *Philadelphia, WB Saunders, 1996.*)

granulomatous prostatitis is blockage of prostatic ducts with stasis of secretions, regardless of the inciting agent.

## BENIGN PROSTATIC HYPERPLASIA

Enlargement of the prostate, commonly referred to as benign prostatic hyperplasia (BPH), consists of overgrowth of the glandular and fibromuscular tissues of the transition zone and periurethral area. It is extremely common, accounting for up to 400,000 prostatectomies annually, making this the most common surgical procedure in American men. Symptoms are caused by interference with muscular sphincteric function and by obstruction of urine flow through the prostatic urethra. BPH consists of variably sized nodules that are usually firm, rubbery, and yellow-gray; these bulge from the cut surface upon sectioning. Prominent epithelial hyperplasia, in addition to stromal hyperplasia, creates soft and spongy nodules that ooze a pale-white watery fluid. If the BPH is predominantly fibromuscular (stromal), there is diffuse enlargement of numerous trabeculations without prominent nodularity. Degenerative changes include calcification and infarction, often with reactive microscopic changes in the epithelium at the periphery, including squamous metaplasia and transitional cell metaplasia. BPH and its associated benign lesions have numerous histologic variants. Some of these can mimic carcinoma microscopically. Atrophy is a common microscopic finding, consisting of small distorted glands with flattened epithelium, hyperchromatic nuclei, and stromal fibrosis. It is usually idiopathic, and the prevalence increases with age. Postatrophic hyperplasia consists of atrophic glands with benign proliferating luminal cells. Basal cell hyperplasia is characterized by proliferation of basal cells, forming two or more cells in thickness at the periphery of prostatic glands and acini, usually occurring in the setting of BPH. Adenoid basal cell tumor consists of basaloid cell nests of varying size infiltrating the stroma without circumscription. Rare cases display perineural invasion and extension into the periprostatic soft tissues, but there have been no reports of metastases or deaths due to these tumors. Cribriform hyperplasia is a histologic variant of BPH that consists of a nodule of glands with a distinctive cribriform pattern with pale to clear cytoplasm and small uniform nuclei with inconspicuous nucleoli.

Atypical adenomatous hyperplasia is a localized proliferation of small glands within the prostate, usually seen in transurethral resection specimens from the transition zone, that may be mistaken microscopically for carcinoma. Atypical adenomatous hyperplasia is distinguished from well-differentiated carcinoma by its inconspicuous nucleoli, infrequent crystalloids, lack of basophilic mucin, and fragmented basal cell layer as demonstrated immunhistochemically with basal cell–specific antikeratin antibodies. The basal cell layer is characteristically discontinuous and fragmented in atypical adenomatous hyperplasia, whereas carcinoma has an absent basal cell layer. This diagnostic feature can be demonstrated immunohistochemically in formalin-fixed sections. The identification of atypical adenomatous hyperplasia should not influence or dictate therapeutic decisions, but close surveillance and follow-up are indicated. Further discussion of this topic is beyond the scope of this section, but most cancers arise in the prostate with concomitant BPH. Cancer is found incidentally in a significant number of transurethral prostatectomy specimens. It is important to exclude the possibility of underlying cancer in patients presenting with symptoms of urinary obstruction presumed due to BPH.

Transurethral prostatic resection (TURP) specimens consist of tissue from the transition zone, urethra, periurethral area, bladder neck, and anterior fibromuscular area.[90] Studies of radical prostatectomies performed after TURP reveal that the resection does not usually include tissue from the central or peripheral zone, and some of the transition zone usually remains. Well-differentiated cancer found incidentally in TURP chips usually represents cancer that has arisen in the transition zone. Such tumors are frequently small and may be completely resected by TURP; however, there is no accurate method to determine the completeness of excision. The optimal number of chips to submit for histologic evaluation from a TURP specimen remains controversial, with some experts advocating complete submission even with large specimens that would require many cassettes. The Cancer Committee of the College of American Pathologists (1994)[91] and the Consensus Committee on Staging and Grading of the American Cancer Society (1992)[92] recommend a minimum of six cassettes for the first 30 g of tissue and one cassette for every 10 g thereafter.

## PROSTATIC INTRAEPITHELIAL NEOPLASIA AND ADENOCARCINOMA

Prostatic intraepithelial neoplasia (PIN) represents the putative precancerous end of the morphologic spectrum of cellular proliferations within prostatic ducts, ductules, and acini.[93] Two grades of PIN, low and high, are identified. Only high-grade PIN is considered a precursor of invasive carcinoma (Fig. 4D-78). The continuum of atypia

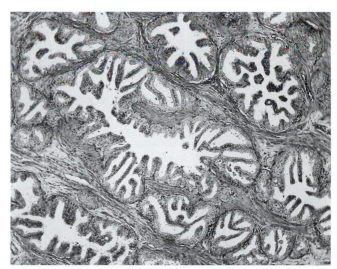

**FIGURE 4D-78.** High-grade prostatic intraepithelial neoplasia (PIN). Acinar spaces are filled with orderly epithelial papillae. Higher-magnification microscopy revealed extreme nuclear atypia, similar to that of invasive carcinoma. (*With permission, from Banks PM, Kraybill WG:* Pathology for the Surgeon. *Philadelphia, WB Saunders, 1996.*)

between high-grade PIN and early invasive cancer is characterized by disruption of the basal cell layer, progressive loss of markers of secretory differentiation, increasing nuclear and nucleolar abnormalities, increasing proliferative potential, and increasing variation in DNA content (aneuploidy). The clinical importance of recognizing PIN is based upon its strong association with carcinoma. Its identification in biopsy specimens of the prostate warrants further search for concurrent invasive carcinoma.

Prostate cancer is the most common cancer among men in the United States and is second only to lung cancer as a cause of cancer death. In 1995 it is estimated that 40,400 men died of prostate cancer and 240,000 new patients were diagnosed. Although most prostatic cancers grow relatively slowly and will not be manifest during the man's lifetime, the clinical course is often unpredictable in its rate of progression. This perhaps is due to the heterogeneity of histologic grade and other factors that influence tumor growth. Despite an autopsy prevalence of up to 80% by age 80, the clinical incidence is much lower, indicating that most men die *with* prostate cancer rather than *of* prostate cancer. Definitive diagnosis of prostate cancer requires confirmative microscopy. About 95% of cancers are adenocarcinomas. Evaluation of glandular proliferations in the prostate can be a challenge, particularly when the specimen or suspected focus is small. Diagnosis relies on a combination of architectural and cytologic findings, which may be aided by ancillary studies such as prostate-specific antigen (PSA) immunohistochemistry. Architectural features include haphazard arrangement of packed glands, irregular glandular contours, and variation in gland size and shape. Comparison with adjacent uninvolved prostatic glands is helpful. Cytologic features include nuclear and nucleolar enlargement, luminal mucin, and crystalloid. The basal cell layer is absent in carcinoma, whereas it is present at the periphery of benign glands. Perineural invasion is common in cancer, but is seen only rarely with benign glands. Microvascular invasion is also an indicator of malignancy.

The combination of an automated spring-loaded 18-gauge needle core biopsy gun with transrectal ultrasound guidance has numerous advantages over the traditional wider 14-gauge needle biopsy performed under digital direction alone. In one study the rate of postbiopsy infection fell from 7.39% to 0.81%, and there was a decline in urinary clot retention from 3.2% to less than 1%. The false-negative rate declined to 11%, and the quality of the tissue sample improved, with little or no compression artifact. Compared with matched prostatectomy specimens, needle core biopsy underestimates tumor grade in 33% to 45% of patients and overestimates grade in 4% to 32%.[94] Grading errors are greatest in biopsies with small amounts of tumor and low-grade tumors and are probably due to tissue sampling error, tumor heterogeneity, and undergrading of needle biopsy samples. FNA remains popular for cytologic examination of the prostate in parts of Europe but is rarely used in the United States, in deference to the ease of the 18-gauge needle core sampling procedure. Both techniques have similar sensitivity in the diagnosis of prostate cancer, and both are limited by small sample size.

The histologic pattern of prostate cancer correlates significantly with biologic malignancy, and many useful systems of grading are available. The most popular system in the United States, the Gleason grading system, is based upon the degree of glandular differentiation,

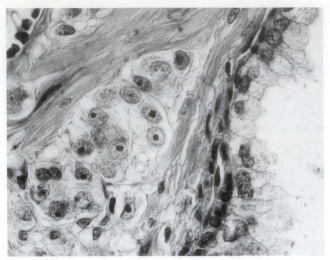

**FIGURE 4D-79.** Invasive high-grade prostatic acinar carcinoma. Tumor cells (left side of field) show large nucleoli in vesicular nuclei, in contrast to delicate features of benign glandular epithelium (right side). (*With permission, from Banks PM, Kraybill WG: Pathology for the Surgeon. Philadelphia, WB Saunders, 1996.*)

reflecting tumor heterogeneity by assigning a primary pattern for the dominant grade and a secondary pattern for the nondominant grade; the histologic score is derived by adding these two patterns together (Fig. 4D-79).[95] The success of the Gleason system is due to four factors:

1. The histologic patterns are identified by their degree of glandular differentiation without relying on morphogenetic or histogenetic models.
2. A simplified and standardized artist's representation of growth patterns in relation to grades was created.
3. The study provided invaluable prospective information that allowed objective development of this self-defining grading system.
4. Unlike any other grading system, the Gleason system provided for tumor heterogeneity by identifying primary and secondary patterns.

## RADICAL PROSTATECTOMY

The completeness of pathologic sectioning of radical prostatectomies affects the determination of pathologic stage. When the results of limited sectioning (sections of palpable tumor and two random sections of apex and base) are compared with complete sectioning (whole organ step-sectioning procedure), the latter approach results in a significant increase in positive surgical margins (12% vs. 59%, respectively) and higher pathologic stage.[96]

Both the American and TNM pathologic stage of prostate cancer is dependent on the best available pathologic data.[97] For patients undergoing radical prostatectomy, careful evaluation of the pathology specimen is required. Complete and careful submission of tissue for histologic evaluation requires the following:

1. Unequivocal orientation of specimen and tumor (left, right; transition zone, peripheral zone; anterior, midposterior; apex, base)
2. Thorough assessment and quantitation of the extent and location of capsular perforation and seminal vesicle invasion
3. Quality control data for the surgeon, particularly in regard to surgical margins in nerve-sparing prostatectomy
4. Postoperative measurement of tumor volume for correlation with imaging studies
5. Complete evaluation of tumor for grading

Several rare benign stromal tumors and tumorlike proliferations arise in the prostate. Malignant soft tissue tumors of the prostate are rare and account for less than 0.1% of primary prostatic neoplasms. One-third of these occurs in children under 10 years of age and most are rhabdomyosarcoma. Leiomyosarcoma is the most common sarcoma in adults and accounts for 26% of all prostate sarcomas. Other rare sarcomas of the prostate have been reported. Recognition of the transition of carcinoma to sarcomatous differentiation as well as immunostaining with cytokeratin may be helpful. Malignant lymphoma and leukemia are rare and usually involve the prostate gland following systemic spread.

Neoplasms arising in the seminal vesicle are rare except for contiguous or metastatic involvement by prostatic adenocarcinoma, observed in about 12% of radical prostatectomy specimens from patients with prostate cancer otherwise confined to the prostate. A variety of rare benign and malignant soft tissue tumors have been described in the seminal vesicles.

## TESTES AND PARATESTICULAR STRUCTURES

The usual presentation of cancer of the testes is a painless swelling or nodule in one gonad. The differential diagnosis should include testicular torsion, epididymitis, or epididymal orchitis. High-resolution ultrasonography will demonstrate whether a mass is intratesticular or extratesticular.[98] Removal of the testis by an inguinal approach remains the definitive procedure for pathologic diagnosis and local treatment of nonseminomatous germ cell tumors. The management of testicular cancer is dependent upon histopathologic evaluation.

## INTRATUBULAR GERM CELL NEOPLASIA AND GERM CELL TUMORS

Intratubular germ cell neoplasia (ITGCN) consists of abnormal germ cells within the seminiferous tubules and is considered the precursor of testicular germ cell tumors (Fig. 4D-80). Intratubular germ cell neoplasia has invasive potential and may occur in the absence of a testicular mass. It is frequently observed in patients with gonadal dysgenesis, in the contralateral testis of patients with invasive germ cell tumor, in patients with cryptorchidism (2% to 8%), and in patients with androgen-receptor disorders. At least 50% of untreated patients with cryptorchidism and ITGCN followed for several years develop invasive germ cell neoplasms, and bilateral testicu-

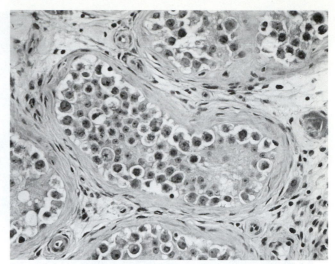

**FIGURE 4D-80.** Intratubular germ cell neoplasia (IGCN) of the testis. Immature vesicular nuclei are abundant and unaccompanied by normal maturation. (*With permission, from Banks PM, Kraybill WG:* Pathology for the Surgeon. *Philadelphia, WB Saunders, 1996.*)

lar biopsy may be of value. Screening biopsies are recommended for those with cryptorchidism between the ages of 18 and 20 years, because negative findings suggest minimal risk. The neoplastic cells of ITGCN react strongly with antibodies to placental alkaline phosphatase (PLAP), a finding that may be useful in microscopic differential diagnosis.

Testicular germ cell tumors are the most common cause (13%) of cancer death in 20- to 34-year-old American males. These tumors are rare among blacks in both the United States and Africa. Risk factors include family history (16% of cases), cryptorchidism (10%), and infection. Germ cell tumors are frequently asymptomatic. Even with enlargement, there may not be associated pain. Other types of tumors can occur in the testicular tunics, rete testis, and other adnexal structures, but these are rare. They include cysts, benign hyperplastic growths, and neoplasms. Serum concentration of germ cell tumor markers should be obtained preoperatively. These markers include β-human chorionic gonadotropin (HCG), α-fetoprotein (AFP), and PLAP. For correct diagnosis and treatment, orchiectomy with removal of the cord is usually indicated. Final treatment depends upon the histology of the primary tumor, the serum concentration of tumor markers after orchiectomy, and the presence and histologic type of metastases.

There are five main types of germ cell tumor: seminoma, embryonal carcinoma, yolk sac tumor, choriocarcinoma, and teratoma. Frequently, mixed tumors are seen, thus dictating the need for adequate histologic sampling and thorough examination. Seminoma is the most common, usually occurring in patients 30 to 50 years of age. In pure seminoma, AFP and HCG levels are negative, but tumor cells contain abundant glycogen (Fig. 4D-81). Cells are aneuploid. Embryonal carcinoma is a primitive germ cell neoplasm of adolescence and adulthood that rarely occurs in pure form, but is seen as a component in about 47% of germ cell tumors; it is not observed in infants

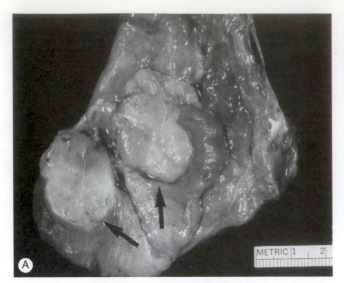

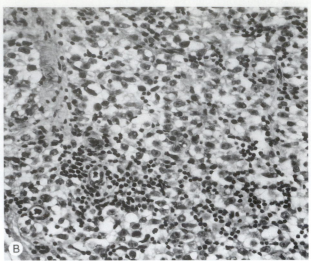

**FIGURE 4D-81.** Testicular seminoma. *A*. Grossly, a solitary uniform nodule has been bisected (arrows). *B*. Microscopically, the tumor cells are uniform and large, with clear cytoplasm. There is a conspicuous infiltration by small, reactive lymphocytes. (*With permission, from Banks PM, Kraybill WG: Pathology for the Surgeon. Philadelphia, WB Saunders, 1996.*)

or children. In pure embryonal carcinoma, there may be marginal elevation of AFP concentration, probably due to inapparent yolk sac tumor elements. HCG is not observed in these cells. Yolk sac tumor, also called endodermal sinus tumor, occurs in infants and children. In pure form, it is rare in adults, but as a component, it is present in about 41% of mixed germ cell tumors. Typical histologic patterns include anastomosing tubuloacinar structures, papillary structures, and Schiller-Duval bodies. AFP is considered a marker of yolk sac tumor. Choriocarcinoma is a rare and aggressive testicular tumor, usually detected clinically as manifestations of metastatic tumor. HCG level is markedly elevated in the serum and present within tumor cells; AFP level is usually negative. Two cell types are observed: syncytiotrophoblastic and cytotrophoblastic. Unlike other testicular germ cell tumors, choriocarcinoma metastasizes by hematogenous as well as lymphatic routes. Teratoma composed exclusively of mature tissues is clinically benign and does not require treatment other than orchiectomy. Most teratomas occurring in prepubertal children are mature and, even when immature, are clinically benign. In adults, teratomas that have areas with immature tissues are considered malignant.

The management of germ cell neoplasms of the testes is initiated with inguinal orchiectomy. The testis and attached tunics and spermatic cord should be weighed, measured, and examined in the fresh state soon after surgical removal. Immersion of the intact specimen in fixative does not allow penetration through the tunics, often resulting in autolysis of the testicular parenchyma. For this reason, rapid processing is essential. If delay in pathologic examination is anticipated, the surgeon should make a single deep incision through the testis to allow penetration of fixative. The cord should be measured and palpated for neoplasm, as should the tunica vaginalis and tunica albuginea. The testis should be bisected, preferably through

the hilum and then serially sliced with parallel cuts. The size, gross appearance, and location of any neoplasms should be recorded, and multiple blocks should be submitted to encompass the entire mass of small tumors or at least 10 blocks of larger tumors. Thorough sectioning is essential to identify heterogeneous elements in many germ cell tumors, recognizing that the presence of even a microscopic field of any other type of tumor within a seminoma alters therapy.

The predictive value for survival among patients with germ cell neoplasms is reflected in the AJCC staging system for testicular tumor, which is unique in incorporating an S component ranging from S0 to S3 according to levels of lactate dehydrogenase (LDH), HCG and AFP (Table 4D-12).

A variety of rare tumors are observed in the testis, testicular tunics, and adnexal structures. These include sex cord–stromal tumors (Leydig cell and Sertoli cell tumors, both usually benign, often presenting with hormone-induced changes such as gynecomastia); malignant lymphoma (the most common testicular tumor in men over 50 years of age); and a variety of benign and malignant soft tissue tumors.

## THE OBSTETRIC AND GYNECOLOGIC SYSTEM

Clinical manifestations of gynecologic neoplasms include such nonspecific complaints as abdominal or pelvic pain, menstrual disturbances, intestinal obstruction, fever, ascites, and pleural effusion. Gynecologic tumors should always be considered in the differential diagnosis of women presenting with pelvic or abdominal symptoms.[99]

**TABLE 4D-12.** AJCC STAGING SYSTEM FOR TESTICULAR TUMORS

Definition of TNM

Primary Tumor (pT): The extent of primary tumor is classified after radical orchiectomy.

pTX    Primary tumor cannot be assessed (if no radical orchiectomy has been performed, TX is used).
pT0    No evidence of primary tumor (e.g., histologic scar in testis).
pTis   Intratubular germ cell neoplasia (carcinoma in situ).
pT1    Tumor limited to the testis and epididymis without vascular/lymphatic invasion; tumor may invade into the tunica albuginea but not the tunica vaginalis.
pT2    Tumor limited to the testis and epididymis with vascular/lymphatic invasion, or tumor extending through the tunica albuginea with involvement of the tunica vaginalis.
pT3    Tumor invades the spermatic cord with or without vascular/lymphatic invasion.
pT4    Tumor invades the scrotum with or without vascular/lymphatic invasion.

Regional Lymph Nodes (N)

Clinical:
NX    Regional lymph nodes cannot be assessed.
N0    No regional lymph node metastasis.
N1    Metastasis with a lymph node mass 2 cm or less in greatest dimension; or multiple lymph nodes, none more than 2 cm in greatest dimension.
N2    Metastasis with a lymph node mass, more than 2 cm but not more than 5 cm in greatest dimension; or multiple lymph nodes, any one mass greater than 2 cm but not more than 5 cm in greatest dimension.
N3    Metastasis with a lymph node mass more than 5 cm in greatest dimension.

Pathologic (pN):
pNX   Regional lymph nodes cannot be assessed.
pN0   No regional lymph node metastasis.
pN1   Metastasis with a lymph node mass, 2 cm or less in greatest dimension and less than or equal to 5 nodes positive, none more than 2 cm in greatest dimension.
pN2   Metastasis with a lymph node mass, more than 2 cm but not more than 5 cm in greatest dimension; or more than 5 nodes positive, none more than 5 cm; or evidence of extranodal extension of tumor.
pN3   Metastasis with a lymph node mass more than 5 cm in greatest dimension.

Distant Metastasis (M):
MX    Distant metastasis cannot be assessed.
M0    No distant metastasis.
M1    Distant metastasis.
      M1a   Nonregional nodal or pulmonary metastasis.
      M1b   Distant metastasis other than to nonregional lymph nodes and lungs.

Serum Tumor Markers (S):
SX    Marker studies not available or not performed.
S0    Marker study levels within normal limits.
S1    LDH $< 1.5 \times$ N and
hCG   (mIu/mL) <5000 and
AFP   (ng/mL) <1000
S2    LDH $1.5$–$10 \times$ N or
hCG   (mIu/mL) 5000–50,000 or
AFP   (ng/mL) 1000-10,000
S3    LDH $>10 \times$ N or

(continued)

**TABLE 4D-12.** (*Continued*)

hCG    (mlu/mL) >**50,000** or
AFP    (ng/mL) >**10,000**
N        Indicates the upper limit of normal for the LDH assay.

Stage Grouping:

| Stage 0 | pTis | N0 | M0 | S0 |
|---|---|---|---|---|
| Stage I | pT1–4 | N0 | M0 | SX |
| Stage IA | pT1 | N0 | M0 | S0 |
| Stage IB | pT2 | N0 | M0 | S0 |
|  | pT3 | N0 | M0 | S0 |
|  | pT4 | N0 | M0 | S0 |
| Stage IS | Any pT/Tx | N0 | M0 | S1–3 |
| Stage II | Any pT/Tx | N1–3 | M0 | SX |
| Stage IIA | Any pT/Tx | N1 | M0 | S0 |
|  | Any pT/Tx | N1 | M0 | S1 |
| Stage IIB | Any pT/Tx | N2 | M0 | S0 |
|  | Any pT/Tx | N2 | M0 | S1 |
| Stage IIC | Any pT/Tx | N3 | M0 | S0 |
|  | Any pT/Tx | N3 | M0 | S1 |
| Stage III | Any pT/Tx | Any N | M1 | SX |
| Stage IIIA | Any pT/Tx | Any N | M1a | S0 |
|  | Any pT/Tx | Any N | M1a | S1 |
| Stage IIIB | Any pT/Tx | N1–3 | M0 | S2 |
|  | Any pT/Tx | Any N | M1a | S2 |
| Stage IIIC | Any pT/Tx | N1–3 | M0 | S3 |
|  | Any pT/Tx | Any N | M1a | S3 |
|  | Any pT/Tx | Any N | M1b | Any S |

Histopathologic Type:

Following the guidelines of the *World Health Organization Histological Classification of Tumors*, germ cell tumors may be either seminomatous or nonseminomatous. Seminomas may be classic type or with syncytiotrophoblasts. Nonseminomatous germ cell tumors may be pure (embryonal carcinoma, yolk sac tumor, teratoma, choriocarcinoma) or mixed. Mixtures of these types (including seminoma) should be noted, starting with the most prevalent component and ending with the least represented. Similarly, gonadal stromal tumors should be classified according to the *World Health Organization Histological Classification of Tumors*.

SOURCE: With permission from the American Joint Committee on Cancer: *AJCC Cancer Staging Manual*, 5th ed, JD Fleming et al (eds). Philadelphia, Lippincott-Raven, 1997.

## OVARY

Although malformations, premature atrophic conditions, and inflammatory diseases occasionally involve the ovary, the most common pathologic conditions are nonneoplastic cysts and benign and malignant neoplasms. A convenient classification schema divides ovarian cysts into those of epithelial inclusion origin and those of follicular origin. The former represent invaginations of the overlying surface epithelium into the ovarian cortex; they accumulate fluid and enlarge to microscopic or clinical size. The latter are derived from one or more layers of the ovarian follicle or corpus luteum. All of these benign cysts tend to be unilocular and filled with clear, colorless, or amber-colored fluid (Fig. 4D-82). An exception is corpus luteum cysts, which are often hemorrhagic and may rupture with hemoperitoneum. The corpus luteum cyst is recognized grossly by the bright yellow to orange color of its wall, analogous to that of the

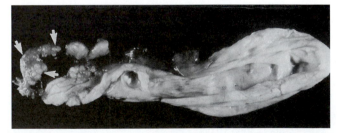

**FIGURE 4D-82.** Benign ovarian cyst. The partially opened cyst is unilocular and thin-walled, with a smooth inner lining. The attached fallopian tube on the left shows a few serosal nodules of endosalpingiosis (arrows). (*With permission, from Banks PM, Kraybill WG:* Pathology for the Surgeon. *Philadelphia, WB Saunders, 1996.*)

normal corpus luteum. Microscopically, germinal inclusion cysts are initially lined by a single layer of flattened to cuboidal epithelial cells. Follicular cysts are lined by a layer of small round granulosa cells surrounded by larger spindled or polygonal theca cells, as in a normal follicle. These cysts can have clinical associations. Multiple follicular cysts with varying degrees of thecal luteinization are a prominent feature of the polycystic ovary syndrome, also known as the Stein-Leventhal syndrome.

Other benign cysts are included in the differential diagnosis of some of the lesions discussed. A simple cyst results when the pressure of the intraluminal contents compresses the lining cells and they are no longer recognizable. Paraovarian or paratubal cysts are lined by Mullerian-type epithelium, usually displaying differentiation into epithelium resembling the normal mucosa of the fallopian tube. Any of the epithelial neoplasms of the ovary discussed subsequently may rarely develop within one of these cysts, the most common being the serous tumor of low malignant potential. The major pitfall for the surgeon is performing unnecessary surgery for a benign, nonneoplastic cyst. Most of the unilateral solitary cysts can be locally excised, sparing the uninvolved ovarian tissue.

## OVARIAN NEOPLASMS

Ovarian neoplasms are one of the most complex topics in gynecologic pathology and indeed in all of surgical pathology. In addition to the numerous tumors that metastasize to the ovaries, there are over 75 separate primary ovarian neoplasms. Most primary ovarian neoplasms are derived from coelomic surface epithelium covering the ovary (epithelial tumors), ovarian stroma (sex cord–stromal tumors) or the germ cells (germ cell tumors). Furthermore, up to 10% of malignant neoplasms of the ovary are metastatic, making this a consideration in the evaluation of any ovarian tumor.[100] Many of these, particularly those derived from the gastrointestinal tract, may clinically mimic primary ovarian neoplasms, with the actual metastatic nature becoming apparent only after microscopic examination. The surgeon encountering bilateral malignant ovarian tumors should explore the pelvis and abdomen to exclude nonovarian origins such as the gastrointestinal tract, since the majority of metastatic ovarian cancers are bilateral.

## EPITHELIAL TUMORS

As a group, epithelial tumors of the ovary are the most common primary ovarian neoplasms, particularly in adults. They represent about 60% of all primary ovarian neoplasms and over 90% of those that are malignant (Table 4D-13).[101] The single most common ovarian tumor, benign cystic teratoma ("dermoid cyst"), is not an epithelial tumor but germ cell in histogenesis. Epithelial tumors are classified by their pathway of differentiation and their degree of benignity or malignancy (Table 4D-14). Most of these tumors are derived from coelomic surface epithelium, which invaginates beneath the ovarian surface, proliferates, and then differentiates into one or more of the epithelial types, most of which are of the Mullerian origin.[102] Thus, tumors that resemble the mucosa of the fallopian

**TABLE 4D-13.** OVARIAN CANCER: COMPILED STATISTICS

| Type of Tumor Survival | Incidence, % | Bilaterality, % | 5-Year, % |
|---|---|---|---|
| Serous borderline tumor | 10–15 | 60[1] | 95[2] |
| Serous carcinoma | 25–35 | 60[1] | 20 |
| Mucinous borderline tumor | 5–10 | 20[1] | 95[2] |
| Mucinous carcinoma | 5–10 | 20[1] | 45 |
| Endometrioid carcinoma | 15–30 | 30[1] | 50 |
| Clear cell carcinoma | 4–6 | 10–30 | 40 |
| Undifferentiated carcinoma | 5–10 | 55 | 10 |
| Yolk sac tumor | <1 | <5 | >50[3] |
| Dysgerminoma | 1–2 | 10–20 | 90 |
| Immature teratoma | <1 | <5 | >50[3] |
| Secondary malignant teratoma | <1 | 0 | 15 |
| Granulosa cell tumor | <5 | 5 | 90[2] |
| Androblastoma | <1 | 5 | 90 |

[1] Approximately half in stage I.
[2] Late recurrence common.
[3] With appropriate chemotherapy.
SOURCE: From Gompel C, Silverberg SG: *Pathology in Gynecology and Obstetrics*, 4th ed. Philadelphia, JB Lippincott, 1994. With permission, from Banks PM, Kraybill WG: *Pathology for the Surgeon*. Philadelphia, WB Saunders, 1996.

tube are designated serous, whereas mucinous tumors display either endocervical or intestinal differentiation, endometrioid tumors contain elements resembling endometrial glands, and Brenner tumors and transitional cell carcinomas contain epithelium resembling urinary bladder mucosa. Many ovarian tumors demonstrate more than one pathway of differentiation, further complicating classification.

In comparison with the other major types, the epithelial neoplasms are more common, more likely to be bilateral, and more likely to be malignant. Likelihood of malignancy increases with age. Invasive carcinomas are rare before the age of 30 and are more frequent with succeeding decades. Sonographic evaluation and serum CA-125 antibody levels are useful in initially distinguishing between benign and malignant ovarian masses; nevertheless, exploration is necessary in many cases that ultimately are found to be benign or even nonneoplastic. Because these pathologic entities may present acutely with rupture, hemorrhage, or torsion, the general surgeon must be aware of the gross appearances of these neoplasms as well as their operative management (Fig. 4D-83). The diagnosis of carcinoma gains credibility if there is local extension of tumor beyond the ovary, with adhesions to or invasion of adjacent organs, or if there is metastatic spread. Even with these findings, however, pelvic inflammatory disease and endometriosis must be considered, since these conditions can be associated with extensive local adhesions or even a "frozen pelvis." Benign conditions such as endometriosis, endosalpingiosis, tuberculosis, and disseminated peritoneal leiomyomatosis can occur with nodules throughout the peritoneal cavity. A careful, directed approach with intraoperative pathology is necessary for decision making.

**TABLE 4D-14.** HISTOGENESIS AND NOMENCLATURE OF DIFFERENTIATED EPITHELIAL TUMORS OF COELOMIC ORIGIN

| PATHWAY OF DIFFERENTIATION | BENIGN TUMOR | BORDERLINE TUMOR | INVASIVE MALIGNANT TUMOR |
|---|---|---|---|
| Tubal | Serous:<br>  Cystadenoma<br>  Adenofibroma<br>  Surface papilloma | Borderline serous tumor | Serous carcinoma |
| Endocervical or intestinal | Mucinous:<br>  Cystadenoma<br>  Adenofibroma* | Borderline mucinous tumor | Mucinous carcinoma |
| Endometrial | Endometrioid<br>  Adenofibroma* | Borderline endometrioid tumor* | Endometroid carcinoma |
| Clear cell (?endometrial) | Clear cell<br>  Adenofibroma*<br>  Brenner tumor | Borderline clear cell tumor<br>Proliferating Brenner tumor* | Clear cell carcinoma<br>Malignant Brenner |

*Rare.
SOURCE: From Gompel C, Silverberg SG: *Pathology in Gynecology and Obstetrics*, 4th ed. Philadelphia, JB Lippincott, 1994. With permission, from Banks PM, Kraybill WG: *Pathology for the Surgeon*. Philadelphia, WB Saunders, 1996.

## MICROSCOPIC APPEARANCES OF EPITHELIAL NEOPLASMS

Because of the variety of ovarian epithelial neoplasms, the microscopic appearances vary considerably. Accordingly, only a few generalities are covered here. In general, benign epithelial neoplasms are either cystic or solid. The cysts are generally paucilocular and lined by a single or pseudostratified layer of cells with minimal atypia (Fig. 4D-84). In the more solid tumors, a dense nonreactive stroma is punctuated by glands and cysts lined by epithelium similar to that previously described.

Invasive carcinomas are characterized by atypical and mitotically active epithelium invading a cellular, reactive stroma. Serous

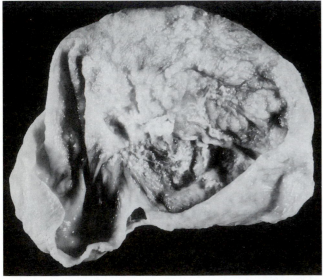

**FIGURE 4D-83.** Ovarian carcinoma. The large cyst is filled with a solid and papillary mass with foci of necrosis. (*With permission, from Banks PM, Kraybill WG:* Pathology for the Surgeon. *Philadelphia, WB Saunders, 1996.*)

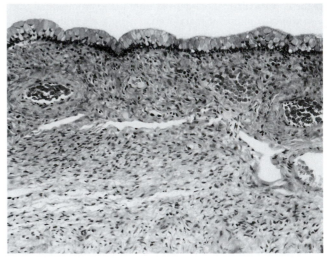

**FIGURE 4D-84.** Mucinous cystadenoma of ovary. In this benign cystic epithelial tumor, the cyst lining is composed of a single layer of mucinous cells displaying endocervical-type differentiation and no cytologic atypia. (*With permission, from Banks PM, Kraybill WG:* Pathology for the Surgeon. *Philadelphia, WB Saunders, 1996.*)

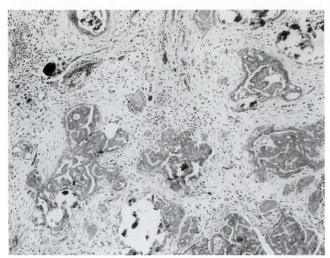

**FIGURE 4D-85.** Invasive serous carcinoma of ovary. Papillary-glandular tumor nests invade a reactive stroma. The black material in this photomicrograph represents microcalcifications known as psammoma bodies. (*With permission, from Banks PM, Kraybill WG: Pathology for the Surgeon.* Philadelphia, WB Saunders, 1996.)

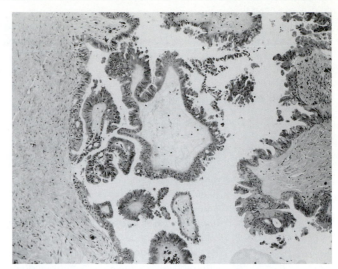

**FIGURE 4D-86.** Serous tumor of low malignant potential ("borderline tumor") of ovary. This tumor is characterized by papillarity, cellular stratification and atypia, but lacks invasion into the underlying stroma. (*With permission, from Banks PM, Kraybill WG: Pathology for the Surgeon.* Philadelphia, WB Saunders, 1996.)

carcinomas have varying amounts of papillary architecture, with papillae more prominent in well-differentiated serous carcinomas than in those that are poorly differentiated (Fig. 4D-85). In mucinous carcinomas, cells showing mucin production line small and large glands, which resemble intestinal epithelium. Endometrioid carcinomas mimic endometrial adenocarcinoma and are composed of small round glands of uniform size and shape frequently associated with sheets of squamous epithelium. Clear cell carcinomas grow in tubules, papillae, or solid sheets of cells and are characterized by an admixture of clear and hobnailed cells. Transitional cell carcinoma of the ovary resembles its more common counterpart in the urinary bladder. Many malignant epithelial tumors show mixed patterns and should be diagnosed as mixed carcinomas, with the specific types and their relative frequencies specified. Roughly 10% of ovarian carcinomas lack significant differentiation and so are called simply undifferentiated carcinoma. In most series, undifferentiated and serous carcinomas carry the worst prognosis, and mucinous and endometrioid carcinomas the best. The prognosis is more a function of extent of tumor than type of tumor—serous and undifferentiated types tend to occur with more advanced disease. The AJCC system for staging ovarian carcinomas corresponds with T system for the tumor staging to that developed by the Federation Internationale de Gynecologic et d'Obstetrique (FIGO) (Table 4D-15). The histologic grade of a malignant epithelial tumor may be more important prognostically than its epithelial type, although prognostic differences between grades diminish when patients are treated with chemotherapy. Between benign epithelial tumors and invasive malignant ones lurk the so-called borderline tumors or tumors of low malignant potential.[103] These are primarily serous and mucinous tumors and are defined by malignant cytologic features without stromal invasion (Fig. 4D-86). These diagnoses must ultimately be based upon permanent sections. Reliance on an intraoperative diagnosis of invasive carcinoma may result in unnecessary surgery, particularly in young women. Again, invasive carcinoma of the ovary is rare in women under 30 years of age, whereas borderline tumors are relatively common.

## SEX CORD–STROMAL TUMORS

Only a few of these tumors are commonly encountered. The most common stromal tumors are the benign fibroma and the thecoma, both of which are solid, firm to hard in consistency, and sharply circumscribed. Of the two, the fibroma is more common and represents from 1% to 5% of all ovarian tumors. Although large ones may cause symptoms related to their size or may even be associated with ascites, fibromas are often asymptomatic and discovered incidentally. In comparison, thecomas often display hormonal function, usually estrogenic but occasionally androgenic. Postmenopausal patients typically present with postmenopausal bleeding. The cut surface of a fibroma is usually white, whereas that of a thecoma is typically yellow, due to its steroid hormone content. Microscopically, both of these tumors are composed of whorled, anastomosing fascicles of uniform cells. Malignant varieties of these tumors are rare. Less common sex cord–stromal tumors include the granulosa cell tumor and the Sertoli-Leydig cell tumor, which are often characterized clinically by hormonal function, the former generally estrogenic and the latter androgenic. The gross appearance of both of these tumors is an admixture of solid and cystic regions. Granulosa cell tumors are composed of small, uniform cells with grooved nuclei, or gyriform patterns or a combination of these. The Sertoli-Leydig cell tumors often contain tubular elements, but when more poorly differentiated are characterized by cordlike arrangements of the Sertoli cells, among

**TABLE 4D-15. STAGING SYSTEM FOR OVARIAN TUMORS**

Definition of TNM:
The definitions of the T categories correspond to the several stages accepted by the Federation Internationale de Gynecologie et d'Obstetrique (FIGO). Both systems are included for comparison.

Primary Tumor (T)

TNM Categories FIGO Stages

| TNM | FIGO | |
|-----|------|---|
| TX | | Primary tumor cannot be assessed. |
| T0 | | No evidence of primary tumor. |
| T1 | I | Tumor limited to ovaries (one or both). |
| T1a | IA | Tumor limited to one ovary; capsule intact, no tumor on ovarian surface. No malignant cells in ascites or peritoneal washings.[1] |
| T1b | IB | Tumor limited to both ovaries; capsules intact, no tumor on ovarian surface. No malignant cells in ascites or peritoneal washings.[1] |
| T1c | IC | Tumor limited to one or both ovaries with any of the following: capsule ruptured, tumor on ovarian surface, malignant cells in ascites or peritoneal washings. |
| T2 | II | Tumor involves one or both ovaries with pelvic extension. |
| T2a | IIA | Extension and/or implants on uterus and/or tube(s). No malignant cells in ascites or peritoneal washings. |
| T2b | IIB | Extension to other pelvic tissues. No malignant cells in ascites or peritoneal washings. |
| T2c | IIC | Pelvic extension (2a or 2b) with malignant cells in ascites or peritoneal washings. |
| T3 and/or N1 | III | Tumor involves one or both ovaries with microscopically confirmed peritoneal metastasis outside the pelvis and/or regional lymph node metastasis. |
| T3a | IIIA | Microscopic peritoneal metastasis beyond pelvis. |
| T3b | IIIB | Macroscopic peritoneal metastasis beyond pelvis 2 cm or less in greatest dimension. |
| T3c and/or N1 | IIIC | Peritoneal metastasis beyond pelvis more than 2 cm in greatest dimension and/or regional lymph node metastasis. |
| M1 | IV | Distant metastasis (excludes peritoneal metastasis). |

Regional Lymph Nodes (N):
NX    Regional lymph nodes cannot be assessed
N0    No regional lymph node metastasis
N1    Regional lymph node metastasis

Distant Metastasis (M):
MX    Distant metastasis cannot be assessed
M0    No distant metastasis
M1    Distant metastasis (excludes peritoneal metastasis)

pTNM Pathologic Classification:
The pT, pN, and pM categories correspond to the T, N, and M categories.

Stage Grouping:

| Stage | T | N | M |
|-------|-----|-----|-----|
| Stage IA | T1a | N0 | M0 |
| Stage IB | T1b | N0 | M0 |
| Stage IC | T1c | N0 | M0 |
| Stage IIA | T2a | N0 | M0 |
| Stage IIB | T2b | N0 | M0 |
| Stage IIC | T2c | N0 | M0 |
| Stage IIIA | T3a | N0 | M0 |
| Stage IIIB | T3b | N0 | M0 |
| Stage IIIC | T3c | N0 | M0 |
| | Any T | N1 | M0 |
| Stage IV | Any T | Any N | M1 |

[1] *Note:* The presence of nonmalignant ascites is not classified. The presence of ascites does not affect staging unless malignant cells are present.
[2] *Note:* Liver capsule metastases are T3/Stage III; liver parenchymal metastasis, M1/Stage IV. Pleural effusion must have positive cytology for M1/Stage IV.
SOURCE: With permission from the American Joint Committee on Cancer: *AJCC Cancer Staging Manual*, 5th ed. JD Fleming et al (eds). Philadelphia, Lippincott-Raven, 1997.

which may be dispersed the large, polygonal, eosinophilic Leydig cells. Both of these should be considered tumors of low malignant potential with 5-year survival rates in the range of 90%.

## GERM CELL TUMORS

Although malignant germ cell tumors of the ovary are uncommon, they are particularly important in the second and third decades of life. The most common is the dysgerminoma, which is analogous to testicular seminoma. This is a fleshy, gray-tan or white tumor that is composed of nests of large, primitive cells separated by a prominent lymphocytic infiltrate within fibrous septa. Like testicular seminoma, dysgerminoma carries a favorable prognosis, with 5-year survival rates well over 90%. The other malignant germ cell tumors—yolk sac tumor (endodermal sinus tumor), embryonal carcinoma, immature teratoma, and choriocarcinoma—are rare. They occur predominantly in young women and are associated with a poorer prognosis than that of dysgerminoma. Most of these tumors will be lethal when treated by surgery alone. Although dysgerminoma is bilateral in 10% of patients, these other tumors are virtually never bilateral. This may allow preservation of the contralateral adnexa in many patients. Benign cystic teratomas (so-called dermoid cysts) are the most common single primary ovarian neoplasm, accounting for 25% of all ovarian tumors. They are most common between 20 and 50 years of age. They are grossly recognizable by their cystic contents of grumous material, oily or clear liquid, tufts of hair, teeth, bone, or cartilage and foci of glial (brain or thyroid) tissue (Fig. 4D-87). Accordingly, the microscopic appearance may include a mixture of almost any tissues of the human body, most commonly cutaneous.

Only rarely is malignancy found in ovarian teratomas; it is of two types. First, immature teratoma is seen in children and young adults; it represents a malignant germ cell tumor with immature malignant tissues, usually of neuroepithelial type, superimposed on an otherwise benign teratoma. Second, older women with benign teratomas may secondarily develop malignant tumors of adult type arising in one of the component tissues. These are usually squamous cell carcinomas, but other carcinomas, sarcomas, melanomas, and other rarer tumor types are occasionally encountered.

## FALLOPIAN TUBES

Pathologic problems associated with the fallopian tubes are most frequently benign. Torsion of the fallopian tube is fairly common in young to middle-aged women as a painful surgical emergency. Salpingitis secondary to bacterial infection is common and must be differentiated from appendicitis and other causes of acute abdominal emergencies. Ruptured ectopic pregnancy is associated with a positive pregnancy test, acute abdomen, and hemodynamic shock.

The fallopian tube gives rise to the smallest number of primary malignant tumors of the female genital tract. To be considered a primary fallopian carcinoma, the tumor must be located in the fallopian tube and not involve either the ovary or the uterus. The most common malignant tumors of the fallopian tubes are adenocarcinomas. Areas of degeneration with hemorrhage and necrosis are commonly seen. Of primary fallopian tube carcinomas, 90% are papillary serous carcinomas. Metastatic disease to pelvic and paraaortic nodes is common.

## UTERINE CORPUS AND CERVIX

Leiomyomas of the uterus occur in approximately 40% of women after the age of 35 years.[104] The tumor is rarely seen before menarche and generally stabilizes or regresses after menopause. It may increase in size during pregnancy or with oral contraception and often shrinks when treated with a gonadotropin-releasing hormone agonist such as leuprolide acetate (Lupron). Leiomyomas may be submucous (immediately beneath the endometrium), intramural, or subserous. Regardless of location the leiomyoma is spherical or ovoid, sharply circumscribed, and firm in consistency (Fig. 4D-88). Microscopically, the typical leiomyoma consists of interlacing fascicles of uniform spindled cells with bland nuclei, separated by variable amounts of fibrous connective tissue and small blood vessels (Fig. 4D-89). There are a number of histologic variants. The presence of hypercellularity, atypia, high levels of mitotic activity, and tumor necrosis distinguish leiomyosarcoma from leiomyoma.

## CARCINOMAS OF THE ENDOMETRIUM AND CERVIX

About 95% of malignant tumors of the uterine corpus are adenocarcinomas, whereas a slightly less dominant majority of cervical cancers are squamous cell carcinomas. The prototype adenocarcinoma of the endometrium is the endometrioid type and is composed of small, round, relatively uniform glands lined by columnar cells with their nuclei oriented perpendicular to the basement membrane.

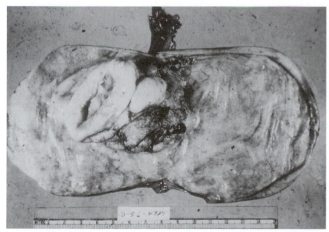

**FIGURE 4D-87.** Benign cystic teratoma ("dermoid cyst") of ovary. This cystic lesion contains sebaceous debris and hair. (*With permission, from Banks PM, Kraybill WG: Pathology for the Surgeon. Philadelphia, WB Saunders, 1996.*)

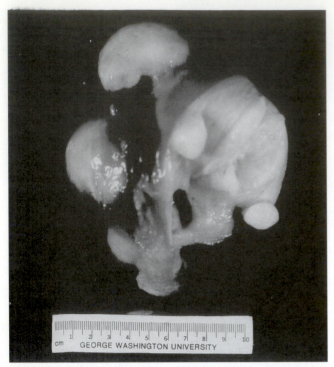

**FIGURE 4D-88.** Uterine leiomyomas. Multiple, well-circumscribed, firm white tumors are present within the myometrium and fungate out from the serosal surface. (*With permission, from Banks PM, Kraybill WG:* Pathology for the Surgeon. *Philadelphia, WB Saunders, 1996.*)

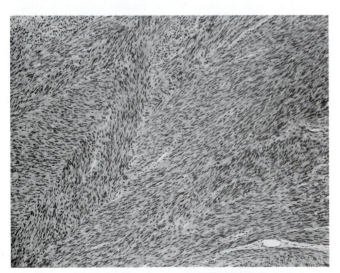

**FIGURE 4D-89.** Leiomyoma of uterus. Typical microscopic appearance with interlacing fascicles of uniform spindled smooth muscle cells. (*With permission, from Banks PM, Kraybill WG:* Pathology for the Surgeon. *Philadelphia, WB Saunders, 1996.*)

They are often accompanied by a minor or major squamous component. The glandular component may also grow in solid sheets of more anaplastic cells. The histologic grade of the tumor is higher with increasing proportions of this solid growth pattern. Although the majority of endometrial carcinomas are well differentiated, the poorly differentiated forms are more likely to metastasize.[105] Other less common types of endometrial adenocarcinoma are the serous and clear cell types that carry a poorer prognosis and a greater likelihood of distant metastases than the usual type of endometroid adenocarcinoma. Endometroid carcinomas can also originate in the ovary and, less frequently, in the endocervix, fallopian tube, and foci of endometriosis anywhere in the pelvis or abdomen.

Of invasive cervical cancers, 85% are of the squamous cell type. Most of the remainder are adenocarcinomas. In contrast to endometrial carcinoma, which is a disease of postmenopausal women, many invasive cervical cancers occur in younger women. Unlike ovarian cancer, which may occur with widespread disease and ascites, the majority of endometrial and cervical cancers occur with localized gynecologic symptoms. Moreover, cervical cancer may be detected while still occult or while in a preinvasive state by routine screening with Pap smears. Minor abnormalities, such as repetitively atypical smears or interpretations as low-grade squamous intraepithelial lesion (LGSIL), require further evaluation. Often condylomas are detected by Pap smear, and certain subtypes of human papillomavirus have been associated more often with both cervical dysplasia and carcinoma. Colposcopy with small directed biopsies can determine whether occult abnormalities are dysplasia or invasive cancer. Occasionally, excisional biopsies such as conization or loop electrosurgical excision are necessary to exclude the presence of invasive cancer. Evaluation of the extent of disease by imaging and biopsy or by careful pathologic evaluation of node dissections from radical hysterectomy specimens are important in defining the prognosis of cervical cancer patients. Tumor grade and depth of myometrial invasion in patients treated for endometrial cancer provide important information with regard to tumor stage and prognosis.

## VAGINA AND VULVA

The vagina and vulva are both lined by squamous epithelium and are therefore susceptible to the same condylomatous, dysplastic, and carcinomatous squamous lesions as is the cervix. A variety of benign tumors may arise in the vagina. Although most are asymptomatic, occasionally dyspareunia may result. These include epidermal inclusion cysts, Mullerian (paramesonephric) cysts, and Gartner's duct (mesonephric) cysts. These cysts should be removed only if they are symptomatic. Rarer tumors are fibroepithelial polyps and leiomyomas.

Primary malignant tumors of the vagina are rare; metastatic or locally extensive lesions from the cervix, vulva, uterine corpus, and rectum are more common. Squamous carcinoma of the vagina arises from the mucosal surface and spreads by local invasion through the lymphatics to the pelvic and inguinal-femoral nodes. Endodermal sinus tumor and embryonal rhabdomyosarcoma are rare primary vaginal tumors of childhood. Vaginal adenocarcinomas of clear cell or endometrioid type are occasionally encountered in women whose mothers received diethylstilbestrol (DES) while pregnant. Far more common are benign microscopic glandular abnormalities (adenosis) and gross anatomic deformities.

Common benign vulvar tumors are condylomas and fibroepithelial polyps. Some 90% of malignant vulvar tumors are squamous cell carcinomas; 5% are melanomas. Grossly these tumors may assume an exophytic, ulcerative, or flat configuration. These cancers generally spread either by direct extension or by embolic metastases to the regional lymph nodes in the groin. Paget's and Bowen's disease are in situ forms of adenocarcinoma and squamous cell carcinoma, respectively. Such lesions are frequently multifocal and may involve the perineum and perianal region as well as the vulva.

## FEMALE PERITONEUM

Many of the same tumors that affect the female genital tract can involve the peritoneum, giving rise to a spectrum of lesions different from those in the male peritoneum. For example, malignant mesothelioma, a diffuse, highly malignant, and invariably lethal tumor of the peritoneum that is frequently associated with asbestos exposure, is seen 10 times more frequently in men than women, whereas primary peritoneal adenocarcinoma is a disease almost exclusively of women. Benign conditions such as endometriosis and endosalpingiosis are also limited to women.

### ENDOMETRIOSIS AND ENDOSALPINGIOSIS. Endometriosis is a common and clinically important benign condition defined as the presence of benign endometrial epithelium and stroma in an ectopic site. It is found throughout the peritoneal cavity, but it is most frequently seen involving the peritoneal surfaces of pelvic structures. The gross appearances are protean and vary with the menstrual cycle. The lesions may be small white or yellow nodules, red-brown or blue cysts or huge hemorrhagic densely adherent masses. The diagnostic features may be obscured by old and recent hemorrhage. Multiple sections may be necessary to demonstrate the diagnostic endometrial epithelium and/or stroma. Marked epithelial atypia may occasionally be observed and probably represents a precarcinomatous change. Endometrioid or clear cell adenocarcinoma or, rarely, endometrioid sarcoma or carcinosarcoma may be a complication of endometriosis. These malignant changes must be sought when firm, focally necrotic tissue is encountered within an otherwise typical focus of endometriosis.

Endosalpingiosis has only lately been recognized as a common female peritoneal lesion. It is defined as any proliferation of Mullerian-type epithelium on a peritoneal surface. Unlike endometriosis, these lesions are rarely symptomatic and are almost always incidental findings. Their significance lies in their distinction from metastatic adenocarcinoma. Lesions occur as small, gray or white, firm, and frequently calcified nodules measuring 1 to 2 mm in diameter. Microscopically, they consist of glands, papillae, or cysts lined by a single layer of cuboidal cells, with transitions to various types of Mullerian epithelium, most commonly resembling tubal mucosa with prominent ciliated cells. Histologically, similar benign glandular inclusions may also be encountered in pelvic and periaortic lymph nodes, again almost exclusively in women.

### ADENOCARCINOMA. Carcinomas in the female peritoneum may be primary or metastatic. Although primary peritoneal adenocarcinoma is the subject of much interest to gynecologic oncologists and pathologists, in most patients carcinoma of the peritoneum is metastatic in nature. Although any malignant tumor can metastasize to the peritoneum, the most common origins are the ovary, endometrium, and large intestine. Peritoneal fluid washings should always be obtained and sent for cytologic examination in any patient being explored for a primary cancer of any abdominal or pelvic organ.

Two types of cancer metastatic to the female peritoneum that are of particular interest are pseudomyxoma peritonei and gliomatosis peritonei. The former term refers to mucinous ascites associated with mucinous tumor of the ovary, appendix, or both. It presents grossly as loculated, yellow-brown, adhesive mucus on peritoneal surfaces, eventuating in dense mucinous adhesions. Microscopically, relatively small numbers of low-grade mucinous tumor cells are found floating in voluminous pools of extracellular mucin. It is currently controversial whether the ovary, the appendix, or the peritoneum is the source of this lesion. In peritoneal gliomatosis, the source of the mature glial implants studding the peritoneum is an immature teratoma of the ovary. The implants generally show a higher degree of maturation into benign-appearing tissues than do the primary ovarian tumors and their behavior is accordingly benign.

The main consideration in the differential diagnosis of metastatic adenocarcinoma, particularly of serous type, in the female peritoneum is primary serous carcinoma of the peritoneum.[106] About 10% of disseminated serous carcinomas are peritoneal rather than ovarian in origin, although the distinction between primary peritoneal serous carcinoma and ovarian serous carcinoma with peritoneal implants is often subjective. The clinical presentation and gross appearance of these lesions are identical to those of metastatic ovarian serous carcinoma, with the exception that the ovaries are absent (having been removed previously for unrelated disease), present but uninvolved with tumor, or present but minimally involved, with their neoplastic burden limited to a coating of their peritoneal surfaces. Although the microscopic appearances of peritoneal serous carcinoma are usually characteristic, various histochemical and immunohistochemical stains may be used to distinguish this lesion from either malignant mesothelioma or reactive proliferations of mesothelium. Among the most useful antigens are carcinoembryonic antigen (CEA), Leu-M1 (CD15), TAG-72 recognized by monoclonal antibody B72.3, and the antigen recognized by monoclonal antibody BER-EP4. All of these are present in most adenocarcinomas (including metastases to the peritoneum) and absent in almost all mesotheliomas.

## THE HEMATOLYMPHOID SYSTEM

Understanding the hematolymphoid system is important to the surgical oncologist for two reasons. First, the oncology patient's

# IN THE SURGICAL PATIENT

## HEMIC
### (Blood, bone marrow)

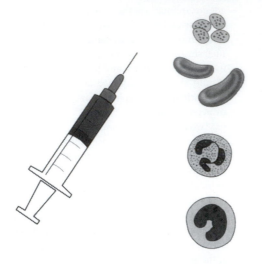

**PLATELETS**
hemostasis, wound healing

**RED BLOOD CELLS**
oxygen transport (tissue
viability, wound healing)

**WHITE BLOOD CELLS**
neutrophils—first line of defense
against bacterial infection (abscess
formation)

monocytes/histocytes—defense
against persistent agents (fungi,
mycobacteria, foreign materials)
with granuloma formation

## LYMPHOID
### (Lymph nodes, spleen, thymus, mucosal lymphoid tissues)

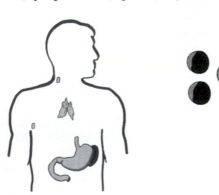

lymphocytes, T-cell—cell mediated
immunity against viruses; transplant
rejection

lymphocytes, B-cell—humoral immunity (antibodies), effective as immune
barrier against some bacterial infections, e.g. Pneumovax® for pneumococcal infections in post-splenectomy
patients

**FIGURE 4D-90.** The functions of hemic and lymphoid cells in surgical patients are represented
in this diagram. Not represented are the nutritional and hydrodynamic functions served by
the blood and lymphatic vascular systems. (*With permission, from Banks PM, Kraybill WG:
Pathology for the Surgeon. Philadelphia, WB Saunders, 1996.*)

management often involves this system. Second, contrary to the
common impression that disorders of this system are "medical" and
not "surgical" in nature, the surgeon typically plays a critical role in
diagnosis and therapeutic management of these patients.[107]

Elements of the blood, formed in the marrow, are critical to
every surgical patient (Fig. 4D-90). Circulating platelets, deriving
from megakaryocytes of the marrow, form the initiating stage in
hemostasis and are necessary for the normal integrity of blood vessels and for wound healing. Red blood cells deliver oxygen to and
remove carbon dioxide from the tissues. White blood cells are me-

diators of the immune defenses. Neutrophils carry out rapid, nonspecific reactions to bacteria with the suppurative tissue response.
Monocytes and their specialized derivatives histiocytes are effective against persistent intracellular agents such as fungi and mycobacteria, with granuloma formation physically isolating such infections. Lymphocytes and plasma cells belong to the highly specific
elements of the immune system, generating cell-mediated and humoral immunity with anamnestic (memory) capacity, preventing
reinfection by previously encountered microbes. Lymphoid cells
are particularly effective against certain infectious agents such as

viruses and derive not only from bone marrow but also from sites strategically localized in relation to pathways of infection. Mucosal surfaces of the gut and upper airway are normally endowed with concentrations of lymphoid apparatus, such as Peyer's patches of terminal ileum and the Waldeyer's ring region of the upper aerodigestive tract. The spleen, acting as the blood's filtering mechanism, is richly laden with lymphoid tissue, and lymph nodes, functioning as sentinels of the lymphatics draining interstitial fluid from peripheral tissues, represent the body's purest concentration of active immune cellularity. Of course, surgical oncologists are familiar with lymph node anatomy because of their function as first barriers to the metastatic spread of neoplasms through the regional lymphatic channels.[108]

## CLINICAL MANIFESTATIONS OF PRIMARY HEMATOLYMPHOID DISORDERS

Because of the importance of normal functions of this system to the oncology patient who is an operative candidate, history and physical examination should include observations that assure its continued supportive roles. For example, is there any history of prolonged bleeding from previous procedures or menstruation, any problem with recurring or persistent infections? On physical examination are there cutaneous or mucosal ecchymoses or petechiae, ulcers, cellulitis, or abscess? Before any major surgery every patient should have blood studied with an automated complete blood count (CBC) to assure normal concentrations of red blood cells, white blood cells, and platelets.[109] Plasma coagulation activity is screened with both prothrombin time (PT) and partial thromboplastin time (PTT).[110] Since neither of these laboratory screens is completely sensitive, specialist consultation from a hematologist is indicated when either history or examination raises unexplained questions.

Leukemias are usually first manifest by signs and symptoms of cytopenias due to bone marrow involvement. Chronic leukemias are indolent, can be of myeloid or lymphoid origin, and microscopically are composed of mature cells. Acute leukemias are immediately life threatening, are often highly responsive to chemotherapy, and microscopically consist of rapidly proliferating blast cells. Acute lymphoblastic leukemia is more common in children and young adults and, generally, is more successfully treated than acute myeloid leukemia, which predominates in older individuals.

Hematolymphoid disorders can effectively mimic tumors of other organ systems. Therefore the surgical oncologist may be the first to suspect or diagnose lymphoma, leukemia, or other lymphoproliferative or myeloproliferative disease. Table 4D-16 lists some of the manifestations of primary hematolymphoid disorders that may result in patient referral to the surgical oncologist.

## DISORDERS REQUIRING SURGICAL INTERVENTION

The most common surgical intervention for hematolymphoid disease is for installation of an intravenous portal. This affords constant access both for evaluation of the blood and for intravenous therapy. Because of difficulty in long-term intravenous access for patients with chronic disease, surgeons are often asked to place central

**TABLE 4D-16.** SIGNS AND SYMPTOMS POSSIBLY RELATED TO HEMATOLYMPHOID DISEASE THAT MAY PROMPT SURGICAL REFERRAL

| GENERAL CATEGORY | SPECIFIC OBSERVATION |
|---|---|
| Lumps and bumps | Σ Lymphadenopathy (peripheral or Waldeyer's ring) |
| | Σ Dermal mass or rash |
| | Σ Subcutaneous mass |
| | Σ Breast mass |
| | Σ Thyroid mass |
| | Σ Salivary gland mass |
| Abdominal mass | Σ Splenomegaly |
| | Σ Hepatomegaly |
| | Σ Retroperitoneal mass |
| | Σ Intraabdominal mass |
| Thoracic mass | Σ Mediastinum (thymus, lymph nodes) |
| | Σ Hilar adenopathy |

SOURCE: With permission, from Banks PM, Kraybill WG: *Pathology for the Surgeon*. Philadelphia, WB Saunders, 1996.

catheters. Such patients often face crises in hemostasis and immunity, so that successful establishment of such a device truly represents a lifeline.[111]

Splenectomy may be indicated for both diagnostic and therapeutic reasons. The spleen's complex anastomosing microstructure functions as a blood filter, normally removing any foreign particulate material, including microbes, and selecting older, less elastic circulating cells out of circulation for biochemical recycling. Any process that clogs the sinuses of the spleen produces excess function, i.e., hypersplenism. If the spleen enlarges beyond a point, its excessive filtering activity becomes irreversible. Although increased bone marrow cellular production can compensate to some extent, in patients with underlying hematolymphoid disease, the marrow reserve may be inadequate. Splenectomy may be necessary to alleviate cytopenias (diminished platelets, white or red cells) or simply to alleviate symptoms of massive splenomegaly. Figure 4D-91 shows a fresh-cut section of massive splenic enlargement due to a chronic myeloproliferative disorder. In such disorders, bone marrow progenitor cells proliferate in the spleen; however, because of their effect in increasing splenic filtering, they actually worsen rather than improve the patient's circulating cell counts. Malignant lymphomas may also show predilection for the spleen (Figs. 4D-92 and 4D-93), but only uncommonly do neoplasms of other systems spread to this organ.

For the pathologist, interpretation of splenic tissue is notoriously difficult. Ancillary methods such as flow cytometry and immunostains are often needed for a definitive diagnosis. When the surgeon is unable to deliver the spleen as a fresh specimen to the laboratory, as for example with splenectomy for traumatic rupture, a small portion

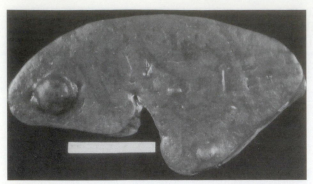

**FIGURE 4D-91.** Massive splenomegaly in a patient with chronic myeloproliferative disorder (agnogenic myeloid metaplasia or so-called myelofibrosis). This spleen weighed nearly 3000 g and was removed for worsening pancytopenia caused by a combination of fibrotic replacement of normal marrow elements and secondary (inappropriate) hypersplenism due to enlargement and congestion from extramedullary hematopoiesis. The nodules at extreme left and bottom right represent concentrations of platelet-producing cell clusters, so-called megakaryocytic plums. (*With permission, from Banks PM, Kraybill WG:* Pathology for the Surgeon. *Philadelphia, WB Saunders, 1996.*)

should be set aside and refrigerated at 4°C (for potential special studies) and the remainder preserved in formalin, after a few slices have been made to assure capsular disruption for penetration of the fixative.

Lymph node biopsy is frequently requested to confirm suspected metastasis or relapse of established malignancies (melanoma, gastrointestinal or pulmonary carcinoma, etc.) or to determine the pathogenesis of lymphadenopathy as a primary clinical manifestation. It is a common fallacy that intraoperative pathology is contraindicated in lymph node biopsy. Assessment by gross examination, cytology preparations, and even frozen sections is an effective means to assure adequacy of sampling for diagnosis and to effectively prioritize allocation of tissue for special study requirements. Although the distinction of lymphoma from reactive hyperplasia is often difficult or impossible intraoperatively, the recognition of major differential diagnostic groupings can be confidently rendered. Therefore, the surgeon should not hesitate to request intraprocedural pathology, and, in fact, may choose to use this strategy to assure that the specimen is examined in a fresh state.

Because lymph nodes and other concentrations of immune tissues must be capable of rapid cellular response to antigenic challenges, benign hyperplasia is capable of achieving alarming size and mimicry of malignancy (Fig. 4D-94). Smaller, more superficial nodes should not be biopsied in preference to larger, deeper ones, since many types of malignancy, most notably Hodgkin's lymphoma, can be limited to only the largest nodes in a group, sparing nearby smaller ones. The pathologist relies on recognizing the microanatomy of a functional immune reaction to diagnose lymph nodes and other lymphoid tissues as benign in nature (Fig. 4D-95).

Malignant lymphomas range greatly in their aggressiveness and potential curability. Low-grade lymphomas are often clinically inapparent but usually at an advanced stage and effectively incurable at diagnosis (see Fig. 4D-92). By contrast, high-grade lymphomas are

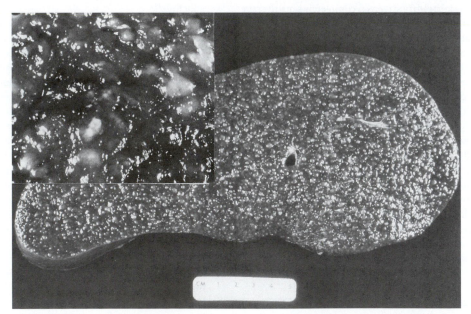

**FIGURE 4D-92.** Spleen showing gross pathologic features typical of a low-grade lymphoma. Massive enlargement is due to universal expansion of lymphoid pulp component (inset at small distance). This appearance reflects homing of well-differentiated lymphomas to normal areas of lymphoid tissues and early systemic spread. (*With permission, from Banks PM, Kraybill WG:* Pathology for the Surgeon. *Philadelphia, WB Saunders, 1996.*)

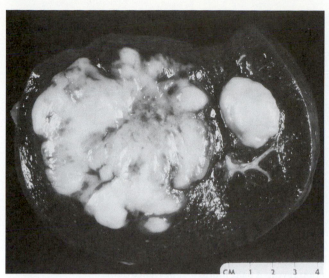

**FIGURE 4D-93.** Gross appearance characteristic of a high-grade lymphoma. In this spleen the rapidly growing tumors have displaced normal tissues rather than selectively involving lymphoid pulp (compare to Fig. 4D-92). High-grade lymphomas are more often localized (early stage) than low-grade lymphomas. (*With permission, from Banks PM, Kraybill WG: Pathology for the Surgeon. Philadelphia, WB Saunders, 1996.*)

aggressive and often difficult to distinguish both clinically and microscopically from other "cancers" (see Fig. 4D-93). Paradoxically, because of their greater proliferative activity, these high-grade neoplasms are often curable. Classification of lymphomas can be based on conventional microscopic findings alone, with discernment of major predictive groupings (Table 4D-17)[112] or more detailed characterization employing immunologic criteria can be used for more precise prognostic assignment.[113] Hodgkin's lymphoma (Hodgkin's

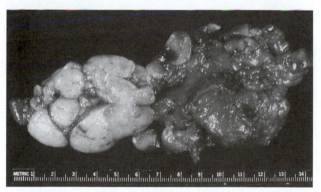

**FIGURE 4D-94.** Massive enlargement of periparotid lymph node due to benign hyperplasia. Pain and tenderness were reported, which are clinical features favoring benign rather than malignant adenopathy. (*With permission, from Banks PM, Kraybill WG: Pathology for the Surgeon. Philadelphia, WB Saunders, 1996.*)

**TABLE 4D-17. CATEGORIZATION OF MALIGNANT LYMPHOMAS (OTHER THAN HODGKIN'S DISEASE) INTO LOW-, INTERMEDIATE-, AND HIGH-GRADE, ACCORDING TO THE WORKING FORMULATION FOR CLINICAL USAGE OF 1982**

Low Grade:
A.  Small lymphocytic (may correspond to chronic lymphocytic leukemia)
B.  Follicular, small cleaved cell
C.  Follicular, mixed (small cleaved cell and large cell)

Intermediate Grade:
D.  Follicular, large cell
E.  Diffuse, small cleaved cell
F.  Diffuse, large cell
G.  Diffuse, large cell*

High Grade:
H.  Diffuse, immunoblastic
I.  Lymphoblastic (may correspond to acute lymphoblastic leukemia)
J.  Small noncleaved cell (Burkitt and Burkitt-like variants)

*Although originally included within the intermediate grade grouping, the diffuse, large cell type has been shown to be difficult to distinguish consistently from diffuse, immunoblastic type, and the survival difference between these two types is not significant.
SOURCE: With permission, from Banks PM, Kraybill WG: *Pathology for the Surgeon*. Philadelphia, WB Saunders, 1996.

disease) is a distinct clinicopathologic grouping of lymphomas characterized microscopically by a hiatus between scattered tumor giant cells (Reed-Sternberg cells) and benign background cellularity. The process progresses predictably along contiguous lymph-node-bearing regions, with predilection for young adults with mediastinal presentation. Prognosis is highly stage dependent.

Staging of lymphomas differs from that of most organ systems in deemphasizing size of the primary tumor, so that in the AJCC system there is no T category (Table 4D-18).

In recent years, considerable insights have been gained regarding distinct clinicopathologic groupings of lymphomas that present in extranodal sites. One of these types, mantle cell type, is particularly resistant to therapy and sometimes presents as widespread mucosal polyps of the gastrointestinal system, so-called lymphomatous polyposis (Fig. 4D-96). By contrast, so-called MALT lymphomas (lymphomas of mucosa-associated lymphoid tissue) remain long localized to their extranodal site of presentation, such as lung, salivary gland, or stomach, and are potentially curable with surgical resection or radiation therapy (see Figs. 4D-64 and 4D-97).[114]

## IMMUNODEFICIENCY STATES

Patients who are therapeutically immunosuppressed or intrinsically immunodeficient represent a challenge to both the surgeon and

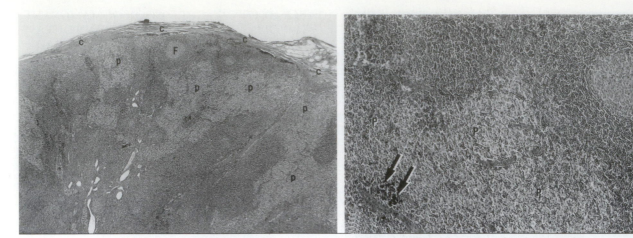

**FIGURE 4D-95.** Low-magnification microscopic appearance of a hyperplastic inguinal lymph node. There are recognizable functional compartments of the immune system: follicles (F), paracortex (p), and a retained, intact capsule. Intermediate magnification reveals a pale, mottled appearance of the paracortex (p) due to interspersed histiocytes, some of which contain dark pigment (arrows). These features are specific for "dermatopathic lymphadenitis," secondary to inflammatory skin conditions, in this case involving the lower extremities. (*With permission, from Banks PM, Kraybill WG:* Pathology for the Surgeon. *Philadelphia, WB Saunders, 1996.*)

## TABLE 4D-18. AJCC STAGING SYSTEM FOR LYMPHOMAS

Stage Grouping:

Stage I     Involvement of a single lymph node region (I) or localized involvement of a single extralymphatic organ or site ($I_E$).

Stage II     Involvement of two or more lymph node regions on the same side of the diaphragm (II), or localized involvement of a single associated extralymphatic organ or site and its regional nodes with or without other lymph node regions on the same side of the diaphragm ($II_E$).*

Stage III     Involvement of lymph node regions on both sides of the diaphragm (III) that may also be accompanied by localized involvement of an extralymphatic organ or site ($III_E$), by involvement of the spleen ($III_S$), or both ($III_{E+S}$).

Stage IV     Disseminated (multifocal) involvement of one or more extralymphatic organs with or without associated lymph node involvement, or isolated extralymphatic organ involvement with distant (nonregional) nodal involvement.

*Note: The number of lymph node regions involved may be indicated by a subscript (e.g., $II_3$).
Source: With permission from the American Joint Committee on Cancer: *AJCC Cancer Staging Manual,* 5th ed. JD Fleming et al (eds). Philadelphia, Lippincott-Raven, 1997.

the pathologist. Opportunistic infections must be suspected and searched for in all samples. Explosive lymphoproliferative disorders driven by the Epstein-Barr virus can mimic and sometimes progress to high-grade lymphomas, both clinically and microscopically.

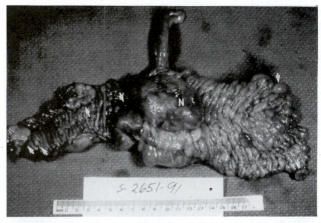

**FIGURE 4D-96.** Mantle cell lymphoma has involved the ileocecal region of this middle-aged male patient as lymphomatous polyposis. A large lymphomatous nodule (N) has necessitated surgery for obstruction of the valve; however, innumerable smaller "polyps" represent expansion of the normal mucosal lymphoid tissue by lymphoma (arrows). (*With permission, from Banks PM, Kraybill WG:* Pathology for the Surgeon. *Philadelphia, WB Saunders, 1996.*)

# COLOR PLATES*

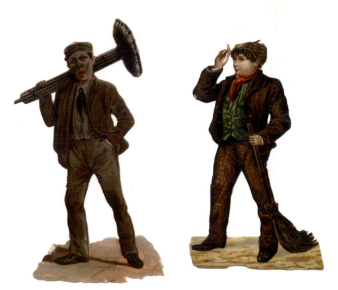

**PLATE 1** (Fig. 1B-1). Nineteenth-century English die-cuts depicting chimney sweeps.

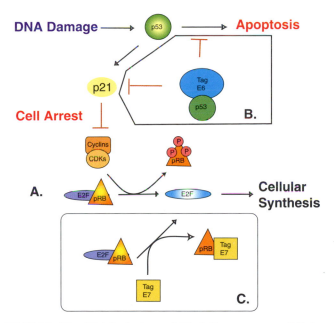

**PLATE 3** (Fig. 1B-14). Actions of Viral Oncogenes on Cellular Tumor Suppressor Proteins. *A.* Phosphorylation of pRB by cellular cyclins and CDKs results in the release of the cellular transcriptional factor E2F, resulting in cellular synthesis. *B.* DNA damage results in the induction of the p53 protein, which can push the cell into apoptosis or can induce p21, which causes the cell to arrest at the $G_1/S$ boundary. The SV40 T antigen (Tag) and papillomavirus E6 protein bind p53, preventing the induction of apoptosis or the p21 protein. *C.* The SV40 Tag or papillomavirus E7 protein bind to hypophosphorylated pRB, resulting in premature release of E2F and the onset of cellular synthesis.

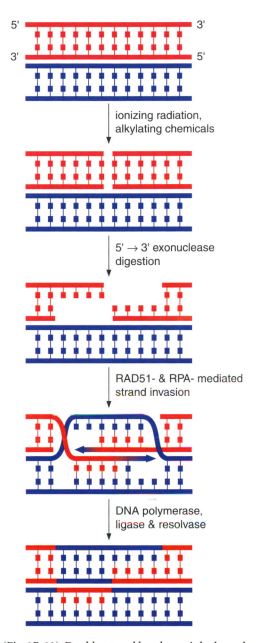

**PLATE 2** (Fig. 1B-11). Double-strand break repair by homologous recombination.

*The figures in parentheses following the Plate numbers have been included in order to indicate the chapter in which they are discussed and the order of their citation therein.

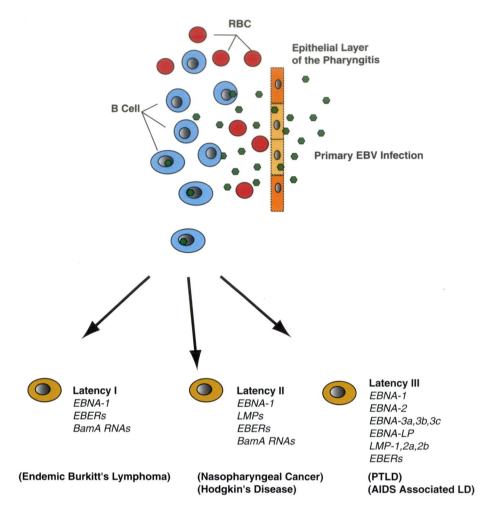

**PLATE 4** (Fig. 1B-15). EBV Replication and Latency. A primary EBV infection of the epithelial layer of the pharynx results in lytic viral replication that spreads to infiltrating B cells. Infected B cells serve as sites of viral latency, which is divided into three types based on viral gene expression.

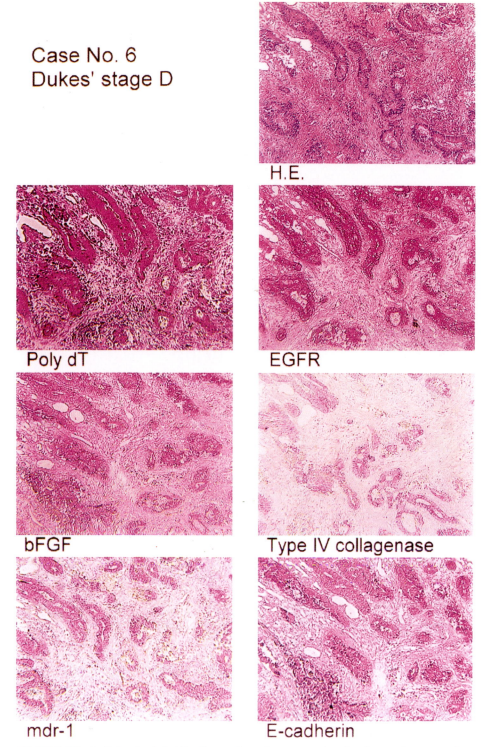

Case No. 6
Dukes' stage D

H.E.

Poly dT

EGFR

bFGF

Type IV collagenase

mdr-1

E-cadherin

**PLATE 5** (Fig. 2-4). In situ hybridization analyses for metastasis-related genes in tumors from patients with *A.* Dukes' stage B (*panel A*) and *B.* Dukes' stage D disease. Tumor cells from patients with Dukes' stage D disease expressed higher levels of metastasis-related genes than patients with Dukes' stage B disease. (H.E., hematoxylin and eosin, ×275.) (*From Kitadai et al.*[196] *Reproduced with permission.*)

Case No. 10
Dukes' stage B

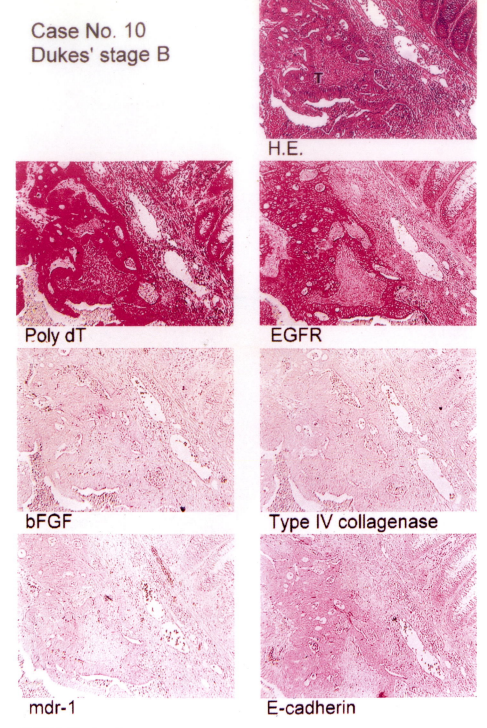

H.E.

Poly dT

EGFR

bFGF

Type IV collagenase

mdr-1

E-cadherin

**PLATE 5** *(Continued)*

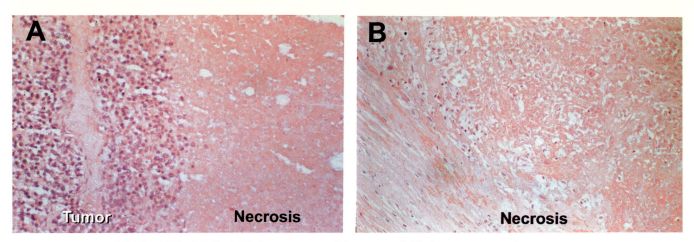

**PLATE 6** (Fig. 3D-4). *A.* Limb sarcoma: partial response. *B.* Limb sarcoma: complete response after isolated limb perfusion.

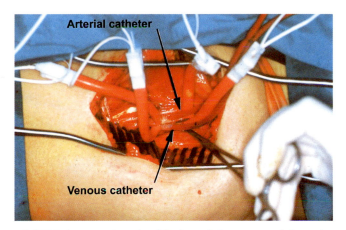

**PLATE 7** (Fig. 3D-6). Isolated limb perfusion: approach from the femoral vessels.

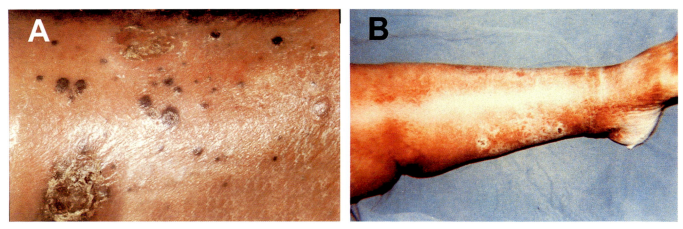

**PLATE 8** (Fig. 3D-7). Stage III melanoma: *A.* before isolated limb perfusion; *B.* after isolated limb perfusion.

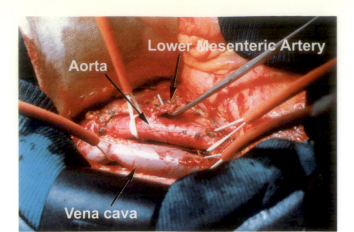

**PLATE 9** (Fig. 3D-9). The aorta, anterior mesenteric artery, and vena cava are dissected before cannulation.

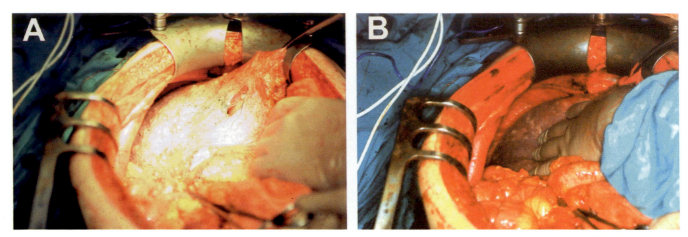

**PLATE 10** (Fig. 3D-16). Peritonectomy procedure: *A.* Upper right quadrant peritoneal stripping; *B.* after procedure.

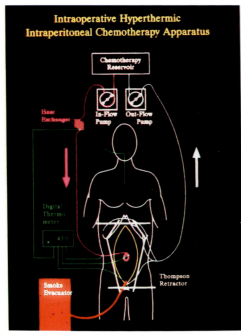

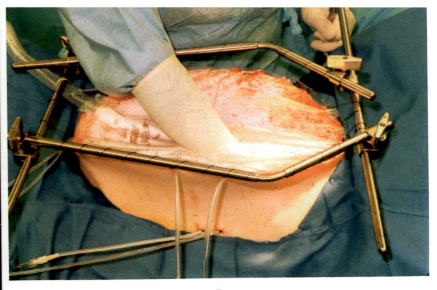

**PLATE 11** (Fig. 3D-18). Intraperitoneal hyperthermic perfusion: *A.* Open abdomen technique (intraoperative view). (*From Sugarbaker.*[100]) *B.* Scheme of intraperitoneal hyperthermic perfusion.

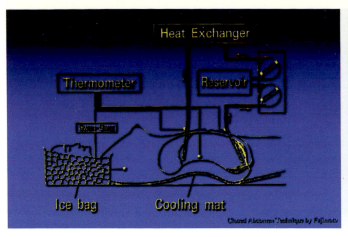

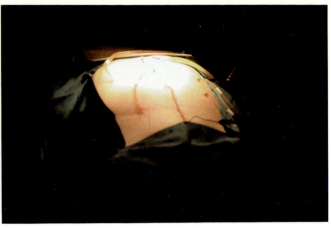

| A | B |

**PLATE 12** (Fig. 3D-19A,B). Intraperitoneal hyperthermic perfusion: *A.* Closed abdomen technique (intraoperative view). *B.* Scheme of intraperitoneal hyperthermic perfusion. (*From Fujimoto.*[105])

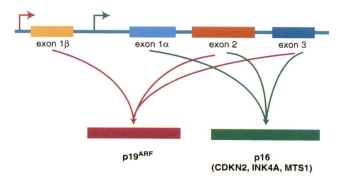

**PLATE 13** (Fig. 3F-3). The p16-p19$^{ARF}$ gene illustrates the process of RNA splicing. Two completely distinct products arise out of a single locus through RNA splicing and the use of different reading frames. p16 is derived from exons 1a, 2, and 3, with a promoter region depicted by the green arrow. The p19$^{ARF}$ transcript, on the other hand, is derived from exons 1b, 2 and 3, with the promoter shown in magenta. Although both transcripts share exons 2 and 3, they have different reading frames, and thus, have no amino acid sequence similarity.

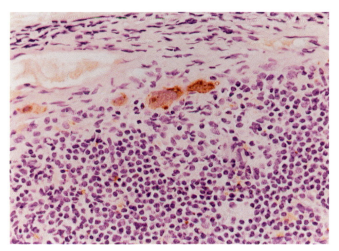

**PLATE 14** (Fig. 3F-13). Photomicrograph of sentinel lymph node removed from a melanoma patient. Routine hematoxylin and eosin (H&E) staining failed to reveal evidence of melanoma. Immunohistochemical staining with S-100 antibody revealed melanoma tumor cells (brown stain). (*Courtesy of Dr. Lori Lowe, Department of Pathology, University of Michigan.*)

**PLATE 15** (Fig. 5B-1). Esophageal cancer.

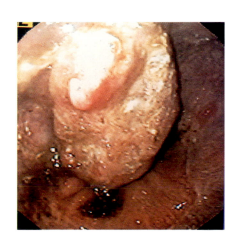

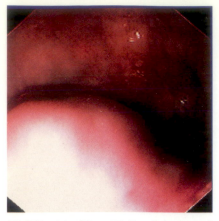

**PLATE 16** (Fig. 5B-2). Submucosal esophageal tumor.

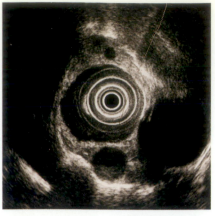

**PLATE 17** (Fig. 5B-4). A large malignant lymph node is seen at the 12:00 and 6:00 position along with a large esophageal tumor extending from the 6:00 to the 12:00 position. At the 4:00 position, the large dark spot represents the aorta.

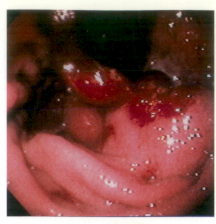

**PLATE 18** (Fig. 5B-5). Carcinoma of stomach at esophagogastric junction.

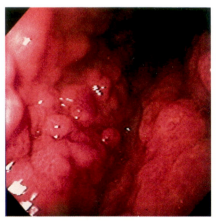

**PLATE 19** (Fig. 5B-6). Endoscopic view of lymphoma of stomach.

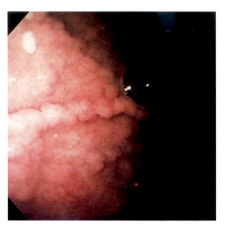

**PLATE 20** (Fig. 5B-7). Endoscopic view of fundic gland polyps of the stomach.

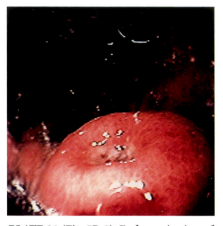

**PLATE 21** (Fig. 5B-8). Endoscopic view of a leiomyoma of the stomach with central depression and ulceration. This area of ulceration can also be a cause of upper gastrointestinal bleeding.

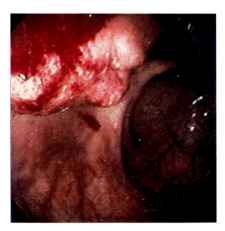

**PLATE 22** (Fig. 5B-9). Endoscopic view of a rectal carcinoma.

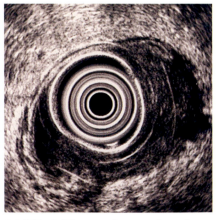

**PLATE 23** (Fig. 5B-10). EUS of rectal carcinoma showing T3 lesion.

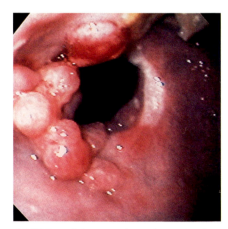

**PLATE 24** (Fig. 5B-11). Endoscopic view of a villous polyp of the rectum. When the polyp size is greater than 1–2 cm in diameter, the incidence of malignancy is between 20% and 40% and increases as the polyp size increases.

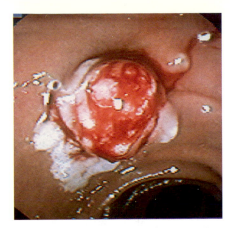

**PLATE 25** (Fig. 5B-14). Endoscopic view of a villous polyp of the ampulla of Vater.

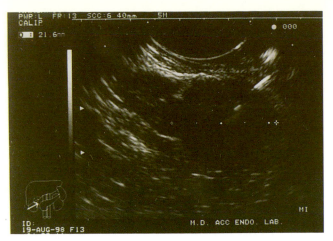

**PLATE 26** (Fig. 5B-15). EUS-guided biopsy of a pancreatic tumor adjacent to the portal vein.

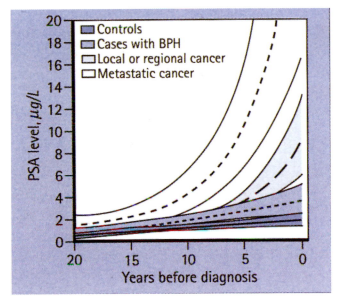

**PLATE 27** (Fig. 17D-6). Changes in PSA level over time before diagnosis of prostate cancer, which is the basis for PSA velocity. Patients eventually diagnosed with prostate cancer have a logarithmic change in PSA as opposed to patients with benign prostatic hyperplasia. (*From HB Carter et al.*[39] *Reproduced with permission.*)

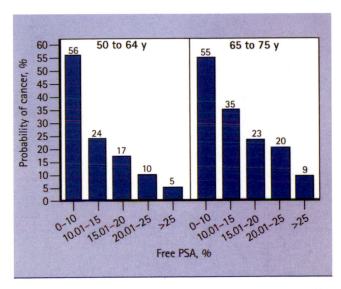

**PLATE 28** (Fig. 17D-7). A. Probability of cancer as calculated by % free PSA and patient age for patients with PSA levels between 4 and 10 ng/mL. (*From WJ Catalona et al.*[43] *Reproduced with permission.*)

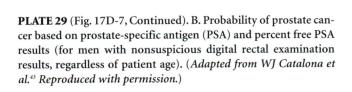

**PLATE 29** (Fig. 17D-7, Continued). B. Probability of prostate cancer based on prostate-specific antigen (PSA) and percent free PSA results (for men with nonsuspicious digital rectal examination results, regardless of patient age). (*Adapted from WJ Catalona et al.*[43] *Reproduced with permission.*)

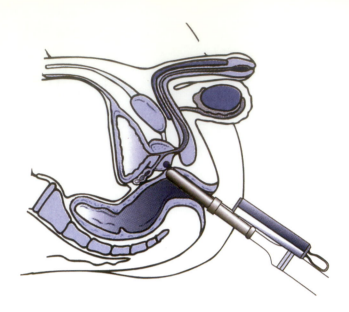

**PLATE 30** (Fig. 17D-9). TRUS-guided prostatic biopsy, using an automated biopsy gun.

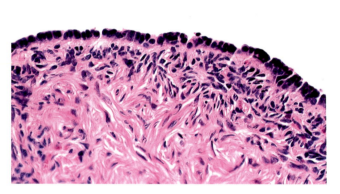

*A*

*B*

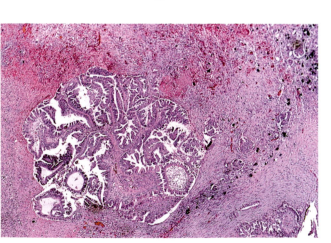

*C*

**PLATE 31** (Fig. 18E-4 A,B,C). The pathologic spectrum of serious ovarian neoplasm: (*a*) A benign serous ovarian tumor. These neoplasms are characterized by being lined by a single layer of serous cells. (*b*) A border line serous ovarian tumor. Epithelial cells covering fibrovascular cores and an absence of invasion into the ovarian stroma characterizes these. (*c*) A serous invasive ovarian carcinoma. Sheets of proliferating cells invading into and replacing the ovarian stroma characterize these.

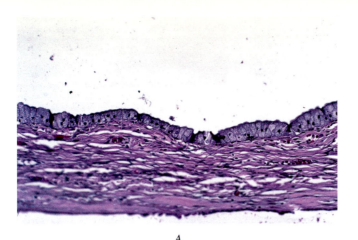 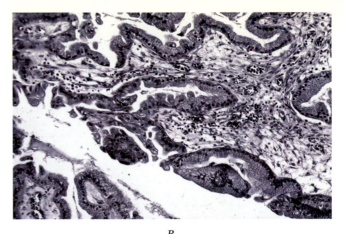

*A*  *B*

**PLATE 32** (Fig. 18E-5 A,B). (*a*) A benign tumor consisting of a single layer of cells. (*b*) A malignant mucinous tumor, consisting of sheets of cells.

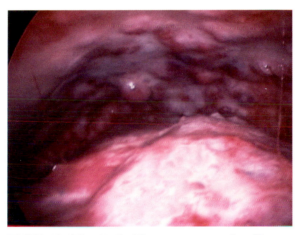

**PLATE 33** (Fig. 22-7). The appearance of malignant mesothelioma at the time of a videothoracoscopic biopsy.

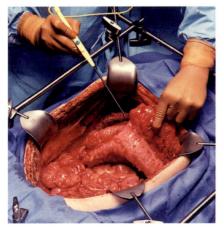 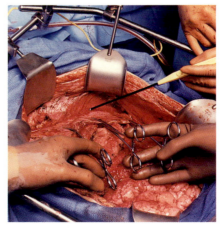

**PLATE 34** (Fig. 24D-2). Abdominal exposure using a self-retaining retractor, complete greater omentectomy and splenectomy.

**PLATE 35** (Fig. 24D-3). Peritoneal stripping from the left diaphragm.

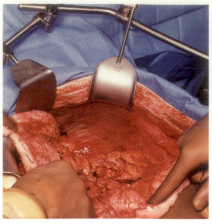

**PLATE 36** (Fig. 24D-4). Left subphrenic peritonectomy completed.

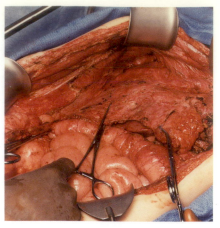

**PLATE 37** (Fig. 24D-5). Peritoneal stripping of the undersurface of the right hemidiaphragm.

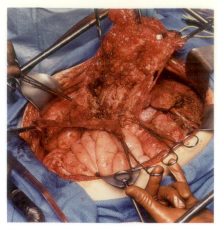

**PLATE 38** (Fig. 24D-6). Stripping of tumor from beneath the right hemidiaphragm, from the right subhepatic space and from the surface of the liver.

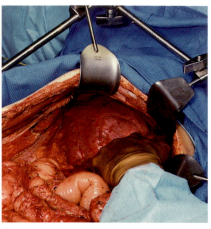

**PLATE 39** (Fig. 24D-7). Completed right subphrenic peritonectomy.

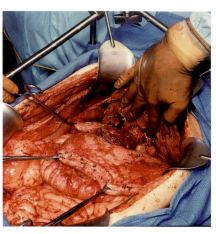

**PLATE 40** (Fig. 24D-8). Lesser omentectomy and cholecystectomy with stripping of the porta hepatis.

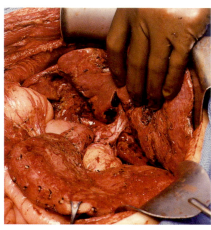

**PLATE 41** (Fig. 24D-9). Stripping of the omental bursa.

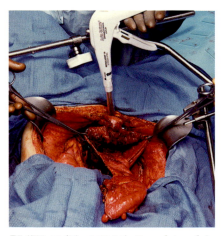

**PLATE 42** (Fig. 24D-10). Complete pelvic peritonectomy.

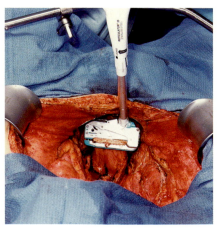

**PLATE 43** (Fig. 24D-11). Resection of rectosigmoid colon and cul-de-sac of Douglas.

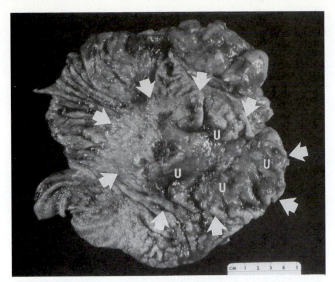

**FIGURE 4D-97.** Low-grade B-cell lymphoma of MALT type arising in a stomach in association with longstanding follicular gastritis due to *Helicobacter pylori* infection. The lymphoma is not clearly demarcated (arrows) due to mucosal changes of gastritis, and there is extensive ulceration (U). (Also see Fig. 4D-64). (*With permission, from Banks PM, Kraybill WG:* Pathology for the Surgeon. *Philadelphia, WB Saunders, 1996.*)

Recognition of such "posttransplantation lymphoproliferative disorders" as distinct from true lymphomas is of more than academic interest, since the former responds to diminished immunosuppression whereas, in direct contrast, the latter requires intensive chemotherapeutic intervention.[115] In HIV-infected individuals, high-grade lymphoma or Kaposi's sarcoma may be the initial definitional manifestation of AIDS. Such tumors often arise in extranodal sites such as gut or tonsils. For identification of opportunistic agents, FNA biopsies can initially be attempted on enlarged nodes. To avoid disruptive cryostat decontamination procedures, cytology scrape-smear preparations can often be used successfully for intraoperative recognition of either malignancy or opportunistic infection.

## SOFT TISSUE TUMORS

### DEFINITION AND PATHOBIOLOGY

Soft tissues are defined as nonepithelial extraskeletal tissues exclusive of the reticuloendothelial system and neural glia. They include muscle, adipose tissue, and supporting vasculature and nerves.[116] The etiology of most soft tissue tumors (STTs) is unknown. Benign lesions have been associated with trauma and foreign materials. Soft tissue sarcomas (STSs) have been associated with several chemical toxins and prior irradiation.[117] Benign and malignant STTs are a component of several familial disorders, including neurofibromato-

sis, Gardner's syndrome, familial retinoblastoma, and Li-Fraumeni familial cancer syndrome.[118]

The biologic potential of both benign and malignant STTs is varied, and at times unpredictable. For example, among benign fibrous proliferations, some lesions, such as nodular fasciitis, proliferate rapidly, whereas others grow insidiously. Although there is considerable variation in the behavior of sarcomas, a few generalizations can be made. Sarcomas tend to "respect" fascial borders unless altered by surgical intervention or advanced growth. Subcutaneous lesions typically expand radially, whereas intramuscular or osseous sarcomas spread longitudinally. Pseudocapsules, although consisting primarily of collagen, fibroblasts, newly formed vessels, and inflammatory elements, will always contain some viable tumor. For this reason, local recurrence invariably follows enucleation of what appeared to be a circumscribed lesion.

The behavior of STSs varies with the histologic type of the tumor, tumor size, and tumor grade. Low-grade STSs rarely metastasize hematogenously, although they may recur locally. High-grade sarcomas may also recur locally, extending along fascial borders, but in addition, they may metastasize hematogenously and occasionally lymphatically. Their propensity to do so is related to their size. Although grading is important, some histologic subtypes independently define the anticipated biologic potential. Although the AJCC staging system exists for STSs, this emphasizes histopathologic classification and grading of the tumor, rather than degree of local or regional spread.[7]

## EVALUATION AND DIAGNOSIS OF PATIENTS WITH SOFT TISSUE TUMORS

The selection of patients with STTs for biopsy is dependent on the clinician's index of suspicion that a given STT may be a malignant, i.e., STS. Factors relevant to the development of that suspicion are described elsewhere. Patients in whom such a suspicion is present should be adequately imaged prior to biopsy. Core needle biopsy offers low cost and minimal tissue damage. It may be used with relatively little concern about wound healing in patients who will subsequently undergo radiation. The accuracy of the core needle biopsy is about 80%, and this method is being used increasingly as the initial biopsy method in patients with STT. However, in tumors having abundant fibrosis, extracellular matrix, necrosis, or heterogeneous composition, needle biopsy may prove nondiagnostic due to sampling error. Of the three biopsy types, fine-needle aspiration (FNA) is the most subject to sampling error. The diagnostic information provided by the pathologist is often of a general nature—malignant or benign. However, some groups with an extensive experience using FNA in STSs have reported this to be very effective in the diagnosis of STS.[119] However, in most hands, FNA is less reliable than core needle biopsy or open biopsy. For these reasons we do not advocate FNA for primary diagnosis of STSs but believe it is useful to document recurrent or metastatic disease. All biopsies, particularly open biopsies, are performed with the ultimate surgical resection in mind. Thus, it is best if the same surgeon plans for both biopsy and potential resection. In the extremities, most incisions are radial. Care should be taken to assure adequate hemostasis and avoid seromas.

In the evaluation of STT, microscopically it is usually best to rely on permanent section evaluation rather than frozen section. This permits careful and thoughtful microscopic consideration of a specimen free of artifact and, if necessary, consultation or repeat biopsy. However, frozen section does have several important roles in evaluation of these difficult tumors. Frozen section permits the pathologist to inform the surgeon intraoperatively whether the tissue sample is of satisfactory quality and quantity. It allows the exclusion of infection as the etiology of the soft tissue mass, and on occasion it may provide help in the assessment of surgical margins. We rarely use frozen-section diagnoses to make major therapeutic decisions, although it may be appropriate in select circumstances; in particular when a patient's differential diagnosis has been narrowed by clinical and radiologic information down to only a few considerations that can be confidently distinguished with frozen-section method. The pathologist should always reserve the right to defer to assessment of permanent sections.

## TREATMENT, PROCESSING, AND ASSESSMENT OF SPECIMENS

In general, specimens should be reviewed with the pathologist for orientation and surgical margins; anatomic landmarks that are obvious in situ are less so following excision. To avoid spurious contamination by tumor, resection surfaces can be painted with India ink, blotted to avoid smearing, and sampled prior to sectioning through the tumor (see Fig. 4D-4). Soft tissue and neurovascular margins are sampled. The tumor is measured for staging. One histologic section for each centimeter of tumor should be sampled. All lymph nodes are submitted for microscopic examination. If special studies are contemplated, fresh tissue either frozen or suspended in media, should be procured. Lymphoma may be in the differential diagnosis and in this circumstance appropriate studies should be done.

One of the most accurate criteria to assess prognosis in these uncommon tumors is microscopic grading. Grading schemes may be two-tiered (low and high) or may have up to four grades. Each system has proven clinical utility. In the United States, use of three grades is the most prevalent approach.[120] The histologic features used in grading schemes include:

1. Degree of tumor differentiation
2. Cellularity
3. Nuclear atypia
4. Cellular pleomorphism (presence of tumor giant cells and bizarre nuclei)
5. Mitotic rate
6. Amount of fibrous stroma and myxoid stroma
7. Presence and amount of inflammation
8. Percent necrosis

This last feature is particularly important. Preoperative therapies, such as radiation, may alter some of these features. Inherent in the very diagnosis of some types of STS are implications regarding high- or low-grade biologic behaviors. These issues must be con-

sidered when making therapeutic decisions on the basis of tumor grade.

## STANDARDIZED REPORTING OF STSs

The pathology report from a resection specimen should include information concerning the following items:

1. Residual tumor
2. Tumor location
3. Histologic type
4. Histologic grade
5. Surgical margins status (actual distance, if margin is close)
6. Presence of tumor deposits in vessels, in lymph nodes, outside of the main mass, in the joint space, or in bone
7. Estimated percent necrosis
8. Tumor size measured from the specimen
9. Results of any special stains used to support diagnosis
10. Comment: Unusual features of the case should be mentioned as well as expected biologic behavior, and if recurrence or metastasis, whether tumor differs in appearance from that of original lesion

The listed information concerning the primary tumor is the responsibility of the pathologist. Physical findings and pertinent radiographic studies can be used for staging, and a treatment plan with input from the surgeon, medical oncologist, and radiation therapist can then be formulated based upon the expected biologic potential of the lesion.

## HISTOLOGIC CLASSIFICATION OF STSs

The WHO currently recognizes 165 histologic types of STT.[121] Tumors are likened to the adult tissue type they resemble. It is beyond the scope of this chapter to discuss type and subtypes in detail. Rather, a relevant description of the major categories and a spectrum of their biologic behaviors will be presented.

**FIBROUS LESIONS.** Fibrous STTs make up a spectrum of disease from nodular fasciitis to fibrosarcoma. The former is the prototype of the pseudosarcomatous benign fibroblastic proliferations. Clinically it presents as a rapidly growing mass in young adults. Because of high cellularity and brisk mitotic activity, nodular fasciitis may be confused with sarcoma with the untoward results of unnecessarily extensive resection (Fig. 4D-98). Local excision is usually curative. The fibromatoses are classified among benign fibrous proliferations (Fig. 4D-99). In the absence of radiation, fibromatoses do not transform to fibrosarcoma. Whereas palmar and plantar fibromatoses are readily treated by local excision, fibromatoses in other sites recur in 25% to 50% of patients, and mesenteric lesions may be fatal. Cases associated with Gardner's syndrome are more aggressive than random cases. Treatment of fibromatoses should balance the need for complete extirpation of the lesion against the morbidity of the procedure. Fibrosarcomas are rare tumors that typically occur in the deep tissues of the lower extremities of adults in the fifth

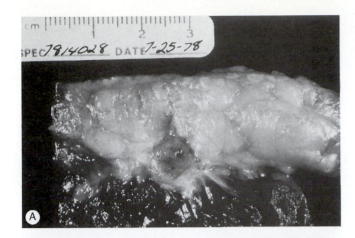

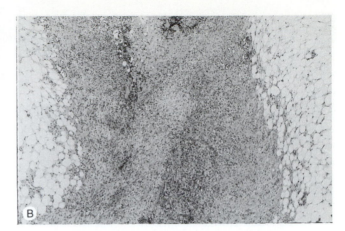

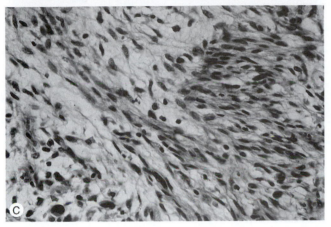

**FIGURE 4D-98.** Nodular fasciitis typically presents as a relatively superficial, small (2- to 3-cm) tumefaction that attains its maximum dimension in a matter of weeks. *A.* Gross specimen shows a nodule at the interface of subcutaneous fat and fascia. It is cured by local excision or may even regress spontaneously. Nodular fasciitis is characterized by a proliferation of myofibroblasts arranged in a loose storiform pattern punctuated by myxoid stroma, chronic inflammatory elements, and extravasated erythrocytes. Although mitoses may be present, the cytologic features are benign (*B.* Low magnification; *C.* High magnification). (*With permission, from Banks PM, Kraybill WG:* Pathology for the Surgeon. *Philadelphia, WB Saunders, 1996.*)

decade. Histologically, they may be confused with either malignant peripheral nerve sheath tumors or synovial sarcomas (Fig. 4D-100). Immunohistochemical stains may be helpful in their differentiation (see Fig. 4D-19).

FIBROHISTIOCYTIC LESIONS. Dermatofibrosarcoma protuberans (DFSP) and malignant fibrous histiocytoma (MFH) make up this group of tumors (Fig. 4D-101). DFSP is regarded as borderline or low-grade malignancy. Metastases occur in only 5% of reported patients. However, this tumor is very prone to local recurrence and requires aggressive surgical resection.[122] The Mohs' technique for dermatologic surgery has been used successfully in some patients with this disease and is indicated in selected tumors located in anatomically "tight" areas. MFH may occur in various high- and low-grade forms, with corresponding biologic behavior. Melanomas, lymphomas, and carcinomas can simulate some forms of MFH with pleomorphic spindle morphology. Immunohistochemical stains are effective in making this important distinction (see Fig. 4D-19).

LIPOMATOUS TUMORS. The spectrum of lipomatous tumors varies from benign lipoma and their variants to various types of poorly differentiated liposarcoma. Lipomas require simple excision. Lipomas deep to the deep fascia must be differentiated from low-grade liposarcomas. Low-grade liposarcomas may attain large size and may dedifferentiate into high-grade sarcomas (Fig. 4D-102). Treatment of low-grade liposarcomas is the same as that of other low-grade sarcomas, with optimal local therapy. High-grade liposarcomas require resection with negative margins and radiation therapy. Large liposarcomas of the retroperitoneum have a particularly ominous long-term prognosis. Chromosomal translocation is present in over 90% of myxoid or round cell liposarcoma [t(12;16) (q13;p11)].[116] Treatment of extremity liposarcoma usually consists of limb salvage therapy.

NEURAL TUMORS. Scwhannomas arise from Schwann cells and fibroblasts ensheathing peripheral nerve. They can occur at any age but predominate within the 20- to 50-year range. They may attain significant size and mimic sarcomas, both clinically and microscopically. They virtually never undergo malignant degeneration. Treatment is local excision. For very large tumors where complete excision is not possible, partial excision may reduce local pressure and still be beneficial to the patient. About 90% of neurofibromas are solitary and occur in young adults (aged 20 to 30). Cases associated with neurofibromatosis (NF) are more likley to arise in large nerve trunks. The plexiform variant of neurofibroma is a neurofibroma that expands and distorts a nerve trunk; these lesions are considered pathognomonic for type I NF (Fig. 4D-103).

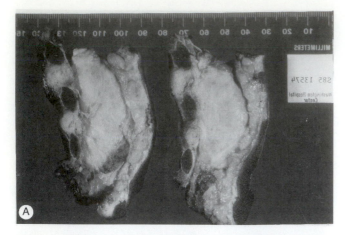

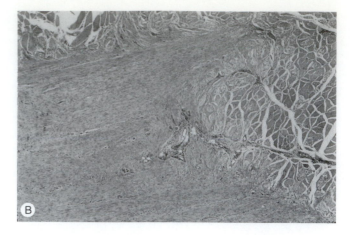

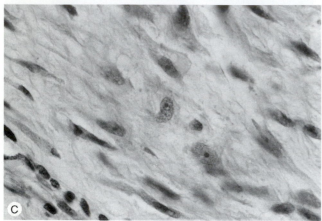

**FIGURE 4D-99.** Fibromatosis. Fibromatoses are typically firm; macroscopically, they may appear deceptively circumscribed. This appearance is somewhat typical of fibromatosis, but it may be observed in any number of sarcomas as well, underscoring the need for pathologic examination. This example of cicatricial fibromatosis, an uncommon form, occurred in a prior thoracotomy scar. *A.* Gross specimen. Although these lesions do not metastasize, they typically infiltrate local structures, often to include skeletal muscle, as shown in the right field of *B* (low magnification). The proliferating fibroblasts have a bland chromatin pattern (*C.* High magnification). (*With permission, from Banks PM, Kraybill WG:* Pathology for the Surgeon. *Philadelphia, WB Saunders, 1996.*)

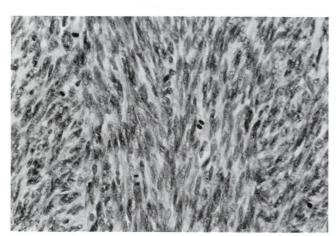

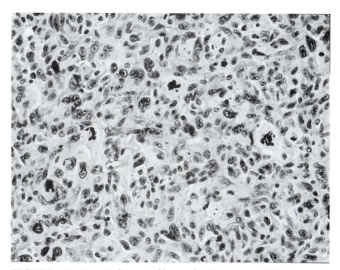

**FIGURE 4D-100.** Fibrosarcoma. This example of a high-grade fibrosarcoma shows the typical herringbone pattern composed of cytologically malignant spindle cells. This example has a brisk mitotic rate (high magnification). (*With permission, from Banks PM, Kraybill WG:* Pathology for the Surgeon. *Philadelphia, WB Saunders, 1996.*)

**FIGURE 4D-101.** Malignant fibrous histiocytoma. This is a typical example of the common pleomorphic form, although several variants have been described. Note haphazardly arranged cells with marked pleomorphism (high magnification). (*With permission, from Banks PM, Kraybill WG:* Pathology for the Surgeon. *Philadelphia, WB Saunders, 1996.*)

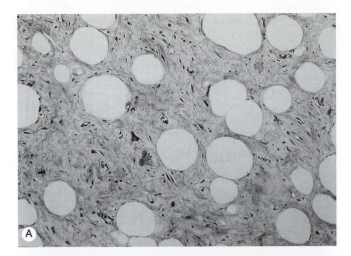

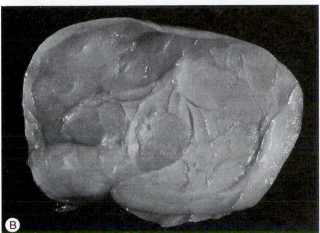

**FIGURE 4D-102.** Well-differentiated liposarcoma often shows mature-appearing fat and enlarged hyperchromatic cells in a background of fibrosis (sclerosis). Lipoblasts may be infrequent. *A*. Intermediate magnification. *B*. Well-differentiated liposarcoma of retroperitoneum, gross specimem. Note that although these tumors appear similar to mature adipose tissue, any fatty tumor of the retroperitoneum should be regarded as liposarcoma until proven otherwise. (*With permission, from Banks PM, Kraybill WG: Pathology for the Surgeon. Philadelphia, WB Saunders, 1996.*)

Treatment consists of excision, but negative margins may be difficult to obtain. Transformation to malignant, often lethal, peripheral nerve sheath tumors occurs almost exclusively in patients with underlying NF.

**SMOOTH MUSCLE TUMORS.** Tumors of smooth muscle may occur in any location where smooth muscle is present. Leiomyomas are benign tumors that occur most commonly in the GI tract in both sexes and in the female genital tract as well. They are uncommon in other areas. Leiomyosarcoma may occur in the subcutaneous tissue, female genital tract, GI tract, and vascular walls. The criteria

for diagnosis of these tumors in the GI tract where they are included within gastrointestinal stromal tumors (GISTs) and the female genital tract vary significantly. Assessing grade in these tumors is often difficult. Management is dependent on the assessment of grade and size. Large high-grade tumors are treated with excision with negative margins and radiation, whereas smaller tumors may be simply widely excised. Large tumors should be considered high-risk tumors and fit into the general category of STS.

**ROUND CELL SARCOMAS ("SMALL-CELL," "BLUE-CELL" OR "BLASTIC" SARCOMAS).** These tumors, which include neuroblastoma, rhabdomyosarcoma, and Ewing's sarcoma, occur in significantly younger patients than most other STSs. The accurate diagnosis of these tumors is important because their treatment is so different, consisting of more aggressive chemotherapy and radiation. Although surgery still has a significant role in some of these patients, especially those with neuroblastoma or rhabdomyosarcoma, chemotherapy assumes a more important role, especially for neuroblastoma, rhabdomyosarcoma in children, and in the Ewing's (EWS-PNET) family of tumors. Hence, the surgeon's role in these rare and interesting tumors is predominantly one of diagnosis, with the significant exceptions noted above.

**MISCELLANEOUS MALIGNANT LESIONS.** Synovial sarcomas represent about 10% of all sarcomas and arise most commonly in the deep soft tissues of the lower extremities of young adults. A characteristic translocation is seen in synovial sarcoma [t(x;18) (q11;q11)]. Most grading schemes categorize all synovial sarcomas as high-grade lesions. For therapeutic purposes, these tumors still behave as high-grade STSs and can metastasize to regional lymph nodes. Appropriate treatment consists of wide local excision with negative margins and radiation therapy. Clear cell sarcoma, also known as malignant melanoma of soft parts,[123] typically occurs in the distal lower extremities. Peak incidence is in the third decade. A chromosomal translocation has been demonstrated that distinguishes it from melanoma [t(12;22)(q13-14;q12)].[124] This tumor is one of the STSs that can metastasize to lymph nodes. Surgical resection with adjuvant radiation is the most effective treatment. Epithelioid sarcomas most commonly occur in the hands and forearms of young adults (third decade). Lymph node metastases are common. The disease is fatal in about one-third of patients. Early aggressive surgical intervention with radiation therapy offers the best chance for cure.[125]

## TUMORS AND TUMORLIKE CONDITIONS OF BONES AND JOINTS

### CLINICAL ASSESSMENT

Only the fundamental principles for the diagnosis and evaluation of bone symptomatology and tumors will be presented.[126] Pertinent patient historical information including age, date of onset and duration of symptoms, severity of pain, and presence of concomitant constitutional symptoms must be collected and reviewed. A history of previous neoplasm or fever should be excluded before

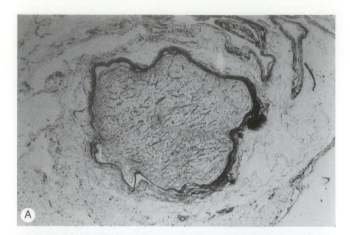

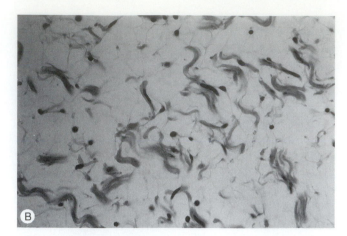

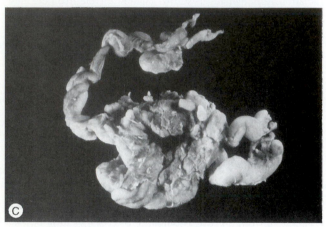

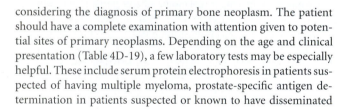

**FIGURE 4D-103.** Neurofibroma. This example of neurofibroma is small and circumscribed, as the proliferation has not expanded beyond the confines of the perineurium. *A*. Low magnification. Note the myxoid stroma and the presence of slender nuclei neatly apposed to slender, kinky bundles of collagen. *B*. High magnification. *C*. Plexiform neurofibroma. These are virtually pathognomonic of neurofibromatosis. The impressive distortion of the nerve trunk by this lesion imparts a tortous configuration likened to a "bag of worms." (also see Fig. 4D-44). (*With permission, from Banks PM, Kraybill WG:* Pathology for the Surgeon. *Philadelphia, WB Saunders, 1996.*)

considering the diagnosis of primary bone neoplasm. The patient should have a complete examination with attention given to potential sites of primary neoplasms. Depending on the age and clinical presentation (Table 4D-19), a few laboratory tests may be especially helpful. These include serum protein electrophoresis in patients suspected of having multiple myeloma, prostate-specific antigen determination in patients suspected or known to have disseminated

prostate cancer, and serum parathyroid hormone level measurement in patients in whom the radiographic features and serum calcium levels suggest hyperparathyroidism. Imaging is very important to the pathologist's review of slides in considering a final diagnosis. The most useful diagnostic test may be plain radiography. Radiographs obtained in two planes at right angles to each other define the anatomic localization, intraosseous extent, distortion of the surrounding soft tissue planes, margination of the tumor, and periosteal reaction. Various tumors of the long bones have distinct predilection to involve certain anatomic regions within such bones (Table 4D-20). Computed tomography (CT) provides better resolution of mineralized or ossified tissue (Fig. 4D-104).[127] Magnetic resonance imaging (MRI) allows accurate determination of local disease and especially soft tissue extension. However, neither CT nor MRI can predict the histogenesis or aggressiveness of the process imaged. For such information, the microscope is needed.

**TABLE 4D-19.** AGE AS A DIAGNOSTIC FACTOR IN BONE TUMORS

| AGE 20 OR BELOW | AGE 20–60 | AGE 60 OR ABOVE |
|---|---|---|
| Osteochondroma | Giant cell tumor | Lymphoma |
| Aneurysmal bone cyst | Hemangioma | Myeloma |
| Simple cyst | Hemangioendothelioma | Metastases |
| Chondroblastoma | Infection | Paget's disease |
| Histiocytosis X | Hyperparathyroidism | |
| Infection | Lymphoma | |
| Osteosarcoma | Fibrosarcoma | |
| Ewing's sarcoma | Chondrosarcoma | |
| Leukemia | | |

SOURCE: With permission, from Banks PM, Kraybill WG: *Pathology for the Surgeon*. Philadelphia, WB Saunders, 1996.

## BIOPSY

The planning and performance of the biopsy of bone neoplasms may be critical to the success of the overall management of the patient. Errors made in this aspect of the care of the patient with a bone tumor may not be correctable. A review of patients who had poorly planned biopsies prior to referral to tertiary oncology centers found significant problems in at least 20%: an adverse effect on prognosis

## TABLE 4D-20. SITE AS A DIAGNOSTIC FACTOR IN BONE TUMORS

| EPIPHYSIS | METAPHYSIS | DIAPHYSIS |
|---|---|---|
| Giant cell tumor | Chondromyxoid fibroma | Hemangioma |
| Chondroblastoma | Aneurysmal bone cyst | Adamantinoma |
| Clear-cell chondrosarcoma | Unicameral bone cyst | Ewing's sarcoma |
| Hyperparathyroidism | Infection | Paget's disease |
| | Osteosarcoma | Lymphoma |
| | Lymphoma | Myeloma |
| | Metastases | Metastases |

SOURCE: With permission, from Banks PM, Kraybill WG: *Pathology for the Surgeon.* Philadelphia, WB Saunders, 1996.

in 8%, and in 5% the biopsy precluded limb-sparing surgery.[128] These figures underscore the need for cooperation and communication among surgeon, radiologist, and pathologist to identify the ideal biopsy site by imaging studies *before* the biopsy is performed. Since the definitive procedure may not necessarily be performed at the same time as the open biopsy, the incision site should be placed so as to allow subsequent removal of the biopsy tract en bloc with the underlying tumor. The advantage of an open biopsy is that sufficient diagnostic material is obtained. The pathologist can confirm the adequacy of the specimen with intraoperative frozen-section assessment. In some circumstances the surgeon can proceed with definitive operative management; however, for most open biopsies the differential diagnosis requires withholding definitive management until the final result is reported. Closed percutaneous needle biopsies are being used more frequently.[129] This is a cost-efficient method for establishing the diagnosis in many patients, especially in those with metastatic disease. The major disadvantages include nondiagnostic aspirates (20%) and the possibility of local recurrence in the needle tract if this is not excised with the primary tumor.[130] Thus the route of needle biopsy should be carefully planned to avoid contaminating critical neurovascular structures. As with other resections, it is very important that the surgeon identify anatomic landmarks on resected specimens and discuss areas of potential concern with the pathologist.

## COMMON MALIGNANT TUMORS OF BONE

The reader who seeks more detailed information concerning bone tumors is referred to textbooks on bone tumors.[126,130] An overview of different groups of tumors will be provided.

Metastatic carcinoma is the most common neoplasm affecting bone. Most patients with metastatic carcinoma are older adults with a history of known primary neoplasm. However, some will present with bony metastasis of unknown origin, though a primary may be suspected. Again, the biopsy must be carefully planned. Immunohistochemistry may be very helpful in identifying the origin of the metastasis. Close communication between the surgeon and pathologist is important so that an adequate and appropriate specimen is provided. Clinical information is useful to the pathologist in selecting special studies to pinpoint the primary.

Myeloma is the most common primary neoplasm of bone and bone pain is its most frequent symptom. Roentgenograms typically

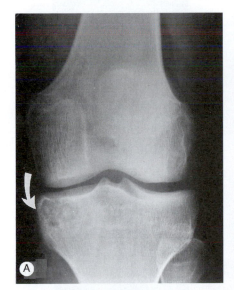 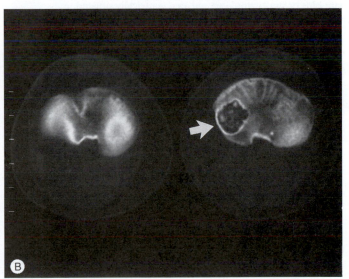

**FIGURE 4D-104.** *A.* Eccentric epiphyseal lesion (arrow) in proximal tibia of a patient at skeletal maturity with progressive closure of epiphyseal plate. *B.* CT reveals a sclerotic rim separating the lesion (arrow) from the host bone and confirms the calcification within the lesion. The anatomic location, age, and radiographic appearance support chondroblastoma, a benign tumor. (*With permission, from Banks PM, Kraybill WG:* Pathology for the Surgeon. *Philadelphia, WB Saunders, 1996.*)

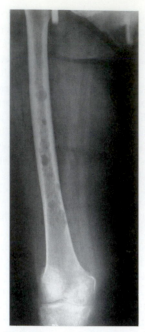

**FIGURE 4D-105.** Roentgenogram showing multiple lytic areas in a patient with plasma cell myeloma. There is no associated sclerosis. (*With permission, from Banks PM, Kraybill WG:* Pathology for the Surgeon. *Philadelphia, WB Saunders, 1996.*)

show multiple, punched-out, purely lytic lesions (Fig. 4D-105). Histologically, myeloma consists of sheets of plasma cells. In most all cases, the plasma cell nature of the neoplasm is apparent by conventional microscopy, at least focally (Fig. 4D-106). The cells have abundant blue or pink cytoplasm and an eccentrically situated nucleus with marginated ("clockface") chromatin. Primary malig-

nant lymphoma is an uncommon bone tumor. It may affect both young and old. As with myeloma, the presentation is usually bone pain. Roentgenograms show a permeative, destructive lesion, typically involving the shaft of a long bone (see Fig. 4D-3). The classic histologic appearance is a mixed lymphoid cell infiltrate that is accompanied and sometimes obscured by delicate fibrosis (see Fig. 4D-3). The subclassification of malignant lymphoma in bone may be difficult, but it is often assisted by special methods, such as immunohistochemistry or (with fresh tissue) flow cytometry phenotyping. Accurate classification is the single most important prognostic factor for malignant lymphoma.[131]

Ewing's sarcoma is a rare bone tumor that affects children and young adults. Any portion of the skeleton may be involved, but in about one-half of patients, long bones are the primary site. Roentgenograms show an extensive permeative lesion, which may involve the entire bone (Fig. 4D-107). The neoplasm is composed of uniform small round cells (Fig. 4D-108). Special stains such as periodic acid-Schiff (PAS) and electron microscopy usually demonstrate glycogen in the cytoplasm and the tumor cells are positive by immunostaining for CD99.

Osteosarcoma is the second most common primary malignant neoplasm of bone, following myeloma. This tumor may be defined simply as a malignant tumor of bone in which the tumor cells produce an osteoid matrix, at least focally. Most frequently, it is a tumor of childhood or adolescence. The tumor usually forms a large area of bony destruction centered on the metaphysis extending into adjacent soft tissue (Fig. 4D-109). There is great variation in the microscopic appearance of osteosarcoma. Approximately 50% will produce large

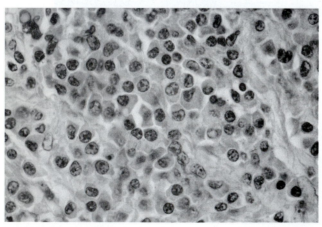

**FIGURE 4D-106.** "Pure culture" appearance of plasma cells in myeloma. Nuclei are eccentric and there is abundant pink cytoplasm. (Hematoxylin and eosin, ×40.) (*With permission, from Banks PM, Kraybill WG:* Pathology for the Surgeon. *Philadelphia, WB Saunders, 1996.*)

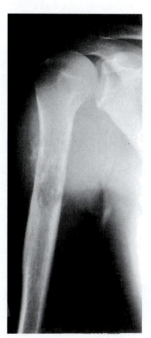

**FIGURE 4D-107.** Ewing's tumor involving proximal humerus. There is a permeative destructive lesion with periosteal new bone formation. (*With permission, from Banks PM, Kraybill WG:* Pathology for the Surgeon. *Philadelphia, WB Saunders, 1996.*)

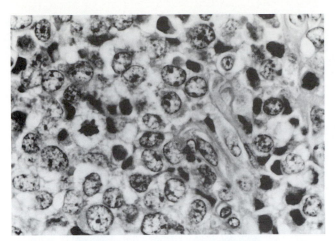

**FIGURE 4D-108.** Ewing's sarcoma showing delicate uniform round cells. (Hematoxylin and eosin, ×100.) (*With permission, from Banks PM, Kraybill WG:* Pathology for the Surgeon. *Philadelphia, WB Saunders, 1996.*)

amounts of osteoid. Chondroid elements or pure spindle cell proliferation may also occur. Because of such heterogeneous composition, chondrosarcoma is usually diagnosed with large incisional biopsies.

Chondrosarcoma is the third most common malignant tumor of bone and is about half as common as osteosarcoma. Like osteosarcoma, it may be divided into distinct clinicopathologic entities. Chondrosarcomas usually affect older adults. Bones of the pelvis and shoulder girdles are commonly involved and, for this reason, any cartilaginous tumor involving the pelvis in an adult patient should be considered chondrosarcoma until proved otherwise. The roentgenographic appearance of chondrosarcoma can be diagnostic. In a long bone, the lesion produces expansion of the bone and thickening of the cortex (Fig. 4D-110). Chondrosarcomas are graded from grade 1 to 3 depending on the cellularity and atypia of the chondrocytes. Behavior relates to tumor grade, with high-grade tumors having an aggressive course.

## BENIGN BONE LESIONS

Although this section concerns primarily malignant tumors of bone, important in the differential diagnosis are benign lesions. Five examples of benign lesions of bone merit mention. Benign giant cell

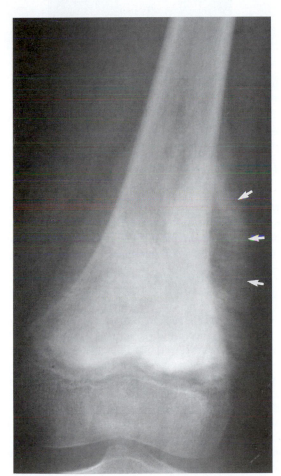

**FIGURE 4D-109.** Densely sclerotic osteosarcoma of distal femur. Tumor extends into soft tissues where it forms a mineralized mass (arrows). (*With permission, from Banks PM, Kraybill WG:* Pathology for the Surgeon. *Philadelphia, WB Saunders, 1996.*)

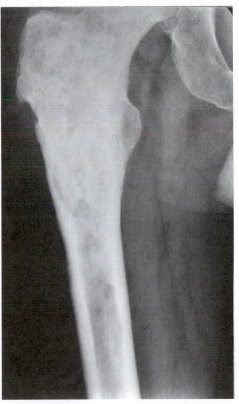

**FIGURE 4D-110.** Chondrosarcoma of the proximal femur showing widening of the bone and thickening of the cortex. (*With permission, from Banks PM, Kraybill WG:* Pathology for the Surgeon. *Philadelphia, WB Saunders, 1996.*)

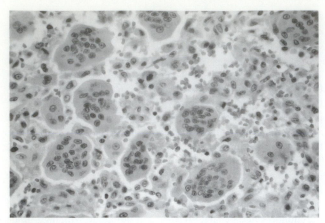

**FIGURE 4D-111.** Microscopic appearance of giant cell tumor. Giant cells are distributed more or less uniformly through the lesion. Nuclei of the mononuclear cells are similar to those of the giant cells. (Hematoxylin and eosin, ×100.) (*With permission, from Banks PM, Kraybill WG:* Pathology for the Surgeon. *Philadelphia, WB Saunders, 1996.*)

tumors occur in skeletally mature individuals around 20 years of age. They are one of the few bone tumors with a predilection for women. Although any site may be involved, the most common sites in order of incidence are the distal femur, proximal tibia, distal radius, and sacrum. Roentgenograms usually show a purely lytic destructive lesion that extends to the articular cartilage. Grossly, the tumor is usually soft with a characteristic dark-brown color. Microscopically, giant cell tumors show a proliferation of benign giant cells containing between 10 and 40 nuclei (Fig. 4D-111). The treatment of this benign tumor is surgical. Curettage should be attempted initially before more extensive procedures such as bone resection are done.

Fracture callus may in certain circumstances be confused with malignant tumors such as Ewing's sarcoma. Roentgenograms showing extensive periosteal new bone formation may be alarming in appearance. The fracture line may not be obvious. Bone scans may show hot spots and roentgenograms a destructive-appearing lesion. This clinical presentation may occur as a stress fracture in athletes or following stress fracture in elderly patients with osteoporosis. Biopsy specimens will show areas of reactive new bone formation, but no tumor formation. Typical roentgenographic and clinical features allow the diagnosis, and the biopsy may thus be avoided altogether.

Enchondromas are benign tumors composed of mature hyaline cartilage that arises within bone. They are important because of the potentially difficult distinction from chondrosarcoma and because they may undergo malignant transformation. Lesions involving the femur, pelvis, and ribs are at greater risk for malignant transformation than tumors at distal sites. Pain may be a sign of malignancy and should stimulate a more aggressive diagnostic approach on the part of the clinician.

The diagnosis of osteomyelitis is usually not difficult. However, both acute and chronic osteomyelitis can mimic a neoplasm (Fig. 4D-112). The systemic symptoms are similar to those of Ewing's sarcoma and chronic localized osteomyelitis can mimic an osteoid osteoma. The roentgenographic appearance of this disease may sug-

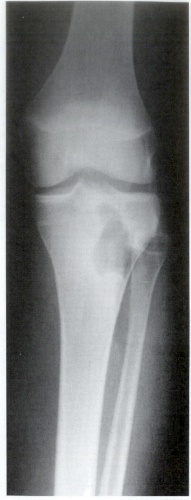

**FIGURE 4D-112.** Chronic osteomyelitis involving proximal tibia. There is a geographic area of destruction with surrounding sclerosis. (*With permission, from Banks PM, Kraybill WG:* Pathology for the Surgeon. *Philadelphia, WB Saunders, 1996.*)

gest a round cell sarcoma. The gross appearance of acute osteomyelitis is typical and when the lesion is entered, frank pus is encountered. However, it is necessary to confirm the diagnosis with a frozen section. Acute osteomyelitis shows a mixture of acute and chronic inflammatory cells and capillary proliferation. Granulomatous osteomyelitis may be difficult to discern because the granulomas may not be well formed and the lesion may be mistaken for a neoplasm, especially lymphoma. Although special stains can sometimes identify organisms, appropriate microbiologic cultures and sensitivity tests are vital for accurate diagnosis and treatment. Patients with chronic osteomyelitis with a chronically draining sinus who develop increased pain and drainage should be rebiopsied. The development of squamous cell cancer in this setting is not uncommon.

Langerhans' cell histiocytosis, historically called histiocytosis X, may be confused with primary bone tumors (see Fig. 4D-20). Radiologically, the findings are those of a destructive lesion with periosteal elevation occurring in over half of patients. Treatment may be with curettage or radiation, depending on location.

## SPECIAL CONSIDERATIONS FOR THE PEDIATRIC PATIENT

Unlike the general surgeon who operates on adult patients suffering from acquired surgical conditions, the pediatric surgeon must be intimately familiar with embryology.[132] In the differential diagnosis of neoplasms in the pediatric age group, problems in embryogenesis must be considered, but are beyond the purview of this brief section. Like other entities of pediatric pathology, many of the neoplasms that occur exclusively in this age group are peculiar in their behavior. In fact, questions remain whether some of these tumors are bona fide neoplasms or whether they represent autonomous aberrant embryogenic proliferations.[133] Examples of this controversy are cystic hygroma of the neck and cutaneous or soft tissue capillary hemangiomas. Although generally considered neoplasms, in most instances they are probably the result of a defect in regulation of normal vascular development. A common characteristic of the more important childhood neoplasms is their microscopic similarity to normal embryonic and fetal tissue.[134] The resemblance of neuroblastoma to normal fetal neuroblasts and triphasic Wilms' tumor to the developing kidney are two examples.[135] Exploration of the events that control the development of childhood neoplasms has therefore improved our understanding of normal embryogenesis, and vice versa.[135]

Because childhood neoplasms are so diverse in their biologic behavior and differ in many respects from most tumors of adults, no AJCC staging systems have been developed for these tumors.[7]

### SELECTED TOPICS FOR DISCUSSION

It is beyond the scope of this section to cover the entire broad topic of pediatric oncologic pathology. However, the basic principles and selected examples will be presented.[133] These include

1. Head and neck masses
2. Intrathoracic cysts and tumors
3. Renal neoplasms and neuroblastomas
4. Germ cell neoplasms
5. Soft tissue neoplasms

**HEAD AND NECK MASSES.** Persistent cervical lymphadenopathy without other clinical manifestations is an indication for lymph node biopsy.[136] If there is any suspicion of infection, microbiologic cultures should be taken at the time of biopsy. If lymphoma, including Hodgkin's lymphoma, is in the differential diagnosis, fresh tissue should be reserved for flow cytometry and fresh-frozen tissue for other potential ancillary studies. Fortunately, the most common finding in a lymph node from a child or an adolescent is benign follicular hyperplasia. Viral infection is suggested by an increased number of immunoblasts. In contrast, toxoplasmosis is associated with a different pattern: parafollicular epithelioid granulomas, fol-

licular hyperplasia, and monocytoid B-cell proliferation. Without going into great detail, suffice it to say that biopsy and assessment of abnormal lymph nodes is a challenging undertaking (see the preceding Hematolymphoid section).

Cysts and multicentric lesions often represent developmental abnormalities, most commonly thyroglossal duct cysts or branchial cleft cysts. When a cystic lesion is multiloculated, especially in an infant, the presumptive diagnosis is "cystic hygroma," i.e., cavernous lymphangioma. Microscopic features useful for differentiating developmental cysts include type of epithelial lining (squamous versus respiratory), presence or absence of subepithelial lymphoid aggregates, and remnants of thyroid follicles. More uncommon types of developmental and neoplastic cysts include solid and cystic teratomas of the neck (which occur as large congenital neck masses), dermoid cysts, and enteric duplication cysts.[137]

Vascular neoplasms, occurring more often in the neck than on the face, constitute as much as 10% of all masses in the head and neck region in children. Lymphangiomas, typically cavernous ("cystic hygromas"), are more common than hemangiomas. They may permeate tissues in an aggressive manner, causing considerable morbidity (Fig. 4D-113). Hemangiomas, particularly in infants, occur as deforming masses. Sites of predilection in younger children are the orbital soft tissues, oral cavity, and parotid gland. Grossly, the tumors are solid and multilobular (Fig. 4D-114). A densely cellular hemangioma with diminutive vascular spaces is recognized by its lobular architecture and the presence of larger vascular spaces usually at the periphery of lobules. In exceptional cases microscopy with immunoperoxidase staining may be necessary to recognize the endothelial elements. It is estimated that 90% of capillary hemangiomas will have undergone involution by the time the child is 10 years old.[138] Other tumors of the head and neck in children include the salivary gland–based neoplasms, nonneoplastic

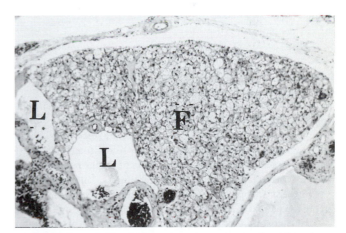

**FIGURE 4D-113.** Cystic hygroma or cavernous lymphangioma with thin-walled vascular spaces surrounding a lobule of immature fat (F) in the soft tissues of the neck in an infant. Note the presence of larger lymphatic spaces (L) pushing the fat aside. (*With permission, from Banks PM, Kraybill WG: Pathology for the Surgeon. Philadelphia, WB Saunders, 1996.*)

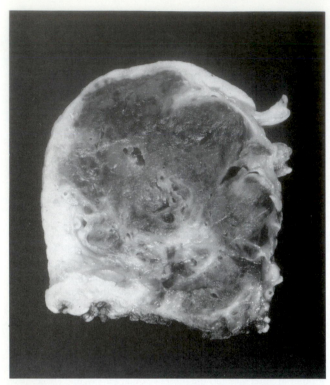

**FIGURE 4D-114.** Capillary hemangioma in the skin and soft tissues of an infant, showing a multinodular, reddish-brown mass with a predominantly solid appearance and focal cystic or cavernous areas. (*With permission, from Banks PM, Kraybill WG:* Pathology for the Surgeon. *Philadelphia, WB Saunders, 1996.*)

hamartomas, neuroectodermal neoplasms, soft tissue neoplasms, and thyroid-based masses.

CHEST WALL TUMORS. The chest wall and thoracic cavity, with their varied anatomy including soft tissues, bones, and visceral organs, are the sites and sources of a number of developmental and neoplastic disorders in children. Most of these conditions are distinctive for this age group. Chest wall masses or lesions in children range from the congenital melanocytic nevus of the so-called bathing trunk or giant type to neoplasms of the soft tissues. Rhabdomyosarcoma infrequently occurs in the soft tissues of the chest wall or thoracic cavity. With the exception of the Ewing's sarcoma–primitive neuroectodermal (EWS-PNET) tumors, most cutaneous and soft tissue neoplasms of the thoracic soft tissues are diagnosed before the patient is 2 years of age.

In 60% or more of patients, solid tumors of the mediastinum are Hodgkin's or non-Hodgkin's lymphoma of the anterior mediastinum or neuroblastic tumor of the posterior mediastinum.[139] Most children with mediastinal lymphoma are over 5 years of age at diagnosis. By contrast, the majority of children with thoracic neuroblastoma are 2 years of age or less. Most neuroblastic tumors in this location have favorable histologic features with evidence of differentiation.

In contrast to adults, neoplasms of the lung are uncommon in children. Inflammatory myofibroblastic tumor (so-called plasma cell granuloma) accounts for 40% to 50% of pulmonary tumors in the pediatric age population.[140] Most occur in children between the ages of 6 and 10 years as a solitary mass in the lower lobe. Although benign, they may be infiltrative. Lobectomy is the treatment of choice. A well-circumscribed, firm, gray-yellow to tan mass with or without grossly visible calcifications occupies the greater part of the resected lobe. Microscopically, there is a spindle cell proliferation representing myofibroblasts, variable numbers of plasma cells and lymphocytes and dense hypocellular collagen. Bronchial carcinoid is the most common primary malignant neoplasm of the lung in childhood. This tumor is not unique to children. In contrast, the rare so-called pleuropulmonary blastoma is seen only in the lung and thoracic cavity of children.[141] This tumor is composed of a complex intermixture of embryonal blastoma cells, spindle cells, immature rhabdomyoblasts, chondrosarcomatous nodules, and individual anaplastic cells. The prognosis for the solid, or predominantly solid, pleuropulmonary blastoma is poor.

RENAL NEOPLASMS AND NEUROBLASTOMA. Primary renal neoplasms (particularly Wilms' tumor) and neuroblastoma account for approximately 75% or more of intraabdominal malignant neoplasms in children. Less common intraabdominal malignancies include non-Hodgkin's malignant lymphoma of the small noncleaved cell type (Burkitt's lymphoma), hepatoblastoma, ovarian malignant germ cell neoplasm, rhabdomyosarcoma, intraabdominal desmoplastic small cell tumor, pancreatoblastoma, and EWS-PNET (pelvis and retroperitoneum).

Approximately 400 to 500 renal neoplasms are newly diagnosed in children each year in the United States. This is Wilms' tumor in 90% of patients.[142] Current therapy includes nephrectomy and chemotherapy with or without adjuvant radiation, depending upon the pathologic stage. The disease-free survival for this tumor is at least 80%. Wilms' tumor consists of a spectrum of renal neoplasms that occur in children. Although some may regress and are clinically inconsequential, others progress to become a malignant process with the potential to recur or metastasize.[143] Two tumor types with poor prognostic implications have emerged: clear cell sarcoma of the kidney (CCSK) and malignant rhabdoid tumor (MRT). Together these two neoplasms represented less than 10% of all renal tumors referred to the National Wilms' Tumor Study.[144] However, CCSK and MRT account for a disproportionate number of treatment failures and tumor-related deaths. Both neoplasms are histogenetically distinct from Wilms' tumor and its congeners. Although the prognosis of CCSK has steadily improved with intensified therapy, MRT remains one of the most treatment-resistant neoplasms of childhood.

Classic Wilms' tumor is a unilateral, circumscribed neoplasm that largely replaces the kidney with an eccentric compressed rim of renal tissue at the periphery of the mass (Fig. 4D-115). These tumors often weigh in excess of 300 g. Wilms' tumor is quite soft and is sometimes cystic and hemorrhagic. For these reasons, resection risks intraoperative rupture and spillage of tumor into the peritoneal cavity—an event that changes a potential stage I (a completely resected Wilms' tumor with an intact renal capsule and coned to the hilar plane) to stage III (an incompletely resected Wilms' tumor).[145]

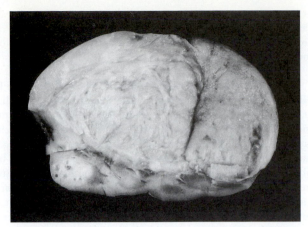

**FIGURE 4D-115.** Wilms' tumor, showing near complete replacement of the kidney by a soft gray-tan mass. (*With permission, from Banks PM, Kraybill WG:* Pathology for the Surgeon. *Philadelphia, WB Saunders, 1996.*)

The nephrectomy specimen should be submitted to the surgical pathology laboratory intact and unopened. Prior to sectioning, the external surface should be marked with India ink. This allows microscopic evaluation for invasion through the capsule.

Studies of the ontogeny of Wilms' tumor have identified a group of microscopic nephroblastic proliferations that are either progenitors of Wilms' tumor or have failed to evolve into a frankly malignant Wilms' tumor. A careful search for these lesions is important because their presence indicates risk for Wilms' tumor in the contralateral kidney (Fig. 4D-116).[143] On histologic grounds, it may be difficult to distinguish between a hyperplastic nephrogenic rest and an early Wilms' tumor.

Mesoblastic nephroma, CCSK, and MRT are the three monophasic neoplasms of the kidney in children.[146] As previously mentioned, the latter two neoplasms have histologic features distinct from those of classic Wilms' tumor. CCSK metastasizes to the skeletal system (40% of patients). In contrast, bony metastases are documented in only 3% to 4% of classic Wilms' tumors.[145] With the recognition of CCSK, an aggressive therapeutic approach has substantially reduced the frequency of bony metastasis, resulting in improved prognosis. In contrast, the MRT, a renal tumor typically diagnosed in children under 2 years of age, continues to be a treatment-resistant neoplasm. Grossly, CCSK and MRT resemble classic Wilms' tumor. Microscopic examination allows distinction. Although Wilms' tumor is composed of diverse elements, including some showing primitive tubule formation, the MRT is composed only of poorly organized plump oval cells with varying amounts of pink cytoplasm. Although it is important for the pathologist to note specific features for pathologic staging

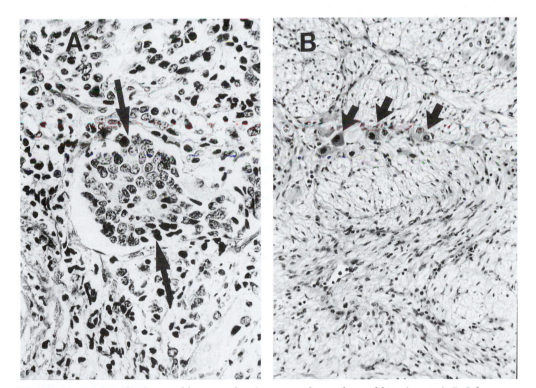

**FIGURE 4D-116.** *A.* Classic neuroblastoma, showing a central nest of neuroblasts (arrows). *B.* Other areas of the tumor, showing neuromatous stroma and ganglion cells (arrows) in various stages of maturation. (*With permission, from Banks PM, Kraybill WG:* Pathology for the Surgeon. *Philadelphia, WB Saunders, 1996.*)

of CCSK and MRT, these are less critical for making a treatment decision.

Congenital mesoblastic nephroma (CMN) was the first of the primary renal neoplasms of childhood to be recognized as an entity separate from classic Wilms' tumor.[146] In the past, CMN was referred to as "congenital Wilms' tumor" or "spindle cell Wilms' tumor." Not all CMNs are congenital, however, most are diagnosed in the first year of life as renal-based abdominal masses. In contrast to Wilms' tumor, the CMN replaces most of the affected kidney as a solitary circumscribed mass whose borders blend into the adjacent parenchyma. Microscopically, the CMN is composed of fascicles of uniform fusiform to ovoid spindle cells with entrapped tubules and glomeruli at the infiltrating interface. Nephrectomy is the treatment of choice. There is only occasional local recurrence, and metastasis is rare. The prognosis is excellent, and adjuvant therapy is rarely indicated.

Neuroblastoma is the second most common solid malignant neoplasm of childhood. It is exceeded in frequency only by brain tumors.[142] In the past 10 years progress has been made in the understanding of neuroblastomas from the perspective of molecular biology.[13,147] Most neuroblastomas show deletion of the short arm of chromosome 1 and amplification of N-*myc* oncogene on chromosome 2. Nuclear aneuploidy in a neuroblastoma connotes a favorable outcome. This is in stark contrast to the ominous implications carried by most aneuploid tumors in adults. Despite the advances in understanding these tumors on a molecular biologic level, the prognosis has not improved over the past 25 to 30 years. A spectrum of neuroblastic tumors exists ranging from poorly differentiated neuroblastoma to mature ganglioneuroblastoma.[148] Approximately 40% of neuroblastic tumors arise in the adrenal gland. The remainder arises in extraadrenal sites: retroperitoneum (25%), posterior mediastinum (15%), pelvis (5%), and neck (5%). A palpable abdominal mass is the most common clinical presentation. Among pediatric malignancies, neuroblastoma is one of the most diagnostically confounding upon presentation and, unfortunately, approximately half of afflicted children have metastatic disease at the time of diagnosis. Neuroblastoma, more than any other solid malignancy of childhood, presents clinically with metastasis and an occult primary source. Bone marrow, bone, lymph nodes, and liver are the most common metastatic sites. Urinary catecholamine levels are elevated in more than 90% of children with neuroblastoma, facilitating preoperative diagnosis.

In contrast to the surgeon's role in the definitive diagnosis and excision of Wilms' tumor, the surgeon's role in the management of patients with neuroblastoma is less clearly defined. Unlike Wilms' tumors, which are often amenable to complete resection, only a minority of cases of neuroblastoma are completely resectable. In most patients, the surgeon is asked to excise residual tumor following nonoperative therapy. Resection of these tumors is often technically demanding due to marked retroperitoneal fibrosis and matting of lymph nodes. Surgical margins are virtually impossible to assess because these tumors are excised piecemeal. Three pathologic indicators of poor prognosis are:

1. Lack of differentiation
2. High mitotic activity
3. Macroscopically visible nodules of neuroblasts surrounded by ganglioneuroma (nodular, stroma-rich neuroblastoma, composite ganglioneuroblastoma) (Fig. 4D-116).[148]

However, the most reliable prognostic indicators are age at diagnosis (less than versus greater than 1 year old) and pathologic stage.[149] A child under 1 year of age with localized resectable tumor has the most favorable outcome.

GERM CELL NEOPLASMS—TERATOMA AND RELATED NEOPLASMS. Growths presumably derived from the primordial germ cells (ovum and spermatogonium) are the quintessential tumors of childhood, with overlapping features of maldevelopment and neoplasia.[150] Attention to detail is critical for proper management. Among congenital neoplasms that are detectable in utero by ultrasonographic examination, the sacrococcygeal teratoma is the most common. Whether in children or adults, germ cell neoplasms are divided into distinct tumor types based upon microscopic features. These include pure teratoma, germinoma, embryonal carcinoma, endodermal sinus tumor, and choriocarcinoma or a mixed pattern with two or more type components.[150] By definition, any germ cell neoplasm with more than one pattern or type is malignant and is therefore designated as a malignant mixed germ cell neoplasm. In children, 65% to 75% of germ cell neoplasms originate in extragonadal locations in the following order of frequency: sacrococcygeum, mediastinum, central nervous system, head and neck, and retroperitoneum. Tumors of the sacrococcygeal and head and neck regions typically occur in children under the age of 2 years, whereas germ cell neoplasms in other extragonadal sites typically occur at a later age. Teratomas of the stomach and pericardium are seen almost exclusively in infants.

Sacrococcygeal teratoma accounts for 40% or more of germ cell neoplasms in children. Females are affected more commonly than males in a ratio of 3:1 to 4:1. A mass is apparent in 65% to 75% of patients at or shortly after birth (Fig. 4D-117). Only 2% to 3% of sacrococcygeal teratomas diagnosed in the neonatal and early infancy period have evidence of malignancy, usually in the form of endodermal sinus tumor (Fig. 4D-118). In contrast, 50% of sacrococcygeal teratomas prove malignant when the tumor is recognized after 1 year of age, and virtually all tumors are malignant if they escape detection until the patient is 4 to 5 years old.[151] Grossly, sacrococcygeal teratomas vary from a 6- to 12-cm mass composed of multiple collapsible cystic structures with mucoid contents to a much smaller cystic and solid or exclusively solid tumor (see Fig. 4D-117). The neuroepithelial component of the tumor corresponds grossly to soft grayish tan to white tissue with cerebroid features. Firm, infiltrative areas of hemorrhage and necrosis should raise concern about malignancy. However, in most cases of neonatal malignant sacrococcygeal teratomas, features indicating malignancy are difficult to appreciate by gross inspection. As is true for all large tumors, thorough sampling of sacrococcygeal teratoma is necessary. In general, one microscopic section is taken for each centimeter of maximum dimension of the tumor. One potential pitfall in the microscopic assessment of these large tumors is missing focal immature teratomatous elements, especially primitive neuroectoderm with foci of embryonic-appearing neural tubes and sheets of neuroblastic cells. These areas may be virtually indistinguishable from neuroblastoma. Some sacrococcygeal teratomas are dominated by immature neuroepithelium. More commonly, there is a mixture of immature and mature elements.

SOFT TISSUE NEOPLASMS. In a review by the Surveillance, Epidemiology, and End Results (SEER) Program, 8.5 soft tissue

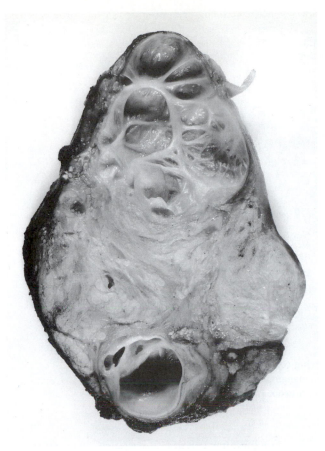

**FIGURE 4D-117.** Sacrococcygeal teratoma, presenting in a newborn female showing solid and cystic features. Many of the solid areas were composed of mature neuroglial tissue. (*With permission, from Banks PM, Kraybill WG: Pathology for the Surgeon. Philadelphia, WB Saunders, 1996.*)

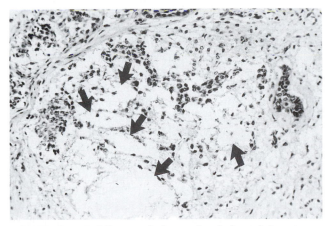

**FIGURE 4D-118.** Microscopic focus of endodermal sinus tumor in a sacrococcygeal teratoma presenting in a neonate. Note long delicate spaces resembling endodermal sinus structures (arrows). (*With permission, from Banks PM, Kraybill WG: Pathology for the Surgeon. Philadelphia, WB Saunders, 1996.*)

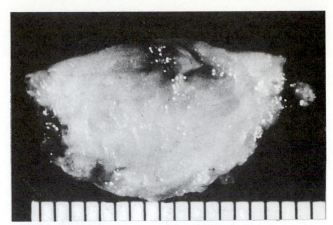

**FIGURE 4D-119.** Infantile myofibromatosis of the neck in an infant. The cut surface has a glistening trabeculated appearance and a nodular periphery. (*With permission, from Banks PM, Kraybill WG: Pathology for the Surgeon. Philadelphia, WB Saunders, 1996.*)

sarcomas per million children between the ages of 0 and 14 years were seen. In the first two decades of life, approximately 30% of all tumors were of vascular origin, consisting principally of capillary hemangiomas and cavernous lymphangiomas.[142] Nerve sheath, fibrous, myofibroblastic, and rhabdomyogenic neoplasms together accounted for 14% of the total. When age at diagnosis was restricted to the first year of life, vascular tumors were still the largest category (34% of patients), with fibrous and myofibroblastic tumors representing 27% of all tumors.[152]

Juvenile fibrous tumors actually encompass several distinct neoplasms that have a predilection for children, especially those who are less than 7 years old. The most common type of juvenile fibrous tumor is infantile myofibromatosis. This lesion occurs in infants as a solitary, firm cutaneous and/or subcutaneous mass measuring 1 to 3 cm in diameter (Fig. 4D-119). Less commonly the lesion is multifocal. The generalized form of infantile myofibromatosis has lesions in multiple organs, in addition to the soft tissues and bone. Obstruction of the pulmonary veins by these nodules may prove lethal. Microscopically, the tumor is composed of compact bundles or fascicles of spindle cells, less cellular areas with hyalinized stroma and, in some tumors, hemangiopericytoma-like foci (Fig. 4D-120). Necrosis and calcification reflect the tendency of these tumors to undergo spontaneous regression.

Rhabdomyosarcoma of the embryonal and alveolar subtypes is the most common soft tissue sarcoma in the first two decades of life.[153] Of childhood sarcomas, 45% to 55% are rhabdomyosarcomas. In the past, the category of "undifferentiated sarcoma" or "malignant small cell tumor of indeterminate histogenesis" was the second most frequent type of soft tissue sarcoma in children. Later studies have permitted the correct identification of most of these tumors as either soft tissue Ewing's sarcoma or primitive neuroectodermal tumor (EWS-PNET). Juvenile rhabdomyosarcomas, in particular the embryonal type (50% to 60% of patients), have a predilection for the head and neck region (45% of patients) and genitourinary tract (25% of patients).[153] Embryonal rhabdomyosarcoma may appear as a polypoid mass (so-called sarcoma botryoides)

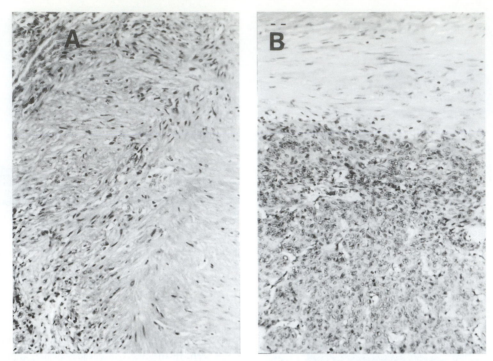

**FIGURE 4D-120.** *A.* Infantile myofibromatosis, showing contiguous spindle cell and hyalinized areas. *B.* Another area of the same tumor showing a hemangiopericytoma-like pattern. (*With permission, from Banks PM, Kraybill WG:* Pathology for the Surgeon. *Philadelphia, WB Saunders, 1996.*)

in the middle ear, nasopharynx, urinary bladder, and vagina, or as a solid mass. Microscopically these neoplasms are composed of delicate blastic cells with subtle patterns produced by polarization of spindling cells and variations in cellular density (Fig. 4D-121). Another distinction is that liposarcoma and malignant fibrous histiocy-

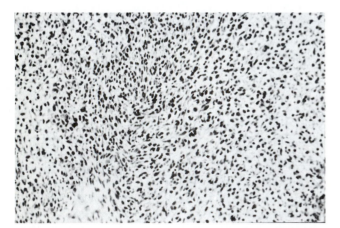

**FIGURE 4D-121.** Embryonal rhabdomyosarcoma of the nasopharynx showing the uniform primitive cellular composition of this neoplasm. (*With permission, from Banks PM, Kraybill WG:* Pathology for the Surgeon. *Philadelphia, WB Saunders, 1996.*)

toma, which constitute 35% to 45% of all adult soft tissue sarcomas, are uncommon in children.

Alveolar rhabdomyosarcoma is a particularly aggressive, potentially lethal type of juvenile rhabdomyosarcoma. Long-term survival is only 40% to 50%. This contrasts with the more favorable embryonal type of rhabdomyosarcoma that has an overall survival of 70%. Patients with the alveolar type of tumor are generally older (late childhood, adolescence, and young adulthood) than children with embryonal rhabdomyosarcoma, who are usually diagnosed before 10 years of age. A small subset of alveolar tumors can present disseminated and can mimic hematopoietic neoplasms with generalized lymphadenopathy, bone lesions, and pleural effusions. A biopsy or needle aspiration sample may be misinterpreted microscopically, since the cells are delicate and uniform and may lack an obvious alveolar pattern. Differential immunohistochemistry and cytogenetics allow recognition as alveolar rhabdomyosarcoma with its expression of myogenous filament proteins and characteristic reciprocal translocation t(2;13) (q35;q14), respectively.

EWS-PNET is now considered a single family of closely related small round cell neoplasms.[13,154] These tumors have a common reciprocal translocation, t(11,22) (q24;q12) in 80% to 90% of patients. Typically, the tumor is greater than 6 to 8 cm and is often cystic and hemorrhagic. Microscopically, there is either a geographic arrangement of cohesive small cells with or without rosette formation or formless sheets or nests of infiltrating cells. When strict microscopic criteria are applied to distinguish between EWS and PNET, the latter is the more aggressive of the two neoplasms. Electron microscopy, immunohistochemistry, and cytogenetics accurately differentiate EWS-PNET from the other small cell neoplasms of childhood. Because EWS-PNETs typically spread hematogenously early in their course, and because of their sensitivity to both radiation and chemotherapy, resection alone is no longer acceptable for clinical management.

## REFERENCES

1. BANKS PM, KRAYBILL WG: *Pathology for the Surgeon.* Philadelphia, Saunders, 1996.
2. FECHNER R: Immediate management of mammographically detected breast lesions. Am J Clin Pathol 100:92, 1993.
3. BANKS PM: Pathology is more than just microscopy. Am J Clin Pathol 103:3, 1995.
4. CULLEN TS: A rapid method of making permanent specimens from frozen sections by the use of formalin. Johns Hopkins Hosp Bull 67, 1895.
5. MacCARTY WC, BRODERS AC: Studies in clinico-pathologic standardization and efficiency. I. Legitimate actual error in diagnosis of mammary conditions. Surg Gynecol Obstet 25:666, 1917.
6. NICHOLS L et al: Are autopsies obsolete? Am J Clin Pathol 110:210, 1998.
7. FLEMING ID et al (eds): *AJCC Cancer Staging Manual,* 5th ed. Philadelphia, Lippincott-Raven, 1997.
8. FRABLE WJ: Fine needle aspiration biopsy, in *Pathology for the Surgeon,* PM Banks, WG Kraybill (eds). Philadelphia, Saunders, 1996, pp 33–45.
9. WICK MR: Special techniques in surgical pathology, in *Pathology for the Surgeon,* PM Banks, WG Kraybill (eds). Philadelphia, Saunders, 1996, pp 20–32.
10. JENNINGS CD, FOON KA: Recent advances in flow cytometry: Application to the diagnosis of hematologic malignancy. Blood 90:2863, 1997.
11. BRIFFOD M et al: Evaluation of breast carcinomas chemosensitivity by flow cytometric DNA analysis and computer-assisted image analysis. Cytometry 13:250, 1992.
12. TALLINI G et al: Combined morphologic and karyotypic study of 28 myxoid liposarcomas. Am J Surg Pathol 20:1047, 1996.
13. DEHNER LP: The evolution of the diagnosis and understanding of primitive and embryonic neoplasms in children: Living through an epoch. Mod Pathol 11:669, 1998.
14. PULITZER DR et al: The skin, in *Pathology for the Surgeon,* PM Banks, WG Kraybill (eds). Philadelphia, Saunders, 1996, pp 46–58.
15. CLARK WH JR et al: A study of tumor progression: The precursor lesions of superficial spreading and nodular melanoma. Hum Pathol 15:1147, 1984.
16. BRESLOW A: Thickness, cross-sectional areas and depth of invasion in the prognosis of cutaneous melanoma. Ann Surg 172:902, 1970.
17. VERONESI U, CASCINELLI N: Narrow excision (1-cm margin): A safe procedure for thin cutaneous melanoma. Arch Surg 126:438, 1991.
18. CASEY TT et al: Stratified approach to fine needle aspiration of the breast. Am J Surg 163:305, 1992.
19. ABRAHAM SC et al: Sampling of grossly benign breast reexcisions. Am J Surg Pathol 23:316, 1999.
20. TETU B et al: p53 and c-erbB-2 as markers of resistance to adjuvant chemotherapy in breast cancer. Mod Pathol 11:823, 1998.
21. TURNER RR et al: Optimal histopathologic examination of the sentinel lymph node for breast carcinoma staging. Am J Surg Pathol 23:263, 1999.
22. RUBIN E et al: Proliferative disease and atypia in biopsies performed for mammographically detected nonpalpable lesions. Cancer 61:2077, 1988.
23. FITZGIBBONS PL et al: Benign breast changes and the risk for subsequent breast cancer: An update of the 1985 consensus statement. Arch Pathol Lab Med 122:1053, 1998.
24. FLEMING JD et al: *American Joint Committee on Cancer: Manual for Staging of Cancer,* 5th ed. Philadelphia, Saunders, 1997.
25. BARNES L, JOHNSON JT: Pathological and clinical considerations in the evaluation of major head and neck specimens resected for cancer, part I, in *Pathology Annual,* Vol 21, SC Somers et al (eds). Norwalk, CT, Appleton-Century-Crofts, 1986, p 173.
26. FRIERSON HF JR, COOPER PH: Prognostic factors in squamous cell carcinoma of the lower lip. Hum Pathol 17:346, 1986.
27. MEDINA JE et al: Verrucous-squamous carcinoma of the oral cavity: A clinicopathologic study of 104 cases. Arch Otolaryngol 110:437, 1984.
28. LOPES MBS et al: The nervous system, in *Pathology for the Surgeon.* PM Banks, WG Kraybill (eds). Philadelphia, Saunders, 1996, pp 99–124.
29. DAUMAS-DUPORT C et al: A histologic and cytologic method for the spatial definition of gliomas. Mayo Clin Proc 62:435, 1987.
30. MARTINEZ AJ et al: Touch preparations in the rapid intraoperative diagnosis of central nervous system lesions: A comparison with frozen sections and paraffin-embedded sections. Mod Pathol 1:378, 1988.
31. KLEIHUES P et al: *Histologic Typing of Tumours of the Central Nervous System,* 2d ed. Berlin, Springer-Verlag, 1993.
32. BURGER PC, SCHEITHAUER BW: Tumors of the central nervous system, in *Atlas of Tumor Pathology,* 3d Series, Fascicle 10. Washington, DC, Armed Forces Institute of Pathology; 1994.
33. ZULCH DJ: *Brain Tumors: Their Biology and Pathology,* 3d ed. Berlin, Springer-Verlag; 1986.
34. ZEIGER MA, HRUBAN RH: Endocrine pathology, in *Pathology for the Surgeon,* PM Banks, WG Kraybill (eds). Philadelphia, Saunders, 1996, pp 125–133.
35. GHARIB H, GOELLNER J: Fine-needle aspiration biopsy of the thyroid: An appraisal. Ann Intern Med 118:282, 1993.
36. GRANT C et al: Long-term follow-up of patients with benign thyroid fine-needle aspiration cytologic diagnoses. Surgery 106:980, 1989.
37. TIELENS ET et al: Follicular variant of papillary thyroid carcinoma: A clinicopthologic study. Cancer 73:424, 1994.
38. EDIS A et al: *Manual of Endocrine Surgery,* 2d ed. New York, Springer-Verlag, 1975, p 238.
39. ARNOLD A et al: Monoclonality and abnormal parathyroid hormone genes in parathyroid adenomas. N Engl J Med 318:658, 1989.
40. AKERSTROM G et al: Surgical anatomy of human parathyroid glands. Surgery 95:14, 1984.
41. OBARA T et al: Functioning parathyroid carcinoma: Clinicopathologic features and rational treatment. Semin Surg Oncol 13:134, 1997.
42. HAKAIM AG, ESSELSTYN CB: Parathyroid carcinoma: 50-year experience at the Cleveland Clinic. Cleveland Clin J Med 60:331, 1993.

43. HERF S et al: Identification and differentiation of surgically correctable hypertension due to primary aldosteronism. Am J Med 67:397, 1979.

44. NOTH R, BIGLIERI E: Primary hyperaldosteronism. Med Clin North Am 72:1117, 1988.

45. VAN SLOOTEN H et al: Morphologic characteristics of benign and malignant adrenocortical lesions. Cancer 55:766, 1985.

46. WEISS L et al: Pathologic features of prognostic significance in adrenocortical carcinoma. Am J Surg Pathol 13:202, 1989.

47. HARRIS NL, WILKINS EW: The mediastinum, in *Pathology for the Surgeon.* PM Banks, WG Kraybill (eds). Philadelphia, Saunders, 1996, pp 135–153.

48. QUINTANILLA-MARTINEZ L et al: Thymoma: Morphologic subclassification correlates with invasiveness and immunohistologic features: A study of 122 cases. Hum Pathol 24:958, 1993.

49. QUINTANILLA-MARTINEZ L et al: Thymoma: Histologic classification predicts clinical behavior. Cancer 74:606, 1994.

50. KAPLAN H: Hodgkin's Disease, 2d ed. Cambridge, MA, Harvard University Press, 1978.

51. JACOBSON J et al: Mediastinal large cell lymphoma: An uncommon subset of adult lymphoma curable with combined modality therapy. Cancer 62:1893, 1988.

52. YOUSEM S et al: Primary mediastinal non-Hodgkins lymphomas: A morphologic and immunologic study of 19 cases. Am J Clin Pathol 83:676, 1985.

53. NATHWANI B et al: Lymphoblastic lymphoma: A clinicopathologic study of 95 patients. Cancer 48:2347, 1981.

54. WICK M: The mediastinum, in *Textbook of Surgical Pathology,* S Sternberg (ed). New York, Raven Press, 1989, pp 1135–1182.

55. COLBY TV, DESCHAMPS C: The lung and pleura, in *Pathology for the Surgeon,* PM Banks, WG Kraybill (eds). Philadelphia, Saunders, 1996, pp 155–168.

56. GAZDAR AF, LINNOILA RL: The pathology of lung cancer: changing concepts and newer diagnostic techniques. Semin Oncol 15:215, 1988.

57. TRAVIS WD et al: Neuroendocrine tumors of the lung with proposed criteria for large-cell neuroendocrine carcinoma: An ultrastructural, immunohistochemical, and flow cytometric study of 35 cases. Am J Surg Pathol 15:529, 1991.

58. MCCAUGHEY WTE et al: Diagnosis of diffuse malignant mesothelioma: experience of a US/Canadian panel. Mod Pathol 4:342, 1991.

59. WOLBER RA, SCUDAMORE CH: The gastrointestinal tract, in *Pathology for the Surgeon,* PM Banks, WG Kraybill (eds). Philadelphia, Saunders, 1996, pp 169–198.

60. WONG HH et al: Comparative features of esophageal and gastric adenocarcinomas: Recent changes in type and frequency. Hum Pathol 17:482, 1986.

61. GOLDSTEIN NS et al: Disparate surgical margin lengths of colorectal resection specimens between *in vivo* and *in vitro* measurements. Am J Clin Pathol 111:349, 1999.

62. HAGGIT RC et al: Prognostic factors in colorectal carcinomas arising in adenomas: Implications for lesions removed by endoscopic polypectomy. Gastroenterol 89:328, 1985.

63. MOERTEL CG et al: Carcinoid tumor of the appendix: Treatment and prognosis. N Engl J Med 317:1699, 1987.

64. NORHEIM I et al: Malignant carcinoid tumors: An analysis of 103 patients with regards to tumor localization, hormone production, and survival. Ann Surg 206:115, 1987.

65. WOTHERSPOON AC et al: Regression of primary low grade B-cell gastric lymphoma of mucosa associated lymphoid tissue type after eradication of *Helicobacter pylori.* Lancet 342:575, 1993.

66. AZAB MB et al: Prognostic factors in primary gastrointestinal non-Hodgkin's lymphoma: A multivariate analysis, report of 106 cases, and review of the literature. Cancer 64:1208, 1989.

67. HJERMSTEAD BM: Stromal tumors of the gastrointestinal tract: Myogenic or neurogenic? Am J Surg Pathol 11:383, 1987.

68. EMORY TS et al: Prognosis of gastrointestinal smooth-muscle (stromal) tumors. Am J Surg Pathol 23:82, 1999.

69. ALBORES-SAAVEDRA J, SNYDER WH: The liver, biliary tract, and pancreas, in *Pathology for the Surgeon,* PM Banks, WG Kraybill (eds). Philadelphia, Saunders, 1996, pp 199–216.

70. CHOI BI et al: Small hepatocellular carcinoma versus small cavernous hemangioma: Differentiation with MR imaging at 2.0 $T_1$. Radiology 176:103, 1990.

71. ISHAK KG et al: Epithelioid hemangioendothelioma of the liver: A clinicopathologic and follow-up study of 32 cases. Hum Pathol 165:839, 1984.

72. WANDS JR, BLUM HE: Primary hepatocellular carcinoma. N Engl J Med 325:729, 1991.

73. YUKI N et al: Hepatitis B virus markers and antibodies to hepatitis C virus in Japanese patients with hepatocellular carcinoma. Dig Dis Sci 37:65, 1992.

74. KANAI T et al: Pathology of small hepatocellular carcinoma. Cancer 60:810, 1987.

75. LACK EE et al: Hepatoblastoma: A clinical and pathologic study of 54 cases. Am J Surg Pathol 6:693, 1982.

76. GANJEI P et al: Histologic markers in primary and metastatic tumors of the liver. Cancer 62:1994, 1988.

77. ASHUR H et al: Calcified gallbladder (porcelain gallbladder). Arch Surg 113:594, 1978.

78. WIESNER RH et al: Diagnosis and treatment of primary sclerosing cholangitis. Semin Liver Dis 5:241, 1985.

79. ALBORES-SAAVEDRA J, HENSON DE: Tumors of the gallbladder and extrahepatic bile ducts, in *Atlas of Tumor Pathology,* 2d series, fascicle 22, WH Hartman (ed). Washington, DC, Armed Forces Institute of Pathology, 1986.

80. EDOUTE Y et al: Preoperative and intraoperative fine needle aspiration cytology of pancreatic lesions. Am J Gastroenterol 86:1015, 1991.

81. WARSHAW AL et al: Pancreatic carcinoma. N Engl J Med 326:455, 1992.

82. URBAN T et al: Detection of c-Ki-ras mutation by PCR/RFLP analysis and diagnosis of pancreatic adenocarcinomas. J Natl Cancer Inst 85:2008, 1993.

83. MILCHGRUB S et al: Intraductal carcinoma of the pancreas: A report of four cases. Cancer 69:651, 1992.

84. ALBORES-SAAVEDRA J et al: The pancreas, in *The Pathology of Incipient Neoplasia,* 2d ed. DE Henson, J Albores-Saavedra (eds). Philadelphia, Saunders, 1993.

85. KLOPPEL G, HEITZ PU: Pancreatic endocrine tumors. Pathol Res Pract 183:155, 1988.

86. BOSTWICK DG, OESTERLING IE: The urologic and male reproductive systems, in *Pathology for the Surgeon,* PM Banks, WG Kraybill (eds). Philadelphia, Saunders, 1996, pp 217–233.

87. EBLE JN (ed): *Tumors and Tumor-like Conditions of the Kidneys and Ureters.* New York, Churchill Livingstone, 1990.

88. MURPHY WM et al: Tumors of the urinary bladder, urethra, ureters, renal pelvis, and kidneys, in *Atlas of Tumor Pathology,* 2nd series, fascicle 11. Washington, DC, Armed Forces Institute of Pathology, 1994.

89. STILLWELL TJ et al: The clinical spectrum of granulomatous prostatitis: A report of 200 cases. J Urol 138:320, 1987.

90. MCNEAL JE, BOSTWICK DG: Anatomy of the prostate: Implications for disease, in *Pathology of the Prostate,* DG Bostwick (ed). New York, Churchill Livingstone, 1990, pp 1–14.

91. HENSON DE et al: Practice protocol for the examination of specimens removed from patients with carcinoma of the prostate gland: A publication of the cancer committee. College of American Pathologists. Arch Pathol Lab Med 118:779, 1994.

92. GRAHAM SD et al: Report of the committee on staging and pathology. Cancer 70(Suppl):359, 1992.

93. BOSTWICK DG: High grade prostatic intraepithelial neoplasia: The most likely precursor of prostatic adenocarcinoma. Cancer 75:1823, 1995.

94. BOSTWICK DG: Gleason grading of prostatic needle biopsies: Correlation with grade in 316 matched prostatectomies. Am J Surg Pathol 18:796, 1994.

95. GLEASON DF: Histologic grading of prostatic carcinoma, in *Pathology of the Prostate,* DG Bostwick (ed). New York, Churchill Livingstone, 1990, pp 83–93.

96. HALL GS et al: Evaluation of radical prostatectomy specimens: A comparative analysis of sampling methods. Am J Surg Pathol 16:315, 1992.

97. BOSTWICK DG et al: Staging of prostate cancer. Semin Surg Oncol 10:60, 1994.

98. RICHIE JP et al: Ultrasonography as a diagnostic adjunct for the evaluation of masses in the scrotum. Surg Gynecol Obstet 154:695, 1982.

99. SILVERBERG SG, Lyn JY: Obstetric and gynecologic pathology, in *Pathology for the Surgeon,* PM Banks, WG Kraybill (eds). Philadelphia, Saunders, 1996, pp 234–251.

100. YOUNG RH, SCULLY RE: Metastatic tumors in the ovary: A problem-oriented approach and review of the recent literature. Semin Diagn Pathol 8:250, 1991.

101. KATSUBE Y et al: Epidemiologic pathology of ovarian tumors: A histopathologic review of primary ovarian neoplasms diagnosed in the Denver Standard Metropolitan Statistical Area, 1 July–31 December 1969 and 1 July–31 December 1979. Int J Gynecol Pathol 1:3, 1982.

102. SCULLY RE: Tumors of the ovary and maldeveloped gonads. *Atlas of Tumor Pathology,* 2d series, fascicle 16. Washington, DC, Armed Forces Institute of Pathology, 1979.

103. BOSTWICK DG et al: Ovarian epithelial tumors of borderline malignancy: A clinical and pathologic study of 109 cases. Cancer 58:2052, 1986.

104. VOLLENHOVEN B et al: Uterine fibroids: A clinical review. Br J Obstet Gynaecol 97:285, 1990.

105. ZAINO RJ et al: The prognostic value of nuclear versus architectural grading in endometrial adenocarcinoma: A Gynecologic Oncology Group study. Int J Gynecol Pathol 13:29, 1994.

106. FROMM GL et al: Papillary serous carcinoma of the peritoneum. Obstet Gynecol 75:89, 1990.

107. BANKS PM, PAGE CP: The hematolymphoid system, in *Pathology for the Surgeon,* PM Banks, WG Kraybill (eds). Philadelphia, Saunders, 1996, pp 267–284.

108. HAAGENSEN CD et al: *The Lymphatics in Cancer,* Philadelphia, PA: Saunders; 1972.

109. KJELDSBERG C et al: Hematopoiesis: Peripheral blood and bone marrow examination, in *Practical Diagnosis of Hematologic Disorders,* C Kjeldsberg (ed). Chicago, ASCP Press, 1991, pp 1–16.

110. HARMENING DM: Introduction to hemostasis: An overview of hemostatic mechanisms, platelet structure and function, and extrinsic and intrinsic systems, in *Clinical Hematology and Fun-*

*damentals of Hemostasis,* DM Harmening (ed). Philadelphia, FA Davis, 1992, pp 415–439.

111. BANKS PM, PAGE CP: The hematolymphoid system, in *Pathology for the Surgeon,* PM Banks, WG Kraybill (eds). Philadelphia, Saunders, 1996, pp 269ff.

112. The Non-Hodgkin's Lymphoma Pathology Classfication Project: National Cancer Institute sponsored study of classifications of non-Hodgkin's lymphomas: Summary and description of a Working Formulation for Clinical Usage. Cancer 49:2112, 1982.

113. HARRIS NL et al: A revised European-American classification of lymphoid neoplasms: A proposal from the International Lymphoma Study Group. Blood 84:1361, 1994.

114. BANKS PM, ISAACSON PG: MALT lymphomas in 1997: Where do we stand? Am J Clin Pathol 111(Suppl):75, 1999.

115. CRAIG FE et al: Posttransplantation lymphoproliferative disorders. Am J Clin Pathol 99:265, 1993.

116. MONTGOMERY EA et al: Soft tissue tumors, in *Pathology for the Surgeon,* PM Banks, WG Kraybill (eds). Philadelphia, Saunders, 1996, pp 285–300.

117. LASKIN WB et al: Postradiation soft tissue sarcomas: An analysis of 53 cases. Cancer 62:2330, 1988.

118. MALKIN D et al: Germline p53 mutations in a familial syndrome of breast cancer, sarcomas, and other neoplasms. Science 250:1233, 1990.

119. SUIT HD et al: Treatment of the patients with stage $M_o$ soft tissue sarcoma. J Clin Oncol 6:854, 1988.

120. COSTA J et al: The grading of soft tissue sarcoma: Results of a clinicopathologic correlation in a series of 163 cases. Cancer 53:530, 1984.

121. WEISS SW: *Histological Typing of Soft Tissue Tumors,* 2nd ed, in *World Health Organization Series of International Histological Classification of Tumours,* LH Sobin (ed). Berlin, Springer-Verlag, 1994.

122. BRABANT B et al: Dermatofibrosarcoma protuberans of the chest and shoulder: Wide and deep excisions with immediate reconstruction. Plast Reconstr Surg 92:459, 1993.

123. ENZINGER FM: Clear cell sarcoma of tendons and aponeuroses: An analysis of 21 cases. Cancer 18:1163, 1965.

124. FLETCHER JA: Translocation (12;22) (q13-14;q12) is a nonrandom aberration in soft tissue clear cell sarcoma. Genes Chromosom Cancer 5:184, 1992.

125. EVANS HL, BAER SC: Epithelioid sarcoma: A clinicopathologic and prognostic study of 26 cases. Semin Diagn Pathol 10:286, 1993.

126. ROCK MG, UNNI KK: Tumors and tumor-like conditions of bones and joints, in *Pathology for the Surgeon,* PM Banks, WG Kraybill (eds). Philadelphia, Saunders, 1996, pp 301–323.

127. DESANTOS LA et al: Computed tomography in the evaluation of musculoskeletal neoplasms. Radiology 128:89, 1978.

128. MANKIN HJ et al: The hazards of biopsy in patients with malignant primary bone and soft-tissue tumors. J Bone Joint Surg (Am) 64:1121, 1982.

129. STOKER DJ et al: Needle biopsy of musculoskeletal lesions: A review of 208 procedures. J Bone Joint Surg (Br) 73:498, 1991.

130. DAHLIN DC, UNNI KK: *Bone Tumors: General Aspects and Data on 8,542 Cases,* 4th ed. Springfield, IL, Charles C Thomas, 1986.

131. OSTROWSKI ML et al: Malignant lymphoma of bone. Cancer 58:2646, 1986.

132. SKANDALAKIS JE, GRAY SW (eds): *Embryology for Surgeons,* 2d ed. Baltimore, Williams & Wilkins, 1994.

133. DEHNER LP: Special considerations for the pediatric patient,

in *Pathology for the Surgeon,* PM Banks, WG Kraybill (eds). Philadelphia, Saunders, 1996, pp 339–359.

134. Bolande RP: Neoplasia of early life and its relationships to teratogenesis. Perspect Pediatr Pathol 3:145, 1976.

135. Coppes MJ et al: Genetic events in the development of Wilms' tumor. N Engl J Med 331:586, 1994.

136. Bodenstein L, Altman RP: Cervical lymphadenitis in infants and children. Semin Pediatr Surg 3:134, 1994.

137. Filston HC: Hemangiomas, cystic hygromas, and teratomas of the head and neck. Semin Pediatr Surg 3:147, 1994.

138. Silverman RA: Hemangiomas and vascular malformations. Pediatr Clin North Am 38:811, 1991.

139. Azarow KS et al: Primary mediastinal masses: A comparison of adult and pediatric populations. J Thorac Cardiovasc Surg 106:67, 1993.

140. Stocker JT, Dehner LP: Acquired neonatal and pediatric diseases, in *Pulmonary Pathology,* 2nd ed, DH Dall, SP Hammar (eds). New York, Springer-Verlag, 1993, pp 191–254.

141. Dehner LP et al: Pleuropulmonary blastoma: A unique intrathoracic-pulmonary neoplasm of childhood. Perspect Pediatr Pathol 18:214, 1995.

142. Robison LL: General principles of the epidemiology of childhood cancer, in *Principles and Practice of Pediatric Oncology,* PA Pizzo, DG Poplack (eds). Philadelphia, Lippincott, 1993, pp 3–21.

143. Beckwith JB et al: Nephrogenic rests, nephroblastomatosis and the pathogenesis of Wilms' tumor. Pediatr Pathol 10:1, 1990.

144. Beckwith JB, Palmer NF: Histopathology and prognosis of Wilms' tumor. Results from the First Wilms Tumor Study. Cancer 41:1937, 1978.

145. Beckwith JB: Renal neoplasms of childhood, in *Diagnostic Surgical Pathology,* 2nd ed. SS Sternberg (ed). New York, Raven Press, 1994, pp 1741–1766.

146. Kissane JM, Dehner LP: Renal tumor and tumor-like lesions in pediatric patients. Pediatr Nephrol 6:365, 1992.

147. Brodeur GM: Molecular biology and genetics of human neuroblastoma, in *Neuroblastoma Tumor Biology and Therapy,* C Pochedly (ed). Boca Raton, FL, CRC Press, 1989, pp 31–42.

148. Dehner LP: Pathologic anatomy of classic neuroblastoma including prognostic features and differential diagnosis, in *Neuroblastoma: Tumor Biology and Therapy,* C Pochedly (ed). Boca Raton, FL, CRC Press, 1989, pp 112–119.

149. Brodeur GM et al: Revisions of the international criteria for neuroblastoma diagnosis, staging and response to treatment. J Clin Oncol 11:1466, 1993.

150. Dehner LP: Gonadal and extragonadal germ cell neoplasms: Teratomas in childhood, in *Pathology of Neoplasia in Children and Adolescents,* M Finegold (ed). Philadelphia, Saunders, 1986, pp 282–298.

151. Schropp KP et al: Sacrococcygeal teratoma: The experience of four decades. J Pediatr Surg 27:1075, 1992.

152. Coffin CM, Dehner LP: Soft tissue tumors in first year of life: A report of 190 cases. Pediatr Pathol 10:509, 1990.

153. Raney RB et al: Rhabdomyosarcoma and the undifferentiated sarcomas, in *Principles and Practice of Pediatric Oncology,* 2nd ed, PA Pizzo, DG Poplack (eds). Philadelphia, Lippincott, 1993, pp 769–782.

154. Delattre O et al: The Ewing family of tumors: A subgroup of small-round-cell tumors defined by specific chimeric transcripts. N Engl J Med 331:294, 1994.

# CHAPTER 5

# SPECIAL DIAGNOSTIC AND THERAPEUTIC TECHNIQUES

## 5A / LAPAROSCOPY IN MALIGNANT DISEASES

*G. Dean Roye and Joseph F. Amaral*

## INTRODUCTION

The origin of laparoscopy can be traced to Bozzini of Frankfurt, who in 1805 placed a tube illuminated by a candle into the urethra of a male to examine the bladder.[1] By 1843, the first effective cystoscope designed by Desormeaux was operational.[2] Jacobaeus, in 1910, used a cystoscope to perform the first laparoscopy and thoracoscopy in a human, 9 years after Keeling had introduced the concept by performing celioscopy in a dog.[3] In the United States, the first laparoscopy was performed by Bernard M. Bernheim[4] at the Johns Hopkins Hospital on a patient with pancreatic cancer on the surgical service supervised by Dr. William Halsted. The patient was correctly staged as having no visible metastatic disease and underwent a pancreatic resection. Despite numerous subsequent breakthroughs in technology such as the development of the Hopkins lens system, fiberoptics, and operative instruments, diagnostic and therapeutic laparoscopy were rarely utilized by general surgeons. Indeed, in 1972, Dr. W. T. Mosenthal[5] noted that it was curious that such a direct and reliable approach was not more widely applied. However, the rapid technologic advancements of the 1980s and early 1990s have brought recognition of the valuable and important role that diagnostic laparoscopy exerts in the management of malignancy. Today, laparoscopy is used to diagnose and stage intraabdominal malignancies, monitor the effectiveness of adjuvant therapy, and provide supportive measures, such as placement of intestinal feeding tubes and intestinal diversion in patients with intraabdominal malignancy.

## GENERAL APPROACH

All patients undergoing laparoscopy should receive perioperative antibiotics, compression stockings, and intraoperative nasogastric, orogastric, and bladder decompression. These measures reduce the morbidity of the procedure. The risk of infection for diagnostic laparoscopy is small. However, initiation of laparoscopy through the potentially unclean umbilicus is a possible source of postoperative infection.[6] The risk of deep venous thrombophlebitis and subsequent pulmonary embolism is also low, but the elevation in intraabdominal pressure during insufflation reduces venous return and thus increases risk.[7] Compression stockings objectively enhance venous return, thereby diminishing venous stasis.[7] Gastric and bladder decompression are simple measures that minimize the risk of gastric and urinary bladder perforation during the initiation of laparoscopy. Furthermore, these measures prevent distention of these organs during the procedure, thereby improving visualization of intraabdominal structures.

Overall, the morbidity and mortality of a diagnostic laparoscopy is very small. The reported incidence of major complications is 0.006%[8] and of minor complications less than 5%.[9] Mortality is extremely rare, with reported incidences of 0.005% to 0.3%.[8–10]

General anesthesia is preferred for these procedures, although local anesthesia is an alternative. Local anesthesia with infiltration of the trocar sites is best tolerated when the procedure is of short duration, the volume of insufflation is small (<1 L of gas) and a 5-mm laparoscope is used. Nitrous oxide is often chosen as the insufflating gas with the local anesthesia technique to minimize the abdominal and shoulder pain that ensues with carbon dioxide insufflation.[11] However, the explosive nature of nitrous oxide obviates the use of electrosurgery or laser surgery. Thus, local anesthesia with or without nitrous oxide is best suited for the brief diagnostic procedure (e.g., simple biopsy) that can be performed with a small volume of insufflation. Unfortunately, a thorough evaluation often cannot be performed under these conditions, and the information gathered may be nondiagnostic. Therefore, we favor general anesthesia.

## TECHNIQUE

An open or closed technique may be used to obtain access to the abdominal cavity. Regardless of technique, additional laparoscopic cannulas are placed under direct vision as needed. Usually, at least two additional cannulas are necessary for complete inspection of the abdominal cavity, intestine, and retroperitoneum. However, biopsy of visible liver masses may be performed using only a percutaneous Trucut biopsy needle without use of auxiliary cannulas. Alternatively, biopsy of the mass can be performed via a 5-mm cannula using biopsy forceps. In either case, these small biopsies usually do not result in significant bleeding or the need for ancillary coagulation methods. When the situation does arise, electrosurgery via a shielded instrument, the ultrasonically activated scalpel, or microfibrillar collagen, alone or in combination, are virtually always effective hemostatic measures.

Cytologic evaluation of ascites is an important method in evaluating the patient with intraabdominal malignancy. Fluid should be procured prior to any technical manipulation that may cause bleeding. If no ascites is present, the abdomen is irrigated with 200 to 300 mL of 0.9% normal saline and aspirated to obtain a fluid specimen for cytology. This can be achieved by attaching a Lueken's trap to the suction tubing. Using cytologic examination, Warshaw et al.[12] showed positive cytology was associated with a low (10%) resectability rate for pancreatic cancer.

Tumor implantation and seeding during laparoscopic surgery should be of serious concern to the operator. Numerous case reports cite tumor implantation at trocar sites for operations of various solid tumors.[13] Experimental tumor implantation in animal models has been observed to be accelerated at sites of peritoneal disruption.[14] However, agents such as heparin, which reduce cell adherence, are noted to diminish tumor implantation in these models. These data suggest that heparin should be added to the irrigant solution when oncologic laparoscopic surgery is conducted. We routinely add 5000 units of heparin to a liter of normal saline. Dilute povodine-iodine (1:10 dilution with saline) has also been shown to eliminate trocar site tumor implantation in laboratory models.[15] To avoid the theoretical risk of tumor seeding, the specimen is placed in one of many commercially available specimen bags and retrieved via one of the cannula sites under direct visualization.

## PORT SITE METASTASIS

Much has been made about port site metastasis in laparoscopy either for unsuspected malignancies or after staging or treatment of cancers with laparoscopy. An increased incidence of port site (wound) metastasis after laparoscopy than after laparotomy has been reported.[16] Because of this, it has been recommended to limit the use of laparoscopy in the treatment of malignancies.[17] Until prospective randomized trials are done, the true risk of wound recurrences from laparoscopy will remain a subject of speculation. Laboratory and clinical work is slowly elucidating the factors that contribute to port site recurrences and the true incidence after laparoscopic intervention for malignant diseases.

Carbon dioxide has been implicated as a potential cause of this phenomenon. In animal models using colon carcinoma, Neuhaus et al.[18] studied the effect of various gases for establishing the pneumoperitoneum on the incidence of port site metastasis. Air, carbon dioxide, and nitrous oxide all had similar incidences of wound recurrences. Helium, on the other hand, was associated with significantly fewer recurrences, suggesting that the insufflating agent is important in the development of wound recurrences. In an elegant study, Mathew et al.[19] instilled viable adenocarcinoma cells into the abdomen of rats undergoing laparoscopy with carbon dioxide pneumoperitoneum. The carbon dioxide was then vented via a tube connecting the first rat with another rat's abdomen. Of the recipient rats, 83% developed tumors at the site of the venting tube connection to their abdomen. A similar study was run with gasless laparoscopy and no tumors were seen in the recipient rats.[19] In addition to the difference seen with the insufflating agent, the trocars were shown to have adherent, viable tumor cells on their surface.[20]

The type of tumor also may have a role in wound recurrence. In animal models, using neuroblastoma, Iwanaka et al.[21] showed that the insufflating agent may not be important with a more aggressive tumor model. There was no difference in carbon dioxide pneumoperitoneum versus wall lift methods in wound recurrence. Interestingly, animals treated with intravenous or intraperitoneal chemotherapy (cyclophosphamide) had decreased recurrences regardless of the operative technique.[21]

Other studies have suggested that there is no difference in recurrences at the wound site with laparoscopy when compared with laparotomy. Paik et al.,[22] using a rat colon carcinoma model, found no increase in the incidence of wound recurrence between laparoscopy and laparotomy. In a prospective randomized trial of humans with colon carcinoma, no difference in wound recurrences was seen. There were 44 laparoscopic-assisted colectomies (LACs) and 47 open colectomies (OCs) performed. No port site or laparotomy recurrences were seen nor was there an increase in intraabdominal recurrence with either technique (16.1% LAC vs. 15% OC).[23]

That port site recurrences occur is indisputable. However, it is controversial that the incidence is greater than incisional recurrence after laparotomy. In fact, in a preliminary report of a prospective randomized trial with 80 patients with colon carcinoma, there were no wound or port site metastases or recurrences in either the LACs or OCs.[24] There were also no differences in the overall recurrence rate between laparoscopic and conventional surgery.[24] The etiology behind port site recurrences is unclear, but it is probably multifactorial. The insufflating agent is involved, but operative technique and avoidance of tumor manipulation and perforation may be more important. Reymond and colleagues[25] accurately point out that wound recurrences have been reported after thoracoscopic procedures as well where no insufflating agent is used. The investigation of laparoscopy in the treatment of malignancies should not be limited based on concerns of port site metastases. However, now that it has been shown to be technically possible to treat many intraabdominal and retroperitoneal tumors with laparoscopic techniques, further investigations should be in the context of prospective randomized trials.

## LAPAROSCOPIC ULTRASOUND

The limitation of laparoscopy in staging lies in the inability of the surgeon to obtain tactile sensations. Despite the increased sensitivity and accuracy of laparoscopy compared to extracorporeal ultrasound, CT scan, and MRI, only the anterior segments and fissures and part of the inferior surface of the liver are visualized using laparoscopy. Deep parenchymal lesions and lesions on the inferior surface will remain undiagnosed. In this regard, flexible and directable laparoscopic ultrasound is proving of significant value in identifying these occult lesions in a manner similar to intraoperative ultrasound. The advantage of laparoscopic ultrasound lies in the ability to place the ultrasound probe directly on the organ of interest, thus utilizing higher-frequency (7.5 to 10-MHz) probes. With the improved resolution from the higher-frequency probes, laparoscopic ultrasound has improved the sensitivity of laparoscopic staging. An additional 29% (57% with laparoscopy and laparoscopic ultrasound) improvement in staging of gastrointestinal malignancies was reported by Hunerbein and associates[26] over the combination of conventional staging and laparoscopy.

Laparoscopic ultrasound is superior to CT at TNM staging for esophageal and gastric cancer: T stage 82% vs. 47%; N stage 92% vs. 70%; M stage 89% vs. 62% accuracy.[27] The combination of laparoscopy and laparoscopic ultrasound in hepatobiliary and pancreatic malignancies showed unsuspected reasons for unresectability in 23% to 65% (median 45%) of patients.[28] John et al.[29] reported on 50 patients with potentially resectable liver tumors with CT staging. An additional 33% of patients with intrahepatic lesions not seen by CT and laparoscopy were found with laparoscopic ultrasound, and it added information to laparoscopy in 42% of patients.[29] Cuesta et al.[30] also reported that additional diagnostic information was obtained in 20 of 25 patients (80%) with established liver lesions, carcinoma of the gallbladder, or pancreatic cancer evaluated with ultrasonography at the time of laparoscopy. These ultrasonographic findings often initiated a change in the surgical approach.

Contemporary laparoscopic ultrasound allows accurate assessment of tumor size and invasion of vascular structures, facilitates target biopsy, and allows identification of lesions that are not evident at laparoscopy. Furthermore, the availability of laparoscopic ultrasound makes laparoscopic cryosurgery possible. Experience with the latter modality is enlarging; early results have documented its feasibility and value.[31]

Laparoscopic ultrasonography requires three trocars (umbilical and right and left subcostal) that will allow access to the entire upper abdomen. Putting the patient in the reverse Trendelenberg position aids in caudal displacement of the small and large bowel. The dome of the liver can be accessed by instilling saline into the right upper quadrant and transducing via the liquid-organ interface or by decreasing the pneumoperitoneum to facilitate contact. Imaging the pancreas from the right and left subcostal ports gives longitudinal images, whereas axial images are obtained from the umbilical port. If the lesser sac is not opened, the pancreas can be visualized via the transgastric approach by instilling saline into the stomach to aid in creating an acoustic window. However, opening the lesser sac and imaging the pancreas with a 10-MHz probe will give superior resolution. The bile duct is imaged longitudinally from the umbilicus and axially from the subcostal ports.[32]

## LYMPHOMA

Laparoscopy is useful in diagnosing Hodgkin's and non-Hodgkin's lymphoma. Lesions of retroperitoneal origin confirmed on CT scan can be explored laparoscopically and biopsied for diagnostic and staging purposes.[33] Appropriate staging for Hodgkin's disease requires splenectomy and liver biopsy. In addition, lymph node biopsies from mesenteric, aortic, and parailiac lymph nodes are also needed. With the development of laparoscopic splenectomy, it became possible to completely stage patients laparoscopically.

Mann et al.[34] reported on 94 patients with suspected or diagnosed lymphoma that underwent diagnostic or staging laparoscopy. Laparoscopy was successfully completed in 85 patients. In only two patients (one false negative, one nonresult) was a diagnosis not correctly obtained. Importantly, in all other patients there was adequate tissue for diagnosis. In 21% of the patients with recurrent or persistent lymphoma, the diagnosis or stage was changed.[34] Ferzli et al.[35] reported on six patients with Hodgkin's disease that were completely staged laparoscopically. No patient was upstaged. Zornig[36] reported a case of recurrent disease that was completely staged laparoscopically. This patient had abdominal disease that was detected with laparoscopy (stage IIIE).

During diagnostic laparoscopy, lymph nodes must be carefully dissected and electrosurgery avoided so that nodal architecture is preserved. The entire lymph node, rather than a needle or piecemeal biopsy, should be obtained and submitted to provide adequate tissue for pathologic diagnosis. Portions of nodes or small pieces of tissue are difficult to interpret because of the importance of nodal architecture.

Traditional staging of Hodgkin's disease necessitated open techniques with intraperitoneal and retroperitoneal dissection or biopsy and splenectomy. Today, staging of Hodgkin's disease, including liver biopsy, celiac and paraaortic lymph node biopsies and splenectomy may be performed laparoscopically.[37] All patients should receive pneumococcal vaccine at least 10 days preoperatively and should have autologous blood available. Routine preoperative measures for laparoscopy (antibiotics, compression stockings, nasogastric tube, and indwelling urinary catheter) also pertain for procedures that are diagnostic or therapeutic for this cancerous state.

Laparoscopic splenectomy is achieved using five cannulas (Fig. 5A-1). Devascularization of the spleen commences at the inferior pole (Fig. 5A-2). Exposure of the hilum is accomplished by retraction of the stomach toward the right side of the patient using a Babcock clamp. Blood vessels are divided between titanium clips or with Laparosonic coagulating shears until the splenic artery and vein are visualized (Fig. 5A-3). Short gastric and superior pole vessels are then divided between titanium clips, leaving only the splenic artery and splenic vein (Figs. 5A-4, 5A-5). These large vessels are

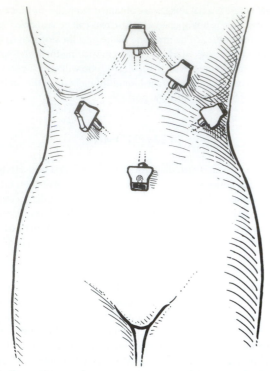

**FIGURE 5A-1.** Location of cannulas for laparoscopic splenectomy. (*From Amaral CP: Diagnostic and therapeutic laparoscopy for malignant diseases, in* Atlas of Surgical Oncology, *Bland KI et al (eds). Philadelphia, WB Saunders, 1995, pp 749–789.*)

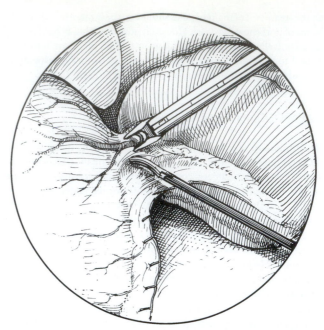

**FIGURE 5A-3.** The vessels are divided between clips or with Laparosonic coagulating shears. (*From Amaral CP: Diagnostic and therapeutic laparoscopy for malignant diseases, in* Atlas of Surgical Oncology, *Bland KI et al (eds). Philadelphia, WB Saunders, 1995, pp 749–789.*)

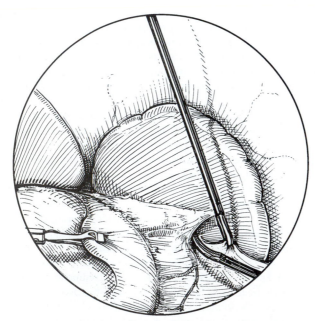

**FIGURE 5A-2.** Devascularization of the spleen commences at the inferior pole. (*From Amaral CP: Diagnostic and therapeutic laparoscopy for malignant diseases, in* Atlas of Surgical Oncology, *Bland KI et al (eds). Philadelphia, WB Saunders, 1995, pp 749–789.*)

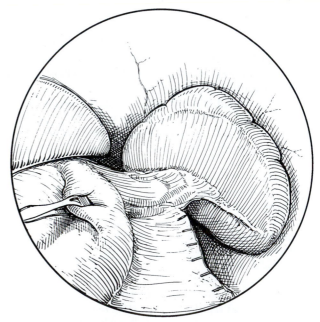

**FIGURE 5A-4.** The short gastric vessels are divided. (*From Amaral CP: Diagnostic and therapeutic laparoscopy for malignant diseases, in* Atlas of Surgical Oncology, *Bland KI et al (eds). Philadelphia, WB Saunders, 1995, pp 749–789.*)

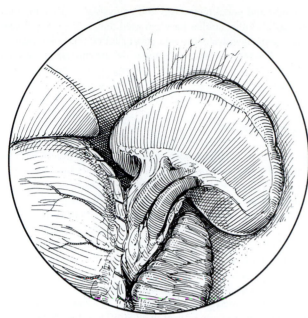

**FIGURE 5A-5.** The splenic artery and vein are mobilized off the pancreas. (*From Amaral CP: Diagnostic and therapeutic laparoscopy for malignant diseases, in* Atlas of Surgical Oncology, *Bland KI et al (eds). Philadelphia, WB Saunders, 1995, pp 749–789.*)

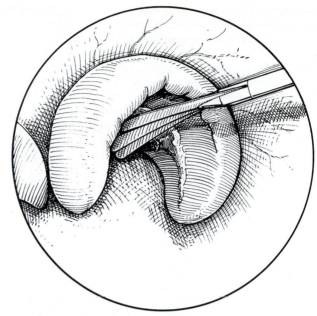

**FIGURE 5A-7.** The spleen is completely detached. It is then placed in a heavy duty bag for extraction via the umbilical incision. (*From Amaral CP: Diagnostic and therapeutic laparoscopy for malignant diseases, in* Atlas of Surgical Oncology, *Bland KI et al (eds). Philadelphia, WB Saunders, 1995, pp 749–789.*)

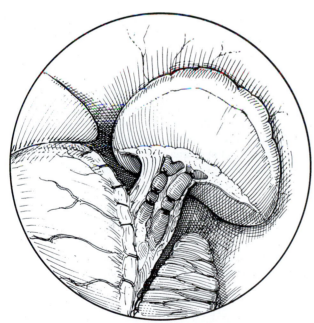

**FIGURE 5A-6.** The splenic artery and vein are ligated with extra-corporeal sutures, twice proximally and once distally. (*From Amaral CP: Diagnostic and therapeutic laparoscopy for malignant diseases, in* Atlas of Surgical Oncology, *Bland KI et al (eds). Philadelphia, WB Saunders, 1995, pp 749–789.*)

suture-ligated twice proximally and once distally prior to division with scissors (Fig. 5A-6). Alternatively, a laparoscopic endoscopic stapler may be used. The spleen should not be grasped during the procedure because the capsule will easily tear. Furthermore, any manipulation of the spleen must be performed gently with forgiving instruments such as a balloon or fan-type retractor. Irrigation is not used until all vessels to the spleen are divided. In this manner an accurate estimate of blood loss can be obtained from the suction canister.

The devascularized intact spleen is placed in a heavy-duty bag and removed via an extended vertical incision through the umbilicus (Fig. 5A-7); 4 cm of length is adequate. Although it is possible to fragment the spleen in the bag to facilitate extraction, we prefer exteriorization of the intact spleen. Not only is the risk of splenosis reduced, accurate pathologic diagnosis is enhanced for the morphologically intact organ, since involvement with Hodgkin's disease may exist in only a few lymphoid nodules of the spleen.[38]

## GASTROINTESTINAL TUMORS

Laparoscopy is effective in confirming the resectability of tumors that are deemed resectable by imaging methods such as CT scan, ultrasonography, and arteriography. These malignancies include liver metastasis and pancreatic, esophageal, and gastric carcinomas. In this regard, laparoscopy has been found to detect accurately upward of 96% of intraabdominal metastases[39] and 90% of liver metastases.[40] Furthermore, numerous studies report that as many as 40% of patients deemed resectable by current diagnostic imaging modalities (e.g., CT scan, ultrasound, and arteriography) will be deemed unresectable or palliative by laparoscopy.[12,40,41] In large part, this enhanced diagnostic probability results from the superiority of laparoscopy to detect 1- to 2-mm hepatic and peritoneal metastases. Resolution imaging of CT scans of lesions less than 1 cm is poor, and a sensitivity rate of 49% is expected for these smaller lesions.[26] Endoscopic ultrasound has shown good results in esophageal, gastric, pancreatic, and rectal cancers with accuracy results of 80% to 90% for T-stage and 70% to 80% for N-stage disease.[42] However, endoscopic ultrasound is still limited by an inability to determine metastatic disease and thus unresectability accurately.

## ESOPHAGEAL CANCER

Historically, 42% of all patients with esophageal carcinoma were not thought to be resectable for cure. Of the 58% resected, only 39% had curative resections, with a 5-year survival of only 4%.[43] Newer chemoradiation protocols have promise of improving survival in those responding to treatment. Accurate staging of patients helps determine candidates for these protocols. However, noninvasive staging modalities are still inadequate. Shandall and Johnson,[40] using laparoscopy, found 16 of 23 patients (70%) with esophageal cancer deemed resectable by noninvasive imaging studies to have nodal and peritoneal spread that precluded resection. Therefore, laparotomy was avoided in over two-thirds of these patients, of whom 74% died in the 18-month follow-up period.

In an extensive comparative study by Watt and colleagues[41] of laparoscopy, ultrasound, and CT for diagnosis of carcinoma of the esophagus and gastric cardia, laparoscopy was significantly more accurate than CT scan or ultrasound for detecting metastases to the liver, lymphatics, and peritoneum (Table 5A-1). In evaluating patients with esophageal carcinoma, laparoscopy offers the benefit of enhancing diagnostic accuracy and providing the opportunity to obtain suspicious tissue samples under direct vision. It is noteworthy that 51% of patients who had upper- and middle-third lesions also had intraabdominal metastasis.[41] This was similar to the 58% of patients with lower-third esophageal and cardiac lesions who harbored intraabdominal metastatic disease.[41] These data suggest that laparoscopy should be performed routinely not only for lower-third adenocarcinoma or squamous cell carcinoma of the esophagus, but also for lesions in the upper and middle thirds of this organ.

This is tempered by results from other reports. Bonavina et al.[44] showed only a 10% change in management with laparoscopy. This was because only 3 of 36 patients had peritoneal or liver metastasis. They concluded that laparoscopy was superior in detecting

**TABLE 5A-1.** ACCURACY (%) OF STAGING IN ESOPHAGEAL AND GASTRIC CARCINOMA

|  | LAPAROSCOPY | ULTRASOUND | CAT SCAN |
|---|---|---|---|
| Hepatic metastases | 96 | 83 | 85 |
| Peritoneal metastases | 72 | 52 | 57 |
| Nodal metastases | 98 | 89 | — |

SOURCE: Reymond MA et al.[20]

peritoneal and nodal metastasis, and equivalent in detecting liver metastasis.[44] Other studies have reported only a 5% to 6% change in management with laparoscopic staging for esophageal malignancies.[45,46] The reasons for the discrepancies are unclear but suggest a role for cautious optimism in applying staging laparoscopy to esophageal cancer.

## GASTRIC CANCER

Laparoscopy is also highly accurate for detection of liver metastasis, peritoneal dissemination, serosal infiltration, and tumor fixation in gastric carcinoma.[47] Despite a high specificity, its value in detecting lymph node metastases in stomach cancer in comparison to liver or peritoneal metastases was less accurate, secondary to a sensitivity of 53%.[47] Overall, these attributes make it beneficial for staging gastric cancer and in planning therapy. It also avoids futile laparotomy in the patient without complications of the disease. Kriplani and Kapur[48] evaluated 40 patients with gastric carcinoma deemed resectable by preoperative ultrasound and CT scan. Laparoscopy revealed unrecognized distant metastatic disease in 12.5%; locally advanced unresectable neoplasia was evident in 27.5%. Thus, the application of staging laparoscopy in this series avoided futile laparotomy in 40% of these patients. Laparoscopy has shown improved accuracy when compared with CT and ultrasound in staging gastric carcinoma. Burke et al.[49] showed the incidence of missed distant metastasis in patients staged with CT to be 28% to 37%, and the accuracy of laparoscopy to be 89% to 94%.[49]

The value of laparoscopy in gastric cancer has been questioned because a percentage of patients with gastric cancer will require palliative surgery for obstruction, perforation, or hemorrhage. Indeed, Shandall and Johnson[40] found 9 of 14 patients with gastric carcinoma to be unresectable for cure; however, 5 of these 9 underwent palliative resection. The assumption that patients with gastric cancer should have palliative resections in the face of metastatic disease to avoid complications is controversial. Patients who do not present with complications are unlikely to develop complications that necessitate an operation. Burke and associates[49] showed that of the 24 patients with laparoscopically proven metastatic disease, none required a subsequent operation. Furthermore, obstruction is not a contraindication to laparoscopic staging provided the patient is a candidate for laparoscopic gastroenterostomy.

More controversial is laparoscopic resection of gastric malignancies. Ballesta-Lopez and co-workers[50] reported on 10 cases of gastric cancer treated by laparoscopic subtotal gastrectomy. The authors were able to perform the resection with a D1 lymphadenectomy and Billroth II reconstruction. Long-term follow-up is needed to determine whether laparoscopic gastrectomy is a sound oncologic procedure.

## PANCREATIC CANCER

Pancreatic cancer has the worst prognosis and smallest percentage of patients who qualify for curative resection. At exploration, 15% of patients with cancer of the pancreas are deemed resectable, 40% have localized but unresectable tumors, and 45% have distant metastatic disease (M1 disease).[51] Pancreatic cancer predominantly metastasizes to the liver and peritoneum.[52] Therefore, unresectability from M1 disease will be accessible to evaluation by laparoscopy. The role of laparoscopy in the evaluation of resectability for cancer of the pancreas has been extensively studied by Warshaw and Cushieri. Warshaw[12,51] evaluated 40 patients with negative ultrasound, CT scan, and arteriography by laparoscopy prior to resection. Of these 40 patients,[14] (35%) had metastatic disease that precluded laparotomy. The remaining 26 patients underwent laparotomy; 23 of the 26 patients had curative pancreatic resections.[12] In a similar study, Cushieri[53] determined that 42 of 51 patients (82%) with pancreatic cancer were unresectable at laparoscopy and 9 were resectable. Laparotomy confirmed the technical inability to resect these 42 patients who were deemed unresectable by laparoscopy. In addition, 5 of the 9 patients deemed resectable by laparoscopy were also unresectable at laparotomy secondary to invasion of the portal vein (4 patients) and previously unrecognized hepatic metastasis. Laparoscopy also allowed histologic confirmation of pancreatic cancer in 92% of these laparoscopy patients.[53]

Although an aggressive approach that includes mobilization and biopsy of the pancreas can be initiated to determine resectability of pancreatic cancer, our standard approach includes inspection of the omentum, liver, and peritoneal surfaces for metastatic disease unrecognized by conventional noninvasive imaging techniques. The abdominal cavity is lavaged with normal saline for cytologic analysis. In addition, the gastrocolic ligament should be divided and the lesser sac entered to inspect the peripancreatic area. Search for nodal disease is best initiated by the Kocher maneuver, because a high percentage of nodal disease for cancer of the head of the pancreas will be anatomically documented in retroduodenal and periduodenal sites.[54] The utility of a laparoscopic Kocher maneuver is questionable, because lymph nodes in the area of resection would not be a contraindication to resection. Therefore, the Kocher maneuver should be done only if laparoscopic resection is planned. Laparoscopic pancreaticoduodenectomy has been shown to be technically feasible; however, concerns over the adequacy of resection, tumor spillage, and morbidity associated with the laparoscopic procedure make it a questionable operation.[55] However, laparoscopic distal pancreatectomy may have a role in the treatment of the patient with a small malignancy in the distal pancreas. It must be stressed that ideal patient selection is recommended prior to undertaking laparoscopic pancreatectomy for malignant disease.

The decision may arise in patients with metastatic pancreatic cancer as to whether one should proceed with operative biliary diversion. Controversy exists as to the best approach for biliary decompression in patients with unresectable pancreatic cancer since operative, endoscopic, and radiologic techniques are available.[42,56–58] To this confusion is added laparoscopic biliary decompression via a cholecystojejunostomy when anatomically and technically appropriate.[59,60] Nagy et al.[61] reported on 10 patients with duodenal obstruction that underwent laparoscopic gastrojejunostomy. The procedure was successful in 9 of 10. One patient also had a cholecystojejunostomy simultaneously.

Our approach to laparoscopic cholecystojejunostomy involves a three-cannula technique including a 10-mm cannula in the umbilicus, a 5-mm cannula in the right midabdomen, and a 12-mm

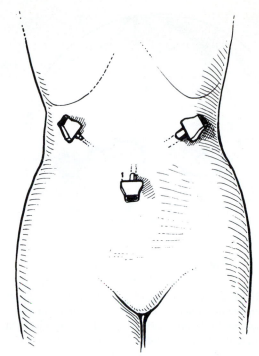

**FIGURE 5A-8.** Location of cannulas for laparoscopic cholecystojejunostomy. (*From Amaral CP: Diagnostic and therapeutic laparoscopy for malignant diseases, in* Atlas of Surgical Oncology, *Bland KI et al (eds). Philadelphia, WB Saunders, 1995, pp 749–789.*)

cannula in the left midclavicular line positioned midway between the ribs and umbilicus (Fig. 5A-8). The ligament of Trietz is identified and the course of the jejunum followed to a point where the cholecystojejunal anastomosis is possible (Fig. 5A-9). The small bowel is anchored to the lateral right abdominal wall near the gallbladder using a percutaneous suture (Fig. 5A-10). An enterotomy and cholecystotomy are created with electrosurgery or the ultrasonically activated scalpel (Fig. 5A-11); the anastomosis is created using a laparoscopic 30-mm intestinal stapler (Figs. 5A-12, 5A-13). The remaining enterotomy is closed with a running 2-0 silk suture tied intracorporeally (Figs. 5A-14, 5A-15). The 2-0 size suture is chosen because the needle is technically simpler to manipulate intracorporeally than needles of smaller sutures.

Gastrojejunostomy can be performed in a similar fashion if gastric outlet obstruction exists. Should biliary obstruction coexist, decompression by cholecystojejunostomy is completed initially. This allows anchoring of the jejunum, which facilitates creation of the gastrojejunostomy. Adequate length of jejunum must be planned and retained proximal to the cholecystojejunostomy such that tension on either anastomosis is avoided.

Gastrojejunostomy may require additional cannulas to retract the liver and to aid in mobilization of the stomach. Usually four cannulas will be needed, including a 5-mm cannula in the right midclavicular line, a 10-mm cannula between the 5-mm cannula and the umbilicus, a 10-mm cannula in the umbilicus, and a 12-mm cannula in the left midclavicular line (Fig. 5A-16).

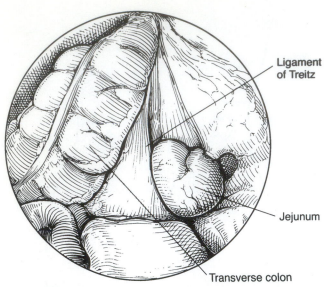

Ligament
of Treitz

Jejunum

Transverse colon

**FIGURE 5A-9.** The ligament of Trietz identified by elevating the transverse colon. (*From Amaral CP: Diagnostic and therapeutic laparoscopy for malignant diseases, in* Atlas of Surgical Oncology, *Bland KI et al (eds). Philadelphia, WB Saunders, 1995, pp 749–789.*)

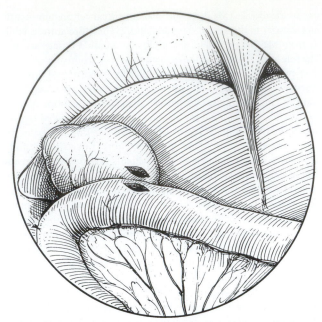

**FIGURE 5A-11.** Jejunostomy and cholecystotomy are performed. (*From Amaral CP: Diagnostic and therapeutic laparoscopy for malignant diseases, in* Atlas of Surgical Oncology, *Bland KI et al (eds). Philadelphia, WB Saunders, 1995, pp 749–789.*)

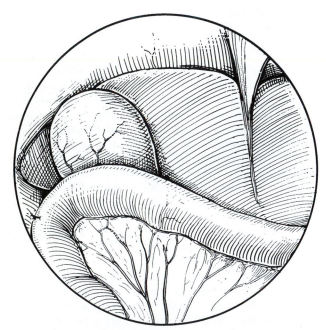

**FIGURE 5A-10.** The jejunum is anchored temporarily to the lateral abdominal wall with percutaneous sutures. (*From Amaral CP: Diagnostic and therapeutic laparoscopy for malignant diseases, in* Atlas of Surgical Oncology, *Bland KI et al (eds). Philadelphia, WB Saunders, 1995, pp 749–789.*)

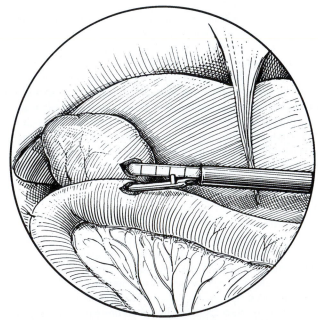

**FIGURE 5A-12.** The endoscopic linear stapler is inserted into the enterotomies. (*From Amaral CP: Diagnostic and therapeutic laparoscopy for malignant diseases, in* Atlas of Surgical Oncology, *Bland KI et al (eds). Philadelphia, WB Saunders, 1995, pp 749–789.*)

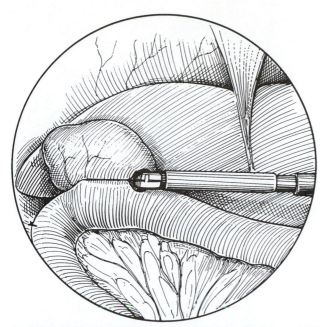

**FIGURE 5A-13.** The endoscopic linear stapler is closed and fired. (*From Amaral CP: Diagnostic and therapeutic laparoscopy for malignant diseases, in Atlas of Surgical Oncology, Bland KI et al (eds). Philadelphia, WB Saunders, 1995, pp 749–789.*)

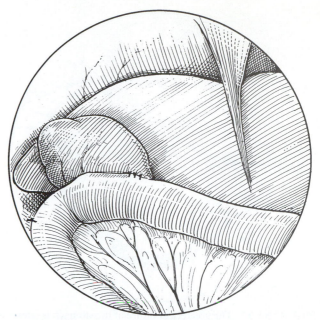

**FIGURE 5A-15.** Completed laparoscopic cholecystojejunostomy. (*From Amaral CP: Diagnostic and therapeutic laparoscopy for malignant diseases, in Atlas of Surgical Oncology, Bland KI et al (eds). Philadelphia, WB Saunders, 1995, pp 749–789.*)

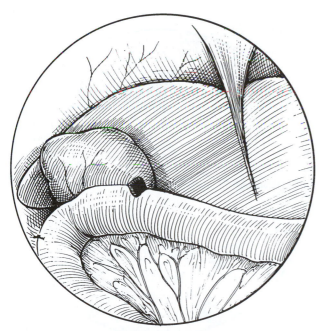

**FIGURE 5A-14.** The enterotomies are closed with a 2-0 silk running suture. (*From Amaral CP: Diagnostic and therapeutic laparoscopy for malignant diseases, in Atlas of Surgical Oncology, Bland KI et al (eds). Philadelphia, WB Saunders, 1995, pp 749–789.*)

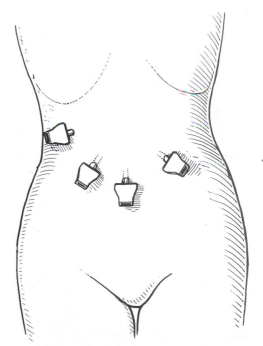

**FIGURE 5A-16.** Location of cannulas for laparoscopic gastrojejunostomy. (*From Amaral CP: Diagnostic and therapeutic laparoscopy for malignant diseases, in Atlas of Surgical Oncology, Bland KI et al (eds). Philadelphia, WB Saunders, 1995, pp 749–789.*)

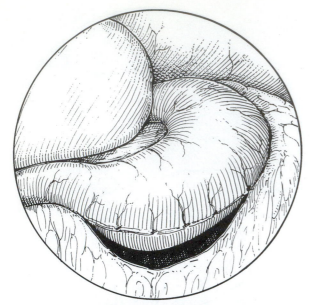

**FIGURE 5A-17.** The greater curvature of the stomach is devascularized. (*From Amaral CP: Diagnostic and therapeutic laparoscopy for malignant diseases, in* Atlas of Surgical Oncology, *Bland KI et al (eds). Philadelphia, WB Saunders, 1995, pp 749–789.*)

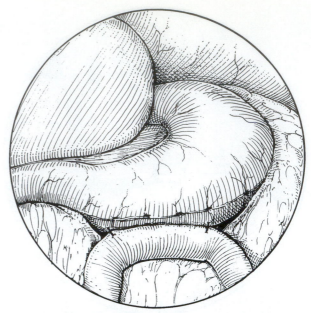

**FIGURE 5A-18.** The jejunum is anchored to the stomach with interrupted sutures. (*From Amaral CP: Diagnostic and therapeutic laparoscopy for malignant diseases, in* Atlas of Surgical Oncology, *Bland KI et al (eds). Philadelphia, WB Saunders, 1995, pp 749–789.*)

The gastrojejunal anastomosis is completed on the greater curvature of the stomach after an adequate area has been devascularized between clips or with the Laparosonic coagulating shears (Fig. 5A-17). The latter modality is preferred because it does not leave clips that can interfere with the subsequent stapled anastomosis. The jejunum is anchored to the stomach distal to the anticipated site of the gastrojejunostomy to facilitate the anastomosis (Fig. 5A-18). A gastrotomy and enterotomy are made using electrosurgery or the ultrasonically activated scalpel (Fig. 5A-19). A 30-mm endoscopic stapler is then placed through the enterotomies and discharged (Figs. 5A-20, 5A-21). The remaining enterotomy is closed with a 2-0 silk running suture using intracorporeal knots (Fig. 5A-22).

## HEPATIC CANCER

Laparoscopy has become an invaluable tool in the management of primary and metastatic hepatic malignancies. Numerous studies have documented a 70% to 80% sensitivity for preoperative extracorporeal ultrasound, CT scan, MRI, or angiography; the combined diagnostic modality rate does not exceed 80%.[62–65] Given these values, from 40% to 70% of patients undergoing laparotomy are deemed unresectable because of unrecognized coexistent disease such as cirrhosis, extrahepatic metastatic disease, or multicentric hepatic lesions. Since survival rates following palliative resections of hepatic metastases are equivalent to those achieved with nonsurgical therapy, enhanced evaluation prior to laparotomy is essential to avoid noncurative exploratory procedures.

Laparoscopy has been known for many years to be vital in the diagnosis of hepatic disease. Early experiences with laparoscopy were

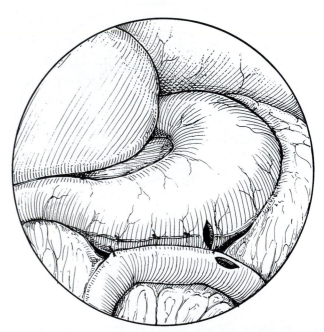

**FIGURE 5A-19.** Enterotomy and gastrotomy are made in preparation for the stapled anastomosis. (*From Amaral CP: Diagnostic and therapeutic laparoscopy for malignant diseases, in* Atlas of Surgical Oncology, *Bland KI et al (eds). Philadelphia, WB Saunders, 1995, pp 749–789.*)

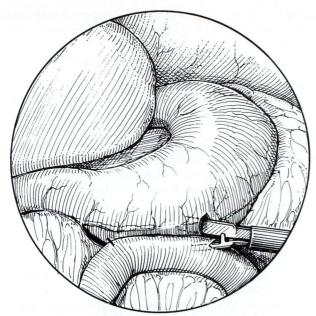

**FIGURE 5A-20.** The endoscopic linear stapler is placed via the 11-mm left midline cannula. (*From Amaral CP: Diagnostic and therapeutic laparoscopy for malignant diseases, in* Atlas of Surgical Oncology, *Bland KI et al (eds). Philadelphia, WB Saunders, 1995, pp 749–789.*)

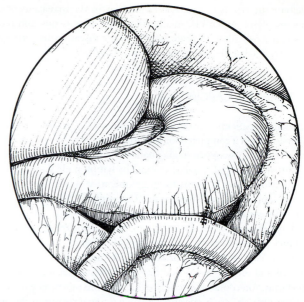

**FIGURE 5A-22.** The enterotomy is closed with 2-0 running silk sutures. (*From Amaral CP: Diagnostic and therapeutic laparoscopy for malignant diseases, in* Atlas of Surgical Oncology, *Bland KI et al (eds). Philadelphia, WB Saunders, 1995, pp 749–789.*)

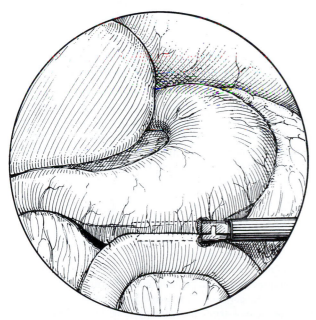

**FIGURE 5A-21.** The endoscopic linear stapler is closed and fired. (*From Amaral CP: Diagnostic and therapeutic laparoscopy for malignant diseases, in* Atlas of Surgical Oncology, *Bland KI et al (eds). Philadelphia, WB Saunders, 1995, pp 749–789.*)

primarily limited to hepatology and best represented in the 5000 patients reported on by Kalk.[3] Recently, Babineau and colleagues[65] reported their experience using laparoscopy as an adjunct for the management of hepatic metastasis. Of 29 patients considered resectable because of favorable CT scan, ultrasound, and arteriography, 14 patients (48%) were deemed unresectable by laparoscopy. Both primary hepatic tumors and metastatic liver tumors were included in this study. Laparoscopy was effective in determining unresectability in both types of tumors. Of 12 patients with primary liver tumors, 8 were unresectable, and 6 of 17 patients with metastasis to the liver were unresectable. This resulted in a reduction of length of hospital stay from 6.6 + 0.5 days for nonresectable laparotomy (historical controls) to 1.2 + 0.5 days for laparoscopy alone.[65]

John et al.[29] reported on 50 consecutive patients with hepatic lesions deemed resectable by ultrasound, CT, and CT portography. Laparoscopy determined 46% of the patients to be unresectable secondary to cirrhosis, multicentricity, or metastatic spread. As a result of laparoscopic staging, resectability rates increased from 58% to 93%.

In summation, all patients who have advanced primary cancer, especially those with cancers that have statistically low cure rates, benefit from diagnostic laparoscopy prior to potentially curative laparotomy. These patients include those with pancreatic, esophageal, and gastric cancer. The procedure adds little time, essentially no morbidity or mortality, and provides accurate assessment of the stage of disease. This information will not only avoid nontherapeutic laparotomy, but it may be of value in reassessing the clinical situation following a period of chemotherapy or radiation therapy. For example, pretherapy evaluation of nodal disease for esophageal carcinoma has been suggested by LoCicero[66] as a means to better evaluate the effects of multimodal therapy in the management of this neoplasm. Much like mediastinoscopy, laparoscopy and thoracoscopy will allow accurate staging of the disease with regard to local, regional, and distant metastasis.

## COLORECTAL CARCINOMA

Virtually all patients with colorectal carcinoma undergo resection or diversion, even if completed for palliative purposes alone. Therefore, the role of laparoscopy in staging patients with colorectal carcinoma is limited. Staging of rectal carcinoma by lymph node sampling has been advocated as a means to guide operative strategy for radical abdominoperineal resection or local excision.[67] However, no data currently exist to support this approach.

Furthermore, laparoscopy has not been reported to date as an adjunct in the follow-up of patients with treated colorectal carcinoma. Persistent pain and/or rising CEA values suggest recurrent disease and are the usual findings that initiate "second-look" laparotomy. Anecdotal reports and evidence from other malignancies such as ovarian carcinoma suggest value for laparoscopy as the first invasive modality in the evaluation of the patient with recurrent colorectal carcinoma (e.g., a suspected recurrence with elevated CEA levels and equivocal or negative noninvasive imaging techniques). However, there are no reported series to date.

An evolving, but as yet undefined, area of applicability for laparoscopy in the management of colorectal carcinoma is resection of the primary lesion via a laparoscopically assisted approach. Three questions are essential to this discussion: (1) What is the feasibility and advantage of laparoscopic or laparoscopically assisted colon surgery over conventional open methods? (2) Does a laparoscopically assisted colon resection yield the same extent of resection as an open resection? (3) Does laparoscopic colon surgery compromise the principles of cancer surgery and lead to reduced long-term survival?

The feasibility of laparoscopic or laparoscopically assisted colon resections has been established by numerous investigators.[68–74] In general, the techniques used for resection are the same as for open surgery, with the important caveat that the former are performed through multiple 5- to 12-mm cannulas under video guidance. The entire gamut of colon procedures from right colectomy to abdominoperineal resection have been reported and technically described. In general, they range from the completely laparoendoscopically performed sigmoid or abdominoperineal resection to the laparoscopically assisted right or transverse colectomy.

Laparoscopic approaches require more operative time than the open alternative (205 min for laparoscopic versus 123 min for open low anterior resection) and are more costly for all but the right colectomy.[74] In contrast, when successfully performed to completion by a laparoscopic approach, passage of flatus, resumption of oral intake, postoperative analgesic requirements, intraoperative blood loss, length of hospital stay, and resumption of normal daily activities are significantly improved in the laparoscopic group.[24,74]

It is also clear that not all patients can successfully undergo laparoscopic or laparoscopically assisted colectomy; conversion rates to open technique in preselected patients range from 17% to 23%. In examining the technical difficulty associated with each type of colectomy, Geis et al.[73] noted right and sigmoid colon resections to be the least difficult technically, whereas left and transverse colon resections were the most difficult. Each of these procedures was rendered more difficult and time consuming if an intracorporeal rather than extracorporeal anastomosis was performed.

The morbidity and mortality of laparoscopic colectomy is difficult to establish since available reports are provided by experienced laparoscopic surgeons and suffer from patient selection biases with high rates of conversion to open technique. Nonetheless, given these caveats, the overall incidence of complications with laparoscopic approaches for colon resection appears comparable to open techniques.

The issue of what constitutes a radical or adequate resection for colon cancer is sometimes based as much on subjective findings as it is on fact. It has been documented that colon and rectal cancer almost always spread to contiguous levels of nodes without "skip" metastatic areas, and that there is no survival difference between high and low ligation of the inferior mesenteric artery.[75] Indeed, the best predictor of recurrence is if the last (highest level) node excised is involved with tumor. Although aggressive approaches such as the "no-touch" technique have been advocated as superior to other approaches, randomized prospective trials have shown no benefit. In this regard, studies of lymph node yield from specimens removed laparoscopically document the same number as those found in specimens from conventional open colectomy.[75] Moreover, the mesentery is ligated at the origin of the primary vascular supply of the colonic segment, resulting in standard lymphatic resections.

The actual survival of patients undergoing laparoscopic approaches for resection of colon cancer is unknown. However, it is not likely that a laparoscopic approach has an adverse effect on patients with Dukes' D lesions, since these lesions are advanced and noncurative with any approach. However, the influence of a laparoscopic approach may make a substantial difference in survival of Dukes' A, B, and C lesions if inadequate node dissection is performed. Clearly, only long-term follow-up in randomized studies will answer this question.

## GENITOURINARY CARCINOMA

As with gastrointestinal carcinoma, genitourinary carcinomas are being staged and treated with minimally invasive techniques. The use of multimodal treatments in advanced genitourinary malignancies mandates accurate staging. Laparoscopy, with the ability to visualize and biopsy lymph nodes and peritoneal implants, offers a unique tool to aid in staging of these malignancies.

### OVARIAN CANCER

There appears to be no role for laparoscopy in the initial management of ovarian carcinoma at the present time. The steps involved with surgical treatment include bilateral salpingo-oophrectomy, hysterectomy, paraaortic and pelvic lymphadenectomy, omentectomy, and serosal stripping. Case reports exist showing the technical feasibility of primary management of patients with ovarian cancer with laparoscopy,[76,77] but the risk of understaging this highly morbid disease with a consequent reduction in disease-free survival is too great.[78] Subjecting all patients with an adnexal mass to laparotomy results in an extremely high percentage of patients with greater length of hospital stay, complications, and convalescence.

For example, 18,703 ovarian masses were analyzed in the 1990 survey of the American Association of Gynecologic Laparoscopists (AAGL). There were a total of 411 malignancies (2.8%) reported by the AAGL, of which all but 53 (13%) were managed either by initial laparotomy or laparoscopy converted to laparotomy following visual inspection of the adnexal mass. These 53 patients had benign-appearing masses removed at laparoscopy that proved malignant at pathologic examination; subsequently, all patients underwent staging laparotomy. In total, 0.3% of all patients studied and 0.4% of all patients undergoing an initial laparoscopy for an ovarian mass had ovarian cancers removed laparoscopically.[79]

The technical concern of laparoscopic resection of an ovarian cancer followed by laparotomy results from an upstaging of stage IA ovarian carcinoma to stage IC following cyst rupture or fluid spillage during laparoscopy.[80] The ominous consequence of cyst rupture as an important prognostic factor in patients with ovarian carcinoma remains controversial. Recent work by Dembo and colleagues[81] seems to disprove this hypothesis. In their two-hospital multivariate analysis of 519 patients, only grade, adherence, and ascitic fluid were associated with a predictive value of prognosis and disease-free and overall survival. Cyst rupture, bilaterality, tumor size, or capsular penetration did not have independent predictive value. However, given the unsettled nature of this controversy, a careful preoperative and intraoperative assessment should be undertaken to exclude all patients with an ovarian malignancy.

Two diagnostic modalities employed in preoperative assessment of ovarian carcinoma are CA 125 and ultrasonography. The positive predictive value of CA 125 in postmenopausal women is 87% to 98%, and the negative predictive value ranges between 68% and 80%.[82] In contrast the positive predictive value in premenopausal women is not as accurate (36% to 67%).[82] Therefore, CA 125 is of considerably greater value in the management of postmenopausal women with ovarian masses than premenopausal women. Parker and Berek[83] have demonstrated 100% accuracy in a pilot study of benign disease in postmenopausal women when CA 125 is less than 35 U/mL and ultrasonography reveals a cyst less than 10 cm with distinct borders and the absence of irregular areas, septae, ascites, or matted bowel. Unfortunately, predictive guidelines for premenopausal women other than ascites, complex ovarian cyst, or evidence of metastatic disease remain uncertain.

The laparoscopic approach to the adnexal mass should begin with aspiration of any peritoneal fluid for cytologic evaluation followed by washings and aspiration. Subsequently, the peritoneum, omentum, serosal surfaces of bowel, and diaphragm should be carefully inspected for evidence of metastatic disease and biopsied if indicated. The ovarian pathology itself should be addressed, with special attention given to any characteristic suggestive of malignancy (e.g., surface irregularities of the cyst or mass). Finally, a biopsy should be obtained for frozen section with care taken to avoid rupture or spillage of the contents of the cyst or mass. Should these analyses confirm or suggest malignancy, the procedure is terminated or converted immediately to laparotomy. If there is no suggestion of malignancy, one can proceed with laparoscopic salpingo-oophorectomy or ovarian cystectomy as deemed appropriate. If the latter is chosen, a biopsy of the ovary should be performed.

Laparoscopic oophorectomy is performed with the patient in modified lithotomy, steep Trendelenberg position, and rotation of the pathologic adnexa upward. The vagina is prepared in the usual

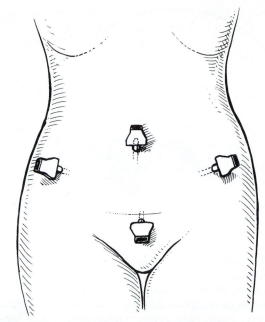

**FIGURE 5A-23.** Location of cannulas for laparoscopic oophorectomy. (*From Amaral CP: Diagnostic and therapeutic laparoscopy for malignant diseases, in* Atlas of Surgical Oncology, *Bland KI et al (eds). Philadelphia, WB Saunders, 1995, pp 749–789.*)

fashion and a uterine manipulator is inserted. Three or four cannulas are used for the procedure: 10-mm umbilical; 12-mm and 5-mm cannulas in the right and left midabdomen at the level of the umbilicus placed lateral to the rectus muscle to avoid the epigastric artery; and a suprapubic midline 5-mm cannula (Fig. 5A-23).

Traction of the uterus anteriorly and away from the area of the procedure via the uterine manipulator facilitates dissection (Fig. 5A-24). The ureter is identified prior to dividing the infundibulopelvic ligament. This ligament may be divided by any one of several means: a triple extracorporeal suture ligature; an endoscopic 30-mm linear stapler; clips and ligating loops; bipolar electrosurgery and ligating loops; or the ultrasonically activated shears and ligating loops (Fig. 5A-25). The broad ligament is divided with electrosurgical or ultrasonically activated shears (Fig. 5A-26). Any of these techniques may be repeated for division of the fallopian tube and the proximal ovarian ligament (Fig. 5A-27). The specimen is then placed in a thick specimen bag and extracted via a trocar site or culpotomy. Once in the bag, the specimen is aspirated if necessary to facilitate removal. Aspiration is performed under careful visualization to avoid perforation of the specimen bag; the cyst fluid is forwarded for pathologic examination. Finally, the abdomen is copiously irrigated with sterile water or saline and aspirated dry.

Laparoscopy is of proven value in the management of advanced epithelial ovarian cancer as a means to assess responses to various chemotherapeutic regimens.[84–86] Indeed, laparoscopy appears ideally suited for "second-look" procedures, since it allows rapid assessment of the extent of disease on an outpatient basis or brief hospital stay, is more accurate than conventional imaging modalities, and is associated with a reduced incidence of de novo adhesion formation when compared to laparotomy.[87] Krafft et al.[86] compared the

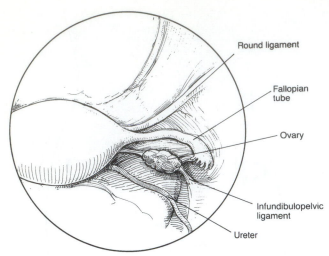

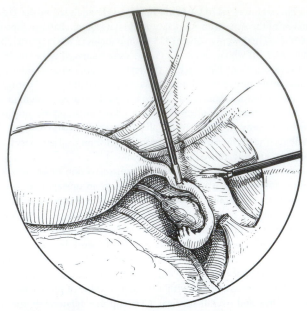

**FIGURE 5A-24.** Exposure of the tuboovarian complex by upward and contralateral displacement of the uterus via the transcervical uterine manipulator. (*From Amaral CP: Diagnostic and therapeutic laparoscopy for malignant diseases, in* Atlas of Surgical Oncology, *Bland KI et al (eds). Philadelphia, WB Saunders, 1995, pp 749–789.*)

**FIGURE 5A-26.** Division of the broad ligament with shears. (*From Amaral CP: Diagnostic and therapeutic laparoscopy for malignant diseases, in* Atlas of Surgical Oncology, *Bland KI et al (eds). Philadelphia, WB Saunders, 1995, pp 749–789.*)

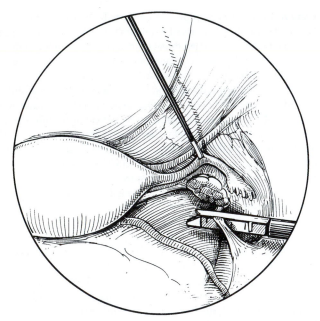

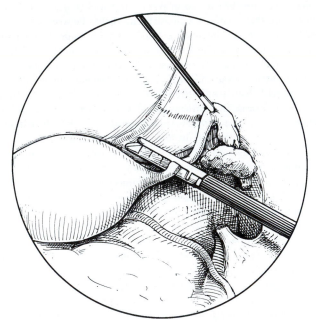

**FIGURE 5A-25.** Division of the infundibulopelvic ligament with endoscopic linear stapler. (*From Amaral CP: Diagnostic and therapeutic laparoscopy for malignant diseases, in* Atlas of Surgical Oncology, *Bland KI et al (eds). Philadelphia, WB Saunders, 1995, pp 749–789.*)

**FIGURE 5A-27.** Division of the proximal fallopian tube and ovarian ligament with endoscopic linear stapler. (*From Amaral CP: Diagnostic and therapeutic laparoscopy for malignant diseases, in* Atlas of Surgical Oncology, *Bland KI et al (eds). Philadelphia, WB Saunders, 1995, pp 749–789.*)

**TABLE 5A-2.** ABILITY (%) OF IMAGING MODALITIES TO DETECT METASTATIC PELVIC NODES
IN CERVICAL CANCER

| IMAGING TECHNIQUE | SENSITIVITY | SPECIFICITY | ACCURACY | FALSE(−) | FALSE(+) |
|---|---|---|---|---|---|
| Lymphangiography | 25–66 | 82–91 | 69–85 | 32 | 10 |
| CT Scan | 60–80 | 86–100 | 76–89 | 13 | 21 |
| MRI | 60 | 91 | 84 | — | — |

SOURCE: Bemelman WA et al.[45]

remission rate for cisplatin-treated ovarian cancer when laparoscopy or laparotomy was used. Remission times were similar regardless of the method used, implying that laparoscopy and laparotomy are equally effective in evaluating patients for recurrent disease. In this regard, laparoscopy is advocated for the evaluation of patients with treated ovarian carcinoma who develop a rise in CA 125 level during follow-up.[88]

## ENDOMETRIAL CANCER

With improvement in laparoscopic instrumentation and techniques and success of laparoscopic-assisted vaginal hysterectomy (LAVH) and laparoscopic lymph node dissections, the feasibility of treatment of oncologic diseases of the uterus became possible. Proper staging for endometrial cancer requires an assessment of whether the disease is confined to the uterus or has extended to contiguous structures or lymph nodes. This can be technically performed laparoscopically. The incidence of lymph node metastases increases with stage. For stage I, only 2% of patients will have lymph node metastases, whereas 50% of stage II patients will have nodal metastases.[89] Treatment usually consists of hysterectomy but, with poor survival for stage III and IV disease, laparoscopic staging may have a role in selecting patients for neoadjuvant protocols. Several small studies have reported success with treatment of early-stage endometrial cancer.

Holub and colleagues[90] compared open versus laparoscopic treatment of stage I endometrial cancer and concluded that the procedure was technically possible and was associated with shorter hospitalizations and more rapid recovery. Mage et al.[91] retrospectively studied 17 patients with stage I disease. Five patients were converted; the remaining 12 patients were successfully treated by laparoscopic means. With a mean follow-up of 22 months, 11 of 12 patients remain disease-free.[91] Despite these successes, experience with treatment and staging is limited and further work needs to be done.

## CERVICAL CANCER

Pretreatment surgical staging of cervical cancer has not been widely employed because laparotomy has been required in the past and the information gained is likely to benefit only a small portion (7%) of the patients.[92] Nonetheless, in 1980, the Gynecologic Oncology Group Cooperative Study reported that when clinical staging was compared to pretreatment surgical staging in 545 patients with cervical cancer, 23% of clinical stage IIB and 64% of stage IIIB were

incorrectly staged.[93] In part, this relates to the lack of precision of modalities in detecting nodal disease (Table 5A-2). In addition to the status of nodal disease, operative staging offers information regarding peritoneal cytologic analysis and adnexal or peritoneal metastatic disease.

This issue is of particular importance when one compares the morbidity of extended field radiation with the need or likelihood for improvement with such treatment. Berman et al.[94] reported that only 4% of patients with surgical stage IB, 13% of stage IIA, and 19% of stage IIB cervical carcinoma will have paraaortic lymph node metastases. Furthermore, the incidence of positive paraaortic lymph nodes is less than 1% if pelvic lymph nodes are negative[95] and 36% if they are positive.[96] Given an unknown status of the paraaortic lymph nodes, the probability that extended field radiation will improve therapy is estimated to be no greater than 4%.[97]

Recent investigations at the Universities of Arizona,[98,99] Minnesota,[92] and in Roubaix, France,[97,100] have established the technique, safety, and efficacy of laparoscopic pelvic and paraaortic lymphadenectomies in the staging of cervical carcinoma. Fowler et al.[92] evaluated 12 patients by laparoscopic pelvic and paraaortic lymphadenectomy followed by immediate laparotomy. Laparoscopy alone yielded 75% of the nodes found by the combination modalities of laparoscopy and laparotomy.[92] No patient with negative nodes at laparoscopy had positive nodes at laparotomy; laparoscopy was a better predictor of lymph node spread than CT. Similarly, Childers and colleagues[98] evaluated 12 patients with stage I cervical carcinoma and 6 patients with stage II or greater. Three of eight stage I patients who were anticipated to need radical hysterectomy were found to have metastatic disease (35% change in planned therapy). Furthermore, laparotomy was utilized for the remaining five patients and yielded only 9% of the total lymph nodes, none of which were positive. Mean length of stay for the laparoscopy-only group was 1.5 days.[98]

Therefore, laparoscopic staging of cervical cancer appears to have an important role in the treatment of patients with clinical stage I disease who are scheduled for radical hysterectomy and may have metastatic disease and benefit from alternative therapy. The procedure is performed with minimal blood loss and complications. The usual advantages of laparoscopy, short hospital stay and convalescence, were noted.

Plante et al.[101] retrospectively reviewed 13 patients with proven or suspected recurrent cervical carcinoma. These patients underwent laparoscopic staging prior to laparotomy. One patient could not be staged laparoscopically. Of the remaining 12 metastatic disease was present in 9. One patient underwent a palliative exenteration. Laparotomy was avoided in 8 of 12 patients.

## RENAL CANCER

Because of the kidneys' retroperitoneal location, laparoscopy is of little use in diagnosing or staging renal malignancies. CT scan and percutaneous biopsy are the standards for diagnosis and staging. Radical nephrectomy (including the adrenal gland, Gerota's fascia, perinephric fat, and regional lymph nodes) is the treatment of choice if the patient has good contralateral renal function. As with malignancies in other organs, laparoscopy is being evaluated in the treatment of renal cell carcinoma. Thus far, only small studies have been done in selected patients with T1 and T2 tumors, but all report good technical success.

Ono[102] reported on 25 patients that underwent laparoscopic nephrectomy. Both transperitoneal (11 patients) and retroperitoneal (14 patients) approaches were used. There were five complications, including one conversion. There were no recurrences with a mean follow-up of 22 months. Himpens[103] reported on three patients successfully treated completely laparoscopically with a 5-day length of stay and no morbidity. When performed completely laparoscopically, an additional incision must be made to remove the specimen. This is usually accomplished by connecting two trocar sites to create a single incision with an overall length of 5 to 6 cm. Hayakawa et al.[104] and Nishiyama and Terunuma[105] each reported a small series of 7 patients treated by a laparoscopically assisted technique. In addition to the laparoscopic incisions, a 7-cm incision was made on the abdomen prior to placement of the trocars. A gasless wall lift technique was used. All nephrectomies were completed using this method.

Use of laparoscopic methods for nephrectomy in patients with renal cell carcinoma can be done safely. To date, no cases of port site recurrences or other oncologic failures of the technique have been reported.

## BLADDER CANCER

Similar to its use in renal malignancies, laparoscopy is in its infancy in the treatment of bladder carcinoma. There are a few case reports of successful treatment in the literature but no series of significance. Transitional cell carcinoma often spreads to the pelvic lymph nodes, and the efficacy of laparoscopic techniques to examine these nodes points to a potential role in the staging of bladder cancer. The poor survival seen in lymph node–positive patients may make them candidates for neoadjuvant protocols. There may also be a role for laparoscopy in palliation of patients with unresectable disease. Puppo et al.[106] reported on three patients (two with prostate cancer, one with bladder cancer) that received laparoscopic bilateral cutaneous ureterostomies for ureteral obstruction secondary to their primary tumors.

Transitional cell carcinoma has been reported in a port site metastasis following laparoscopic staging of recurrent disease.[107] The usual concerns regarding tumor dissemination during laparoscopy may limit the treatment of bladder carcinoma if transitional cell carcinoma has a propensity to implant in trocar sites. This has been noted in a review by Elbahnasy et al.[108] They reported that the incidence of port site metastasis after staging lymphadenectomy for transitional cell carcinoma of the bladder was fortyfold greater than that

**TABLE 5A-3.** ACCURACY (%) OF DIAGNOSTIC PROCEDURES FOR STAGING PELVIC LYMPH NODES IN PROSTATE CANCER

| | SENSITIVITY | SPECIFICITY | ACCURACY |
|---|---|---|---|
| CAT scan | 80–100 | 50–70 | 83–92 |
| MRI | — | — | 83–89 |
| Lymphangiography | — | — | 80 |

SOURCE: Cushieri A.[53]

for staging lymphadenectomy for prostate cancer (4% vs. 0.1%). Clearly, the data are preliminary and scant, but caution must be advised.

## PROSTATE CANCER

The staging of prostate carcinoma is of utmost importance in determining appropriate therapy, since no advantage is provided by radical prostatectomy for patients with metastatic disease. Unfortunately, current noninvasive imaging modalities are not precise enough to determine accurately the presence of positive lymph nodes (Table 5A-3). Large pelvic lymph nodes may harbor no malignant tissue, whereas small, normal-size nodes may possess micrometastases. Similarly, pedal lymphangiography commonly does not demonstrate micrometastases, inconsistently opacifies the internal iliac and obturator chains, and does not differentiate metastatic nodes smaller than 5 mm.[109]

Until recently, surgical staging of prostate cancer has been objectively determined by laparotomy. However, the pioneering efforts of Winfield[110] and Schuessler[111] with the laparoscopic approach has led to widespread acceptance of this modality by urologic oncologists. Its applicability is defined by the following patient population with known prostate cancer: (1) patients considered candidates for radical retropubic prostatectomy who have a PSA level of 40 ng or greater; (2) Gleason score 8 or greater; (3) stage B2, C, or D0 disease; and/or (4) a negative CT-directed needle biopsy for lymphadenopathy determined by CT scan.[112] Patients scheduled for radiation therapy because of age, concurrent illness, or other factors should not be subjected to laparoscopic staging. Furthermore, patients with stage A1, A2, or B2 disease with a PSA below 20 ng/dL, and Gleason score of less than 6 rarely have positive nodes and probably do not benefit from lymphadenectomy.

Evidence supporting a laparoscopic approach includes earlier oral intake, earlier hospital discharge (1.7 vs. 5.4 days), earlier return to normal activities (4.94 vs. 42.9 days), and a reduction in blood loss (100 vs. 212.5 mL).[112] The diagnostic superiority of laparoscopy to preoperative CT was reported by Taillandier et al.[113] who observed 23 of 48 patients (48%) with normal CT scans had metastatic lymph nodes at laparoscopic evaluation.

Comparison of lymph node harvest performed by laparoscopy or laparotomy shows no statistical difference when the former procedure was performed by experienced surgeons. Parra and colleagues[114] randomized a group of 24 men with prostate cancer to either open or laparoscopic lymphadenectomy. The average total number of lymph

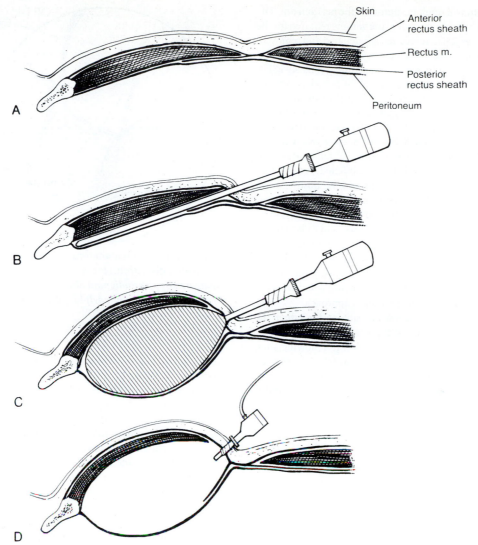

**FIGURE 5A-28.** *A.* Sagittal anatomy of rectus sheath. *B.* Placement of balloon introducer above posterior rectus sheath and below the rectus muscle. *C.* Balloon distends the extraperitoneal space. *D.* Balloon is removed and the space filled with carbon dioxide gas. (*From Amaral CP: Diagnostic and therapeutic laparoscopy for malignant diseases, in Atlas of Surgical Oncology, Bland KI et al (eds). Philadelphia, WB Saunders, 1995, pp 749–789.*)

nodes was 11+5.7 in the laparotomy group and 10.7+5.7 in the laparoscopy group. Furthermore, no additional lymphatic tissue was obtained in any of the patients undergoing open staging; there was no morbidity in either group.[114]

## LAPAROSCOPIC PELVIC LYMPHADENECTOMY

Laparoscopic pelvic lymphadenectomy is performed with the patient supine and in steep Trendelenberg position with rotation toward the ipsilateral side to be dissected first. Either a transperitoneal or extraperitoneal approach is used. The transperitoneal approach as described previously is initiated with either a Veress needle or

an open technique. The abdomen is insufflated to 15 mmHg and dissection begun by dividing the peritoneum.

The total extraperitoneal approach, as the name implies, involves the creation of an extraperitoneal space for insufflation and surgery.[115,116] This is done by using a balloon dissector (GSI or Origin) to create the space. A 10-mm infraumbilical midline incision is completed with exposure of the anterior rectus sheath. This fascial sheath is divided transversely, exposing the rectus abdominis muscle and the posterior rectus sheath (Fig. 5A-28A). The balloon dilator is inserted below the anterior rectus sheath and superficial to the posterior rectus sheath (Fig. 5A-28B). Placement above the anterior sheath will result in creation of a subcutaneous space that is anatomically of no value to the procedure; placement below the posterior rectus sheath will result in rupture of the peritoneum. The balloon is insufflated with saline or air to the volume required for the specific balloon (Fig. 5A-28C); thereafter, it is deflated and removed. A laparoscopy cannula is then placed in the umbilical incision and the extraperitoneal space insufflated to 8 to 15 mmHg (Fig. 5A-28D).

The advantages of the extraperitoneal approach over the transperitoneal method are related to the intact peritoneum in the extraperitoneal approach. Since the procedure is performed completely out of the peritoneal cavity, the risk of visceral injury is negligible. Visualization of the urinary bladder is improved with the extraperitoneal method because small volumes of fat are dissected away with the peritoneum as the balloon is inflated. As gas does not enter the peritoneal cavity during the procedure, postoperative shoulder pain is reduced. Anatomic structures are more easily recognized because they are not invested with peritoneum. Finally, there is no interference from the bowel during a subsequent radical retropubic prostatectomy because the peritoneum remains intact. Should the peritoneum be left open following the transperitoneal approach, the bowel may herniate into the operative field during subsequent prostatectomy. Therefore, closure of the peritoneum with sutures or clips is recommended with the transperitoneal approach.

Cannula placement and dissection are similar for either the transperitoneal or the extraperitoneal approach. Three or four cannulas are used for the procedure and include the following sites: 10- or 12-mm umbilical; two 5-mm cannulas in the right and left midabdomen about the level of the umbilicus and lateral to the rectus muscle to avoid the epigastric artery; and finally, a suprapubic midline 10-mm cannula (Fig. 5A-29). The node dissection com-

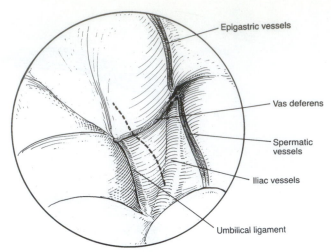

**FIGURE 5A-30.** Pelvic anatomy and location of incision for pelvic lymph node dissection. (*From Amaral CP: Diagnostic and therapeutic laparoscopy for malignant diseases, in* Atlas of Surgical Oncology, *Bland KI et al (eds). Philadelphia, WB Saunders, 1995, pp 749–789.*)

mences on the side most likely to yield positive nodes: demonstrable nodes on CT scan, the ipsilateral side of a single positive prostate biopsy, or the side with the higher Gleason score when evaluating bilateral disease.

In the transperitoneal approach, a peritoneal incision is completed lateral to the umbilical ligament near the level of the internal inguinal ring, curving inferiorly toward the iliac pulsation (Fig. 5A-30). This incision is extended to approximately the iliac bifurcation. Opposing retraction of the peritoneal leaves with graspers, held in lateral directions, exposes the space to be dissected (Fig. 5A-31). The extraperitoneal approach obviates this step.

The vas deferens is identified and transected between titanium clips. The pubic tubercle and Cooper's ligament are identified and dissection is begun laterally and away from the bladder (Fig. 5A-32). Bladder perforation is a recognized complication; thus care should be taken to assure bladder fat is not being dissected. The medial surface of the external iliac vein is identified following meticulous medial dissection of the external iliac artery. The pulsation of this vessel serves as a useful anatomic landmark. The vein is skeletonized along its length by gentle blunt medial dissection. The circumflex vein identifies the anterior extent of the dissection. An aberrant obturator vein also may be encountered in the midpoint of the iliac vein dissection; this structure may be divided or preserved. As the nodal packet is swept medially from the iliac vein, the obturator nerve will be encountered running obliquely to enter the obturator foramen. This marks the deep margin of dissection. The nodal packet is then dissected inferiorly to the bifurcation of the iliac vessels, where dissection of the obturator chain is completed. The packet, which generally measures 2 × 5 cm, is removed in a specimen bag for immediate pathologic analysis.

Thereafter, the ipsilateral iliac nodal chain is dissected. The transperitoneal approach requires extension of the peritoneal incision over the iliac artery toward the aortic bifurcation (Fig. 5A-33). The

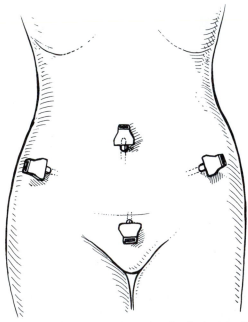

**FIGURE 5A-29.** Location of cannulas for laparoscopic pelvic lymph node dissection. (*From Amaral CP: Diagnostic and therapeutic laparoscopy for malignant diseases, in* Atlas of Surgical Oncology, *Bland KI et al (eds). Philadelphia, WB Saunders, 1995, pp 749–789.*)

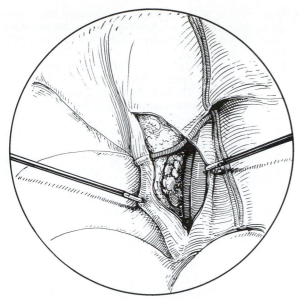

**FIGURE 5A-31.** Dissection of the peritoneum off underlying structures and lateral retraction of the peritoneal leaves exposes the space. (*From Amaral CP: Diagnostic and therapeutic laparoscopy for malignant diseases, in* Atlas of Surgical Oncology, *Bland KI et al (eds). Philadelphia, WB Saunders, 1995, pp 749–789.*)

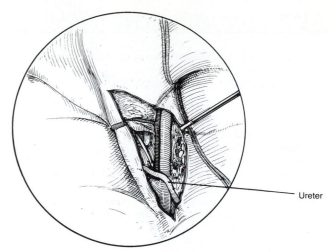

**FIGURE 5A-33.** Extension of the peritoneal incision to reveal the bifurcation of the internal and external iliac arteries and the crossing ureter. (*From Amaral CP: Diagnostic and therapeutic laparoscopy for malignant diseases, in* Atlas of Surgical Oncology, *Bland KI et al (eds). Philadelphia, WB Saunders, 1995, pp 749–789.*)

ureter must be identified. The fatty tissue lying lateral to the external iliac artery is dissected bluntly with lateral retraction until the genitofemoral nerve is encountered (Fig. 5A-34). The fatty tissue interposed between the external iliac artery and the genitofemoral nerve is bluntly dissected from approximately the level of the iliopubic tract to the site at which the ureter crosses the iliac vessels. At the superior margin of dissection, care should be taken to avoid injury to the circumflex iliac and epigastric vessels. This completes the dissection of the iliac nodes, which are then placed within a specimen bag and forwarded to pathology. In the absence of pathologically positive nodes, the procedure is repeated on the contralateral side.

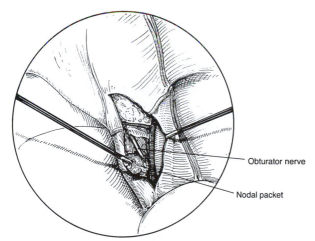

**FIGURE 5A-32.** The vas deferens is divided. The pelvic lymph node packet is swept off the iliac vein. The circumflex vein signals the superior part of the dissection. (*From Amaral CP: Diagnostic and therapeutic laparoscopy for malignant diseases, in* Atlas of Surgical Oncology, *Bland KI et al (eds). Philadelphia, WB Saunders, 1995, pp 749–789.*)

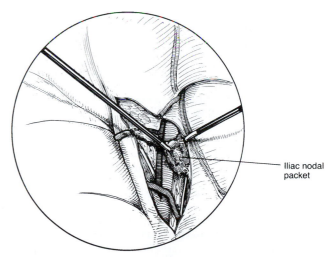

**FIGURE 5A-34.** Dissection of the node bearing tissue lateral to the iliac artery to expose the genitofemoral nerve. (*From Amaral CP: Diagnostic and therapeutic laparoscopy for malignant diseases, in* Atlas of Surgical Oncology, *Bland KI et al (eds). Philadelphia, WB Saunders, 1995, pp 749–789.*)

## REFERENCES

1. PARASKEVA PA et al: The evolution of laparoscopic surgery. Min Inv Ther 369, 1994.

2. DAVIS CJ: A history of endoscopic surgery. Surg Laparosc Endosc 2:16, 1992.

3. ROCK JA, WARSHAW JR: The history and future of operative laparoscopy. Am J Obstet Gynecol 170:7, 1994.

4. BERNHEIM B: Organoscopy: Cystoscopy of the abdominal cavity. Ann Surg 53:764, 1911.

5. MOSENTHAL WT: Peritoneoscopy: A neglected aid in the diagnosis of the general medical and surgical disease. Am J Surg 123:421, 1972.

6. PIER A et al: Laparoscopic appendectomy in 625 cases: From innovation to routine. Surg Laparosc Endosc 1:8, 1991.

7. MILLARD JA et al: Intermittent sequential pneumatic compression in prevention of venous stasis associated with pneumoperitoneum during laparoscopic cholecystectomy. Arch Surg 128:914, 1993.

8. CHAMBERLAIN G, BROWN SC: The report of the working party of the confidential inquiry into gynecological laparoscopy—London. Royal College of Obstetricians and Gynecologists, 1978.

9. CUSHIERI A: Value of laparoscopy in hepatobiliary disease. Br J Surg 57:33, 1975.

10. RIEDEL HH et al: The frequency of distribution of various pelviscopic operations, including complication rates—Statistics of the Federal Republic of Germany in the years 1983–85. Zentralbl Gynakol 111:78, 1989.

11. SACKIER JM et al: Elective diagnostic laparoscopy. Am J Surg 161:326, 1991.

12. WARSHAW AL et al: Laparoscopy in the staging and planning of therapy for pancreatic cancer. Am J Surg 151:76, 1986.

13. NDUKA CC et al: Abdominal wall metastases following laparoscopy. Br J Surg 81:648, 1994.

14. GOLDSTEIN DS et al: Inhibition of peritoneal tumor-cell implantation: model for laparoscopic cancer surgery. J Endourol 7:237, 1993.

15. NEUHAUS SJ et al: Efficacy of cytotoxic agents for the prevention of laparoscopic port site metastases. Arch Surg 133:762, 1998.

16. FERNANDEZ-DEL CASTILLO C, WARSHAW AL: Laparoscopy for staging pancreatic carcinoma. Surg Oncol 2(suppl 1):25, 1993.

17. EGAN C et al: Port site recurrences: A current review of the literature. Surg Endosc 11:196, 1997.

18. NEUHAUS SJ et al: Wound metastasis after laparoscopy with different insufflation gases. Surgery 123:579, 1998.

19. MATHEW G et al: The effect of laparoscopy on the movement of tumor cells and metastasis to surgical wounds. Surg Endosc 11:1163, 1997.

20. REYMOND MA et al: The incidence of port-site metastases might be reduced. Surg Endosc 11:902, 1997.

21. IWANAKA T et al: Mechanism and prevention of port-site tumor recurrence after laparoscopy in a murine model. J Pediatr Surg 33:457, 1998.

22. PAIK PS et al: Abdominal incision tumor implantation following pneumoperitoneum laparoscopic procedure vs. Standard open incision in a syngeneic rat model. Dis Colon Rectum 41:419, 1998.

23. LACY AM et al: Port site metastases and recurrence after laparoscopic colectomy. Surg Endosc 12:1039, 1998.

24. MILSOM JW et al: A prospective, randomized trial comparing laparoscopic versus conventional techniques in colorectal cancer surgery: a preliminary report. J Am Coll Surg 187:46, 1998.

25. REYMOND MA et al: Pathogenesis of puncture site metastases after laparoscopy. Zentralbl Chir 122:387, 1997.

26. HUNERBEIN M et al: The role of staging laparoscopy for multimodal therapy of gastrointestinal cancer. Surg Endosc 12:921, 1998.

27. FINCH MD et al: Laparoscopic ultrasonography for staging gastroesophageal cancer. Surgery 121:10, 1997.

28. GOUMA DJ et al: Laparoscopic ultrasonography for staging of gastrointestinal malignancy. Scand J Gastroenterol 31(suppl 218): 43, 1996.

29. JOHN TG et al: Superior staging of liver tumors with laparoscopy and laparoscopic ultrasound. Ann Surg 220:711, 1994.

30. CUESTA MA et al: Laparoscopic ultrasonography for hepatobiliary and pancreatic malignancy. Br J Surg 80:1571, 1993.

31. SOTOMAYOR R, RAVIKUMAR TS: Cryosurgery on the treatment of hepatic tumors. Cancer Control 3:414, 1996.

32. VANDELDEN OM et al: Laparoscopic ultrasonography for abdominal tumor staging: technical aspects and imaging findings. Abdom Imaging 22:125, 1997.

33. SALKY BA et al: The use of laparoscopy in retroperitoneal pathology. Gastroint Endosc 34:227, 1988.

34. MANN GB et al: Emerging role of laparoscopy in the diagnosis of lymphoma. J Clin Oncol 16:1909, 1998.

35. FERZLI G et al: Laparoscopic staging of Hodgkins disease. J Laparoendosc Adv Surg Tech A 7:353, 1997.

36. ZORNIG C et al: Staging laparoscopy in Hodgkin's disease. A valid alternative to staging laparotomy. Dtsch Med Wochenschr 118:1401, 1993.

37. LEFOR AT et al: Laparoscopic staging of Hodgkin's disease. Surg Oncol 2:217, 1993.

38. DEARTH JC et al: Partial splenectomy for staging Hodgkin's disease: Risk of false-negative results. N Engl J Med 299:345, 1978.

39. BRADY PG et al: Role of laparoscopy in the evaluation of patients with suspected hepatic or peritoneal malignancy. Gastrointest Endosc 37:27, 1991.

40. SHANDALL A, JOHNSON C: Laparoscopy or scanning in esophageal and gastric carcinoma? Br J Surg 72:449, 1985.

41. WATT I et al: Laparoscopy ultrasound and computed tomography in cancer of the esophagus and gastric cardia. Br J Surg 76:1036, 1989.

42. ROSCH T: Endoscopic techniques in gastrointestinal oncology. Curr Opin Oncol 6:413, 1994.

43. EARLAM R, CUNHA-MELO JR: Oesophageal squamous cell carcinoma: I. A critical review of surgery. Br J Surg 67:381, 1980.

44. BONAVINA L et al: Preoperative laparoscopy in management of patients with carcinoma of the esophagus and of the esophagogastric junction. J Surg Oncol 65:171, 1997.

45. BEMELMAN WA et al: Laparoscopy and laparoscopic ultrasonography in staging of carcinoma of the esophagus and gastric cardia. J Am Coll Surg 181:421, 1995.

46. VAN DIJKUM EJ et al: The efficacy of laparoscopic staging in patients with upper gastrointestinal tract tumors. Cancer 79:1315, 1997.

47. POSSIK RA et al: Sensitivity, specificity and predictive value of laparoscopy for the staging of gastric cancer and for the detection of liver metastases. Cancer 58:1, 1986.

48. KRIPLANI AK and KAPUR BM: Laparoscopy for preoperative

staging and assessment of operability in gastric carcinoma. Gastrointest Endosc 37:441, 1991.

49. BURKE EC et al: Laparoscopy in the management of gastric adenocarcinoma. Ann Surg 225:262, 1997.

50. BALLESTA-LOPEZ C et al: Laparoscopic Billroth II distal subtotal gastrectomy with gastric stump suspension for gastric malignancies. Am J Surg 171:289, 1996.

51. WARSHAW AL: Implications of peritoneal cytology for staging of early pancreatic cancer. Am J Surg 161:26, 1986.

52. FERNANDEZ-DEL CASTILLO C, WARSHAW AL: Peritoneal metastasis in pancreatic cancer. Hepatogastroenterology 40:430, 1993.

53. CUSHIERI A: Laparoscopy for pancreatic cancer: Does it benefit the patient? Eur J Surg Oncol 14:41, 1988.

54. CUBILLA AL et al: Lymph node involvement in carcinoma of the head of the pancreas area. Cancer 41:880, 1978.

55. GAGNER M, POMP A: Laparoscopic pylorus-preserving pancreatoduodenectomy. Surg Endosc 8:408, 1994.

56. LAI EC et al: Choice of palliation for malignant hilar biliary obstruction. Am J Surg 163:208, 1992.

57. HAVENSTEIN KH et al: Percutaneous interventions on the bile duct in obstructive jaundice. A meaningful or excruciating prolongation of life? Radiology 32:13, 1992.

58. GORDON RL et al: Malignant biliary obstruction: Treatment with expandable metallic stents. Radiology 182:697, 1992.

59. FLETCHER DR, JONES RM: Laparoscopic cholecystojejunostomy as palliation for obstructive jaundice in inoperable carcinoma of pancreas. Surg Endosc 6:147, 1992.

60. SHIMI S et al: Laparoscopy in the management of pancreatic cancer: endoscopic cholecystojejunostomy for advanced disease. Br J Surg 79:317, 1992.

61. NAGY A et al: Laparoscopic gastroenterostomy for duodenal obstruction. Am J Surg 169:539, 1995.

62. GUVEN P et al: Preoperative imaging of liver metastasis. Ann Surg 202:573, 1985.

63. WARD BA et al: Prospective evaluation of hepatic imaging studies in the detection of colorectal metastases: Correlation with surgical findings. Surgery 105:180, 1989.

64. FORSE RQA et al: Laparoscopy/thoracoscopy for staging. Semin Surg Oncol 9:51, 1993.

65. BABINEAU TJ et al: Role of staging laparoscopy in the treatment of hepatic malignancy. Am J Surg 167:151, 1994.

66. LOCICERO J III: Laparoscopy/thoracoscopy for staging: II. Pretherapy nodal evaluation in carcinoma of the esophagus. Semin Surg Oncol 9:56, 1993.

67. MILSOM JW et al: Preoperative biopsy of pararectal lymph nodes in rectal cancer using endoluminal ultrasonography. Dis Colon Rectum 37:364, 1994.

68. FOWLER DL, WHITE SA: Laparoscopically-assisted sigmoid resection. Surg Endosc Laparosc 1:183, 1991.

69. MONSON JR et al: Prospective evaluation of laparoscopic-assisted colectomy in an unselected group of patients. Lancet 340:831, 1992.

70. BEART RW: Laparoscopic colectomy: Status of the art. Dis Colon Rectum 37:S47, 1994.

71. JACOBS M et al: Minimally invasive colon resection (laparoscopic colectomy). Surg Laparosc Endosc 1:144, 1991.

72. SCOGGIN SD et al: Laparoscopic assisted bowel surgery. Dis Colon Rect 36:747, 1993.

73. GEIS WP et al: Sequential psychomotor skills development in laparoscopic colon surgery. Arch Surg 129:206, 1994.

74. TATE JJT et al: Prospective comparison of laparoscopic and conventional anterior resection. Br J Surg 80:1396, 1993.

75. GABRIEL WB et al: Lymphatic spread in cancer of the rectum. Br J Surg 23:395, 1935.

76. NEZHAT C et al: Laparoscopic radical hysterectomy with paraaortic and pelvic lymph node dissection. Am J Obstet Gynecol 166:864, 1992.

77. REICH H et al: Laparoscopic management of stage I ovarian cancer. A case report. J Reproductive Med 35:601, 1990.

78. YOUNG RC et al: Staging laparotomy in early ovarian cancer. JAMA 250:3072, 1983.

79. HULKA JF et al: Management of ovarian masses. AAGL 1990 survey. J Reproductive Med 37:599, 1992.

80. WEBB MJ et al: Factors influencing survival in stage I ovarian cancer. Am J Obstet Gynecol 116:222, 1973.

81. DEMBO AJ et al: Prognostic factors in patients with stage I epithelial ovarian cancer. Obstet Gynecol 75:263, 1990.

82. ALVAREZ RD et al: Staging ovarian cancer diagnosed during laparoscopy: accuracy rather than immediacy. South Med J 86:1256, 1993.

83. PARKER WH, BEREK JS: Management of selected cystic adnexal masses in postmenopausal women by operative laparoscopy: A pilot study. Am J Obstet Gynecol 163:1574, 1990.

84. LAMBERT HE et al: A randomized trial comparing cancer: a North Thames Ovary Group study. J Clin Oncol 11:440, 1993.

85. NICOLETTO MO et al: Phase I-II intraperitoneal mitoxantrone in advanced pretreated ovarian cancer. Eur J Cancer 29A:1242, 1993.

86. KRAFFT W et al: Second-look Operation oder Second-look Laparoskopie zur Sicherung der kompletten Remission beim Ovarialkarzinom. Zentralbl Gynakol 112:767, 1990.

87. OPERATIVE LAPAROSCOPY STUDY GROUP: Postoperative adhesion development after operative laparoscopy: Evaluation at early second-look procedures. Fert Steril 55:700, 1991.

88. HOGBERG T, KAGEDAL B: Long-term follow-up of ovarian cancer with monthly determinations of serum CA 125. Gynecol Oncol 46:191, 1992.

89. HAMMOND CB: Malignant diseases of the uterus, in Textbook of Surgery, DC Sabiston (ed). Philadelphia, WB Saunders, 1991, pp 1422–1423.

90. HOLUB Z et al: A comparison of laparoscopic surgery with open procedure in endometrial cancer. Eur J Gynaecol Oncol 19:294, 1998.

91. MAGE G et al: Treatment of endometrial clinical stage I adenocarcinoma by laparoscopic surgery. Seventeen cases. J Gynecol Obstet Biol Reprod (Paris) 24:485, 1995.

92. FOWLER JM et al: Lymph node yield from laparoscopic lymphadenectomy in cervical cancer: a comparative study. Gynecol Oncol 51:187, 1993.

93. LAGASSE LD et al: Results and complications of operative staging in cervical cancer: Experience of the Gynecologic Oncology Group. Gynecol Oncol 9:90, 1980.

94. BERMAN M et al: Survival and patterns of recurrence in cervical cancer metastatic to para-aortic lymph nodes. Gynecol Oncol 19:8, 1984.

95. MARTIMBEAU P et al: Stage IB Carcinoma of the cervix: The Norwiegian Hospital: Results when pelvic lymph nodes are involved. Obstet Gynecol 60:215, 1982.

96. DOWNEY G et al: Pretreatment surgical staging in cervical carcinoma: Therapeutic efficacy of pelvic lymph node resection. Am J Obstet Gynecol 160:1055, 1989.

97. QUERLEU D: Laparoscopic paraaortic node sampling in

gynecologic oncology: a preliminary experience. Gynecol Oncol 49:24, 1993.

98. CHILDERS JM et al: The role of laparoscopic lymphadenectomy in the management of cervical carcinoma. Gynecol Oncol 47:38, 1992.

99. CHILDERS JM, SURWIT EA: Combined laparoscopic and vaginal surgery for the management of two cases of stage I endometrial cancer. Gynecol Oncol 45:46, 1992.

100. QUERLEU D et al: Laparoscopic pelvic lymphadenectomy in the staging of early carcinoma of the cervix. Am J Obstet Gynecol 164:579, 1991.

101. PLANTE M, ROY M: Operative laparoscopy prior to a pelvic exenteration in patients with recurrent cervical cancer. Gynecol Oncol 69:94, 1998.

102. ONO Y et al: Laparoscopic radical nephrectomy: The Nagoya experience. J Urol 158:719, 1997.

103. HIMPENS J et al: Operative strategy in laparoscopic nephrectomy. Eur Urol 26:276, 1994.

104. HAYAKAWA K et al: A trial of laparoscopic assisted radical nephrectomy. Nippon Hinyokika Gakkai Zasshi 88:801, 1997.

105. NISHIYAMA T, TERUNUMA M: Laparoscopy-assisted radical nephrectomy in combination with mini-laparotomy: report of initial 7 cases. Int J Urol 2:124, 1995.

106. PUPPO P et al: Laparoscopic bilateral cutaneous ureterostomy for palliation of ureteral obstruction caused by advanced pelvic cancer. J Endourol 8:425, 1994.

107. ANDERSEN JR, STEVEN K: Implantation metastasis after laparoscopic biopsy of bladder cancer. J Urol 153:1047, 1995.

108. ELBAHNASY AM et al: Laparoscopic staging of bladder tumor: concerns about port site metastases. J Endourol 12:55, 1998.

109. KOEHLER PR: Current status of lymphangiography in patients with cancer. Cancer 37 (suppl 1):503, 1976.

110. WINFIELD HN et al: Laparoscopic pelvic lymph node dissection for genitourinary malignancies: indications techniques and results. J Endourol 6:103, 1992.

111. SCHUESSLER WW et al: Transperitoneal endosurgical lymphadenectomy in patients with localized prostate cancer. J Urol 145:988, 1991.

112. KERBL K et al: Staging pelvic lymphadenectomy for prostate cancer: A comparison of laparoscopic and open techniques. J Urol 150:396, discussion 399, 1993.

113. TAILLANDIER J et al: Pelvic lymphadenoscopy. A simple reliable method for the staging of pelvic cancers. Int Surg 77:208, 1992.

114. PARRA RO et al: Staging laparoscopic pelvic lymph node dissection: Comparison of results with open pelvic lymphadenectomy. J Urol 147:875, 1992.

115. VILLERS A et al: Extraperitoneal endosurgical lymphadenectomy with insufflation in the staging of bladder and prostate cancer. J Endourol 7:229, 1993.

116. GAUR DD: Laparoscopic operative retroperitoneoscopy: Use of a new device. J Urol 148:1137, 1992.

# 5B / ENDOSCOPY IN CANCER: DIAGNOSTIC AND THERAPEUTIC ASPECTS

*Rosario Vecchio and Bruce V. MacFadyen, Jr.*

## INTRODUCTION

Although several attempts at viewing the internal lumen of hollow viscera were performed before 400 B.C., this became practical only after the development of fiberoptic technology by J. C. Baird and C. W. Hansell in 1927 and its adaptation to gastroscopy by Heinuck Lamm in 1930[1] and later utilized in 1958 by Hirschowitz.[2] The first fiberoptic examination is credited to Hirschowitz, who in 1957 performed gastroscopy on himself as a demonstration at the American Gastroscopic Society. Interest in flexible endoscopy increased, and later its use expanded into the colon by means of a modified gastroscope.[3] Flexible sigmoidoscopy and colonoscopy, however, were later popularized only after the development in Japan and the United States of four-way tip deflection and increased endoscope flexibility. Overholt[4,5] first described his clinical experience with colonoscopy in 1968 and again in 1970. Williams[3] described the technique of hot biopsy for the treatment of small polyps, and in 1979, Shinya and Wolff[6] reported a large series of colonoscopies and polypectomies.

Diagnostic and therapeutic applications of endoscopy in oncology have increased with the development of several endoscopic techniques including video image enhancement, reflectance spectometry, and ultrasound and ultrasonic mucosal blood flow mapping.[7–9] Endoscopy is now a reliable and safe outpatient procedure for the diagnosis and treatment of neoplasms of the stomach, small intestine, colon, and biliopancreatic regions.

## CURRENT STATUS

### ENDOSCOPY IN ESOPHAGEAL TUMORS

**DIAGNOSTIC ENDOSCOPY.** Esophageal cancer of either the squamous cell or adenocarcinoma type has a poor prognosis with a 5-year survival ranging from 5% to 25%. Diagnosis is usually made when the disease becomes symptomatic with the onset of dysphagia, retrosternal pain, and weight loss. Endoscopy is the most effective diagnostic tool because it enables the physician to obtain a definitive pathologic diagnosis by means of endoscopic biopsy and cytology. The mucosal extent of the disease can be evaluated by endoscopic ultrasound, as can the depth of transmural tumor infiltration and the occurrence of periesophageal and mediastinal lymph node metastasis.

Macroscopically, esophageal cancer is friable and exophytic and the lumen is often stenotic (Fig. 5B-1). Macroscopic diagnosis is 70% to 75% accurate, and endoscopic biopsy and cytology increase the diagnostic accuracy to 95% to 100%.[10,11] Six or more biopsies and cytology should be obtained from a nonulcerated area in order to avoid nondiagnostic necrotic tissue. In cases of severe tumor stenosis, it may be necessary to perform endoscopic dilatation first so that the endoscope can be advanced into a nonnecrotic region and thus decrease the potential of esophageal perforation. The proximal and distal mucosal extent of esophageal cancer can be predicted endoscopically by staining the mucosa with Lugol's solution. However, since esophageal cancer frequently skips through the submucosa, total esophagectomy is often performed, thus minimizing the usefulness of the staining technique.

Submucosal esophageal tumors are diagnostically more challenging for the endoscopist since they present with an intraluminal mass and overlying normal mucosa (Fig. 5B-2). Intramural lipomas often can be suspected because of the display of the "pillow sign," consisting of persistent depression of the soft mass when probed with a catheter, whereas benign cystic masses show a smooth, rounded endoscopic appearance that is fluctuant when probed. The most common tumor is a leiomyoma, which when greater than 3 cm is more likely malignant. In the majority of submucosal masses, a histologic diagnosis can be obtained by performing repeated biopsies in the same site (tunneling technique), thus allowing the endoscopist to obtain deep submucosal tissue.

Endoscopic ultrasound (EUS) can be very helpful in defining the type of esophageal tumor. This technique uses high-frequency ultrasound (7.5 to 12 MHz) and images are obtained with a 360° radial scanner that permits detailed anatomy up to a depth of 29 mm. The wall of the esophagus is imaged in five layers, which shows a close correlation with the visceral anatomy (Fig. 5B-3).[12,13] The first two layers are related to the mucosa, the third layer is the submucosa, and the fourth layer is the muscularis propria. In the stomach, duodenum, colon, and rectum, the fifth layer is the serosa or adventitia.

The most important advantage of esophageal EUS is in its ability to stage esophageal cancer by defining the intramural extent of infiltration of the tumor according to the TNM classification (Table 5B-1).[14] With submucosal lesions, determining whether the tumor is truly submucosal or extrinsic is important. Direct extension

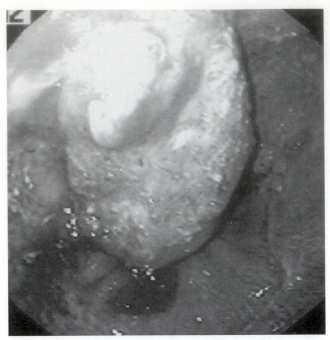

**FIGURE 5B-1.** Esophageal cancer. (See also Plate 15.)

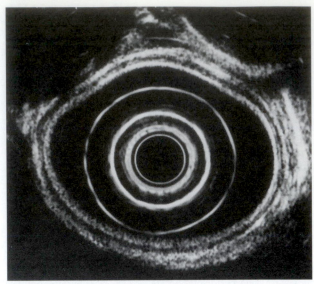

**FIGURE 5B-3.** Endoscopic ultrasound of esophagael tumor: mucosa—inner dark layer; submucosa—white layer; muscularispropria. In the rest of the gastrointestinal tract, a fourth layer would be the serosa and would be dark.

of the esophageal tumor through the esophageal wall and identifying lymph node metastasis greater than 5 mm in size can be demonstrated by showing the hypoechoic pattern and irregular borders (Fig. 5B-4). Confirmation of tumor involvement can be obtained by EUS-guided fine-needle aspiration cytology.

The sensitivity and specificity of EUS in staging transmuralinfiltration and regional metastases of esophageal cancer are higher than those reported for CT scan and traditional ultrasound with an overall sensitivity and specificity of 84% and 77%, respectively.[15,16] The performance of endoscopic ultrasound fine-needle aspiration improves the accuracy of determining nodal involvement to 90%,[17,18] but the accuracy of EUS is lower in T4 lesions invading the tracheobronchial tree, the pleural cavity, and the vertebral spine, where

**TABLE 5B-1. CLASSIFICATION AND CORRELATION OF THE DEPTH OF TUMOR INFILTRATION OF THE ESOPHAGUS**

| | |
|---|---|
| EUS-T1: | Hypoechoic tumor localized in the first (mucosa type), second, or third echo layer (submucosa type). |
| EUS-T2: | Hypoechoic tumor in the first three echo layers, extending into the fourth layer. |
| EUS-T3: | Hypoechoic transmural tumor (first, second, third, and fourth structures), with penetration into the fifth layer. |
| EUS-T4: | Hypoechoic transmural tumor with penetration into adjacent structures such as pericardium, descending aorta, tracheobronchial tree, diaphragm (curva diaphragmatica), or liver. Accurate definition of penetration into adjacent structures should be described as follows: no clear demarcation between the tumor and the adjacent organ irregularities of the organ contour, e.g., aorta, jugular vein, tracheobronchial tree, etc. |

SOURCE: Tio TL.[14] Reproduced with permission.

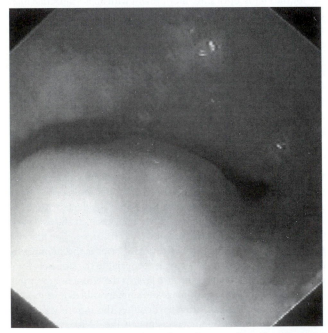

**FIGURE 5B-2.** Submucosal esophageal tumor. (See also Plate 16.)

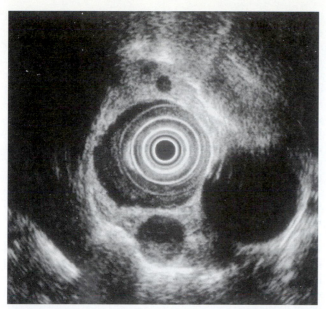

**FIGURE 5B-4.** A large malignant lymph node is seen at the 12:00 and 6:00 position along with a large esophageal tumor extending from the 6:00 to the 12:00 position. At the 4:00 position, the large dark spot represents the aorta. (See also Plate 17.)

definition is very difficult because of the reverberation phenomena of the ultrasound waves over bone and cartilage.[14]

**THERAPEUTIC ENDOSCOPY.** In general, esophageal cancer has a poor prognosis because the majority of patients first present with symptoms and already have regional and distant disease and only palliative treatment can be considered. In a collected series of 83,783 patients by Earlam and Cunha-Melo,[19] surgery was performed in 58% of the patients, and in only 39% of these was resection possible. The survival of the resected patient group at 1-, 2-, and 3-year follow-up was only 18%, 9%, and 4%, respectively. Although if earlier diagnosis occurs, survival can be increased to 10% to 15% at 5 years.[20] Palliation remains the mainstay treatment in approximately 50% of the esophageal cancer patients, and endoscopic treatment is the method of choice since surgery for palliation has a higher morbidity and mortality rate.

Endoscopic techniques have been proposed for early-stage cancer patients who refuse surgery or ones who are at high surgical risk.[21] Endoscopic mucosectomy with a wire snare of an early-stage tumor has proven to be successful, with a 5-year survival of 90%, 84%, and 56% in tumors limited to the mucosa, submucosa, and muscularis mucosa, respectively. Neodymium:yttrium-aluminum garnet (Nd:YAG) laser and photodynamic therapy have also been used to ablate early esophageal cancers.[22,23] In the latter technique, a chemical photosensitizer, hematoporphyrin derivative (HPD), is administered 2 to 4 hours prior to the procedure. The HPD is selectively concentrated in the cancer cell, and when the endoscope is inserted into the esophagus, the surface of the tumor is illuminated with a laser light with a wavelength of 640 nm and oxygen free radicals are

produced that destroy neoplastic tissue. Although these techniques are promising treatment for early esophageal cancer, further studies assessing long-term results as well as complications such as strictures, perforations, and local and distant recurrences are needed.

The goal of endoscopic treatment for palliation of advanced esophageal cancer consists of relieving dysphagia and symptoms related to a tracheoesophageal fistula and improving nutritional status. Several endoscopic techniques can be used, including tumor dilatation, placement of an endoscopic esophageal stent, use of the Nd:YAG laser, photodynamic therapy, bipolar tumor probe (bicap) therapy, local injection therapy, and brachytherapy.[24] The choice of the most suitable method for each patient is dictated by the patient's functional status and compliance and the stage and characteristics of the tumor. Patients with a poor functional status or short life expectancy are candidates for endoscopic procedures such as dilatation and stent placement for immediate relief of dysphagia. The location as well as the longitudinal and circumferential extent of the tumor are also important where short and mid to distal esophageal lesions are best treated with a stent. Stent placement is not recommended in cervical esophageal stenosis because of the risk of airway compression. A bipolar tumor probe and photodynamic therapy are more effective in long circumferential tumors, whereas laser therapy is more effective for asymmetrical short tumors. Physician expertise plays an important role, since the best palliative results are achieved by an experienced team.

Endoscopic dilatation of a malignant stricture is a simple procedure that is performed using either a tapered Eder-Puestow, Savary, or balloon dilator. The dysphagia improves for 1 to 3 months and repeated dilations are required. Chest pain often occurs during the procedure. Perforation of the diseased esophagus is the most frequent complication of this technique and has been described in approximately 5% of patients. Bleeding, transient bacteremia, and chest pain have been described.[25] Therefore, endoscopic dilatation should be considered only in patients with a short life expectancy.

Transtumoral stent placement has been used for several decades to palliate esophageal tumors. Before the era of flexible endoscopy, esophageal stents were usually placed during surgery by means of a combined endoscopic and laparotomy pull-through technique or using a rigid endoscope to perform a push-through technique. In 1977, Atkinson and Ferguson[26] introduced a new technique that involved transtumoral placement of a Celestin tube that was advanced by means of a pusher device called a Nottingham pusher. In this technique, a guidewire was initially placed endoscopically across the tumor and the stent, which was positioned by the Nottingham pusher, so that the stent extended 2 to 3 cm above and below the tumor. These stents provided temporary relief of the obstruction, but stent obstruction and migration often occurred, requiring frequent endoscopic removal of luminal debris and tumor or repositioning of the stent.

Over the years, numerous modifications have been made with new introducers and prostheses so as to make the procedure simpler and safer. The Nottingham pusher has been abandoned, and in many institutions the Savary-Guillard pusher and rigid stent are used. This pusher allows intubation in patients with cervical arthrosis, since it is more flexible and has been successfully placed in selected patients with tumor stenosis of the cervical esophagus.[27] Rigid stents surrounded by a self-inflating foam-covered cuff have been used in esophageal perforation, tracheoesophageal fistulas, and in severe bleeding from the esophageal tumor.[28]

Expandable covered esophageal wire mesh stents are now the most commonly used stents for palliative management of esophageal cancer, since they are more easily placed and are associated with a lower morbidity and mortality rate.[29] The stent can be introduced through the endoscope over a guidewire in a compressed size and then allowed to expand to a diameter of 20 mm, thus dilating the tumor in a radial direction. The major complication associated with these stents is reobstruction secondary to tumor ingrowth through the wire mesh stent, although this complication can be minimized if either a self-expanding coil stent or a silicone-coated stent is used.[24] These covered expandable stents have also been successfully used in tracheoesophageal fistulas. If an obstruction of the stent occurs, insertion of a second expandable stent inside the first stent is performed, since the removal of the first stent is impossible due to its fixation into the esophageal tissue. The incidence of complications is noted in a review by Shimi[29] and includes stent migration (29% to 50%), tumor ingrowth (5% to 36%), tumor overgrowth (<10% with stent length >10 cm), poststent reflux (6% to 19%), hemorrhage (6% to 9%), pain (3% to 5%), and pulmonary aspiration (<5%).

Nd:YAG laser therapy is another effective method to relieve dysphagia in advanced esophageal cancer. The laser fiber is introduced through the working channel of the endoscope and under direct vision the tumor is vaporized and the lumen reestablished. Usually three to five treatment sessions are needed, and the success rate ranges from 69% to 100%, with the best results achieved in short midesophageal stenosis with prominent intraluminal growth.[30] Complications have been reported in 5% to 20% of cases and include perforation, fistula formation, and bleeding. This technique is more effective than other methods in extensive infiltrating tumors and perforation is uncommon, but other complications such as nausea, fever, pleural effusion, and sunburn of the skin secondary to the photosensitivity from the HPD have been described. Bicap (bipolar electrocautery) is another palliative method of treatment that requires several endoscopic sessions and is recommended in long circumferential esophageal tumors.[31] Tracheoesophageal fistulas and hemorrhage are the major complications. Local injection of ethanol and brachytherapy have also been used for palliation of esophageal tumor stenosis, and the early results in small series of patients are promising.[32,33]

## ENDOSCOPY IN THE SCREENING OF ESOPHAGEAL CANCER.

Although both adenocarcinoma and squamous cell carcinoma of the esophagus are aggressive tumors, their prognosis is good if the disease is detected when limited to the mucosa or submucosa (5-year survival greater than 90%), thereby emphasizing early detection. Several studies have recognized Barrett's esophagus as a risk factor for the development of severe dysplasia and adenocarcinoma of the esophagus where the malignancy rate increases from 30 to 125 times over that of the normal population.[34] Others have noted this incidence as being 1 in 208 patient-years.[35] This risk for malignant transformation in Barrett's esophagus is closely associated with the development of intestinal metaplasia, whose detection should be used as a criterion for an oncologic screening program.[36,37] Annual or biannual screening endoscopy with multiple esophageal biopsies should be carried out as soon as the diagnosis of Barrett's esophagus with intestinal metaplasia is made. Four quadrant biopsies of the

lesion and biopsies of the esophagus every 2 cm from the cervical esophagus to 2 cm below the esophagogastric junction are necessary. Destruction of the Barrett's mucosa and regrowth of normal mucosa has occurred using an endoscopic laser and photodynamic therapy in the presence of total acid suppression.[38,39] The impact of this therapy on the prevention of malignant transformation still needs to be addressed, and long-term follow-up is required to assess whether regression is maintained and cancer risk decreased. Follow-up screening and biopsy for dysplasia and intestinalization of the mucosa is recommended every 6 months for 1 year and then every 1 to 3 years. For high-grade dysplasia, surgery is indicated or routine screening should be performed every 6 months.[40]

Screening methods for squamous cell carcinoma have been carried out on a large scale in northern China with promising results.[41,42] In China, methods for screening include endoscopy, cytology, detection of occult blood in the stomach, and biopsies. Topical Lugol's solution is used as a marker for malignant transformation, and biopsies are taken from these marked areas. However, similar screening programs in heavy smokers and drinkers in the United States have not been proven to be cost-effective, and therefore the issue is still under debate.

## ENDOSCOPY IN GASTRIC TUMORS

**DIAGNOSTIC ENDOSCOPY.** Gastric cancer still remains the leading cause of death for malignant disease in Japan, eastern Europe, and South America. However, in the United States, its incidence has decreased over the past 60 years, but interestingly, the incidence of newly diagnosed proximal gastric and gastroesophageal adenocarcinomas have increased in the last 15 years.[43] The prognosis for gastric cancer in the United States is poor, with a 5-year survival rate ranging from 5% to 15%, probably reflecting the fact that diagnosis is often late, thus implying the need for early detection. Endoscopy is the most accurate diagnostic method and should be used routinely for initial evaluation and staging. It provides a better assessment of the location, size, and extent of tumor growth and permits the performance of biopsies for pathologic analysis with an accuracy approximating 95%. On the other hand, barium studies yield a positive diagnosis for 5- to 10-mm lesions of only 75% when the double contrast technique is used.[44] Advanced gastric cancers usually appear as ulcerative endoluminal exophytic masses or as a stenosing tumor (Fig. 5B-5). Linitis plastica spreads submucosally involving the entire stomach wall, and results in loss of wall distensibility. In this advanced form, endoscopic diagnosis is accurate using 6 to 10 biopsy samples and cytology.[45]

Endoscopic diagnosis of early gastric cancer is more challenging, but detection of tumors in the early stage has been rewarding, as observed in Japan where patient survival has been improved through an increased early-diagnosis program. Small lesions of the stomach are often difficult to interpret endoscopically, and only 60% of these lesions are correctly diagnosed at initial examination. Small neoplastic ulcers can be easily confused with benign lesions, since initial biopsies can be negative and healing of the lesion may be observed. It is important to note that healing in malignant lesions is transient, and an endoscopic follow-up with repeated biopsies performed 4 to 8 weeks after the initial examination will demonstrate the malignant changes in almost every patient.

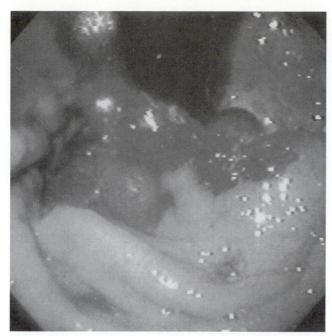

**FIGURE 5B-5.** Carcinoma of stomach at esophagogastric junction. (See also Plate 18.)

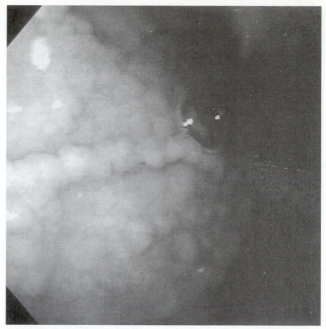

**FIGURE 5B-7.** Endoscopic view of fundic gland polyps of the stomach. (See also Plate 20.)

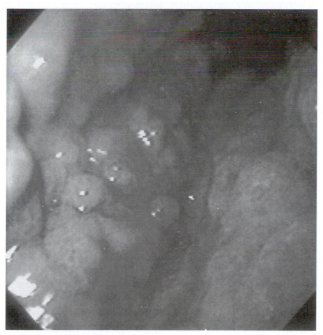

**FIGURE 5B-6.** Endoscopic view of lymphoma of stomach. (See also Plate 19.)

The endoscopic diagnosis of gastric lymphoma is also challenging (Fig. 5B-6). Although large folds associated with decreased motility are indirect endoscopic signs, the definitive diagnosis is sometimes difficult and occasionally diagnostic laparotomy or laparoscopy is re-

quired. Since the lesion is submucosal, endoscopic biopsies are often inadequate and, therefore, multiple large biopsies using the tunneling technique are necessary for establishing immunohistochemical analysis. EUS can also be used to diagnose this lesion. A less malignant form of this is related to MALT (mucosa-associated lymphoid tissue) tumors, which have been associated with *Helicobacter pylori*. Recent studies have indicated tumor regression with eradication of the *H. pylori*.[46,47] Endoscopic follow-up is very important to rule out tumor progression to a high-grade lymphoma.

Among benign tumors, gastric polyps can be recognized by endoscopy. Hyperplastic polyps or fundic gland polyps are the most common, and some of these will cause upper gastrointestinal bleeding (Fig. 5B-7). All polyps should be excised, and those greater than 2 cm in diameter have a greater potential for developing malignancy. If the polyp is completely excised, repeat endoscopy should be performed in 6 to 12 months, and if this endoscopy is negative, surveillance endoscopy can be done every 2 to 3 years.

Although patients with familial adenomatous polyposis (FAP) most frequently present with colon polyps or cancer, gastric and duodenal polyps do occur, with an incidence ranging from 33% to 100%.[48,49] Gastric polyps are usually the fundic gland type and are not premalignant, whereas duodenal polyps are often adenomas and are most frequently located in the ampullary and periampullary region. Malignancy can occur, particularly in the ampullary region, and is the most common cause of death from FAP outside the colon. Sometimes, small lesions can be excised endoscopically if they are not in the periampullary region. However, surgery is often necessary for large periampullary adenomas. Follow-up endoscopic surveillance is indicated every 2 to 3 years.

Although gastric cancer has been reported in patients who have had previous surgery for benign peptic ulcer disease (4% to 6%),[50]

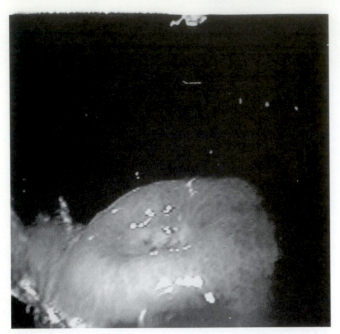

**FIGURE 5B-8.** Endoscopic view of a leiomyoma of the stomach with central depression and ulceration. This area of ulceration can also be a cause of upper gastrointestinal bleeding. (See also Plate 21.)

these data have not been confirmed in a large population-based study.[51]

Benign tumors are often submucosal and include leiomyomas, lipomas, and fibromas. Definitive diagnosis is difficult, since mucosal biopsies are often negative. The endoscopic appearance of a leiomyoma is often cylindrical and there is a central depression that often causes bleeding (Fig. 5B-8). This lesion should be excised completely and pathologic examination for mitotic figures recorded to differentiate it from a leiomyosarcoma. At times these lesions can be diagnosed by removing the overlying mucosa with an endoscopic snare, elevating the tumor with saline injections, and excising the lesion with the snare. Potentially, this technique can cause perforation, especially in lesions larger than 1 to 2 cm, and in these cases, transgastric laparoscopic excisional biopsy should be considered.

Endoscopic ultrasound has been extensively used in gastric cancer to assess the depth of tumor penetration and lymph node metastasis. Its overall accuracy is higher than CT in diagnosing regional lymph nodes (71%), with a sensitivity and specificity of 86% and 47%, respectively.[25] EUS has been found to be of help in linitis plastica, where the characteristic features include thickness of the submucosa two to four times that of the normal gastric wall and the presence of hypoechogenic infiltration. The mucosa may also show diffuse nodules that can be selectively biopsied, thus improving the diagnostic accuracy.

**THERAPEUTIC ENDOSCOPY.** In early gastric cancer, endoscopic strip biopsies can be performed using submucosal injections of saline to elevate the mucosa in the area corresponding to the early tumor. Using a two-channel endoscope, the malignant mucosa is elevated by means of an endoscopic forceps and removed with an endoscopic snare passed through the second channel of the endoscope. Lambert[52] compared the results of this technique with open surgery and found similar 5-year survival rates of 84% and 89%, respectively.

Placement of an endoscopic prosthesis and laser therapy have been used successfully to palliate carcinoma of the gastroesophageal junction. However, the risk of perforation is high and relief of gastric obstruction is seldom achieved. Covered expandable metal mesh stents are preferred and can also be used to treat obstruction of the gastric outlet and duodenum. Microwave irradiation and laser photocoagulation can also be used for relief of obstruction and bleeding.[53]

**ENDOSCOPY IN THE SCREENING OF GASTRIC CANCER.** In Japan, the incidence of gastric cancer is high (100:100,000 population) and is a major cause of death. Mass screening programs have been successful using a double contrast barium upper gastrointestinal x-ray and endoscopy. The rate of discovering newly diagnosed early gastric cancer has increased 40%, and this has improved the rate of cure. In the United States and western Europe, mass screening studies have not been as effective and cost beneficial since the incidence of the disease has markedly decreased in the last 10 to 20 years, except in high-risk groups such as those with previous partial gastrectomy, patients with atrophic gastritis with metaplasia, and in those with dysplasia found on routine screening. These patients should have endoscopy every 1 to 3 years. In addition, patients with *H. pylori* and intestinal metaplasia in adenomatous polyps are also at an increased risk for the development of malignancy.[54,55] In patients with gastric adenomatous polyps and in patients with FAP and Gardner's syndromes, yearly endoscopy should be performed, especially in gastric adenomatous polyps greater than 2 cm, which are at high risk for malignant transformation. Since carcinoma of the periampullary duodenum is now the leading cause of death in patients with FAP who have already had a colectomy, gastroduodenoscopy is recommended every 1 to 2 years.[55]

## ENDOSCOPY IN COLORECTAL TUMORS

**DIAGNOSTIC ENDOSCOPY.** Colorectal cancer is one of the most common malignancies in the United States and western Europe, where approximately 1 in 20 people will develop adenocarcinoma of the large bowel in his or her lifetime, with 155,000 new cases of colorectal cancer diagnosed each year in the United States. Colonoscopy has the preeminent role in the diagnosis of this disease when biopsies and cytology are utilized.

Endoscopically, adenocarcinoma of the colon or rectum usually appears as an ulcerative exophytic lesion that can present with bleeding and colon obstruction (Fig. 5B-9). When probed with biopsy forceps, it feels hard, is friable, and easily bleeds. Sometimes, however, it can be small, and the possibility of missing the lesion is present. Neoplasms located in the cecum or in the rectum are at risk of not being detected, and the reason for missing these tumors is usually related to an inadequate biopsy technique or inability to reach the cecum during the exam. Occasionally small cancers can appear as reddened areas or a thickened suspicious fold, and in these cases, multiple biopsies and careful identification of tumor location should be done. In many instances, the endoscopic appearance of

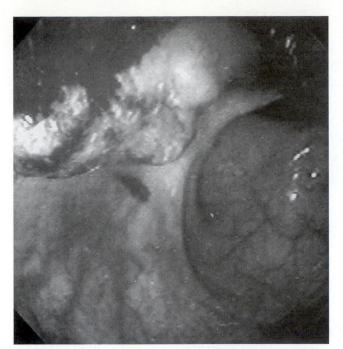

**FIGURE 5B-9.** Endoscopic view of a rectal carcinoma. (See also Plate 22.)

the lesion is typical, since the tumor has an irregular surface and is fixed to the underlying bowel wall.

EUS is used to stage colorectal tumors, but the staging accuracy is less than 60% in the colon, and has been reported to be as high as 80% in the rectum (Fig. 5B-10).[56] EUS is reliable in correctly assessing the depth of tumor infiltration, node metastasis, and delineation of proximal and distal tumor-free margins, which is important information prior to performing a radical tumor resection (see Fig. 5B-10). It can also be helpful in villous adenomas to detect malignant transformation with invasion of the submucosa or muscularis propria layers.[57] EUS staging of colorectal tumors has been defined by Tio,[14] but overstaging in rectal carcinoma can occur due to peritumoral inflammation, abscesses, and previous irradiation, and in patients with intramucosal carcinoma.

**THERAPEUTIC ENDOSCOPY.** Colonic polypectomy is the most common therapeutic endoscopic procedure. The progression of benign adenomatous polyps to adenocarcinoma is well recognized, and polypectomy should be performed when a polyp is detected, as its impact in lowering the incidence of colorectal cancer has been documented in the United States National Polyp Study.[58] From this study, there was noted to be a significant reduction to 0.5% in the incidence of colorectal cancer in patients undergoing removal of one or more polyps as compared to the expected rate of cancer of 1.18% to 3.73%.

The classification of colon and rectal tumors and polyps is listed in Table 5B-2.[59] Submucosal tumors such as lipomas, lymphomas, and fibromas are most commonly seen in the cecal region, whereas carcinoid tumors are most frequently located in the appendix (35% to 40%) and are also seen in the colon (10%) and rectum (15%). Rectal carcinoids may have a benign clinical course, especially if they

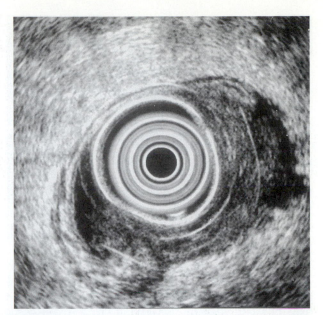

**FIGURE 5B-10.** EUS of rectal carcinoma showing T3 lesion. (See also Plate 23.)

are under 2 cm in size, and some authors have recommended that these tumors be removed locally through the endoscope if adequate margins can be obtained. In this situation, a transanal endoscopic resection may be the preferred treatment to remove the mucosa and muscularis, and if necessary, full-thickness removal of the rectal wall with closure may be performed up to 20 to 25 cm from the anal verge.

**TABLE 5B-2.  CLASSIFICATION OF BENIGN AND MALIGNANT TUMORS AND POLYPS OF THE COLON AND RECTUM**

Submucosal Lesions
    Lipomas
    Carcinoid tumors
    Pneumatosis cystoides intestinalis
    Lymphoma
    Metastatic neoplasms
    Fibromas

Mucosal Lesions
    Nonneoplastic
        Hyperplastic polyps
        Juvenile polyps
        Inflammatory polyps (pseudopolyps)
    Neoplastic
        Benign
            Tubular adenomas
            Tubulovillous adenomas
            Villous adenomas
    Malignant
        Carcinomas in situ
        Invasive carcinomas

Source: Imbembo AL, Lefor AT.[59] Reproduced with permission.

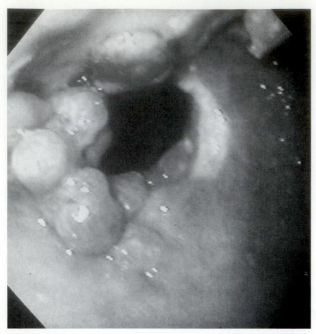

**FIGURE 5B-11.** Endoscopic view of a villous polyp of the rectum. When the polyp size is greater than 1–2 cm in diameter, the incidence of malignancy is between 20% and 40% and increases as the polyp size increases. (See also Plate 24.)

Hyperplastic polyps are a common finding on colonoscopy and are usually multiple and less than 5 mm in diameter. They are not premalignant and have an orderly papillary configuration of the mucosa with normal mitosis and maturation. Follow-up colonoscopy should be recommended as in the normal population.

Juvenile polyps are often found in children less than 10 years of age, and 75% are located in the rectum. This type of polyp is a hamartoma and sometimes called a retention polyp, and it often presents with bleeding and prolapse of the polyp through the anus. There is no malignant potential in the polyp, but it should be removed for relief of symptoms.

Neoplastic mucosal lesions include adenomatous and villous polyps, which can develop malignant changes (Fig. 5B-11). Tubular adenomas are the most common histologic variety (60% to 80%) and they often have a long stalk and are less than 10 mm in diameter, whereas the villous adenoma is sessile with a broad base. Of adenomatous polyps, 20% have severe atypia but only 5% have carcinoma.

Tubulovillous and villous adenomas contain branching glands in fingerlike projections. The tubulovillous tumors are most likely 10 to 20 mm in diameter, whereas pure villous tumors are usually greater than 20 mm. The risk of malignancy increases with the amount of villous component, and a tumor with a villous polyp over 20 mm has a 40% chance of malignancy. Other potential complications of colorectal neoplastic polyps include bleeding and obstruction.

The adenoma-carcinoma sequence is considered one of the major mechanisms for the development of colon carcinomas, since the incidence of these polyps parallels the development of malignancy. The sequence is described in Fig. 5B-12. In general, patients with adenomas are 5 to 7 years younger than patients with colorectal cancer, and larger polyps have been noted to show varying degrees of atypia, abnormal chromosomal patterns, dysplasia, and carcinoma. One proposed mechanism for cancer development is the loss of the tumor suppressor gene function, which has been identified at the FAP focus on chromosome 5q, including the mutation in colon cancer (*MCC*) and the adenomatosis polyposis coli (*APC*) genes. The *APC* site mutations have been recorded in 60% of polyps smaller than 5 mm and may lead to hyperproliferative epithelium.

Another considered mechanism is the K-*ras* oncogene on chromosome 12p, which has been found to be mutated in 9% of adenomatous polyps smaller than 10 mm. The mutation rate increases to 58% in adenomas over 10 mm, and this mutation incidence has been observed in 47% of cancer patients.[60]

A third possibility is the deleted in colon cancer (*DCC*) tumor suppressor gene located on chromosome 18q, which has also been implicated in the etiology of colon cancer. Mutations of this gene have been observed in 75% of colorectal cancers and 47% of large adenomas. The p53 tumor suppressor gene located on the 17p chromosome has also been observed in the sequence from adenoma to cancer and has been found in 75% of colon cancer patients.

These risk factors necessitate complete colonoscopy and polypectomy. If a polyp(s) is removed, colonoscopy should be repeated in 3 to 6 months to assure clearance. Once the colon is negative, colonoscopy should be performed in 2 years, and if negative, a repeat colonoscopy can be done every 3 to 5 years.

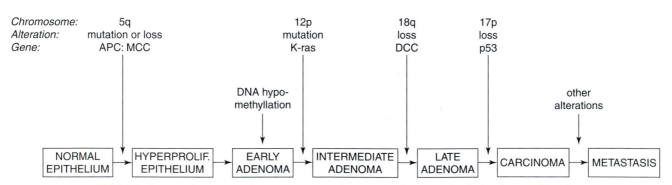

**FIGURE 5B-12.** Adenoma-carcinoma sequence of tumor development. (Redrawn from *Sabiston's Textbook of Surgery.* Philadelphia, WB Saunders, 1997, 993.)

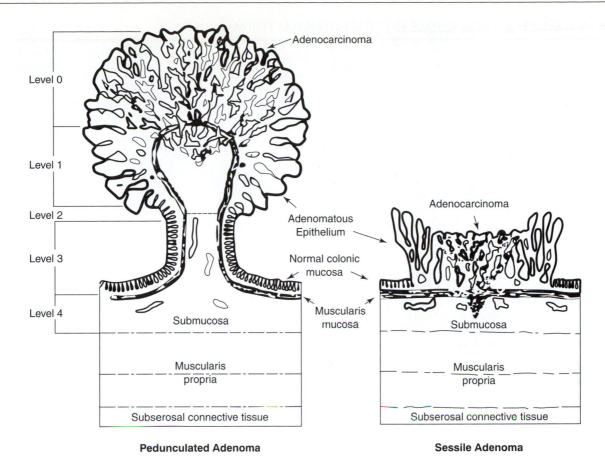

**FIGURE 5B-13.** Schematic drawing showing invasion of a polyp with carcinoma. The incidence of lymph node metastasis is approximately 35% in level 4 invasion. (Redrawn from Gastroenterology 1985; 89:328.)

Several multiple polyposis syndromes have been described, and their potential for malignancy is noted in Table 5B-3.

Endoscopic polypectomy can be accomplished using several techniques. Small polyps under 5 mm in diameter are removed using a "hot biopsy" forceps, which consists of cauterization of the base of the polyp as the special forceps entrap the polyp. The snare cautery technique is used for polyps greater than 5 mm in diameter. In this technique, a wire loop snare is passed around the polyp base, which is then transected by cauterization. This is more easily accomplished with a pedunculated polyp that has a small polyp base and a long stalk. For large sessile polyps with a broad base, submucosal saline injections can be used to elevate the polyp, and then the polyp is removed in a piecemeal technique. When there is suspicion of invasive cancer, the polyp site can be injected with sterile India ink so as to allow future identification of the colon segment at repeat endoscopy or surgery. Major complications of endoscopic polypectomy are low, and include bowel perforation and hemorrhage with an incidence of 0.11% and 2.16%, respectively.[61]

Overall, malignancy may be found in 5% of adenomatous polyps, but is under 1% in polyps less than 10 mm and 10% in those 10 to 20 mm in diameter. This incidence increases with villous polyps to 10% in those smaller than 10 mm and increases to 40% to 50% when the polyp size is greater than 20 mm. The depth of invasion, the grade of differentiation, lymphatic invasion, and a positive or close polypectomy margin are the most important factors to consider in predicting local recurrence or node metastasis of the malignancy, which would then necessitate surgical colon resection (Fig. 5B-13).[61] Several studies have suggested that polypectomy alone can cure almost all patients with well or moderately differentiated cancer that is limited to the head of a pedunculated adenomatous polyp with a clear margin on the stalk and no evidence of lymphatic invasion. The detection of invasive cancer in a sessile polyp is an indication for definitive resectional colon surgery.

Therapeutic endoscopy can be used to palliate bleeding or obstructing colon cancers in patients with disease that is not suitable for surgery. Using Nd:YAG laser coagulation, bleeding from tumors can be controlled and colon obstruction relieved with vaporization of the tumor tissue.[62] It is the treatment of choice in the palliative endoscopic management of colorectal tumors, and successful palliation of obstructing rectal tumors has been reported to range from 85% to 95% of patients. However, multiple endoscopic sessions are necessary to open the bowel lumen and maintain bowel patency, and

**TABLE 5B-3. POLYPOSIS SYNDROMES AND THE POTENTIAL FOR MALIGNANCY**

| SYNDROME | CHARACTERISTICS | LOCATION | TYPE OF POLYP | THERAPY | MALIGNANCY POTENTIAL |
|---|---|---|---|---|---|
| 1. Familial adenomatous polyposis (FAP) | 1/10,000–1/30,000 births Age of onset 25 years 40–60% have polyps in stomach and duodenum 20% have FAP in family Autosomal dominant | Stomach, duodenum, colon; periampullary polyps are cancer prone | Multiple adenomatous polyps (<5 mm) | Proctocolectomy and ileoanal anastomosis | 100% |
| 2. Gardner's syndrome | Familial multiple GI adenomas with osteomas of mandible, skull, long bone, and soft tissue lesions including sebaceous cysts, fibromas, lipomas, and desmoid tumors Autosomal dominant | Stomach, duodenum, small bowel and periampullary: colon is primary site | Adenomas | Proctocolectomy and ileoanal anastomosis | 10%–12% |
| 3. Turcot syndrome | Inherited colonic polyposis and highly malignant brain tumors Autosomal recessive | Colon | Adenomas | Remove involved colon, treat brain tumor | Can develop cancer of colon but brain tumor usually presents first and is fatal. |
| 4. Cronkite-Canada syndrome | Noninherited polyps, hyperpigmentation alopecia, protein-losing enteropathy, diarrhea, weight loss, and dystrophy of fingernails | Diffuse GI polyposis | Hamartomas | Polyp removal for bleeding and or obstruction | 0% |
| 5. Cowden's disease | Multiple hamartomas, microcutaneous lesions, breast lesions (fibrocystic disease to cancer) multinodular goiter, thyroid cancer, lipomas, ovarian cysts | GI tract | Hamartomas | Symptomatic | 0% |
| 6. Basal cell nevus syndrome | Hamartomas and basal cell cancer | Colon | Hamartomas | Symptomatic | 0% |
| 7. Neurofibromatosis type I | Submucosal neurofibromas of GI tract, café-au-lait spots, long bone abnormalities, neurofibromas of central and peripheral nerves | Stomach, jejunum, colon—25% incidence of stomach and jejunum are primary sites Jejunum—secondary site | Neurofibromas | Symptomatic | Potential malignant transformation of neurofibromas |
| 8. Peutz-Jeghers syndrome | Mucocutaneous pigmentation of lips, bucal mucosa, nostrils, hands, feet, and perianal area and GI polyposis Autosomal dominant | GI—most frequently small bowel | Hamartomas with some adenomatous characteristics | For complications of intussusception, bowel obstruction, and bleeding | 50% incidence of duodenum, small bowel, colon, and extraintestinal cancer Increased incidence of breast, pancreas, gallbladder, and bile duct cancer *(continues)* |

**TABLE 5B-3.** (*Continued*)

| SYNDROME | CHARACTERISTICS | LOCATION | TYPE OF POLYP | THERAPY | MALIGNANCY POTENTIAL |
|---|---|---|---|---|---|
| 9. Juvenile polyposis syndrome | Three familial types Autosomal dominant | Three types—stomach, colon, or diffuse GI tract | Hamartomas | Symptomatic | Increased risk of colon cancer when combined with adenomatous polyps |

with each endoscopic treatment, there is the risk of bowel perforation. Transanal endoscopic resection of inoperable rectal tumors or of large rectal adenomas has been reported to have a success rate of 90% to 95%.[63] Endoscopic implantation of expandable mesh stents for palliative treatment of obstructive rectal cancer has been described.[64] Although stent obstruction and tumor ingrowth can occur, metallic Endocoil or silicone-coated mesh stents have a lower incidence of these complications.

**ENDOSCOPIC SCREENING OF COLORECTAL CANCER.**
The early detection of colorectal cancer is associated with a significant reduction of tumor-related deaths, thus emphasizing the importance of endoscopic screening in high-risk patients. However, the cost-effectiveness of this method is continuing to be evaluated, especially in the general population, with an average risk of developing colorectal cancer. The American Cancer Society and the World Health Organization (WHO) recommend the performance of screening for colorectal cancer in average-risk patients over 50 years using yearly fecal occult blood test on three consecutive days combined with flexible sigmoidoscopy every 3 to 5 years. Recommendations from the U.S. Preventive Service Task Force differ, and suggest a fecal occult blood test or sigmoidoscopy yearly for asymptomatic subjects over the age of 50 years.[65] Screening colonoscopy or double contrast barium enema is not recommended, since the cost-effectiveness is not acceptable. However, it is noteworthy that in a study on asymptomatic subjects, colonoscopy was able to detect adenomatous polyps at a rate that was twice that expected from flexible sigmoidoscopy alone.[66] Almost all authors agree that colonoscopy should be performed if the fecal occult blood test is positive, since data from a recent trial have shown that approximately 50% of subjects with positive occult blood test have either adenomatous polyps or polyposis (82%) or cancer (12%).[66] Flexible sigmoidoscopy only evaluates the rectum and descending colon, and, therefore, 25% to 45% of colon cancers and polyps may be missed. A complete colonoscopy should be performed if any neoplastic lesion is found during screening sigmoidoscopy, since patients with a rectosigmoid polyp or cancer may have synchronous lesions.

Patients at high risk of developing colorectal cancer include those with longstanding ulcerative colitis, a family history of colorectal cancer, FAP, and a personal history of a previous cancer and/or polyp. Ulcerative colitis is associated with at least a 20 times greater risk of developing colorectal cancer than in normal subjects, and this risk increases with the duration and extent of the disease, the onset of the disease at an earlier age, and in patients with fulminant disease. In these patients, colonoscopy with multiple biopsies taken every 5 cm is recommended every 1 to 2 years.[61] Since a history of colorectal cancer in one or more first-degree relatives is associated with an increased risk of colorectal cancer, screening colonoscopy in asymptomatic persons with a positive family history has been recommended.[67] Although screening guidelines in this subset of subjects are still debated, it is now believed that in autosomal dominant cancer families (Lynch syndrome), screening should start at the age of 30 years with a colonoscopy, and a double contrast barium enema every 3 to 5 years. Since polyp growth has been observed to be approximately 1 cm every 2 years, some investigators have suggested colonoscopy surveillance every 2 to 3 years. A screening program starting at the age of 35 to 40 years is also appropriate in those with a positive family history other than Lynch syndrome. These tests should include a fecal occult blood test every year and flexible sigmoidoscopy every 3 to 5 years.

Siblings of patients with FAP have an almost 100% risk of developing colorectal cancer. Gene abnormalities responsible for this syndrome have been localized to the long arm of chromosome 5, and detection of this gene combined with the identification of congenital hypertrophy of the retinal pigment of the eyes should be helpful in selecting family members who are at risk of developing colorectal polyposis. Screening should be started by the age of 20 years with fecal occult blood tests and colonoscopy, and these tests should be continued at least every 1 to 2 years. When a diagnosis of polyposis is made, these patients should undergo resection of the colon and rectum with an ileoanal anastomosis. If the rectum is retained and a ileorectal anastomosis performed, the rectum should be examined every 6 to 12 months with fulguration of any developing polyps. Genetic screening identifying a proband is also important to determine which patients are at high risk of developing colon cancer.

Patients with a personal history of colon cancer or adenomatous polyps are at risk of developing metachronous colon cancers and polyps with a rate approximating 5% to 10% and 60%, respectively. The National Polyp Study found that in most patients who had an adenomatous polyp removed, a 3-year-interval screening colonoscopy was appropriate to reduce the mortality from colorectal cancer.[58] Similar guidelines have been advocated by the American College of Gastroenterology,[68] the WHO Collaborating Centre,[69] and the American Society of Gastrointestinal Endoscopy[70] (Table 5B-4). Patients with multiple polyps, especially the villous type, will require a more aggressive screening, with a 1-year-interval colonoscopy to be sure the colon is clear of polyps, and then repeat

**TABLE 5B-4.** SUMMARY OF THE ASGE COLON SURVEILLANCE

| PERSONAL HISTORY | SURVEILLANCE RECOMMENDATION |
|---|---|
| **I. PATIENTS WITH SIGNIFICANT PERSONAL HISTORY** | |
| Prior colorectal cancer | Colonoscopy at 3 years after curative resection and clearance of the remainder of the colon at or around the time of resection, then at 3- to 5-year intervals to detect metachronous neoplasia. |
| Prior colonic adenomas | After clearance, surveillance colonoscopy at 3- to 5-year intervals. |
| Ulcerative pancolitis of 8 years' duration | Surveillance colonoscopy every 1–3 years with systematic biopsies to |
| Left-sided colitis of >15 years' duration | detect dysplasia. |
| **II. PATIENTS WITH SIGNIFICANT FAMILY HISTORY** | |
| Familial adenomatous | |
|   FAP with positive genetic test in proband | Offer genetic testing with genetic counseling; if positive, annual sigmoidoscopy beginning at age 10–12 years with colectomy when polyps develop. If no polyps, annual colonoscopy to age 40, then every 2–5 years thereafter. |
|   FAP with negative genetic test in proband | Sigmoidoscopy in all potentially affected relatives performed as above. |
| Hereditary nonpolyposis colorectal cancer syndrome | Colonoscopy every 2 years beginning at age 25, or 5 years younger than the earliest age of diagnosis of colorectal cancer, whichever is earlier. Annual screening after age 40. |
| First-degree relatives with sporadic colorectal cancer or adenomas before the age of 60 or multiple first-degree relatives with colorectal cancer or adenomas | Colonoscopy every 3–5 years beginning at age 10 years earlier than the youngest affected relative. |

colonoscopy every 2 years. On the other hand, it has been argued that similar endoscopic surveillance is probably not necessary after removal of a tubular adenomatous polyp under 10 mm in size.

After colorectal cancer resection, colonoscopy is mandatory to detect metachronous adenomas or cancers and should be performed 3 to 6 months after resection and then every 2 years. In patients who have had surgery for an obstructing cancer, a synchronous cancer and adenoma may be detected with an incidence of 2.2% and 27%, respectively.[71] Subsequent surveillance colonoscopy has been performed by many investigators at a 6- to 24-month interval with the aim of detecting neoplastic growth and to diagnose recurrent tumor at the anastomosis.[72] Metachronous cancers are usually slow-growing tumors, and some have suggested a longer interval, with colonoscopy performed 1 year after surgery and then every 2 to 5 years. It is important that the surgeon make a definitive schedule and follow it consistently.

## ENDOSCOPY IN TUMORS OF THE BILE DUCTS AND PANCREAS

**DIAGNOSTIC ENDOSCOPY.** Although less invasive imaging of the pancreas and bile ducts is available, endoscopic retrograde cholangiopancreatography (ERCP) has been extensively utilized in the diagnosis of biliopancreatic tumors to visualize the biliary and pancreatic ducts. Although the introduction of magnetic resonance cholangiopancreatography (MRCP) will probably change the diagnostic approach to biliopancreatic diseases,[73] the role of ERCP will

remain relevant because of its combined diagnostic and therapeutic potential, especially in patients with malignant strictures. Moreover, EUS has been used in the diagnosis and staging of esophageal, gastric, and rectal cancers and provides more information in staging biliopancreatic tumors than CT, MRI, and angiography.[74] However, the potential complications of ERCP include bleeding, biliary infection, pancreatitis, and bowel and bile duct perforation, and the incidence ranges from 3% to 8% in most endoscopy centers.[75] However, since MRCP has very few if any complications, it may replace diagnostic ERCP as the primary diagnostic modality.

ERCP is performed using a side-viewing duodenoscope that is advanced through the stomach into the second part of the duodenum and positioned en face to the papilla of Vater. A 5.5 French cholangiocatheter or papillotome is advanced through the working channel of the endoscope and is directed into both the common bile duct orifice at the 11 o'clock to 12 o'clock position of the papilla and the pancreatic duct orifice at the 3 o'clock position. If the papillary openings are strictured, a guidewire can be advanced through the catheter and through the stricture, thus allowing complete access of the cholangiocatheter or papillotome into the bile and pancreatic ducts. Approximately 5% of the patients may require a precut papillotomy prior to successful bile duct cannulation, but this technique should only be used if there are concomitant therapeutic indications. Once the catheter is positioned in the bile duct or pancreatic duct, contrast medium is injected under fluoroscopic guidance and radiographs are taken.

Tumors arising in and around the papilla of Vater can be easily visualized with the lateral-viewing duodenoscope and biopsies

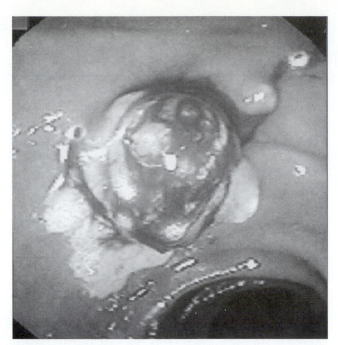

**FIGURE 5B-14.** Endoscopic view of a villous polyp of the ampulla of Vater. (See also Plate 25.)

and cytology can be obtained to establish the final diagnosis (Fig. 5B-14). Pancreatic cancers are suspected if pancreatic duct obstruction is demonstrated during pancreatography; however, the radiologic distinction between pancreatic cancer and chronic pancreatitis can sometimes be difficult and a tissue diagnosis is necessary.[76] On the other hand, the specificity of endoscopic pancreatography is high, and if a normal pancreatogram with smooth first- and second-order pancreatic branches is demonstrated, the likelihood of a pancreatic cancer is very low. The occurrence of a stricture in both the bile and pancreatic ducts (double duct sign) is pathognomonic of a tumor in the head of the pancreas. ERCP is limited in its ability to diagnose tumors of the uncinate process and in hypersecreting mucin tumors of the pancreas that produce excessive intraductal mucin. This limits the diagnostic accuracy in the dilated pancreatic duct.

Tumors of the bile ducts are usually visualized as strictures with partial or complete obstruction. When posttraumatic or iatrogenic bile duct strictures are excluded, these findings are most commonly associated with bile duct tumors, primary sclerosing cholangitis, and postinflammatory strictures secondary to bile duct stones, chronic pancreatitis or recurrent pyogenic cholangitis. Diagnosis may be difficult, and brushing cytology and biopsy are necessary to make the diagnosis. The accuracy rate of these procedures is 80% to 85%. With EUS and FNA, 5- to 10-mm pancreatic lesions can be diagnosed with a high degree of accuracy.

Although ERCP is technically challenging, its success should approach 90% to 95% in experienced centers. Unsuccessful ductal cannulation may occur in patients with periampullary diverticula, duodenal invasion by pancreatic cancer, postgastrectomy Billroth II diversion, and pancreas divisum. With less manipulation of the

papilla, small-quantity and low-pressure injection of contrast medium into the pancreatic duct, and appropriate endoscopic drainage after an ERCP in the presence of an obstructed bile duct, the complication rate of the procedure will decrease. Endoscopic sphincterotomy (ES) is often used for easier access to the bile duct and for stent placement to relieve obstruction secondary to tumor.

*Cholangioscopy and pancreatoscopy* have recently been introduced with the development of small miniscopes (daughter scopes) that can be passed through the accessory channel of a large-diameter duodenoscope into the papilla, bile duct, and pancreatic duct. This technique requires a sphincterotomy, since the daughter scopes are 3 to 4 mm in diameter. Although these endoscopes have an operating channel and a deflectable tip and can be maneuvered in the appropriate ducts, they are very expensive, susceptible to breakage, and require two endoscopists to perform the procedure, thus limiting their usefulness.

EUS has emerged as a very useful technique in patients with pancreatic and biliary cancer to determine tumor staging and surgical resectability (Fig. 5B-15).[77] Since many biliopancreatic cancers are unresectable at the time of diagnosis and nonsurgical palliation is available for these advanced tumors, EUS is an important tool to avoid an unnecessary surgical exploration. Moreover, real-time EUS-guided FNA of a pancreatic mass or a peripancreatic lymph node is important in making a pathologic diagnosis. Both radial and linear array echoendoscopes can be used to visualize the pancreaticobiliary region, but local staging according to TNM classification is usually performed with the radial echoendoscope.[78] A specially designed needle catheter aspiration system is passed through the working channel of the echoendoscope, and under ultrasound guidance is advanced into the lesion. Both radial and linear echoendoscopes can be used, but the FNA with a radial array is technically more difficult.

The accuracy of combined EUS and FNA is high, with a sensitivity and specificity in pancreatic cancer of 83% to 90% and 85% to 100%, respectively.[79] This technique is especially useful in the

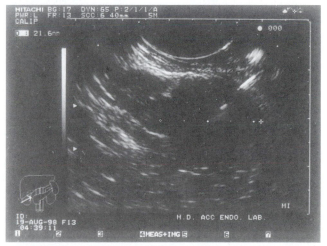

**FIGURE 5B-15.** EUS-guided biopsy of a pancreatic tumor adjacent to the portal vein. (See also Plate 26.)

diagnosis of pancreatic tumors less than 4 cm in size, and the most common complications are pancreatitis and infection (14%). The risk of malignant seeding has not been described thus far, and it is reasonable to suppose that this risk should be lower than the risk of tumor seeding following percutaneous transabdominal FNA, since with the EUS technique, the needle tract is shorter and is included in the surgical specimen if a resection is performed. With the transabdominal FNA, there has been only one report of tumor seeding in the skin in a series of 10,766 patients in a multicenter trial.[80]

When EUS is compared to CT, MRI, and angiography in ampullary tumors, EUS has a greater accuracy (78%) in T staging as opposed to CT (24%) and MRI (46%) and N staging is 68%, 59%, and 77% accurate, respectively.[81] Angiography has been noted by Rosch[82] to be less sensitive than EUS in the detection of portal venous infiltration in pancreatic and ampullary cancers. However, EUS is less sensitive than angiography in detecting celiac nodal involvement. Angiography is highly specific for visualizing portosplenic involvement (88%), whereas EUS was 100% specific in ruling out peritumor invasion of the portosplenic vessels. It should be noted that there is a trend toward EUS T understaging when a transpapillary stent is in place (72% vs. 84%).[81] This issue is significant because T1 lesions can be 100% accurately staged in ampullary carcinoma and, therefore, ampullectomy may be the preferred treatment. Understaging in T2 and T3 lesions may also occur, and thus lead to less invasive surgical treatment and decreased long-term survival. This problem is emphasized by the fact that lymph node metastasis is 0% in T1 lesions and 46% in T2 tumors.[83] It has also been demonstrated that bile duct wall thickness increases 100% in only 2 weeks of endostenting, thus producing bile duct wall inflammation and fibrotic thickening that leads to difficulty in distinguishing T1, T2, and T3 lesions.[84]

In pancreatic cancers, EUS is approximately 87% accurate in determining resectability in regard to malignant vascular invasion.[85] When EUS is compared to CT, EUS is better in staging than CT when tumors are less than 4 cm in size. T-stage accuracy with EUS is 73% for pancreatic tumors and 83% for ampullary cancers, whereas N-stage accuracy is 69% and 100% for pancreatic and ampullary lesions. Overall, EUS accurately stages pancreatic cancers 82% of the time and ampullary cancers 86%, and lymph node involvement is assessed accurately in 72% of patients. Small hepatic and peritoneal implants are difficult to detect, but the use of laparoscopy improves this aspect of preoperative staging.[86]

THERAPEUTIC ENDOSCOPY. Since the median survival in unresectable pancreaticobiliary malignancies ranges from 4 to 7 months,[87] endobiliary stenting is the least invasive palliation for jaundice and sepsis. In pancreatic malignancies, placement of stents has been proposed to relieve pain, but this role is still unclear.[88] In unresectable tumors of the ampulla of Vater, endoscopic laser therapy has been successfully used to ablate or open an obstructed papilla. This procedure should be combined with endobiliary stenting and may need to be repeated several times if restenosis occurs. One of the most common immediate complications of ERCP-ES is postprocedure bleeding, which can be controlled by epinephrine injections into the papilla and balloon tamponade. Brachytherapy with iridium 192 inserted endoscopically into the tumors has been used, but controlled studies are not available.

**TABLE 5B-5.** ENDOSCOPIC PALLIATION IN PATIENTS WITH MALIGNANT BILIARY OBSTRUCTION AT THE AMPULLARY, DISTAL COMMON BILE DUCT, HILAR REGIONS

| TUMOR OBSTRUCTION | AMPULLARY | DISTAL CBD | HILAR |
|---|---|---|---|
| Success, % | 96–97 | 84–90 | 88–96 |
| Complications | 8–32 | 10–19 | 8–60 |
| 30-day mortality, % | 1–3 | 10–17 | 10–33 |
| Late jaundice, % | 36 | 37 | 40–68 |
| Duodenal obstruction, % | 23 | 5–17 | — |
| Median survival, months | 9–14 | 4–6 | 2–6 |

SOURCE: Shields SJ et al.[91] Reproduced with permission.

When the technique of endoscopic stent placement is utilized, an 8- to 10-mm papillotomy is performed and a 0.035-inch guidewire is inserted into the bile duct under fluoroscopic guidance. Over the wire, a guiding catheter is inserted and a 10 to 11.5 French polyethylene or Teflon endobiliary stent is advanced and positioned across the stenosis. Occasionally, presenting balloon dilation of the stricture is helpful for placement of larger stents. Sometimes an expandable metal mesh stent can be used. A typical plastic stent has a tendency to clog in 4 to 6 months, and for this reason almost 30% of patients will need more than one stent replacement,[89] whereas the expandable silicone-covered metal stent will remain patent for a longer period of time.[90] However, metal stents cannot be removed and their cost ranges from $1000 to $1500 per stent as opposed to polyethylene, which is $200 to $300 per stent. More recently, Teflon stents without side holes (Tannebaum stents) have been proposed for their potential advantage of longer patency. However, patency studies have not confirmed this finding.

Table 5B-5 compares the clinical results for endobiliary stenting in ampullary, distal common bile duct, and hilar regions.[91] Stent placement in ampullary tumors has the best success in terms of ease of placement, relief of jaundice, and hospital mortality. Hilar lesions are often difficult to stent endoscopically, and a combined percutaneous transhepatic wire placement across the tumor into the duodenum allows for endoscopic grasping of the wire and endobiliary stent advancement through the endoscope over the wire. With this technique, successful endoscopic stent placement can increase to 95%.

Early complications related to endoscopic stent placement in biliary and pancreatic malignancies are low and are related to bleeding, pancreatitis, cholangitis, and perforation. The success rate in relieving obstructive jaundice has been reported to be 70% to 90%. In a review of several series,[92] early complications occurred less frequently following endoscopic treatment when compared to palliative surgical treatment. Late complications from stent clogging include recurrent obstructive jaundice and cholangitis, which may develop in 20% to 25% of patients, and duodenal stenosis may develop secondary to continued tumor growth in up to 10% to 25% of patients. The overall mortality from endobiliary stenting is low when compared to surgical palliation with a choledochojejunostomy and gastrojejunostomy (Table 5B-6).[93] Since median survival is short (4 to 7 months), endobiliary stenting is the preferred treatment.

**TABLE 5B-6.** A SERIES OF RANDOMIZED CONTROLLED TRIALS OF ENDOSCOPIC VS. SURGICAL PALLIATION IN THE MANAGEMENT OF MALIGNANT BILIARY OBSTRUCTION

| | MIDDLESEX STUDY | | | WESSEX STUDY | | |
| --- | --- | --- | --- | --- | --- | --- |
| | ENDOSCOPY | | SURGERY | ENDOSCOPY | | SURGERY |
| Patients, N | 100 | * | 101 | 23 | | 25 |
| Success, % | 95 | * | 94 | 91 | | 92 |
| Complications, % | 11 | * | 29 | 33 | | 56 |
| Mortality—proced, % | 3 | | 14 | Not indicated | | |
| Mortality—30 day, % | 8 | | 15 | 9 | | 20 |
| Duodenal obstruction, % | 19 | | 18 | 9 | * | 4 |
| Initial hospital, days | 8 | * | 13 | 5 | * | 13 |
| Median survival, weeks | 21 | | 26 | 22 | | 18 |
| Stent exchange | 36 | * | 0 | 43 | * | 0 |

*$P < 0.05$
SOURCE: Shields SJ et al.[92] Reproduced with permission.

In conclusion, flexible endoscopy can be used accurately for diagnosing and staging of gastrointestinal malignancies. It is cost-effective and allows the surgeon to visualize the tumor and perform therapeutic treatments that can palliate and resect small tumors, particularly early gastric malignancies and carcinoma in a colon polyp. As the instrumentation and techniques continue to develop, including endoscopic suturing and stapling, it may be possible to perform larger endoscopic tumor resections. There is already an endoscopic sewing machine available that can approximate the full thickness of the gastric wall but what place this technology will play in the future is not known. With economic concerns, rapid efficient diagnosis and treatment are important and flexible endoscopy has a significant role in the management of malignant disease.

## REFERENCES

1. LAMM H: Biegsame optische Gerate. Z Instrumentenk 50:579, 1930.
2. HIRSCHOWICZ BL et al: Demonstration of a new gastroscope: The "fibrescope." Gastroenterology 35, 1958.
3. WILLIAMS G: History and development of endoscopy of the colon, rectum and anus, in *Endoscopy of the Colon, Rectum and Anus*, JM Church (ed). New York, Igaku-Shoin, 1995, pp 1–10.
4. OVERHOLT BF: Clinical experience with the fibersigmoidoscope. Gastrointest Endosc 15:27, 1968.
5. OVERHOLT BF: Description and experience with flexible fibersigmoidoscopes. *Proceedings of the Sixth National Cancer Conference (1968)*. Philadelphia, JB Lippincott, 1970, pp 443–446.
6. SHINYA H, WOLFF WI: Morphology, anatomic distribution and cancer potential of colonic polyps: An analysis of 7,000 polyps endoscopically removed. Am Surg 190:679, 1979.
7. REY JF et al: Electronic video endoscopy: Preliminary results of image modification. Endoscopy 20:8, 1988.
8. COTHREN RM et al: Gastrointestinal tissue diagnosis by laser-induced fluorescence spectroscopy at endoscopy. Gastrointest Endosc 36:105, 1990.
9. GANA TJ et al: A controlled study of human resting gastric mucosal blood flow by endoscopic laser-Doppler flowmetry. Gastrointest Endosc 36:264, 1990.
10. FENNERTY M: Tissue staining. Gastrointest Endosc Clin North Am 4:296, 1994.
11. TYGAT G: Diagnosis and differential therapy of malignant esophageal stenosis. Internist 23:251, 1982.
12. GRIMM H et al: Ultrasonic esophagoprobe (prototype 1). Gastrointest Endosc 38:490, 1992.
13. CALETTI G et al: Endoscopic ultrasonography: A summary of the conclusions of the working party for the Tenth World Congress of Gastroenterology, Los Angeles, California. October 1994. Am J Gastroenterol 89:S138, 1994.
14. TIO TL: *Gastrointestinal TNM Cancer Staging by Endosonography*. New York, Igaku-Shoin, 1995.
15. BOTET JF et al: Preoperative staging of esophageal cancer: Comparison of endoscopic US and dynamic CT. Radiology 2:419, 1991.
16. ROSCH T: Endosonographic staging of esophageal cancer: A review of literature results. Gastrointest Endosc Clin North Am 5:537, 1995.
17. VILMANN P et al: Endoscopic ultrasonography-guided fine needle aspiration biopsy of lesions in the upper gastrointestinal tract. Gastrointest Endosc 41:230, 1995.
18. WIERSEMA MJ et al: Endosonography-guided real-time fine needle aspiration biopsy. Gastrointest Endosc 40199, 1994.
19. EARLAM RJ, CUNHA-MELO JR: Esophageal squamous cell carcinoma: A critical review of surgery. Br J Surg 67:381, 1980.
20. CONSOLI A et al: Our experience in palliative endoscopic prosthesis placement in patients with esophageal and cardiac carcinoma. Atti 89 Cong
21. ENDO M: Endoscopic resection as local treatment of mucosal cancer of the esophagus. Endoscopy 25:672, 1993.
22. YANG GR et al: Endoscopic Nd:YAG laser therapy in patients with early superficial carcinoma of the esophagus and the gastric cardia. Endoscopy 26:681, 1994.
23. SIBILLE A et al: Long term survival after photodynamic therapy for esophageal cancer. Gastroenterology 108:337, 1995.
24. PONEC RJ, KIMMEY MB: Endoscopic therapy of esophageal cancer. Surg Clin North Am 77:1197, 1997.
25. LUNDELL L et al: Palliative endoscopic dilation in carcinoma of

the esophagus and esophagogastric junction. Acta Chir Scand 155:179, 1989.

26. Atkinson M, Ferguson R: Fibreoptic endoscopic palliative intubation of inoperable esophagogastric neoplasms. Br Med J 1:266, 1977.

27. Loizou LA et al: Treatment of malignant strictures of the cervical esophagus by endoscopic intubation using modified endoprostheses. Gastrointest Endosc 38:158, 1992.

28. Lux G et al: A cuffed tube for the treatment of esophageal-bronchial fistula. Endoscopy 19:28, 1987.

29. Shimi SM: Self-expanding metallic stents in the management of advanced esophageal cancer: A review. Semin Laparosc Surg 6:1, 1999.

30. Lightdale CJ et al: Photodynamic therapy with porphorym sodium versus thermal ablation therapy with Nd:YAG laser for palliation of esophageal cancer: A multicenter randomized trial. Gastrointest Endosc 42:507, 1995.

31. Johnston JH et al: Palliative bipolar electrocoagulation therapy of obstructing esophageal cancer. Gastrointest Endosc 33:349, 1987.

32. Payne-James JJ et al: Use of ethanol-induced tumor necrosis to palliate dysphagia in patients with esophagogastric cancer. Gastrointest Endosc 36:43, 1990.

33. Low DE, Pagliero KM: Prospective randomized clinical trial comparing brachytherapy and laser photoablation for palliation of esophageal cancer. J Thorac Cardiovasc Surg 104:173, 1992.

34. Spechler SJ, Goyal RK: Barrett's esophagus. N Engl J Med 315:362, 1986.

35. Drewitz DJ et al: The incidence of adenocarcinoma in Barrett's esophagus: A prospective study of 170 patients followed 48 years. Am J Gastroenterol 92:212, 1997.

36. Ortiz A et al: Conservative treatment versus antireflux surgery in Barrett's esophagus: Long term results of a prospective study. Br J Surg 83:274, 1996.

37. Riddell RH: Early detection of neoplasia of the esophagus and gastroesophageal junction. Am J Gastroenterol 91:853, 1996.

38. Sampliner RE et al: Regression of Barrett's esophagus by laser ablation in an acid environment. Dig Dis Sci 38:365, 1993.

39. Overholt B et al: Photodynamic therapy for treatment of early adenocarcinoma in Barrett's esophagus. Gastrointest Endosc 39:73, 1993.

40. Patti MG et al: Barrett's esophagus: A surgical disease. J Gastrointest Surg 3:397, 1999.

41. Li FP, Shiang EL: Screening for esophageal cancer in 62,000 Chinese. Lancet 2:804, 1979.

42. Dawsey SM et al: Squamous dysplasia and early esophageal cancer in the Linzian region of China: Distinctive endoscopic lesions. Gastroenterology 105:1333, 1993.

43. Salvon-Harman JC et al: Shifting proportions of gastric adenocarcinomas. Arch Surg 129:381, 1994.

44. Kurihara M et al: Diagnosis of small early gastric cancer by x-ray, endoscopy and biopsy. Cancer Detect Prev 4:377, 1981.

45. Graham DY et al: Prospective evaluation of biopsy number in the diagnosis of esophageal and gastric carcinoma. Gastroenterology 82:228, 1982.

46. Parsonnet J et al: Helicobacter pylori infection and gastric lymphoma. N Engl J Med 330:1267, 1994.

47. Weber DM et al: Regression of gastric lymphoma of mucosa-related lymphoid tissue with antibiotic therapy for Helicobacter pylori. Gastroenterology 107:1835, 1994.

48. McGannon E: Gastric and duodenal polyps in familial adenomatosis polyposis: A prospective study of the nature and prevalence of upper gastrointestinal polyps. Gut 28:306, 1987.

49. Beckwith PS et al: Prognosis of symptomatic duodenal adenomas in familial adenomatosis polyposis. Arch Surg 126:825, 1991.

50. Domellof L, Janunger KG: The risk for gastric carcinoma after partial gastrectomy. Am J Surg 134:581, 1977.

51. Ross AHM et al: Late motality after surgery for peptic ulcer. N Engl J Med 307:519, 1982.

52. Lambert R: Endoscopic treatment of esophagogastric tumors. Endoscopy 26:28, 1994.

53. Maunoury V et al: Palliative treatment of esophagogastric cancer by laser photoablation. Gastroenterol Clin Biol 11:371, 1987.

54. Munoz N: Is Helicobacter pylori a cause of gastric cancer? An appraisal of the serological evidence. Cancer Epidermiol Biomarkers Prev 3:445, 1994.

55. Kurtz RC et al: Upper gastrointestinal neoplasia in familial polyposis. Dig Dis Sci 32:459, 1987.

56. Rosch T, Classen M: Colonoscopic ultrasonography. Semin Colon Rectal Surg 3:49, 1992.

57. Tio TL: Endosonography of colorectal disease. Endoscopy 2:99, 1992.

58. Winawer SJ et al: Randomized comparison of surveillance intervals after colonoscopic removal of newly diagnosed adenomatous polyps. N Engl J Med 328:901, 1993.

59. Imbembo AL, Lefor AT: Benign neoplasms of the colon, including vascular malformations, in Sabiston's Textbook of Surgery, 15th ed, DC Sabiston, HK Lyerly (eds). Philadelphia, WB Saunders, 1997, pp 993–1001.

60. Vogelstein B et al: Genetic alterations during colorectal tumor development. N Engl J Med 319:525, 1988.

61. Haggitt RC et al: Prognostic factors in colorectal carcinomas arising in adenomas: Implications for lesions removed by endoscopic polypectomy. Gastroenterology 89:328, 1985.

62. Eckhauser ML et al: The role of pre-resectional laser recanalization for obstructing adenocarcinoma of the rectum: Comparison of costs and complications. Gastrointest Endosc 21:81, 1989.

63. Steele RJC et al: Transanal endoscopic microsurgery. Initial experience from three centres in the United Kingdom. Br J Surg 83:207, 1996.

64. Dohmoto M et al: Application of rectal stents for palliation of obstructing rectosigmoid cancer. Surg Endose 11:758, 1997.

65. U.S. Preventative Service Task Force: Guidelines of the U.S. Preventative Service Task Force. Baltimore, Williams & Wilkins, 1996.

66. Rex DK et al: Screening colonoscopy in asymptomatic average-risk persons with negative fecal occult blood test. Gastroenterology 100:64, 1991.

67. Rex DK: Colonoscopy: A review of its yield for cancers and adenomas by indication. Am J Gastroenterol 90:353, 1995.

68. Bond JH: Polyp guideline: Diagnosis, treatment and surveillance for patients with nonfamilial colorectal polyps (from the Practice Parameters Committee of the American College of Gastroenterology). Ann Intern Med 119:836, 1993.

69. Winawer SJ et al: Prevention of colorectal cancer: Guidelines based on new data. Bull WHO 73:7, 1995.

70. American Society for Gastrointestinal Endoscopy: Colonoscopy in the screening and surveillance of individuals at increased risk for colorectal cancer. Gastrointest Endosc 48:676, 1998.

71. CARLSSON G et al: The value of colonoscopy surveillance after curative resection for colorectal cancer or synchronous adenomatous polyps. Arch Surg 122:1261, 1987.

72. JUHL G et al: Six-year results of annual colonoscopy after resection of colorectal cancer. World J Surg 14:255, 1990.

73. YAMAGUCHI K et al: Comparison of endoscopic retrograde and magnetic resonance cholangiopancreatography in the surgical diagnosis of pancreatic diseases. Am J Surg 175:203, 1998.

74. PALLAZZO L et al: Endoscopic ultrasonography in the diagnosis and staging of pancreatic adenocarcinoma. Endoscopy 25:143, 1993.

75. CHUNG SC: Biliary endoscopy. Curr Opin Gastroenterol 8:770, 1992.

76. FOCKENS P, HUIBREGTSE K: Staging of pancreatic and ampullary cancer by endoscopy. Endoscopy 25:52, 1993.

77. SNADY H et al: Endoscopic ultrasonographic criteria of vascular invasion by potentially resectable pancreatic tumors. Gastrointest Endosc 40:326, 1994.

78. BHUTANI MS et al: Endoscopic ultrasound guided fine needle aspiration of malignant pancreatic lesions. Endoscopy 29:854, 1997.

79. GRESS F et al: Endoscopic ultrasound (EUS) guided fine needle aspiration (FNA) biopsy utilizing linear array and radial scanning endosonography: Results of diagnostic accuracy and complications (abstract). Gastrointest Endosc 47:421, 1997.

80. FORNARY F et al: Complications of ultrasonically guided fine needle abdominal biopsy. Scand J Gastroenterol 24:949, 1989.

81. CANNON ME et al: EUS compared with CT, magnetic resonance imaging, and angiography and the influence of biliary stenting on staging accuracy of ampullary neoplasms. Gastrointest Endosc 50:27, 1999.

82. ROSCH T et al: Staging of pancreatic and ampullary carcinoma by endoscopic ultrasonography. Gastroenterology 102:188, 1992.

83. BOTTGER TC et al: Clinicopathologic study for the assessment of resection for ampullary carcinoma. World J Surg 21:379, 1997.

84. TAMADA K et al: Influence of biliary drainage catheter on bile duct wall thickness as measured by intraductal ultrasonography. Gastrointest Endosc 47:28, 1998.

85. BUSCAIL L et al: Role of EUS in the management of pancreatic and ampullary carcinoma: A prospective study assessing resectability and prognosis. Gastrointest Endosc 50:34, 1999.

86. WARSHAW AL, FERNANDEZ-DEL-CASTILLO C: Medical progress: Pancreatic carcinoma. N Engl J Med 326:455, 1992.

87. CONLON KC et al: Long-term survival after curative resection for pancreatic ductal adenocarcinoma: Clinical pathologic analysis of 5-year survivors. Ann Surg 223:273, 1996.

88. COSTAMAGNA G et al: Treatment of obstructive pain by endoscopic drainage in patients with pancreatic head carcinoma. Gastrointest Endosc 39:774, 1993.

89. SHERMAN S et al: Therapeutic biliary endoscopy. Endoscopy 26:93, 1994.

90. WAGNER HJ et al: Plastic endoprostheses versus metal stents in the palliative treatment of malignant biliary obstruction: A prospective and randomized trial. Endoscopy 25:213, 1994.

91. SHIELDS SJ et al: Endoscopic management of malignant biliary obstruction, in *Endosurgery*, J Toouli et al (eds). New York, Churchill Livingstone, 1996, pp 563–572.

92. WATANABA P, WILLIAMSON RCN: Surgical palliation for pancreatic cancer: Developments during the past two decades. Br J Surg 79:8, 1992.

93. LILLEMOE KD: Surgical and non-surgical palliation. J Am Coll Surg 4:429, 1998. Paper presented at Pancreatic Cancer: 1998 Update (symposium).

# 5C / CRYOSURGERY FOR SOLID TUMORS

*Andrew A. Gage*

Cryosurgery is a method that uses freezing temperatures to achieve specific responses in tissues. The word *cryotherapy*, often used interchangeably with the word *cryosurgery*, has broader connotations that include the use of cold temperatures for any therapeutic use, ranging from the application of cold packs to relieve the pain and swelling caused by trauma to the use of apparatus for the purpose of treating disease by freezing. Cryosurgery is a form of cryotherapy that uses freezing techniques to produce a tissue response, either inflammatory or destructive. The destructive properties of freezing tissue are of prime interest in the cryosurgical treatment of tumors. Cryosurgery provides a method of freezing tumors in situ. The devitalized tissue sloughs or is absorbed, depending on location in the body. Since no excision is needed, little or no hemorrhage is caused. In accessible lesions, need for anesthesia is reduced. The intraoperative dissemination of cancer cells is avoided. These advantages reduce surgical risk to a minimum, even when operative exposure is required. An important limitation of cryosurgery is the absence of a surgical specimen in order to examine the margins of treatment for viable cancer cells. Therefore cryosurgery is limited in part by the surgeon's ability to define the extent of disease, just as is true of any method of therapy.

## HISTORY

### THE BEGINNING

Freezing temperatures were first used for the treatment of tumors in 1845 to 1851 when James Arnott described the benefits of local applications of cold for the treatment of a wide variety of illnesses, ranging from headaches to advanced cancers. For the treatment of cancer, Arnott used solutions of salt containing crushed ice at a temperature in the range of $-18°$ to $-24°$C to freeze incurable cancers in accessible sites, such as the breast and uterine cervix. The treatment was given with irrigation devices that Arnott developed for these special purposes. In the patients with cancer, the benefits that were described included relief of pain, reduction in the size of the tumor, and lessening of bleeding and malodorous discharge.

Arnott's apparatus was cumbersome to use to treat advanced cancer and had only limited applicability since it could be used only on accessible tissues and had minimal freezing capability. Arnott later focused on the anesthetic properties of cold and now is recognized as a pioneer in refrigeration anesthesia.[1] Although the usefulness of

cold application for the relief of pain was acknowledged by physicians in those years, further development of cryosurgery had to await advances in technology, especially the availability of better cryogenic agents.

Late in the nineteenth century, scientists were able to liquefy atmospheric gases and the term *cryogen* came into use. As the century ended, liquid air and solid carbon dioxide were available for the treatment of localized skin disease. The initial clinical application of liquid air ($-190°$C) was by A. C. White[2] of New York City, who used the cryogen, applied topically with a cotton swab or by spray, to treat a variety of skin diseases, including epitheliomas. Solidified carbon dioxide ($-78.5°$C), commonly called dry ice, was introduced into clinical practice for the treatment of skin diseases by W. Pusey[3] of Chicago, who favored this agent because of its ready availability in comparison to liquid air. Stimulated by these initial reports, many physicians made use of the freezing techniques for the treatment of skin diseases. The course of events after freezing of skin lesions, which were bulla formation followed by superficial crusting, the formation of an eschar, and healing to form a superficial scar, were well described in the medical reports published in these years. Bowen and Towle[4] reviewed the literature in 1907, defined the value of pressure on the lesion to control depth of freezing, and concluded that liquid air, although a valuable agent, was impractical because of lack of ready availability. Liquid air was little used after 1910. Solid carbon dioxide was the most popular cryogenic agent in the early 1900s. The techniques of forming solid carbon dioxide into various shapes for specific uses were described in Low's book, which was published in 1911.[5]

In the 1930s and 1940s, efforts were made to widen the usefulness of solid carbon dioxide by the development of new instruments and techniques. Lortat-Jacobs and Solente[6] in the monograph "La Cryotherapie," perhaps the first use of the word *cryotherapy*, described the use of copper tips of various sizes and shapes cooled by solid carbon dioxide for use in the treatment of skin diseases, chronic cervicitis, and cervical erosions. These instruments offered little advantage over the use of the simple stick of solid carbon dioxide, a cryogen that had a measure of usefulness in therapy, but lacked the freezing capability needed to treat neoplasms.

The work of T. Fay[7] with the local and general refrigeration of patients with cancer and other illnesses in the years 1936 to 1940 is of interest, although the investigation did not contribute to the development of cryosurgery. Fay treated patients having large symptomatic incurable carcinomas with irrigations of cold solution and application of ice packs, producing tissue temperatures of about

−5°C and a limited local freezing. Fay also implanted metal capsules (connected to an external cold irrigation system) in the brain for the treatment of tumors and abscesses by cold irrigation, producing freezing. The tissue response featured reduction in tumor size and lessening of symptoms, just as described by Arnott so many years earlier. Fay's work was interrupted by World War II and never resumed thereafter.

More than Fay's work, experimental studies during the 1940s and 1950s in which tissue lesions were produced by freezing for the purpose of gaining information pertinent to the pathophysiology of disease are important to the later development of cryosurgery. Hass and Taylor[8] described a technique of producing sharply defined necrotic lesions in the brain, the liver, and the kidneys by freezing those tissues with apparatus cooled by pressurized carbon dioxide. The absence of suppuration and the slow uncomplicated healing process were noteworthy. Other investigators used devices cooled by liquid nitrogen (−196°C) or solid carbon dioxide to produce cerebral lesions. These investigations showed that focal lesions could be produced in the brain, that varying degrees of hemorrhage and edema developed about the lesions, and that the freezing procedures were controllable and safe.[9–11] The clinical significance of these experiments was recognized and led to investigation of freezing techniques for the destruction of brain tumors. In 1959, using a cannula that permitted circulation of 95% alcohol through a mixture of solid carbon dioxide and acetone, Rowbotham and his associates[12] produced localized freezing in the brains of three patients with inoperable gliomas. The treatments of the gliomas did not produce any lasting benefit, but the absence of immediate deleterious effects of freezing brain tissue in situ gave some assurances about the safety of the procedure.

## THE MODERN ERA

Cryosurgery as it is used today began with the development by Cooper and Lee[13] in 1961 of automated cryosurgical apparatus cooled by liquid nitrogen. The vacuum-insulated probes, which could be cooled to any temperature down to about −170°C, were designed for freezing the basal ganglia for the treatment of Parkinson's disease. Cooper[14,15] recognized that the apparatus could be used to destroy neoplasms, performed experimental work on freezing various tissues in animals, and treated some cancers. He interested physicians in other medical specialties in clinical trials of the freezing techniques, now being termed cryogenic surgery or cryosurgery.

A substantial amount of experimental and clinical work with cryosurgical techniques quickly followed. Probes longer and more suitable for the treatment of cancer than Cooper's small (about 3 mm in diameter) brain probe were devised. In many reports published in the years 1964 to 1970, reports of the use of cryosurgery in the treatment of tumors in many sites were described.[16–34] Most of the clinical applications were in easily accessible sites for a wide range of different types of diseases including tumors (Table 5C-1). Many applications were intended only for palliation of distressing symptoms and control of neoplastic growth, but others were intended to cure the disease. During these years, other types of cryosurgical apparatus, cooled by several kinds of cryogenic agents, differing in freezing capability, were developed. In general, a promising new therapy for

### TABLE 5C-1. APPLICATIONS OF CRYOSURGERY, 1965–1970

| NON-NEOPLASTIC | TUMORS OF |
|---|---|
| Skin diseases | Skin |
| Parkinsonism | Brain |
| Retinal detachment | Eye |
| Ménière's disease | Oral cavity |
| Hypertrophic rhinitis | Pharynx |
| Nasal polyps | Larynx |
| Mucosal diseases | Bronchus |
| Chronic cervicitis | Lung |
| Cervical dysplasia | Esophagus |
| Hemorrhoids | Rectum |
| Anal fissures | Prostate |
| Condylomata | Uterus |
| Pilonidal disease | Bone |

the treatment of tumors was accorded high expectations and a quick trial.

By the mid-1970s, the initial enthusiasm for cryosurgery had waned, at least in some applications. Use of cryosurgery for prostatic disease gradually decreased because of the prolonged catheter drainage required after operation and the high incidence of complications. Nevertheless, some interest persisted in the cryosurgical treatment of prostatic cancer because of the potential benefit from a favorable immunologic response as suggested by experimental work and by reports of remission of metastatic cancer after freezing.[35,36] Oral cancers, easily accessible for cryosurgery, continued to be treated in clinical trials in a few medical centers but did not attract wide interest.[37–39] The competition of lasers reduced the use of cryosurgery for cervical intraepithelial neoplasia, but the results achieved with the two methods of therapy were about the same. Cryosurgery for skin cancer, commonly given by handheld devices cooled by liquid nitrogen, became accepted practice.[40,41] Although cryosurgery had undergone evaluation in these years and its original promise had been readjusted, a considerable amount of experimental work defining the effects of freezing on various tissues was done in this period.

In the 1980s, progress was slow. Cryosurgical techniques came into use in ophthalmic surgery for the treatment of diverse diseases, including tumors.[42,43] Use in treating cervical intraepithelial neoplasia continued and cryosurgery was considered a standard therapy.[44–48] Interest in cryosurgery for prostatic cancer was maintained in only a few medical centers, although reports from Bonney and his associates[49,50] showed a survival rate that they compared favorably with radical prostatectomy. Cryosurgery was used for liver tumors, including metastatic colorectal cancer, but the lack of ability to visualize the deep lesions permitted only occasional clinical applications that were of uncertain benefit. Cryosurgery was applied to selected patients with bone tumors, generally benign locally aggressive tumors.[51] In thoracic disease, the palliative treatment of obstructing tracheobronchial tumors was beneficial.[52–54] However, as the 1980s ended, although cryosurgical techniques had become a standard treatment in specialties such as dermatology and gynecology, cryosurgery was a minor therapeutic tool for most tumors and was considered only for palliative treatment of easily accessible advanced cancers or was used when surgical excision was not applicable because of surgical risk, including patients with a coagulopathy.[55]

Technological advances in three areas renewed interest in cryosurgery late in the 1980s. Intraoperative ultrasound was developed and its usefulness in relation to cryosurgery of the liver and the prostate was described by Onik and his associates.[56,57] The ultrasound image identified the site of the lesion, guided the placement of the cryoprobe into the lesion, and monitored the process of freezing. In addition, the development of endoscopic and percutaneous access devices facilitated the use of cryosurgery for visceral tumors. In the same years, improvements in liquid nitrogen–cooled cryosurgical apparatus provided enhanced freezing capability.[58,59] These advances and their potential for usefulness in visceral tumors, provided new enthusiasm for freezing techniques as cryosurgery moved into the 1990s.

## CRYOBIOLOGY

An understanding of the nature of cryogenic injury is important to the use of cryosurgery. Two different mechanisms cause cell and tissue death in severe cold injury. These are the following:

1. The direct effects of freezing on cells, such as crystallization of water, high intracellular concentration of solutes, and irreversible changes in cell membranes.
2. The vascular stasis that develops in the tissue after thawing.

The tissue damage from the direct effects on the cells occurs during the act of freezing, whereas that due to the vascular stasis occurs after thawing. Each mechanism is capable of causing necrosis by itself, so definition of the relative importance of each is difficult.

### DIRECT CELL INJURY

During the freezing of cells, the cornerstone of injury is the formation of ice crystals and the consequent withdrawal of water from the metabolism. As the temperature falls and the tissue freezes, water turns to ice. In biologic tissues, the temperature may be reduced as low as $-10°$ to $-15°C$ before ice crystals form, a phenomenon known as supercooling. The ice crystals form first in the extracellular spaces and are barred from entering the cell by the cell membrane. As the temperature falls below $-10°$ to $-15°C$, the increase in solute concentration depresses the freezing point of the remaining unfrozen water. With further cooling, the extracellular ice crystals grow in size and intracellular ice formation is likely. Certain formation of intracellular ice requires temperatures colder than $-40°C$.[58]

The distribution of ice crystals is dependent upon the cooling rate. During slow cooling, that is, of the order of about $5°C$ per minute, ice crystals form in the extracellular spaces and increase in size and number as the temperature falls. Water is withdrawn from the cells in response to the increased concentration of solutes in the extracellular space and the cells shrink. Although intracellular ice crystals do not form, the concentration of solutes and cellular dehydration are injurious. On thawing, the water moves back into the cells, which become swollen and rupture. This sequence of events has been termed *solution effects*.[60] Rapid cooling, about $50°C$ or more per minute, does not allow sufficient time for water to leave the cells, so the ice crystal formation is intracellular and extracellular. Intracellular ice is lethal for cells under cryosurgical conditions. Rapid cooling injures the cell membranes, distorting the rough endoplasmic reticulum, and disturbing the structure and function of mitochondria and other cell organelles.

Thawing is an important mechanism of injury in cryosurgery. During slow thawing, small ice crystals coalesce to form large crystals, a process called recrystallization. The large crystals produce mechanical injury to cell membranes, especially in tissues with cells packed tightly. Injury from cell dehydration and toxic concentration of electrolytes is also operative at this time. For these reasons, slow thawing is an integral part of cryosurgical technique.

### DAMAGE DUE TO VASCULAR STASIS

Damage directly to the cells during freezing and thawing is enhanced by the effect of freezing on the circulation. With thawing, the circulation returns and a hyperemic response is evident for a brief period. Then microcirculatory failure begins and generally is complete in 30 to 40 min. Endothelial cell damage causes increased permeability of the small blood vessels, edema forms, the circulation slows, and microthrombi from platelet aggregation form. The loss of blood supply deprives all cells in the previously frozen tissue of any possibility of survival. The result is uniform necrosis of tissue, except at the periphery of the previously frozen area. Vascular stasis is clearly an important factor in cell death.

### THE CRYOGENIC LESION

The tissue injury is characterized by necrosis that is sharply demarcated and closely corresponds to the volume of frozen tissue. As thawing occurs, the previously frozen tissue becomes swollen due to edema and discolored due to congestion and perivascular hemorrhage. Edema is progressive over the first 24 hours after injury. Sharply demarcated necrosis is apparent in about 2 days.

The subsequent events vary in different types of tissue and depend in large part upon the stroma. Highly cellular tissue in an exposed location, such as the rectal lumen or oral cavity, will slough in 7 to 10 days. In closed locations, such as deep in the liver, the necrotic tissue will not be absorbed for several months. Skin, with its abundant fibrous stroma, resists change, and the necrotic tissue requires about 2 weeks to slough. Devitalized cartilage resists slough. Bone, devitalized by freezing, appears unchanged after freezing and thawing.

### WOUND HEALING

Repair of the cryogenic wound is ordinarily favorable. Although the tissues are devitalized by freezing, the matrix may be little changed and the preservation of this architecture is important to the later repair. For example, the resistance of the collagen fibers in skin to damage from freezing is responsible for the favorable healing reported in experiments and in the treatment of skin disease.[61,62] Delay in healing is characteristic of cryosurgical wounds. Time is required to clear the necrotic tissue whether by slough or by absorption, so healing is slow in comparison to excision and primary suture of a wound.

Tissue response to cryogenic injury is related to structure and function. Ductal structures commonly form strictures in healing. Nerves temporarily lose their function, but although the axons and Schwann cells degenerate, the structure of the perineurium is preserved. The intact perineurium serves as a pathway for regrowth of axons, leading eventually to a return of nerve function. Large arteries and veins, devitalized by freezing, undergo repair while continuing to function as conduits of blood. Bone maintains form and function as the devitalized bone is slowly resorbed and replaced with new bone in a lengthy healing process. The bone is weakened and susceptible to fracture in the first 2 months after injury, when bone resorption is maximal.

## EQUIPMENT

Cryosurgery requires the use of refrigerating apparatus and a cryogenic agent. Some basic information is provided in this section. Additional information on the engineering aspects of cryosurgery, including refrigeration methods and the design and operation of cryosurgical apparatus, may be found in detailed reports on these subjects.[63–65]

### CRYOGENIC AGENTS

The cryogenic agents provide a range of temperatures and different freezing capabilities (Table 5C-2). In current cryosurgical practice, liquid nitrogen, argon, nitrous oxide, or carbon dioxide is used. The latter three gases are commonly used in pressurized states to cool by the Joule-Thomson effect. The temperature that each of these agents produces at the point of application to the tissue is less than the temperatures cited in Table 5C-2. The variations in operating

### TABLE 5C-2. CRYOGENS USED IN CRYOSURGERY

| CRYOGEN | BOILING POINT AT ATMOSPHERIC PRESSURE, °C |
|---|---|
| Dichlorotetrafluoromethane (Freon 114) | 3.8* |
| Dichlorodifluoromethane (Freon 12) | −29.8 |
| Chlorodifluoromethane (Freon 22) | −40.8 |
| Carbon dioxide, solid | −78.5† |
| Nitrous oxide, liquid | −89.5 |
| Argon, liquid | −185.7 |
| Nitrogen, liquid | −195.8 |

*When sprayed on tissue, the fluorinated hydrocarbons yield colder temperatures (Freon 114 about −30°C, Freon 12 about −80°C, Freon 22 about −70°C).
**Sublimes at 1 atm.

temperature are due in large part to the engineering characteristics of the different types of delivery apparatus.

Liquid nitrogen is a clear, odorless, nonflammable fluid with a boiling point of 195.8°C at 1 atm pressure. This cryogen expands about 700 times its volume as it changes to a gas. For use in clinics, liquid nitrogen commonly is stored in a vacuum-insulated container with a capacity of 15 to 35 L. Liquid nitrogen will evaporate at a rate of a few percent per day, so provision is made in the container for pressure relief. When the liquid nitrogen is transferred from the container to the cryosurgical instrument, spillage or splashing on the skin or in the eyes must be avoided by adequate protective measures. In automated cryosurgical apparatus, liquid nitrogen commonly provides probe freezing surface temperature of −160° to −190°C, depending upon the size of the probe and engineering features of the apparatus. In handheld apparatus, a spray of liquid nitrogen is directed onto the tissue.

Nitrous oxide is a colorless nonflammable gas, commonly available in hospitals in E cylinders that hold 2.72 kg (6 lb) of liquid $N_2O$ (−89.5°C) at a pressure of 740 lb/in$^2$ gauge (psig). The withdrawal of the nitrous oxide gas diminishes the pressure in the E cylinder, and this reduces the cooling efficiency of the apparatus and the rate of freezing. In the use of this apparatus, care must be taken to exhaust the nitrous oxide safely from the room because excessive concentrations in the room air expose personnel to ill effects, such as impaired cognition and performance. In cryosurgical apparatus, nitrous oxide provides probe tip (freezing surface) temperatures of about −70°C.

Carbon dioxide is a colorless gas that is used as a cryogen in solid and gaseous forms. Solid carbon dioxide (−78.5°C) has been used in various forms for direct application to tissue for about 100 years. Carbon dioxide is also available as a compressed gas contained in E cylinders. In cryosurgical apparatus, it provides probe temperatures (freezing surface) of about −60°C.

Argon is a colorless, odorless, tasteless inert gas that condenses to a liquid at −185.8°C. Argon is available as a compressed gas contained in cylinders. In cryosurgical apparatus, argon provides probe freezing surface temperatures in the range of −90° to 130°C, depending upon the size of the probe. During use, the pressure in the cylinder falls and capacity to freeze is reduced.

Fluorinated hydrocarbons, commonly called Freon, are a group of chemicals with different boiling points at 1 atm pressure and different cooling capacity. In simple cryosurgical apparatus, these agents can be sprayed onto a tissue surface or used to cool a probe. When sprayed onto a surface, the fluorinated hydrocarbons yield colder temperatures than their boiling points. These compounds have little usefulness in the treatment of neoplasms. Ethyl chloride sprays and other minor cryogens have been used for cold analgesia and not for destructive freezing.

### APPARATUS

Cryosurgical apparatus is available in a wide variety of types that provide different tissue-freezing capabilities. The equipment, whether simple or complex, uses one of several refrigeration methods, which are the following:

1. The change in phase of the cryogen, that is, evaporation (or sublimation) of a liquid or solid.

2. The expansion of a compressed gas after passage through a restriction orifice (Joule-Thomson effect).
3. Thermoelectric cooling (Peltier effect) produced by passing a direct current through dissimilar metal junctions (thermocouples).

Liquid nitrogen–cooled apparatus uses the method of change of phase of the cryogen. The devices range from automated expensive apparatus suitable for the treatment of visceral tumors to inexpensive handheld units that are little more than Thermos bottles with simple controls for the flow of the cryogen. In dermatologic practice, the handheld devices that provide a spray of liquid nitrogen are popular. They usually have a storage capacity of 250 to 500 mL and weigh about 1 kg when empty. When filled with liquid nitrogen, they are easier to use as a spray device than with a probe, especially since they do not have a heater to release the probe from the tissue. Portable tabletop cryosurgical apparatus is well suited to office or clinical use. Such devices have a flexible feed line that leads to a lightweight probe for application to the lesion. The greater size of the reservoir provides increased treatment time, sufficient for multiple small tumors. The freezing of deeply located tumors, such as those of viscera, is performed with automated apparatus and flexible vacuum-insulated cryogen transfer lines leading to the probe. The temperature of the probes can be adjusted to selected levels, which is important in some clinical applications, such as cancer of the prostate. A heating element speeds release of the probe from the tissue at the conclusion of freezing. Recent improvements in liquid nitrogen–cooled equipment features the use of liquid nitrogen cooled to about $-204°C$ by new technology, so that the probes are colder than earlier devices. In addition, the new probes are thinner and suitable for percutaneous use and multiple probes can be cooled simultaneously with individual temperature controls.[59]

Cryosurgical apparatus cooled by the Joule-Thomson principle are lightweight, portable, and quickly responsive in cooling or warming. The pressurized gas, which can be a number of different gases, including nitrogen, argon, nitrous oxide, and carbon dioxide, is passed through a restrictive orifice and expands, producing a drop in temperature. The pressure required for maximal cooling varies with the different gases. For example, argon requires a pressure of about 6000 lb/in$^2$, whereas carbon dioxide requires about 830 lb/in$^2$. With a fall in pressure in the cylinders during use, the freezing efficiency falls. The agent most commonly used in this type of apparatus is nitrous oxide, which is easily available in many clinical settings.

Devices that use thermoelectric cooling have limited freezing capability and can provide a probe tip temperature of only $-20°$ to $-30°C$ at a low cooling rate. These devices have been satisfactory for ophthalmologic use but not for the treatment of tumors. The efficiency of this method may be improved by combining the technology of heat pipes, which is reported to provide probe temperatures of $-50°$ to $-60°C$.[66] Although this may have some uses for nonneoplastic diseases, applicability to neoplasms is unlikely.

In the past few years, the choice of apparatus has become more complex because the number of manufacturers has increased and different refrigerating methods are being promoted. The choice is easier when the planned use of the apparatus is defined. In the treatment of cancer, cell destruction must be certain. To facilitate heat transfer from the tissue, the probe must be as cold as possible. The coldest cryogen is liquid nitrogen; this is the best agent to use for invasive cancer.

## BASIC TECHNIQUE

In the treatment of tumors, cryosurgery must be performed in a manner that produces a predictable destructive response. The same volume of tissue must be destroyed by freezing that would have been removed if local excision had been used. Therefore an appropriate margin of apparently normal tissue around the tumor must be included in the frozen volume. To achieve certainty of destruction of the tumor, cryosurgical techniques require careful attention to the freeze-thaw cycles and to efficient heat transfer from the tissue. The basic features of cryosurgical technique are the same for all neoplasms. The modifications of these basic techniques required for neoplasms in special sites are described in the later sections of this chapter.

The important features in basic technique are the following:

1. A cryogen suitable for the lesion should be chosen.
2. Appropriate freezing method (probe, spray, pour) should be selected.
3. The freezing rate should be as rapid as possible.
4. A lethal temperature must be produced in the tissue.
5. The frozen tissue should be allowed to thaw slowly.
6. The freeze-thaw cycle should be repeated after thawing is complete.
7. An adequate margin of normal tissue about the tumor should be included in the frozen volume.
8. The frozen volumes should be overlapped if the tumor is too large to be frozen from one probe application site. (Several probes may be used simultaneously, overlapping frozen volumes.)

### CHOICE OF CRYOGEN

The freezing of tumors in situ is produced by the removal of heat from the tissue. The flow of heat is facilitated by a large gradient between the tissue and the heat sink, usually a probe. The cryogen commonly used in cryosurgery for neoplasms is liquid nitrogen, which has sufficient freezing capability for the treatment of invasive cancer. The other cryogens have limited freezing capability and are best suited to nonneoplastic disease, although nitrous oxide has been used in the treatment of bronchial tumors, and little data are available on the efficacy of pressurized argon. Therefore with a few exceptions, the recommendations made in this chapter are based on the use of liquid nitrogen as the cryogen.

### CHOICE OF TECHNIQUE

The basic techniques of cryosurgery fall into two major groups, the applications of the cryogen directly on the tissue by spraying or pouring and the use of the cryogen in a closed system to cool a metal probe that is applied to the tissue. The choice is based on the nature, size, and location of the tumor. Spray techniques, commonly used on the skin surface for superficial lesions, are versatile and can easily freeze wide, irregular areas. Pour techniques are useful in cavities, such as following curettement of bone tumors. Other than skin cancers, almost all tumors are treated by cryoprobe techniques that can be used to freeze from the tumor surface or can be inserted into the tumor for deep freezing.

Efficient transfer of heat from the tissue requires good contact with the cryogen, whether used as a spray or in a probe. Heat is removed from the tissue at a rate dependent upon the temperature of the probe or spray, the area of contact, and the duration of application. The cooling rate is rapid in the tissue in close contact with the cryogen. As the distance increases, the cooling rate slows. Within the frozen volume, a steep gradient of temperature is present, reaching about 0°C at the border of the frozen volume. The volume of tissue frozen expands as time passes until thermal equilibrium is reached, that is, a balance between heat lost from the tissue and heat brought to the area by the circulation of blood is established. At that time the frozen volume no longer increases, so commonly freezing is halted and the tissue is allowed to thaw.

## CRYOPROBE TECHNIQUE

The probe techniques are closed systems in which the cryogen is used to cool a metal probe with a freezing surface at its tip (Fig. 5C-1). Various sizes and shapes of probes are available (Fig. 5C-2). Common sizes range from 3 to 10 mm in diameter and the freezing surface usually varies from 1 to 4 cm in length. The tip may be pointed for insertion into the tissue or flattened for surface application. Practically all probes are rigid. Small probes (2 mm), which may be flexible, are in development, but these may not be useful in the treatment of neoplastic disease because the small cryogen feed line has only limited freezing capability.

Probes are used in surface contact and penetration techniques. With surface contact technique, the freezing surface of the probe is applied to the lesion without penetration, pressing firmly to ensure good heat exchange. If the tissue is dry, the contact is improved by the use of water-soluble hospital lubricating jelly between the probe and the tissue. With penetration technique, the pointed probe is inserted into the tumor, which causes a wound and creates a chance of bleeding. Surface contact techniques are commonly used for easily accessible tumors, whereas penetration techniques are needed for bulky or deeply placed tumors.

To freeze the tissues, the probe is applied to the tumors and is cooled as rapidly as possible. As its temperature falls below 0°C, the probe becomes adherent to the tissue. Care must be taken to avoid motion of the probe because a fracture in the bond between probe and tissue would interfere with heat exchange. The probe is used as cold as possible because a rapid rate of cooling of the tissue is desired.

With surface freezing, as the tissues turn frosted white and hard, the extent of freezing can be judged by inspection and palpation. The shape of the frozen volume is hemispheric, so the depth of freezing can be judged to be about the same as the lateral spread of freezing from the probe. With penetration techniques, which bury the freezing surface of the probe into the tumor, the frozen

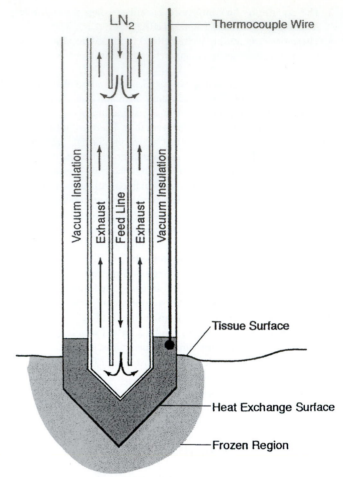

**FIGURE 5C-1.** Diagram of a typical vacuum-insulated cryosurgical probe, showing the central flow channel for liquid nitrogen, the heat exchange surface where tissue freezing occurs, and the cryogen exhaust line. Some modern probes have several ports in the feed line, such as shown on the diagram, to increase the cooling efficacy. The thermocouple wires in the shaft, which are present in some probes, terminate near the heat exchange surface and provide a measurement of the temperature of the probe. Many probe shapes and sizes, ranging from 1 mm (not insulated) to several centimeters in diameter, are available. The choice of probe depends upon the nature, size, and location of the lesion.

volume will be circular or spherical, depending upon the length of the heat exchange surface of the probe. Since the freezing is not visible, monitoring of the frozen volume by the measurement of tissue temperature with thermocouples and/or by the image provided by ultrasound is necessary.

Heat transfer from the tissue is related to the temperature of the probe, the surface area of contrast between the probe and tissue, and the thermal conductivity of probe and tissue. The volume and shape of the frozen tissue is affected also by heat brought to the area by blood vessels. Large probes, usually colder than small probes and with larger heat transfer area, will freeze greater volumes of tissue

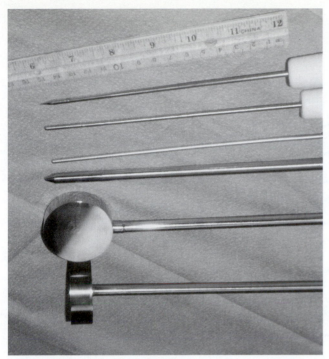

**FIGURE 5C-2.** Many probe shapes and sizes, ranging from 1 mm (not insulated) to several centimeters in diameter, are available. The choice of probe depends upon the nature, size, and location of the lesion. This photograph shows six typical probes. The probe at the top is 3.4 mm in diameter, has a freezing surface 1 cm in length at the probe tip, and is pointed for ease of insertion into the tissues. The adjacent 3.4-mm probes have blunt tips with freezing surfaces 1 cm and 4 cm in length, respectively. The fourth probe from the top is 8 mm in diameter with a freezing surface 4 cm long. The two probes at the bottom have flat freezing surfaces 5 cm in diameter and are useful for freezing of tissue surfaces.

than small probes. For example, a 3-mm probe with a 1-cm-long freezing surface cooled to about −165° to −170°C, will produce a rounded, circular frozen volume about 4 cm in diameter in about 15 min. An 8-mm probe with a 4-cm-long freezing surface cooled to −190°C will produce an ellipsoid frozen volume about 7 cm in diameter in about 15 min. When required, the use of several small probes simultaneously compensates for this difference.

## SPRAY AND POUR TECHNIQUES

Spray techniques are commonly used in the treatment of skin disease, including cancers. Liquid nitrogen sprayed from the nozzle of a handheld device is an efficient method of producing rapid shallow freezing of tissue over a wide area, especially over irregularly contoured surfaces. The use of plastic cones to confine the spray is a good technique that is well suited to many skin cancers.[67] The pour technique is simply pouring liquid nitrogen onto the lesion. Its

usefulness is limited to cavitary lesions, which provide a receptacle to limit the runoff of the cryogen. The pour technique has been used after curettage of bone tumors.

## THE FREEZE-THAW CYCLES

Tissue injury may be produced by any of the diverse components of the freeze-thaw cycles, such as cooling rate, warming rate, and temperature produced in the tissue.

**THE FREEZING RATE.** Rapid freezing produces the lethal intracellular ice, but this occurs only close to the heat sink. The further away from the probe, the slower is the cooling rate. At a distance of 1 cm from a probe, the cooling rate is relatively slow (Fig. 5C-3). Fortunately even slow cooling rates have lethal properties due to cellular dehydration and related effects.

**TISSUE TEMPERATURE.** Care must be taken to produce in all areas of the tumor a temperature certainly lethal for cells. As the temperature falls through the freezing ranges, cells die in increasing numbers from progressive physicochemical changes. At a tissue temperature of −20° to −30°C, substantial damage is caused to cells and tissue. However, some cells survive and safety demands colder tissue temperatures. In the treatment of cancer, a tissue temperature of −50°C in all parts of the tumor must be produced to be certain of cell death.[68] A thermocouple placed in the apparently normal tissue 1 cm beyond the border of the cancer should show a tissue temperature of at least −40°C and that will provide for the safe margin required in cancer surgery when a 1-cm margin is required. This means that the frozen border must extend beyond the 1-cm margin. The isotherms in a frozen volume of tissue are steep, more so in small volumes than in large ones. This is important to recognize when only ultrasound is used to monitor the freezing process.

**DURATION OF FREEZING.** The tissue should be held in the frozen state for several minutes, perhaps 10 to 15 minutes, although the optimal duration is not known. The increased time in the frozen state allows time for ice crystals to grow by recrystallization and cause cell injury.

**THE THAWING RATE.** The thawing rate should be slow and unassisted. During slow warming, small ice crystals grow by recrystallization, which takes place largely in the 0° to −40°C temperature range. The large ice crystals cause mechanical disruption of cells. For maximal damage, the tissue should be allowed to thaw completely, that is, the entire volume of frozen tissue is above 0°C, which may take many minutes, depending upon the volume of tissue frozen.

**REPETITION OF THE FREEZE-THAW CYCLE.** This important facet of the technique increases the certainty of cell destruction. It is best done after complete thawing of the previously frozen tissue. It might be better to wait for an even longer interval, but the optimal interval between freeze-thaw cycles is not known. However, complete thawing is time consuming, so some surgeons wait only until the periphery of the frozen tissue has thawed before repeating the freeze-thaw cycle. This technique is based on the thought that

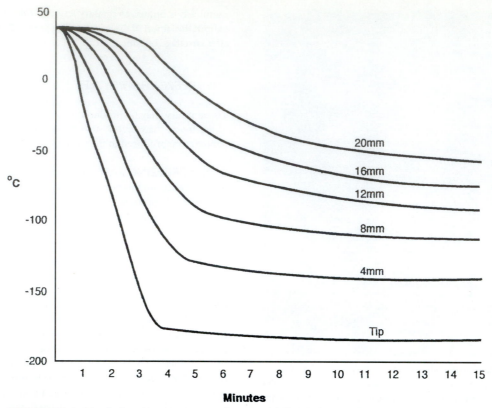

**FIGURE 5C-3.** Graph showing temperature changes at different distances from a cryosurgical probe 8 mm in diameter, cooled by liquid nitrogen, during performance testing. The "tip" thermocouple shows the temperature on the freezing surface of the probe. The cooling rate of the surface of the probe and adjacent tissue is rapid. The cooling rate and duration of freezing, as well as thawing rate, differ depending on the distance from the probe. Close to the probe, the tissue cooling rate is fast. The further from the probe, the slower is the cooling rate. The duration of freezing and the lowest tissue temperature reached also vary with distance. These differences are characteristic of cryosurgery and must be considered when performing cryosurgical procedures.

cell survival is most likely at the border of the frozen volume and therefore only this region need be frozen twice. Some physicians have advocated only a single freeze-thaw cycle, but this variant in technique is not good cryosurgical practice for cancer. Repetitive freeze-thaw cycles, producing a temperature of at least −50°C in all of the cancer tissue, separated by complete thawing, will maximize tissue destruction and introduce the margin of safety required in cancer cryosurgery.[69,70]

## CRYONECROSIS—THE BORDER ZONE

Even with the best cryosurgical technique, the cryogenic lesion will have a peripheral zone of partial destruction (Fig. 5C-4). In this border zone, at the margin of the previously frozen tissue where the temperature has ranged from 0°C to −40°C, some cells will survive, more so close to 0°C than close to −40°C. Many cells in this region have been partially damaged and some will die in the following days. If care has been taken to move this zone well outside of the neoplastic

tissue, then the cancer will not recur in the treated area. However, if cancer cells are in this area, then recurrence is possible. Therefore, maneuvers to increase destruction in the border zone are important. In effect, one is trying to remove the possibility of survival of partially damaged cells. Increased destruction in the border zone, perhaps as close as the −20°C isotherm, is produced by repetition of the freeze-thaw cycle, by holding the tissue in the frozen state for about 15 min, and by increasing the interval between freeze-thaw cycles. Adjunctive treatment by cancer chemotherapeutic drugs and radiotherapy is also likely to be effective against partially damaged cells.

## MONITORING—THERMOCOUPLES AND ULTRASOUND

Both tissue temperature measurements and ultrasound imaging are used as methods of monitoring tissue freezing during cryosurgery. Each method has special areas of usefulness, each provides a different type of information, and each has advantages and disadvantages in cryosurgery.

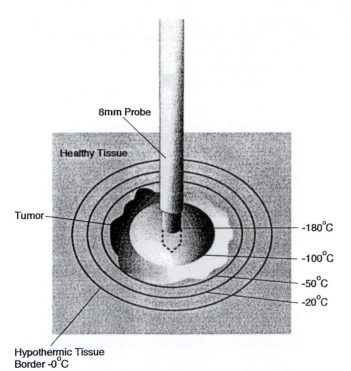

8mm Probe

Healthy Tissue

Tumor

-180°C

-100°C

-50°C

-20°C

Hypothermic Tissue
Border -0°C

**FIGURE 5C-4.** The diagram depicts the isotherms that develop in a tumor with the cryosurgical probe cooled to −180°C. Close to the probe, the cooling rate is fast and lethal temperatures are attained. The tumor within the −50°C isotherm will certainly be destroyed. The cells in the 0° to −20°C range are likely to survive. A repetition of the freeze-thaw cycle, which is most effective after complete thawing, increases the lethality of the treatment and moves the border of destruction closer to the −20°C isotherm.

**THERMOCOUPLES.** Tissue temperature is measured by the placement of needle-mounted thermocouples in appropriate places (i.e., at the border of a lesion) about the target tissue. Thermocouples are formed by the junction of two dissimilar metals, commonly iron and constantan or copper and constantan, in a closed electric circuit. The metal junction is mounted in the tip of a hypodermic needle (as small as 25 gauge). The conductors generate an electromotive force (emf) proportional to the temperature. An instrument, such as a potentiometer or pyrometer, is used to measure the emf and provide a readout in terms of temperature. Copper-constantan (type T) thermocouples, which can be used over the temperature range of +37° to −200°C, are satisfactory for cryosurgery. They should be calibrated at intervals to be certain that their function is satisfactory. The accurate positioning of the thermosensor is of obvious great importance. A 1-mm variation in thermocouple placement in the tissue represents about 10° to 15°C difference in the temperature recorded in the usual cryosurgical freeze-thaw cycles.[71]

A thermocouple measures the temperature only in the site in which it is placed, so that inferences must be made about the temperature elsewhere. However, knowing the temperature of the probe tip and the temperature wherever measured in the frozen tissue permits an estimation of the temperature elsewhere in the area, since the growth of the frozen volume of tissue tends to be symmetrical (altered, of course, by the proximity of large blood vessels). The use of multiple thermocouples increases the information available and enhances the control of the freezing process.

The thermosensor should be placed in the position that is critical to evaluation of the freezing cycle. One important position is in the normal tissue at an appropriate distance from the border of the tumor. For example, in a liver tumor, this position would be 1 cm from the edge of the tumor because that distance is the usually recommended margin for surgical excision. Then, in freezing, care should be taken to achieve lethal temperatures at that site.

**ULTRASOUND.** Intraoperative ultrasound provides a real-time image of the frozen volume of tissue. Since ultrasound provides a more global view of the frozen tissue than do thermosensors, this imaging technique has come into wide use for monitoring the freeze-thaw cycle. Frozen tissue is hypoechoic, so the ultrasonic image is black (Fig. 5C-5). The edge of the frozen tissue is hyperechoic and appears as a bright line. As freezing continues and the volume of frozen tissue increases, the hyperechoic rim moves away from the probe, leaving the hypoechoic zone behind it. Therefore the process of tissue freezing can be observed during the cryosurgical procedure. Good correlation between the ultrasound image and the actual diameter of the frozen tissue has been demonstrated, but it has also become evident that ultrasound overestimates the volume of tissue frozen. Much of the frozen volume is obscured by distortions and reflections of the image. Sonography does not provide an image beyond the near edge of the ice; therefore, complete posterior acoustic shadowing is present.[72–75] Some compensation for this limitation can be obtained by viewing the frozen volume from another angle. Until recently, ultrasound is unable to provide a three-dimensional image, but progress is being made in that direction, at least for prostatic cryosurgery.[76]

The correlation between tissue temperature and the ultrasound image is of considerable importance. The location of the isotherms, especially the critical −40°C isotherm, in the ultrasonic image must be known, but one cannot determine the temperature of frozen tissue from its ultrasonic appearance.[77] The tissue temperature must be estimated from a knowledge of probe temperature, of the probe performance in terms of growth of ice formation around it in relation to time, and of the temperature at the outer edge of the hyperechoic rim. The temperature gradient between the probe surface and the border of the frozen zone is steep. The advancing edge of the freezing tissue, which appears on the ultrasonic image as a hyperechoic border, is about 0°C. The inner edge of the rim, which is 2 mm inside of the leading edge, is about −20°C.[78] In a frozen volume about 3 cm in diameter, the isotherm of −40°C is about 5 to 8 mm into the hypoechoic "black" zone in commonly used cryosurgical freeze-thaw cycles.[79,80] Whatever tissue temperature goal is chosen during treatment, position of that isotherm will shift with the variances in the heat transfer and, therefore, the physician should move in the direction of aggressive freezing technique whenever possible in the treatment of cancer.

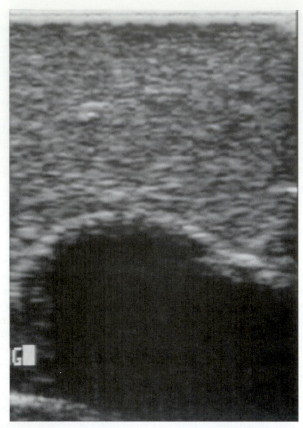

**FIGURE 5C-5.** Typical ultrasonic image during the freezing of tissue. The ice front is seen as a narrow hyperechoic line, which is at a temperature of about 0°C. The ultrasound waves are practically totally reflected at the ice border. Beyond the line, the frozen tissue is hypoechoic and the status of freezing in this area is obscured in the dark shadow; therefore, only the ice front can be monitored. This one-dimensional view should be supplemented by views from other directions to gain a more accurate evaluation of the volume of frozen tissue.

## CLINICAL APPLICATION

Cryosurgical techniques have been used to treat solid tumors in almost every part of the body. In many sites, cryosurgery has been used as a final effort to control neoplastic disease when all else has failed. In some sites, cryosurgery is used as primary treatment with the intent to cure, and therefore the technique is competing with other methods of local treatment. The purpose of cryosurgical treatment should be defined in advance of therapy, that is, whether the intent is to cure the disease or only provide palliation of symptoms. The intent to cure requires accurate assessment of the limits of the tumor and careful attention to the freeze-thaw cycles. The treatment for the palliation of symptoms of incurable cancer is a less exacting technique. The palliative benefits of cryosurgery are the same wherever used and include reduction in tumor bulk, relief of pain, and lessening of bleeding and malodorous discharge.

In the following sections of this chapter, the use of cryosurgery to treat diverse tumors will be described. In sites where cryosurgery is commonly used, the factors in case selection, complications, results, and comparison with other therapy are given. However, practically no controlled comparative trials of cryosurgery have been performed, so the results of cryosurgery must be evaluated in terms of knowledge of the biologic behavior of the cancer and the results achieved by commonly used methods of therapy. In many sites, cryosurgery is chosen only when conventional surgery cannot be used because of age, coagulopathy, or other factors increasing the patient's surgical risk. The basic techniques already described apply to every disease site, so only special features in technique will be described in sections on different organs. This includes the monitoring techniques, commonly either ultrasound or thermosensors, that differ in usefulness in diverse situations. Wherever cryosurgery is used, clinical judgment is the most important method of controlling the process of tissue freezing.

Biologic tissue resists freezing injury and the freezing capacity of cryosurgical apparatus is limited in comparison to the size of many tumors. Therefore in many locations, especially for large tumors, adjunctive therapy is used. This may take the form of partial excision, perhaps using electrocoagulation, to remove most of the tumor before freezing the remainder, or may consist of radiotherapy or the administration of cancer chemotherapeutic drugs. One or more of these methods of treatment are commonly used with cryosurgery.

## CRYOSURGERY—ADJUNCT TO SURGICAL EXCISION

Cryosurgery has considerable value as an adjunct to surgical excision. One adjunctive use is the cryosurgical treatment of tumors remaining in the organ after excision of metastatic tumors in the liver. Another important form of adjunctive use is for the treatment by freezing (probe, spray, or pour technique) of the margins of excision for the purpose of destroying remaining neoplastic cells and improving the possibility of cure. This is a good technique after curettage of selected bone tumors. It is also useful in the management of liver cancers when the margin of excision is inadequate because of the proximity of important structures or the presence of cancer cells in the wound edge. The third form of adjunctive use is termed cryoassisted excision. By functioning as a traction device, the cryoprobe is used to facilitate excision of a tumor. The cryoprobe is inserted into the tumor and freezing is performed to a predetermined margin. The ice ball is then maintained during excision of the frozen tissue. This provides the possibility of excision of a geometrically shaped volume of tissue, and the avoidance of spread of cancer cells by manipulation. Cryoassisted excision has been used in the removal of tumors in several sites, such as the brain, the eye, and the liver.[81–83]

## SKIN CANCER

The common treatments of skin cancer, excepting melanomas, are surgical excision, irradiation, Mohs' therapy, and cryosurgery. The great majority of skin cancers are small, that is, less than 2 cm in diameter on the skin surface, and many do not extend more than

3 mm below the surface of the skin. These characteristics have made skin cancers suitable for cryosurgery, a technique that has become accepted as a standard therapy in dermatologic practice in the past 20 and more years.

## SELECTION CRITERIA

Basal cell carcinoma or squamous cell carcinoma may be treated by cryosurgery. The histologic cell type makes no difference as far as destruction of the local lesion by freezing is concerned, but the potential for metastatic spread is greater with squamous cell cancer and therefore it requires somewhat more aggressive freezing. The morphea type of basal cell carcinoma, with its narrow strands of cancer cells embedded in an abundant fibrous stroma, also requires aggressive freezing. The nature of the disease should be established by biopsy before starting therapy. Skin cancers of any size from small to large, including advanced and recurrent disease, are amenable to cryosurgery. However, a decision should be made in advance of therapy as to whether the treatment is to be given with the intent to cure or only for palliation of symptoms.

Cryosurgery is most commonly used for small superficial lesions that also could be treated easily by excision. Special reasons to use cryosurgery in preference over excision include the following:

1. Multiple small skin cancers. Treatment can be given to many cancers in quick sequence.
2. Cancers arising in irradiated skin. This permits conservation of tissue, which is important in damaged skin.
3. Cancers overlying bone. The effect of freezing extends into the bone and destroys any cancer cells that may have invaded.
4. Cancers about the nose and ears. Excision and surgical closure without skin grafting is sometimes difficult in these areas.

An important factor in selection is the ability to define the limits of the cancer, which ordinarily can be done rather easily. If the border is indefinite, cryosurgery should not be used.

Cryosurgery should be used with caution in heavily pigmented skin because freezing will result in some hypopigmentation. It also should be used with caution around the lips and ala nasi because of deformity after healing (lip retraction, nasal notching), and on the eyelids (especially near the lacrimal duct) because of the danger of cancer spreading into the orbit.

Cryosurgery can also be used for control of tumor growth and palliation of symptoms in large incurable cancers, either of primary origin in the skin or from other tissues, when no other treatment can be used. Repetitive treatment at a frequency of every several months is needed to maintain control of the growth of the cancer.

## TECHNIQUE

Cryosurgery is well suited for skin cancer because the lesion is accessible and the process of freezing and healing can be readily observed. The cryosurgical techniques used for small to moderate-sized skin cancers are well developed and vary chiefly in choice of spray or probe and in the use of curettage as a preliminary step to facilitate freezing of the base of the cancer. The patient is positioned for treatment. Little or no anesthesia is required because the freezing process desensitizes the nerves. However, for patient comfort, especially if thermocouple needles are to be inserted, a local anesthetic agent can be injected. Physicians experienced in cryosurgery often use clinical judgment only to control the extent of freezing, but this is not the most accurate technique. The temperature of frozen tissue cannot be determined by its appearance; therefore, the use of a thermocouple to supplement clinical judgment is a wise precaution.

The margins of the cancer are outlined with a skin marking pen. Another line is drawn 5 mm outside of the cancer outline—the freezing should extend at least as far as the outer line. The treatment is commonly given with a handheld device containing liquid nitrogen by one of three techniques, including open spray, a spray confined by a plastic cone, and the probe. The choice depends on the size, shape, and location of the disease, but the personal preference of the physician is a factor. A spray technique is commonly used. The freezing must include the entire tumor, and a sufficient margin of apparently healthy tissue around it. A margin of 5 mm around the cancer is advised, if that distance can be obtained in the anatomic site. As treatment is given, the surface frosting is easily visible, but the depth of freezing must be estimated by palpation unless a thermocouple has been placed beneath the lesion to measure tissue temperature. A tissue temperature of at least $-50°C$ in all the cancer area is desirable. After freezing and thawing, the freezing cycle is repeated. After treatment, the treated area becomes edematous within an hour, the wound becomes discolored, and serous exudation develops. The exudate dries to form an eschar in about a week and the wound heals completely in about another 2 weeks, the time depending upon the extent of the injury.

Variants in the technique feature preliminary partial excision before freezing. By removing the bulk of the tumor, the burden on freezing is reduced and the volume of frozen tissue that must slough is lessened. For small to large superficial skin cancers, cryosurgery may be combined with preliminary partial removal by curettage, converting thick into shallow lesions, thus facilitating freezing. Bulky tumors may require partial removal by excision or electrocoagulation and the use of freezing at appropriate intervals, guiding subsequent freezing by biopsies of the ulcerated wound to detect residual disease before allowing healing to occur. Advanced cancers, sometimes recurrent after previous surgical excision or irradiation, yet still localized and perhaps curable, may also benefit by these combined techniques.

## RESULTS

As the wound completes the healing process, including the return of pigmentation, the final cosmetic result is usually favorable. Some degree of hypopigmentation is common and the skin is usually thinned in the treated area. Commonly hair does not return. The cosmetic result is directly related to the size of the lesion and the extent of cryogenic injury, so the treatment of small lesions yields better cosmetic results than large ones. The complications that have occurred include hyperpigmentation of the skin, neuropathy from nerve damage, retraction of tissue in some locations (lips, eyelids, ala nasi), and nitrogen gas insufflation. The latter is an unusual event that might follow a spray of liquid nitrogen into an open wound, such as would result from preliminary curettage.

Data on the efficacy of cryosurgery for the treatment of skin cancer has been reported in several large series. These reports, based on at least 5 years of follow-up, show a success rate of about 98% in small to moderate-sized skin cancers, most of which were basal cell carcinomas.[84–88] The squamous cell carcinomas in these reports had practically the same results. Persistent disease was usually evident in the first year after treatment, but occasionally was detected some years later, as long as 5 years after treatment. From these data showing a high success rate, one can conclude that cryosurgery is an effective method of therapy. When used for skin cancers recurrent after other treatment, the success rate is good in selected cases.[87,89]

Cryosurgery has also been used for the management of advanced skin cancers. Survival data are not available, except as case reports on small numbers of patients in whom good results were achieved in difficult problems in management, such as large cancers, perhaps invading bone, often persistent after other methods of therapy. The palliation of symptoms of incurable cancers involving the skin, including breast cancers, rectal cancers, sarcomas, and melanomas, may yield worthwhile benefits, but life is not prolonged.[90–92]

## COMPARISON WITH OTHER THERAPY

Comparison of the relative efficacy of cryosurgery with the other methods of treatment is difficult because of lack of controlled studies and diverse factors in selection of patients. The high success rate of cryosurgery with small skin cancers (less than 2 cm on the surface) is similar to what can be achieved by surgery or other methods of therapy. The advantages of cryosurgery are in its simplicity, adaptability to multiple lesions, and usefulness in the special situations that were described earlier. The generally favorable cosmetic result is also noteworthy. The disadvantages are the slow healing of the wound and the lack of a surgical specimen on which to make a judgment on the adequacy of treatment.

## MELANOMA

Melanomas of the skin require excision that provides a specimen for examination to judge adequacy of excision and for staging. Cryosurgery should not be used for melanomas. Nevertheless, on an experimental basis, cutaneous malignant melanomas have been treated by cryosurgery by Breitbart,[93] who reported no recurrences in a small series of patients with early disease (stage 1, TNM classification). His primary interest has been in investigation of immunostimulation by freezing the melanoma in situ.[93] No clinical benefits on an immunologic basis have been demonstrated. Cryosurgery has been used to produce palliative benefits in advanced disease by control of tumor growth to relieve distressing symptoms, just as it has been used for incurable cancers elsewhere in the body.

Noncutaneous melanomas arise in the eye and in the mucosa in almost any location. Ocular melanomas were treated in the past by enucleation, but in recent years radiation has gained wide acceptance. The interest in a more conservative method of management is evident.[94] The sensitivity of melanosomes to cold

injury, demonstrated by Hidayat and his associates[95] in the freezing of uveal melanomas, encourages thought of application of cryosurgery in some cases. In the treatment of melanomas of the conjuctiva, Jacobiec and his associates[43] excised the melanoma nodules, then treated the base of the tumor by cryosurgery, which apparently extended the possibility of a cure. Melanomas arising from mucosa should be excised if possible. For those lesions that are not operable, cryosurgery is an option and will provide control of tumor growth and related benefits by repeated use.[96]

## EYE TUMORS

Cryosurgery has a limited role in the treatment of ocular tumors. The usefulness of the technique was first investigated by Lincoff and his associates,[24] who treated retinoblastomas, melanomas, and metastatic carcinomas of the eye. The results of the treatment of retinoblastoma encouraged further trials, but the applications to the other cancers did not suggest chance of benefit. In the following years this judgment has held firm, although cryosurgery as an adjunct to surgical excision has been useful in reducing the recurrence rate of malignant epithelial tumors of the conjunctiva.[97] Cryoassisted excision has been useful in the management of orbital tumors.[98,99] A cryoextraction technique for the extraction of cavernous hemangiomas anywhere in the orbit has been reported to be beneficial.[100]

Experience has shown that cryosurgery has merit in the treatment of retinoblastoma, the most common primary tumor of the eye in children. Enucleation of the eye has been the standard treatment, but often the disease is bilateral, and that encourages efforts to save at least one eye. In recent years alternative treatments, such as radiotherapy, photocoagulation, and cryosurgery, have become useful in therapy. Shields and his associates[101] have defined the indication for cryosurgery as being a tumor confined to the sensory retina (without evidence of vitreous seeding), less than 3.5 mm in diameter and less than 3.0 mm thick.[101] Tumors located anterior to the equator are easier to treat than those in the equatorial region and beyond. Treatment is given with a cryoprobe cooled by nitrous oxide. The tumor's small size requires only brief freezing (10 to 15 s) and repeated freeze-thaw cycles are used. Effective treatment results in a flat demarcated scar with variable pigmentation. Shields and his associates[101] reported successful treatment of 53 of 67 tumors (79%) and consider cryosurgery to be an effective method of management of selected retinoblastomas.

## BRAIN TUMORS

Tumors of the brain are commonly treated by surgical excision, radiotherapy, or chemotherapy. In the problem cases, cryosurgery has had a limited trial. Early in the modern era of cryosurgery, Cooper and Stellar[81] reported on the cryosurgical treatment of 12 patients with inoperable brain tumors of diverse types. They emphasized freezing the tumor and excision while still frozen (cryoassisted excision), but in some cases, the tumor was frozen and left in situ. Rand[102] described two patients in whom complete surgical excision of brain tumors was not possible, but destruction was successfully completed by freezing the remaining tumor in situ and long-term survival was achieved. Nevertheless, little progress in cryosurgery for brain tumors was possible because the neuroimaging techniques were not sufficiently developed to permit accurate localization of intracranial lesions.

Taking advantage of advances in stereotactic and imaging techniques in recent years, Maroon and his associates[103] reported on the cryosurgical treatment of 71 patients with diverse types of tumors of the brain, spinal cord, and orbit. Cryosurgery was used to facilitate surgical excision in 64 patients and was used to destroy residual tumor after incomplete excision in 7 patients. The cryoassisted excision facilitated the operation. The cryoablation procedures were successful, at least as far as freedom from complications was concerned. Judging from this and several other reports, cryoassisted extraction of tumors of the orbit, spinal cord, and brain is an effective adjunctive technique.[98–100,104] Other than the cryoassist technique, the long-term value of cryosurgery for brain tumors remains to be determined. However, cryoablation in situ with stereotactic placement of the probes merits trial use for tumors in surgically inaccessible sites and for selected cases of disease that recurs after excision.

## ORAL CANCER

Cancers of the oral cavity are treated by excision or radiotherapy, often with adjunctive chemotherapy. Nevertheless, selected cancers may be considered for cryosurgery. Lesions of the oral cavity are well suited to cryosurgical treatment because of ease of access, low operative risk, and the possibility of close observation in the postoperative period. Follow-up by biopsy is easily performed, and treatment may be repeated whenever necessary to control the disease. In addition, cryosurgery offers the advantage of conservation of bone of the oral cavity and permits avoidance of bone-sacrificing operations and their attendant sequelae. Cryosurgery has been used as primary treatment of oral cancer, for the treatment of residual disease, and for the palliation of advanced disease.

### SELECTION CRITERIA

**PRIMARY TREATMENT BY CRYOSURGERY.** The selection of cryosurgery as the primary treatment may be considered when the cancer is small to moderate in size and no cervical lymphadenopathy is present (T1-2 N0 M0). In addition the patient should be at high surgical risk because of extensive cardiopulmonary disease or blood coagulopathy. Cryosurgery is especially suited for cancers overlying bone because the bone limits the depth of the tumor. In my opinion, when the above-cited factors in selection are present and when the cancer is adjacent to bone so that excision would require removal of a portion of the mandible or palate, cryosurgery is a good choice.

The choice of cryosurgery as a primary method of treating oral cancer requires some thought on the management of the cervical lymph nodes. If the cervical lymph nodes are not enlarged, in high-surgical-risk patients, consideration should be given to the use of radiotherapy to the cervical lymph nodes after cryosurgery has established control of the primary lesion. When the cervical lymph nodes are already enlarged when first seen, cryosurgery may be given to the primary lesion, followed by radical lymph node dissection about a month later. This later major surgery negates some of the advantages of cryosurgery because of the need for general anesthesia and its attendant risk.

**TREATMENT OF RESIDUAL CANCER.** Often after surgical excision or radiotherapy, disease persists. Usually further surgical excision is not possible and additional radiotherapy may not be tolerable. In some patients, only a small amount of cancer is obvious. For such patients, in the absence of metastases, cryosurgery may be able to destroy the remaining local cancer. Since pain is often present, even if cure is not achieved, pain relief is a probable benefit.

**PALLIATION OF ADVANCED ORAL CANCER.** Pain, bleeding, and difficulty in mastication and deglutition are common symptoms of advanced oral cancer. Reduction in the bulk of the tumor and desensitization of nerves by cryosurgery offers a good chance for palliation of the symptoms. The patients selected for cryosurgery should be those in whom the disease is still localized, though bulky, and preferably in the anterior part of the oral cavity. Large bulky cancers in the posterior part of the oral cavity are not good choices for cryosurgery. Although reduction in tumor bulk can be achieved, the threat to the airway will necessitate a tracheostomy, and the presence of large necrotic masses will interfere with food intake. Radiotherapy is a better choice in most circumstances.

### TECHNIQUE

The cryosurgical treatment is given in the clinic or hospital operating room, using sterile equipment and technique. In selected patients, local anesthesia or field block anesthesia can be used, but commonly, general anesthesia is advisable to ensure the comfort of the patient during manipulation. Cryosurgical equipment cooled by liquid nitrogen is required. To measure tissue temperature during freezing, needle-mounted thermocouples are placed in the normal tissue at the periphery of the tumor about 1 cm from its border.

Surface contact freezing is almost always used in the oral cancer. To ensure efficient heat transfer, maintenance of good contact between the cryoprobe and the tumor is facilitated by using water-soluble hospital lubricating jelly between the probe and the tumor. Occasionally, when the tumor is soft and bulky, insertion of the probe into the tumor promotes faster and deeper freezing. Each freezing site requires about 5 to 7 min in the first freeze-thaw cycle, depending upon the size of the tumor. Cancer larger than 3 cm in diameter will require several freezing sites, overlapping the frozen areas. After thawing, the freezing is repeated so that completion of treatment commonly requires 30 to 40 min. The freezing should be given without regard to damage to teeth or to bone because the primary obligation is to cure the cancer.

In cryosurgery for palliation, commonly a large mass of tissue must be frozen. Since cure is not the goal, the freezing can be confined to the tumor and not extended into normal tissue. Clinical observation of the extent of freezing is sufficient to guide the treatment. Surface contact freezing is most often used, although occasionally penetration of the tumor to achieve greater depth is necessary, especially if pain is a dominant symptom or if the tumor is bulky. Large tumors commonly require the application of the probe to multiple sites. Cryosurgical treatment may be repeated as often as necessary to maintain control of tumor growth.

## POSTOPERATIVE CARE

The edema that follows thawing and the later necrosis of the tissue establish the requirements of postoperative care. Small tumors, especially on the buccal mucosa, palate, or anterior floor of the mouth, generally require little care except mouthwashes and analgesics. However, when large volumes of tissue are frozen, interference with speech, mastication, and swallowing may result and cause troublesome problems in care. The edema that follows the freezing of tongue cancer can be substantial. Freezing of tumors in the posterior third of the tongue results in edema that can threaten the airway.

In about a week, when the necrotic tissue begins to slough, there is some chance of bleeding, commonly not serious, which may require control by suture or electrocoagulation. The wound usually has a clean granulating base in about 3 weeks and then should be inspected carefully for persistent disease. At this time, tissue that is suspected of being persistent tumor should be biopsied. If tumor is still present, cryosurgery should be repeated or a choice of alternate therapy should be made. Careful follow-up is necessary in order to detect recurrence at the earliest possible time.

The extent of freezing required by many oral cancers causes extensive soft tissue loss and prolonged healing. If bone is exposed as a result of soft tissue loss, final healing may take many months. Bone that has been devitalized in the course of treatment will require months for complete healing. Sequestration of bone has occurred and probably is most likely to occur if the bone has been damaged by previous radiotherapy. This bone loss has been minor, so the use of cryosurgery should not be avoided because of this occasional complication.

## RESULTS

Cryosurgery has not been widely used for the primary treatment of oral cancer. No controlled comparative studies have been performed, but the results of treatment of carefully selected patients provide some understanding of the potential of the technique. The results of cryosurgery, using selection criteria defined earlier, are demonstrated in a series of 82 patients treated in the years 1964 to 1975.[105,106] The 5-year survival rate was 83% (25 of 30 patients) in stage 1 disease. None of the deaths in this group were from cancer. In stage 2 disease, the 5-year survival rate was 50% (18 of 36 patients), but the common cause of death was associated disease. The survival rate was better in patients in whom the cancer was overlying bone because the underlying bone limited the depth of penetration of the cancer, creating a clinical situation favorable for cryosurgery. Less favorable results were achieved in the posterior one-third of the oral cavity where earlier metastatic spread was possible. The results in

advanced cancers, that is, those in the third and fourth stages of the disease, were poor and, therefore, it is best not to use cryosurgery for such patients. The results showed that cryosurgery was most effective in small to moderate-sized cancers in patients without cervical lymphadenopathy. The method was suited to high-surgical-risk patients and the technique permitted avoidance of bone-sacrificing operations.

The experience of other physicians has been similar. Weaver and Smith,[107] treating a series of 50 patients with oral cancer, achieved local control of the cancer for more that 2 years in 90% of patients.[107] In a later report, they concluded that cryosurgery was effective for small cancers and not very satisfactory for large invasive ones. They also concluded that cryosurgery was useful in patients with associated diseases causing high risk for surgery and that the possibility of preserving the mandible or maxilla was a principal benefit of cryosurgery.[108] The same conclusion, that cryosurgery is best suited for small oral cancers that are not good candidates for conventional treatment, was reached by other physicians.[109–111]

The use of cryosurgery in tongue cancer, a site which is easily accessible, was reported by Wang and by Li. Wang[112] described the cryosurgical treatment of 80 patients with tongue carcinoma in diverse stages of disease but principally early lesions. In the follow-up period of 6 months to 7 years, the early control rate of the primary lesion was 95%, but the recurrence rate was 11% and 18 patients died with cervical lymph node metastases that appeared after cryosurgery. Of 32 patients followed more than 3 years, the survival rate was 72%. The experience of Li,[113] who described the cryosurgical treatment of 50 patients followed for 3 to 10 years, is similar. These reports endorsed the use of cryosurgery for tongue cancer, but also pointed out the need to plan treatment for the regional lymph nodes.

Several reports have described the treatment of new and recurrent oral cancers by combining cryosurgery with radiotherapy and chemotherapy and have achieved good results in some cases.[110,114,115] In these reports, the degree of benefit is difficult to evaluate because of the diversity of treatment. Nevertheless, reports that focus on the use of cryosurgery as a method of treating recurrent oral cancer when all else has failed have achieved a measure of success as was evidenced by long-term survival without evidence of cancer.[114,116,117]

The results of the treatment of incurable cancer for palliation of symptoms are sometimes good, often not. Tumor bulk reduction is easy to achieve. Benefit from reduction in tumor bulk is most obvious in the anterior part of the oral cavity where the ability to eat, swallow, and talk may be restored. Benefits in the posterior part of the oral cavity are more difficult to provide because the production of a mass of necrotic tissue in this area causes problems with the airway from edema and later from the slough of necrotic tissue. Relief of pain is sometimes substantial, more commonly incomplete, and occasionally not successful.

Although cryosurgery seems well suited for selected patients with oral cancer, currently the technique is used by only a few physicians, usually for advanced disease in conjunction with chemotherapy or radiotherapy. Little interest has been shown in the application to early stages of the disease. However, the advances in cryosurgical equipment and imaging techniques encourage new trials of the technique.

## CANCER OF THE PHARYNX

Pharyngeal cancers readily infiltrate the adjacent tissues and are not easily treated by surgical techniques. Experience with cryosurgery in this area is small. The use of cryosurgery has been limited to the palliation of disease and generally radiotherapy or chemotherapy have been combined with cryosurgery. The most favorable area in the pharynx for attempted salvage is the tonsillar area, but the freezing of bulky tumors anywhere in the pharynx is associated with postoperative edema and a threat to the airway. In general, radiotherapy and chemotherapy are better choices than cryosurgery. Combined therapy has been reported for carcinoma of the nasopharynx with a favorable short-term follow-up.[118] In this work the cryosurgery was considered helpful in eliminating the bulk of the tumor at the original site, and the physicians also believed that the cryosurgery increased the effectiveness of the radiotherapy given 2 weeks later.

## CANCER OF THE LARYNX

Cancer of the larynx is best treated by surgical excision or radiotherapy. Cryosurgery has practically no applicability to early cancer because of the difficulty in defining the extent of the disease and the consequences of edema and sloughing necrotic tissue in this area. Cryosurgery may provide palliation of symptoms of advanced laryngeal cancer, relieving obstruction by control of tumor growth. However, other techniques, including laser therapy, are better in most cases.

## TRACHEOBRONCHIAL TUMORS

Advanced bronchial tumors threaten life by airway obstruction, hemorrhage, and infection. Endobronchial therapy can palliate symptoms, may prolong life, and in a few patients provide time for preparation of definitive therapy. The options in palliative endobronchial therapy are multiple, which suggests that no one therapy fits all clinical circumstances.[119,120] Cryosurgery is one option in clinical use. Interest in the cryosurgical treatment of tracheobronchial tumors developed in the 1970s and slowly evolved into an effective technique in a few medical centers. Although some clinical trials are in progress on the cryosurgical treatment of microinvasive bronchial cancer, the major clinical experience has been for the relief of obstructions of the trachea and bronchi due to inoperable cancer.

### TECHNIQUE

Treatment is given via endoscopy, using either rigid or fiberoptic bronchoscopes to visualize the tumor. Rigid, semirigid, and flexible probes are available, but the greatest experience is with rigid probes. Flexible probes are not yet well developed. A suction catheter is needed to clear the bronchus of secretions before freezing the tumor and to clear the area of frozen water vapor during freezing of the tumor, thus promoting good visualization. The most commonly used cryogen for endoscopic therapy has been nitrous oxide, which is adequate for palliative purposes. The use of a probe cooled by liquid nitrogen provides greater freezing capability. The treatment is given under general anesthesia with appropriate monitoring of cardiac function and oxygen saturation. A cryosurgical probe is passed through the bronchoscope and is applied to the neoplasm with firm pressure. The probe is then cooled until an appropriate amount of tissue freezing has been accomplished.

Homasson[121] uses an impedance-measuring device to supplement clinical judgment about the extent of freezing. Maiwand[122] has used thermocouple needles to record temperature during treatment. Knowledge of the performance of the probe, that is, the volume of tissue frozen in a given time, is important in this area where visualization of freezing is not easy. After freezing to an appropriate extent, the probe is allowed to thaw completely and then the lesion is refrozen. Large lesions require application of the probe to multiple sites. For continued control of tumor growth, the treatment must be repeated as needed at intervals of several months.

### RESULTS

Extensive experience with this technique has been reported by Maiwand and Homasson,[122] who achieved benefits in about 70% of a large number of patients with inoperable tracheobronchial cancer. The noteworthy benefits included relief of dyspnea, cough, stridor, and hemoptysis. Pulmonary function tests were improved in 30% to 40% of patients. The elimination of the airway obstruction by cryosurgery avoided local complications, improved survival, and permitted safer and more effective radiotherapy. Similar beneficial results have been reported by others.[123–125]

In comparison with other therapies, laser therapy is a principal competitor of cryotherapy. Laser is faster in removing obstructing tissue, but it is best at removing protruding tumors. Cryosurgery has much the same capability of providing relief of obstruction, although the effect is slower, so that 7 to 10 days is required for the necrotic tissue to clear the bronchus. As an advantage, cryosurgery penetrates the tissue at an easily controllable rate and produces a depth of necrosis that can destroy infiltrating cancer. A disadvantage of cryosurgery is the present-day need for use of the rigid cryoprobe in most cases. The further development of flexible cryoprobes, useful via fiberoptic bronchoscopy, will increase the applicability of cryosurgery to bronchial disease, including benign tumors, dysplastic disease, and advanced cancer.

## TUMORS OF THE LIVER

Primary tumors and metastatic cancers of the liver are best managed by excision, which offers the chance of longer survival and possibly cure. Primary liver cancer, uncommon in the United States in comparison to the incidence in Asia, can be resected in only about 20% of patients, yielding long-term survival in about 20% of those resected. The outlook for cancer metastatic to the liver is only slightly better. When the liver is the sole site of metastasis, about 20% of patients can be considered for partial hepatic resection, and the long-term survival in this select group of patients treated by surgical excision is about 25%.[126] The large majority of cancers of the liver, whether primary or secondary to cancer originating elsewhere, are not suitable for surgical excision. One reason for this is related to location of the tumor, perhaps in more than one lobe (multiple lesions) or in such close proximity to a major vascular structure that excision has a high risk. Another reason is the coexistence of other disease, such as cirrhosis or severe associated disease in other organs, which increases the risk of excisional surgery. These are the candidates for other methods of therapy, including cryosurgery.

Cryosurgery of liver tumors, based on extensive experimental work, has been used in occasional clinical cases for many years, but its development in past years was hindered by the inability to detect disease deep in the liver. Greater clinical interest followed the report of Onik and his associates[127,128] in 1984 on the feasibility of monitoring the tissue-freezing process by sonography and the demonstration of clinical applicability. Since then, cryosurgery has come into increasing use for the treatment of tumors of the liver.

## SELECTION CRITERIA

Cryosurgery is used for liver tumors in several clinical circumstances. Commonly the technique has been used for those patients considered to have unresectable tumors because of multiple lesions, perhaps in several segments, and perhaps in close proximity to major blood vessels. Cryosurgery has also been used for patients in whom surgical excision has transected the tumor, leaving disease in the wound margin. Less commonly, cryosurgery has been used for the treatment of liver tumors, ordinarily resectable, in patients with severe associated disease, such as cirrhosis, which increased surgical risk. Careful preoperative evaluation, including the extent of disease as shown by imaging techniques, is required to demonstrate freedom from extrahepatic cancer and the suitability of the patient for hepatic surgery. A decision to choose cryosurgical treatment can be made at this time, but often cryosurgery is chosen as part of the management because the extent of disease is evaluated early in the operation.

## TECHNIQUE

Cryosurgery has most commonly been performed via laparotomy, using a right subcostal incision that can be extended as needed. Recently, some cryosurgical operations have been done via laparoscopy, a technique that is attractive for the high-surgical-risk patient.[129] Whether or not effective treatment is compromised by the percutaneous approach remains to be determined. With either technique, accurate determination of the location of the tumors is necessary. The patient is prepared in a manner appropriate for major hepatic surgery. To maintain body temperature during the procedure, the patient should be placed on a warming blanket. After anesthesia is produced, the liver is exposed by laparotomy and the extent of the disease is evaluated. After mobilization of the liver, it is examined manually and by the use of several linear-array (5.0- to 7.5-MHz) ultrasound probes.[130] The size, number, and location of the hepatic lesions are evaluated in relation to choice of excision or cryosurgery,

or perhaps to determine that nothing can be done. Extrahepatic disease eliminates any consideration of curative surgery.

Most single lesions will be excised if possible. If not possible, cryosurgery may be considered. Commonly excisional surgery is combined with cryosurgery, that is, the tumors in favorable areas are excised and the tumors in less accessible areas are frozen. Those lesions that have been considered unsuitable for surgical resection generally are located near large blood vessels or in multiple lobes, or severe associated disease may coexist. In high-surgical-risk patients, cryoablation may be chosen for all of the lesions in preference to excision. In considering cryosurgery, most surgeons will limit the number of tumors to a maximum of 6 and will limit the size of a lesion to a maximum of about 8 cm. However, no absolute limitation has been established. Many surgeons will set smaller number and size limits. Some surgeons have frozen numbers and sizes of lesions greater than the figures just cited.[131,132] The diversity of opinion about size, number, and location of lesions in relation to suitability for cryoablation will be resolved somewhat as experience increases. Many surgeons are wary of treating tumors in close proximity to major blood vessels (inferior vena cava, portal vein) or to major bile ducts.

Tumors on the surface of the liver are treated by application of a large flat probe, so that penetration of the liver does not occur. This has the advantage of avoiding a wound that may bleed but is associated with cracking or fissuring of the liver surface during freezing, which becomes obvious in the thawing period, and bleeding may be troublesome. The large flat probe is also useful for the treatment of the surface of the wound in the liver when the surgical margins after excision still contain cancer cells and further excision is not practical. Freezing the wound to an appropriate depth, perhaps 2 cm may improve the chance of cure.

Deep lesions require the insertion of the cryoprobe into the tumor. The size of probe and the number of probes depends on the size of the tumor. A tumor about 2 cm in diameter can be treated by a single 3-mm probe. A tumor about 4 cm in diameter can be treated with a single 8-mm probe. Large tumors, that is, those 5 cm or greater in diameter, will require the use of more than one probe for effective freezing, and these probes should be spaced in a manner that will ensure freezing to encompass the entire lesion and an appropriate volume of adjacent normal liver. Multiple lesions may be treated simultaneously, although care must be taken not to compromise the monitoring by ultrasound.

The probes may be placed directly into the tumor under ultrasound guidance, a technique that is practical, especially for lesions placed anteriorly. However, the preferred technique is placement of the probe into the tumor by a Seldinger-type technique involving the insertion of a needle into the tumor under ultrasound guidance, followed by a J guide wire, and a dilator and sheath in sequence. Care should be taken to avoid injury to major blood vessels and bile ducts. Once in place, the guide wire and dilator are withdrawn, leaving the sheath in place. The probe is inserted via the sheath, which is then withdrawn sufficiently to expose the freezing surface of the probe. The probe is placed in a position to form a frozen volume encompassing the tumor and a margin (1 cm) of apparently normal tissue. When the probe is properly positioned and fixed in place by cooling, the freezing cycle is initiated by cooling the probe rapidly to about −190°C. As the tissue freezes and the process is monitored by ultrasound from several perspectives, the advancing frozen border is seen as a hyperechoic zone with complete acoustic shadowing. The frozen tissue is hypoechoic. To achieve a lethal temperature within the tumor and a margin of adjacent normal tissue, the ultrasound image of frozen tissue must extend more than 1 cm beyond the tumor. For any one probe, depending upon the size of the tumor, the freezing period is commonly about 15 min. If the tumor cannot be frozen in that time, usually the probe should be thawed for placement in a new site or multiple probes should be used.

The tissue is allowed to thaw, which requires at least as much time as the freezing cycle. A common practice is to allow only enough time for the border to thaw, which may be as short as 10 min, which prevents dislodgement of the still-frozen probe. After partial thaw, the entire freeze-thaw cycle is repeated. As tissue thaws, bleeding, often due to blood vessel injury by the penetration of the probe into the liver, must be controlled. The identification of major blood vessels by sonography during probe placement helps to avoid vascular injury and major bleeding. Troublesome bleeding can also result from the fissuring of the frozen area due to thermal stress. Control of bleeding is obtained by the insertion of a hemostatic agent, such as Gelfoam (Upjohn) or Surgicel (Johnson & Johnson) into the probe tract and by sutures placed across bleeding tissues. After hemostasis is obtained, the wound is closed.

The close proximity of major blood vessels and large bile ducts to hepatic lesions is a concern. Experiments have shown that the large arteries and veins may be included in the frozen mass without later loss of function. Usually, because the flowing blood is a heat sink, the entire blood vessel does not freeze. Even if blood flow is shut off and the vessel freezes, no permanent damage to the blood vessel results. Nevertheless, in clinical practice, tumors next to major vessels are approached with a measure of caution. To ensure cell death in tumors adjacent to major vessels, the blood flow to the liver can be occluded temporarily during freezing. No ill effects, such as late hemorrhage, have been reported in the cases in which this has been done. On the other hand, the major bile ducts are susceptible to freezing injury, which takes the form of stricture formation as the injury heals.[133] In the freezing of tumors in close proximity to major bile ducts, a measure of protection can be provided by perfusion of the duct with warm normal saline.[134]

Although complete thawing of the frozen tissue between the two freezing cycles is more destructive and should be standard technique for cancer therapy, it commonly is not used in hepatic cryosurgery. The greater destructive effect of complete thawing before repetition of the freezing cycle increases the severity of the coagulopathy and the possibility of postoperative complications.[131,135–137] Therefore many surgeons allow only a partial thawing.

## POSTOPERATIVE CARE

The basic features of patient care in the postoperative period are the same as those provided after any major abdominal operation. The major risks are related to disturbances in blood coagulation and kidney function. Coagulopathy requires the administration of the appropriate blood products. The prevention of renal failure requires the administration of mannitol, low-dose dopamine to produce a high output of urine, and sodium bicarbonate to alkalinize the urine during and after the operation.

Postoperative complications occur in 5% to 10% of patients. The postoperative complications are those associated with any intra-abdominal operation and those characteristic of cryosurgery, which includes a group of special problems. Right pleural effusion, occasionally requiring thoracentesis, is common. Elevations of results of liver function tests are transient. Platelet counts are depressed and coagulation is prolonged in proportion to the volume of liver frozen. The activated partial thromboplastin time and the prothrombin time are prolonged. In general the postoperative mortality has been low, but the rate has ranged from 0% to 4%. Deaths have been related to severe coagulopathy, perhaps with intraabdominal bleeding, and multisystem organ failure. Bile duct injuries have occurred and myoglobinuria has been reported.[131,137]

## RESULTS

Serial determinations of tumor markers, such as carcinoembryonic antigen (CEA) level and contrast-enhanced CT scans are performed in the months after operation. With successful treatment, the CEA reading falls to a normal level. Rising levels indicate that disease is still present.[138] The CT scans after cryosurgery commonly show a well-defined area of necrosis, manifested by an image of lower attenuation than the normal liver.[139–142] The image of the treated area should be larger than the original lesion and should include the tumor within its volume (Fig. 5C-6). Gas bubbles are often seen in the cryolesions, but generally these disappear in several weeks. An increase in the number and size of gas bubbles suggests the development of an abscess, but this is not a common occurrence. If the tumor was treated successfully, the image slowly shrinks as healing progresses. The image on CT persists for several months, the duration dependent upon the volume of liver frozen. Small cryogenic lesions may disappear. If the image enlarges, concern about residual cancer should lead to a biopsy.

The results of cryosurgery, as detailed in several reports, indicate a generally favorable experience, whether used for primary or metastatic tumors or only to assist resection. In the treatment of primary liver cancer, the long experience of Zhou and his associates[143] in Shanghai, China, has been noteworthy. They used cryosurgery for patients with severe liver cirrhosis in whom resection was contraindicated, for patients with residual tumor when the resection was incomplete, and for patients with recurrent tumor after major hepatic resection. No operative mortality or severe complications occurred. They reported a 5-year survival rate of 22% in a series of 107 patients and consider cryosurgery to be safe and effective therapy for unresectable hepatic cancer. Evaluation by others in a small number of patients has led to a similar conclusion.[144]

In the treatment of cancer metastatic to the liver, the recent reports are beginning to provide survival data. Ravikumar and his associates[145] in 1994 described 21 patients with liver cancer (17 with colorectal metastatic cancer) treated by cryosurgery. At a median follow-up period of 16 months, 24% were apparently disease-free. The rate of recurrence at the operative site was about 10%.[145] Shafir and his associates[132] reported the cryoablation of diverse types of liver cancers in 39 patients. In a mean follow-up of 14 months, 65% of the patients were alive and 51% were apparently free of the disease. In a series of 47 patients with metastatic colorectal

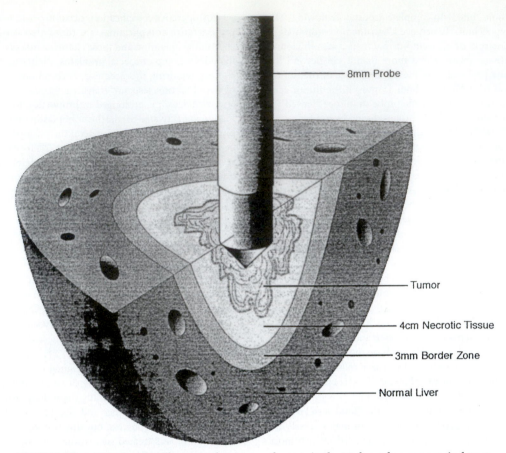

8mm Probe

Tumor

4cm Necrotic Tissue

3mm Border Zone

Normal Liver

**FIGURE 5C-6.** This drawing illustrates the course of events in the 10 days after cryosurgical treatment of a liver tumor that was about 2 cm in diameter. The devitalized tumor is at the center of the necrotic tissue, which is about 4 cm in diameter. The cryosurgery produced the required 1-cm margin of destruction around the tumor. The border zone, which is 3 mm wide, was at the periphery of the previously frozen tissue where the tissue temperature was in the 0°C to −20°C range. In this zone of partial destruction, wound healing begins.

cancer to the liver treated by cryoablation, performing excision also in some cases, Weaver and his colleagues[131] reported a 2-year survival rate of 62%. Preketes and his associates[146] achieved increased survival in patients with liver metastases from colorectal cancer treated with cryosurgery when adjunctive chemotherapy was given via the hepatic artery. However, more commonly the drug has been given systemically via a peripheral vein. Since cryosurgery is a local treatment only, adjunctive chemotherapy seems warranted, but the choice of drug and the method of delivery is an unsettled question.[129]

Recent reports stress the safety of hepatic cryosurgery, the value of tumor marker levels in follow-up, the favorable influence on short-term survival, and the need for longer follow-up to better define the value of the therapy.[130,147–149] Short-term results of cryosurgery suggest that about 25% of patients will benefit, at least to the point of increased survival. When one considers the fact that the patients selected for cryosurgery are those who are considered to be inoperable or unsuited for excisional surgery, this increased survival and

perhaps a chance of cure is a good result. In comparison with excision, no controlled studies have been done, but Steele[150] reported that survival in his 70 patients following cryosurgery equaled that achieved by surgical resection in the Gastrointestinal Tumor Group series and that the major advantages of cryoablation were conservation of liver tissue and lessened morbidity.

Cryosurgery for liver tumors, including indications for its use and the technique, is still in evaluation. The results to date suggest that cryosurgery will be complementary to surgical excision of selected primary and secondary tumors of the liver. Cryosurgery extends the curative potential of excisional surgery in tumors of the liver and will have value in the treatment of some unresectable tumors, especially those with metastases in several lobes or those that occur in patients with severe associated disease and resultant high surgical risk. Cryoablation will also prove useful in the management of other difficult problems in the therapy of metastatic cancer in the liver, including the palliative care of patients with metastatic functioning neuroendocrine tumors.

## CANCER OF THE PANCREAS

Cryosurgery has no place in the treatment of pancreatic tumors at this time but some interest has been shown in developing a technique for this purpose, a possibility that is supported by experimental work with animals. Limited pancreatic freezing has been done in animals without mortality. The effect on the pancreas featured an inflammatory response, including a sharp rise in serum pancreatic enzyme levels for several days, followed by progressive changes ending in complete destruction of the normal architecture and healing with fibrous tissue formation.[151–154] Freezing the major blood vessels in the region of the pancreas has been well tolerated. More serious consequences from pancreatic freezing were seen in the experiments of McIntosh and his associates,[155] who, freezing 50% of the pancreas in dogs, caused acute hemorrhagic pancreatitis in all animals with a 38% mortality rate. None of the surviving animals developed pancreatic functional insufficiency. These experiments suggested that cryosurgical techniques may be applicable to pancreatic cancer.

### SELECTION CRITERIA

Cryosurgery has been used for a few selected patients with incurable cancer for palliation of symptoms, principally pain. Application for the cure of pancreatic cancer is unlikely; potentially curable cancers are treated by excision. However, cryosurgery may be useful for the treatment of multicentric functioning islet-cell pancreatic tumors.

### TECHNIQUE

Selected cases of pancreatic cancer have been treated by a minimal operation, that is, application of the cryoprobe to lesions of the body and tail of the pancreas without establishing any bypasses. Freezing cancer of the head of the pancreas is more complex and may require biliary and intestinal bypasses similar to those constructed in excisional surgery. However, the use of bypasses only to facilitate cryosurgery takes the scope of the operation beyond that justifiable for palliative purposes.

The technique requires either application of the probe to the surface of the tumor or penetration of the tumor from the surface of the gland by several small probes. In the treatment of tumors of the head of the pancreas, intraduodenal irrigation with warm saline and appropriate placement of needle-mounted thermocouples will help prevent duodenal injury. Freezing of the pancreatic duct will be associated with stricture formation, but generally the duct is already obstructed by the cancer. The freezing of the celiac plexus of nerves should improve the chance of palliation of pain.

### RESULTS

Some surgeons have used or are considering the use of cryosurgery for pancreatic cancer, but few reports have yet been made of these trials. In Russia, Patiutko and associates[156] in 1991 described the cryosurgical treatment and adjunctive radiotherapy in 30 patients with locally advanced pancreatic cancer. Relief of pain, improved health, and increased survival were reported. Pertinent also is the point that cryosurgery has been used for the relief of pain due to chronic pancreatitis. In Russia, Komkova has reported good results in 28 of 32 patients.[157,158] Nevertheless, given the paucity of experience with pancreatic cancer, the place for cryosurgery is uncertain.

## CANCER OF THE RECTUM

Cancer of the rectum is best treated by excision. Nevertheless, cryosurgery has been used for the treatment of localized rectal cancer that is possibly curable and for the palliative treatment of incurable cancer.

### SELECTION CRITERIA

When used for small cancers that are localized and are possibly curable, the selection of patients is based on indications that are similar to those used for conservative local excision or destruction by electrocoagulation. The appropriate patients are those of high surgical risk because of associated disease. The appropriate lesion is a cancer within reach of the examining finger and on the posterior or lateral walls of the rectum. Superficial or polypoid tumors, well-differentiated lesions 10 cm or less from the anal verge and about 3 to 4 cm in surface diameter, are well suited to cryosurgery. The incidence of regional lymph node involvement in such cases is about 10%. Rectal ultrasound or other imaging techniques may prove useful in evaluating the size and depth of the primary lesion. Cancers on the anterior wall are not appropriate for cryosurgery because of the risk of fistula formation.

When used for the palliative treatment of advanced rectal cancer that is incurable because of extent of disease, cryosurgery may be chosen to relieve distressing symptoms, such as obstruction, tenesmus, and bleeding. The selection of patients is based on the presence of these symptoms, a problem in management for any therapeutic method. Some patients have previously untreated disease, whereas others have had previous resection and other therapy.

### TECHNIQUE

Cryosurgical treatment of rectal cancer is commonly an outpatient or day hospital procedure. Those patients who are ill because of bowel obstruction, bleeding, or other serious problems must be hospitalized for general care and preparation for the procedure. Commonly no anesthesia is needed, especially for palliative treatment. However, a minority of patients, especially those who have lesions at the dentate line, who have low discomfort thresholds, or who cannot cooperate during therapy, require general or spinal anesthesia. The preoperative preparation is principally bowel cleansing. Depending upon the location of the tumor, the patient is placed in the lithotomy or Sims position.

For the small lesions in the rectum, the probe is applied to the tumor under direct vision through a large proctoscope. Repeated freeze-thaw cycles, using a large cryosurgical probe cooled by liquid nitrogen, are used. Commonly about 30 to 40 min is needed for the treatment. Monitoring the treatment with ultrasound or with thermocouples placed at the base of the cancer is possible, but more important is control of the treatment by clinical judgment of the extent of the cancer and knowledge about the probe performance in terms of how much tissue will be frozen in a given time. The frozen mass of low-lying lesions can be evaluated by palpation.

Treatment for palliation is given by the same technique but with different goals. The common objectives are the relief of obstruction, thus avoiding a colostomy, or relief of tenesmus or bleeding. The tumor is commonly bulky and often the residual lumen is small. Usually the probe can be inserted easily into the tumor for more effective freezing. Low-lying tumor is treated via proctoscopy. A sigmoidoscope can be used to treat tumor at the rectosigmoid junction, but the risk of perforation into the peritoneal cavity is high when the necrotic tumor sloughs.

The cryosurgical treatment of those patients who have recurrence of cancer in the perineum after abdominoperineal resection is easy because the cancer is on the external surface. Such lesions extend deep into the pelvis, so cure is not possible and even pain relief is difficult. Often little or no anesthesia is needed. Freezing must be extensive and repeated at intervals of about a month, depending on the rapidity of growth and on the need to relieve discomfort. With repeated treatments, a large wound eventually develops, but it is ordinarily free of discomfort.

## POSTOPERATIVE CARE AND COMPLICATIONS

Postoperative care is minimal. The necrotic tumor will slough quickly into the bowel lumen. Special requirements in care relate principally to the correction of the effects of obstruction or bleeding that preceded cryosurgery. The incidence of postoperative complications following rectal cryosurgery is about 10% and these chiefly consist of hemorrhage, strictures, and fistulas. These complications are more commonly associated with the freezing of large volumes of tissue. The bleeding is associated with the slough of necrotic tissue and usually is controlled easily. Strictures may follow circumferential freezing and fistulas may be associated with freezing above the peritoneal reflection.

## RESULTS

Biggers and co-workers[159] reported on the treatment by diverse local techniques in 282 patients with carcinoma of the rectum within 12 cm of the dentate line. Selected patients, those with well-differentiated lesions, particularly those less than 3 cm in diameter, were managed by local treatment, which frequently can be curative. In their series, local excision was commonly used, but 46 patients had tumor destruction by other methods, including cryosurgery, fulguration, and laser. No clear difference in survival was noted in the patients treated by these diverse techniques.

Heberer and his associates[160] reported on the use of cryosurgery for local palliation in 268 patients with rectal cancer. Colostomy was avoided in 80% of the patients. The results were best in patients with cancers no greater than 3 cm in diameter. In this small select group, 77% had no evidence of disease later and the complication rate was low. For this group of patients, the success rate was considered comparable to other methods of therapy such as local excision or electrocoagulation. In the large series of inoperable cancers reported by Geissler and his associates,[161] cryosurgery was considered a worthwhile method of maintenance of the lumen of the rectum. Of 213 patients, only 23 required a later colostomy for obstruction. Similar benefits were described by Orth and his co-workers.[162] Substantial reduction in the size of the tumor or complete destruction of the tumor were produced in 70% of patients.

## COMPARISON WITH OTHER THERAPY

Small well-differentiated cancers in the rectum, best treated by local excision, also can be treated effectively by cryosurgery, which is especially suitable for patients with severe associated disease and consequent high risk for surgery. For inoperable cancer, cryosurgery reduces tumor bulk in a safe and effective manner and palliation of distressing symptoms is provided in a high percentage of patients. Obstruction is relieved and colostomy avoided for months. As the tumor regrows, treatment must be repeated at intervals to maintain control. The same palliative benefits can be provided by other methods of therapy. Limited excision is associated with a high morbidity rate and usually is not practical for this type of patient. Electrocoagulation via endoscopy can provide the same benefit as cryosurgery and has been widely used for this purpose.[163] Laser therapy provides quick results and is the preferred treatment of some physicians.[164,165] The slower response to cryosurgery is a factor contributing to its safety.

## CANCER OF THE PROSTATE

For many years, the usual treatment in an attempt to cure carcinoma of the prostate gland has been radical excision or radiotherapy, often combined with hormonal therapy. In recent years, as a result of earlier detection of disease and improved evaluations of the results of standard treatment, differences in opinion have become evident regarding the efficacy of current methods of management and the new options in therapy. Cryosurgical ablation, a technique that had clinical trials and was abandoned in the 1970s, has emerged again in the past 5 years in new clinical trials featuring improved techniques.

## SELECTION CRITERIA

In the course of clinical trial, gaining experience with the techniques, physicians have used cryosurgery to treat all stages of prostatic cancer. Cryosurgery is best chosen for those patients who have early cancer (stages T1 to T2), especially if their general health precludes consideration of excision, but cryosurgery has been used also for extensive local disease (stage T3). Some physicians use cryosurgery only for those patients in whom irradiation has failed to cure the cancer, which often is the case in extensive local disease. Patients with advanced disease (stage T4) may be treated by cryosurgery for local control of cancer and relief of symptoms caused by obstruction, but there is little chance for cure.

## TECHNIQUE

After evaluation of the clinical data and after careful explanation of all of the treatment options, when cryosurgery is chosen, a decision must be made as to whether or not to use androgen ablation therapy to decrease the size of the prostate gland before cryosurgery. Although some difference in opinion exists on the need of shrinking the gland, a small gland is easier to freeze completely than a large gland, so decreasing the size of the prostatic cancer by endocrine management prior to any treatment is reasonable. The preoperative management includes standard bowel-cleansing procedures and prophylactic administration of antibiotics, such as neomycin and erythromycin, on the day before operation and intravenous gentamycin and cefazolin or ampicillin just before operation. Spinal or general anesthesia is used. The necessary manipulations (lithotomy position, draping, cystoscopy, suprapubic tube placement) are done. A urethral warming catheter is placed through the urethra into the bladder to permit the circulation of warm saline (38° to 40°C) to reduce the chance of damage to the urethra and urinary sphincters during freezing of the prostate. The administration of intravenous mannitol will benefit kidney function during and after operation.

The cryoprobes, five or more in number, each about 3 mm in diameter with a freezing surface 4 cm long at the end of the probe, are placed through the skin of the perineum and into the prostate. The placement of the probes in appropriate position, that is, generally two anteriorly, two posterolaterally, and one posteriorly, is performed with ultrasound guidance. After the probes are fixed in place by initial cooling to a moderate degree, deep freezing of the prostate is done. The probes can be cooled individually, in sequence, or simultaneously in any combination so that the frozen volume conforms to the desired shape and extent. Usually the anterior probes are activated first and the two lateral probes are cooled last. This sequence allows for better definition of the freezing action of the individual probes. The process is monitored by a biplane ultrasound device placed in the rectum. Special care is taken to avoid freezing through the rectal wall. After thawing, the freeze-thaw cycle is repeated. Greater detail on the technique of prostatic cryosurgery is available in reports on the subject.[166–168]

Some physicians monitor the cryosurgical procedure with thermocouples as well as ultrasound. The thermocouples are used to monitor the tissue temperatures in critical locations where cancer may persist after freezing, such as the neurovascular bundles and the seminal vesicles. Thermocouples may also be placed in the tissue between the rectum and the prostate to avoid rectal freezing. The measurement of tissue temperature in conjunction with ultrasound monitoring increases the control of prostatic cryosurgery and should improve results.[76,77,169,170]

## POSTOPERATIVE CARE

After operation, the suprapubic tube provides drainage of the bladder and the tube is removed when the postvoid residual volume is less than 100 mL. Oral antibiotics are continued until the suprapubic tube is removed. Hormone-suppressive therapy, if begun before operation, is discontinued. The patient generally leaves the hospital in 48 hours. In the follow-up period, the prostate-specific antigen (PSA) level is determined every 3 months. Multiple prostatic biopsies should be performed yearly, although some physicians will choose to rely on the PSA to determine if and when biopsies should be done.

## RESULTS

The morbidity after prostatic cryosurgery is low. The warming of the urethra during freezing reduced the incidence of urethral slough to less than 5% of patients. Minor complications, such as edema of the scrotum, have been common. The major complications are impotence, urinary incontinence, and urethrorectal fistula. Almost all patients are impotent after prostatic cryosurgery because the neurovascular bundle posterior to the prostate is frozen. The incidence of return of potency varies in different reports, but if the patient was potent before operation, there is a chance of return of potency several months after operation. Incontinence occurs in a small percentage of patients, but develops more commonly in those who had previous radiation therapy.[171] Urethrorectal fistula occurs in about 1% or less of patients. The incidence of urethrocutaneous fistula is slightly higher.

The results of ultrasound-guided prostatic cryosurgery, currently short term in view of the biologic behavior of prostatic cancer, are best evaluated in terms of PSA level and prostatic biopsies. The PSA reading should remain at low levels (0.4 ng/mL or less, preferably undetectable); this is an indication of successful cryoablation. A later rise in the PSA is a signal that the cancer persists and is progressing.[172] In the report of Cohen and his associates,[173] the positive biopsy rate was 18.1% (21 of 116 patients in all stages of disease, including those who received androgen deprivation therapy) 2 years after cryosurgery.[173] In previously untreated patients with clinical stage T1 and T2 disease, the positive biopsy rate about 6 months after cryosurgery was 12.8%. Others have reported about the same results.[174–176]

These reports show that with increasing experience, the treatment becomes more effective and the positive biopsy rate lessens and that patients who are failures of radiation treatment have a higher positive biopsy rate than previously untreated patients. In general the short-term results of prostatic cryosurgery suggest that the long-term results may be competitive with other well-established types of therapy in selected patients. The short-term use has demonstrated that morbidity is low and that effective early local control is provided. Data on the long-term curative efficacy of cryoablation of prostatic cancer is not yet available.

## BONE TUMORS

The use of cryosurgery in bone tumors has been principally adjunctive to conventional surgical techniques, principally curettage. In this use, the intent is to reduce the incidence of recurrence by extending the curative potential of the curettage. Occasionally, cryosurgery has been used alone, usually for palliative benefits, such as the relief of pain due to metastatic cancer.

## SELECTION CRITERIA

Four types of clinical conditions have been treated by cryosurgical techniques.

1. Benign bone tumors, such as giant cell tumors and ameloblastoma that are locally aggressive and prone to recurrence after curettage
2. Sarcomas of bone
3. Cancer metastatic to bone
4. Aneurysmal bone cysts, keratocystic bone lesions, and other benign bone lesions

## TECHNIQUE

Since cryosurgery is adjunctive therapy in treating bone tumors, the technique is the same for the different clinical circumstances. The tumor is removed by curettage and then the resultant cavity is frozen, which devitalizes an additional 1 or 2 cm of bone. In this way, cryosurgery extends the curative potential of the conventional curettage. The freezing has been done by pouring or spraying liquid nitrogen into the cavity, but probe techniques have been used also, especially in areas not suitable for the pour or spray techniques. When the pour technique is used, it is commonly necessary to limit the runoff of liquid nitrogen from the cavity into adjacent tissues. This can be done by the use of a wide-mouth funnel or a cone-shaped device, sealing the area of contact to the rim of the cavity with Gelfoam or hospital lubricating jelly. When the cavity can be positioned appropriately to hold the fluid, the liquid nitrogen can be poured into the cavity without using the funnel. In some locations, the probe technique, using a probe (or several probes) as large as possible for the size of the bone cavity, is necessary. The cavity should be filled with water-soluble hospital lubricating jelly before freezing to improve contact between the bone and the probe and to facilitate heat transfer. During freezing, the use of thermocouples to monitor temperature in the tissues is desirable. The thermocouple should be placed in the normal bone 1 cm from the edge of the curetted cavity. Tissue temperatures of $-40°C$ should be achieved at this site. After thawing, the freeze-thaw cycle should be repeated.

When the cryosurgical treatment is complete, the bone cavity is reinforced with bone grafts or acrylic cement, the choice depending in part on the location and size of the tumor. Because of bone weakness consequent to the tumor and its treatment, bone support (casts, braces, intramedullary rods, etc.) is desirable in order to reduce the chance of fracture. Good soft tissue coverage of the treated bone is essential.

## POSTOPERATIVE CARE

The principal complication is postoperative fracture. The bone is weakened by the tumor, the curettage, and the freezing. Because bone healing is slow, fractures at the treatment site are common. Avoidance of stress on the treated bone is often necessary for several months while healing progresses. A rare complication is gas embolism, which may result when liquid nitrogen is poured or sprayed into the open wound.[177] This complication can be avoided entirely by use of the probe technique.

## RESULTS

Curettage and adjunctive cryosurgery has had only limited use. Malawer and Dunham[178] reported a local control rate of 96% in their series of 25 patients with giant cell tumors, chondroblastomas, and aneurysmal bone cysts. Marcove and associates[179] described the use of curettage and cryosurgery for giant cell tumors of the sacrum in seven patients. Two patients developed local recurrence and were treated by a repeat curettage and cryosurgery. In long follow-up, all patients are disease-free.[179] The local control rate of giant cell tumors after curettage and cryosurgery is better than 90%, especially if care is taken to detect recurrence at an early stage so that treatment can be repeated. This control rate appears to be somewhat better than provided by curettage and cement alone, although this too is effective therapy.

Others have reported favorable experience with the adjunctive use of cryosurgery in selected bone tumors, including cancers metastatic to bone.[180–182] Malignant bone tumors are not often treated by cryosurgery with the intent to cure, but chondrosarcoma is an example of a low-grade malignant bone tumor successfully managed by curettage and cryosurgery.[183,184] In selected cases, cryosurgery can provide palliative benefits by relief of pain, which is immediate after freezing.

The use of curettage and cryosurgery for other bone lesions is also reported. Salmassy and Pogrel[185] reported on the treatment of mandibular lesions, including amelioblastomas, myxomas, and odontogenic keratocysts in 20 patients, which showed the importance of bone grafting to decrease the possibility of fracture. Aneurysmal bone cysts and other cystic benign lesions have also been treated successfully by similar cryosurgical techniques.[186]

## TUMORS OF THE UTERUS

With regard to neoplastic disease of the uterus, cryosurgery has principally been used for cervical intraepithelial neoplasia (CIN). Advanced cancers of the cervix have been treated for palliation of symptoms, including bleeding. Recently investigations into the usefulness for uterine fibroids has begun. Each merits a brief description.

### CERVICAL INTRAEPITHELIAL NEOPLASIA

Selection of appropriate patients is based on careful colposcopic examination and histologic diagnosis from specimens obtained at biopsy. Care must be taken to detect invasive carcinoma. The cryosurgical treatment is commonly given under cervical block anesthesia. A cryosurgical probe with a freezing surface shaped to fit the uterine cervix and cooled by either nitrous oxide or liquid nitrogen is applied to the diseased tissue. Freezing to a depth of at least 5 mm in a double freeze-thaw cycle is necessary.[187]

In the postoperative course, as the necrotic tissue sloughs, a vaginal discharge occurs for about 10 days. Healing is ordinarily favorable, but the complications are cervical stenosis and rarely pyometra. The results are satisfactory in about 90% of patients. The rate of persistence of disease is about 10%.[188–190] The treatment of failures raises questions about the accuracy of evaluation of the extent of disease and the adequacy of the cryosurgical technique. Instances of invasive carcinoma emphasize the need for careful diagnosis, treatment, and long-term follow-up examinations.[191,192]

Laser therapy is a strong competitor of cryosurgery in the treatment of CIN. Ferenczy,[193] in a comparative study of cryosurgery and laser therapy, reported that with either technique, the cure rate was about 90% after one treatment and about 95% after two treatments. Cryosurgery was considered as good as laser therapy in treating lesions less than 3 cm in diameter, but laser therapy was preferable for large lesions because of speed of treatment. Persistence of disease was similar with both methods of therapy.[193] In a randomized study by Berget and associates,[194] laser therapy and cryosurgery were judged highly acceptable to the patients. The results of treatment were satisfactory in 96% of the laser-treated patients and in 93% of the patients treated with cryosurgery.

## ADVANCED CANCERS OF THE UTERUS

Advanced cancers of the uterus and vagina in patients who are not candidates for excisional surgery have been treated by cryosurgery to control tumor growth and relieve symptoms. The techniques are the same as for advanced cancers in other accessible locations. A liquid nitrogen–cooled probe is applied to the cancer and extensive freezing is done. Certainly the bulk of the tumor will be reduced and control of bleeding, infection, and malodorous discharge is likely. Relief of pain may be achieved. Treatment is repeated as often as needed to maintain control of the local tumor.

## LEIOMYOMAS

Cryosurgical techniques currently are under investigation for the treatment of leiomyomas, also known as myomas. Depending in part on size and location, myomas cause pain, abnormal bleeding, uterine enlargement, obstructive symptoms due to pressure on adjacent organs, and may cause infertility. The interest in cryosurgery is centered on the desire to avoid removal of the uterus, thereby avoiding the complications of excisional surgery and perhaps permitting later pregnancy. The factors in appropriate selection of myomas for cryosurgery, that is, size, number, and location, are not yet known. However, large myomas, greater than about 10 cm in diameter, may not be best treated with cryosurgery.

In preparation for cryosurgery, the patients are treated with gonadotropin-releasing hormone agonistic for about 2 months before operation to reduce the size of the uterus and the myoma. Before surgery, the usual diagnostic procedures, including pelvic or vaginal ultrasound and CT or MRI examinations, are performed to aid in determining the size and location of the myomas. The cryosurgical technique will vary with the location of the myoma, but the basic principles of technique are the same in the uterus as they are for benign tumors elsewhere in the body.

Two methods of gaining access to the myomas in the subserous and intramural position are currently in use, namely laparotomy and laparoscopy. To perform the cryosurgery via laparoscopy is attractive (minimally invasive). Whatever the approach, the cryosurgical procedure is the same. The cryoprobe (4.8 mm or smaller, perhaps pointed for direct insertion without using a sheath) is placed in the myoma and the tissue freezing is performed. Since myomas are not malignant, the tissue should be frozen only to the limits of the myoma. The tissue-freezing process is monitored via the laparoscope, and in some cases by transrectal ultrasound. If the size of the myoma precludes adequate freezing from one site, the probe is repositioned to permit treatment of the unfrozen tissue. Repetition of freezing is not as critical for benign tumors as it is in cancer.

Myomas in the submucous position may be treated via hysteroscopy. Experience with this approach is small. Under anesthesia, the cervix is dilated and a curettage is done. Operative hysteroscopy is performed to examine the uterine cavity and the myoma. Transrectal ultrasound is used to place the probe in the myoma and to monitor the freezing process, which is done in the usual manner. The patient may expect to be sent home on the day of the procedure. The follow-up visits include ultrasound examinations at 6 months, 1 year, and 2 years after treatment to measure reduction in size of the myoma.

Comparison with other methods of treatment, which include hysterectomy, myomectomy, and myolysis, is not practical at this time because experience with cryomyolysis is just beginning. However, the early results in terms of relief of symptoms and reduction in size of myomas encourages continued trial.

The advantages of cryosurgery for myomas include the low risk of a minimally invasive procedure, the preservation of the uterus, the quick return to normal activity, and the possibility of discontinuing the use of gonadotropin-releasing hormone-agonistic analog.

## TUMORS IN OTHER SITES

In other locations in the body, a wide diversity of tumors has been treated in the past years. In some locations, experience is just beginning, and in other locations, only a few patients have been treated.

Application to kidney tumors is just beginning. Recent experimental studies have shown the practicality of the technique for treating this organ.[195,196] The few clinical reports have demonstrated that cryosurgery to kidney tumors may be done by open operative or laparoscopic techniques.[197,198] Nevertheless, the potential place for cryosurgery in renal tumors remains to be determined. Most renal cell cancers should be excised because that therapy offers the best chance of cure. In selected patients in need of kidney-conserving therapy, such as patients in whom partial nephrectomy is often chosen, cryosurgery may prove to be a safer therapeutic option. The current clinical trials feature minimally invasive ultrasound-monitored techniques for small tumors (2 cm or less in diameter) as the use of cryosurgery develops with an appropriate measure of caution.

Tumors of the esophagus, breast, lung, and connective tissues, including sarcomas in diverse sites, have been treated by cryosurgery.[55,199–205] In some reports, the treatment has been given for the palliation of advanced cancer, but in other reports, sometimes with partial excision, the treatment is intended to cure the disease. The techniques used in these new or infrequent applications do not differ in any important way from those already described. These reports show that the scope of cryosurgery is likely to expand.

## FUTURE DIRECTIONS

The need for research leading to a better understanding of the effects of freezing on tissue and to more effective methods of producing a cryogenic injury of appropriate dimensions is critical to further development of cryosurgical technique. In many tumors, adjunctive therapy, either chemotherapy or radiotherapy, directed at the border zone of the cryogenic lesion, is needed to improve the results. Investigation into these adjunctive therapies is important. The question of an immunologic response to cryosurgery of tumors remains unanswered, although speculation stimulated by results with experimental tumor systems persists.

Advances in the technology of imaging, including MRI-compatible cryoprobes, and continued development of cryosurgical apparatus, especially in the direction of disease-specific devices, will broaden the usefulness of cryosurgical techniques. Cryosurgery already has a place in surgical practice in situations in which conventional excisional surgery cannot be used, including those patients who have severe associated disease. Cryosurgery also may find a place as a less invasive procedure with the associated reduction in risk and costs, advantageous features that may make cryosurgical techniques competitive with excisional surgery in the treatment of selected tumors.

## REFERENCES

1. BIRD H: James Arnott, M.D. (Aberdeen) 1797–1883: A pioneer in refrigeration analgesia. Anaesthesia 4:10, 1949.
2. WHITE AC: Liquid air: Its application in medicine and surgery. Med Rec 56:109, 1899.
3. PUSEY W: The use of carbon dioxide snow in the treatment of nevi and other lesions of the skin. JAMA 49:1354, 1907.
4. BOWEN J, TOWLE H: Liquid air in dermatology. Boston Med Surg J 157:561, 1907.
5. LOW RC: *Carbonic Acid Snow as a Therapeutic Agent in the Treatment of Disease of the Skin.* New York, Wm. Wood, 1911.
6. LORTAT-JACOBS L, SOLENTE G: *La Cryotherapie.* Maisson et Cie, Paris, 1930.
7. FAY T: Early experiences with local and generalized refrigeration of the human brain. J. Neurosurg 16:239, 1959.
8. HASS G, TAYLOR C: A quantitative hypothermal method for the production of local injury of tissue. Arch Pathol 45:563, 1948.
9. CLASEN R et al: The production by liquid nitrogen of acute closed cerebral lesions. Surg Gynecol Obstet 96:605, 1953.
10. KLATZO I et al: The relationship between edema, blood-brain barrier and tissue elements in a local brain injury. J Neuropath Exp Neuro 17:548, 1958.
11. ROSOMOFF H: Experimental brain injury during hypothermia. J Neurosurg 16:177, 1959.
12. ROWBOTHAM G et al: Cooling cannula for use in the treatment of cerebral neoplasms. Lancet 1:12, 1959.
13. COOPER I, LEE A: Cryostatic congelation: A system for producing a limited controlled region of cooling or freezing of biologic tissues. J Nerv Ment Dis 133:259, 1961.
14. —— Cryogenic surgery. A new method of destruction or extirpation of benign or malignant tumors. N Engl J Med 268:743, 1963.
15. —— Cryogenic surgery for cancer. Fed Proc 24:S237, 1965.
16. CAHAN W: Cryosurgery of malignant and benign tumors. Fed Proc 24:S241, 1965.
17. GONDER M et al: Experimental prostate cryosurgery. Invest Urol 3:372, 1964.
18. —— et al: Cryosurgical treatment of the prostate. Invest Urol 3:372, 1966.
19. GAGE A et al: Cryotherapy for cancer of the lip and oral cavity. Cancer 18:1646, 1965.
20. SMITH M et al: Cryosurgical techniques in removal of angiofibroma. Laryngoscope 84:1071, 1964.
21. RAND R et al: Stereotactic cryo-hypophysectomy. JAMA 189:255, 1964.
22. WILSON C et al: Stereotaxic cryosurgery of the pituitary gland in carcinoma of the breast and other disorders. JAMA 198:587, 1966.
23. CONWAY L, COLLINS W: Results of trans-sphenoidal cryohypophysectomy for carcinoma of the breast. N. Engl J Med 281:1, 1969.
24. LINCOFF H et al: Cryosurgical treatment of intraocular tumors. Am J Ophthalmol 63:389, 1967.
25. JORDAN W et al: Cryotherapy of benign and neoplastic tumors of the prostate. Surg Gynecol Obstet 125:1265, 1967.
26. CRISP W et al: Application of cryosurgery to gynecologic malignancy. Obstet Gynecol 30:668, 1967.
27. GAGE A et al: Cancer cryotherapy. Mil Med 132:55, 1967.
28. GAGE A: Cryotherapy for inoperable rectal cancer. Dis Colon Rectum 11:36, 1968.
29. GAGE A: Cryotherapy for oral cancer. JAMA 204:565, 1968.
30. GAGE A, ERICKSON R: Cryotherapy and curettage for bone tumors. J Cryother 1:60, 1968.
31. MARCOVE R, MILLER T: The treatment of primary and metastatic localized bone tumors by cryosurgery. Surg Clin North Am 49:421, 1969.
32. MILLER D, METZNER D: Cryosurgery for tumors of the head and neck. Trans Am Acad Ophthalmol Otolaryngol 73:300, 1969.
33. ZACARIAN S: *Cryosurgery of Skin Cancer.* Springfield, IL, Charles C Thomas, 1969.
34. CAHAN W: Cryosurgery: The management of massive recurrent cancer. In *Cryogenics in Surgery,* H von Leden, W Cahan (eds): Flushing, NY, Medical Examination Publishing, 1971, pp 182–234.
35. SOANES W et al: Remission of metastatic lesions following cryosurgery in prostatic cancer: Immunologic considerations. J Urol 104:154, 1970.
36. GURSEL E et al: Regression of prostate cancer following sequential cryotherapy to the prostate. J Urology 108:928, 1972.
37. WEAVER A, SMITH D: Cryosurgery for head and neck cancer. Am J Surg 128:466, 1974.
38. SMITH D, WEAVER A: Cryosurgery for oral cancer—A six-year retrospective study. J Oral Surg 34:245, 1976.
39. BENSON J: Combined chemotherapy and cryosurgery for oral cancer. Am J Surg 130:596, 1975.
40. ZACARIAN S: *Cryosurgical Advances in Dermatology and Tumors of the Head and Neck,* Springfield, IL, Charles C Thomas, 1977.

41. TORRE D et al: Cryosurgical treatment of basal cell carcinomas. Prog Dermatol 12:11, 1978.

42. SHEILD J et al: The role of cryotherapy in the management of retinoblastoma. Am J Ophthalmol 108:260, 1989.

43. JACOBIEC F et al: Cryotherapy for conjunctival primary acquired melanosis and malignant melanoma—Experience with 62 cases. Ophthalmology 95:1058, 1988.

44. TOWNSEND D, RICHART R: Cryotherapy and carbon dioxide laser management of cervical intraepithelial neoplasia: a controlled comparison. Obstet Gynecol 61:75, 1983.

45. CREASEMAN W et al: Cryosurgery in the management of cervical intraepithelial neoplasia. Obstet Gynecol 63:145, 1984.

46. FERENCZY A: Comparison of cryo and carbon dioxide laser therapy for cervical intraepithelial neoplasia. Obstet Gynecol 66:793, 1985.

47. BENEDET J et al: The results of cryosurgical treatment of cervical intraepithelial neoplasia at one, five, and ten years. Am J Obstet Gynecol 157:268, 1987.

48. ANDERSEN E et al: The results of cryosurgery for cervical intraepithelial neoplasia. Gynecol Oncol 30:21, 1988.

49. BONNEY W et al: Cryosurgery in prostate cancer: survival. Urology 19:37, 1982.

50. BONNEY W et al: Cryosurgery in prostate cancer: Elimination of local lesion. Urology 22:8, 1983.

51. MARCOVE R: A 17-year review of cryosurgery in the treatment of bone tumors. Clin Orthop 163:231, 1982.

52. RODGERS B et al: Endotracheal cryotherapy in the treatment of refractory airway strictures. Ann Thorac Surg 35:52, 1983.

53. HOMASSON J et al: Bronchoscopic cryotherapy for airway strictures caused by tumors. Chest 90:159, 1986.

54. MAIWAND M: Cryotherapy for advanced carcinoma of the trachea and bronchi. Br Med J 293:181, 1986.

55. GAGE A: Cryosurgery in the treatment of cancer. Surg Gynecol Obstet 174:73, 1992.

56. ONIK G et al: Sonographic monitoring of hepatic cryosurgery in an experimental animal model. Am J Roentgenol 144:1043, 1985.

57. ONIK G et al: Characteristic of frozen prostate. Radiology 168:629, 1988.

58. BAUST J, CHANG Z: Underlying mechanisms of damage and new concepts in cryosurgical instrumentation, in Cryosurgery. Mechanism and Applications, Paris, International Institute of Refrigeration, 1995, pp 21–36.

59. BAUST J et al: Minimally invasive cryosurgery—Technological advances. Cryobiology 34:373, 1997.

60. MAZUR P et al: A two-factor hypothesis of freezing injury: evidence from Chinese hamster tissue culture cells. Exper Cell Res 71:345, 1972.

61. SHEPHERD J, DAWBER R: Wound healing and scarring after cryosurgery. Cryobiology 21:157, 1984.

62. LI A et al: Differences in healing of skin wounds caused by burn and freeze injuries. Ann Surg 191:244, 1980.

63. GARAMY G: Engineering aspects of cryosurgery, in Cryosurgery, R Rand et al (eds). Springfield, IL Charles C Thomas 1968, pp 92–132.

64. BALD W, FRASER J: Cryogenic surgery. Rep Prog Phys 45:138, 1982.

65. ORPWOOD R: Biophysical and engineering aspects of cryosurgery. Phys Med Biol 26:555, 1981.

66. HAMILTON A, HU J: An electronic cryoprobe for cryosurgery using heat pipes and thermoelectric coolers: a preliminary report. J Med Engin Technol 17:104, 1993.

67. TORRE D: Cryosurgical treatment of epitheliomas using cone—Spray technique. J Dermatol Surg Oncol 3:432, 1977.

68. NEEL H et al: Requisites for successful cryogenic surgery for cancer. Arch Surg 102:45, 1971.

69. GAGE A: Basic technique, in Cryosurgical Treatment of Skin Cancer, E Kuflik, A Gage (ed). New York, Igaku-Shoin Publishers, 1990, pp 65–82.

70. GAGE A: Experimental cryosurgery, in Cryosurgery, Mechanism and Applications. Paris International Institute of Refrigeration, 1995, pp 37–44.

71. GAGE A et al: A comparison of instrument methods of monitoring freezing in cryosurgery. J Dermatol Surg Oncol 9:209, 1983.

72. LITTRUP P et al: Prostatic cryotherapy: Ultrasonic and pathologic correlation in the canine odel. Urology 44:175, 1994.

73. LAM C et al: Ultrasonic characterization of hepatic cryolesions. Arch Surg 130:1068, 1995.

74. GRAMPAS S et al: Salvage radical prostatectomy after failed transperineal cryotherapy: Histologic findings from prostate wholemount specimens correlated with intraperative transrectal ultrasound images. Urology 45:9536, 1995.

75. SALIKEN J et al: Laboratory evaluation of ice formation around a 3 mm Accuprobe. Cryobiology 32:285, 1995.

76. CHIN JL et al: Three-dimensional prostate ultrasound and its application to cryosurgery. Techniques Urol 2:187, 1997.

77. STEED J et al: Correlation between thermosensor temperature and transrectal ultrasonography during prostate cryoablation. Can Assoc Radiol J 48:186, 1997.

78. LEE F et al: US-guided percutaneous cryoablation of prostate cancer. Radiology 192:769, 1994.

79. AUGUSTINOWICZ S, GAGE A: Temperature and cooling rate variations during cryosurgical probe testing. Int J Refrig 8:198, 1985.

80. GAGE A: Correlations of electrical impedance and temperature in tissue during freezing. Cryobiology 16:56, 1979.

81. COOPER I, STELLAR S: Cryogenic freezing of brain tumors for excision or destruction in situ. J Neurosurg 20:921, 1963.

82. FRAUNFELDER F et al: No-touch technique for intraocular malignant melanomas. Arch Ophthalmol 95:1616, 1977.

83. POLK W et al: A technique for the use of cryosurgery to assist hepatic resection. J Am Coll Surg 180:171, 1995.

84. ZACARIAN S: Cryosurgery of cutaneous carcinomas: an 18 year study of 3022 patients with 4228 carcinomas. J Am Acad Dermatol 9:947, 1983.

85. KUFLIK E, GAGE A: The five-year cure rate achieved by cryosurgery for skin cancer. J Am Acad Dermatol 24:1002, 1991.

86. GRAHAM G: Cryosurgery. Clin Plast Surg 20:131, 1993.

87. KUFLIK E, GAGE A: Cryosurgical Treatment for Skin Cancer. Igaku-Shoin Medical Publishers, New York, 1990, pp 245–249.

88. LINDGREN G, LARKO O: Long-term follow-up of cryosurgery of basal cell carcinoma of the eyelid. J Am Acad Dermatol 36:742, 1997.

89. KUFLIK EG, GAGE AA: Recurrent basal cell carcinoma treated with cryosurgery. J Am Acad Dermatol 37:82, 1997.

90. GAGE AA: Cryosurgery for difficult problems in cutaneous cancer. Cutis 16:465, 1975.

91. KUFLIK E: Cryosurgery for palliation. J Dermatol Surg Oncol 11:867, 1985.

92. GONCALVES J: Cryosurgery of advanced cancer of the extremities. Skin Cancer 1:211, 1986.

93. BREITBART E: Cryosurgery in the treatment of cutaneous malignant melanoma. Clin Dermatol 8:96, 1990.

94. RENNIE I: Diagnois and treatment of ocular melanomas. Br J Hosp Med 46:144, 1991.

95. HIDAYAT A et al: The effect of rapid freezing of uveal melanomas. Am J Ophthalmol 103:66, 1987.

96. SCALA M et al: Cryosurgery alone or in combination with radiotherapy and hyperthermia in the treatment of head and neck mucosal and cutaneous melanoma. J Exp Clin Cancer Res 13:243, 1994.

97. PEKSAYER G et al: Long-term results of cryotherapy on malignant epithelial tumors of the conjunctiva. Am J Ophthalmol 107:337, 1989.

98. HURWITZ JJ, MISHKIN SK: The value of cryoprobe-assisted removal of orbital tumor. Ophthalmic Surg 19:94, 1988.

99. GEYER O et al: Transconjunctival approach for intraorbital tumors. Arch Ophthalmol 106:14, 1988.

100. LOEWENSTEIN A et al: Cavernous haemangioma of the orbit: treatment by transconjunctival cryoextraction (letter). Eye 7:597, 1993.

101. SHIELDS J et al: Cryotherapy for retinoblastoma. Int Ophthalmol Clin 33:101, 1993.

102. RAND R: Cryosurgery in neurosurgery, in Cryogenics in Surgery, H Von Leden, W Cahan (eds). New York, Examination Publishing, 1971, pp 235–251.

103. MAROON J et al: Cryosurgery re-visited for the removal and destruction of brain, spinal and orbital tumors. Neurol Res 14:294, 1992.

104. ENDO S et al: Cryoretraction in the removal of intracranial vascular tumors—Technical note. Neuro Med Chir (Tokyo) 33:44, 1993.

105. GAGE A: Five-year survival following cryosurgery for oral cancer. Arch Surg 111:990, 1979.

106. GAGE A: Treatment of malignant soft tissue lesions of oral cavity, pharynx, face and scalp, in Cryosurgery of the Maxillofacial Region, P Bradley (ed). CRC Press, Boca Raton, 1986, pp 1–30.

107. WEAVER A, SMITH D: Cryosurgery for head and neck cancer. Am J Surg 128:466, 1974.

108. SMITH D, WEAVER A: Cryosurgery for oral cancer—A six-year retrospective study. J Oral Surg 34:245, 1976.

109. HAUSAMEN J: The basis, technique and indication for cryosurgery in tumors of the oral cavity and face. J Max-fac Surg 3:41, 1975.

110. HOHKI A et al: Cryosurgery of head and neck malignant tumors. Prog Clin Biol Res 107:827, 1982.

111. LUNDQUIST P, KUYLENSTIERNA R: The clinical use of cryosurgery in tumor treatment. J Laryngol Otol 97:431, 1983.

112. WANG S: Cryosurgery in 80 cases of tongue carcinoma. Chin Med Soc 97:131, 1984.

113. LI ZY: Cryosurgery in 50 cases of tongue carcinoma. J Oral Maxillofac Surg 49:504, 1991.

114. BENSON J: Combined chemotherapy and cryosurgery for oral cancer. Am J Surg 130:596, 1975.

115. AIROLDI M et al: Combined cryosurgical, chemotherapeutic, and radiotherapeutic management of T1-4N0M0 oral cavity cancers. Cancer 56:424, 1985.

116. CHANDLER J: Cryosurgery for recurrent cancer of the head and neck. Otolaryngol Clin North Am 7:193, 1974.

117. MEYZA J, TOWPIK E: Surgical and cryosurgical salvage of oral and oropharyngeal cancer recurring after radical radiotherapy. Eur J Surg Oncol 17:567, 1991.

118. SHENG H, JIA H: Combined therapy for carcinoma of the nasopharynx: A report of 49 cases. J Laryngol Otol 107:201, 1993.

119. BECKER H: Options and results in endobronchial treatment of lung cancer. Min Invas Ther Allied Technol 5:165, 1996.

120. SUTEDJA G, POSTMUS P: Bronchoscopic treatment of lung tumors. Lung Cancer 11:1, 1994.

121. HOMASSON J: Tracheo-bronchial endoscopic cryotherapy, in Cryotherapy in Chest Medicine, J Homasson, N Bell (eds). Paris, Springer-Verlag, 1992, pp 36–45.

122. MAIWAND M, HOMASSON J: Cryotherapy for tracheobronchial disorders. Int Pulmonol 16:427, 1995.

123. VERGNON J et al: Initial combined cryotherapy and irradiation for unresectable non-small cell lung cancer. Chest 102:1436, 1992.

124. MARASSO A et al: Cryosurgery in bronchoscopic treatment of tracheobronchial stenosis. Chest 103:472, 1993.

125. MATHUR P et al: Fiberoptic bronchoscopic cryotherapy in the management of tracheobronchial obstruction. Chest 110:718, 1996.

126. BLUMGART L, FONG Y: Surgical options in the treatment of hepatic metastasis from colorectal cancer. Curr Probl Surg 32:336, 1995.

127. ONIK G et al: Ultrasonic characteristics of frozen liver. Cryobiology 21:321, 1984.

128. RAVIKUMAR T et al: Hepatic cryosurgery with intraoperative ultrasound monitoring for metastatic colon carcinoma. Arch Surg 122:403, 1987.

129. RAVIKUMAR T: The role of cryotherapy in the management of patients with liver tumors. Adv Surg 30:281, 1997.

130. LEE F JR et al: Hepatic cryosurgery with intraoperative US guidance. Radiology 202:624, 1997.

131. WEAVER M et al: Hepatic cryosurgery in treating colorectal metastases. Cancer 76:210, 1995.

132. SHAFIR M et al: Cryoablation of unresectable malignant liver tumors. Am J Surg 171:27, 1996.

133. GAGE AA et al: Freezing injury to large blood vessels in dogs. With comments on the effect of experimental freezing of bile ducts. Surgery 61:748, 1967.

134. SILVERSTEIN JC et al: Thermal bile duct protection during liver cryoablation. J Surg Oncol 64:163, 1997.

135. COZZI PJ et al: Thrombocytopenia after hepatic cryotherapy for colorectal metastases: correlates with hepatocellular injury. World J Surg 18:774, 1994.

136. STEWART GJ et al: Hepatic cryotherapy: Double-freeze cycles achieve greater hepatocellular injury in men. Cryobiology 32:215, 1995.

137. ONIK G: Cryosurgery. Crit Rev Oncol Hematol 23:1, 1996.

138. MORRIS DL et al: Cryoablation of hepatic malignancy: An evaluation of tumor marker data and survival in 110 patients. GI Cancer 1:247, 1996.

139. MCLOUGHLIN R et al: CT of the liver after cryotherapy of hepatic metastases: imaging findings. 165:329, 1995.

140. LAM C et al: Ultrasonic characterization of hepatic cryolesions. Arch Surg 130:1068, 1995.

141. KUSZYK B et al: Hepatic tumors treated by cryosurgery: normal CT appearance. 166:363, 1996.

142. KING J et al: Computed tomography changes following cryotherapy for hepatic cancer. Australasien Radiol 41:112, 1997.

143. ZHOU X et al: The role of cryosurgery in the treatment of hepatic cancer: A report of 113 cases. J Cancer Res Clin Oncol 120:100, 1993.

144. ZHAO J et al: Cryotherapy for hepatocellular carcinoma. Asian J Surg 20:140, 1997.

145. RAVIKUMAR T et al: Intraoperative ultrasonography of liver: detection of occult liver tumors and treatment by cryosurgery. Cancer Detect 18:131, 1994.

146. PREKETES A et al: Effect of hepatic artery chemotherapy on survival of patients with hepatic metastases from colorectal carcinoma treated with cryotherapy. World J Surg 19:768, 1995.

147. MCKINNON J et al: Cryosurgery for malignant tumors of the liver. Can J Surg 39:401, 1996.

148. ADAM R et al: Place of cryosurgery in the treatment of malignant liver tumors. Ann Surg 225:39, 1997.

149. YEH K et al: Cryosurgical ablation of hepatic metastases from colorectal carcinomas. Am Surg 63:63, 1997.

150. STEELE G: Cryoablation in hepatic surgery. Semin Liver Dis 14:120, 1994.

151. MYERS RS et al: Cryosurgery of primate pancreas. Cancer 25:411, 1970.

152. MYERS RS et al: Cryosurgical necrosis of the head of the pancreas. Ann Surg 171:413, 1970.

153. NEEL HB et al: Alteration of blood sugar and plasma insulin after cryosurgery of functioning islet cell tumor. J Surg Oncol 4:511, 1972.

154. MCINTOSH G et al: In situ freezing of the pancreas and portal vein in the pig. Cryobiology 22:183, 1985.

155. MCINTOSH G: Alternative to radical pancreatic excision. Gut 23:A440, 1992.

156. PATIUTKO L et al: The combined treatment of locally disseminated pancreatic cancer using cryosurgery. Vopr Onkol 37:695, 1991.

157. KOMKOVA T: Cryosurgery of pancreas due to chronic painful pancreatitis, in Cryosurgery, AS Kogan (ed). Irkutsk, The USSR Ministry of Health. Institute for Doctor's Advancement of Irkutsk. 1987, pp 80–84.

158. KOMKOVA T: Results of treatment of chronic pancreatitis with cryosurgery. Vestn Khir 145:21, 1990.

159. BIGGERS O et al: Local excision of rectal cancer. Dis Colon Rectum 29:374, 1986.

160. HEBERER G et al: Local procedures in the management of rectal cancer. World J Surg 11:499, 1987.

161. GEISSLER N et al: Ergebnisse der kryochirurgie bei der behandlung inoperabler Tumor—stenosen der Anus and Rektums. Zentralbl Chir 116:319, 1991.

162. ORTH K et al: Cryotherapy in rectal cancer: A palliative local tumor treatment. Chirurg 63:421, 1992.

163. MADDEN J, KANDALAFT S: Electrocoagulation of rectal cancer, Am J Surg 22:347, 1971.

164. ZAMAN A et al: Superiority of ND:YAG laser to cryosurgery in the treatment of rectal carcinoma. J Clin Laser Med Surg 12:79, 1994.

165. MATHUS-VLIEGEN E, TYTGAT G: Laser photocoagulation in the palliation of colorectal malignancies. Cancer 57:2212, 1986.

166. ONIK G et al: Transrectal ultrasound-guided percutaneous radical cryoablation of the prostate. Cancer 72:1291, 1993.

167. VON ESCHENBACH A et al: Technique of cryosurgery of the prostate. Atlas Urol Clin North Am 2:127, 1994.

168. BAHN D et al: Prostate cancer: US guided percutaneous cryoablation. Radiology 194:551, 1995.

169. WONG W et al: Cryosurgery as a treatment for prostate carcinoma. Cancer 79:963, 1997.

170. LEE F et al: Cryosurgery of prostate cancer. Use of adjuvant hormonal therapy and temperature monitoring—A one year follow-up. Anticancer Res 17:1511, 1997.

171. CESPEDES R et al: Long term follow-up of incontinence and obstruction after salvage cryosurgical ablation of the prostate: Results in 143 patients. J Urol 157:237, 1997.

172. SHINOHARA K et al: Cryosurgical ablation of prostatic cancer: patterns of cancer recurrence. J Urol 158:2206, 1997.

173. COHEN J et al: Cryosurgical ablation of the prostate: two year prostate specific antigen and biopsy results. Urology 47:395, 1996.

174. WAKE R et al: Cryosurgical ablation of the prostate for localized adenocarcinoma: a preliminary experience. J Urol 155:1663, 1996.

175. CARROLL P et al: Focal therapy for prostate cancer 1996: Maximizing outcome. Urology 49:84, 1997.

176. LEE F et al: Cryosurgery of prostate cancer: use of adjuvant hormonal therapy and temperature monitoring—A one year followup. Anticancer Res 17:1511, 1997.

177. SCHREUDER H et al: Venous gas embolism during cryosurgery for bone tumors. J Surg Oncol 60:196, 1995.

178. MALAWER M, DUNHAM W: Cryosurgery and acrylic cementation as surgical adjuncts in the treatment of aggressive (benign) bone tumors. Analysis of 25 patients below the age of 21. Clin Orthop 262:42, 1991.

179. MARCOVE R et al: Conservative surgery for giant cell tumors of the sacrum. Cancer 74:1253, 1994.

180. ABOULAFIA A et al: Treatment of large subchondral tumors of the knee with cryosurgery and composite reconstruction. Clin Orthop Rel Res 307:189, 1994.

181. MELLER I et al: Cryosurgery. Clin Orthop India 10:115, 1995.

182. ALKALAY D et al: Giant cell tumors with intraarticular fracture. Two-stage local excision, cryosurgery and cementation in 5 patients with distal femoral tumor followed for 2–4 years. Acta Orthop Scand 67:291, 1996.

183. MARCOVE R et al: The use of cryosurgery in the treatment of low and medium grade chondrosarcoma. Clin Orthop 122:147, 1977.

184. MARCOVE R et al: Cryosurgery in osteogenic sarcoma: Report of three cases. Compr Ther 10:52, 1984.

185. SALMASSY D, POGREL A: Liquid nitrogen cryosurgery and immediate bone grafting in the management of aggressive primary jaw lesions. J Oral Maxillofac Surg 53:784, 1995.

186. MARCOVE R et al: The treatment of aneurysmal bone cyst. Clin Orthop Rel Res 311:157, 1995.

187. BOONSTRA H et al: Analysis of cryolesions in the uterine cervix: Application techniques, extension and failures. Obstet Gynecol 75:232, 1990.

188. CREASMAN W et al: Cryosurgery in the management of cervical intraepithelial neoplasia. Obstet Gynecol 63:145, 1984.

189. KWIKKEL H et al: Laser or cryotherapy for cervical intraepithelial neoplasia: a randomized study to compare efficacy and side effects. Gynecol Oncol 22:23, 1985.

190. BENEDET J et al: The results of cryosurgical treatment of cervical intraepithelial neoplasia at one, five, and ten years. Am J Obstet Gynecol 157:268, 1987.

191. SEVIN B et al: Invasive cancer of the cervix after cryosurgery. Obstet Gynecol 53:465, 1979.

192. TOWNSEND DE et al: Invasive cancer following outpatient evaluation and therapy for cervical disease. Obstet Gynecol 57:145, 1981.

193. FERENCZY A: Laser treatment of patients with condylomata and squamous carcinoma precursors of the lower female genital tract. CA 37:334, 1987.

194. BERGET A et al: Outpatient treatment of cervical intra-epithelial

neoplasia: The $CO_2$ laser therapy versus cryotherapy, a randomized trial. Acta Obstet Gynecol Scand 66:531, 1987.

195. STEPHENSON R et al: Renal cryoablation in a canine model. Urology 47:772, 1996.

196. COZZI P et al: Renal cryotherapy in a sheep model: A feasibility study. J Urol 157:710, 1997.

197. UCHIDA M et al: Percutaneous cryosurgery for renal tumors. Br J Urol 75:132, 1995.

198. DELWORTH M et al: Cryotherapy for renal cell carcinoma and angiomyolipoma. J Urol 155:252, 1996.

199. STAREN E et al: Cryosurgery of breast cancer. Arch Surg 132:28, 1997.

200. SALIKEN JC et al: CT for monitoring cryosurgery. AJR 166:853, 1996.

201. DEVRIES J et al: Cryosurgical treatment of sacrococcygeal chordoma. Cancer 58:2348, 1986.

202. MONTES LF et al: Response of leiomyosarcoma to cryosurgery: clinicopathological and ultrastructural study. Clin Exp Dermatol 20:20, 1995.

203. VAN SONNENBERG E et al: Therapeutic cryosurgery guided by MRI and ultrasound for haemangiomas in erector muscles of the back. Min Invas Ther Allied Technol 6:343, 1997.

204. UHLSCHWID G et al: Cryosurgery of pulmonary metastases. Cryobiology 16:171, 1979.

205. XIE DY et al: Cryosurgery and anaerobic corynebacterium vaccine in disseminated lung cancer. Report of 50 cases. Chin Med J 96:691, 1983.

# 5D / LASERS, CAVITRON ULTRASONIC SURGICAL ASPIRATION, AND PHOTODYNAMIC THERAPY FOR SOLID TUMORS

*David Fromm, Mark Herman, and David Kessel*

## LASERS

### LASER THEORY

The theoretical groundwork for the laser was laid by Einstein in 1917.[1] A single electron in its ground state, or lowest orbital shell, is able to absorb energy, raising it to a higher shell. The electron will subsequently return to its ground state, spontaneously emitting the previously absorbed energy as an electromagnetic wave. If the electron in its higher shell is again stimulated by energy of the same wavelength, it will return to the ground state faster. This results in the emission of an electromagnetic wave, which is additive to the initial stimulating energy and travels in the same direction. This *stimulated emission* then excites other electrons to higher shells, or acts as the second stimulus to previously excited electrons. This continues until more electrons are in their higher shells than in the ground state, a condition known as *population inversion*. When this condition is met, lasing can occur.

This process occurs not only with electrons but also with molecules and ions. The nature of the medium used thus determines the nature of the emitted electromagnetic wave. Most commonly it is light of the visible or infrared spectrum. The term *laser* is hence an acronym for *l*ight *a*mplification by the *s*timulated *e*mission of *r*adiation. The use of a mirror and a partially reflecting lens allows the light to be focused into a high-energy beam with a unique wavelength and minimal divergence. Several good reviews of surgical laser physics and tissue interactions are available.[2–4]

The first laser was successfully constructed in 1960 by Maiman,[5] and the first medical use was in 1967 by Goldman,[6] who treated port-wine stains. Treatment of human tumors began in 1972,[7] and subsequent years brought rapid development of multiple types of lasers as well as broad applications in oncology. Four types of lasers are commonly used in surgical oncology: $CO_2$, neodymium:yttrium-aluminum garnet (Nd:YAG), argon, and dye. Although lasers have been applied to virtually every imaginable type of tumor, there is a clear niche in the management of esophageal and colorectal cancers as well as a developing niche for interstitial and percutaneous treatment of solid organ and breast cancers.

### SURGICAL LASERS

Choosing the proper type of laser depends primarily upon the desired tissue effect, which may range from incising and dissecting like a knife, coagulation of blood or lymphatic vessels, local hyperthermia, vaporization, and nonthermal activation of photosensitizing drugs (photodynamic therapy). A host of local tissue factors combines with properties of the laser beam to determine the effect.[3,4] Light is absorbed by different pigments or substances in tissue depending upon its wavelength. The wavelength also determines the depth of penetration, with longer wavelengths penetrating better. The four surgical lasers—$CO_2$, Nd:YAG, argon, and dye—vary primarily in their wavelength, and are thus used for different purposes (Table 5D-1).

The $CO_2$ laser has a mid-infrared wavelength of 10,600 nm. However, extensive absorption by water molecules limits penetration to less than 0.5 mm. It is primarily used as a knife, since a small zone of coagulation necrosis allows for a relatively dry dissection. Vaporization of larger surfaces is easily done by using a widened beam, although this technique should only be performed when a histologic specimen is not necessary. Delivery of the beam to the tissues has been a problem in the past due to lack of fiberoptic capabilities for the $CO_2$ laser, necessitating articulated mechanical arms.

The Nd:YAG laser emits 1,064-nm light of the near-infrared spectrum. Absorption in tissue is very nonspecific, with water and blood being only moderately affected. Penetration is in excess of 5 mm, which is the deepest of the surgical lasers. Light delivery is simple and versatile, with a range of flexible fiberoptic cables and beam-focusing fiber tips available. The Nd:YAG laser has been recently described as the most versatile of the surgical lasers.[8] It can function to incise, deeply coagulate, thermally ablate, or vaporize tumor in a number of settings, ranging from cutaneous, endoscopic, open surgical, or percutaneous.

Argon lasers emit blue light at 488 or 514 nm. At these wavelengths, light is primarily absorbed by pigment such as melanin and hemoglobin, and it penetrates to depths of 1 mm. Its use is primarily limited to photocoagulation of tissue. Hemangiomas, both internal cavernous and cutaneous port-wine types, are thus amenable to treatment with the argon laser.[3]

**TABLE 5D-1.** CHARACTERISTICS OF COMMON LASERS IN SURGICAL ONCOLOGY

| LASER | WAVELENGTH, nm | SPECTRUM | ABSORPTION | DEPTH, mm | FUNCTION |
|---|---|---|---|---|---|
| $CO_2$ | 10,600 | Mid-infrared | Water | <0.5 | Knife, vaporization |
| Nd:YAG | 1064 | Near-infrared | Nonspecific | 5 | Multiple |
| Argon | 488 or 514 | Visible, blue | Melanin, Hgb | 1 | Coagulation |
| Dye | Variable (633)* | Visible (red)* | Photosensitizer | 2–15 | PDT |

* Kiton red and rhodamine B are commonly used dyes for PDT, both of which produce 633-nm red light.

Lastly, dye lasers consist of a stream of liquid dye that circulates across the beam of a pump laser. When the pump laser excites the liquid, it also lases. The wavelength produced is adjusted by changing the type of dye. The output is coupled to a fiberoptic device, allowing for delivery to any tissues. A common setup, and the one used at our institution, is an argon laser pumping a red dye (Kiton red or rhodamine B) that emits at 633 nm.[9] In this manner, either endogenous or exogenous photosensitizing agents can be activated for the purpose of photodynamic therapy (PDT).

## ESOPHAGEAL CANCER

Cure for esophageal cancer remains surgical; however, only 39% of patients are resectable.[10] Palliation of dysphagia is thus the goal for the majority of patients. The laser was first used for the palliation of esophageal cancer by Fleischer in 1982.[11] As a novel approach to a problem with no good solutions, laser ablation of esophageal cancers was heavily explored during the following decade. Several types of lasers have been used, including argon and Nd:YAG. Due to its versatility, fiberoptic capability for endoscopy, and deep tissue penetration, the Nd:YAG laser has proven to be superior and is currently the laser of choice for these lesions.[12–14] The technique of endoscopic laser recanalization of the esophagus has been well described.[12,13,15] Retrograde ablation of the tumor is the preferred method. This involves sequential vaporization of the tumor mass beginning at its most distal end, working in a circumferential manner until the proximal extent is reached. Since the esophageal lumen is often too narrow to allow distal passage of the scope, the tumor must be dilated first. This can be done with smaller scopes, including pediatric sizes; however, dilation over a guide wire is preferred. An adequate lumen for scope passage has also been established using biopsy forceps, although with added risk of perforation due to inability to judge the location of the potential lumen.[12] Failure or inability to create a lumen for retrograde ablation might lead one to perform a prograde recanalization, whereby the tumor is vaporized beginning at its proximal margin. False channels and perforations occur more frequently with this method.[13,16] Finally, the technical goal is to deobstruct, not to debulk. Failure to keep this in mind is likely to result in perforations or tracheoesophageal fistulas due to overaggressive destruction of esophageal wall.

The results of Nd:YAG laser palliation must be compared to previously established modes of palliation, namely surgery, radiation, and dilation. Relief of dysphagia following surgery occurs in 85% of patients.[17] Because of this high rate of success, surgery is still preferred for good-risk patients.[18] However, operation carries a mortality rate ranging from 7% to 30%,[10,15,16] with an average of 10% to 20%.[19] High morbidity is another problem, occurring in 41% of patients after esophageal resection and 57% after bypass, with dysphagia improving in 73% and 71% of patients, respectively.[16] External beam radiation improves dysphagia to a degree comparable to that of surgery[16,18]; however, considerable time is required for improvement to become manifest, and some patients may actually experience worsening dysphagia due to esophagitis. Although morbidity is 10%, approximately one-half of irradiated patients will subsequently require dilation procedures for recurrent symptoms.[20] Dilation as the sole means of palliation works very well, with 90% of patients experiencing improved swallowing.[21] Overall morbidity is approximately 8%, most of that occurring secondary to perforation, which is reported in 2% to 9% of patients.[21] The primary drawback of dilation is that relief is extremely short-lived, necessitating multiple procedures.[18] In one series, patients were dilated an average of 27 times.[21] This raises questions regarding the utility of this procedure for terminal patients whose comfort and quality of life should not be interrupted by frequent hospital visits.

The Nd:YAG laser was extensively studied in the 1980s as an alternative to these traditional techniques, and it was soon apparent that the laser is limited in terms of technical success, something that is not typically reported for other modalities. The ability to reestablish an esophageal lumen is not indicative of successful elimination of dysphagia.[22] Multiple reviews have established a technical success rate of 93% to 100% (average 95%),[13–16,23,24] with success usually defined as establishment of a lumen greater than 11 mm.[14] Successful treatment of dysphagia, defined by an improved score of at least 1 on a 4- to 6-point dysphagia scale,[15] is reported by 50% to 100% of patients (average 75%). Overall morbidity ranges from 2% to 10%, and mortality is 1% or less. Specific complications attributable to these figures include perforation (most commonly), as well as tracheoesophageal fistula, delayed hemorrhage, bacteremia and sepsis, and aspiration. Patients undergoing laser palliation require monthly follow-up, average 2.5 to 7.3 treatments each,[14,15] and experience dysphagia-free intervals lasting 6 to 11 weeks.[14,16] Although survival figures following laser ablation are frequently reported, these are often misleading given the palliative nature of the procedure. Despite initial criticism that laser technology is expensive and limited in availability, it is now deemed to be relatively cost effective given the fact that fewer procedures are necessary compared to dilation. For many, it has evolved into the treatment of choice for malignant dysphagia.[14]

The insertion of a rigid plastic stent across malignant esophageal strictures has been a widely accepted practice since the mid-1800s, especially when used to occlude a tracheoesophageal fistula.

However, when used for dysphagia, a high complication rate of up to 48% and a mortality up to 16%[12,15,18,25,26] has led to criticism. The most frequent and significant of these complications is perforation (2% to 15%), which likely is caused at least partially by the dilation required prior to insertion of the stent. Other complications include stent migration, tumor overgrowth, pressure necrosis, and hemorrhage.[27] Although long-lasting improvement in dysphagia can result, most agree that swallowing capability is limited to liquids and purees and cannot be normal given the narrow diameter of the stent lumen (approximately 11 mm). When rigid stenting was compared to the Nd:YAG laser in a prospective, randomized fashion,[28] complications were higher in the laser group, with 15% suffering a perforation, whereas there were none in the stented group. The laser did improve swallowing to a significantly greater extent, but at the expense of longer hospital stay and more procedures. The authors concluded that the two techniques are complementary.

The use of self-expanding metal stents is a more recent development, and appears to be replacing the use of traditional rigid plastic stents.[18] They are technically easier to insert, usually do not require prior dilation, and are able to expand to create a lumen up to 18 to 20 mm. Successful insertion thus approaches 100%, although 80% to 90% of patients report improved dysphagia.[18] The complication rate is also quite low at 0% to 9%, with perforations occurring in up to 9%.[26,29] The primary concerns regarding the metal stents are high cost and rapid tumor ingrowth, although this latter complication can be avoided by using a plastic-coated metal stent. The best study comparing metal stents to the Nd:YAG laser involved the prospective randomization of 60 patients who had received no prior palliation of any kind.[29] All patients were followed until death, with complications occurring in 5% of the laser group and 11% of the stent group, and with one death in each group. The stented patients, however, had a significantly greater improvement in their dysphagia, leading the authors to conclude that metal stents should be the preferred method of palliation. Others agree, stating the higher cost is outweighed by the low morbidity and mortality rates compared to plastic stents and by the better swallowing achieved compared to laser treatment.[30] Troublesome tumor ingrowth of an expandable stent can be treated with PDT.

## COLORECTAL CANCER

Laser technology has similarly been applied to colorectal cancers. Initial reports preferred the use of the $CO_2$ or argon laser because of their shallow depth of penetration, minimizing the risk of perforating an endoscopically dilated and thin-walled colon. As experience with the Nd:YAG laser has grown, it has become the laser most commonly used.[31] Primary indications for use of the laser are for the palliation of bleeding and/or obstructing tumors, ablation of adenomatous polyps, the primary treatment of early carcinomas in nonoperative candidates, and the diagnosis of dysplastic or neoplastic regions by laser-induced fluorescence. The technique used to treat obstruction is similar to that used for esophageal tumors, namely retrograde vaporization or coagulation following passage of the endoscope beyond the most proximal margin of the tumor. Although used for very tight lumens, the prograde approach is generally not preferred.

Symptoms amenable to laser palliation are bleeding and obstruction. Other symptoms such as pain and tenesmus have not responded as well to the laser, most likely because they are manifestations of extracolonic extension of the tumor. Successful control of bleeding is reported for 85% to 100% of patients, whereas obstruction is relieved in 86% to 97%.[14,23,31,32] Some reports quote an overall morbidity up to 19%,[31] but larger series generally accept a 2% to 3% morbidity rate and a mortality rate of 1% or less.[14,23,32] The most common complication is perforation, although early and delayed hemorrhage, abscess, fistula, and stenosis may also occur.

Comparison of laser treatment to surgical palliation is difficult. The laser has largely been restricted to use in those patients whose medical condition prohibits surgery or those who refuse surgery. Proponents of the laser state that surgery is associated with more complications (21%), greater mortality rate (2.5%), and higher cost,[16,32–34] leading one large series to conclude that the laser should be the palliative treatment of choice.[14] However, the outcome depends a lot on patient selection. Laser recanalization of an obstructing tumor can be used prior to surgical resection.[35,36] This allows for preoperative preparation of the colon and avoids a two-stage procedure involving a preliminary, decompressive colostomy. Mortality is zero following the laser procedure, and the perforation rate is less than 3.5%.

Another indication for laser surgery involves ablation of adenomatous polyps. Since laser ablation does not allow the submission of a specimen, multiple biopsies are required prior to the procedure for confirmation of the diagnosis. Despite having multiple biopsies, the major danger involved is missing an invasive carcinoma at the base of the polyp. Successful eradication of adenomas is accomplished in about 84% to 93% of patients, and is based upon a 38-month follow-up.[14,23,32] The success rate is better for adenomas less than 1 cm in diameter, but it is as low as 64% for those over 4 cm. Although the morbidity rate is very low, 1% to 5%, and the mortality rate approaches zero, the progression to invasive cancer ranges from 5.7% to 9.1% of patients. Because of the lack of a biopsy specimen, and because of the possibility of missing even one invasive tumor, laser ablation of sessile adenomas should be strictly limited to nonoperative candidates with small adenomas who have no other option.[32]

The laser is also being used for the primary treatment of early invasive carcinomas. Success in this arena arose from patients undergoing palliative laser treatment and were coincidentally found to be free of disease on subsequent biopsies.[32] One small series reported successful treatment of adenocarcinoma in 93.5% of patients based upon a 37-month follow-up.[37] All lesions were invasive, but none extended beyond the submucosal layer, as defined by endoscopic ultrasound or biopsy. Morbidity and mortality rates were both zero, and the 5-year survival rate was 62%, despite the poor medical condition of the patients. Naturally, only nonoperative patients would be candidates for this type of procedure.

An investigational application involves laser-induced fluorescence spectroscopy (LIF), which involves the endoscopic irradiation of tissue with low-intensity laser light from a helium, cadmium, argon, or dye laser. This induces tissue fluorescence, the intensity and spectrum of which is detected by the same optical probe that carries the laser beam. Different cellular properties or cellular architecture result in different spectra,[38] allowing for rapid differentiation between normal and dysplastic or neoplastic tissue. The initial use of

LIF on colonic tissue was able to differentiate normal mucosa from adenomatous polyps in 100% of the specimens tested.[39] Although this was an in vitro study, subsequent in vivo clinical work, using a blinded approach, has detected dysplasia with a sensitivity rate, specificity rate, and positive predictive value of 90%, 95%, and 90%, respectively.[40]

Advantages of LIF, aside from its reported accuracy, include the ability to identify areas of dysplasia or cancer that would otherwise not be able to be seen endoscopically, near instantaneous diagnosis, and the ability to perform guided rather than random biopsies. Fewer directed biopsies may result in lower endoscopy costs.[40,41] These readily apparent advantages and the impressive statistics reported must be weighed against the fact that the studies to date have largely focused on colonic polyps, which are usually readily visible at endoscopy and will still require histologic analysis. The future of LIF lies in detecting and guiding biopsies of regions housing invisible disease.[42] This would include monitoring for neoplastic transformation in patients with longstanding ulcerative colitis or Crohn's disease, Barrett's dysplasia, margins of a surgical resection, and anastomotic recurrences.

A technique similar to LIF that is currently under investigation is photodynamic diagnosis (PDD). Rather than relying on tissue autofluorescence, PDD requires the administration of a drug that is stimulated by the laser to fluoresce. Its primary advantage is the ability to couple it to PDT of the diagnosed lesion.[9,43] Side effects of the fluorescent drugs, which may include prolonged skin sensitivity to light, might preclude their use in patients undergoing simple diagnostic or screening procedures.

## INTERSTITIAL LASER HYPERTHERMIA

Laser treatment of tumors is not limited to cutaneous or endoscopically accessible lesions. Advances in fiberoptics have allowed for the treatment of solid organ tumors by inserting the laser fiber directly into the interstitium of the tumor.[8,44] Local hyperthermia generated at the fiber tip results in tumor coagulation and necrosis. Insertion of the fiber(s) can be done via an open or a percutaneous approach, the latter generally being preferred because it avoids the complications inherent in general anesthesia and open abdominal surgery. With either approach, proper fiber positioning within the tumor as well as the extent of hyperthermic injury must be closely monitored, preferably in real time, in order to prevent injury to surrounding normal tissue. Monitoring techniques include ultrasound,[45–49] color-coded duplex ultrasound,[8,50] computed tomographic (CT) scanning,[46,48,49] magnetic resonance imaging,[50,51] and thermistor probes,[47,49,52] alone or in combination. Repeat imaging over time, sometimes combined with biopsies, is performed to follow tumor regression (or progression).

Interstitial laser hyperthermia (ILH) has been applied in a variety of tumor locations; however, liver tumors, especially metastatic colorectal malignancy, have been the most widely studied. This is because they are easily imaged and readily accessible by percutaneous techniques. Since surgical resection remains the treatment of choice for hepatic metastases from colorectal cancer, only patients deemed unresectable have been candidates for ILH. Initial studies using real-time ultrasound (US) to visualize hyperthermic changes

during percutaneous treatment have shown a 44% tumor response rate documented by necrosis as seen on CT scan up to 6 months after treatment.[46] Partial responses of 82% have been reported, with 100% response for tumors under 3.5 cm in diameter.[48] Better success with smaller tumors has been reported elsewhere, with responses of 69% and 44% at 6 and 12 months, respectively, for lesions under 2.0 cm. Lesions over 2.0 cm showed 41% and 27% responses at 6 and 12 months, respectively.[51] Complications have been limited to mild pain and discomfort, with the exception of one study that reported subcapsular hematomas in 19% of patients and pleural effusions in 21%, although they were asymptomatic and discovered incidentally on follow-up scans.[48] Mortality rate approaches zero.[45,47–49,51,52] Unresectable pancreatic tumors have been another target for ILH, but reported complications of bile duct obstruction and fatal hemorrhagic pancreatitis, as well as fears of acute pancreatitis, fistula, and infection of necrosed pancreatic tissue have limited further attempts until the response of pancreatic tissue to hyperthermia is better studied.[46]

Comparison of ILH to other treatment modalities for hepatic metastasis from colorectal cancer is difficult since no comparative studies have been performed, and the current nonrandomized studies contain relatively few select patients with short follow-up. Nevertheless, it has been touted as superior to ethanol ablation because the diffusion of the ethanol through the tumor tissue is neither controllable nor predictable, and may be associated with significant pain.[45–47] Local intraarterial chemotherapy produces a response in 40% to 60% of patients, with questionable survival benefit and requires a laparotomy. Systemic chemotherapy has a lower response rate of 17% to 21%.[48,53–56] Cryoablation is a method that is growing in popularity and is closely related to ILH in that it allows for treatment under US guidance and real-time monitoring of tissue changes. Mean survival following cryotherapy ranges from 21 to 24 months,[57,58] but comparative trials with long-term follow-up are lacking. The biggest disadvantages of cryotherapy are the need for a laparotomy and specific complications such as myoglobinuria, renal failure, biliary fistula, hepatic hemorrhage, and hepatic abscess,[59,60] none of which have yet been reported following ILH. ILH holds promise not only for future palliation of hepatic metastases from colorectal cancer but also for cure. Cure is realistic once the extent of tumor necrosis can be matched closely to tumor volume.[46]

## BREAST CANCER

Considering current trends toward less invasive surgery and breast conservation, it is not surprising that the laser has surfaced as an option for breast cancer treatment. Laser use in this setting is primarily limited to aiding traditional dissections. However, other uses include wound sterilization for the prevention of local recurrence as well as primary treatment of small lesions by a percutaneous approach.[61]

The scalpel has been replaced by the laser (both the $CO_2$ and Nd:YAG) for performing all types of breast surgery, including simple biopsy, lumpectomy or segmentectomy, radical and modified radical mastectomy, and reconstructions. Proponents for laser dissection boast significantly less intraoperative bleeding, shorter operative time, fewer postoperative seromas, less pain, shorter hospitalization, earlier return to normal activities, and no complications when compared to scalpel dissection.[62,63] Similarly, others have reported decreased bleeding but found increased operative time and a seroma rate of 53%, paralleling that seen following scalpel dissection.[64] The only prospective, randomized study in this area compared the Nd:YAG laser and scalpel in performing modified radical mastectomy, using outcomes similar to previous studies.[65] The laser was found to result in significantly less intraoperative blood loss and in longer operative times. With all other outcomes being equal, the use of the laser for breast surgery was not recommended.

Laser proponents further argue that the wound should be sterilized following removal of the specimen.[61] This is performed by gently heating the margins of resection using a slightly defocused beam at a lower power setting, such that no vaporization or carbonization occurs. The resulting local thermal effect decreases the incidence of local tumor recurrence, as shown in animal models.[66] No good clinical evidence exists for this technique, and it cannot be recommended for use until prospective clinical trials compare its efficacy with that of established means of controlling local disease such as external beam radiation therapy.

Future laser breast surgery may involve the application ILH,[44] whereby a Nd:YAG laser fiber with a diffusing tip is percutaneously inserted into a solid tumor using radiographic (usually US) guidance. This technique has been shown to result in tumor necrosis in a small cohort of patients,[46] and models for the combination of ILH and stereotactic biopsy of small breast cancers are being developed.[67] This would allow for minimally invasive diagnosis and treatment of selected breast tumors, although not precluding the use of radiation or chemotherapy. If cost-effective, the treatment algorithm could potentially change in favor of ILH rather than lumpectomy prior to radiation.

## CAVITRON ULTRASONIC SURGICAL ASPIRATOR (CUSA)

The CUSA consists of an ultrasonic vibrating tip contained within a handpiece connected by an electrical cord to a control console. Vibration (oscillation) of the tip, which is a hollow titanium tube that moves longitudinally at a fixed rate of approximately 23,000 times per second,[68,69] is initiated by an alternating electric current passing through a coil around a transducer located in the handpiece. The maximal stroke of the oscillating (vibrating) tip is 308 $\mu$m, or 1/12,000 in[70] and is adjustable from 0 to 10 calibration (or 0% to 100% of maximal output). The resulting oscillatory mechanical motion fragments tissue as the cells implode.[71] The handpiece system combines this fragmentation with aspiration and irrigation. Suction pressure at the tip is adjustable from 0–610 mmHg. Aspiration is facilitated by irrigation, which serves as a diluent. It is supplied from the console and passes through a plastic flue surrounding the proximal portion of the titanium tip.[70] The control console contains a suction trap, the contents of which permits histologic confirmation of pathologic tissue using a variety of histologic techniques.[68,72,73]

The friction created by direct contact of the tissue with the vibrating tip transfers heat, which can be used to spontaneously cauterize small vessels (diameter less than 2 mm). However, hemostasis depends on the stroke length, time of tissue contact, and irrigation.[70] Increasing stroke length and greater time of contact increase heat generation, but irrigation has a cooling effect. Thus, effective hemostasis requires adjustment of these three factors. However, some irrigation must be supplied or a literal meltdown of the handpiece occurs. The bulky handpiece used in open abdominal applications is now available in a size suitable for laparoscopic surgery.[74,75]

The advantage of the CUSA is that the ultrasonic vibrations of the tip permit fragmentation of tissue in a precise manner. The precision of tissue fragmentation depends exclusively on the variation of the stroke, with a shorter stroke enabling more precise dissection. However, the efficiency of the instrument is related to the proportion of water content in the target tissue; there is relative sparing of collagen-rich tissues.[68] Larger vascular structures and the ureter, which are less water dense and more elastic, are less easily injured by the vibrating tip, providing that contact is superficial and brief. This permits isolation of major vessels (e.g., during liver resection) and dissection of metastatic adenocarcinoma, including lymph nodes, away from major vessels and ureters.[68] However, major bile ducts and the ureters are not immune from injury.[76,77]

There are also several disadvantages of the CUSA. Its rapidly oscillating tip with a short stroke fragments tissue in a radius of 1 to 2 mm,[78] and the volume of fragmentation is limited to 1 mL from the vibrating tip.[79] Thus, dissection of large tumor masses can be tedious and slow. The instrument also has limited value in removing dense fibrous tumors. Although suction removes most of the emulsion of tissue and irrigation fluid, some of the latter spills into the operative field. Experimental studies show that the fluid contains morphologically viable tumor cells,[72,80,81] a finding that is not significantly altered by CUSA settings at 40% or 100% of its maximal output.[80] A retrospective study suggests that the CUSA may be associated with an increased incidence of intraoperative development of disseminated intravascular coagulation (DIC) during cytoreductive surgery for ovarian cancer.[82] However, this was not substantiated by a prospective randomized study.[83] Tissue damage is not confined to the point of contact with the probe tip. Neural damage occurs within a 1-mL volume radius of the tip.[72,79,84,85]

The CUSA has been used in a variety of procedures, including the central nervous system, liver, spleen, pancreas, intestinal tract, kidney, neck, and gynecologic tract.[71,85,86] The instrument is rarely used alone in abdominal procedures but rather in conjunction with traditional methods for tumor excision. The instrument is useful as the primary means for dissection of hepatic substance during resection of small residual metastatic deposits, especially in debulking ovarian metastases.[87–89] A small prospective randomized study of ovarian cancer suggested that CUSA was more effective in cytoreduction by measuring $\alpha$ tumor marker (CA 125) but not by gross estimate of residual disease.[83] Most find the CUSA can be used to destroy ovarian metastatic deposits in almost any location (including splenic capsular metastases, intestinal serosa),[89,90] but others find argon beam coagulator more efficient for destruction of metastases on comparatively large surface areas such as diaphragm, liver, and mesentery.[90] The vibration setting generally has to be adjusted from patient to patient because of variations in tumor consistency. We find a stetting of 7 to 8 to be most applicable for adenocarcinomas in any location and for liver resections.

The CUSA can be particularly helpful during hepatic resection because it facilitates definition of major hepatic veins. However, use of the CUSA is more tedious than the finger fracture method. The consistency of a cirrhotic liver renders the CUSA less effective.[91] A canine study of liver resection concluded that CUSA was better than Nd:YAG laser and standard blunt dissection for delineation of blood vessels and bile ducts and caused significantly less tissue damage.[92] We also find the CUSA advantageous in debriding necrotic tumors, especially those adherent to retroperitoneal structures.

Blood loss using the CUSA may be less than what is lost during standard resectional approaches. Whether or not the CUSA decreases blood loss compared to finger fracture during hepatectomy is controversial.[78,93,94] Significantly less blood loss has also been reported during cytoreductive surgery for ovarian cancer, but the difference amounted to 200 mL.[83] In the same study, the number of operative organ injuries was not significantly different in the absence of using the CUSA, but it is unclear how many of the injuries were a result of the CUSA or standard operative approach.

## PHOTODYNAMIC THERAPY

Photodynamic therapy (PDT) is a relatively new and potentially important form of primary and adjuvant treatment for a variety of cancers. Treatment initially involves the preferential accumulation of a photosensitizing compound by malignant tissue. A suitable photodynamic sensitizer exhibits no spontaneous toxicity until excited by a wavelength of light corresponding to one of its absorbance band(s). Excitation of the photosensitizer leads to cellular destruction, primarily mediated by singlet oxygen.[9,95–101] This form of molecular oxygen is toxic and results in both direct tumor cell kill as well as lethal effects due to vascular occlusion.[102,103]

A number of reports indicate that PDT is effective in treating malignant tumors in experimental animals. There also are an increasing number of reports describing the use of PDT for the treatment of human tumors, including carcinoma of the oral cavity, esophagus, stomach, rectum, biliary tract, tracheobronchial tree, lung, skin, breast, brain, bladder, female genital tract, Kaposi's sarcoma, retroperitoneal sarcomas, mesothelioma, and carcinomatosis of the peritoneal cavity.[95,104–119] However, many of these reports are anecdotal and/or preliminary.

Advantages of PDT include the low incidence of side effects; tumor responsiveness does not appear to be compromised by previous treatment with x-radiation and/or chemotherapy; treatment does not preclude the subsequent use of x-ray therapy and/or chemotherapy, and treatment can be repeated in multiple successive sessions. Furthermore, photosensitizing agents are fluorescent, so that tumor localization is also feasible with a suitable imaging system.[43,120]

## PHOTOSENSITIZATION

Photosensitization of tumors is accomplished by either an exogenous or endogenous means. The exogenous approach involves administration of a photoreactive compound intravenously and relies on selective uptake of the drug by the target tissue, or tumor. With endogenous photosensitization, the target tissue converts a "precursor drug" into a photoreactive compound.

## EXOGENOUS PHOTOSENSITIZERS

**HPD/PHOTOFRIN.** Although demonstrations of tumor localization by porphyrins had been previously made, the modern era of PDT was initiated by Dougherty and associates[99] with their 1975 report of efficacy of the photosensitizer hematoporphyrin derivative (HPD), an unstable mixture of porphyrins derived from hematoporphyrin. HPD is a mixture of porphyrin monomers and higher oligomers joined by ether and ester linkages.[121–123] All of these porphyrins are potent photosensitizers in cell-free systems except for hematoporphyrin, which is too hydrophilic to cross cell membranes.[124] The monomers can photosensitize intact cells, but are either insufficiently selective or persist for such a short time that they are essentially inactive in vivo. The active ingredients in HPD consist of the dimeric and trimeric porphyrin esters and ethers, with sec-OH or vinyl groups on the periphery.[125]

More recently, a uniform and stable form of HPD has become available, Photofrin, a somewhat purified proprietary preparation of HPD. Photofrin is an effective photosensitizer but has the undesirable side effect of prolonged cutaneous photosensitization. This requires keeping patients out of sunlight or bright incandescent lighting for as long as 4 to 6 weeks or more after receipt of the drug. Moreover, the efficiency of conversion of light to cytotoxic products is low, the degree of tumor localization is inferior to that obtained with some of the newer sensitizers, and the wavelength of light required can only penetrate tissue to about 1 cm depth.[126,127] Photofrin, which is activated by red light (630 nm) has been approved for specific clinical procedures by government regulatory groups in the United States, Canada, Netherlands, and Japan.

A number of newer sensitizers have been formulated with a view toward minimizing instability and persistent skin photosensitization, and to provide a more efficient conversion of light to cytotoxic products at wavelengths that offer better tissue penetration (i.e., agents with high extinction coefficients at wavelengths >650 nm). It is not yet clear just how much more tumor depth kill occurs with the longer wavelengths of light[128] corresponding to the absorbance bands of second-generation photosensitizers [chlorins, purpurins, tetra(m-hydroxyphenyl)chlorin, phthalocyanines, benzoporphyrins, texaphyrins].

**CHLORINS.** The chlorins are porphyrins with one reduced double bond, resulting in a substantially greater absorbance at a wavelength farther in the red, so that tissue penetration of light is enhanced. To date, the bulk of clinical studies have been carried out with NPe6, an aspartyl derivative of chlorin-e6. This agent has proved efficacious in clinical trials, and animal toxicity studies are complete.[129]

**PURPURINS.** The tin etiopurpurin SnET2 has a substantial absorbance band at 660 nm, so that its efficacy will be greater than that of the porphyrins.[130,131] SnET2 is weakly soluble in water and needs formulation via liposomes or in an emulsion. Canine studies indicate that this agent may also be useful for photodynamic treatment of prostate cancer and prostatic hypertrophy.[132]

**m-THPC.** Tetra(m-hydroxyphenyl)chlorin (m-THPC) exhibits a large extinction coefficient in the near infrared region and appears to be a very potent PDT sensitizer. Preclinical studies indicate that the substantial absorbance of the drug results in a very effective agent that can yield tumor eradication in experimental animals using very low drug and light doses.[133,134]

PHTHALOCYANINES. The phthalocyanine structure is a modification of the porphyrin skeleton, with N atoms in the bridges joining the four heterocyclic components; this results in enhanced long-wavelength absorbance. The phthalocyanines are commonly used as dyes, notably in ballpoint pen inks. There is a substantial literature on the phthalocyanines and a related series of compounds, the naphthalocyanines. The latter have even longer absorbance bands and values as high as 800 nm have been reported. Because of the very high extinction coefficients in the red, some phthalocyanines are extremely potent PDT agents.[135,136]

BENZOPORPHYRINS. This agent shows absorbance at 690 nm, where there is a window between the absorbance of hemoglobin and that of water. Benzoporphyrin D has been the subject of a series of preclinical tests against different animal tumor systems and is undergoing clinical trials. Like Sn etiopurpurin 2, there are formulation problems because of poor water solubility.[137]

TEXAPHYRINS. An expanded porphyrin structure, termed texaphyrins, has recently been described and is stabilized by insertion of a lanthanide in the center of the ring system. One such product, bearing a lutetium atom, has a strong absorbance at 732 nm and can be used to treat successfully a variety of experimental animal tumors.[138,139] If a gadolinium atom is inserted into the texaphyrin ring, the resulting product can be used to enhance magnetic resonance imaging of neoplastic tissues.[140]

## ENDOGENOUS PHOTOSENSITIZATION

The only current means of endogenous photosensitization involves the oral administration of 5-aminolevulinic acid (ALA), which is absorbed into the bloodstream and converted by cellular enzymes to protoporphyrin IX (PpIX). ALA is a naturally occurring amino acid and is the first committed intermediate in the heme biosynthetic pathway located in mitochondria.[141,142] ALA per se is not a photosensitizer but rather its end product, PpIX, is photoreactive.

Heme inhibits the activity of ALA synthase, the first and rate-limiting enzyme of the PpIX biosynthetic pathway, thereby preventing normal cells from drowning in excess production of its own porphyrins. This negative-feedback control can be bypassed in certain types of malignant cells exposed to an excess amount of ALA, which is continuously metabolized, leading to an overproduction of PpIX (Fig. 5D-1). Excess accumulation of PpIX occurs because of the enzyme makeup of certain malignant cells. The enzyme ferrochelatase catalyzes the insertion of an iron atom into PpIX. This

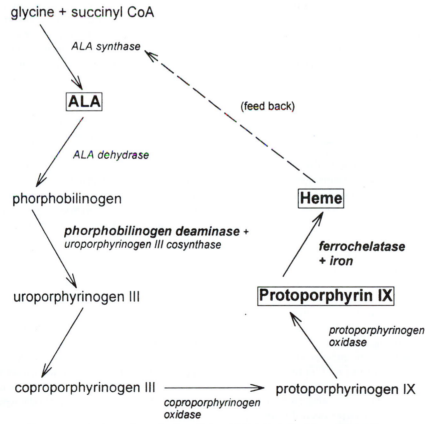

**FIGURE 5D-1.** Pathway for aminolevulinic acid (ALA)–induced synthesis of protoporphyrin IX. (*From Webber J et al, reproduced with permission from the publisher.*)

forms heme, which is not photoreactive. However, cancer cells have a relatively low activity of ferrochelatase,[143–147] which leads to an excess accumulation of PpIX. Another factor leading to augmented PpIX synthesis is the increased activity of the rate-limiting enzyme porphobilinogen deaminase in various malignant tissues.[95,151–153] Furthermore, hepatic synthesis of PpIX from ALA is quite efficient, and it is likely that there is subsequent transport of PpIX by the bloodstream to peripheral sites. PpIX is activated by a wavelength of light identical to Photofrin.

## MODES OF TUMOR LOCALIZATION

Based on reports that photosensitizers show affinity for circulating low-density lipoprotein (LDL) and those indicating that neoplastic cells often exhibit high levels of surface LDL receptors, it was proposed that LDL-directed localization was a major mechanism of photosensitizer localization.[118–120] This theory could also explain the concentration of many sensitizers in normal tissues with high receptor levels: adrenal cortex, liver, spleen, sites of wound-healing, and embryonic tissues. However, later evidence indicated that the LDL-mediated localization hypothesis could not explain many examples of sensitizer biodistribution.[121,154]

PDT is effective in the treatment of rodent,[99] dog, and cat tumors,[154,155] species with substantially higher high-density lipoprotein (HDL) levels, and lower LDL levels than humans. However, many effective sensitizers show little or no capacity for LDL binding, and instead prefer HDL and/or albumin (e.g., NPe6, SnET2, and the texaphyrins). There may be HDL receptors on tumor cell surfaces, or other hitherto unknown factors. It has been proposed that tumor-associated macrophages may play an important role in the accumulation of sensitizers that tend to aggregate in plasma or become bound to large macromolecules that are engulfed by these cells.[123]

## PHOTOACTIVATION

Upon irradiation of cells containing a photosensitizer with a specific wavelength of light corresponding to an absorbance maximum of the sensitizer, the electronic configuration of the sensitizer is raised to a higher energy level, or excited state. This excess energy can be converted to heat, to fluorescence emission, or via an intersystem crossing to the triplet state from which energy can be transferred to oxygen in tissues. This results in the formation of singlet molecular oxygen, a highly reactive, short-lived (half life = $10^{-6}$ s) cytotoxic agent.[151–158] The latter reacts with amino acids, unsaturated fatty acids, and nucleic acids, resulting in cell damage.[95] Other reactive oxygen species can be formed (superoxide, hydrogen peroxide, and the hydroxyl radical),[159–161] but PDT effects on tumor tissue appear to be mediated largely by singlet oxygen.[161,162] The yield of singlet oxygen depends on the oxygen concentration in the tissues.[163] Isolated cells are completely insensitive to PDT in the absence of oxygen.[163]

The light source most frequently used to activate a photosensitizer is a laser, not only because of its sharply defined wavelength, but also because the light bundle of a laser shows little divergence, making it possible to focus sharply. Specific laser photoactivation of

sensitized cells acts like a switch to activate the sensitizer rather than photocoagulation or photothermal ablation (vaporization).[164,165] The optimal dose of light used to activate a photosensitizer in human cancers is not known and consideration of this issue is complex. Light dose is expressed as the delivered quantity in joules per square centimeter ($J/cm^2$), but the absorbed dose depends on the spectrum of the light source, irradiation geometry, depth of penetration, light scattering in the tissue, concentration of the photosensitizer in the tissue, hemorrhage within the tumor, as well as other factors,[127,166] making the absorbed dose difficult to calculate.

The PDT response is dependent on both the drug concentration and the light dose (conc × $J/cm^2$).[135,167–169,136] A threshold PDT dose must be exceeded for necrosis to occur. Since photosensitizers are degraded (bleached) by light, a weaker response occurs at low drug concentrations. In order to obtain a PDT response at lower cellular drug concentrations, the light exposure must be increased. If a proper photosensitizer dose is used, then differential uptake by tumor should allow destruction of tumor and protection of normal tissue even at very high light doses because the level of photosensitizer in normal tissue would be below the photodynamic threshold for necrosis.[170] Thus there are at least three variables: degradation of the sensitizer (bleaching), differential tissue uptake, and threshold effects.

## MECHANISM OF CELLULAR INJURY

The oxidative injury mediated by PDT involves various subcellular targets. PDT increases the expression of stress proteins and heme-oxygenase (a rate-limiting enzyme in heme metabolism) as well as the release or increased production of eicosanoids, tumor necrosis factor, interleukins, serotonin, and histamine.[102,103,170,171] Depending on the photosensitizer used, PDT can affect mitochondria and lysosomes, but lysosomal hydrolases are inactivated by photochemical treatment before escaping the lysosomal compartment.[172] Photodamage can also be detected at the plasma and endoplasmic reticulum (ER) membranes, and can affect DNA, resulting in the rapid initiation of apoptosis.[103,173–180] Photofrin appears to mediate oxidative stress through protein kinase–mediated signal transduction pathway(s) to activate early-response genes.[181] ALA-induced porphyrin formation is more specifically localized to the mitochondria of certain types of normal and malignant cells in laboratory animals, and this includes mitochondria of endothelial cells of tumor tissue.[143] However, various photosensitizers act differently as a result of different patterns of intracellular localization of the sensitizers,[103] since singlet oxygen reacts at its sites of origin. The subcellular distribution of sensitizers has been studied mainly in in vitro systems, although it has been proposed that patterns of biodistribution matter little with respect to in vivo effectiveness.[102] A substantial fraction of PpIX in cells incubated with ALA is bound to proteins. During light exposure these binding sites are destroyed and PpIX molecules appear to move to different binding sites believed to be more vital for cell survival. Photodamage induced at these new binding sites is more lethal for cells than photodamage at the primary binding sites.[182]

Eventual vessel occlusion seems to be a general phenomenon associated with PDT using Photofrin.[102] The time frame for a decrease in blood levels is variable, ranging from within 10 s to 10 min in experimental tumors.[183,184] It is not clear if this range is due to characteristics of the specific tumor model and/or technical features related to the application of PDT. Nevertheless, phototoxicity from Photofrin appears to involve the destruction of the tumor vasculature, an effect that appears to be selective, even in regions of tumor where the photosensitizer concentration is similar to that in normal adjacent tissue.[103] Thus, the effect of Photofrin may be mainly an indirect one, derived from the destruction of the tumor vasculature.[185] Vascular destruction itself, without any contribution from direct tumor cell kill, can lead to cures of experimental tumors. Given the importance of oxygen availability on phototoxicity, the rapid formation of hypoxic cells resulting from vascular damage increases the likelihood that some tumor cells will escape direct photodestruction.[186,187] If a photodynamic agent has primarily vascular effects, there is a theoretical disadvantage of hypoxic, but still viable, cells persisting at the interface of necrotic regions and surrounding well-perfused regions.[188]

A proposed advantage of chemically induced porphyria with ALA is that the phototoxic effect relies primarily on direct cell kill, whereas other photosensitizing agents appear to rely more on vascular effects.[164,189–191] However, it is becoming apparent that ALA has definite vascular effects, but the data are difficult to compare because of the number of confounding technical variables involved in these studies. For example, the vascular effects are related to the duration and intensity of the light source used to activate PpIX derived from ALA.[192] Adding to the controversy are magnetic resonance spectroscopic studies suggesting that direct cellular damage from PDT per se occurs well before the changes observed with tumor hypoxia, which usually occur later and are mostly attributable to vascular damage.[193] If this is the case, it suggests that cellular destruction caused by PDT occurs by a dual synergistic mechanism.

Reports that PDT could rapidly induce apoptosis, both in vitro[174,194] and in vivo,[195] have provided new information on phototoxicity. Malignant cell types often exhibit an impaired ability to undergo apoptosis, an effect associated with an enhanced ability to survive chemotherapy with many common antitumor agents.[197–199] The apoptotic response to these drugs may determine whether or not cell death will occur.[200] If apoptosis is a primary mode of phototoxicity, the broad responsiveness pattern of PDT suggests that PDT induces apoptosis in almost any cell, perhaps at such a stage that circumvents survival signals.[196]

## PDT EFFECTS ON NORMAL TISSUE

Photosensitizers are not completely specific for malignant tissue. As a result, there will always be some photosensitization of normal tissues. In the case of ALA, this effect is mainly caused by the relatively slow conversion of PpIX to heme. However, photodestruction can be avoided by relying on bleaching of the photosensitizer. Most sensitizers undergo rapid photobleaching; upon irradiation, they catalyze formation of singlet oxygen that can destroy both malignant cells and sensitizers. A low concentration of a photosensitizer can be photobleached before the photodynamic threshold for tissue damage occurs. This phenomenon makes it possible to "overdose" the treatment field to get maximum light penetration without causing serious damage to normal tissue. However, malignant cells will only be destroyed if sufficient sensitizer accumulates so that there is a loss of viability before photobleaching can reduce the sensitizer concentration to a nontoxic level.[135,142,163,168,170] Thus, an efficient photosensitizer will have a much greater concentration in the target tissue compared to surrounding normal tissue in order to avoid significant damage to the latter.

## TIME OF PDT APPLICATION

There is greater flexibility in the timing of PDT treatment with exogenously administered photosensitizers because they do not require conversion by the target tissue into a photoreactive substance. For example, it is recommended that primary application of PDT using Photofrin be done 40 to 50 hr after administration of the drug and secondary application can be done 96 to 120 hr after injection. In contrast, endogenous photosensitization, for example with ALA, relies on tumor synthesis of the photoreactive substance and the time of peak accumulation varies among patients.[201] Thus, a very practical issue is knowing when the concentration of PpIX in the target tissue reaches not only a sufficient level for PDT to be effective but also a level substantially greater than the surrounding normal tissue. Actual tissue concentrations of PpIX after administration of ALA indicate that the time of peak PpIX levels occurring in both normal and malignant tissues can vary by several hours among patients.[201] The importance of this observation is that it may explain why some adenocarcinomas of the gastrointestinal tract appear to be unresponsive to PDT using ALA.[101] Serial measurements of actual PpIX tissue concentrations prior to PDT treatment are impractical because of the involved time for such determinations. However, advantage can be taken of the fact that photosensitizers fluoresce. PpIX fluoresces to a salmon pink color in response to blue light. In humans, it has been shown that more than 96% of fluorescing porphyrin after administration of ALA is PpIX.[108,202]

Gross visualization of porphyrin fluorescence does not always correlate with the actual tissue concentrations.[203] This is related to tissue pigmentation, fluorescence quenching, and the lack of quantitative sensitivity of the human eye. However, changes in tissue concentrations of PpIX can be quantitated in humans by applying spectrophotometric methodology.[108] The advantage of the latter is that it offers a practical means for determining the most favorable time for starting PDT because relative changes in fluorescent signals correlate with changes in tissue concentrations of PpIX.[108] Spectrophotometric detection of peak Photofrin levels in tissue is impractical because this agent consists of several porphyrins and the specific active species in Photofrin is controversial.[204]

It is not yet known if the ratios between tumor and normal tissue concentrations can be improved in humans with intravenously administered ALA, although experimental studies show that the temporal kinetics of either oral or intravenous administration are similar.[202] Presently, oral intake of ALA by patients is preferable to intravenous administration because the latter requires buffering to avoid adverse side effects. ALA is also poorly soluble in water and is chemically unstable at pH 7.4. However, there are several experimental ways to increase PpIX synthesis in response to ALA,[117,166] which may ultimately become clinically applicable. Among potential vehicles for drug delivery are liposomes, oil emulsion systems, lipoproteins, and monoclonal antibody conjugates.[109] Intravenous administration of pure PpIX is also presently impractical because PpIX is only slightly soluble in water at physiologic pH.[142]

## LIMITATIONS OF PDT

The major limiting factor in using PDT is the depth of tumor kill. The depth of penetration of 630-nm light (used for Photofrin and ALA) in tissue ranges from 0.2 to 2 cm.[103,110,117,205,206] The mean depth of destruction of rectal and sigmoid adenocarcinomas in patients receiving Photofrin amounts to 0.6 cm with a range of 0.3 to 1.5 cm following intraluminal insertion of an optical fiber 1 mm into the tumor.[207] Among factors that limit light penetration are the presence of blood clot and necrosis within the tumor and absorption of light by the photosensitizer itself (a phenomenon called "self-shielding"). Precise depths of tumor destruction are difficult to determine because of sloughing, and the actual extent of destruction may be variable due to the effects of PDT on blood flow. However, given the relatively small extent of tumor destruction, it appears that the main benefit of PDT at present for tumors may be fourfold.

1. Local control of microscopic deposits remaining after what appears to be a curative resection.
2. Removal of relatively small deposits remaining after debulking surgery
3. Primary treatment for small lesions
4. Palliative treatment.

More promising are newer experimental photoreactive agents that are sensitive to longer wavelengths of light (>660 nm). This will result in deeper tissue penetration than the 630- to 633-nm wavelength required to activate Photofrin and PpIX, but just how much greater depth of tumor kill may result is unclear. The therapeutic depth may in fact be greater than the depth of light penetration, a phenomenon that may relate to additional vascular injury.[208]

Another limitation is the expense not only of purchase but also maintenance of the equipment (especially lasers) necessary to apply PDT. However, as photodiode technology advances to the point that more powerful sources are available, the equipment costs will lessen. Although photodiodes do not have sharply defined wavelengths as lasers, this may be of some advantage. For example, activation of PpIX results in the formation of a photoproduct, photoprotoporphyrin, which is photoreactive at a wavelength around 670 nm.[209] This and the 630-nm absorbance band could be incorporated within photodiode wavelengths.

## TOXICITY OF PHOTOSENSITIZERS

The toxicity of PDT is site-specific and dependent upon the organ being irradiated and the selectivity of the photosensitizer for target tissue over normal tissue. However, there are also reactions related to the sensitizer per se that are independent of those related to the treatment site. A universal and clinically important adverse effect of

PDT is skin photosensitization that can lead to sunburns.[106] Most photosensitizing agents are not concentrated in the skin per se, but low concentrations can be found in the skin for several weeks. For example, Photofrin cannot be bleached sufficiently to achieve photoprotection of the skin.[210] Although the mean duration of photosensitization following Photofrin injection is 4 to 6 weeks, Photofrin can be found in human serum 1 year or more after administration.[211] It is not known if this is associated with any risk. In contrast, ALA-induced PpIX is almost completely cleared from human plasma by 48 hr after oral administration.[201] An occasional patient has been reported to develop mild cutaneous phototoxicity as late as 48 hr after receiving ALA.[212] Cutaneous phototoxic reactions in patients taking ALA can be avoided by exposure to only subdued light for 48 hr, preventing more than momentary exposure to photodiode monitors (e.g., a pulse oximeter)[213] and filtering operating room lights to prevent nonspecific photoactivation of PpIX.[201] Oral intake of ALA causes mild nausea or vomiting in almost a quarter as well as transient and variable abnormalities of liver "function" tests in about a third of patients.

## APPLICATION OF PRINCIPALS OF PDT TO TUMOR DETECTION

Excitation of a photosensitizer by an incident photon produces re-emission of a fluorescent photon, which can be used to localize the reaction.[106] This might enable detection of metastases not ordinarily evident.[105] There appears to be a correlation between the presence of local tumor and local fluorescence. Success has been reported in examining potential treatment fields exposed to Photofrin using UV light.[105,112,142] Gross detection of fluorescence using UV light works with Photofrin and ALA-induced PpIX, but this requires subjective assessment using the eye, and the UV spectrum does not include the peak excitation wavelength (410 nm) of PpIX.[214] More sensitive detection of PpIX can be accomplished in patients using spectrophotofluorometric technology using specific excitation wavelengths.[43] Application of this principle may ultimately lead to a relatively simple method for detecting tumor spread and directing site-specific, rather than random, biopsies in order to more accurately determine the stage of the tumor. However, the intensity of the fluorescent signal produced from tissue containing PpIX is affected by several variables, which include blood flow, desmoplasia, pigment distribution, and keratin thickness.[43]

## CURRENT STATE

The clinical use of PDT is still very much in its infancy. The majority of treated tumors respond with unpredictable depths of necrosis using a variety of photosensitizers. Apparent complete responses and palliation with variable short-term follow-up have been reported for a variety of tumors involving the head and neck,[215,216] gastrointestinal tract,[212,217–224] urinary bladder,[225,226] respiratory tract,[224,227] extrahepatic bile ducts,[228] brain,[208] skin,[229–232] and accessible metastases from breast cancer.[113,233] In a review of 34 reports involving skin tumors and those of the head and neck, brain, eye, lung and bronchus, esophagus, stomach, urinary bladder, and gynecologic organs with variable follow-up, complete responses ranged from 10% to 100%.[234] As the sole modality of treatment, PDT is currently limited to tumors only a few millimeters thick.[113,212,229] PDT also has been reported to be of benefit in palliation of obstructing esophageal and bronchial tumors.[113,212,219–222,224] A small randomized trial of PDT and Nd:YAG laser treatment of esophageal cancer found that a greater duration of response followed PDT.[220] PDT has also been variously successful in the treatment of Barrett's dysplasia of the esophagus,[224,235,236] which appears to preferentially accumulate PpIX following ALA administration.[236] Despite its success, PDT is not without complications related to the field of treatment. Hemorrhage may occur after treatment of gastrointestinal tumors.[207,220] Fistulas, pleural effusion, fever, fibrosis of the urinary tract, dysuria, urgency, interstitial cystitis, bladder contracture, and esophageal stricture are among other reported complications.[108,212,223–226,235,237–239]

PDT is clearly effective for small cancers, but it is not known if such treatment is any more effective than other currently acceptable approaches. As data from current and future clinical trials become available, a clearer perspective of just where PDT fits in the treatment of cancers will occur. Many issues regarding pharmacokinetic data of photosensitizers, newer technology involved in light sources, optimal treatment regimens that take advantage of the pharmacophysiology of photoablation and light dosimetry still require solution. One can foresee application of differing sensitizers and light sources depending upon the specific clinical situation.

## REFERENCES

1. EINSTEIN A: Zur quantentheorie der strahlung. Physiol Z 18:121, 1917.
2. ARNOFF BL, JUDY MM: Lasers in oncology, in *Fundamentals of Surgical Oncology,* RJ McKenna, GP Murphy (eds). New York, Macmillan, 1986, pp 955–964.
3. FULLER TA: Fundamentals of lasers in surgery and medicine, in *Surgical Application of Lasers,* 2d ed, JA Dixon (ed). Chicago, Year Book, 1987, pp 16–33.
4. ——— Fundamentals of laser surgery, in *Surgical Lasers—A Clinical Guide,* TA Fuller (ed). New York, Macmillan, 1987, pp 1–17.
5. MAIMAN TH: Stimulated optical radiation in ruby. Nature 187:493, 1960.
6. GOLDMAN L: Treatment of port wine marks by an argon laser. J Dermatol 2:385, 1972.
7. JAKO GJ: Laser surgery of the vocal cords. Laryngoscope 82:2204, 1972.
8. PHILIPP CM et al: Nd:YAG laser procedures in tumor treatment. Semin Surg Oncol 11:290, 1995.
9. FROMM D: Feasibility of photodynamic therapy using endogenous photosensitization for colon cancer. Arch Surg 131:667, 1996.
10. EARLAM R, CUNHA-MELO JR: Oesphageal squamous cell carcinoma: A critical review of surgery. Br J Surg 67:381, 1980.
11. FLEISCHER D et al: Endoscopic Nd:YAG laser therapy for carcinoma of the esophagus: A new palliative approach. Am J Surg 143:280, 1982.

12. KLASS A: Lasers in diseases of the digestive tract, in *Surgical Lasers—A Clinical Guide,* TA Fuller (ed). New York, Macmillan, 1987, pp 170–193.
13. OVERHOLT BF: Laser and photodynamic therapy of esophageal cancer. Semin Surg Oncol 8:191, 1992.
14. SPINELLI P et al: Endoscopic treatment of gastrointestinal tumors: Indications and results of laser photocoagulation and photodynamic therapy. Semin Surg Oncol 11:307, 1995.
15. NARAYAN S, SIVAK MV: Palliation of esophageal carcinoma—Laser and photodynamic therapy. Chest Surg Clin N Amer 4:347, 1994.
16. QUINTON A, LAMOULIATTE H: Laser applications in gastrointestinal cancer, in *Gastrointestinal Oncology,* JD Ahlgren, JS MacDonald (eds). Philadelphia, JB Lippincott, 1992, pp 593–605.
17. ELLIS H JR: Cancer of the esophagus and cardia: Role of surgery in palliation. Postgrad Med 75:139, 1984.
18. KHANDELWAL M: Palliative therapy for carcinoma of the esophagus. Comprehensive Ther 21:177, 1995.
19. MULLER JM et al: Surgical therapy of esophageal carcinoma. Br J Surg 77:845, 1990.
20. EARLAM R, CUNHA-MELO JR: Oesphageal squamous cell carcinoma: A critical review of radiotherapy. Br J Surg 67:457, 1980.
21. MOSES FM et al: Palliative dilation of esophageal carcinoma. Gastrointest Endosc 31:61, 1985.
22. MELLOW MH, PINKAS H: Endoscopic therapy for esophageal cancer with Nd:YAG laser: Prospective evaluation of efficacy, complications, survival. Gastrointest Endosc 30:334, 1984.
23. SPINELLI P et al: Current role of laser and photodynamic therapy in gastrointestinal tumors and analysis of a 10-year experience. Semin Surg Oncol 8:204, 1992.
24. MACIEL J et al: Nd:YAG laser as a palliative treatment for malignant dysphagia. Eur J Surg Oncol 22:69, 1996.
25. HAHL J et al: Comparison of endoscopic Nd:YAG laser therapy and oesophageal tube in palliation of oaesophagogastric malignancy. Scand J Gastroenterol 26:103, 1991.
26. KNYRIM K et al: A controlled trial of an expansile metal stent for palliation of esophageal obstruction due to inoperable cancer. N Engl J Med 329:1302, 1993.
27. MEHRAN RJ, DURANCEAU A: The use of endoprosthesis in the palliation of esophageal carcinoma. Chest Surg Clin North Am 4:331, 1994.
28. CARTER R et al: Laser recanalization versus endoscopic intubation in the palliation of malignant dysphagia: A randomized prospective study. Br J Surg 79:1167, 1992.
29. ADAM A et al: Palliation of inoperable esophageal carcinoma: A prospective randomized trial of laser therapy and stent placement. Radiology 202:344, 1997.
30. STURGESS RP, MORRIS AI: Metal stents in the esophagus. Gut 37:593, 1995.
31. ENDRES JC, STEINHAGEN RM: Lasers in anorectal surgery. Surg Clin North Am 74:1415, 1994.
32. BRUNETAUD JM et al: Lasers in rectosigmoid tumors. Semin Surg Oncol 11:319, 1995.
33. MELLOW MH: Endoscopic laser therapy as an alternative to palliative surgery for adenocarcinoma of the rectum—comparison of costs and complications. Gastrointest Endosc 35:283, 1989.
34. BRUNETAUD JM et al: Endoscopic laser treatment for rectosigmoid villous adenoma-factors affecting the results. Gastroenterology 97:272, 1989.
35. KIEFHABER P et al: Preoperative neodynium-YAG laser treatment of obstructive colon cancer. Endoscopy 18(Suppl 1):44, 1986.

36. Eckhauser ML et al: The role of pre-resectional laser recanalization for obstructing carcinomas of the colon and rectum. Surgery 106:710, 1989.

37. Mathus-Vliegen EMH. Laser ablation of early colorectal malignancy. Endoscopy 25:462, 1993.

38. Römer TJ et al: Laser-induced fluorescence microscopy of normal colon and dysplasia in colonic adenomas: implications for spectroscopic diagnosis. Am J Gastroenterol 90:81, 1995.

39. Kapadia CR et al: Laser-induced spectroscopy of human colonic mucosa. Gastroenterology 99:150, 1990.

40. Cothren RM et al: Detection of dysplasia at colonoscopy using laser-induced fluorescence: A blinded study. Gastrointest Endosc 44:168, 1996.

41. Bohorfoush AG: Tissue spectroscopy for gastrointestinal diseases. Endoscopy 28:372, 1996.

42. Van Dam J: Laser-induced fluorescence spectroscopy: Somewhere over the rainbow. Gastroenterology 110:643, 1996.

43. Webber J et al: On-line fluorescence of human tissues after oral administration of 5-aminolevulinic acid. J Photochem Photobiol B:Biology 38:209, 1997.

44. Bown SG. Phototherapy of tumors. World J Surg 7:700, 1983.

45. Steger AC et al: Interstitial laser hyperthermia: A new approach to local destruction of tumors. Br Med J 299:362, 1989.

46. Masters A, Bown SG: Interstitial laser hyperthermia. Semin Surg Oncol 8:242, 1992.

47. Nols e CP et al: Interstitial hyperthermia of colorectal liver metastases with a US-guided Nd:YAG laser with a diffuser tip: A pilot clinical study. Radiology 187:333, 1993.

48. Amin Z et al: Hepatic metastases: Interstitial laser photocoagulation with real-time US monitoring and dynamic CT evaluation of treatment. Radiology 187:339, 1993.

49. Tranberg KG et al: Interstitial laser treatment of malignant tumors: Initial experience. Eur J Sur Oncol 22:47, 1996.

50. Saxton RE et al: Laser photochemotherapy: A less invasive approach for treatment of cancer. Semin Surg Oncol 11:283, 1995.

51. Vogl TJ et al: Malignant liver tumors treated with MR imaging-guided laser-induced thermotherapy: Technique and prospective results. Radiology 196:257, 1995.

52. Hahl J et al: Laser-induced hyperthermia in the treatment of liver tumors. Lasers Surg Med 10:319, 1990.

53. Grage TB et al: Results of a prospective randomized study of hepatic artery infusion with 5FU versus intravenous 5FU in patients with hepatic metastasis from colorectal cancer. Surgery 86:550, 1979.

54. Chang AE et al: A prospective randomized trial of regional versus systemic continuous 5-fluorodeoxyuridine chemotherapy in the treatment of colorectal liver metastases. Ann Surg 206:685, 1987.

55. Cunningham D: Cytotoxic drugs for gastric and colorectal cancer. Br Med J 299:1479, 1989.

56. Martin JK et al: Intraarterial floxuridine vs systemic fluorouracil for hepatic metastases from colorectal cancer. Arch Surg 125:1022, 1990.

57. Ravikumar TS et al: Experimental and clinical observations on hepatic cryosurgery for colorectal metastases. Cancer Res 51:6323, 1991.

58. Onik G et al: Ultrasound-guided hepatic cryosurgery in the treatment of metastatic colon carcinoma: Preliminary results. Cancer 67:901, 1991.

59. Fong Y et al: Surgical treatment of colorectal metastases to the liver. CA Cancer J Clin 45:50, 1995.

60. Blumgart LH, Fong Y: Surgical options in the treatment of hepatic metastasis from colorectal cancer. Curr Probl Surg 32:340, 1995.

61. Lanzafame RJ: Applications of laser technology in breast cancer therapy. Semin Surg Oncol 11:328, 1995.

62. Ansanelli VW: $CO_2$ laser in cancer surgery of the breast: a comparative clinical study. Lasers Surg Med 6:470, 1986.

63. Wang YH: Laser operation for breast cancer. Int Surg 72:208, 1987.

64. Wyman A, Rogers K: Radical breast surgery with a contact Nd:YAG laser scalpel. Eur J Surg Oncol 18:322, 1992.

65. ——— Randomized trial of laser scalpel for modified radical mastectomy. Br J Surg 80:871, 1993.

66. Lanzafame RJ et al: Comparison of local tumor recurrence following excision with the $CO_2$ laser, Nd:YAG laser, and argon beam coagulator. Lasers Surg Med 8:515, 1988.

67. Robinson DS et al: Stereotactic uses beyond core biopsy: model development for minimally invasive treatment of breast cancer through interstitial laser hyperthermia. Am Surg 62:117, 1996.

68. Deppe G et al: Debulking surgery for ovarian cancer with the Cavitron Ultrasonic Surgical Aspirator (CUSA)—A preliminary report. Gynecol Oncol 31:223, 1988.

69. ——— et al: Debulking of pelvic and para-aortic lymph node metastases in ovarian cancer with the cavitron ultrasonic surgical aspirator. Obstet Gynecol 76:1140, 1990.

70. Derderian GP et al: Ultrasonic surgical dissection in the dog spleen. Am J Surg 143:269, 1982.

71. Epstein F: The Cavitron ultrasonic aspirator in tumor surgery. Clin Neurosurg 31:497, 1983.

72. Thomson MA et al: Structural and function integrity of ovarian tumor tissue obtained by ultrasonic aspiration. Cancer 67:1326, 1991.

73. Wu AY et al: Pathologic evaluation of gynecologic specimens obtained with the Cavitron Ultrasonic Surgical Aspirator (CUSA). Gynecol Oncol 44:28, 1992.

74. Yahata H et al: Laparoscopic transhiatl esophagectomy for advanced thoracic esophageal cancer. Surg Laparosc Endosc 7:13, 1997.

75. Kato K et al: An ultrasonically powered instrument for laparoscopic surgery. J Laparoendosc Surg 5:31, 1995.

76. Millat B et al: Prospective evaluation of ultrasonic surgical dissectors in hepatic resection. HPB Surg 5:135, 1992.

77. Sonnino RE, Laberge JM: A problem with the use of the Cavitron Ultrasonic Aspirator (CUSA) in the resection of neuroblastomas (letter). J Pediatr Surg 25:585, 1990.

78. Hardy KJ et al: Hepatic resection: Value of operative ultrasound and ultrasonic dissection. Austral NZJ Surg 59:621, 1989.

79. Epstein FJ, Farmer JP: Trends in surgery: Laser surgery, use of the cavitron, and debulking surgery. Neurol Clin 9:307, 1991.

80. Oosterhuis JW et al: Viability of tumor cells in the irrigation fluid of the Cavitron Ultrasonic Surgical Aspirator (CUSA) after tumor fragmentation. Cancer 56:368, 1985.

81. Richmond IL, Hawksley CA: Evaluation of the histopathology of brain tumor tissue obtained by ultrasonic aspiration. Neurosurgery 13:414, 1983.

82. Donovan JT et al: Cytoreductive surgery for ovarian cancer with the Cavitron Ultrasonic Surgical Aspirator and the development of disseminated intravascular coagulation. Obstet Gynecol 83:1011, 1994.

83. van Dam PA et al: Ultraradical debulking of epithelial ovarian cancer with ultrasonic surgical aspirator. Am J Obstet Gynecol 174:943, 1996.

84. GLEESON MJ et al: A morphological study of the effect of the Cavitron ultrasonic surgical aspirator system near human peripheral nerves. Arch Otolaryngol Head Neck Surg 13:530, 1987.

85. MOWRY R, HENGRER AS: The ultrasonic scalpel in head and neck surgery. Otolaryngol Head Neck Surg 90:305, 1982.

86. ADELSON M: Ultrasonic surgical aspirator in cytoreduction of splenic metastases to avoid splenectomy. J Reproduct Med 37:917, 1992.

87. DEPPE G et al: Use of Cavitron surgical aspirator for debulking of diaphragmatic metastases in patients with advanced carcinoma of the ovaries. Surg, Gynecol Obstet 68:455, 1989.

88. ADELSON MD et al: Cytoreduction of ovarian cancer with the Cavitron ultrasonic surgical aspirator. Obstet Gynecol 72:140, 1988.

89. PATSNER B, ROSE PG: CUSA splenorraphy for ovarian cytoreductive surgery. Gynecol Oncol 41:28, 1991.

90. EISENKOP SM et al: Peritoneal implant elimination during cytoreductive surgery for ovarian cancer: Impact on survival. Gynecol Oncol 51:224, 1993.

91. FARID HM, O'CONNELL T: Hepatic resections. Am Surg 60:748, 1994.

92. TRANBERG KG et al: Liver resection. Am J Surg 151:368, 1986.

93. LITTLE JM, HOLLANDS MJ: Impact of the CUSA and operative ultrasound on hepatic resection. HPB Surg 3:271, 1991.

94. RAU HG et al: A comparison of different techniques for liver resection. Eur J Surg Oncol 21:183, 1995.

95. WILSON JHP et al: Photodynamic therapy for gastrointestinal tumors. Scand J Gastroenterol 188(Suppl 26):20, 1991.

96. KONIG K et al: Variation in the fluorescence decay properties of hematoporphyrin derivative during its conversion into photoproducts. J Photochem Photobiol B:Biol 8:103, 1990.

97. WEISHAUPT KR et al: Identification of singlet oxygen as the cytotoxic agent in photo-inactivation of a murine tumor. Cancer Res 36:2326, 1976.

98. FOOTE CS: Mechanisms of photosensitized oxidation. Science 162:963, 1968.

99. DOUGHERTY TJ et al: Photoradiation therapy. II. Cure of animal tumors with hematoporphyrin and light. J Natl Cancer Inst 55:115, 1975.

100. MOAN J et al: The mechanism of photodynamic inactivation of human cells in vitro in the presence of hematoporphyrin. Br J Cancer 39:398, 1979.

101. REGULA J et al: Photosensitisation and photodynamic therapy of oesophageal, duodenal and colorectal tumours using 5 aminolaevulinic acid induced protoporphyrin IX— A pilot study. Gut 36:67, 1995.

102. HENDERSON BW, DOUGHERTY TJ: How does photodynamic therapy work? Photochem Photobiol 55:145, 1992.

103. MOAN J, BERG K: Photochemotherapy of cancer: Experimental research. Photochem Photobiol. 55:931, 1992.

104. KENNEDY JC et al: Photodynamic therapy with endogenous protoporphyrin IX: Basic principles and present clinical experience. J Photochem Photobiol B:Biol 6:143, 1990.

105. HERRERA-ORNELAS L et al: Photodynamic therapy in patients with colorectal cancer. Cancer 57:677, 1986.

106. EVRARD S et al: Intra-abdominal photodynamic therapy: From theory to feasibility. Br J Surg 80:298, 1993.

107. GRANT WE et al: Photodynamic therapy of oral cancer: Photosensitization with systemic aminolaevulinic acid. Lancet 342:147, 1993.

108. DELANEY TF et al: Phase I study of debulking surgery and photodynamic therapy for disseminated intraperitoneal tumors. Int J Radiation Oncol Biol Phys 25:445, 1993.

109. SINDELAR WF et al: Technique of photodynamic therapy for disseminated intraperitoneal malignant neoplasms. Arch Surg 126:318, 1991.

110. EDELL ES, CORTESE DA. Photodynamic therapy in the management of early superficial squamous cell carcinoma as an alternative to surgical resection. Chest 102:1319, 1992.

111. PASS HI et al: Intrapleural photodynamic therapy: Results of a phase I trail. Ann Surg Oncol 1:28, 1994.

112. NAMBISAN RN et al: Intraoperative photodynamic therapy for retroperitoneal sarcomas. Cancer 61:1248, 1988.

113. DOUGHERTY TJ et al: Photoradiation therapy for the treatment of malignant tumors. Cancer Res 38:2628, 1978.

114. BENSON RC JR: The use of hematoporphyrin derivative (Hpd) in the localization and treatment of transitional cell carcinoma (TCC) of the bladder, in *Porphyrin Localization and Treatment of Tumors*, DR Doiron, CJ Gomer (eds). New York, Alan R. Liss, 1984, pp 795–804.

115. SUTEDJA T et al: Photodynamic therapy as an alternative treatment for surgery in a patient with lung cancer undergoing bone marrow transplantation. Chest 103:1908, 1993.

116. MCCAUGHAN JD et al: Photodynamic therapy for esophageal tumors. Arch Surg 124:74, 1989.

117. SCHOENFELD N et al: Protoporphyrin biosynthesis in melanoma B16 cells stimulated by 5-aminolevulinic acid and chemical inducers: Characterization of photodynamic inactivation. Int J Cancer 56:106, 1994.

118. IMAMURA S et al: Photodynamic therapy and/or external beam radiation therapy for roentgenologically occult lung cancer. Cancer 73:1608, 1994.

119. GOSSNER L et al: Oral administration of 5-aminolaevulinic acid for photodynamic therapy in patients with gastrointestinal carcinomas: Preliminary results. (abstr) Gastroenterology 106:387, 1994.

120. PROFIO AE et al: Fluorescence bronchoscopy for localization of carcinoma in situ. Med Phys 10:35, 1983.

121. DOUGHERTY TJ: Studies on the structure of porphyrins contained in Photofrin II. Photochem Photobiol 46:569, 1987.

122. KESSEL D et al: Probing the structure and stability of the tumor-localizing derivative of hematoporphyrin by reductive cleavage with LiAlH$_4$. Cancer Res 47:4642, 1987.

123. BONNET R: Photosensitizers of the porphyrin and phthalocyanine series for photodynamic therapy. Chem Soc Rev 24:19, 1995.

124. KESSEL D: Transport and binding of hematoporphyrin derivative and related porphyrins by murine leukemia L1210 cells. Cancer Res 41:1318, 1981.

125. PANDEY RK, DOUGHERTY TJ: Synthesis and photosensitizing activity of a di-porphyrin ether. Photochem Photobiol 47:769, 1988.

126. DOIRON DR et al: Light dosimetry in tissue: Application to photoradiation therapy, in *Advances in Experimental Medicine and Biology*, D Kessel, TJ Dougherty (eds). New York, Plenum Press, 1983, pp 63–77.

127. PROFIO AE, DOIRON DR: Dosimetry considerations in phototherapy. Med Phys 8:190, 1981.

128. VAN HILLEGERSBERG R et al: Current status of photodynamic therapy in oncology. Drugs 48:510, 1994.

129. ALLEN R et al: Photodynamic therapy of superficial malignancies with NPe6 in man, in *Photodynamic Therapy and*

*Biomedical Lasers,* P Spinelli et al (eds). New York, Elsevier Science, 1992, pp 441–445.

130. MORGAN AR et al: New photosensitizers for photodynamic therapy: a study of combined effects of metalopurpurin derivatives and light on transplantable bladder tumors. Cancer Res 48:194, 1988.

131. MORGAN AR et al: Tin (IV) etiopurpurin dichloride: An alternative to DHE? Proc SPIE 847:172, 1987.

132. SELMAN SH, KECK RW: The effect of transurethral light on the canine prostate after sensitization with the photosensitizer tin (II) etiopurpurin dichloride: a pilot study. J Urol 152:2129, 1994.

133. BONNET R et al: Hydroporphyrins of the mesotetra (hydroxyphenyl)porphyrin series as tumour photosensitizers. Biochem J 261:277, 1989.

134. VAN GEEL IPJ et al: Photosensitizing efficacy of mTHPC compared to Photofrin-PDT in the RIF1 mouse tumour and normal skin. Int J Cancer 60:388, 1995.

135. BARR H et al: Photodynamic therapy in the normal rat colon with phthalocyanine sensitisation. Br J Cancer 56:111, 1987.

136. BOWN SG et al: Photodynamic therapy with porphyrin and phthalocyanine sensitisation in normal rat liver. Br J Cancer 54:43, 1986.

137. RICHTER A et al: Preliminary studies on a more effective phototoxic agent than hematoporphyrin. J Natl Cancer Inst 79:1327, 1987.

138. YOUNG SW et al: Lutecium texaphyrin (PCI-0123): A near-infrared, water-soluble photosensitizer. Photochem Photobiol 63:892, 1996.

139. WOODBURN KW et al: Localization of efficacy analysis of the phototherapeutic lutetium texaphyrin (PCI-0123) in the murine EMT-6 sarcoma model. Photochem Photobiol 65:410, 1997.

140. YOUNG SW et al: Preclinical evaluation of gadolinium (III) texaphyrin complex. Invest Radiol 29:330, 1994.

141. REBEIZ N et al: Photodestruction of tumor cells by induction of endogenous accumulation of protoporphyrin IX: Enhancement by 1,10-phenanthroline. Photochem Photobiol 55:431, 1992.

142. KENNEDY JC, POTTIER RH: Endogenous protoporphyrin IX, a clinically useful photosensitizer for photodynamic therapy. J Photochem Photobiol B: Biol 14:275, 1992.

143. PENG O et al: Distribution and photosensitizing efficiency of porphyrins induced by application of exogenous 5-aminolevulinic acid in mice bearing mammary carcinoma. Int J Cancer 52:433, 1992.

144. VAN HILLEGERSBERG R et al: Selective accumulation of endogenously produced porphyrins in a liver metastasis model in rats. Gastroenterology 103:647, 1992.

145. EL-SHARABASY MMH et al: Porphyrin metabolism in some malignant diseases. Br J Cancer 65:409, 1992.

146. DAILY HA, SMITH A: Differential interaction of porphyrins used in photoradiation therapy with ferrochelatase. Biochem J 223:441, 1986.

147. SCHOENFELD N et al: The heme biosynthetic pathway in lymphocytes of patients with malignant proliferative disorders. Cancer Lett 43:43, 1991.

148. LEIBOVICI L et al: Activity of porphobilinogen deaminase in peripheral blood mononuclear cells of patients with metastatic cancer. Cancer 62:2297, 1988.

149. LAHAV M et al: Increased porphobilinogen deaminase activity in patients with malignant lymphoproliferative disease. JAMA 257:39, 1987.

150. NAVONE NM et al: Heme biosynthesis in human breast cancer-mimetic "in vitro" studies and some heme enzymatic activity levels. Int J Biochem 22:1407, 1990.

151. JORI G et al: Evidence for a major role of plasma lipoprotein as hematoporphyrin carriers in vivo. Cancer Lett 24:291, 1984.

152. KESSEL D: Porphyrinlipoprotein association as a factor in porphyrin localization. Cancer Lett. 33:183, 1986.

153. REYFTMANN JP et al: Interactions of human serum low density lipoproteins with porphyrins: A spectroscopic and photochemical study. Photochem Photobiol 40:721, 1984.

154. KESSEL D et al: Lipoprotein-mediated distribution of N-aspartyl chlorin e6 in the mouse. Photochem Photobiol 56:51, 1992.

155. DOUGHERTY TJ et al: Interstitial photoradiation therapy for primary solid tumors in pet cats and dogs. Cancer Res 41:401, 1981.

156. KORBELIK M et al: Distribution of Photofrin between tumour cells and tumour associated macrophages. Br J Cancer 64:508, 1991.

157. CINCOTTA L et al: Novel photodynamic effects of a benzophenothiazine on two different murine sarcomas. Cancer Res 54:1249, 1994.

158. TRUSCOTT TG et al: Detection of haematoporphyrin derivative and haematoporphyrin excited states in cell environments. Cancer Lett 41:31, 1980.

159. VASVARI G et al: Physico-chemical modeling of the role of free radicals in photodynamic therapy. II. Interactions of ground state sensitizers with free radicals studied by chemiluminescence spectrometry. Biochem Biophys Res Commun 197:1536, 1993.

160. SPIKES JD, STRAIGHT R: Sensitized photochemical processes in biological systems. Annu Rev Phys Chem 18:409, 1967.

161. SPIKES JD: Photochemotherapy: molecular and cellular processes involved. Adv Photochemother Proc SPIE 997:92, 1988.

162. ORTEL B et al: Lethal photosensitization by endogenous porphyrins of PAM cells-modification by desferrioxamine. J Photochem Photobiol B: Biol 17:273, 1993.

163. LOH CS et al: Photodynamic therapy of normal rat stomach: a comparative study between di-sulfonated aluminum phthalocyanine and 5-aminolaevulinic acid. Br J Cancer 66:452, 1992.

164. SLINEY DH, TROKEL SL: *Medical Lasers and Their Safe Use.* New York, Springer-Verlag, 1992.

165. SVAASAND LO, ELLINGSEN R: Optical penetration in human intracranial tumors. Photochem Photobiol 41:73, 1985.

166. BARR H et al: Photodynamic therapy for colorectal disease. Int J Colorect Dis 4:15, 1989.

167. HENDERSON BW, FINGER VH: Relationship of tumor hypoxia and response to photodynamic treatment in an experimental mouse tumor. Cancer Res 47:3110, 1987.

168. MOAN J: Effect of bleaching of porphyrin sensitizers during photodynamic therapy. Cancer Lett 33:45, 1986.

169. POTTER WR et al: The theory of photodynamic therapy dosimetry: consequences of photodestruction of sensitizer. Photochem Photobiol 46:97, 1987.

170. NSEYO UO et al: Urinary cytokines following photodynamic therapy for bladder cancer. A preliminary report. Urology 36:167, 1990.

171. EVANS S et al: Effect of photodynamic therapy on tumor necrosis factor production by murine macrophages. J Natl Cancer Inst 82:34, 1990.

172. BERG K et al: Photochemical treatment with the lysosomally localized dye tetra(4-sulfonatophenyl)porphine results

in lysosomal release of the dye but not of b-N-acetyl-D-glucosaminidase activity. Biochem Biophys Acta 1158:300, 1993.

173. KESSEL D: Sites of photosensitization by derivative of hematoporphyrin. Photochem Photobiol 44:489, 1986.

174. AGARWAL ML et al: Photodynamic therapy induces rapid cell death by apoptosis in L5178Y mouse lymphoma cells. Cancer Res 51:5993, 1991.

175. GOMER CJ et al: Properties and applications of photodynamic therapy. Radiat Res 120:1, 1989.

176. GOMER CJ et al: Increased transcription and translation of heme oxygenase in Chinese hamster fibroblasts following photodynamic therapy or Photofrin incubation. Photochem Photobiol 53:275, 1991.

177. GOMER CJ et al: Glucose regulated protein (GRP-78) induction and cellular resistance to oxidative stress mediated by porphyrin photosensitization. Cancer Res 51:6574, 1991.

178. PENNING LC et al: Calcium mediated PGE2 induction reduces haematoporphyrin-derivative-induced cytotoxicity of T24 human bladder transitional carcinoma cells in vitro. Biochem J 292:237, 1993.

179. HENDERSON BW, DONOVAN JM: Release of prostaglandin E2 from cells by photodynamic treatment in vitro. Cancer Res 49:6896, 1989.

180. WEBBER J et al: An apoptotic response to photodynamic therapy with endogenous protoporphyrin in vivo. J Photochem Photobiol B:Biol 35:209, 1996.

181. LUNA MC et al: Photodynamic therapy mediated induction of early response genes. Cancer Res 54:1374, 1994.

182. MOAN J et al: Photobleaching of protoporphyrin IX in cells incubated with 5-aminolevulinic acid. Int J Cancer 70:90, 1997.

183. WEIMAN TJ et al: Effect of photodynamic therapy on blood flow in normal and tumor vessels. Surgery 104:512, 1988.

184. SELMAN SH et al: Acute blood flow changes in transplantable FANFT-induced urothelial tumors treated with hematoporphyrin derivative and light. Surg Forum 34:676, 1983.

185. STAR WM et al: Destruction of rat mammary tumor and normal tissue microcirculation by hematoporphyrin derivative photoradiation observed in vivo in sandwich observation chambers. Cancer Res 46:2532, 1986.

186. HENDERSON BW, FINGAR VH: Oxygen limitation of direct tumor cell kill during photodynamic treatment of a murine tumor model. Photochem Photobiol 49:299, 1989.

187. VAN GEEL IPJ et al: Changes in perfusion of mouse tumors after photodynamic therapy. Int J Cancer 56:224, 1994.

188. THOMLINSON RH, GRAY LH: The histological structure of some human lung cancers and the possible implication for radiotherapy. Br J Cancer 9:539, 1955.

189. MATTIELO J et al: Effect of photodynamic therapy on RIF-1 tumor metabolism and blood flow examined by 31P and 2H NMR spectroscopy. NMR Biomed 3:64, 1990.

190. WEST CML et al: A comparison of the sensitivity to photodynamic treatment of endothelial and tumour cells in different proliferative states. Int J Radiat Biol 58:145, 1990.

191. LEUNIG M et al: Photodynamic therapy-induced alterations in interstitial fluid pressure, volume and water content of an amelanotic melanoma in the hamster. Br J Cancer 69:101, 1994.

192. ROBERTS DJH et al: Tumour vascular shutdown following photodynamic therapy based on polyhaematoporphyrin or 5-aminolaevulinic acid. Int J Oncol 5:763, 1994.

193. BREMNER JCM et al: Magnetic resonance spectroscopic studies on 'real-time' changes in RIF-1 tumour metabolism and blood flow during and after photodynamic therapy. Br J Cancer 69:1083, 1994.

194. HE XY et al: Photodynamic therapy with Photofrin II induces programmed cell death in carcinoma cell lines. Photochem Photobiol 59:468, 1994.

195. ZAIDI SIA et al: Apoptosis during photodynamic therapy-induced ablation of RIF-1 tumors in C3H mice: Electron microscopic, histopathologic and biochemical evidence. Photochem Photobiol 58:771, 1993.

196. RAFF MC: Social controls on cell survival and death. Nature 356:397, 1992.

197. CHAPMAN RS et al: The suppression of drug-induced apoptosis by activation of v-ABL tyrosine kinase. Cancer Res 54:5131, 1994.

198. FISHER TC et al: bcl-2 Modulation of apoptosis induced by anticancer drugs: Resistance to thymidylate stress is independent of classical resistance pathways. Cancer Res 53:3321, 1993.

199. HICKMAN JA et al: Apoptosis and cancer chemotherapy. Phil Trans R Soc Lond B 345:319, 1994.

200. DIVE C, HICKMAN JA: Drug-target interactions: Only the first step in the commitment to a programmed cell death? Br J Cancer 64:192, 1991.

201. WEBBER J et al: Side effects and photosensitization of human tissues after aminolevulinic acid. J Surg Res 68:31, 1997.

202. LOH CS et al: Oral versus intravenous administration of 5-aminolaevulinic acid for photodynamic therapy. Br J Cancer 68:41, 1993.

203. GOMER CJ, DOUGHERTY TJ: Determination of [3H]- and [14C]hematoporphyrin derivative distribution in malignant and normal tissue. Cancer Res 39:146, 1979.

204. VAN DER VEEN N et al: In vivo fluorescence kinetics and photodynamic therapy using 5-aminolaevulinic acid-induced prophyrin: Increased damage after multiple irradiations. Br J Cancer 70:867, 1994.

205. ABULAFI AM, WILLIAMS NS: Photodynamic therapy for cancer: Still awaiting rigorous evaluation. Br Med J 304:589, 1992.

206. VAN GEMERT JC et al: Wavelength and light-dose dependence in tumour phototherapy with haematoporphyrin derivative. Br J Cancer 52:43, 1985.

207. BARR H et al: Photodynamic therapy for colorectal cancer: A quantitative pilot study. Br J Surg 77:93, 1990.

208. POPOVIC EA et al: Photodynamic therapy of brain tumors. J Clin Laser Med Surg 14:251, 1996.

209. STRECHKYTE G et al: Photomodification of ALA-induced protoporphyrin IX in cells in vitro. SPIE 2325:58, 1994.

210. ROBERTS WG et al: Skin photosensitivity and photodestruction of several photodynamic sensitizers. Photochem Photobiol 49:431, 1989.

211. BELLNIER DA, DOUGHERTY TJ: A preliminary pharmacokinetic study of intravenous Photofrin$^R$ in patients. J Clin Laser Med Surg 14:311, 1996.

212. SIBILLE A et al: Long-term survival after photodynamic therapy for esophageal cancer. Gastroenterology 108:337, 1995.

213. FARBER NE et al: Skin burn associated with pulse oximetry during perioperative photodynamic therapy. Anesthesiology 84:983, 1996.

214. GOFF BA et al: Effects of photodynamic therapy with topical application of 5-aminolevulinic acid on normal skin of hairless guinea pigs. J Photochem Photobiol B:Biol 15:239, 1992.

215. BIEL MA: Photodynamic therapy and the treatment of head and neck cancers. J Clin Laser Med Surg 14:239, 1996.

216. HOPPER C: The role of photodynamic therapy in the management of oral cancer and precancer. Oral Oncol Eur J Cancer 32B:71, 1996.

217. JIN ML et al: Analysis of haematoprophyrin derivative and laser photodynamic therapy of upper gastrointestinal tumours in 52 cases. Lasers Med Sci 2:51, 1987.

218. KATO H et al: Evaluation of photodynamic therapy in gastric cancer. Lasers Med Sci 1:67, 1986.

219. MCCAUGHAN JS JR et al: Photodynamic therapy for esophageal tumors. Arch Surg 124:74, 1989.

220. KRASNER N et al: Photodynamic therapy of tumours in gastroenterology—A review. Lasers Med Sci 5:233, 1990.

221. HEIER SK et al: Photodynamic therapy for obstructing esophageal cancer: Light dosimetry and randomized comparison with Nd:YAG laser therapy. Gastroenterology 109:63, 1995.

222. ORTH K et al: Intraluminal treatment of inoperable oesophageal tumours by intralesional photodynamic therapy with methylene blue. Lancet 345:519, 1995.

223. WANG KK, GELLER A: Photodynamic therapy for early esophageal cancers: Light versus surgical might. Gastroenterology 108:593, 1995.

224. MCCAUGHAN JS JR et al: Photodynamic therapy to treat tumors of the extrahepatic biliary ducts. Arch Surg 126:111, 1991.

225. NSEYO UO: Photodynamic therapy in the management of bladder cancer. J Clin Laser Med Surg 14:271, 1996.

226. KRIEGMAIR M et al: Integral photodynamic treatment of refractory superficial bladder cancer. J Urol 154:1339, 1995.

227. KATO H et al: Photodynamic therapy for early state bronchogenic carcinoma. J Clin Laser Med Surg 14:235, 1996.

228. MCCAUGHAN JS JR: Photodynamic therapy of endobronchial and esophageal tumors: An overview. J Clin Laser Med Surg 14:223, 1996.

229. KENNEDY JC et al: Photodynamic therapy (PDT) and photodiagnosis (PD) using endogenous photosensitization induced by 5-aminolevulinic acid (ALA): Mechanisms and clinical results. J Clin Laser Med Surg 14:289, 1996.

230. WOLF P et al: Photodynamic therapy for mycosis fungoides after topical photosensitization with 5-aminolevulinic acid. J Am Acad Dermatol 31:678, 1994.

231. FIJAN S et al: Photodynamic therapy of epithelial skin tumours using delta-aminolevulinic acid and desferrioxamine. Brit J Dermatol 133:282, 1995.

232. CAIRNDUFF F et al: Superficial photodynamic therapy with topical 5-aminolaevulinic acid for superficial primary and secondary skin cancer. Br J Cancer 69:605, 1994.

233. KOREN H et al: Photodynamic therapy—An alternative pathway in the treatment of recurrent breast cancer. Int J Radiation Oncol Biol Phys 28:464, 1994.

234. ROSENTHAL DI, GLATSTEIN E: Clinical applications of photodynamic therapy. Ann Med 26:405, 1994.

235. OVERHOLT BF, PANJEHPOUR M: Photodynamic therapy in Barrett's esophagus. J Clin Laser Med Surg 14:245, 1996.

236. BARR H et al: Eradication of high-grade dysplasia in columnar-lined (Barrett's) oesophagus by photodynamic therapy with endogenously generated protoporphyrin IX. Lancet 348:584, 1996.

237. GROSJEAN P et al: Photodynamic therapy for cancer of the upper aerodigestive tract using tetra($m$-hydroxyphenyl)chlorin. J Clin Laser Med Surg 14:281, 1996.

238. LUKETICH JD et al: Brochoesophagopleural fistula after photodynamic therapy for malignant mesothelioma. Ann Thorac Surg 62:283, 1966.

239. LEVEKCKIS J et al: Kinetics of endogenous protoporphyrin IX induction by aminolevulinic acid: Preliminary studies in the bladder. J Urol 152:550, 1994.

# CHAPTER 6

# NUTRITION AND CANCER

*Michael H. Torosian*

## INTRODUCTION

Malnutrition is very common in cancer patients and occurs secondary to the disease process as well as to all forms of antineoplastic therapy. Numerous metabolic, biochemical, and nutritional abnormalities that result in significant weight loss and tissue catabolism have been documented in cancer patients. Abnormalities in protein, carbohydrate, lipid, and energy metabolism have been documented in patients with a variety of malignancies.[1–3] Weight loss, low serum albumin levels, and malnutrition in general are important prognostic factors associated with reduced survival in this patient population.[4,5]

Despite numerous retrospective studies that suggest reduced morbidity in cancer patients receiving nutritional support, the use of nutrient supplements in these patients remains controversial. The subsequent prospective, randomized studies that have been performed to evaluate objectively the use of nutritional support in cancer patients have, in general, failed to document a significant reduction in morbidity and mortality in this clinical population.[1,2,6] The only group of patients in whom nutritional support can be objectively found to improve survival are the severely malnourished cancer patients undergoing aggressive antineoplastic therapy.[7,8] This subset of cancer patients represents only about 5% of the total cancer patient population. Secondly, although the potential to stimulate tumor growth and metastasis has been demonstrated in animal models, few clinical studies support this clinical concern.[9,10] Finally, the use of specific nutrients may be used to prevent specific complications under certain clinical conditions. The use of specific nutrients to improve host immunity to combat infectious complications and to maintain the integrity of critical organ systems (e.g., bone marrow, gastrointestinal tract) is an area of active investigation. The efficacy of nutritional support in the cancer patient will be critically reviewed in this chapter.

## ETIOLOGY OF CANCER CACHEXIA

The etiology of cancer cachexia is complex and multifactorial. Cancer cachexia is a clinical syndrome consisting of anorexia, weight loss, severe tissue wasting, asthenia, and organ dysfunction. Both disease- and treatment-related factors contribute to the development of cachexia in the cancer patient, and metabolic and nutritional abnormalities function as both the cause and result from the effects of cachexia. In general, two major mechanisms work in the development of cachexia in the cancer patient. A local effect of the tumor can cause obstruction, preventing the adequate intake of nutrients and resulting in weight loss and cachexia. Many of the effects of malnutrition in patients with an obstructive etiology for cachexia can be reversed by tumor resection or by providing nutrients in a way that bypasses the local point of obstruction. A more common mechanism of cancer cachexia is the nonobstructive form that results from circulating factors elaborated by the tumor or induced from host tissues by the presence of cancer.[12,13] Provision of nutrients is ineffective in reversing malnutrition in this patient population, and successful treatment of malnutrition is dependent upon effective anticancer therapy. Significant reduction or ablation of malignancy is required to diminish significantly or eliminate the production of catabolic factors associated with nonobstructive cancer cachexia.

Although numerous theories have been postulated to explain its etiology, the mechanism of cancer cachexia remains unknown. Widespread aberrations in energy, carbohydrate, lipid, and protein metabolism have been documented in patients with malignancy.[1–3,13] Aberrations in energy expenditure and inefficient energy utilization have been commonly demonstrated.[14,15] It was initially hypothesized that increased energy expenditure in the cancer patient accounted for progressive weight loss and host tissue wasting. However, clinical measurements of energy expenditure in the cancer patient have found that energy expenditure can be normal, increased, or decreased in the individual cancer patient. Thus, hypermetabolism (i.e., increased energy expenditure) is not directly associated with weight loss in these patients. Knox et al.[16] measured energy expenditure in 200 malnourished cancer patients with gastrointestinal malignancy. Only 41% of cancer patients exhibited normal resting energy expenditure, whereas decreased and increased resting energy expenditure were observed in 33% and 26% of patients, respectively. Thus, although abnormalities in energy expenditure were found in 59% of cancer patients, weight loss cannot be explained by hypercatabolism alone. In fact, severe catabolism and weight loss are present in patients with increased, decreased, or normal energy expenditure.

Inefficient energy utilization has also been documented in the tumor-bearing host. Holroyde and Reichard[17] reported increased Cori cycle activity in patients with cancer, particularly those patients with progressive weight loss. The Cori cycle is a futile cycle in which glucose is broken down to lactic acid and subsequently reconverted to glucose in the liver. This is an energy-wasting cycle consuming energy for a biochemical reaction that produces no net synthesis of a biologic molecule. The highest level of Cori cycle activity was observed in patients with the greatest degree of weight loss in this study. The Cori cycle is only one example of many futile cycles that can function to consume energy abnormally in the cancer patient. Futile cycles exist in the body for purposes of fine metabolic regulation and control of thermogenesis. However, pathophysiologic disturbances of such futile cycles can lead to a cascade of abnormalities induced by creating a deficit of high-energy compounds. Another example of inefficient bioenergenics in cancer patients is the elevated rate of anaerobic glycolysis that occurs in tumor cells.[18] In comparison with oxidative metabolism, anaerobic glycolysis represents an extremely inefficient process for utilizing glucose. Abnormalities in carbohydrate metabolism include glucose intolerance, impaired insulin sensitivity, decreased glucose oxidation, and increased rates of gluconeogenesis and glucose recycling.[13,17] In response to a glucose challenge by either the oral or intravenous route, hyperglycemia results.[17,18] This state of glucose intolerance is associated with impaired insulin release from the pancreas as well as peripheral tissue resistance to circulating insulin levels.[19,20] Even with high-dose insulin infusion, peripheral glucose uptake remains impaired. These metabolic changes are typically associated with advanced stages of cancer.

Shaw and Wolfe[21] studied patients with gastrointestinal tumors and documented increased rates of basal hepatic glucose production. In this study, a direct relationship between tumor burden and the increased rate of gluconeogenesis was observed. With curative tumor resection, a decrease in the rate of gluconeogenesis was observed. Finally, glucose oxidation rates are decreased in patients with cancer.[13,17] Therefore, although cancer patients do not metabolize glucose efficiently, glucose production continues because of elevated Cori cycle activity and the increased rate of gluconeogenesis. This combination of derangements in carbohydrate metabolism causes a deleterious effect on the host by consuming energy to synthesize glucose at a time when glucose utilization by peripheral tissues is impaired.

Increased rates of protein turnover also result in significant energy loss in the cancer patient.[22] The drive for increased gluconeogenesis results in the breakdown of skeletal muscle to provide substrates for glucose synthesis.[19,23] This is perhaps the most harmful of the metabolic derangements occurring in cancer patients, since it is the protein component of the body that is the goal for all routes of nutritional repletion. Improved visceral and somatic protein synthesis is the clinical endpoint for a successful nutrition support regimen. Protein breakdown is associated with increased morbidity and mortality in many clinical situations including cancer. In noncancer patients with reduced nutrient intake, the rate of gluconeogenesis typically falls as glucose utilization is replaced by fat fuel metabolism by normal adaptive mechanisms. In the cancer patient, these adaptive mechanisms are blunted and continued glucose production occurs and is associated with progressive protein breakdown.[13,21]

Lipid metabolic alterations in the cancer patient include changes in body composition and substrate metabolism. Lipid catabolism is a prominent feature of the clinical syndrome of cancer cachexia. However, peripheral fat depletion does not occur in a uniform manner. Early reports in cancer patients indicate that specific lipid fractions, including phospholipid and free cholesterol, were increased in cancer patients despite severe loss of total body fat.[11] Thus, body composition is altered in the face of severe total body lipid depletion. Oxidation rates of lipids are increased in the cancer patient with clinical studies documenting increased mobilization of endogenous fat stores and increased utilization of exogenously administered fat emulsions.[20,24] The increased rate of lipid metabolism has been found in both the fasting and fed states. During periods of glucose administration, normal individuals suppress lipid mobilization and preferentially utilize glucose as a fuel source. In contrast, cancer patients continue to break down peripheral fat stores and oxidize free fatty acids despite glucose administration.[20] Thus, normal control mechanisms for metabolic processes are deranged in the cancer patient and lack the normal feedback mechanisms for adapting to regulatory stimuli.

Additional changes in body composition include increased extracellular fluid and total body sodium levels and decreased intracellular fluid and total body potassium levels.[25] Antineoplastic therapy (including surgery, chemotherapy, and radiation therapy) also adversely affects the nutritional and metabolic abnormalities found in the cancer patient. The nutritional and metabolic consequences of cancer therapy exacerbate and contribute to the ongoing development of cancer cachexia.

The etiology of cancer cachexia remains unknown. However, two classes of cachexia mediators believed to be important in pathogenesis are cytokines and regulatory hormones. The systemic effects of the circulating factors cause a myriad of catabolic effects with the end result being the clinical syndrome of cancer cachexia. Cytokines are soluble proteins secreted by host tissues in response to malignancy, sepsis, and other pathophysiologic events. Cytokines function by multiple mechanisms of action including autocrine (i.e., same cell), paracrine (i.e., adjacent cells) or systemic (i.e., distant) effects. Tumor necrosis factor (TNF), interferon-α, interleukin 1 (IL-1), and interleukin 6 (IL-6) are specific cytokines that have been implicated in the development of cancer cachexia.[26,27] TNF or cachectin is a 17,000-dalton protein.[12] This protein is secreted by macrophages in response to malignancy, endotoxins, and other stimuli. In animals treated with TNF, documented effects include anorexia, weight loss, skeletal muscle loss, depletion of fat stores, hypoproteinemia, and increased level of total body water.[12] However, the complete syndrome of cancer cachexia cannot be reproduced with TNF administration alone. There are certainly other mediators involved in the development of the complex syndrome of cancer cachexia. Furthermore, pharmacologic and not physiologic levels of TNF are often needed to cause the effects typically associated with cancer cachexia. Clinically, it is extremely difficult to detect circulating levels of TNF in cancer patients, even those with advanced malignancy and severe degrees of cachexia. IL-1 is secreted by macrophages in response to endotoxin exposure. IL-1 causes anorexia, pyrexia, hypotension, decreased systemic vascular resistance, and increased cardiac output.[28] Alterations in hepatic protein synthesis induced by IL-1 are similar to those seen in the tumor-bearing state.[29] IL-6 is secreted by macrophages stimulated by TNF or IL-1.[30] Elevated levels of IL-6 have been documented in tumor-bearing animals and cause many of the same effects seen with TNF or IL-1.[28,30] Thus, these cytokines appear to contribute to the development of cancer cachexia—however, the relative importance of these cytokines and other yet undiscovered circulating proteins remains to be determined.

Regulatory hormones also play an important role in the catabolism associated with malignancy. Patients with cachexia from cancer, sepsis, and other pathophysiologic stimuli often demonstrate decreased insulin and increased glucagon levels.[31] The insulin-glucagon ratio is an index of host anabolism and a reduction in this ratio indicates a catabolic hormonal environment. This catabolic state promotes weight loss, muscle breakdown, and depletion of peripheral fat stores. Insulin administration alone cannot reverse the total body catabolism due to an offsetting compensatory rise in circulating glucagon levels. In fact, frequently there is an overshooting of the glucagon response that results in a further reduction in the insulin-glucagon ratio. In an animal model, our laboratory has found that providing insulin combined with the somatostatin analogue octreotide can dramatically increase the insulin-glucagon ratio.[32] Octreotide is administered to prevent the compensatory increase in glucagon levels associated with insulin administration. With a triple combination of insulin, octreotide, and growth hormone, we previously demonstrated increased carcass weight and improved host nutritional status in tumor-bearing animals. These host effects occurred without stimulating tumor growth. However, further investigation is required to elucidate thoroughly the biologic mechanisms and to develop effective treatment strategies to treat cancer cachexia.

## METHODS OF NUTRITION SUPPORT

Nutrition support can be administered by the oral, enteral, or parenteral route. The goal of nutrition support is to promote host anabolism and to reverse the weight loss and negative nitrogen balance characteristic of cancer cachexia. As described previously, nutrition support alone can reverse some of the nutritional abnormalities if a major component of cachexia is caused by obstruction preventing adequate nutrient intake. In the majority of cancer patients, however, cachexia is caused by the distant metabolic effects of cytokines and abnormalities in regulatory hormone levels. In this group of patients, nutrition support alone is unable to reverse significantly the catabolic effects of cachexia and tumor resection, or effective chemotherapy or radiation therapy is necessary to treat the associated cachexia successfully.

Although the oral route of administering nutrients is preferred when possible, oral supplementation alone is rarely sufficient to combat cancer cachexia effectively. A variety of commercially available supplements can be used in patients with mild or moderate degrees of cachexia, but long-term success with such formulas is rarely achieved. Anorexia and taste fatigue of such products oftentimes prevents adequate oral intake with resultant ongoing cachexia.

Enteral nutrition support provides nutrients by a catheter or tube into the gastrointestinal tract. Access to the intestinal tract can be provided by a nasoenteric tube, a gastrostomy, or a jejunostomy feeding tube.[33] For short-term feeding, a nasoenteric tube can be used. If enteral nutrition support is to be continued for more than 4 weeks, it is suggested that an endoscopically placed or surgically placed gastrostomy or jejunostomy tube be inserted. The route and duration of nutrition support depends upon many clinical factors, including the patient's nutritional and general medical status, patient prognosis, clinical stage and site of the cancer, and the obstructive or nonobstructive nature or malnutrition.

Many commercial formulas are available for enteral feedings.[34] Many of these formulas can provide complete nutrition support with adequate provision of protein and calories. Carbohydrates typically represent the major source of calories, with fat supplied as triglycerides or vegetable oils. Disease-specific formulas are available for patients with renal, cardiac, or hepatic insufficiency.

Specialized nutrient formulas are currently being investigated in an attempt to reduce specific complications in the cancer patient. Arginine, glutamine, omega-3 fatty acids, nucleotides, specific lipid moieties, and anabolic hormones are currently under clinical and basic science investigation.[35–37] The goal of this research is to develop specific nutrient formulations to eliminate or dramatically reduce the incidence of organ- or site-specific morbidity or to alter tumor growth and metastasis in the cancer patient.

Glutamine is the most abundant amino acid in the body, plays an important role in regulating amino acid metabolism, and functions to maintain the anatomic and physiologic integrity of the gastrointestinal tract. Glutamine comprises over 60% of the free intracellular amino acid pool and is currently lacking from parenteral nutrient solutions because of its instability in solution.[38] Enteral nutrient formulas containing glutamine supplements have shown promising results in animal studies. In glutamine-supplemented animals receiving chemotherapy or radiation therapy, numerous studies have demonstrated a marked decrease in morbidity and mortality.[39,40] Glutamine is an important substrate for the gastrointestinal tract and can significantly improve the anatomic, metabolic, and functional integrity of the gastrointestinal tract.[41] With glutamine supplementation, bacterial translocation by the intestinal route may be reduced. In this way, it has been hypothesized that glutamine supplementation may reduce the incidence of sepsis and multisystem organ dysfunction that is a major source of morbidity in patients receiving chemotherapy or radiation therapy. Clinical trials of glutamine supplementation in the cancer patient undergoing aggressive chemotherapy and radiation therapy are currently under way.

Immunomodulation with specific nutrients has been studied in critically ill and cancer patients in an attempt to prevent infectious complications in these patient populations. The combination of arginine, nucleotides, and omega-3 fatty acids has been found to stimulate the immune response significantly in several studies.[42,43]

Arginine functions as a nonspecific stimulant of both humoral and cellular immunity, improves nitrogen balance, and promotes polyamine synthesis required for cellular proliferation.[44] Nucleotides are clearly required for cellular proliferation because they are the purine and pyrimidine building blocks of DNA and RNA.[45,46] Omega-3 fatty acids, or fish oils, are immunostimulatory, in contrast to omega-6 fatty acids, or vegetable oils, which depress the immune system.[47] Thus, by increasing the omega-3–omega-6 fatty acid ratio, it is possible to stimulate host immunity.

Several early studies demonstrated the efficacy of enteral nutrition supplemented with arginine, nucleotides, and omega-3 fatty acids to stimulate the immune system. Cerra et al.[43] found in critically ill patients that improved lymphocyte activation by concanavalin A and phytohemagglutinin improved delayed hypersensitivity, and maintenance of nutritional status could be achieved with supplements of arginine, nucleotides, and omega-3 fatty acids. Daly et al.[42] conducted a prospective trial of 60 patients with upper gastrointestinal tract malignancies randomized to receive a standard enteral diet or enteral nutrition supplemented with arginine, nucleotides, and omega-3 fatty acids. Significant reductions in postoperative infections and hospital length of stay were reported in the group receiving the supplemented diet.[36,42] In a large clinical trial of patients undergoing major elective upper abdominal surgery, similar improvements were noted in immune function in the supplemented group with a significant reduction in infectious complications.[48] The beneficial effects of these supplemented enteral nutrients were demonstrated in patients who received enteral nutrition by tube feeding in the early postoperative period. Preoperative oral supplementation with immunonutrients in gastrointestinal cancer patients failed to stimulate the immune response significantly in patients undergoing major surgery. Therefore, the route and timing of enteral nutrient supplements are important factors in determining the efficacy of such formulas.[49]

Specific lipid substrates can significantly influence tumor and host metabolism as demonstrated by numerous animal studies. Lipids are important structural components of cell membranes and are incorporated into tumor cells following exogenous administration. Lipid moieties can significantly alter the physiochemical properties of tumor cell membranes, including permeability, distensibility, and sensitivity to chemotherapy or radiation therapy.[50]

In animal studies differential effects on tumor growth and metastasis have been shown with long-chain triglycerides, medium-chain triglycerides, and omega-3 fatty acids.[51,52] In general, these studies show increased tumor growth and metastasis with long-chain fatty acids, and reduced tumor growth with medium-chain triglycerides and omega-3 fatty acids. Interestingly, long-chain fatty acids are those typically used in conventional nutrition support regimens. Structured lipids can be specifically designed with a glycerol backbone and selected fatty acid side chains. Studies using structured lipids composed of glycerol with medium-chain fatty acid and omega-3 fatty acid side chains have demonstrated reduced tumor growth rates with maintenance of nutritional status.[53] These exciting areas of basic and clinical investigation indicate the tremendous potential for use of specific lipid components to affect tumor growth and host metabolism differentially.

In the future total metabolic support of the cancer patient will require more than providing protein and calories in the form of carbohydrates and lipid; it will likely also require the use of anabolic hormones, cytokines, anticytokines, and other substrates known to alter host metabolic pathways. For example, the use of growth hormone in the cancer patient may significantly reverse catabolism but must be studied cautiously because of its theoretic potential to stimulate tumor growth. Many tumors have cells that express receptors for growth hormone on their surface and, thus, may exhibit increased growth when exposed to exogenous growth hormone. However, growth hormone can reverse many of the catabolic effects typically observed in the patient with advanced malignancy. Numerous animal studies have demonstrated that growth hormone can increase total body weight, increase fat-free mass, and increase whole body and muscle protein content.[32,54–57] Despite the concern of stimulating tumor growth, either no effect or decreased tumor growth has generally been observed in animal studies.[32,54–57] In acromegalic patients, there is the clinical finding of an increased incidence of gastrointestinal tumors and polyps.[58] In children with growth hormone deficiency states treated with growth hormone chronically, an increased risk of leukemia (twofold) has been observed.[59] Although a possible relationship between growth hormone and these tumors exists, the causal effect between growth hormone and other factors in these patients has not been elucidated.

The combination of growth hormone, insulin, and somatostatin in tumor-bearing animals has been shown to treat cancer cachexia selectively in animals bearing a mammary adenocarcinoma.[32,60] Growth hormone supplementation alone led to a 10% increase in carcass weight in the protein-fed state of tumor-bearing animals and a 33% decrease in tumor growth in the protein-starved state— yielding a significant reduction in tumor-carcass ratio in both dietary groups.[57] The mechanism of tumor growth inhibition with growth hormone supplements in protein-starved animals is unknown. Growth hormone was then combined with somatostatin and insulin therapy in order to improve multiple aspects of glucose and protein metabolism in the tumor-bearing host.[32] Since insulin administration alone leads to a hypercompensatory rise in glucagon, somatostatin was added to prevent this exaggerated glucagon release so that a significant increase in the insulin-glucagon ratio (an anabolic index) could be effectively established. This combined hormone therapy led to an 18% increase in carcass weight and a 14% reduction in tumor weight. There was a significant decrease in tumor protein content and in the S-phase fraction of tumor cells observed on flow cytometry. By using growth hormone and increasing the insulin-glucagon index, a favorable metabolic environment was created for the host to compete with tumor cells for limited circulating substrates. It is hypothesized that selective deprivation of nutrients to tumor cells caused the reduction in tumor growth and allowed host tissues to be nutritionally supported. These studies demonstrated for the first time that the host could be supported nutritionally in a selective fashion at the expense of tumor growth. Further clinical investigation is clearly warranted to study this phenomenon.

## CLINICAL EFFICACY OF NUTRITION SUPPORT

Retrospective studies initially suggested that morbidity and mortality can be reduced in surgical patients receiving nutrition support. In general, however, subsequent prospective randomized studies have conflicted with the earlier retrospective reports and show limited efficacy to reduce postoperative complications except in severely malnourished patients. Heatley et al.[61] prospectively studied 74 patients with upper gastrointestinal cancer who underwent surgical resection. In patients receiving total parenteral nutrition, the only significant finding was a reduction in postoperative wound infections. No difference in incidence of other major complications or mortality was observed in patients receiving nutrition support compared to the control group. Limited or no effect on postoperative complications and mortality have similarly been observed in the majority of prospective randomized trials of nutrition support in surgical patients.[62] Critical analysis of these studies demonstrates that many of these clinical studies are flawed by study design, including too few patients analyzed to detect a significant difference in outcome, too short duration of preoperative nutrition support, heterogeneous patient populations with disparate prognostic and complication risks, and no stratification for the extent of preoperative malnutrition. All of these clinical parameters can certainly influence the results of surgical outcome studies designed to detect incidence and effect of nutrition support on postoperative morbidity and mortality.

Mueller et al.[7] in 1982 reported a dramatic effect of 10 days of preoperative nutrition support in patients undergoing elective gastrointestinal surgery. Postoperative morbidity in patients receiving total parenteral nutrition was approximately one-half that compared to the control group (17% vs. 32%). Mortality rate was reduced from 16% in the control group to 4% in the nutritionally supplemented group. However, this study was criticized for its failure to provide standard antibiotic prophylaxis in the perioperative period and, despite dramatic differences between the patients receiving nutrition and the control group, an alarmingly high incidence of complications and mortality was observed in this study. Perhaps the best and one of the largest studies performed on elective abdominal and thoracic surgical patients was the Veterans Administration Cooperative Study.[63] Postoperative complications were analyzed in surgical patients that were randomized to receive 7 to 10 days of preoperative total parenteral nutrition or the control group. In this study, only the severely malnourished group of patients demonstrated fewer noninfectious complications (5%) versus control patients (43%). In borderline or mildly malnourished patients, infectious complications were actually higher in the group receiving total parenteral nutrition. Perhaps the presence of a central venous catheter, the presence of parenteral nutrients that may impair host immune response, or the obligatory preoperative hospital stay to receive parenteral nutrition contributed to the higher incidence of infectious complications in these patients. The conclusion from the series of studies performed over the past few decades to evaluate nutrition support in surgical patients is that a significant benefit can only be documented in patients with severe malnutrition in whom a major abdominal or thoracic surgical procedure is planned.

In cancer patients receiving chemotherapy, the use of nutrition support is similarly controversial. Despite the majority of animal studies that show that nutrition support can significantly reduce chemotherapy-related morbidity and mortality, clinical trials have failed to reproduce these laboratory-based results.[64] It is clear from observational studies that increased chemotherapy toxicity correlates with increased severity of malnutrition. It was thus hypothe-

sized that the use of nutrition support to improve nutritional status might effectively prevent or minimize chemotherapy-related toxicities. Numerous interventional trials of nutrition support in patients receiving chemotherapy were subsequently undertaken. Gastrointestinal, hematologic, and infectious complications were monitored in patients with a variety of malignancies including colonic, testicular, lung, hematologic, and other cancers. The majority of these trials reported no difference in chemotherapy-related toxicity between control patients and those receiving nutrition support.[2,6] Marginal improvement in gastrointestinal and hematologic tolerance to chemotherapy were counterbalanced in other studies showing increased toxicity in patients receiving parenteral nutrition. At the current time, colony-stimulating factors can dramatically reduce the period of bone marrow suppression from chemotherapy and can selectively reduce hematologic and infectious complications independent of host nutritional status.

An important exception to these studies is the use of nutrition support in bone marrow transplant patients.[8] In this group of patients, total parenteral nutrition has been found to improve overall survival, improve disease-free survival, and decrease the rate of relapse compared to control patients. As chemotherapy regimens become more aggressive and toxic, additional select groups of patients may be identified who will benefit from the use of nutrition support.

Radiation therapy can exacerbate the development of cancer cachexia by causing xerostomia, decreased taste sensation, esophagitis, enteritis, fistula formation, and intestinal strictures. All of these effects can cause decreased nutrient intake and/or decreased nutrient assimilation. Despite these adverse clinical effects, trials of nutrition support in patients receiving radiation therapy have generally showed limited efficacy to prevent ongoing cachexia.[65] No significant difference in treatment-related toxicity has been observed in multiple prospective randomized trials of total parenteral nutrition performed in patients receiving radiation therapy. One consistent observation in these studies is an increase in body weight in patients receiving total parenteral nutrition. It is believed that the majority of weight gain in patients receiving total parenteral nutrition during radiation therapy treatment is due to fluid retention. This explanation is plausible since the increase in body weight is not clinically associated with reduction in radiation-related toxicity. Thus, routine use of nutrition support in patients undergoing radiotherapy is not indicated to reduce adverse treatment-related effects.

## SUMMARY

The clinical efficacy of nutrition support to reduce morbidity and mortality in cancer patients undergoing surgery, chemotherapy, and radiation therapy is limited. Prospective randomized trials have demonstrated benefit to nutrition support only in severely malnourished patients undergoing extensive surgical resection or bone marrow transplant patients receiving aggressive chemotherapy regimens. Further research is currently under way to develop innovative methods of nutritional and metabolic support to prevent both disease- and treatment-related complications in the cancer patient.

## REFERENCES

1. TOROSIAN MH, DALY JM: Nutritional support in the cancer-bearing host. Cancer 58:1915, 1986.
2. BRENNAN MF: Total parenteral nutrition in the cancer patient. N Engl J Med 305:375, 1981.
3. LUNDHOLM K et al: Metabolism in peripheral tissues in cancer patients. Cancer Treat Rep 65(Suppl):79, 1981.
4. STUDLEY HO: Percentage of weight loss: A basic indicator of surgical risk in patients with chronic peptic ulcer. JAMA 106:458, 1936.
5. MULLEN JL: Consequences of malnutrition in the surgical patient. Surg Clin North Am 61:465, 1981.
6. KORETZ RL: Parenteral nutrition: Is it oncologically logical? J Clin Oncol 2:534, 1984.
7. MUELLER J et al: Perioperative parenteral feeding in patients with gastrointestinal carcinoma. Lancet 1:68, 1982.
8. WEISDORF SA et al: Positive effect of prophylactic total parenteral nutrition on long-term outcome of bone marrow transplantation. Transplantation 43:833, 1987.
9. TOROSIAN MH et al: Alteration of tumor cell kinetics by total parenteral nutrition: Potential therapeutic implications. Cancer 53:1409, 1984.
10. POPP MB et al: Host and tumor responses to increasing levels of intravenous nutritional support. Surgery 94:300, 1983.
11. THEOLOGIDES A: Cancer cachexia. Cancer 43:2004, 1979.
12. BEUTLER B, CERAMI A: Cachectin and tumor necrosis factor as two sides of the same biological coin. Nature 320:584, 1986.
13. BRENNAN MH: Uncomplicated starvation versus cancer cachexia. Cancer Res 37:2359, 1977.
14. YOUNG VR: Energy metabolism and requirements in the cancer patient. Cancer Res 37:2336, 1977.
15. GUNDERSON GH: The basal metabolism in myelogenous leukemia and its relation to the blood findings. Boston Med Surg J 185:785, 1921.
16. KNOX LS et al: Energy expenditure in malnourished cancer patients. Ann Surg 197:152, 1983.
17. HOLROYDE CP, REICHARD GA: Carbohydrate metabolism in cancer cachexia. Cancer Treat Rep 65(Suppl):55, 1981.
18. MACBETH RAL, BEKESI JE: Oxygen consumption and anaerobic glycolysis of human malignant and normal tissue. Cancer Res 22:244, 1962.
19. SCHEIN PS et al: Cachexia of malignancy: Potential role of insulin in nutritional management. Cancer 43:2070, 1979.
20. WATERHOUSE C, KEMPERMAN JH: Carbohydrate metabolism in subjects with cancer. Cancer Res 31:1273, 1971.
21. SHAW JH, WOLFE R: Glucose and urea kinetics in patients with early and advanced gastrointestinal cancer: The response to glucose infusion, parenteral feeding, and surgical resection. Surgery 101:181, 1987.
22. EDEN E et al: Whole-body tyrosine flux in relation to energy expenditure in weight-losing cancer patients. Metabolism 33:1020, 1984.
23. GOLD J: Cancer cachexia and gluconeogenesis. Ann NY Acad Sci 230:86, 1974.
24. EDMONSTON JH: Fatty acid mobilization and glucose metabolism in patients with cancer. Cancer 19:277, 1966.
25. DALY JM et al: Nutritional support in the cancer patient. J Parenter Enteral Nutr 14:244S, 1990.
26. NAKAHARA W: A chemical basis for tumor host relations. J Natl Cancer Inst 24:77, 1960.
27. LANGSTEIN H et al: Reversal of cancer cachexia by antibodies to interferon-gamma but not cachectin/tumor necrosis factor. Surg Forum 40:408, 1989.
28. WOLOSKI BMRNJ, FULLER GM: Identification and partial characterization of hepatocyte stimulating factor from leukemia cell lines: Comparison with interleukin 1. Proc Natl Acad Sci 82:1443, 1985.
29. DINARELLO CA: Interleukin 1 and the pathogenesis of the acute phase response. N Engl J Med 311:1413, 1984.
30. POWANDA MC, BEISEL WR: Hypothesis: Leukocyte endogenous mediator/endogenous pyrogen/lymphocyte activating factor modulates the development of nonspecific and specific immunity and affects nutritional status. Am J Clin Nutr 35:762, 1982.
31. UNGER RH: Glucagon and the insulin:glucagon ratio in diabetes and other catabolic illness. Diabetes 20:834, 1981.
32. BARTLETT DL et al: Growth hormone, insulin and somatostatin therapy of cancer cachexia. Cancer 73:1499, 1994.
33. SHIKE M: Enteral feeding, in *Modern Nutrition in Health and Disease,* 8th ed, ME Shils et al (eds). Philadelphia, Lea & Febiger, 1994, pp 1417–1429.
34. BLOCH AS, SHILS ME: Appendix, in *Modern Nutrition in Health and Disease,* 8th ed, ME Shils et al (eds). Philadelphia, Lea & Febiger, 1994, pp A182–A183.
35. DALY JM et al: Immune and metabolic effects of arginine in the surgical patient. Ann Surg 208:512, 1988.
36. DALY JM et al: Enteral nutrition during multimodality therapy in upper gastrointestinal cancer patients. Ann Surg 221:327, 1995.
37. KLIMBERG VS et al: Glutamine facilitates chemotherapy while reducing toxicity. J Parenter Enteral Nutr 16(Suppl 6):83S, 1992.
38. SOUBA WW et al: The role of glutamine in maintaining a healthy gut and supporting the metabolic response to injury and infection. J Surg Res 48:383, 1990.
39. FOX AD et al: The effect of a glutamine-supplemented enteral diet on methotrexate-induced enterocolitis. J Parenter Enteral Nutr 12:325, 1988.
40. SOUBA WW et al: Glutamine nutrition in the management of radiation enteritis. J Parenter Enteral Nutr 14:106S, 1990.
41. ROMBEAU JL. A review of the effects of glutamine-enriched diets on experimentally induced enterocolitis. J Parenter Enteral Nutr 14:100S, 1990.
42. DALY JM et al: Enteral nutrition with supplemental arginine, RNA, and omega-3 fatty acids in patients after operation: Immunologic, metabolic and clinical outcome. Surgery 112:57, 1992.
43. CERRA FB et al: Improvement in immune function in ICV patients by enteral nutrition supplemented with arginine, RNA and menhadein oil independent of nitrogen balance. Nutrition 7:193, 1991.
44. BARBUL A: Arginine, biochemistry, physiology and therapeutic implications. J Parenter Enteral Nutr 10:227, 1986.
45. RUDOLPH FB et al: Involvement of dietary nucleoties in T lymphocyte function. Adv Exp Med Biol 165B:175, 1984.
46. FANSLOW FC et al: Effect of nucleotide restriction and supplementation on resistance to experimental murine cadidiasis. J Parenter Enteral Nutr 12:49, 1988.
47. GOTTSCHLICH M et al: Differential effects of three enteral dietary regimens on selected outcome variables in burn patients. J Parenter Enteral Nutr 14:225, 1990.
48. GIANOTTI L et al: Effect of route of delivery and formulation of postoperative nutritional support in patients undergoing major operations for malignant neoplasms. Arch Surg 132:1222, 1997.

49. McCARTER MD et al: Preoperative oral supplement with immunonutrients in cancer patients. J Parenter Enteral Nutr 22:206, 1998.
50. SPECTOR AA, BURNS CP: Biological and therapeutic potential of membrane lipid modification in tumors. Cancer Res 47:4529, 1987.
51. BARTLETT D et al: Differential effect of median- and long-chain triglycerides on tumor growth and metastasis. J Parenter Enteral Nutr 16(Suppl):55S, 1992.
52. CAVE WT JR: Dietary n-3 (w-3) polyunsaturated fatty acid effects on animal tumorigenesis. FASEB J 5:2160, 1991.
53. MENDEZ B et al: Effects of different lipid sources in total parenteral nutrition on whole body protein kinetic and tumor growth. J Parenter Enteral Nutr 16:545, 1992.
54. WOLF RF et al: Effect of growth hormone on tumor and host in an animal model. Ann Surg Oncol 1:314, 1994.
55. NG B et al: Growth hormone administration preserves lean body mass in sarcoma-bearing rats treated with doxorubicin. Cancer Res 53:5483, 1993.
56. NG B, ENG HE et al: Insulin-like growth factor I preserves host lean tissue mass in cancer cachexia. Am J Physiol 262:R426, 1992.
57. BARTLETT DL et al: The effect of growth hormone and protein intake on tumor growth and host cachexia. Surgery 117:260, 1995.
58. PINES A et al: Gastrointestinal tumors in acromegalic patients. Am J Gastroenterol 80:266, 1985.
59. FRADKIN JE et al: Risk of leukemia after treatment with pituitary growth hormone. JAMA 270:2829, 1993.
60. TOROSIAN MH, DONOWAY RB: Growth hormone inhibits tumor metastasis. Cancer 67:2280, 1991.
61. HEATLEY RV et al: Preoperative intravenous feeding: A controlled trial. Postgrad Med J 55:541, 1979.
62. KLEIN S et al: Nutrition support in clinical practice: Review of published data and recommendations for future research directions. J Parenter Enteral Nutr 21:133, 1997.
63. Perioperative total parenteral nutrition in surgical patients. The VA total parenteral nutrition co-operative study group. N Engl J Med 325:525, 1991.
64. TOROSIAN MH et al: Reduction of methotrexate toxicity with improved nutritional status in tumor-bearing animals. Cancer 61:1731, 1988.
65. DONALDSON SS: Nutritional support as an adjunct to radiation therapy. J Parenter Enteral Nutr 8:302, 1984.

# PART II

# ORGAN SYSTEM CANCER

# CHAPTER 7

# NEOPLASMS OF THE SKIN

## 7A / PRECANCEROUS LESIONS AND CARCINOMA IN SITU, SQUAMOUS CELL CARCINOMA (EPIDERMOID CARCINOMA), AND BASAL CELL CARCINOMA

*Charles J. McDonald, Michelle Krause, Raymond G. Dufresne, and Leslie Robinson-Bostom*

### INTRODUCTION

Malignant neoplasms of the skin are the most common malignancies in all geographic regions inhabited by Caucasians. The most common skin cancers are classified as nonmelanoma skin cancer, which includes basal cell carcinoma (BCC), squamous cell carcinoma (SCC), and carcinoma in situ (Bowen's disease, erythroplasia of Queyrat, and keratoacanthoma). This chapter will address the epidemiology, causative factors, diagnosis, staging, and treatment of nonmelanoma skin cancer as well as precancerous conditions.

### INCIDENCE AND EPIDEMIOLOGY

Nonmelanoma skin cancer is the most common malignancy in the United States.[1] The projected incidence of nonmelanoma skin cancer in the United States was estimated to be 900,000 to 1,200,000 cases for 1994 alone.[2] The rates are even higher in Australia, where the incidence is the highest in the world. The standardized incidence of treated nonmelanoma skin cancers in Australia in 1984 was 827 per 100,000 versus the 19 per 100,000 world average.[3] There is a profound north-to-south gradient in incidence of nonmelanoma skin cancer due primarily to differences in exposure to ultraviolet (UV) light (Table 7A-1). Caucasian individuals living in the southern United States have a higher incidence of nonmelanoma skin cancer than those living in the northern states. The incidence of nonmelanoma skin cancer also appears to be rising. In British Columbia from 1973 to 1987, the incidence of BCC increased by 60.6% in men and 48.4% in women, and SCC increased by 59.2% in men and 67.4% in women.[4] Significant increases have also been observed in

the United Kingdom. From 1978 to 1991, BCC was found to have increased by 235% (1:1 male to female ratio) and SCC by 153% (3:2 ratio).[5]

### ETIOLOGY

#### EXTERNAL FACTORS

It is almost universally accepted that UV light is the single most important etiologic agent in the development of skin cancer.[6–11] UV light acts as a tumor initiator and promoter, causing DNA mutations associated with immune suppression.

It has been well established that sunburn and carcinogenesis are induced by UV radiation in the spectrum of UV light B and C (UV-B and UV-C, 250 to 320 nm). Ultraviolet light A (UV-A, 320 to 440 nm) can also produce sunburn and augment the sunburn effects of UV-B, but it is approximately 1000 to 10,000 times less mutagenic than either UV-B or UV-C.[12,13]

Absorption of UV light by DNA produces an excited state that induces the formation of pyrimidine dimers. These are usually rectified by excisional repair.[8] These repair mechanisms are eventually overwhelmed and become ineffective under conditions of constant UV bombardment, such as repeated sunburn. Ineffective excisional repair leads to partial defect repair, mutation and carcinogenesis, altered metabolism, or cell death. After decades of faulty DNA repair, cutaneous malignancies can develop in susceptible individuals. It has been suggested that skin cancer induction by UV-B is initiated by early and initial DNA repair.[14,15] Cells survive the repair but now have abnormal replication mechanisms that favor errors in DNA replication, which promote neoplastic change. Inherent defective

**TABLE 7A-1.** INCIDENCE OF BASAL AND SQUAMOUS CELL CARCINOMA AMONG CAUCASIANS

| 1970S AND 1980S | LATITUDE | YEAR | BASAL CELL CARCINOMA INCIDENCE [NO. ($10^5$) YR] | | | | SQUAMOUS CELL CARCINOMA INCIDENCE [NO. ($10^5$) YR] | | | |
|---|---|---|---|---|---|---|---|---|---|---|
| | | | CASES | MEN | WOMEN | MALE-TO-FEMALE RATIO | CASES | MEN | WOMEN | MALE-TO-FEMALE RATIO |
| Kauai, Hawaii | 22°N | 1983–87 | 242 | 576 | 298 | 1.9 | 58 | 153 | 92 | 1.7 |
| New Orleans, LA | 30°N | 1977–78 | 2114 | 410 | 215 | 1.9 | 653 | 153 | 49 | 3.1 |
| Dallas–Ft. Worth, TX | 33°N | 1971–72 | 2442 | 394 | 205 | 1.9 | 776 | 145 | 54 | 2.7 |
| Atlanta, GA | 34°N | 1977–78 | 3214 | 423 | 229 | 1.8 | 836 | 131 | 53 | 2.5 |
| New Mexico: | 33–37°N | 1977–78 | 2549 | 346 | 205 | 1.7 | 638 | 98 | 42 | 2.3 |
|   Caucasian | 37°N | 1977–78 | 2376 | 495 | 279 | 1.8 | 600 | 143 | 55 | 2.6 |
|   Hispanic American | 37°N | 1977–78 | 173 | 64 | 48 | 1.3 | 38 | 13 | 12 | 1.1 |
| San Francisco–Oakland, CA | 38°N | 1977–78 | 5355 | 239 | 145 | 1.6 | 1010 | 56 | 18 | 3.1 |
| | | 1971–72 | 2103 | 198 | 117 | 1.7 | 427 | 52 | 16 | 3.3 |
| Utah | 37–42°N | 1977–78 | 2610 | 327 | 198 | 1.7 | 817 | 123 | 46 | 2.7 |
| Iowa | 41–44°N | 1971–72 | 1489 | 123 | 69 | 1.8 | 507 | 51 | 14 | 3.6 |
| Detroit, MI | 42°N | 1977–78 | 3871 | 142 | 97 | 1.5 | 634 | 30 | 11 | 2.7 |
| Vermont and New Hampshire | 43–45°N | 1979–80 | 2022 | 159 | 87 | 1.8 | 285 | 32 | 8 | 4.0 |
| Rochester, MN | 45°N | 1976–84 | 657 | 175 | 124 | 1.4 | 169 | 63 | 23 | 2.8 |
| Minneapolis–St. Paul, MN | 45°N | 1977–78 | 2939 | 213 | 144 | 1.5 | 382 | 37 | 12 | 3.1 |
| | | 1971–72 | 1018 | 165 | 102 | 1.6 | 175 | 37 | 12 | 3.1 |
| Portland, OR | 46°N | 1960–86 | — | — | — | — | 1874 | 81 | 24 | 3.4 |
| Seattle, WA | 48°N | 1977–78 | 1810 | 210 | 125 | 1.7 | 325 | 47 | 16 | 2.9 |
| British Columbia | 49–60°N | 1973 | 1684 | 71 | 62 | 1.1 | 344 | 17 | 9 | 1.8 |
| | | 1980 | 2736 | 96 | 81 | 1.2 | 622 | 26 | 13 | 2.0 |
| | | 1987 | 4152 | 120 | 92 | 1.3 | 963 | 31 | 17 | 1.8 |

repair mechanisms may predispose individuals to nonmelanoma skin cancers. Individuals with a history of BCC exhibited decreased DNA repair after exposure to UV radiation[16] and more frequent basal cell replication than normal controls.[17] The exact relationship between these observations and the development of skin cancer in a susceptible host is not entirely clear. UV light also causes mutations in the p53 tumor suppressor gene, which is found in SCCs. This protein acts as a tumor suppressor by promoting apoptosis of cells with DNA damage.[18,19] Additional support for the role of UV light in development of nonmelanoma skin cancer is the site distribution of these lesions. By far the most frequent location of nonmelanoma skin cancer in Caucasians for both genders is the face, followed by the neck, trunk, upper extremities, and lower extremities.[20,21]

UV-B, as well as UV-A, also appears to promote tumor formation by selective immunosuppression.[7] UV irradiation appears to affect the host's cell-mediated immune system by shifting to the suppressor T cell pathway over the helper T cell pathway, thereby altering immunologic surveillance and rejection of tumor cells.[22,23] The helper T lymphocyte/suppressor T lymphocyte ratio is abnormally low, and the absolute T suppressor count is high, in individuals with a history of heavy UV exposure and multiple nonmelanoma skin cancer.[22] Contact hypersensitivity, also a cell-mediated process, is also inhibited by UV exposure.[23]

Although UV-A is carcinogenic, especially in combination with UV-B, UV-A exposure may be protective to the skin because it stimulates the production of melanin, decreasing the risk of sunburn.[12]

There is good evidence, however, that exposure to 8-methoxypsoralen and UV-A (PUVA) is mutagenic as well as immunosuppressive.[24–28] Patients who have been exposed to long-term PUVA are at significantly increased risk of developing nonmelanoma skin cancer, particularly if the number of exposures is above 100 and the dose is greater than, or equal to, 250 J/cm$^2$.[24,25]

UV-C (wavelengths less than 290 nm) is effectively filtered by the ozone layer in the stratospheric atmosphere and does not reach the surface of the earth. Depletion of the ozone layer by physical (high-altitude supersonic aircraft) and chemical (volatile hydrocarbons) means has raised concerns about increased exposure to all wavelengths of UV light.[29,15] The most recent theoretical estimate for increased risk of nonmelanoma and melanoma skin cancers is that a 1% decrease in stratospheric ozone may increase nonmelanoma and melanoma skin cancers by 2.3%.[30]

X-irradiation produces cutaneous malignancies in a manner similar to UV-induced carcinogenesis. In the past, many of these cancers occurred as a result of chronic occupational exposure. Exposure of patients to direct x-irradiation and physicians and technicians to scattered x-irradiation has been greatly reduced since the turn of the century, and the incidence of these tumors has decreased dramatically. However, skin cancer is still seen as a late sequela of therapeutic radiation, such as past treatment for acne or skin cancers.

Numerous potential chemical carcinogens have been extensively studied; these include polycyclic and aromatic hydrocarbons, and, to a lesser extent tar, pitch, soot, creosol, asphalt, and diesel oils, among others.[31] The actual incidence of carcinomas attributable to these substances is unknown. Cutaneous malignancies, particularly SCC, have long been associated with arsenic exposure through medicines as well as pesticides. This has been especially problematic in Asian countries where arsenic was used in proprietary medications[32–34] and may be an underrecognized factor in this country.[35] Arsenic exposure is associated with internal malignancies, especially of the lung and bladder, that classically present after the skin cancers are apparent.[35]

## HOST FACTORS

Skin color is the single most important host factor in the development of nonmelanoma skin cancer. Melanin gives skin its color and is our principal cutaneous sun protector. Individuals with the lowest concentration of melanin tend to be of Celtic origin. These very fair Caucasians are prone to severe sunburn after relatively short sun exposure and are at increased risk of developing cutaneous neoplasms. In contrast, native black Africans have skin that is rich in melanin, burn only after extensive sun exposure, and rarely develop sun-related neoplasms. Kricker[36] found for Australians that an increased risk of BCC was strongly associated with fair skin color, inability to tan, birth or early age of arrival in Australia, northern European ancestry, presence of multiple nevi, and presence of solar elastosis (cutaneous sun damage).

A "sun-reactive skin typing system" proposed by Pathak[12] is used frequently in dermatology as a counseling tool to educate patients about the harmful effects of sun exposure and sunburn protection. Skin types are based on genetically determined melanin content of skin, skin color, facultative skin color (ability of skin to produce protective melanin and tan). Skin types I and II generally describe persons of northern European extraction; types III and IV describe southern Europeans, northern Mongolians, and Mediterraneans; and types V and VI describe African, darker Mediterraneans, and southern Mongolians.

Immunosuppression, whether from UV exposure or otherwise, increases the risk for nonmelanoma skin cancer. This has been especially well studied among renal transplant patients.[37–39] The overall risk of developing nonmelanoma skin cancer is 40% at 20 years after renal transplant.[38] The risk is 43.8% at 7 years after heart transplant.[40] Risk is further increased in both cases in light skin types and with a history of prolonged UV exposure. Increased risk of nonmelanoma skin cancer has also been associated with chronic corticosteroid treatment and altered immune states, such as lymphomas and leukemia.[39]

Human papillomavirus infection has also been associated with nonmelanoma skin cancer, especially in immunosuppressed individuals. Human papillomavirus is frequently found in precancerous lesions and squamous cell carcinomas in renal transplant patients.[41–43] This association is not as dramatic in the general population. Human papillomavirus type 16 has been associated with Bowen's disease and SCC of the fingers, while virus types 16 and 18 have been associated with SCC of the genital tract.[44–46] The association between human papillomavirus and nonmelanoma skin cancers on other areas of the body is less clear in a normal host. However, epidermodysplasia verruciformis is a disorder in which widespread infection with human papillomavirus, primarily types 5 and 8, produces multiple flat warts, which tend to develop into SCC.[47] Widespread nonmelanoma skin cancers, several of which were positive for type 16 or 18 papillomavirus, have been reported in a patient after 10 years of PUVA therapy for psoriasis.[48]

In addition to epidermodysplasia verruciformis, other cutaneous disorders that have an increased risk of nonmelanoma skin cancer include xeroderma pigmentosum, basal cell nevus syndrome, and albinism. The classic inherited disease of defective DNA repair is xeroderma pigmentosum. By the second decade of life, these patients have typically developed hundreds of cutaneous malignancies, primarily in sun exposed areas, that are attributable to faulty DNA repair.[11,49] Individuals with basal cell nevus syndrome (Gorlin syndrome), an autosomal dominant disorder, develop numerous BCCs starting in the second decade of life. Other defects seen in this genodermatosis include palmar pits, dental cysts, bifid ribs, spinal cord defects, broad nasal root, hypertelorism, and myriad disorders of the central nervous system, gastrointestinal system, bones, and other organs. It has been associated with noncutaneous tumors such as fibrosarcoma, medulloblastoma, rhabdomyosarcoma, meningioma, ovarian fibroma, and cardiac fibroma. The gene for Gorlin syndrome has been cloned and mapped to 9q22.3. A point mutation is present, and loss of the second allele leads to tumor formation.[50,51] An association between UV exposure and malignancy has not been established in these patients.[52] Albinos lack skin pigment, are unable to tan, and are at increased risk of developing skin cancers.[53]

## METHODS OF TREATING SKIN CANCERS

The cost of treating skin cancers and precancers is significant, primarily because of the high incidence of these tumors. Multiple modalities are available, and proper selection of techniques can result in a high cure rate and relative cost effectiveness (Table 7A-2). Algorithms for treating nonmelanoma skin cancer have been

**TABLE 7A-2. TREATMENT OF PRECANCERS AND CANCERS**

Topical:
  5-Fluorouracil
  Retinoids

Surgical:
  Excision
  Mohs' surgery
  Electrodessication and curettage
  Cryosurgery
  Dermabrasion
  Laser abrasion

Other:
  Systemic retinoids
  Interferon
  Photodynamic therapy

described[54,55] based on the many factors involved in selecting a technique. Excisional surgery needs no description in this text and is the "gold standard" of therapy. However, to avoid redundancy later in this chapter, several common techniques will be reviewed, including topical 5-fluorouracil (5-FU), electrodessication and curettage, laser vaporization, cryosurgery, interferon, retinoids, photodynamic therapy, and Mohs' micrographic surgery.

5-FU blocks DNA synthesis by inhibiting thymidylate synthetase. In the 1960s, it was noted that actinic keratoses respond to systemically administered 5-FU.[56] Solutions and creams (of 1% to 20% concentration) were formulated and used as topical therapy for skin cancers and precancers. Precancers and very superficial small cancers responded best, but high recurrence rates were reported in the routine use of this method of treatment for skin cancers. The length of treatment is usually 3 to 4 weeks, that is, until necrosis of the tumor occurs. This form of treatment must be done under supervision and entails long-term re-evaluation.

Electrodessication and curettage can be a highly effective procedure for treating lower-risk tumors, with a cure rate of approximately 93% in basal cell carcinoma.[57] It is a quick and highly cost effective treatment requiring minimal equipment. In general, the tumor is debulked with a curette and the tissue desiccated for further destruction. The cycle is repeated, generally three times, to achieve a tumorless plane. The defect is allowed to heal over a few weeks, usually with a minor scar and dyschromia. Carbon dioxide ($CO_2$) laser vaporization can also be used as a destructive tool instead of the electrosurgery unit. The $CO_2$ lasers allow better visualization of tissue with less char and possibly better healing because of less adjacent tissue injury.[58]

Using cryosurgery, high lesion cure rates have been reported; a recent review reports 92.5% complete response at 5 years.[57] In cryotherapy, the tissues are quickly cooled to 50°C, preferably with liquid nitrogen. Tumor cells are more sensitive to cold than normal cells, so a semiselective destruction occurs. In small superficial tumors, an open spray can be used. In larger tumors, a thermocouple is used to measure the temperature at the desired depth and lateral margins of destruction. In highly skilled hands, cryosurgery can be effective, even in large tumors.

Intralesional interferon, primarily α interferon, has been reported as effective in the treatment of actinic keratoses, Bowen's disease, BCC, SCC, and keratoacanthoma.[59] Interferon induces both antitumor and potentially immunomodulating effects.[60–62] Interferon is limited in use because of the cost,[62] the numerous injections required to cause an effect, the number of associated systemic symptoms and side effects, and some evidence suggesting less effectiveness than traditional methods. In combination with systemic retinoids, systemic interferon has also been used as an adjunct in aggressive or widespread disease.

Retinoids, topically and systemically, can be used both as a preventative measure and, at times, as a treatment. Retinoids have several effects, including potent antiproliferative and differentiation-inducing effects. Topical isotretinate can be used to diminish the number of precancers and the development of new lesions, and in combination with 5-FU,[63] or combined with systemic retinoids, to control disease in patients with numerous lesions.[64] Systemic retinoids, and etretinate, have been used prophylactically in patients such as those with basal cell nevus syndrome or xeroderma pigmentosa,[65] and as a treatment in patients with numerous lesions,

prior organ transplantation,[64] or aggressive local lesions, and as a modulating therapy in patients with metastatic disease.

Photodynamic therapy is based on the selective excitation of cells that have taken up a photosensitizer and are then excited by a local light source. In cutaneous oncology, this has been accomplished using the systemic administration of substances such as porphyrins. Systemic photosensitization has led to the evaluation of other materials, including topical aminolevulinic acid. In reports of small series, both systemic and topical therapy has been reported to be successful in treating Bowen's disease, basal cell carcinoma, and squamous cell carcinoma.[66] The indications, and limitations, of this technique have not been fully evaluated, and responses are reported as having variable success.[67,68] A patient with numerous, superficial lesions, such as the basal cell nevus syndrome, may be the best candidate.[69]

Mohs' micrographic surgery is a variant of excision that is reported to have the highest 5-year cure rate of the commonly used surgical methods: 97% to 98% for BCCs and approximately 95% for primary SCC.[57,70,71] By means of a technique of fully evaluating the margins of the excision during surgery, the procedure, which is usually performed in a special facility, offers high cure rates of contiguously growing tumors such as BCCs and most SCCs. Because there is better margin control, which allows tissue conservation, more conservative margins can be utilized without compromising the cure. The procedure is limited by its availability, its higher cost than a destructive procedure or simple excision, and its being less applicable to tumors that grow in a noncontiguous manner. A large number of cutaneous tumors have been treated with Mohs' surgery.[70,71]

## PRECANCEROUS LESIONS AND CARCINOMA IN SITU

BCCs have no known precancerous lesions. However, common precursors to SCC include actinic keratoses, actinic cheilitis, and SCC in situ. Bowen's disease and erythroplasia of Queyrat (Bowen's of the glans penis) are designated carcinoma in situ because they appear histologically to have greater malignant potential than other precancerous lesions.

The potential for malignant change depends on the lesion in question. In a study of the malignant potential of actinic keratoses, 60% of SCCs diagnosed arose from actinic keratoses documented in the previous year.[72] Malignant transformation, if it does occur, requires 6 to 10 years, although it can vary significantly. Although the relative frequency of malignant degeneration in any individual keratosis is low, susceptible individuals may develop hundreds of these lesions in a lifetime. The risk of malignant degeneration is significant in Bowen's disease. If left untreated, 50% of Bowen's tumors will eventually undergo malignant change; 10% of actinic keratoses will do the same.[73]

**ACTINIC KERATOSIS.** Actinic keratoses are the most common epithelial precancerous lesion.[10,72,74,75] They develop almost exclusively in Caucasians. Actinic keratoses occur more frequently in older individuals, likely secondary to cumulative sunlight exposure and latitude of residence. Marks et al. reported a prevalence of 59.2% in an Australian study with subjects age 40 and older.[75] In contrast, the prevalence was found to be 23% in a Welsh study with subjects age 60 and older.[76]

Actinic keratoses are located predominantly on sun-exposed skin. The vast majority occur on the face, head, and neck followed by the upper extremities, trunk, and lower extremities.[10] Risk factors for developing actinic keratoses include older age, high cumulative UV-B exposure, pale eyes, childhood freckling, and propensity toward sunburn.[10]

Actinic cheilitis is a lesion of the lower lip that is analogous to actinic keratosis. As with actinic keratoses, it is widely accepted that this lesion is caused by excessive sun exposure. The lesion occurs almost exclusively on the lower lip, predominantly at the vermillion border because of its direct angle with the sun. There is a higher incidence in fair-skinned individuals. Chronic skin irritation (i.e., from tobacco, poor hygiene, ill-fitting dentures) has also been associated with increased risk of actinic cheilitis.[77]

As with actinic keratoses, actinic cheilitis has been associated with malignant transformation into SCC. The relative risk is estimated at 2.5.[78]

Premalignant lesions, such as actinic keratoses and actinic cheilitis, occur more frequently in genodermatoses that exhibit decreased UV filtration or defective DNA repair. Although almost unheard of in normal blacks, actinic keratoses are common in black albinos. In a study of Tanzanian albinos, 91% of patients over the age of 20 years were found to have actinic keratoses.[53] The youngest child in this study with actinic keratoses was 8 years old. Individuals with xeroderma pigmentosum develop actinic keratoses in childhood secondary to defective DNA repair.[79]

Immunosuppression also increases the risk of developing actinic keratoses. Organ transplant patients who are chronically immunosuppressed have an increased incidence of actinic keratoses.[80–82] One study comparing heart and kidney transplant patients found a higher incidence of actinic keratoses in heart transplant patients.[81] The difference was attributed to older age at transplant and more profound immunosuppression.

*CLINICAL MANIFESTATIONS.* Actinic keratoses may start out as ill-defined pink to red macules or papules with telangiectasias (Fig. 7A-1). As they progress, they develop adherent scale that is difficult to remove. Removal of the scale may produce bleeding points. Left untreated, the scale becomes hypertrophic. A cutaneous horn may eventually develop. These lesions predominate on sun-exposed areas such as the head, face, neck, and upper extremities.

Actinic cheilitis may present early as persistent lip erythema (Fig. 7A-2). Later xerosis and scaling develop and may involve the entire lower lip. Some areas may develop white thickening known as leukoplakia. Ill-defined vermillion border, atrophy, ulceration, and nodularity are warning signs for malignant transformation, although apparently insignificant surface change may represent carcinoma. These lesions occur almost exclusively on the lower lip.

*HISTOLOGY OF ACTINIC KERATOSES.* Actinic keratoses demonstrate disordered epithelial maturation, nuclear atypia, pyknosis, dyskeratosis, and suprabasilar mitoses[83] (Fig. 7A-3). Follicular epithelium is usually spared. Solar elastosis is seen in the dermis. Subtypes of actinic keratoses include acantholytic (adenoid), atrophic, hypertrophic, pigmented, and bowenoid types.[84]

*TREATMENT.* Multiple modalities are available for the treatment of actinic keratoses. Cryosurgery with liquid nitrogen is a

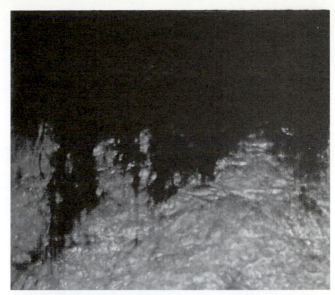

**FIGURE 7A-1.** Actinic keratosis: An ill-defined papule with adherent scale.

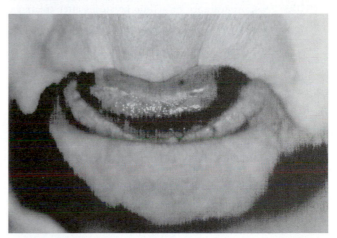

**FIGURE 7A-2.** Lower lip xerosis and scaling characteristic of actinic cheilitis.

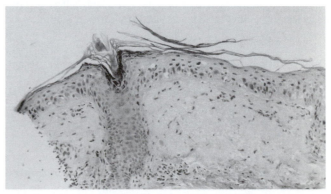

**FIGURE 7A-3.** Actinic keratosis: One observes disordered epithelial maturation, nuclear atypia, pyknosis, and dyskeratosis.

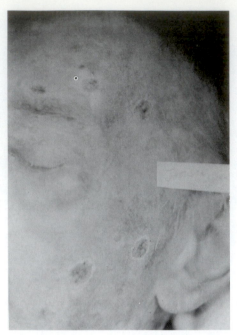

**FIGURE 7A-4.** Appearance of actinic keratoses after treatment with $CO_2$ laser.

highly effective method. In thicker hyperkeratotic lesions, curettage with or without desiccation may be helpful to remove the thicker material. In widespread lesions, topical 5-FU (available as 1% to 5% cream and solutions) for 3 to 4 weeks will result in a significant reduction of a precancerous lesion. In exceptional refractory and extensive cases, medium-depth chemical peeling,[85] dermabrasion,[86] and $CO_2$ laser resurfacing[87] (Fig. 7A-4) can be utilized. As an adjunctive therapy, daily sunscreen alone appears to modulate the number that develop into skin cancer. Topical retinoids (isotretinate) are reported to decrease the number of actinic keratoses.[88] Photodynamic therapy with 5-aminolevulinic acid is highly effective.[89] Systemic retinoids can be selectively used in severe and extensive cases.

The treatment of actinic cheilitis is similar to actinic keratoses.[90] Focal treatment with a destructive approach such as electrodestruction or cryosurgery is appropriate and highly effective (79% success).[91,92] However, actinic cheilitis tends to be a multifocal disease. Topical 5-FU offers palliative responses but not histologic elimination of tumor.[93,94] In most cases, $CO_2$ laser resurfacing results in histologic and clinical responses and is described as having fewer side effects than traditional vermilionectomy.[90] Delayed healing of the lip is a major disadvantage of laser vermilionectomy. Vermilionectomy is the standard in severe refractory actinic cheilitis and allows confirmation of the diagnosis and exclusion of invasive SCC.[95–100]

**BOWEN'S DISEASE.** Bowen's disease, or SCC in situ, is a premalignant neoplasm that occurs on both sun-exposed and non-sun-exposed areas of the body. Body site distribution of Bowen's disease is a topic of debate. Kossard et al.[101] found in Australian patients the most common sites for Bowen's disease were the head and neck. In contrast, in Hawaii and the United Kingdom, the most common body sites were found to be the extremities.[102,103] Bowen's disease is typically a disease of elderly Caucasians but may occur as early as the third decade.[101] Bowen's disease has been reported in black patients.[104,105] It probably goes underdiagnosed in black patients because it may look like other dermatoses and tends to be asymptomatic.

Bowen's tumors are known to be associated with chronic trivalent arsenic exposure from medicinal and environmental sources.[104,106,32] In a recent study of Chinese patients with Bowen's disease attributed to arsenic exposure, the mean length of exposure was 6.4 years. The site distribution of lesions in these patients were in non-sun-exposed areas such as the trunk and palms, as well as sun-exposed areas such as the extremities.[32] When there is a history of chronic arsenic ingestion, there is a strong relationship between Bowen's disease and associated internal malignancies.[107,73,106]

*CLINICAL MANIFESTATIONS.* Clinically the lesions appear as sharply demarcated red to brown plaques with very fine scale or crust (Fig. 7A-5). Little or no surface elevation is present and induration is usually absent. As the lesions transform into malignancies, they become indurated and the surface tends to be irregular. When the lesions occur on the fingers, they may mimic eczema and are often treated unsuccessfully with eczema treatments.

*DIAGNOSIS.* Biopsy is necessary to confirm the diagnosis and is done by shave biopsy or preferably punch biopsy. An adequate specimen to the depth of the dermis is often needed to distinguish this lesion from SCC.

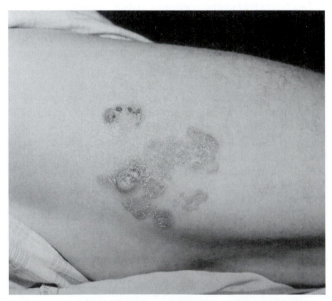

**FIGURE 7A-5.** Bowen's tumor on the thigh showing sharp demarcation, irregular shape, and scale.

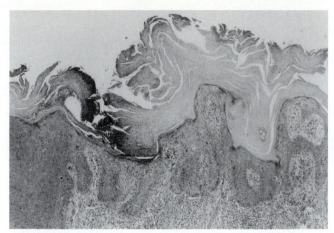

**FIGURE 7A-6.** Bowen's disease: Full-thickness epidermal atypia with "windblown" appearance. The epidermis is acanthotic with elongation of the rete ridges. The stratum corneum is hyperkeratotic and parakeratotic.

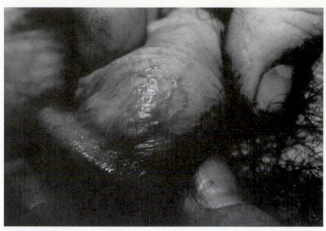

**FIGURE 7A-7.** An ill-defined, red, friable, velvety plaque characteristic of erythroplasia of Queyrat.

*HISTOLOGY.* Bowen's disease or SCC in situ is characterized histologically by disordered keratinocytes with little or no maturation (Fig. 7A-6). This full-thickness keratinocyte atypia results in a "windblown" appearance of the epidermis. Hyperchromatic nuclei, dyskeratotic cells, pyknotic cells, and mitoses are frequent and randomly dispersed. The epidermis is often acanthotic with elongation and thickening of the rete ridges. Vacuolization of the upper spinous and granular cell layers may be seen. The stratum corneum is hyperkeratotic and parakeratotic. In SCC in situ, the basement membrane zone remains intact; however, atypical keratinocytes may deeply involve hair follicles and other adnexal structures.[108]

In some examples of Bowen's disease, nests of atypical keratinocytes are seen in an otherwise normal epidermis. This has been previously termed the intraepidermal epithelioma of Borst-Jadassohn.[109]

*STAGING.* Clinical staging is not followed in Bowen's disease.

*TREATMENT.* For a small localized area, topical 5-FU, simple destruction with cryosurgery, electrodestruction, or $CO_2$ laser vaporization can be sufficient.[110] However, microinvasion or spread down hair follicles results in a variable response. Because of the high risk of focal invasion, excision may be the treatment of choice in larger lesions. Mohs' surgery can be selectively employed in recurrent, poorly defined tumors or if wide resection is not desired, such as in the case of a digit.[111] Interferon has been used successfully in Bowen's disease.[66,67] Photodynamic therapy can be used either with systemic or topical sensitizers.[69] A combination of isotretinoin and interferon has been reported in extensive multiple lesions.[112]

ERYTHROPLASIA OF QUEYRAT. Erythroplasia of Queyrat (EQ) is a precancerous lesion, SCC in situ, that occurs principally on the glans penis. Although EQ is histologically indistinguishable from Bowen's disease, it tends to be more invasive. EQ was found to be invasive in 14% of cases, whereas Bowen's disease was invasive in 5% of cases.[104] However, EQ does not have the association with internal malignancy noted with Bowen's disease. This disease is seen almost exclusively in uncircumcised males.[113]

*CLINICAL MANIFESTATIONS.* These lesions present as red, friable, velvety, oozing plaques (Fig. 7A-7). As a rule they do not have a crust. On occasion they may present as dry, darkly pigmented plaques or papular, verrucous plaques. Ulceration suggests that dermal invasion may have occurred.

*DIAGNOSIS.* Biopsy is necessary to confirm the diagnosis and is done by shave biopsy or punch biopsy. If ulceration is present, biopsy of the ulcerated portion is necessary to rule out an invasive tumor.

*HISTOLOGY.* The histology of EQ has the same appearance as Bowen's disease. Please refer to the above description.

*TREATMENT.* The treatment of EQ is similar to that for the other noninvasive cancers or precancers. Focal lesions can be addressed with destructive techniques including cryosurgery,[114] electrodesiccation and curettage, $CO_2$ laser vaporization, and topical 5FU.[115,116] These destructive techniques are associated with several weeks of recovery. Excision is important in refractory cases and when the possibility of invasion is of concern. Mohs' surgery has been employed for tissue conservation.[117,118] Excision may be combined with a circumcision. The use of isotretinoin has been described anecdotally.[119]

KERATOACANTHOMA. Keratoacanthoma is a relatively common, rapidly growing tumor of the elderly with a clinical and histologic pattern similar to that for SCC. These tumors rarely progress to SCCs and tend to resolve spontaneously. They are grouped into solitary and multiple types.

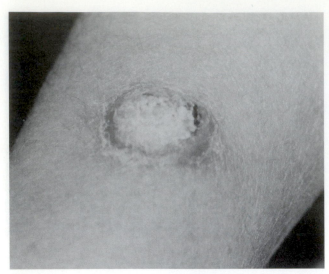

**FIGURE 7A-8.** Keratoacanthoma: Rapidly growing, domed plaque with central keratotic plug on the forearm.

UV light probably plays a role in the genesis of these lesions since the majority occur on sun-exposed skin.[120] The face, extensor surface of the hands, and forearms are the most common sites.[121,122] Tumors of the lower leg are found almost exclusively in women. Tumors of the hands are more common in men.[121]

Keratoacanthomas occur more frequently in men than women.[121] Like SCC, these lesions occur most frequently in older individuals with fair skin.[121,123] The peak incidence occurs during the fifth and sixth decades.[121,122]

An increased risk of keratoacanthomas has been associated with Muir-Torre syndrome. This is a rare autosomal disorder characterized by multiple tumors, keratoacanthomas, and adenocarcinoma of the colon. These cases usually present during the fifth and sixth decades.[124,125] Individuals with xeroderma pigmentosum also have an increased risk of keratoacanthomas with presentation early in life.[6,49,79]

Immunosuppressed patients are at increased risk of developing keratoacanthomas as well as other cutaneous malignancies.[126–128]

*CLINICAL MANIFESTATIONS.* Solitary keratoacanthomas present as rapidly growing, dome-shaped papules or nodules (Fig. 7A-8). These lesions usually present initially as a small, domed papule with a central keratotic umbilication that grows rapidly over a period of 6 to 8 weeks. Most keratoacanthomas measure 1.0 to 2.5 cm. Mature nodules exhibit a smooth pink to red surface with telangiectasias. The center contains a horny plug. The majority of lesions spontaneously resolve over a period of 3 to 6 months with a resultant atrophic scar.

Three clinical variants of the solitary keratoacanthoma include the giant keratoacanthoma, keratoacanthoma centri fugum marginatum, and subungual keratoacanthoma. Giant keratoacanthomas are solitary keratoacanthomas on the nose and eyelids that grow to 5 cm or greater. They tend to resolve spontaneously.[129,130] Keratoacanthoma centrifugum marginatum is a solitary keratoacanthoma

on the hands or legs that may grow up to 20 cm in diameter. Unlike the other solitary keratoacanthomas, it tends not to resolve spontaneously.[129,131,132] Subungual keratoacanthomas develop under the distal fingernail. They are painful and tend not to resolve spontaneously.[133–135]

Multiple keratoacanthomas, also known as the Ferguson Smith type, are identical to solitary keratoacanthomas but develop several lesions at any one time. The lesions appear suddenly, involute spontaneously, and recur periodically. Unlike solitary keratoacanthomas, these lesions occur in younger individuals, usually during early adulthood.[129,136]

A subtype of multiple keratoacanthomas includes eruptive keratoacanthomas of Grzybowski. In this disease, hundreds to thousands of 2- to 3-mm domed papules with central keratotic plugs occur in a disseminated distribution. Pruritus is a common feature. The palms and soles are usually spared. Lesions spontaneously resolve without scarring.[136,137]

*DIAGNOSIS.* The clinical presentation of keratoacanthoma is distinctive. Biopsy is confirmative and allows the exclusion of invasive SCC. To establish depth of invasion, if it exists, punch or excisional biopsy is preferred over shave biopsy.

*HISTOLOGY.* Keratoacanthomas are dynamic tumors that demonstrate proliferative, fully developed, and involuting stages[138] (Fig. 7A-9). Histology varies with the stage of growth. The classic histology is described in fully developed tumors. The architecture is characterized by a central keratin-filled crater surrounded by a lip of acanthotic epidermis without significant cytologic atypia. The epidermis proliferates irregularly at the base of the crater and is composed of eosinophilic glassy keratinocytes. Neutrophil microabscesses may be seen within these lobules. Dense inflammation is also typically present. The tumor does not usually extend below the level of the eccrine glands. Perineural invasion has been reported.[139]

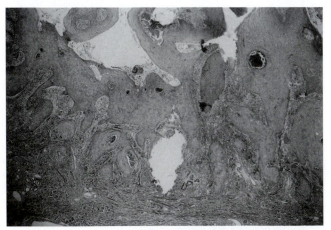

**FIGURE 7A-9.** Keratoacanthoma: Central keratin-filled crater with strands of atypical epidermis extending irregularly into the dermis.

Some authors categorize fully developed keratoacanthoma as a well-differentiated SCC (grade 1).[140] The early proliferative stage of keratoacanthoma mimics moderately differentiated SCC with strands of atypical epidermis extending irregularly into the dermis. Individual cell keratinization, dyskeratosis, and atypical mitoses may be seen, with a central keratin-filled crater.[138]

During involution, the borders of the crater are thin. Lichenoid inflammation, apoptotic keratinocytes, and fibrosis are observed at the crater's base. Flattening of the crater gradually occurs.[139]

*TREATMENT.* The treatment of keratoacanthoma is essentially the same as for SCC. In an early lesion, cryosurgery and electrodesiccation and curettage can be used with good reported success.[141] Although a keratoacanthoma will follow a self-limited course and regress spontaneously, the behavior cannot be predicted and many act like a SCC, including rapid growth and regional spread and metastasis. Excision is generally the treatment of choice. Mohs' surgery is reported to have a very low recurrence rate of 2.4%.[142]

These tumors are very sensitive to radiation, which, if used, may avoid local deformity.[143] Intralesional interferon has great appeal, but larger studies need to be performed.[144] There have been reports of intralesional treatment and response to numerous agents, including 5-FU, methotrexate, and bleomycin.[145–147] Systemic retinoids have been reported as helpful in patients with multiple lesions.[148]

## SQUAMOUS CELL CANCER (EPIDERMOID CARCINOMA)

Squamous cell cancer (SCC) is the second most common skin neoplasm in Caucasians and accounts for 20% of skin cancers.[149] The incidence among Australians is 201 per 100,000.[74] In the nonwhite races, SCC is the most common skin cancer. SCC is generally a disease of the middle-aged and elderly.

Most SCCs that occur in Caucasians arise on sun-exposed areas, principally the head, neck, and extremities.[149] In general, in African Americans SCCs occur on sun-protected areas.[150] However, in a study of 163 black patients treated at Charity Hospital in New Orleans, Mora and Perniciaro[151] found that the most common sites of squamous cell tumors were the face and lower extremities. Sunlight exposure may have contributed to the frequency of facial tumors at 33.9%. Collectively, the predisposing condition to cancers at the other sites was a history of scarring. Similar observations have been recorded in reports from India[152] and Singapore.[153]

**ETIOLOGY AND PATHOGENESIS.** The development of SCC is strongly associated with prolonged sunlight exposure and fair complexions. This is evident in Caucasians with excessive sun exposure, such as residents of Australia and New Zealand,[154–156] as well as in sailors, fishermen, ranchers, and farmers.[10]

The incidence of cutaneous SCC is markedly increased in immunosuppressed patients. This is particularly apparent in transplant patients who are on immunosuppresive agents for extended periods of time. Renal transplant patients are at 250 times increased risk of developing cutaneous SCC.[38] Literally hundreds of SCCs may be found on all areas of the body, with a predilection for sun-exposed areas. Although the incidence of BCC is also increased in this population, the normal ratio of BCC–SCC is reversed, and SCCs predominate. These tumors are also more aggressive.

Cutaneous SCC has also been associated with the human papillomavirus. Epidermodysplasia verruciformis is a rare familial disorder in which the face, neck, hands, and knees are covered with multiple, domed-shaped warts. Papillomavirus types 5 and 8 have been isolated from these lesions. Nonmelanoma skin cancers develop in sun-exposed areas in 25% of these individuals.[47] The Buschke-Löwenstein tumor, or verrucous carcinoma, is a rare tumor of the genital and perianal regions. It occurs most frequently on the glans or prepuce of uncircumcised males. This tumor has been associated with human papillomavirus types 6 and 11 in both its benign and premalignant stages.[157–159]

Although it occurs rarely, SCC is the most common cutaneous malignant lesion among African Americans. It is 20% more common than BCC.[151] Black albinos are at markedly increased risk of developing SCCs.[160,53] Blacks with vitiligo, however, are not at increased risk of developing SCC.[160] External factors such as exposure to chemical carcinogens, delayed effects of x-irradiation exposure, and possibly burns, scars, and chronic ulcers (Marjolin's ulcer) play a significant role in the carcinogenesis of SCCs in black individuals.[151,152,160,161] These factors play only a minor role in carcinogenesis in Caucasians.

Unusual skin cancers associated with chronic skin irritation and direct trauma are seen in the Kashmir region of northern India. In this frigid region, earthenware pots full of hot coals and leaves are held against the abdomen for warmth. Skin exposed to the pots develops chronic dermatitis, burns, and eventually scars. SCCs, or Kangri cancers, tend to develop in areas of scarring.[162] Additional evidence linking SCC with scarring was presented by Oettle,[163] who described SCC developing in chronic leg ulcers and following trauma, especially burns, in the South African black population.

**MODES OF SPREAD.** As with BCC, SCC initially is locally invasive and destructive. Spread can occur intraepithelially by skipping in a discontinuous manner through the skin and soft tissue. Local invasion can occur by lymphatic, perineural, and, rarely, intravascular means. All are associated with a significantly worsened prognosis.

Metastatic and nodal spread is common. Initial metastasis is by lymphatic invasion. Regional lymph nodes become enlarged and firm. Cancerous cells eventually metastasize to surrounding tissues. Distant metastases to the lungs, chest, or brain generally occur by hematologic spread. Distant metastases occur rarely, in long neglected cancers.

Several factors affect the prognosis of SCC, including the presence of a precancerous lesion, anatomic location, depth of invasion, and histologic grade. Tumors associated with actinically damaged skin tend to be slow growing and rarely metastasize. Estimates for rates of metastases in these lesions range from less than 0.1% of cases[164] to less than 2.6%.[165] Tumors that arise from apparently normal skin or from precancerous lesions other than actinic keratoses act more malignant and frequently metastasize. They are more invasive and frequently involve surrounding tissues, producing large, firm nodules. The rate of metastasis also depends on the location of the tumor. By meta-analysis, the overall rate of metastasis for SCC is 5.2%; the rate for ear and lip lesions is 11% and 13.7%, respectively.[157]

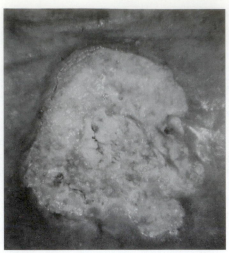

**FIGURE 7A-10.** A squamous cell carcinoma showing elevation, vegetation, and ulceration.

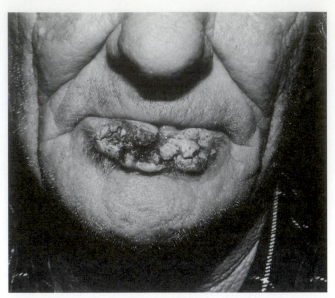

**FIGURE 7A-12.** Long-neglected squamous cell carcinoma on the lower lip.

Lesions occurring on the head and neck area tend to invade locally and extend along peripheral nerves.[166] Perineural tumor may be associated with symptoms, such as pain, but usually is initially asymptomatic. Recurrences are very common, and a high mortality rate is associated with perineural squamous cell carcinoma. Poorly differentiated tumors and deeply invasive tumors also have a worse prognosis.

**CLINICAL MANIFESTATIONS.** The clinical presentation of SCCs depends on the site of origin and type of precursor lesion (Figs. 7A-10, 7A-11). Cutaneous SCCs are usually asymptomatic.

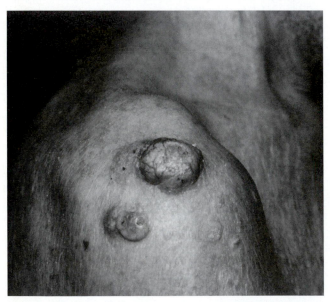

**FIGURE 7A-11.** Two smooth-domed squamous cell carcinomas on the shoulder of an elderly male.

Tumors that evolve from actinic keratoses appear red, are slightly elevated, and have scaling plaques. They are differentiated from actinic keratoses by the presence of induration, which is not a feature of actinic keratoses. As these tumors enlarge, they become firm and occasionally smooth. Telangiectasias and irregular pigmentation are characteristic, as well as surrounding xerotic skin. Eventually, they may, with minimal trauma, ulcerate and bleed. At this stage, because they rise above the surrounding normal skin, the tumors are usually well defined. Early SCCs are freely mobile. As they invade surrounding tissues, they become more indurated and fixed.

SCC of the lip is frequently subtle (Fig. 7A-12). Palpable induration is not a prominent feature of this tumor and is not as helpful in assessing for malignancy as it is in SCC of other sites. If induration is present, it is a sign of long-standing disease. These tumors often present early as an innocuous white patch with a small fissure or ulceration.

Tumors arising in burn scars tend to occur on the periphery of the scars in hyperkeratotic areas. Multiple SCCs can occur in former radiation ports and in individuals exposed to chemical carcinogens. Tumors arising in chronic ulcers and along sinus tracts can be diagnostic dilemmas. They may be essentially indistinguishable from benign tumors. They may also hide in sinus tracts or beneath ulcer debris.

Certain tumors are at risk of local recurrence. Recurrent tumors, tumors in the mid-facial-embryonic fold, large tumors greater than 2 cm, tumors greater than 4 mm in depth, poorly differentiated or spindle cell variants, and neurotrophic tumors are all at higher risk of recurrence (Table 7A-3).

Metastasis can be in-transit to local nodes and occasionally distant to the lungs. Risk factors for metastasis include many of the factors for recurrence. Location is a particularly important prognostic factor. Lips and ears are well-defined locations with a higher

**TABLE 7A-3. NONMELANOMA TUMORS AT RISK OF RECURRENCE**

Basal cell and squamous cell carcinoma:
  Recurrent tumor
  Large tumor, deep tumor
  Perineural tumor
  Mid face/embryonic plane

Basal cell carcinoma:
  Morpheaform-infiltrating
  Multifocal-multicentric
  Basosquamous-metatypical
  Micronodular

Squamous cell carcinoma:
  Poorly differentiated
  >4 mm depth

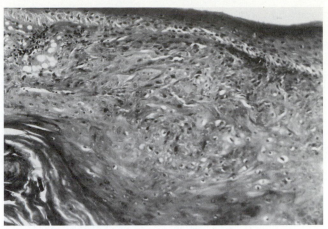

**FIGURE 7A-13.** Squamous cell carcinoma invading lobules of anaplastic cells with hyperchromatic nuclei, atypical mitoses, individual cell keratinization, and loss of intercellular bridges.

tendency for metastasis. Tumors arising from old scar or inflammation, such as the Marjolin ulceration, are at particularly high risk of metastasis.[167] Deep tumors, that is, those greater than 10 mm (Wanebo)[167] or Clark level IV or V, are at risk of regional or distant spread.

DIAGNOSIS. Biopsy of the skin is necessary for a definitive diagnosis. Punch biopsy should provide adequate tissue for diagnosis, except in the case of lesions within scars and ulcerations. In these situations, a large tissue sample is necessary to reveal the pattern of tumor growth and cellular architecture sufficient to differentiate the tumor from pseudoepitheliomatous hyperplasia, which is a benign hyperplasia that may occur at the margins of a chronic ulcer.

HISTOLOGY. In SCC, anastomosing lobules and cords of polygonal epithelial cells irregularly proliferate through the dermoepidermal junction into the dermis (Fig. 7A-13). Invading lobules are composed of varying amounts of normal epithelial cells and anaplastic cells with hyperchromatic nuclei, atypical mitoses, individual cell keratinization, and loss of intercellular bridges.

Broders[168] has histologically graded SCC by estimating the rate of differentiated (keratinizing cells) to undifferentiated cells. Broders's grade 1 SCCs are well-differentiated tumors with abundant keratinization, keratinocytes with glassy eosinophilic cytoplasm, and intercellular bridges. Tumor cells invade the dermis in a jagged pattern.[168] Some authors categorize keratoacanthoma as a subtype of grade 1 SCC.[140]

Broders's grades 2 and 3 tumors, or moderately differentiated SCC, are more deeply invasive with less keratinization, less glassy cytoplasm, more nuclear atypia, and increased mitoses. Necrosis en masse and intravascular, intralymphatic and perineural invasion may be detected.

Broders's grade 4 tumors are poorly differentiated or spindle cell variants with deep infiltration without keratinization or obvious intercellular bridges. Keratinocytes are anaplastic and pleomorphic with abundant atypical mitoses.[168] Lobules are confluent with irregular borders. Perineural and intralymphatic invasion are more common.

Aggressive histologic variants of SCC include acantholytic (pseudoglandular), small-cell, spindle cell, and pleomorphic.[169,170] Verrucous carcinoma is an indolent variant of SCC that rarely metastasizes.[171]

Some authors recommend that pathology reports should include tumor grade, thickness, presence or absence of perineural invasion, and skeletal muscle invasion.[172] In SCC of the lip, tumors less than 2 mm in thickness rarely metastasize.[173] Perineural invasion is associated with local recurrence after apparently complete surgical excision.

STAGING. Patients may be grouped into three stages. Stage I (localized) includes those patients with a primary tumor without evidence of metastasis. Stage II (regional) includes those patients with regional nodal metastases. Stage III (systemic) includes those with distant metastases.

TREATMENT. The treatment of SCC is primarily surgical. Small, thin actinically derived tumors in low-risk sites are amenable to a destructive approach, but excision is the standard treatment. With standard excisions, minimal margins are in the 4- to 5-mm range and should be increased according to the clinical risk of the situation.[174] Wide margins are needed in more aggressive tumors because of skipping of tumor or in-transit metastasis.

Mohs' micrographic surgery may be helpful to define the tumor and offers a cure of primary tumors in approximately 95% of cases.[71,70] Tissue conservation is noted in early lesions of the ear and lip with cures of 100%[175] and 95%, respectively. However, in aggressive, extensive cases, an additional margin after the Mohs' resections is recommended.

Tumor with perineural invasion is a particular problem, with recurrence being a common sequela[176] occurring in 14% to 36% of such squamous cell carcinomas. Both the risks of metastasis and local recurrence are increased. Recurrence is reported as 47%. Mohs' surgery may be helpful to defined perineural tumors with up to a 12% local recurrence.[177] However, adjuvant radiation is a good option in this situation.

In the aggressive tumor, clinical and radiographic screening (CT scanning, MRI)[178] should be performed for nodal spread. Clinical staging of the local nodes is a very important predictor of outcome.[179] In head and neck lesions, suspicious nodes can be addressed with needle biopsy or surgical node evaluation. Neck dissection is indicated in cases with evidence of local spread. Radiation may offer additional control as an adjunct to neck dissection, either prior to or after surgery,[180] and chemosensitization can be used as an adjunctive method.[181] In the absence of nodal spread, but with high-risk tumors, such as deep tumors, especially on the extremities,[167] lip,[182] and ear,[183] nodal dissection or adjunctive radiation may be prudent. Control studies are needed to further evaluate and define the indications and effectiveness of this treatment.

Intralesional interferon has been used, with complete responses and low recurrence rates reported. Ikuc[59] reported that only 2 out of 31 SCCs reoccurred after being treated intralesionally. Interferon has been used subcutaneously with 13-cis-retinoic acid for refractory inoperable tumors, with a 93% response.[184] In distantly spread tumor, partial regional response and one complete response was reported.

Refractory or metastatic disease has been treated with retinoids, traditional chemotherapy, radiation, and interferon. Systemic retinoids have been reported to have a modulating effect on both refractory and metastatic disease,[185] with temporary regression of tumor. Chemotherapy is predominantly cis-platinum–based, with the addition of 5-FU, bleomycin,[186,187] or doxorubicin, and offers palliative response. Radiation can be used as a sole agent or as adjuvant to aggressive tumor.[188]

## BASAL CELL CARCINOMA

BCC is the most common neoplasm of Caucasians, and the incidence is increasing.[4,189,190] It is uncommon among African Americans.[191] The head and neck areas are by far the most frequent sites of BCC in both men and women, with 80% of lesions occurring here.[4] BCCs have been reported to occur in non-sun-exposed areas.[192,193]

BCCs do occur in nonwhite races, but are less common than SCCs.[150,153,161] In a comprehensive study of skin cancer in African Americans conducted in 1988 at Howard University, 89% of BCCs were found to be on sun-exposed areas.[150] Most lesions occur at or after age 50.[150,194]

### ETIOLOGY AND PATHOGENESIS. It is widely accepted that UV light plays a crucial role in the pathogenesis of BCC. However, some lesions cannot be completely explained by prolonged sun exposure. BCCs are known to occur at sites protected from sun exposure such as behind the ear and the inner canthus. BCCs have even been reported on the vulva.[193] In some studies an association between cumulative sun exposure and risk of BCC was not found.[190,195] Genetic factors also affect risk of developing BCC. A markedly increased risk of developing BCC is associated with Gorlin syndrome. First BCCs may occur in the second decade of life.

Individuals with xeroderma pigmentosum have defective DNA excisional repair and are therefore at increased risk of sunlight-induced nonmelanoma skin cancers, starting at the mean age of 8 years.[79] Because of their tendency toward light skin, blue eyes, freckling, and inability to tan, people of Irish, English, and Welsh descent are also at increased risk of developing BCCs.

Exposure to chemical carcinogens and ionizing radiation has also been associated with an increased risk of BCC, although to a lesser degree than SCC. There is substantial evidence linking BCC with ingestion of trivalent arsenic and exposure to therapeutic x-irradiation.[32,196] BCCs have been reported to occur in scars induced by burns, vaccination, chickenpox, and chronic leg ulcers.[197–200]

### MODES OF SPREAD. BCCs originate in the epidermis and tend to grow slowly and remain confined to this area. BCCs are often referred to as basal cell epitheliomas or nonorganic (nonorganoid) hamartomas instead of carcinomas because of their indolent nature.[201] Over decades, these tumors do have the potential to become deeply invasive into soft tissue and to erode into blood vessels, bone, cartilage, and sinuses. Certain prognostic factors (see Table 7A-3) based on clinical criteria and histologic criteria are well described. Recurrent tumors tend to be more aggressive than primary tumors. These tumors usually have a worse histologic subtype, grow in irregular patterns, and have a higher risk of recurrence. Large tumors (greater than 2 cm) and tumors arising in a midfacial location are at higher risk of recurrence. Infiltrating BCCs (morpheaform-sclerotic, micronodular, adenocytic, metatypical-basosquamous, and superficial "multifocal" types) are associated with a higher risk of recurrence. Perineural spread occurs and is a risk factor for recurrence, but it is not associated with the mortality of perineural SCC.

Metastatic BCC is rare but reported.[202–205] Sites of metastases include the bloodstream, regional lymph nodes, bone, lung, liver, and other viscera.[206–215] Metastases occur at an incidence of 0.1%.[206]

### CLINICAL MANIFESTATIONS. Patients frequently complain of bleeding or crusting lesions that may heal partially but tend to recur. Most BCCs occur on sun-exposed regions such as the head and neck area. BCCs are categorized in subtypes that have characteristic clinical presentations. These categories include nodular, morpheaform, superficial, and pigmented.

Nodular BCCs present as translucent, pearly papules of various sizes that are traversed by tortuous telangiectatic blood vessels (Figs. 7A-14 through 7A-16). As the lesion ages, the center becomes flat and potentially crusted, and the peripheral borders become raised and pearly. The thickened borders are produced by vertical rather than horizontal spread of the tumor. The center may eventually ulcerate, producing a rodent ulcer. Nodulocystic tumors may have the appearance of pustules or epidermal cysts.

Morpheaform BCCs present as ill-defined, white, waxy, and sclerotic plaques (Fig. 7A-17). They are usually devoid of telangiectasias and may be only slightly raised above the surrounding normal skin. The lesions tend to be firm, depressed, and smooth. They are less likely to have pearly features than nodular BCC. They often resemble scars or scleroderma.

Horizontal spread, rather than vertical, occurs in superficial BCC (Fig. 7A-18). These lesions present as ill-defined, erythematous,

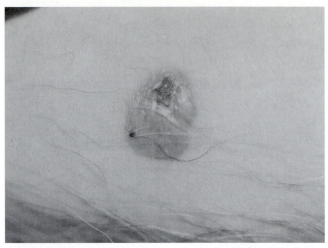

**FIGURE 7A-14.** Ill-defined pearly papule with tortuous telangiectasias and erosion characteristic of nodular basal cell carcinoma.

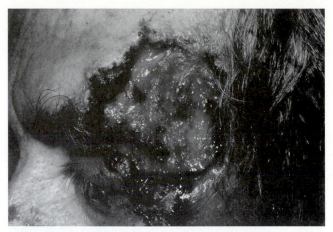

**FIGURE 7A-16.** Long-neglected, ulcerated basal cell carcinoma.

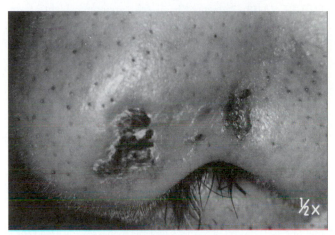

**FIGURE 7A-17.** Morpheaform basal cell carcinoma. Ill-defined, sclerotic, waxy papule with erosions on the nose.

scaling plaques without telangiectasias. These tumors are potentially confused with Bowen's disease or localized eczema.

Pigmented BCCs are identical to nodular BCCs, except for pigmentation (Fig. 7A-19). They may be sprinkled with pigment or may be entirely pigmented. These occur more frequently in people with dark skin types. They are easily confused with malignant melanoma.

DIAGNOSIS. Biopsy is done by simple excision, shave biopsy, or punch biopsy and is confirmatory.

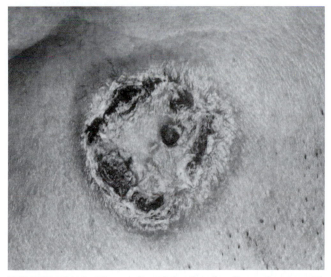

**FIGURE 7A-15.** Ulcerated nodular basal cell carcinoma with domes, borders, and irregular telangiectasias.

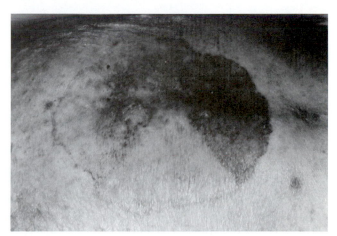

**FIGURE 7A-18.** Superficial basal cell carcinoma: Thin, ill-defined, scaling, erythematous plaque without telangiectasias.

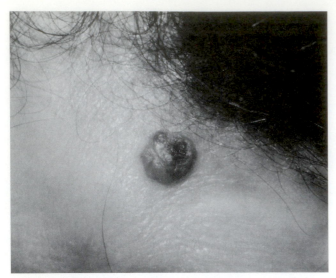

**FIGURE 7A-19.** Pigmented basal cell carcinoma: Light-brown, pearly papule with areas of "floating" pigment.

**HISTOLOGY.** Histologically, BCCs can be divided into tumors that show differentiation toward cutaneous appendages (hair, sebaceous glands, and eccrine glands) and those with no obvious differentiation.[216] The latter can be subdivided into circumscribed and infiltrative patterns. Examples of circumscribed histologic subtypes include solid (nodular) and nodulocystic. Morpheaform-sclerotic, micronodular, and metatypical-basosquamous BCCs are infiltrative subtypes with more aggressive clinical courses. Some of these will be described in greater detail.

Nodulocystic BCC, the most common type, is composed of dermal nodules connected to the epidermis by narrow or broad cords (Fig. 7A-20). Typical cells are basophilic with large, oval nuclei and scant cytoplasm. Mitoses are variable. Although there is some re-

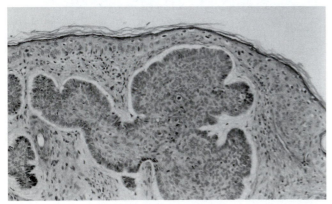

**FIGURE 7A-20.** Nodular basal cell carcinoma demonstrating basophilic cells with large oval nuclei and scant cytoplasm. Peripheral palisading and clefting are present.

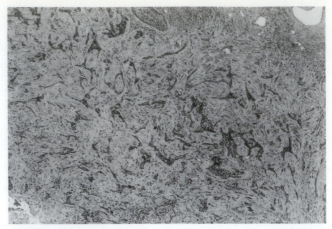

**FIGURE 7A-21.** Morpheaform basal cell carcinoma with cords and strands of basophilic cells embedded in a dense stroma.

semblance to the basal cells of the epidermis, intercellular bridges are not observed in BCC. The peripheral cells of the nodules are aligned at right angles to those in the center (peripheral palisading). The surrounding stroma is myxoid, and tumor cell clusters characteristically exhibit retraction clefts from the surrounding dermis. Central necrosis of the nodules results in cysts, both clinically and histologically.[217]

Of the more aggressive subtypes, the infiltrative subtype is composed of small cords and strands of several layers thick with little palisading. There is more nuclear variability without significant increase in stromal density.[218]

The morpheaform, or sclerotic, subtype demonstrates narrow cords and strands of tumor cells embedded in a dense stroma (Fig. 7A-21). Deep dermal extension is characteristic.

Although not uniformly accepted by all pathologists, metatypical or basosquamous cell carcinomas are considered to represent a transition tumor with cellular features of both BCCs and SCCs.[219] These tumors show a higher tendency to metastasize than BCC.

Superficial-multifocal BCC is characterized by buds of tumor cells attached to the epidermis with little penetration into the dermis (Fig. 7A-22). However, in long-standing tumors, invasion may occur focally. Although superficial BCCs demonstrate a multifocal growth pattern when examined in routine histologic sections, computerized three-dimensional reconstruction confirms a unicentric origin.[220]

The cell of origin of BCC is still under debate; however, current view points toward pluripotential cells that form continuously during life and are analogous to the embryonic primary epithelial germ cells.[221] These cells have the potential to form hair, sebaceous glands, and apocrine glands.

Stromal factors are important in the development of BCC. Autotransplants of BCCs only survive experimental transplantation when stroma is included. Furthermore, BCCs lack autonomy when transplanted into athymic nude mice.[222] These findings are consistent with the low incidence of metastases.

**STAGING.** Clinical staging is not followed in basal cell cancer.

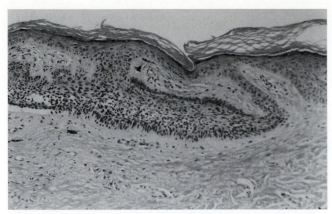

**FIGURE 7A-22.** Superficial basal cell carcinoma: Buds of basophilic cells with peripheral palisading and retraction clefts attached to epidermis.

**TREATMENT.** All of the previously described techniques of skin cancer treatment have been reported as effective. Algorithms for selection of modalities based on location, histology, size, tumor history, and other factors have been described.[54] Destructive techniques, such as cryosurgery and electrodessication and curettage, are indicated in many of the uncomplicated tumors, with an effectiveness of approximately 93%.[57] Radiation therapy is quite effective in BCC.[223,224] Excisional surgery is the standard to which all modalities need to be compared. All of the above techniques offer 5-year cure rates in the low 90% range.[57] In tumors at risk for recurrence, as defined above, intraoperative fresh frozen or Mohs' micrographic surgery offers an improved cure rate. Mohs' surgery is well documented with exceptional cures of 97% to 99% for all BCCs in several large university series and prior Mohs' citation[225,226] (Figs. 7A-23 and 7A-24). This high cure rate is maintained in recurrent tumors and tumors at risk of recurrence based on location (e.g., midface and ears) and histology (morpheaform, infiltrating, micronodular, and multicentric); therefore, Mohs' surgery is the treatment of choice for these problematic tumors.

Topical 5-FU is limited by the depth of penetration and has a high failure rate in all but the most superficial lesions. Radiation is effective in primary and recurrent tumors and offers a nonsurgical, nonmultilating method, and thus some believe it should be the treatment of choice.[223,224] However, long-term problems may occur after radiation therapy, including radiation scar, scar contraction, radiation dermatitis, and occasional secondary radiation-induced tumors, which limit the use of radiation in younger patients.

Subtotally resected tumor is a common occurrence in clinical practice. Selection of proper margins is essentially based on location, histology types, and other considerations. The significance of residual tumor is debated, but it is clear that some histology types such as infiltrating or multicentric types are at higher risk of recurrence,[227] as are tumors of the midfacial area and the ears. Observation can be used in a low-risk location and situation, but reexcision or Mohs' surgery[228] should be used in a patient with risk factors for recurrence. Adjunctive radiation has also been used in this situation.

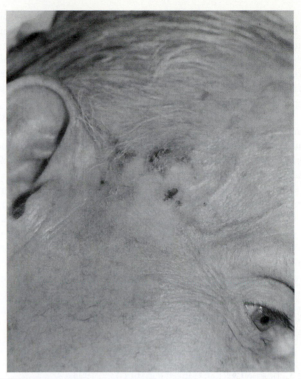

**FIGURE 7A-23.** Preoperative photo of morpheaform basal cell carcinoma of right temple.

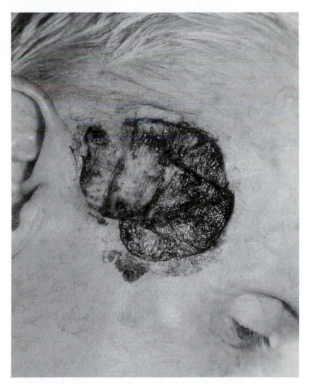

**FIGURE 7A-24.** Postoperative defect of same patient after Mohs' micrographic surgery.

In small series, intralesional interferon has been reported to have a high clinical response of 67% to 96%.[59,229] In more aggressive tumors, the response rate is lower, with 27% complete response and 33% partial response.[230] The cosmetic outcomes are excellent, and a nonsurgical approach is appealing. However, the cost, the side effects of interferon, a lower cure rate, and less documented experience than the traditional approach limit the usage of interferon in BCC.

Systemic retinoids (isotretinate and etretinate) modulate the course of BCC. In patients with multiple lesions, regression of tumors occurs. Used prophylactically in the high-risk patients,[231] such as those having the basal cell nevus syndrome or xeroderma pigmentosa, significant long-term improvement has been reported.

Photodynamic therapy is undergoing evaluation and offers some promise in extensive disease. Early reports have been promising, with up to 88% complete response.[232] Topical 5-aminolevulinic acid is effective.[233] Indications, limitations, and parameters are not yet fully developed. At this time, patients with numerous superficial tumors may prove to be the best candidates for this therapy, although recurrent and other higher-risk tumors have been treated with this modality.

# REFERENCES

1. Boring CL et al: Cancer statistics 43:7, 1993.
2. Miller DL, Weinstock MA: Nonmelanoma skin cancer in the United States: Incidence. J Am Acad Dermatol 30:774, 1994.
3. Stenbeck KD et al: Patterns of treated non-melanoma skin cancer in Queensland: The region with the highest incidence rates in the world. Med J Aust 153:511, 1990.
4. Gallagher RP et al: Trends in basal cell carcinoma, squamous cell carcinoma, and melanoma of the skin from 1973 through 1987. J Am Acad Dermatol 23:413, 1990.
5. Walton S et al: The emerging epidemic of skin cancer. Br J Dermatol 130:269, 1994.
6. Cleaver JE: Defective repair replication of DNA in xeroderma pigmentosum. Nature 218:652, 1968.
7. Kripke ML: The role of UVR-induced immunosuppression in experimental photocarcinogenesis, in Progress in Dermatology, vol 16, E Epstein Jr (ed). Evanston, IL, Dermatology Foundation, 1982.
8. Painter RR, Cleaver JE: Repair replication, unscheduled DNA synthesis, and the repair of mammalian DNA. Radiat Res 37:451, 1969.
9. Moan J, Dahlback A: The relationship between skin cancers, solar radiation and ozone depletion. Br J Cancer 65:916, 1992.
10. Vitasa BC et al: Association of nonmelanoma skin cancer and actinic keratosis with cumulative solar ultraviolet exposure in Maryland watermen. Cancer 65:2811, 1990.
11. Kraemer KH et al: The role of sunlight and DNA repair in melanoma and nonmelanoma skin cancer. Arch Dermatol 130:1018, 1994.
12. Pathak MA: Sunscreens: Topical and systemic approaches for protection of human skin against harmful effects of solar radiation. J Am Acad Dermatol 7:285, 1982.
13. Setlow RV et al: Wavelengths effective in induction of malignant melanoma. Proc Natl Acad Sci USA 90(14):6666, 1993.
14. Epstein JH: Ultraviolet carcinogenesis, in Photophysiology, vol 5, AC Geise (ed). New York, Academic, 1970.
15. Adams R et al: Occupational skin cancer, in Occupational Skin Disease, 2d ed, RA Adams (ed). Philadelphia, Saunders, 1990, p 136.
16. Alcalay J et al: Excision repair of pyrimidine dimers induced by simulated solar radiation in the skin of patients with basal cell carcinomas. J Invest Dermatol 95(5):506, 1990.
17. Gregg K, Mansbridge J: Epidermal characteristics related to skin cancer susceptibility. J Invest Dermatol 79:178, 1982.
18. Brash DE et al: A role for sunlight in skin cancer: UV-induced p53 mutations in squamous cell carcinoma. Proc Natl Acad Sci USA 88(22):10124, 1991.
19. Ziegler A et al: Sunburn and p53 in the onset of skin cancer. Nature 372(6508):773, 1994.
20. Franceschi S et al: Site distribution of different types of skin cancer: new aetiological clues. Int J Cancer 67:24, 1996.
21. Magnus K: The Nordic profile of skin cancer incidence: A comparative epidemiological study of the three main types of skin cancer. Int J Cancer 47:12, 1991.
22. Frentz G et al: Increased number of circulating suppressor T-lymphocytes in sun-induced multiple skin cancers. Cancer 62:294, 1988.
23. Kripke ML: Immunosuppressive effects of ultraviolet (280–320 nm) radiation and psoralen plus ultraviolet (320–400 nm) radiation in mice. J Natl Cancer Inst 69(1):171, 1982.
24. Stern RS et al: Non-melanoma skin cancer occurring in patients treated with PUVA five to ten years after first treatment. J Invest Dermatol 91:120, 1988.
25. Morison WL et al: In-vivo effects of PUVA on lymphocyte function. Br J Dermatol 104:405, 1981.
26. Morison WL et al: Abnormal lymphocyte function following long term PUVA for psoriasis. Br J Dermatol 108:448, 1983.
27. Ree K: Reduction of Langerhans cells in human epidermis during PUVA therapy: A morphometric study. J Invest Dermatol 78:488, 1982.
28. McKenna KE et al: Cutaneous neoplasia following PUVA therapy for psoriasis. Br J Dermatol 134:639, 1996.
29. Czarnecki D et al: Age and multiple basal cell carcinomas in Australia. Int J Dermatol 30:713, 1991.
30. Kricker A et al: Measurement of skin cancer incidence. Health Reports 5(1):63, 1993.
31. Brookes P (ed). Chemical carcinogens. Br Med Bull 36:1, 1980.
32. Wong SS et al: Cutaneous manifestations of chronic arsenicism: Review of seventeen cases. J Am Acad Dermatol 38:179, 1998.
33. Yu HS et al: Alterations of mitogenic responses of mononuclear cells by arsenic in arsenical skin cancers. J Dermatol 19(11):710, 1992.
34. Yu HS et al: Alterations in skin-associated lymphoid tissue in the carcinogenesis of arsenical skin cancer. Pro Natl Sci Counc Repub China (B) 16(1):17, 1992.
35. Maloney ME: Arsenic in dermatology. Dermatol Surg 22(3):301, 1996.
36. Kricker A et al: Pigmentary and cutaneous risk factors for non-melanocytic skin cancer: A case control study. Int J Cancer 48:650, 1991.
37. Liddington M et al: Skin cancer in renal transplant recipients. Br J Surg 76(10):1002, 1989.
38. Hartevelt MM et al: Incidence of skin cancer after renal transplantation in the Netherlands. Transplantation 49(3):506, 1990.

39. DINEHART SM et al: Immunosuppression in patients with metastatic squamous cell carcinoma. J Dermatol Surg Oncol 16(3):271, 1990.

40. ESPAÑA A et al: Skin cancer in heart transplant recipients. J Am Acad Dermatol 32:458, 1995.

41. EUVRARD S et al: Association of skin malignancies with various and multiple carcinogenic and noncarcinogenic human papillomaviruses in renal transplant recipients. Cancer 72:2198, 1993.

42. DE VILLIERS EM et al: Prevailing papillomavirus types in non-melanoma carcinomas of the skin in renal allograft recipients. Int J Cancer 73:356, 1997.

43. TIEBEN LM et al: Detection of epidermodysplasia verruciformis-like human papillomavirus types in malignant and premalignant skin lesions of renal transplant recipients. Br J Dermatol 131:226, 1994.

44. KAWASHIMA M et al: Premalignant lesions and cancers of the skin in the general population: Evaluation of the role of human papillomaviruses. J Invest Dermatol 95:537, 1990.

45. ELIEZRI YD et al: Occurrence of human papillomavirus type 16 DNA in cutaneous squamous and basal cell neoplasms. J Am Acad Dermatol 23(5 Pt 1):836, 1990.

46. FORSLUND O et al: DNA analysis indicates patient-specific human papillomavirus type 16 strains in Bowen's disease on fingers and in archival samples from genital dysplasia. Br J Dermatol 136:678, 1997.

47. MAJEWSKI S, JABLONSKA S: Epidermodysplasia verruciformis as a model of human papillomavirus-induced genetic cancer of the skin. Arch Dermatol 131(11):1312, 1995.

48. WEINSTOCK MA et al: Human papillomavirus and widespread cutaneous carcinoma after PUVA photochemotherapy. Arch Dermatol 131:701, 1995.

49. KRAEMER KH et al: DNA repair protects against cutaneous and internal neoplasia: evidence from xeroderma pigmentosum. Carcinogenesis 5(4):511, 1984.

50. GAILANI MR et al: Developmental defects in Gorlin syndrome related to putative tumor suppressor gene on chromosome 9. Cell 69:111, 1992.

51. SHANELY SM et al: Fine deletion mapping on the long arm of chromosome 9 in sporadic and familial basal cell carcinomas. Hum Mol Genet 4:129, 1995.

52. GORLIN RJ et al: The multiple basal cell nevus syndrome. Cancer 18:88, 1965.

53. LOOKINGBILL DP et al: Actinic damage and skin cancer in albinos in northern Tanzania: Findings in 164 patients enrolled in an outreach skin care program. J Am Acad Dermatol 32:653, 1995.

54. ALBRIGHT SD: Treatment of skin cancer using multiple modalities. J Am Acad Dermatol 7(2):143, 1982.

55. GEISSE JK: Comparison of treatment modalities for squamous cell carcinoma. Clin Dermatol 13(6):621, 1995.

56. FALKSON G, SCHULZ EJ: Skin changes in patients treated with 5-fluorouracil. Br J Dermatol 74:229, 1962.

57. ROWE DE et al: Long-term recurrence rates in previously untreated (primary) basal cell carcinoma: implications for patient follow-up. J Dermatol Surg Oncol 15(3):315, 1989.

58. FITZPATRICK RE et al: Clinical advantage of the $CO_2$ laser superpulsed mode: Treatment of verruca vulgaris seborrheic keratoses, lentigines, and actinic cheilitis. J Dermatol Surg Oncol 20(7):449, 1994.

59. IKIC D et al: Interferon reduces recurrences of basal cell and squamous cell cancers. Int J Dermatol 34(1):58, 1995.

60. STADLER R et al: Interferons in dermatology. J Am Acad Dermatol 20(4):650, 1989.

61. BARON S et al: The interferons. Mechanisms of action and clinical applications. JAMA 266(10):1375, 1991.

62. SHIELL A: Consideration of the cost of interferon alfa-2b in the treatment of basal cell carcinoma. Australas J Dermatol 35(2):71, 1994.

63. ROBINSON TA, KLIGMAN AM: Treatment of solar keratoses of the extremities with retinoic acid and 5-fluorouracil. Br J Dermatol 92:703, 1975.

64. ROOK AH et al: Beneficial effect of low-dose systemic retinoid in combination with topical tretinoin for the treatment and prophylaxis of premalignant and malignant skin lesions in renal transplant recipients. Transplantation 59(5):714, 1995.

65. KRAEMER KH et al: Prevention of skin cancer in xeroderma pigmentosum with the use of oral isotretinoin. N Engl J Med 318(25):1633, 1988.

66. CALZAVARA-PINTON PG: Repetitive photodynamic therapy with topical delta-aminolaevulinic acid as an appropriate approach to the routine treatment of superficial non-melanoma skin tumors. J Photochem Photobiol B 29(1):53, 1995.

67. ROBERTS DJ, CAIRNDUFF F: Photodynamic therapy of primary skin cancer: a review. Br J Plast Surg 48(6):360, 1995.

68. CAIRNDUFF F et al: Superficial photodynamic therapy with topical 5-aminolaevuliniocid for superficial primary and secondary skin cancer. BR J Cancer 69(3):605, 1994.

69. ALLISON RR et al: Photodynamic therapy for the treatment of nonmelanatous cutaneous malignancies. Semin Cutan Med Surg 17(2):153, 1998.

70. NELSON BR et al: Mohs' micrographic surgery for non-melanoma skin cancers. Clin Plast Surg 24(4):705, 1997.

71. SWANSON NA: Mohs' surgery. Technique, indications, applications, and the future. Arch Dermatol 119(9):761, 1983.

72. MARKS R et al: Malignant transformation of solar keratoses to squamous cell carcinoma. Lancet 1(8589):795, 1988.

73. GRAHAM JH, HELWIG EB: Cutaneous precancerous conditions in man. Natl Cancer Inst Monogr 10:323, 1963.

74. MARKS R et al: The incidence of non-melanocytic skin cancers in an Australian population: Results of a five-year prospective study. Med J Aust 150(9):475, 1989.

75. MARKS R et al: Spontaneous remission of solar keratoses: The case for conservative management. Br J Dermatol 115(6):649, 1986.

76. HARVEY I et al: Non-melanoma skin cancer and solar keratoses. I. Methods and descriptive results of the South Wales skin cancer study. Br J Cancer 74:1302, 1996.

77. DUFRESNE JR, CURLIN MU: Actinic chelitis: A treatment review. Dermatolog Surg 23:15, 1997.

78. BAKER SR: Risk factors in multiple carcinomas of the lip. Otolaryngol Head Neck Surg 88:248, 1980.

79. KRAEMER KH et al: Xeroderma pigmentosum: Cutaneous, ocular, and neurologic abnormalities in 830 published cases. Arch Dermatol 123(2):241, 1987.

80. JENSEN P et al: Cutaneous complications in heart transplant recipients in Norway 1983–1993. Acta Derm Venereol 75(5):400, 1995.

81. EUVRARD S et al: Comparative epidemiologic study of premalignant and malignant epithelial cutaneous lesions developing after kidney and heart transplantation. J Am Acad Dermatol 33:222, 1995.

82. FERRANDIZ C et al: Epidermal dysplasia and neoplasia in kidney transplant recipients. J Am Acad Dermatol 33:590, 1995.

83. BROWNSTEIN MH, RABINOWITZ AD: The precursors of cutaneous squamous cell carcinoma. Int J Dermatol 18:1, 1979.

84. WADE TR, ACKERMAN AB: The many faces of solar keratoses. J Dermatol Surg Oncol 14:730, 1978.

85. MONHEIT GD: The Jessner's + TCA peel: A medium-depth chemical peel. J Dermatol Surg Oncol 15(9):945, 1989.

86. WINTON GB, SALASCHE SJ: Dermabrasion of the scalp as a treatment for actinic damage. J Am Acad Dermatol 14(4):661, 1986.

87. TRIMAS SJ et al: The carbon dioxide laser. An alternative for the treatment of actinically damaged skin. Dermatol Surg 23:885, 1997.

88. PECK GL: Topical tretinoin in actinic keratosis and basal cell carcinoma. J Am Acad Dermatol 15(4):829, 1986.

89. JEFFES EW et al: Photodynamic therapy of actinic keratosis with topical 5-aminolevulinic acid: A pilot dose-ranging study. Arch Dermatol 133(6):727, 1997.

90. DUFRESNE RG JR, CURLIN MU: Actinic cheilitis: A treatment review. Dermatol Surg 23:15, 1997.

91. DIWAN R, SKOUGE JW: A comparison of electrosurgery and the carbon dioxide laser for the treatment of actinic cheilitis. J Dermatol Surg Oncol 16:80, 1990 (abstr).

92. LUBRITZ RR, SMOLEWSKI SA: Cryosurgery cure rate of premalignant leukoplakia of the lower lip. J Dermatol Surg Oncol 9:235, 1983.

93. WARNOCK GR et al: Evaluation of 5-fluorouracil in the treatment of actinic keratosis of the lip. Oral Surg Oral Med Oral Pathol 52:501, 1981.

94. ROBINSON JK: Actinic cheilitis: A prospective study comparing four treatment methods. Arch Otolarynogol Head Neck Surg 115:848, 1989.

95. BURKET J: Vermilionectomy for lower leukoplakia. Arch Dermatol 95:397, 1967.

96. BIRT BD: The lip shave operation for premalignant conditions and microinvasive carcinoma of the lower lip. J Otolaryngol 6:407, 1977.

97. BRUFAU C et al: Our experience in the surgical treatment of cancer and precancerous lesions of the lower lip. J Dermatol Surg Oncol 11:908, 1985.

98. SANCHEZ-CONEJO-MIR J et al: Follow-up of vermilionectomies: evaluation of the technique. J Dermatol Surg Oncol 12:180, 1986.

99. FERNANDEZ VOZMEDIANO JM et al: Vermilionectomy using the w-plasty technique. J Dermatol Surg Oncol 15:627, 1989.

100. FIELD LM: Improved design for vermilionectomy with a mucous-membrane advancement flap. J Dermatol Surg Oncol 17:833, 1991.

101. KOSSARD S, ROSEN R: Cutaneous Bowen's disease: An analysis of 1001 cases according to age, sex, and site. J Am Acad Dermatol 27:406, 1992.

102. COX NH: Body site distribution of Bowen's disease. Br J Dermatol 130:714, 1994.

103. REIZNER GT et al: Bowen's disease (squamous cell carcinoma in situ) in Kauai, Hawaii. J Am Acad Dermatol 31:596, 1994.

104. GRAHAM JH, HELWIG EB: Bowen's disease and its relationship to systemic cancer. Arch Dermatol 83:738, 1961.

105. MORA RG, BURRIS R: Cancer of the skin in blacks: A review of 128 patients with basal cell carcinoma. Cancer 47:1436, 1981.

106. MIKI Y et al: Cutaneous and pulmonary cancers associated with Bowen's disease. J Am Acad Dermatol 6:26, 1982.

107. CALLEN JP, HEADINGTON J: Bowen's and non-Bowen's squamous intraepidermal neoplasia of the skin. Arch Dermatol 116:422, 1980.

108. STRAYER DS, SANTA CRUZ DJ: Carcinoma in situ of the skin: A review of histopathology. J Cutan Pathol 7:244, 1980.

109. STEFFEN C, ACKERMAN AB: Intraepidermal epithelioma of Borst-Jadassohn. Am J Dermatopathol 7:5, 1985.

110. GORDON KB et al: Bowen's disease of the distal digit: Outcome of treatment with carbon dioxide laser vaporization. Dermatol Surg 22(8):723, 1996.

111. BARAN RL, GORMELY DE: Polydactylous Bowen's disease of the nail. J Am Acad Dermatol 17:201, 1987.

112. GORDON KB et al: Treatment of multiple lesions of Bowen disease with isotretinoin and interferon alfa: Efficacy of combination chemotherapy. Arch Dermatol 133(6):691, 1997.

113. GOETTE DK: Erythroplasia of Queyrat. Arch Dermatol 100:271, 1974.

114. SONNEX TS et al: Treatment of erythroplasia of Queyrat with liquid nitrogen cryosurgery. Br J Dermatol 106(5):581, 1982.

115. GREENBAUM A et al: A carbon dioxide laser treatment of erythroplasia of Queyrat. J Dermatol Surg Oncol 15:747, 1989.

116. LEWIS RJ, BENDL BJ: Erythroplasia of Queyrat: Report of a patient successfully treated with topical 5-fluorouracil. J Can Med Assoc 104(2):148, 1971.

117. BROWN MC et al: Penile tumors: their management by Mohs micrographic surgery. J Dermatol Surg Oncol 13:1163, 1987.

118. MORITZ DL, LYNCH WS: Extensive Bowen's disease of the penile shaft treated with fresh tissue Mohs micrographic surgery in two separate operations. J Dermatol Surg Oncol 17(4):374, 1991.

119. HARRINGTON KJ et al: Erythroplasia of Queyrat treated with isotretinoin. Lancet 342(8877):994, 1993.

120. RANK BK, DIXON PL: Another look at keratoacanthoma. Australia and New Zealand J Surg 49:654, 1979.

121. KINGMAN J, CALLEN JP: Keratocanthoma: A clinical study. Arch Dermatol 120:736, 1984.

122. CHUANG TY et al: Keratoacanthoma in Kauai, Hawaii: The first documented incidence in a defined population. Arch Dermatol 129(3):317, 1993.

123. SCHWARTZ RA: Keratoacanthoma. J Am Acad Dermatol 30:1, 1994.

124. SCHWARTZ RA, TORRE DP: The Muir-Torre syndrome: A 25-year retrospect. J Am Acad Dermatol 33(1):90, 1995.

125. COHEN PR et al: Muir-Torre syndrome. Dermatol Clin 13(1):79, 1995.

126. MARSHALL V: Premalignant and malignant skin tumors in immunosuppressed patients. Transplantation 17:272, 1974.

127. DANGOISSE C et al: Multiple eruptive keratoacanthoma and immunity disorders. Dermatology 186(4):313, 1993.

128. WASHINGTON CV JR, MIKHAIL GR: Eruptive keratoacanthoma en plaque in an immunosuppressed patient. J Dermatol Surg Oncol 13(12):1357, 1987.

129. SCHALLER M et al: Multiple keratoacanthomas, giant keratoacanthomas and keratoacanthoma centrifugum marginatum: Development in a single patient and treatment with oral isotretinoin. Acta Derm Venereol 76(1):40, 1996.

130. PICKERELL K et al: Giant keratoacanthomas. Ann Plast Surg 3(2):172, 1979.

131. PETEIRO MC et al: Keratoacanthoma centrifugum marginatum versus low-grade squamous cell carcinoma. Dermatologica 170(5):221, 1985.

132. WEEDON D, BARNETT L: Keratoacanthoma centrifugum marginatum. Arch Dermatol 111(8):1024, 1975.

133. BARAN R, GOETMANN S: Distal digital keratoacanthoma: A report of 12 cases and a review of the literature. Br J Dermatol 139(3):512, 1998.

134. ALLEN CA et al: Subungual keratoacanthoma. Histopathology 75:181, 1994.

135. OLIWIECKI S et al: Subungual keratoacanthoma: A report of four cases and review of the literature. Clin Exp Dermatol 19(3):230, 1994.

136. YOUNG SK et al: Generalized eruptive keratoacanthoma. Oral Surg Oral Med Oral Pathol 62(4):422, 1986.

137. KAVANAGH GM et al: A case of Grzybowski's generalized eruptive keratoacanthomas. Australas J Dermatol 36(2):83, 1995.

138. KIRKHAM N: Keratoacanthoma, in *Lever's Histopathology of the Skin,* 8th ed, D Elder et al (eds). Philadelphia, Lippincott-Raven, 1997, pp 732–733.

139. LAPINS NA, HELWIG EB: Perineural invasion by keratoacanthoma. Arch Dermatol 116:791, 1986.

140. HODAK E et al: Solitary keratoacanthoma is a squamous cell carcinoma: three examples with metastases. Am J Dermatopathol 15:332, 1993.

141. NEDWICH JA: Evaluation of curettage and electrodesiccation in treatment of keratoacanthoma. Australas J Dermatol 32(3):137, 1991.

142. LARSON PO: Keratoacanthomas treated with Mohs' micrographic surgery (chemosurgery): A review of forty-three cases. J Am Acad Dermatol 16:1040, 1987.

143. DONAHUE B et al: Treatment of aggressive keratoacanthomas by radiotherapy. J Am Acad Dermatol 23:489, 1990.

144. GROB JJ et al: Large keratoacanthomas treated with intralesional interferon alfa-2a. J Am Acad Dermatol 29:237, 1993.

145. EUBANKS SW et al: Treatment of multiple keratoacanthomas with intralesional fluorouracil. J Am Acad Dermatol 7(1):126, 1982.

146. MELTON JL et al: Treatment of keratoacanthomas with intralesional methotrexate. J Am Acad Dermatol 25(6):1017, 1991.

147. SAYAMA S, TAGAMI H: Treatment of keratoacanthoma with intralesional bleomycin. Br J Dermatol 109(4):449, 1983.

148. SCHALLER M et al: Multiple keratoacanthomas, giant keratoacanthoma and keratoacanthoma centrifugum marginatum: Development in a single patient and treatment with oral isotretinoin. Acta Derm Venereol 76(1):40, 1996.

149. KWA RE et al: Biology of cutaneous squamous cell carcinoma. J Am Acad Dermatol 26:1, 1992.

150. HALDER RM, BANG KM: Skin cancer in blacks in the United States. Dermatol Clin 6(3):397, 1988.

151. MORA RG, PERNICIARO C: Cancer of the skin in blacks: I. Review of 163 black patients with cutaneous squamous cell carcinoma. J Am Acad Dermatol 5:535, 1981.

152. MULAY DM: Skin cancer in India. Natl Cancer Inst Monogr 10:215, 1963.

153. SHANMUGARATNAM K, LABROOY EB: Skin cancer in Singapore. Natl Cancer Inst Monogr 10:127, 1963.

154. BELISARIO JC: *Cancer of the Skin.* London, Butterworths, 1959.

155. EASTCOTT DF: Epidemiology of skin cancer in New Zealand. Natl Cancer Inst Monogr 10:141, 1963.

156. TENSELDAM REJ: Skin cancer in Australia. Natl Cancer Inst Monogr 10:153, 1963.

157. ROWE DE et al: Prognostic factors from local recurrence, metastasis, and survival rates in squamous cell carcinoma of the skin, ear, and lip: Implications for treatment modality selection. J Am Acad Dermatol 26(6):976, 1992.

158. GISSMANN L et al: Analysis of human genital warts (condylomata acuminata) and other genital tumors for human papillomavirus type 6 DNA. Int J Cancer 29(2):143, 1982.

159. CHU QD et al: Giant condyloma acuminatum (Buschke-Lowenstein tumor) of the anorectal and perianal regions: Analysis of 42 cases. Dis Colon Rectum 37(9):950, 1994.

160. OETTLE AG: Geographical and racial differences in the frequency of Kaposi's sarcoma as evidence of environmental or genetic causes. ACTA Un Int Cancer 18:330, 1962.

161. PRINGGOUTOMO S: Skin cancer in Indonesia. Natl Cancer Inst Monogr 10:191, 1963.

162. CHOWDRI NA, DARZI MA: Postburn scar carcinomas in Kashmiris: Burns. 22(6):477, 1996.

163. OETTLE AG: Skin cancer in Africa. Natl Cancer Inst Monogr 10:197, 1963.

164. LUND HZ: How often does squamous cell carcinoma of the skin metastasize? Arch Dermatol 92:635, 1965.

165. KATZ AD: The frequency and risk of metastases in squamous cell carcinoma of the skin. Cancer 10:1162, 1957.

166. COTTELL WI, PROPER S: Mohs' surgery, fresh tissue technique: Our technique with a review. J Dermatol Surg Oncol 8:576, 1982.

167. FRIEDMAN HI et al: Prognostic and therapeutic use of microstaging of cutaneous squamous cell carcinoma of the trunk and extremities. Cancer 56:1099, 1985.

168. BRODERS AC: Squamous cell epithelioma of the skin. Ann Surg 73:141, 1921.

169. KUWANO H et al: Atypical fibroxanthoma distinguishable from spindle cell carcinoma in sarcoma-like skin lesion. Cancer 55:172, 1985.

170. LICHTIGER B et al: Spindle-cell variant of squamous cell carcinoma: A light and electron microscopic study of 13 cases. Cancer 26:1311, 1970.

171. KAO GF et al: Carcinoma cuniculatum (verrucous carcinoma of the skin): a clinicopathologic study of 46 cases with ultrastructural observations. Cancer 49:2395, 1982.

172. WEEDAN D et al: Histology review of squamous cell carcinoma. Cosmetic Dermatol 10, 5:45, 1997.

173. SAYWELL M et al: Histologic correlates of metastasis in primary invasive squamous cell carcinoma of the lip. Aust J Dermatol 37:193, 1996.

174. BRODLAND DG, ZITELLI JA: Surgical margins for excision of primary cutaneous squamous cell carcinoma. J Am Acad Dermatol 27(2 Pt 1):241, 1992.

175. MEHREGAN DA, ROENIGK RK: Management of superficial squamous cell carcinoma of the lip with Mohs micrographic surgery. Cancer 66:463, 1990.

176. GOEPFERT H et al: Perineural invasion in squamous cell skin carcinoma of the head and neck. Am J Surg 148:542, 1984.

177. LAWRENCE N, COTTEL WI: Squamous cell carcinoma of skin with perineural invasion. J Am Acad Dermatol 31(1):30, 1994.

178. VAN DEN BREKEL MW et al: Magnetic resonance imaging vs. palpation of cervical lymph node metastasis. Arch Otolaryngol Head Neck Surg 117(12):1410, 1991.

179. KRAUS DH et al: Regional lymph node metastasis from cutaneous squamous cell carcinoma. Arch Otolaryngol Head Neck Surg 124(5):582, 1998.

180. BARTELINK H et al: The value of postoperative radiotherapy as an adjuvant to radical neck dissection. Cancer 52(6):1008, 1983.

181. SLOTMAN GJ et al: Preoperative combined chemotherapy and radiation therapy plus radical surgery in advanced head and neck cancer: Five year results with impressive complete response rates and high survival. Cancer 69(11):2736, 1992.

182. CRUSE CE, RADOCHA RF: Squamous cell carcinoma of the lip. Plast Reconstr Surg 80(6):787, 1987.

183. BYERS R et al: Squamous carcinoma of the external ear. Am J Surg 146(4):447, 1983.

184. LIPPMAN SM et al: 13-cis-Retinoic acid and interferon alpha-2a: Effective combination therapy for advanced squamous cell carcinoma of the skin. J Natl Cancer Inst 84(4):235, 1992.

185. LIPPMAN SM, MEYSKENS FL JR: Treatment of advanced squamous cell carcinoma of the skin with isotretinoin. Ann Intern Med 107(4):499, 1987.

186. SADEK H et al: Treatment of advanced squamous cell carcinoma of the skin with cisplatin, 5-fluorouracil, and bleomycin. Cancer 66(8):1692, 1990.

187. GUTHRIE TH JR et al: Cisplatin-based chemotherapy in advanced basal and squamous cell carcinomas of the skin: Results in 28 patients including 13 patients receiving multimodality therapy. J Clin Oncol 8(2):342, 1990.

188. GEOHAS J et al: Adjuvant radiotherapy after excision of cutaneous squamous cell carcinoma. J Am Acad Dermatol 30(4):633, 1994.

189. MARKS R: An overview of skin cancers. Cancer 75:607, 1995.

190. GALLAGHER RP et al: Sunlight exposure, pigmentary factors, and risk of nonmelanocytic skin cancer. I. Basal cell carcinoma. Arch Dermatol 131(2):157, 1995.

191. HALDER RM, BRIDGEMAN-SHAH S: Skin cancer in African Americans. Cancer 75:667, 1995.

192. URBACH F et al: Ultraviolet radiation and skin cancer in man, in Advances in Biology of Skin: Carcinogenesis, vol 2, W Montagna, RL Dobson (eds). New York, Pergamon, 1966, p 195.

193. MILLER ES et al: Vulvar basal cell carcinoma. Dermatol Surg 23(3):207, 1997.

194. ALTMAN A et al: Basal cell epithelioma in black patients. J Am Acad Dermatol 17:741, 1987.

195. DIFFY BL et al: Solar dosimetry of the face: The relationship of natural ultraviolet radiation exposure to basal cell carcinoma localization. Phys Med Biol 24:931, 1979.

196. DINEHART SM et al: Basal cell carcinoma in young patients after irradiation from childhood malignancy. Med Pediatr Oncol 19(6):508, 1991.

197. BURNS DA, CALNAU CD: Basal cell carcinoma in a chronic leg ulcer. Clin Exp Dermatol 3:443, 1978.

198. HAZELRIGG OE: Basal cell carcinoma arising in a vaccination scar. Int J Dermatol 17:723, 1978.

199. HENDRICKS WM: Basal cell carcinoma arising in a chicken pox scar. Arch Dermatol 116:1304, 1980.

200. WHITE SW: Basal cell carcinoma arising in a burn scar: Case report. J Dermatol Surg Oncol 9:159, 1983.

201. ELDER E et al: Tumors and cysts of the epidermis, in Lever's Histopathology of the Skin, 8th ed, D Elder et al (eds). Philadelphia, Lippincott-Raven, 1997, p 730.

202. FARMER ER, HELWIG EB: Metastatic basal cell carcinoma: A clinicopathologic study of seventeen cases. Cancer 46:748, 1980.

203. SAFAI B, GOOD RA: Basal cell carcinoma with metastasis: Review of the literature. Arch Pathol Lab Med 101:327, 1977.

204. STANLEY MW et al: Basal cell carcinoma metastatic to the salivary glands: Differential diagnosis in fine-needle aspiration cytology. Diagn Cytopahtol 16(3):247, 1997.

205. DEGNER RA et al: Metastatic basal cell carcinoma: Report of a case presenting with respiratory failure. Am J Med Sci 301(6):395, 1991.

206. VON DOMARUS H, STEVENS PJ: Metastatic basal cell carcinoma: Report of five cases and review of 170 cases in the literature. J Am Acad Dermatol 10(6):1043, 1984.

207. RIEFKOHL R et al: Metastatic basal cell carcinoma. Ann Plast Surg 13(6):525, 1984.

208. SMITH JM, IRONS GB: Metastatic basal cell carcinoma: Review of the literature and report of three cases. Ann Plast Surg 11(6):551, 1983.

209. BAKER PB, BERGGREN R: Metastatic basal cell carcinoma: Review and report of a case. Ann Plast Surg 11(5):428, 1983.

210. STALEY TE et al: Metastatic basal cell carcinoma of the scrotum. J Urol 130(4):792, 1983.

211. JARCHOW RC, RHODES MF: Metastatic basal cell carcinoma: Report of a case. Laryngoscope 93(4):481, 1983.

212. SCANLON EF et al: Metastatic basal cell carcinoma. J Surg Oncol 15(2):171, 1980.

213. FARMER ER, HELWIG EB: Metastatic basal cell carcinoma: A clinicopathologic study of seventeen cases. Cancer 46(4):748, 1980.

214. LARSON DL et al: Metastatic basal cell carcinoma of the lung. South Med J 73(5):647, 1980.

215. STELL JS et al: Basal cell carcinoma metastatic to the bone. Arch Dermatol 93(3):338, 1966.

216. KIRKHAM N: Basal cell carcinoma, in Lever's Histopathology of the Skin, 8th ed, D Elder et al (eds). Philadelphia, Lippincott-Raven, 1997, pp 720–731.

217. REIDBORD HE et al: Ultrastructural study of basal cell carcinoma and its variants with comments on histogenesis. Arch Dermatol 104:132, 1971.

218. MEHREGAN AH: Aggressive basal cell epithelioma on sunlight-protected skin. Am J Dermatopathol 5:221, 1983.

219. BOREL DM: Cutaneous basosquamous carcinoma: Review of the literature and report of 35 cases. Arch Pathol 95:293, 1973.

220. LANG PG JR et al: Three dimensional reconstruction of the superficial multicentric basal cell carcinoma. Am J Dermatopathol 9:198, 1987.

221. PINKUS H: Premalignant fibroepithelial tumors of the skin. Arch Dermatol Syph 67:598, 1953.

222. VAN SCOTT EJ, REINERTSON RP: The modulating influence of stromal environment on epithelial cells studied in human autotransplants. J Invest Dermatol 36:109, 1961.

223. WILDER RB et al: Recurrent basal cell carcinoma treated with radiation therapy. Arch Dermatol 127(11):1668, 1991.

224. WILDER KB et al: Basal cell carcinoma treated with radiation therapy. Cancer 68(10):2134, 1991.

225. SAWNSON NA: Mohs' surgery: The technique, indications, applications, and the future. Arch Dermatol 119:761, 1983.

226. TROMOVITCH TA, STEGMAN SJ: Microscopic-controlled excision of cutaneous tumors: Chemosurgery, fresh tissue technique. Cancer 41:653, 1978.

227. FRIEDMAN H et al: Recurrent basal cell carcinoma in margin-positive tumors. Ann Plast Surg 38(3):232, 1997.

228. SWANSON NA et al: A novel method of re-excising incompletely excised basal cell carcinomas. J Dermatol Surg Oncol 6:438, 1980.

229. CHIMENTI S et al: Use of recombinant interferon alfa-2b in the treatment of basal cell carcinoma. Dermatology 190(3):214, 1995.

230. STENQUIST B et al: Treatment of aggressive basal cell carcinoma with intralesional interferon: Evaluation of efficacy by Mohs' surgery. J Am Acad Dermatol 27(1):65, 1992.

231. PECK GL et al: Treatment and prevention of basal cell carcinoma with oral isotretinoin. J Am Acad Dermatol 19(1):176, 1988.

232. WILSON BD et al: Photodynamic therapy for the treatment of basal cell carcinoma. Arch Dermatol 128(12):1597, 1992.

233. WOLF P et al: Topical photodynamic therapy with endogenous porphyrins after application of 5-aminolevulinic acid: An alternative treatment modality for solar keratoses, superficial squamous cell carcinomas, and basal cell carcinomas? J Am Acad Dermatol 28(1):17, 1993.

# 7B / MALIGNANT MELANOMA

*Constantine P. Karakousis, Kirby I. Bland, and Charles M. Balch*

## INCIDENCE

The incidence of malignant melanoma has increased dramatically. In the United States, the lifetime risk in 1930 was 1 per 1500, in 1981 it was 1 per 250, in 1985 1 per 150, and in 1996, it rose to 1 per 87 (1 per 70 for white males).[1] There are about 47,700 new invasive cases diagnosed annually, and 20,000–40,000 in situ cases.[1] The lifetime risk is 1/74 for the year 2000. This increase in melanoma incidence is a worldwide phenomenon, and it is real and not artifactual. The death rate from melanoma has continued to rise about 2% annually, although the annual increase in melanoma is 6%. The survival rates for people with localized melanoma have improved from 50% in the 1950s to about 90% today.[2] Therefore, although there is an increase in the absolute death rates due to the larger number of cases, this has not kept pace with the incidence, in recent years, primarily as a result of earlier diagnosis and consequently higher survival.

## ETIOLOGY

The major etiologic factor involved in the causation of malignant melanoma is ultraviolet (UV) radiation exposure. Owing to its capacity to cause erythema, it is presumed that the 290- to 320-nm UV-B range of UV radiation may be the range that tends to cause melanoma, although studies on users of sun-tanning beds (UV-A, 320 to 400 mm) suggest that the UV-A range also may contribute.[3] The evidence that solar radiation is implicated derives from epidemiologic studies showing an increase in the incidence of melanoma as the latitude decreases, in the coastal areas, and for people spending their vacations in sunny climates. Both latitude and altitude affect the intensity of exposure to sunlight. There is a considerable time lag between repeated sunlight exposures, which induce and then promote melanoma, and the subsequent clinical appearance of this neoplasm. Apparently, bursts of UV-B exposure early in one's life present a higher risk than simply chronic long-term exposure. The gradual depletion of the ozone layer may be another factor, since this layer is estimated to have decreased by 3% to 7% since 1969. Apparently, each 1% decrease in stratospheric ozone results in a 1% increase in the incidence of melanoma.[4]

Partly because of its degree of efficacy as a filter for solar radiation, the degree of skin pigmentation of an individual or race is another factor affecting the incidence of melanoma. Whites have a higher incidence of melanoma than nonwhites. Thus, whites have 10 times the incidence of melanoma as blacks. In blacks, melanomas arise more commonly in less pigmented skin areas, for example, the palms, soles, and mucous membranes.

About 8% to 12% of melanomas occur within families, which indicates the role of heredity for these patients. Initially, it was Clark[5] who described the association between the clinical entity of multiple nevi with unique clinical and histopathologic characteristics described as the "B-K mole" syndrome ("B-K" were the initials of the first 2 patients with this syndrome) and a higher risk of developing malignant melanoma. The term *familial atypical multiple mole melanoma (FAMMM)* was later proposed, and more recently, the condition has been called the *dysplastic nevus (DN)* syndrome. Patients with DN may be associated with familial cutaneous melanoma, but the majority of these patients do not have such a history. They often have numerous and sometimes hundreds of atypical moles. Histologically, DN manifest disordered proliferation of atypical melanocytes in a lentiginous epidermal pattern. About 1.8% to 7% of all whites, and 30% to 50% of patients with melanoma, have DN. Persons with sporadic DN have a 6% lifetime risk of developing melanoma. This risk approaches 100% for those with DN and a history of familial melanoma.[6] A series of sequential biologic changes from the normal melanocyte to metastatic melanoma provide the opportunity for early detection and therapeutic intervention (Table 7B-1).[7]

## PREVENTIVE MEASURES

Measures to prevent malignant melanoma involve public education programs emphasizing the risk for developing skin cancer by excessive exposure to sunlight, particularly for those with fair skin. Reducing exposure to sunlight through avoidance of such exposure, the wearing of protective clothing, and the use of sunscreens is an important goal. Sunscreen products that offer a broad spectrum of protection (that is, also filtering, to some extent, UV-A) and a rating of at least 15 are recommended. However, this is the long-term approach, since at the present, the benefit of reducing the degree of exposure to sunlight will not manifest itself for a few decades, given the long time required between induction and promotion to the clinical appearance of melanoma. Increasing early detection of this neoplasm by increasing public and professional awareness of this condition represents the short-term approach in reducing mortality.

**TABLE 7B-1. BIOLOGIC CHANGES IN MELANOMA PROGRESSION**

| Normal melanocyte/Nevus | → | Sun-damaged nevus | → | Nevus with atypical changes | → | Melanoma in situ | → | Thin, invasive melanoma | → | Thick, invasive melanoma | → | Metastatic disease |
|---|---|---|---|---|---|---|---|---|---|---|---|---|

## CLINICAL MANIFESTATIONS

There are usually no subjective symptoms associated with the appearance of a localized malignant melanoma, with the exception of occasional itching in the area of the mole. The characteristics suggestive of a melanoma for a specific skin lesion can be memorized through the use of the mnemonic ABCDE (Table 7B-2): A (asymmetry), B (border irregularity), C (color variegation), D (diameter larger than 6 mm), and E (evolution, that is, showing relatively rapid change in the course of weeks or a few months). When the history is reliable, the last characteristic is important because benign moles remain stable and change only slightly over the course of years, whereas melanomas change perceptibly in the course of a few weeks (3 to 12) or months. Mole changes that are suspicious of melanoma include: a change in color or shape, an increase in diameter, a surface that becomes more raised and irregular, and a lesion that bleeds (Fig. 7B-1). Ulceration of the surface epithelium of a mole is also a suspicious sign. Itching is a symptom in 20% to 46% of the lesions.[8]

The four major growth patterns of melanomas are superficial spreading melanoma (SSM), nodular melanoma (NM), lentigo maligna melanoma (LMM), and acral lentiginous melanoma (ALM). SSM is the most common lesion (in about 70% of cases), occurring as a pigmented, flat lesion that often arises in a preexisting mole that initially tends to spread radially and only later may develop nodules within its perimeter. NM, the second most common variety of melanoma (15% to 30% of the lesions), is biologically aggressive, often arising de novo and presenting a raised, domed surface that may resemble a blood blister or a hemangioma with different hues of color. LMM (4% to 10% of cases) is a distinct variety of flat, tan-brown lesions, typically located in the face of elderly individuals and slowly evolving over several years from the precursor form (lentigo maligna). ALM (2% to 8% of cases) is usually located in the plantar or palmar surfaces of the skin of older people; this type tends to have a worse prognosis than SSM or LMM. Although still useful to the clinician, the categorization of melanomas according to

**TABLE 7B-2. CLINICAL FEATURES DIFFERENTIATING BENIGN MOLES FROM MELANOMA**

| FEATURE | BENIGN MOLE | MELANOMA |
|---|---|---|
| Asymmetry | No | Yes |
| Border irregularity | No | Yes |
| Color variegation | No | Yes |
| Diameter | Usually <6 mm | Often >6 mm |
| Evolution | Stable | Rapid change |

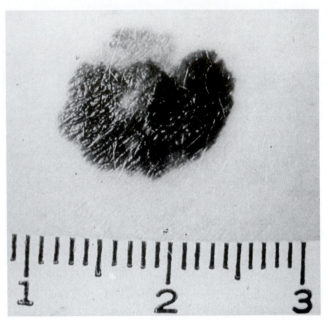

**FIGURE 7B-1.** Typical melanoma showing irregularity of the border, surface, color, and large diameter.

growth pattern has been superseded largely with regard to prognostic implications by the microstaging methods concerning the primary lesion. Subungual melanoma is a rare form of cutaneous melanoma presenting as a brown-black discoloration of the nail bed that may be confused with hematoma. Lacking a clear history of trauma or failure for this discoloration to clear within 2 to 4 weeks should lead to biopsy, usually by removing a portion of the nail plate. Pigmentation of the adjacent cuticle or skin supports the clinical diagnosis of subungual melanoma.

About 5% of NMs and 10% of subungual melanomas may lack pigment (amelanotic), in which cases the suspicion of a neoplastic lesion is raised by the general appearance of a growth. Approximately 4% of melanomas appear in the subcutaneous tissue, a nodal basin, or other sites without any known primary skin site. In these patients, either the primary skin site existed at some point and regressed spontaneously unbeknown to the patient or these melanoma sites in other than skin areas represent primary growth sites from ectopic melanocytes to these areas which underwent malignant degeneration.

## DIAGNOSIS

A clinically suspicious mole should be subjected to biopsy. This can be an incisional or punch biopsy of the most suspicious area of

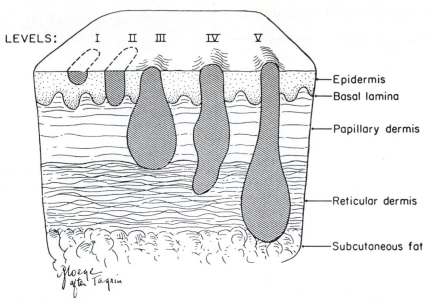

**FIGURE 7B-2.** Schematic illustrating Clark's method of classification of the depth of involvement in the primary lesion.

the mole, particularly if the mole is big and cosmetic considerations are involved. However, in general, it is preferable to perform an excisional biopsy, since the entire lesion can thus be examined, which eliminates sampling errors and allows more accurate determination of the level of invasion and thickness of the lesion. The orientation of the elliptical incision that is to be used for excisional biopsy should have its long axis pointing toward the regional nodal basin. This means that for melanomas involving the entremity, the ellipse should be longitudinal, not transverse, on the skin of the extremity around the presumed melanoma. In the trunk, the ellipse should again point toward the nearest regional nodal basin unless otherwise indicated by skin availability for primary closure. The reasons for this recommendation are twofold: (1) any melanomatous cells within the lymphatics adjacent to the lesion will tend to migrate along such lymphatics toward the regional nodal basin and are more likely to be included in a wide-excision ellipse pointing toward the nodal basin and (2) given the longitudinal course of lymphatics in the extremities, transverse incisions interrupt more lymphatics and therefore tend to increase the incidence of lymphedema, particularly in the lower extremity when added to a groin dissection. Finally, transverse biopsy incisions require more often the use of a skin graft than longitudinal biopsy incisions at the time of wide excision.

## PATHOLOGY—MICROSTAGING

Microstaging the primary lesion (classifying it with the use of a microscope) is a significant tool for the clinician because it allows the physician to make accurate prognostic correlations with the expected recurrence and survival rates and to rationalize the application of the surgical treatment. Developed by Clark,[9] the method

recognizes levels of invasion according to the layer of skin involved by the melanoma process. Thus (Fig. 7B-2)[9]:

1. Melanomas confined to the epidermis (in situ) are level I.
2. Those penetrating the basement membrane into the papillary dermis are level II.
3. Those reaching the interface of the papillary and reticular dermis are level III.
4. Those penetrating into the reticular dermis are level IV.
5. Those extending into the subcutaneous fat are level V.

In the method proposed by Breslow,[10] the greatest thickness of the lesion is measured on cross section with an ocular micrometer determining the total vertical height from the granular layer of the epidermis to the point of deepest penetration. Both Clark's and Breslow's methods are used and are believed to be complementary, although the general consensus is that Breslow's method is a more accurate prognostic indicator.[11–13] The presence or absence of ulceration on the surface of the lesion is another important prognostic indicator—ulcerated lesions having a worse prognosis.[11–12] With localized melanomas, additional prognostic parameters are the gender of the patient, the anatomic location of the lesion, and the age of the patient (women, involvement of an extremity, and younger age are all factors having a better prognosis).[14] The various prognostic factors and corresponding survival rates are given in Table 7B-4 on page 509.[15]

## STAGING OF THE DISEASE

Initially, a three-stage system for melanoma was employed. Stage I was that of localized melanoma, stage II that of regional metastases,

**TABLE 7B-3.** STAGE GROUPINGS FOR CUTANEOUS MELANOMA

| 0 | Tis | N0 | M0 |
|---|---|---|---|
| IA | T1a | N0 | M0 |
| IB | T1b | N0 | M0 |
| | T2a | N0 | M0 |
| IIA | T2b | N0 | M0 |
| | T3a | N0 | M0 |
| IIB | T3b | N0 | M0 |
| | T4a | N0 | M0 |
| IIC | T4b | N0 | M0 |
| IIIA | any T1-4a | N1b(C); N1a(P) | M0 |
| IIIB | any T1-4a | N2b(C); N1b(P) | M0 |
| | | N2a(P) | M0 |
| IIIC | any T | N2c(C); N2b, N2c(P) | M0 |
| | any T | N3 | M0 |
| IV | any T | any N | any M |

C: Clinical staging includes microstaging of the primary melanoma and clinical/radiologic evaluation for metastases.
P: Pathologic staging includes clinical staging and pathologic information about the regional lymph nodes after partial or complete lymphadenectomy.

and stage III that of distant metastases. Although a simple system, this was a crude prognostic instrument, since in stage I, in which 85% of the patients are currently diagnosed, the risk varies widely according to the thickness of the primary lesion. This staging system has largely been abandoned.

A second staging system proposed by the M.D. Anderson Hospital in Houston distinguished a stage I disease as that of a localized melanoma; stage II that of local recurrence; stage IIIA that of in-transit metastases; stage IIIB that of regional nodal metastases; stage IIIAB that of both IIIA and IIIB recurrences; and stage IV that of distant disseminated disease, with IVA denoting cutaneous metastases only and IVB any visceral metastases.[16] This system is still in use, because it distinguishes between in-transit and regional nodal recurrences, which may have different management. Therefore, when the focus is on the differential management of these two types of recurrences, this system may still be used.

In the latest proposed staging system for malignant melanoma, Tis is melanoma in situ. T1 is a lesion ≤1 mm—a, without ulceration; b, with ulceration or Level IV or V. T2 is a lesion, 1–2 mm thick. T3 is a lesion 2.01–4 mm thick. A T4 lesion is >4 mm thick. Each T category is subdivided into: a, without ulceration, and b, with ulceration. N1 is a one lymph node involvement at the regional basin—a, with micrometastases; b, with macrometastases. N2 is a state of 2–3 lymph node involvement (a, with micrometastases; b, with macrometastases; c, in transit metastases or satellites without metastatic lymph nodes. N3 is four or more metastatic lymph nodes or a combination of in-transit metastases, satellites, or ulcerated melanoma and metastatic lymph nodes. M1 is the state of distant skin, subcutaneous, or lymph node metastases with a normal LDH; M2, lung metastases with normal LDH; M-3, all other visceral or distant metastases with normal or elevated LDH.

## TREATMENT OF LOCALIZED MELANOMA (STAGES I AND II)

### PRIMARY SITE

In the past, at the primary site, 4- to 5-cm margins of excision were recommended and practiced for any invasive melanoma. Since the mid-1970s, it has become evident that for thin melanomas (stage IA), margins of 1 cm were adequate. The overall rate of recurrence for such melanomas has been shown to be only 1%.[17] The standard margin now recommended for melanomas <1 mm thick is 1 cm. In European studies, it has been found that a 1-cm margin is sufficient for lesions <2 mm thick.[18] Following publication of the results of the multi-institutional surgical trial, in a prospective randomized setting, it was established that a 2-cm excision margin provides as good local control as a 4-cm margin in intermediate-thickness melanomas (1 to 4 mm) and therefore is the recommended margin.[19,20] A 2-cm margin provides the opportunity of primary closure for the majority of the patients and results in improved cosmesis and reduced morbidity. For melanomas thicker than 4 mm, a 2- to 3-cm margin is recommended, although hard data are lacking for this minority of lesions among currently diagnosed melanomas and the issue of local control becomes secondary for these thick lesions, which recur predominantly at regional and distant sites.

In performing the wide excision, when primary closure is anticipated, an ellipse is made with the radius of the short axis that of the recommended margin and a long axis pointing toward the regional nodal basin. The lateral margin is measured from the center of the biopsy incision. The skin incision is then carried vertically through the subcutaneous fat to the level of the investing fascia. The fascia may or may not be removed at the discretion of the surgeon. Then, if it looks like a primary closure can be done, the flaps can be undermined at the level of the fascia as necessary in order to permit primary closure. When it is expected that a skin graft will be required, a circle is outlined around the primary site with a radius equal to the recommended margin. After the skin incision is made, the dissection proceeds obliquely through the subcutaneous fat and reaches the fascia at a circle wider than the circle made in the skin so that more subcutaneous fat is removed than skin. The skin edge is then approximated with a subcuticular suture to the fascia. Removing part of the subcutaneous fat around the circular skin edge makes for a smooth transition between the skin with subcutaneous fat of normal height and the level of the skin graft.

For patients presenting with stage III melanoma, the primary site should be dealt with as in stages I and II, along with surgical treatment of the regional recurrence(s). For those diagnosed for the first time in stage IV, the primary site may receive only excisional biopsy, unless surgical treatment of the distant recurrences also is planned. Unknown primary melanoma presenting in the subcutaneous tissue or a nodal basin without any other evidence of distant dissemination should be treated with wide resection or radical nodal dissection, respectively, since the 5-year survival rate thus obtained is equivalent to that of patients with regional recurrence from a known and controlled primary cutaneous site.[21]

The treatment of anal canal melanomas may be individualized. Thin lesions may be treated with wide excision, whereas thicker

**TABLE 7B-4.** PROGNOSTIC FACTORS AND SURVIVAL FOR PATIENTS WITH LOCALIZED MELANOMA

| TUMOR THICKNESS (MM) | ANATOMIC SITE | ULCERATION | CLARK'S LEVEL | SEX | 5-YR SURVIVAL RATE (%) | 10-YR SURVIVAL RATE (%) |
|---|---|---|---|---|---|---|
| <0.76 | | | | | | |
| | Extremity | — | II | — | 99 | 97 |
| | Extremity | — | Other | — | 97 | 94 |
| | Axial | — | II | — | 96 | 92 |
| | Axial | — | Other | — | 91 | 84 |
| 0.76–1.49 | | | | | | |
| | Extremity | No | II | — | 98 | 97 |
| | Extremity | No | Other | — | 93 | 89 |
| | Extremity | Yes | II | — | 94 | 91 |
| | Extremity | Yes | Other | — | 82 | 72 |
| | Axial | No | II | — | 95 | 93 |
| | Axial | No | Other | — | 85 | 77 |
| | Axial | Yes | II | — | 88 | 81 |
| | Axial | Yes | Other | — | 64 | 49 |
| 1.50–2.49 | | | | | | |
| | Extremity | No | — | — | 86 | 81 |
| | Extremity | Yes | — | — | 76 | 69 |
| | Axial | No | — | — | 76 | 67 |
| | Axial | Yes | — | — | 61 | 49 |
| 2.50–3.99 | | | | | | |
| | Extremity | No | — | Female | 80 | 72 |
| | Extremity | No | — | Male | 73 | 62 |
| | Extremity | Yes | — | Female | 74 | 64 |
| | Extremity | Yes | — | Male | 74 | 51 |
| | Axial | No | — | Female | 73 | 63 |
| | Axial | No | — | Male | 63 | 51 |
| | Axial | Yes | — | Female | 65 | 52 |
| | Axial | Yes | — | Male | 53 | 39 |
| 4.00–7.99 | | | | | | |
| | — | No | II/III | — | 80 | 73 |
| | — | No | IV/V | — | 68 | 58 |
| | — | Yes | II/III | — | 67 | 57 |
| | — | Yes | IV/V | — | 51 | 38 |
| ≥8.00 | | | | | | |
| | — | — | — | — | 43 | 25 |

SOURCE: Adapted with permission from Ref. 15.

lesions may require an abdominoperineal resection, although the survival rate of such patients is generally poor.[22]

## REGIONAL NODES

**ELECTIVE DISSECTION.** When the regional nodes are clinically negative, the issue of elective node dissection arises. In the past, simple intuition suggested that eradication of microscopic disease in the regional nodes might improve survival by preventing growth and further dissemination of the disease from the regional nodes. Indeed, many retrospective studies supported this notion.[11–13] However, three prospective randomized studies showed no survival difference between patients treated with wide excision plus observation as compared with patients treated with wide resection plus elective node dissection.[23–24a] Elective dissection should be considered in the context of the thickness of the primary lesion, because the thickness provides the single most important prognostic indicator of the likelihood of microscopic regional node involvement. On the basis of the

**TABLE 7B-5.** INCIDENCE OF REGIONAL MICROMETASTASES IN PATIENTS WITH CLINICALLY LOCALIZED MELANOMA (STAGES I AND II)

|          | LOCATION AND THICKNESS (MM) OF PRIMARY LESION | RISK OF OCCULT REGIONAL METASTASES ONLY (%) |
|----------|-----------------------------------------------|---------------------------------------------|
| Female   | Extremity:                                    |                                             |
|          | <0.76                                         | 2                                           |
|          | 0.76–1.49                                     | 5–7                                         |
|          | 1.50–3.99                                     | 7–19                                        |
|          | ≥4.0                                          | 0                                           |
| Male     | Extremity:                                    |                                             |
|          | <0.76                                         | 2                                           |
|          | 0.76–1.49                                     | 22–24                                       |
|          | 1.50–3.99                                     | 24–29                                       |
|          | ≥4.0                                          | 0                                           |
| Female   | Axial:                                        |                                             |
|          | <0.76                                         | 8                                           |
|          | 0.76–1.49                                     | 14–17                                       |
|          | 1.50–3.99                                     | 17–21                                       |
|          | ≥4.0                                          | 0                                           |
| Male     | Axial:                                        |                                             |
|          | <0.76                                         | 9                                           |
|          | 0.76–1.49                                     | 27–28                                       |
|          | 1.50–3.99                                     | 28–30                                       |
|          | ≥4.0                                          | 0                                           |

available prognostic parameters, one may estimate fairly accurately the risk of microscopic nodal involvement only (i.e., without occult distant metastases) for a given patient (Table 7B-5).[25] Thus, elective dissection need not be considered for lesions <1 mm thick, since the risk of microscopic involvement of the regional nodes for those thin lesions is minimal. Some simple calculations help to put this issue in perspective. In data culled from retrospective reviews, the survival rate of patients with microscopic involvement of the regional nodes has been estimated to be 25% higher than that of patients with palpable involvement of these nodes.[26] Since the risk of microscopic regional disease for intermediate (1- to 4 mm-thick lesions) is about 20%,[26] it follows that the survival benefit for this subgroup of lesions may be realized in 25% of the 20%, that is, 5% of the patients subjected to elective dissection. Therefore, even if we accept that patients with microscopic nodal involvement (elective dissection) have, on the average, a 5-year survival rate that is 25% higher than those with palpable nodal involvement (therapeutic dissection)—something disputed by certain investigators who believe that there is no substantial survival difference between the two groups—it is still obvious that we are dealing with a small minority of patients for whom a survival benefit may be derived through elective node dissection. Therefore, the question arises as to which subset of patients, if any, may benefit from elective node dissection.

The latest and largest prospective randomized study, conducted largely in the United States, showed no difference in the overall sur-

vival rate of patients treated with wide excision and observation or wide excision plus elective dissection.[27] In this study, patients treated with observation whenever they developed regional palpable adenopathy were subjected to therapeutic lymphadenectomy. Although there was no difference in the overall survival rate between the two treatment groups, there was a significant survival rate improvement, according to actual treatment or randomized intent with elective node dissection, (1) for patients <60 years of age, (2) for those with lesions 1 to 2 mm thick, (3) for patients with extremity lesions, and (4) especially significant improvement ($P = 0.003$) for patients <60 years of age with lesions 1 to 2 mm thick.[27] In the last update of this trial, it was concluded that elective lymph node dissection (ELND) significantly improved survival for patients with nonulcerated melanomas, this feature being the key factor in making recommendations for ELND.[27a] Given that the two previous prospective studies, as well as the latest one, were negative for overall survival, the last study's positive results on specific subsets have been received with some skepticism. However, we may conclude that for patients who have nonulcerated melanomas, there is now justification in considering elective node dissection when sentinel node biopsy is not applicable or is unsuccessful.

SENTINEL NODE BIOPSY. In what is now known as intraoperative lymphatic mapping, or *sentinel node biopsy* (SNB), it was the pioneering work of Morton and co-workers[26] which showed, that there is a single node (occasionally two) in the regional nodal basin that is specific for each anatomic skin area and that first receives the lymphatic drainage from that area. This is the node to first receive and trap by filtration any melanomatous cells that may have escaped from the primary lesion and have travelled into the regional nodal basin. The sentinel node may be identified with the use of a blue dye, isosulfan blue (lymphazurin), injected intradermally near the primary biopsy site. According to the original description by Morton, 0.5 to 1.0 mL of the dye is injected intradermally on either side of the biopsy incision. This area is gently massaged for about 5 min; an incision is then made over the regional nodal basin, and a flap is raised toward the direction of the primary site. Blue-stained lymphatic channels are identified and are traced to the blue-stained (sentinel) node. This node is removed and subjected to frozen section. Additional dissection is performed in order to rule out the possibility of a second or third blue-stained lymph node (sentinel), which must be removed if present. While awaiting the results of the frozen section, one may proceed with the closure of the incision by using a subcutaneous layer of closure with absorbable material followed by skin approximation. The use of a suction drain is optional, depending on the extent of the dissection that was required for the identification of the sentinel node. If a suction drain is used, the exit point is placed in the same line as that of the incision. Should the frozen section report be positive, an elliptical incision is made around the previous incision and the drain exit point. Flaps are raised, and the node dissection is completed without ever entering the plane and cavity created by removing the sentinel node(s), which is potentially contaminated with tumor cells. One usually has time to complete the wide excision of the primary site while waiting for the results of the frozen section. Lately, it is believed that it is best to wait for the results of permanent sections since a small microscopic focus may be lost in the process of freezing. The SNB should be performed in the same sitting, immediately before the wide excision of the primary site. A previous wide excision may distort the lymphatic drainage of the site previously occupied by the melanoma and render unreliable the identification of the correct sentinel node. In the authors' experience, with a previous wide excision and primary closure, the site originally occupied by the melanoma can be estimated to be reasonably close to the center of the wide excision incision, and therefore the SNB procedure can be performed with satisfactory reliability, as judged by the ability to find the sentinel node, being also the sole positive regional node in several of such cases. However, when a rotation flap has been used to cover the defect of the wide excision, one can no longer approximate the primary site with any accuracy.

In his original paper, Morton recommended the intradermal injection of 0.5 to 1.0 mL of the blue dye, because larger injections tended to diffuse into the subcutaneous fat, which in feline experiments led to tracking of the dye along the lymphatic channels coursing along the major blood vessels. He therefore advised repeating the intradermal injection every 20 min as necessary until the sentinel node is found. The problem with the approach of repeated injections is that following the initial dissection in the nodal basin to identify the blue-stained lymphatic channels, if no such channels are found, repeated injections at the primary site may no longer be helpful if the lymphatic channels deriving from the melanoma site have been already divided at the nodal basin. One of the authors (CPK) prefers to inject 3 mL of the dye, as much of it intradermally as possible, always near the side or the corner of the biopsy incision facing the nodal basin, to elevate the injected site for 5 min (by lifting this area, when feasible, or tilting the operating table) in order to allow gravity to facilitate the flow of dye to the nodal basin, and finally to use sharp dissection along a single plane from the skin incision to the surface of the lymph nodes, that is, without making flaps (Fig. 7B-3), and intently observing for a colored lymphatic channel and/or a blue-stained lymph node.[28]

Lymphoscintigraphy is of crucial importance prior to SNB.[29] The zone of ambiguity separating the cutaneous drainage areas of the axilla and groin on each side is much broader than Sappey's line would suggest, which extends between the umbilicus anteriorly to the level of the L2 vertebra posteriorly. Trunk lesions, particularly those close to the midline or those located between the axilla and groin, may exhibit drainage to two nodal basins. Although extremity melanomas drain predictably in the axilla or groin depending on their location in the upper or lower extremity, they occasionally may show drainage to an epitrochlear or popliteal node. Technetium 99m sulfur colloid is injected intradermally at the melanoma site, and scanning of the relevant nodal basins is made within 2 hr after injection. This radioactive material persists in the regional nodes for several hours. The procedure of intraoperative lymphatic mapping can be facilitated with the use of an intraoperative probe that detects radioactivity. Since there is considerable difference in the half-life of various preparations used in lymphoscintigraphy, the surgeon should be familiar with the specifics of the material used at his or her hospital if the injection of the radioactive material is done on the day of the operation so that it can be appropriately timed in relation to the procedure. There is still some debate as to which may be the optimal radioactive tracer.[30] Although with some experience the sentinel node can be identified accurately in over 90% of the patients with the blue dye alone, the use of an intraoperative probe following lymphoscintigraphy done in the morning prior to the operation facilitates the dissection and removal of the sentinel node in several ways. Prior to making the incision in the nodal basin, the probe, covered with a sterile sheath, is applied successively along the length of the intended incision on the nodal basin. The point of the highest radioactive count lies directly over the sentinel node. Thus, the incision along the same line as that of a node dissection can be smaller and centered over the point of highest radioactivity. As the dissection proceeds through the subcutaneous fat, it can be further directed by the use of the probe. Once the blue-stained lymphatic channels and a blue-stained lymph node are identified, and the node is excised, the radioactivity count of the sentinel node is documented ex vivo, and the count over the nodal basin is again recorded. If the latter falls to or near the background levels, one is assured that the sentinel node has been correctly identified and removed and there are no other "sentinel" nodes in the regional basin. Therefore, the use of the probe reduces the need for further dissection to rule out the presence of additional sentinel node(s). The blue dye method is still important, because it sharply delineates the sentinel node(s). The two methods appear to be complementary,

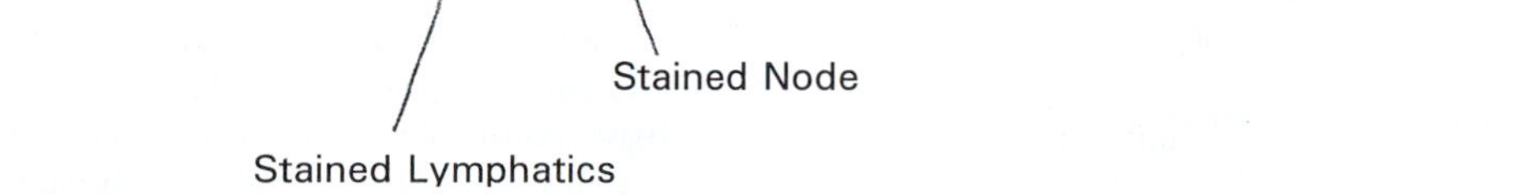

Primary Site

Nodal Basin

Skin

Subcutaneous Fat

Chain of Lymph Nodes

Stained Node

Stained Lymphatics

**FIGURE 7B-3.** In identifying the sentinel node and the associated lymphatic channel, a direct approach toward the surface of the nodes (---) may be more expeditious than raising a flap and insisting on finding the blue-stained lymphatic channel first ( . . .).

and with their combined use, the rate of successful identification of the sentinel node(s) should be close to 100%.

For patients who show a microscopically positive sentinel node, either on frozen or permanent section, a complete node dissection should be performed, because about 37% of such patients are found to have additional positive nodes in the specimen of node dissection.[26] A rate of 29% of additional positive nodes, found in the specimen of complete lymphadenectomy when the sentinel node was originally positive, was also reported in another study.[31] In order to identify all patients with microscopic disease in the regional nodes, it is important for the pathologist to perform immunohistochemistry (i.e., S100 protein and HMB45) in addition to routine hematoxylin-eosin staining of the preparation.[26] Newer assays using tyrosinase reverse transcription-polymerase chain reaction (RT-PCR) on preparations from lymph nodes are extremely sensitive in detecting micrometastases.[32] Rarely, despite the apparently successful identification of a sentinel node that is found to be negative, a palpable positive node appears later in the same basin, which suggests a false-negative result for the initial sentinel biopsy, unless an intervening local or in-transit recurrence provides a probable origin for this nodal recurrence. This probably occurs as a result of technical problems in identifying all "sentinel" nodes at the initial biopsy, and according to Morton's original report, it may occur in 1% of the patients.[26] Therefore the reliability of this method in accurately staging the nodal basin appears to be close to 99%. This information is important not only for its staging prognostic value but also because of the need to consider adjuvant therapy for patients with regional node metastases. Whether this method, by identifying the patients with microscopic nodal disease for whom a selective lymphadenectomy is performed, will have an impact on survival remains to be seen. This is one of the objectives of a multicenter prospective study, under the leadership of Donald Morton, in which patients with melanomas ≥1 mm or those with level IV or V melanomas, regardless of thickness, are randomized between wide excision alone or wide excision plus intraoperative lymphatic mapping.

The surgical treatment of localized melanoma (stages I and II) is summarized in Table 7B-6 and in the form of an algorithm (stages I to III) given in Fig. 7B-4. Given that elective node dissection does not appear to affect survival, except for the substantial numerical group of younger patients with 1- to 2-mm-thick melanomas, and that the procedure of SNB biopsy has not yet been proved to have an impact on survival, some melanoma specialists consider that observation of the regional nodes is a legitimate option.[33] However,

**TABLE 7B-6.** MARGINS OF RESECTION AND MANAGEMENT OF REGIONAL LYMPH NODES IN PATIENTS WITH PRIMARY CUTANEOUS MELANOMA

| TUMOR THICKNESS | MARGIN | OPTIONS FOR LYMPH NODES |
|---|---|---|
| <1.0 mm* | 1 cm | Observation |
| 1.0–2.0 mm | 2 cm | SNB |
| 2.01–4.0 mm | 2 cm | SNB |
| >4.0 cm | 2–3 cm | SNB |

* Patients with Clark's level IV or deeper may be considered for SNB, even for lesions <1 mm thick.

the recent finding of an adjuvant therapy (interferon α2b) with a modest but significant effect on disease-free survival for patients with metastases to the regional nodes has promoted the use of the SNB for its staging value, so that, at present, in melanoma clinics, observation of the regional nodes is no longer an option for lesions ≥1 mm in thickness, except for patients who owing to advanced age or other infirmities, are not eligible for adjuvant therapy. The reliability of the SNB in staging the regional nodes seems to be well established.

## TREATMENT OF LOCOREGIONAL RECURRENCE

### LOCAL RECURRENCE AND IN-TRANSIT METASTASES

Local recurrence of malignant melanoma has been variously defined. Older definitions have included any recurrence within 5 cm from the surgical scar of the primary lesion. In the multi-institutional surgical trial, a 2-cm boundary around the surgical scar was accepted as one defining a local recurrence. Lesions occurring beyond the 2-cm limit are called *in-transit lesions*. The overall incidence of local recurrence is low, occurring in 4% of patients with intermediate-thickness lesions in the above-mentioned trial.[20] The prognosis associated with this type of recurrence is ominous, because 80% of such patients succumb to their disease.[20] However, several investigations have pointed to a crucial distinction. It appears that this poor outlook is associated with patients having a discontinuous recurrence from the surgical scar, providing a visible demonstration of the ability of the particular melanoma cells to metastasize within lymphatic vessels. On the other hand, local recurrence within, or continuous with, the margin of the primary surgical scar does not have this poor prognosis, because 80% of such patients may attain a 5-year survival.[34,35] Although there is no provision in the current AJCC staging system specifically for local recurrence, local recurrence discontinuous from the primary site has a similar prognosis as in-transit disease and therefore may be subsumed under stage III disease.

When there are multiple lesions around the primary site scar, all within 2 cm, the term *satellitosis* has been employed. Lesions occurring beyond 2 cm of the primary scar are by definition in-transit lesions, since they are caused by trapping of melanoma cells, in either subcutaneous or dermal lymphatics, which were in transit along the lymphatic flow to the regional nodes. When these lesions are intradermal, they produce visible, pigmented lesions that are conspicuous, however, when they are subcutaneous, in the beginning of their clinical onset, they are not visible but are detectable on careful palpation of the extremity from the primary site to the regional nodes. One may then feel one or more pea-size or smaller nodules in the subcutaneous fat. Occasionally, they occur distal to the primary site, and because these are more frequent after node dissection, particularly groin dissection for positive nodes, the alternate term of stasis lesions has been employed for this type of recurrence. Since they appear in multiple sites of the involved extremity, in-transit lesions occur not only in a longitudinal direction between the primary site and the regional nodal basin but also finally circumferentially involve the entire extremity and later progress to the skin and subcutaneous fat of the adjacent trunk.

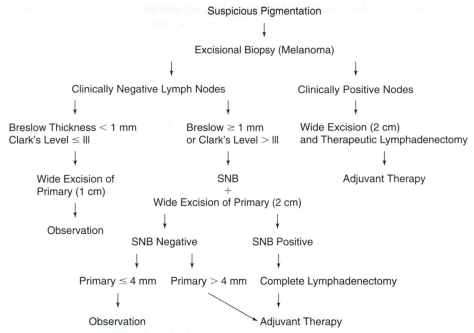

**FIGURE 7B-4.** Algorithm for the surgical treatment of localized melanoma (stages I and II).

Both discontinuous local recurrences and in-transit lesions have an ominous prognosis, because the majority of such patients harbor distant microscopic metastases at the time of locoregional recurrence. However, the majority of (50% to 80%), rather than all, patients with such recurrences have distant subclinical metastases, a fact that determines the type of their treatment. Since systemic treatments at the present stage of their development produce a complete and permanent regression in only 5% or less of these patients, this type of treatment cannot be relied on to eradicate locoregional disease that may be curable in more than 30% of the cases. Therefore, local treatments have taken precedence historically. Wide excision of local recurrences or of in-transit lesions is the simplest treatment.[36] With multiple in-transit lesions, integumentectomy, that is, the en-bloc removal of all in-transit lesions and the intervening skin as a wide strip of skin and subcutaneous fat, has been practiced. The extreme version of integumentectomy for heavy involvement of the extremity is the so-called Charles or Kondoleon procedure, in which the entire skin and subcutaneous fat is removed from the extremity, followed by skin grafting. The latter procedure has not been practiced extensively owing to the unsightly result and morbidity for the extremity. In the past, major amputations of the extremity were practiced for in-transit disease, with a reported 20% to 30% 5-year survival rate.[37] Intralesional injections of bacille Calmette-Guérin (vaccine) (BCG) or other inflammatory agents have produced complete regressions of the injected lesions in immunoreactive patients.[38] Thus, for purified protein derivative–positive patients or those becoming positive after one or two intradermal injections of BCG, the rate of complete regression of cutaneous in-transit lesions was reported to be 90%. However, the rate of regression of subcutaneous in-transit lesions was only about 30%, and the use of multiple BCG injections carried the risk of systemic infection and required

systemic antituberculous treatment. Intralesional injections are now used infrequently. Since the late 1950s, isolation perfusion and, since the late 1960s, hyperthermic isolation limb perfusion (HILP) have been used extensively for the treatment of in-transit lesions of the extremity. Initially, melphalan was used, either alone or in combination with actinomycin D and/or nitrogen mustard. More recently, the combination of melphalan with tumor necrosis factor and interferon γ has resulted in complete regression rates of 90%. Therefore, hyperthermic isolation perfusion has become the most effective treatment for the control of extremity in-transit lesions.[39] Unfortunately, there is a considerable rate of local recurrence following complete regression, and thus the full impact of the new combinations used in HILP has not been definitely assessed on long-term follow-up.

Regional drug infusion, that is, intraarterial infusion, has the advantage over perfusion of simplicity (the catheter is percutaneously placed) and of repeat administration of several courses. Its disadvantage lies in low drug concentrations in the tissues of the infused area and lower response rates than those achieved by perfusion. The technique of tourniquet infusion achieves as high drug concentrations in the tissues as perfusion,[40] and an objective response rate of 67% has been noted,[41] but in the current state of development of this technique, drug concentrations are not as homogeneous as in perfusion. Certainly further clinical work using the newer agents with this technique is needed.

## THERAPEUTIC NODE DISSECTIONS

When the regional nodes become palpable in the follow-up period and the metastatic work-up remains negative, a therapeutic node dissection is indicated. Given the absence of infection in the regional area that may account for a reactive, hyperplastic enlargement of the regional nodes, palpability of recent onset in the regional nodal basin of a patient with a history of melanoma usually signifies neoplastic involvement by the tumor. On clinical examination, a hyperplastic node retains its fusiform shape and is flat and soft, whereas a tumor-involved node tends to be more spherical and firm. Often one can make the differentiation on clinical grounds and proceed with node dissection when the palpable node is suspicious. Under these circumstances, the clinical diagnosis will be correct in over 90% of the patients. With nodal enlargement, which is clinically dubious, particularly in the area of the groin (with the risk of lymphedema after groin dissection), it may be prudent to proceed with needle aspiration of the node and, if negative, with an excisional biopsy. When the latter method is used, the biopsy incision should be made in the line of the routine lymphadenectomy incision. When the biopsy is positive, the puncture site or biopsy incision is encompassed by an elliptical incision which allows the en-bloc resection of the biopsy track and the underlying lymph nodes.

GROIN DISSECTION. In the case of the groin, when the inguinal nodes are palpable, there is about 40% chance that the deep nodes (iliac and/or obturator) will also be involved.[42,43] When the inguinal nodes are only microscopically involved, the chance of involvement of the deep nodes drops to 20%.[43] Some workers believe that if the deep nodes are involved, this amounts to distant dissemination of the disease. Several articles support this notion, given 5-year survival rates of 0% to 9% following ilioinguinal dissection with findings of involved deep nodes.[44–47] Patients with clinical involvement of the inguinal nodes, but with negative deep nodes, may be expected to have a 5-year survival rate of about 50%.[43] However, patients with involvement of the inguinal as well as the deep nodes in our series have a 5-year survival rate of about 30% and a 10-year survival rate of about 20%.[48] It appears, therefore, that an appreciable percentage of patients with involvement of the deep nodes may enjoy a long-term survival after a complete ilioinguinal dissection, including the inguinal, iliac, and obturator nodes, preferably

in continuity with division of the inguinal ligament for improved exposure. Some workers, in an effort to limit the procedure to a superficial groin dissection, have used biopsy of Cloquet's node as an indicator of the positivity of the deep nodes.[49] If this node situated at the femoral ring is negative on biopsy, it suggests that the deep nodes also are negative, whereas if it is positive, a high likelihood of involvement of the deep nodes is suggested. At any rate, if one performs a superficial groin dissection for clinically involved inguinal nodes, the program of follow-up should include a periodic computed tomographic (CAT) scan of the pelvis.

Immediate postoperative complications following groin dissection are as follows:

1. Skin edge necrosis, which should occur rarely if one is careful to avoid excessively thin flaps; the flaps should be made 2 to 3 mm thick for 3 to 4 cm from the skin incision and then progressively thicker as the base of the flaps is approached with care to avoid dissection of the flaps beyond the recommended boundaries.
2. Wound infection, occurring in 20% of the patients, often in the form of cellulitis, which responds quickly to intravenous antibiotics, usually antistaphylococcal agents.
3. Lymphocele following removal of the suction drains, which is treated with periodic aspiration in the clinic until it ceases to reaccumulate. For lymphoceles persistently recurring after 2 weeks of such management, a Penrose drain may be inserted in the dependent portion of the lymphocele and left in place until the drainage ceases, which may require 1 to 3 weeks.

In patients having ilioinguinal dissection with division of the inguinal ligament, the theoretic risk of an incisional hernia arises. However, this risk appears to be negligible, that is, less than 1%, if one repairs the inguinal ligament and sutures it lateral to the vessels to the iliac fascia and medial to the vessels to Cooper's ligament (Figs. 7B-5 to 7B-7). The most significant long-term risk after groin dissection (superficial or radical) is the development of permanent lymphedema of the ipsilateral extremity. This occurs in 20%

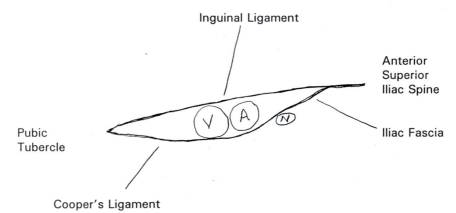

**FIGURE 7B-5.** Cross section at the level of the inguinal ligament shows the relationship between the inguinal ligament and Cooper's ligament medial to the vessels (V and A) and between the inguinal ligament and iliac fascia lateral to the vessels with the femoral nerve (N) posterior to the fascia.

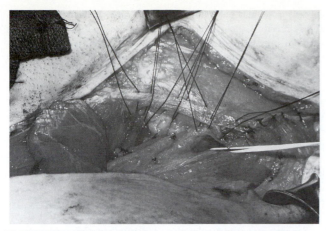

**FIGURE 7B-6.** Placement of sutures between the inguinal ligament and Cooper's ligament medial to the vessels and lateral portion of inguinal ligament and iliac fascia lateral to the vessels. The vessel loop is around the femoral nerve.

to 30% of the patients for the area below the knee, although nearly all patients have localized edema of the anteromedial thigh. Obviously, in the majority of patients, collateral lymphatic circulation around the posterior thigh-buttock and along the internal iliac vessels proves to be sufficient for the drainage of the distal part of the lower extremity.

Factors that may prevent or diminish the incidence or extent of lymphedema are as follows:

- Use of a longitudinal (rather than transverse) incision in the groin.
- Avoidance of excessively thin or wide flaps.
- Restriction of the procedure to a superficial rather than an ilioinguinal dissection.
- Avoidance of transverse incisions in the wide excision of the primary site, if the latter is localized in the lower extremity.
- Avoidance of wound infection in the groin.

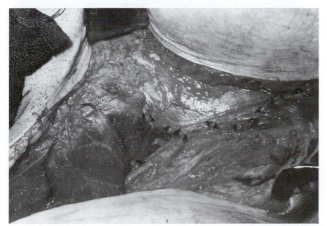

**FIGURE 7B-7.** The sutures have been tied, thus securely repairing the inguinal area following radical groin dissection.

- Elevation of the extremity at night, starting in the immediate postoperative period and for 2- to 3-half-hour intervals during the day, with continuation of this practice as a life-long routine.
- The use of custom-made elastic stocking.

For patients who develop frank lymphedema, daily treatment with sequential pneumatic compression stockings may be helpful.

AXILLARY DISSECTION. In the axilla, a transverse incision between the border of pectoralis major and that of latissimus dorsi is made at two fingerbreadths below the axillary fold. In melanoma, a complete node dissection to level III nodes is preferred. When dealing with palpable axillary nodes, there should be no hesitation to include in the dissection the lymph nodes and adipose tissue above the level of the axillary vein, thus exposing the brachial plexus, whose trunks become visible through their sheath, which is usually left intact. The axillary vein may be skeletonized by entering its sheath.

When the lymph nodes extend to the supraclavicular area, the dissection may be continued to include a supraclavicular node dissection, with removal of a segment of clavicle when necessary in order to remove completely and in continuity the axillary and supraclavicular nodes. When the axillary vein is involved by adjacent lymph nodes, it may be resected without replacement, particularly if its distal portion is involved. When the nodes are fixed, adjacent muscles such as the pectoralis major, latissimus dorsi, or serratus anterior may have to be resected. Despite the extensive involvement of the axilla in patients such as the above, 15% may attain a 5-year survival.[50] Although the majority of them succumb to their disease, palliation in terms of prolongation of survival or avoidance of symptomatic ulcerated growths in the nodal basin is achieved in the majority of patients.

Skin edge necrosis is extremely rare following axillary dissection. The wound infection rate is about 10%. Lymphoceles may be treated with aspiration and, if persistently recurring, with the insertion of a Penrose drain. Neurapraxia in the distribution of the musculocutaneous nerve, reversible within 3 weeks, may be observed if one fastens and leaves the extremity attached to an ether screen throughout the procedure. This complication should not occur if one leaves the extremity, prepped and draped with a stockinette, resting on an arm board. The extremity then is brought over the chest by the assistant for brief periods of time during the procedure, thus relaxing the pectoralis major as the apex of the axilla is dissected.

The incidence of lymphedema of the ipsilateral extremity following axillary dissection such as is done for melanoma is very low (about 2%).

Survival following axillary dissection is significantly better when the disease in the axilla is subclinical, as opposed to palpable, and diminishes further according to the degree of involvement.

POPLITEAL NODE DISSECTION. The popliteal nodes are infrequently involved by malignant melanoma. It appears that these nodes directly drain only a small area of skin in the upper portion of the calf, and that their filtering capacity and number of actual nodes is low, so that, in comparison with the inguinal nodes, they infrequently become involved. A rough estimate of the frequency of their clinical involvement in comparison with that of the inguinal nodes is about 1:20. When they become clinically involved, dissection of these nodes is indicated in the absence of detectable distant metastatic disease. The technique of popliteal dissection involves dissecting the tibial and common peroneal nerves and the popliteal vessels, thus allowing the removal of the popliteal nodes.[51] The concomitant presence of in-transit lesions or inguinal adenopathy suggests the additional removal of the in-transit lesions and groin dissection, since occasional patients with such involvement become cured.

Elective node dissection or SNB in the popliteal area may be indicated in patients in whom lymphoscintigraphy shows a definite uptake of the radioactive material, injected at the primary site, by these nodes.

NECK DISSECTION. Usually a modified radical neck dissection or a modification thereof is performed. For clinical involvement of these nodes, a radical neck dissection may be advisable. In SNB, intraoperative lymphatic mapping of the nodal group in the anterior or posterior neck triangle is further specified and localized by the preoperative lymphoscintigram and the transcutaneous detection of the point of highest radioactivity by applying the probe on successive areas of the skin immediately prior to making the skin incision, which is centered over that point.

Significant prognostic factors on multivariate analysis for patients with regional lymph node metastases are the number of tumor-containing lymph nodes (the strongest predictor of survival) and the thickness and site (extremity versus axial) of the primary lesion.[52]

## ADJUVANT THERAPY

Given the various prognostic parameters of malignant melanoma, of which the most prominent is the stage of the disease, it has been possible for at least the last 15 years to provide an accurate prognosis for each patient. As a result, numerous attempts have been made in the past to identify an effective adjuvant treatment for the high-risk groups. All these efforts have been largely negative, with the exception of a recently completed and reported prospective randomized study in which patients with primary lesions thicker than 4 mm or positive regional nodes were treated with interferon α2b or observation following the surgical treatment. Both the overall and disease-free survival rates were significantly better for the treated group as compared with the observation group in this study.[53] The 5-year improvement in disease-free survival was 12%. Interferon α2b became the standard adjuvant therapy for such patients. However, in a follow-up study there was again significant improvement in the disease-free survival for the interferon α2b group, but no significant difference in overall survival.[53a] A third study reaffirmed the beneficial effect of interferon α2b for both disease-free and overall survival for patients with IIB–III melanoma.[53b] Vaccine therapy is being actively evaluated at the present.

## TREATMENT OF STAGE IV DISEASE

In this stage, according to AJCC classification, patients with heavy involvement (large fixed or matted nodes) in the regional node basin are also included. However, patients with such metastases, particularly those with long disease-free intervals (exceeding 1 and prefer-

ably 2 years), may enjoy long tumor-free intervals after dissection and removal of such metastases and certainly all are palliated in terms of preventing tumor ulceration and bleeding from its surface or compression of the adjacent neurovascular bundle with its attendant symptomatology.

Some investigations consider involvement of two nodal basins as equivalent to hematogenous disease. In the absence of detectable visceral disease, dissection of both nodal basins as a way to forestall complications from the nodal basins and as a measure likely to prolong the patient's life is advised.

Prognostic factors in stage IV disease are the number of metastatic lesions (the smaller the better), their location (cutaneous and subcutaneous sites do better), stage of disease preceding distant metastases (stage I or II does better than stage III), and the prior disease-free interval (>18 months is better than ≤18 months).[52]

For patients with an isolated or small number of visceral metastasis, particularly those occurring after a disease-free interval of 1 year or longer, resection of the metastasis, particularly when this is not technically complicated, may be advisable, since about a 20% 5-year survival rate has been noted in several series.[54,55] This approach may become more applicable in the future since various biologic therapies are being developed that seem to be more effective in suppressing microscopic rather than bulky disease. If the patient's overall condition and prognosis permit this approach, palliative resection of a solitary brain metastasis, followed by radiation or resection of symptomatic gastrointestinal (GI) tract metastases causing symptoms of periodic intussusception (Fig. 7B-8) or GI bleeding, is indicated.[56,57]

## SYSTEMIC THERAPY

Chemotherapy of malignant melanoma historically has resulted in a modest overall response rate of about 20%.[58] The main drug has been dacarbazine (dimethyltriazenyl imidazole carboxamide, DTIC), which as a single agent causes tumor regression in about 20% of patients. Combinations of dacarbazine, with other drugs have not caused a substantial increase in the response rate, including

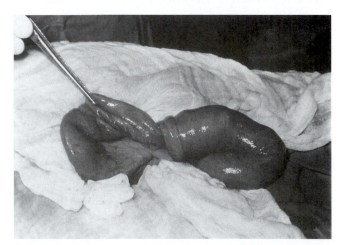

**FIGURE 7B-8.** Intussusception due to malignant melanoma metastatic to the small bowel.

the combination of dacarbazine, 1,3-bis-[2-chloroethyl]-1-nitrosourea (BCNU), cisplatin, and tamoxifen initially reported to produce overall response rates of about 46%.[59]

Biologic therapies, such as high doses of interleukin 2 (IL-2) or IL-2 with lymphokine-activated killer (LAK) cells, initially produced exciting results, with occasional, durable complete regressions. However, as they were studied more extensively, the overall response rate was found to be about 20%[58] and substantial toxicity was encountered. The combination of IL-2 with tumor-infiltrating lymphocytes resulted in objective response rates of about 35%.[58] Combinations of chemotherapy with biologic agents have also been employed with encouraging results.

Recently, considerable interest and effort has been focused on the development of tumor vaccines, both as a therapeutic and adjuvant modality in melanoma with promising initial results.[60] The full impact of such immunologic approaches, however, is not likely to materialize until further progress defines what may be the optimal methods of stimulating an effective immune response by the patient against the weak tumor-associated antigens.

## REFERENCES

1. RIGEL DS, CARUCCI JA: Malignant melanoma: Prevention, early detection, and treatment in the 21st century. CA Cancer J Clin 50:215, 2000.
2. PARKER SC et al: Cancer statistics, 1996. CA Cancer J Clin 46:7, 1996.
3. WALTER SD et al: The association of malignant melanoma with the use of sunbeds and sunlamps. Am J Epidemiol 131:232, 1990.
4. GRIN-JORGENSEN CM et al: The worldwide incidence of malignant melanoma, in Cutaneous Melanoma, 2d ed, CM Balch et al (eds). Philadelphia, Lippincott, 1992, pp 27–39.
5. CLARK WH Jr et al: Origin of familial malignant melanomas from heritable melanogetic lesions: "The B-K mole syndrome." Arch Dermatol 114:732, 1978.
6. ALBERT LS, SOBER AJ: The dysplastic nevus as precursor and marker of increased risk for melanoma, in Cutaneous Melanoma, 2d ed, CM Balch et al (eds). Philadelphia, Lippincott, 1992, pp 59–69.
7. ALBINO AP et al: Molecular biology of cutaneous malignant melanoma, in Cancer: Principles & Practice of Oncology, 5th ed, VT DeVita Jr, et al (eds). Philadelphia, Lippincott, 1977, pp 1935–1946.
8. SOBER AJ et al: Detection of "thin" primary melanomas. CA Cancer J Clin 33:160, 1983.
9. CLARK WH Jr et al: The histogenesis and biologic behavior of primary human malignant melanomas of the skin. Cancer Res 29:705, 1969.
10. BRESLOW A: Thickness, cross-sectional areas and depth of invasion in the prognosis of cutaneous melanoma. Ann Surg 172:901, 1970.
11. BALCH CM et al: A multifactorial analysis of melanoma: prognostic histopathologic features comparing Clark's and Breslow's staging methods. Ann Surg 188:732, 1978.
12. BALCH CM et al: Tumor thickness as a guide to surgical management of clinical stage I melanoma patients. Cancer 43:883, 1979.
13. BALCH CM et al: A comparison of prognostic factors and surgical results in 19,786 patients with localized (stage I) melanoma treatment in Alabama, USA, and New South Wales, Australia. Ann Surg 196:677, 1982.
14. KARAKOUSIS CP, DRISCOLL DL: Prognostic parameters in localized melanoma. Gender versus anatomical location. Eur J Cancer 31A:320, 1995.
15. SOONG S-J, WEISS HL: Predicting outcome in patients with localized melanoma, in Cutaneous Melanoma, 3rd ed. CM Balch et al (ed), St. Louis, Quality Medical Publishing, 1998, pp 51–61.
16. KETCHAM AS et al: Classification and staging, in Cutaneous Melanoma, 2d ed, CM Balch et al (eds). Philadelphia, Lippincott, 1992, pp 213–220.
17. KONSTADOULAKIS M et al: Survival of patients with stage IA malignant melanoma. Surg Oncol 4:101, 1995.
18. VERONESI U, CASCINELLI N: Narrow excision (1 cm margin): A safe procedure for thin cutaneous melanoma. Arch Surg 126:438, 1991.
19. BALCH CM et al: Efficacy of 2 cm surgical margins for intermediate-thickness melanomas (1 to 4 mm): Results of a multi-institutional randomized surgical trial. Ann Surg 218:262, 1993.
20. KARAKOUSIS CP et al: Local recurrence in malignant melanoma: Long-term results of the multi-institutional randomized surgical trial. Ann Surg Oncol 3:446, 1996.
21. LOPEZ R et al: Malignant melanoma with unknown primary site. J Surg Oncol 19:151, 1982.
22. KONSTADOULAKIS MM et al: Malignant melanoma of the anorectal region. J Surg Oncol 58:118, 1995.
23. SIM FH et al: A prospective randomized study of the efficacy of routine elective lymphadenectomy in management of malignant melanoma. Cancer 41:948, 1978.
24. VERONESI U et al: Inefficacy of immediate node dissection in stage I melanoma of the limbs. N Engl J Med 297:627, 1977.
24a. CASCINELLI N et al: Immediate or delayed dissection of regional nodes in patients with melanoma of the trunk. A randomized trial. Lancet 351:793–796, 1998.
25. BALCH CM et al: Elective lymph node dissection: Pros and cons, in Cutaneous Melanoma, 2d ed, CM Balch et al (eds). Philadelphia, Lippincott, 1992, pp 345–366.
26. MORTON DL et al: Technical details of intraoperative mapping for early stage melanoma. Arch Surg 127:392, 1992.
27. BALCH CM et al: Efficacy of an elective regional lymph node dissection of 1 to 4 mm thick melanomas for patients 60 years of age and younger. Ann Surg 224:255, 1996.
27a. BALCH CM et al: Long term results of a multi-institutional randomized trial comparing prognostic factors and surgical results for intermediate thickness melanomas (1.0 to 4.0 mm). Ann Surg Oncol 7:89, 2000.
28. KARAKOUSIS CP, GRIGOROPOULOS P: Sentinel node biopsy before and after wide excision of the primary melanoma. Annals of Surg Oncol 6:785–789, 1999.
29. NORMAN J et al: A redefinition of skin lymphatic drainage by lymphoscintigraphy for malignant melanoma. Am J Surg 162:432, 1991.
30. McCARTHY WH et al: Invited commentary. Arch Surg 130:659, 1995.
31. KRAG DN et al: Minimal access surgery for staging of malignant melanoma. Arch Surg 130:654, 1995.
32. MORTON DL, THOMPSON JF, ESSNER R, ELASHOFF R, et al: Validation of the accuracy of intraoperative lymphatic mapping and sentinel lymphadenectomy for early-stage melanoma. A multicenter trial. Annals of Surg 230:453–465, 1999.

33. Urist MM: Surgical management of primary cutaneous melanoma. CA Cancer J Clin 46:217, 1996.

34. Brown CD, Zetelli JA: The prognosis and treatment of true local cutaneous recurrent malignant melanoma. Dermatol Surg 21:285, 1995.

35. Drzewiecki KT, Andersson AP: Local melanoma recurrences in the scar after limited surgery for primary tumor. World J Surg 19:346, 1995.

36. Karakousis CP et al: Biologic behavior and treatment of in-transit metastasis of melanoma. Surg Gynecol Obstet 150:29, 1980.

37. Turnbull A et al: Recurrent melanoma of an extremity treated by major amputation. Arch Surg 106:496, 1973.

38. Morton DL et al: BCG immunotherapy of malignant melanoma: Summary of a 7 year experience. Ann Surg 180:635, 1976.

39. Lienard D et al: High dose of rTNF-$\alpha$ in combination with IFN-gamma and melphalan in isolated perfusion of the limbs for melanoma and sarcoma. J Clin Oncol 122:52, 1991.

40. Karakousis CP et al: Tourniquet infusion versus hyperthermic perfusion. Cancer 49:850, 1982.

41. Bland KI et al: A phase II study of the efficacy of di-amminedichloroplatinum (cisplatin) for the control of locally recurrent and in-transit malignant melanoma of the extremities using tourniquet outflow-occlusion techniques. Ann Surg 209:73, 1989.

42. Karakousis CP et al: Groin dissection in malignant melanoma. Am J Surg 152:491, 1986.

43. Karakousis CP et al: Survival after groin dissection for malignant melanoma. Surgery 109:119, 1991.

44. McCarthy JG et al: The role of groin dissection in the management of melanoma of the lower extremity. Ann Surg 179:156, 1974.

45. Coit DG, Brennan MF: Extent of lymph node dissection in melanoma of the trunk or lower extremity. Arch Surg 124:162, 1989.

46. Finck SJ et al: Results of ilioinguinal dissection for stage II melanoma. Ann Surg 196:180, 1982.

47. Fortner JG et al: Results of groin dissection for malignant melanoma in 220 patients. Surgery 55:485, 1964.

48. Karakousis CP, Driscoll DL: Positive deep nodes in the groin and survival in malignant melanoma. Am J Surg 171:421, 1996.

49. Coit DG: Extent of groin dissection for melanoma. Surg Oncol Clin North Am 1:271, 1992.

50. Karakousis CP et al: Axillary node dissection in malignant melanoma. Am J Surg 162:202, 1991.

51. Karakousis CP: The technique of popliteal lymph node dissection. Surg Gynecol Obstet 151:420, 1980.

52. Morton DL et al: Malignant melanoma, in Cancer Medicine, 4th ed, JF Holland et al (eds). Baltimore, Williams & Wilkins, 1997, pp 2467–2499.

53. Kirkwood JM et al: Interferon alfa-2b adjuvant therapy of high-risk resected cutaneous melanoma: The Eastern Cooperative Oncology Group Trial EST 1684. J Clin Oncol 14:7, 1996.

53a. Kirkwood JM et al: High- and low-dose interferon alfa-2b in high-risk melanoma: First analysis of intergroup trial E1690/S9111/C9190. J Clin Oncol 18:2444, 2000.

53b. Kirkwood JM, Ibrahim J, Sondak VK, Sosman JA, Ernstoff MS: Relapse-free and overall survival are significantly prolonged by high-dose IFN alpha 2b (HDI) compared to vaccine GM2-KLH with QS21 (GMK, Progenics) for high-risk resected stage IIB–III melanoma: Results of the Intergroup Phase II study E 1694/S9512/C503801. Annals of Oncol 11(Suppl 4): 4, 2000.

54. Karakousis CP et al: Metastasectomy in malignant melanoma. Surgery 115:295, 1994.

55. Wronom IL III et al: Surgery as palliative treatment for distant metastases of melanoma. Ann Surg 204:181, 1986.

56. Madajewicz S et al: Malignant melanoma brain metastases: Review of Roswell Park Memorial Institute experience. Cancer 53:2550, 1984.

57. Goodman PL, Karakousis CP: Symptomatic gastrointestinal metastases from malignant melanoma. Cancer 48:1058, 1981.

58. Del Prete SA et al: Combination chemotherapy with cisplatin, carmustine, dacarbazine and tamoxifen in malignant melanoma. Cancer Treat Rep 68:1403, 1984.

59. Rosenberg SA: Principles of cancer management: biologic therapy, in Cancer: Principles & Practice of Oncology, 5th ed, VT DeVita et al (eds). Philadelphia, Lippincott, 1997, pp 349–373.

60. Morton DL, Barth A: Vaccine therapy for malignant melanoma. CA Cancer J Clin 46:225, 1996.

# CHAPTER 8

# CANCERS OF THE HEAD AND NECK

*Joseph Espat, John F. Carew, and Jatin P. Shah*

## INTRODUCTION

Cancer of the head and neck is a relatively uncommon disease, representing less than 5% of all cancers in the United States and responsible for 21,500 cancer deaths in 1998[1] (Fig. 8-1). Head and neck cancer ranks as the sixth most common cancer worldwide, defining it as a major healthcare problem.[2]

The term "head and neck cancer" encompasses a wide spectrum of diseases with varied histology and site of origin, as well as diverse biologic behavior. However, more than 90% of these tumors are squamous cell carcinomas (SCC) arising from the mucosa of the upper aerodigestive tract (oral cavity, oropharynx, hypopharynx, and larynx).[3,4] The risk factors most implicated for the development of head and neck cancer are tobacco and alcohol use (Fig. 8-2). Alcohol potentiates tobacco-related carcinogenesis and is an independent risk factor.[5–9] There is a strong epidemiologic association between smokeless tobacco and oral carcinogenesis.[10,11] Despite the well-publicized risk factors and a concentrated effort to educate the public on the negative health risks associated with these behaviors, SCC continues to be a growing problem. In fact, a large portion of the population at risk fails to obtain early diagnosis, and, as such, many present with advanced-stage disease.

Occupational risk factors for the development of head and neck cancer have also been identified and include nickel refining, woodworking, and exposure to textile fibers.[12,13] Previous radiation exposure has also been implicated as a risk factor.[14] Carotenoid (contained in yellow to deep red-colored vegetables) may provide a protective role in that there is an inverse relationship between the consumption of fruits and vegetables and the incidence of head and neck cancer.[15–17] Thus, dietary habits also play a role in the etiology of SCC.

There is increasing evidence that viruses contribute to the development of head and neck cancer.[18–20] DNA from papillomavirus has been detected in malignant tissue from the head and neck. Furthermore, Epstein-Barr virus is closely associated with nasopharyngeal cancer (NPC), a cancer that is rare in the United States but is more common in Asian and North African countries.[20]

Genetic predisposition to head and neck cancers is suggested by its sporadic occurrence in young adults and in nonusers of tobacco and alcohol.[21] Mutagen-induced chromosomal fragility is an independent risk factor itself and correlates with the prospective development of second primary tumors.[22–25]

In this chapter, we discuss cancers of the head and neck arising in the upper aerodigestive tract, thus including tumors of the nasopharynx, oral cavity, oropharynx, larynx, and hypopharynx. Tumors of the salivary glands, which are divided into major and minor glands, are also presented. The role and recommended approach for neck dissection is also discussed. In addition, the roles for radiotherapy and chemotherapy as adjuvant or neoadjuvant treatment modalities are presented.

## TUMORS OF THE ORAL CAVITY, PHARYNX, AND LARYNX

### THE ORAL CAVITY

The oral cavity is the most common site of cancers in the head and neck.[1] As with other head and neck tumors, oral cavity tumors are predominantly SCCs that are usually related to tobacco and alcohol exposure.[5–9] It is estimated that oral cavity cancer will account for 30,200 new cases and 7,800 cancer related deaths in the United States in 2000.[26] The disease is the most prevalent in the fifth and sixth decades of life.

The most common sites within the oral cavity are the tongue and floor of mouth, sites that account for over half of all tumors in this

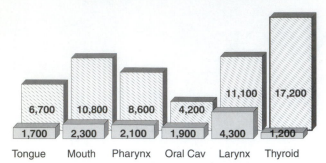

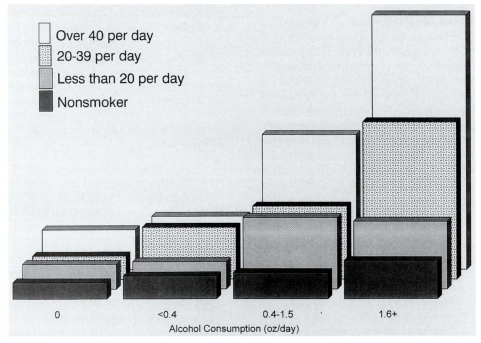

**FIGURE 8-1.** Incidence of new cases and deaths from cancers of the head and neck in the United States. (*Data adapted from American Cancer Society statistics, CA, January 1998.*)

region (Fig. 8-3). Within these sites, over 90% of tumors are SCCs, with the preponderance occurring in males. Tumors can also arise in other sites throughout the oral cavity, including the lips, upper or lower gingiva, buccal mucosa, retromolar trigone, and hard palate. While the majority of tumors in these sites are also SCCs, other tumor histologies can be seen that often reflect the make-up of the mucosa and soft tissue in that region. For example, minor salivary

gland tumors are commonly found on the hard palate, which has the greatest density of minor salivary glands in the upper aerodigestive tract. In addition, unique practices found in some parts of the world may alter the distribution of SCCs in the sites throughout the oral cavity. For example, chewing tobacco or betel nut increases the proportion of tumors seen in the buccal mucosa and retromolar trigone. The following section highlights the clinical presentation and management of tumors of the oral cavity. This is limited primarily to SCCs of the oral cavity and most often the tongue and floor of the mouth.

CLINICAL ASPECTS. The tongue and related structures of the oral cavity serve a vital function in both mastication and articulation. When these structures are involved with tumor, their respective functions are impaired. Hence, patients with oral cavity tumors will often present with complaints of difficulty eating and speaking. The most common signs and symptoms in patients with oral tongue lesions are localized pain (45%) and the presence of an ulcer (50%).[27] Patients also may present with an asymptomatic lesion that they or their dentist has noticed. Often, these are seen when patients brush their teeth or inspect their oral cavity. Because of the early symptoms and the relative accessibility for examination, over half of patients with oral cancer will present with early-stage disease. Sixty-five percent of patients present with stage I or II disease.

Several aspects of the physical examination are critical to the accurate assessment of oral cavity tumors. The first is the relationship of the tumor to the mandible. Initially, this can often be assessed during the history, since most patients with mandibular involvement

**FIGURE 8-2.** Relative risk of oropharyngeal cancer in relation to smoking and alcohol consumption. (*Data derived from Rothman K, Keller A: The effect of joint exposure to alcohol and tobacco on risk of cancer of the mouth and pharynx.* J Chronic Dis 25:711–716, 1972.)

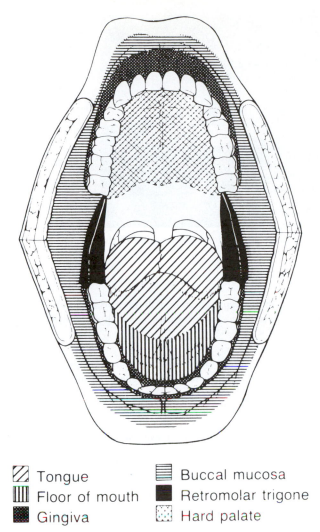

Tongue  Buccal mucosa
Floor of mouth  Retromolar trigone
Gingiva  Hard palate

**FIGURE 8-3.** Anatomic sites for primary cancers in the oral cavity.

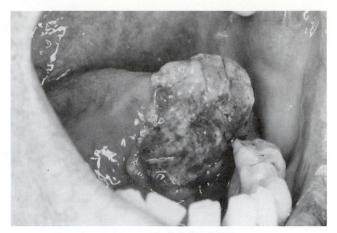

**FIGURE 8-4.** Exophytic carcinoma of the oral tongue.

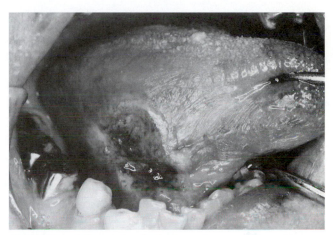

**FIGURE 8-5.** Ulcerated endophytic carcinoma of the oral tongue.

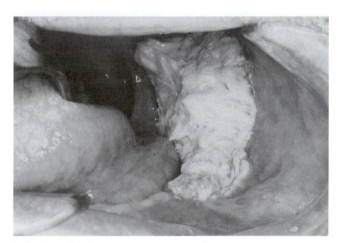

**FIGURE 8-6.** Verrucous carcinoma of the lower gum.

experience pain and difficulty with mastication. On physical examination, the proximity of the lesion to the mandible and the mobility of the tumor over the mandible should be noted. Palpation of the lesion, including bimanual palpation when the lesion extends to the floor of mouth or elsewhere, is also a critical part of the examination of the oral cavity.

The clinical appearance of a lesion can often suggest the histologic diagnosis (Figs. 8-4 through 8-6). The most important aspect of the clinical appearance is whether it is a mucosal or submucosal lesion. The vast majority of SCCs are mucosal. In contrast, submucosal masses may result from a vast array of histologies, including minor salivary gland tumors and soft tissue tumors.

Several ominous signs can be seen in patients presenting with advanced oral cavity tumors: (1) The first is trismus, which suggests that the pterygoid, temporalis, or masseter muscles are involved. (2) The second ominous sign is reduced tongue mobility, which suggests involvement of the deep musculature of the tongue or the hypoglossal nerve. (3) Finally, if the tumors display a deeply

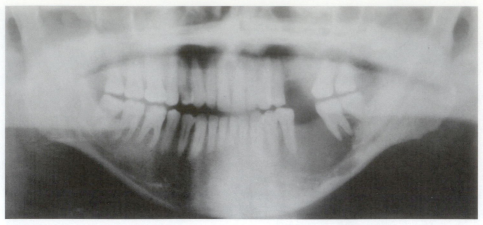

**FIGURE 8-7.** Panoramic x-ray of the mandible showing bone destruction with invasion of the inferior alveolar canal by cancer of the lower gum.

infiltrative pattern of growth rather than an exophytic pattern, survival usually is poor.

Patients with SCC of the upper aerodigestive tract have a high rate of both synchronous and metachronous multiple primary cancers. For this reason, any patient found to have a SCC of the oral cavity should have a complete head and neck examination. Likewise, a high index of suspicion is warranted in a patient with a history of previous SCC of the upper aerodigestive tract who has complaints originating in the oral cavity or upper aerodigestive tract.

A radiologic evaluation should be performed in a patient with an oral cavity tumor that is in close proximity to, abuts, or is fixed to the mandible. The initial and most simple test is the panoramic x-ray (Panorex) (Fig. 8-7). This film provides information regarding the entire mandible but is limited in its ability to evaluate the symphysis and lingual cortex. If a lesion is close to these areas, the Panorex may be supplemented with dental occlusal films and intraoral dental x-rays. CT scanning of the mandible can be used in selected cases where the Panorex and dental films are inadequate (Figs. 8-8, 8-9).

A cross-sectional representation of the entire mandible may be seen using a software package, Dentascan, which reconstructs the CT image (Fig. 8-10).

MANAGEMENT. The initial step in treating any tumor of the oral cavity is obtaining a histologic diagnosis. As mentioned earlier in this chapter, the majority of tumors will turn out to be SCCs. An incisional biopsy at the periphery of the lesion, where tumor meets grossly normal appearing mucosa, will usually render the diagnosis. Occasionally, in lesions with extensive keratinization or verrucous forms of SCC, on a superficial biopsy, the histologic diagnosis may be difficult, and thus deep biopsies must be taken. Submucosal masses also may prove difficult to diagnose, unless deep biopsies are taken with samples of representative tissue from the center of the lesion. If a lesion is clinically suspicious, biopsies should be repeated until an accurate diagnosis is made. Even when adequate tissue is obtained, the histologic distinction between benign and malignant may be difficult in some tumors. One example is pseudoepitheliomatous

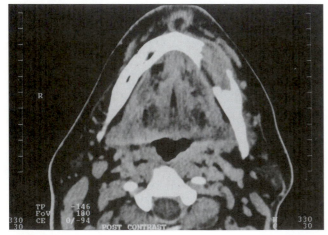

**FIGURE 8-8.** Axial view of a CT scan of the oral cavity (soft tissue window) showing invasion of the mandible.

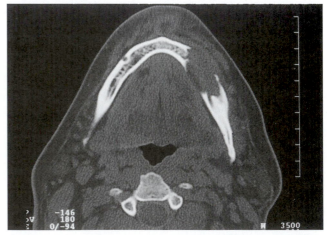

**FIGURE 8-9.** Axial view of the CT scan of the oral cavity (bone window) showing the extent of bone destruction of the mandible.

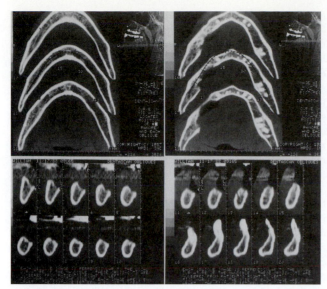

**FIGURE 8-10.** A Dentascan showing multiple sections of the axial view of a mandible showing bone invasion by a cancer of the lower gum.

**TABLE 8-1.** AJCC/UICC* STAGING OF ORAL CAVITY TUMORS

| PRIMARY | NECK |
|---------|------|
| Tis: Carcinoma in situ | |
| T1: Tumor <2 cm | N0: No clinically palpable nodes |
| T2: Tumor >2 cm <4 cm | N1: Single ipsilateral node <3 cm |
| T3: Tumor >4 cm | N2a: Single ipsilateral node 3–6 cm |
| T4: Tumor invades adjacent | N2b: Multiple ipsilateral nodes <6 cm |
| structures (e.g., through | N2c: Bilateral or contralateral |
| cortical bone, into deep | nodes <6 cm |
| extrinsic muscle, skin) | |
| | N3: Node >6 cm |

**DISTANT METASTASIS**

| MX | Distant metastasis cannot be assessed |
|----|---------------------------------------|
| M0 | No distant metastasis |
| M1 | Distant metastasis |

**STAGE GROUPING**

| Stage 0 | Tis | N0 | M0 |
|---------|-----|----|----|
| Stage I | T1 | N0 | M0 |
| Stage II | T2 | N0 | M0 |
| Stage III | T3 | N0 | M0 |
| | T1 | N1 | M0 |
| | T2 | N1 | M0 |
| | T3 | N1 | M0 |
| Stage IVA | T4 | N0 | M0 |
| | T4 | N1 | M0 |
| | Any T | N2 | M0 |
| Stage IVB | Any T | N3 | M0 |
| Stage IVC | Any T | Any N | M1 |

*Union Internationale Contre le Cancer (International Union Against Cancer).

hyperplasia, in which squamous cells can be seen extending down into the minor salivary glands, which may be difficult to distinguish from invasive carcinoma.

Once histologic diagnosis is confirmed, and the patient is properly staged, the treatment can be planned. Staging oral cavity tumors is relatively simple. The current American Joint Committee on Cancer (AJCC) staging is shown in Table 8-1. As mentioned earlier, over half of the patients with oral cavity tumors present with early-stage disease. In this cohort of patients, single modality therapy in the form of surgery or radiation therapy will yield favorable results, provided there is no evidence of neck disease. The choice between these two modalities depends on multiple factors related to the patient and tumor. If a patient has significant medical comorbidities precluding an operative approach, external beam radiation therapy offers a good treatment option. However, radiation therapy for primary tumors in the oral cavity results in significant xerostomia along with a risk of osteoradionecrosis of the mandible. For this reason, if a patient is a surgical candidate and the planned resection is not expected to result in a significant aesthetic or functional defect, surgery is the treatment of choice. Currently at the author's institution fewer than 10% of patients are treated with definitive radiation alone for oral tongue lesions.[27–30] If radiation therapy is utilized as the primary treatment modality, brachytherapy may be added to improve local control of more advanced primaries. The majority of oral tongue tumors can be resected by an approach through the open mouth. For lesions more posterior in the oral cavity, a variety of surgical approaches are available to achieve greater access (Fig. 8-11).

For advanced-stage lesions, multidisciplinary treatment in the form of surgery and external beam irradiation is the optimal therapy. However, with bulky primary lesions, a significant aesthetic and functional deficit may result. In the past two decades, free tissue transfer has greatly improved our ability to reconstruct these defects. However, the functional results are at times suboptimal. Realizing

this, if a patient has advanced-stage disease and a large primary tumor that would require an operation resulting in significant functional morbidity, consideration should be given to a nonsurgical treatment option of combined chemotherapy and radiation therapy. Treatment results of concurrent chemotherapy with radiation therapy for advanced-stage oral cavity tumors have been reported in only a limited number of patients.[31] In this report, 86% of patients had a complete clinical response and 2-year survival was 71%. However, in this study, only eight patients had primary tumors in the oral cavity. With the limited number of patients in preliminary studies and the lack of randomized prospective trials, this treatment paradigm for advanced-stage oral cavity tumors remains investigational. It should be realized, however, that patients opting for this nonsurgical treatment approach for advanced-stage oral cavity tumors may experience significant treatment-related morbidity with regard to deglutition and speech. An organ-preserving approach to chemotherapy and radiation therapy may not necessarily be a function-preserving approach.

A critical aspect of treating oral cavity cancer is the management of the mandible. The clinical assessment of the relationship of the tumor to the mandible, with regard to its proximity and fixation to the

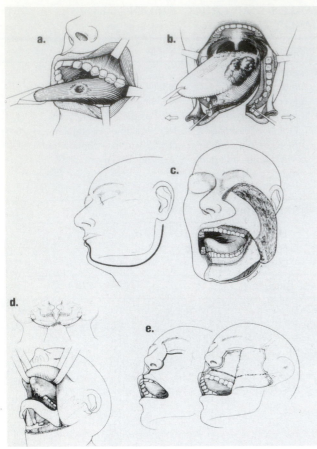

**FIGURE 8-11.** Surgical approaches for oral cancer. *A.* Oral approach; *B.* mandibulotomy approach; *C.* lower cheek flap approach; *D.* visor flap approach; *E.* upper cheek flap (Weber-Ferguson incision) approach.

mandible, yields the majority of the needed information. Additional information, however, can sometimes be gleaned from radiographic studies, including Panorex films, dental films, CT scan, and Dentascans. The necessity of mandibular resection depends in part on the site of the primary tumor. Mandibulectomy is seldom required for oral tongue lesions (1.6% of cases) but is often required for gum lesions (93% of cases).[28,30] Mandibular resection is primarily determined, however, by the relationship of the tumor to the mandible. The extent of the mandibulectomy is dictated by the depth of bone invasion. If a tumor abuts the mandible with minimal involvement of the periosteum or cortical bone, a marginal mandibulectomy, in which the continuity of the jaw is preserved, can be performed. Pathologic examination of the non-irradiated mandible has demonstrated that SCC usually invades through the occlusal surfaces, thus giving a rationale for the conservative marginal resection of the mandible that preserves continuity.[32] This has obvious functional and aesthetic advantages. In mandibles that have been previously irradiated, the pattern of invasion is less predictable and warrants a segemental resection.[33] For larger tumors with more extensive bone invasion, a segmental mandibulectomy is needed to provide an

oncologically sound resection. Recent dental extraction at the site of the tumor opens a portal for tumor spread into the mandible and thus usually requires a segmental mandibulectomy. When the tumor has invaded deeply into the mandible, such that it involves the inferior alveolar canal, an aggressive mandibulectomy from the entry of the inferior alveolar nerve to the mental foramen should be performed to minimize local recurrence. With the advent of microsurgical reconstruction over the past two decades, free tissue transfer of osseocutaneous grafts now provides excellent aesthetic reconstruction of these segmental mandible defects. These patients, however, require aggressive rehabilitation postoperatively to minimize functional deficits in speech and deglutition.

A key member of the multidisciplinary team taking care of patients with tumors of the oral cavity is the dentist. Often, the dentist is the first person to notice and identify a suspicious lesion. Preoperatively, dental films and Panorex films aid in the evaluation of oral cavity tumors. In additional, preoperative dental treatment and counseling can minimize the sequelae of adjuvant postoperative radiation therapy. Finally, the dentist is critical to the proper fitting of any dental appliance or prosthesis for oral rehabilitation.

**CERVICAL LYMPH NODES IN ORAL CANCER.** The risk of occult metastasis is relatively high for most primary tumors in the oral cavity. For this reason, all but the earliest lesions should have elective treatment of the neck in the form of external beam radiation or supraomohyoid neck dissection. The risk of occult metastasis from an oral tongue or floor-of-mouth lesion is directly related to the thickness of the primary tumor and increases significantly in lesions greater than 2 mm thick.[30] This information can be used preoperatively to determine which patients have the highest risk of harboring occult neck disease and may benefit from elective neck dissection. In addition to the risk of regional lymph node metastasis, survival has also been shown to be related to tumor thickness.[30] When possible, only one treatment modality should be used; thus if the primary tumor is treated surgically, then the neck should be treated surgically. Likewise, if the primary tumor is being treated with definitive radiation therapy, then the clinically negative neck that has a significant risk of occult metastasis should also be treated electively with external beam irradiation. When a neck at risk for occult lymph node metastasis is treated electively with radiation therapy, regional control rates exceeding 90% are claimed.[34] It should be noted, however, that only about 30% of these necks actually harbor occult microscopic disease and thus regional control in pathologically positive necks is less than 90%. In contrast, if the primary tumor is treated surgically, the neck should be treated surgically. It has been shown that levels I, II, and III lymph nodes are at greatest risk for occult metastasis from oral cavity primaries.[35,36] A supraomohyoid neck dissection, which encompasses levels I to III, therefore is an adequate oncologic procedure for elective treatment of the neck. In patients undergoing elective supraomohyoid neck dissection, approximately 24% to 31% will have histologic evidence of lymph node metastasis.[37,38] In these patients with pathologically node-positive necks, regional failure is observed in 7% to 15% of patients. Adjuvant postoperative radiation therapy is given to these patients if there is evidence of extracapsular spread or multiple positive nodes.

In patients with clinical evidence of cervical lymph node metastasis, a therapeutic neck dissection that includes levels I to V in the neck is performed. Usually, a therapeutic neck dissection for SCC is a modified but comprehensive neck dissection that includes levels I to V, the internal jugular vein, and the sternocleidomastoid muscle but, when oncologically feasible, spares the spinal accessory nerve. Again, adjuvant radiation therapy is given if there is evidence of extracapsular spread or multiple pathologically positive nodes.

At our institution, over 90% of patients with early-stage SCC of the oral cavity are treated with surgery alone. Utilizing this approach, 5-year determinate survival for early-stage disease (stages I and II) was 77% to 88%.[27,29] Advanced-stage disease was treated using a combination of surgery with adjuvant postoperative radiation radiotherapy, with a 5-year determinate survival of 24% to 34% for stage IV disease.[27–29]

**ADJUVANT RADIATION THERAPY.** The indications for adjuvant radiation therapy for SCC of the oral cavity include the following: (1) invasion of muscle, bone, and skin; (2) perineural invasion; (3) gross residual tumor after surgical resection; (4) residual microscopic tumor or positive margins; (5) advanced-stage disease; (6) regional lymph node metastasis, and (7) evidence of extracapsular spread in lymph node metastasis. When adjuvant radiation therapy was used in patients with stage III and IV oral tongue tumors, local regional control increased from 57% to 71%.[27] In addition, in patients with oral cavity and oropharynx primary tumors, with close or positive surgical margins, the use of postoperative radiation therapy at a dose greater than or equal to 60 Gy yielded local control rates exceeding 90%.[39] The oral tongue, however, was the worst subsite in this study, with only one-half of patients achieving locoregional control when adjuvant radiation therapy was given in the setting of positive margins.[39]

**SECOND PRIMARY TUMORS.** Patients with SCC of the oral cavity who have a high incidence of tobacco and alcohol use are at risk for developing second primary tumors. Nearly one-quarter of patients with oral tongue tumors followed for a minimum of 5 years, developed second primary tumors.[27] Three-quarters occurred metachronously, with almost 60% arising in the head and neck and just over 10% arising in the lungs. Therefore, patients with oral cavity tumors require lifelong surveillance following treatment. In addition, cessation of tobacco and alcohol use will reduce the risk of developing a second primary.[40]

## THE NASOPHARYNX

Although malignancies of the nasopharynx are comprised predominantly of tumors arising from the epithelium (as with other sites in the upper aerodigestive tract), they have several unique characteristics. This includes their clinical presentation, histologic subtypes, treatment response, and surgical treatment. These defining characteristics of nasopharyngeal carcinoma (NPC) are presented in this section.

**DEMOGRAPHICS.** NPC occurs in two forms: the endemic variety found in southern China and the nonendemic variety found in the other parts of the world including the United States. These two forms differ in their predominant histologic type, etiology, and clinical behavior. The endemic form has the highest incidence, which approaches 50 per 100,000 population, in the Guangdong province in southern China.[41] Histologically, according to the World Health Organization (WHO), NPC is classified into three types. WHO type 1 is keratinizing SCC, which is similar in appearance to SCC in other sites throughout the upper aerodigestive tract. This type occurs in 25% to 50% of patients in the United States and fewer than 5% in endemic areas.[41,42] WHO type 1 carries the worst prognosis. The other two types of NPC, WHO type 2 (transitional cell) and WHO type 3 (undifferentiated), are nonkeratinizing and represent less differentiated forms of NPC. These undifferentiated forms, WHO types 2 and 3, are more common in the endemic regions.

There is epidemiologic as well as laboratory data that suggest that the high rate of NPC in the endemic area is related to dietary, genetic, and viral factors. In the endemic regions, a major component of the diet is smoked fish. High levels of the known class of carcinogen, nitrosamines, are found within smoked fish. In these endemic regions, the high rate of NPC has been associated with intake of salted fish.[43] People who have moved from these endemic areas and have changed their diet have a partially lowered risk of NPC, but this does not decrease to the level seen in the nonendemic areas.[44] This partial decrease in risk suggests that there are both dietary as well as genetic factors contributing to the development of NPC. This is further supported by the epidemiologic data showing that subsequent generations of emigrants from the endemic areas retain a portion of their increased risk, despite the adoption of a western diet.[44] In addition, familial clustering and association with certain human leukocyte antigens has been observed and further supports the genetic link in NPC.[45]

There has also been an association between the Epstein-Barr virus (EBV) and NPC. A high prevalance of elevated titers of EBV early antigen and viral capsid antigen has been found in the patients who developed NPC. More recently, advances in molecular techniques and use of polymerase chain reaction have shown a high rate of EBV DNA detection within the NPC tumor cells. The EBV genome is the same in each NPC tumor cell of a single patient, suggesting a clonal process.[46] Other studies have demonstrated the presence of EBV DNA in pre-neoplastic lesions, such as severe dysplasia and carcinoma in situ, thus suggesting that the EBV enters the tumor cells early in the transformation process.[47] Further investigations have shown that the EBV DNA usually does not incoporate into the host cell DNA and thus is episomal.[48] The rate of EBV DNA detection was 100% in WHO types 2 and 3, but only 14% in WHO type 1 NPC, in one study.[49] In another study, however, EBV DNA was found in all NPC tumors, even in nonendemic populations.[50] The role of EBV in the nonendemic form of NPC is thus uncertain. Aside from the viral data, the development of WHO type 1 NPC has also been linked to tobacco usage.[51,52]

Anti-EBV serology has been used as a tool for screening patients for NPC in endemic regions. In one study, anti-EBV viral capsid antigen IgA was used to screen over 42,000 patients in an endemic region. Of the 2800 with an elevated EBV viral capsid antigen titer, between 3% and 5% were found to develop NPC over a 2-year period.[53] The incidence of NPC was highest in the middle-aged male patients, suggesting that this population may be the best suited for EBV serologic screening in endemic regions. As with other tumors of the upper aerodigestive tract, a male predominance, with a male to

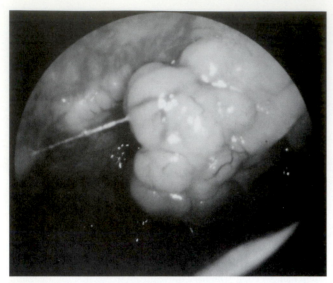

**FIGURE 8-12.** Endoscopic view of a cancer of the nasopharynx.

female ratio of 3:1, is seen in NPC. In the endemic regions, the mean age of patients with NPC is lower (40 to 50 years of age) than in the patients in nonendemic regions. In addition, a bimodal age incidence has been seen, with a significant peak in the young adult age group.[54]

**CLINICAL PRESENTATION.** NPC arises most commonly from the fossa of Rosenmüller, which is located along the posterolateral wall of the nasopharynx, just above the orifice of the eustachian tube (Fig. 8-12). Tumor growth in this region leads to symptoms of a sensation of ear fullness, unilateral serous otitis media, conductive hearing loss, otalgia, nasal obstruction, hyposmia, and epistaxis. With more advanced disease, cranial nerve deficits may develop and are found in 15% to 20% of patients at presentation.[41] Cranial nerves V and VI are most commonly involved. However, the most common symptom experienced by a patient with a NPC is a neck mass. This highlights both the difficuly in diagnosing these indolent tumors as well as the propensity for early lymph node metastasis. In a series of over 5000 patients with NPC, regional lymph node involvement was found in over 90% of patients at presentation.[55] Whenever a patient presents with nodal metastasis in the high posterior triangle from an unknown primary tumor, consideration should be given to the possibility of a nasopharyngeal primary tumor. In addition, an adult with a persistent unilateral otitis media with effusion should have a careful examination of the nasopharynx.

With improvement of diagnostic tools, such as the fiberoptic and rigid nasal endoscopes, previous difficulties in visualizing the nasopharynx have now been overcome. Despite the excellent view of the nasopharynx afforded by nasal endoscopes, NPC continues to ocassionally be difficult to diagnose, even with adequate visualization. For this reason, NPC may account for a proportion of patients presenting with neck metastasis from an unknown primary source. Often, these neck metastases are bulky and high in the posterior triangle of the neck. In the vast majority of cases of NPC, however, there will be evidence of a tumor mass or ulceration in the nasopharynx that is easily seen on nasal endoscopy.

The rate of distant metastasis at time of presentation in patients with NPC is higher than in patients with epithelial tumors at other sites in the head and neck. In a prospective study evaluating the rate of distant metastasis in patients with N3 disease, subclinical evidence of distant metastsis was seen in 40% of patients.[56] However, this study involved an aggressive work-up for distant metastases that included a bone marrow biopsy.

**RADIOGRAPHIC EVALUATION.** Although the extent of nasopharyngeal disease is often apparent from the history and physical examination, current radiographic techniques, including high-resolution computed tomography (CT) and magnetic resonance imaging (MRI), offer invaluable information regarding extension into the paranasopharyngeal region and skull base. Not only does this have prognostic significance, but it also allows sophisticated conformal, multiplanar image-based treatment planning, which maximizes locoregional control while minimizing the sequelae of external beam irradiation. Interestingly, by allowing a more precise mapping of the planned treatment volume, the increased accuracy of radiographic assessment has indirectly led to an improvement in survival in patients with NPC.[57]

**STAGING.** The staging of patients with NPC has been the subject of controversy. This is in part due to the disparate forms of this tumor seen in endemic and nonendemic regions. In addition, in large studies in endemic regions, factors that have been shown to be related to prognosis, such as disease in the supraclavicular region, were not incorporated into the AJCC system until the most recent edition of the staging manual.[58] The current AJCC/UICC staging system for NPC, shown in Table 8-2, reflects the incorporation of factors such as the significance of disease low in the neck.

**TABLE 8-2.** AJCC/UICC STAGING OF NASOPHARYNGEAL CARCINOMA

| PRIMARY | NECK |
|---|---|
| T1: Tumor confined to the nasopharynx. | N0. No regional lymph node metastasis. |
| T2: Tumor extends to the soft tissues of the oropharynx and/or nasal fossa. | N1: Unilateral lymph node metastasis <6 cm and above supraclavicular fossa. |
| T2A: (−) Parapharyngeal extension. | N2: Bilateral lymph node metastasis <6 cm and above supraclavicular fossa. |
| T2A: (+) Parapharyngeal extension. | N3A: Lymph node metastasis >6 cm. |
| T3: Tumor invades bony structures and/or paranasal sinuses. | N3A: Lymph node metastasis in supraclavicular fossa. |
| T4: Intracranial extension and/or involvement of cranial nerves, infratemporal fossa, hypopharynx, or orbit. | |

**PROGNOSTIC FACTORS.** Survival in patients with NPC is related to patient factors, primary tumor factors, and regional lymph node factors. With regard to patient factors, females and younger patients tend to have a better prognosis.[59] Several tumor factors, including histology, size, and local extension, affect survival. Patients with WHO types 2 and 3 histologies have a significantly higher 5-year survival rate (60% to 70%) compared to patients with WHO type 1, keratinizing SCC (20% 5-year survival).[60,61] Not surprisingly, bulkier tumors with cranial nerve involvement or intracranial extension have a poor outcome.[59,62]

The factor that has the most profound impact on survival, however, is the presence and characteristic of regional lymph node involvement. The mere presence of regional lymph node involvement, specifically nodal involvement that is bulky, low in the neck or fixed, is associated with a poor survival.[63]

**TREATMENT.** NPC is a relatively radiosensitive tumor and, for this reason, is usually treated by primary radiation therapy. CT scans and MRI allow sophisticated treatment plans compensating for paranasopharyngeal and retropharyngeal extension. The primary tumor and regional lymph nodes are included in the radiation portals. With conventional radiation therapy schedules, locoregional control rates range from 46% to 71% and 5-year survival ranges from 35% to 53%.[55,64–68] With advances in external beam radiation therapy delivery techniques, the results continue to improve.[69] Rates of distant failure in these series range from 24% to 60% and are significantly higher than in other tumors of the upper aerodigestive tract.[55,64–68]

The relatively high rate of distant metastasis and chemosensitivity of NPC has made it an ideal candidate for neoadjuvant and adjuvant chemotherapy. Recently, a prospective randomized study in the United States demonstrated an increase in survival in those patients with locoregionally advanced NPC who received neoadjuvant cisplatin-based chemotherapy with radiation therapy (80% 2-year survival) compared to those who received external beam radiation therapy alone (55% 2-year survival).[70] Other reports have also documented the benefits of neoadjuvant chemotherapy in locoregionally advanced NPC.[71–73]

As discussed earlier, approximately one-half of patients with NPC will fail locally or regionally. In most patients, a second course of radiation therapy is given, with reported survival ranging from 32% to 41% for recurrent T1 and T2 lesions.[74–76] Re-irradiation of the nasopharynx, however, can result in significant morbidity and therefore must be considered carefully. The other treatment option in patients with locoregionally recurrent NPC is surgical resection. The location of the nasopharynx at the central skull base combined with the proximity of both internal carotid arteries and a previously irradiated field makes this approach challenging. Nevertheless, in the highly select group of patients with resectable disease, surgery has yielded some long-term survivors.[77–80]

## THE LARYNX AND HYPOPHARYNX

As with other sites in the head and neck, over 90% of larynx and hypopharynx cancers are SCCs. The larynx is the second most common site within the head and neck, and it is estimated that larynx cancer will account for 10,100 new cases and 3,900 cancer-related deaths in the United States in 2000.[26]

**GENERAL CONSIDERATIONS.** The larynx can be subdivided into glottic, supraglottic, and subglottic anatomic regions (Fig. 8-13). SCCs of the larynx are found most commonly in the glottic larynx (56%), followed by the supraglottic larynx (31%) and rarely the subglottis (1%).[81] It is important to realize that tumors within these subsites have different clinical behaviors and risks of regional lymph node metastasis. Supraglottic tumors, for example, have a higher rate of occult and bilateral regional lymph node metastasis when compared to glottic primary tumors.[82,83] As a result, rates of regional failures for patients with supraglottic primary tumors are higher than those for patients with similarly staged glottic primary tumors.[81] Due to the high risk of regional dissemination, patients with supraglottic primary tumors have a worse 5-year disease-free survival rate when compared to patients with glottic primary tumors.[81]

The hypopharynx, which lies in close proximity to the larynx, includes the pyriform sinus, postcricoid region, and posterior pharyngeal wall. The vast majority of hypopharyngeal tumors occur in the pyriform sinus and are closely related to the larynx. Since many of the issues relevant to larynx cancer are also relevant to hypopharyngeal cancer, they are presented together here. Differences between hypopharynx cancer and larynx cancer are highlighted throughout this section. From the outset, however, it should be noted that patients with hypopharyngeal carcinomas have a worse prognosis and have a higher rate of regional metastasis than patients with laryngeal primary tumors. In addition, the surgical procedure required to resect most advanced hypopharyngeal tumors is a total laryngopharyngectomy and thus necessitates some form of reconstruction of the pharynx.

In addition to the site of origin of the primary, survival for patients with laryngeal and hypopharyngeal cancer is also affected by the stage of the disease. Patients with stage I or II laryngeal cancer have a 5-year disease-specific survival ranging from 78% to 91%, while those with stage III or IV disease have survivals ranging from 42% to 67%.[81] Patients with hypopharyngeal cancer have survival rates that are lower than those with laryngeal primary tumors. The percentage of patients presenting with advanced-stage disease is also greater with hypopharyngeal tumors since their symptoms are often insidious. Presently, the AJCC staging system for laryngeal and hypopharyngeal cancer is based on the local extent of the tumor (T stage) and the status of regional lymph nodes (N stage).[58] Although survival has been related to both T stage and N stage, it is most profoundly affected by the nodal status of the patient.[81,82,84] It has long been known that in head and neck cancer patients, regional lymph node involvement decreases survival by approximately 50%.[82,84] The present staging AJCC system groups both patients with locally advanced tumors (T3N0) and patients with regional lymph node metastasis (T1–3N1) together into stage III.[58] This may arbitrarily group two subsets of patients together who have a widely different prognosis. Therefore, when interpreting results from the treatment of larynx and hypopharynx cancer, both the stage and the nodal status must be considered.

**HISTORICAL REVIEW.** Treatment of cancer of the larynx and hypopharynx was initially limited by the inability to adequately

# Supraglottis

# Glottis

# Subglottis

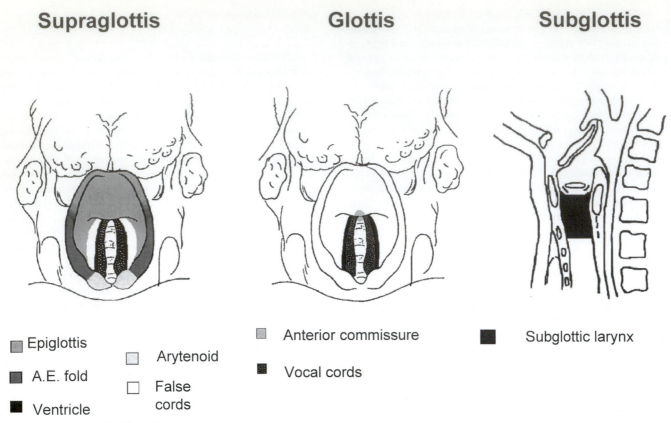

■ Epiglottis

■ A.E. fold

■ Ventricle

□ Arytenoid

□ False cords

□ Anterior commissure

▨ Vocal cords

■ Subglottic larynx

**FIGURE 8-13.** Anatomic regions and sites of the larynx.

examine this region. In mid-1800s, a singing teacher by the name of Manuel Garcia used a mirror to indirectly visualize his own vocal folds.[85] Later in the 1800s, Kirstein performed the first direct visualization of the endolarynx by direct laryngoscopy.[85] Tools used to visualize the interior of the larynx have evolved substantially over the past 100 years. Recently, the widespread use of the fiberoptic laryngoscope has allowed unparalleled visualization of the larynx and hypopharynx in the outpatient setting. In the operating room, the use of the 0°, 30° and 70° telescopes has also allowed improved visualization of areas that had been previously difficult to examine, such as the subglottis.

In the mid- and late 1800s, early attempts at curative treatment of laryngeal cancer were primarily directed at surgical approaches. Performed by Buck in 1851, the first surgical approach was a laryngofissure, in which the thyroid cartilage was split in the midline to gain access to the tumor.[85] Twenty-five years later, in 1876, Billroth performed the first total laryngectomy.[86] Several years later, Billroth also performed the first vertical partial laryngectomy. Late in the nineteenth century, Solis-Cohen described diverting the tracheal remnant to the skin, and Sorensen reported a single-stage pharyngeal closure.[85] Over the ensuing decades, the morbidity and mortality rates from these procedures fell as experience grew. In the early twentieth century, Gluck[87] and Sorenson reported 160 total

laryngectomies, with no mortalities in the last 63 consecutive cases. Surgery remained the mainstay of treatment of cancer of the larynx and hypopharynx until the 1920s, when Coutard advocated fractionated external beam radiation therapy as a definitive treatment modality.[88] The use of megavoltage radiation further improved results and led to its widespread application in the 1950s. From this time onward, external beam radiation therapy has remained an effective form of definitive treatment of early-stage laryngeal and hypopharyngeal cancer as well as an option for definitive or adjuvant treatment of advanced-stage cancer of the larynx and pharynx. During most of the mid-twentieth century, external beam radiation therapy was the primary modality of treatment of laryngeal cancer.

However, surgical approaches saw a resurgence in the second half of the twentieth century. Much of this could be attributed to an improved understanding of the predictability of local growth and spread of laryngeal tumors, as described by Kirchner in his whole-organ laryngeal sectioning studies.[89] This knowledge was applied in further refinements in partial laryngeal surgery as popularized by Alonzo and Ogura.[90–92] In the later half of the twentieth century, conservation laryngeal surgery reached its limits with the description of the near-total laryngectomy by Pearson[93] and the supracricoid subtotal laryngectomy by Laccourreye.[94]

Another approach to conservation surgery of the larynx evolved as a result of Jako's[95] popularization of the laser as a tool for laryngeal surgery. The laser has allowed resection of lesions through the laryngoscope while maintaining hemostasis. Surgeons are now able to resect T2 and T3 laryngeal tumors through an endoscopic approach using the laser, as reported by Steiner[96] and Zeitels and associates.[97]

Over the last century, attempts to improve the ability to speak after treatment of cancer of the larynx and hypopharynx have proceeded on two fronts. First, as described above, surgical techniques that spare as much of the larynx and hypopharynx as oncologically possible have evolved. Second, improved methods of voice rehabilitation following total laryngectomy have been exploited. With the most significant of these, popularized by Blom and Singer,[98] a fistula is created between the trachea and the esophagus. A small, duck-billed prosthesis is then placed in this fistula, which allows the production of lung-powered speech that is often quite satisfactory. Over the last decade, combined chemotherapy-radiotherapy treatment programs have allowed the preservation of the larynx in many patients with chemoresponsive tumors.

Despite the many advances in the treatment of larynx and hypopharynx cancers witnessed over the last century, survival in patients with advanced cancer of the larynx has improved little in the last 25 years.[1]

CLINICAL PRESENTATION. The majority of patients presenting with cancer of the larynx and hypopharynx have a history of prolonged tobacco and alcohol use. Males outnumber females, and the majority of patients present in their sixth and seventh decade. The most common presenting symptom for patients with tumors of the larynx is a change in voice. The vibratory characteristics of the epithelium of the vocal fold is disrupted early in the process of tumor invasion in patients with cancer of the glottic larynx. In addition, patients are very sensitive to changes in or loss of their voice. For these reasons, most patients with vocal cord cancer present with early-stage disease (Fig. 8-14). In contrast, symptoms related to supraglottic larynx and hypopharyngeal primaries, such as dysphagia, odynophagia, and otalgia, tend to occur late in the disease process. With this insidious tumor growth, a high percentage of patients present with advanced-stage disease (Fig. 8-15).

GOALS OF TREATMENT. Maximizing survival continues to be the ultimate goal in treating patients with advanced-stage laryngeal and hypopharyngeal cancer. Recently, however, due to the lack of improvement in survival, significant efforts have been made to improve the quality of life in these patients. Paramount to this is preservation of a functional larynx. Toward this goal, treatment options have been formulated with the hope of increasing laryngeal preservation while not sacrificing survival. Multimodality therapy, in the form of neoadjuvant chemotherapy, radiation therapy (RT), and surgical salvage, has emerged as a viable treatment option allowing anatomic preservation of the larynx without sacrificing survival.[99] Results from similar studies in patients with hypopharyngeal cancer have been less encouraging.[100–104] Nevertheless, in this cohort, chemotherapy and RT offer a useful treatment option.

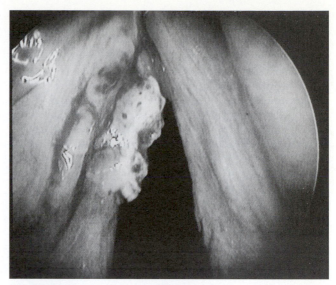

**FIGURE 8-14.** Carcinoma of the right true vocal cord.

Now that a method of laryngeal preservation has been established, future goals in treatment are directed at increasing the rates of both laryngeal preservation and survival.

TREATMENT OPTIONS. In the last two decades, the 5-year survival rate of patients with laryngeal and hypopharyngeal cancer has not changed dramatically.[1] In a recent study of 16,213 patients with laryngeal cancer, overall 5-year disease-specific survival was

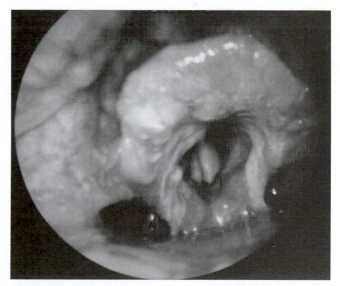

**FIGURE 8-15.** Carcinoma of the supraglottic larynx (arytenoepiglottic fold).

75%.[81] Of these patients, fewer than 40% presented with advanced-stage disease (stage III or IV).[81] With the majority of patients presenting with early-stage disease (stage I or II), high local control and survival is achieved with single modality therapy consisting of either external beam RT or surgery.[81,105] The debate as to the optimal treatment modality for early-stage larynx and hypopharynx cancer continues to evolve. Those in favor of using RT for early-stage larynx cancer argue that a superior voice quality is obtained after RT as compared to after surgery. Advocates of surgery claim similar voice results, with the possibility of better locoregional control.

Advanced-stage SCC of the larynx and hypopharynx requires multimodality therapy. Until the early 1980s, conventional treatment of advanced-stage laryngeal and hypopharyngeal cancer consisted of surgery and external beam RT. In the early 1980s, stimulated by several trials demonstrating a high rate of tumor response to chemotherapy in patients with SCC of the head and neck, treatment paradigms using induction chemotherapy followed by RT evolved.[106,107] The goal of these strategies was to develop a treatment program for laryngeal cancer that preserved laryngeal function while not adversely affecting survival. In the early 1990s, a prospective, randomized trial of patients treated at Veterans Affairs hospitals with stage III and stage IV SCC of the larynx, comparing conventional treatment of surgery and postoperative RT, with induction chemotherapy followed by RT was performed.[99] In this study, patients in the chemotherapy-RT arm who did not display at least a 50% response to induction chemotherapy, or who showed persistent or recurrent disease following RT, were salvaged with surgery. This landmark study demonstrated survival rates that were not statistically different between treatment arms (68% for both), but allowed 64% of patients within the chemotherapy-RT arm to preserve their larynx.[99] Therefore, the combination of chemotherapy and RT offers a treatment option for patients with advanced-stage laryngeal cancer.

Alternatively, surgical procedures emphasizing conservation can be used to treat carefully selected patients with cancer of the larynx. Oncologically, these conservation procedures are based on the study of the anatomic barriers and routes of tumor spread, which allow an en bloc tumor resection while preserving the function of the larynx. In selected patients, conservation surgical procedures can be employed for advanced-stage tumors, often in combination with adjuvant radiation therapy to improve locoregional control. Conservation surgical procedures continue to evolve and, in combination with postoperative RT, remain an effective form of treatment for selected patients with advanced-stage laryngeal ancer.

In patients with bulky laryngeal primary tumors or significant cartilage invasion, the efficacy of a combination of chemotherapy with radiation has yet to be established. The patients who have a high rate of locoregional recurrence may benefit from a surgical approach combined with adjuvant external beam RT.

In general, hypopharyngeal cancers, with their high rate of submucosal spread, are poor candidates for conservation surgical procedures. In selected patients, however, partial laryngopharyngectomy may be feasible. A significant number of patients, however, are not suitable candidates for laryngeal conservation procedures either because of oncologic concerns or patient factors such as inadequate pulmonary reserve. In these patients, the standard surgical treatment is a total laryngopharyngectomy, which leaves a significant pharyngeal defect. Reconstruction of these defects is challenging and often requires free tissue transfer with jejunum.

*CHEMOTHERAPY RT.* The combination of induction chemotherapy and RT has emerged as a treatment option that allows preservation of the larynx in nearly two-thirds of patients.[99] Despite the convincing results of this prospective randomized trial, many controversies exist regarding this study and its application to all patients with advanced-stage laryngeal cancer.

Detecting patients who fail to respond to induction chemotherapy or who display persistent or recurrent disease after RT, is critical to successful early surgical salvage. Often the post-treatment changes seen in the mucosa of the upper aerodigestive tract hamper the detection of persistent or recurrent disease. Once persistent or recurrent disease has been identified, early salvage surgery is the only curative option.

In a recent report encompassing 9334 patients with laryngeal cancer treated in the United States between 1990 and 1992, only 8.2% and 11% of patients with stage III and stage IV laryngeal cancer, respectively, were treated with the combination of chemotherapy and RT.[81] Although these patients were treated during the time that the Veterans Affairs Larynx Cancer Study Group (VALCSG) report was published, it illustrates the point that as recently as 5 years ago, only approximately 10% of patients with advanced-stage larynx cancer were treated with chemotherapy-RT. Currently, at the authors' institution, Memorial Sloan-Kettering Cancer Center, the vast majority of patients with advanced-stage laryngeal cancer who would require total laryngectomy if treated surgically and selected patients with hypopharyngeal cancer are being treated on a larynx-preserving protocol of chemotherapy and RT. It has become apparent that concurrent administration of chemotherapy and RT is superior to sequential treatment, although treatment-related toxicity is higher. Future directions and current studies in the multimodality treatment of larynx cancer include evaluating the benefit and role of chemotherapy in chemotherapy-RT protocols, patient selection, biologic markers predicting survival, and finally the continued efforts toward improving survival via innovative regimens, delivery systems, and novel therapeutic modalities. Overall, at this time, chemotherapy remains investigational in the treatment of cancer of the larynx and pharynx.

## HYPOPHARYNX AND EXTRALARYNGEAL SITES

With the encouraging results from the various trials using the combination of induction chemotherapy and RT for advanced laryngeal cancer, similar trials have been applied to other sites that, if treated conventionally, would require total laryngectomy. The majority of this work has been done in treating hypopharyngeal cancer. Hypopharyngeal, and most commonly pyriform sinus, tumors, have shown lower rates of larynx preservation (29% to 38%), locoregional control (39% to 60%) and survival (19% to 41%) in comparison to laryngeal primary tumors.[100–104] In the largest randomized prospective trial, equal survival rates were seen in the conventional surgical-RT arm when compared to the induction chemotherapy-RT arm, as reported by Lefebvre.[100] These results have been corroborated by results from retrospective studies.[100,104] However, a recent study demonstrated an improved 5-year survival rate in patients receiving induction chemotherapy, surgical resection, and postoperative RT (37%) when compared to patients receiving induction chemotherapy and RT (19%).[102] It should be noted, however, that the patients who did not respond to induction chemotherapy went on to definitive RT, rather than opting for early surgical salvage as in the VALCSG trial.[102] Controversy continues to exist regarding the optimal treatment of hypopharyngeal cancer, and improvements in locoregional control and survival are awaited.

It should not be forgotten, however, that while the protocols of chemotherapy and RT have defined the role of these options in the treatment of advanced-stage laryngeal cancer, conservation surgery that preserves the function of the larynx still remains an excellent treatment option in selected patients. Recently, the supracricoid partial laryngectomy with either cricohyoidopexy or cricohyoido-epiglottopexy has extended the ability to resect advanced laryngeal lesions with acceptable functional outcome and survival.[94]

Overall, treatment protocols using chemotherapy-RT to preserve organ function have successfully demonstrated their ability to anatomically preserve the larynx in a percentage of patients. However, one aspect of these protocols that is often underappreciated is the functional capacity of the retained organs. Few investigators have clearly documented the functional sequelae of chemotherapy and RT. Recently, Lazarus and colleagues[108] retrospectively studied patients being treated with chemotherapy and RT and found that 40% had swallowing difficulties. Clinical evidence of disorders in the pharyngeal phase of swallowing has been demonstrated in patients who have undergone chemotherapy and RT for tumors of the upper aerodigestive tract. Specifically, reduced laryngeal closure, reduced laryngeal elevation, and reduced posterior tongue base movement relative to age-matched controls have been documented.[108] Certainly, patients who successfully undergo chemotherapy-RT treatments to preserve their larynx have a much-improved quality of life relative to patients requiring total laryngectomy. Nevertheless, it should be realized that anatomic preservation does not always result in functional preservation.

CONCLUSION.  Early-stage laryngeal and hypopharyngeal cancer can be efficiently treated with single-modality treatment. For patients with chemosensitive tumors, the combination of induction chemotherapy with external beam RT is an effective means of treating selected patients with advanced-stage laryngeal cancer. Alternatively, in selected patients, conservation surgery of the larynx offers a useful treatment option. Finally, when applied to hypopharyngeal cancer, chemotherapy-RT strategies yield less promising results. The cooperation of the head and neck surgeon, radiation oncologist, and medical oncologist is paramount to the successful application of multidisciplinary treatment programs. The goal, however, remains to improve survival in these patients with advanced-stage disease.

## SALIVARY GLAND TUMORS

Historically, tumors of the salivary glands have been treated with surgery alone. The importance of adjuvant RT in the management of salivary tumors has become evident over the last decade.

Surgeons assuming the responsibility of patients with salivary gland tumors should possess a complete understanding of the varied pathologies and growth characteristics of these tumors. Planning an appropriate procedure that encompasses the primary tumor and the potential routes of metastasis requires a detailed knowledge of the complex anatomy.[109]

Tumors of the major salivary glands include those arising in the parotid and submandibular glands. Although the majority of diseases are glandular in origin, the proximity of tissues arising from all three embryonic layers enables the potential for both salivary and nonsalivary tumors to be present in the salivary glands.[110]

### THE PAROTID GLAND

Early in the first fetal trimester, the parotid gland arises from the epithelial lining of the oral cavity.[110] This epithelial cord develops appendages, recannulates, and becomes a hollow structure as it intimately associates with branches from the facial nerve. Risk for the development of parotid gland tumors is associated with previous radiation exposure. However, occupation, nutrition, and genetic factors have also been implicated in the development of salivary gland carcinomas. Patients with benign tumors or masses present for more than 10 years are at increased risk for developing malignant transformation.

Tumors of the parotid gland can be divided into primary benign, malignant, and mixed malignant tumors (Table 8-3). Metastatic lesions to the parotid can occur from breast, thyroid, larynx, colon, prostate, and lung primary tumors. Classification systems presently in use are based on the system first described by Foote and Frazell[111] in 1953.

BENIGN TUMORS.  Three-fourths of all tumors of the parotid gland are benign (Fig. 8-16). With the exception of Warthin's tumors, benign parotid tumors are more frequent in women than in men.[112,113]

### TABLE 8-3.  TUMORS OF THE PAROTID GLAND

Benign tumors:
    Pleomorphic adenoma (mixed benign tumor)
    Monomorphic adenoma
    Papillary cystadenoma lymphomatosum (Warthin's tumor)

Malignant tumors:
    Mucoepidermoid carcinoma
    Acinic cell carcinoma
    Adenoid cystic carcinoma
    Adenocarcinoma
    Epidermoid carcinoma (SCC)
    Small cell carcinoma
    Lymphoma

Malignant mixed tumors:
    Carcinoma ex pleomorphic adenoma (carcinosarcomas)

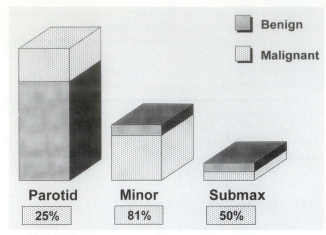

**FIGURE 8-16.** Distribution of benign and malignant tumors in major and minor salivary glands.

Non-neoplastic infiltrative processes, cysts, or inflammation account for approximately 25% of surgically resected parotid masses.[114] Salivary gland hypertrophy and other granulomatous diseases, including actinomycosis, mycobacterial diseases, or sialosis, are other common benign causes of parotid prominence.[114]

*Pleomorphic adenomas* (benign mixed tumors) are the most common type of parotid neoplasm, making up over 80% of parotid lesions.[113] Clinical presentation is that of a discrete, firm, slowly enlarging parotid mass located in the lower portion of the lateral lobe of the parotid that is rarely accompanied by pain or facial paralysis. Pleomorphic adenomas demonstrate both epithelial and mesenchymal components. Surgical treatment consists of superficial parotidectomy for lesions in the superficial lobe, or conservative (facial nerve sparing) total parotidectomy for tumors of the deep lobe. The recurrence rate with appropriate excision is 1% to 5%; however, a 30% to 50% recurrence rate is noted after simple enucleation.[115]

*Monomorphic adenomas* are rare benign tumors composed of a single cell type. The most common are basal cell adenomas. Myoepitheliomas, membranous adenomas, and clear cell tumors of the sebaceous elements are less common.[116] These adenomas are characterized as slow growing, with infrequent recurrence following adequate excision.

*Papillary cystadenoma lymphomatosum* (Warthin's tumors) are the second most common benign tumor of the parotid gland, comprising only 3% to 18% of parotid neoplasms.[117–119] Extremely rare instances of malignant transformation (0.3%) have been reported.[120] Clinical presentation is usually that of a discrete, painless, soft to semifirm mass located in the lower pole of the parotid. Histology reveals a cystic morphology lined by eosinophilic epithelium and filled with a yellow to brown material. Heterotopic salivary tissue in lymphoid centers is the proposed tissue of origin. As previously stated, a male predominance for this tumor is observed.[121] Warthin's tumor is the most common bilateral benign neoplasm of the parotid (up to 10%).[122] Extraparotid involvement in the subdigastric lymph nodes has been described in up to 8% of patients.[123] Surgical treatment consists of complete excision of the tumor, which may require

superficial parotidectomy for lesions of the superficial lobe and total conservative (facial nerve sparing) parotidectomy for tumors of the deep lobe.

**MALIGNANT TUMORS.** Malignant tumors of the parotid gland represent less than half of all parotid tumors.[116] Histologic types within this group include mucoepidermoid, acinic cell, adenocarcinoma, adenoid cystic, epidermoid, and small cell carcinomas.

*Mucoepidermoid carcinoma* is the most common malignancy of the parotid gland.[123] This tumor can appear at any age, although the highest incidence is during the third to fifth decades of life.[124,125] Prognosis for mucoepidermoid carcinoma is directly related to the degree of cellular differentiation and nodal status.[126] Characteristically, this tumor is composed of a variety of cell types within a single lesion and consists mainly of epidermoid and secretory cells.

Low-grade tumors demonstrate minimal local invasion and nodal metastasis. In this group, good survival outcome has been observed, with 5-year survival rates greater than 90%. In contrast, high-grade tumors have a local recurrence up to 78%. In addition, regional node metastasis is seen in 40% or more, and clinically evident distant metastases in 15% to 20% of patients.[125,127–130] The 5-year survival rate for patients without regional node involvement is about 70%. However, almost half of the intermediate-grade and high-grade tumors have positive lymph nodes at initial presentation. The presence of positive lymph nodes carries a negative prognostic value since the 5-year survival rate for these patients is less than 10%.[126] As would be expected, the treatment outcome for patients with mucoepidermoid carcinoma is strongly influenced by tumor grade.[131]

Mucoepidermoid carcinomas in the submandibular gland demonstrate more aggressive behavior. They grow rapidly, are painful, and present with a high rate of regional metastasis. High-grade tumors appear in the submandibular gland twice as often as in the parotid.[124,127,128]

*Acinic cell carcinoma* occurs almost exclusively in the parotid gland and accounts for 12% to 17% of malignant parotid tumors.[114,132,133] This tumor is more common in women and can present as a bilateral and multicentric neoplasm.[134,135] Acinic cell carcinoma morphologically resembles an enlarged salivary gland lobule or acini with a benign appearance; however, this is a malignant process. Nerve invasion is infrequent, but local recurrence is seen in about one-third of patients.[136–138] The 5- and 10-year survival rates are reported as 82% and 68%, respectively.[139] Facial nerve sacrifice is indicated only if it is essential to tumor extirpation. Neck dissection is only indicated in the presence of clinically positive nodes.[140] Regional node involvement is infrequent, and distant metastasis occurs only in patients with extensive local disease.[132,134–136]

*Adenocarcinoma* represents up to 10% of malignant parotid tumors.[114,126] About one-third (36%) of patients present with regional lymph node metastasis. These lesions vary in histologic pattern and grade such that prognosis is directly correlated with grade.[126] Grade I tumors have a 75% 5-year survival rate, while the more advanced grades approach 20%.[126] Patients with well-differentiated adenocarcinoma of the parotid gland have a longer disease-free survival and develop fewer distant metastases than patients with higher grades of tumor.[141]

Local disease control at 5 years was statistically better (80%) for patients who received combined modality therapy than for those treated by surgery (33%) or radiation (18%) alone. Radical parotidectomy, often requiring facial nerve sacrifice and therapeutic radical neck dissection, is the recommended treatment for high-grade tumors.[142]

Adenocarcinoma of the submandibular gland is often poorly differentiated and has a dismal prognosis.[143]

*Adenoid cystic carcinoma* represents a small fraction of parotid tumors (7%), but is more common in the submandibular and minor salivary glands (35%).[114,126] Age at presentation for these patients is 40 to 70 years old, with an equal gender distribution. Adenoid cystic carcinoma has a predilection for perineural invasion. In a reported series, 20% of patients had symptoms of pain and paresthesias and 25% had nerve dysfunction at the time of their initial presentation.[126]

The morphologic architecture is characterized by patterns of cystic spaces surrounded by malignant cells. Four patterns are described: tubular, cylindromatous, cribriform, and solid.[116] Adenoid cystic tumors are classified into grades according to relative cellular composition:[144]

1. Grade I: Tumors with tubular or cribriform areas without solid components.
2. Grade II: Cribriform tumors that are either pure or mixed, with less than 30% solid areas.
3. Grade III: Tumors with a predominantly solid pattern.

The cribriform histologic subtype is associated with multiple local recurrences, local aggressiveness, and a worsened salvage rate than the tubular subtype.[145] Overall prognosis in terms of distant metastasis and survival, however, is worse for the solid subtype.[145] The fifteen-year survival rate is reported as 39% for grade I tumors, 26% for grade II, and 5% for grade III. One-third to one-half of patients with adenoid cystic carcinoma of the parotid gland develop distant metastases late in the patient's course, despite local control at the primary site; hence long-term follow-up is necessary.[146–148]

Postoperative irradiation is recommended for patients with perineural or soft tissue involvement and for patients with positive surgical margins. Local tumor clearance is essential, since postoperative radiotherapy is not effective for gross residual tumor.[149–150]

*Epidermoid carcinoma* (primary SCC) of the parotid and other major salivary glands is quite rare. Epidermoid carcinoma accounts for less than 1% for the parotid and about 4% for the submandibular gland carcinomas.[126] The 30-year experience from Memorial Sloan-Kettering Cancer Center indicates that locoregional failure is the most significant problem. Radical surgical resection with preservation of the facial nerve when possible is recommended as the most effective approach.[152] Many of the patients required concurrent neck dissection, total parotidectomy, and sacrifice of the facial nerve. The authors made every effort to spare the nerve, unless it was directly involved with, or surrounded by, tumor. Despite aggressive therapy, survival rates at 5, 10, and 15 years were 21%, 15%, and 13%. The absolute 10-year survival rate for stage I squamous carcinoma of the parotid and submandibular gland was 75%; whereas for stages II and III, it was 11%.[151,152]

*Small cell carcinoma* arises from two different cell types in the parotid gland: duct cells or neuroendocrine cells. The duct-cell type exhibits prominent cell junctions and mature desmosomes. The neuroendocrine type is similar to Merkel's cell tumors of the skin, with granule-bearing dendritic processes and primitive attachment sites. Both types of tumor are composed of small, undifferentiated cells. While neoplasms of duct-cell origin rarely metastasize, those of neuroendocrine origin have a very aggressive course and must be treated accordingly.[153]

*Lymphoma* should be included in the differential diagnosis of parotid gland masses, since the head and neck is the third most common site of lymphoma.[154] When the entire parotid gland is enlarged and there are other palpable regional lymph nodes, lymphoma should be suspected. These nodes can then be biopsied in lieu of a formal parotidectomy.[155]

Clinically, there is generalized enlargement of the gland, with a "rubbery" consistency and normal facial nerve function. Patients with lymphoma require surgery only to establish tissue diagnosis and occasionally for staging. Definitive treatment is by chemotherapy and/or radiotherapy.[155–157]

**MALIGNANT MIXED TUMORS.** Malignant mixed tumors comprise the majority of malignant tumors of the parotid gland.[158] Presentation is that of an asymptomatic mass, present for years with subsequent rapid enlargement. Tumors can either be high-grade (ductal, undifferentiated, true malignant mixed) or low-grade (terminal duct). Carcinoma ex pleomorphic adenomas describe a tumor where the epithelial component is malignant in a carcinoma arising in a mixed tumor.[158]

Three distinct histologic types of malignant mixed tumors are described. (1) Carcinosarcoma with chondrosarcoma histology is by far the most common, although fibrosarcoma and occasionally metastasizing pleomorphic adenoma have been reported.[159] (2) A second type is a histologically benign primary tumor with malignant potential for metastasis.[159,160] (3) Third, true malignant mixed tumors (carcinosarcomas) are relatively rare. They contain both epithelial and mesenchymal components, are malignant, and demonstrate distant metastasis. Prognosis depends on the extent of invasion and histologic subclassification.[161] The 5-year survival rate for true malignant mixed tumors has been reported as 55%, with a 10-year survival rate of 31%. Aggressive surgery plus postoperative irradiation is the recommended treatment for these tumors. Death is usually due to metastatic disease.

**CLINICAL ASPECTS.** The preoperative evaluation and initial workup of a suspected parotid tumor should include the following:

1. History and physical examination
2. Radiographic evaluation (selected patients)
3. Needle biopsy (selected patients)
4. Frozen section (if indicated)

*HISTORY AND PHYSICAL EXAMINATION.* The patient's history often gives clues to the type of parotid disease present. The most common symptoms are a mass (81%), pain (12%), and facial nerve paralysis (12% to 20%).[131] Facial nerve paralysis associated with ear pain and sensory loss in the second and third divisions of the trigeminal nerve heralds a dismal prognosis and indicates a high probability of an advanced malignant lesion, even in the presence of normal findings on noninvasive studies.[131,161–163] Intraparotid facial nerve neurofibroma[164] and traumatic neuromas[165] can cause facial nerve dysfunction and must be differentiated from facial nerve neoplasms. It should be noted that half of the patients with parotid tumors have symptoms for a year before they seek medical attention; however, 10% trace their complaints 10 years back or longer.[131]

The possibility of a deep lobe tumor should be evaluated by intraoral examination with particular attention to the tonsillar fossa, soft palate, and lateral pharyngeal wall. Stensen's duct opposite the upper second molar should be inspected for character of salivary flow (clarity, consistency, and purulence) as well as for redness, bulging, and irritation of the ductal orifice. The entire oral cavity, oropharynx, and neck should be thoroughly evaluated for other primary lesions or nodal disease.

Recurrent attacks of pain and swelling incited by eating are generally indicative of obstructive sialopathy due to stone disease and not tumor. Repeated inflammatory processes (e.g., sialectasia, chronic sialadenitis) also can be manifested as generalized enlargements of the gland and are not related to meals.

*RADIOLOGIC EVALUATION.* Plain x-ray films of the parotid or submandibular areas are sometimes useful in ruling out stone disease. High-resolution CT, with or without contrast, can clearly define lesions of both the superficial and deep lobe of the parotid[166] (Fig. 8-17). MRI may be equivalent to CT scans in accuracy and may even indicate what type of tumor is present.[167] In general terms, magnetic resonance tomography shows the mass in greater contrast to surrounding tissue, but with less adjacent tissue detail than CT scans[168] (Figs. 8-18 and 8-19). Anatomic evaluation by CT or MRI is recommended for the following:[169]

1. Malignant aspiration cytology
2. Warthin's tumor aspirate (suspicion of bilateral disease)
3. Clinical suspicion of deep lobe involvement
4. Facial paralysis
5. Parotid mass fixation
6. Possible lymphadenopathy

*FINE-NEEDLE ASPIRATION.* Eneroth,[170] a proponent of fine-needle aspiration (FNA) biopsy of salivary gland masses, reports

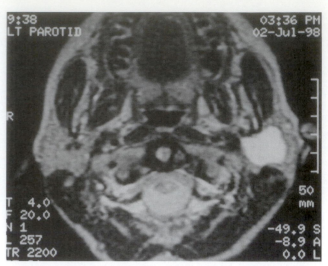

**FIGURE 8-18.** Axial view of an MRI scan showing a deep-lobe benign mixed tumor of the left parotid gland.

92% accuracy in diagnosing parotid tumors. The technique requires the active participation of a cytopathologist specifically trained and interested in salivary neoplasms. Only positive diagnoses should be accepted as accurate. Occasionally, a suspicious lymph node may be a more superior biopsy choice than the parotid mass itself. Several investigators have found a good correlation (90% to 94%) between diagnosis of FNA and final histologic diagnosis.[171,172] Aspiration cytology is thus cost-effective, accurate and safe.

SURGICAL APPROACH. Superficial parotidectomy is the treatment of choice for most benign tumors and many stage I (T1N0 and T2N0) malignant lesions.[173] For larger tumors or when there is a clinical suspicion of cancer, a biopsy is indicated to better prepare the patient and the surgeon for the appropriate operation.

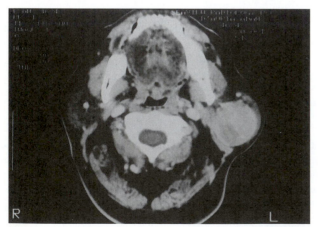

**FIGURE 8-17.** Axial view of the CT scan of a patient with Warthin's tumor of the left parotid gland (note cystic areas within the lesion).

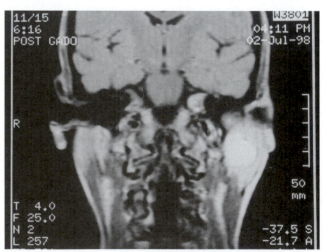

**FIGURE 8-19.** Coronal view of an MRI scan showing a deep-lobe benign mixed tumor of the left parotid gland.

When no definite diagnosis can be made, the nodes in the upper jugular chain can be biopsied early in the dissection. Should malignancy be diagnosed, the decision regarding the facial nerve is made intraoperatively based on gross invasion or the proximity of tumor of the nerve. A total parotidectomy is indicated for invasive tumors and for those originating in, or extending into, the deep lobe. In any case, confirmation of malignancy should be obtained prior to deciding the fate of the seventh nerve.

By definition, deep lobe tumors are seated deep to the facial nerve and make up approximately 10% to 12% of parotid tumors.[173,174] The most common presenting sign is an asymptomatic swelling in the preauricular area with a few patients who may have swelling of the palate or tonsil. CT or MRI can help evaluate the extent of the tumor in these patients.

Surgical treatment consists of a standard parotidectomy sparing the facial nerve. Most serious complications of parotid surgery stem from damage to the facial nerve. Other less common problems include seroma, hematoma, and infection.[175]

## ADJUVANT THERAPY

*RADIATION THERAPY.* In the past, on the basis of its record with large lesions and inadequate energy, irradiation was believed to be ineffective for the management of salivary gland tumors. Surgery alone is adequate therapy for low-grade and most intermediate-grade malignant lesions. However, subclinical aggregates of cancer cells are radiosensitive,[176] and the addition of irradiation will be of benefit when treating aggressive high-grade cancers.[177]

The indications for postoperative irradiation for salivary gland tumors include the following:[178]

1. Highly malignant tumors by histology
2. Invasion of muscle, bone, skin, and temporomandibular joint
3. Perineural invasion
4. Regional lymph node metastasis
5. Recurrent tumor after surgical resection
6. Malignant tumors involving the deep lobe
7. Gross residual tumor after surgical resection
8. Possible residual microscopic tumor adjacent to the facial nerve

Several authors have achieved excellent local control and improved survival rates with combined surgery and irradiation.[179–183]

Using chemotherapy to treat salivary gland cancer is a relatively recent, and not particularly successful, modality demonstrating short, incomplete responses with poor control rates. Locoregional disease seems to be more susceptible to chemotherapeutic agents than distant spread; lung metastases have shown the best response.[184,185]

Tumor histology is the main factor affecting response to chemotherapeutic drugs. The adenocarcinoma-like cancers (adenoid cystic, adenocarcinoma, carcinoma ex pleomorphic adenoma, and acinic cell tumors) respond best to doxorubicin (Adriamycin) and cisplatin/5-FU, while epidermoid-like tumors (SCC and mucoepidermoid carcinoma) are more responsive to methotrexate and cisplatin.[186] This differential response appears to correlate well with the bicellular theory of salivary gland tumor histogenesis, i.e., that adenocarcinoma-like cancers arise from the stem cells of the intercalated ducts, and mucoepidermoid-squamous cell cancers originate from the stem cells of the excretory ducts.[187]

PROGNOSTIC FACTORS. The major determinants of survival in malignant parotid gland neoplasms are tumor histology and clinical stage. Byers and colleagues[188] noted that a poor prognosis correlates with the following:

1. Poor cytologic differentiation
2. Nodal metastases
3. Nerve invasion
4. Locally invasive disease

*HISTOPATHOLOGY.* Low-grade adenocarcinoma, mucoepidermoid, and acinic cell carcinomas have 100% survival rates at 5 years, but various high-grade tumors have 5-year survival rates ranging from 23% to 39%.[189] Eneroth[191] has reported 15-year survival rates of 80% for low-grade mucoepidermoid carcinoma, 73% for acinic cell carcinoma, 25% for adenoid cystic, and 20% for poorly differentiated carcinoma.

*CLINICAL STAGE.* Tumor size and nodal status are also prognostically significant. Stage I patients with tumors of all histologic types have an overall 5-year survival rate of approximately 60%, whereas stage III patients demonstrate less than 10% survival. Patients with cervical node metastasis at admission have the lowest survival rate (9%), while those who never had cervical node metastasis have a much better chance, 41% survival at 5 years. If the patient progresses to have nodal disease, the 5-year survival rate is 25%.[189,190]

The importance of tumor size (stage) as an isolated factor in prognosis is equivocal. Spiro[126] noted an 85% 5-year survival when the tumors were less than 3 cm in diameter, compared to 67% for tumors 3.1 to 6 cm in size, but Fu and associates[180] record 68% and 64% 5-year survival, respectively, for stage I and stage II tumors.

*LOCAL INVASION.* The prognostic significance of facial nerve involvement has been discussed previously. Parotid cancers only invade the skin when the primary tumor is massive (T3 and T4 lesions) and/or highly aggressive.

*OTHER FACTORS.* The value of pain as an independent prognostic factor is unclear. Eneroth[191] did not attach any particular meaning to it, yet others[126,192] have noted a survival advantage of greater than 30% for asymptomatic patients. This may suggest that pain is likely a sign of neural invasion by tumor, and as such heralds a poor prognosis.

## SUBMANDIBULAR GLAND NEOPLASMS

In the majority of patients, the finding of a mass in the submandibular gland is due to ductal obstruction from calculi. Submandibular gland tumors account for 10% to 15% of all salivary gland malignancies.[112,113] Malignant submandibular tumors occur in a reported 38% to 50% of previously untreated patients.[112,113] As such, a tumor in the submandibular gland has twice the likelihood of being malignant as compared to the parotid gland.

With history and physical examination, submandibular tumors can be differentiated from inflammatory processes. Submento-vertex and occlusal radiographs aid in examining the floor of the mouth for possible calculi. Mandibular x-rays are not diagnostically significant if negative for stones, in which case CT scans and MRI are useful in delineating the anatomic extent of disease. If the process is benign and calculi are seen, intraoral removal of stones is occasionally adequate, but most patients will require excision of the gland.

Primary malignant tumors of the submandibular gland require surgical excision and postoperative irradiation, when indicated. Small T1 or T2 lesions without involvement of cranial nerves (V, VII, or XII), the mandible, or regional lymph nodes should be treated with dissection of submandibular triangle. The indicators of a poor prognosis include the following:

1. Nerve invasion
2. Local or regional lymph node metastases
3. Periglandular soft tissue invasion
4. High-grade mucoepidermoid carcinoma and adenoid cystic carcinoma
5. Tumor invasion of the mandible

In most cases, the submandibular mass can be diagnosed by needle biopsy before surgery. If aspiration does not yield a diagnosis, submandibular triangle dissection will serve as biopsy and treatment.[132]

## NECK DISSECTION FOR CANCER OF THE HEAD AND NECK

Head and neck malignancies arise from a wide range of epithelial tissues; however, greater than 90% of patients have SCC. As such, the focus of this section is on the management of the cervical lymph nodes in patients with SCC.

The most important prognostic factor for patients with SCC of the upper aerodigestive tract is the pathologic status of the cervical lymph nodes. To the cervical lymph nodes, the negative prognostic value of having metastatic disease has long been recognized. Patients with positive cervical nodes demonstrate a cure rate that is roughly half of their node negative counterparts.[3] At the present time, despite technical and diagnostic advances, as well as the use of combination therapies, the most important prognostic indicator for patients with SCC of head and neck remains the status of the cervical lymph nodes.

### LYMPHATIC ANATOMY OF THE NECK

Initially described by Rouviere[193] and later by others,[194] there are several different methods describing the location of the different cervical lymph nodes. The most widely used and easily reproducible system was described by the Head and Neck Service at Memorial Sloan-Kettering Cancer Center (MSKCC).[195] Cervical lymph node beds are described as separate nodal groups or levels I to V (Fig. 8-20).

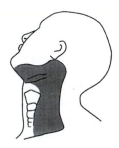

Radical Neck Dissection

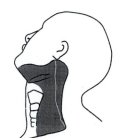

Preserved: Spinal accessory nerve

Modified
Radical Neck Dissection - Type I

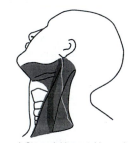

Preserved: Sternocleidomastoid muscle,
Internal jugular vein and Spinal accessory nerve

Modified
Radical Neck Dissection - Type III

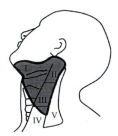

Supraomohyoid Neck Dissection

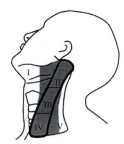

Antero-lateral (Jugular) Neck Dissection

**FIGURE 8-20.** The most commonly employed neck dissections for cervical lymph node metastasis.

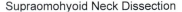

1. **Level I.** *Submental group:* Refers to the nodal tissue located between the anterior belly of the digastric muscle and above the hyoid bone. *Submandibular group:* Refers to nodal tissue in the triangular area bounded by the anterior and posterior bellies of the digastric muscle and the inferior border of the mandible.

2. **Levels II, III, and IV** correspond to the upper, middle, and lower third of the deep jugular chain lymph nodes of the neck.

3. **Level II.** *Upper jugular group:* Refers to nodal tissue around the upper portion of the internal jugular vein (IJV) and the upper spinal accessory nerve. The upper extent of the tissue is the skull base, and the inferior limit is at the level of the bifurcation of the carotid artery (the hyoid bone is the clinical landmark). The posterior limit is bounded by the posterior border of the sternocleidomastoid muscle (SCM), and the anterior boundary is the lateral border of the sternohyoid muscle.

4. **Level III.** *Middle jugular group:* Refers to nodal tissue around the middle third of the IJV from the inferior border of level II to the omohyoid muscle (the cricothyroid membrane is the clinical landmark). The anterior and posterior borders are the same as those for level II.

5. **Level IV.** *Lower jugular group:* Refers to nodal tissue around the inferior third of the IJV from the inferior border of level III to the clavicle. The anterior and posterior borders are the same as for level II and III.

6. **Level V.** *Posterior triangle group:* Refers to nodal tissue around the lower portion of the spinal accessory nerve and along the transverse cervical vessels; that is, tissue within the triangle formed by the clavicle, posterior border of the SCM, and anterior border of the trapezius muscle.

7. **Level VI.** Tracheoesophageal groove lymph nodes.

8. **Level VII.** Superior mediastinal lymph nodes.

## SURGICAL MANAGEMENT OF CERVICAL LYMPH NODE METASTASIS

The treatment of clinically evident cervical lymph nodes has traditionally been surgical. However, in recent decades a combined surgical and radiotherapeutic approach has evolved. Butlin[196] was the first surgeon to describe the systematic removal of the cervical lymph nodes by excising the tissue in the submandibular triangle in continuity with a primary lesion of the oral tongue. However, this technique did not remove all tissue at risk for subsequent metastasis. It was not until the radical neck dissection was described by Crile[197] in 1906 and later popularized by Martin and colleagues[198] that systematic removal of the cervical lymph nodes became routine. Radical neck dissection (RND) attains comprehensive clearance of the cervical lymph nodes by removing the SAN, IJV, and SCM, along with the nodal beds contained from the mandible to the clavicle and from the anterior cervical midline to the anterior border of the trapezius muscle. As would be anticipated, this operation carries a significant postoperative morbidity, including compromise of ipsilateral shoulder function as a consequence of the spinal accessory nerve removal and aesthetic deformity resulting from resection of the SCM and excision of the internal jugular vein, particularly when the RND is performed on both sides, which results in marked facial edema and has potential for neurologic impairment. The adverse effects following classic RND are compounded when patients are subsequently treated with adjuvant radiotherapy.

Although clearance of all cervical lymph node beds is achieved through RND, there is no rationale to support this procedure and accept its resultant morbidity. For this reason, Bocca and colleagues[199] as well as Byers and others[200,201] have proposed modifications of this technique. Bocca's group proposed the "functional" cervical lymph node dissection, which aimed to remove all five levels of cervical nodes while sparing the spinal accessory nerve, IJV, and SCM. In comparing the recurrence rates for patients undergoing functional neck dissection to historical controls that had undergone RND, the recurrence rates were similar in patients with a clinically negative neck or limited neck disease. However, in patients with multiple positive nodes, the recurrence rates were higher. These studies also failed to provide a rationale or explanation to justify removal of all five cervical lymph node levels in the clinically negative neck.

More recently, further modifications to RND have been proposed that not only spare the nonlymphatic structures in the neck (SAN, IJV, SCM) but also do not remove all of the lymphatic tissue in the clinically negative neck. These dissections have been termed *selective* or *limited* and are based on observations that cancers of the head and neck tend to metastasize in predictable patterns based on the location of the primary tumor.[35] Therefore, selective node dissection, in which only tissues at risk for metastatic disease are removed, has emerged. Surgeons who practice selective node dissection also advocate postoperative radiotherapy, should multiple positive lymph nodes or extracapsular spread be noted within the specimen.

## NECK DISSECTIONS

The proposed classification of neck dissection by the American Academy of Otolaryngology, Head, and Neck Surgery is as follows:[195]

1. *Radical neck dissection (RND)* is defined as the standard basic neck dissection, and all other procedures are considered to be modifications of RND. RND is defined as the comprehensive removal of lymph node levels I to V, along with the SAN, IJV, and SCM.

2. *Modified RND (MRND)* includes removing lymph node levels I to V and preserving one or more of the nonlymphatic structures normally removed during RND. MRND is further subdivided to define which structures are preserved: (a) *MRND type 1* preserves the spinal accessory nerve (MRND I). (b) *MRND type 2* preserves the spinal accessory nerve and the IJV (MRND II). (c) *MRND type 3* preserves the spinal accessory nerve, IJV, and SCM (MRND III).

3. *Selective neck dissection* consists of the selective removal of one or more lymph node groups with preservation of the spinal accessory nerve, IJV, and SCM. Common selective neck dissections include the following: (a) *Supraomohyoid neck dissection (SOHND)*, in which levels I to III are removed. (b) *Lateral neck dissection (LND) (jugular node dissection)*, in which levels II to IV are removed. (c) *Posterolateral neck dissection (PLND)*, in which lymph node levels II to V are removed.

The most frequently employed modifications in comprehensive neck dissections, and selective neck dissections are shown in Fig. 8-20.

## PATTERNS OF NODAL METASTASIS

In patients with tumors of the head and neck, the clinical examination is relatively inaccurate, since up to 30% of clinically node negative patients harbor occult metastasis.[202] For this reason, systematic evaluation has been performed to describe the patterns of nodal metastasis for the formulation of treatment strategies.

Lindberg[36] demonstrated that for lesions of the oral tongue, floor of the mouth, retromolar trigone–anterior faucial arch, and soft palate, the incidence of cervical node metastasis increased with increasing size of the primary lesion. The incidence of nodal metastasis, however, did not correlate with size when the primary tumor was in the tonsillar fossa, base of the tongue, supraglottic larynx, or hypopharynx.[36]

SCC of the upper aerodigestive tract metastasizes in a predictable pattern. The most common site of metastasis for all tumors is the level II nodes. Tumors that lie anterior to the circumvallate papilla of the tongue tend to metastasize to the level I and upper jugular chain level II. Level III nodes are seldom involved, and levels IV and V almost never. Tumors of the oropharynx have a low propensity to metastasize to level I, but commonly go to level II, and, with decreasing frequency, to levels III and IV and only rarely to level V nodes. A similar pattern of metastasis is noted for tumors of the supraglottic larynx and hypopharynx. Nasopharyngeal tumors are unique in that they favor wide metastasis to nodes in levels II to V. However, nasopharyngeal tumors rarely metastasize to the level I area. Contralateral metastasis is infrequent with tumors of the floor of the mouth, oral tongue, hypopharynx, and retromolar trigone and anterior faucial arch. In contrast, tumors of the nasopharynx, base of tongue, oropharyngeal walls, soft palate, supraglottic larynx, and tonsil have substantial rates of contralateral metastasis. These data provided valuable information about the patterns of nodal metastasis in patients with clinically evident disease, but no information on the patterns of spread for patients with occult metastasis.

In order to fully assess all of the lymph nodes at risk for a specific primary tumor site, Shah[35] presented a series of patients who underwent RND for SCC of the upper aerodigestive tract. These operations included elective RND in 343 patients with clinically negative necks, and therapeutic RND in 776 patients with clinically palpable disease. Metastasis was confirmed pathologically in 82% of the clinically apparent nodes and in 33% of the clinically negative group. In patients undergoing therapeutic RND for oral cavity tumors, the majority of metastatic nodes were in levels I to III, level IV was involved in only 20% of patients, and level V an infrequent 4%. Tumors of the oropharynx demonstrated a metastatic preponderance to levels II to IV, with levels I and V demonstrating a 17% and 11% rate of metastasis, respectively. Similarly, tumors of the hypopharynx spread to levels II to IV, and the level I and V frequency of metastasis was 10% and 11%, respectively. Primary lesions of the larynx again demonstrated an increased prevalence to metastasize to levels II to IV nodes, with levels I and V demonstrating positive nodes 8% and 5%, respectively (Table 8-4).

In patients undergoing elective RND in the setting of a clinically negative neck, the patterns of nodal metastasis just noted were found to be consistent in those patients with pathologically determined occult metastasis. In patients undergoing elective RND for oral cavity tumors, the majority of metastatic nodes were in levels I to III, level

## TABLE 8-4. THERAPEUTIC RND FOR CLINICALLY EVIDENT DISEASE (% INVOLVEMENT OF VARIOUS LEVELS)

| PRIMARY SITE | LEVEL I | LEVEL II | LEVEL III | LEVEL IV | LEVEL V |
|---|---|---|---|---|---|
| Oral cavity | 61 | 57 | 44 | 20 | 4 |
| Oropharynx | 17 | 85 | 50 | 33 | 11 |
| Hypopharynx | 10 | 78 | 75 | 47 | 11 |
| Larynx | 8 | 68 | 70 | 35 | 5 |

IV was involved in only 9% of patients, and level V an infrequent 2%. Tumors of the oropharynx demonstrated a metastatic preponderance to levels II to IV, with levels I and V each demonstrating a 7% rate of metastasis. Similarly, tumors of the hypopharynx spread to levels II to IV, with no identified metastases to the level I and V nodes. Primary lesions of the larynx again demonstrated an increased prevalence to metastasize to level II to IV nodes, with levels I and V demonstrating positive nodes 14% and 7%, respectively (Table 8-5).

These data suggest that for an oral cavity primary tumor with an N0 neck, the cervical nodes at risk would be adequately sampled by a supraomohyoid lymph node dissection (levels I, II, and III). For the patient with an N0 neck and a primary tumor of the oropharynx, hypopharynx, or larynx, a lateral (jugular, levels II, III, and IV) neck dissection would be appropriate. There is a very small risk for there to be subclinical disease in the remaining nodal tissue; however, in the elective setting this disease should be microscopic and responsive to radiotherapy. As such, in the N0 patient, the role of the selective node dissection is that of a staging operation.[203] The morbidity of the RND procedure is avoided for two-thirds of the patients who will have a negative specimen. In those patients (one-third) found to have metastasis, the decision to proceed with radiotherapy is based on pathologic results.

The frequency of metastasis to the level V nodes has also been examined.[204] Metastasis was found to be present in the level V nodes in 3% of all the patients undergoing neck dissection. Level V metastases were highest in patients with primary tumors of the hypopharynx and oropharynx: 7% and 6%, respectively. Of the 40 patients identified with level V metastasis, only 3 patients had N0 clinical neck examinations. Thus, the incidence of level V metastasis is small and almost nonexistent in the patient with an N0 neck. Neck dissections and their indications are presented in Table 8-6.

## TABLE 8-5. ELECTIVE RND FOR CLINICALLY NEGATIVE DISEASE (%)

| PRIMARY SITE | LEVEL I | LEVEL II | LEVEL III | LEVEL IV | LEVEL V |
|---|---|---|---|---|---|
| Oral cavity | 58 | 51 | 26 | 9 | 2 |
| Oropharynx | 7 | 80 | 60 | 27 | 7 |
| Hypopharynx | 0 | 75 | 75 | 75 | 0 |
| Larynx | 14 | 52 | 55 | 24 | 7 |

**TABLE 8-6.** NECK DISSECTIONS AND THEIR INDICATIONS

| DISSECTION TYPE | LEVELS DISSECTED | STRUCTURES PRESERVED | INDICATIONS |
|---|---|---|---|
| RND | I–V | None | Metastatic tumor from any primary where the SAN is involved by tumor and cannot be dissected free; or in the presence of previous radiotherapy or surgery to the neck. |
| MRND I | I–V | SAN | Metastatic carcinoma at any site except differentiated thyroid cancer, with a SAN free of disease. |
| MRND III | I–V | SAN | Metastatic differentiated thyroid cancer. |
| SOHND | I–III | SAN IJV, SCM | Elective neck dissection in cases of SCC of the oral cavity or oropharynx (include level IV) and malignant melanoma with primary site anterior to the ear (including parotidectomy) for facial and scalp lesion. |
| LND (JND) | II–IV | SAN IJV, SCM | Elective neck dissection for SCC of the hypopharynx and larynx. |
| PLND | II–V | SAN IJV, SCM | Elective neck dissection for malignant melanoma of the posterior scalp or neck. |

## METASTATIC SCC WITH AN OCCULT PRIMARY TUMOR

Metastatic SCC with an unknown primary tumor accounts for fewer than 10% of head and neck cancers. Most commonly, these tumors metastasize to the level II nodes. Because the location of the primary is unknown, it is not possible to predict the patterns of metastasis. Since the lymph nodes at risk cannot be identified, the neck dissection in these patients should be comprehensive, with preservation of the spinal accessory nerve, if it is not grossly involved by disease, at the discretion of the surgeon.

## SALIVARY GLAND CARCINOMA

Primary carcinoma of the salivary glands rarely metastasizes to the cervical lymph nodes. The potential for metastasis of these tumors is based on the size and histologic type of the primary tumor.[205] The relatively infrequent risk of metastasis from salivary carcinoma metastasis does not warrant a recommendation for elective lymph node dissection. When therapeutic neck dissection is indicated for clinically evident disease, a comprehensive neck node dissection with sparing of the spinal accessory nerve (if possible) is advocated.

## CUTANEOUS MELANOMA OF THE HEAD AND NECK

Elective node dissection for cutaneous melanoma of the head and neck remains a controversial issue. In general, patients with intermediate thickness melanoma draining to one side of the neck should be considered for a regional lymph node dissection. The patterns of metastatic spread influence the extent of the dissection.[206] An imaginary coronal plane at the top of the helix separates the drainage into two regions. Lesions located anterior to this plane seldom drain into the posterior triangle. As such, elective lymph node dissection anterior to this line should include parotidectomy and dissection of lymph node levels I to III. Lesions posterior to this line should have a posterolateral lymph node dissection, including the occipital nodes and levels II to V. Patients with clinically apparent nodes should have a comprehensive neck dissection with ipsilateral parotidectomy if the preauricular nodes are in the drainage area of the primary lesion.

## DISSECTION OF THE LEVEL VI (TRACHEOESOPHAGEAL) LYMPH NODES

The lymph nodes present in the tracheoesophageal groove are termed level VI.[195] Nodes in this bed are commonly affected by carcinoma of the thyroid gland and cancers of the subglottic and transglottic larynx and cervical esophagus. Dissection in this area requires careful attention to preservation of the recurrent laryngeal nerve and may require sacrifice of the ipsilateral parathyroid glands.

This dissection is indicated for clinically evident disease in the treatment of thyroid cancer and cutaneous melanoma. When performed for thyroid cancer, it is possible to preserve and reimplant the ipsilateral parathyroid glands if frozen-section confirmation of the glands is obtained.

In cases of subglottic and transglottic SCC where total laryngectomy is indicated, the level VI nodes should be cleared; with a low postoperative incidence of hypocalcemia, preservation of the RLN can be disregarded and the ipsilateral parathyroids can be discarded.

SCC of the cervical esophagus can be approached similarly, depending on whether or not it is necessary to perform a total laryngectomy.

## REFERENCES

1. LANDIS SK et al: Cancer Statistics, 1998. CA Cancer J Clin 48:6, 1998.
2. PARKIN DM et al: Global burden of cancer, in *Biannual Report 1986–87*, World Health Organization and International Agency for Research on Cancer. Lyon, France, IARC, 1987, p 11.

3. SHAH JP, ANDERSEN PF: The impact of patterns of nodal metastasis on modifications of neck dissection. Ann Surg Oncol 1:521, 1994.

4. SHAH JP: Cancer of the upper aerodigestive tract, in *The Practice of Cancer Surgery,* AE Alfonso, B Gardner (eds). New York, Appleton-Century-Crofts, 1982.

5. DECKER J, GOLDSTEIN JC: Risk factors in head and neck cancer. N Engl J Med 306:1151, 1982.

6. JACOBS CD: Etiologic considerations for head and neck squamous cancers, in *Carcinomas of the Head and Neck: Evaluation and Management,* C Jacobs (ed). Boston, Kluwer Academic, 1990, pp 265–282.

7. WINN DM et al: Mouthwash use and oral conditions in the risk of oral and pharyngeal cancer. Cancer Res 51:3044, 1991.

8. FALK RT et al: Effect of smoking and alcohol consumption on laryngeal cancer risk in coastal Texas. Cancer Res 49:4024, 1989.

9. NAM J et al: Cigarette smoking, alcohol, and nasopharyngeal carcinoma: A case-control study among U.S. whites. J Natl Cancer Inst 84:619, 1992.

10. WINN DM et al: Snuff dipping and oral cancer among women in the southern United States. N Engl J Med 304:745, 1981.

11. BROWN LM et al: Occupational risk factors for laryngeal cancer on the Texas Gulf Coast. Cancer Res 48:1960, 1988.

12. MUSCAT JE, WYNDER EL: Tobacco, alcohol, asbestos, and occupational risk factors for laryngeal cancer. Cancer 69:2244, 1992.

13. STOCKWELL HG, LYMAN GH: Impact of smoking and smokeless tobacco on the risk of cancer of the head and neck. Head Neck Surg 9:104, 1986.

14. FRANCESCHI S et al: Maize and risk of cancers of the oral cavity, pharynx, and esophagus in northeastern Italy. J Natl Cancer Inst 82:1407, 1990.

15. PETO R et al: Can dietary beta-carotene materially reduce human cancer rates? Nature 290:201, 1981.

16. MCLAUGHLIN JK et al: Dietary factors in oral and pharyngeal cancer. J Natl Cancer Inst 80:1237, 1988.

17. LA VECCHIA C et al: Dietary indicators of laryngeal cancer risk. Cancer Res 50:4497, 1990.

18. SHILLITOE EJ et al: Antibody to early and late antigens of herpes simplex virus type 1 in patients with oral cancer. Cancer 54:266, 1984.

19. WATTS SL et al: Human papilloma virus DNA types in squamous cell carcinomas of the head and neck. Oral Surg Oral Med Oral Pathol 71:701, 1991.

20. HENLE G, HENLE W: Epstein-Barr virus-specific IgA serum antibodies as an outstanding feature of nasopharyngeal carcinoma. Intl J Cancer 17:1, 1976.

21. LUND VJ, HOWARD DJ: Head and neck cancer in the young: A prognostic conundrum? J Laryngol Otol 104:544, 1990.

22. SPITZ MR et al: Chromosome sensitivity to bleomycin-induced mutagenesis, an independent risk factor for upper aerodigestive tract cancers. Cancer Res 49:4626, 1989.

23. SCHANTZ SP et al: Young adults with head and neck cancer express increased susceptibility to mutagen-induced chromosome damage. J Am Med Assoc 262:3313, 1989.

24. SCHANTZ SP et al: Mutagen sensitivity in patients with head and neck cancers: a biologic marker for risk of multiple primary malignancies. J Natl Cancer Inst 82:1773, 1990.

25. SHIELDS PG, HARRIS CC: Molecular epidemiology and the genetics of environmental cancer. J Am Med Assoc 266:681, 1991.

26. GREENLEE RT et al: Cancer Statistics 2000. CA 50:7, 2000.

27. FRANCESCHI D et al: Improved survival in the treatment of squamous carcinoma of the oral tongue. Am J Surg 166:360, 1993.

28. SOO KC et al: Squamous carcinoma of the gums. Am J Surg 156:281, 1988.

29. SHAHA AR et al: Squamous cell carcinoma of the floor of mouth. Am J Surg 148:455, 1984.

30. SPIRO RH et al: Predictive value of tumor thickness in squamous carcinoma confined to the tongue and floor of mouth. Am J Surg 152:345, 1986.

31. KOCH W et al: Chemoradiotherapy for organ preservation in oral and pharyngeal carcinoma. Arch Otolaryngol Head Neck Surg 121:974, 1995.

32. MCGREGOR AD, MACDONALD G: Routes of entry of squamous cell carcinoma of the mandible. Head Neck Surg 10:294, 1988.

33. ———— Patterns of spread of squamous cell carcinoma of the ramus of the mandible. Head Neck Surg 15:440, 1993.

34. MILLION RR: Elective neck irradiation for TxN0 squamous carcinoma of the oral tongue and floor of mouth. Cancer 34:149, 1974.

35. SHAH JP: The pattern of cervical lymph node metastasis from squamous cell carcinoma of the head and neck. Am J Surg 160:405, 1990.

36. LINDBERG R: Distribution of cervical lymph node meatstases from squamous cell carcinoma of the upper respiratory and digestive tracts. Cancer 29:1446, 1972.

37. SPIRO JD et al: Critical assessment of supraomohyoid neck dissection. Am J Surg 156:286, 1988.

38. SPIRO JD et al: Supraomohyoid neck dissection. Am J Surg 172:650, 1996.

39. ZELEFSKY MJ et al: Postoperative radiation therapy for squamous cell carcinomas of the oral cavity and oropharynx: Impact of therapy on patients with positive surgical margins. Int J Radiat Oncol Biol Phys 25:17, 1993.

40. MOORE C: Cigarette smoking and cancer of the mouth, pharynx and larynx: A continuing study. JAMA 218:553, 1971.

41. ALTUN M et al: Undifferentiated nasopharyngeal cancer (UCNT): current diagnostic and therapeutic aspects. Int J Rad Oncol Biol Phys 32:859, 1995.

42. FANDI A, CVITKOVIC E: Biology and treatment of nasopharyngeal cancer. Cur Opinion Oncol 7:255, 1995.

43. ZHENG YM et al: Environmental and dietary risk factors for nasopharyngeal carcinoma: A case control study in Zangwu County, Guangxi, China. Br J Cancer 69:508, 1994.

44. GRULICH AE et al: Cancer incidence in Asian migrants to New South Wales, Australia. Br J Cancer 71:400, 1995.

45. BURT RD et al: Association between human leukocyte antigen type and nasopharyngeal carcinoma in caucasians in the United States. Cancer Epidemiology, Biomarkers Prevention 5:879, 1996.

46. LIEBOWITZ D: Nasopharyegeal carcinoma: the Epstein-Barr virus association. Semin Oncol 21:376, 1994.

47. PATHMANATHAN R et al: Clonal proliferation of cells infected with Epstein-Barr virus in preinvasive lesions related to nasopharyngeal carcinoma. N Engl J Med 333:693, 1995.

48. KIRPALANI-JOSHI S, LAW HY: Identification of integrated Epstein-Barr virus in nasopharyngeal carcinoma using pulse field gel electrophoresis. Int J Cancer 56:187, 1994.

49. HORDING U et al: Nasopharyngeal carcinoma: Histopathologic types and association with Epstein-Barr virus. Oral Oncol Eur J Cancer 29:137, 1993.

50. RAAB-TRAUB N et al: The differentiated form of nasopharyngeal carcinoma contains Epstein-Barr virus DNA. Int J Cancer 39:25, 1987.

51. CHOW WH et al: Tobacco use and nasopharyngeal carcinoma in a cohort of US veterans. Int J Cancer 55:539, 1993.

52. ZHU K et al: A population based case-control study of the relationship between cigarette smoking and nasopharyngeal cancer. Cancer Causes Control 6:507, 1995.

53. ZONG YS et al: Immunoglobulin A against viral capsid antigen of Epstein-Barr virus and indirect mirror examination of the nasopharynx in the detection of asymptomatic nasopharyngeal carcinoma. Cancer 69:3, 1992.

54. APPLEBAUM E et al: Lymphoepithelioma of the nasopharynx. Laryngoscope 92:510, 1982.

55. LEE AW et al: Retrospective analysis of 5037 patients with nasopharyngeal carcinoma treated during 1976–1985: Overall survival and patterns of failure. Int J Rad Oncol Biol Phys 23:261, 1992.

56. MICHEAU C et al: Bone marrow biopsies in patients with undifferentiated carcinoma of nasopharyngeal type. Br J Radiol 60:2459, 1987.

57. CELAI E et al: Computed tomography in nasopharyngeal carcinoma. Part II impact on survival. Int J Rad Oncol Biol Phys 19:1177, 1990.

58. AMERICAN JOINT COMMITTEE ON CANCER: *AJCC Cancer Staging Manual*, 5th ed. Philadelphia, Lippincott-Raven, 1997.

59. TANG SGJ et al: Prognostic factors of nasopharyngeal carcinoma: A multivariate analysis. Int J Radiat Oncol Biol Phys 19:1143, 1990.

60. CHEN WZ et al: Long-term observation after radiotherapy for nasopharyngeal carcinoma. Int J Radiat Oncol Biol Phys 16:311, 1989.

61. HOPPE RT et al: Carcinoma of the nasopharynx: The significance of histology. Int J Radiat Oncol Biol Phys 4:199, 1978.

62. PEREZ CA et al: Carcinoma of the nasopharynx: Factors affecting prognosis. Int J Radiat Oncol Biol Phys 23:271, 1992.

63. SHAM JST et al: Nasopharyngeal carcinoma: The significance of neck node involvement in relation to the pattern of distant failure. Br J Radiol 63:108, 1990.

64. MARCIAL VA et al: Concomitant cisplatin chemotherapy and radiation therapy in advanced mucosal squamous cell carcinoma of the head and neck. Cancer 66:1861, 1990.

65. LARAMORE GE et al: Nasopharyngeal carcinoma in Saudi Arabia: A retrospective study of 166 cases treated with curative intent. Int J Radiat Oncol Biol Phys 15:1119, 1988.

66. WANG CC: Accelerated hyperfractionated radiation therapy for carcinoma of the nasopharynx. Cancer 63:2461, 1989.

67. GEARA FB et al: Carcinoma of the nasopharynx treated by radiotherapy alone: Determinants of distant metastasis and survival. Radiother Oncol 43:53, 1997.

68. SANGUINETTI G et al: Carcinoma of the nasopharynx treated by radiotherapy alone: Determinants of local and regional control. Int J Radiat Oncol Biol Phys 37:985, 1997.

69. CMELAK AJ et al: Radiosurgery for skull base malignancies and nasopharyngeal carcinoma. Int J Radiat Oncol Biol Phys 37:997, 1997.

70. AL-SARRAF M et al: Superiority of chemo-radiotherapy vs radiotherapy in patients with locally advanced nasopharyngeal cancer. Proc Am Soc Clin Oncol (ASCO) 15:abstr 882, 1996.

71. CVITKOVIC E: Neoadjuvant chemotherapy (NACT) with epirubicin, cisplatin and bleomycin (BEC) in undifferentiated nasopharyngeal carcinoma type: Preliminary results of an international phase III trial. International Nasopharynx Study Group. Proc Am Soc Clin Oncol (ASCO) 13:abstr 915, 1994.

72. HUANG SC et al: Nasopharyngeal cancer: Study III. A review of 1206 patients treated with combined modalities. Int J Radiat Oncol Biol Phys 11:1789, 1985.

73. INTERNATIONAL NASOPHARYNX STUDY GROUP: Preliminary results of a randomized trial comparing neoadjuvant chemotherapy (cisplatin, epirubucin, bleomycin) plus radiotherapy with radiotherapy alone in undifferentiated nasopharyngeal carcinoma: A positive effect of progression-free survival. International Nasopharynx Study Group VUMCA I trial. Int J Radiat Oncol Biol Phys 35:463, 1996.

74. YAN J et al: Radiation therapy of recurrent nasopharyngeal carcinoma: Report of 219 patients. Acta Radiol Oncol 22:23, 1983.

75. WANG CC: Reirradiation of recurrent nasopharyngeal carcinoma: Treatment techniques and results. Int J Radiat Oncol Biol Phys 13:953, 1987.

76. PRYZANT RM et al: Retreatment of nasopharyngeal carcinoma in 53 patients. Int J Radiat Oncol Biol Phys 22:941, 1992.

77. FEE WE et al: Long-term survival after surgical resection for recurrent nasophayngeal cancer after radiotherapy failure. Arch Otolaryngol Head Neck Surg 117:1233, 1991.

78. TU G et al: Salvage surgery for nasopharyngeal carcinoma. Arch Otolaryngol Head Neck Surg 114:328, 1988.

79. WEI WI et al: Surgical resection for nasopharynx cancer, in *Head and Neck Cancer*, vol III, JT Johnson, MS Didolkar (eds). Amsterdam, Elsevier Science, 1993, pp 465–478.

80. HSU MM et al: Salvage surgery for recurrent nasopharyngeal carcinoma. Arch Otolaryngol Head Neck Surg 123:305, 1997.

81. SHAH JP et al: Patterns of care for cancer of the larynx in the United States. Arch Otolaryngol Head Neck Surg 123:475, 1997.

82. MEYERS EM, ALVI A: Management of carcinoma of the supraglottic larynx: Evolution, current concepts and future trends. Laryngoscope 106:559, 1996.

83. LEVENDAG P et al: The problem of neck relapse in early stage supraglottic carcinoma. Cancer 63:345, 1989.

84. NGUYEN TD et al: Advanced carcinoma of the larynx: Results of surgery and radiotherapy without induction chemotherapy (1980–1985): A multivariate analysis. Int J Radiat Oncol Biol Phys 36:1013, 1996.

85. TUCKER HM: *The Larynx*, 2d ed. New York, Thieme Medical, 1993.

86. GUSSENBAUER C: Uber die erst durch Th. Billorth am menschen ausgefuhrte kehlkopf exterpation. Arch Clin Chir 17:343, 1872.

87. GLUCK T: Die chirurgische therapie des kehlkopfkarzinoms. Jahreshurse Artzt Fortbild 2:20, 1912.

88. COUTARD H: Roentgentherapy of epitheliomas of the tonsillar region, laryngopharynx and larynx from 1920 to 1926. Am J Roentgenol 28:313, 1921.

89. KIRCHNER JA, Som ML: Clinical and histological observations of supraglottic cancer. Ann Otol Laryngol Rhinol 80:638, 1971.

90. ALONZO JM: Conservation surgery for cancer of the larynx. Trans Am Acad Ophthalmol Otolaryngol 51:633, 1947.

91. OGURA JH: Supraglottic subtotal laryngectomy and radical neck dissection for carcinoma of the epiglottis. Laryngoscope 68:983, 1958.

92. OGURA JH et al: Conservation surgery for epidermoid carcinoma of the supraglottic larynx. Laryngoscope 85:1810, 1975.

93. PEARSON BW: Subtotal laryngectomy. Laryngoscope 91:1904, 1981.

94. LACCOURREYE O et al: Glottic carcinoma with a fixed true vocal cord: Outcomes after neoadjuvant chemotherapy and

supracricoid partial laryngectomy with cricohyoidoepiglot-topexy. Otolaryngol Head Neck Surg 114:400, 1996.

95. Jako GJ: Laser surgery of the vocal cords: An experimental study with carbon dioxide lasers on dogs. Laryngoscope 82:2204, 1972.

96. Steiner W: Experience in endoscopic laser surgery of malignant tumors of the upper aerodigestive tract. Adv Otorhinolaryngol 39:135, 1988.

97. Zeitels SM et al: Endoscopic management of early supraglottic cancer. Ann Otol Rhinol Laryngol 99:951, 1990.

98. Singer MI, Blom ED: Tracheoesophageal puncture: A surgical prosthetic method for post laryngectomy speech restoration. Proceedings of the Third International Symposium on Plastic Reconstructive Surgery of the Head and Neck, 1979.

99. The Department of Veterans Affairs Laryngeal Cancer Study Group: Induction chemotherapy plus radiation in patients with advanced laryngeal cancer. N Engl J Med 324:1685, 1991.

100. Lefebvre J et al: Larynx preservation in pyriform sinus cancer: Preliminary results of a European Organization for Research and Treatment of Cancer phase III trial. J Natl Cancer Inst 88:890, 1996.

101. Beauvillain C et al: Final results of a randomized trial comparing chemotherapy plus radiotherapy with chemotherapy plus surgery plus radiotherapy in locally advanced resectable hypopharyngeal carcinomas. Laryngoscope 107:648, 1997.

102. Kraus DH et al: Larynx preservation with combined chemotherapy and radiation therapy in advanced hypopharynx cancer. Otolarynogol Head Neck Surg 11:31, 1994.

103. Kraus DH et al: Combined surgery and radiation therapy for squamous cell carcinoma of the hypopharynx. Otolaryngol Head Neck Surg 116:637, 1997.

104. Zelefsky MJ et al: Combined chemotherapy and radiotherapy versus surgery and postoperative radiotherapy for advanced hypopharyngeal cancer. Head Neck 18:405, 1996.

105. Mendenhall WM et al: The role of radiation therapy in laryngeal cancer. CA Cancer J Clin 40:150, 1990.

106. Hong WK et al: Induction chemotherapy in advanced head and neck cancer with high dose cisplatin and bleomycin infusion. Cancer 44:19, 1979.

107. Weaver A et al: Superior clinical responses and survival with initial bolus of cisplatin and 120 hour infusion of 5-fluorouracil before definitive therapy for locally advanced head and neck cancer. Am J Surg 144:445, 1982.

108. Lazarus CL et al: Swallowing disorders in head and neck cancer patients treated with radiotherapy and adjuvant chemotherapy. Laryngoscope 106:1157, 1996.

109. Close LG: Tumors of the salivary glands, in Surgical Oncology, EM Copeland III (ed). New York, Wiley, 1983, pp 153–166.

110. Nussbaum M et al: Parotid space tumors of non-salivary origin. Ann Surg 183:10, 1976.

111. Foote FW, Frazell EL: Tumors of the major salivary glands. Cancer 6:1065, 1953.

112. Richardson GS et al: Tumors of salivary glands: An analysis of 752 cases. Plast Reconstruct Surg 55:131, 1975.

113. Spiro RH: Salivary neoplasms: Overview of a 35-year experience with 2,807 patients. Head Neck Surg 8:177, 1986.

114. Snyderman NL, Johnson JT: Salivary gland tumors: Diagnostic characteristics of the common types. Postgrad Med 82:105, 1987.

115. Conley J et al: Analysis of 115 patients with tumors of the submandibular gland. Ann Otolaryngol 81:323, 1972.

116. Batsakis JG et al: The pathology of head and neck tumors: Salivary glands, part 3. Head Neck Surg 1:260, 1979.

117. Skolnik EM et al: Tumors of the major salivary glands. Laryngoscope 87:843, 1977.

118. Eneroth CM: Incidence and prognosis of salivary-gland tumours at different sites: A study of parotid, submandibular and palatal tumours in 2,632 patients. Acta Otolaryngol 263:174, 1970.

119. Hugo NE et al: Management of tumors of the parotid gland. Surg Clin N Am 53:105, 1973.

120. Lesser RW, Spector JG: Facial nerve palsy associated with Warthin's tumor. Arch Otolaryngol 111:548, 1985.

121. Eveson JW, Cawson RA: Warthin's tumor (cystadeno-lymphoma) of salivary glands: A clinicopathologic investigation of 278 cases. Oral Surg 61:256, 1986.

122. Lamelas J et al: Warthin's tumor: Multicentricity and increasing incidence in women. Am J Surg 154:347, 1987.

123. Synderman C et al: Extraparotid Warthin's tumor. Otolaryngol Head Neck Surg 94:169, 1986.

124. Jakobsson PA et al: Mucoepidermoid carcinoma of the parotid gland. Cancer 22:111, 1968.

125. Spiro RH et al: Mucoepidermoid carcinoma of salivary gland orgin. Am J Surg 136:461, 1978.

126. Spiro RH et al: Cancer of the parotid gland: A clinicopathologic study of 288 primary cases. Am J Surg 130:452, 1975.

127. Eneroth CM et al: Malignant tumors of the submandibular gland. Acta Otolaryngol 263:174, 1970.

128. Spiro RH et al: Cancer of the parotid gland: A clinicopathologic study of 288 primary cases. Am J Surg 130:452, 1975.

129. Healey WV et al: Mucoepidermoid carcinoma of salivary gland origin: Classification, clinical-pathologic correlation and results of treatment. Cancer 26:368, 1970.

130. O'Brien CJ et al: Malignant salivary tumors: Analysis of prognostic factors and survival. Head Neck Surg 9:82, 1986.

131. Mustard RA, Anderson WM: Malignant tumors of the parotid. Ann Surg 159:291, 1964.

132. Byers RM et al: Malignant tumors of the submaxillary gland Am J Surg 126:458, 1973.

133. Perzin KH et al: Adenoid cystic carcinomas arising in salivary glands. Cancer 42:265, 1978.

134. Blanck C et al: Poorly differentiated solid parotid carcinoma. Acta Radiol Ther Physics Biol 13:17, 1974.

135. Illes RW, Brian MB: A review of the tumors of the salivary gland. Surg Gynecol Obstet 163:399, 1986.

136. Levin JM et al: Acinic cell carcinoma. Arch Surg 110:64, 1975.

137. Skolnik E et al: Tumors of the major salivary glands. Laryngoscope 87:843, 1977.

138. Spiro RH et al: Acinic cell carcinoma of salivary origin. Cancer 41:924, 1978.

139. Chong GC et al: Surgical management of acinic cell carcinoma of the parotid gland. Surg Gynecol Obstet 138:65, 1974.

140. Eneroth CM et al: Acinic cell carcinoma of the parotid gland. Cancer 19:1761, 1966.

141. Hickman RE et al: The prognosis of specific types of salivary gland tumors. Cancer 54:1620, 1984.

142. Beahrs OH, Chong GC: Management of the facial nerve in parotid gland surgery Am J Surg 124:473, 1972.

143. Matsuba HM et al: Adenocarcinomas of major and minor salivary gland origin: A histopathologic review of treatment failure patterns. Laryngoscope 98:784, 1988.

144. Batsakis JG, Regesi JA: The pathology of head and neck tumors: Salivary glands, part 4. Head Neck Surg 1:340, 1979.

145. SZANTO PA et al: Histologic grading of adenoid cystic carcinoma of the salivary glands. Cancer 54:1062, 1984.

146. MATSUBA HM et al: Adenoid cystic salivary gland carcinoma: A histopathologic review of treatment failure patterns. Cancer 57:519, 1986.

147. ——— et al: Adenoid cystic carcinoma of major and minor salivary gland origin. Laryngoscope 94:1316, 1984.

148. VIKRAM B et al: Radiation therapy in adenoid-cystic carcinoma. Int J Rad Oncol Biol Phys 10:221, 1984.

149. AMPIL FL, MISRA RP: Factors influencing survival of patients with adenoid cystic carcinoma of the salivary glands. J Oral Maxillofacial Surg 45:1005, 1987.

150. SHINGAKI S et al: Adenoid cystic carcinoma of the major and minor salivary glands: A clinicopathological study of 17 cases. J Maxillofacial Surg 14:53, 1986.

151. SPIRO RH et al: Tumors of the submaxillary gland. Am J Surg 132:463, 1976.

152. SHEMEN LJ et al: Squamous cell carcinoma of salivary gland origin. Head Neck Surg 9:235, 1987.

153. LEIPZIG B, GONZLAES-VITALE JC: Small cell epidermoid carcinoma of salivary glands: Pseudo-oat cell carcinoma. Arch Otolaryngol 108:511, 1982.

154. SHIKHANI A et al: Primary lymphoma in the salivary glands: Report of five cases and review of the literature. Laryngoscope 97:1438, 1987.

155. NIME FA et al: Primary malignant lymphomas of the salivary glands. Cancer 37:906, 1976.

156. NICHOLS RD et al: Lymphoma of the parotid gland. Laryngoscope 92:365, 1982.

157. SCHUSTERMAN MA et al: Lymphoma presenting as a salivary gland mass. Head Neck Surg 10:411, 1988.

158. TORTOLEDO ME et al: Carcinomas ex pleomorphic adenoma and malignant mixed tumors: Histomorphologic indexes. Arch Otolaryngol 110:172, 1984.

159. STEPHEN J et al: True malignant mixed tumors (carcinosarcoma) of salivary glands. Oral Surg 61:597, 1986.

160. CHEN KTK et al: Carcinosarcoma of the salivary gland. Am J Otolaryngol 5:415, 1984.

161. BIORKLUND A, ENEROTH CM: Management of parotid gland neoplasms. Am J Otolaryngol 1:155, 1980.

162. ENEROTH CM: Facial nerve paralysis: A criterion of malignancy in parotid tumors. Arch Otolaryngol 95:300, 1972.

163. BRODERICK JP et al: Facial paralysis and occult parotid cancer: A characteristic syndrome. Arch Otolaryngol Head Neck Surg 114:195, 1988.

164. SULLIVAN MJ et al: Intraparotid facial nerve neurofibroma. Laryngoscope 97:219, 1987.

165. SNYDERMAN C et al: Facial paralysis: Traumatic neuromas vs facial nerve neoplasms. Otolaryngol Head Neck Surg 98:53, 1988.

166. WITTICH GR et al: Ultrasonography of the salivary glands. Radiol Clin North Am 23:29, 1985.

167. SWARTZ JD et al: High resolution computed tomography, part 2: The salivary glands and oral cavity. Head Neck Surg 7:150, 1984.

168. SCHAEFER SD et al: Evaluation of NMR versus CT for parotid masses: A preliminary report. Laryngoscope 95:945, 1985.

169. RICE DH, BECKER T: Magnetic resonance imaging of the salivary glands: A comparison with computed tomographic scanning. Arch Otolaryngol Head Neck Surg 113:78, 1987.

170. ENEROTH CM et al: Aspiration biopsy of salivary gland tumors: A critical review of 910 biopsies. Acta Cytol 11:470, 1967.

171. BERG HM et al: Correlation of fine needle aspiration biopsy and CT scanning of parotid masses. Laryngoscope 96:1357, 1986.

172. FRABLE MA, FRABLE WJ: Fine-needle aspiration biopsy revisited. Laryngoscope 92:1414, 1982.

173. WOODS JE: Parotidectomy versus limited resection for benign parotid masses. Am J Surg 149:749, 1985.

174. NIGRO MF, SPIRO RH: Deep lobe parotid tumors. Am J Surg 134:523, 1977.

175. BAKER DC, CONLEY J: Surgical approach to retromandibular parotid tumors. Ann Plastic Surg 3:304, 1979.

176. RICHARDSON GS et al: Tumors of salivary glands: An analysis of 752 cases. Plastic Reconstruct Surg 55:131, 1975.

177. WANG CC: The management of parotid lymph node metastases by irradiation. Cancer 50:223, 1982.

178. GUILLAMONDEGUI OM et al: Aggressive surgery in treatment for parotid cancer: The role of adjunctive postoperative radiotherapy. Am J Roentgenol 123:49, 1975.

179. BYERS RM: Treatment of malignant tumors of the parotid and submaxillary glands. Resident Staff Physician 28:52, 1982.

180. FU KK et al: Carcinoma of the major and minor salivary glands: Analysis of treatment results and sites and causes of failures. Cancer 40:2882, 1977.

181. CHUNG CT et al: The changing role of external-beam irradiation in the management of malignant tumors of the major salivary glands. Radiology 145:175, 1982.

182. MATSUBA HM et al: High-grade malignancies of the parotid gland: Effective use of planned combined surgery and irradiation. Laryngoscope 95:1059, 1985.

183. REDDY SP, MARKS JE: Treatment of locally advanced high-grade malignant tumors of major salivary glands. Laryngoscope 98:450, 1988.

184. RENTSCHLER R et al: Chemotherapy of malignant major salivary gland neoplasms: A 25-year review of M.D. Anderson Hospital experience. Cancer 40:619, 1977.

185. SUEN JY, JOHNS ME: Chemotherapy for salivary gland cancer. Laryngoscope 92:235, 1982.

186. KAPLAN MJ et al: Chemotherapy for salivary gland cancer. Otolaryngol Head Neck Surg 95:165, 1986.

187. BATSAKIS JG, REGEZI JA: The pathology of head and neck tumors. Salivary glands, part I. Head Neck Surg 1:59, 1978.

188. BYERS RM et al: Malignant parotid tumors in patients under 20 years of age. Arch Otolaryngol 110:232, 1984.

189. ENEROTH CM: Salivary gland tumors in the parotid gland, submandibular gland and the palate region. Cancer 27:1415, 1971.

190. SPIRO RH et al: Adenoid cystic carcinoma of salivary origin: A clinicopathologic study of 242 cases. Am J Surg 128:512, 1974.

191. ENEROTH CM: Histological and clinical aspects of parotid tumors. Acta Otolaryngol Supplement (Suppl):191, 1963.

192. MUSTARD RA, ANDERSON W: Malignant tumors of the parotid. Ann Surg 159:291, 1964.

193. ROUVIERE H: Anatomy of the Human Lymphatic System. Edwards Brothers, Ann Arbor, MI, 1938.

194. HAAGENSEN CD et al (eds): The Lymphatics in Cancer. Philadelphia, Saunders, 1972.

195. ROBBINS KT et al: Standardizing neck dissection terminology. Arch Otolaryngol Head Neck Surg 117:601, 1991.

196. BUTLIN HI, SPENCER WG: Diseases of the Tongue, 2d ed. London, Cassell, 1900.

197. CRILE G: Excision of cancer of the head and neck with special reference to the plan of dissection based on one hundred and thirty-two operations. J Am Med Assoc 47:1780, 1906.

198. MARTIN H: The treatment of cervical metastatic cancer. Ann Surg 114:972, 1944.

199. BOCCA E et al: Functional neck dissection: An evaluation and review of 843 cases. Laryngoscope 94:942, 1984.

200. BYERS RM: Modified neck dissection: A study of 967 cases from 1970 to 1980. Am J Surg 150:414, 1985.

201. BYERS RM et al: Rationale for modified neck dissection. Head Neck Surg 10:160, 1988.

202. TEICHGAEBER JF, CLAIRMONT AA: Incidence of occult metastases for cancer of the oral tongue and floor of mouth: Treatment rationale. Head Neck Surg 7:15, 1984.

203. SPIRO JD et al: Critical assessment of supraomohyoid neck dissection. Am J Surg 156:286, 1988.

204. DAVIDSON BJ et al: Posterior triangle metastases of squamous cell carcinoma of the upper aerodigestive tract. Am J Surg 166:395, 1993.

205. ARMSTRONG JG et al: The indication of elective treatment of the neck in cancer of the major salivary glands. Cancer 69:615, 1992.

206. SHAH JP et al: Patterns of regional lymph node metastasis from cutaneous melanoma of the head and neck. Am J Surg 162:320, 1991.

# CHAPTER 9

# NEOPLASMS OF THE LUNG

*Nael Martini and Robert J. Ginsberg*

## PRIMARY LUNG CANCERS

In the United States, lung cancer is the leading cause of cancer death in both men and women. The American Cancer Society projects the lung cancer incidence to be 164,100 new cases for the year 2000,[1] with a male-to-female ratio of 1.2:1. Despite our best efforts, the overall 5-year survival rate has remained low, and is again estimated for this year to be less than 10%.

Approximately 85% of all lung cancers occur in cigarette smokers. Despite the concerted efforts to curtail smoking by establishing smoke-free environments in public transportation, department stores, hospitals, and restaurants, and despite preventing cigarette advertising on radio and television, more than 50 million Americans smoke. The United States remains the leading exporter of tobacco in the world. Extensive lobbying by tobacco companies from states whose economy and viability depend on the tobacco industry continues to undermine efforts to curtail cigarette smoking.

With few exceptions, prognosis in lung cancer is influenced by the stage of the disease at presentation and by the treatment that can be rendered (Fig. 9-1). Curative treatment requires earlier detection and effective control of the primary tumor before metastasis occurs. Surgical treatment of lung cancer is still regarded as the most effective method of cure, provided a complete resection is possible and the risks of the procedure are low. It is the therapy of choice for early-stage non–small cell lung cancer.

Lung cancers, as classified by the World Health Organization, encompass non–small cell cancers that include squamous cell carcinomas, adenocarcinomas, and large cell carcinomas, and small cell lung cancers.[2] In North America, adenocarcinoma is currently the most frequent histologic type and makes up nearly one-half of all cases, squamous cell carcinoma accounts for one-third, and large cell carcinoma about 15%. In the rest of the world, squamous cell carcinoma continues to be the most prevalent.

It is now standard practice to carefully stage all lung cancers at the time of their initial presentation. The American Joint Committee for Cancer's TNM Staging System has been used since 1972 and the International Staging System since 1986.[3] Both were revised

in 1997.[4,5] Briefly stated, tumors confined to lung without any metastasis, regional or distant, are classified as stage I. All other localized tumors are classified as stage II or III disease, and tumors presenting with distant metastases (M1) are classified as stage IV tumors (Tables 9-1 and 9-2).

More than 90% of lung tumors can be diagnosed and staged accurately without thoracotomy by one or more of the following procedures: percutaneous fine-needle aspiration, bronchoscopy, mediastinoscopy or mediastinotomy, thoracoscopy, and biopsy of accessible metastases, for instance, cervical lymph nodes. This approach has become particularly important when preoperative therapy is under consideration. Histologic documentation of mediastinal lymph node involvement will currently prompt serious consideration for combined modality treatment. Failing a pretreatment diagnosis and staging of patients, an exploratory thoracatomy is advised. This occurs in less than 10% of patients. The use of positron emission tomography (PET) scanning in diagnosis and staging is currently being investigated.

Surgical treatment is generally offered to all patients with stage I or II disease and to specific groups of patients with stage II disease.

In discussing therapy, we will refer to our own experience, which is consistent with other reports in the literature, and will indicate those areas where controversy still exists.

### OCCULT CARCINOMAS

Very few patients with lung cancer are diagnosed before the cancer becomes apparent on chest roentgenogram, accounting for less than 1% of the lung cancer population.[6] In this "occult" group, diagnosis usually is established on sputum cytology or by bronchoscopy in patients presenting with an unexplained cough or hemoptysis and a normal chest roentgenogram.

For cancers detected on sputum cytology, the source of the cancer cells must be identified. For instance, cancer cells may originate from a head and neck primary tumor or from other upper aerodigestive sources. After a negative head and neck evaluation, localization of

**TABLE 9-1.** TNM DESCRIPTORS FROM THE REVISED INTERNATIONAL STAGING SYSTEM FOR LUNG CANCER—1997

### T—PRIMARY TUMOR

| | |
|---|---|
| TX | Primary tumor cannot be assessed, or tumor proven by the presence of malignant cells in sputum or bronchial washings but not visualized by imaging or bronchoscopy. |
| T0 | No evidence of primary tumor |
| Tis | Carcinoma in situ |
| T1 | Tumor 3 cm in greatest dimension, surrounded by lung or visceral pleura, without bronchoscopic evidence of invasion more proximal than the lobar bronchus |
| T2 | Tumor with any of the following features of size or extent:<br>>3 cm in greatest dimension<br>Involves main bronchus, 2 cm distal to the carina<br>Invades the visceral pleura<br>Associated with atelectasis or obstructive pneumonitis that extends to the hilar region but does not involve the entire lung. |
| T3 | Tumor of any size that directly invades any of the following: chest wall (including superior sulcus tumors), diaphragm, mediastinal pleura, parietal pericardium; or tumor in the main bronchus <2 cm distal to the carina, but without involvement of the carina; or atelectasis or obstructive pneumonitis of the entire lung. |
| T4 | Tumor of any size that invades any of the following: mediastinum, heart, great vessels, trachea, esophagus, vertebral body, carina; separate tumor nodule(s) in the same lobe; tumor with a malignant pleural or pericardial effusion. |

### N—REGIONAL LYMPH NODES

| | |
|---|---|
| NX | Regional lymph nodes cannot be assessed |
| N0 | No regional lymph node metastasis |
| N1 | Metastasis in ipsilateral peribronchial and/or hilar lymph nodes and intrapulmonary nodes, including involvement by direct extension |
| N2 | Metastasis in ipsilateral mediastinal and/or subcarinal lymph nodes(s) |
| N3 | Metastasis in contralateral mediastinal, contralateral hilar, ipsilateral or contralateral scalene, or supraclavicular lymph node(s) |

### M—DISTANT METASTASIS

| | |
|---|---|
| MX | Distant metastasis cannot be assessed |
| M0 | No distant metastasis |
| M1 | Distant metastasis, includes separate tumor nodule(s) in a different lobe (ipsilateral or contralateral) |

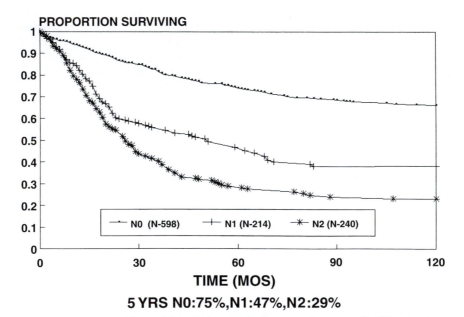

**FIGURE 9-1.** Survival by nodal status in completely resected non–small cell lung cancer.

**TABLE 9-2.** STAGE GROUPING BY TNM SUBSETS (REVISED INTERNATIONAL STAGING SYSTEM FOR LUNG CANCER—1997)

| STAGE | TNM SUBSET |
|---|---|
| 0 | Carcinoma in situ |
| | TXN0M0 |
| IA | T1N0M0 |
| IB | T2N0M0 |
| IIA | T1N1M0 |
| IIB | T2N1M0 |
| | T3N0M0 |
| IIIA | T3N1M0 |
| | T1N2M0 |
| | T2N2M0 |
| | T3N2M0 |
| IIIB | T4N0M0 |
| | T4N1M0 |
| | T4N2M0 |
| | T1N3M0 |
| | T2N3M0 |
| | T3N3M0 |
| | T4N3M0 |
| IV | Any T any N M1 |

occult lung tumors is accomplished by fiberoptic bronchoscopy. If a lesion is seen, a biopsy is obtained for confirmation. If a lesion is not seen, repeated positive brushings from an isolated segment are acceptable for localization. Otherwise, diagnosis is deferred and bronchoscopy repeated in 2 to 3 months.[6,7] Recently, fluorescent staining of bronchial mucosa with hematoporphyrin derivatives and laser-induced autofluorescence have improved bronchoscopic localization.[8,9]

Histologically, 90% of occult lung cancers are squamous carcinomas, and 10% are either adenocarcinomas or large cell carcinomas.[6,7] Surgical treatment is curative in this small group of patients. After localization, the treatment of choice is removal of the primary tumor by lobectomy, pneumonectomy, or segmentectomy. Frequently, sleeve resections combined with these procedures can be used to preserve lung function. Because most occult lung cancers are located in major airways, wedge resections usually are not possible. Although recurrent tumor after resection is extremely rare, the risk of a patient developing a *new* lung cancer is as high as 45%, suggesting "field cancerization" in such cases.[6]

Photodynamic therapy using transbronchoscopic laser-induced photoexcitation of hematoporphyrin derivative has been shown to be effective in eradicating occult in situ endobronchial lung cancers and can be considered as an alternative therapy, especially in patients who cannot tolerate a surgical resection.[10–12] Once invasive carcinoma has been identified, treatment with hematoporphyrin is not curative, and primary resection is necessary. Historically, patients

treated solely by external irradiation ultimately died of recurrent disease. In patients unable to tolerate a surgical approach, endoluminal brachytherapy and/or three-dimensional conformal high-dose external radiotherapy is appropriate.

## STAGE I LUNG CANCER

This is the most common form of early lung cancer seen by most physicians. Many cases are detected on routine chest films in patients that present for unrelated medical conditions. Most are discrete peripheral tumors. Computed tomographic (CT) scans are routinely done on these patients to assess the mediastinum, the liver, and the adrenal glands. Full-organ scanning as a screening for metastases beyond the CT scan has not been shown to be cost-effective. Routine mediastinoscopy remains controversial if the CT scan is negative.[13] If no mediastinal nodal involvement is suspected, these patients are recommended to undergo surgical therapy.

The new TNM classification subdivides stage I tumors into stage IA for those 3 cm in diameter or less but without visceral pleural invasion and to stage IB for tumors greater than 3 cm in diameter or tumors of any size associated with visceral pleural involvement.

For all patients with clinical stage I disease, surgical resection is the treatment of choice whenever possible. However, at the time of final pathologic staging, despite all preoperative efforts, a significant number of patients are found to have been understaged. In a prospective validation of the International Union Against Cancer TNM Classification, the data of 3823 patients were analyzed for concordance with clinically and pathologically confirmed TNM stages. The agreement in stage I disease was only 61%.[14]

For many stage I patients, lobectomy is the surgical treatment of choice because it encompasses all disease and preserves lung function. Infrequently, with more proximal tumors, pneumonectomy is required, although, a sleeve lobectomy often is sufficient for cure and allows preservation of functioning pulmonary tissue.

Limited resection (i.e., wedge resection or segmentectomy) is not recommended as standard therapy in the management of stage I lung cancer. This treatment is reserved for patients who cannot tolerate a lobectomy but who can be resected completely by this lesser operation.[15]

In a recent review of our experience at Memorial Sloan-Kettering Cancer Center with complete resection of stage I non–small cell lung cancer, 598 patients were analyzed.[16,17] T1 tumors (stage IA) were found in 49% of the patients and T2 tumors (stage IB) in 51%. Lobectomy was performed in 85% of the patients, pneumonectomy in 4%, and wedge resection or segmentectomy in 11%. Of the last group, nearly 90% had T1 tumors. A mediastinal lymph node dissection was carried out in 560 patients (94%) and lymph node sampling in 38 (6%). Almost all (99%) of the patients were observed for a minimum of 5 years or until death (median follow-up: 91 months). The 30-day surgical mortality rate was 2.3%.

The overall 5- and 10-year survival rates were 75% and 67%. Survival of patients with T1 tumors (stage IA) was 82% at 5 years and 74% at 10 years, compared with 68% at 5 years and 60% at 10 years for those with T2 tumors ( $p < 0.0004$ ) (Fig. 9-2). Because the exact diameter of each resected tumor was recorded, each subset (T1 and T2) was analyzed further by tumor size. We found that

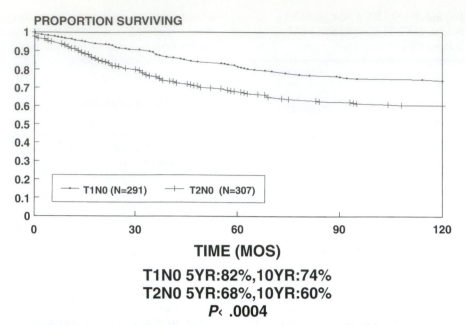

**PROPORTION SURVIVING**

T1N0 5YR:82%,10YR:74%
T2N0 5YR:68%,10YR:60%
$P < .0004$

**FIGURE 9-2.** Survival after resection in stages Ia and Ib non–small cell lung cancer.

tumor size significantly influenced survival among the following groups: tumors less than 1 cm, 1 to 3 cm, greater than 3 to 5 cm, and greater than 5 cm. Patients with T2 tumors involving the visceral pleural but up to 3 cm in diameter had survival rates comparable to patients without visceral pleural involvement. Based on our experience, the validity of classifying these patients as IB versus IA by virtue of visceral pleural involvement alone is questionable.

During the course of follow-up, 159 patients (27%) developed recurrence, most within 5 years of treatment, although 9% developed a recurrence later than 5 years.[16] The first sites of recurrence were mostly distant and were not influenced by histology (local, 20%; regional, 8%; and distant, 72%). The most common site of distant metastasis was the brain.

Resection less extensive than lobectomy and no lymph node dissection had adverse effects on recurrence. Of patients who had wedge resection or segmentectomy, 50% had a recurrence ($p = 0.00002$), half of which were local or regional recurrences. Of patients who had no formal lymph node dissection, 55% had recurrences ($p = 0.00008$), 71% of which were local recurrences. Only 5% of all recurrences were local or regional in patients who had mediastinal lymph node dissection.

The Lung Cancer Study Group completed a randomized clinical trial of lobectomy versus a lesser resection by wedge or segmentectomy in stage I carcinomas presenting as small peripheral tumors.[15] There was a threefold increase in the incidence of local recurrence in patients treated by lesser resections than lobectomy.

The Memorial Sloan-Kettering experience confirms other reports[18–20] that patients undergoing a pulmonary resection less extensive than a lobectomy had a poorer survival and higher local recurrence rate, with the 5- and 10-year survival rates for pneumonectomy or lobectomy being 77% and 70%, respectively, compared with 59% and 35% in patients with lesser resections ($p = 0.026$).

The incidence of recurrence was influenced also by the T factor and by tumor size. This experience was statistically significant between T1 and T2 tumors ($p = 0.0004$). An interesting observation was the number of second primary cancers occurring in the surviving patients. There were 206 patients who had second cancers, an overall incidence of 34%. This was similar among histologies. One-third of the second tumors were lung cancers.

Other than tumor stage, there have been no other confirmed predictors of survival. In the past, vascular or lymphatic invasion and tumor differentiation were implicated without substantiation.[21] Recently, blood vessel invasion has been reported to be a main predictor of recurrence in T1N0M0 non–small cell lung cancers.[22] Recent interest in genetic markers has suggested that K-*ras* oncogene expression in tumors (especially adenocarcinoma) may be a negative predictor of survival.[23] Other predictors that have yet to be substantiated include the presence of blood group antigen A, a deletion of the p53 gene, and the presence of aneuploidy. Although there are reports that note that DNA assessment is valuable, it was not prognostic in our experience,[24,25] nor in that of the Lung Cancer Study Group[18] (LCSG).

Because vitamin A and retinoids inhibit epithelial cancer progression in experimental carcinogenesis, several randomized studies have been completed or are currently in progress to assess the merits of retinoids with 13 *cis*-retinoic acid (isotretinoin) or vitamin A in preventing secondary aerodigestive cancer or recurrence in patients cured of lung cancer.[26,27] Chemoprevention studies with vitamin A have shown an adverse effect. The data for retinoids are still viewed as preliminary but show promise and will require several years of follow-up before definitive conclusions can be drawn. At this time, it is recommended that retinoids be offered only in protocol settings.

Radiation therapy is considered an alternative treatment to surgery in patients who cannot undergo or refuse treatment by surgery.[28] Only a limited number of reports in the literature refer to the results of radiation therapy with curative intent in early lung cancer. Smart and Hilton[29] reported the results of external radiation therapy in 33 patients with good performance status, technically resectable lesions, and no evidence of mediastinal node involvement. The 5-year survival rate was 33%. In 1976, Schumacher[30] reported his experience with external radiation therapy in stage I and II patients. His 5-year survival rate was 31% (13 of 42 patients). Cooper et al.[31] reported a 5-year survival rate of 6% for patients with operable lung cancer treated by radiation alone (4 of 67). It should be noted that none of these reports treated patients with doses now considered to be adequate. As well, current treatment concepts include adding chemotherapy as a radiation sensitizer.[32,33]

Chemotherapy alone as primary treatment in this stage of disease is not recommended. The role of adjuvant radiotherapy, chemotherapy, or a combination of both after surgical resection for stage I lung cancer is also unclear. Several randomized trials in the past two decades have failed to show a survival benefit when adjuvant therapy is added to surgical resection. A host of immunopotentiators and chemotherapeutic agents have been tested as adjuvants in resected stage I disease. A survival advantage was noted initially in patients treated with intrapleural bacille Calmette-Guérin (BCG).[34] However, this benefit was not confirmed in a large multicenter study by the LCSG.[35] Other immunotherapeutic approaches were intradermal BCG, oral levamisole, and intravenous *Corynebacterium parvum*. They also have not been shown to be effective. In a study by the LCSG, patients with completely resected T2N0 tumors were randomized to receive either CAP [cyclophosphamide, adriamycin (doxorubicin), cisplatin] chemotherapy or no further treatment.[36] There was no benefit demonstrated for the CAP chemotherapy. A recent metaanalysis of all studies confirms this disappointing result.[37]

At this time, no adjuvant treatment is recommended for patients with stage I disease after resection, although ongoing phase III trials are being conducted.

## T1N1 AND T2N1 TUMORS

Tumors confined to the lung or bronchus with involvement of bronchopulmonary or hilar lymph nodes as the sole site of tumor spread (T1–2N1 disease) make up less than 5% of the lung cancer population and less than 10% of all resected lung cancers.[17,38] We reviewed our experience at Memorial Sloan-Kettering Cancer Center on the surgical treatment of these patients.[39] From 1973 to 1989, 214 patients had undergone a complete resection with a mediastinal lymph node dissection. Of these, 35 patients had T1N1 lesions (stage IIA) and 179, T2N1 (stage IIB) tumors. The male-female ratio was 2:1, and the median age was 62 years. There were 116 adenocarcinomas and 98 squamous cancers.

Lobectomy was the procedure of choice in most patients. A lobectomy was performed in 68%, pneumonectomy in 31%, and a wedge resection or segmentectomy in 1%. Interestingly, one-half of the patients had only a single N1 node involved and 85% of the patients had involvement at a single N1 nodal level (i.e., hilar vs. bronchial vs. segmental).

The overall survival rate after resection (Kaplan-Meier) was 47% at 5 years.[40] There was no difference in survival rates between T1 and T2 tumors (Fig. 9-3). Favorable prognostic factors included the number of involved nodes (one versus more than one) and the size of the primary lesion. There was a significant difference in survival between those with tumors 3 cm or smaller in diameter and those 5 cm or greater. Moreover, the survival rate following resection in patients with involvement of a single lymph node was 45% compared with 31% in patients with multiple lymph node

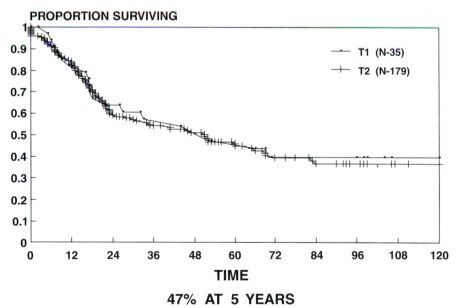

**47% AT 5 YEARS**

**FIGURE 9-3.** Survival following complete resection in T1N1M0 and T2N1M0 non–small cell lung cancer.

involvement. The best survival rate was obtained in patients with small tumors (≤3 cm) and a single N1 node, and the worst survival rate was obtained in those with large tumors (≥5 cm) and multiple N1 nodes (52% vs. 37%). The location of the primary tumor, the location of the N1 nodes, histology, and the presence or absence of visceral pleural involvement had no appreciable impact on survival.

There were more local or regional recurrences in patients with squamous cancers and more distant metastases in patients with adenocarcinoma. The incidence of local or regional recurrence was reduced in our series by the administration of postoperative mediastinal irradiation. However, there was no impact on survival by the addition of postoperative radiation therapy. Recurrence rates were high despite resection. Most patients who did not respond to the initial therapy ultimately developed distant metastases, suggesting the need for an effective systemic treatment, but the specific regimens that benefit this group of patients are still undetermined.

The LCSG randomized 189 patients with resected T1N1 or T2N1 tumors by histology to receive adjuvant treatments. Those with resected squamous cancers were treated by postoperative external radiation or received no further treatment. This study concluded that in squamous carcinoma, postoperative radiation therapy reduced local and regional recurrence but had no impact on survival.[41] In resected stage II adenocarcinomas, postoperative adjuvant trials of chemotherapy, immunotherapy, or combinations of the two have had no effect on survival in randomized studies.[42] A recent meta-analysis of adjuvant radiotherapy suggests an adverse effect of adjuvant radiotherapy.[43]

In another trial comparing postoperative irradiation with chemoirradiation, the LCSG reported some advantages in lengthening the time to recurrence of combined adjuvant radiation and chemotherapy in adenocarcinoma, but no survival benefit.[44] However, this study did not compare or assess adjuvant treatment with chemotherapy alone to no adjuvant treatment in stage II adenocarcinoma. More data are necessary to assess the role and type of adjuvant treatment in these patients.

A Finnish study utilizing CAP chemotherapy as adjuvant treatment but for a longer period of time than any of the LCSG trials has demonstrated an improved survival in the treated group.[45] As well, a Japanese study using oral 5-fluorouracil (5FU) long-term (1 year) shows a favorable effect.[46] Recently, an American cooperative trial (Intergroup 0115) completed a study comparing postoperative radiotherapy to postoperative concomitant chemoradiotherapy for patients with completely resected stage II and stage III disease.[47] We will have to await the results of this trial to see if survival can be improved with simultaneous chemoradiotherapy.

Because most patients die as a result of metastases to distant sites, and since more than 50% of patients with this stage of disease are not cured by surgery alone, or with adjuvant therapy, the role of preoperative (induction) chemotherapy prior to surgery is now being investigated in a multicenter phase II trial in North America[48] and a phase III trial in France.[49]

## TREATMENT OF T3N0M0 TUMORS

Under the new TNM classification, T3N0M0 tumors are stage IIB tumors. In the absence of any regional lymph node metastases

(N1 or N2), this group includes all tumors extending to chest wall, mediastinum, or diaphragm, or tumors in proximity to carina without carinal invasion.

TUMORS INVADING CHEST WALL. Cancers of the lung that invade the chest wall are usually peripheral in position. Hilar or mediastinal lymph node metastases are less likely to occur in this group of patients. These tumors extend to invade the parietal pleura, but some involve the muscles and ribs of the chest wall. Despite the presence of chest wall invasion, significant numbers of these patients are amenable to treatment by resection. Factors that influence survival in this group of patients are:

1. Complete resectability of the tumor
2. The extent of invasion of the chest wall
3. The presence or absence of regional lymph node metastases

In 1985, we reviewed 111 patients with carcinoma of the lung invading the chest wall who were treated surgically.[50] Of these, 67% had a complete resection with an overall 5-year survival rate of 40%. In patients where resection was incomplete (macroscopic or microscopic disease) or not possible, the survival time did not extend beyond 2.5 years. Postoperative radiation therapy in this group of patients did not affect their survival. These results have been confirmed at the Mayo Clinic[51] and by other centers[52] (Table 9-3).

In our experience, the depth of chest wall involvement by the tumor also affected survival. In patients in whom the tumor extended to the parietal pleura but did not penetrate into the soft tissues of the chest wall and the ribs, the 5-year survival rate following complete resection was better than in patients with deeper involvement of the chest wall[50,50a] (62% vs. 35% in patients with T3N0M0 disease). Whether or not en bloc resection of chest wall (versus parietal pleura only) is required in every instance remains controversial.

We favor chest wall reconstruction with a Marlex mesh and methyl methacrylate sandwich technique whenever there is a suspicion of chest wall instability, but rarely find this necessary with resection of fewer than three contiguous rib segments.[53] For such smaller defects, Marlex mesh patch closure ensures acceptable cosmetic results and chest wall stability. Others prefer a Gore-Tex patch for large defects.[54] Very small defects may require no reconstruction, especially if situated posteriorly beneath large muscles or scapula.

## TABLE 9-3. RESULTS OF RESECTION OF BRONCHOGENIC CARCINOMA INVOLVING CHEST WALL

| SERIES | YEAR | n | POSTOPERATIVE MORTALITY RATE, % | 5-YEAR SURVIVAL RATE, % |
|---|---|---|---|---|
| Patterson et al.[52] | 1982 | 35 | 8.5 | 38 |
| Trastek et al.[51a] | 1984 | 73 | 12.3 | 40 |
| McCaughan et al.[50] | 1985 | 125 | 4.0 | 40 |
| Allen et al.[52a] | 1991 | 52 | 3.8 | 26 |
| Albertucci et al.[52b] | 1992 | 37 | 10.8 | 30 |

Like other stages of non–small cell lung cancer, there is no evidence that preoperative radiation therapy benefits patients with tumors invading the chest wall.[50,52] Although postoperative radiation therapy is usually advised in patients with residual disease in an attempt to decrease local recurrence, the efficacy of this treatment as an adjuvant to complete resection has not been addressed in formal trials.

**SUPERIOR SULCUS TUMORS.** Superior sulcus tumors (Pancoast tumors) represent a subset of carcinomas of the lung invading the chest wall. By reason of their location in the pleural apex, they invade adjoining tissues early in their course. These patients are generally symptomatic from the outset. Early invasion of the lower brachial plexus, especially the T1 nerve root, is common. Shoulder and arm pain radiating to the inner aspect of the upper arm (T1), and less often the ulnar distribution in the fourth and fifth fingers of the hand (C8), is a common presenting symptom.[55] Extension to the stellate ganglion with a consequent Horner's syndrome is seen in at least one-third of the patients. Extension to the ribs or vertebrae is also common.

Most superior sulcus tumors are initially diagnosed histologically or cytologically by a percutaneous needle biopsy performed under fluoroscopic or CT guidance. Diagnostic bronchoscopy is less helpful in establishing a tissue diagnosis in this group of patients because of the peripheral position of the lesion, although transbronchoscopic biopsy using image intensification has been successful. The majority of tumors are squamous carcinomas or adenocarcinomas, but 3% to 5% are small cell carcinomas with different therapeutic implications, hence the importance of a tissue diagnosis before treatment.

Shaw[56] and Paulson[57] first advocated the combined use of preoperative radiation and resection and demonstrated a 31% 5-year survival rate. The current standard therapy for this group of patients is a combination of preoperative radiation followed by resection. Therapy begins by a preoperative course of external radiation therapy to a dose of 3000 to 4500 cGy to the tumor. This can be given in 300-cGy fractions over 2 weeks[58] or 1000 cGy per week for a period of $4^1/_2$ weeks.[59] The radiation port generally includes the primary tumor, the adjacent mediastinum, and the ipsilateral supraclavicular area. Following a rest period of 1 month, these patients are assessed for surgery. If no distant disease is evident, they are then offered surgical exploration for removal of the residual tumor.

In most of our patients in whom the tumor is incompletely resected or unresectable, interstitial implantation of radioisotopes (brachytherapy) was used to complete the radiation therapy of the tumor, although additional postoperative radiotherapy may be just as effective.

Having popularized the technique of intraoperative brachytherapy, our center first reported the results of the use of intraoperative brachytherapy combined with preoperative radiotherapy and surgery in the treatment of these tumors in 1971,[60] and updated that report in 1987.[61] It was concluded that preoperative radiotherapy increased the resectability rate, decreased locoregional failure, and improved survival in those patients with complete resection. In patients with incomplete resection, it appeared that partial resection added no benefit to intraoperative brachytherapy alone without resection. Those patients treated in this latter fashion, despite no resection, achieved a 15% 5-year survival rate.

We recently analyzed the results of surgical treatment of all patients presenting with untreated superior sulcus tumors between 1974 and 1991.[55] Most patients received preoperative radiotherapy. Thoracotomy was performed in 124 patients, and 100 patients underwent resection. The overall 5-year survival rate was 26% for all patients. Those patients receiving a complete resection achieved a 41% 5-year survival rate. The best single group were those patients undergoing a lobectomy (versus wedge resection) and en bloc chest wall resection (60% 5-year survival rate). We were unable to demonstrate an advantage for the use of intraoperative brachytherapy in those patients with complete resection. For those patients with incomplete resection treated with brachytherapy combined with preoperative or postoperative external radiation therapy, a 9% 5-year survival rate was observed. Locoregional failure was significant both in patients with complete resection and in patients with incomplete resection. Adverse prognostic factors included Horner's syndrome, N2 and N3 disease, T4 disease, and incomplete resections. We concluded that complete resection of the tumor by en bloc chest wall resection combined with lobectomy and adequate nodal staging remains the surgical treatment of choice.

Whether radiotherapy is used prior to or following surgery is a moot point. We have used both approaches without any evidence of advantage to either. Most recently, to address low resectability and both distant and local failures, a North American phase II trial of induction chemoradiation therapy has been instituted.[62] This study represents the first prospective trial ever initiated for patients with superior sulcus tumors.

**TUMORS IN PROXIMITY TO CARINA.** Another subset of stages IIB and IIIA lung cancers that benefit from surgical management are patients with central tumors that extend within 2 cm of the carina. In many instances, the carina itself is not involved and complete surgical extirpation of the tumor is possible. In patients in whom resection can be undertaken, despite the proximity of the lesion to the carina but without involvement, the 5-year survival rate following resection is reported at 36%.[63–66]

A pneumonectomy is generally required to encompass all of the tumor protruding from a lobal orifice into a main bronchus and to provide clear margins of resection. However, a sleeve lobectomy is a worthwhile alternative and has lower morbidity and mortality rates than pneumonectomy.[67] When complete excision is feasible, curability by sleeve lobectomy is comparable to that obtained by pneumonectomy.

Those extensive lesions that invade the carina (T4) have a much poorer prognosis. Some surgeons advocate pneumonectomies with tracheal sleeve resections in young patients who are good surgical risks.[68] Best results for this procedure approach a 20% 5-year survival rate, but often in the face of a 15% to 30% operative mortality rate. Selectivity is important prior to offering surgical therapy as extensive as this, with good results only occurring in clinical N0 patients. More advanced disease (e.g., T4N1–2, T3N1–2) should be treated with combined modality therapy without surgery since the results of surgery for these locally advanced primary tumors with lymph nodes metastases is poor.

**TUMORS INVADING MEDIASTINUM.** Patients with tumors invading the mediastinum generally do poorly if treated by surgery alone. This is because two-thirds of these patients also have mediastinal lymph node metastases (T3N2). From 1974 to 1984, 225 patients underwent thoracotomy at Memorial Sloan-Kettering Cancer Center for non–small cell lung cancer invading only the mediastinum (T3).[69] Of these, only 49 (22%) underwent complete resection of all intrathoracic disease, and the 5-year survival rate in this group was a disappointing 9% despite successful surgery. There were no 5-year survivors among patients who underwent partial resection or brachytherapy without resection.

We recently reviewed the results of surgical treatment in patients with non–small cell lung cancer invading the mediastinum by direct extension.[70] We excluded those who had N2 disease to eliminate the adverse prognostic effect of this nodal subset. There were 58 T3 tumors invading the mediastinal pleura or fat, phrenic nerve, vagus nerve, pericardium, or pulmonary vessels, and 44 T4 lesions invading aorta, vena cava, esophagus, trachea, spine, or atrium. Complete resection was possible in less than half of the patients (46/102).

The overall survival rate was 19% at 5 years with a median survival time of 18 months. The extent of mediastinal involvement (T3 vs. T4) influenced resectability and survival ($p = 0.06$). Factors found to significantly affect survival were complete resectability and histology. With complete resection the 5-year survival rate was 30%. Patients with adenocarcinoma or large cell cancers had a 5-year survival rate of 30% compared to 14% in patients with squamous carcinomas ($p = 0.002$).

We concluded that most patients with non–small cell lung cancer and mediastinal invasion, regardless of nodal status, do poorly with primary surgical treatment. We believe that this group of patients should also be considered for induction chemotherapy or chemoradiotherapy before surgical resection following the promising results of combined modality therapy in patients with N2 disease (see below).

## TREATMENT OF STAGE IIIA TUMORS (T1–3N2M0 AND T3N1M0)

**T1–3N2M0 TUMORS.** A major factor affecting the prognosis of patients undergoing surgery for stage IIIA non–small cell lung cancer is the presence of mediastinal lymph node metastases as the sole site of extrapulmonary spread, seen in an estimated 40,000 patients annually. This is nearly 50% of all non–small cell lung cancer presenting as localized disease.[71] Only 20% have localized disease that is operable or resectable and 80% are either not operable or do poorly with surgery as their primary treatment. It is in this group of patients that induction therapy with chemotherapy alone or with irradiation has proven most beneficial.

Patients with N2 disease treated primarily by surgery are usually individuals with peripheral tumors and a normal-appearing mediastinum on CT scan and bronchoscopy, and those explored following a negative mediastinoscopy but incidentally found to have minimal N2 disease at thoracotomy.[72,73] There is some consensus that all those who have surgical exploration for whatever reason and are found to have previously unsuspected N2 disease should have a complete resection that encompasses all regional lymph nodes by a systematic dissection whenever technically possible (Fig. 9-4). The 5-year survival rate following resection in this group of patients ranges from 20% to 30%[73–81] (Table 9-4). Like earlier-stage disease, adjuvant therapies have failed to improve survival.[82] On the other hand, those patients preoperatively identified to have N2 disease (clinical N2) are rarely cured by primary surgery[71] (Fig. 9-5).

Until recently, in most centers, patients with clinical N2 disease have not been offered surgery but have been treated by primary radiation therapy. In our own experience, the 5-year disease-free survival rate in patients with clinical N2 disease treated by primary surgery was 0%. Patients in good performance status presenting

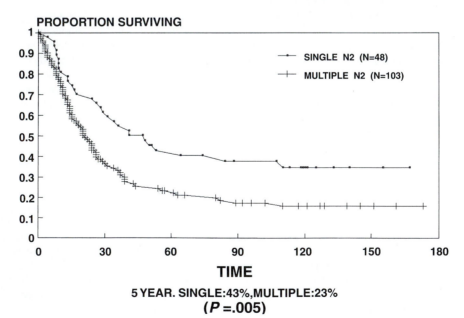

**FIGURE 9-4.** Completely resected stage IIIa (N2) lung cancer—survival by number of N2 nodes (1974–1981).

## TABLE 9-4. SURVIVAL RESULTS WITH PRIMARY SURGERY IN STAGE IIIA (N2) LUNG CANCER*

| AUTHOR | YEAR | NUMBER OF PATIENTS | 5-YEAR SURVIVAL RATE, % |
|---|---|---|---|
| Pearson[72] | 1982 | 76 | 15–41 |
| Kirsh[75] | 1982 | 136 | 21 |
| Mountain[79] | 1985 | 92 | 26 |
| Martini[71] | 1987 | 151 | 30 |
| Naruke[78] | 1988 | 242 | 19 |
| Watanabe[81] | 1991 | 84 | 24 |
| LeVasseur[76] | 1993 | 191 | 25 |
| Schirren[80] (Vogt-Moykopf) | 1993 | 131 | 18 |
| Goldstraw[74] | 1994 | 127 | 20 |
| Total | | 1230 | |

*Complete resection; single institution; ≥75 patients per series.

with preoperatively identified N2M0 disease now are being offered preoperative chemotherapy or chemoradiotherapy with cisplatin-based regimens. Of these, 60% to 75% demonstrate major response to this induction treatment and then are offered surgery to resect all residual disease.[37,83–86] Complete resection following major response to induction therapy is possible in 60% to 80% of the patients with apparent improved long-term survival.

We have recently reported our cumulative experience with the use of induction chemotherapy in this stage of disease. From 1984 to 1991, 136 consecutive patients with clinical stage IIIA (N2) disease received two to three cycles of MVP (mitomycin plus vindesine or vinblastine plus high-dose cisplatin) chemotherapy.[38] All patients had "clinical N2" disease, defined as bulky mediastinal lymph node metastases or multiple levels of lymph node involvement in the ipsilateral mediastinum or subcarinal region on chest roentgenograms, CT scans, and usually proven at mediastinoscopy. After chemotherapy, patients were surgically explored and complete resection was carried out whenever possible. After operation, two additional cycles of chemotherapy were planned. Mediastinal irradiation was recommended to patients with viable tumor in N2 nodes at pathologic examination. Survival was calculated from start of chemotherapy.

The overall major response rate to chemotherapy was 77% (105/136). Complete responses occurred in 13 patients, and 92 patients had partial responses (>50%). The overall complete resection rate was 65% (89/136), with a complete resection rate of 78% (82/105) in patients with a major response to chemotherapy. There was no histologic evidence of tumor in the resected specimens of 19 patients. The overall survival rate was 28% at 3 years and 17% at 5 years (median, 19 months). For patients who had a complete resection, the median survival was 27 months and the 3-year and 5-year survivals were 41% and 26%, respectively (Fig. 9-6). There were seven treatment-related deaths, five of which were postoperative deaths. To date, 33 patients, all of whom had complete resection, have had no recurrence after treatment. These results demonstrate that: (1) preoperative chemotherapy with MVP produces high response rates in stage IIIA (N2) disease, (2) high complete resection rates occur after chemotherapy, and (3) survival is longest in patients who have a complete resection after major response to chemotherapy and all long-term survivors are in this group. Similar encouraging

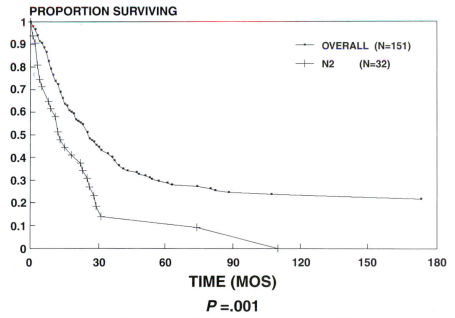

**FIGURE 9-5.** Stage IIIa(N2) non–small cell lung cancer—survival following resection by clinical N.

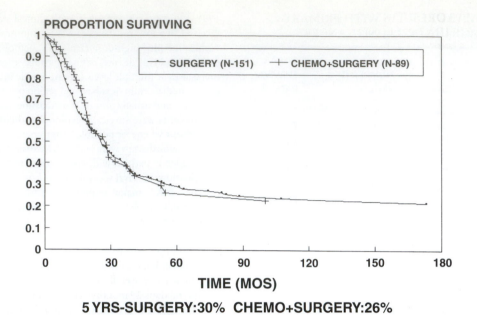

**FIGURE 9-6.** Stage IIIa(N2) non–small cell lung cancer—survival following complete resection in clinically presumed N0–N1 tumors ($n = 151$) versus survival with induction chemotherapy followed by complete resection in major responders ($n = 89$).

results have been reported with chemotherapy combined with radiation therapy[87–92] (Table 9-5).

Initial trials of induction therapy were phase II studies and nonrandomized. Three randomized trials of induction chemotherapy plus surgery compared to primary surgery have been completed and support the observations of nonrandomized experience demonstrating prolonged survival for patients treated with induction chemotherapy approach[93–95] (Table 9-6).

Radiation oncologists have also tested induction chemotherapy before thoracic irradiation as primary treatment in patients

with stage III non–small cell lung cancer. Using a cisplatin plus vinca alkaloid regimen similar to the ones used in many surgical trials before thoracic irradiation, investigators of the Cancer and Leukemia Group B (CALGB) demonstrated significant improvements in response, median survival, and 5-year survival for patients receiving this combined therapy in a multicenter randomized trial.[32] A 5-year survival rate of 17% was observed. The results were confirmed with a second randomized trial of similar design.[96,97]

Because of the similarity of the results with a "surgical" versus a "nonsurgical" approach, the North American intergroup has begun to assess the optimal postinduction treatment: surgery or thoracic irradiation.[47] The criteria of admissibility to the trial include stage IIIA (N2M0) patients with non–small cell lung cancer. These patients are randomized to receive chemotherapy with cisplatin plus etoposide plus concomitant external radiation therapy followed by further external radiation therapy or the same induction regimen followed by surgery. Accession of 512 patients is planned over 6 years.

In summary, with the advent of induction therapy, a significant proportion of patients presenting with N2 disease are currently being treated effectively with some expectations of long-term survival and cure rather than palliation. Despite variance in selection criteria, some conclusions can be drawn:

1. Every effort should be made preoperatively to identify N2 disease.
2. Most resected cases that do well with surgery alone have peripheral tumors with one nodal station of N2 disease or enlarged but well-encapsulated lymph nodes, usually found unexpectedly at surgery.
3. Any patient surgically explored and found to have previously unsuspected N2 disease should have a complete resection whenever

**TABLE 9-5.** RESULTS OF INDUCTION CHEMORADIOTHERAPY AND SURGERY IN STAGE IIIA NON-SMALL CELL LUNG CANCER

| YEAR | N | RESPONSE RATE, % | % RESECTED | MEDIAN, MONTHS |
|---|---|---|---|---|
| **NONRANDOMIZED** | | | | |
| 1990 Rush (Faber/Bonomi)[88] | 85 | 70 | 68 | 22 |
| 1992 CALGB (Strauss)[92] | 41 | 51 | 61 | 16 |
| 1994 SWOG (Rusch)[90] | 74 | 88 | 74 | 13 |
| 1989 Dana Farber (Skarin)[91] | 41 | 72 | 88 | 32 |
| 1994 MGH (Choi)[87] | 35 | 91 | 80 | 24 |
| **RANDOMIZED** | | | | |
| 1994 Intergroup 0139[47] Target enrollment: 512 Accrual as of 9/98: 270 | Chemotherapy + Radiation therapy vs. Chemotherapy + Radiation therapy + Surgery | | | |

**TABLE 9-6.** RESULTS OF INDUCTION CHEMOTHERAPY AND SURGERY IN STAGE IIIA NON–SMALL CELL LUNG CANCER

| YEAR | N | CHEMO RESPONSE, % | % RESECTED | MEDIAN SURVIVAL, MONTHS | | P VALUE |
|------|---|------|------|------|------|------|
| | | | | COMBINATION | SURGERY ONLY | |
| **NONRANDOMIZED** | | | | | | |
| 1993 MSKCC (Martini)[38] | 136 | 77 | 65 | 19 | | |
| 1994 Toronto (Burkes)[83] | 55 | 71 | 51 | 21 | | |
| 1993 Italy (Darwish)[84] | 46 | 82 | 62 | 24 | | |
| 1990 France (Pujol)[86] | 33 | 70 | 55 | 10 | | |
| **RANDOMIZED VS. SURGERY ALONE** | | | | | | |
| 1992 NCI (Pass)[93] | 27 | 62 | 85 | 28 | 15 | .095 |
| 1994 MD A (Roth)[94] | 60 | 35 | 39 | 64 | 11 | <.008 |
| 1994 Spain (Rosell)[95] | 60 | 60 | 77 | 26 | 8 | <.001 |

possible, including a systematic mediastinal lymph node dissection. (At thoracotomy, every effort is made to carry out a complete resection even when N2 disease is found, but assiduous preoperative staging for N2 disease is urged.)

4. Both surgery and radiotherapy can be effective treatments following induction therapy for clinical N2 disease but fare less well as single modality primary treatment.

**T3N1M0 TUMORS.** Although patients with non–small cell lung cancer with invasion of mediastinum, chest wall, carina, or diaphragm, but without evidence of any regional lymph node metastases, are presumed to have favorable prognosis after resection, those with involvement of hilar or peribronchial lymph nodes do less well.[50] This latter category remains classified under stage IIIa disease. In most instances the N1 involvement is not documented histologically, preoperatively, or confirmed radiographically. Because of this, most patients with clinical T3N1 disease are recommended for surgical exploration on a first instance unless the primary tumor is considered too large and its resection questionable. Mediastinoscopy in these patients helps to rule out N2 disease but rarely confirms the presence of N1 involvement.

Very few patients present with T3N1 disease, although their outcome following resection is generally as poor as those patients who also have N2 lymph node involvement. In the absence of currently effective adjuvant treatments for non–small cell lung cancer, selection of postoperative radiation and/or chemotherapy is generally individualized. We favor no further adjuvant treatment if the resection was complete despite the presence of N1 involvement. Most publications to date encompass T3N1 tumors under stage IIIa tumors, but point to their less favorable outlook compared to patients with no regional lymph node involvement despite extension of the disease into chest wall, mediastinum, or carina.[50,54]

Several centers now recommend induction therapy for patients with T3N0 tumors, and the subset of patients with N1 involvement will probably be encompassed under these new approaches. We currently do not favor treatment options confined to T3N1 tumors but prefer to group them under the more common stage IIIa tumors.

## TREATMENT OF STAGE IIIB TUMORS (T4, N ANY, M0 AND T ANY, N3M0)

Patients presenting with supraclavicular or contralateral mediastinal lymph node metastases (N3), as well as patients with tumors invading spine, carina, esophagus, aorta, or heart (T4) and those associated with malignant pleural effusions, are currently classified under stage IIIb disease and are usually considered inoperable. Most of these patients are treated with primary external radiation therapy or chemoradiation. Few are currently considered for surgical treatment even after response to nonsurgical modes of therapy.[90] However, there is a small group of patients usually identified at thoracotomy to have T4 disease that can undergo a complete resection (e.g., minimal vascular adventitial involvement).

Most patients with stage IIIb disease are symptomatic and generally inoperable.[98] Patients presenting with superior vena caval syndrome are also classified under stage IIIb disease. They usually present with widening of the mediastinum as the most frequent abnormality on chest x-rays and CT scans. Chest radiography and CT scans are the most useful noninvasive imaging techniques to depict tumor extension and mediastinal involvement. Nuclear magnetic resonance imaging is helpful when invasion of spine is suspected or to better define the involvement of the subclavian vessels and the brachial plexus in superior sulcus tumors.[99] However, if T4 involvement is in doubt, the tumor should be classified as T3—not as T4!

Since the vast majority of stage IIIb tumors are inoperable, radiation therapy can play an important role in controlling some of these tumors, although this treatment is usually palliative and the long-term survival rate with radiation therapy alone does not exceed 5%.[100–104] More recently, intensive multidrug chemotherapy combined with external radiation therapy has been favored as the treatment of choice for stage IIIb tumors. Exclusive of tumors associated with malignant effusions, many patients are currently treated with three-dimensional conformal external radiation therapy with more effective delivery of radiation significantly reducing damage to normal structures and allowing higher doses to be applied.[105] This treatment approach is still investigational and is limited to those centers with such equipment. For T4 tumors resected completely, most centers advocate postoperative irradiation.

## TREATMENT OF SOLITARY SYNCHRONOUS RESECTABLE METASTASES (MI)

Most patients presenting with metastases have multiple sites of involvement, but 7% present with solitary metastases to brain, lung, liver, bone, or adrenal tissue.[106] Resection of the primary tumor and the solitary site of metastasis has yielded long-term survivors in up to 20% of such individuals.[107,108] Because induction therapy in stage IIIa disease is proving to be beneficial, the role of preoperative chemotherapy plus resection is under investigation in patients with potentially resectable primary tumors who present with non–small cell lung cancer and a solitary resectable synchronous metastasis. More recently, there has been enthusiasm for treating selected brain metastases with stereotactic radiosurgery.[109]

In those presenting with a symptomatic solitary brain metastasis, a craniotomy is recommended first.[110] In all other patients with a solitary synchronous metastasis, either lesion can be approached first, depending on the clinical situation.

## ROLE OF SURGERY IN THE TREATMENT OF SMALL CELL LUNG CANCER

Small cell lung cancer accounts for 20% of all lung cancers. Early dissemination to regional lymph nodes and/or distant metastases are present in most patients at the time of initial presentation.

Early reports of surgical treatment for limited (locoregional) small cell carcinoma were disappointing. Although surgical resection was employed, in reality few were resectable and few if any were alive at 5 years.[111,112]

The same was true with external radiation therapy.[113,114] With the advent of effective systemic treatment, surgery was abandoned as a treatment modality and chemotherapy with irradiation has become the treatment of choice.[115–117]

The rationale for surgery in limited small cell carcinoma stems from the fact that 85% of patients fail to respond to treatment, mostly in the chest, whether they receive radiation or chemotherapy. However, the role of surgery in patients who fail to respond to chemotherapy or those who recur locally after initial response is still unclear.[118,119]

It is now well accepted that surgical resection used alone is not usually curative in small cell lung cancer.[120] Moreover, there is no clear benefit from surgery in the presence of regional lymph node metastases. There is a role for surgery if the tumor presentation is that of an isolated peripheral pulmonary nodule provided careful staging is done. Surgery is indicated if the tumor is classified as a T1N0M0 or T2N0M0 lesion by CT scan and/or mediastinoscopy. Adjuvant chemotherapy is included as an integral part of treatment.

A small number of patients are also treated surgically at the outset because of unknown or mistaken histology. This group should receive postoperative chemotherapy (and irradiation if nodal disease is present). The overall survival rate of these patients is similar to that seen in patients who were not operated upon but were treated by primary chemoradiotherapy.[118,120,121]

Induction chemotherapy followed by surgery has been tested in locally advanced disease. The results of this approach are no better than standard chemoradiation without surgery.

At present we recommend surgery with postoperative chemotherapy to patients with peripheral clinical T1N0 or T2N0 tumors and postoperative chemotherapy and radiation if the tumor is more advanced at final staging (stages II and IIIa), or are only diagnosed as small cell carcinoma at thoracotomy. Neoadjuvant chemotherapy followed by surgery and irradiation as well as surgery for local recurrence are currently reserved for patients in study protocols.

## LESS COMMON PRIMARY TUMORS

Less common tumors of bronchial origin include benign tumors and low-grade malignant neoplasms that arise from the epithelium, ducts, and glands of the tracheobronchial tree and account for approximately 0.5% to 1% of all bronchopulmonary tumors. Included in this group are carcinoid tumors, adenoid cystic carcinomas, and mucoepidermoid tumors.

### BENIGN TUMORS

Less than 1% of lung tumors are benign.[122] They are derived from all cell types and may be parenchymal or endobronchial in location (Table 9-7).

The most common benign tumor is the hamartoma. This name was first used to denote abnormalities of the liver and bile ducts, and by definition, represents an overgrowth of normal tissue that serves no useful purpose. It is most commonly an overgrowth of cartilage and is pathologically designated as a "chrondroma" or a "chondromyxoid hamartoma." Arrigoni and associates[123] reported that hamartomas make up 77% of all benign tumors of the lungs.

## TABLE 9-7. TYPES OF BENIGN LUNG TUMORS

I. Hamartoma-chondromyxoid
II. Tumors of epithelial origin
   Benign mixed tumor
   Papilloma
   Polyp
   Tumorlet
   Benign teratoma
III. Tumors of mesenchymal origin
   Lipoma
   Fibroma
   Leiomyoma
   Rhabdomyoma
   Neuroma
   Hemangioma
   Lymphangioma
   Benign histiocytoma
IV. Tumors of lymphoid origin
   Plasmacytoma
   Plasma cell granuloma
   Lymphocytoma

Of these lesions, 90% present as a solitary peripheral mass. They are most common in the middle-aged adult, although no age group is exempt, and they occur twice as often in men as in women.[124]

Most patients with peripherally located lesions are asymptomatic. Only those few patients who have an endobronchial lesion have symptoms, including cough, hemoptysis, and repeated or persistent pulmonary infection.

Roentgenographically, the peripheral lesion appears as a smooth and well-circumscribed mass; at times the margins appear lobulated. Calcifications have been reported to be present in 10% to 30% of these lesions evaluated by CT.

Although bronchoscopy is indicated in most patients with a pulmonary lesion, it is unrewarding in those with a peripheral lesion. Percutaneous needle aspiration biopsy yields are variable and depend on the expertise of the cytopathologist.[125] Cartilage is more often demonstrated by standard histologic examination of the aspirated material and is diagnostic. Most recently, when excision is indicated, video-assisted thoracoscopy is preferred, and the lesion is excised for diagnosis and treatment.

When the diagnosis is known or highly suspected in a patient with a peripherally located hamartoma, the patient may be observed without surgical intervention. Incision of the pleura and enucleation of the mass can be readily carried out, although a wedge resection is acceptable. Extensive sacrifice of lung tissue is unnecessary. When the hamartoma is endobronchial, a lobectomy or segmentectomy is required. Recurrence after excision of a hamartoma is practically unknown.

**OTHER BENIGN TUMORS.** Other benign tumors of the lung are rarely encountered.[122] *Fibrous polyps* and *papillomas* originate from the bronchial mucosa and are confined to the bronchial lumen. They may be removed endoscopically, although occasionally a bronchotomy or bronchial sleeve resection may be necessary.

*Lymphocytoma* is a benign lymphoid hyperplasia that develops in lung parenchyma. Its histologic significance lies in its differential diagnosis from the more malignant forms of lymphoid tumors. Tumors that interfere with the bronchial lumen are usually symptomatic and are associated with cough, hemoptysis, dyspnea, and wheezing. When the diagnosis is certain and the obstruction reversible, one should perform a sleeve resection of the involved bronchus with its endobronchial tumor without sacrificing lung parenchyma. When the bronchial obstruction is total and longstanding, secondary damage to the obstructed portions of the lung may necessitate a major pulmonary resection, that is, a lobectomy or a pneumonectomy.

*Leiomyomas* are reported to account for 2% of the benign tumors of the lung. They may present in trachea or bronchus or may be parenchymal.[123] The frequency of occurrence in a tracheobronchial or parenchymal location is essentially the same. The tumor is most often seen in adults of any age and is more common in women than in men. Surgical resection is the treatment of choice.

*Lipomas* arise most often in the upper airways and are more common in men than in women. Local excision, or a bronchial sleeve resection, is sufficient to remove all the tumor. *Fibromas* as well as *benign neurogenic tumors* rarely appear in the lungs.

*Pseudotumors,* also known as plasma cell granuloma, fibroma, or fibrous histiocytoma, are also benign lung tumors.[126] They oc-

cur at any age and without sex predilection. Most are asymptomatic and are detected fortuitously on chest films as solitary nodules. Surgical resection is diagnostic and curative. *Sclerosing hemangiomas* and *sugar tumors,* also known as *Castleman's disease,* are rare benign tumors of the lung and their excision is generally curative.[127,128]

Countless extremely rare benign tumors are also reported to originate in lung. Except for their differential diagnosis from malignant neoplasms, they represent unique curiosity findings.

## CARCINOID TUMORS

Bronchial carcinoids constitute less than 1% of all lung tumors. Most tumors are confined to the lung or bronchus, but 10% to 15% of patients have regional lymph node metastases at diagnosis.[129,130] A smoking history is rare (vis-à-vis lung cancer). Although bronchial carcinoids can occur at any age, typical carcinoids usually occur at a younger age than primary lung cancer (median 42 years versus 62 years). Rarely do patients with typical carcinoids present older than 55 years of age.

Bronchial carcinoids were previously called adenomas but are now recognized as malignant tumors because of their potential to metastasize. There has been considerable controversy regarding the nomenclature that best reflects this group of patients. Typical and atypical carcinoids appear to share with small cell lung cancer a common neuroectodermal stem cell.[123] Electron microscopic findings and biochemical markers common in carcinoid tumors, as well as in small cell cancer, have led to the postulation of a neoplastic continuum among these tumors.[131,132] As a result, some have suggested that these tumors be called KCC I, II, and III to reflect their origin from Kulchitsky cells.[133] Others have opted to refer to them as neuroendocrine carcinomas of different degrees of differentiation. There is now mounting evidence that nuclear deoxyribonucleic acid studies can be helpful in differentiating the typical and atypical carcinoid tumors from small cell carcinomas.[134,135]

Clinically, carcinoid tumors and small cell lung cancer are distinctly separate entities.[129] Bronchial carcinoids are generally uncommon cancers, and their natural history is long, whereas small cell cancers represent nearly 15% to 20% of all lung cancers and patient survival is measured in months. We favor the term carcinoid tumor (typical or atypical) over the terms neuroendocrine carcinoma or KCC that group small cell lung cancer with carcinoid.[136]

No correlation exists between the history of smoking and the development of carcinoid tumors. The primary treatment is surgical when the disease is confined to the chest. Surgical resection is the accepted treatment even when mediastinal nodal metastases are present. No study has addressed whether adjuvant treatment after resection is either necessary or helpful. They are generally considered unresponsive to radiation or chemotherapy, and the long-term prognosis is excellent for both typical and atypical carcinoid tumors treated with resection.

**CLINICAL FEATURES.** The symptoms and physical findings depend on the location of the tumor. The peripheral tumors are most often asymptomatic, presenting as solitary pulmonary nodules on roentgenographic studies of the chest. Those presenting endobronchially are usually symptomatic. Cough, hemoptysis, and recurrent bouts of infection are the common symptoms. Because of the small size and slow growth of these tumors, symptoms may persist for many years before the underlying cause is discovered. A history of wheezing or recurrent infection dating back many years is common.[137] These tumors frequently masquerade clinically as bronchial asthma, chronic bronchitis, or bronchiectasis, particularly if the tumor produces incomplete obstruction and is located in the trachea or proximal portions of the bronchial tree. Stridor can be the presenting symptom in tracheal or main stem bronchial tumors. Recurrent hemoptysis results from ulceration of the hyperemic mucosa overlying the tumor or simply from chronic inflammation distally. This is most commonly seen in carcinoid tumors and in women has been noted to be accentuated during times of menstrual flow.

The carcinoid syndrome occurs infrequently and almost exclusively in patients with hepatic metastases. Fine-needle aspiration biopsy of peripheral lesions can be accurate, but histologic examination of tumor tissue is the only completely reliable means of diagnosis. None of the radiologic techniques accurately differentiates these tumors from other benign and malignant neoplasms.

CT scans are helpful in staging bronchial carcinoids, but mediastinoscopy is not essential once a carcinoid diagnosis is established. Fewer than 15% of cases have nodal involvement; more importantly, even if lymph node metastases exist, their presence does not preclude surgical treatment because long-term survival is still possible. In our experience with 23 surgically treated patients with nodal involvement, 75% were alive at 5 years, and local control was effective in 22 of 23 patients.

**DIAGNOSIS.** With the exception of bronchoscopy and octreotide scans,[138] no other diagnostic modality is available that reliably detects carcinoid tumors.[139] Many patients have normal chest roentgenograms, and sputum cytology tests are rarely positive for malignant cells. However, the diagnosis can often be suspected in patients who have repeated bouts of pneumonia associated with hemoptysis and wheezing.

Bronchoscopy remains the most reliable method of diagnosing endobronchial tumors. Since most carcinoid tumors occur centrally, a submucosal polypoid mass is nearly always visualized, and biopsies are positive in nearly 85% of cases. A negative biopsy report does not exclude these neoplasms, since nearly all are covered by an intact mucous membrane, which may prevent actual sampling of the tumor. Since these tumors present submucosally, they do require deeper biopsies than other malignant bronchial neoplasms. Massive bleeding with biopsy has been reported, but in our experience it is an infrequent occurrence. Frozen-section examination of the biopsy material may be misleading.

Peripheral tumors can be diagnosed by fine-needle aspiration biopsy. Because of their similarity to small cell carcinoma, carcinoid tumors have occasionally been misdiagnosed by this technique.

**TREATMENT.** Both typical and atypical carcinoids, though malignant, are far more favorable tumors prognostically than any histologic type of lung cancer with nodal involvement. Resection remains the only effective treatment for this group of tumors, despite the presence of nodal metastases.[140]

Controversy exists regarding the extent of resection necessary to obtain the most favorable results.[141–144] Provided there is sufficient

pulmonary reserve, we recommend a complete pulmonary resection with mediastinal lymph node dissection in patients with lymph node involvement.[129] This provides excellent local control and results in long-term survival for bronchial carcinoids even in the presence of regional lymph node metastases. Recurrence is generally late and in distant sites and appears more dependent on histologic subset (typical vs. atypical) than on nodal status. There is no indication that postoperative radiation therapy is beneficial for local control or overall survival. The merits of systemic adjuvants are not assessable, since too few patients had effective systemic treatment.

In summary, bronchial carcinoid neoplasms are extremely slow growing. Prognosis is excellent; fully 90% of all patients are alive and well 5 years after definitive treatment. Survival, however, varies with the specific type of neoplasm. Based on the Mayo Clinic experience, patients with the typical bronchial carcinoid tumors have a 5-year postsurgical survival rate of 94%, 10-year survival rate of 87%, 20-year survival rate of 76%, and 25-year survival rate of 66%. If lymph nodes are involved with metastases, 71% of patients are alive at 5 years. Patients with atypical bronchial carcinoids, on the other hand, have a 5-year postsurgical survival rate of only 57%.

## ADENOID CYSTIC CARCINOMA

**CLINICAL FEATURES.** This malignant tumor, also called cylindroma, is a slowly growing malignant lesion arising from bronchial mucous glands and is similar in most respects to adenoid cystic carcinoma of the major and minor salivary glands. It is much less common (one-tenth as common) than carcinoid tumors, much more aggressive, and has a poorer prognosis. As with carcinoid tumors, there is an equal sex incidence and similar age range, the commonest incidence occurring in the fifth decade of life.[145]

**PATHOLOGY.** Unlike carcinoid tumors, adenoid cystic carcinomas occur most frequently in the lower trachea at the level of the carina and the orifices of the main bronchi. Rarely are they situated peripherally. In general, most of the peripheral tumors prove to be metastatic from another primary site, usually salivary glands.

Although distant metastases tend to occur late in the course of the disease, approximately one-third of patients have evidence of metastases at the time of first treatment, to regional lymph nodes, or distally to liver, bone, and kidneys. Bronchoscopically, the tumor appears as a broad-based mass with an intact mucosa overlying it. Microscopically, these tumors are identical to those in the salivary glands.[146]

**TREATMENT.** Because adenoid cystic carcinomas are of low-grade malignancy but are locally invasive, the aims of curative therapy include a generous en bloc excision of the tumor. Preservation of as much normal lung tissue as possible is another goal of treatment. If complete excision is impossible, therapy should be aimed at local control of the tumor to relieve airway obstruction.

Bronchoscopic removal is not curative but can be used effectively in relieving airway obstruction before definitive surgery or as palliation when surgery is contraindicated because of the extent of the disease. Endoscopic laser ablation is extremely effective in relieving the obstruction and has replaced mechanical debridement as the bronchoscopic procedure of choice.[147] Long-term palliation in inoperable cases can be achieved by repeated endoscopic removal of tumor. Frequently, this is used conjointly with radiation therapy and/or endobronchial stent placement.

For complete excision, a tumor arising in lobar or main stem bronchi can be dealt with by lobectomy, sleeve resection, or a combination of both. Because of the high incidence of submucosal extension and lymph node metastases, wide local excision, including peribronchial tissue and a hilar node dissection, should be performed. Frozen-section examination of the margins of resection is mandatory.

Lesions occurring in the trachea and carina are challenging surgical problems. Modern techniques of mobilization and reconstruction of the trachea allow up to 8 cm of tracheal length to be excised with end-to-end anastomoses.[148]

Perelman and Koroleva[149] proposed the following principles in the management of these tumors:

1. Routine preoperative biopsies are performed at different levels around the tumor, including submucosa, to determine proximal and distal spread. Preoperative endoscopic biopsy proximal and distal to the tumor can help guide the surgeon as to the extent of resection.
2. If the tumor is believed to be circumscribed, sleeve resection should be performed with frozen-section guidance.
3. If extensive submucosal involvement is detected at preoperative endoscopy or intraoperatively before tracheal resection, serious consideration should be given to abandoning the attempt at resection. However, palliative resections can allow for long-term freedom from airway compromise.

Although tracheal prostheses have been used to extend the length of tracheal resection, these prostheses are fraught with complications and should be avoided wherever possible, as Pearson and colleagues[150] have noted. Postoperative radiotherapy is recommended following surgical resection.

A single pulmonary metastasis with a localized endotracheal or endobronchial tumor does not necessarily contraindicate a surgical approach. The solitary metastasis can be removed as part of the surgical procedure.

**RADIATION THERAPY.** Although adenoid cystic carcinomas are fairly radiation resistant, those occurring in the airway have been treated successfully and appear to be more sensitive than those occurring in other salivary gland sites. Perelman and Koroleva[149] found that these tumors are more sensitive to radiation than squamous cell carcinomas of the trachea.

Radiation therapy should be considered in all inoperable patients as part of the palliative approach. Rostom and Morgan[151] reported that radiation doses in the curative range (greater than 5500 rads) are required and the response is usually slow. Munsch and associates[152] suggested that before irradiation, if airway obstruction is a problem, laser ablation of the tumor is warranted. Ryan and associates[153] reported that the combination of intraluminal brachytherapy and external beam irradiation allows higher doses of radiation therapy to the tumor.

Although surgical therapy remains the treatment of choice, a radiation therapy approach can lead to long-term survival and occasionally to cure.

If residual tumor remains after resection, postoperative irradiation is indicated. As Pearson[150] and Grillo[148] noted, the question of whether preoperative or postoperative irradiation, or both, is valuable has not been answered. The role of chemotherapy in this disease is undefined and at present of little known value.

In summary, adenoid cystic carcinoma is inherently a more malignant tumor than the carcinoid tumor. Because of its tendency to permeate lymphatics and metastasize to regional lymph nodes, this tumor is prone to recur locally unless adequately excised. Its natural history, however, is prolonged, and long-term survival, measured in decades, with persistent disease is common. Before modern tracheal surgical techniques were developed, only 30% of patients could be expected to survive without recurrent disease. Grillo,[148] however, reported that 12 of 16 patients were disease-free after five years. Similarly, Pearson[150] reported that 50% of patients were disease-free 2 to 18 years after tracheal resection. Perelman and Koroleva[149] reported a 65% 5-year and 56% 10-year survival rate in resected patients.

Owing to its low biologic activity, even after incomplete surgical excision, long survival periods can occur even with persisting or recurrent disease. For this reason, aggressive treatment of these tumors, palliative or curative, is warranted.

## MUCOEPIDERMOID CARCINOMAS

These carcinomas are extremely rare bronchial tumors. They are seen most commonly in persons in the fifth decade of life, but have been reported in patients as young as 10 and as old as 75 years of age. Sex incidence is approximately equal.

**PATHOLOGY.** Reichle and Rosemond[154] reported that mucoepidermoid carcinomas are found in the same location as carcinoid tumors. As with other mucoepidermoid tumors, those arising in the bronchial tree may be either of high- or low-grade malignancy, most of them being of the latter variety. Endoscopically, the tumor appears either as a polypoid submucosal mass located in the main stem or peripheral bronchi or as an infiltrative mass.

Microscopically, the tumors resemble those found in the salivary glands. They are composed of three characteristic cell types—mucous, squamous, and intermediate cells. The three types are seen in varying proportions in different tumors. The low-grade tumors have a high proportion of mucous cells, whereas the high-grade tumors have a high proportion of squamous cells. The tumor may have a predominantly solid growth pattern or mixed solid and cystic pattern.

The low-grade variety can infiltrate the bronchial wall but does not invade vessels or metastasize to lymph nodes. The high-grade variety metastasizes to regional lymph nodes and distantly like other bronchial carcinomas.

**TREATMENT.** The principles of treatment outlined for carcinoid tumors apply to the mucoepidermoid variety, low-grade type. These procedures should include complete removal of tumor with preservation of as much normal lung tissue as possible.

Segmentectomy, lobectomy, or, rarely, pneumonectomy with or without sleeve resection may be required. Preoperative bronchial biopsies and intraoperative surgical staging of lymph nodes should be performed to identify the more malignant variety.

The high-grade malignant mucoepidermoid carcinoma should be investigated and managed with the same philosophy as that used for other non–small cell carcinomas, the treatment depending upon the local and regional extent of disease.

The low-grade malignant mucoepidermoid tumor can be completely cured by adequate surgical removal. Although few high-grade mucoepidermoid carcinomas have been reported, the results of surgical therapy seem to be similar to those seen for bronchial carcinoma, according to the local and distant spread of the disease at the time of treatment.

## PRIMARY SARCOMAS AND LYMPHOMAS OF THE LUNG

Primary malignant tumors of nonepithelial origin are rare, representing less than 1% of primary pulmonary malignancies. In this group are included tumors that arise from mesenchymal structures or sarcomas and tumors that arise from the reticuloendothelial system or lymphomas (Table 9-8).

SARCOMAS. It is estimated that sarcomas occur in lung in 0.2% to 0.013% of cases.[155,156] Sarcomas generally arise from the stromal elements of the bronchial wall or lung parenchyma. Rarely do they invade and break through the bronchial epithelium. As a result, these tumors do not exfoliate, and a diagnosis by cytologic examination of bronchial secretions is unlikely. When peripherally located, they appear on chest roentgenogram as sharply defined masses and they may invade pleura or chest wall. They generally spread by local invasion and metastases to distant organs are usually late manifestations of the disease. The poorly differentiated or high-grade sarcomas are often indistinguishable histologically from the common anaplastic cancers. The symptoms and radiologic appearance of sarcomas are similar to those seen with carcinomas of the lung. They occur at any age and with equal frequency in either sex. Many are asymptomatic and are detected only on a routine chest roentgenogram. Sarcomas are usually solitary and confined to one lung. Calcification is not a feature in lung sarcomas. Those obstructing a bronchus may be associated with chest pain, dyspnea, cough, or hemoptysis.

In central sarcomas, bronchoscopy and bronchial biopsy can establish the diagnosis, but in those that are peripherally located, the diagnosis is usually established at thoracotomy or recently at thoracoscopy. It is important to note that limited biopsy material or frozen sections are insufficient for accurate diagnosis in most cases.

It is often impossible to differentiate histologically between a primary and a metastatic sarcoma. A sarcoma is considered to arise in the lung only if there is no sarcoma elsewhere in the body. Careful evaluation of the patient and long-term follow-up are necessary to rule out metastatic sarcoma from other sites. Moreover, the specific histologic classification of sarcomas is difficult, even though they may be recognized to be sarcomas at the initial examination. The correct type-specific identification is of great importance in myosarcomas in particular, since the prognosis with leiomyosarcomas is far better than other forms of sarcomas and the prognosis with rhabdomyosarcomas is worse than other forms of sarcomas.

Early detection of the tumor by chest roentgenogram and bronchoscopy followed by surgical resection when feasible is the only effective method of controlling these tumors. Long-term survival with external radiation therapy or chemotherapy alone is extremely rare.

Soft tissue sarcomas arising in lung are best treated with complete resection when possible. The survival rate correlates closely with tumor stage and grade of malignancy, as for any sarcomas of soft tissue origin. Combined modality therapy should be used when good results have been obtained in treating similar tumors at other sites.

The type of resection depends on the location of the tumor. Leiomyosarcomas have an excellent prognosis when resected early. Nearly one-half of the patients survive over 5 years and many live more than 15 to 20 years after resection. On the other hand, patients with rhabdomyosarcoma have an extremely poor prognosis and the majority die in less than a year in spite of treatment. With the exception of sarcomas of muscle origin, most patients with sarcoma generally succumb to the disease within 3 years.

**TABLE 9-8.** MEMORIAL SLOAN-KETTERING EXPERIENCE WITH PRIMARY LYMPHOMAS AND SARCOMAS OF THE LUNG (1926–1986)

| LYMPHOMA | NO. PATIENTS | SOFT TISSUE SARCOMA | NO. PATIENTS |
|---|---|---|---|
| Lymphosarcoma | 11 | Leiomyosarcoma | 16 |
| Reticulum cell sarcoma | 8 | Rhabdomyosarcoma | 5 |
| Lymphoma | 13 | Spindle cell sarcoma | 13 |
| Lymphocytoma | 2 | Angiosarcoma | 2 |
| Plasmacytoma | 1 | Malignant fibrous histiocytoma | 3 |
| | | Fibrosarcoma | 2 |
| | | Hemangiopericytoma | 1 |
| | | Blastoma | 1 |
| Total | 35 | Total | 43 |

The following excerpts from the published Memorial Sloan-Kettering experience are worthy of note:[156] *Malignant fibrous histiocytoma* was diagnosed in three patients. All three received surgery. One is alive and free of disease at 6 years, two died at 7 and 17 months, respectively. *Primary angiosarcoma* was resected in one patient who died of disease at 3 years; another was treated with radiation therapy and survived 22 months. *Pulmonary blastoma* was resected by pneumonectomy in one patient who remained free of disease at 12 years. One patient had a *hemangiopericytoma* resected by lobectomy followed with chemotherapy but died of disease 13 months after surgery.

LYMPHOMAS. Malignant lymphomas arising in lung make up 0.34% to 0.45% of all lymphomas. A lymphoma in the lung is considered of primary origin only when it meets the following criteria as described by Saltzstein[157] and L'Hoste[158]:

1. The lymphoma must involve the lung or bronchus; there may or may not be hilar or mediastinal lymph node involvement.
2. There should be no evidence of extrathoracic lymphoma at the time of diagnosis nor on long-term follow-up. If the patient dies, autopsy findings are used to ensure that the lymphoma involved the lung primarily.

Most *lymphocytomas* are benign; however, if histologic elements that suggest potential malignancy are identified, they are classified under lymphomas. *Plasmacytoma* is considered potentially malignant and classified under lymphomas since its histologic picture and that of multiple myeloma are identical. Although some tumors of lymphoid origin produce no symptoms, systemic manifestations of malaise, fatigue, fever, and weight loss are prominent in malignant lymphomas. Symptoms secondary to lung irritation are related to the location of the tumor and are no different from the symptoms of carcinomas arising in lung.

It is worthy of note that patients who present with lymphoma confined to the lung have a better prognosis than those with other lung cancers or with lymphomas at other sites.

In our series of 32 patients with primary pulmonary lymphomas, 13 had lymphoma, 11 had lymphosarcoma, and 8 had reticulum cell sarcoma.[155,156] Of 14 patients resected for cure, 12 survived disease-free for 11 to 18 years. Twelve patients were treated with radiation therapy alone; of these, nine died of their disease 5 months to 8 years after treatment; two are alive 4 and 27 years, respectively, after treatment; five patients received chemotherapy alone or combined with radiation therapy or surgery. All are alive 1 to 14 years after treatment. One patient presented with far advanced disease and received no treatment.

Two lymphocytomas that had histologic elements suggesting potential malignancy and one plasmacytoma were treated by resection and survived free of disease from 10 to 16 years after surgery.

In summary, malignant lymphomas as well as plasmacytomas should be viewed as systemic diseases. Although local control can be achieved by resection or irradiation, systemic therapy is usually necessary and appropriate and early medical oncology consultations should be obtained. The majority of patients with solitary plasmacytomas eventually develop multiple myeloma, and close surveillance for detection of their systemic manifestations must be incorporated in their follow-up.

## METASTATIC CANCERS TO LUNG

### HISTORICAL REVIEW

Pulmonary metastases are very common with advanced cancers. Nearly one-third of all patients dying of cancer have pulmonary metastases.[159] More importantly, 15% to 25% of metastases are confined to the lungs and frequently to one lung.

Treatment of metastases by resection is not a new concept.[160,161] The first resection of pulmonary metastases at some distance from the primary tumor was carried out in 1882 by Weinlechner.[162] While resecting a large sarcoma of the ribs, he opened the pleural cavity widely and found two small metastatic nodules in the upper lobe, which he excised. Unfortunately, the patient died the day after surgery from shock. Kronlein,[163] in 1883, operated on a recurrent chest wall sarcoma and discovered a metastatic nodule in lung tissue at some distance from the chest wall tumor and removed it by wedge resection. His patient lived for 7 years after her pulmonary resection, eventually dying from recurrent cancer.

Divis[164] is credited with the first report (1927) of resection of a pulmonary metastasis performed as a separate procedure in 1926; he published the report in the Scandinavian literature. In the American literature, Torek,[165] in 1930, was the first to report on resection of a pulmonary metastasis from the right lower lobe. He operated on a woman 2 years after she had a hysterectomy for an adenocarcinoma of the uterus.

The Barney and Churchill[166] report in 1939 is the most quoted early case. A lobectomy for a solitary tumor proved to be metastatic renal cell carcinoma. This patient remained alive and well for 23 years and died of coronary disease with no evidence of tumor at autopsy.[167,168]

In 1947 John Alexander and Cameron Haight[169] reported on a total of 24 patients treated surgically for solitary lung metastases. Alexander and Haight were also the first to set criteria for resection of pulmonary metastases. They believed that metastatic tumors should be resected if the primary tumor had been removed, no other metastases were evident, and the patient was in good enough condition to have the operation.

Until 1965, for the most part, surgery was offered only to select patients with one or two metastases and a long disease-free interval after treatment of their primary tumor.[170–176] Surgical treatment of pulmonary metastases began in earnest in 1965.[177] From 1965 to the present over 400 publications have addressed the results of surgical treatment of pulmonary metastases from a variety of primary tumors and tumor sites, tempered by the advent of effective systemic treatments.[178,179]

### CLINICAL PRESENTATION

Since most pulmonary metastases are peripheral, most patients have no symptoms at the time of the diagnosis of their metastases. Symptoms usually result from delay in diagnosis or generally reflect endobronchial disease, pleural involvement, or compromise of the lung by a large bulky tumor or by extensive multiplicity of the metastases. Routine bronchoscopy is generally unrewarding. In the presence of multiple lesions, preoperative biopsy usually is not necessary. In the instance of a solitary lesion, differential diagnosis necessarily includes benign lesions of the lung and a new primary lung tumor. Hence, tissue diagnosis becomes essential. In general, a solitary lung lesion is more likely to be metastatic if the primary tumor is a sarcoma or a melanoma. It is more likely to be a new lesion if the known primary tumor is of head and neck, lung, or breast origin. In patients with cancers at other sites, there is an equal chance for a solitary lesion to be a new lung cancer or a benign lesion as opposed to a metastasis.

Adkins[180] and associates reported on 50 patients presenting with a solitary lung nodule following treatment of a malignancy elsewhere in the body. The mass was benign in 9 patients, a new primary lung carcinoma in 9, and a metastasis in 32.

In 1984, Casey[181] reported that 3% of 1416 patients with breast cancer had presented with a solitary pulmonary nodule (synchronous or metachronous), and half of these were primary cancers, 5% were benign, and the rest were metastases from breast carcinoma.

## PRETREATMENT WORKUP

The extent of metastatic workup depends largely on tumor type. Sarcomas have a tendency to metastasize to the lungs, and chest radiography has become an integral part of the workup and the follow-up of all patients with sarcoma. In this group of tumors, most metastases occur within the first 2 years; hence very close radiologic surveillance is done every 1 to 2 months for the first year, every 3 months for the second year, and every 6 months thereafter. Once metastases are detected on plain chest films, computer tomographic (CT) scan of the chest is done routinely to determine the number and location of the lesions. The workup in patients with metastatic sarcoma need not be too extensive, since these tumors rarely metastasize to other organs (Table 9-9). The majority of sarcomas present for surgical treatment with multiple pulmonary metastases. In our experience two-thirds of patients treated by pulmonary resection for metastatic sarcoma had multiple lesions.

With metastatic carcinomas and with melanoma the problem is somewhat different.[182] First, with the exception of those who have testicular tumors, the majority of the patients considered for pulmonary resection have solitary metastases, and nearly 80% undergo one thoracotomy. Second, for the lungs to contain the only metastases is uncommon. Unlike sarcomas, carcinomas usually metastasize to lung and to other organs, notably liver, brain, and bone. Hence, it is essential to conduct a thorough search for other foci of active disease before formulating a treatment plan. Lastly, surgical

## TABLE 9-9. ADVERSE PROGNOSTIC FACTORS IN METASTATIC SARCOMAS TO LUNG

1. High grade of tumor
2. Inadequate or no resection
3. Local recurrence

treatment of multiple metastases in carcinomas or melanoma is not as effective as when there is a solitary metastatic lesion.

Carcinoma metastases to lung are very apt to also metastasize to the regional lymph nodes, especially with melanomas. As well, patients with colon, breast, renal, and thyroid metastases have commonly associated regional lymph node involvement. In general, sarcomas do not metastasize to mediastinal lymph nodes. We have seen, on occasion, cases of metastatic liposarcoma or synovial sarcoma with metastases in mediastinal lymph nodes; this very rarely occurs in osteogenic sarcoma.

## TREATMENT

Surgical resection is the procedure of choice for most patients with a solitary metastasis to the lung. However, this group constitutes 10% or less of all patients with pulmonary metastases. As a rule, surgical treatment of metastases is offered to patients who are good operative risks and whose primary tumor is controlled, no extra thoracic metastases are present, no effective nonoperative therapy is available, and a complete excision of all metastases is anticipated. In simultaneous presentations, surgical treatment of the pulmonary metastases may be recommended first, particularly if major ablative surgery is considered for the primary site. If the lungs can be cleared of tumor, the primary is resected. The reverse sequence is entertained when resectability of the primary tumor is in question and pulmonary metastases are limited to one or two lesions in a single lung.

Surgical treatment is also offered for multiple and even bilateral lesions if effective nonoperative treatments are not available. Clearly patients with multiple metastases do more poorly than patients presenting with solitary lesions. However, we have not been able to identify the specific number of metastases beyond which attempts at resection become unrewarding. For the surgical treatment of pulmonary metastases to be effective and justified, two considerations are paramount. The first is removal of all gross tumor, and the second is maximal conservation of functioning lung tissue. However, the extent of resection depends on the location of the metastases. In many, the metastases, though multiple, are small and peripheral and so are easily removed by multiple small excisions. We have in such instances removed as many as 20, 30, or more lesions. On the other hand, excision of a deep-seated tumor or a central lesion, though solitary, may require a lobectomy or pneumonectomy, which may not be possible owing to the patient's limited pulmonary reserve or not justified if metastases are multiple.

Since the majority of patients with lung metastases are asymptomatic, surgical treatment must aim for prolonged survival and cure. We have found that complete resection has been possible in over 90% of the patients accepted for thoracotomy. The 1% operative mortality rate made it feasible to offer an operation as an alternative, even in patients with a short tumor doubling time. However, palliative resection is limited to symptomatic patients without other palliative options.

It is often necessary to consider re-resection for recurrent pulmonary metastases. As long as the risks are low and preservation of adequate lung tissue is possible, resection is offered if nonsurgical alternatives are not available and total metastasectomy is anticipated.

Tumor doubling time of less than 40 days has been suggested as a contraindication to resection,[183] but when the lungs contain the only metastatic tumor, and this tumor can be resected, waiting for any length of time to ascertain doubling time may be counterproductive, as it is demonstrated in many patients with metastatic sarcoma of the lung.

If the lung lesion and another distant primary lesion are discovered at the same time, one must determine whether the two lesions are related. When they are not related, one must decide which of the two lesions is more threatening to the life of the patient, and if surgical intervention is decided upon, in what sequence the two operations would be better tolerated. The simultaneous occurrence of solitary bilateral lesions or multiple lesions in the same lung poses a difficult therapeutic decision, and individualization must be the rule.

The following course of action is recommended when a metastatic pulmonary lesion or lesions develop after adequate treatment of the primary tumor. If the primary tumor is known to be sensitive to chemotherapy, as in lymphomas or myeloid tumors, the appropriate chemotherapeutic regimen is given. The role of external radiation therapy in metastatic disease to the lung has been limited to the rare instance in which the treatment could be applied through a limited portal. If little or no response is noted after treatment by radiation therapy or chemotherapy, surgical resection is indicated. Implantation of radioactive iodine seeds at the time of thoracotomy in nonresectable lesions has been useful in controlling the metastasis, with prolonged survival in some patients. Since no effective nonsurgical treatment is available for most sarcomas and carcinomas, surgical treatment of metastases in this group of patients becomes an important modality.

Wedge resection is the procedure of choice when multiple lesions are present. In general, most patients (60% to 70%) are treated by wedge resection, a few (20% to 25%) by lobectomy, and less than 5% by pneumonectomy. This last procedure is done when metastases are solitary and central and when complete resection can be effective with minimal risk. Enucleation is reserved for the small, deep-seated, multiple or solitary tumors in patients with impaired pulmonary reserve.

In surgical resection of a solitary lesion, lobectomy is recommended when the known primary is a carcinoma and a new primary tumor of lung cannot be excluded. Diagnosis by frozen section is often unsatisfactory in differentiating primary from metastatic disease. Permanent pathologic diagnosis may be needed to confirm that the new lesion is not a second primary carcinoma of the lung. In this group of patients, mediastinal exploration and lymph node dissection are also recommended, since this may be a primary lung tumor. If the solitary pulmonary lesion is a sarcoma, a wedge resection or segmentectomy is sufficient, unless the lesion is central and precludes excision without performing lobectomy. A lobectomy is only indicated when a lesser resection will not completely remove the metastatic lesion. Only in select instances where cure is anticipated is a pneumonectomy justified for a solitary metastasis that cannot be removed with a lesser resection.

## THE ROLE OF ADJUVANT THERAPY

Nearly one-third of all patients presenting with pulmonary metastases as the only site of disease may benefit from resection of their metastases. Moreover, prolonged survival and apparent cure of select patients following the surgical removal of pulmonary metastases seems well established.

With the advent of effective chemotherapy, the initial reaction was to treat all patients with lung metastases by chemotherapy alone without considering the necessity for surgical treatment. We now know that combined efforts by surgery and chemotherapy are necessary in many tumors if better survival results are to be achieved. In some of the patients, chemotherapy has shown to be of benefit in preventing metastases and in effectively treating metastases when they do occur. There continues to be a need for surgical treatment to ascertain the viability of the tumor in lesions that show partial or no response, as well as to help reduce the tumor burden in patients with extensive disease otherwise controllable with chemotherapy.[179]

Testicular carcinomas are a unique group of tumors in many respects, because the majority of patients are young and, since the 1970s, effective chemotherapy has led to gratifying remissions and prolonged survival. Chemotherapy is now their primary form of treatment. It is the treatment of choice for pulmonary metastatic lesions of choriocarcinoma, with remission rates exceeding 85% for isolated pulmonary nodules. Surgery is only recommended when there is no response or continued progression of the disease in the face of active chemotherapy, or when there are residual nodules despite return of tumor markers to a normal range. In these instances, thoracotomy is done to assess the histologic nature of these metastases, to rule out benign transformations such as seen in maturing teratomas, and to resect all residual viable tumors. The use of tumor markers has proven to be very useful in the management of testicular carcinomas but not in other forms of neoplasms. Elevated carcinoembryonic antigen (CEA) readings do not usually occur with only pulmonary metastases nor are the readings consistent enough to be dependable.

A special treatment plan is used for those patients with osteogenic sarcoma who present with pulmonary metastases. Patients with diffuse bilateral pulmonary metastases are first treated with intensive chemotherapy. Any residual pulmonary disease not responding to the chemotherapy is then surgically removed. Patients presenting with one solitary metastasis or a few of similar size are candidates for an initial thoracotomy followed by adjuvant, but intensive, chemotherapy. The pathologic specimen in these resected metastases frequently shows "mature bone," indicating the chemotherapeutic response.

Except for osteogenic sarcoma, chemotherapy for sarcomas is still unsatisfactory, with a 30% favorable response at best. As noted earlier, the workup need not be extensive and a disease-free interval per se is not important. The extent of resection relates to the number and location of the metastases, the majority of which are treated by wedge resection.

Metastatic breast carcinoma has always merited special attention. We have found that the lungs are seldom the sole site of metastatic disease in these patients, and a meticulous search for other metastases is merited. The response of these patients to chemotherapy or hormonal manipulation is well documented. Surgical intervention is reserved for those rare instances of solitary metastases or when the tumor becomes refractory to other treatment modalities and a finite number of nodules persist only in the lung.

In primary colon carcinoma, renal cell cancers, and melanomas, no effective chemotherapy is as yet available and the search continues for a better systemic approach. Resection of metastases continues to be offered when other treatment is ineffective and the tumors are completely resectable.

## OTHER CONSIDERATIONS

The interval from treatment of the primary tumor to the diagnosis of pulmonary metastases varies from zero, when the lesions are diagnosed simultaneously, to nearly 30 years. As a rule, testicular tumors have the shortest disease-free intervals and many patients have pulmonary metastases at the time of the diagnosis of their primary tumor. Disease-free interval and tumor doubling time have not, in our experience, affected survival in patients where complete resection of all visible tumor was possible. The ultimate prognosis is relative to site of origin and its specific tumor type and not so much to the tumor's doubling time. Early and complete eradication of all known tumor offers the best chance for long-term survival.

The classic, often-noted paper on the significance of doubling time is the one by Morton and associates[184] in 1973; 60 consecutive patients were analyzed. Patients with tumor doubling times of less than 20 days did poorly compared with those with tumor doubling times of greater than 40 days. An interesting observation to note in their report was the fact that patients with pulmonary metastases treated by surgical resection had done better than patients who had primary bronchogenic carcinoma, and that the results of surgical resection for patients with multiple metastases rivaled those reported in patients with solitary lesions.

The absolute number of metastases resectable is variable. In our experience the specific number of metastases per se is no guideline for patient selection for surgical treatment, but complete resectability is. Setting the limit of resectability for cure to four or fewer tumors as reported by some is not in accord with our experience where neither number nor disease-free interval have limited survival in patients with completely resected metastases.

## SURGICAL APPROACHES

There are essentially five surgical approaches to resect pulmonary metastases: a posterolateral thoracotomy, a median sternotomy, a bilateral anterior thoracotomy, a clamshell incision, and a video-assisted thoracoscopy (VATS).

The principle advantage of a standard posterolateral thoracotomy is the excellent exposure to the entire hemithorax, including all lobes. It provides an excellent view of all lesions and palpation of peripheral as well as central lesions as small as 1 mm not discernable on CT scans. It also provides an excellent means of palpation and removal of all gross tumor. The disadvantage is the large incision necessary with more pain, and the need for a second operation for bilateral disease.

The median sternotomy provides a simultaneous access to both lungs, detects occult metastases not suspected in the contralateral lung, and is less painful.[185] The disadvantages of a median sternotomy are the difficult access to posterior and central lesions, the difficult exposure to the left lower lobe, and the need for a single lung ventilation.

The bilateral clamshell incision, also known as a bilateral anterior thoracotomy with a transverse sternotomy, provides excellent access to bilateral disease. It is associated with less patient discomfort than sequential thoracotomies and is a cosmetic incision.[186] The main disadvantage is the need to sacrifice both internal mammary arteries. This is obviated when bilateral anterior thoracotomies are performed without transverse sternotomies.

The VATS has the advantage of an excellent visualization of the lung surface, less patient discomfort than the previous three approaches, and a shorter hospital stay.[187,188] It is an excellent procedure for biopsy and is helpful in determining resectability. Its main disadvantages, however, are the inability to feel, detect, and resect all metastases completely, and also the inability to detect deep-seated metastases. Recently, tumor implantation along the thoracoscopy incisions have been reported, with a consequent risk of early local recurrence.[188a]

For patients presenting with solitary or multiple unilateral pulmonary metastases, the posterolateral or anterior thoracotomy approach is preferred. Thus, access to all metastases is possible, and complete removal of all tumor is more certain. In patients with bilateral lung metastases, a median sternotomy is preferred by some and a staged lateral thoracotomy by others.[189] Since the advent of CT scanning, a more accurate assessment of the number of metastases has prompted the necessity for exploration of both lungs at initial treatment. A single operation is desirable whenever possible, but must be balanced against the need for complete removal of all tumor. Centrally placed lesions and those in the left lower lobe, particularly if multiple, are difficult to resect from a sternotomy approach. When the bilateral metastases are few, peripheral, and anteriorly placed, a median sternotomy with single lung anesthesia is very effective. More recently in our center, bilateral clamshell incisions with or without transverse sternotomy have been used for better access to all metastases with less morbidity than sequential posterolateral thoracotomies or sternotomies.

Extension of pulmonary metastases to mediastinum, chest wall, or diaphragm, and effusion are poor prognostic signs, since neither adequateness of resection nor prolonged survival is usually attained in this group of patients.

It is often necessary to consider resection for recurrent pulmonary metastases. As long as the risks are low and preservation of adequate lung tissue is possible, resection is offered if nonsurgical alternatives are not available. The overall 5-year survival rate in resected metastases from all types of sarcoma and from carcinomas is 25%, with little difference in survival among the various histologic types.[53] The overall morbidity rate is low, and the postoperative mortality rate remains around 1%, justifying the surgical treatment in the absence of alternatives. In 1971, we reported a 27% long-term survival rate.[190] In 1984, Mountain and associates[191] reported their 20-year experience. They reported a 33% long-term survival rate for single and multiple metastases.

## COMMENTS AND CONCLUSIONS

From 1965 to the present, over 400 reports have addressed the results of surgical treatment of pulmonary metastases from a variety of primary tumors and tumor sites. Except for germ cell tumors, the expectation of overall 5-year survival rate in patients with most tumors following treatment of pulmonary metastases is less than 50%, despite treatment by surgery, chemotherapy, or both. Until sustained responses to systemic treatment become uniformly possible by novel treatment regimens, pulmonary metastasectomy will remain an essential consideration in their treatment.[192]

The advent of thoracoscopy has refocused our attention on the impact of complete resection for lung metastases. Some advocates of thoracoscopy believe that complete resection of multiple metastases is a myth, and that concern about missing very small lesions that are not seen on CT scans or visualized at thoracoscopy but are palpable at thoracotomy does not necessarily imply a greater likelihood of prolonged survival in those patients with lesions that might be missed by thoracoscopy. The problem will necessarily resolve itself if effective systemic treatment becomes available for those tumors currently nonresponsive or partially responsive to chemotherapy.

The prognosis of patients with solitary pulmonary metastases is favorable. The 5-year survival for such patients when treated by surgical resection approximates the overall 5-year survival results of primary lung cancer adequately treated by resection. None of the long-term survival rates approach those achieved after resection of a primary stage I lung cancer.

The prognosis of patients with multiple pulmonary metastases is poor. Our overall survival results lead us to conclude that one-third of the patients die within 1 year of surgical treatment of metastases. Because of effective chemotherapy, we believe that the prognosis can be improved by combining surgery and chemotherapy. Therefore, a diligent watch for pulmonary metastases in all cancer patients and a positive approach when they are found will continue to improve the survival statistics.

Unfortunately, most retrospective reviews of results of resection for pulmonary metastases contain too few patients to analyze subsets of patients for prognosis. An International Registry of Lung Metastases was established in 1991 to assess the long-term results of pulmonary metastasectomy.[193] The registry gathered 5206 cases from 18 departments of thoracic surgery in Europe ($n = 13$), the United States ($n = 4$), and Canada ($n = 1$). Of these patients, 4572 (88%) had undergone complete surgical resection. The primary tumor was epithelial in 2260 patients, sarcoma in 2173, germ cell in 363, and melanoma in 328. Single metastases accounted for 2383 patients and multiple lesions for 2726. The mean follow-up was 46 months.

The overall operative mortality was 1%. Sarcomas and melanomas had a higher probability of relapse: 64% compared with 46% in epithelial primaries and 25% in germ cell tumors.[194] Primary sarcomas had a 66% intrathoracic relapse rate; melanoma reoccured in other distant sites 73% of the time. Incidence of repeat thoracotomies was highest with sarcomas, an experience that is consistent with that of most centers.

The three parameters with prognostic significance were resectability, disease-free interval, and number of metastases (1 vs. >1) (Table 9-10). The actuarial survival after complete metastasectomy was 36% at 5 years and 26% at 10 years. Multivariate analysis showed a better prognosis for patients with germ cell tumors, disease-free intervals of 36 months or more, and single metastases.

The International Registry demonstrated that long-term survival is achievable by pulmonary metastasectomy. It also confirmed that complete removal of all metastases is mandatory and that current

**TABLE 9-10.** FAVORABLE PROGNOSTIC FACTORS IN SELECTING RESECTION FOR PULMONARY METASTASES

1. Disease-free interval <36 months
2. Single metastasis
3. Resectability

radiologic staging is inaccurate. Intraoperative exploration is required in all patients to detect all metastases.

## REFERENCES

1. AMERICAN CANCER SOCIETY: *Cancer Facts and Figures—2000.* Atlanta, American Cancer Society, 2000.
2. WORLD HEALTH ORGANIZATION: The W.H.O. histologic typing of lung tumors. Am J Clin Pathol 77:123, 1982.
3. MOUNTAIN CF: The new international staging system for lung cancer. Surg Clin North Am 67:925, 1987.
4. FLEMING ID et al (eds): *AJCC Cancer Staging Manual,* 5th ed. Philadelphia, Lippincott-Raven, 1997, chap 19, pp 127–138.
5. INTERNATIONAL UNION AGAINST CANCER. *TNM Classification of Malignant Tumours,* 5th ed. New York, Wiley-Liss, 1997, pp 91–97.
6. MARTINI N, MELAMED MR: Occult carcinomas of the lung. Ann Thorac Surg 30:215, 1980.
7. SANDERSON DR et al: Bronchoscopic localization of radiographically occult lung cancer. Chest 65:608, 1974.
8. EDELL ES, CORTESE DA: Bronchoscopic localization and treatment of occult lung cancer. Chest 96:919, 1989.
9. LAM S et al: Detection of dysplasia and carcinoma in situ with a lung imaging fluorescence endoscopic device. J Thorac Cardiovasc Surg 105:1035, 1993.
10. CORTESE DA et al: Roentgenographically occult lung cancer. A ten-year experience. J Thorac Cardiovasc Surg 86:373, 1983.
11. HAYATA Y et al: Photoradiation therapy with hematoporphyrin derivative in early and stage I lung cancer. Chest 86:169, 1984.
12. OHO K et al: Indications for endoscopic Nd-YAG laser surgery in the trachea and bronchus. Endoscopy 15:302, 1983.
13. RAMSDELL JW et al: Multiorgan scans for staging lung cancer. J Thorac Cardiovasc Surg 73:653, 1977.
14. BULZEBRUCK H et al: New aspects in the staging of lung cancer. Prospective validation of the International Union Against Cancer TNM classification. Cancer 70:1102, 1992.
15. GINSBERG RJ, RUBINSTEIN LV: Randomized trial of lobectomy versus limited resection for T1N0 non–small cell lung cancer. Ann Thorac Surg 60:615, 1995.
16. MARTINI N et al: Incidence of local recurrence and secondary primary tumors in resected stage I lung cancer. J Thorac Cardiovasc Surg 109:1, 1995.
17. MARTINI N, GINSBERG RJ: Treatment of stage I and II disease, in *Comprehensive Textbook of Thoracic Oncology,* J Aisner et al (eds). Baltimore, Williams & Wilkins, 1996, pp 339–350.
18. GAIL MN et al: Prognostic factors in patients with resected stage I non-small cell lung cancer: A report from the Lung Cancer Study Group. Cancer 54:1802, 1984.
19. PAIROLERO PC et al: Post-surgical stage I bronchogenic carcinoma: Morbid implications of recurrent disease. Ann Thorac Surg 38:331, 1984.

20. THOMAS P, RUBINSTEIN L: Lung Cancer Study Group. Cancer recurrence after resection: T1 N0 non–small cell lung cancer. Ann Thorac Surg 49:242, 1990.

21. SHIELDS TW: Prognostic significance of parenchymal lymphatic vessel and blood vessel invasion in carcinoma of the lung. Surg Gynecol Obstet 157:185, 1983.

22. MACCHIARINI P et al: Blood vessel invasion by tumor cells predicts recurrence in completely resected T1 N0 M0 non–small-cell lung cancer. J Thorac Cardiovasc Surg 106:80, 1993.

23. SLEBOS RJC et al: K-ras oncogene activation as a prognostic marker in adenocarcinoma of the lung. N Engl J Med 323:561, 1990.

24. CIBAS ES et al: The effect of tumor size and tumor cell DNA content on the survival of patients with stage I adenocarcinoma of the lung. Cancer 63:1552, 1989.

25. RICE TW et al: Prognostic significance of flow cytometry in non-small-cell lung cancer. J Thorac Cardiovasc Surg 106:210, 1993.

26. LIPPMAN SC, HONG WK: Not yet standard: Retinoids versus second primary tumors (editorial). J Clin Oncol 11:1204, 1993.

27. PASTORINO U et al: Adjuvant treatment of stage I lung cancer with high-dose vitamin A. J Clin Oncol 11:1216, 1993.

28. HILARIS BS et al: Results of radiation therapy in stage I and II unresectable non-small-cell lung cancer. Endocuriether Hyperther Oncol 2:15, 1986.

29. SMART J, HILTON G: Radiotherapy of cancer of the lung. Results in a selected group of cases. Lancet 270:880, 1956.

30. SCHUMACHER W: The use of high-energy electrons in the treatment of inoperable lung and bronchogenic carcinoma, in *High-Energy Photons and Electrons: Clinical Applications in Cancer Management*, S Kramer et al (eds). New York, Wiley, 1976, pp 255–284.

31. COOPER JD et al: Radiotherapy alone for patients with operable carcinoma of the lung. Chest 87:289, 1985.

32. DILLMAN RO et al: Improved survival in stage III non-small-cell lung cancer: Seven-year follow-up of cancer and leukemia group B (CALGB) 8433 trial. J Natl Cancer Inst 88:1210, 1996.

33. KOMAKI R et al: Randomized study of chemotherapy/radiation therapy combinations for favorable patients with locally advanced inoperable nonsmall cell lung cancer: Radiation Therapy Oncology Group (RTOG) 92-04. Int J Radiat Oncol Biol Phys 38:149, 1997.

34. McKNEALLY MF et al: Regional immunotherapy of lung cancer with BCG. Lancet 21:377, 1976.

35. MOUNTAIN CF, GAIL MH: Surgical adjuvant intrapleural BCG treatment for stage I non-small cell lung cancer: Preliminary report of the National Cancer Institute Lung Cancer Study Group. J Thorac Cardiovasc Surg 82:649, 1981.

36. FELD R et al: Lung Cancer Study Group. Sites of recurrence in resected stage I non-small cell lung cancer: A guide for future studies. J Clin Oncol 2:1352, 1985.

37. NON–SMALL CELL LUNG CANCER COLLABORATIVE GROUP: Chemotherapy in non–small cell lung cancer: A meta analysis using updated data on individual patients from randomized clinical trials. Br Med J 311:899, 1995.

38. MARTINI N et al: Preoperative chemotherapy for stage IIIA (N2) lung cancer: The Sloan-Kettering experience with 136 patients. Ann Thorac Surg 55:1365, 1993.

39. MARTINI N et al: Survival after resection in stage II non-small cell lung cancer. Ann Thorac Surg 54:460, 1992.

40. KAPLAN EL, MEIER P: Nonparametric estimation from incomplete observations. J Am Stat Assoc 53:457, 1958.

41. WEISENBURGER TH: Lung Cancer Study Group. Effects of postoperative mediastinal radiation on completely resected stage II and stage III epidermoid cancer of the lung. N Engl J Med 315:1377, 1986.

42. HOLMES EC, GAIL M: Lung Cancer Study Group. Surgical adjuvant therapy for stage II and III adenocarcinoma and large cell undifferentiated carcinoma. J Clin Oncol 4:710, 1986.

43. PORT META-ANALYSIS TRIALISTS GROUP: Postoperative radiotherapy in non-small-cell lung cancer: Systematic review and metaanalysis of individual patient data from nine randomised controlled trials. Lancet 352:257, 1998.

44. LAD T et al: The benefit of adjuvant treatment for resected locally advanced non-small cell lung cancer. J Clin Oncol 6:9, 1988.

45. NIIRANEN A et al: Adjuvant chemotherapy after radical surgery for non-small cell lung cancer: A randomized study. J Clin Oncol 10:1927, 1992.

46. WADA H et al: Postoperative adjuvant chemotherapy for non-small-cell lung cancer. West Japan Study Group for Lung Cancer Surgery. The Japan Lung Cancer Research Group on Postsurgical Adjuvant Chemotherapy. Oncology 11(9 Suppl 10):98, 1997.

47. RUSCH V: A phase III comparison between concurrent chemotherapy plus radiotherapy, and concurrent chemotherapy plus radiotherapy followed by surgical resection for stage IIIa(N2) non–small cell lung cancer (CALGB 9592/RTOG 93-09) (personal communication).

48. PISTERS K et al: Phase II trial of induction paclitaxel/carboplatin (PC) in early stage (T2N0), T1-2N1, and selected T3N0-1 non-small cell lung cancer (NSCLC). Proceedings of the Eight World Conference on Lung Cancer, Dublin, Ireland, August 10–15, 1997.

49. DEPIERRE A: Neo-adjuvant chemotherapy (NCT) in non-small cell lung cancer (NSCLC): Hope for progress. Lung Cancer 21(suppl): S24, 1998.

50. McCAUGHAN BC et al: Chest wall invasion of carcinoma of the lung: Therapeutic and prognostic implications. J Thorac Cardiovasc Surg 89:836, 1985.

50a. DOWNEY R et al: Extent of chest wall invasion and survival in patient with lung cancer. Ann Thorac Surg 68:188, 1999.

51. PIEHLER JM et al: Bronchogenic carcinoma with chest wall invasion: Factors affecting survival following en bloc resection. Ann Thorac Surg 34:684, 1982.

51a. TRASTEK VF et al: En bloc (non-chest wall) resection for bronchogenic carcinoma with parietal fixation. Factors affecting survival. J Thorac Cardiovasc Surg 87:352, 1984.

52. PATTERSON GA et al: The value of adjuvant radiotherapy in pulmonary and chest wall resection for bronchogenic carcinoma. Ann Thorac Surg 34:692, 1982.

52a. ALLEN MS et al: Bronchogenic carcinoma with chest wall invasion. Ann Thorac Surg 51:948, 1991.

52b. ALBERTUCCI M et al: Surgery and the management of peripheral lung tumors adherent to the parietal pleura. J Thorac Cardiovasc Surg 103:8, 1992.

53. McCORMACK PM et al: Methods of skeletal reconstruction following resection of lung carcinomas invading the chest wall. Surg Clin North Am 67:979, 1987.

54. PAIROLERO PC, ARNOLD PG: Chest wall tumors: Experience with 100 consecutive patients. J Thorac Cardiovasc Surg 90:367, 1985.

55. GINSBERG RJ et al: Influence of surgical resection and intra-operative brachytherapy in the management of superior sulcus tumor. Ann Thorac Surg 57:1440, 1994.

56. SHAW RR et al: Treatment of the superior sulcus tumor by irradiation followed by resection. Ann Surg 154:29, 1961.

57. PAULSON DL: Carcinomas in the superior pulmonary sulcus. J Thorac Cardiovasc Surg 70:1095, 1975.

58. PAULSON DL: The "superior culcus" lesion, in *International Trends in General Thoracic Surgery,* vol 1, NC Delarue, H Eschapasse (eds). Philadelphia, WB Saunders, 1985, pp 121–131.

59. HILARIS BS, MARTINI N: Multimodality therapy of superior sulcus tumors, in *Advances in Pain Research and Therapy,* J Bonica (ed). New York, Raven Press, 1982, p 113.

60. ——— et al: Integrated irradiation and surgery in the treatment of apical lung cancer. Cancer 27:1369, 1971.

61. ——— et al: Treatment of superior sulcus tumors (Pancoast tumor). Surg Clin North Am 67:965, 1987.

62. RUSCH V: Induction chemoradiotherapy followed by surgical resection for non-small cell lung cancer involving the superior sulcus (Pancoast tumors): A phase II intergroup trial. (personal communication.)

63. DESLAURIERS J: Involvement of the main carina, in *International Trends in General Thoracic Surgery,* vol 1. NC Delarue, H Eschapasse (eds). Philadelphia, WB Saunders, 1985, pp 139–145.

64. DESLAURIERS J et al: Long term clinical and functional results of sleeve lobectomy for primary lung cancer. J Thorac Cardiovasc Surg 92:871, 1986.

65. FABER LP et al: Results of sleeve lobectomy for bronchogenic carcinoma in 101 patients. Ann Thorac Surg 37:279, 1984.

66. VOGT-MOYKOPF I et al: Bronchoplastic and angioplastic operation in bronchial carcinoma: Long-term results of a retrospective analysis from 1973 to 1983. Int Surg 71:211, 1986.

67. MATHISEN DJ, GRILLO HC: Carinal resection for bronchogenic cancer. J Thorac Cardiovasc Surg 102:16, 1991.

68. JENSIK RJ et al: Survival in patients undergoing tracheal sleeve pneumonectomy for bronchogenic carcinoma. J Thorac Cardiovasc Surg 84:489, 1982.

69. BURT ME et al: Results of surgical treatment of stage III lung cancer invading the mediastinum. Surg Clin North Am 67:987, 1987.

70. MARTINI N et al: Management of non-small cell lung cancer with direct mediastinal involvement. Ann Thorac Surg 58:1447, 1994.

71. MARTINI N, FLEHINGER BJ: The role of surgery in N2 lung cancer. Surg Clin North Am 67:1037, 1987.

72. PEARSON FG et al: Significance of positive superior mediastinal nodes identified at mediastinoscopy in patients with resectable cancer of the lung. J Thorac Cardiovasc Surg 83:1, 1982.

73. MARTINI N et al: Results of resection in non-oat cell carcinoma of the lung with mediastinal lymph node metastases. Ann Surg 198:386, 1983.

74. GOLDSTRAW P et al: Surgical management of non-small cell lung cancer with ipsilateral mediastinal node metastasis (N2 disease). J Thorac Cardiovasc Surg 107:19, 1994.

75. KIRSCH MM, SLOAN H: Mediastinal metastasis in bronchogenic carcinoma: Influence of postoperative irradiation, cell type and location. Ann Thorac Surg 33:459, 1982.

76. LEVASSEUR PH, REGNARD JF: Long term results after surgery for N2 non-small cell lung cancer. Presented at the IASLC Workshop, Bruges, Belgium, June 17–21, 1990.

77. MOUNTAIN CF: Expanded possibilities for surgical treatment of lung cancer. Survival in stage IIIa disease. Chest 97:1045, 1990.

78. NARUKE T et al: Prognosis and survival in resected lung carcinoma based on the new international staging system. J Thorac Cardiovasc Surg 96:440, 1988.

79. NARUKE T et al: The importance of surgery to non-small cell carcinoma of the lung with mediastinal lymph node metastasis. Ann Thorac Surg 46:603, 1988.

80. SCHIRREN J et al: N2 surgery in bronchial carcinoma: Indications, technique and results. Gen Thorac Surg 32, 1993.

81. WATANABE Y et al: Aggressive surgical intervention in N2 non-small cell cancer of the lung. Ann Thorac Surg 51:253, 1991.

82. PISTERS K et al: Randomized trial comparing postoperative chemotherapy with vindesine and cisplatin plus thoracic irradiation alone in stage III (N2) non-small cell lung cancer. J Surg Oncol 56:236, 1994.

83. BURKES R et al: Induction chemotherapy with mitomycin, vindesine and cisplatin for stage III unresectable non-small cell lung cancer: Results of Toronto phase II trial. J Clin Oncol 10:580, 1992.

84. DARWISH S et al: Neoadjuvant cisplatin and etoposide for stage IIIA (clinical N2) non-small cell lung cancer. Am J Clin Oncol 17:64, 1994.

85. KRIS MG et al: Preoperative and adjuvant chemotherapy in patients with locally advanced non-small cell lung cancer. Surg Clin North Am 67:1051, 1987.

86. PUJOL JL et al: Pilot study of neoadjuvant ifosfamide, cisplatin and etoposide in locally advanced non-small cell lung cancer. Eur J Cancer 26:798, 1990.

87. CHOI N et al: Preoperative accelerated radiotherapy and concurrent chemotherapy for stage IIIA (N0) non-small cell lung cancer: Improved survival by enhanced local tumor control (abstract). Proc Am Soc Ther Radiol Oncol 32:198, 1995.

88. FABER LP, BONOMI PD: Neodajuvant treatment in locally advanced non-small cell lung cancer. Semin Surg Oncol 6:225, 1990.

89. FABER LP et al: Preoperative chemotherapy and irradiation for stage III non-small cell lung cancer. Ann Thorac Surg 47:669, 1989.

90. RUSCH VW et al: Surgical resection of stage IIIA and stage IIIB non-small cell lung cancer after concurrent induction chemoradiation therapy: A Southwest Oncology Group Trial. J Thorac Cardiovasc Surg 105:97, 1993.

91. SKARIN A et al: Neoadjuvant chemotherapy in marginally resectable stage III M0 non-small cell lung cancer: Long term follow-up in 41 patients. J Surg Oncol 40:266, 1989.

92. STRAUSS GM et al: Neoadjuvant chemotherapy and radiotherapy followed by surgery in stage IIIA non-small cell carcinoma of the lung: Report of cancer and leukemia group B phase II study. J Clin Oncol 10:1237, 1992.

93. PASS HI et al: Randomized trial of neoadjuvant therapy for lung cancer: Interim analysis. Ann Thorac Surg 53:992, 1992.

94. ROTH JA et al: A randomized trial comparing preoperative chemotherapy and surgery with surgery alone in resectable stage IIIA non-small cell lung cancer. J Natl Cancer Inst 86:673, 1994.

95. ROSELL R et al: A randomized trial comparing preoperative chemotherapy plus surgery with surgery alone in patients with non-small cell lung cancer. N Engl J Med 330:153, 1994.

96. DILLMAN RO et al: A randomized trial of induction chemotherapy plus high-dose radiation versus radiation alone in stage III non-small-cell lung cancer. N Engl J Med 323:940, 1990.

97. SAUSE WT et al: Radiation Therapy Oncology Group (RTOG) 88-08 and Eastern Cooperative Oncology Group (ECOG) 4588: Preliminary results of a phase III trial in regionally advanced, unresectable non-small cell lung cancer. J Natl Cancer Inst 87:198, 1995.

98. LE CHEVALIER T, ARRIAGADA R: Therapeutic options in locally advanced non-small cell lung cancer (stage IIIB), in Comprehensive Textbook of Thoracic Oncology, J Aisner et al (eds). Baltimore, Williams & Wilkins, 1996, pp 388–415.

99. HEELAN R et al: Carcinomas involving the hilum and mediastinum: Computed tomographic and magnetic resonance evaluation. Radiology 156:111, 1985.

100. DAMSTRUP L et al: Review of the curative role of radiotherapy in the treatment of non small cell lung cancer. Lung Cancer 11:153, 1994.

101. PEREZ CA et al: Impact of tumor control on survival in carcinoma of the lung treated with irradiation. Int J Radiat Oncol Biol Phys 12:539, 1986.

102. PEREZ CA et al: Long term observations of the patterns of failure in patients with unresectable non-oat cell carcinoma of the lung treated with definitive radiotherapy. Cancer 59:1874, 1987.

103. SAUNDERS MI et al: Primary tumor control after radiotherapy for carcinoma of the bronchus. Int J Radiat Oncol Biol Phys 10:499, 1984.

104. STANLEY K et al: Patterns of failure in patients with inoperable carcinoma of the lung. Cancer 47:2725, 1981.

105. LICHTER AS: Three-dimensional conformal radiation therapy: A testable hypothesis. Int J Radiat Oncol Biol Phy 21:853, 1991.

106. BURT ME et al: Prospective evaluation of unilateral adrenal metastases in patients with operable non-small cell lung cancer: Impact of magnetic resonance imaging. J Thorac Cardiovasc Surg 107:584, 1994.

107. BURT ME et al: Resection of brain metastases from non-small cell lung carcinoma: Results of therapy. J Thorac Cardiovasc Surg 103:399, 1992.

108. PATCHELL RA et al: A randomized trial of surgery in the treatment of single metastases to brain. N Engl J Med 322:494, 1990.

109. PHILLIPS MH et al: Stereotactic radiosurgery: A review and comparison of methods. J Clin Oncol 12:1085, 1994.

110. MARTINI N: Rationale for surgical treatment of brain metastasis in non-small-cell lung cancer. Ann Thorac Surg 42:357, 1986.

111. MARTINI et al: Oat cell carcinoma of the lung. Clin Bull 5:144, 1975.

112. SHIELDS TW et al: Surgical resection in the management of small cell carcinoma of the lung. J Thorac Cardiovasc Surg 84:481, 1982.

113. MEDICAL RESEARCH COUNCIL OF GREAT BRITAIN: Working party on the evaluation of different methods of therapy in carcinoma of the bronchus. Comparative trial of surgery and radiotherapy for the primary treatment of small-celled, or oat-celled carcinoma of the bronchus. Lancet 2:979, 1966.

114. FOX W, SCADDING JG: Medical Research Council comparative trial of surgery and radiotherapy for primary treatment of small-celled or oat-called carcinoma of the bronchus. Ten-year follow-up. Lancet 2:63, 1973.

115. AISNER J et al: Role of chemotherapy in small cell lung cancer: A consensus report of the International Association for the Study of Lung Cancer Workshop. Cancer Treat Rep 67:37, 1983.

116. LIVINGSTON RB: Current chemotherapy of small cell lung cancer. Chest 89:2585, 1986.

117. PIGNON J-P et al: A meta-analysis of thoracic radiotherapy for small-cell lung cancer. N Engl J Med 327:1618, 1992.

118. GINSBERG RJ: Surgery and small cell lung cancer—An overview. Lung Cancer 5:232, 1989.

119. SHEPHERD FA et al: Reduction in local recurrence and improved survival in surgically treated patients with small cell lung cancer. J Thorac Cardiovasc Surg 86:498, 1983.

120. SHEPHERD FA et al: Surgical treatment for limited small-cell lung cancer. J Thorac Cardiovasc Surg 101:385, 1991.

121. WARDE P, PAYNE D: Does thoracic irradiation improve survival and local control in limited-stage small-cell carcinoma of the lung? A meta-analysis. J Clin Oncol 10:890, 1992.

122. SHIELDS TW, ROBINSON PG. Benign and less common malignant tumors of the lung, in General Thoracic Surgery, 3d ed, TW Shields (ed). Philadelphia, Lea & Febiger, 1989, pp 935–950.

123. ARRIGONI MG et al: Atypical carcinoid tumors of the lung. J Thorac Cardiovasc Surg 64:413, 1972.

124. HAMPER UM et al: Pulmonary hamartoma: Diagnosis by transthoracic needle aspiration biopsy. Radiology 155:15, 1985.

125. MARTINI N, BEATTIE ER JR: Less common tumors of the lung, in General Thoracic Surgery, 2d ed, TW Shields (ed). Philadelphia, Lea & Febiger, 1982, pp 770–779.

126. BERARDI RS et al: Inflammatory pseudotumors of the lung. Surg Gynecol Obstet 156:89, 1983.

127. LIEBOW AA, CASTLEMAN B: Benign "clear cell" tumors of the lung (abstract). Am J Pathol 43:13a, 1963.

128. KATZENSTEIN AL et al: Sclerosing hemangioma of the lung: A clinicopathologic study of 51 cases. Am J Surg Pathol 4:343, 1982.

129. MARTINI N et al: Treatment and prognosis in bronchial carcinoids involving regional lymph nodes. J Thorac Cardiovasc Surg 107:1, 1994.

130. PAIROLERO PC et al: Carcinoid tumors of the lung, in International Trends in General Thoracic Surgery, vol 5, N Martini, I Vogt-Moykopf (eds). St. Louis, CV Mosby, 1989, pp 258–262.

131. BENSCH KG et al: Oat-cell carcinoma of the lung: Its origin and relationship to bronchial carcinoid. Cancer 22:1163, 1968.

132. DECARO LF et al: Typical and atypical carcinoids within the pulmonary APUD tumor spectrum. J Thorac Cardiovasc Surg 86:528, 1983.

133. WAIN JC et al: Immunohistochemistry and new trends in the diagnosis of carcinoids, in International Trends in General Thoracic Surgery, vol 5, N Martini, I Vogt-Moykopf (eds). St. Louis, CV Mosby, 1989, pp 249–257.

134. EL-NAGGAR AK et al: Typical and atypical bronchopulmonary carcinoids: A clinicopathologic and flow cytometric study. Am J Clin Pathol 95:828, 1991.

135. LARISMONT D et al: Characterization of the morphonuclear features and DNA ploidy of typical and atypical carcinoids and small cell carcinomas of the lung. Am J Clin Pathol 94:379, 1990.

136. MCCAUGHAN BC et al: Bronchial carcinoids. J Thorac Cardiovasc Surg 89:8, 1985.

137. OKIKE N et al: Carcinoid tumours of the lung. Ann Thorac Surg 22:271, 1976.

138. TEMECK BK et al: Somatostatin analogue in the localization

and treatment of bronchial carcinoid tumors. J Surg Oncol 5:195, 1996.

139. BLONDAL T et al: Argyrophil carcinoid tumors of the lung. Chest 78:840, 1980.

140. OKIKE N et al: Bronchoplastic procedures in the treatment of carcinoid tumors of the tracheobronchial tree. J Thorac Cardiovasc Surg 76:281, 1978.

141. JENSIK RJ et al: Bronchoplastic and conservative resectional procedures for bronchial adenoma. J Thorac Cardiovasc Surg 68:556, 1974.

142. LAWSON RM et al: Bronchial adenoma. Review of an 18 year experience at the Brompton Hospital. Thorax 31:245, 1976.

143. TODD TR et al: Bronchial carcinoid tumors. J Thorac Cardiovasc Surg 79:532, 1980.

144. WILKINS EW et al: Changing times in the management of bronchial carcinoid tumors. Ann Thorac Surg 38:339, 1984.

145. GINSBERG RJ et al: Bronchial adenoma, in *General Thoracic Surgery*, 3d ed, TW Shields (ed). Philadelphia, Lea & Febiger, 1989, pp 875–889.

146. BALAZS M: Adenoid cystic (cylindromatous) carcinoma of the trachea: An ultrastructural study. Histopathology 10:425, 1986.

147. PERSONNE C et al: Inductions and technique for endoscopic laser resection in bronchology. J Thorac Cardiovasc Surg 91:710, 1986.

148. GRILLO HC: Tracheal tumours: Diagnosis and management, in *Thoracic Oncology*, NC Choi, HC Grillo (eds). New York, Raven Press, 1983, pp 271–278.

149. PERELMAN MI, KOROLEVA NS: Primary tumours of the trachea, in *International Trends in General Thoracic Surgery*, vol 2, NC Delarue, H Eschapasse (eds). Philadelphia, WB Saunders, 1987.

150. PEARSON FG et al: Experience with primary neoplasms of the trachea and carina. J Thorac Cardiovasc Surg 88:511, 1984.

151. ROSTOM AY, MORGAN RL: Results of treating primary tumours of the trachea by irradiation. Thorax 33:387, 1978.

152. MUNSCH C et al: Urgent treatment for a nonresectable, asphyxiating tracheal cylindroma. Ann Thorac Surg 43:663, 1987.

153. RYAN KL et al: Management of adenoid cystic carcinoma. Chest 89:503, 1986.

154. REICHLE FA, ROSEMOND GP: Mucoepidermoid tumours of the bronchus. J Thorac Cardiovasc Surg 51:443, 1966.

155. MARTINI N et al: Primary sarcoma of the lung. J Thorac Cardiovasc Surg 61:33, 1971.

156. McCORMACK PM, MARTINI N: Primary sarcomas and lymphomas of lung, in *International Trends in General Thoracic Surgery*, vol 5, N Martini, I Vogt-Moykopf (eds). St Louis, CV Mosby, 1989, pp 269–274.

157. SALTZSTEIN SI: Pulmonary malignant lymphomas and pseudo lymphomas: Classification, therapy and prognosis. Cancer 16:928, 1963.

158. L'HOSTE RJ JR et al: Primary pulmonary lymphomas. Cancer 54:1397, 1984.

159. MARTINI N, McCORMACK PM: Evolution of surgical management in pulmonary metastases. Chest Surg Clin North Am 8:13, 1998.

160. MEADE RH: *A History of Thoracic Surgery*. Springfield, IL, Charles C Thomas, 1961.

161. ATTINGER B et al: The first successful lung resection (German). Schweizerische Rundschau Medizin Praxis 82:435, 1993.

162. WEINLECHNER JW: Zur Kasuistik der Tumoren an der Brustwand und deren Behandlung (Resektion der Rippen, Eroffnung der Brusthohle, partielle Entfernung der Lunge). Wien Med Wchnschr 32:589, 1882.

163. KRONLEIN RU: Ueber Lungenchirurgie. Berl Klin Wchnschr 21:129, 1884.

164. DIVIS G: Ein Beitrag Zur Operativen Behandlung der Lungeschwulste. Acta Chir Scandinav 62:329, 1927.

165. TOREK F: Removal of metastatic carcinoma of the lung and mediastinum. Arch Surg 21:1416, 1930.

166. BARNEY JD, CHURCHILL EJ: Adenocarcinoma of the kidney with metastasis to the lung cured by nephrectomy and lobectomy. J Urol 42:269, 1939.

167. BARNEY JD, CHURCHILL EJ: Twelve-year cure following nephrectomy for adenocarcinoma and lobectomy for solitary metastasis. J Urol 52:406, 1944.

168. NAEF AP: *The Story of Thoracic Surgery: Milestones and Pioneers.* Toronto, Hogrefe and Huber, 1990.

169. ALEXANDER J, HAIGHT C: Pulmonary resection for solitary metastatic sarcomas and carcinomas. Surg Gynecol Obstet 85:129, 1947.

170. EDWARDS AT: Malignant disease of the lung. J Thorac Surg 4:107, 1934.

171. EHRENHAFT J et al: Pulmonary resections for metastatic lesions. A M A Arch Surg 77:606, 1958.

172. GLIEDMAN ML et al: Lung resection for metastatic cancer: 29 cases from the University of Minnesota and a collected review of 264 cases. Surgery 42:521, 1957.

173. HANSEN JL: Operative treatment of pulmonary metastases and pulmonary processes with suspected metastases. Ugesk-Laeger 120:1045, 1958.

174. MANNIX EP JR: Resection of multiple pulmonary metastases fourteen years after amputation for osteochondrogenic sarcoma of tibia: Apparent freedom from recurrence two years later. J Thorac Surg 26:544, 1953.

175. SEILER HH et al: Pulmonary resection for metastatic malignant lesions. J Thorac Surg 19:655, 1950.

176. SOMMER GNJ JR: Resection of the bony thoracic wall for solitary hematogenous metastatic tumors. Cancer Jan Um 4:120, 1951.

177. THOMFORD NR et al: The surgical treatment of metastatic tumors in the lungs. J Thorac Cardiovasc Surg 49:357, 1965.

178. MARCOVE RC et al: Osteogenic sarcoma under the age of 21: A review of 145 operative cases. J Bone Joint Surg 52A:411, 1970.

179. McCORMACK PM, MARTINI N: The changing role of surgery for pulmonary metastases. Ann Thorac Surg 28:139, 1979.

180. ADKINS PC et al: Thoracotomy on the patient with previous malignancy: Metastasis or new primary? J Thorac Cardiovasc Surg 56:351, 1968.

181. CASEY JJ et al: The solitary pulmonary nodule in the patient with breast cancer. Surgery 96:801, 1984.

182. McCORMACK PM et al: Pulmonary resection in metastatic carcinoma. Chest 73:163, 1978.

183. JOSEPH WL et al: Prognostic significance of tumor doubling time in evaluating operability in pulmonary metastatic disease. J Thorac Cardiovasc Surg 61:23, 1971.

184. MORTON DL et al: Surgical resection and adjunctive immunotherapy for selected patients with multiple pulmonary metastases. Ann Surg 178:360, 1973.

185. JOHNSTON MR: Median sternotomy for resection of pulmonary metastases. J Thorac Cardiovasc Surg 85:516, 1983.

186. BAINS MS et al: The clamshell incision: An improved approach to bilateral pulmonary and mediastinal tumor. Ann Thorac Surg 58:30, 1994.

187. BRAIMBRIDGE MV: The history of thoracoscopic surgery. Ann Thorac Surg 56:610, 1993.

188. LANDRENEAU RJ et al: Thoracoscopic resection of 85 pulmonary lesions. Ann Thorac Surg 54:415, 1992.

188a. DOWNEY R et al: Dissemination of malignant tumors after video-assisted thoracic surgery: A report of twenty-one cases. J Thorac Cardiovasc Surg 111:954, 1996.

189. ROTH JA et al: Comparison of median sternotomy and thoracotomy for resection of pulmonary metastases in patients with adult soft tissue sarcomas. Ann Thrac Surg 42:134, 1986.

190. MARTINI N et al: Multiple pulmonary resections in the treatment of osteogenic sarcoma. Ann Thorac Surg 12:271, 1971.

191. MOUNTAIN CF et al: Surgery for pulmonary metastasis: A 20-year experience. Ann Thorac Surg 38:323, 1984.

192. PUTNAM JB JR, ROTH JA: Prognostic indicators in patients with pulmonary metastases. Semin Surg Oncol 6:291, 1990.

193. PASTORINO U et al: Long-term results of lung metastasectomy: Prognostic analyses based on 5206 cases. The International Registry of Lung Metastases. J Thorac Cardiovasc Surg 113:37, 1997.

194. PASTORINO U et al: A new staging proposal for pulmonary metastases. The results of analysis of 5206 cases of resected pulmonary metastases. Chest Surg Clin North Am 8:197, 1998.

# CHAPTER 10

# NEOPLASMS OF THE MEDIASTINUM

*Christine L. Lau and R. Duane Davis, Jr.*

## HISTORICAL ASPECTS

The neoplasms found in the mediastinum are a diverse group of tumors, which include thymic lesions, lymphomas, germ cell tumors, neurogenic tumors, endocrine tumors, and other rare tumors. Successful surgical treatment of mediastinal tumors required the introduction of endotracheal anesthesia and closed pleural drainage. Prior to these developments mediastinal surgery was limited to attempts involving lesions in the anterior mediastinum. Complications such as pneumothorax often proved fatal. The history of mediastinal tumors is really one of the individual neoplasms. Notable landmarks are listed in Table 10-1.

Recently advances have been made in the surgical treatment and the medical management of the diverse group of tumors confined in the borders of the mediastinum. Multimodality treatment has significantly improved survival in many of these neoplasms. Improvement in diagnostic techniques has decreased the need for unnecessary surgical procedures. Newer less invasive surgical techniques have decreased the morbidity of surgery in many cases.

This chapter will focus on neoplasms seen primarily in the mediastinum, excluding those found in the mediastinum as metastases from other sites or by direct extension. This chapter also will not include the cystic lesions that represent 25% of the mediastinal masses in many series.

## ANATOMIC LANDMARKS

The borders of the mediastinum are superiorly the thoracic inlet, inferiorly the diaphragm, anteriorly the sternum, posteriorly the vertebral column, and laterally the parietal pleura. There are several ways of dividing the mediastinum into compartments. The division into compartments is done because certain tumors have a predilection to occur in an anatomic compartment. Although most tumors are commonly located in one compartment, lymphoma can be found in all three. This chapter utilizes the three-compartment nomenclature consisting of the anterosuperior compartment, the middle compartment, and the posterior compartment. Each of these has various boundaries as shown in Fig. 10-1. Table 10-2 shows the various tumors found primarily in the mediastinum.

The location of a mediastinal tumor gives a valuable clue about its diagnosis. Table 10-3 shows the common locations of most mediastinal neoplasms.

## INCIDENCE

Mediastinal tumors most frequently present in the third to fifth decades of life. Azarow and colleagues[1] compared primary mediastinal tumors in adults and children. In the pediatric population the most frequent tumors were neurogenic (47%), thymic (28%), lymphoma (9%), and germ cell (9%). In the adult population thymic neoplasms were the most frequent (31%), followed by lymphoma (26%), neurogenic tumors (15%), and germ cell tumors (15%). Davis et al.[2] looked at 2399 patients across multiple studies combining pediatric and adult populations and found an overall incidence of mediastinal neoplasms as seen in Table 10-4. The distribution of tumors in the various compartments for adults and children is seen in Table 10-5.

The incidence of malignancy varies with age, as seen in Fig. 10-2. In adults (>20 years old) approximately 43% of tumors are malignant.[2] Grosfeld[3] reported a series of 201 children with mediastinal tumors and reported 73% of these were malignant and 27% were benign. This compares to an earlier study by the same authors where 76% were malignant and 24% benign.[4] From the Duke series across all age groups, malignant tumors constitute 42% of mediastinal neoplasms and cysts.[2] According to this study masses in the

## TABLE 10-1. LANDMARKS IN MEDIASTINAL TUMORS

| | |
|---|---|
| 1832 | Hodgkin's disease was first described before the Medical and Chirurgical Society by Dr. Thomas Hodgkin. Sternberg and Reed did not describe the multinuclear cells that define this neoplasm for 70 more years. |
| 1893 | Bastianelli excised a dermoid cyst in the anterior mediastinum by resecting the manubrium. |
| 1932 | Drs. Cope and Churchill at Massachusetts General Hospital successfully removed a mediastinal parathyroid adenoma. The now famous patient, Captain Charles Martel, had previously undergone six negative neck explorations when, based on anatomical principles, Drs. Cope and Churchill decided to explore the mediastinum. |
| 1939 | Dr. Alfred Blalock presented a paper on the use of thymectomy in the treatment of myasthenia gravis. In this paper Blalock reported the successful removal of a 6 × 5 × 3 cm thymic tumor from a 19-year-old female. Follow-up of this patient over a 3-year time period demonstrated significant improvement in her symptoms of myasthenia.[141] |
| 1966 | McNeill and Chamberlain introduced anterior mediastinotomy (Chamberlain procedure).[142] |
| 1977 | Einhorn and Donohue introduced the cisplatin, vinblastine, and bleomycin (PVB) chemotherapeutic regimen for the treatment of nonseminomatous germ cell tumors.[143] |

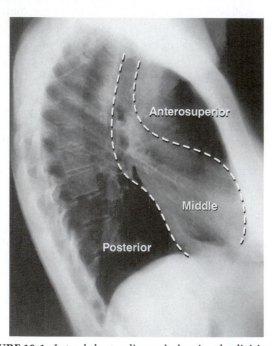

**FIGURE 10-1.** Lateral chest radiograph showing the division into the three mediastinal compartments: anterosuperior, middle, and posterior.

## TABLE 10-2. CLASSIFICATION OF PRIMARY MEDIASTINAL TUMORS AND CYSTS

**Neurogenic Tumors**
Neurofibroma
Neurilemoma
Neurosarcoma
Ganglioneuroma
Neuroblastoma
Chemodectoma
Paraganglioma

**Thymoma**
Benign
Malignant

**Lymphoma**
Hodgkin's disease
Lymphoblastic
Large-cell diffuse growth
 pattern
 T-immunoblastic sarcoma
 B-immunoblastic sarcoma
 Sclerosing follicular cell

**Germ-Cell Tumors**
Teratodermoid
 Benign
 Malignant
 Seminoma
Nonseminomas
 Embryonal
 Choriocarcinoma
 Endodermal

**Primary Carcinomas**

**Mesenchymal Tumors**
Fibroma/Fibrosarcoma
Lipoma/Liposarcoma
Leiomyoma/Leiomyosarcoma
Rhabdosarcoma
Xanthogranuloma
Myxoma
Mesothelioma
Hemangioma
Hemangioendothelioma
Hemangiopericytoma
Lymphangioma
Lymphangiomyoma
Lymphangiopericytoma

**Endocrine Tumors**
Intrathoracic thyroid
Parathyroid adenoma/
 carcinoma
Carcinoid

**Cysts**
Bronchogenic
Pericardial
Enteric
Thymic thoracic duct
Nonspecific

**Giant Lymph Node Hyperplasia**
Castleman's disease

**Chondroma**

**Extramedullary Hematopoiesis**

SOURCE: From Davis RD et al.[82] Reprinted with permission.

anterosuperior mediastinum are more likely to be malignant (59%) than those found in the middle mediastinum (29%) or posterior mediastinum (16%).

## SYMPTOMS AND SIGNS

The symptoms and signs found in patients with mediastinal tumors depend on a number of factors, including the patient's age, the malignant status of the tumor, the tumor's location and size, and associated systemic or paraneoplastic syndromes associated with the tumor.

A 56-year experience at Duke University Medical Center found 62% of patients (adults and children) presented with symptoms from mediastinal neoplasms or cysts.[2] Malignant tumors had a significantly higher incidence of symptoms (85%) compared to benign

**TABLE 10-3.** ANATOMIC LOCATION OF PRIMARY TUMORS AND CYSTS OF THE MEDIASTINUM IN 400 PATIENTS

| TYPE | % |
|---|---|
| **ANTEROSUPERIOR MEDIASTINUM ($n = 215$)** | |
| Thymic neoplasms | 30 |
| Lymphomas | 20 |
| Germ cell | 18 |
| Carcinoma | 13 |
| Cysts | 7 |
| Mesenchymal | 5 |
| Endocrine | 5 |
| Other | 2 |
| **MIDDLE MEDIASTINUM ($n = 82$)** | |
| Cysts | 60 |
| Lymphomas | 21 |
| Mesenchymal | 9 |
| Carcinoma | 7 |
| Other | 3 |
| **POSTERIOR MEDIASTINUM ($n = 103$)** | |
| Neurogenic | 53 |
| Cysts | 34 |
| Mesenchymal | 9 |
| Endocrine | 2 |
| Other | 2 |

SOURCE: From Davis RD et al.[2] Reprinted with permission.

lesions (46%). However, the increased use of radiographic techniques and screening has led to an increase in asymptomatic presentations of malignant mediastinal masses.

Infants and young children are more likely to be symptomatic than adults. Two-thirds of children with tumors have symptoms. Symptoms of airway compromise, including cough, dyspnea, and stridor, may be seen. Respiratory compromise during induction of general anesthesia can be a life-threatening emergency, especially

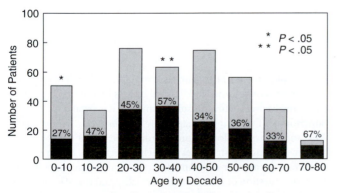

**FIGURE 10-2.** Age distribution and incidence of malignancy relative to age. (*From Davis et al.[2] Reprinted with permission.*)

with large mediastinal masses. Shamberger and colleagues[5] prospectively evaluated 31 children with anterior mediastinal masses and recommended using tracheal area, as assessed by CT imaging, and peak expiratory flow rate as measures to assess safety of general anesthesia. General anesthesia was uneventful in this study in patients with tracheal area and peak expiratory flow rates greater than 50% of predicted.

Typically symptoms can be explained by the location and size of the neoplasm, for example, facial fullness and plethora related to superior vena caval obstruction in an anterosuperior mediastinal mass. Cardiac tamponade may occasionally be seen with middle mediastinal masses. Posterior mediastinal masses with spinal cord involvement may present with symptoms of spinal cord compression. Table 10-6 shows the most common presenting symptoms of mediastinal neoplasms.

Elevated levels of various hormones and serum markers are seen in patients with various mediastinal tumors. For example, in young males with anterior mediastinal masses α fetoprotein and β human chorionic gonadotropin levels can provide additional evidence in cases of suspected nonseminomatous germ cell tumors. In fact, these tumor markers should be measured in all male patients under 50 years of age who present with a mediastinal neoplasm.

Often systemic symptoms arise from hormones secreted from primary mediastinal neoplasms, for example, hypercalcemia from elevated hyperparathyroid hormone production that is seen in patients with mediastinal parathyroid adenomas. Children with posterior mediastinal masses suspicious for a neuroblastoma or ganglioneuroblastoma should be screened for excessive norepinephrine, epinephrine, and ferritin production. Examples of systemic syndromes arising from hormone release from various mediastinal tumors include thyrotoxicosis, the Doege-Potter syndrome, and Cushing's syndrome. The Doege-Potter syndrome describes the episodic hypoglycemic episodes seen in patients with neurogenic tumors and large mesenchymal tumors. Systemic syndromes associated with mediastinal tumors and their hormones are described in Tables 10-7 and 10-8.

When a patient initially presents with a mediastinal mass, a careful history and physical exam should be performed. Symptoms such as chest pain, dyspnea, fever, chills, night sweats, cough, fatigue, weight loss, myasthenia, and dyspnea should be noted. Additionally, signs on physical exam such as lymphadenopathy, facial fullness and plethora, and testicular masses should be carefully evaluated. In cases of suspected myasthenia gravis, the neurologic examination can provide evidence with signs of proximal muscle weakness, ptosis, and diplopia. When these neurologic signs are present, confirmation of myathenia gravis can be obtained from measuring levels of circulating antibodies to acetylcholine receptors, the Tensilon test, or electromyelogram.[6,7]

## DIAGNOSTIC RADIOLOGIC EVALUATION

Standard posteroanterior and lateral chest radiographs provide valuable information concerning the anatomic location of the tumor and size. The location of the mass provides important information regarding the diagnosis. A chest CT scan is now routine in the evaluation of a mediastinal mass, because it provides additional

**TABLE 10-4. PRIMARY MEDIASTINAL TUMORS AND CYSTS IN 2399 PATIENTS**

| TYPE | SABISTON & SCOTT 1952[144] | HEIMBURGER ET AL 1963[145] | BURKELL ET AL 1969[145a] | FONTENELLE ET AL 1971[145b] | BENJAMIN ET AL 1972[145c] | CONKLE & ADKINS 1972[146] | RUBUSH ET AL 1973[147] |
|---|---|---|---|---|---|---|---|
| Neurogenic | 20 | 21 | 13 | 17 | 49 | 8 | 36 |
| Thymoma | 17 | 10 | 12 | 17 | 34 | 11 | 42 |
| Lymphoma | 11 | 9 | 12 | 16 | 32 | 10 | 14 |
| Germ cell neoplasm | 9 | 10 | 3 | 7 | 27 | 2 | 14 |
| Primary carcinoma | 10 | 11 | 0 | 2 | 0 | 10 | 3 |
| Mesenchymal tumor | 1 | 4 | 4 | | 24 | 2 | 10 |
| Endocrine tumor | 2 | 8 | 4 | | 24 | 0 | 13 |
| Other | 14 | | | | | | |
| Cyst | | | | | | | |
| Pericardial | 2 | 4 | 4 | 2 | 3 | 0 | 10 |
| Bronchogenic | 5 | 12 | 9 | 13 | 11 | 0 | 6 |
| Enteric | 2 | 5 | 0 | 4 | 1 | 0 | 2 |
| Other | 8 | 3 | 0 | 4 | 4 | 0 | 3 |
| Total | 101 | 97 | 61 | 90 | 209 | 43 | 153 |

| TYPE | VIDNE & LEVY 1973[148] | OVRUM & BIRKELAND 1979 | NANDI ET AL 1980 | ADKINS ET AL 1984[149] | PARISH ET AL 1984 | DAVIS & SABISTON 1986 | TOTAL | INCIDENCE (%) |
|---|---|---|---|---|---|---|---|---|
| Neurogenic | 9 | 19 | 27 | 8 | 212 | 57a | 496 | 20.7 |
| Thymoma | 9 | 10 | 18 | 4 | 206 | 67 | 458 | 19.1 |
| Lymphoma | 6 | 11 | 4 | 7 | 107 | 62 | 301 | 12.5 |
| Germ cell neoplasm | 3 | 5 | 7 | 11 | 99 | 42 | 239 | 10 |
| Primary carcinoma | 2 | 9 | 0 | 5 | 25 | 34a | 111 | 4.6 |
| Mesenchymal tumor | 4 | 4 | 2 | 0 | 60 | 24 | 143 | 6.0 |
| Endocrine tumor | 2 | 21 | 6 | 2 | 56 | 12b | 154 | 6.4 |
| Other | 1 | 2 | 1 | 1 | 36 | 3 | 58 | 2.4 |
| Cyst | | | | | | | | |
| Pericardial | 2 | 7 | 2 | 0 | 72 | 36c | 144 | 6.0 |
| Bronchogenic | 2 | 0 | 0 | 0 | 54 | 39b | 151 | 6.3 |
| Enteric | 1 | 0 | 0 | 0 | 29 | 11 | 55 | 2.3 |
| Other | 3 | 3 | 7 | 0 | 41 | 13 | 89 | 3.7 |
| Total | 45 | 91 | 74 | 38 | 997 | 400 | 2,399 | 100 |

[a]Significance: $p < 0.005$.

[b]Significance: $p < 0.025$.

[c]Significance: $p < 0.05$.

SOURCE: "Reprinted with permission from the Society of Thoracic Surgeons (The Annals of Thoracic Surgery 1987, Vol. 44, pp. 234–235.)"[2]

information not available from a chest radiograph. More specific information concerning tumor size and location to various vital structures is provided. Mediastinal adenopathy can be appreciated. Further specific information about the tumor can be obtained by CT scanning, such as the consistency of the tumor, that is, whether it is solid or cystic. The margins of the tumor, whether they are encapsulated or diffuse, can also be appreciated. Obliteration of surrounding fat planes indicates invasiveness; however, adhesion of the tumor without invasion may complicate the reading.[8,9]

Magentic resonance imaging (MRI) provides little additional information over CT scanning. It may be useful in certain situations and it avoids the contrast agents used in CT scanning. It may be useful with certain posterior mediastinal masses in terms of evaluating their involvement with the spinal canal. It has been shown to be superior to CT scanning in diagnosing various cysts.[10] Additionally, MRI may provide information regarding the tumor's involvement with major vascular structures and help detect if the tumor is actually a vascular abnormality. Angiographic studies may be required if there is a question of a vascular abnormality and the MRI is unable to determine vessel involvement.

Recently, positron emission tomography (PET) scanning has played an adjunctive role in evaluation of mediastinal neoplasms.

## TABLE 10-5. INCIDENCE OF MEDIASTINAL TUMORS IN EACH COMPARTMENT IN ADULTS AND CHILDREN

| COMPARTMENT | ADULT | CHILDREN |
|---|---|---|
| Anterior | 54% | 44% |
| Middle | 20% | 20% |
| Posterior | 26% | 36% |

Kubota et al.[11] found FDG [2-deoxy-2-(18F)fluoro-D-glucose] to be helpful with PET in determining the malignant potential of a mediastinal mass. In this paper they reported the sensitivity and specificity of CT scanning and PET scanning in diagnosing tumor invasion and found PET scanning to be superior (sensitivity 90%, specificity 92%, accuracy 91%) to CT scanning (sensitivity 70%, specificity 83%, accuracy 77%). With thymic neoplasms high FDG uptake was reflective of invasiveness; high FDG uptake was seen in thymic carcinomas and invasive thymomas.

Single-photon emission computerized tomography (SPECT) using gallium 67 has a role in evaluating tumor recurrence and residual disease in malignant lymphoma, but its use as an adjunct in mediastinal tumor diagnosis is limited because the uptake of gallium 67 is nonspecific.[12–14] Thallium 201 SPECT has been used to detect thymomas, but it does not differentiate between benign and malignant disease.[15]

If concern about the possibility of a intrathoracic thyroid lesion is present, the use of thyroid scans can help make the diagnosis.[16] If this study is being considered, it should be performed prior to CT scanning with contrast medium because the iodinylated contrast medium used during the CT scan may interfere with the results from the thyroid scanning. Meta-iodobenzylguanidine, a precursor of catechol, can be used to scan for possible neurogenic tumors.[17]

## TISSUE-OBTAINING TECHNIQUES

The ability to treat patients with mediastinal masses successfully depends on obtaining the correct tissue diagnosis. Cure of these tumors depends on the proper choice of surgery, chemotherapy, and radiation therapy. For most of these tumors tissue can be obtained by several techniques, including minimally invasive techniques such

## TABLE 10-6. COMMON SYMPTOMS AT PRESENTATION OF A MEDIASTINAL NEOPLASM

Chest Pain
Fevers and Chills
Dyspnea
Cough
Weight loss
Myasthenia gravis
Superior vena caval obstruction
Fatigue
Dysphagia

## TABLE 10-7. SYSTEMIC SYNDROMES CAUSED BY MEDIASTINAL NEOPLASM HORMONE PRODUCTION

| SYNDROME | TUMOR |
|---|---|
| Hypertension | Pheochromocytoma, chemodectoma, ganglioneuroma, neuroblastoma |
| Hypoglycemia | Mesothelioma, teratoma, fibrosarcoma, neurosarcoma |
| Diarrhea | Ganglioneuroma, neuroglastoma, neurofibroma |
| Hypercalcemia | Parathyroid adenoma/carcinoma, Hodgkin's disease |
| Thyrotoxicosis | Thyroid adenoma/carcinoma |
| Gynecomastia | Nonseminomatous germ cell tumors |
| Precocious puberty | Nonseminomatous germ cell tumors |

SOURCE: From Davis RD et al.[82] Reprinted with permission.

## TABLE 10-8. SYSTEMIC SYNDROMES ASSOCIATED WITH MEDIASTINAL NEOPLASMS

| TUMOR | SYNDROME |
|---|---|
| Thymoma | Myasthenia gravis |
| | Red blood cell aplasia |
| | White blood cell aplasia |
| | Aplastic anemia |
| | Hypogammaglobulinemia |
| | Progressive system sclerosis |
| | Hemolytic anemia |
| | Megaesophagus |
| | Dermatomyositis |
| | Systemic lupus erythematosus |
| | Myocarditis |
| | Collagen vascular disease |
| Lymphoma | Anemia, myasthenia gravis |
| Neurofibroma | von Recklinghausen's disease |
| Carcinoid | Cushing's syndrome |
| Carcinoid, thymoma | Multiple endocrine adenomatosis |
| Thymoma, neurofibroma, neurilemoma, mesothelioma | Osteoarthropathy |
| Enteric cysts | Vertebral anomalies |
| Hodgkin's disease | Alcohol-induced pain Pel-Ebstein fever |
| Neuroblastoma | Opsomyoclonus Erythrocyte abnormalities |
| Enteric cysts | Peptic ulcer |

SOURCE: From RD Davis et al.[82] Reprinted with permission.

as fine-needle aspiration or core needle biopsy, minor surgical techniques such as open mediastinal biopsy, mediastinoscopy, and thoracoscopy, or by major surgical procedures including median sternotomy, thoracotomy, or less commonly clamshell incisions.

The CT scan is used as a guide to determine the most appropriate technique to use to obtain tissue. Fine-needle aspiration and core-needle biopsy techniques have proven useful in the evaluation of mediastinal lesions. Material from these needle biopsies can be evaluated cytologically, histologically, immunohistochemically, and by electron microscopy. These biopsy techniques can be combined with special immunohistochemical stains, often allowing even subtyping of lymphomas. Needle biopsies are best performed by an interventional radiologist with expertise in this area and significant clinical judgment because errors in diagnosis can occur. In 189 fine-needle aspiration (FNA) biopsies of mediastinal lesions using 22-gauge needles, Singh et al.[18] reported that 14.8% were nondiagnostic. Of the satisfactory FNA specimens in this series with histologic correlation, 6% were discordant. Gunther,[19] in a recent series of 142 CT-guided core-needle biopsies with 14- to 22-gauge needles, reported that the sensitivity was 98.9% and the specificity was 100% with this technique. In only 0.7% of patients was inadequate material obtained. Zafar and Moinuddin[20] reported a retrospective study of 141 mediastinal needle biopsies with biopsy needles ranging from 18 to 22 gauge under fluoroscopic or CT guidance, and found adequate material for diagnosis was obtained in 92% of patients. All cases of benign tumors were accurately diagnosed, and only one case of malignant lymphoma was misdiagnosed by needle biopsy as a malignant germ cell tumor. Thirteen patients in this series had inadequate material for diagnosis, and in four of these, the nodular sclerosis variant of Hodgkin's disease was found at mediastinoscopy or thoracotomy. In only two of six Hodgkin's lymphoma patients was adequate tissue obtained by needle biopsy. Pneumothorax was the most frequent reported complication in this series, occurring in 14% of patients. This figure is in agreement with other large studies, which found 8% to 23% of patients with pneumothorax. Other complications reported from needle biopsies of mediastinal masses include hemoptysis (up to 10%), and more rarely, hemopericardium and cardiac tamponade.[21] Pneumothorax can be minimized by the use of 20 to 40 mL of saline injected to displace the pleura and widen the mediastinum.[19]

Contraindications, which may be relative, to needle biopsy of mediastinal lesions include uncontrollable cough, previous pneumonectomy, severe chronic obstructive pulmonary disease (COPD), pulmonary arterial hypertension, suspected vascular lesion, bleeding abnormality, or an uncooperative patient.[22] Mediastinoscopy is used to approach mediastinal masses located in the middle mediastinum and in the superior aspect of the anterosuperior mediastinum. When this technique is used, care must be taken to obtain uncrushed biopsy material. Particular attention needs to be given to the biopsy samples when the presumed diagnosis is Hodgkin's disease because the sclerotic surface of the tumor may make it difficult to sample. An extended cervical mediastinoscopy may occasionally be useful in evaluating an anterior mass or lymphadenopathy located in the aorticopulmonary window.

Parasternal or anterior mediastinotomy (Chamberlain procedure) is frequently used to obtain tissue in anterosuperior mediastinal masses, especially when the mass abuts the anterior chest wall. This technique may also be useful in cases when needle biopsy is nondiagnostic. If any doubt over the tissue being biopsied exists, a 20-gauge needle aspiration of the tissue prior to sampling can be performed to prevent inadvertent major vascular injury.

Thoracoscopic surgery is a recent addition to the armamentarium of possible biopsy techniques. This technique, although minimally invasive, does require placement of a dual lumen endotracheal tube, a lateral decubitus position of the patient, and three small holes, and therefore is less advantageous than an anterior mediastinotomy, which requires only a single 2-cm incision in a supine patient. Well-encapsulated, smaller mediastinal masses are more amenable to thoracoscopic surgery. Occasionally this technique may provide easier access to tissue, most frequently in cases where there is a question of a residual mass in a lymphoma patient.[23] This technique may also be useful in the diagnosis of neurogenic tumors located in the posterior mediastinum, and tumors in the middle mediastinum below the level of the carina that are inaccessible to cervical mediastinoscopy or anterior mediastinotomy.

Median sternotomy or thoracotomy may occasionally be necessary to obtain a tissue diagnosis, but in general the least invasive technique should be attempted first. These techniques may still be necessary to assess whether a lesion is resectable. Surgery is still the treatment of choice for most mediastinal neoplasms, but nonsurgical therapies, including chemotherapy and radiation, are playing an increasingly important role in treating many patients.

## THYMIC NEOPLASMS

Thymic neoplasms are a diverse group of lesions and have undergone multiple classifications schemes. As detailed by Shimosato and Mukai,[24] these tumors were initially classified in 1916 by Ewing and later in 1961 by Bernatz; the latter classification was widely used until 1976 when classifications by Rosai and Levine[25], followed by Wick et al.[26] and Lewis et al.[27], were instituted. More recently, Snover et al.,[28] Suster and Rosai,[29] Marino and Müller-Hermelink,[30] and Shimosato and Mukai[24] have proposed classification schemes of thymic tumors. Shimosato and Mukai[24] classified thymic tumors as seen in Table 10-9, and this is the classification used in this chapter.

### THYMOLIPOMA

Thymolipomas are rare tumors comprising 2% to 9% of thymic tumors. Usually they are asymptomatic and therefore grow to large sizes before being detected. They occur equally in men and women, and usually are seen in patients in the 20- to 30-year-old age range. Thymolipomas are radiolucent masses. CT scanning, ultrasound, or MRI imaging showing fat density in the correct location suggests the diagnosis. An association between these tumors and various paraneoplastic syndromes has been reported, including Grave's disease, Hodgkin's lymphoma, chronic lymphoid leukemia, aplastic anemia, hypogammaglobulinemia, and myasthenia gravis. Mature fat and thymic tissue are seen on histologic examination. Treatment is surgical removal and the prognosis, except in patients with an associated syndrome, is excellent.

**TABLE 10-9.** CLASSIFICATION OF THYMIC NEOPLASMS

Thymolipoma and hamartomotous tumor

Tumors of thymic epithelium
  Thymoma
    By extent:
      circumscribed
        encapsulated
        nonencapsulated (invasive but confined to within thymus)
      invasive (invading neighboring organs)
      with implantation or metastasis

    By histology: lymphocyte predominant mixed lymphocytic
        and epithelial
      epithelial cell predominant

    By cell type: spindle cell
      mixed spindle cell and polygonal cell
      polygonal-oval cell

    By cell atypia: absent, slight, moderate,
      and marked

  Thymic carcinoma
    Squamous cell carcinoma (well, moderately, and
      poorly differentiated)
    Basaloid carcinoma
    Mucoepidermoid carcinoma
    Adenosquamous carcinoma
    Adenocarcinoma
    Small cell or neuroendocrine carcinoma
    Lymphoepithelioma-like carcinoma
    Large cell carcinoma
      Clear cell carcinoma
    Sarcomatoid carcinoma

  Tumors composed of other elements
    Carcinoid tumor
    Germ cell tumors
    Malignant lymphomas

SOURCE: From Shimosato Y, Mukai K.[24] Reprinted with permission.

## HAMARTOMATOUS LESIONS

Rare ectopic hamartomatous thymomas are usually found in the supraclavicular or suprasternal regions, occur in adulthood, usually in males, and are often present for significant time prior to presentation. Surgical resection effectively removes the ectopic tissue without recurrence of disease.[24]

## THYMIC EPITHELIAL NEOPLASMS

Based on histologic appearance and biology, thymic epithelial neoplasms are divided into three general categories: benign thymomas, malignant thymomas, and thymic carcinoma. Thymomas are cytologically benign-appearing tumors that may be noninvasive (benign) or invasive (malignant), whereas thymic carcinomas are cytologically malignant lesions.[31]

THYMOMAS (SEE FIG. 10-3). Thymomas most commonly occur in adulthood between the ages of 40 and 60, and the male-female ratio is equal. In patients with myasthenia gravis, however, female patients predominate. Patients with myasthenia gravis also present with thymomas at an earlier age than those without myasthenia. Thymomas were the most common mediastinal tumors seen in the Duke series, representing 17% of mediastinal masses.[2] By far the most common location of thymomas is the anterior mediastinum, but ectopic locations have been reported.

Symptoms from thymomas are variable. These tumors may be asymptomatic, or signs and symptoms may be present from local, systemic, or autoimmune phenomena accompanying these tumors. Myasthenia gravis is the most common presentation followed by asymptomatic patients detected by routine chest x-ray. Up to 30% to 40% of patients with thymic lesions have symptoms suggestive of myasthenia gravis; 5% of patients have other autoimmune diseases, including red cell aplasia, hypogammaglobulinemia, systemic lupus erythematosus (SLE), SIADH, and Cushing's disease.[7] In the Duke series one patient presented with Sjögren's syndrome and an anterior mediastinal mass.[2] Local symptoms due to the effect of the tumor mass are less common than the above presentations, but they do occur as the tumor enlarges and can include chest pain, cough, dyspnea, and symptoms from compression of vital mediastinal structures.

Routine chest radiographs are the initial study used to evaluate the mediastinum. Often a thymoma is better demonstrated on the lateral radiograph. In patients with myasthenia gravis, CT scanning is the diagnostic radiologic procedure of choice. It has an ability to detect thymomas as small as 0.3 to 0.5 cm in size, and accurately localize and characterize (e.g. as cystic, solid, or calcified) these tumors. On CT scans thymomas tend to appear as solid, usually rounded masses, with a tendency to be on one side of midline.[32] Hemorrhage, cystic areas, and calcification may be detected, although calcification is present in only a minority of these lesions. IV contrast medium administration helps define the degree of involvement of the tumor with mediastinal structures. The degree of invasion may be identifiable on CT scans. If surrounding fat planes are well defined, usually the tumor is well encapsulated, whereas complete obliteration of the surrounding fat plane is a strong indicator of invasiveness.[8] Intrathoracic metastatic lesions can be identified in the lungs, pleura, etc.

MRI may provide additional information in evaluating thymomas, especially in determining invasion into vascular structures. On MRI both benign and malignant thymomas have a signal intensity slightly greater than muscle on T1-weighted images. On T2-weighted images an increased signal intensity is also seen with both benign and maligant thymomas, but malignant thymomas are inhomogeneous in signal intensity on T2-weighted images. Malignant thymomas on T2-weighted images also tended to have a lobulated border and internal architecture.[33] More recently PET scanning has been used in evaluation of thymomas. High FDG uptake of thymic lesions on PET scanning appears to reflect invasiveness or malignant nature.[11]

Biopsy of the anterior mediastinal mass by FNA may be diagnostic, but if additional tissue is required, anterior mediastinotomy (Chamberlain) may be useful. Although FNA can be used to make

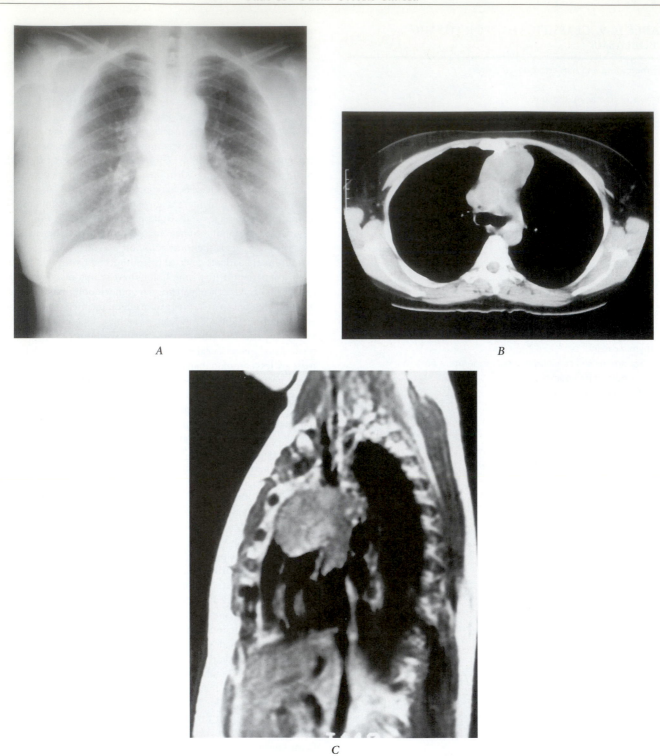

**FIGURE 10-3.** *A.* Chest radiograph of patient with benign thymoma. *B.* CT scan of patient with benign thymoma. *C.* Magnetic resonance imaging (MRI) of patient with benign thymoma. *D1* and *D2.* Chest radiographs of patient with recurrent malignant thymoma.

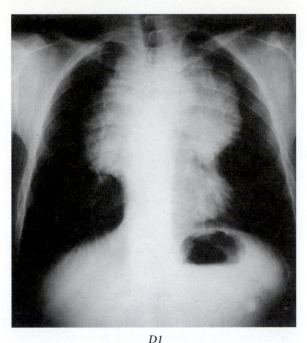

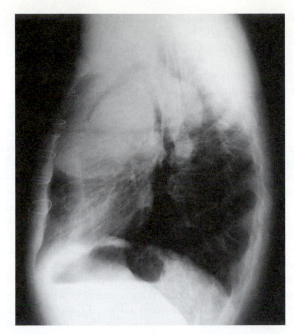

*D1*                                                              *D2*

**FIGURE 10-3.** *Continued.*

the diagnosis with an 87% sensitivity and a 94% specificity, the determination of benign versus malignant is based on gross and microscopic findings at surgery. Well-encapsulated lesions are benign. Local invasion into the surrounding capsule, adjacent structures, or mediastinal fat is evidence of malignancy. Although the surgeon determines gross involvement of structures at the time of surgery, the pathologist determines microscopic involvement of capsule or mediastinal fat.

The histologic appearance of thymomas consists of epithelial cells, lymphocytes, and spindle cell elements. Lymphocytes are present and may be in the majority but are not the neoplastic component. Thymomas may be distinguished from lymphomas by staining for cytokeratin. Thymic neoplasms may be classified as lymphocytic, epithelial predominant, or mixed. Lymphocytic tumors contain more than 66% lymphocytes. Epithelial tumors contain less than 33% lymphocytes, and mixed are in between.

Other histologic classifications for thymomas exist. Marino and Müller-Hermelink[30] devised a classification based on cell type. They described cortical, mixed, and medullary types of thymomas. Cortical thymomas have medium to large epithelial cells with oval or round nuclei with poorly defined cytoplasm. The cortical cell type has potential for malignant spread. Medullary thymomas are composed of cells that are small or medium in size with irregular or spindle-shaped nuclei and tend to have a benign course. Mixed cell types contain areas of mixtures of both cortical and medullary thymomas.

The Masaoka et al.[34] staging system, as seen in Table 10-10, is the most widely used for staging of thymomas.

Wide surgical excision is the primary therapy for all well-encapsulated thymomas and invasive thymomas that can be sur-

gically removed. Wilkins and colleagues[35] have recommended median sternotomy, inspection of both pleural sacs, total thymectomy, extended resection for stage III disease, and removal of all pleural implants in stage IVA disease. Jaretzki et al.[36] recommend en bloc transcervical-transternal "maximal" thymectomy in order to remove all thymic tissue. Fischer et al.[37] also described an aggressive surgical approach for thymectomy as a treatment for myasthenia gravis. In this paper they described the technique as a median sternotomy and thymectomy with removal of all possible mediastinal fat between phrenic nerves and from diaphragm to the superior border of the thymus. Patterson[38] in a review discusses bilateral anterolateral thoracotomies and transverse sternotomy as a technique of providing excellent exposure to the mediastinum, both pleural spaces, and the lower neck. This surgical exposure is especially advantageous

**TABLE 10-10. MASAOKA STAGING OF THYMOMAS**

| Stage I | Mascroscopically completely encapsulated and microscopically no capsular invasion |
|---|---|
| Stage II | 1. Macroscopic invasion into surrounding fatty tissue or mediastinal pleura, or |
| | 2. Microscopic invasion into capsule |
| Stage III | Macroscopic invasion into neighboring organ, i.e. pericardium, great vessels, or lung |
| Stage IVa | Pleural or pericardial dissemination |
| Stage IVb | Lymphogenous or hematogenous metastasis |

SOURCE: From A Masaoka et al.[34] Reprinted with permission.

for patients with pleural disease. These studies site the embryologic development of the thymus, with frequent evidence of thymic tissue in the mediastinal fat as the indication for a more aggressive approach.

Yagi et al.[39] recommend an aggressive surgical approach for invasive thymomas, including angioplasty and vascular reconstruction when the superior vena cava or brachiocephalic vein is invaded. They reported a significant difference in 5-year survival rates in patients with stage III thymomas who had complete resections (94%) versus the 5-year survival rate of 35% in the group with incomplete resection. Nakahara et al.[40] also recommend radical resection and replacement of the superior vena cava or its branches in patients with stage III disease in addition to thymectomy and postoperative radiation, and this group reported 100% 5-year and 95% 10-year survival rates. Patients with thymomas frequently have recurrences, and reoperation for recurrent disease has been recommended.[39] Additionally, surgical exploration of initially unresectable thymomas may be indicated after a response to multimodality therapy.

Wilkins and colleagues[35] recommend postoperative radiation for patients with stage II and higher thymomas because of their propensity for recurrence. They recommend a dose 50 Gy to the mediastinum and operative field. Others have also shown the benefit of postoperative radiation in preventing recurrence and prolonging survival in patients with invasive thymomas. Curran et al.[41] looked at 26 patients with invasive thymomas that had been completely resected and found no recurrence in the 5 of the total 26 patients in the study who had postoperative irradiation. In contrast, 8 of 21 patients who did not undergo postoperative irradiation had mediastinal relapse.

Preoperative radiation has been suggested for large, invasive, bulky thymomas to decrease tumor size and prevent seeding of tumor during the operative procedure. Shamji et al.[42] stated that preoperative irradiation may prevent thoracic dissemination of tumor cells during surgery. Yagi et al.[39] used preoperative irradiation when infiltration of other organs was suspected, and they stated that the reduction in tumor size made complete resection possible in some patients. Further studies are necessary to define the role of preoperative irradiation in the treatment of thymomas.

Chemotherapy may be used in locally advanced and metastatic thymomas, with the best results seen with cisplatin-based regimens. With cisplatin-based chemotherapy, overall response rates of 85% have been seen. Fornasiero et al.[43] reported a series of 32 patients with stage III of IV thymomas treated with a chemotherapeutic combination of cisplatin, doxorubicin, vincristine, and cyclophosphamide. This prospective single institution trial reported complete remission in 47% of patients and an overall response rate of 91%. Fifteen months was the median overall survival time in this study. The Eastern Cooperative Oncology Group (ECOG) in 1995 presented results of a prospective trial of 23 patients with unresectable thymomas treated with four cycles of PAC (cisplatin, doxorubicin, and cyclophosphamide) followed by radiation therapy consisting of 54 Gy. This intergroup study reported an overall response rate of 70% with 5 complete responses and 11 partial responses and a 5-year overall survival rate calculated to be 52.5%.

Neoadjuvant cisplatin regimens have been used to treat patients with unresectable, locally invasive thymomas.[44,45] Macchiarini et al.[44] reported a series of seven patients with stage III thymomas treated

## TABLE 10-11. RESECTABILITY, RECURRENCE, AND SURVIVAL ACCORDING TO THE MASAOKA STAGING SYSTEM

| STAGE | n | RESECTION | | | RECURRENCE, (5 YR) | SURVIVAL | |
| | | CR | PR | BX | | 5 YR | 10 YR |
|---|---|---|---|---|---|---|---|
| I | 25 | 100% | ... | ... | 4% | 95% | 86% |
| II | 41 | 73% | 10% | 17% | 21% | 70% | 55% |
| III | 43 | 56% | 30% | 14% | 47% | 50% | ... |
| IVa | 9 | 78% | 11% | 11% | 80% | 100% | ... |

ABBREVIATIONS: Bx = biopsy; CR = complete resection; PR = partial resection.
SOURCE: From Blumberg D et al.[46] Reprinted with permission.

preoperatively with cisplatin, etoposide, and epirubicin. All patients responded partially and underwent surgical exploration followed by postoperative radiation. Four of seven were able to undergo complete resections.

In summary, the Masaoka stage directs treatment strategies. Complete surgical resection for stage I is sufficient treatment. A complete surgical resection followed by postoperative radiation therapy is recommended for stage II and III thymomas. For patients with unresectable invasive or incompletely resected stage III or IV thymomas, the therapeutic strategy is less defined. Multimodality therapy consisting of surgical debulking, chemotherapy with cisplatin-containing drugs, and radiotherapy seems to be the most reasonable approach in a patient who is healthy at diagnosis. Since thymomas have been reported to have late recurrence, cure rates should be based on 10-year follow-up data. Blumberg et al.[46] reported resectability, recurrence, and survival according to the Masaoka staging system as seen in Table 10-11.

**MYASTHENIA GRAVIS AND THYMECTOMY.** Association of thymic neoplasms with myasthenia gravis is not well understood. In a Massachusetts General Hospital series, 60% of patients had improvement in their myasthenic symptoms if a thymoma was present and removed. If no thymoma was present at resection, 84% had improvement with removal of thymic tissue.[47] Recent improvements in preoperative care of patients with myasthenia gravis have resulted in near-zero mortality figures for surgical thymectomy. Currently patients with myasthenia gravis do not do significantly worse from thymectomies than their nonmyasthenic counterparts. Current preoperative strategy consists of plasmapheresis and maximization of preoperative medications. Indications for thymectomy in myasthenia gravis are to improve symptoms and possibly induce remission.

**THYMIC CARCINOMA.** Thymic carcinomas are much less commonly seen compared to benign and malignant thymomas. As seen in Table 10-9, there are multiple histologic types of thymic carcinomas, the most common being squamous cell carcinoma and lymphoepithelioma-like carcinoma. At the Mayo Clinic only 20 patients were documented over a 75-year period by Wick et al.[26] In 60 patients diagnosed with thymic carcinoma, a study by Suster and Rosai[29] found that 33% had low-grade histologic pattern and the other 66% had a high-grade histology. The low-grade histologic type, most commonly well-differentiated keratinizing squamous cell carcinoma, was associated with a more benign clinical course compared to the high-grade histologic pattern, which most commonly consisted of the lymphoepithelioma-like carcinoma. Interestingly, paraneoplastic syndromes, including myasthenia gravis, are not associated with thymic carcinomas.

Fukai et al.[48] noted the use of monoclonal antibodies to cytokeratin 7 as an aid in differentiating among keratinizing squamous cell carcinomas of thymic origin versus lung origin with involvement of the mediastinum. In this study the immunohistochemical reactivity on frozen sections of keratinizing squamous cell carcinomas of thymic origin and lung origin were examined. Although 9/9 (100%) of the thymic carcinomas reacted with antibody specific for cytokeratin 7, none (0/5) of the lung carcinomas showed reactivity. This immunohistochemical finding may be used to differentiate thymic from lung keratinizing squamous cell carcinoma. Differentiation between the two may be useful in treatment, because thymic carcinomas tend to have a better prognosis compared with lung carcinomas with mediastinal extension. In some thymic carcinomas chromosomal translocations between chromosomes 15 and 19 have been reported.[49,50] Additionally, Epstein-Barr virus infection has been implicated as a possible associated factor in thymic carcinomas in some patients.[51,52]

Treatment of these tumors consists of cisplatin-based regimens, but few data have been published. Weide et al.[53] reported on five patients with thymic carcinoma treated with cisplatin-based chemotherapeutic regimens. Two of five achieved complete responses, and one obtained a partial response. In the two patients with complete responses, relapse occurred at 10 and 12 months.

## THYMIC CARCINOID

Thymic carcinoids arise from the Kulchitsky cells located in the thymus, and therefore are usually located in the anterosuperior mediastinum. They can occur in association with a variant of the multiple endocrine neoplasia (MEN) syndromes. These tumors possess neuroendocrine features and histologies similar to carcinoids that occur in the gastrointestinal tract and the bronchi. A strong male predominance of these tumors is seen, and they tend to occur in adulthood.

One-third of thymic carcinoids are asymptomatic and detected on routine chest radiograph. Often, however, these tumors are hormonally active, and production of adrenocorticotropic hormone (ACTH) resulting in Cushing's syndrome may be seen. Surprisingly, carcinoid syndrome has not been described. Myasthenia and other syndromes associated with thymomas are also not seen. In patients with hormonally inactive tumors, symptoms resulting from the enlarging tumor may be seen.

Although hormonally inactive tumors are easily seen on routine chest x-ray due to their large size, hormonally active tumors may not be detected. CT scanning can help in the diagnosis.

Histologically these tumors are composed of solid nests of small to medium polygonal cells arranged in a pattern suggestive of an endocrine tumor. On electron microscopy these tumors have membrane-bound dense-core neurosecretory granules. Immunohistochemical staining may be positive for ACTH as well as other hormones such as cholecystokinin.[54]

The best chance for cure is surgical excision; however, local invasion or metastatic spread often precludes complete excision. Metastatic spread of these lesions, often to the bones, lung, and lymph nodes, is frequent, occurring in one series in 73% of patients.[55] For all but the well-encapsulated tumors, postoperative radiotherapy with or without chemotherapy is recommended. Patients with paraneoplastic syndromes have a poor prognosis. In general these tumors have a worse outcome than carcinoid tumors in other organs. Additionally, late recurrences may occur.

## NEUROGENIC TUMORS

Neurogenic tumors are the most common tumors found in the posterior mediastinum. Most of these tumors are found in a paravertebral location along the sympathetic chain or associated with a spinal or intercostal nerve. However, less commonly they can be associated with the vagus or phrenic nerves. Rarely these tumors are found in the middle mediastinum in association with the great vessels, the pericardium, or the heart.

In the series from Duke, neurogenic tumors represented 14% of primary mediastinal tumors or cysts.[2] Neurogenic tumors are divided into three categories (Table 10-12):

1. Tumors of nerve sheath origin
2. Tumors of sympathetic ganglia
3. Tumors of parasympathetic ganglia

**TABLE 10-12.** TUMORS OF THE THORACIC PERIPHERAL NERVOUS SYSTEM[a]

| ORIGIN | BENIGN | MALIGNANT |
|---|---|---|
| Nerve sheath | Neurilemoma (schwannoma) | Malignant schwannoma |
| | Neurofibroma[b] | Malignant schwannoma[b] |
| Sympathetic ganglia | Ganglioneuroma | Ganglioneuroblastoma[c] |
| Paraganglion system | | |
| Chromaffin secreting | Pheochromocytoma | Malignant pheochromocytoma |
| Non-chromaffin-secreting | Paraganglioma | Malignant paraganglioma |

[a]Askin tumor not included
[b]Also seen with von Recklinghausen's disease
[c]Most frequent in childhood
SOURCE: From Nelems B.[150] Reprinted with permission.

In adults neurogenic tumors are more commonly of nerve sheath origin, whereas sympathetic ganglia tumors are more commonly seen in children. Tumors of the parasympathetic ganglia are rare. In adults over 90% of neurogenic tumors are benign, whereas in children approximately 50% are malignant. Adults are usually asymptomatic and the tumor is found on routine chest x-ray. When symptoms occur in adults from neurogenic tumors, they usually consist of chest and back pain caused by compression of nerve fibers. Cough and dyspnea may be present as a result of compression or displacement of the tracheobronchial tree as the tumor enlarges. Hoarseness, Horner's syndrome, or spinal cord compression are occasional presenting symptoms.

Children are more likely to present with symptoms. Benign and malignant lesions may present with chest pain, cough, dyspnea, and dysphagia. Children with malignant neurogenic tumors often have associated constitutional symptoms including fever, weight loss, and lassitude. Horner's syndrome may be present from invasion of sympathetic ganglia. Symptoms from invasion of the brachial plexus in Pancoast's tumors and paraplegia from invasion of the spinal canal are occasionally seen. Systemic symptoms may be present as a result of the release of neurohormonal agents, for example, hypertension and headaches from the release of catecholamines. Patients suspected of having neurogenic tumors should have measurements made of vanillylmandelic and homovanillic acid in their urine. The levels of these degradation products of catecholamine synthesis, when elevated, fall to normal values with successful removal of the tumor, and rising levels after resection may indicate recurrence. The Doege-Potter syndrome is the presence of episodic hypoglycemia associated with neurogenic tumors as the result of the release of an insulin-like factor or an insulin-releasing factor. Diarrhea can be seen with ganglioneuromas and neuroblastomas as the result of the release of vasoactive intestinal peptide. Opsoclonus-polymyoclonus syndrome, a peculiar symptom complex consisting of cerebellar and truncal ataxia with a type of abnormal eye movement known as "dancing eyes" may occasionally be seen in infants presenting with neuroblastomas. An autoimmune mechanism may be the cause of this syndrome, and resolution of symptoms usually follows successful removal of the tumor or corticosteroid treatment.

The term "dumbbell-shaped" tumor has been used to describe neurogenic tumors with both a mediastinal and an intraspinal component connected by a narrowed segment in the intervertebral foramen. Akwari et al.[56] found a 9.8% incidence of dumbbell tumors in a series of 706 neurogenic tumors. In more than 60% of patients with an intraspinal component, neurologic symptoms are present. It is more common for benign neurogenic tumors to have an intraspinal component, with only 10% of malignant tumors being dumbbell tumors. Of dumbbell tumors, 70% are nerve sheath in origin, whereas only 30% are of sympathetic nerve origin. It is important to identify these dumbbell tumors prior to surgical treatment. Either removal of the thoracic component or the intraspinal component alone can result in permanent neurologic sequelae due to hemorrhage at the foramen, which may be difficult to control.

Radiographically, neurogenic tumors in adults usually appear as smooth, spherical, and well-defined posterior masses occurring most commonly in a paraspinal location. Lobulations and calcifications may be present. Bony erosions secondary to growth pressures from the tumor are commonly seen in both benign and malignant lesions. When concern of spinal canal extension is present, an MRI should be obtained in addition to the routine radiographic studies. In children, neurogenic tumors, as seen in a radiograph, often have less-defined borders because of their malignant nature and rapid growth. In children compression of vital structures occurs more commonly because these lesions are proportionally larger. Areas of calcification and necrosis may also be seen.

The histopathologic findings of individual neurogenic tumors are discussed separately with each neoplasm. Immunohistochemical analysis of tissue from neurogenic tumors may reveal the presence of neuron-specific enolase and synaptophysin.[57,58] Neurosecretory granules can be seen on electron microscopic examination.

Surgical removal remains the mainstay of treatment for most neurogenic tumors, usually via a thoracotomy incision. Malignant tumors require a multimodal approach to treatment consisting of various combinations of chemotherapy, radiotherapy, and surgery. According to Luketich and Ginsberg,[7] the indications for surgical removal of a neurogenic tumor in an adult include when the diagnosis is in question, lesions that are enlarging or greater than 5 cm, symptomatic lesions, or dumbbell tumors where neurologic symptoms might develop. During the surgical procedure after obtainment of adequate exposure, the pleura overlying the tumor is incised, and the tumor carefully dissected free. If possible, the tumor is removed without division of the nerve of origin, but often the nerve root must be transected. More recently thoracoscopic removal of these posterior mediastinal tumors has been performed with more rapid postoperative recovery in the thoracoscopic group compared to those undergoing standard posterolateral thoracotomies. In a series by Bousamra et al.,[59] two patients out of six treated thoracoscopically experienced transient ptosis.

If there is an intraspinal component to the tumor, a combined neurosurgical and thoracic one-staged surgical approach is recommended. Grillo and colleagues[60] recommend a single skin incision that allows direct visualization for mobilization of both the intraspinal and the intrathoracic components (Fig. 10-4). After

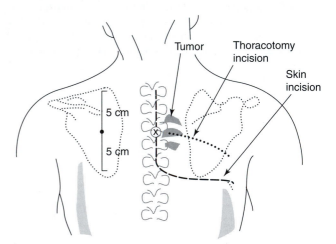

**FIGURE 10-4.** Skin incision. The vertical component, which permits laminectomy, is centered at the level of the involved foramen (X) and extends for about 10 cm. It curves forward to join the anterior portion of the thoracotomy incision. The dotted line indicates the thoracotomy beneath the flap. (*From Grillo et al.*[60] *Reprinted with permission.*)

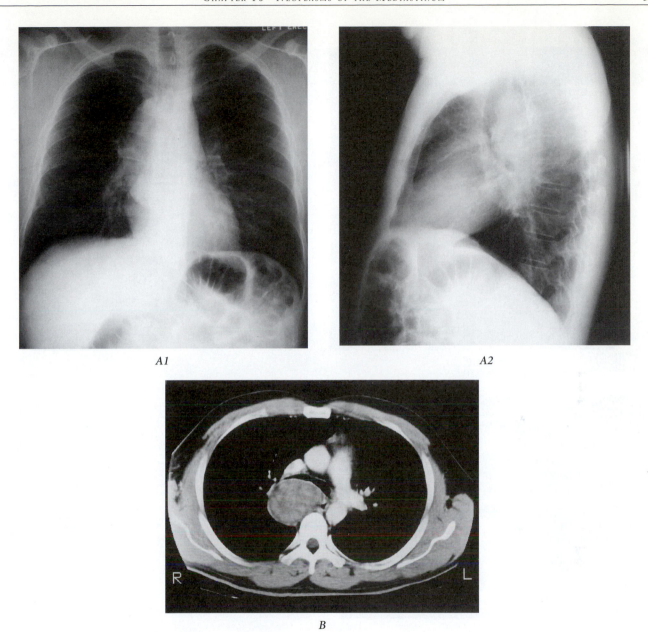

*A1*                                                                    *A2*

*B*

**FIGURE 10-5.** *A1* and *A2*. Chest radiographs of patient with middle mediastinal schwannoma. *B*. CT scan of the tumor. *C1* and *C2*. Chest radiographs of patient with posterior mediastinal schwannoma. *D*. CT scan of the tumor in the posterior mediastinum. *E*. Histopathologic examination of schwannoma showing the highly cellular Antoni A areas and the less cellular Antoni B areas (hematoxylin and eosin, ×68).

mobilization of the intrathoracic component, the neurosurgical team mobilizes the intraspinal component. Sometimes the tumor is completely extradural, but if not, the dura is opened laterally to the tumor and the tumor is gently removed from the spinal cord using microsurgical techniques. The nerve root associated with the neoplasm is divided. Following the removal of the tumor, the dura is closed, and if possible a pleural patch is used to close the foramen, thus preventing a cerebrospinal fluid leak. Shields[61] also recommends a one-staged approach, performing the hemilaminectomy

and intraspinal mobilization first followed by the intrathoracic mobilization. Heltzer and colleagues[62] used the combined neurosurgical and thoracic approach, but performed the thoracic procedure thoracoscopically.

## TUMORS OF NERVE SHEATH ORIGIN (FIG. 10-5)

These tumors consist of neurilemomas (benign schwannomas) and neurofibromas, which are benign tumors of nerve sheath origin,

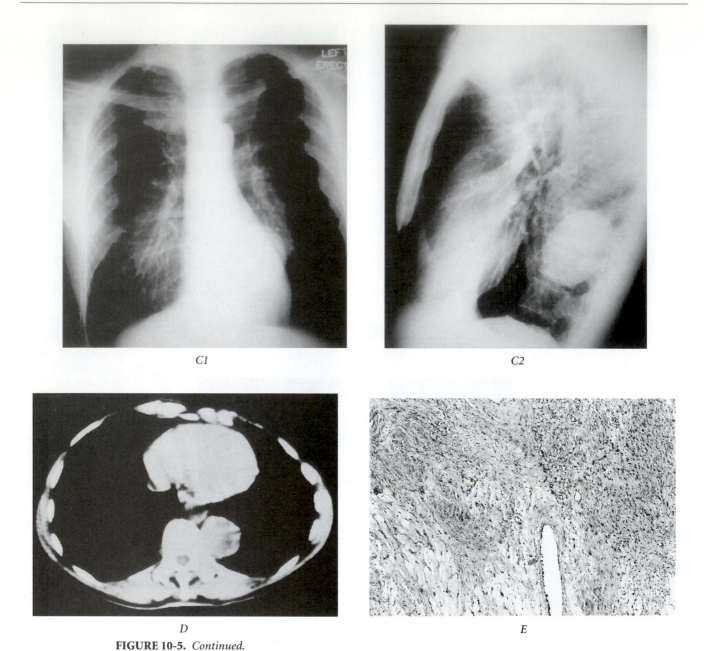

*C1*

*C2*

*D*

*E*

**FIGURE 10-5.** *Continued.*

and malignant neurosarcomas, also known as malignant schwannomas. The benign schwannoma and neurofibroma are more common, and they compose 90% of mediastinal neurogenic tumors in adults. Benign tumors of nerve sheath origin are most common in the third, fourth, and fifth decades, but can be seen in children, most commonly adolescents. They have an equal sex distribution. Schwannomas are more common than neurofibromas. Most benign tumors of nerve sheath origin are asymptomatic at presentation. Malignant tumors of nerve sheath origin occur most commonly in two age groups—patients younger than 20 and older than 50. Neurosarcomas are less commonly seen than benign nerve sheath tumors.

There is a strong association between mediastinal neurofibromas and neurofibromatosis. Of patients presenting with neurofibromas, 30% to 45% have neurofibromatosis. Multiple neurogenic tumors or the presence of a single plexiform neurofibroma is pathognomonic of neurofibromatosis. Multiple schwannomas are not, however, pathognomonic of neurofibromatosis. In patients with neurofibromatosis, the age at presentation of neurofibromas is younger, and there is a higher likelihood of malignant degeneration. Brasfield and Gupta[63] described a series of 110 patients with von Recklinghausen's neurofibromatosis and found 4.5% (5 patients) had mediastinal neurogenic tumors. The number of malignant nerve sheath tumors in patients with von Recklinghausen's disease is increased.

On gross examination schwannomas are well-encapsulated, solitary, circumscribed, grayish-tan tumors with areas of degeneration. The nerve root of origin is often compressed to one side by the tumor. Histologically these tumors retain their encapsulated appearance and have areas of high and low cellularity referred to as Antoni A and Antoni B areas, respectively (See Fig. 10-5E).

On gross examination, neurofibromas appear grayish-colored and are firm and bosselated. Not uncommonly these tumors are multiple. Although these tumors appear encapsulated, histologically neurofibromas are unencapsulated. They are composed in a loose, disorganized pattern of spindle cells with elongated nuclei. In neurofibromas the nerve root of origin has nerve fibers scattered throughout the tumor. A variant of neurofibroma known as plexiform neurofibroma infiltrates along the entire nerve trunk.

Neurosarcomas infiltrate adjacent structures and may have distant metastatic disease at presentation. Histologically these are cellular tumors composed of spindle cells. The cells have pleomorphic nuclei, and multiple mitotic figures are usually appreciated.

Treatment of benign tumors of nerve sheath origin is complete surgical resection via either thoracoscopy or thoracotomy. Recurrence is rare following surgical resection. Treatment of neurosarcomas consists of complete surgical excision if possible and postoperative irradiation. Recurrence and metastatic spread are frequent with neurosarcomas and long-term prognosis is usually poor.

## SYMPATHETIC GANGLIA TUMORS

### GANGLIONEUROMAS (FIG. 10-6).

Ganglioneuromas usually occur in childhood, and they are the most common neurogenic tumors occurring in this age group. Usually patients are asymptomatic at presentation. Chest x-rays often show these tumors as elongated or triangular paraspinal masses. They are benign, well-encapsulated tumors composed of mature ganglion cells and nerve fibers from sympathetic nerves. Usually these tumors are attached to a sympathetic or intercostal nerve trunk. Often areas of cystic degeneration and calcification are seen. Surgical excision provides cure.

### NEUROBLASTOMA (FIG. 10-7).

These highly malignant tumors are most commonly seen in the retroperitoneum, but in 10% to 20% of patients they are primary in the mediastinum. Neuroblastomas most commonly present in childhood, usually in children under 3. Infrequently they can occur in adults. Neuroblastomas are very invasive and frequently metastatic at diagnosis. Frequent sites of metastasis are regional lymph nodes, bone, brain, lung, and liver. Usually these tumors are symptomatic at diagnosis, with one-third of children having neurologic symptoms. The biology of neuroblastoma is incompletely understood, with reports of spontaneous regression.[64]

Grossly these are vascular, reddish-appearing tumors. On histologic examination neuroblastomas are composed of small round cells in a rosette pattern. These cells have a scant amount of cytoplasm and dark hyperchromatic nuclei. Calcification is common, as are areas of degeneration.

Staging for neuroblastomas and ganglioneuroblastomas is based on the Evans et al.[65] staging system as seen in Table 10-13.

Treatment is based on stage. For stage I and II complete surgical resection if possible is recommended, with postoperative radiation therapy for stage II tumors. A dose of 30 Gy has been recommended except in children under 2 where 20 Gy is preferred to prevent subsequent treatment-related sequelae.[66] Multimodality therapy, consisting of chemotherapy and possibly radiotherapy and surgery, is recommended for stage III and IV tumors. Chemotherapeutic regimens consist of combinations of cisplatin, vincristine, doxorubicin, cyclophosphamide, or etoposide. In patients who fail to respond to conventional chemotherapy or who relapse, high-dose chemotherapy with autologous bone marrow transplantation has been used with some success. Although surgical treatment for stage IV-S disease is controversial, Martinez and colleagues[67] have reported improved survival in patients with stage IV-S disease after surgical removal of the primary tumor. Overall survival with neuroblastomas has been reported as 22%, but 80% of patients with stage I disease are long-term survivors.[68] Mediastinal neuroblastomas have a better prognosis than other sites, and younger children with early-stage disease do better. Poor prognostic indicators are increasing age at presentation, more invasive disease, and, according to Shamberger et al.,[69] N-*myc* gene amplification and protein expression.

### GANGLIONEUROBLASTOMA (FIG. 10-8).

These neurogenic tumors are intermediate in malignant potential between benign ganglioneuromas and the highly malignant neuroblastoma. They tend to be seen in a slightly younger age group than ganglioneuromas. Patients are usually symptomatic at presentation. They are composed of immature and mature ganglion cells. Histologically two types are seen: composite, consisting of predominantly mature ganglion cells with focal areas of immature ganglion cells, and diffuse, consisting of a mixture of neuroblasts. Commonly they are attached to a nerve trunk, and a capsule may be recognizable. Calcification is usually appreciated in the tumor. Staging is the same as for neuroblastomas. Treatment is similar to neuroblastoma, except that stage II disease can be treated with surgical excision alone if the patient is less than 3 years old and has a diffuse histologic type. Patients with the composite histologic subtype have a significantly higher percentage of metastatic spread, 65% to 75%, compared with that of the diffuse histologic type, which is 5%. Age is an important predictor of outcome, with children over 3 having a worse prognosis. Other predictors of poor prognosis include stage III or IV disease or composite histologic type. Overall, patients with ganglioneuroblastoma do better than those with neuroblastomas, with long-term survival rates of 88%, including all stages reported.[70]

## TUMORS OF PARASYMPATHETIC ORIGIN

### PARAGANGLIOMAS.

Paragangliomas, or extraadrenal pheochromocytomas, are rare tumors representing only 1% of mediastinal masses. Glenner and Grimley[71] described four broad categories of paragangliomas: brachiometric, intravagal, aorticosympathetic, and visceral-autonomic, depending on anatomic distribution, histochemical features, and innervation. The brachiometric and aorticosympathetic types are found in the mediastinum. Brachiometric tumors include the mediastinal aorticopulmonary paragangliomas associated with the great vessels in the anterior mediastinum.

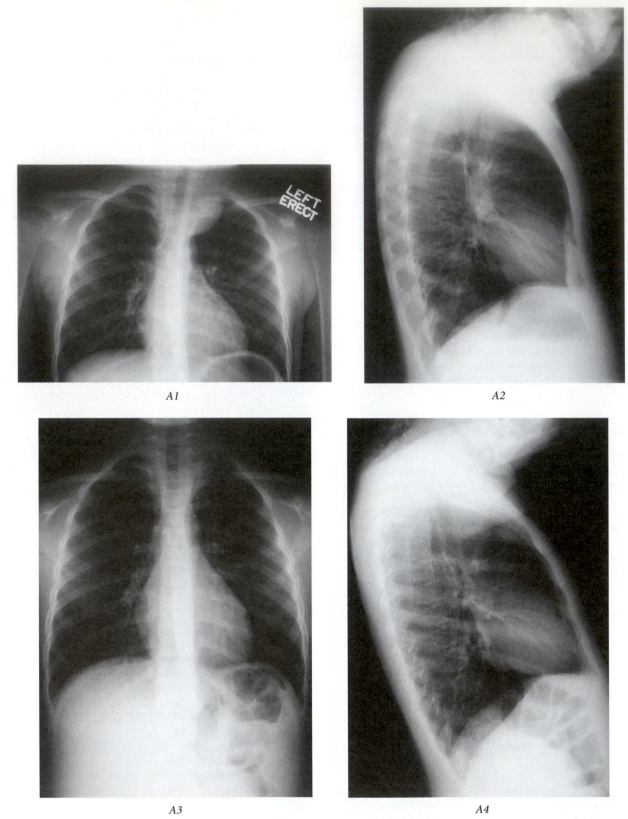

*A1*

*A2*

*A3*

*A4*

**FIGURE 10-6.** *A1* and *A2.* Chest radiographs of patient with a ganglioneuroma before and *A3* and *A4* after surgical resection. *B.* Histopathologic examination of ganglioneuroma (hematoxylin and eosin, ×68).

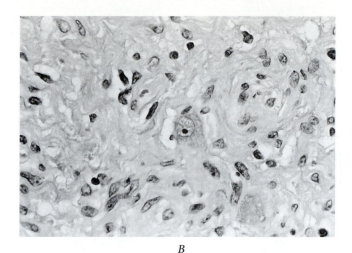

*B*

**FIGURE 10-6.** *Continued.*

Aorticopulmonary paragangliomas may also be referred to as chemodectomas, which are specific tumors of the aortic body. Aorticopulmonary paragangliomas occur in patients with an average age of 49 years and have a slight female predominance (1.5:1).[72]

Mediastinal aorticosympathetic paragangliomas are also known as paravertebral paragangliomas. These tumors are part of the sympathetic autonomic nervous system and are found in the posterior mediastinum anatomically with the sympathetic chain in the costovertebral sulcus. Compared to aorticopulmonary paragangliomas, paravertebral paragangliomas occur at an earlier average age of 29, more often in men (60%), and are more common.[73] Both of these categories of paragangliomas are rare, with only 3 seen in a series of 1064 mediastinal neoplasms from the Mayo Clinic.[74] Of these three, two were paravertebral and one was aorticopulmonary.

Paragangliomas can behave malignantly with the potential to be invasive and metastasize. As a general rule, these tumors should be approached with the idea that they are aggressive lesions. Para-

### TABLE 10-13. EVANS STAGING OF NEUROBLASTOMA

| | |
|---|---|
| Stage I: | Tumor confined to the organ or structure of origin |
| Stage II: | Tumors extending in continuity beyond the organ or structure of origin but not crossing the midline. Regional lymph nodes on the homolateral side may be involved. |
| Stage III: | Tumors extending in continuity beyond the midline. Regional lymph nodes may be involved bilaterally. |
| Stage IV: | Remote disease involving skeleton, organs, soft tissues, or distant lymph node groups, etc. (See IV-S.) |
| Stage IV-S: | Patients who would otherwise be stage I or II, but who have remote disease confined only to one or more of the following sites: liver, skin, or bone marrow (without radiographic evidence of bone metastases on complete skeletal survey.) |

SOURCE: From Evans AF et al.[65] Reprinted with permission.

gangliomas can secrete catecholamines, and therefore patients may present with symptoms similar to patients with adrenal pheochromocytomas. Unlike adrenal pheochromocytomas, which secrete epinephrine and norepinephrine, paragangliomas rarely secrete epinephrine. Nearly half of paravertebral paragangliomas secrete cathecholamines, in comparison with only 3% of aorticopulmonary paragangliomas.[73] Malignant paragangliomas are less likely to secrete catecholamines.[75] Paragangliomas may also synthesize enkephalins.[76] The aorticopulmonary paragangliomas are more likely to present with symptoms secondary to their location and size in relation to vital structures. Paravertebral paragangliomas can rarely present with spinal cord compression[77] or Horner's syndrome. Aorticopulmonary paragangliomas are more likely to be invasive and metastatic compared to paravertebral paragangliomas. Paragangliomas may be associated with multiple endocrine neoplasia (MEN II) syndrome and other associated syndromes. Of patients with paravertebral paragangliomas, 20% have more than one tumor.[73]

Radiologically paragangliomas appear as opaque, rounded, or irregularly shaped masses on routine chest x-ray. Spizarny et al.[78] reported these tumors to be the most common CT-enhancing mediastinal tumors because of their vascularity. MRI might be superior to CT scanning because of its multiplane imaging ability, and its better ability to differentiate tumor from blood vessels. The meta-iodobenzylguanidine ($^{131}$I-MIBG) scan may play an additional role in diagnosis and may allow detection of additional unknown tumors in cases with multiple paragangliomas. Angiography may further evaluate vascularity, and as MIBG does, help detect smaller tumors. In 30% of cases a tumor blush may be appreciated during thoracic arteriography.

Macroscopically, paragangliomas appear as bloody tumors that are firm, reddish-pink to brown in color, with areas of focal necrosis. The usual size of aorticopulmonary paragangliomas is 7.5 cm, whereas paravertebral paragangliomas tend to be slightly smaller, at 6 cm.[73] Although paravertebral paragangliomas are more frequently partially encapsulated, aorticopulmonary tumors are commonly invasive. Histologically both categories of paragangliomas consist of polygonal cells arranged in tightly grouped nests of the same size. This configuration is known as Zellballen, and although found in both paragangliomas types, it is less defined in the aorticopulmonary type. Generally the cells have round or slightly irregularly shaped nuclei. These nests of tumor cells are surrounded by a highly vascular stroma. Mitosis is not a frequent finding. Immunohistochemical staining is positive for neuron-specific enolase, chromogranin, and serotonin of the tumor cells. Electron microscopic examination of these tumors shows them to be composed of two types of cells. The polygonal tumor cells are arranged in the Zellballen configuration as described, and these cells contain neurosecretory granules. Surrounding these cells is another cell type, the sustentacular cells, which do not contain neurosecretory granules. The microscopic appearance of the tumors is not a reliable predictor of the metastatic potential of these tumors, although Kliewer and Cochran[79] reported a decrease in the sustentacular cells in more aggressive lesions. Additionally, tumor ploidy may eventually aid in differentiating benign from malignant lesions.

Both types of paragangliomas are treated by aggressive surgical resection. Aorticopulmonary paragangliomas are commonly

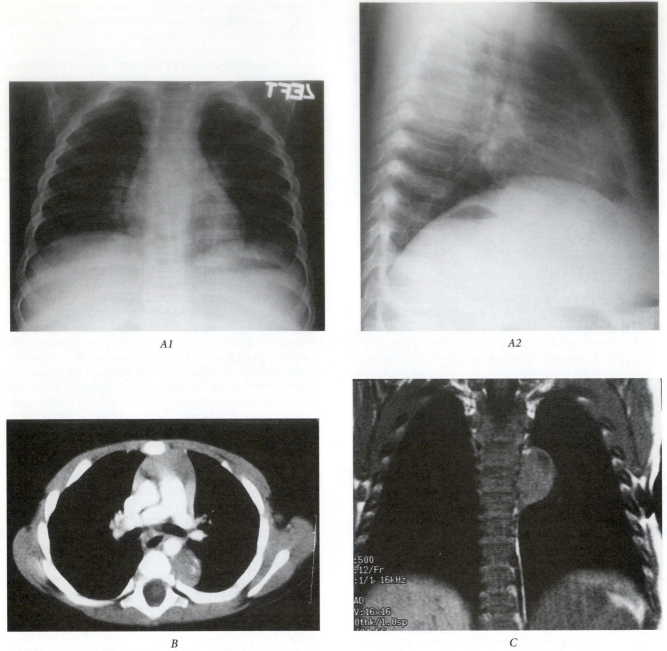

**FIGURE 10-7.** *A1* and *A2*. Chest radiographs of patient with neuroblastoma. *B*. CT scan of tumor. *C*. Coronal MRI of tumor.

unresectable because of their invasive nature and closeness to major thoracic vessels. Because of their dangerous location they also have a 5% to 10% operative mortality. Lamy et al.[80] strongly recommend a median sternotomy, and if necessary cardiopulmonary bypass to obtain complete surgical resection. In their retrospective study of the world literature, they found the survival rate following complete resection of aorticopulmonary paragangliomas to be 84.6% compared with 50% for patients without complete resection and

adjuvant treatment. Aorticopulmonary paragangliomas also were found to have a high local recurrence rate (55.7%) and a 26.6% incidence of metastasis. Paravertebral paragangliomas, on the other hand, because of their location, are less difficult to resect in their entirety, and wide local resection is recommended. They also have only a 14.6% chance of metastasis.[80]

There appears to be little benefit from traditional chemotherapeutic regimens. Radiation therapy appears only partially beneficial,

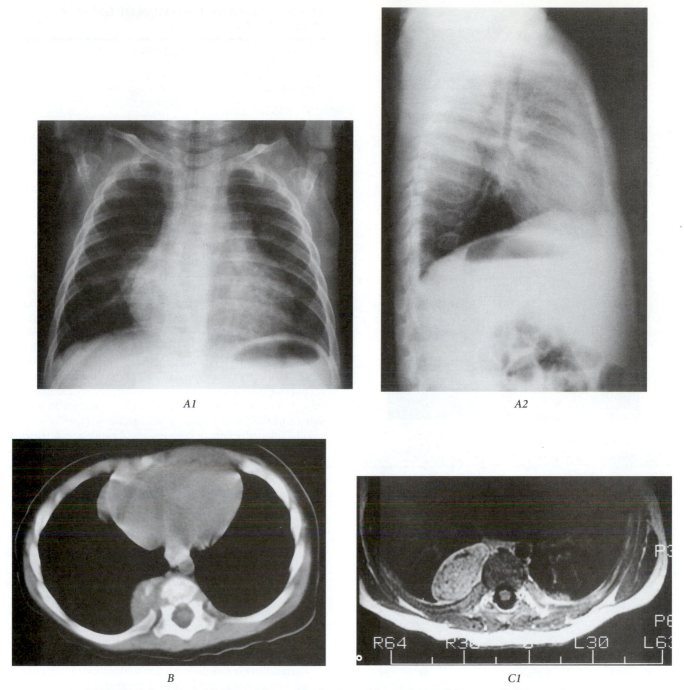

**FIGURE 10-8.** *A1* and *A2*. Chest radiographs of patient with ganglioneuroblastoma. *B*. CT scan of tumor. *C*. MRIs, cross-sectional (1) and sagittal (2), of tumor. *D*. Histopathologic examination of ganglioneuroblastoma showing mature component of tumor (hematoxylin and eosin, ×250).

mostly slowing the growth of the tumor. More recently [131]I-MIBG has been used as adjunct to surgical therapy and as a treatment for metastatic disease.[81] Patients with metastatic disease symptoms from catecholamine release can variably be controlled with α-methyl tyramine, which inhibits catecholamine synthesis.[82]

## GERM CELL NEOPLASMS

Primary mediastinal germ cell neoplasms are a diverse group of tumors with a wide range in their biologic aggressiveness. They range

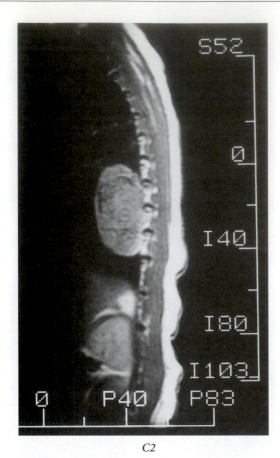

*C2*

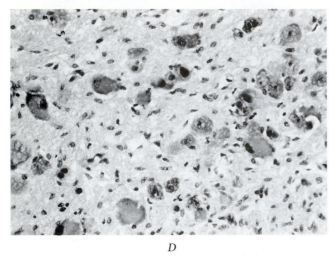

*D*

**FIGURE 10-8.** *Continued.*

---

from the benign teratoma, which is virtually 100% curable by surgical excision, to the highly malignant nonseminomatous group of tumors, with only a 50% long-term cure rate despite high-dose chemotherapy and resection. These tumors are classified in Table 10-14.

**TABLE 10-14. CLASSIFICATION OF GERM CELL TUMORS**

| BENIGN | MALIGNANT |
|---|---|
| Mature teratomas | Seminomas |
| Dermoid cysts | Nonseminomatous germ cell tumors |
| |    immature teratoma |
| |    teratoma with malignant components |
| |    choriocarcinomas |
| |    embryonal cell carcinomas |
| |    endodermal cell (yolk sac) tumors |
| |    mixed germ cell tumors |

Advances in treatment over the last several decades have improved tremendously the outcome for patients with these tumors, especially those in the nonseminomatous germ cell group. These tumors represent malignant transformation of primordial germ cells that failed to complete their migration from the urogenital range. Although evidence that mediastinal germ cell tumors were metastatic lesions from occult testicular tumors came from reports of occasional findings of testicular scars in autopsies of patients with mediastinal or retroperitoneal germ cell tumors, evidence by Luna and Valenzuela-Tamariz[83] of autopsy data from 20 patients with mediastinal germ cell neoplasms found only 1 patient with an occult testicular primary tumor and one with a testicular scar. Additional support for these mediastinal tumors being primary and not metastatic comes from cures without testicular recurrence in patients with mediastinal tumors treated with mediastinal field irradiation. Finally, autopsy reports of large groups of patients with testicular germ cell primary tumors have shown the rarity of isolated mediastinal metastases.[84,85] Current belief, therefore, is that mediastinal germ cell tumors are not metastatic lesions.

Primary mediastinal germ cell tumors are rare; only 1% to 2% of all germ cell tumors arise at extragonadal sites.[86] The mediastinum is the most common extragonadal site, with other sites being the retroperitoneum and more rarely the pineal and presacral areas. In the mediastinum primary germ cell tumors represent 10% of all mediastinal tumors, 15% of anterior mediastinal tumors in adults, and 24% of anterior mediastinal tumors in children.[82,87] Only 3% to 8% of mediastinal germ cell neoplasms are seen in the posterior mediastinum.[74,88] The frequency of benign mediastinal germ cell tumors is equal in adult men and women, but greater than 90% of malignant tumors occur in men. In children benign and malignant lesions occur equally in males and females.

Germ cell tumors are the most common tumors occurring in men between the ages of 15 and 35 years and primary mediastinal disease is usually seen in third decade of life. Of germ cell tumors isolated to the mediastinum, approximately one-third are seminomas and two-thirds are nonseminomatous, including teratomas. The distinction between the two is important in terms of treatment and prognosis. The nonseminomatous mediastinal germ cell tumors have a poorer prognosis than their gonadal counterparts, even though histologically the two are identical.

As many as half the patients with benign tumors are asymptomatic. Large tumors can cause symptoms from local compression of vital structures, such as chest pain, dyspnea, cough, or recurrent episodes of pneumonitis. Teratomas can have unique and even pathognomonic presentations, for example, cough productive of hair (trichoptysis) or sebaceous material, providing evidence of communication with the airways. Rupture into the bronchus, pericardium, or pleura can rarely occur as a result of digestive enzymes secreted from the intestinal or pancreatic tissue in the teratoma. Unusual presentations can occur with pericardial tamponade from compression or recurrent pericarditis from rupture into the pericardium. With ruputre into the pleura, respiratory distress may occur as a result of the irritative properties of the cystic fluid.

In contrast to benign tumors, malignant primary mediastinal germ cell tumors are symptomatic in greater than 90% of patients. The symptoms are most frequently chest pain, cough, and dyspnea. Systemic symptoms of weight loss and fever may be seen, and occasionally symptoms from metastatic disease may be present. Metastasis is most common to the lungs, mediastinal lymph nodes, liver, bone, retroperitoneum, and heart.

Usually few abnormal findings are evident on physical examination. Decreased breath sounds from a large mass or pleural effusion may be evident. With tumor invasion or rupture into the pericardium, a pericardial effusion may be appreciated as muffled heart sounds. In 10% to 20% of large tumors, superior vena cava (SVC) obstruction can occur, resulting in facial plethora, fullness, and distended upper body veins. Extrathoracic spread should be looked for such as supraclavicular adenopathy or other metastatic disease. A thorough testicular examination is required in patients presenting with presumed primary mediastinal germ cell tumors to rule out metastatic spread. Biopsy of testicular masses may be required, and ultrasound of the testes may be used if physical examination is insufficient to rule out a testicular primary.

As noted above, germ cell tumors are usually located in the anterosuperior mediastinum. Radiographic findings are abnormal in over 95% of cases. Chest CT scan provided additional valuable information regarding the location, extent, and nature of the tumor. Abdominal CT scan may be performed to assess for liver metastasis and to rule out retroperitoneal disease. Brain and bone scans are obtained only if symptoms are suggestive of metastatic disease.

Serum tumor markers should be measured in all cases of suspected mediastinal germ cell tumors. β human chorionic gonadotropin (β-HCG), α fetoprotein (AFP), and lactate dehydrogenase measurements should be obtained. Elevation in levels of serologic markers is not seen in patients with benign teratomas. Patients with seminomas do not show elevation in AFP levels, but 10% may show mild elevation in β-HCG level, with values usually less than 100 mIU/mL. Significant elevation in AFP or β-HCG level is diagnostic of nonseminomatous tumors. The marker level most commonly elevated in nonseminomatous tumors is AFP, occurring in 80% of patients, whereas β-HCG level is elevated in 30% of patients.[89] Levels of β-HCG, which is secreted by the syncytiotrophoblasts, are elevated with choriocarcinomas and in some patients with embryonal cell carcinomas. AFP level is most commonly elevated in patients with embryonal cell carcinoma and yolk sac tumors. These serum markers are also useful in assessing response to therapy and subsequent recurrence. The plasma half-life of AFP is 5 days and β-HCG is 12 to 24 hr.

FNA for cytologic evaluation and staining for tumor markers can be used to establish the diagnosis. When additional tissue is required to determine the histologic subtype, a Chamberlain procedure (anterior mediastinotomy) is usually the preferred technique for an anterior mediastinal mass. If a supraclavicular lymph node is enlarged, biopsy of it may provide the diagnosis. Cervical mediastinoscopy is usually avoided because the area it provides access to is rarely involved by germ cell tumors.[90]

Moran et al.[91] have reommended a clinical staging system as seen in Table 10-15. This scheme may have value in assessing prognosis and possibly planning treatment, but it has only recently been proposed.

**TABLE 10-15. CLINICAL STAGING OF MEDIASTINAL GERM CELL TUMORS**

| Stage I | Well-circumscribed tumor with or without focal adhesions to the pleura or pericardium but without microscopic evidence of invasion into adjacent structures |
|---|---|
| Stage II | Tumor confined to the mediastinum with macroscopic and/or microscopic evidence of infiltration into adjacent structures (such as the pleura, pericardium, and great vessels) |
| Stage III | Tumor with metastases |
| Stage IIIA | With metastases to intrathoracic organs (the lymph nodes, lung, etc.) |
| Stage IIIB | With extrathoracic metastases |

SOURCE: Moran CA et al.[91] Reprinted with permission.

## TERATOMATOUS LESIONS (FIG. 10-9)

Teratomas are the most commonly found primary mediastinal germ cell tumors, making up approximately 70% of adult and 60% of childhood cases of mediastinal germ cell tumors in the literature.[92] In contrast to previous studies, Moran et al.[91] reported 322 patients with mediastinal germ cell tumors and found only 44% of these were teratomatous lesions. Of these, 63% were mature teratomas, 33% contained a malignant component, and 4% were immature lesions. Additionally, in this study the overwhelming majority of teratomatous lesions were found in men. Of the 138 patients, 136 were men and only 2 were women. The average age was 42 years, with most cases occurring in the third and fourth decades. Only 10% of patients in this series presented with asymptomatic masses; more commonly patients presented with chest pain, cough, or shortness of breath.

On chest x-ray teratomas usually are round, well-defined masses that contain solid and cystic components. Up to 26% have calcifications, and confirmation of a teratoma is seen if the presence of a tooth is detected on chest x-ray, but this is rare.[92] CT scan showing the predominance of fatty material with denser portions containing bone and teeth and a cystic cavity is relatively specific for a teratoma. Despite these findings the diagnosis depends on tissue examination.

On gross examination teratomas are described as tan, soft tumors with cystic areas. Hair and bone may be found, mostly in mature teratomas. Immature teratomas often contain areas of hemorrhage and

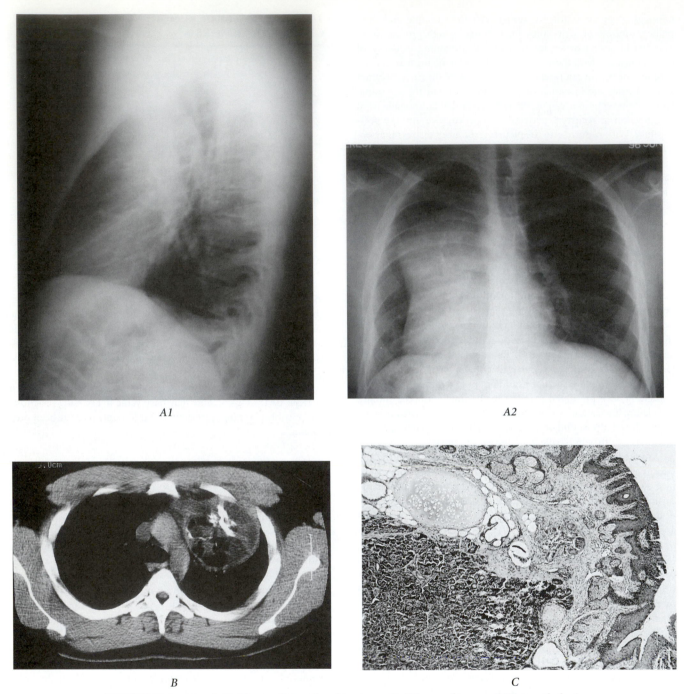

*A1*

*A2*

*B*

*C*

**FIGURE 10-9.** *A1* and *A2.* Chest radiographs of teratoma. *B.* CT scan of tumor. *C.* Histopathologic examination of benign teratoma (hematoxylin and eosin, ×520).

necrosis. These tumors are classified histologically. A dermoid cyst, also called teratodermoid, is predominantly composed of the epidermal layer. Often noted on microscopic examination is the presence of dermal and epidermal glands, hair, and/or sebaceous material. Teratomas are more complex, consisting of at least two and usually all three layers, ectoderm, mesoderm, and endoderm. Multiple tissue types can be present, including bone, cartilage, teeth, connective tissue, fibrous and lymphoid tissue, nerve, thymus, mucous and salivary gland, squamous and glandular epithelium, lung, liver, and pancreas. Differentiation of malignant from benign types is based on the presence of primitive or embryonic tissue. Any primitive or embryonic tissue represents evidence of malignancy. Immature teratomas contain combinations of mature epithelial and connective tissues with immature areas of mesenchymal and neuroectodermal tissues. Teratomas with malignant components are divided into categories based on the elements present. Moran et al.[91] subclassified these into those with malignant components containing sarcomatous elements, another germ cell tumor, an epithelial neoplasm, or a combination of any of these. The most common presentation was teratoma with another germ cell tumor, most commonly a yolk sac tumor.

Treatment for mature teratomatous lesions is complete surgical excision. Successful relief of symptoms and possible prevention of recurrence can be seen in partial resection of benign lesions that are large and unable to be completely removed. Chemotherapy and radiotherapy are not part of the treatment for benign lesions. Chemotherapeutic regimens combined with surgical excision and radiation in the treatment of malignant teratomas are individualized for the type of malignant components contained in the tumors. Late sequelae seen in patients with teratomas are impaired spermatic function and decreased levels of testosterone and luteinizing hormone.[93]

## SEMINOMAS (FIG. 10-10)

At presentation these malignant tumors are usually symptomatic, owing to their size. Presenting symptoms of cough, lethargy, weight loss, and SVC syndrome may be seen. Up to 10% to 20% of patients may present with SVC syndrome. Seminomas usually remain intrathoracic, and local extension to adjacent structures is commonly seen. When seminomas metastasize, the first sites usually are in the regional basin lymphatics with hematogenous spread occurring subsequently. Extrathoracic spread is late, most commonly to bone or lung, although liver, brain, spleen, tonsil, and subcutaneous tissue can also develop metastases. Histologically, these tumors have large seminomatous cells with abundant glycogen, scant cytoplasm, and round nuclei.

Therapy for seminomas is based on stage of the disease and remains somewhat controversial. Mediastinal seminomas, like their testicular counterparts, are exquisitely sensitive to radiation and systemic chemotherapy.[94] Smaller tumors detected on routine chest x-ray may be treated with surgical resection followed by radiation. Radiation is megavoltage to a mediastinal field including supraclavicular and neck regions. The supraclavicular and neck regions are incorporated because they are the site of initial lymphatic spread. When evidence of involvement of cervical lymph nodes is present, the field is expanded to include the axilla, which is the site of next lymphatic spread. Radiation therapy usually consists of 45 to 50 Gy over a 6-week period.

Multimodal chemotherapy has been successfully used in the treatment of seminomas in patients with locally advanced disease and metastatic spread, and currently consists of cisplatin-based chemotherapy. Jain et al.[95] in a nonrandomized study demonstrated superior results with combination chemotherapy compared to radiation in patients with localized mediastinal seminomas. Currently four to six cycles of cisplatin, vinblastine or etoposide, and bleomycin are used. Pulmonary function tests should be obtained before and after chemotherapy, inlcuding assessment of diffusion capacity to assess for any bleomycin-associated lung injury.[96] Radiation therapy has been used after chemotherapy, especially with large, bulky tumors initially or with residual disease.

As discussed below with nonseminomatous mediastinal germ cell tumors, any residual disease should be surgically resected after chemotherapy. Excellent long-term survival has been seen with mediastinal seminoma, with most studies reporting survival rates of 60% to 100%. Follow-up with CT scans at regular intervals is required to detect recurrence.

## NONSEMINOMATOUS TUMORS (FIG. 10-11)

These malignant tumors, which include choriocarcinomas, embryonal cell carcinoma, immature teratomas, teratomas with malignant components, and endodermal (yolk sac) tumors, are more aggressive tumors than seminomas. Malignant teratomas have already

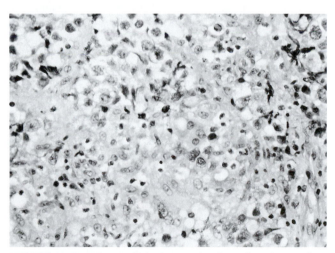

**FIGURE 10-10.** Histopathologic examination of seminoma (hematoxylin and eosin, ×325).

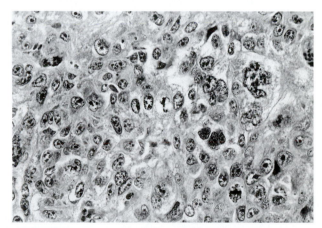

**FIGURE 10-11.** Histopathologic examination of embryonal cell carcinoma (hematoxylin and eosin, ×400).

been discussed with other teratomatous lesions. Moran and colleagues[91] found yolk sac tumors to be the most common type among mediastinal nonseminomatous, nonteratomatous tumors. Nonseminomatous tumors are a mixture of these tumor types in 40% of patients. Frequently they are disseminated at diagnosis. Most patients are symptomatic at presentation with complaints of chest pain, dyspnea, weight loss, cough, hemoptysis, fever, chills, and in 20% of patients, SVC syndrome. The most common presentation is in males in the third to fourth decades of life. When seen in children, the presentation may be precocious puberty. Metastatic spread outside the mediastinum is frequently seen, often to brain, lungs, liver, bones, and the lymphatic system, particularly to the supraclavicular nodes. Chest wall involvement is common. Pulmonary stenosis and coarctation of the aorta may also be seen.

Radiographic findings are usually of a large anterior mediastinal mass. Frequently there is extension into the lung parenchyma, and adjacent mediastinal structures.

Surgical resection of these tumors is often not possible following diagnosis because of their large size, local invasiveness, and metastatic spread. In patients with elevated levels of serum markers of AFP and β-HCG, tissue is obtained only to confirm histologic diagnosis. The endodermal histology is associated with the worst prognosis. Treatment of these nonseminomatous tumors is by multiagent chemotherapy containing cisplatin followed by surgical resection of residual masses. Other frequently used chemotherapy agents are vinblastine, bleomycin, methotrexate, etoposide, and doxorubicin. Hidalgo et al.[98] noted BEP (bleomycin, etoposide, and cisplatin) to be the chemotherapeutic regimen of choice outside a clinical trial. Bower et al.[99] reported the use of POMB/ACE (cisplatin, vincristine, methotrexate, bleomycin, actinomycin D, cyclophosphamide, and etoposide) followed by elective surgical resection of residual masses in the treatment of mediastinal germ cell tumors and noted a complete response in 92% (11/12) and a disease-free 5-year survival rate of 73% in the nonseminomatous germ cell tumor (NSGCT) group. Rarely are these tumors radiosensitive. Serum markers AFP and β-HCG are followed to assess response to treatment, and when levels of these markers normalize, the patient is taken to the operating room and removal of as much of the remaining tumors as possible is performed. The presence of residual disease after chemotherapy portends a poor outcome and the need for additional chemotherapy. If the tumor markers do not normalize, a second course of chemotherapy is begun with new agents. Overall, 60% of patients who undergo chemotherapy have normalization of their tumor marker levels and good long-term response. When on surgical exploration after chemotherapy a benign teratoma is found, a good prognosis is conferred; 20% to 80% of patients experience a complete response with the combination of chemotherapy and surgical resection. Long-term survival following chemotherapy and surgery is 36%.[100]

As opposed to testicular NSGCT tumors where salvage therapies have achieved cures in 30% to 40% of patients with relapsing or refractory disease, these same salvage treatment protocols have been disappointing in mediastinal NSGCT. Saxman et al.[101] reported on a series of 73 patients with extragonadal NSGCT treated with salvage chemotherapeutic regimens, and at the time of their report found only 5% to be without evidence of disease. Similar disappointing results have been seen by Motzer et al.[102] with high-dose carboplatin, etoposide, and cyclophosphamide. Motzer et al.[103] reported the use of paclitaxel as a salvage therapy in patients with previously treated germ cell tumors, and found it to have antitumor activity in germ cell tumors. Of 31 patients treated previously with cisplatin-based regimens, this study found that 8 patients (26%) achieved either a partial ($n = 5$) or complete ($n = 3$) response. Broun et al.[104] reported attempts at treating recurrent or refractory NSGCTs with high-dose chemotherapy and autologous bone marrow transplant without improvement in survival. Once relapse occurs, mean survival despite aggressive chemotherapeutic regimens is only 6 months. Options available for salvage therapy include paclitaxel, or cisplatin, ifosfamide, and either etoposide or vinblastine.[103,106,107] High-dose carboplatin and etoposide regimens with autologous bone marrow transplantation have also been used.[107-109]

There is an association seen between NSGCTs, karyotypic abnormalities, and hematologic malignancies. Klinefelter's syndrome has been associated with the development of mediastinal NSGCTs. A prospective study by Nichols and colleagues[110] found 18% of patients with mediastinal germ cell tumors to have the karyotype 47, XXY. An additional X chromosome may also be seen in the malignant cells of the mediastinal NSGCT and not in the somatic karyotype.

The association of NSGCT and hematologic malignancies has been reported.[111] The median time to diagnosis of hematologic malignancy is 5 to 6 months after diagnosis of the germ cell tumor. The most common hematologic malignancies reported in the literature are acute nonlymphocytic leukemia, acute megakaryocytic leukemia, malignant histiocytosis, myeloproliferative disorder, and refractory thrombocytopenia. These hematologic malignancies do not appear to be related to the chemotherapeutic regimens used to treat these patients, since patients treated similarly for testicular NSGCT do not develop these hematologic malignancies. Additionally, the average time, 6 months, between the appearance of mediastinal germ cell tumor and hematologic malignancies is too short compared to the 25- to 60-month interval between the appearance of most treatment-related hematologic malignancies. Finally, cisplatin-based chemotherapy has not been found to be leukemogenic. Instead of being a treatment-related cause, there appears to be a biologic association between the two tumors. One explanation, and probably the most plausible, for this association is that the hematologic malignancy results from the multipotential differentiation ability of the germ cell tumors.[112] Supporting this hypothesis is the finding by Woodruff and colleagues[113] of the isochromosome 12, i(12p), in both the mediastinal germ cell tumor cells and the leukemic cells in the bone marrow of a patient. The i(12p) karyotype is known to be associated with germ cell tumors and is a useful clinical marker for these tumors. In the same patient, Woodruff and colleagues reported trisomy 8 and XY +X in the germ cell tumor and in the hematologic malignancy. The simultaneous finding of XY +X, i(12p), and trisomy 8 in both lines suggests a common progenitor cell.

## LYMPHOMA (FIG. 10-12)

Primary mediastinal lymphomas, defined as lymphoma isolated clinically and radiographically to the mediastinum, represents approximately 20% of mediastinal masses in adults and 50% in

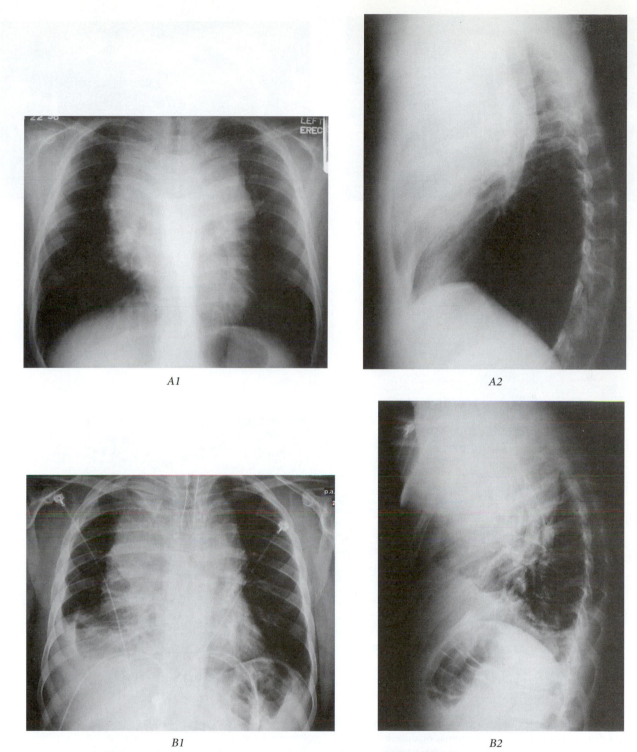

*A1*

*A2*

*B1*

*B2*

**FIGURE 10-12.** *A1* and *A2.* Chest radiographs of patient with Hodgkin's lymphoma. *B1* and *B2.* Chest radiographs of Hodgkin's lymphoma with tracheal stent in place to prevent tracheal collapse by tumor compression. *C.* CT scan prior to tracheal stent placement showing critical tracheal compression. *D.* CT scan after stent placement. *E.* Gallium scan of Hodgkin's lymphoma after 72 hr of uptake. *F.* Histopathologic examination of Hodgkin's lymphoma showing characteristic Reed-Sternberg cell (hematoxylin and eosin, ×520).

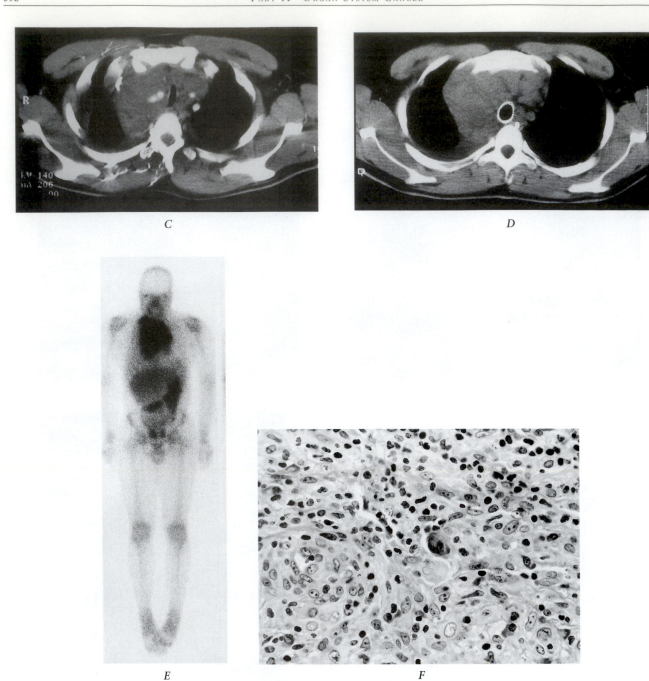

*C*

*D*

*E*

*F*

**FIGURE 10-12.** *Continued.*

children. Over 90% of primary mediastinal lymphomas are Hodgkin's disease, lymphoblastic lymphoma, or diffuse large cell non-Hodgkin's lymphomas. Each has unique characteristics as seen in Table 10-16, and it is important to classify the type of lymphoma for prognostic and treatment reasons.[114] Although lymphoma isolated solely to the mediastinum is uncommon (<5%), mediastinal involvement from an extrathoracic tumor is frequently seen occurring in 40% to 70% of patients sometime during the course of the disease.

At presentation, symptoms are usually present, especially with non-Hodgkin's lymphomas (NHLs) (lymphoblastic lymphoma, diffuse large cell lymphoma). Of patients with NHL at initial presentation, 85% have advanced disease. Constitutional symptoms including fever, night sweats, and weight loss may be present, and are important for staging of Hodgkin's. Symptoms from local mass effect of the tumor, including cough, chest pain, dyspnea, dysphagia, hoarseness, pleural effusion, and SVC syndrome are frequently present. The classical symptoms of Hodgkin's disease, Pel Epstein fevers (cyclical

**TABLE 10-16.** PRINCIPAL CHARACTERISTICS OF PRIMARY MEDIASTINAL LYMPHOMA

| DISEASE | AGE | SEX | SYMPTOMATOLOGY NONE | REGIONAL | SVC OBSTRUCTION | B SYMPTOMS | CLINICAL EXTRANODAL EXTENSION | CNS & BONE MARROW | PATTERN OF PROGRESSION | PHENOTYPE |
|---|---|---|---|---|---|---|---|---|---|---|
| Hodgkin's disease | Early adult | F > M | <20% | >80% | Rare | <30% | <30% | Rare | Commonly localized. Spleen and upper abdominal nodes <30% pretreatment | Nonclonal |
| Lymphoblastic lymphoma | Late-teens, early adult | M > F | Rare | Unusual | Not uncommon | 30%–50% | Common | Common | Rapid systemic progression if untreated; BM and sanctuary sites (CNS, testis) | Immature T-cell |
| Mediastinal large cell lymphoma | Adult, median 30–35 yr | F > M | <20% | >80% | 30%–60% | >50% | >50% | Rare | Progression in retroperitoneal nodes, kidney, pancreas, liver, adrenal | Follicular B-cell (variable differentiation); mature T-cell |

*The characteristics noted represent broad generalizations. Statements within individual reports may vary based on heterogenicity within series and case referral bias.
SOURCE: From Sutcliffe SB.[114] Reprinted with permission.

fevers) and chest pain after consumption of alcohol, may occasionally be seen. Extranodal disease occurs more commonly with NHL. Rarely, lymphomas, both Hodgkin's and NHL, can encase the pulmonary artery, causing symptoms related to pulmonary stenosis.

Although lymphomas can occur in any of the three compartments, the characteristic radiographic appearance is an anterosuperior mass or a hilar fullness in the middle mediastinum. CT scan or MRI is useful because often these will detect mediastinal lymphadenopathy appearing as separate masses suggesting the diagnosis of lymphoma.

The role of surgery in the treatment of mediastinal lymphoma is limited in most cases to obtaining a diagnosis. An adequate surgical biopsy is extremely important in correctly subclassifying lymphomas, and needle biopsies often do not provide sufficient tissue. The decision on the type of surgical procedure performed to obtain adequate tissue if a needle biopsy is inconclusive is decided based on the location of the tumor as determined on radiographic films. Mediastinoscopy, anterior mediastinotomy, partial or complete median sternotomy, thoracoscopy, or thoracotomy can all provide adequate amounts of tissue. An adequate amount of tissue needs to be obtained in case a special procedure, such as immunohistochemistry, cytochemistry, flow cytometric analysis, or electron microscopy study, is needed. A pathologist should be closely collaborating with the operating surgeon at the time of biopsy to confirm adequate tissue, amount, and preservation techniques.[114]

An additional role played by the surgeon at the time of diagnosis, if permitted by the incision, is identification of any additional mediastinal involvement as well as possible performance of biopsies as needed to identify spread patterns. Currently there is no role for attempted complete surgical excision or lymph node dissection.

The role of staging laparotomy in Hodgkin's disease is less important currently than it was in the past. Staging laparotomy is only performed presently if it will change the treatment strategy by altering the stage. Thus it is now used when a patient with clinical stage IA or IIA disease and favorable prognostic indicators presents and consideration is given to using radiotherapy as opposed to multimodal therapy. The staging laparotomy consists of splenectomy, wedge biopsy of the right lobe of the liver, needle biopsy of both lobes of the liver, and biopsy of any suspicious liver lesions. Biopsy of all suspicious nodes should be performed, including samples from paraaortic, splenic hilar, portahepatic, and celiac regions. In addition, careful inspection of the entire abdomen should be undertaken.[115]

Another potential role of the surgeon in mediastinal lymphoma is obtaining tissue following treatment in patients with residual radiologic abnormalities. Residual abnormalities are seen on radiologic studies in 30% to 90% of patients with bulky mediastinal disease, and in most cases represent scarring and not residual disease.[114] Evidence that these abnormalities represent sclerotic tissue as opposed to viable disease has been seen in reports of pathology from tissue biopsies of these lesions and by patterns of recurrence seen in patients with these residual abnormalities.[114] Gallium scanning may play an adjunctive role in determining whether viable disease remains after treatment, but to prevent false negatives, scanning should not be performed until approximately 6 weeks after treatment. The use of MRI in determination of tumor viability versus scarring has been investigated, with evidence suggesting changes in signal intensity may indicate response to therapy, but confirmation of its role has yet to be determined.[116,117] Since intrathoracic relapse, especially with bulky disease, is 20%, it at times remains useful to confirm pathologically that a residual abnormality seen on radiographic studies is not viable tumor. This tissue biopsy needs to be obtained using the same principles as the initial tissue diagnosis, and special care needs to be taken in obtaining tissue after initial treatment due to loss of normal tissue planes.[114]

Finally, the treatment of complications arising from lymphoma or from its treatment may require operative intervention. Figure 10-12 shows a tracheal stent placed in a patient with Hodgkin's lymphoma who presented in respiratory distress. Examples of treatment-related complications that may require surgical intervention include constrictive pericarditis and the early coronary artery disease seen in survivors previously treated with mediastinal irradiation, which may require revascularization.[114]

## HODGKIN'S LYMPHOMA

There is a bimodal age distribution in Hodgkin's disease, with one peak occurring in adolescence and early adulthood, and the second peak occurring after age 50. The mediastinal-predominant form of Hodgkin's tends to occur at an earlier age. The sex distribution in Hodgkin's disease presenting in the mediastinum is equal, but in the subtype of nodular sclerosing Hodgkin's, women present twice as frequently as men. Involvement of the thymus is more common in men.[118]

Hodgkin's lymphoma is classified by the Revised European-American Lymphoma (REAL) system, which was introduced in 1994 by the International Lymphoma Study Group.[119] This updated classification system replaces the previous Rye classification and divides Hodgkin's disease into two main groups: nodular lymphocytepredominant disease and classic Hodgkin's disease. Classic Hodgkin's disease is composed of nodular sclerosing, mixed cellularity, lymphocyte-rich (classic type), and lymphocyte-depleted disease types. The nodular sclerosing type is the most frequent Hodgkin's lymphoma seen in the mediastinum, occurring 55% to 75% of the time, followed by the lymphocyte-predominant type. Nodular sclerosing lymphoma has a predilection for the thymus, whereas other variants tend to affect mediastinal lymph nodes and are not seen as commonly as an isolated mediastinal mass.

Radiographically, MRI does not appear to be superior to CT scanning in detecting mediastinal disease. Gallium 67 has been used along with CT scanning of the chest to detect intrathoracic disease, but the main role of gallium 67 scanning appears to be in detecting early treatment failures. Weiner et al.[120] performed gallium 67 scans before and after chemotherapy treatment with nitrogen mustard, vincristine, procarbazine, and prednisone (MOPP) or with doxorubicin, bleomycin, vinblastine, and dacarbazine (ABVD). After treatment, 18 of 21 previously positive scans converted to negative results. Of these 18 patients, 11 had CT scans negative for residual disease and 7 had residual abnormalities on chest CT. Biopsies performed on all 7 patients were negative for residual disease. All three patients with residual positivity on their gallium 67 scans after treatment had residual Hodgkin's disease. A negative result, however, does not guarantee absence of residual disease, and reports of false positives are seen with hilar uptake and thymic hyperplasia.

The staging of Hodgkin's disease is important because it determines the treatment. Currently the Cotswold Classification,[121] a modification of the Ann Arbor Classification, is used for staging, as seen in Table 10-17.

Treatment of Hodgkin's lymphoma depends on the stage at diagnosis and the prognostic factors related to the patient and the tumor. Patients with clinical stage IA or IIA and pathologic stage IA and IIA with favorable prognostic factors may be considered for radiation therapy alone either to mantle field or mantle, paraaortic, and splenic regions. Total doses of radiation of 30 to 36 Gy are usually employed with areas of gross involvement receiving 40 Gy. Care should be taken that the heart does not receive more than 30 Gy. For patients pathologically staged with laparotomies, prognostic factors that appear to suggest an increased risk of relapse include bulky mediastinal disease, age 40 or older, and the presence of significant weight loss and fevers in the B symptom category. For patients staged clinically without laparotomies, adverse prognostic factors include male sex, age, elevated erythrocyte sedimentation rate, multiple sites involved, bulky mediastinal disease, B symptoms, and mixed cellularity or lymphocyte-depleted histology. When the presence of adverse prognostic factors is seen, treatment with chemotherapy or chemotherapy and radiation has been recommended. When combination chemotherapeutic therapies including adriamycin and radiation are used, care should be taken that the heart does not receive more than 25 Gy.[115]

Patients with more advanced disease at presentation or adverse prognostic factors are treated with chemotherapy alone or multimodality treatment. These chemotherapeutic regimens consists of various combinations: MOPP, MVPP, ChlVPP (chlorambucil, vinblastine, procarbazine, and prednisone), BCVPP (vinblastine, cyclophosphamide BCNU, procarbazine, and prednisone), ABVD, MOPP + ABVD, and MOPP + ABV selected on an individual basis with attention to toxicity of each regimen. If possible, a four-drug combination should be selected for initial therapy. When bulky mediastinal disease is present, involved-field or regional-field irradiation can be added. Failure of these regimens can be salvaged with conventional-dose salvage combination regimens or with intense chemotherapeutic regimens and marrow or peripheral blood stem cell support. Patients who fail salvage therapy can be tried in clinical protocols on experimental treatments. Long-term relapse-free rates of 80% and survival rates of 90% are currently obtained with appropriate treatment.[115]

## NON-HODGKIN'S LYMPHOMA

NHLs are seen in all age groups, but frequently patients are older, with a median age at presentation of 55 years. Men are diagnosed with NHL slightly more often than women.[122] As previously noted there are two distinct types of NHL occurring primarily in the mediastinum, lymphoblastic lymphoma and large cell lymphoma. Like Hodgkin's, NHL is classified by the REAL system.[119]

**LYMPHOBLASTIC LYMPHOMA.** Lymphoblastic lymphoma occurs predominantly in children, adolescents, and young adults, and represents 60% of mediastinal NHL. These tumors usually arise from the thymus, and patients often present with respiratory difficulties from a rapidly enlarging anterior mediastinal mass. This disease is two to four times more common in men and has an aggressive course with rapid dissemination to the central nervous system, bone marrow involvement that often progresses to a leukemic phase, gonads, and other visceral sites. There appears to be a close

**TABLE 10-17.** COTSWOLD STAGING CLASSIFICATION FOR HODGKIN'S DISEASE

| STAGE | DESCRIPTION |
|---|---|
| I | Involvement of a single lymph node region or a lymphoid structure (e.g., spleen, thymus, Waldeyer's ring) or involvement of a single extralymphatic site (IE) |
| II | Involvement of two or more lymph regions on the same side of the diaphragm (hilar nodes, when involved on both sides, constitute stage II disease): localized contiguous involvement of only one extranodal organ or site and lymph node region on the same side of the diaphragm (IIE). The number of anatomic sites should be indicated by a subscript (e.g., II$_5$) |
| III | Involvement of lymph node regions on both sides of the diaphragm (III), which may be accompanied by involvement of the spleen (III$_5$) or by localized contiguous involvement of only one extranodal organ site (IIIE) or both (IIISE) |
| III$_1$ | With or without involvement of splenic, hilar, celiac, or portal nodes. |
| III$_2$ | With involvement of paraaortic, iliac, and mesenteric nodes |
| IV | Diffuse or disseminated involvement of one or more extranodal organs or tissues, with or without associated lymph node involvement. |

| DESIGNATIONS APPLICABLE TO ANY DISEASE STAGE | |
|---|---|
| A | No symptoms |
| B | Fever (temperature >38°C), drenching night sweats, unexplained loss of >10T of body weight within the preceding 6 months |
| X | Bulky disease (a widening of the mediastinum by more than one third or the presence of a nodal mass with a maximal dimension greater than 10 cm) |
| E | Involvement of a single extranodal site that is contiguous or proximal to the known nodal site |
| CS | Clinical stage |
| PS | Pathologic stage (as determined by laparotomy) |

SOURCE: From DeVita VT et al.[115] Reprinted with permission.

relationship between lymphoblastic lymphoma and T-cell acute lymphoid leukemia. Since lymphoblastic lymphoma infiltrates the thymus and is diffuse in appearance, it can be confused with a lymphocyte-predominant thymoma if not carefully studied.[24]

Of lymphoblastic lymphomas, 20% are from B-cell precursors; the remainder are from T-cell precursors and phenotypically express various stages of T-cell differentiation. High levels of terminal deoxynucleotidyl transferase (TdT) activity is often present in lymphoblastic lymphoma. Histologically these tumors are divided into convoluted, nonconvoluted, and large cell subtypes according to the appearance of the neoplastic cells' nuclei. The convoluted type is present in 80% of patients, and the convoluted and nonconvoluted types preferentially involve the mediastinum.

**LARGE CELL LYMPHOMA.** Large cell NHLs of the mediastinum are a diverse group of lymphomas arising from both B-cell and T-cell lineage. These tumors are subdivided into primary mediastinal (thymic) large B-cell lymphoma and anaplastic large cell lymphomas of T- and null cell types. Recently additional variants of mediastinal large cell lymphomas have been identified, large cell lymphoma with marked tropism for germ centers and the low-grade mucosa-associated lymphoma of the thymus (MALT).[123]

The mediastinal (thymic) large B-cell lymphoma is by far the most common of the large cell lymphomas seen in the mediastinum.

Chim et al.,[124] in a retrospective study of 24 patients over a 10-year period, reported a slight female predominance and a median age of 34 years. Bulky mediastinal disease was present in 58% of patients. Patients mainly reported symptoms from mediastinal involvement, with 33% presenting with SVC syndrome. In 38% of patients, B symptoms were present. Primary B-cell lymphomas are located in the anterior mediastinum, and they may originate from a specific population of B cells located in the thymus.[125] These tumors have a tendency to remain intrathoracic. Histologically, mediastinal large B-cell lymphoma tumors are composed of large cells, which often appear compartmentalized by associated connective tissue. Because of this compartmentalization pattern, large cell lymphomas can be mistaken for seminomas, thymic undifferentiated carcinomas, or Hodgkin's lymphoma, based on light microscopic appearance. The degree of B-cell differentiation found in these tumors varies, ranging from early B cells that are negative for surface immunoglobulin to well-differentiated surface-immunoglobulin (usually IgG or IgA)–positive cells.[24] Primary B-cell lymphoma of the mediastinum stains positive for L26 (CD20).[124]

The anaplastic large cell lymphoma of T- and null cell types was initially recognized by its expression of antigen for the Ki-1 (CD30) antibody.[119] These tumors have only rarely been located primarily in the mediastinum; however, up to 75% of patients with these tumors have bulky mediastinal involvement in addition to their extrathoracic disease.[123] Histologically these tumors are composed of large cells and show marked nuclear pleomorphism.

Treatment of NHLs consists of aggressive doxorubicin-containing chemotherapeutic regimens. Following intensive chemotherapy, consolidation radiotherapy may be given.[125] In lymphoblastic lymphoma, central nervous system prophylaxis is given in conjunction with the standard chemotherapeutic regimen and consists of intrathecal chemotherapy, with or without cranial irradiation. Prophylactic treatment of the central nervous system is not needed in large cell lymphoma because of its infrequent involvement.

Lazzarino et al.[125] studied 106 patients with primary mediastinal B-cell lymphoma and reported pericardial effusion and Eastern Cooperative Oncology Group (ECOG) performance status ≥2 as predictive factors of poor outcome. Poor response to initial doxorubicin-containing chemotherapy was a predictor of nonresponsiveness to subsequent chemotherapies. Bulky mediastinal disease at presentation and residual abnormality after initial chemotherapy were risk factors for relapse. Recurrent lymphoma can be treated with high-dose chemotherapy, and either autologous bone marrow or peripheral stem cell transplantation.[126] With an aggressive approach cure rates of 50% and greater have been achieved with NHLs.

## ENDOCRINE TUMORS

### PARATHYROID TUMORS

Mediastinal parathyroid tissue represents approximately 1% of mediastinal masses (3/400 in the Duke series). In 80% to 90% of patients, the mediastinal parathyroid tissue is an adenoma, most of the rest are parathyroid hyperplasia, and less than 1% are parathyroid cancers.[127] Of all parathyroid adenomas, 10% occur in the mediastinum. This percentage increases after unsuccessful neck surgery to 20% to 50%.[128] These lesions are most commonly seen in older women who have had previous unsuccessful neck surgery for hyperparathyroidism. These lesions are found in the anterosuperior mediastinum 80% of the time, usually associated with the thymus gland. Usually the inferior parathyroid glands, which share their embryologic origin with the thymus, developing from the third brachial pouch, are ectopically found in the anterosuperior mediastinum. The adenoma is found 20% of the time in the posterior mediastinum, usually in an ectopic superior mediastinal gland. This relationship occurs most commonly when a thyroid goiter expands and the superior parathyroids, which share a common origin with the thyroid, developing from the fourth brachial pouch, remain associated with the goiter and descend with it.[82] Figure 10-13 shows the common locations of mediastinal parathyroid tissue.

Clinical manifestations from these lesions usually result from hyperparathyroidism. Mass effect from these small tumors is rare. Hyperparathyroidism can result in multiple symptoms, including asymptomatic hypercalcemia, urolithiasis, and lethargy.

Mediastinal parathyroid adenomas are uncommonly detected on routine chest radiograph. On CT scans they may be identified, and 25% will enhance with administration of IV contrast medium. Mediastinal MRI may aid in the diagnosis, detecting 50% to 75% of these lesions. Parathyroid adenomas show increased signal intensity with T2-weighted images and with gadolinium-enhanced T1-weighted

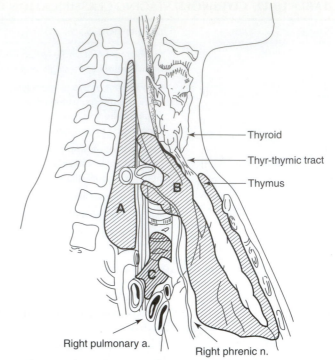

**FIGURE 10-13.** The three regions in which mediastinal ectopic parathyroid glands are found. *A.* Retroesophageal and paraesophageal region, which spans both the neck and the upper mediastinum down to the level of the carina (ectopic upper parathyroid IV). *B.* Anterior mediastinum, including thymus and posteriorly the pericardium, the aortic arch, and the great vessels of the upper mediastinum (ectopic lower parathyroid III). *C.* Midmediastinal compartment in front of the carina and mainstem bronchi. Note close proximity anteriorly of the right pulmonary artery. This area extends out of view along the left main bronchus underneath the aortic arch into the aortopulmonary window. (*From Bredenberg CE, et al.*[127] *Reprinted with permission.*)

images.[122] Technetium 99m–sestamibi scintigraphy can also be used to help identify the location of the ectopic gland. Selective arteriography occasionally is useful in preoperative localization, and venous angiography with selective sampling can help determine the side of the parathyroid gland. Using these techniques, preoperative localization can be made in approximately 80% of patients.

Histologically, mediastinal parathyroid adenomas are identical to their cervical counterparts. They are round, small (usually <3 cm), well-encapsulated masses.[122] If possible, preoperative localization is performed with subsequent surgical excision. Usually after a negative neck exploration the mediastinal parathyroid adenoma can be removed through the cervical incision. Most commonly the vascular supply to the gland is from cervical vessels. Only 15% of mediastinal parathyroid adenomas require median sternotomy. A median sternotomy should be performed following attempted preoperative localization in patients who have residual symptomatic hyperparathyriodism after cervical exploration and identification of four normal glands.[129] If preoperative localization fails to identify the gland, and after an exhaustive search in the mediastinum the location of the gland remains unknown, the pleura and pericardium should be incised and a search made. If the location of the gland is still uncertain, the thymus and parathymic fat should be removed. If necessary, cryopreservation of the excised parathyroid tissue should be done. When a median sternotomy is required, the reported failure rate is approximately 30%.[130]

More recently, successful angiographic ablation of mediastinal adenomas with single-feeding arteries have been performed with infusion of contrast material or alcohol. Cure rates with these techniques of angiographic ablation have been reported as 67% to 68%. Severe sequelae from this technique have been reported, but newer technology has resulted in the most significant complication being hypoparathyroidism, occurring in 6% to 11%. Heller et al.[128] suggest avoidance of this technique when concern exists over the possibility of a parathyroid carcinoma and in patients with a high likelihood of subsequent hypoparathyroidism. Subsequent hypoparathyroidism was more likely in patients with two or more parathyroids removed at the initial operation.[128]

Parathyroid carcinomas are rare, but they do occur in the mediastinum. They often are hormonally active and patients present with more severe symptoms of hypercalcemia. Complete surgical resection if possible is the treatment of choice.[82]

## THYROID TUMORS

Katlic et al.[131] described an intrathoracic goiter as a lesion where the majority of thyroid tissue was found beneath the thoracic inlet. Mediastinal thyroid goiters are most common in women in the fifth to seventh decades. Reeve et al.[132] reported an incidence of 1 in 5040 in the general population and 1 in 2030 in women over 45. Most commonly these tumors are a result of expansion of a cervical goiter into the mediastinum. The vast majority of these lesions arise in the neck, and therefore have a cervical blood supply. As cervical goiters grow, they usually expand along the pretracheal plane, and thus they are usually located in the anterosuperior compartment. As the goiter expands into the mediastinal, it may be shifted to the right by the aortic arch. Rarely thyroid tissue can arise from an ectopic focus within the mediastinum, and in these cases the blood supply may arise from mediastinal vessels. These lesions, like the cervical thyroid tissue that extends into the mediastinum, tend to arise in the anterior mediastinum. Posterior mediastinal thyroid tissue does occur in 10% of patients, with the presentation usually of a posterior mediastinal mass. DeAndrade[133] analyzed 128 instances of posterior mediastinal thyroid tissue, and found these lesions most commonly were located either retrotracheal, lateral to the esophagus, or between the esophagus and the vertebral column goiters. In all 128 patients, the tumor arose from cervical extension.[134]

Symptoms from intrathoracic goiters usually arise from compression of vital structures, particularly at the level of the thoracic inlet. Symptoms from this compression, such as respiratory compromise, dysphagia, or SVC obstruction, are often slow to progress and therefore are advanced by the time they are seen. Mitchell and Donnelly[134] compiled the results of several recent series and found a 53% incidence of respiratory symptoms such as dyspnea, stridor, wheezing, and cough. This respiratory compromise may be positional, being worse when the patient is supine, or, as described by Pemberton,[135] when the patient's arms are raised. Hemorrhage into the thyroid tissue can occur, resulting in the acute presentation of

respiratory distress. Dysphagia can occur from esophageal compression. Symptoms of hyperthyroidism are occasionally appreciated at presentation.[134]

Signs may be present on physical examination. A neck mass representing the cervical component of the thyroid goiter was noted in 53% of the compiled series reported by Mitchell & Donnelly.[134] Dysphagia was seen in 29%, thyrotoxicosis in 13%, and SVC obstruction in 5% of patients. Facial plethora, fullness, and upper thorax superficial venous prominence can be seen in cases of SVC obstruction. In this review, 13% of patients were entirely asymptomatic at presentation; the goiter was usually detected on routine chest x-ray.

Several studies can aid in the diagnosis. Although results of thyroid function tests are usually normal, they should be obtained. Thyroid function tests performed on 228 patients in the review by Mitchell and Donnelly[134] showed 87% to be euthyroid or less commonly hypothyroid, and only 13% to be hyperthyroid. The routine chest x-ray often provides information suggesting the diagnosis of intrathoracic goiter in an anterosuperior mass with focal calcifications and a smooth or slightly nodular border. Further evidence of the diagnosis is seen with compression of the trachea and reflection of the mediastinal pleura below the mass. The appearance of mediastinal goiters on CT scans has been previously described.[136,137] Often extension from a cervical goiter is seen on the CT scan. The presence of punctuate, ringlike, or coarse calcifications; a heterogeneous mass; a mass with well-defined borders; and a mass that enhances on CT following administration of iodinated contrast medium further suggest the diagnosis. Although less important since the universal use of CT scanning, thyroid scanning with [131]I may provide confirmation of suspected mediastinal thyroid tissue. If thyroid scanning is considered, it should be performed prior to the CT scan, because the iodinated contrast agents used in the CT scan can confound the results of the thyroid scan by interfering with uptake of the radioactive iodine by the thyroid tissue. FNA of the cervical mass may be performed, but should not be done on the mediastinal mass because the amount of additional information obtained does not justify the risk associated with a mediastinal biopsy. Pulmonary function tests should be performed to assess the degree of airway compromise, because clinically the amount of compromise is often underestimated.[134]

The vast majority of substernal goiters are multinodular. According to a recent review by Mitchell and Donnelly[134] across several series, the incidence of multinodular goiter was 70%. The results from this review are seen in Table 10-18.

Because of the high likelihood of these lesions causing symptoms, surgical removal of intrathoracic goiters is recommended. Medical treatment consisting of hormone replacement or [131]I radioablation is reserved only for those patients unwilling or unfit to undergo a surgical procedure. Most substernal goiters are removable by a cervical incision. More than 95% of posterior mediastinal goiters are amendable to cervical excision.[133] In certain cases a partial sternotomy incision is recommended. As described by Sand et al,[138] indications for a sternotomy include cases when excessive traction is necessary on the recurrent laryngeal nerves or the intrathoracic vessels, previous surgery for intrathoracic goiter, the presence of thyroid carcinoma, uncertainty in diagnosis, SVC obstruction, or airway obstruction necessitating emergency surgery. In the 10% of patients with posterior mediastinal thyroid goiters, a posterolateral thoracotomy may provide superior

**TABLE 10-18.** GENERAL ASPECTS OF RETROSTERNAL THYROID

| | LAMKE (1979), n = 29 | ALLO & THOMPSON (1983), n = 50 | SAND & McELVEIN (1983), n = 31 | KATLIC & GRILLO (1985), n = 80 | BRADPIECE & MICHEL (1988), n = 34 | MITCHELL & DONNELLY (1990), n = 31 | TOTALS n = 255 |
|---|---|---|---|---|---|---|---|
| Mean age | 58 | 66 | 58 | 56 | 61 | 66 | 60.3 |
| Men | 16 | 12 | 6 | 30 | 12 | 13 | 89 (34.9%) |
| Women | 13 | 38 | 25 | 50 | 22 | 18 | 166 (65.1%) |
| Previous thyroid surgery | 4 | 4 | 5 | 15 | 1 | 7 | 36 (14.1%) |
| No. of posterior mediastinal goiters | NR | 0 | 1 | 7 | 4 | 7 | 19 (8.4%) |
| Histology | | | | | | | |
| Multinodular | 22 | NR* | 27 | 41 | 26 | 28 | 144 (70.2%) |
| Follicular adenoma | 5 | | 0 | 33 | 4 | 2 | 44 (21.5%) |
| Hashimoto's | 0 | | 1 | 4 | 0 | 0 | 5 (2.4%) |
| Carcinoma present | 1 | | 3 | 2 | 4 | 1 | 11 (5.4%) |
| Unknown | 1 | | 0 | 0 | 0 | 0 | 1 |

ABBREVIATION: NR = Not recorded.
*Breakdown of histology not given.
SOURCE: From Mitchell JD, Donnelly RJ.[134] Reprinted with permission.

exposure over a median sternotomy in the rare situation that the intrathoracic thyroid cannot be removed by the standard cervical incision. Alternatively, as described by DeAndrade,[133] an anterior thoracotomy incision may provide additional exposure along with a cervical incision at very little added morbidity. The mortality rate for surgical removal of intrathoracic goiters is less than 1%. Postoperatively, patients with intrathoracic goiters need regular follow-up to identify recurrence. The use of thyroid hormones to prevent recurrent thyroid goiters remains controversial.[134]

## PRIMARY CARCINOMA

Primary mediastinal carcinoma is an uncommon neoplasm occurring in 9% of a series of 400 patients at Duke and 4.6% of the collected series.[2] Its origin is unknown, but differentiation from other poorly differentiated mediastinal tumors and extrathoracic neoplasms metastatic to the mediastinum is important due to substantial differences in optimal treatment. There is an equal sex distribution. Most patients with primary carcinoma are symptomatic at presentation owing to the extensive mediastinal involvement. Metastatic disease outside the mediastinum is also frequent at presentation. Immunohistochemical staining with specific markers and electron microscopy may aid in differentiating primary carcinoma from other tumors, decreasing the number of diagnostic possibilities because of better characterization. Treatment is surgical excision, but this is rarely possible. Chemotherapy and radiation therapy may be attempted, but usually the tumors have little response. The prognosis is poor; most patients die within a year of diagnosis.[82]

## MESENCHYMAL TUMORS

Mesenchymal tumors consist of connective tissue tumors including fibrous, fatty, muscle, blood vessels, and lymphatic tissues. These tumors occur equally in both sexes, are slightly more common

in children, and account for approximately 7% of mediastinal tumors. These tumors are more common at other sites. They have the same biologic behavior in the mediastinum as at other locations. Approximately one-half of the soft tissue tumors are benign, and 70% to 90% of the vascular tumors are benign.[61] The mesenchymal tumors can be divided into tumors of soft tissues and tumors derived from vessels. The soft tissue tumors are shown in Table 10-19.

### SOFT TISSUE TUMORS

These tumors are composed of elements of fibrous tissue, fat, or muscle. Fibromas are tumors of fibroblasts and are rare in the mediastinum. These are benign tumors and treatment is surgical resection. Recurrence is common if resection is not complete. Fibrosarcomas are the malignant counterparts of fibromas and are aggressive tumors. They are invasive and usually symptoms are present at presentation secondary to size and invasiveness of the tumor. The Doege-Potter syndrome has been associated with large fibrosarcomas. Treatment is complete surgical resection, but this is rarely possible.[61]

Lipomas are benign fatty tumors, more common in adults, and more common in men. Approximately half the patients are asymptomatic at presentation. Treatment is surgical resection. Liposarcoma is the malignant counterpart of lipomas. These tumors are rare in the mediastinum and usually occur in adulthood in an equal sex distribution. Most patients are symptomatic at presentation. Histologically there are four types: well differentiated, round cell, pleomorphic, and myxoid. Treatment is surgical excision, and prognosis is based on how advanced the tumor is at presentation, histology of the tumor, and the ability to resect it completely.[61]

Leiomyomas and leiomyosarcomas are tumors of smooth muscle origin and are believed to arise from the media of blood vessels and therefore may best be categorized under tumors of blood vessels. Leiomyomas are more common in women and usually present in adulthood. Leiomyosarcomas are rare in the mediastinum. These

**TABLE 10-19.** PRIMARY MESENCHYMAL TUMORS OF THE MEDIASTINUM

Tumors of adipose tissue
  Thymolypoma
  Thymolyposarcoma
  Lipoma
  Liposarcoma

Tumors of blood vessel origin
  Hemangioma
  Angiosarcoma
  Benign and malignant hemangioendothelioma
  Benign and malignant hemangiopericytoma
  Leiomyoma
  Leiomyosarcoma

Tumors of lymph vessel origin
  Lymphangioma—cystic hygroma

Tumors of fibrous tissue
  Fibroma
  Fibrosarcoma
  Malignant fibrous histiocytoma

Tumors of muscular origin
  Rhabdomyoma
  Rhabdomyosarcoma

Tumors of pluripotential mesenchyme
  Benign mesenchymoma
  Malignant mesenchymoma

Other tumors
  Localized benign or malignant fibrous tumor
  Synovial sarcoma
  Meningioma
  Xanthoma
  Extraskeletal sarcoma

SOURCE: From Shields TW.[61] Reprinted with permission.

tumors are treated by surgical excision and some recommend adjuvant radiation, but its role is unknown. Rhadomyoma and rhabdomyosarcoma are tumors of striated muscle. Rhadomyomas are extremely rare in the mediastinum. Rhabdomyosarcomas in the mediastinum are seen most commonly in children. Treatment of rhabdomyosarcomas is with radiation, possibly with chemotherapy.[61]

## TUMORS OF BLOOD VESSEL AND LYMPHATIC ORIGIN

The tumors of blood vessel and lymphatic origin are most commonly benign. The vascular tumors are seen in all ages and have an equal sex distribution; 90% are benign and half of the benign tumors are asymptomatic. The malignant tumors of blood vessels, in contrast, are usually symptomatic. Benign hemangiomas are by far the most common. Histologically hemangiomas are either capillary or cavernous. Treatment is surgical excision, if symptomatic or compressing vital structures, but asymptomatic children and young

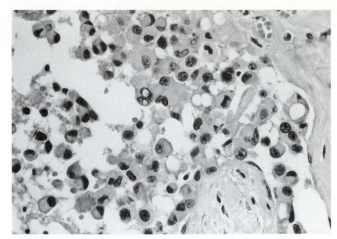

**FIGURE 10-14.** Histopathologic examination of hemangioendothelioma (hematoxylin and eosin, ×400).

adults with hemangiomas may be observed because in this group there have been reports of their spontaneous regression.[139] Angiosarcomas are malignant tumors of blood vessel origin and except when associated with the heart, pericardium, or great vessels, they are not seen in the mediastinum. Intermediate to the benign hemangioma and the malignant angiosarcoma are hemangioendotheliomas. These blood vessel tumors are derived from endothelial cells (Fig. 10-14). Enzinger and Weiss[140] described three histologic types: epithelioid, spindle cell, and the Dabska tumor. Wide surgical excision, including metastatic disease and local lymph nodes, is the recommended treatment. Recurrences are also treated by excision. Radiation or chemotherapy may be added for metastatic disease and recurrence. Hemangiopericytomas are rare blood vessel tumors in the mediastinum. They originate from pericytes in the blood vessel walls. Malignant hemangiopericytomas are differentiated from benign ones based on histologic appearance, including increased number of mitoses and increased cellular pleomorphism. Treatment is surgical excision.[61]

The lymphangioma (Fig. 10-15), also referred to as cystic lymphangioma, lymphatic cyst, cystic hygroma, or hygroma, is the most

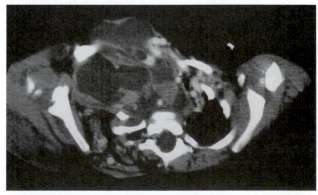

**FIGURE 10-15.** CT scan of cystic hygroma in a 15-month-old. The mediastinal deviation and tracheal compression is evident.

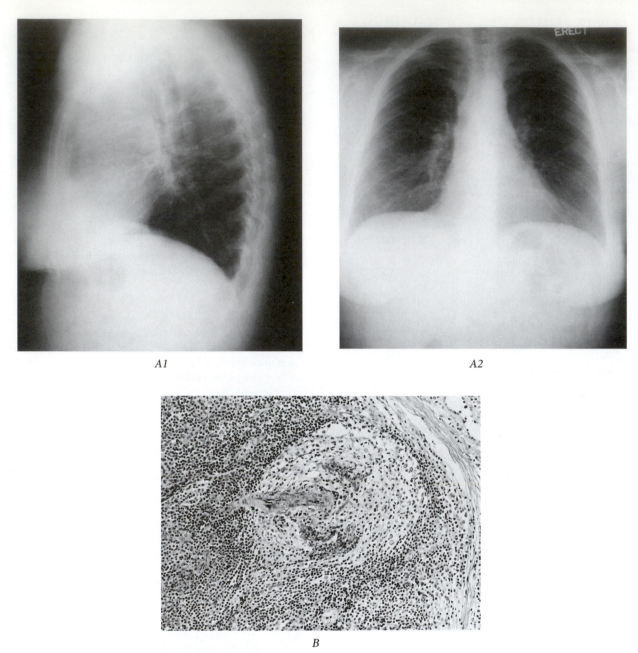

*A1*

*A2*

*B*

**FIGURE 10-16.** *A1* and *A2*. Chest radiographs of patient with Castleman's disease, relatively un-remarkable. *B*. Histopathologic examination of Castleman's disease, hyaline vascular type, showing characteristic follicle (hematoxylin and eosin, ×170).

frequently encountered lymphatic tumor. These are benign tumors of the lymphatic vessels, and they are felt to be a congenital developmental malformation, although some have argued that they are hamartomatous or neoplastic in origin. The most common location is not the mediastinum. They are more common in the cervical region (75%) and axillary regions (20%), but 10% extend from these locations into the mediastinum.[122] Usually these tumors are diagnosed at birth or in childhood, with 90% discovered by age 2. In the

mediastinum, however, they may be asymptomatic and can present in adulthood from symptoms of their size, recurrent pneumonia, chylothorax, or chylopericardium. These tumors can also occur as part of a generalized lymphangiomatosis syndrome. Chest x-ray and CT scanning can aid in the diagnosis with the appearance of a benign, homogeneous, lobulated, rounded-appearing cystic structure. On CT scanning cystic hygromas may show mild enhancement with IV contrast.[122] Histologically these lesions are composed of dilated lymphatic spaced lined by endothelium that contain lymphocytes and erythrocytes in a matrix of loose collagenous tissue. Treatment is surgical excision when possible. Although benign, they often are difficult to resect completely. The local ingrowth of the vessels and the fibrotic reaction to these tumors obscure tissue planes. Recurrence is seen with incomplete resection and multiple procedures may be required. Radiation therapy after surgical excision does play a role in blood vessel tumors, but is less valuable in lymphatic and soft tissue tumors.

## CASTLEMAN'S DISEASE (FIG. 10-16)

Castleman's disease, also known as angiofollicular or giant lymph node hyperplasia, is most commonly found in the mediastinum but can be located at other sites. It was originally described by Castleman in 1956. Usually this hyperplastic lymphoid process presents in the anterosuperior mediastinum as a rounded discrete mass. There are two types of Castleman's disease: a localized type that is seen 90% of the time and less commonly a generalized, multicentric type. The multicentric type is a more aggressive disease, often associated with other malignancies.[24]

Histologically, a hyaline vascular type, a plasma cell type, and an intermediate or mixed type are seen. The hyaline vascular type is the most common. This type occurs in all age groups, with a median age of occurrence of 33 years and it appears equally in men and women. Patients usually present with an asymptomatic mass or with symptoms from compression of vital structures. The hyaline vascular type usually is a solitary, well-defined mass that histologically is composed of abnormal small follicles with germinal centers and a vascular surrounding interfollicular area. Lymphocytes are prominent in the mantle zone of the follicles. These lymphocytes phenotypically express CD5.[24]

The plasma cell type also occurs in all age groups and equally in men and women, but has an earlier mean age of occurrence of 22 years. With the plasma cell type, systemic symptoms are often present. Polyclonal gammopathies, fevers, night sweats, laboratory abnormalities, and anemias may also be seen with this type of Castleman's disease. The plasma cell type may present as a group of matted nodes or a larger mass with surrounding nodes and histologically is composed of larger follicles than are seen with the hyaline vascular type. Plasma cells are present in intervening sheets.[24]

Treatment for both the hyaline vascular and the plasma cell types is complete surgical resection. The hyaline vascular type has the potential to bleed profusely if biopsied during surgery. The constitutional signs and symptoms and the immunologic phenomena seen with the plasma cell type disappear after surgical removal of the tumor.[24]

## CHORDOMA

These are rare, aggressive tumors that are derived from the primitive notochord. They are located in the posterior mediastinum and present with symptoms from compression of vital structures such as cough, dyspnea, chest pain, and spinal cord. These tumors occur more commonly in men, usually at age 40 to 60 years. The only valuable treatment is wide surgical resection and long-term results are poor because distant metastatic disease is common.[82]

## REFERENCES

1. AZAROW KS et al: Primary mediastinal masses. J Thorac Cardiovasc Surg 106:67, 1993.
2. DAVIS RD et al: Primary cysts and neoplasms of the mediastinum: recent changes in clinical presentation, methods of diagnosis, management, and results. Ann Thorac Surg 44:229, 1987.
3. GROSFELD JL: Primary tumors of the chest wall and mediastinum in children. Semin Thorac Cardiovasc Surg 6:235, 1994.
4. ——— et al: Primary mediastinal neoplasms in infants and children. Ann Thorac Surg 12:179, 1971.
5. SHAMBERGER RC et al: Prospective evaluation by computed tomography and pulmonary function tests of children with mediastinal masses. Surgery 118:468, 1995.
6. PHILLIPS LH, MELNICK PA: Diagnosis of myasthenia gravis in the 1990's. Semin Neurol 10:62, 1990.
7. LUKETICH JD, GINSBERG RJ: The current management of patients with mediastinal tumors. Adv Surg 30:311, 1997.
8. CHEN J et al: Computed tomography and pathologic correlations of thymic lesions. J Thorac Imaging 3:61, 1988.
9. RENDINA EA et al: Computed tomographic staging of anterior mediastinal neoplasms. Thorax 43:441, 1988.
10. NAKATA H et al: MRI of bronchogenic cysts. J Comput Assist Tomogr 17:267, 1993.
11. KUBOTA K et al: PET imaging of primary mediastinal tumours. Br J Cancer 73:882, 1996.
12. FRONT D et al: The dilemma of a residual mass in treated lymphoma: The role of gallium-67 scintigraphy, in *Nuclear Medicine Annual*, LM Freeman (ed). New York, Raven Press, 1991, pp 211–220.
13. TSAN MF, SCHEFFEL U: Mechanism of gallium-67 accumulation in tumours. J Nucl Med 27:1215, 1986.
14. CHANDRAMOULY BS et al: Uptake of gallium in the mediastinum. Semin Nucl Med 19:247, 1989.
15. TONAMI N et al: Detection of thymic abnormality in myasthenia gravis with thallium-201 SPECT. J Nucl Med 34:223, 1993.
16. PARK HM et al: Efficacy of thyroid scintigraphy in the diagnosis of intrathoracic goiter. AJR 148:527, 1987.
17. SPIES WG: Radionuclide studies of the mediastinum, in *Mediastinal Surgery*, TW Shields (ed). Malvern, PA: Lea & Febiger, 1991, pp 50–61.
18. SINGH HK et al: Diagnostic pitfalls in fine-needle aspiration biopsy of the mediastinum. Diagn Cytopathol 17:121, 1997.
19. GUNTHER RW: Percutaneous interventions in the thorax: Seventh Annual Charles Dotter Memorial Lecture. J Vasc Interv Radiol 3:379, 1992.
20. ZAFAR N, MOINUDDIN S: Mediastinal needle biopsy: A 15 year experience with 139 cases. Cancer 76:1065, 1995.
21. WEISBROD GL et al: Percutaneous fine-needle aspiration biopsy of mediastinal lesions. AJR 143:525, 1984.
22. WEISBROD GL et al: Percutaneous fine-needle aspiration biopsy of the mediastinum. Clin Chest Med 8:27, 1987.
23. KAISER LR: Thoracoscopic resection of mediastinal tumors and the thymus. Chest Surg Clin North Am 6:41, 1996.

24. Shimosato Y, Mukai K: *Atlas of Tumor Pathology*, 3d series, fascicle 21. Washington, DC, Armed Forces Institute of Pathology, 1997, p 35.

25. Rosai J, Levine GD: Tumors of the thymus, in *Atlas of Tumor Pathology*, 2d series, fascicle 13. Washington, DC, Armed Forces Institute of Pathology, 1976.

26. Wick MR et al: Primary thymic carcinomas. Am J Surg Pathol 6:613, 1982.

27. Lewis JE et al: Thymoma: a clinicopathologic review. Cancer 60:2727, 1987.

28. Snover DC et al: Thymic carcinoma: five distinctive histological variants. Am J Surg Pathol 6:451, 1982.

29. Suster S, Rosai J: Thymic carcinoma: a clinico-pathologic study of 60 cases. Cancer 67:1025, 1991.

30. Marino M, Müller-Hermelink HK: Thymoma and thymic carcinoma: relation of thymoma epithelial cells to the cortical and medullary differentiation of thymus. Virchows Arch 407:119, 1985.

31. Walker AN et al: Thymomas and thymic carcinomas. Semin Diagn Pathol 7:250, 1990.

32. Morgenthaler TI et al: Thymoma. Mayo Clin Proc 68:1110, 1993.

33. Kushihashi T et al: Magnetic resonance imaging of thymic epithelial tumors. Crit Rev Diagn Imaging 37:191, 1996.

34. Masaoka A et al: Follow-up study of thymomas with special reference to their clinical stages. Cancer 48:2485, 1981.

35. Wilkins EW et al: Role of staging in prognosis and management of thymoma. Ann Thorac Surg 51:888, 1991.

36. Jaretzki A et al: "Maximal" thymectomy for myasthenia gravis. J Thorac Cardiovasc Surg 95:747, 1988.

37. Fischer JE et al: Aggressive surgical approach for drug-free remission from myasthenia gravis. Ann Surg 205:496, 1987.

38. Patterson GA: Thymomas. Semin Thorac Cardiovasc Surg 4:39, 1992.

39. Yagi K et al: Surgical treatment for invasive thymoma, especially when the superior vena cava is invaded. Ann Thorac Surg 61:521, 1996.

40. Nakahara K et al: Results with complete resection and adjuvant postoperative irradiation in 141 consecutive patients. J Thorac Cardiovasc Surg 95:1041, 1988.

41. Curran WJ et al: Invasive thymoma: The role of mediastinal irradiation following complete or incomplete surgical resection. J Clin Oncol 6:1722, 1988.

42. Shamji F et al: Results of surgical treatment for thymoma. J Thorac Cardiovasc Surg 87:43, 1984.

43. Fornasiero A et al: Chemotherapy of invasive thymoma. J Clin Oncol 8:1419, 1990.

44. Macchiarini P et al: Neoadjuvant chemotherapy, surgery and postoperative radiation therapy for invasive thymoma. Cancer 68:706, 1991.

45. Rea F et al: Chemotherapy and operation for invasive thymoma. J Thorac Cardiovasc Surg 106:543, 1993.

46. Blumberg D et al: Thymoma: a multivariate analysis of factors predicting survival. Ann Thorac Surg 60:908, 1995.

47. Wilkins EW: Thymoma, in *Thoracic Surgery*, FG Pearson et al (eds). New York, Churchill Livingstone, 1995, pp 1419–1427.

48. Fukai I et al: Differential diagnosis of thymic carcinoma and lung carcinoma with the use of antibodies to cytokeratins. J Thorac Cardiovasc Surg 110:1670, 1995.

49. Kuzume T et al: Establishment and characterization of a thymic carcinoma cell line (Ty-82) carrying t(15;19)(q15;13) chromosome abnormality. Int J Cancer 50:259, 1992.

50. Lee ACW et al: Disseminated mediastinal carcinoma with chromosomal translocation (15;19). Cancer 72:2273, 1993.

51. Leyvraz S et al: Association of Epstein-Barr virus with thymic carcinoma. N Engl J Med 312:1296, 1985.

52. Patton DF et al: Thymic carcinoma with a defective Epstein-Barr virus encoding the BZLF1 *trans*-activator. J Infect Dis 170:7, 1994.

53. Weide LG et al: Thymic carcinoma: a distinct clinical entity responsive to chemotherapy. Cancer 71:1219, 1993.

54. Wick MR, Scheithauer BW: Thymic carcinoid: a histologic, immunohistochemical, and ultrastructural study of 12 cases. Cancer 53:475, 1984.

55. Wick MR et al: Primary mediastinal carcinoid tumors. Am J Surg Pathol 6:195, 1982.

56. Akwari OE et al: Dumbbell neurogenic tumors of the mediastinum: Diagnosis and management. Mayo Clin Proc 53:353, 1978.

57. Marangos PJ, Schmechel D: The neurobiology of the brain enolase, in *Essays in Neurochemistry and Neuropharmacology*, vol 4, MBH Youdin et al (eds). New York, Wiley 1980, p 211.

58. Gould VE et al: Synaptophysin expression in neuroendocrine neoplasms as determined by immunocytochemistry. Am J Pathol 126:243, 1987.

59. Bousamra M et al: A comparative study of thoracoscopic vs open removal of benign neurogenic mediastinal tumors. Chest 109:1461, 1996.

60. Grillo HC et al: Combined approach to "dumbbell" intrathoracic and intraspinal neurogenic tumors. Ann Thorac Surg 36:402, 1983.

61. Shields TW: Primary lesions of the mediastinum and their investigation and treatment, in *General Thoracic Surgery* vol 1, TW Shields (ed). Baltimore, Williams & Wilkins, 1994, pp 1724–1769.

62. Heltzer JM et al: Thoracoscopic excision of a posterior mediastinal "dumbbell" tumor using a combined approach. Ann Thorac Surg 60:431, 1995.

63. Brasfield RD, Gupta TKD: Von Recklinghausen's disease: A clinicopathological study. Ann Surg 175:86, 1972.

64. Gross RE et al: Neuroblastoma sympatheticum: A study and report of 217 cases. Pediatrics 23:1192, 1959.

65. Evans AE et al: A proposed staging for children with neuroblastoma: children's cancer study group A. Cancer 27:374, 1971.

66. Zajtchuk R et al: Intrathoracic ganglioneuroblastoma. J Thorac Cardiovasc Surg 80:605, 1980.

67. Martinez DA et al: Resection of primary tumor is appropriate for children with stage IV-s neuroblastoma: an analysis of 37 patients. J Pediatr Surg 27:1016, 1992.

68. Carlsen NL et al: Prognostic factors in neuroblastoma treated in Denmark from 1943 to 1980: A statistical estimate of prognosis based on 253 cases. Cancer 58:2726, 1986.

69. Shamberger RC et al: Surgical management of stage III and IV neuroblastoma: Resection before or after chemotherapy. J Pediatr Surg 26:1113, 1991.

70. Adam A, Hochholzer L: Ganglioneuroblastoma of the posterior mediastinum: a clinicopathologic review of 80 cases. Cancer 47:373, 1981.

71. Glenner GG, Grimley PM: Tumors of the extra-adrenal paraganglion system (including chemoreceptors), in *Atlas of Tumor Pathology*, second series, fascicle 9. Washington, DC, Armed Forces Institute of Pathology, 1974.

72. WICK MR, ROSAI J: Neuroendocrine neoplasms of the mediastinum. Semin Diagn Pathol 8:35, 1991.

73. GALLIVAN MVE et al: Intrathoracic paravertebral malignant paraganglioma. Arch Pathol Lab Med 104:46, 1980.

74. WYCHULIS AR et al: Surgical treatment of mediastinal tumors: a 40 year experience. J Thorac Cardiovasc Surg 62:379, 1971.

75. ODZE R, BEGIN LR: Malignant paraganglioma of the posterior mediastinum. Cancer 65:564, 1990.

76. DELELLIS RA et al: Leu-enkephalin-like immunocreactivity in proliferative lesions of the human adrenal medulla and extra-adrenal paraganglia. Am J Surg Pathol 7:29, 1983.

77. NOORDA RJP et al: Nonfunctioning malignant paraganglioma of the posterior mediastinum with spinal cord compression. Spine 21:1703, 1996.

78. SPIZARNY DL et al: CT evaluation of enhancing mediastinal masses. J Comput Assist Tomogr 11:990, 1987.

79. KLIEWER KE, COCHRAN AJ: A review of the histology, ultrastructure, immunohistology, and molecular biology of extra-adrenal paragangliomas. Arch Pathol Lab Med 113:1209, 1989.

80. LAMY AL et al: Anterior and middle mediastinum paraganglioma: complete resection is the treatment of choice. Ann Thorac Surg 57:249, 1994.

81. BALL ABS et al: Treatment of metastatic para-aortic paraganglioma by surgery, radiotherapy and 1-131 mIBG. Eur J Surg Oncol 17:543, 1991.

82. DAVIS RD et al: The mediastinum, in Surgery of the Chest, vol 1, DC Sabiston, FC Spencer (eds). Philadelphia, WB Saunders, 1995, pp 576–611.

83. LUNA MA, VALENZUELA-TAMARIZ J: Germ-cell tumors of the mediastinum, postmodern findings. Am J Clin Pathol 1976;65:450.

84. LYNCH MJG, BLEWETT GL: Choriocarcinoma arising in the male mediastinum. Thorax 8:157, 1953.

85. LUNA MA, JOHNSON DE: Postmodern findings in testicular tumors, in Testicular Tumors, DE Johnson (ed). New York, Medical Examination Publishing, 1975.

86. COLLINS DH, PUGH RCB: Classification and frequency of testicular tumors. Br J Urol 36(Suppl):1, 1964.

87. MULLEN B, RICHARDSON JD: Primary anterior mediastinal tumors in children and adults. Ann Thorac Surg 42:338, 1986.

88. WEINBERG B et al: Posterior mediastinal teratoma (cystic dermoid): Diagnosis by computerized tomography. Chest 77:694, 1980.

89. NICHOLS CR et al: Primary mediastinal non-seminomatous germ cell tumors—a modern single institution experience. Cancer 64:1641, 1990.

90. GINSBERG RJ: Mediastinal germ cell tumors: the role of surgery. Semin Thorac Cardiovasc Surg 4:51, 1992.

91. MORAN CA et al: Primary germ cell tumors of the mediastinum II. Mediastinal seminomas—a clinicopathologic and immunohistochemical study of 120 cases. Cancer 80:691, 1997.

92. LEWIS BD et al: Benign teratoma of the mediastinum. J Thorac Cardiovasc Surg 86:727, 1983.

93. LAHDENNE P: Late sequelae of gonadal, mediastinal and oral teratomas in childhood. Acta Paediatr 81:235, 1992.

94. BUKOWSKI RM et al: Alternating combination chemotherapy in patients with extragonadal germ cell tumors. Cancer 71:2631, 1993.

95. JAIN KK et al: The treatment of extragonadal seminoma. J Clin Oncol 2:820, 1984.

96. WAID-JONES MI, COURSIN DB: Perioperative considerations for patients treated with bleomycin. Chest 99:993, 1991.

97. MORAN CA, SUSTER S: Primary germ cell tumors. I. Analysis of 322 cases with special emphasis on teratomatous lesions and a proposal for histopathologic classification and clinical staging. Cancer 80:68, 1997.

98. HIDALGO M et al: Mediastinal non-seminomatous germ cell tumours (MNSGCT) treated with cisplatin-based combination chemotherapy. Ann Oncol 8:555, 1997.

99. BOWER M et al: POMB/ACE chemotherapy for mediastinal germ cell tumours. Eur J Cancer 33:838, 1997.

100. DARTEVELLE PG et al: Long-term follow-up after prosthetic replacement of the superior vena cava combined with resection of mediastinal-pulmonary malignant tumors. J Thorac Cardiovasc Surg 102:259, 1991.

101. SAXMAN SB et al: Salvage chemotherapy in patients with extragonadal nonseminomatous germ cell tumors: the Indiana University experience. J Clin Oncol 12:1390, 1994.

102. MOTZER RJ et al: High-dose carboplatin, etoposide, and cyclophosphamide for patients with refractory germ cell tumors: treatment results and prognostic factors for survival and toxicity. J Clin Oncol 14:1098, 1996.

103. MOTZER RJ et al: Phase II trial of paclitaxel shows antitumor activity in patients with previously treated germ cell tumors. J Clin Oncol 12:2277, 1994.

104. BROUN ER et al: Salvage therapy with high-dose chemotherapy and autologous bone marrow support in the treatment of primary nonseminomatous mediastinal germ cell tumors. Cancer 68:1513, 1991.

105. MOTZER RJ et al: Ifosfamide-based chemotherapy for patients with resistant germ cell tumors: The Memorial Sloan-Kettering Cancer Center experience. Semin Oncol 19:8, 1992.

106. EINHORN LH et al: Second line chemotherapy with vinblastine, ifosfamide, and cisplatin after nitial chemotherapy with cisplatin, VP-16 and bleomycin (PVB16B) in disseminated germ cell tumors (GCT): Long term follow-up. Proc Am Soc Clin Oncol 11:196, 1992.

107. MOTZER RJ et al: Phase I trial with pharmacokinetic analyses of high-dose carboplatin, etoposide, and cyclophosphamide with autologous bone marrow transplantation in patients with refractory germ cell tumors. Cancer Res 53:3655, 1993.

108. NICHOLS C et al: Dose-intensive chemotherapy in refractory germ cell cancer: a phase I/II trial of high-dose carboplatin and etoposide with autologous bone marrow transplantation. J Clin Oncol 7:932, 1989.

109. BROUN ER et al: Long-term outcome of patients with relapsed and refractory germ cell tumors treated with high-dose chemotherapy and autologous bone marrow rescue. Ann Intern Med 117:124, 1992.

110. NICHOLS CR et al: Klinefelter's syndrome associated with mediastinal germ cell neoplasms. J Clin Oncol 5:1290, 1987.

111. NICHOLS CR et al: Hematologic malignancies associated with primary mediastinal germ cell tumors. Ann Intern Med 102:603, 1985.

112. NICHOLS CR et al: Mediastinal germ cell tumors: clinical features and biologic correlates. Chest 99:472, 1991.

113. WOODRUFF K et al: The clonal nature of mediastinal germ cell tumors and acute myelogenous leukemia. Cancer Genet Cytogenet 79:25, 1995.

114. SUTCLIFFE SB: Primary mediastinal malignant lymphoma. Semin Thorac Cardiovasc Surg 4:55, 1992.

115. DeVita VT et al: Hodgkin's disease, in *Cancer: Principles & Practice of Oncology,* vol 1, VT DeVita et al (eds). Philadelphia, Lippincott-Raven, 1997, pp 2242–2283.

116. Nyman RS et al: Residual mediastinal masses in Hodgkin's disease: prediction of size with MR imaging. Radiology 170:435, 1989.

117. Webb WR: M.R. imaging of treated mediastinal Hodgkin's disease (editorial). Radiology 170:315, 1989.

118. Strollo DC et al: Primary mediastinal tumors part I: Tumors of the anterior mediastinum. Chest 112:511, 1997.

119. Harris NL et al: A revised European-American classification of lymphoid neoplasms: A proposal from The International Lymphoma Study Group. Blood 84:1361, 1994.

120. Weiner M et al: Gallium-67 scans as an adjunct to computed tomography scans for the assessment of a residual mediastinal mass in pediatric patients with Hodgkin's disease. Cancer 68:2478, 1991.

121. Lister TA et al: Report of a committee convened to discuss the evaluation and staging of patients with Hodgkin's disease: Cotswold Meeting. J Clin Oncol 7:1630, 1989.

122. Strollo DC et al: Primary mediastinal tumors part II: Tumors of the middle and posterior mediastinum. Chest 112:1344, 1997.

123. Suster S, Moran CA: Pleomorphic large cell lymphomas of the mediastinum. Am J Surg Pathol 20:224, 1996.

124. Chim CS et al: Primary B cell lymphoma of the mediastinum. Hematol Oncol 14:173, 1996.

125. Lazzarino M et al: Treatment outcome and prognostic factors for primary mediastinal (thymic) B-cell lymphoma: A multicenter study of 106 patients. J Clin Oncol 15:1646, 1997.

126. Kessinger A et al: High-dose therapy and autologous peripheral stem cell transplantation for patients with bone marrow metastases and relapsed lymphoma: An alternative to bone marrow purging. Exp Hematol 19:1013, 1991.

127. Bredenberg CE, Hiebert CA: Parathyroids, in *Thoracic Surgery,* FG Pearson et al (eds). New York, Churchill Livingstone, 1995, pp 1465–1474.

128. Heller HJ et al: Angiographic ablation of mediastinal parathyroid adenomas: Local experience and review of the literature. Am J Med 97:529, 1994.

129. Wang C et al: Mediastinal parathyroid exploration: A clinical and pathologic study of 47 cases. World J Surg 10:687, 1986.

130. Conn JM et al: The mediastinal parathyroid. Am Surg 57:62, 1991.

131. Katlic MR et al: Substernal goiter: Analysis of eighty Massachusetts General Hospital cases. Am J Surg 149:283, 1985.

132. Reeve TS et al: The investigation and management of intrathoracic goiter. Surg Gynecol Obstet 115:223, 1962.

133. DeAndrade MA: A review of 128 cases of posterior mediastinal goiter. World J Surg 1:789, 1977.

134. Mitchell JD, Donnelly RJ: Retrosternal thyroid. Semin Thorac Cardiovasc Surg 4:34, 1992.

135. Pemberton J: Surgery of substernal and intrathoracic goiters. Arch Surg 2:1, 1921.

136. Glazer GM et al: CT diagnosis of mediastinal thyroid. Am J Radiat 138:495, 1982.

137. Bashist B et al: Computed tomography of intrathoracic goiters. Am J Radiat 140:455, 1983.

138. Sand ME et al: Substernal and intrathoracic goiter: reconsideration of surgical approach. Am Surg 49:196, 1983.

139. Moran CA, Suster S: Mediastinal hemangiomas: A study of 18 cases with emphasis on the spectrum of morphological features. Hum Pathol 26:416, 1995.

140. Enzinger FM, Weiss SW: *Soft Tissue Tumors,* 2d ed. St. Louis, CV Mosby, 1988.

141. Blalock A et al: Myasthenia gravis and tumors of the thymic region. Ann Surg 110:544, 1939.

142. McNeill TM, Chamberlin JM: Diagnostic anterior mediastinotomy. Ann Thorac Surg 2:532, 1966.

143. Einhorn L, Donohue J: Cis diamminodichloroplatinum, vinblastine and bleomycin combination chemotherapy in disseminated testicular cancer. Ann Intern Med 87:293, 1977.

144. Sabiston DC, Scott HW: Primary neoplasms and cysts of the mediastinum. Ann Surg 136:777, 1952.

145. Heimburger IL, Battersby JS: Primary mediastinal tumors of childhood. J Thorac Cardiovasc Surg 50:92, 1965.

145a. Burkell CC et al: Mass lesions of the mediastinum. Curr Prob Surg 2:57, 1969.

145b. Fontenelle LJ et al: Asymptomtic mediastinal mass. Arch Surg 102:98, 1971.

145c. Benjamin SP, McCormack LJ, Effler DB: Primary lymphatic tumors of the mediastinum. Cancer 30:708, 1972.

146. Conkle DM, Adkins RB: Primary malignant tumors of the mediastinum. Ann Thorac Surg 14:553, 1972.

147. Rubush JL et al: Mediastinal tumors: review of 186 cases. J Thorac Cardiovasc Surg 65:216, 1973.

148. Vidne B, Levy MJ: Mediastinal tumors. Surgical treatment in forty-five consecutive cases. Scand J Thorac Cardiac Surg 7:59, 1973.

149. Adkins RB et al: Primary malignant mediastinal tumors. Ann Thorac Surg 38:648, 1984.

150. Nelems B: Neurogenic tumors, in *Thoracic Surgery,* FG Pearson et al (eds). New York, Churchill Livingstone, 1995, pp 1475–1482.

# CHAPTER 11

# CARCINOMA OF THE ESOPHAGUS

*Nasser K. Altorki*

Esophageal cancer is relatively uncommon in the United States, with approximately 10,000 to 12,000 cases reported yearly. Unfortunately, in the majority of patients, the disease is often fatal due to its advanced stage at the time of diagnosis. Despite significant advances in operative and perioperative techniques and the advent of a variety of novel chemotherapeutic agents, the overall 5-year survival rate remains in the 5% to 10% range.

## PREVALENCE AND INCIDENCE

### SQUAMOUS CELL CARCINOMA

Squamous cell carcinoma of the esophagus demonstrates a remarkable variability in prevalence worldwide. The disease is relatively uncommon outside Asia but is among the leading causes of cancer death in Central and Southeast Asia. A high-incidence esophageal cancer belt seems to extend from the Caspian littoral region of northern Iran, across the southern republics of Central Asia, and into northern China.[1] The highest incidence rates are reported in Iran and northern China. The national mortality rate for esophageal cancer in the Peoples' Republic of China is 19.6 cases per 100,000 individuals for men and 9.8 per 100,000 for women.[2] The disease accounts for 23% of all deaths from cancer.[2] Some of the areas of highest incidence are in the three northern Chinese provinces of Hunan, Shanxi, and Hebey, where the average incidence exceeds 100 per 100,000 of the population per year. Within the Asian continent, carcinoma of the esophagus is also common in Sri Lanka, the Indian subcontinent, and among people of Chinese descent in Singapore.[3–5] In the African continent, a high incidence is found among the Zulu and Bantu tribes of the Cape province and the Transkie regions of South Africa.[6] Squamous cell cancer of the esophagus is relatively uncommon in most of Europe and the Americas. High incidence areas are nestled in northwestern France, mainly Brittany

and Normandy, as well as the northeastern regions of Italy.[7] Within the continental United States, the national incidence of squamous cell carcinoma is approximately 6 cases per 100,000 individuals per year and has remained stable since the mid 1980s. Squamous cell carcinoma of the esophagus accounts for nearly 70% of all esophageal tumors in the United States. High incidence rates are observed in the low country of the Carolinas and in major metropolitan centers such as Los Angeles, New York, Detroit, and Washington, D.C., where the incidence approaches 28 cases per 100,000.[8,9] The incidence of esophageal cancer has remained relatively stable among white men older than 30 years but has nearly tripled over the same period among black men.[10] Esophageal cancer is now the second leading cause of death from cancer among black men younger than 55 years.[10]

### ADENOCARCINOMA

No longer a medical curiosity, adenocarcinoma of the esophagus currently accounts for 30% of all esophageal tumors in the United States.[11] Blot and colleagues[11] reported that the incidence of adenocarcinoma of the esophagus and cardia increased at 10% per year during the 1980s, thus exceeding the increases in cutaneous melanoma, non-Hodgkin's lymphoma, and lung cancer. The epidemiologic reasons for this rising incidence are unknown but are likely related to the reported increased incidence of Barrett's metaplasia, a known premalignant condition.[12] The incidence of malignant degeneration in patients with Barrett's esophagus is estimated at 1 in 200 persons per year of follow-up. These estimates are 30- to 40-fold higher than the expected incidence of esophageal cancer among Caucasian men in North America. The incidence of esophageal adenocarcinoma may be underestimated by the apparent dismissal of most tumors of the gastroesophageal junction as being of gastric origin. Careful pathologic examination of resected specimens reveals evidence of residual Barrett's metaplasia in nearly 70% of cases.[13,14] The combined incidence of adenocarcinoma of the esophagus and cardia is currently estimated at 5.8 per 100,000, ranking this tumor among the top 15 cancers of white men in the United States.[15]

## EPIDEMIOLOGY

### SQUAMOUS CELL CANCER

In the Western Hemisphere, epidemiologic evidence has strongly implicated alcohol and tobacco consumption as predisposing factors for squamous cell carcinoma of the esophagus. Tobacco is one of the important sources of nitrosamines, by-products of which are known potent esophageal carcinogens.[16] Cohort and case control studies in the United States, western Europe, and South America show that smokers are at high risk for squamous cell carcinoma of the esophagus.[17–19] The risk is strongly dose related, with ex-smokers showing a reduced relative risk compared to current smokers. Paradoxically, smoking does not seem to play an important role in the pathogenesis of esophageal cancer in the high-risk areas of the world, where dietary and environmental factors seem to predominate. The ingestion of a diet containing a high level of secondary amines, such as fermented fish, fungus-infested corn, or pickled vegetables, may be a more prominent predisposing factor in the high-incidence areas of the world.[20–22]

Consumption of alcohol has also been strongly associated with esophageal squamous cell carcinoma in the Americas and Europe.[23–25] Regular drinkers display an increased hazard for esophageal carcinoma. The combination of smoking and drinking seems to exert a multiplicative rather than an additive effect.[26] The synergy between alcohol ingestion and tobacco consumption may be secondary to the ease of diffusion of tobacco-related carcinogens through the esophageal wall by alcoholic beverages. Notably, alcohol consumption does not appear to be an important risk factor in the high-incidence areas of northern China and among the Moslem population of Northern Iran.

Environmental factors believed to predispose to esophageal carcinoma include asbestos or radiation exposure and the ingestion of silica fragments. A possible viral cause has also been suggested when papillomavirus particles were found in esophageal cancer cells.[27]

### ADENOCARCINOMA

Among all adenocarcinomas of the cardia and esophagus seen at our institution (Cornell Medical Center), almost 50% are associated with residual benign columnar metaplasia. In the other patients, benign mucosa may have been completely overgrown by the tumor. Careful histologic examination of specimens resected for Barrett's adenocarcinoma often reveal multiple dysplastic lesions associated with invasive carcinoma.[13,14] Furthermore, cell cycle studies using flow cytometry have shown that most patients with Barrett's adenocarcinoma have multiple aneuploid populations that often extend beyond the site of the invasive cancers.[28] These pathologic

and molecular findings suggest that the entire mucosal lining is exposed to a carcinogen that may precipitate cellular transformation. Since most studies have shown that approximately 60% to 70% of patients with confirmed Barrett's adenocarcinoma have a long-standing history of gastroesophageal reflux, the latter has become a prime suspect as the carcinogen involved in induction of the malignant phenotype. However, the exact component of the refluxate contributing to malignant degeneration is unknown. Recent clinical evidence suggests that patients with combined increased acid and alkaline esophageal exposure are more prone to the complications of Barrett's esophagus, including dysplasia, than those with acid reflux only.[29,30] Work in our laboratory has shown the potentially oncogenic effect of both conjugated and unconjugated bile acids in vitro. Exposure of esophageal cell lines to bile acids resulted in a dramatic induction of the cyclooxygenase-2 gene (COX-2), an inducible form of cyclooxygenase that has been implicated in tumor formation in both animals and humans.[31] Furthermore, animal studies have shown that esophageal exposure to unrestricted biliary and pancreatic contents results in the development of a Barrett's-like condition and subsequent adenocarcinoma.[32,33] Despite the experimental evidence demonstrated by in vitro and animal studies, the clinical evidence incriminating reflux in the genesis of esophageal adenocarcinoma remains indirect and largely circumstantial.

## PREMALIGNANT LESIONS

### BARRETT'S ESOPHAGUS

The premalignant nature of Barrett's esophagus has been confirmed by various studies since Morson and Belcher[34] reported on an esphageal adenocarcinoma arising in a columnar lined esophagus. The frequency and tempo of progression from metaplasia to dysplasia and finally carcinoma remain largely unknown. Patients with Barrett's esophagus should be included in a surveillance program aimed at early detection of high-grade dysplasia and early adenocarcinoma. Several studies have now clearly shown that when tumors are detected in patients included within a surveillance program, they are usually early-stage lesions where surgical resection is associated with cure rates in excess of 80%.[35,36] The cost effectiveness of surveillance for patients with Barrett's esophagus remains a controversial issue. At least one study has shown that endoscopic surveillance for Barrett's esophagus compares favorably with the common practice of surveillance mammography to detect early breast cancer.[37] Endoscopic surveillance of 149 patients with benign Barrett's esophagus was performed for a total of 510 patient-years, during which time 7 patients developed adenocarcinoma, an incidence of one case per 73 patient-years of follow-up. In the same study, occult breast cancer was detected in 50 of 12,537 mammograms, a detection rate of 0.4%. A cost analysis in each case including the cost of detection and subsequent treatment showed that the cost per life-per year saved was $4151 for adenocarcinoma in Barrett's esophagus and $57,926 for breast cancer. The authors concluded that the practice should be considered as cost effective as surveillance mammography, a commonly practiced method for early detection of breast cancer.

## ACHALASIA

The first report of esophageal carcinoma associated with achalasia was by Fagge[38] in 1872. Several authors have since confirmed that association and prevalence rates vary between 0% and 20%.[39–41] This wide range is probably due to confusion of "incidence" and "prevalence" and the variability in the length of follow-up periods reported in each study. In one of the few prospective studies, 195 patients with confirmed achalasia treated with pneumatic dilation underwent esophagoscopy and biopsy on a biannual basis.[41] Carcinoma of the esophagus developed in 3 patients an average of 5.8 years since the diagnosis of achalasia and 17 years since the onset of symptoms. The incidence was noted to be 33-fold higher than that expected in the general population. Squamous cell carcinoma is the most common type and is usually located in the middle esophageal third. Unfortunately, tumors are quite advanced by the time the diagnosis is made due to the insidious nature of the symptoms, which are often indistinguishable from the symptoms of achalasia. Approximately 80% of tumors are unresectable by the time the diagnosis is established.

## CHRONIC ESOPHAGITIS

The high prevalence of chronic esophagitis among the population in areas of high risk for esophageal cancer strongly suggests that esophagitis is precursor lesion for squamous cell carcinoma of the esophagus. In the high-risk area of Huixian in northern China, the prevalence of esophagitis approaches 50%, while it is only 17% in the neighboring areas with a lower incidence of esophageal cancer.[42] An epidemiologic study conducted in France suggested that esophagitis was positively correlated with cigarette smoking and frequent consumption of butter.[43] Studies from South America have also associated the presence of esophagitis or dyplasia with cigarette smoking, alcohol consumption, and maté drinking.[44] It appears that whatever the noxious agent, the esophageal response to injury is an inflammatory reaction that may progress to various degrees of dysplasia and eventually carcinoma.

## TYLOSIS

Tylosis (keratopalmar keratosis) is an autosomal inherited defect of keratinization associated with a very high risk for squamous cell carcinoma of the esophagus.[45] In affected individuals, the risk of developing malignant degeneration approaches 95% by the age of 65. Although hyperkeratosis of the palms and sole is a clinical characteristic of the disease, the esophageal epithelium does not usually manifest clinically significant abnormalities of keratinization.

## PLUMMER-VINCENT SYNDROME

This syndrome is characterized by webs of the cervical esophagus, iron deficiency anemia, stomatitis, pharyngitis, and dystrophic changes in the nail bed.[46] An increased incidence of cervical esophageal cancer has been observed and is possibly linked to various nutritional deficiencies implicated in the pathogenesis of the disorder.

## CAUSTIC STRICTURES

The propensity of caustic strictures to undergo malignant degeneration is well recognized.[47] Following lye ingestion, the latent period prior to development of carcinoma may be as long as 40 years. All patients with lye strictures should undergo endoscopic or cytologic surveillance to detect early tumors. When surgical intervention is required for palliation of dysphagia in patients without associated carcinoma, serious consideration should be given to resection of the esophagus and reconstruction rather than simple bypass because a carcinoma can still develop in the excluded portion of the esophagus.[48]

## CLINICAL PRESENTATION

Dysphagia is the presenting symptom in most patients with esophageal carcinoma. Unfortunately, dysphagia occurs late in the course of the disease. The lack of serosal coat allows the esophagus to distend and accommodate an intraluminal growth without noticeably impeding deglutition. Dysphagia occurs when the tumor encroaches on 60% to 80% of the esophageal circumference. Solid-food dysphagia may then rapidly progress to total dysphagia. Odynophagia is experienced by 20% of patients and is occasionally the only symptom. Persistent chest pain or discomfort unrelated to meals is an ominous sign that may indicate mediastinal penetration. Weight loss occurs in most patients, but cachexia is rarely seen in western countries. A variety of symptoms may indicate extraesophageal spread of the tumor, including the following: hoarseness secondary to recurrent laryngeal nerve invasion; aspiration resulting from an esophagobronchial fistula; and occasionally, massive hematemesis resulting from major vessel invasion. At the time the diagnosis is made, approximately half of the patients have locally unresectable disease or distant metastases.

## DIAGNOSIS

### BARIUM SWALLOW

A barium esophagogram is usually the initial study performed in the examination of patients with dysphagia. It is essential that the study include the cervical esophagus as well as the stomach and duodenum. A single contrast study will readily reveal structural abnormalities such as strictures, ulcerations, or masses; however, it is likely to miss small lesions confined to the mucosa and submucosa. Double contrast studies provide a more precise definition of the mucosal pattern, allowing detection of early tumors.

### ESOPHAGOSCOPY

Esophagoscopy is an essential diagnostic modality that not only allows a tissue diagnosis but also permits the surgeon to map out the extent of the lesion. An abnormally placed squamocolumnar junction in association with Barrett's metaplasia or the presence of satellite lesions are carefully sought. Surgeons should be familiar with the appearance of early malignant lesions such as mild erythema, induration, and small ulcerations. When findings are equivocal, vital stains such as Lugol's iodine or toluidine blue should be used to guide endoscopic biopsies. The esophagus is initially washed with 1% acetic acid, followed by the vital stain of choice, and then decolorized by a second application of acetic acid. With toluidine blue, malignant lesions retain the dye but remain unstained with Lugol's iodine. In each case, staining allows directed biopsies. When encountered, strictures are dilated to allow passage of an endoscope. Multiple biopsies are obtained because a positive yield increases with the number of biopsy specimens. In the event that a stricture cannot be safely dilated, then a brush cytologic examination is performed because on occasion a diagnosis is established with this technique. The combined diagnostic accuracy of brushing and biopsy exceeds 90%. If a diagnosis cannot be established despite dilation and brushing, then the patient is treated with a presumptive diagnosis of esophageal cancer.

## STAGING

The existing staging system for esophageal cancer adopted by the American Joint Committee on Cancer (AJCC) and the Union Internationale Contre le Cancer (UICC) emphasizes the degree of wall penetration through the esophageal wall, the presence or absence of nodal metastases, and the presence or absence of visceral metastases as the most important determinants of survival. The current tumor-node-metastasis (TNM) staging system has been recently reviewed by the UICC and adopted for another 10 years. However, staging of nodal disease remains fairly nebulous. A single N1 descriptor encompasses all possible sites of nodal spread. An emerging body of evidence suggests that survival rates may be negatively correlated with the number of involved nodes as well as the location of metastatic nodes. A recent study analyzed survival with respect to the number and location of nodal metastases in 216 patients with esophageal carcinoma. Survival was significantly better in patients with peritumoral nodal disease compared to those in whom the sites of metastatic nodal involvement was distant from the primary site, a group currently included in the M descriptor.[49] Similarly, the number of lymph nodes involved with metastatic carcinoma appeared to be an important determinant of survival, with most series suggesting that the survival rate in patients with four or fewer positive nodes is superior to that in whom metastatic carcinoma involves five or more nodes.[50–52] The current TNM staging system and group staging are shown in Tables 11-1 and 11-2.

### STAGING MODALITIES

**COMPUTED TOMOGRAPHY.** Computed tomography (CT) of the chest and upper abdomen is routinely performed in patients with esophageal carcinoma. The primary tumor is usually marked by a thickening of the esophageal wall. Although on occasion a blurring of the contour of the esophagus in the region of the tumor may indicate full-thickness penetration, the overall ability of CT to predict T (tumor) status is suboptimal. Similarly, the ability of CT scanning to predict nodal involvement is unreliable. Diagnostic accuracy is only 50% because false-negative rates frequently occur with small nodes. The criteria that determine invasion of adjacent structures by the primary tumor are also not well defined. Aortic invasion is predictable when the tumor encroaches on more than 90° of the aortic circumference, but the diagnostic accuracy of this sign is poor with lesser degrees of encroachment. CT criteria for gross airway invasion include distortion of the airway anatomy or an obvious endoluminal extension of the tumor. Nonetheless, CT signs of early invasion of the airway are not uniformly reliable and should not prevent exploration in an otherwise operable patient. We currently continue to use CT scanning to define the presence or absence of distant metastases, such as hepatic or adrenal metastases and also to evaluate gross evidence of unresectability of the primary tumor.

**ENDOSCOPIC ULTRASONOGRAPHY.** Endoscopic ultrasonography has emerged over the past decade as a useful modality in the clinical staging of esophageal cancer. The procedure should be

### TABLE 11-1. TNM SYSTEM

**Primary tumor**

| | |
|---|---|
| TX | Primary tumor cannot be assessed |
| T0 | No evidence of primary tumor |
| Tis | Carcinoma in situ |
| T1 | Tumor invades lamina propria or submucosa |
| T2 | Tumor invades muscularis propria |
| T3 | Tumor invades adventitia |
| T4 | Tumor invades adjacent structures |

**Lymph node**

| | |
|---|---|
| NX | Regional nodes cannot be assessed |
| N0 | No regional lymph node metastasis |
| N1 | Regional lymph node metastasis |

**Distant metastasis**

| | |
|---|---|
| M0 | No distant metastasis |
| M1 | Distant metastasis (including positive celiac nodes) |

### TABLE 11-2. TUMOR STAGES

| Stage 0 | Tis | N0 | M0 |
|---|---|---|---|
| Stage I | T1 | N0 | M0 |
| Stage IIA | T2 | N0 | M0 |
| | T3 | N0 | M0 |
| Stage IIB | T1 | N1 | M0 |
| | T2 | N1 | M0 |
| Stage III | T3 | N1 | M0 |
| | T4 | Any N | M0 |
| Stage IV | Any T | Any N | M1 |

considered as an adjunct rather than a substitute for CT. Although on occasion a metastatic lesion in the left lobe of the liver may be readily visible by the endoscopic ultrasound, the detection of disseminated disease is beyond the capability of this technique. However, endoscopic ultrasonography is superior to CT scanning in predicting the extent of mural penetration by the primary tumor (T status) as well as in predicting the presence or absence of metastatic disease to the lymph nodes (N status).[53,54] The accuracy of preoperative T staging approaches 80% and is particularly accurate for predicting T3 and T4 lesions. The accuracy of predicting submucosal and intramuscular tumors is problematic and may lead to overstaging in some cases. The endoscopic assessment of lymph node metastases has also been shown to be more accurate than CT scanning and is usually in the 60% to 70% range.[55] Unlike CT scan, the endoscopic ultrasound can provide additional information regarding the lymph node shape, border characteristics, and internal echogenicity. However, micrometastases that are currently detectable only by histologic evaluation may not provide enough echogenic patterns to be detectable by current endoscopic ultrasounds. Perhaps the most important predictor of the frequency of nodal metastasis is increasing degrees of wall penetration by the primary tumor. The presence of nodal disease increases steadily from 15% in submucosal tumors to nearly 70% to 80% when the tumor traverses the entire thickness of the esophageal wall. Current technology allows for endoscopic ultrasound-guided fine-needle aspiration of suspected lymph nodes.

**BRONCHOSCOPY.** Bronchoscopy is always done in patients with carcinoma of the cervical as well as the upper and middle thirds of the thoracic esophagus. The mobility of the vocal cords is carefully evaluated. A mere bulge into the membranous trachea or mainstem bronchi does not necessarily indicate malignant invasion. However, erythema and edema are ominous signs of airway invasion, and biopsy specimens and cytologic samples are retrieved from suspicious areas. A recent study prospectively evaluated the bronchoscopic findings of airway invasion in 16 patients with potentially operable esophageal cancer.[56] In patients with esophageal cancer above the tracheal bifurcation, 32% of patients showed some macroscopic abnormality at bronchoscopy. A mobile protrusion of the posterior tracheal wall was the most frequent abnormality. When compared with histologic results, normal macroscopic appearance of the trachea and main bronchi had a negative predictive value of 98%, but the positive predictive value of all macroscopic abnormalities for the diagnosis of airway invasion was low, particularly in patients who received preoperative radiation therapy. It has not been our practice to exclude patients from consideration for surgical resection unless there is unmistakable evidence of macroscopic involvement of the posterior membranous trachea or unless preoperative bronchoscopic biopsies show evidence of malignant infiltration.

**MISCELLANEOUS.** Invasive measures such as mediastinoscopy, cervical node biopsy, thoracoscopy, laparoscopy, and occasionally laparotomy should be liberally utilized. Although thoracoscopic-laparoscopic staging for esophageal cancer has recently been advocated by some groups,[57] we found the procedure to be time-consuming and frequently the available information has little impact on treatment planning. We currently restrict the use of

**TABLE 11-3. TREATMENT OPTIONS FOR ESOPHAGEAL CARCINOMA**

1. Primary surgical resection
2. Primary radiotherapy
3. Chemotherapy followed by a planned operation
4. Radiotherapy followed by a planned operation
5. Chemoradiation followed by a planned operation
6. Primary chemoradiation

thoracoscopy and laparoscopy to the confirmation of distant metastases or locally unresectable disease if either were strongly suggested by other staging modalities such as CT scanning or endoscopic ultrasonography.

## TREATMENT

The generally poor outcome of patients with esophageal cancer has generated considerable controversy among medical oncologists and surgeons as to what constitutes the standard therapy. The available options are outlined in Table 11-3. We believe that, to date, primary surgical resection remains the standard of care if patients are considered suitable surgical candidates. Most of the evidence accumulated from a number of random assignment trials seems to suggest that the use of various modalities of induction therapy provide little or no advantage over primary surgical resection alone. Patients not considered suitable for an esophagectomy should receive definitive chemoradiation, which is a superior alternative to radiation therapy alone.[58]

### SURGICAL THERAPY

Resection of the thoracic esophagus can be accomplished by a variety of surgical approaches. Worldwide, the most commonly used approach is a right thoracotomy and laparotomy, as initially proposed by Lewis.[59] A modification was proposed by McKeown,[60] whereby an additional cervical incision allows the anastomosis to be performed in the neck, thus avoiding the potential hazards of an intrathoracic anastomosis. A less commonly used incision for esophageal resection is the left thoracotomy. Preferred by Sweet and others,[61] this approach was gradually abandoned because of the significant increase in pulmonary morbidity incurred by the radial incision of the diaphragm required for exposure of the upper abdomen. The technique can be modified by adopting a peripheral semilunar incision located approximately 1.5 inches from the chest wall, thus preserving diaphragmatic innervation. This exposure is popular in China and is our exposure of choice for tumors of the gastroesophageal junction and intraabdominal portion of the esophagus.

As initially proposed and performed by Denk[62] in 1913, resection without thoracotomy has been reintroduced and popularized by Orringer.[63] The operation can be performed through an upper abdominal and cervical incision without the need for a thoracotomy. However, surgeons who use this approach should be willing and capable of performing a thoracotomy to deal with the potential but rare intrathoracic vascular or tracheal injuries that might occur during esophageal resection.

Tumors of the cervical esophagus are exposed through a generous collar or U-shaped incision. Additional exposure can be obtained through an upper sternal split, a technique that is potentially useful in exposing tumors that extend into the thoracic inlet. Laryngectomy and a terminal tracheostomy are also performed. Reconstruction is achieved by advancing the stomach or an isoperistaltic segment of colon. A free jejunal graft may also be used for reconstruction.

TRANSHIATAL ESOPHAGECTOMY. This operation is best suited for resection of carcinoma of the cardia, but it is also used for resection of carcinoma of the intrathoracic esophagus. Perhaps the largest single experience with transhiatal esophagectomy is that of Orringer and colleagues.[64] They reported on 417 patients with carcinoma of the esophagus and cardia resected with this technique over a 15-year period. The overall hospital mortality rate was 5%, and complications were no more clinically significant than those encountered with standard transthoracic resection. The overall 5-year survival rate was 27% and did not vary greatly with cell type or tumor location. Tumor stage was the only statistically significant determinant of survival. Gelfand and coworkers[65] reported on 160 patients who underwent transhiatal esophagectomy for carcinoma of the lower esophagus and cardia. Most tumors were adenocarcinoma and most presented in earlier stages. Survival rates at 1, 2, and 5 years were 62%, 40%, and 21%, respectively. Gertsch reported on 100 patients with esophageal carcinoma who were uniformly treated with transhiatal esophagectomy without adjuvant therapy over a 10-year period.[66] The hospital mortality rate was 3% and the morbidity rate was 68%. The median survival was 18 months and the overall 5-year survival rate was 23%. Survival was better for patients with T1 and T2 lesions (63% 5-year survival rate). Vigneswaran and coworkers[67] reported on 131 patients who underwent transhiatal resection with an operative mortality rate of 2%. The overall 5-year survival rate was 21%. Survival was significantly better for patients with stage I disease, 47.5% of whom were alive at 5 years, compared to patients with stage III disease, who had a 5.8% 5-year survival rate. In the latter study, the 5-year survival rate for adenocarcinoma was 27%. None of the patients with squamous cell carcinoma were alive at 5 years.

Proponents of transhiatal esophagectomy maintain that overall survival rates are not significantly different from those achievable with standard transthoracic resection or even extended resections and that occasional cures are possible in only a few patients with superficial tumors and without nodal metastases (T1-T2N0). However, critics of transhiatal esophagectomy argue that a complete lymphadenectomy is a necessary component of resection for carcinoma, primarily for staging and possibly for curative purposes. There is an increasing body of evidence suggesting that nodal metastases occur in 25% to 50% of patients in whom the tumor is limited to the submucosa, thus lending support to the argument favoring a more aggressive lymphadenectomy.[68,69] Extended resections in these situations can result in a 5-year survival rate in the range of 50% to 60%.[70,71]

STANDARD TRANSTHORACIC ESOPHAGECTOMY. Standard transthoracic esophagectomy is performed through either a right or left thoracotomy, depending on the preference of the surgeon and the location of the tumor. Generally, a right thoracotomy is reserved for tumors located in the middle third of the esophagus in close proximity to the tracheal bifurcation or the arch of the aorta. A fifth-interspace right thoracotomy provides excellent exposure of these structures. Single lung ventilation greatly enhances the exposure. On the other hand, a left thoracotomy is reserved for tumors located within the abdominal portion of the esophagus or gastroesophageal junction or within the lower third of the esophagus. A left sixth-interspace thoracotomy provides excellent exposure of the lower mediastinum, and semilunar division of the diaphragm approximately 1 inch from the costal margin allows access to the upper abdomen with excellent exposure of the hiatus and the left upper quadrant. In either case, the esophagus is mobilized from its mediastinal bed, and mobilization is carried proximally to the thoracic inlet and distally to the hiatus. All easily accessible periesophageal nodes are removed with the specimen, but no attempt is made toward a radical dissection of the lymph nodes in the mediastinum and the upper abdomen. Patients operated on through a right thoracotomy will obviously need a laparotomy in order to prepare the esophageal substitute, which is then passed to the neck either through the posterior mediastinum or through a retrosternal tunnel for a cervical anastomosis. When the procedure is performed through a left thoracotomy, the esophagus is mobilized from under the aortic arch and along its course in the supraaortic posterior mediastinum and freed well into the neck. The prepared gastric tube is then passed under the aortic arch and attached to the esophageal stump; both are tucked into the prevertebral cervical space. The diaphragm is reattached and the thoracotomy is closed. With the patient in the supine position, a small cervical incision is performed and dissection is carried to the prevertebral space where the esophageal stump and the gastric tube are encountered and easily delivered into the neck for a cervical anastomosis.

Several studies have shown little difference in the operative mortality and morbidity rates between transthoracic and transhiatal esophagectomy.[72–74] Chu reported a randomized controlled trial comparing transhiatal and transthoracic resection in patients with esophageal cancer.[72] Thirty-nine patients with carcinoma of the lower third of the esophagus were prospectively randomized to receive either a transhiatal esophagectomy or a transthoracic resection. There was no significant difference between the groups in the amount of blood loss, postoperative ventilatory requirements, cardiopulmonary complication rates, and mean hospital stay. Median survival rates were 16 months after transhiatal esophagectomy and 13.5 months following transthoracic resections. Other investigators also compared transhiatal and transthoracic resections and appreciated no significant differences in perioperative morbidity or mortality rates.[73,74] Survival rates reported with transthoracic resections were essentially identical to those reported after transhiatal resection.

EN BLOC RESECTION. En bloc resection of carcinoma of the cardia and lower esophagus was originally proposed in 1963 by Logan,[75] who reported on 250 patients who underwent resection with the en bloc technique with a 16% 5-year survival rate but a formidable operative mortality of 21%.[75] The technique was modified in 1969 and later extended to resections of carcinoma of the thoracic and cervical esophagus.[76] The basic principle of en bloc resection is the extirpation of the esophagus within an envelope of adjoining normal tissue. This includes the posterior pericardium and both pleural surfaces where they abut the tumor-bearing esophagus as well as all the lymphovascular tissue (including the thoracic duct) wedged dorsally between the esophagus and the spine (Fig. 11-1). This "mesoesophagus" is probably the remnant of the embryonic esophageal mesentery that determines the pathway of vascular supply and lymphatic drainage of the esophagus. Because the esophagus lacks a defined serosal coat, both pleural surfaces and the pericardium are construed as serosal counterparts, especially because the lower esophageal longitudinal muscle layer is partly attached to the subpleural and pericardial fibrous layers. For tumors of the cardia and intraabdominal esophagus, a 1-inch cuff of diaphragm is resected en bloc with the specimen. Upper abdominal and mediastinal lymphadenectomy completes the procedure. The gastrointestinal tract is divided approximately 10 cm on either side of the tumor, and gastrointestinal continuity is established with the esophageal substitute of choice. We have recently reported our experience with 78 patients who underwent en bloc resection and compared their outcome with 50 patients who underwent standard resection.[77] The hospital mortality rate following en bloc resection was 3.9%, compared to 5.4% in patients undergoing a standard transthoracic esophagectomy. Overall survival for all 128 patients was 25%. The four-year survival rate for the 50 patients undergoing limited transthoracic resection was 8%, compared with 41% for the en bloc group. Significantly, in the subgroup of patients with stage III disease, en bloc esophagectomy resulted in a superior median and 5-year survival rate (Fig. 11-2). Thirty-three patients who underwent an en bloc esophagectomy had a median survival of 27 months and a 5-year survival rate of 34%, compared with a median survival of 12 months and a 5-year survival rate of 11% for 21 patients who underwent a more limited resection. The difference in survival between the groups was statistically significant. When survival analysis was performed based on N status, the survival rate of patients with node-negative disease was 68% following en bloc esophagectomy, compared to 27% in patients undergoing a less radical operation. The mean number of resected nodes in patients with node-negative disease was 36 nodes per patient after en bloc resection and nearly 20 nodes per patient after limited resection. Eighty-six patients had metastatic carcinoma in their lymph nodes. The three-year survival rate for 47 patients who underwent en bloc esophagectomy was 34%, with a median of 23 months (Fig. 11-3). In the patients with node-positive disease who underwent a limited resection, the corresponding survival figures were 13% and 12.6 months, respectively. It is clear that the more extensive lymphadenectomy offered by the en bloc technique allows better staging, as evidenced by the improved survival rate among patients with node-negative disease treated by en bloc resection compared with similar patients undergoing a more standard resection. Undoubtedly, a significant number of patients treated by a limited resection had their disease understaged. This stage migration has been shown by other investigators.

THREE-FIELD LYMPHADENECTOMY. The surgical strategy of Japanese surgeons has always emphasized the need for a subtotal esophagectomy with resection of the thoracic duct and extensive me-

diastinal and upper abdominal lymphadenectomy (two-field lymphadenectomy). Despite the impressive survival rates reported by Japanese investigators, large follow-up studies indicated that as many as 30% to 40% of patients had recurrences in the cervical nodes.[78] This has prompted a multi-institutional trial between 1983 and 1989, whereby patients with esophageal cancer underwent esophagectomy with three-field lymph node dissection that included the cervical, mediastinal, and abdominal lymph nodes.[79] The results of this study were reported by Isono and coworkers[79] and are summarized as follows:

1. Metastases to the cervical nodes occurred in almost 30% of 1791 patients treated with three-field lymphadenectomy. Although the incidence of nodal metastases was highest when the tumor was located in the upper third of the thoracic esophagus (42%), almost 20% of patients with cancer of the lower third had metastases to the cervical lymph nodes.

2. The frequency of nodal metastases increased with the depth of tumor penetration through the esophageal wall. While none of the patients with intramucosal carcinoma had positive nodes, tumor invasion into the submucosa (T1) signaled a 50% probability of nodal metastases. Patients with T2 or T3 tumors had a 60% to 80% probability of nodal disease.

3. The cervical nodes most frequently involved with metastatic carcinoma included the chain of nodes along the right and left recurrent nerves, as well as the deep cervical nodes along the posterior aspect of the proximal extent of the internal jugular vein. Involvement of the supraclavicular nodes was infrequent and often associated with extensive nodal disease.

4. In the mediastinum, the location of nodal metastases from carcinoma of the thoracic esophagus varied with the location of the tumor. Nonetheless, the most commonly involved nodes were those along the right recurrent nerve, which represented a continuum of nodes into the neck. The left paratracheal, periesophageal, subcarinal, and right paratracheal nodes were involved in approximately 20% of patients.

5. Within the abdomen, nodal metastases were predominantly located along the cardia, the lesser curvature, the left gastric trunk, and the celiac axis—a pattern defined by Akiyama in the early 1980s.[80]

It is clear from these data that a large number of tumors will be inaccurately staged after isolated mediastinal and abdominal lymphadenectomy. Most studies of three-field lymph node dissection have shown a consistent improvement in survival rates beyond those obtained with two-field lymphadenectomy in patients without nodal metastases. Isono and coworkers[79] reported that the survival after two- and three-field lymph node dissection was significantly better in patients without nodal metastases after three-field lymph node dissection (56% versus 45%). This finding suggested the presence of occult cervical nodal metastases in patients who underwent two-field lymphadenectomy. Similarly, Kato reported on 79 patients who underwent transthoracic esophagectomy with mediastinal, abdominal, and bilateral cervical lymphadenectomy with an operative mortality rate of 3.8%.[81] The overall survival rate for 57 patients with positive nodes was 33.6%. Patients with cervical nodal metastases had a 30% five-year survival rate, suggesting that the cervical nodal basin

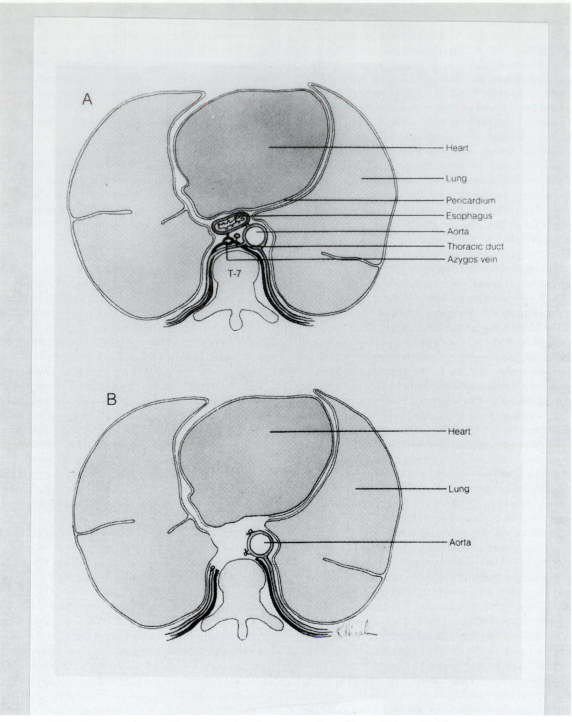

**FIGURE 11-1.** Diagramatic cross-sectional representation of boundaries of enbloc resection. *A*, Anterior view. *B*, Posterior view.

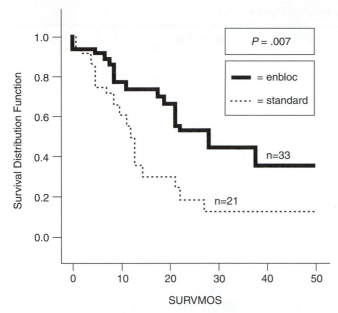

**FIGURE 11-2.** Superior survival advantage for stage III patients treated by enbloc resection compared to standard transthoracic resection.

should be considered a regional (N1) rather than a distant (M1) site of spread. Similar results were reported by Akiyama and coworkers[82] on 538 patients. The 5-year survival rate for patients with positive nodes was 42% after three-field dissection, compared with 28% after

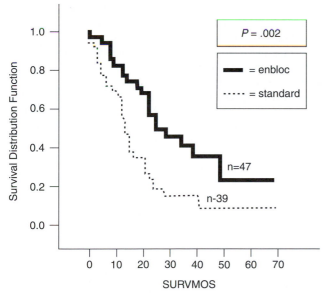

**FIGURE 11-3.** Survival in patients with node-positive disease. Three- and five-year survival rate of 34% after enbloc resection and 13% after standard transthoracic resection.

two-field lymphadenectomy. Despite the excellent survival rates reported for extensive lymph node dissection, the operation carried a significant morbidity rate when performed in centers without extensive experience in esophageal surgery. The principal morbidity was the risk of injury to the recurrent nerves, which occurred in nearly 20% to 50% of patients. The high morbidity rate and the risk of recurrent nerve injury have dissuaded a number of western surgeons from adopting a similar approach. Since 1994, we have embarked on a prospective study evaluating three-field lymph node dissection in patients with invasive cancer of the thoracic esophagus. En bloc resection with three-field dissection was performed in 58 patients with either squamous cell carcinoma or adenocarcinoma. The hospital mortality rate was 5% and morbidity was 45%, not dissimilar to those encountered following two-field lymphadenectomy. Injury to the recurrent nerve occurred in 8% of patients, none of whom required tracheostomy. Among 40 patients with positive nodes, almost half had previously unsuspected nodal metastases to the cervical lymph nodes, particularly those along the right and left recurrent nerves. The actuarial 5-year survival rate for the entire group was 55%. Patients without nodal metastases had an 80% 5-year survival rate, compared to 45% for those with nodal disease. In the subgroup of patients with cervical nodal metastases, the actuarial 5-year survival rate was 25%. Approximately 28% of patients with carcinoma of the lower third of the esophagus had previously unsuspected metastatic carcinoma in the cervical lymph nodes. Metastases to cervical nodes appear to occur independent of cell type or tumor location. These data are in agreement with those from Japan and indicate that a substantial number of patients treated by isolated two-field lymphadenectomy are likely to have residual disease at the conclusion of the operation. Since the ability to perform a complete or R-0 resection seems to be an important determinant of survival, it is likely that the presence of residual disease at the time of the initial surgery would have a detrimental effect on long-term patient outcome.

## RADIATION THERAPY

**DEFINITIVE RADIOTHERAPY.** Many authors have reported results of external beam radiation therapy alone for esophageal carcinoma.[83–85] Most series include patients with unfavorable features, such as clinical T4 lesions, positive lymph nodes, and unresectable disease. The use of radiation therapy as a potentially curative modality requires doses of at least 5000 cGy at 180 to 200 cGy per fraction. Given the large size of many unresectable esophageal cancers, doses of 6000 cGy or greater are probably required. The overall 5-year survival rate of patients with carcinoma of the esophagus treated with radiation therapy alone is approximately 10%.

**PREOPERATIVE RADIOTHERAPY.** Five randomized trials of preoperative radiation therapy for esophageal cancer have been performed (Table 11-4).[86–90] The total dose of preoperative radiation therapy varied from 20 to 35 cGy. Overall there was no difference in the resectability rates between patients who received preoperative radiation therapy and those who underwent primary surgical resection. Local failure rates were reported in two of these studies. The study by Mei et al.[86] showed no significant difference in the

**TABLE 11-4.** RANDOMIZED TRIALS OF PREOPERATIVE RADIOTHERAPY

| AUTHOR | n | RT DOSE (GY) | OP MORT (%) | 5-YR SURVIVAL RATE (%) | p VALUE |
|---|---|---|---|---|---|
| Lanuois (1981)[88] | S 57 | — | 11 | 11.5 | ns |
| | RT 67 | 40 | 14 | 9.5 | |
| Gignoux (1987)[87] | S 114 | — | 19 | 9 | ns |
| | RT 115 | 33 | 24 | 10 | ns |
| Mei (1989)[86] | S 102 | — | 5 | 30 | ns |
| | RT 104 | 40 | 5 | 35 | |
| Nygaard (1992)[90] | S 41 | — | 13 | 9 (3 yr) | ns |
| | RT 48 | 35 | 11 | 21 (3 yr) | ns |

ABBREVIATIONS: ns = not stated, RT = radiation therapy, S = surgery, n = number of patients.

local failure rate; however, that by Gignoux and coworkers[87] reported a statistically significant difference in the locoregional failure rate in favor of preoperative radiotherapy (67% versus 46%). With the exception of one study,[90] none of the remaining five has shown a significant difference in survival favoring preoperative radiation. A recently published analysis updated individual patient data from all properly randomized trials, comprising 1147 patients from five randomized trials.[92] With a median follow-up of 9 years, a hazard ratio of 0.89 suggested an overall reduction in the risk of death by 11% and an absolute survival benefit of 3% at 2 years and 4% at 5 years. These results were not statistically significant. The authors concluded that there is no clear evidence that preoperative radiation improved the survival of patients with potentially resectable cancer.

POSTOPERATIVE RADIOTHERAPY. The rationale for postoperative radiation therapy in clinically resectable esophageal cancer is based on the high incidence of locoregional failure following surgical resection alone. The incidence of local recurrences in the surgical control arms of preoperative radiation therapy randomized trial ranges between 12% and 67%. Therefore, although most patients with cancer of the esophagus die of distant metastases, the incidence of locoregional failure following surgical excision alone in patients with clinically resectable disease is high enough to support the use of adjuvant radiation therapy. However, the only randomized trial that tested that proposition failed to show any benefit for postoperative radiotherapy.[92] In fact, the median survival of patients assigned to receive postoperative radiation was 8.5 months compared to 15 months in the surgery-alone arm. The majority of deaths in the experimental arm were radiation related. It has not been our practice to give patients adjuvant radiation therapy since the local failure rate after radical esophagectomy is 5%.

PREOPERATIVE CHEMOTHERAPY

Several phase II trials have been performed using preoperative chemotherapy followed by a planned operation.[93–95] Most utilized cis-platinum–based combination chemotherapy given in two to four cycles. A major clinical response (complete response + partial response) was observed in approximately 40% to 60% of patients, with a complete pathologic response noted in approximately 5% to 10%. Nearly 70% to 80% of tumors were resectable an preoperative chemotherapy did not seem to adversely affect the operative mortality rate. Some studies suggested that responders, particularly patients with a complete pathologic response, seem to enjoy an improved survival. However, phase III trials of preoperative chemotherapy have been discouraging. Five randomized trials compared preoperative chemotherapy followed by a planned operation with primary surgical resection alone (Table 11-5).[96–100] The largest of these studies was the Intergroup North American Trial, where nearly 440 patients were randomly assigned to receive two cycles of 5-fluorouracil (5-FU) and cis-platinum followed by esophagectomy or primary surgical resection alone.[99] The median survival rate and the 2-year survival rate were similar in both groups. A more recent study randomized patients with squamous cell carcinoma of the esophagus to receive preoperative 5-FU and cis-platinum followed by surgery versus surgery alone.[100] There was no difference in the overall survival rate between the two groups. Patients exhibiting a major objective response to chemotherapy had a significantly better survival rate than the surgical group, while the nonresponders had a significantly worse survival rate at 5 years. Interestingly, a subgroup of patients in the surgery-alone arm, in whom a complete R0 resection was possible, had comparable survival rates to that of the responders. The bulk of the current evidence thus strongly implies that preoperative chemotherapy has no impact on survival in patients with esophageal cancer and should not be advocated except in the context of a controlled clinical trial.

PREOPERATIVE CHEMORADIATION

Most preoperative chemoradiation therapy trials have used cis-platinum or mitomycin C in combination with 5-FU given by continuous infusion. Radiation therapy was given in doses ranging from 20 to 45 cGy, usually given concurrently with chemotherapy. The initial trials with preoperative chemoradiation were conducted by the Southwestern Oncology Group (SWOG) and the Radiation Therapy Oncology Group (RTOG), who jointly conducted a large-scale phase II trial of treatment of epidermoid carcinoma.[101,102] The SWOG trial evaluated the treatment of 106 patients who were

**TABLE 11-5. PREOPERATIVE CHEMOTHERAPY: PHASE III TRIALS**

| AUTHOR | n | CHEMOTHERAPY | OPERATIVE MORTALITY RATE (%) | 5-YR SURVIVAL RATE (%) | MEDIAN SURVIVAL (MO) |
|---|---|---|---|---|---|
| Roth et al (1988)[96] | 36 | CDDP-BL-VDS | S—0 | 5 | 9 |
| | | | CT—12 | 25 | 9 |
| Schlag (1988)[97] | 69 | CDDP-FU | S—12 | ns | 9 |
| | | | CT—21 | ns | 8 |
| Kelsen et al* (1990)[98] | 96 | CDDP-FU | RT + S—13.5 | ns | 12.4 |
| | | | CT + S—11.1 | ns | 10.4 |
| Law et al (1998) | 147 | CDDP-FU | S—8.7 | 31 (2 yr) | 13 |
| | | | CT—8.3 | 44 (2 yr) | 16.8 |
| Kelsen et al (1999) | 440 | CDDP-FU | S—6 | 37 (2 yr) | 16.1 |
| | | | CT—6 | 35 (2 yr) | 14.9 |

ABBREVIATIONS: CDDP = cis-platinum, BL = bleomycin, VDS = vindesine, FU = 5-fluorouracil, ns = not stated.
* Preoperative chemotherapy versus preoperative radiotherapy.

deemed operable at the entry into the study. Following induction chemoradiation, 60% were considered operable and only 49% of the patients underwent resection. The operative mortality rate was 11%. Pathologic complete response rates were seen in 17% of patients, and the median survival time of all patients was only 12 months. The RTOG study of 41 patients had similar results. Naunheim and coworkers[103] reported the results of treatment of 47 patients who received preoperative radiotherapy and concurrent 5-FU and cis-platinum followed by esophagectomy. Thirty-nine patients underwent surgical excision, and the pathologic response rate was 21%. The overall treatment mortality rate was 5%, with a median survival time of 23 months and a 3-year actuarial survival rate of 40%.

Using a different surgical technique, Forastiere and coworkers[104] conducted a study of an intensive 21-day preoperative trial of 5-FU and cis-platinum given by continuous IV infusion in combination with 45 cGy of radiation therapy delivered concurrently.[104] Forty-three patients were entered into the study including both epidermoid carcinoma and adenocarcinoma. The operability rate was 95%, and 91% of the tumors were resectable. An R0 resection was achievable in 84% of patients. There was only one postoperative death. A major response was seen in 42% of patients, and the pathologically complete response rate was 24%. The median survival rate was 29 months, and a 5-year actuarial survival rate was 34%. Because of the encouraging survival results in this and other phase II trials of preoperative chemoradiotherapy, several randomized trials have been conducted evaluating the efficacy of preoperative chemoradiation.[105–108] Four published randomized trials were performed (Table 11-6). Four of these studies showed no significant difference in either median survival rate or 3-year survival rate between the surgery-alone arm and the combined-modality arm. One of the more recent

**TABLE 11-6. PREOPERATIVE CHEMORADIATION: PHASE III TRIALS**

| AUTHOR | n | RT DOSE (GY) | CHEMOTHERAPY | OPERATIVE MORTALITY (%) | COMPLETE PATHOLOGIC RESPONSE (%) | MEDIAN SURVIVAL TIME (YR) | SURVIVAL RATE (%) |
|---|---|---|---|---|---|---|---|
| LePrise et al (1994)[107] | 86 | 20 (Seq) | CDDP-FU | S—7 | ns | ns | 42 (1 yr) |
| | | | | CTRT—8.5 | ns | ns | 42 (1 yr) |
| Urba et al (1997)[108] | 100 | 45 (Con) | CDDP-BL-VBL | S—ns | ns | ns | 33 (3 yr) |
| | | | | CTRT—ns | ns | ns | 18 (3 yr) |
| Walsh et al (1996)[106] | 113 | 40 (Con) | CDDP-FU | S—3.6 | — | 11 | 32 (3 yr) |
| | | | | CTRT—8.6 | 25% | 6 | 6 (3 yr) |
| Bosset et al (1997)[105] | 297 | 18.5 (Seq) | CDDP | S—3.6 | — | 18.6 | 38 (3 yr) |
| | | | | CTRT—12.3 | 26% | 18.6 | 38 (3 yr) |

ABBREVIATIONS: CDDP = cis-platinum, FU = 5-fluorouracil, ET = etoposide, BL = bleomycin, VBL = vinblastine, Con = concurrent, Seq = sequential, ns: not stated, CTRT = chemotherapy radiotherapy.

studies compared multimodality therapy and surgery for esophageal adenocarcinoma.[106] Fifty-eight patients were assigned to a multimodality therapy that included two cycles of cis-platinum and 5-FU given concurrently with 40 cGy of radiotherapy prior to planned resection. Of the 58 patients assigned to preoperative chemoradiation, 48 underwent esophagectomy for an operability rate of 87%. At the time of surgery, 42% of the patients treated with preoperative multimodality therapy had positive nodal metastases as compared to 82% of patients who underwent surgery alone. A complete response was noted in 25% of patients in the preoperative chemoradiation group. The median survival time of patients assigned to multimodality therapy was 16 months, compared to 11 months in those assigned to the surgery-alone arm. The 3-year survival rate was significantly better at 32% in the preoperative chemoradiation arm compared to only 6% in the surgery-alone arm. Interestingly, using the same regimen in patients with squamous cell carcinoma of the esophagus, the same group was unable to demonstrate a survival advantage of preoperative chemoradiation. Despite several criticisms of this study, it remains the only study that has shown a significant survival advantage in patients receiving chemoradiation prior to esophagectomy. At the present time, a nationwide intergroup trial is in progress using the same preoperative regimen in an attempt to reproduce the results obtained by the latter study using a larger number of patients. As is the case with preoperative chemotherapy, preoperative chemoradiation should still be considered an investigational approach and should only be performed within the context of controlled clinical trials.

## PRIMARY CHEMORADIATION

Radiation therapy with concurrent chemotherapy as definitive nonoperative therapy has been the subject of many single-arm trials. Coia and coworkers[109] reviewed the experience over a 10-year period in 57 patients treated with continuous infusion of 5-FU and mitomycin given for two cycles concurrently with high-dose radiation therapy. The median survival time was 18 months, and 18% of the patients survived 5 years. Eventually, local failure occurred in 48% of patients, and 72% had some component of distant failure.

An important phase III random assignment trial evaluated 120 patients assigned to receive either radiation therapy alone or radiation with concurrent 5-FU and platinum.[58] Systemic side effects, which consisted of nausea, vomiting, and myelosuppression, occurred more frequently in the combined arm, while local side effects were similar in both groups. With a minimum follow-up time of 5 years for all patients, the median survival time was 14 months and the 5-year survival rate was 27% in the combined modality group, while the median survival time was 9.3 months with no patients alive at 5 years in the radiation therapy–alone group.[58] An additional 69 patients were treated with the same combination therapy regimen. The results of the last group confirmed all of the results of combined chemoradiation therapy in the randomized trial with median survival duration of 17 months and a 3-year survival rate of 30%.[110] This RTOG study strongly indicates that concurrent chemotherapy and radiation therapy is superior to radiation therapy alone for the treatment of locally advanced esophageal carcinoma.

## REFERENCES

1. WATERHOUSE J et al: Cancer incidence in five continents. International Agency for Research on Cancer, vol 4, Lyon 42:1, 1982.
2. OFFICE OF RESEARCH ON CANCER PREVENTION AND TREATMENT OF THE MINISTRY OF HEALTH: Atlas of Cancer Mortality of the Peoples' Republic of China. Ministry of Health, China, Beijing, China, 1980.
3. STEPHEN SJ, URAGODA CG: Some observations on oesophageal cancer in Ceylon, including its relation to betel chewing. Br J Cancer 24:11, 1970.
4. JUSSAWALLA DJ: Esophageal cancer in India. J Cancer Res Clin Oncol 99:29, 1981.
5. DEJONG UW et al: Aetiological factors in oesophageal cancer in Singapore Chinese. Int J Cancer 13:291, 1974.
6. ROSE EF, MCGLASHAN ND: The spatial distribution of oesophageal cancer in Transkei, South Africa. Br J Cancer 31:197, 1979.
7. TUYNS AJ, MASSE G: Cancer of the esophagus: An incidence study in Ille-et-Vilaine. Int J Epidemiol 4:55, 1975.
8. BLOT WJ, FRAUMENI JF: Geographic epidemiology of cancer in the United States, in Cancer Epidemiology and Prevention, D Schotterfeld, J Fraumeni (eds). Saunders, Philadelphia, 1982, p 179.
9. FRAUMENI JF, BLOT WJ: Geographic variation in esophageal cancer mortality in the United States. J Chron Dis 30:759, 1977.
10. BLOT WJ, FRAUMENI JF JR: Trends in esophageal cancer mortality among US blacks and whites. Am J Public Health 77:296, 1987.
11. ——— et al: Rising incidence of adencocarcinoma of the esophagus and gastric cardia. JAMA 265(10):1287, 1991.
12. CAMERON AJ et al: Prevalence of columnar-lined (Barrett's) esophagus. Gastroenterol 99:918, 1990.
13. HAMILTON S et al: Prevalence and characteristics of Barrett's esophagus in patients with adenocarcinoma of the esophagus or the esophagogastric junction. Human Pathol 19:942, 1988.
14. KALISH RJ et al: Clinical, epidemiological and morphologic comparison between adenocarcinomas arising in Barrett's esophageal mucosa and in the gastric cardia. Gastroenterol 86:461, 1984.
15. BLOT WJ et al: Continuing climb in rates of esophageal adenocarcinoma: An update. JAMA 270:1320, 1993(lett).
16. BARTSCH J, MONTESANO R: Relevance of nitrosamines to human cancer. Carcinogenesis 5:1381, 1984.
17. HAMMOND EC: Smoking in relation to death rates of one million men and women. Natl Cancer Inst Monogr 19:127, 1966.
18. ROGOT E, MURRAY JL: Smoking and causes of death among U.S. veterans: 16 years of observation. Public Health Rep 95:213, 1980.
19. DE STEFANI E et al: Mate drinking, alcohol, tobacco, diet, and esophageal cancer in Uruguay. Cancer Res 50:426, 1990.
20. YANG J et al: Preliminary studies on the etiology and conditions of carcinogenesis of the esophagus in Linxian, Experimental Research on Esophageal Cancer, J Yang, J Gao (eds). Renmin Weisheng Publishers, Beijing, China, 1980, p 82.
21. DEPARTMENT OF CHEMICAL ETIOLOGY OF CICAMS AND LRTPTEC: Preliminary investigation on the carcinogenicity of extracts of pickles in Linxian. Res Cancer Prev Treatment 2:46, 1977.
22. LU SH et al: Unrinary excretion of N-nitrosamino acids and nitrate by high and low esophageal risk populations in

northern China: Endogenous formation of *N*-nitrosproline and its inhibition by vitamin C. Cancer Res 46:1485, 1986.

23. MIMIC Y et al: Tobacco, alcohol, diet, occupation and cancer of the esophagus. Cancer Res 48:3843, 1988.

24. WYNDER EL, BROSS IJ: A study of etiological factors in cancer of the esophagus. Cancer 14:389, 1961.

25. POTTERN LM et al: Esophageal cancer among black men in Washington DC. I. Alcohol, tobacco and other risk factors. JNCI 67:777, 1981.

26. TUYNS AJ et al: Le cancer de l'oesophage en Ille-et-Vilaine en fonction des niveaux de consommation d'alcool et de tabac: des risques qui se multiplient. Bull Cancer 64:63, 1977.

27. HILLE JJ et al: Human papillomavirus and carcinoma of the esophagus. N Engl J Med 312:1707, 1985 (lett).

28. RABINOVITCH PS et al: Progression to cancer in Barrett's esophagus is associated with genomic instability. Lab Invest 60:65, 1988.

29. DEMEESTER TR et al: Surgical therapy in Barrett's esophagus. Ann Surg 212:528, 1990.

30. VAEZI MF, RICHTER JE: Bile reflux in columnar-lined esophagus. Gastroenterol Clin North Am 26:565, 1997.

31. ZHANG F et al: Dihydroxy bile acids activate the transcription of cyclooxygenase-2. J Biol Chem 273:2424, 1998.

32. IRELAND AP et al: Gastric juice protects against the development of esophageal adenocarcinoma in the rat. Ann Surg 224:358, 1996.

33. GOLDSTEIN SR et al: Development of esophageal metaplasia and adenocarcinoma in a rat surgical model without the use of a carcinogen. Carcinogenesis 18:2265, 1997.

34. MORSON BC, BELCHER JR: Adenocarcinoma of the oesophagus and ectopic gastric mucosa. Br J Cancer 6:127, 1953.

35. LERUT T et al: Surgical treatment of Barrett's carcinoma: Correlations between morphologic findings and prognosis. J Thorac Cardiovasc Surg 107:1059, 1994.

36. PETERS JH et al: Outcome of adenocaricnoma arising in Barrett's esophagus in endoscopically surveyed and nonsurveyed patients. J Thorac Cardiovasc Surg 108:813, 1994.

37. STREITZ JM et al: Endoscopic surveillance of Barrett's esophagus: A cost effectiveness comparison and mammographic surveillance for breast cancer. Am J Gastroenterol 93:911, 1998.

38. FAGGE CH: A case of simple stenosis of the oesophagus followed by epithelioma. Guy's Hosp Rep 17:413, 1872.

39. CHUONG JJ et al: Achalasia as a risk factor for esophageal carcinoma: A reappraisal. Dig Dis Sci 29:1105, 1984.

40. AGGESTRUP S et al: Does achalasia predispose to cancer of the esophagus? Chest 102:1013, 1992.

41. MEIJSSEN MAC et al: Achalasia complicated by oesophageal squamous cell carcinoma: A prospective study in 195 patients. Gut 33:155, 1992.

42. CHANG-CLAUDE JC et al: An epidemiological study of precursor lesions of esophageal cancer among young persons in a high-risk population in Huixian, China. Cancer Res 50:2268, 1990.

43. JACOB JH et al: Prevalence survey of precancerous lesions of the oesophagus in a high-risk population for oesophageal cancer in France. Eur J Cancer Prev (England) 2:53, 1993.

44. CASTELLETTO R et al: Pre-cancerous lesions of the oesophagus in Argentina: Prevalence and association with tobacco and alcohol. Int J Cancer 51:34, 1992.

45. HOWELL-EVANS W et al: Carcinoma of the oesophagus with keratosis palmaris et plantaris (tylosis): A study of two families. Q J Med 27:413, 1958.

46. VINSON PP: Hysterical dysphagia. Minn Med 5:107, 1992.

47. CSIKOS M et al: Late malignant transformation of chronic corrosive oesophageal strictures. Langenbeck's Arch Chir 365:231, 1985.

48. IMRE J, KOPP M: Argument against long-term conservative treatment of oesophageal strictures due to corrosive burns. Thorax 27:594, 1972.

49. KORST RJ et al: Proposed revision of the staging classification for esophageal cancer. J Thorac Cardiovasc Surg 115:660, 1998.

50. LIEBERMAN MD et al: Carcinoma of the esophagus. Prognostic significance of histologic type. J Thorac Cardiovasc Surg 109:130, 1995.

51. MATSUBARA T et al: How extensive should lymph node dissection be for cancer of the thoracic esophagus? J Thorac Cardiovasc Surg 107:1073, 1994.

52. KATO H et al: Evalution of the new (1987) TNM classification for thoracic esophageal tumors. Int J Cancer 53:220, 1993.

53. LIGHTDATE CJ: Staging of esophageal cancer. I. Endoscopic ultrasonography. Semin Oncol 21:438, 1994.

54. CHANDAWARKAR RY et al: Endosonography for preoperative staging of specific nodal groups associated with esophageal cancer. World J Surg 20:700, 1996.

55. ALTORKI NK et al: Endosonography for cancer of the esophagus and cardia: Is it worthwhile? Dis Esophagus 9:1998, 1996.

56. RIEDEL M et al: Preoperative bronchoscopic assessment of airway invasion by esophageal cancer: A prospective study. Chest 113:687, 1998.

57. KRASNA MJ et al: Combined thoracoscopic/laparoscopic lymph node staging for lung and esophageal cancer. Oncology 793, 1996.

58. HERSKOVIC A et al: Combined chemotherapy and radiotherapy compared with radiotherapy alone in patients with cancer of the esophagus. N Engl J Med 326:1593, 1992.

59. LEWIS I: The surgical treatment of carcinoma of the oesophagus with special reference to a new operation for growths in the middle third. Br J Surg 34:18, 1946.

60. MCKEOWN KC: Total three-stage oesophagectomy for cancer of the oesophagus. Br J Surg 63:259, 1976.

61. SWEET RH: Surgical management of carcinoma of the mid thoracic esophagus. N Engl J Med 233:1, 1945.

62. DENK W: Zur Radikaloperation des oesophaguskarzinoms (Vorlaufige Mitteilung). Zentralbl f Chir 40:1065, 1913.

63. ORRINGER MB, SLOAN H: Esophagectomy without thoracotomy. J Thorac Cardiovasc Surg 76:643, 1978.

64. ORRINGER MB et al: Transhiatal esophagectomy for benign and malignant disease. J Thorac Cardiovasc Surg 105:265, 1993.

65. GELFAND GA et al: Transhiatal esosphagectomy for carcinoma of the esophagus and cardia: Experience with 160 cases. Arch Surg 127:1164, 1992.

66. GERTSCH P et al: Long-term results of transhiatal esophagectomy for esophageal carcinoma: A multivariate analysis of prognostic factors. Cancer 72:2312, 1993.

67. VIGNESWARAN WT et al: Transhiatal esophagectomy for carcinoma of the esophagus. Ann Thorac Surg 56:838, 1993.

68. NAGAWA H et al: The relationship of macroscopic shape of superficial esophageal carcinoma to depth of invasion and regional lymph node metastasis. Cancer 75:1061, 1995.

69. SABIK JF et al: Superficial esophageal carcinoma. Ann Thorac Surg 60:896, 1995.

70. HOLSCHER AH et al: Early adenocarcinoma in Barrett's oesphagus. 84:1470, 1997.

71. KORST RJ, ALTORKI NK: Extent of resection of lymphadenectomy in early Barrett's cancer. Dis Esophagus 10:172, 1997.

72. CHU KM et al: A prospective randomized comparison of transhiatal and transthoracic resection for lower-third esophageal carcinoma. Am J Surg 174:320, 1997.

73. HORSTMAN O et al: Transhiatal oesophagectomy compared with transthoracic resection and systematic lymphadenectomy for the treatment of oesophageal cancer. Eur J Surg 161:557, 1995.

74. GOLDMINC M et al: Oesophagectomy by a transhiatal approach or thoracotomy: A prospective randomized trial. Br J Surg 80:367, 1993.

75. LOGAN A: The surgical treatment of carcinoma of the esophagus and cardia. J Thorac Cardiovasc Surg 46:150, 1963.

76. SKINNER DB: En-bloc resection for neoplasms of the esophagus and cardia. J Thorac Cardiovasc Surg 85:59, 1983.

77. ALTORKI NK et al: En bloc esophagectomy improves survival for stage III esophageal cancer. J Thorac Cardiovasc Surg 114:948, 1997.

78. ISONO K et al: Recurrence of intrathoracic esophageal cancer. Jpn J Clin Oncol 15:49, 1985.

79. ISONO K et al: Results of nationwide study on the three-field lymph node dissection of esophageal cancer. Oncology 48:411, 1991.

80. AKIYAMA H: Surgery for cancer of the esophagus. Curr Probl Surg 17:53, 1980.

81. KATO H et al: Lymph node metastasis in thoracic esophageal carcinoma. J Surg Oncol 48:106, 1991.

82. AKIYAMA H et al: Systematic lymph node dissection for esophageal cancer—effective or not? Dis Esophagus 7:1, 1994.

83. DE-REN S: Ten-year follow-up of esophageal cancer treated by radical radiation therapy: Analysis of 869 patients. Int J Radiation Oncol Biol Phys 16:329, 1989.

84. NEWAISHY GA et al: Results of radical radiotherapy of squamous cell carcinoma of the esophagus. Clin Radiol 33:347, 1982.

85. OKAWA T et al: Results of radiotherapy for inoperable locally advanced esophageal cancer. Int J Radiat Oncol Biol Phys 17:49, 1989.

86. MEI W et al: Randomized clinical trial on the combination of preoperative irradiation and surgery in the treatment of esophageal carcinoma: Report on 206 patients. Int J Radiat Oncol Biol Phys 16:325, 1989.

87. GIGNOUX M et al: The value of preoperative radiotherapy in esophageal cancer: Results of a study of the E.O.R.T.C. World J Surg 11:426, 1987.

88. LAUNOIS B et al: Preoperative radiotherapy for carcinoma of the esophagus. Surg Gynecol Obstet 153:690, 1981.

89. ARNOTT SJ et al: Low dose preoperative radiotherapy for carcinoma of the oesophagus: Results of a randomized clinical trial. Radiother Oncol 24:108, 1993.

90. NYGAARD K et al: Pre-operative radiotherapy prolongs survival in operable esophageal carcinoma: A randomized, multicenter study of pre-operative radiotherapy and chemotherapy. The second Scandinavian trial in esophageal cancer. World J Surg 16:1104, 1992.

91. ARNOTT SJ et al: Preoperative radiotherapy in esophageal carcinoma: A meta-analysis using individual patient data (Oesophageal Cancer Collaborative Group). Int J Radiat Oncol Biol Phys 41:579, 1998.

92. FOK M et al: Postoperative radiotherapy for carcinoma of the esophagus: A prospective, randomized controlled study. Surgery 113:138, 1993.

93. SCHLAG P et al: Preoperative chemotherapy in esophageal cancer: A phase II study. Acta Oncol 27:811, 1988.

94. AJANI JA et al: Intensive preoperative chemotherapy with colony-stimulating factor for resectable adenocarcinoma of the esophagus or gastroesophageal junction. J Clin Oncol 11:22, 1993.

95. ILSON DH et al: Neoadjuvant therapy of esophageal cancer. Surg Oncol Clin North Am 6:723, 1997.

96. ROTH JA et al: Randomized clinical trials of preoperative and postoperative adjuvant chemotherapy and cisplatin, vindesine, and bleomycin for carcinoma of the esophagus. J Thorac Cardiovasc Surg 96:242, 1988.

97. SCHLAG P: Randomisierte Studie zur praoperativen chemotherapy beim plattenepithelcarcinom des oesphagus. Chirurg 63:709, 1992.

98. KELSEN DP et al: Preoperative therapy for esophageal cancer: A randomized comparison of chemotherapy versus radiation therapy. J Clin Oncol 8:1352, 1990.

99. KELSEN DP et al: Chemotherapy followed by operation versus operation alone in the treatment of patients with localized esophageal cancer: A preliminary report of intergroup study 113 (RTOG 89-11) (abstract). Meeting of the American Society of Clinical Oncology (ASCO), Denver, 1997.

100. LAW S et al: Preoperative chemotherapy versus surgical therapy alone for squamous cell carcinoma of the esophagus: A prospective randomized trial. J Thorac Cardiovasc Surg 114:203, 1997.

101. POPLIN E et al: Combined therapies for squamous cell carcinoma of the esophagus: A Southwest Oncology Group Study (SWOG-8037). J Clin Oncol 5:622, 1987.

102. SEYDEL HG et al: Preoperative radiation and chemotherapy for localized squamous cell carcinoma of the esophagus: A RTOG study. Int J Radiat Oncol Biol Phys 14:33, 1988.

103. NAUNHEIM KS et al: Preoperative chemotherapy and radiotherapy for esophageal carcinoma. J Thorac Cardiovasc Surg 5:887, 1992.

104. FORASTIERE AA et al: Preoperative chemoradiation followed by transhiatal esophagectomy for caricnoma of the esophagus: Final report. J Clin Oncol 11:1118, 1993.

105. BOSSET JF et al. Randomized phase III clinical trials comparing surgery alone versus pre-operative combined radiochemotherapy (XRT-CT) in stage I–II epidermoid cancer of the esophagus. Preliminary analysis: A study of the FFCD (French group) no. 8805 and EORTC no. 40881. Proc Am Soc Clin Oncol 13:197, 1994.

106. WALSH TN et al: A comparison of multimodal therapy and surgery for esophageal adenocarcinoma. N Engl J Med 35:462, 1996.

107. LE PRISE E et al: A randomized study of chemotherapy, radiation therapy, and surgery versus surgery for localized squamous cell carcinoma of the esophagus. Cancer 73:1779, 1994.

108. URBA S et al: A randomized trial comparing surgery to preoperative concomitant chemoradiation plus surgery in patients with resectable esophageal cancer: Update analysis. Proc Am Soc Clin Oncol 6:227, 1997.

109. COIA LR et al: Long-term results of infusional 5-FU, mitomycin-C and radiation as primary management of esophageal carcinoma. Int J Radiat Oncol Biol Phys 20:29, 1992.

110. AL-SARRAF M et al: Progress report of combined chemoradiotherapy alone in patients with esophageal cancer: An intergroup study. J Clin Oncol 5:277, 1997.

# CHAPTER 12

# NEOPLASMS OF THE STOMACH

*D. Scott Lind and Stephen B. Vogel*

## INTRODUCTION

looseness1A variety of benign and malignant neoplasms are found in the stomach. The widespread use of endoscopy has increased the detection of gastric neoplasms. Leiomyoma is the most common benign gastric tumor, and adenocarcinoma is the most common gastric malignancy.[1] Although the incidence of gastric adenocarcinoma has decreased substantially in the United States, it remains a significant problem worldwide.[2] Surgery is the primary treatment for most gastric neoplasms. Although novel chemotherapy regimens have produced significant response rates for patients with advanced gastric adenocarcinoma, the results of well-designed clinical trials are required before adjuvant chemotherapy can be incorporated into standard clinical practice. Knowledge of the molecular biology of gastric cancer is still in its infancy, but future molecular-based diagnostic and therapeutic approaches may provide some optimism in the management of this challenging malignancy.

## POLYPS

Gastric polyps are relatively rare compared to colonic polyps. Although gastric polyps may be the source of gastrointestinal blood loss, most polyps are discovered incidentally by endoscopy or by radiologic evaluation of the stomach. Gastric polyps are classified histologically as hyperplastic, inflammatory, or adenomatous. Hyperplastic gastric polyps account for 75% of all gastric polyps. Hyperplastic polyps are not true neoplasms but represent a regenerative response to injury and, therefore, they have low malignant potential.[3]

Inflammatory polyps are usually located in the antrum and they consist histologically of a fibroblast matrix with inflammatory infiltrate. Inflammatory polyps have little or no malignant potential.

Adenomatous polyps are true neoplasms with a distinct malignant potential. Like their colonic counterparts, adenomatous polyps are classified histologically as tubular, villous, or tubulovillous. Pure villous adenomas of the stomach are very uncommon. The incidence of malignancy in an adenomatous gastric polyp is proportional to size, with polyps larger than 2 cm having a greater malignant potential.[3] Adenomatous gastric polyps may be associated with the polyposis syndromes such as familial adenomatous polyposis, Gardner's syndrome, and Peutz-Jegher's syndrome. Complete endoscopic polypectomy is the treatment of choice for most adenomatous gastric polyps; however, large polyps and multiple polyps may require gastric resection.

## ADENOCARCINOMA

More than 90% of gastric malignancies are adenocarcinomas. In this country, gastric adenocarcinoma has traditionally been considered a highly lethal malignancy with little chance for cure. The consistently poor 5-year survival rate for gastric cancer during the past 25 years has fueled this pessimism. The delay in diagnosis of gastric adenocarcinoma in this country has resulted in an overall 5-year survival rate of 10% to 15%.[4] On the other hand, the incidence and age-adjusted death rate of gastric cancer in the United States have decreased substantially in the last 60 years. In 1930, there were approximately 30 gastric cancer deaths per 100,000 in this country, whereas in 1990 this rate decreased to 6 and 3 per 100,000 for males and females, respectively. This rate compares favorably with the 65 to 70 gastric cancer deaths per 100,000 in Japan, Chile, and Costa Rica. In contrast to the poor survival statistics in the United States, the 5-year survival rate for gastric cancer in Japan is greater than 50%. The improved survival rate is primarily the result of earlier detection, with approximately 40% to 50% of all gastric cancers diagnosed as early gastric cancer (i.e., tumor confined to mucosa and/or submucosa), with a 5-year survival rate of greater than 80%.[5]

## RISK FACTORS

The factors responsible for the dramatic decline in the incidence of gastric cancer in this country have not been defined. The fact that the incidence of gastric cancer in Japanese immigrants decreases with successive generations that remain in the United States suggests that environmental factors be involved. Whether improvements in nutrition or changes in socioeconomic and occupational conditions have contributed to the declining incidence of this disease remain speculative.

A number of factors are associated with an increased risk for the development of gastric adenocarcinoma. Adenomatous gastric polyps may be considered premalignant and they should be completely removed. Patients with a history of gastric polyps should also undergo periodic radiologic or endoscopic surveillance.

Patients with chronic atrophic gastritis, pernicious anemia, and patients who have undergone a prior gastric resection (15 to 20 years previously) may be at increased risk for gastric adenocarcinoma. Some investigators have proposed a pathway from injury to chronic atrophic gastritis with intestinal metaplasia as a maladaptive response, progressing to dysplasia, and finally invasive carcinoma.[6] Although the precise risk of gastric cancer is not well defined, patients with pernicious anemia are definitely at increased risk and may benefit from periodic endoscopic surveillance. Whether the frequency of carcinoma is increased in the gastric remnant following gastric resection for benign disease remains controversial. Therefore, routine endoscopic screening of postgastrectomy patients is probably unwarranted. Nevertheless the presence of symptoms referable to the upper gastrointestinal tract warrants immediate evaluation in this group of patients. Endosocopic screening of the general population is not cost-effective because of the declining incidence of gastric cancer in the United States.

The frequency with which cancer arises in a benign gastric ulcer is probably less than 1%.[7] Nevertheless, the presence of a nonhealing gastric ulcer should raise the suspicion of malignancy. The old adage, "cancers frequently ulcerate but ulcers never cancerate," holds true. In other words, a nonhealing gastric ulcer was probably malignant from the outset.

The gram-negative microaerophilic spiral bacterium, *Helicobacter pylori*, is involved in the pathogenesis of peptic ulcer disease. The prevalence of this organism in patients with chronic atrophic gastritis and gastric adenocarcinoma suggests an association between *H. pylori* and gastric adenocarcinoma, but a causal relationship has not been established.[8] Potential oncogenic mechanisms of action for *H. pylori* are speculative. It is unlikely, however, that the bacterium is a direct carcinogen but rather acts as a promoter in the complex process of gastric carcinogenesis. Further studies are needed to determine if antibiotic treatment of *H. pylori* reduces the subsequent incidence of gastric adenocarcinoma.

In the absence of specific recommendations for screening high-risk groups, clinicians should make individual assessments of high-risk patients to determine the need for endoscopic or radiologic investigation. The lack of tumor markers specific for gastric cancer makes it unlikely that clinicians in this country will be able to diagnose gastric cancer at an earlier stage, particularly in an era of cost containment and managed competition.

## PATHOLOGIC FINDINGS AND STAGING

Gastric adenocarcinoma is most commonly located on the lesser curve of the distal stomach. It appears, however, that the incidence of proximal gastric cancer is increasing, particularly in young white males.[9] Numerous pathologic classification systems have been described for gastric cancer. The Borrmann classification is based on gross morphology and includes type I (polypoid lesion with no ulceration), type II (fungating, ulcerating lesion with distinct borders), type III (ulcerating lesion with indistinct borders), and type IV (diffuse infiltrating lesion). Type IV corresponds to the appearance of *linitis plastica,* producing a rigid, nondistensible gastric wall. Broder's classification system categorizes gastric cancer according to the degree of differentiation (i.e., grade 1 is most differentiated, grade 4 is least differentiated). The histopathologic classification of Lauren describes two types of gastric malignancy: diffuse and intestinal (Table 12-1). The Lauren histopathologic classification has epidemiologic and prognostic significance. The intestinal type is more prevalent in the high-risk regions of the world and has a better prognosis, whereas the diffuse type is more common in geographic areas with a low incidence of gastric cancer and has a poorer prognosis. In the United States, approximately 50% of all gastric cancers are of the diffuse type, 40% are of the intestinal type, and 10% have a mixed histologic pattern.[10]

Although the staging of gastric cancer has undergone numerous modifications, currently the preferred staging method is the American Joint Commission on Cancer tumor-node-metastasis (TNM) system (Tables 12-2A and 12-2B). Recently, the TNM staging

### TABLE 12-1. HISTOLOGIC CLASSIFICATION OF GASTRIC CARCINOMAS

|  | INTESTINAL | DIFFUSE |
|---|---|---|
| Epidemiology | Environmental association more likely | Genetic association more likely, e.g., blood group A or familial |
| Age | Older patients | Young and middle-aged patients |
| Site | Antrum and cardia | Body |
| Gross features | Circumscribed | Diffuse, linitis plastica |
| Cell type | Well-differentiated, intestinal (glandular) type | Poorly differentiated, polygonal or signet-ring type |
| Precancerous states | Pernicious anemia, atrophic gastritis, intestinal metaplasia, dysplasia | None |
| Prognosis | Better | Poorer |

**TABLE 12-2A.** TUMOR-NODE-METASTASIS STAGING OF GASTRIC CANCER

| T | PRIMARY TUMOR |
|---|---|
| T1 | Tumor limited to mucosa or submucosa regardless of extent or location |
| T2 | Tumor extends to the serosa |
| T3 | Tumor penetrates serosa |
| T4 | Tumor involves contiguous structures |

| N | LYMPH NODE INVOLVEMENT |
|---|---|
| N0 | No metastases in regional lymph nodes |
| N1 | Metastases in 1–6 regional lymph nodes |
| N2 | Metastases in 7–15 regional lymph nodes |
| N3 | Metastases in >15 regional lymph nodes |

| M | DISTANT METASTASIS |
|---|---|
| M0 | No distant metastases |
| M1 | Distant metastases |

| R | SURGICAL RESULTS |
|---|---|
| R0 | No residual tumor |
| R1 | Microscopic residual tumor |
| R2 | Macroscopic residual tumor |

**TABLE 12-2B.** STAGE GROUPING OF CARCINOMA OF THE STOMACH

|  | | | |
|---|---|---|---|
| Stage 0 | Tis | N0 | M0 |
| Stage IA | T1 | N0 | M0 |
| Stage IB | T1 | N1 | M0 |
| | T2 | N0 | M0 |
| Stage II | T1 | N2 | M0 |
| | T2 | N1 | M0 |
| | T3 | N0 | M0 |
| Stage IIIA | T2 | N2 | M0 |
| | T3 | N1 | M0 |
| | T4 | N0 | M0 |
| Stage IIIB | T3 | N2 | M0 |
| | T4 | N1 | M0 |
| Stage IV | T4 | N2 | M0 |
| | Any T | Any N | M1 |

SOURCE: From American Joint Committee on Cancer. *Manual for Staging*, 5th ed, 1997.

system was revised to reflect the importance of the number of lymph nodes that contain metastases.[11] The ratio of involved to examined nodes may be of even more importance than the absolute number of involved lymph nodes. For example, 1 positive lymph node out of a total of 5 lymph nodes removed may not carry the same prognosis as a single positive lymph node out of 25 lymph nodes removed. Various modifications have also occurred in the stage grouping of gastric cancer. Table 12-2B describes a practical approach in which all T1 lesions without nodal involvement or distant metastases are considered stage I. Stage II includes all T2 and T3 lesions without nodal involvement or metastases, and stage III lesions involve all T1 to T3 lesions with N1 or N2 involvement. Modifications of this system have subdivided stage I into IA, involving T1 lesions without nodal involvement, and IB, including T1 lesions with N1 nodal involvement or T2 lesions without either nodal involvement or distal metastases.

Unfortunately, most gastric cancers in the United States are diagnosed at an advanced stage. Overall 5-year survival rates in the United States for patients whose cancer is resected for "potential cure" range from 20% to 35%. Patients in western countries with T1 and T2 lesions have survival rates ranging from 30% to 75%, respectively, compared with Japanese patients with similar lesions, whose survival rates range from 70% to 98%. The differences in survival statistics between the two countries appear to be multifactorial but may be the result of stage migration due to the more extensive node dissections and the more intensive pathologic assessment of gastric cancer performed in Japan. The term *early gastric cancer* has been used by Japanese clinicians to describe gastric malignancies involving only the mucosa and/or submucosa. Overall 5-year survival rates of 90% to 97% and 80% to 95% have been documented for lesions involving the mucosa and submucosa, respectively. In Japan, early gastric cancer represents up to 40% of all gastric cancer in contrast to the United States, where early gastric cancer only accounts for approximately 10% to 15% of all gastric cancer. Early gastric cancer may represent a distinct pathologic entity that remains confined to the mucosa or submucosa for a prolonged time period prior to penetration through the gastric wall.

## MOLECULAR BIOLOGY

Understanding the molecular basis of gastric cancer is essential to developing more effective methods of primary prevention, secondary prevention (early diagnosis), and treatment. Although the molecular mechanisms involved in gastric carcinogenesis have not been completely delineated, some important advances in the molecular biology of gastric cancer have been made.[12] Several abnormalities in oncogenes, tumor suppressor genes, and growth factor expression have been identified in gastric cancer. p53 is a tumor suppressor gene located on the short arm of chromosome 17 that plays a key role in regulating the cell cycle. Advanced gastric cancers have a higher rate of p53 mutations than early gastric cancers, suggesting a role for p53 expression in prognosis. Overexpression of the *ras* protein, p21, has also been identified in gastric cancer. In addition, the *bcl*-2 protooncogene that plays a critical role in programmed cell death (apoptosis) is also associated with gastric cancer. Furthermore, abnormalities of several growth factors and growth factor receptors have been detected in gastric cancer patients, including fibroblast growth factor, transforming growth factor, and epidermal growth factor receptor (EGFR). EGFR overexpression is associated with aneuploidy, a high proliferation rate, and lymph node metastases in gastric cancer. Certainly, our understanding of the molecular biology of gastric cancer is in its infancy and future research efforts will translate into clinical advances.

## DIAGNOSIS

The initial symptoms of gastric cancer tend to be vague and non-specific, such as early satiety, dyspepsia, and heartburn. Since these symptoms are common in the general population and they are frequently treated with over-the-counter medications, clinicians sometimes fail to pursue radiologic or endoscopic evaluation of these symptoms. Patients with more advanced gastric cancer often present with anorexia, weight loss, and epigastric discomfort. In addition, dysphagia may be the first marked symptom of gastric carcinoma involving the cardia.

A barium-contrast upper gastrointestinal series has been the standard test for the radiologic diagnosis of gastric cancer. Accuracy rates of 80% to 90% for contrast studies reflect the high incidence of advanced lesions at presentation in this country. Small nonulcerating mucosal lesions may be missed by contrast studies. Most patients with persistent upper gastrointestinal symptoms now undergo upper gastrointestinal endoscopy. The combination of endoscopy and multiple biopsies yields accuracy rates up to 95% in the diagnosis of gastric cancer. Contrast studies can also complement endoscopy and may be useful as a roadmap for surgeons who don't perform endoscopy. Endoscopic ultrasonography accurately predicts the depth of invasion of a cancer through the layers of the stomach wall. Although endoscopic ultrasonography can image adjacent organs and lymph nodes, it cannot reliably distinguish between lymph nodes that are enlarged due to inflammation versus those lymph nodes that are enlarged secondary to metastatic tumor. Furthermore, small lymph nodes may also contain metastatic tumor.[13]

Almost all patients with gastric cancer undergo computed tomography (CT) scan. CT accurately identifies lymph nodes greater than 1.0 cm in diameter, liver lesions greater than 1.0 to 2.0 cm, and involvement of adjacent organs.[14] Laparoscopy may be superior to CT in identifying peritoneal carcinomatosis or surface hepatic metastases less than 1.0 cm in diameter.[15] Laparoscopic ultrasonography and laparoscopic peritoneal cytology may further improve the usefulness of this staging procedure. Laparoscopy may avoid laparotomy in unresectable patients and may aid in planning an operation in those patients that are resectable.

## SURGICAL PLANNING

In general, patients with multiple hepatic metastases, peritoneal carcinomatosis, or with other sites of distant disease are not surgical candidates unless they require surgical palliation. The surgeon should not be deterred, however, from an aggressive approach in patients presenting with locally advanced disease. The mainstay of surgical treatment includes en bloc resection of the gastric tumor and lymphadenectomy to include one level beyond the presence of obvious lymph node metastases. The Japanese have developed a detailed classification system for the nodal stations around the stomach that includes 16 separate nodal stations (Table 12-3).[16] The radicality (R value, R1, R2, R3, R4) of the dissection is determined by the extent of the gastric resection and the extent of the lymphadenectomy (some authors use a D prefix instead of an R to indicate the extent of the resection). For example, an R0 dissection involves gastric resection plus incomplete removal of the N1 lymph nodes (lymph

**TABLE 12-3.** NODAL STATIONS FOR GASTRIC ADENOCARCINOMA

| STATION | LOCATION |
| --- | --- |
| 1 | Right cardiac lymph nodes |
| 2 | Left cardiac lymph nodes |
| 3 | Lesser curvature lymph nodes |
| 4 | Greater curvature lymph nodes |
| 5 | Suprapyloric lymph nodes |
| 6 | Infrapyloric lymph nodes |
| 7 | Left gastric artery lymph nodes |
| 8 | Common hepatic artery lymph nodes |
| 9 | Celiac artery lymph nodes |
| 10 | Splenic hilar lymph nodes |
| 11 | Splenic artery lymph nodes |
| 12 | Hepatoduodenal ligament lymph nodes |
| 13 | Retropancreatic lymph nodes |
| 14 | Root of mesentery lymph nodes |
| 15 | Middle colic artery lymph nodes |
| 16 | Paraaortic lymph nodes |

node stations 1 to 6), whereas an R1 dissection involves complete removal of the N1 lymph nodes. The R2, R3, and R4 dissections involve complete removal of all lymph nodes through levels N2, N3, and N4, respectively (i.e., R4 dissection includes N1, N2, N3, and N4 lymph nodes). The effectiveness of an extended lymphadenectomy for gastric cancer is controversial in this country. Some studies have demonstrated an increased incidence of postoperative complications related to extended lymphadenectomy,[17] whereas other studies have found no increase in the morbidity and mortality.[18] It also appears that the level of experience of the surgeon influences complication and overall survival rates.[19]

Figure 12-1 describes the various types of lymphadenectomy performed in the presence of a distal prepyloric tumor. An R1 lymphadenectomy is indicated in the absence of clinically positive lymph nodes, whereas an R2 or R3 lymphadenectomy is performed when N1 and N2 lymph nodes are clinically involved with tumor. An R3 lymphadenectomy usually includes the spleen and splenic hilum lymph nodes; however, routine splenectomy is not indicated unless the tumor is in close proximity to the splenic hilum or invades it directly. The extent of gastric resection (i.e., total gastrectomy versus subtotal gastrectomy) is based primarily on the location of the tumor. Middle and upper-third gastric lesions require near-total or total gastrectomy in order to obtain histologically tumor-free margins and to perform an adequate lymphadenectomy. Figure 12-2 describes the R1 and R2 dissection for distal, middle-, and upper-third gastric cancers. As described in Fig. 12-2, however, the R1 operation for upper-third lesions and the R2 lymphadenectomy for middle- and upper-third lesions usually include total gastric resection. The R2 dissection for middle- and upper-third lesions includes all R1 lymph nodes plus splenic hilar, paraesophageal, left gastric, and hepatic lymph nodes. Cancers that involve contiguous organs, such as the spleen, distal pancreas, or transverse colon, should undergo en bloc resection to include adjacent organs. The decision regarding the type of gastric reconstruction should be based on

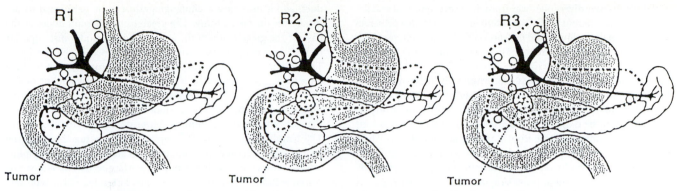

**FIGURE 12-1.** The extent of lymphadenectomy in the presence of a distal prepyloric tumor. A standard R1 lymphadenectomy is performed in the absence of obvious lymph node involvement. R2 and R3 lymphadenectomy procedures are performed for N1 and N2 nodal involvement, respectively. (*Redrawn from Shiu M-H et al: Tumors of the stomach, in* Gastrointestinal Cancer, *SJ Winawer, RC Kurtz [eds]. New York, Gower Medical, 1992, p 2.14.*)

recognition of the patterns of local recurrence for gastric cancer. Locally recurrent gastric cancer often involves the duodenum, the proximal gastric margin, or either the afferent or efferent limb of a Billroth II reconstruction. Therefore, a Billroth II gastroenterostomy is preferred over a Billroth I gastroduodenostomy because of the proximity of the duodenal margin to the tumor and greater potential for anastomotic recurrence. A "Pólya-type" anastomosis may lessen the potential for obstruction due to tumor recurrence at the suture line. The performance of a distal (25 cm from the gastroenterostomy) Braun enteroenterostomy between the afferent and

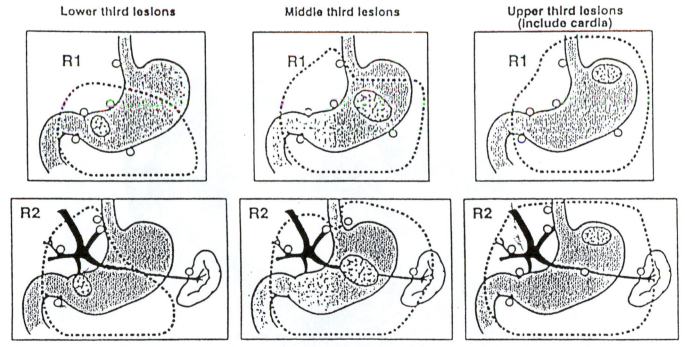

**FIGURE 12-2.** The extent of lymphadenectomy for distal-, middle-, and upper-third gastric carcinomas. Subtotal gastrectomy can be performed for distal lesions. Near-total and total gastrectomy are performed for the appropriate R-stage lymphadenopathy for middle- and upper-third lesions. (*Redrawn from Shiu M-H et al: Tumors of the stomach, in* Gastrointestinal Cancer, *SJ Winawer, RC Kurtz [eds]. New York, Gower Medical, 1992, p 2.15.*)

efferent limbs may divert bile away from the gastric remnant and decompresses the afferent limb. The enteroenterostomy also preserves gastrointestinal continuity and may prevent afferent or efferent loop syndrome in cases of recurrent anastomotic tumor at the gastroenterostomy.

Following a total or near-total gastrectomy, the preferred type of reconstruction is either a Roux-en-Y esophagojejunostomy or anastomosis of the Roux limb to the small gastric remnant. To divert bile away from the esophagus, the distal enteroenterostomy is constructed approximately 50 cm from the proximal anastomosis. There is no advantage to preserving the distal stomach and performing an esophagogastrostomy for small cancers in the cardia of the stomach. Although this operation appears simpler than a total gastrectomy and esophagojejunostomy, esophagogastrostomy is associated with significant reflux of bile into the esophagus.

## SURGICAL TECHNIQUE

Following a midline abdominal incision, thorough exploration of the entire abdominal cavity is performed. In the absence of obvious metastatic disease, the surgeon should evaluate the primary tumor with respect to penetration through the serosa, and involvement of lymph nodes or contiguous organs. In the presence of a distal tumor without obvious lymph node involvement, a subtotal gastric resection with the R1 lymphadenectomy is planned. Figure 12-3 denotes the location of the appropriate lymph nodes to be included in the various operations. The nodes inferior to the pylorus can be included in the specimen only by transecting the duodenum 3 to 4 cm distal to the pylorus. The surgeon should palpate the ampulla of Vater to avoid injury to the distal common bile

duct, and if necessary, a cholangiogram can be performed to delineate the ductal anatomy. The greater-curve lymph nodes at the base of the greater omentum and the lymph nodes just superior to the lesser curve of the stomach are included in the specimen. The proximal line of resection should be approximately 6 to 7 cm away from gross tumor. The transverse anastomosis stapling device (TA-90, U.S. Surgical Corp., Norwalk, CT) can be used to transect the proximal stomach, whereas the duodenum is divided distally using the gastrointestinal anastomosis (GIA) stapling device (Fig. 12-4). The lymph nodes for an R1 lymphadenectomy together with the greater and lesser omentum and the right gastric and gastroepiploic arteries are included with the specimen. Margins may be assessed by frozen section. A standard side-to-side, antecolic, Pólya-type gastroenterostomy is performed using either the GIA-60 or 80 stapling device (Figs. 12-5 and 12-6). In cases of a wide gastric remnant, the GIA-60 device is used twice to perform an anastomosis that extends from the greater to the lesser curve of the gastric remnant. The anastomosis can be performed either anteriorly or posteriorly, but should be at least 1 cm from the TA-90 staple line to avoid an ischemic anastomosis. A distal enteroenterostomy is constructed using the GIA-60 stapling device approximately 25 cm from the gastroenterostomy. As previously described, in the presence of N1 nodal involvement, the lymphadenectomy is broadened to include the R2 resection and the next level of grossly uninvolved lymph nodes.

In most cases of proximal or midgastric carcinomas, a near-total or total gastrectomy is necessary. For a near-total or total gastrectomy, the division of the duodenum is similar to the transection performed for a subtotal gastrectomy. Proximally, the esophagus is mobilized for at least 4 to 5 cm, requiring division of the anterior and posterior trunks of the vagus nerve.

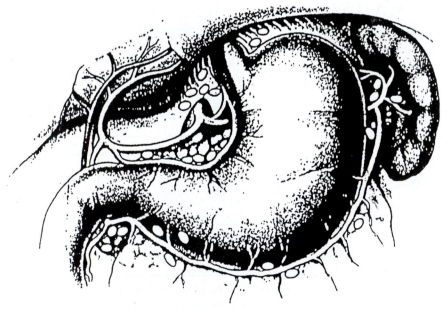

**FIGURE 12-3.** The approximate location of perigastric and paraesophageal lymph nodes, with their relationship to blood vessels and anatomic structures.

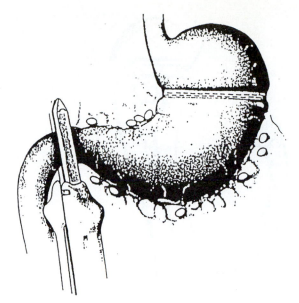

**FIGURE 12-4.** Transection of the postpyloric duodenum and proximal stomach using stapling devices. The lymph nodes along the lesser and greater curve are removed with the lesser and greater omentum.

Following mobilization of the greater and lesser omentum, the stomach is displaced anteriorly, and the left gastric artery is transected at its origin. A lymphadenectomy encompassing the hepatic and left gastric arteries is performed in continuity with the specimen.

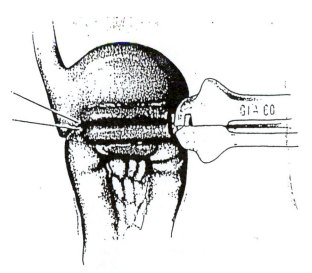

**FIGURE 12-5.** A standard anterior side-to-side gastrojejunostomy performed using the gastrointestinal anastomosis (GIA) stapling device.

The spleen is mobilized to remove all splenic hilar lymph nodes. If the body or tail of the pancreas is grossly involved with tumor, the pancreas should be removed en bloc with the specimen. Transection of the pancreas can be performed using the TA-55 stapling device. Following a pancreatic resection, a closed-suction drain is placed in the left upper quadrant to provide drainage for any pancreatic leak. There are several techniques for gastrointestinal reconstruction following a near-total or total gastrectomy. The surgeon must take care not to devascularize the distal esophagus because ischemia may lead to anastomotic disruption. One method of restoring gastrointestinal continuity involves the creation of a side-to-side esophagojejunostomy using the GIA stapler. This technique may result in an improved anastomotic blood supply compared to an end-to-side anastomosis. The side-to-side esophagojejunostomy functions clinically as an end-to-end esophagojejunostomy. Figures 12-7 and 12-8 describe two techniques using the GIA stapler to create a side-to-side esophagojejunostomy. In Fig. 12-7, the stomach is used as a "handle" to provide traction during mobilization of the distal esophagus and during construction of the esophagojejunal anastomosis. The Roux-en-Y jejunal limb is created by transecting the jejunum with a GIA stapler just distal to the ligament of Treitz. The jejunal limb is then brought up to the transected end of the esophagus and the two blades of the GIA stapling device are inserted separately into a small hole in both the esophagus and the Roux-en-Y jejunal limb. After firing the GIA stapler to create the anastomosis, the remaining hole is closed using the TA-55 stapler. An enteroenterostomy is performed at least 50 cm away from the esophagus to divert bile and prevent alkaline reflux esophagitis. Finally, the stomach is transected and sent to pathology. In Fig. 12-8, the stomach is transected prior to performance of the anastomosis. Stay sutures are placed in the distal esophagus, and the esophagojejunostomy is performed in a side-to-side fashion using the GIA stapler.

Figure 12-9 describes a stapled end-to-side esophagojejunostomy after performing total gastrectomy. Following mobilization of the esophagus and transection of the 50-cm Roux limb, the end-to-end anastomosis (EEA) stapling device is placed through the open end of the Roux limb. The correct-size EEA stapling device is chosen based on the diameter of the distal esophageal lumen. The proximal anvil of the EEA stapler is placed in the distal end of the esophagus and a purse-string suture is tied to hold the device in the distal esophagus (Fig. 12-10). The trocar tip of the main instrument is now advanced through the side of the Roux limb by turning the wing nut on the end of the EEA device. After removal of the trocar, the anvil is inserted into the main instrument. The two ends of the device are then brought together snugly by screwing the wing nut. The EEA device is then fired and an end-to-side anastomosis is created. The wing nut is then turned in the opposite direction and the device is gently removed through the anastomosis. Prior to closure of the open end of the jejunum with a TA-55 stapler, the integrity of the esophagojejunostomy can be tested with air or fluid. Creating an enteroenterostomy 50 cm from the esophagojejunostomy restores gastrointestinal continuity. Although the aforementioned emphasis has been on stapled anastomoses, a hand-sewn esophagojejunostomy is certainly acceptable technique.

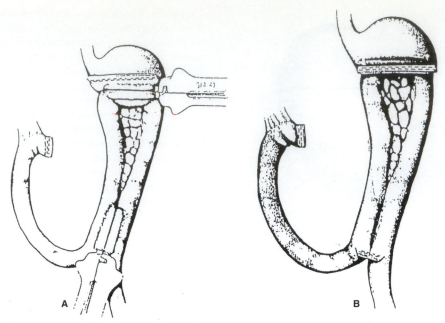

**FIGURE 12-6.** *A*. A posterior antecolic side-to-side gastrojejunostomy. *B*. A distal (25-cm) enteroenterostomy constructed between the afferent and efferent limbs of the Billroth II anastomosis.

Whether the creation of a gastric replacement pouch or jejunal reservoir (i.e., Hunt-Lawrence pouch) improves the nutritional consequences of total gastrectomy has not been conclusively proven. Figure 12-10 illustrates the creation of a jejunal pouch following total gastrectomy. Following the end-to-side procedure with the EEA device, the blades of the GIA stapling device are inserted in the open end of the Roux limb and through a separate enterotomy in the downstream Roux limb. The GIA-60 or GIA-80 stapling device can be used in performing this procedure. A double firing of the GIA produces a 10- to 15-cm pouch. Following the side-to-side anastomosis, the openings are closed using the TA-55 stapler.

If it can be performed with an acceptable morbidity and mortality, gastrectomy offers the best palliation for patients who cannot be resected for cure. If, however, at the time of operation the tumor is unresectable, a stapled esophagojejunal bypass may relieve obstruction from a proximal gastric cancer. Figure 12-11 demonstrates a side-to-side Roux-en-Y esophagojejunostomy that is performed with the GIA stapler, leaving stomach and tumor in their original positions. The esophagus proximal to the adherent tumor is mobilized after incision of the peritoneal reflection or incision of the diaphragm. The esophagus is then encircled with a Penrose drain and the Roux limb is placed side by side with the mobilized esophagus and a side-to-side anastomosis is created using the staplers as previously described. This procedure usually restores gastrointestinal continuity and allows the patient to swallow secretions and maintain a moderate oral intake throughout the course of the disease. Performing a stapled gastroenterostomy proximal to the tumor can palliate patients with unresectable distal obstructing cancers. Minimally invasive techniques, such as laparoscopic gastroenterostomy, may provide palliation without the morbidity and longer hospital stay associated with laparotomy. Alternative palliative procedures for obstructing gastric cancers include surgical or endoscopic placement of intraluminal devices (Celestin tube, self-expanding metallic stents, etc.), but the precise role of these palliative procedures has not been determined. Some studies suggest that palliative chemotherapy may prolong survival and improve the quality of life (i.e., relief of symptoms and improved performance status). Further studies are necessary to determine the optimal method of palliation for patients with gastric cancer.

## MULTIMODAL THERAPY

Although surgery offers the best chance for cure, many patients with gastric cancer initially present with advanced disease and are not candidates for a potentially curative resection. Even those patients who undergo a complete resection have a high relapse rate. Therefore, additional therapies such as radiation therapy and chemotherapy have been investigated to improve upon the relatively disappointing results obtained from surgery alone.

Although postoperative chemotherapy for patients at high risk for recurrence is considered the standard of care in Japan, adjuvant chemotherapy for gastric cancer is not widely accepted in the United States. Clinical trials performed in this country have failed to demonstrate convincingly a survival benefit for adjuvant chemotherapy in gastric cancer.[20] Many of these trials have suffered from poor study design and other methodological flaws that may have limited their ability to demonstrate any efficacy from adjuvant chemotherapy. The timing and route of administration and type of chemotherapy have all varied significantly in the treatment

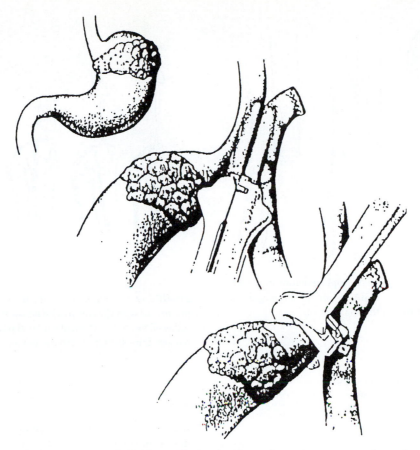

**FIGURE 12-7.** A standard side-to-side Roux-en-Y esophagojejunostomy performed using the gastrointestinal anastomosis (GIA) stapling device. The stomach and tumor are removed following the anastomosis.

of gastric cancer. Relatively recent data from trials of neoadjuvant (preoperative) chemotherapy employed for patients with advanced disease have provided some encouraging response rates. A few studies comparing neoadjuvant chemotherapy and complete tumor resection to primary resection show a trend toward improved survival in those patients receiving neoadjuvant chemotherapy.[21–23] Caution must be used, however, in interpreting data from neoadjuvant trials because some studies employed suboptimal pretherapeutic staging and have inadvertently included patients with small peritoneal implants. The Japanese have utilized hyperthermic intraperitoneal chemotherapy administered immediately postoperatively in an effort to reduce peritoneal recurrences in patients with gastric cancer.[24] Intraperitoneal chemotherapy may have its greatest benefit in patients at greatest risk for peritoneal spread (i.e., transmural tumors). Further studies examining alternative and combined routes for the administration of chemotherapeutic agents (i.e., intraarterial, intraperitoneal, and systemic) are required.

Some of the encouraging chemotherapy regimens for gastric cancer include etoposide, Adriamycin, and 5-fluorouracil (ELF); and 5-fluorouracil, Adriamycin, and methotrexate (FAMTX). Ongoing studies are attempting to define clinicopathologic predictors of re-

sponse to chemotherapy as well as evaluating chemotherapy regimens incorporating newer agents such as Taxotere and irinotecan.[25]

Local relapse of gastric cancer either alone or in combination with systemic disease is a significant problem after a potentially curative resection. Therefore, radiation therapy has been used in gastric cancer in an effort to reduce local and regional recurrences. The use of external beam radiation is somewhat limited by the large target volume and dose-limiting toxicities to the structures in the upper abdomen (i.e., small bowel, kidneys, liver, and spinal cord). Unfortunately, clinical trials involving radiotherapy have suffered from methodological flaws similar to those seen in chemotherapy clinical trials.[27] Intraoperative radiotherapy has been applied to gastric cancer to try to maximize the dose of radiation delivered to the sites at greatest risk while reducing the dose to critical structures. Studies suggest improved local control rates with intraoperative radiation, but the local toxicity (i.e., bleeding, perforation) rates are high.[28]

Radiation therapy may be recommended for patients with positive margins after extirpative surgery, but it cannot be recommended for adjuvant use except in the context of a controlled clinical trial.

Combined chemoradiation has also been applied to gastric cancer to take advantage of some potential synergism between the two

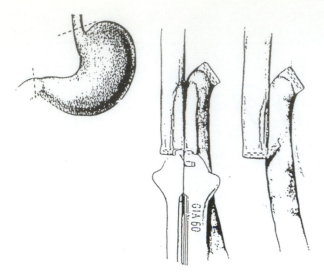

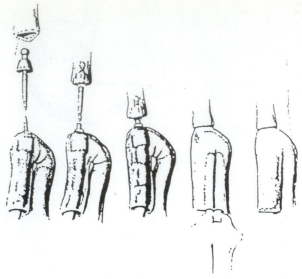

**FIGURE 12-8.** A standard Roux-en-Y esophagojejunostomy with the gastrointestinal anastomosis (GIA) 60 or 80 stapling device. The stomach is removed prior to the anastomosis.

**FIGURE 12-10.** The end-to-side Roux-en-Y esophagojejunostomy performed with the end-to-end anastomosis (EEA) stapling device, followed by construction of a jejunal pouch using the gastrointestinal anastomosis (GIA) stapling device.

modalities.[28] Concomitant chemotherapy and radiotherapy results in significant toxicity, and data from ongoing and future trials are needed to assess fully the benefits of aggressive chemoradiation for gastric cancer.

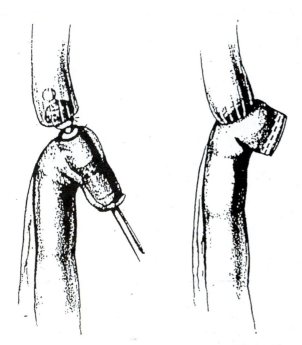

**FIGURE 12-9.** A standard Roux-en-Y end-to-side esophagojejunostomy performed using the end-to-end anastomosis stapling (GIA) device through the open end of the Roux limb.

## LYMPHOMA

Although primary gastric non-Hodgkin's lymphoma is the second-most-common malignant gastric tumor, it only accounts for 5% of all gastric malignancies. Unfortunately, however, the incidence of primary gastric lymphoma is increasing. The stomach is the most common site of primary extranodal non-Hodgkin's lymphoma, and the stomach may also be involved secondarily by systemic nodal lymphoma. Symptoms related to gastric lymphoma include early satiety, vague epigastric pain, and obstructive symptoms and weight loss. Patients with gastric lymphoma may also present with constitutional symptoms such as fever and night sweats. Since gastric lymphomas develop submucosally, it may be difficult to make a histologic diagnosis by routine endoscopic biopsy. Multiple, deep, submucosal needle biopsies or newer endoscopic biopsy techniques that permit a larger biopsy specimen may aid the endoscopist in obtaining a tissue diagnosis. Nevertheless, even with adequate tissue, it may still be difficult for the pathologist to tell poorly differentiated adenocarcinoma from lymphoma.

Endoscopic ultrasound may be helpful in pretreatment staging, but its precise role in the management of gastric lymphoma remains to be defined. A CT scan of the abdomen and chest will aid in the assessment of additional organ (i.e., liver and spleen) and abdominal or mediastinal lymph node involvement. Additional staging studies may include a peripheral blood smear and bone marrow aspirate to determine if disseminated disease is present.

Most primary gastric non-Hodgkin's lymphomas are B-cell–derived and are classified as low- or high-grade lesions. Occasionally, T-cell and Hodgkin's lymphomas may arise in the stomach. The staging system most commonly used to classify gastric lymphomas is the Ann Arbor staging system (Table 12-4). In an effort to standardize

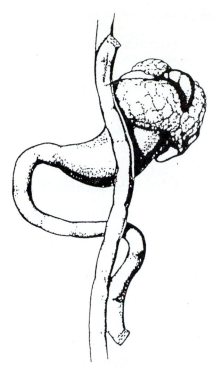

**FIGURE 12-11.** An unresectable proximal gastric cancer bypassed using a gastrointestinal anastomosis stapling device to do a side-to-side Roux-en-Y esophagojejunostomy anastomosis.

cancer staging, the TNM system has recently been applied to gastric lymphomas (Tables 12-5A and 12-5B).

There is no consensus on the most effective therapy for gastric lymphoma. The low frequency of occurrence of gastric lymphoma has limited the ability to perform well-designed, prospective clinical trials, and data from retrospective trials suffer from selection bias.

Although surgery is generally recommended for patients with disease confined to the stomach, some studies have demonstrated that nonsurgical therapy is equivalent to surgical therapy for early-stage disease. It appears from retrospective reviews that single-modality therapy is effective for early-stage disease. A recently

### TABLE 12-4. ANN ARBOR STAGING SYSTEM OF PRIMARY GASTRIC LYMPHOMA

| STAGE | DESCRIPTION |
|-------|-------------|
| IE | Involvement of the stomach only |
| II1E | Involvement of the stomach and continuous lymph nodes |
| II2E | Involvement of the stomach and noncontiguous, subdiaphragmatic lymph nodes |
| IIIE | Involvement of stomach, nodes on both sides of the diaphragm, or spleen |
| IV | Diffuse involvement of the stomach and extralymphatic sites |

### TABLE 12-5A. TUMOR-NODE-METASTASIS (TNM) STAGING OF PRIMARY GASTRIC LYMPHOMA

| T | PRIMARY TUMOR |
|---|---------------|
| T1 | Tumor invades the lamina propria or submucosa |
| T2 | Tumor invades the muscularis propria |
| T3 | Tumor invades the subserosa |
| T4 | Tumor penetrates the serosa, no invasion of adjacent structure |
| T5 | Tumor invades adjacent structures |

| N | LYMPH NODE INVOLVEMENT |
|---|------------------------|
| N0 | No metastases in regional lymph nodes |
| N1 | Metastases in perigastric lymph nodes within 3 cm of the primary tumor |
| N2 | Metastases to regional lymph nodes more than 3 cm from the primary tumor including the lymph nodes along the left gastric, hepatic, splenic, and celiac arteries |
| N3 | Metastases to the paraaortic, hepatoduodenal pancreatic, and mesenteric lymph nodes |
| N4 | Metastases to lymph nodes beyond N3 |

| M | DISTANT METASTASIS |
|---|--------------------|
| M0 | No distant metastases |
| M1 | Distant metastases |

### TABLE 12-5B. STAGE GROUPING OF PRIMARY GASTRIC LYMPHOMA

| STAGE | TUMOR (T) | NODE (N) | METASTASES (M) |
|-------|-----------|----------|----------------|
| I | T1 | N0,N1 | M0 |
| II | T1 | N2 | M0 |
| | T2, T3 | N0, N1, N2 | M0 |
| III | T4, T5 | Any N | M0 |
| | Any T | N3, N4 | M0 |
| IV | Any T | Any N | M1 |

published randomized prospective trial involving 75 patients found a statistically significant improvement in survival with no difference in treatment-related complications for patients given multimodal therapy.[30]

The lack of a nonsurgical group in this trial makes assessment of the contribution of gastric resection to combined-modality therapy difficult. A recent metaanalysis showed improved survival for patients receiving surgery, either alone or as part of combined therapy, over patients treated without surgery. The results of this review should be interpreted with caution, however, because patients who undergo resection may have a more favorable prognosis. In the absence of conclusive data, chemotherapy should be considered for patients with nodal involvement or other extragastric disease.

Radiotherapy should also be considered for those patients with positive margins, nodal disease, and adjacent organ involvement to reduce the risk of local failure. Unfortunately, there remains no consensus on the exact indications for combined-modality therapy for gastric lymphoma. Well-designed, prospective, multiinstitutional trials are needed to answer a number of important questions surrounding the treatment of gastric lymphoma.

Some investigators advocate gastric resection prior to chemotherapy or radiotherapy for patients with advanced disease to avoid the possibility of treatment-related gastric perforation or hemorrhage. Initial studies may have overestimated the risk of gastric perforation or hemorrhage in this setting. Other investigators have attempted to identify factors that might predispose patients to these complications. The risk of perforation may be greatest in the subgroup of patients with high-grade tumors that involve the entire gastric wall.

Gastric lymphomas that arise from mucosa-associated lymphoid tissue (MALT) are a distinct clinicopathologic entity. In the past, these lesions were referred to as pseudolymphomas. Gastric MALT lymphomas are low-grade tumors that may remain indolent for prolonged periods of time. There is some evidence to suggest an association between chronic gastric infection with *H. pylori* and the development of gastric MALT lymphomas. Furthermore, antibiotic treatment to eradicate *H. pylori* infection may lead to regression of low-grade, B-cell gastric MALT lymphomas. This finding certainly raises the possibility of a causal relationship between *H. pylori* infection and some gastric lymphomas. Tumors that fail to respond to *Helicobacter* eradication require additional therapy. The development of an oral vaccine against *H. pylori* might prevent subsequent *H. pylori* infection and its associated diseases.

## MESENCHYMAL TUMORS

The stomach is the site of 50% of all gastrointestinal stromal cell tumors. Leiomyomas are the most common benign mesenchymal gastric tumors. They usually present as solitary, well-circumscribed, submucosal gastric masses. Most of these tumors are asymptomatic, but large lesions may produce symptoms of obstruction and hemorrhage.

Leiomyosarcoma is the malignant variant of leiomyoma. These tumors tend to be broad-based and often outgrow their blood supply, leading to ulceration and occasionally massive hemorrhage. Pathologists now consider gastric leiomyomas and leiomyosarcomas as part of a group of neoplasms referred to as gastrointestinal stromal cell tumors (GISTs). These lesions demonstrate a spectrum of malignant potential depending upon tumor size, grade, and mitotic index. Tumors greater than 5 cm in size with more than five mitoses per high-power field have a worse prognosis. Surgical therapy is dictated in part by tumor size and location (cardia, corpus, antrum, prepyloric area, lesser or greater curve, etc.). In general, wedge resection with a 1- to 2-cm margin of normal gastric wall is adequate therapy. Although formal lymphadenectomy is not necessary, local invasion of adjacent organs requires wide en bloc resection of involved structures.

The surgeon must keep in mind the possibility of multiple gastric lesions. Laparoscopic resection of benign stromal cell tumors has recently been described, and with technological advances, minimally invasive approaches to these tumors will become increasingly employed.

There is no proven role for adjuvant radiation or chemotherapy following resection of stromal cell tumors. A recently described syndrome that occurs primarily in young women referred to as Carney's triad consists of gastric epitheloid leiomyosarcoma, pulmonary chondroma, and functional extraadrenal paraganglionoma. It is important to consider this syndrome because of the possible consequences of catecholamine release from an unrecognized functional paraganglioma at the time of gastric resection.

## CARCINOID TUMORS

Gastric carcinoid tumors account for only 2% to 3% of all carcinoid tumors. Carcinoid tumors rise from the enterochromaffin cells of the gastric epithelium. Since gastrin is a mitogen for enterochromaffin cells, gastric carcinoids may arise in the setting of hypergastrinemia associated with pernicious anemia, chronic atrophic gastritis, achlorhydria, and Zollinger-Ellison syndrome. Most gastric carcinoids associated with gastrinomas occur in the setting of multiple endocrine neoplasia (MEN) 1 syndrome (i.e., gastrinoma, parathyroid hyperplasia, and pituitary adenoma). Long-term inhibition of acid secretion with proton pump inhibitors such as omeprazole may also lead to enterochromaffin cell hyperplasia and gastric carcinoids. Immunohistochemical staining for chromogranin or neuron-specific enolase may aid the pathologist in securing a diagnosis of carcinoid. Treatment of gastric carcinoids is based on tumor size, number, and gastrin level. Elimination of hypergastrinemia may lead to regression of the gastric carcinoids. Sporadic carcinoids that occur in patients with normal serum gastrin levels have a more malignant behavior. These more aggressive lesions require gastric resection and lymphadenectomy. Small lesions may be treated with endoscopic polypectomy and periodic surveillance endoscopy.

## METASTATIC TUMORS

Extragastric malignancies infrequently metastasize to the stomach. Some of the more common tumors that may secondarily involve the stomach include melanoma, breast cancer, and lung cancer. The treatment of tumors metastatic to the stomach is almost always palliative and is dictated primarily by the presence and severity of symptoms.

## REFERENCES

1. SIEWERT JR et al: Gastric cancer. Curr Probl Surg 34:835, 1997.
2. SAWYERS JL: Gastric carcinoma. Curr Probl Surg 32:101, 1995.
3. ORLOWSKA J et al: Malignant transformation of benign epithelial gastric polyps. Am J Gastroenterol 10:108, 1995.
4. AUDISIO RA et al: Gastric cancer. Crit Rev Oncol Hematol 27:143, 1998.
5. KARPEH MS JR, BRENNAN MF: Malignant disease of the stomach and duodenum, part I: Adenocarcinoma, in *Current Practice of Surgery,* vol 2, BA Levine et al (eds). New York, Churchill Livingstone, 1993.

6. RUGGE M et al: Gastric epithelial dysplasia. How clinicopathologic background leads to management. Cancer 76:376, 1993.

7. LONGMIRE WP JR, GRAY GF JR: Carcinoma of the stomach, in *Surgery of the Stomach, Duodenum, and Small Intestine.* HW Scott Jr, JL Sawyers (eds). Chicago, Blackwell Scientific, 1987.

8. TALLY NJ et al: Gastric adenocarcinoma and Helicobacter pylori infection. J Natl Cancer Inst 83:1734, 1991.

9. RAKIC S et al: Increasing incidence of adenocarcinoma of the proximal stomach. Eur J Surg Oncol 18:340, 1992.

10. LAUREN P: The two histologic types of gastric carcinoma: diffuse and so-called intestinal-type carcinoma. Acta Pathol Microbiol Scand 64:31, 1965.

11. BEARHS OH et al: *Manual for Staging of Cancer (American Joint Committee on Cancer)*, 5th ed. Philadelphia, Lippincott, 1997.

12. TAHARA E: Molecular biology of gastric cancer. World J Surg 19:484, 1995.

13. LIGHTDALE CJ: Endoscopic ultrasound for the staging of esophageal and gastric cancer. Principals Pract Oncol Updates 9:1, 1995.

14. CHO JS et al: Preoperative assessment of gastric carcinoma: value of two-phase dynamic CT with mechanical infusion of i.v. contrast material. Am J Roentgenol 163:69, 1994.

15. BURKE EC et al: Laparoscopy in the management of gastric adenocarcinoma. Ann Surg 225:262, 1997.

16. JAPANESE RESEARCH SOCIETY FOR GASTRIC CANCER: The general rule for gastric cancer study in surgery and pathology. Jpn J Surg 11:127, 1981.

17. CUSCHERI A et al: Prospective morbidity and mortality after D1 and D2 resections for gastric cancer. Preliminary results of the MRC randomised controlled clinical trial (the Surgical Cooperative Group). Lancet 347:995, 1996.

18. SIEWERT JR et al: Relevant prognostic factors in gastric cancer; ten year results of a German gastric cancer study. Ann Surg 228:449, 1998.

19. BRENNAN MF: Lymph node dissection for gastric cancer. N Engl J Med 340:956, 1999.

20. SCHIPPER DL, WAGENER DJT: Chemotherapy of gastric cancer. Anti-Cancer Drugs 7:137, 1996.

21. WILS J: Treatment of gastric cancer. Curr Opin Oncol 10:357, 1998.

22. ROUKOS DH: Current advances and changes in treatment strategy may improve survival and quality of life in patients with potentially curable gastric cancer. Ann Surg Oncol 6:61, 1999.

23. LOWY AM et al: Response to neoadjuvant chemotherapy best predicts survival after curative resection. Ann Surg 229:303, 1999.

24. FUKUSHIMA M: Adjuvant therapy of gastric cancer: the Japanese experience. Semin Oncol 23:369, 1996.

25. AJANI JA: Chemotherapy for gastric carcinoma; new and old options. Oncology (Huntington) 12(suppl 7):44, 1998.

26. MINSKY BD: The role of radiation therapy in gastric cancer. Semin Oncol 23:390, 1996.

27. AVIZONIS VN et al: Treatment of adenocarcinoma of the stomach with resection, intraoperative radiotherapy, and adjuvant external beam radiation: A phase II study from the RTOG 85-04. Ann Surg Oncol 2:295, 1995.

28. KELSEN D: Neoadjuvant therapy for upper gastrointestinal tract cancers. Curr Opin Oncol 8:321, 1996.

29. STEPHENS J, SMITH J: Treatment of primary gastric lymphoma and gastric mucosa-associated lymphoid tissue lymphoma. J Am Coll Surg 187:312, 1998.

# CHAPTER 13

# EXOCRINE NEOPLASMS OF THE PANCREAS

*Tara M. Breslin, Peter W.T. Pisters, Jeffrey E. Lee, James L. Abbruzzese, and Douglas B. Evans*

## INTRODUCTION

Adenocarcinoma of the pancreas is responsible for approximately 27,000 deaths per year in the United States and 50,000 deaths per year in Europe (excluding the former USSR). Because of aggressive tumor biology, the advanced stage of disease at diagnosis, and the lack of effective systemic therapies, only 1% to 4% of patients with adenocarcinoma of the pancreas survive 5 years after diagnosis. In the United States in 2000, pancreatic cancer will be the fifth leading cause of adult deaths from cancer (after lung, colorectal, breast, and prostate cancers) and will be responsible for close to 5% of all cancer-related deaths.[1]

A number of environmental risk factors are associated with the development of pancreatic cancer. The most firmly established risk factor associated with pancreatic cancer is tobacco use.[2] Experimental models of pancreatic cancer have been developed through long-term administration of tobacco-specific *N*-nitrosamines or by parenteral administration of other *N*-nitroso compounds. These carcinogens are metabolized to electrophiles that readily react with DNA, leading to miscoding and activation of specific oncogenes such as K-*ras*. Numerous case-control and cohort studies have reported an increased risk of pancreatic cancer for cigarette smokers in both the United States and Europe. Current estimates suggest that approximately 30% of pancreatic cancer cases are related to cigarette smoking. The risk of pancreatic cancer increases as the amount and duration of smoking increase, consistent with experimental data demonstrating higher levels of DNA adducts (lipid peroxidation products) in patients with pancreatic cancer.

Chronic pancreatitis has long been suspected to be associated with an increased risk of pancreatic cancer. However, the magnitude of this risk remains uncertain. Clinical studies have suggested that the chronic forms of pancreatitis accompanied by pancreatic calcifications are most closely associated with the subsequent development of pancreatic cancer. Calculation of a general estimate of population-attributable risk has suggested that chronic pancreatitis may explain as many as 5% of pancreatic cancer cases.[3] Recently, the gene for familial pancreatitis has been identified. The gene, located on chromosome 7q, codes for cationic trypsinogen.[4] Mutation of this gene at residue 117 leads to a protein product that is resistant to cleavage and inactivation. Loss of this cleavage site results in an excess of activated trypsin within the pancreas and autodigestion. Families with hereditary pancreatitis have an increased incidence of pancreatic cancer; however, there remains no objective data to link the chronic inflammation of pancreatitis to the dysplasia-carcinoma sequence.

Attempts to identify premalignant ductal lesions of the pancreas in humans have been limited to autopsy studies. A spectrum of histopathologic changes in proliferating ductal epithelium can be identified, from nonpapillary ductal hyperplasia to papillary hyperplasia, atypical papillary hyperplasia, and carcinoma in situ. These studies have revealed specific point mutations at codon 12 of the K-*ras* oncogene in 75% to 90% of pancreatic adenocarcinoma specimens. The identification of mutated K-*ras* DNA in the majority of patients with invasive pancreatic cancer has provided a possible tool with which these hyperproliferative states can be assessed for their malignant potential based on the frequency of K-*ras* mutations.[5] The *ras* protein is an important signal-transduction mediator for receptor protein tyrosine kinases. Signaling is initiated by the recruitment of guanine nucleotide exchange proteins promoting hydrolysis of GTP to GDP. *ras* bound to GTP is maintained in an active configuration that triggers other enzymatic second messengers leading to nuclear signals resulting in cellular division and proliferation. The mutated *ras* oncogene is not able to convert GTP to inactive GDP. The result is a constitutively active *ras* protein product, unregulated cellular proliferation signals, and susceptibility to malignant

**TABLE 13-1.** ONCOGENES AND TUMOR SUPPRESSOR GENES IN PANCREATIC CANCER

| GENE | FUNCTION | CHROMOSOME | MECHANISM OF INACTIVATION | % MUTATED OR DELETED |
|------|----------|------------|---------------------------|----------------------|
| K-ras | Protooncogene | 12p | Point mutation codons 12,13 | 75–90 |
| p53 | Tumor suppressor | 17p | LOH + IM | 50–75 |
| DPC4 | Tumor suppressor | 18q | LOH + IM, homozygous deletion | 50 |
| p16 | Tumor suppressor | 9p | LOH + IM, homozygous deletion, hypermethylation | 82 |
| hMSH2, hMLH1, PMS1, PMS2 | DNA repair | 2p, 3p, 7p, 2q | Point mutation, deletions | 50 |
| c-erbB-2 (HER-2-neu) | Cell surface receptor | 13q | Point mutation, deletions | 45–90 |

ABBREVIATIONS: LOH + IM = loss of heterozygosity and internal mutation.

transformation. K-*ras* mutations can be detected in the DNA isolated from pancreatic juice, bile, and stool of patients with pancreatic adenocarcinoma.[6] However, translating this information into effective techniques for screening and early diagnosis has proven more difficult.

The *p53* gene is located on chromosome 17p and encodes for a nuclear phosphoprotein, which is responsible for regulation of transcription and cell proliferation. Mutations in this gene are found in a wide variety of tumor types including adenocarcinomas, leukemias, and sarcomas. Studies in pancreatic cancer evaluating the impact of *p53* status on patient outcome have been conflicting; a mutation in *p53* does not imply early tumor recurrence in all patients.[7] In addition, activation of K-*ras* may be accompanied by mutation of *p53*.

Additional genetic alterations (Table 13-1) have been described in human pancreatic cancer. These candidate tumor suppressor genes, appropriately termed deleted in pancreatic cancer *(DPC)*, include *DPC1/2* on chromosome 13q12 (the region of the *BRCA2* gene), *DPC3 (p16/MTS-1)* on chromosome 9q21, and *DPC4* on chromosome 18q21.1.[8] *DPC4* may function as a transcription factor in the transforming growth factor β (TGF-β) receptor-mediated signal transduction pathway. A functional role for *DPC4* was suggested by its peptide sequence, which is similar to those of the *Drosophila melanogaster* Mad protein and the *Caenorhabditis elegans* Mad homologues sma-2, sma-3, and sma-4. Mad proteins have been linked to the TGF-β superfamily of cytokines that regulate cell differentiation and are potent inhibitors of cellular proliferation for most normal cells. The gene for the p16 protein belongs to a class of cyclin-dependent kinase (CDK)–inhibitory proteins (including *p21/WAF1/Cip1*). The p16 protein inhibits the cyclin D/CdK-4 complex, which normally acts by phosphorylating the RB protein. Phosphorylation of *RB* results in the transcription of genes that promote cell cycle progression.[9] Inactivation of *p16* could therefore lead to unregulated cell growth. Allelic deletions involving *p16* were found in 85% of human pancreatic xenografts, and current evidence suggests that the majority of exocrine pancreatic cancers may contain an inactive *p16* tumor suppressor gene.[10] Based on the frequency with which mutations in K-*ras, p53, p16, and DPC4* are found, a model of pancreatic carcinogenesis has been suggested whereby the malignant clone evolves from cells driven by a dominant oncogene

(K-*ras*) with subsequent deregulation of cell growth precipitated by abnormal cell-cycle control resulting from mutations in *p53, p16, and/or DPC4*.

The recent emergence of the importance of inherited genetic abnormalities in gastrointestinal tract neoplasia has led to investigation of the potential role for heritable factors in pancreatic cancer. One case-control study estimated that 3% of pancreatic cancers had a hereditary origin. Evaluation of approximately 30 extended families with presumed familial pancreatic cancer has suggested that transmission occurs in an autosomal dominant pattern. Patient characteristics, tumor histopathology, and overall survival of persons affected by pancreatic cancer in these families are reported to be similar to those of persons with pancreatic cancer in the general population.[11] Continued study of these patients and their families may provide insight into the critical molecular genetic abnormalities leading to familial pancreatic cancer. Familial genetic abnormalities may then provide insight into the process of pancreatic carcinogenesis for patients with sporadic pancreatic cancer and provide opportunities for early detection and chemoprevention.

## CLINICAL MANIFESTATIONS

The lack of obvious clinical signs and symptoms delays diagnosis in most patients. Jaundice, due to extrahepatic biliary obstruction, is present in approximately 50% of patients at diagnosis and may be associated with a less advanced stage of disease than are other signs or symptoms. Tumors located in the pancreatic head or uncinate process may obstruct the intrapancreatic portion of the common bile duct while still relatively small and potentially resectable. In the absence of extrahepatic biliary obstruction, few patients present with localized, potentially resectable disease, because symptoms due to tumor bulk are often vague and nonspecific.[12] The characteristic pain of locally advanced pancreatic cancer is due to tumor invasion of the celiac ganglia and mesenteric nerve plexus. This pain is a dull, fairly constant pain of visceral origin localized to the region of the middle and upper back. Vague, intermittent epigastric pain occurs in some patients; its etiology is less clear. Fatigue, weight loss, and anorexia are common even in the absence of mechanical gastric outlet obstruction. Obstruction of the pancreatic duct may result in malabsorption and steatorrhea due to pancreatic exocrine insufficiency.

The majority of patients with pancreatic cancer have glucose intolerance. Although the exact mechanism of hyperglycemia remains unclear, both altered β-cell function and impaired tissue insulin sensitivity are present. Diabetes mellitus has been implicated as both an early manifestation of pancreatic carcinoma and a predisposing factor. Pancreatic cancer is known to induce peripheral insulin resistance. The argument that longstanding diabetes mellitus is also a risk factor for pancreatic cancer is supported by a recent cohort study showing that after an initial hospitalization for diabetes, patients had an increased risk of developing pancreatic cancer and that this risk persisted for more than a decade.[13] In addition, a metaanalysis of studies published between 1975 and 1994 showed that pancreatic cancer occurred with increased frequency in patients with longstanding diabetes.[14] The mechanisms underlying the association between pancreatic cancer and diabetes, if one exists, remain poorly defined.

## CLINICAL STAGING AND PRETREATMENT DIAGNOSTIC EVALUATION

A standardized system for the clinical and pathologic staging of pancreatic cancer does not currently exist in the United States. The system modified from the American Joint Committee on Cancer (AJCC) and the TNM Committee of the International Union Against Cancer appears in Table 13-2.[15] However, this staging system is most applicable to the pathologic evaluation of resected specimens as accurate measurement of tumor size is difficult to obtain radiographically, and lymph node status cannot be determined without surgical treatment. Pathologic staging can be applied only to patients who undergo pancreatectomy; in all other patients, only clinical staging, based on radiographic examinations, can be done. Treatment and prognosis are based on whether the tumor is potentially resectable, locally advanced, or metastatic, definitions that do not directly correlate with TNM status. For example, both potentially resectable and locally advanced tumors may be stage T4 based on the extent of vascular involvement. As will be discussed later in this chapter, isolated involvement of the superior mesenteric vein (SMV) or portal vein in the absence of tumor extension to the superior mesenteric artery (SMA) or celiac axis is amenable to en bloc resection at the time of pancreaticoduodenectomy. In contrast, patients with tumor extension to the SMA or celiac axis are not considered to have potentially resectable disease. Therefore, a system for clinical staging such as the one illustrated in Table 13-3 is useful to practicing medical oncologists, surgeons, and radiation oncologists.[16]

Advances in diagnostic imaging, surgical technique, and interventional endoscopy have significantly changed the diagnostic and treatment algorithms for patients with malignant obstruction of the extrahepatic bile duct secondary to exocrine pancreatic cancer. Laparotomy is no longer necessary for diagnosis or palliative biliary decompression in the majority of patients. Local tumor resectability can be accurately predicted based on high-quality computed tomography (CT) images, and in patients with unresectable disease, a cytologic diagnosis can be obtained with fine-needle aspiration (FNA).

### TABLE 13-2. TNM STAGING SYSTEM

**PRIMARY TUMOR (T)**

| | |
|---|---|
| TX | Primary tumor cannot be assessed |
| T0 | No evidence of primary tumor |
| T1 | Tumor limited to the pancreas 2 cm or less in greatest dimension |
| T2 | Tumor limited to the pancreas more than 2 cm in greatest dimension |
| T3 | Tumor extends directly to any of the following: duodenum, bile duct, or peripancreatic tissues |
| T4 | Tumor extends directly to any of the following: stomach, spleen, colon, or adjacent large vessels |

**REGIONAL LYMPH NODES (N)**

| | |
|---|---|
| NX | Regional lymph nodes cannot be assessed |
| N0 | No regional lymph node metastasis |
| N1 | Regional lymph node metastasis |
| | 1a  single regional lymph node |
| | 1b  multiple regional lymph nodes |

**DISTANT METASTASIS (M)**

| | |
|---|---|
| MX | Presence of distant metastasis cannot be assessed |
| M0 | No distant metastasis |
| M1 | Distant metastasis |

**STAGE GROUPING**

| Stage I | T1 | N0 | M0 |
|---|---|---|---|
| | T2 | N0 | M0 |
| Stage II | T3 | N0 | M0 |
| Stage III | T1–3 | N1 | M0 |
| Stage IVA | T4 | Any N | M0 |
| Stage IVB | Any T | Any N | M1 |

SOURCE: Beahrs OH et al (eds): *American Joint Committee on Cancer Manual for Staging of Cancer*, 5th ed. Philadelphia, JB Lippincott, 1997, pp 122–123.

Biliary decompression, if necessary, can be achieved with endoscopic or laparoscopic techniques. Laparotomy can thereby be reserved for carefully selected patients with localized disease amenable to pancreaticoduodenectomy as part of a multimodality treatment program that includes systemic chemotherapy and external-beam radiation therapy.

However, many surgeons still believe that intraoperative evaluation is the most sensitive method of determining resectability in all patients with presumed nonmetastatic pancreatic cancer. At the time of surgical exploration for pancreatic head cancer, a Kocher maneuver is the first procedure performed to assess the relationship of the tumor to the SMA by palpation (Fig. 13-1). The close proximity of the pancreatic head (tumor) to the SMA makes assessment by palpation of this vital tumor-vessel relationship an unrealistic expectation. Patients are frequently judged to be resectable or unresectable by intraoperative palpation at the time of the Kocher maneuver.

**TABLE 13-3.** CLINICAL (RADIOGRAPHIC) STAGING OF PANCREATIC CANCER

| STAGE | CLINICAL/RADIOGRAPHIC CRITERIA |
|---|---|
| I | Resectable (T1–3, selected*T4, NX, M0) |
| | No evidence of tumor extension to the celiac axis or SMA |
| | Patent SMPV confluence |
| | No extrapancreatic disease |
| II | Locally advanced (T4, NX–1, M0) |
| | Arterial encasement (celiac axis or SMA) or venous occlusion (SMPV) |
| | No extrapancreatic disease |
| III | Metastatic (T1–4, NX–1, M1) |
| | Metastatic disease (typically to liver and peritoneum and occasionally to lung) |

ABBREVIATIONS: SMA = superior mesenteric artery; SMPV = superior mesenteric–portal vein.
*Resectable T4 tumors include those with isolated involvement of the superior mesenteric vein, portal vein, or hepatic artery without tumor extension to the celiac axis or SMA.

Direct intraoperative assessment of the extent of retroperitoneal tumor growth in relation to the SMA origin is not completed until the final step in tumor resection, after gastric and pancreatic transection, when the surgeon has committed to resection even if all of the tumor cannot be safely removed.[17] The high incidence of positive-margin resections reported in most surgical series of patients who underwent pancreaticoduodenectomy supports our contention that intraoper-

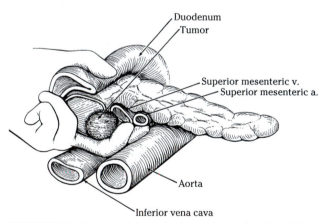

**FIGURE 13-1.** Intraoperative palpation to determine the relationship of the tumor to the mesenteric vessels at the time of the Kocher maneuver; the tumor is palpated with the left hand. The close proximity of the pancreatic head (tumor) to the SMA makes assessment by palpation of the tumor–SMA/SMV relationship an unrealistic expectation. As seen in Figs. 13-3 and 13-5, the relationship of the tumor to the mesenteric vessels is best appreciated preoperatively by high-quality contrast-enhanced CT scans. (*From Cusack JC et al.[18] Reproduced with permission.*)

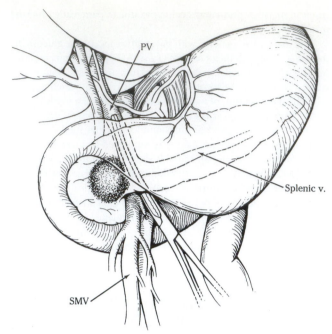

**FIGURE 13-2.** Illustration demonstrating the tumor-free plane between the anterior surface of the superior mesenteric–portal vein confluence and the posterior surface of the pancreas. This plane can often be developed despite fixation of the tumor to the lateral wall of the superior mesenteric vein. (PV = portal vein; SMV = superior mesenteric vein.)

ative palpation of the tumor-SMA margin is inaccurate. Therefore, the relationship of the tumor of the SMA and celiac axis should be the main focus of the preoperative radiographic evaluation.

The second intraoperative maneuver performed to assess local tumor resectability is to develop a plane of dissection between the anterior surface of the superior mesenteric–portal vein (SMPV) confluence and the posterior surface of the neck of the pancreas. Tumor encasement of this region, in the opinion of most surgeons, precludes resection (Fig. 13-2). For surgeons not trained in venous resection and reconstruction at the time of pancreaticoduodenectomy, this technique for intraoperative evaluation has also proven to be inaccurate, and many patients are incorrectly judged to be resectable. Tumors of the pancreatic head or uncinate process are prone to invade the lateral or posterior wall of the SMPV confluence. The anterior wall is rarely involved in the absence of encasement of the celiac axis or SMA origin (as seen in locally advanced tumors of the pancreatic neck or body). The true relationship of a pancreatic head tumor to the lateral and posterior walls of the SMPV confluence can be determined only after gastric and pancreatic transection.[18] Preoperative contrast-enhanced CT demonstrating loss of the normal fat plane between the tumor and the SMV (Fig. 13-3) should alert the surgeon to the potential for direct tumor invasion of the vessel wall: high-quality CT correctly predicts the need for venous resection in approximately 85% of patients. If the tumor is inseparable from the lateral wall of the SMV on preoperative CT scans, surgery should not be undertaken unless the surgeon has developed

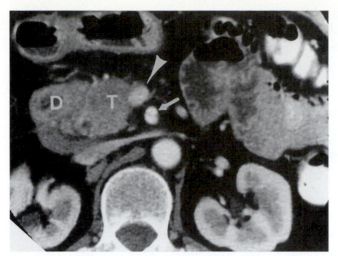

**FIGURE 13-3.** Contrast-enhanced CT scan demonstrating a resectable adenocarcinoma of the pancreatic head (T) with loss of the normal fat plane between the tumor and the superior mesenteric vein (arrowhead). This would commonly require a segmental resection of the superior mesenteric vein. Note the normal fat plane between the tumor and the superior mesenteric artery (arrow). (D = duodenum.)

a technical strategy for the intraoperative management of this condition. The inability to intraoperatively perform a reliable assessment of the relationship of a pancreatic head tumor to the SMA and SMPV confluence prior to gastric and pancreatic transection mandates that these critical tumor-vessel relationships be accurately imaged preoperatively.

Therefore, our recommended diagnostic algorithm is based on high-resolution, contrast-enhanced, helical CT (Fig. 13-4). Accurate preoperative assessment of resectability increases resectability rates and minimizes positive-margin resections. The accuracy of CT in predicting unresectability is well established; state-of-the-art imaging has eliminated the use of laparotomy to assess local tumor resectability. Based upon a fundamental knowledge of the three-dimensional anatomy of the upper abdomen, objective preoperative radiographic criteria for resectability have been established. CT criteria for resectability include: (1) the absence of extrapancreatic disease, (2) a patent SMPV confluence, and (3) no direct tumor extension to the celiac axis or SMA (Fig. 13-5).[17] Patients whose tumors are deemed unresectable by these radiographic criteria are not considered to be candidates for a potentially curative pancreaticoduodenectomy and, therefore, do not undergo laparotomy. Tumor extension to the SMA or celiac axis or occlusion of the SMPV confluence is evidence of locally advanced, unresectable disease (Fig. 13-6). Palliative surgery in patients with pancreatic cancer should be avoided when possible; it can result in a perioperative morbidity rate of 20% to 30%, an average hospital stay of as much as 14 days, and a median survival after surgery of only 6 months.[12] Further, patients whose tumors are resected with positive margins have a survival duration less than 1 year.[17] This survival duration is no different than that achieved with palliative chemotherapy and irradiation in patients with locally advanced, unresectable disease. Therein lies the rationale for accurate pretreatment staging to clearly image the relationship of the pancreatic tumor to the celiac axis, SMA, and SMPV confluence.

## CT-RESECTABLE DISEASE

Patients with a potentially resectable pancreatic mass (based on the CT criteria previously described) and no evidence of extrapancreatic disease undergo endoscopic ultrasound (EUS) and EUS-guided FNA. Preoperative pancreatic biopsy is performed only in patients who are candidates for protocol-based neoadjuvant therapy.[19,20] If a low-density mass is not seen on CT scans, patients undergo diagnostic and therapeutic endoscopic retrograde cholangiopancreatography (ERCP) and EUS. A malignant obstruction of the intrapancreatic portion of the common bile duct is characterized by the double-duct sign (proximal obstruction of the common bile and pancreatic ducts), which can often be accurately differentiated from choledocholithiasis and the long, smooth, tapering stricture seen with chronic pancreatitis. Endoscopic biliary stents are placed to prevent cholangitis in patients who undergo diagnostic cholangiography in the setting of extrahepatic biliary obstruction. This procedure is useful both for relief of jaundice in patients undergoing neoadjuvant therapy and for palliation in those deemed to be unresectable. EUS can identify hypoechoic lesions in the pancreatic head as well as assess the relationship of the tumor to the SMV and SMA.

## CT-UNRESECTABLE DISEASE

For patients with locally advanced or metastatic disease, operation for palliation is rarely needed. Multiple studies have attempted to compare surgical biliary bypass with endoscopic stent placement in patients with jaundice due to malignant obstruction of the intrapancreatic portion of the common bile duct. The higher initial morbidity and mortality rates and longer hospital stay associated with laparotomy are countered by the higher frequency of hospital readmission for recurrent stent occlusion and cholangitis with endoscopic stent placement.[21] Recent innovations in stent construction and the development of the expandable 10-mm metal stent have improved stent patency rates making previous studies less applicable to patient management decisions of today. Patients with liver metastases or ascites have a median survival of less than 6 months, making endoscopic stent placement (with a polyethylene stent) an obvious choice. Patients with locally advanced disease treated with chemoradiation have a median survival of 10 to 12 months, with 20% surviving 2 years; the added expense of a metal stent is justified in this patient population. Patients with a superior performance status at diagnosis often survive longer, yet it is difficult in most patients to predict, at the time of diagnosis, the tempo of disease progression. Currently, we reserve operative (open or laparoscopic) biliary bypass for patients who survive long enough, with minimal disease progression and a good performance status, to experience recurrent stent occlusion. In such patients, the potential morbidity of laparotomy is justified by the apparent favorable tumor biology and longer survival duration.

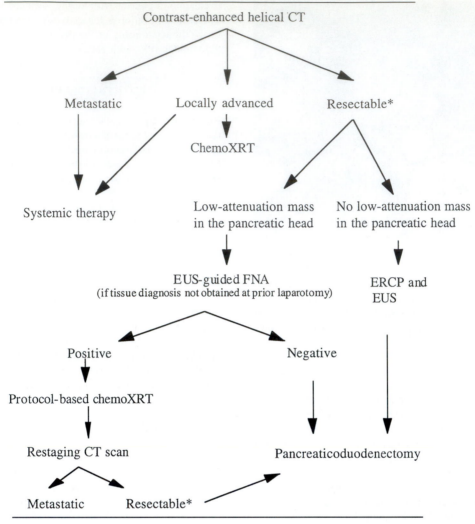

*No extrapancreatic disease, no evidence of tumor extension to the celiac axis or SMA, patent superior mesenteric-portal vein confluence.

**FIGURE 13-4.** Management algorithm employed at our institution for patients with suspected or biopsy-proven (from previous laparotomy prior to referral) adenocarcinoma of the pancreatic head. Angiography is performed in patients who have undergone a previous biliary bypass involving the common bile duct to define hepatic arterial anatomy prior to reoperative pancreaticoduodenectomy. Laparoscopy is performed selectively based upon clinical and CT findings.

## LAPAROSCOPY AND ANGIOGRAPHY

Laparoscopy and angiography are used selectively in the current management of patients with periampullary carcinoma according to our suggested diagnostic schema. Laparoscopy has been used for patients with radiographic evidence of localized disease to detect extrapancreatic tumor not seen on CT scans. If extrapancreatic dis-

ease is found, laparotomy is avoided, thereby increasing resectability rates. As expected, the more advanced the stage of disease, the greater the yield of positive findings at laparoscopy. If laparoscopy is performed early in the diagnostic sequence, or following poor-quality CT, it will have a higher yield of positive findings. In contrast, if it is used only after high-quality, contrast-enhanced CT in patients with localized, potentially resectable disease (as defined by objective radiographic criteria), it will have a much lower rate of positive

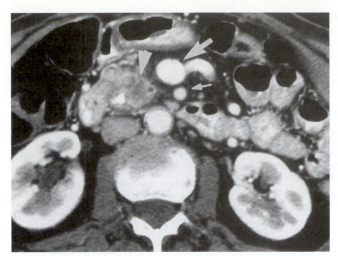

**FIGURE 13-5.** Contrast-enhanced CT scan demonstrating a resectable adenocarcinoma of the pancreatic head (arrowhead). Note the normal fat plane between the tumor and both the superior mesenteric artery (small arrow) and the superior mesenteric vein (large arrow). The intrapancreatic portion of the common bile duct contains a stent, which was endoscopically placed for biliary drainage.

findings. Contrast-enhanced, helical CT can accurately assess the important tumor-vessel relationships, is less invasive, and therefore less costly than laparoscopy, which still requires general anesthesia in most centers and, therefore, remains the initial study of choice for determining whether a patient has potentially resectable, locally advanced, or metastatic disease. Laparoscopy will prevent unnec-

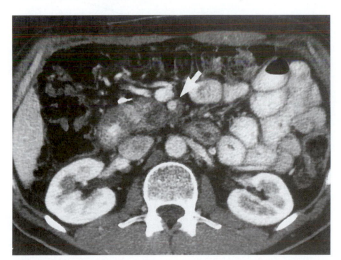

**FIGURE 13-6.** Contrast-enhanced CT scan demonstrating (in the opinion of the authors) an unresectable adenocarcinoma of the pancreatic head. Note the loss of the normal fat plane between the low-density tumor and the superior mesenteric artery (arrow); tumor is seen to be inseparable from the posterior and left lateral walls of the SMA. The superior mesenteric vein appears uninvolved.

essary laparotomy in approximately 10% to 15% of patients with presumed localized, potentially resectable pancreatic cancer following high-quality CT.[22–24] It should be used prior to laparotomy in any patient whose radiographic images or clinical presentation suggests extrapancreatic disease. The routine use of laparoscopy prior to laparotomy in all patients with potentially resectable disease is reasonable assuming both procedures are planned under the same anesthetic.

Contrast-enhanced, helical CT has also reduced the role of preoperative angiography, which only provides details of the vessel lumen; the surrounding tumor and soft tissue cannot be evaluated. The critical anatomic information that is needed to determine the anatomic relationship between the tumor and the SMA is provided by high-quality, contrast-enhanced CT or magnetic resonance imaging (MRI). We limit the use of angiography to reoperative cases, in which identification of aberrant hepatic arterial anatomy may prevent iatrogenic injury during portal dissection when there is extensive scarring from a previous biliary procedure.

## PANCREATICODUODENECTOMY

Our recommended technique for pancreaticoduodenectomy utilizes a bilateral subcostal incision. The liver and peritoneal surfaces are carefully examined to exclude the presence of metastatic disease, and intraoperative ultrasonography of the liver and pancreas is performed. We would not proceed with pancreaticoduodenectomy in the setting of a histologically positive peritoneal or liver metastasis. Random lymph node sampling is not done.

The surgical resection is divided into the following six clearly defined steps, which are performed in a clockwise direction (Fig. 13-7).[25]

### 1. EXPOSURE OF THE INFRAPANCREATIC SMV

The lesser sac is entered by removing the greater omentum from the transverse colon. The right colon is mobilized in the fashion of Cattell and Braasch and the hepatic flexure taken down. When complete, this maneuver allows cephalad retraction of the right colon and small bowel, exposing the third and fourth portions of the duodenum. Mobilization of the retroperitoneal attachments of the mesentery is necessary if venous resection and reconstruction is to be performed. The middle colic vein is identified, ligated, and divided prior to its junction with the SMV (Fig. 13-8). Routine division of the middle colic vein allows greater exposure of the infrapancreatic SMV and prevents iatrogenic traction injury during dissection of the middle colic vein–SMV junction.

### 2. KOCHER MANEUVER

The Kocher maneuver is begun at the junction of the ureter and right gonadal vein (Fig. 13-9). The gonadal vein is ligated and divided, and all fibrofatty and lymphatic tissue is removed medial to the right kidney and anterior to the inferior vena cava. The gonadal

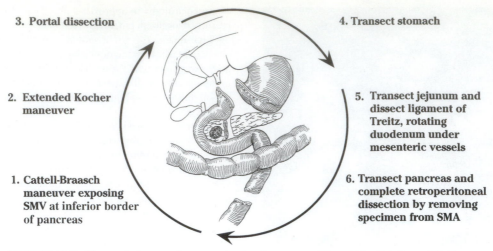

**3. Portal dissection**

**2. Extended Kocher maneuver**

**1. Cattell-Braasch maneuver exposing SMV at inferior border of pancreas**

**4. Transect stomach**

**5. Transect jejunum and dissect ligament of Treitz, rotating duodenum under mesenteric vessels**

**6. Transect pancreas and complete retroperitoneal dissection by removing specimen from SMA**

**FIGURE 13-7.** Six surgical steps of pancreaticoduodenectomy. (*From Tyler DS, Evans DB: Reoperative pancreaticoduodenectomy. Ann Surg 219:214, 1994. Reproduced with permission.*)

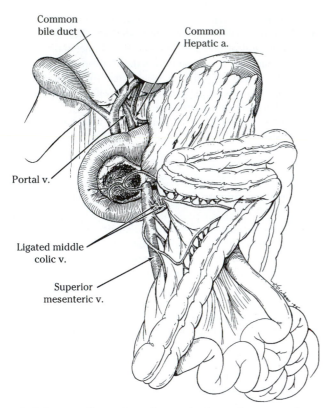

Common bile duct

Common Hepatic a.

Portal v.

Ligated middle colic v.

Superior mesenteric v.

**FIGURE 13-8.** Illustration of step 1 in the performance of pancreaticoduodenectomy. The colon has been completely mobilized in the fashion of Cattell and Braasch and the lesser sac entered. The infrapancreatic superior mesenteric vein is exposed at the inferior border of the pancreas. The middle colic vein (and usually the gastroepiploic vein) is divided. Occasionally, the middle colic and gastroepiploic veins share a common trunk. Modified from Ref. 25.

vein is again ligated at its entrance into the inferior vena cava. The Kocher maneuver is continued to the left lateral edge of the aorta, with careful identification of the left renal vein. Traditionally, the relationship of the tumor to the SMA would be assessed by manual palpation following a completed Kocher maneuver. As previously stated, preoperative contrast-enhanced CT is a more precise way of assessing this critical tumor-vessel relationship.

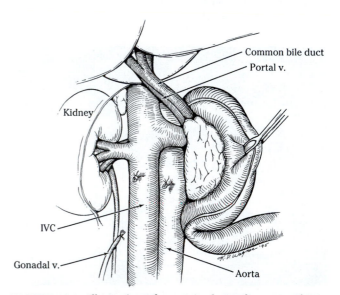

Common bile duct

Portal v.

Kidney

IVC

Gonadal v.

Aorta

**FIGURE 13-9.** Illustration of step 2 in the performance of pancreaticoduodenectomy. An extended Kocher maneuver has been performed, thereby removing all fibrofatty and lymphatic tissue anterior to the inferior vena cava (IVC) and aorta. Note the extension of the Kocher maneuver to the left lateral border of the aorta. Modified from Ref. 25.

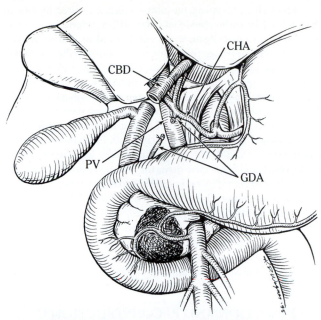

**FIGURE 13-10.** Illustration of step 3 in the performance of pancreaticoduodenectomy. Dissection of the porta hepatis begins with dissection of the common hepatic artery (CHA) and ligation and division of the gastroduodenal artery (GDA). The hepatic duct or common bile duct (CBD) is divided and the gallbladder removed from the liver bed. With the CHA reflected medially, the underlying portal vein (PV) is easily exposed. Modified from Ref. 25.

## 3. PORTAL DISSECTION

The portal dissection is initiated by exposing the common hepatic artery proximal and distal to the gastroduodenal artery. The gastroduodenal artery is then ligated and divided (Fig. 13-10). Two large lymph nodes are commonly encountered during portal dissection: one along the inferior border of the common hepatic artery, and one behind the portal vein (PV) seen after transection of the common bile duct. Removal of these lymph nodes is necessary to adequately mobilize the hepatic artery and PV. However, they rarely contain metastatic disease in the setting of a localized, otherwise resectable primary tumor. Lymph node metastases from pancreatic cancer are commonly small and are usually found by the pathologist rather than the surgeon. The gallbladder is dissected free from the liver bed, and the common bile duct is transected just cephalad to its junction with the cystic duct. The anterior wall of the PV is easily exposed following division of the common hepatic duct and medial retraction of the common hepatic artery. Loose connective tissue anterior to the PV is divided in a caudal direction to the junction of the PV and the neck of the pancreas. A constant venous tributary, the posterior superior pancreaticoduodenal vein, can be located at the superolateral aspect of the PV. Bleeding caused by traction injury to this venous tributary may be difficult to control at this time in the operation. The PV should be identified but not extensively mobilized until step 6, at which time the stomach and pancreas have been divided; iatrogenic injury to the SMV or PV prior to gastric

and pancreatic transection may result in excessive operative blood loss due to inadequate vascular exposure.

Variations in hepatic arterial circulation can complicate portal dissection. Rarely, the hepatic artery (distal to the origin of the gastroduodenal artery) courses posterior to the PV. More commonly, an accessory or replaced right hepatic artery arises from the proximal SMA and lies posterolaterally to the PV. The common hepatic artery may arise from the SMA (type IX hepatic arterial anatomy); fatal hepatic necrosis can result if this is unrecognized and the vessel is sacrificed. Identification of aberrant arterial anatomy is generally not difficult except in reoperative portal dissections; preoperative arteriography (to define arterial anatomy) is helpful in such cases.

## 4. GASTRIC TRANSECTION

The stomach is transected with a GIA (blue) tissue stapler at the level of the third or fourth transverse vein on the lesser curvature and at the confluence of the gastroepiploic veins on the greater curvature. The omentum is divided at the level of the greater curvature transection.

## 5. LIGAMENT OF TREITZ DISSECTION

The jejunum is also transected with a GIA stapler (white) approximately 10 cm distal to the ligament of Treitz, and its mesentery is sequentially ligated and divided (Fig. 13-11). The duodenal mesentery

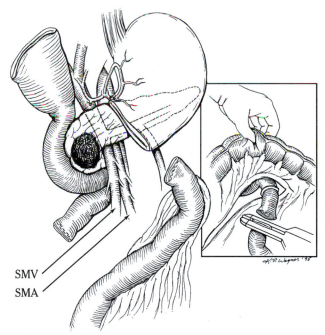

**FIGURE 13-11.** Illustration of step 5 in the performance of pancreaticoduodenectomy. Transection of the jejunum is followed by ligation and division of its mesentery. The duodenum and jejunum are reflected underneath the mesenteric vessels after dissection of the ligament of Treitz. (SMA = superior mesenteric artery; SMV = superior mesenteric vein.) Modified from Ref. 25.

is similarly divided to the level of the aorta, and the duodenum and jejunum are then reflected beneath the mesenteric vessels. Division of the jejunum at least 10 cm distal to the ligament of Treitz leaves one with a very mobile proximal jejunum, preventing unnecessary tension on the pancreaticojejunostomy at the time of pancreatico-biliary reconstruction.

## 6. RETROPERITONEAL DISSECTION

Step 6 is the most important step in the operation, and should be the main focus of surgical education with regard to the technical aspects of pancreaticoduodenectomy. After traction sutures are placed on the superior and inferior borders of the pancreas, the pancreas is transected with an electrocautery at the level of the PV. If there is evidence of tumor adherence to the PV or SMV, the pancreas can be divided at a more distal location in preparation for segmental ve-nous resection. The specimen is separated from the SMV by ligating and dividing the small venous tributaries to the uncinate process and pancreatic head (Fig. 13-12). Complete removal of the uncinate process combined with medial retraction of the SMPV confluence facilitates exposure of the SMA, which is then dissected to its ori-gin at the aorta. Visual exposure of the SMA is critically important

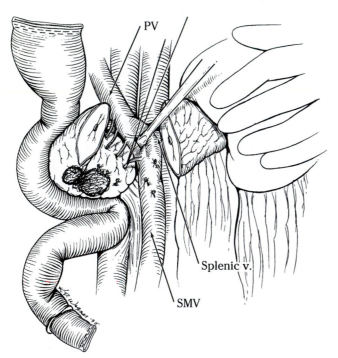

**FIGURE 13-12.** Illustration of step 6 in the performance of pan-creaticoduodenectomy; the most critical and technically challeng-ing part of the operation. The pancreas has been divided at the level of the portal vein and reflected laterally, allowing identification of small venous tributaries to the portal (PV) and superior mesenteric (SMV) veins, which are ligated and divided. Modified from Ref. 25.

(Fig. 13-13); it avoids iatrogenic injury and ensures direct ligation of the inferior pancreaticoduodenal artery (IPDA) or arteries. Control of the IPDA in a mass ligature without direct identification is likely the cause of hemorrhage (requiring reoperation) in the early post-operative period (Fig. 13-14). Further, lack of direct identification of the IPDA suggests that exposure of the SMA was inadequate and probably associated with an incomplete retroperitoneal dissection. The high incidence of local recurrence following standard pancre-aticoduodenectomy mandates that greater attention be paid to the retroperitoneal margin. Perineural invasion involving the mesen-teric plexus at the SMA origin and tumor cell infiltration of lym-phatic vessels and connective tissue may extend beyond the confines of the palpable tumor. A more extensive retroperitoneal dissection with full mobilization of the SMPV confluence and dissection of all soft tissue off of the proximal SMA is necessary to obtain a negative retroperitoneal margin. As is true for other solid tumors, adequate local-regional control of pancreatic cancer requires a negative mar-gin of excision. In addition, clear identification of the SMA avoids the potential for iatrogenic injury.

## RESECTION AND RECONSTRUCTION OF THE SMV AND/OR SMPV CONFLUENCE

Following pancreatic transection, segmental resection of the SMPV confluence is performed when, in the opinion of the surgeon, the tumor is inseparable from the lateral wall of the SMV or PV. Impor-tantly, routine resection of the SMPV confluence, as performed in re-gional pancreatectomy,[26] is not done; the SMV or SMPV confluence is resected only when deemed necessary to complete a negative-margin pancreaticoduodenectomy. When tumor invasion of the SMV or PV prevents mobilization and medial retraction of the SMPV confluence from the pancreatic head and uncinate process, access to the SMA origin and completion of the retroperitoneal dis-section can be achieved in one of two ways: (1) ligation and division of the splenic vein or (2) venous resection and reconstruction. Early in our experience with segmental resection of the SMV or SMPV confluence, division of the splenic vein was routine. Division of the splenic vein at its junction with the SMPV confluence allows access to the origin of the SMA medial to the SMV (Fig. 13-15) and pro-vides increased mobility of the PV, usually enabling a primary venous anastomosis to be constructed between the PV and SMV without tension (Fig. 13-16). If the segment of SMPV confluence to be re-sected is 3 to 4 cm or greater, an internal jugular vein interposition graft is usually required.

Splenic vein ligation, while usually a safe maneuver, occasion-ally resulted in gastrointestinal hemorrhage due to sinistral portal hypertension. Therefore, we began trying to preserve the splenic vein–PV confluence when technically possible. However, maintain-ing an intact splenic vein–PV junction significantly limits the mo-bilization of the PV and prevents primary anastomosis between the SMV and PV unless excision of the SMV is less than 2 cm. Further, an intact splenic vein prevents direct access to the proximal SMA, making completion of the retroperitoneal dissection impossible in most patients. This difficulty is circumvented by performing venous resection and reconstruction with autologous internal jugular vein

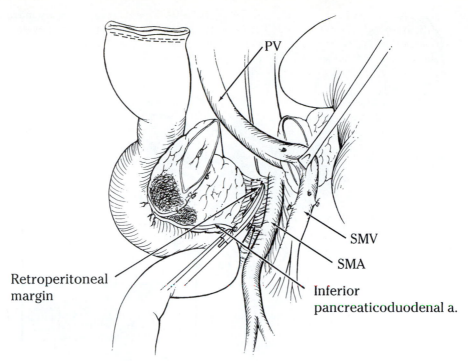

**FIGURE 13-13.** Illustration of the continuation of step 6, and the final step in resection of the specimen. Full mobilization and medial retraction of the superior mesenteric–portal vein confluence facilitates dissection of the soft tissues adjacent to the lateral wall of the proximal superior mesenteric artery (SMA); this site represents the retroperitoneal margin. The inferior pancreaticoduodenal artery(s) is identified at its origin from the SMA, ligated, and divided. (PV = portal vein; SMV = superior mesenteric vein; a. = artery.) (*From Fuhrman GM et al.*[17] *Reproduced with permission.*)

prior to completion of the retroperitoneal dissection and removal of the specimen (Fig. 13-17).[27] However, vascular reconstruction prior to specimen removal can be more difficult due to the limited exposure created by the specimen remaining in situ. In preparation for venous resection, low-dose systemic heparin is administered. When interposition grafting is performed, the SMA is temporarily cross-clamped prior to venous occlusion. This maneuver serves to prevent venous congestion and edema of the small bowel.

## PATHOLOGIC EVALUATION OF THE PANCREATICODUODENECTOMY SPECIMEN

Similar to the radiographic criteria used to determine resectability, standardized criteria are needed for the pathologic analysis of pancreaticoduodenectomy specimens to allow accurate interpretation of survival statistics (Table 13-4).[28] The surgeon and pathologist should evaluate each pancreaticoduodenectomy specimen together. Dissection of the specimen begins with frozen-section examination of the common bile duct transection margin and the pancreatic transection margin; re-resection is performed if either of these margins is positive. The retroperitoneal margin is evaluated by permanent

**TABLE 13-4.** PATHOLOGIC EVALUATION OF THE PANCREATICODUODENECTOMY SPECIMEN

A. Frozen-Section Analysis
  1. Bile duct transection margin
  2. Pancreatic transection margin
B. Permanent-Section Analysis
  1. Retroperitoneal margin
  2. Tumor histopathologic type
  3. Degree of differentiation (tumor histopathologic grade)
  4. Tissue of origin (pancreas, distal bile duct, ampulla of Vater, duodenum)
  5. Maximal transverse tumor diameter
  6. Histologic evidence of invasion:
       Vascular
       Lymphatic
       Perineural
       Superior mesenteric or portal vein (when applicable)
  7. Standard pathologic evaluation of lymph node status (anatomic dissection board)
  8. Grade of chemoradiation effect (when applicable)

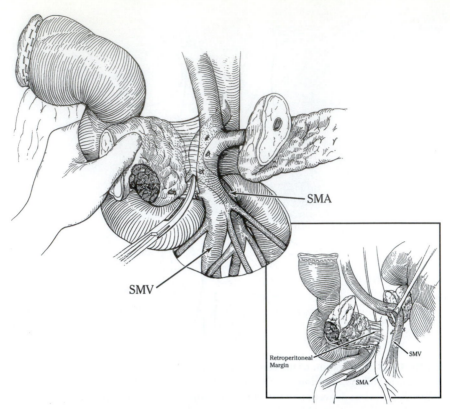

**FIGURE 13-14.** Illustration demonstrating the potential for arterial injury during the final step in pancreaticoduodenectomy if the retroperitoneal dissection is performed without direct visualization of the lateral wall of the superior mesenteric artery (SMA). Lateral traction on the specimen can cause lateral displacement of the proximal SMA making arterial injury possible. In contrast (see insert), complete medial mobilization of the superior mesenteric–portal vein confluence and direct visualization of the SMA will avoid iatrogenic arterial injury and allow the performance of a more complete retroperitoneal dissection. (SMV = superior mesenteric vein.) (*From Pisters PWT et al. Standard forms of pancreatic resection, in* Pancreatic Cancer Pathogenesis, Diagnosis, and Treatment, *HA Reber (ed). Totowa, NJ, Humana Press, 1998, pp 181–200. Reproduced with permission.*)

section and is defined as the soft-tissue margin directly adjacent to the proximal 3 to 4 cm of the SMA (Fig. 13-18). At the time of initial gross inspection of the specimen, this margin is either inked, or a 2- to 3-mm full-face (en face) section of the margin is taken. This margin represents the soft tissue margin most likely to be positive and specifically reflects the extent of tumor growth posterior and medial to the SMPV confluence. Identification of the retroperitoneal margin of resection is not possible once the gross examination of the specimen has been completed. The retroperitoneal margin is the most frequent site of margin positivity following pancreaticoduodenectomy and accurate analysis of this margin is critical when performing outcome studies using survival duration or local tumor control as primary study endpoints. Samples of multiple areas of each tumor, including the interface between tumor and adjacent uninvolved tissue, are submitted for paraffin-embedded histologic examination (5 to 10 blocks). Sections 4 $\mu$m are cut and stained with hematoxylin and eosin. Final pathologic evaluation of perma-

nent sections includes a description of tumor histology and differentiation; gross and microscopic evaluation of the tissue of origin (pancreas, bile duct, ampulla of Vater, or duodenum); and assessments of maximal transverse tumor diameter, lymph node status, and the presence or absence of perineural, lymphatic, and vascular invasion. When segmental resection of the SMV is required, the area of presumed tumor invasion of the vein wall is serially sectioned and examined in an attempt to discriminate benign fibrous attachment from direct tumor invasion.

The method for classifying subsets of regional lymph nodes in pancreaticoduodenectomy specimens is based on the work of Cubilla.[29] The soft fibrofatty tissue containing regional lymph nodes is divided into six regions as outlined on the anatomic pathology dissection board (Fig. 13-19). If lymph nodes are not identified, fat or other potentially neoplastic tissue is submitted for microscopic examination. Previous work from our institution has demonstrated that the number of lymph nodes identified in the surgical specimen

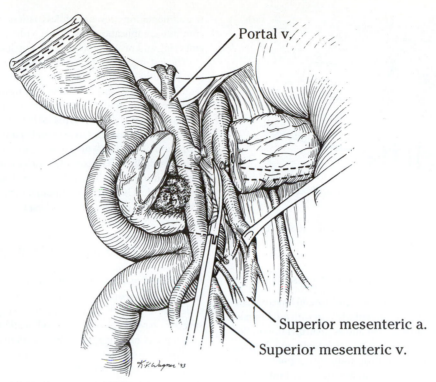

Portal v.

Superior mesenteric a.

Superior mesenteric v.

**FIGURE 13-15.** Illustration of the final step in pancreaticoduodenectomy when segmental venous resection and splenic vein ligation is required. In preparation for segmental resection of the superior mesenteric vein, the splenic vein has been divided and the superior mesenteric artery identified. The retroperitoneal dissection is completed by dissecting the specimen free from the lateral wall of the artery. The tumor is then attached only by the superior mesenteric–portal venous confluence. (*From Cusack JC et al.*[18] *Reproduced with permission.*)

is increased by the use of a standardized system of specimen analysis. The dissection board provides a simple means of improving lymph node identification and documenting the location of histologically confirmed lymph node metastases. As the use of multimodality treatment strategies for pancreatic cancer becomes more common, it will be critical to standardize pathologic assessment of tumor specimens.

## PANCREATIC, BILIARY, AND GASTROINTESTINAL RECONSTRUCTION

Reconstruction proceeds in a counterclockwise direction incorporating the following three steps (Fig. 13-20)[25]:

### 1. PANCREATICOJEJUNOSTOMY

The pancreatic remnant is mobilized from the retroperitoneum and splenic vein for a distance of 2 to 3 cm; failure to adequately mobilize the pancreatic remnant results in poor suture placement. The transected jejunum is brought retrocolic through a defect in the transverse mesocolon to the left of the middle colic vessels. We prefer

to bring the jejunum retrocolic rather than retroperitoneal (posterior to the mesenteric vessels in the bed of the resected duodenum). A two-layer, end-to-side, duct-to-mucosa pancreaticojejunostomy is performed over a small Silastic stent (Dow Corning, Midland, MI) (Fig. 13-21). If the pancreatic duct is not dilated, a stent is not necessary. Following completion of the posterior row of interrupted 4-0 Proline seromuscular sutures, a small full-thickness opening in the bowel is made. The anastomosis between the pancreatic duct and the small bowel mucosa is completed with 4-0 or 5-0 monofilament absorbable sutures (PDS). Each stitch incorporates a generous bite of the pancreatic duct and a full-thickness bite of the jejunum. The posterior knots are tied on the inside and the lateral and anterior knots on the outside. Prior to the anterior sutures being tied, the stent is placed across the anastomosis so that it extends into the pancreatic duct and small bowel for a distance of approximately 2 to 3 cm. The anastomosis is completed with placement of an anterior row of 4-0 seromuscular sutures.

### 2. HEPATICOJEJUNOSTOMY

A single-layer biliary anastomosis is performed using interrupted, 4-0 absorbable monofilament sutures. It is important to align the

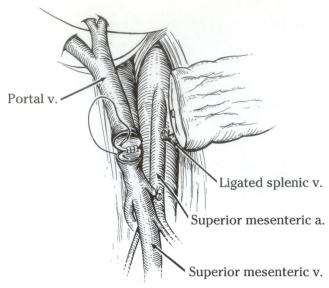

Portal v.

Ligated splenic v.

Superior mesenteric a.

Superior mesenteric v.

**FIGURE 13-16.** Illustration of a primary end-to-end anastomosis of the portal vein and the superior mesenteric vein with 6-0 Prolene suture. Transection of the splenic vein allows identification of the SMA, located medial to the SMV, while also providing adequate length for a primary venous anastomosis following segmental vein resection. If the splenic vein–portal vein junction is left intact, the portal vein remains relatively nonmobile, making reconstruction of the SMV (following segmental resection) difficult or impossible without interposition grafting (see Fig. 13-17). (*From Cusack JC et al.[17] Reproduced with permission.*)

jejunum with the bile duct to avoid tension on the pancreatic and biliary anastomoses. We also leave enough room between the two anastomoses so that the falciform ligament can be placed between the hepatic artery [at the level of the gastroduodenal artery (GDA) origin] and the afferent jejunal limb. A stent is not used in the construction of the hepaticojejunostomy.

## 3. GASTROJEJUNOSTOMY

An antecolic, end-to-side gastrojejunostomy is constructed in two layers. Starting from the greater curvature, 6 to 8 cm of the gastric staple line is removed. A posterior row of 3-0 sutures is followed by a running, monofilament, full-thickness inner layer; the anterior row of 3-0 sutures complete the anastomosis. The distance between the biliary and gastric anastomoses should allow the jejunum to assume its antecolic position (for the gastrojejunostomy) without tension 40–50 cm. The jejunal limb should be aligned so that the efferent limb is adjacent to the greater curvature of the stomach.

Gastrostomy and feeding jejunostomy tubes are placed using the Witzel technique, and then two closed-suction drains are placed. Delayed gastric emptying is common after this operation. Placement of an 18 French gastrostomy tube for intermittent drainage and placement of a 10 French jejunal feeding tube for postopera-

tive alimentation prevent needless patient morbidity from the most common complications associated with this operation: poor gastric emptying and resulting inadequate nutritional support.

The last maneuver performed prior to closure of the abdomen is to place the falciform ligament over the stump of the GDA. This requires a mobile length of falciform ligament, which may not be available in reoperative patients (in which case omentum is used). The vascularized falciform is placed between the GDA stump and the afferent limb of jejunum to prevent hepatic artery pseudoaneurysm formation at the GDA origin with resulting arterioenteric fistula. This complication is usually due to a leak at the pancreaticojejunostomy resulting in localized infection or abscess formation extending to involve the GDA stump. Although infrequent, this complication is usually fatal; prevention is the best treatment.

## PYLORUS PRESERVATION

Preservation of the antropyloroduodenal segment in combination with pancreaticoduodenectomy was first described by Traverso and colleagues[30] in 1978. Since then, increasing numbers of pancreatic surgeons have employed this modification of the procedure. This technique is mainly applicable to patients with benign disease or small periampullary lesions. Proponents of the technique argue that preservation of the antropyloric pump mechanism results in improved long-term upper gastrointestinal tract function.[31] Detractors of this modification of the procedure counter that the reported improvements in gastrointestinal and nutritional functions are small, if any, and that they come at the expense of an increased incidence of early postoperative delayed gastric emptying.[32] Further, in some patients, leaving the distal stomach and duodenum may compromise margins of excision. Pylorus preservation should not be performed for patients with bulky tumors of the pancreatic head, duodenal tumors involving the first or second portions of the duodenum, or lesions in which pyloric and peripyloric lymph nodes are grossly positive.

The steps in pylorus-preserving pancreaticoduodenectomy are identical to those in standard pancreaticoduodenectomy except in the approach to the antrum, pylorus, and duodenum (steps 3 and 4). During the portal dissection, it is important to avoid unnecessary division of the right gastric artery or injury to the nerves of Laterjet. This is the fundamental technical difference in the pylorus-preserving procedure and is essential in facilitating a well-vascularized duodenojejunostomy and avoiding postoperative gastroparesis. The duodenum is divided approximately 2 to 3 cm beyond the pylorus. If tumor encroachment prevents creation of a well-vascularized segment, the surgeon should either create the duodenojejunostomy closer to the pylorus to ensure its vascularity or proceed with a distal gastrectomy. The duodenojejunostomy is performed in an end-to-side fashion using a single-layer technique with monofilament absorbable sutures.

## ADJUVANT OR NEOADJUVANT TREATMENT

External-beam radiation therapy (EBRT) and concomitant 5-FU chemotherapy (chemoradiation) were shown to prolong survival in

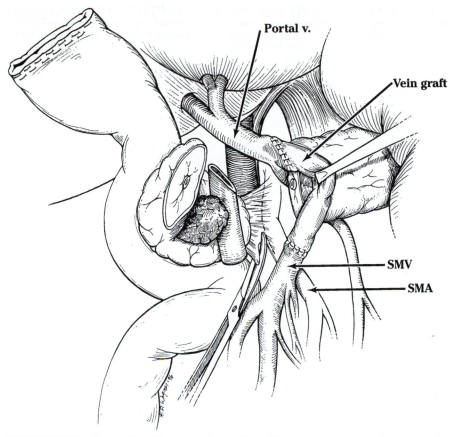

**FIGURE 13-17.** Illustration of segmental resection of the superior mesenteric–portal vein confluence with splenic vein preservation. With the splenic vein intact, exposure is often inadequate to separate the specimen from the lateral aspect of the proximal superior mesenteric artery (SMA). Therefore, the graft is usually placed prior to completing the retroperitoneal dissection. The reconstructed superior mesenteric–portal vein confluence can then be retracted medially, allowing the specimen to be removed from the proximal SMA under direct vision. When interposition grafting is performed, the SMA is temporarily cross-clamped (not shown) to prevent vascular congestion of the small bowel. (SMV = superior mesenteric vein; v. = vein.) (*From Leach SD et al.*[27] *Reproduced with permission.*)

patients with locally advanced adenocarcinoma of the pancreas.[33] Those data were the foundation for a Gastrointestinal Tumor Study Group (GITSG) prospective randomized study of adjuvant chemoradiation (500 mg/m$^2$ per day of 5-FU for 6 days and 40 Gy of radiation) following pancreaticoduodenectomy (Table 13-5).[34–41] That trial also demonstrated a survival advantage from multimodality therapy compared to resection alone. Because of a prolonged recovery from surgery, adjuvant therapy was delayed as long as 10 weeks in 5 (24%) of the 21 patients in the adjuvant chemoradiation arm. This, despite the obvious selection bias in patient accrual; the patients likely to be considered for protocol entry were those who recovered rapidly from surgery and had a good performance status. Similar findings have recently been reported from the European Organization for Research and Treatment of Cancer (EORTC). The EORTC initiated a study in 1987 comparing adjuvant 5-FU–based chemora-

diation following pancreatectomy with surgery alone. Between 1987 and 1995, 218 patients were randomized to receive either chemoradiation or no further treatment following pancreaticoduodenectomy for adenocarcinoma of the pancreas (55%) or periampullary region (45%). Of those randomized to receive chemoradiation, 22% did not receive intended therapy due to postoperative complications or patient refusal.[42]

Despite the selection bias likely in effect when attempts are made to retrospectively compare patients who received postoperative adjuvant chemoradiation with patients who were treated only with pancreaticoduodenectomy, recently reported data from Yeo and colleagues[38] at Johns Hopkins University add further support to the use of multimodality therapy. Those investigators reviewed all patients who underwent pancreaticoduodenectomy for adenocarcinoma of the pancreatic head during a 4-year period; 120 patients

**TABLE 13-5.** RECENT CHEMORADIATION STUDIES IN PATIENTS WITH RESECTABLE PANCREATIC CANCER

| FIRST AUTHOR (YEAR) | NO. PATIENTS* | EBRT DOSE, GY | CHEMOTHERAPY AGENT | MEDIAN SURVIVAL, MONTHS |
|---|---|---|---|---|
| POSTOP (ADJUVANT) | | | | |
| Kalser (1985)[34] | 21 | 40 | 5-FU | 20 |
|    Surgery alone | 22 | — | — | 11 |
| GITSG (1987)[35] | 30 | 40 | 5-FU | 18 |
| Whittington (1991)[36] | 28 | 45–63 | 5-FU | 16 |
| Foo (1993)[37] | 29 | 35–60 | 5-FU | 23 |
| Yeo (1997)[38] | 120 | >45 | 5-FU | 20 |
|    Surgery alone | 53 | — | — | 14 |
| PREOP (NEOADJUVANT) | | | | |
| Hoffman (1998)[39] | 24 | 50.4 | 5-FU, Mito-C | 16 |
| Staley (1996)[40] | 39 | 30–50.4 | 5-FU | 19 |
| Pisters (1998)[41] | 20 | 30 | 5-FU | 25 |

*All patients underwent a pancreatectomy with curative intent.
ABBREVIATIONS: EBRT = external beam radiation therapy; 5-FU = 5-fluorouracil; Mito-C = mitomycin C.

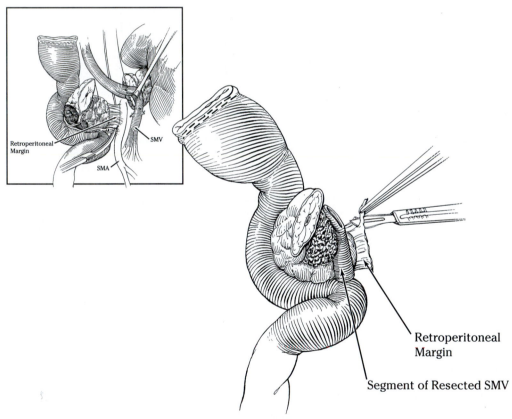

**FIGURE 13-18.** Illustration of the retroperitoneal margin as defined at the time of tumor resection. A 2- to 3-mm full-face (en face) section of the margin is taken at the time of initial specimen analysis. Alternatively, the retroperitoneal margin can simply be linked at the time of gross evaluation and histologically evaluated on permanent-sections of the specimen. This specimen is shown with a segment of superior mesenteric vein (SMV) removed with the pancreatic head; the retroperitoneal margin is defined the same way when pancreaticoduodenectomy does not require vein resection (insert). This margin reflects the extent of tumor growth posterior and medial to the SMPV confluence along the right lateral border of the superior mesenteric artery (SMA).

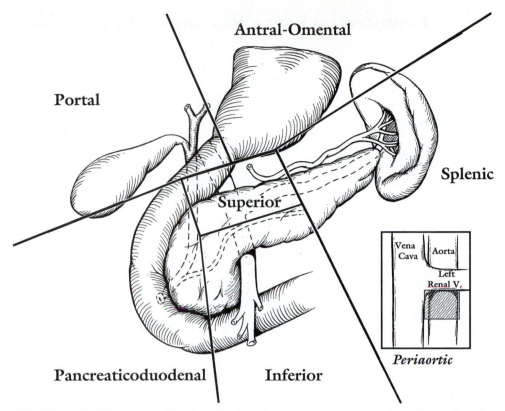

**FIGURE 13-19.** Illustration of the dissection board used to separate the specimen into regions for lymph node analysis (V. = vein).

received adjuvant chemoradiation, and 53 underwent pancreaticoduodenectomy alone. Median survival for those receiving adjuvant therapy was 19.5 months compared with 13.5 months for the group who received surgery alone.

The risk of delaying adjuvant therapy, combined with small published experiences of successful pancreatic resection following EBRT, prompted many institutions to initiate studies in which chemoradiation was given in a preoperative or neoadjuvant setting for patients with potentially resectable (or locally advanced) adenocarcinoma of the pancreas. The preoperative use of chemoradiation is supported by the following considerations[12,43]:

1.  Radiation therapy is more effective on well-oxygenated cells that have not been devascularized by surgery.
2.  Peritoneal tumor cell implantation due to the manipulation of surgery may be prevented by preoperative chemoradiation.
3.  Because chemotherapy and irradiation will be given first, delayed postoperative recovery will have no effect on the delivery of multimodality therapy.
4.  The high frequency of positive-margin resections recently reported supports the concern that the retroperitoneal margin of excision, even when negative, may be only a few millimeters.
5.  Patients with disseminated disease evident on restaging studies after chemoradiation (up to 25%) will not be subjected to laparotomy.

In patients who receive chemoradiation prior to surgery, a repeat staging CT scan after chemoradiation reveals extrapancreatic disease in approximately 25% of patients. If these patients had undergone pancreaticoduodenectomy at the time of diagnosis, it is probable that the liver metastases would have been subclinical; these patients would therefore have undergone a major surgical procedure only to have liver metastases found soon after surgery. In the M. D. Anderson Cancer Center trails, patients who were found to have disease progression at the time of restaging had a median survival of only 7 months.[44] The avoidance of a lengthy recovery period and the potential morbidity of pancreaticoduodenectomy in patients with such a short expected survival time represents a distinct advantage of preoperative over postoperative chemoradiation. When delivering multimodality therapy for any disease, it is beneficial, when possible, to deliver the most toxic therapy last, thereby avoiding morbidity in patients who experience rapid disease progression not amenable to currently available therapies.

Because of the documented low response rates to systemic therapy in patients with advanced disease, there is ongoing work toward understanding the molecular basis of chemosensitivity and metastasis. New agents are being investigated in order to combine conventional chemoradiation and surgery with the systemic or regional delivery of novel agents that inhibit essential steps in tumor cell growth. The evolution of preoperative or neoadjuvant

# Counterclockwise Reconstruction

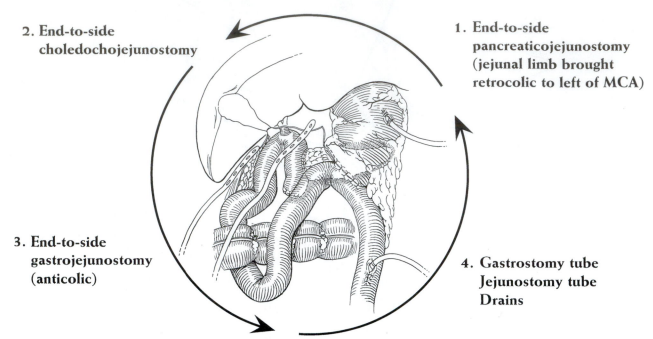

**2. End-to-side choledochojejunostomy**

**1. End-to-side pancreaticojejunostomy (jejunal limb brought retrocolic to left of MCA)**

**3. End-to-side gastrojejunostomy (anticolic)**

**4. Gastrostomy tube Jejunostomy tube Drains**

**FIGURE 13-20.** Four surgical steps of reconstruction following pancreaticoduodenectomy. Following pancreaticobiliary and gastric reconstruction, gastrostomy and jejunostomy tubes are routinely placed along with one or two closed suction drains. MCA = middle colic artery. (*From Tyler DS, Evans DB: Reoperative pancreaticoduodenectomy. Ann Surg 219:214, 1994. Reproduced with permission.*)

multimodality therapy for patients with potentially resectable pancreatic cancer appears in Fig. 13-22.

## TREATMENT OF LOCALLY ADVANCED DISEASE

Patients with clear evidence of encasement of the celiac axis or SMA or occlusion of the SMPV confluence on contrast-enhanced helical CT do not require laparotomy to confirm that the tumor is unresectable; cytologic confirmation of malignancy can be achieved with FNA performed under the guidance of either EUS or CT. This fundamental advance in pretreatment diagnosis for patients with pancreatic cancer will improve the quality of patient survival and reduce health care costs by avoiding the morbidity and prolonged recovery associated with palliative pancreatic cancer surgery.

A pilot trial of 5-FU and supervoltage radiation therapy in patients with locally advanced adenocarcinoma of the pancreas served as the foundation for a subsequent study of 5-FU–based chemoradiation by the GITSG.[45] All patients were surgically staged; only patients with disease confined to the pancreas and peripancreatic organs, regional lymph nodes, and regional peritoneum were eligible for treatment. Radiation therapy was delivered as a split course

with 20 Gy given over 2 weeks followed by a 2-week rest. Patients received a total of either 40 or 60 Gy. 5-FU was delivered intravenously at a bolus dose of 500 mg/m$^2$ per day for the first 3 days of each 20-Gy cycle and given weekly (500 mg/m$^2$) following the completion of chemoradiation. Patients were randomized to receive 40 Gy plus 5-FU, 60 Gy plus 5-FU, or 60 Gy without chemotherapy. Median survival was 10 months in each of the chemoradiation groups and 6 months for patients who received 60 Gy without 5-FU. Additional chemotherapy beyond 5-FU–based chemoradiation increased toxicity without apparent therapeutic benefit.

All patients were entered in the GITSG studies following laparotomy, at which time the disease was deemed unresectable by the operating surgeon. Chemoradiation was reasonably well tolerated following major surgery. Approximately 80% of patients completed chemoradiation, and the two fatal septic events were believed not to be treatment related. The most frequent toxic effects were nausea and vomiting, which were seldom severe. The significant morbidity reported with palliative pancreatic surgery suggests that only patients with a high-performance status could have recovered rapidly enough to be eligible for these studies. Thus, although surgical staging made for a more uniform study population, it also introduced significant selection bias: only rapidly recovering patients were

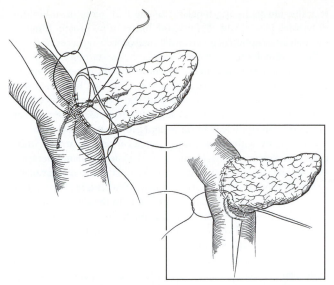

**FIGURE 13-21.** Illustration of step 1 in the reconstruction after pancreaticoduodenectomy. A two-layer, end-to-side, duct-to-mucosa pancreaticojejunostomy is performed over a small stent. The stent (4- to 5-cm long) is sewn to the pancreatic duct with absorbable suture.

considered for treatment. Comparison of future studies to these data must account for this selection bias.

Currently, continuous-infusion 5-FU in dosages of 250 to 300 mg/m$^2$ per day for 5 or 7 days a week has been given during EBRT [50 to 55 Gy in 5.5 weeks (1.8 Gy per fraction)]. In patients with locally advanced pancreatic cancer, treatment can be administered in the outpatient setting, and 5-FU is given through a portable pump attached to a percutaneous central venous catheter. Acute side effects include nausea, diarrhea, vomiting, weight loss, fatigue, and hand/foot syndrome, but rarely is leukopenia encountered. Acute toxicity during 5-FU chemoradiation is decreased by administering 5-FU for 5 days a week rather than 7 days a week. The late effects of combined-modality therapy do not appear to be increased compared to those seen with EBRT alone. Paclitaxel and gemcitabine represent two new radiation enhancers that are currently under clinical evaluation.

The increased length of survival for patients treated with chemoradiation is limited largely to patients with higher performance status. Therefore, a program of 5-FU–based chemoradiation is justified in fully ambulatory patients with locally advanced disease who have minimal symptoms. Systemic therapy with gemcitabine also represents a reasonable alternative in these patients. For patients with poor performance status, chemoradiation is probably not indicated. Current pharmacologic and interventional techniques for

# Multimodality therapy of potentially resectable pancreatic cancer

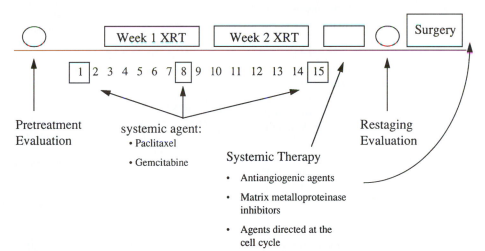

**FIGURE 13-22.** The future of multimodality therapy for patients with potentially resectable adenocarcinoma of the pancreatic head. Treatment schemas emphasize the importance of minimizing toxicity and treatment duration while attempting to improve therapeutic efficacy. Cytotoxicity is enhanced by combining radiation therapy with more potent radiation-sensitizing agents. Systemic therapy is continued after both chemoradiation and surgery with systemic agents of low toxicity directed at specific molecular events involved in pancreatic tumorigenesis [i.e., inhibition of angiogenesis, the use of protease inhibitors (matrix metalloproteinase inhibitors), or inhibition of ras-dependent signal transduction].

pain control, including percutaneous injection of alcohol into the celiac plexus, have proven highly successful in patients with pancreatic cancer. Further, adequate pain control improves performance status and quality of life, which may translate into increased length of life. The limited therapeutic options available for patients with locally advanced disease and the modest impact of current treatments on survival rates provide the rationale for the entry of patients into trials examining novel systemic agents.

## TREATMENT OF METASTATIC AND RECURRENT DISEASE

Most studies of single-agent or combination chemotherapy in patients with advanced adenocarcinoma of the pancreas have documented low response rates and little reproducible impact on patient survival or quality of life. Response rates as high as 15% to 30% occasionally seen in pilot studies of novel agents or combinations have not been reproduced, suggesting that patient selection often accounts for apparent differences between study results. The inherent difficulty in accurately applying bidimensional measurements to pancreatic masses and the problem of interobserver variations in the measurement of metastatic disease may contribute to the poor reproducibility of clinical trials in patients with locally advanced or metastatic pancreatic cancer.

Gemcitabine (2',2'-difluorodeoxycytidine, Gemzar) is a deoxycytidine analogue with structural and metabolic similarities to cytarabine. In both preclinical and clinical testing, gemcitabine demonstrated activity in solid tumors greater than that of cytarabine. Following phase I study, gemcitabine was evaluated in a multicenter trial of 44 patients with advanced pancreatic cancer.[46] Although only five objective responses were documented, the investigators noted frequent subjective symptomatic benefit, often in the absence of an objective tumor response. Based on these observations, two subsequent trials of gemcitabine in patients with advanced pancreatic cancer have been completed.[47,48] In one randomized trial, gemcitabine was compared to 5-FU in previously untreated patients. Patients treated with gemcitabine had a median survival of 5.65 months compared to 4.41 months ($p = 0.0025$) in those treated with 5-FU. Of patients treated with gemcitabine, 24% were alive at 9 months compared with 6% of patients treated with 5-FU. In addition, more clinically meaningful effects on disease-related symptoms (pain control, performance status, weight gain) were seen with gemcitabine (23.8% of patients) than with 5-FU (4.8% of patients). Similar systemic effects and demonstrable disease responses were documented in patients who were treated with gemcitabine after experiencing disease progression while receiving 5-FU.

Despite the recent encouraging results with gemcitabine, however, median survival for patients with metastatic disease continues to be less than 6 months, with very few patients achieving long-term disease stabilization. Some of the effects attributed to chemotherapy may not be substantially different from what can be achieved with aggressive supportive care alone. Study of novel chemotherapeutic agents based on our improved understanding of the pathobiology of pancreatic cancer represent exciting areas of research. A number of general areas of clinical investigation may yield favorable results including interruption or modulation of growth factors and signal transduction pathways, blockade of the EGF receptor, inhibition of tyrosine kinase, and chemical inhibition of *ras* protein function through interruption of posttranslational processing necessary to localize *ras* proteins to the plasma cell membrane (farnesyl transferase inhibitors). A second general approach utilizes genetic strategies to inhibit dominant oncogene function. The high frequency with which K-*ras* is altered in exocrine pancreatic cancer and its central function in signal transduction suggest that inhibiting production of this protein could lead to significant growth-inhibitory effects.

For patients with metastatic pancreatic cancer who present with a good performance status, treatment with systemic chemotherapy is appropriate. In view of the limited impact of the currently available agents on survival, continued enrollment of patients in phase II trials of new agents or combinations is essential. In the absence of access to a phase II trial, treatment with gemcitabine appears to be the evolving standard. However, it must be recognized that the primary impact of gemcitabine is on disease-related symptoms. Continued evaluation of novel agents, especially those targeted against specific molecular events important in the pathogenesis of pancreatic cancer, is crucial.

## REFERENCES

1. Greenlee RT et al: Cancer Statistics, 2000. CA Cancer J Clin 50:13, 2000.
2. Silverman DT et al: Cigarette smoking and pancreas cancer: A case-control study based on direct interviews. J Natl Cancer Inst 86:1510, 1994.
3. Lowenfels AB et al: Pancreatitis and the risk of pancreatic cancer. N Engl J Med 328:1433, 1993.
4. Whitcomb D et al: A gene for hereditary pancreatitis maps to 7q35. Gastroenterology 110:1975, 1996.
5. Almoguera C et al: Most human carcinomas of the exocrine pancreas contain mutant c-K-ras genes. Cell 53:549, 1988.
6. Abbruzzese JL et al: Detection of mutated c-Ki-ras in the bile of patients with pancreatic cancer. Anticancer Res 17:795, 1997.
7. Bold RJ et al: Prognostic factors in resectable pancreatic cancer: p53 and bcl-2. J Gastrointestinal Surg 3:263, 1999.
8. Hahn SA et al: DPC4 a candidate tumor suppressor gene at human chromosome 18q21.1. Science 271:350, 1996.
9. Massague J: TGF signaling: Receptors, transducers, and mad proteins. Cell 85:947, 1996.
10. Caldas C et al: Frequent somatic mutations and homozygous deletions on the p16 (MTS1) gene in pancreatic adenocarcinoma. Nat Genet 8:27, 1994.
11. Hruban RH et al: Genetics of pancreatic cancer. From genes to families. Surg Oncol Clin North Am 7(1):1, 1998.
12. Evans DB et al: Cancer of the pancreas, in *Cancer: Principles and Practice of Oncology*, ed 5. VT De Vita Jr et al (eds). Philadelphia, Lippincott, 1997.
13. Chow WH et al: Risk of pancreatic cancer following diabetes mellitus: a nationwide cohort study in Sweden. J Natl Cancer Inst 87:930, 1995.
14. Everhart J, Wright D: Diabetes mellitus as a risk factor for pancreatic cancer. A meta-analysis. JAMA 273:1605, 1995.
15. Fleming ID et al (eds): *American Joint Committee on Cancer Manual for Staging of Cancer*, 5th ed. Philadelphia, Lippincott, 1977, pp 121–126.
16. Evans DB et al: Cancer of the Pancreas, in *UICC Manual of*

*Clinical Oncology*, 7th ed. RE Pollock (ed). New York, John Wiley, 1999, pp 453–475.

17. FUHRMAN GM et al: Thin-section contrast enhanced computed tomography accurately predicts the resectability of malignant pancreatic neoplasms. Am J Surg 167:104, 1994.

18. CUSAK JC et al: Managing unsuspected tumor invasion of the superior mesenteric-portal venous confluence during pancreaticoduodenectomy. Am J Surg 168:352, 1994.

19. BRESLIN TM et al: Neoadjuvant chemoradiation for adenocarcinoma of the pancreas. Front Biosci 3:193, 1998.

20. MILLER AR et al: Neoadjuvant chemoradiation and pancreaticduodenectomy for adenocarcinoma of the pancreas. Surg Oncol Clin North Am 7:183, 1998.

21. SMITH AC et al: Prospective randomized trial of bypass surgery versus endoscopic stenting in patients with malignant obstructive jaundice. Gut 30:A1513, 1989.

22. ANDREN-SANDBERG A et al: Computed tomography and laparoscopy in the assessment of the patient with pancreatic cancer. J Am Coll Surg 186:35, 1998.

23. FRIESS H et al: The role of diagnostic laparoscopy in pancreatic and periampullary malignancies. J Am Coll Surg 186:675, 1998.

24. HOLZMAN MD et al: The role of laparoscopy in the management of suspected pancreatic and periampullary malignancies. J Gastrointest Surg 1:236, 1997.

25. NYHUS LM et al (eds): Pancreaticoduodenectomy (Whipple operation) and total pancreatectomy for cancer, in *Mastery of Surgery*, 3d ed. Boston, Little, Brown 1233, 1997.

26. FORTNER J: Technique of regional subtotal and total pancreatectomy. Am J Surg 150:593, 985.

27. LEACH SD et al: Survival following pancreaticoduodenectomy with resection of the superior mesenteric-portal vein confluence for adenocarcinoma of the pancreatic head. Br J Surg 85:611, 1998.

28. STALEY C et al: Need for standardized pathologic staging of pancreaticoduodenectomy specimens. Pancreas 12:373, 1996.

29. CUBILLA AL et al: Lymph node involvement in carcinoma of the head of the pancreas area. Cancer 41:880, 1978.

30. TRAVERSO LW, LONGMIRE WP: Preservation of the pylorus in pancreaticoduodenectomy. Surg Gynecol Obstet 146:959, 1978.

31. GRACE PA et al: Pylorus preserving pancreaticoduodenectomy: an overview. Br J Surg 77:968, 1990.

32. PATEL AG et al: Pylorus-preserving Whipple resection for pancreatic cancer. Arch Surg 130:838, 1995.

33. GASTROINTESTINAL TUMOR STUDY GROUP: A multi-institutional comparative trial of radiation therapy alone and in combination with 5-fluorouracil for locally unresectable pancreatic carcinoma. Ann Surg 189:205, 1979.

34. KALSER MH, ELLENBERG SS: Pancreatic cancer: Adjuvant combined radiation and chemotherapy following curative resection. Arch Surg 120:899, 1985.

35. GASTROINTESTINAL TUMOR STUDY GROUP: Further evidence of effective adjuvant combined radiation and chemotherapy following curative resection of pancreatic cancer. Cancer 59:2006, 1987.

36. WHITTINGTON R et al: Adjuvant therapy of resected adenocarcinoma of the pancreas. Int J Radiat Oncol Biol Phys 21:1137, 1991.

37. FOO ML et al: Patterns of failure in grossly resected pancreatic ductal adenocarcinoma treated with adjuvant irradiation + 5-fluorouracil. Int J Radiat Oncol Biol Phys 26:483, 1993.

38. YEO C et al: Pancreaticoduodenectomy for pancreatic adenocarcinoma postoperative adjuvant chemoradiation improves survival. Ann Surg 225:621, 1997.

39. HOFFMAN J et al: Phase II trial of preoperative radiation therapy and chemotherapy for patients with localized, resectable adenocarcinoma of the pancreas. An Eastern Cooperative Oncology Group study. J Clin Oncol 16:317, 1998.

40. STALEY C et al: Preoperative chemoradiation, pancreaticoduodenectomy, and intraoperative radiation therapy for adenocarcinoma of the pancreatic head. Am J Surg 171:118, 1996.

41. PISTERS PWT et al: Rapid-fractionation preoperative chemoradiation, pancreaticoduodenectomy, and intraoperative radiation therapy for resectable pancreatic adenocarcinoma. J Clin Oncol 16:3843, 1998.

42. KLINKENBIJL J et al: Radiotherapy and 5-FU after curative resection for cancer of the pancreas and peri-ampullary region: A phase III trial of the EORTC CITCCG (abstract). Eur J Cancer 33(S8):1239, 1997.

43. EVANS DB et al: Preoperative chemoradiation and pancreaticoduodenectomy for adenocarcinoma of the pancreas. Arch Surg 127:1335, 1992.

44. SPITZ F et al: Preoperative and postoperative chemoradiation strategies in patients treated with pancreaticoduodenectomy for adenocarcinoma of the pancreas. J Clin Oncol 15:928, 1997.

45. MOERTEL CG et al: Therapy of locally unresectable pancreatic carcinoma: a randomized comparison of high dose (6000 rads) radiation alone, moderate dose radiation and 5-fluorouracil. Cancer 48:1705, 1981.

46. CASPER ES et al: Phase II trial of gemcitabine (2,'2'-difluorodeoxycytidine) in patients with adenocarcinoma of the pancreas. Invest New Drugs 12:29, 1994.

47. BURRIS HA 3d et al: Improvements in survival and clinical benefit with gemcitabine as first-line therapy for patients with advanced pancreas cancer: a randomized trial. J Clin Oncol 15:2403, 1997.

48. ROTHENBERG ML et al: Gemcitabine effective palliative therapy for pancreas patients failing 5-FU (abstract). Proc Ame Soc Clin Oncol 14:198, 1995.

# CHAPTER 14

# HEPATOBILIARY NEOPLASMS

## 14A / PRIMARY HEPATIC NEOPLASMS

*Ravi S. Chari, David P. Foley, and William C. Meyers*

Benign and malignant liver tumors are increasing in frequency throughout the world. This increase may be, in a large part, due to the vast improvements and availability of diagnostic technology. The observation that malignant lesions still greatly outnumber benign neoplasms suggests that other features besides improved diagnosis are involved. If improved diagnosis were the only explanation, then one would expect a relative disproportion of benign lesions. Possible other explanations include an increase in the incidence of both hepatitis B and C as well as an increasing role of environmental carcinogens.

At the same time, improved surgical management of liver neoplasms has generated enthusiasm for strategies designed to cure patients. Advances in the correlation of pathologic features with the clinical course of some tumors have contributed to the progress in treatment. This chapter reviews the clinical features of benign and malignant primary hepatic tumors, with emphasis on recent advances in the understanding and treatment of these lesions.

## BENIGN HEPATIC NEOPLASMS

Benign tumors of the liver occur in about 1% of autopsies. CT and MRI are considerably more sensitive than autopsy, finding some form of liver lesion in about 5% of patients. Benign tumors are classified as true neoplasms, hamartomas, and pseudotumors. Nonbiliary hepatic neoplasms of the liver are classified as hepatocellular, cholangiocellular, vascular, and other nonvascular lesions (Table 14A-1). This section discusses the most common benign lesions and their characteristic features.

### HEPATIC ADENOMA

Hepatic adenomas arise in otherwise normal livers. They appear as focal abnormalities or masses. Literature reports probably do not accurately reflect the true incidence of the disease. However, the occurrence of hepatic adenoma probably increased after 1960. There were only eight cases of hepatic adenoma reported between 1940 and 1960. Between 1960 and 1977, 36 cases of liver cell adenomas appeared in medical journals. Although hepatic adenomas can occur in males or females, in children or adults, over 90% develop in women in the third to fifth decades of life.

The introduction of oral contraceptives (OCPs) in 1960 presumptively caused an increase in the frequency of hepatic adenomas in young women after that time. This temporal association strongly suggests a causal relationship between the oral ingestion of estrogens and the development of these benign hepatocellular neoplasms[1] and, statistically, 90% of patients with hepatic adenomas have used oral contraceptives. Annual incidence among oral contraceptive users appears to be 3 to 4 per 100,000 in users of more than 2 years. The risk of developing hepatic adenoma increases with the ratio and strength of the OCP preparation. Experimental and clinical evidence suggests that sex hormones are promoters rather than initiators of hepatocellular neoplasms.[2] Adenomas are also associated with noncontraceptive estrogen use, androgenic steroid use, diabetes, glycogen storage diseases, and iron overload.

CLINICAL MANIFESTATIONS. About half of patients with hepatic adenomas have abdominal pain. Some patients experience chronic or episodic mild upper abdominal pain; others have repeated, acute attacks of severe pain, caused by hemorrhage into the tumor or adjacent liver. A third pain syndrome is caused by rupture and resulting hemoperitoneum, which produces hemorrhage and frequently shock. The latter syndrome occurs in 10% to 30% of patients with adenomas. About 27% to 30% of patients sense an abdominal mass, which is palpable in about one-third. The remainder of hepatic adenomas are discovered incidentally at autopsy, laparotomy, or during radiologic evaluation of another condition. Other physical findings that can be associated with hepatic adenomas

**TABLE 14A-1.** HISTOLOGIC CLASSIFICATION OF BENIGN LIVER TUMORS

| *Hepatocellular:* | *Others:* |
|---|---|
| Hepatic adenoma | Mesenchymal hamartoma |
| Focal nodular hyperplasia | Leiomyoma |
| Nodular regenerative hyperplasia | Fibroma |
| | |
| *Cholangiocellular:* | Lipoma |
| Bile duct adenoma | Lymphangiomatosis |
| Biliary cystadenoma | Adrenal rest tumor |
| | |
| *Vascular:* | Pancreatic heterotopia |
| Hemangioma | Inflammatory pseudotumor |
| Infantile hemangioendothelioma | "Focal fatty sparring" |
| (capillary endothelioma) | |
| Hereditary hemorrhagic telangiectasia | |

include abdominal tenderness and signs of blood loss or shock. Pregnancy is reported to stimulate adenomas and the development of complications.

DIAGNOSIS. Clinical information may suggest the diagnosis but is not definitive. The imaging studies most commonly used to detect the hepatic mass are ultrasound, and multiphasic, helical computerized tomography (CT); arteriography, positron emission tomography (PET scan) and magnetic resonance imaging (MRI) have also been advocated. Differentiating between benign and malignant lesions may be difficult, especially if only one imaging modality is used. Therefore, a combination of imaging modalities is preferred. Adenomas characteristically display heterogeneous echo patterns on ultrasound and lesions as small as 1 or 2 cm in diameter can be detected. Conventional CT generally yields little specific diagnostic information. However, multiphasic, helical CT, including both arterial and portal venous phases, identifies the hypervascular adenoma quite well. Similarly, on gadolinium-enhanced MRI, these lesions are easily identified. On arteriography, the lesion is typically hypervascular, with some hypovascular regions representing areas of hemorrhage or necrosis. Hepatic adenomas usually exhibit centripetal blood flow. Due to recent improvements and the noninvasive nature of CT and MRI technology, arteriography is largely unnecessary in the evaluation of these lesions.

When radiologic studies show the characteristic inhomogeneous, hypervascular mass with internal echos, one must strongly consider the diagnosis of a hepatocellular tumor, particularly if there is no evidence of a primary malignancy elsewhere. MRI or erythrocyte-labeled isotope liver scan can effectively exclude the diagnosis of hemangioma. Although percutaneous needle biopsy or fine-needle aspiration for cytodiagnosis may help, even experienced pathologists have difficulty distinguishing between well-differentiated hepatocellular carcinoma and adenoma, and sometimes between adenoma and pseudotumor. For this reason, there is little to no utility for needle aspiration or biopsy in this and other hepatic lesions.

Recent work has shown that PET scan is useful in differentiating malignant tumor from benign lesions.[3] Because most malignant cells contain a relatively low level of glucose-6-phosphatase, they accumulate and trap [18F] fluorodeoxyglucose (FDG) intracellularly, allowing the visualization of increased uptake compared to normal cells. In one study, 110 patients with hepatic lesions >1 cm were evaluated for potential resection and underwent PET imaging. All (100%) liver metastases from adenocarcinoma and sarcoma primaries in 66 patients and all cholangiocarcinomas in 8 patients had increased uptake of FDG. Hepatocellular carcinoma (HCC) had increased uptake in 16 of 23 patients (70%). All benign hepatic lesions ($n = 23$), including adenoma and focal nodular hyperplasia, had poor uptake. Overall, the combination of abdominal pain, falling hematocrit, and a liver tumor in young females should strongly suggest a diagnosis of adenoma.

HISTOLOGY. Hepatic adenomas are usually solitary and round, but not usually encapsulated. They may vary in size up to 30 cm in diameter. Adenomas often bulge from the surface of the liver and contain several large blood vessels. Occasionally, they are pedunculated. The cut surface is yellow or tan and has areas of hemorrhage and necrosis. Microscopically, the adenomas are closely approximated cords of hepatocytes that *lack* surrounding bile ducts and have vacuolated sinusoidal borders. Centers of the adenomas may undergo degenerative changes. The hepatocytes are often paler than normal because of increased glycogen or fat content. Ultrastructurally, adenoma cells are similar to normal hepatocytes but have fewer organelles and canaliculi. Approximately 10% of surgically excised hepatic adenomas harbor foci of HCC.[4]

TREATMENT. Most commonly, hepatic adenoma is present as an undiagnosed liver mass. Only a minority of patients present with intraperitoneal bleeding. For those patients in the latter group, the differential diagnosis includes ruptured ectopic pregnancy (less likely in women taking birth control pills), bleeding visceral artery aneurysm, and ruptured spleen. Emergency ultrasound confirms the presence of a hepatic mass, and peritoneal lavage is occasionally performed to document intraabdominal bleeding. During evaluation, the patient with suspected hemorrhage from a hepatic tumor should receive vigorous blood transfusions with hemodynamic monitoring. Operation is best performed following the initial resuscitation, and control of bleeding is usually best achieved by removal of the tumor.

For those patients with a hepatic mass in whom adenoma is suspected, resection is the best treatment option for the following reasons: (1) Nonoperative discrimination between hepatic adenoma and hepatocellular carcinoma is difficult. (2) Hepatic adenomas sometimes harbor foci of cancer and may be premalignant lesions. (3) Hepatic adenomas often produce symptoms and sometimes life-threatening hemorrhage. Resection can usually be performed electively with lower morbidity and mortality rates compared to emergent resection in the hemodynamically unstable patient. With the discovery of a hepatocellular neoplasm, oral contraceptive use should cease immediately. Several case reports document regression of liver cell tumors after discontinuation of birth control pills. Furthermore, cessation of OCP will not change the frequency of cancer: development of HCC in the site of adenoma regression has been reported. In those patients who are pregnant at the time of diagnosis, the adenoma should be removed electively during the second trimester. Liver transplantation is another reported therapy for adenomas or adenomatosis.

## FOCAL NODULAR HYPERPLASIA

Focal nodular hyperplasia (FNH) is an unusual hepatic lesion that is frequently confused with adenoma. The documented incidence of FNH is increasing, probably because of the increase in abdominal imaging. Many lesions are still found incidentally at laparotomy or autopsy. Nearly 90% of FNH cases occur in women, primarily in the second and third decades, but the disease also affects older women and a small number of men and children. Between 1960 and 1967, only 37 cases of FNH were described in medical journals.

FNH can occur in any portion of the liver, and 12% to 13% of patients have multiple lesions. FNH probably represents a hyperplastic response of the hepatic parenchyma to a preexisting arterial malformation rather than a true neoplasm. No convincing evidence links OCP use to the development of FNH. However, oral contraceptive use may foster growth of FNH and a tendency for an established FNH to bleed. Very few cases of FNH have been reported to regress after discontinuation of birth control pills.

CLINICAL MANIFESTATIONS. In contrast to hepatic adenomas, FNH is generally a benign process that does not cause symptoms. Hemorrhage, rupture or other problems such as malignant changes are exceedingly rare. Only 10% of patients with FNH have symptoms, which usually consist of mild, chronic, intermittent abdominal pain. Acute symptoms are rare.

DIAGNOSIS. Most imaging techniques cannot reliably establish the diagnosis of FNH. Arteriography is highly sensitive but lacks specificity. A central scar is a characteristic feature of FNH and may be seen on CT scan, ultrasound, or MRI (Figs. 14A-1 and 14A-2). Of note, a central scar can also be seen in fibrolamellar hepatocellular carcinoma, hemangioma, and lymphoma. More than 80% of arteriograms show a sharply delineated hypervascular mass with intense venous staining. One-half to two-thirds of arteriograms show a single central artery and centrifugal filling of the vessels. Focal liver masses that appear hypervascular with intense venous-phase staining during arteriography and that lack evidence of hemorrhage within the tumor most commonly represent FNH. Typical CT findings for FNH include early hypodensity with subsequent isodensity and hypodensity. Technetium-labeled cholescintigraphy is also useful in identifying FNH. Criteria required for a diagnosis of FNH include hypoperfusion during the early phase (1 min), no or positive contrast during the parenchymal phase, and trapping of radioactivity during the late phase (>90 min). In 92 patients with histologic confirmation of FNH, preoperative cholescintigraphy plus ultrasound and CT led to the imaging diagnosis of FNH in 82 patients (89.1%).[5]

HISTOLOGY. FNH consists of one or more grossly visible, localized nodules in an otherwise normal liver, most frequently formed at the surface of the liver. The nodules are usually several centimeters in size, but occasionally grow to be much larger. In one series, 84% were less than 5 cm in diameter and only 3% were over 10 cm.

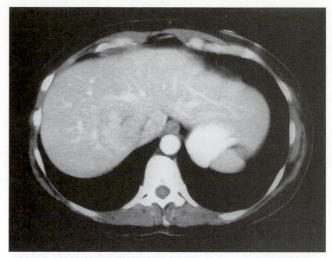

**FIGURE 14A-1.** Spiral CT scan in hepatic venous phase. This demonstrates the presence of a focal nodular hyperplastic lesion at the dome of the liver (segments 7 and 8), pushing the right hepatic vein anteriorly and wrapping around it. There is a black area in the center of this, consistent with central scar, suggesting the diagnosis of FNH.

Grossly, FNH appears as a well-circumscribed but nonencapsulated lesion with a central scar and stellate radiations that account for the nodular and sometimes umbilicated appearance. It is usually lighter in color than the surrounding normal parenchyma.

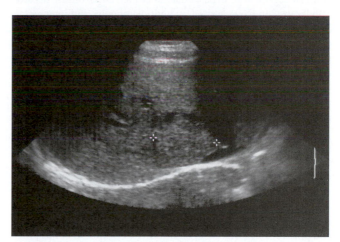

**FIGURE 14A-2.** Intraoperative ultrasound of patient with a liver lesion wrapped around the right hepatic vein and abutting the middle hepatic vein. Because of patient characteristics and history suggestive of a malignant process, this patient was brought to the operating room for assessment of a mass (see Fig. 14A-1). Intraoperative ultrasound was performed and demonstrated the presence of this mass, which had isoechoic features compared to the normal liver. Serial biopsies failed to ensure the diagnosis, and resection was undertaken. FNH was confirmed on postoperative pathologic sectioning of the mass lesion.

Histologically, this lesion has a central stellate scar and no true encapsulation and the cells, which are slightly different in color, usually blend with normal hepatic parenchyma. The ultrastructure of the hepatocytes in nodular hyperplasia is similar to that of normal hepatocytes. Microscopically FNH consists of many normal hepatic cells mixed with bile ducts or ductules and divided by fibrous bands, or septa, into nodules. The fibrous septa contain numerous bile ducts and a moderate predominantly lymphocytic infiltration. There is usually some evidence of mild cholestasis. The blood supply to areas of focal nodular hyperplasia is quite different from that of hepatic adenomas, with most of the supply arising centrally rather than peripherally.

TREATMENT. Treatment of a patient with FNH depends primarily on the certainty of the diagnosis. If malignancy or an adenoma remain as possible diagnoses, the patient should undergo a laparotomy. Small superficial masses are easily removed with local excision. Excisional biopsy is also usually recommended for symptomatic, larger lesions, even if excision requires a major liver resection. If FNH is conclusively diagnosed, and the patient is asymptomatic, the mass usually should be left undisturbed. One must also be aware that FNH occasionally occurs in the vicinity of hepatocellular carcinoma, in which case multiple biopsies may avoid sampling errors. Whenever the diagnosis remains in doubt after biopsy, the lesion should be removed, if the procedure can be done safely.

## NODULAR REGENERATIVE HYPERPLASIA

Nodular regenerative hyperplasia is a noncirrhotic, diffuse hepatocellular process characterized by multiple nodules and intervening areas of hepatic atrophy. It is frequently associated with portal hypertension. The primary distinction between nodular regenerative hyperplasia and cirrhosis is the *absence* of severe fibrosis. This condition is rare, but because the confusion between this entity and cirrhosis exists, its exact incidence is quite variable, depending on the observer. It is similar to FNH in that both are not true neoplasms.

Nodular regenerative hyperplasia most likely has a variety of causes, in light of the wide variety of associated nonhepatic chronic diseases. These include myeloproliferative disorders, lymphoproliferative disorders, and collagen vascular diseases. The pathology of nodular regenerative hyperplasia is similar to that of lesions produced experimentally and clinically by a number of drugs, including the experimental carcinogens, ethionine, aflatoxin B, Thorotrast, and dimethylnitrosamine. In addition, the association of this process with many chronic diseases implicates an association with drug therapy. The primary theories concerning pathogenesis involve neoplasia, drug-induced pathogenesis, or a vascular pathogenesis.

CLINICAL MANIFESTATIONS. The primary clinical effects of nodular regenerative hyperplasia are related to portal hypertension, although ascites is unusual. Occasionally, a nodule may rupture, causing hemoperitoneum similar to hepatocellular adenoma. The lesion may be discovered coincidentally at laparotomy. Treatment is usually directed toward correcting the portal hypertension. Occasionally, patients are good candidates for liver transplantation.

HISTOLOGY. The hepatocytes themselves are usually somewhat enlarged, and their cytoplasm is slightly pale. Larger nodules or groups of nodules may displace vascular structures, particularly the portal triads. Portal hypertension probably results from obstruction of the portal venous inflow by the nodules themselves or from an independent pathophysiology.

TREATMENT. Treatment is usually directed toward correcting the portal hypertension. Occasionally, patients are good candidates for liver transplantation. In cases where diagnosis is in question, resection is appropriate to exclude the absence of malignancy.

## HEMANGIOMAS

About 2% of autopsied livers contain cavernous hemangiomas, making this lesion the most common benign liver tumor. Most hemangiomas are small and do not cause symptoms. However, they may be large and when associated with diffuse hemangiomatosis can nearly replace the liver. The lesion occurs in all age groups and is probably more common in women. The pathology is similar to that of hemangiomas in other parts of the body. There is usually a dominant solitary mass and the size is extremely variable.

CLINICAL MANIFESTATIONS. Most hepatic hemangiomas produce no symptoms. Fewer than half that are over 4 cm in diameter are associated with symptoms of a full feeling or upper abdominal pain. Occasional lesions rupture spontaneously as a result of trauma. About 10% of patients with clinically detectable lesions are febrile. Hepatomegaly or an abdominal mass is the most common physical finding. These lesions demonstrate no malignant potential.

DIAGNOSIS. Radiologic imaging studies may play a key role in diagnosis, although laparotomy is occasionally necessary to make the diagnosis.[6] Percutaneous needle biopsy of suspected lesions is almost never recommended. On ultrasound, cavernous hemangiomas usually appear as well-defined, solitary, homogeneously echogenic, smooth masses with faint acoustic enhancement. Although ultrasound consistently reveals some features of hepatic hemangiomas, this modality rarely establishes the diagnosis definitively. In the past, hepatic angiography was considered the most accurate radiologic test available for hemangiomas, despite the disadvantage of a slightly higher risk compared to the other imaging studies. Time-sequence CT scans obtained with a rapid and intravenous (IV) injection of a radiographic contrast agent permit accurate diagnosis of most hemangiomas more than 3 cm in diameter. The primary entity in the differential diagnosis is hypervascular malignancy. A finding of globular enhancement or areas of pooling of contrast in the periphery of the lesion is a sign that differentiates hemangioma from hepatic metastases by helical CT scan (Fig. 14A-3). In a recent study evaluating the diagnostic efficiency of various imaging modalities in diagnosing 238 patients with hemangiomas, a combination of ultrasound, contrast (bolus)-enhanced CT, and a blood pool study with single-photon emission CT (SPECT) for hemangioma led to an imaging diagnosis in 136 patients (91%).[5] MRI is a very accurate technique for the detection and characterization of hepatic hemangiomas, with multiple studies demonstrating sensitivity, specificity,

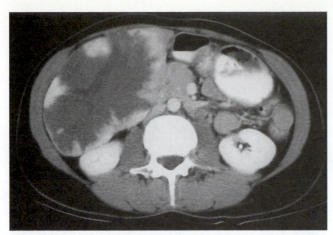

**FIGURE 14A-3.** Giant hemangioma of the liver extending well below the costal margin. This lesion was found in an otherwise asymptomatic 33-year-old female. In the early arterial phase of her four-phase CT scan, the peripheral enhancement of this lesion is consistent with the contrast density seen in the aorta. Through progression of the scan, there remains peripheral pooling of the dye and puddling. These features make it essentially diagnostic on CT scan for a hemangioma.

and diagnostic accuracy between 92% and 100%. MRI with long T2 weighting and dynamic, enhanced T1 weighting is probably the most sensitive, specific modality for hemangioma diagnosis.

TREATMENT. Most hepatic hemangiomas have a benign course. The risk of malignancy or of continued growth is negligible and spontaneous hemorrhage is rare. Therefore, most hepatic hemangiomas should remain undisturbed, provided that diagnostic uncertainty can be eliminated. Surgical resection is indicated in the following circumstances:

1. If a hemangioma produces persistent, bothersome symptoms such as pain or fever.
2. If intraperitoneal or intrahepatic rupture of the lesion is suspected.
3. If a lesion is considered large enough to be at high risk for traumatic rupture. Those lesions below the costal margin are particularly at risk for rupture.
4. If malignancy is suspected, and imaging cannot definitively establish the diagnosis of hemangioma.

In the case of multiple lesions, resection generally should be limited to the hemangioma causing the problem. Mortality and morbidity rates for operation for hepatic hemangiomas remain low, and patients can anticipate full functional recovery and normal life expectancy following removal of hepatic hemangiomas.

## INFANTILE HEMANGIOENDOTHELIOMA

Infantile hemangioendotheliomas are capillary hemangiomas similar to lesions that commonly occur in infancy in skin and mucous membranes. The incidence of this tumor in the liver is difficult to determine because many lesions probably involute before diagnosis. The cutaneous variety is reported to occur in 0.5% of neonates. Nearly all cases occur in infancy. Females outnumber males by a 2:1 ratio. The center of the lesion is necrotic, and the periphery contains proliferating vascular channels. Some lesions appear more aggressive histologically and may be confused with angiosarcoma. However, metastases from such lesions have been reported.

CLINICAL MANIFESTATIONS. Most affected patients are asymptomatic. Symptomatic patients may have high-output congestive failure secondary to severe arterial venous shunting. Rupture, pain, and symptoms related to the size of the mass are more unusual. In most cases, the tumor acts benignly, going through various stages of proliferation, maturation, involution, and disappearance. Symptoms are associated with a 67% mortality rate. Causes of death include congestive heart failure, hepatic failure, or rupture. Hepatic artery ligation, embolization, radiation therapy, steroids, and transplantation have been used with some success.

## OTHER BENIGN SOLID TUMORS

Other benign solid tumors that may appear in the liver include lipomas, fibromas, leiomyomas, myxomas, teratomas, carcinoid tumors, and mesenchymal hamartomas. The most commonly known benign tumors of the liver are bile duct hamartomas. These are small nodules found on the liver surface with benign hypoplastic bile ductular epithelium on microscopic evaluation. Carcinoid tumors are exceedingly rare primary liver tumors associated with the carcinoid syndrome. Mesenchymal hamartomas are rare but important to recognize because they grow to an extremely large size in an infant or young child and require surgical resection. Biliary cystadenomas and bile duct adenomas are also rare and may cause pain or extrahepatic biliary obstruction. There is a risk of malignancy, so these should be resected. Other, even rarer benign biliary tumors include meningioma, fibroma, and granular cell myoblastoma. Another lesion that is usually of little pathologic significance but is relatively common is focal fatty change.

Some benign conditions that can be confused with hepatic neoplasm include hereditary hemorrhagic telangiectasia, peliosis hepatis, and hepatic pseudotumor. Hereditary hemorrhagic telangiectasia is a diffuse telangiectatic process of the liver with numerous arterial venous fistulas. It is rare, associated with fibrosis, and considered by some to be a form of cirrhosis. Peliosis hepatis is also a rare lesion characterized by variably sized blood lakes. The most common association is with anabolic steroid therapy, but this process has also been seen with other drugs in chronic wasting diseases. The lesion is thought to be associated with toxic damage to sinusoidal or hepatic venous endothelium. Rarely is this condition clinically important. Over 50 cases of inflammatory pseudotumor have been reported, most probably resulting from healed abscesses. Hepatic pseudotumors are overgrowths of chronic inflammatory tissue which most likely result from healed abscesses (Fig. 14A-4).

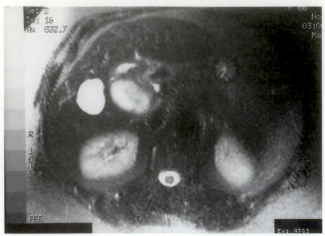

**FIGURE 14A-4.** Hepatic pseudotumor. This elderly lady presented with a newly diagnosed mass lesion in her liver. She was completely asymptomatic but had the ultrasound performed for vague abdominal complaints. Following demonstration of this on a CT scan, this MRI was taken. This T2-weighted image demonstrates the lesion to be closely related to the bile duct and superior to the fundus of the gallbladder. On exploratory laparotomy, it was found that this lesion was, in fact, a posterior perforation of the gallbladder into the liver, with fibrotic inflammatory response. Resection of the gallbladder and resection of this portion of segments 5 and 6 removed this lesion entirely and confirmed the benign nature of this lesion.

## PRIMARY MALIGNANT LIVER TUMORS

Primary malignant neoplasms of the liver arise from hepatocytes, bile ductular epithelium, or mesenchymal hepatic elements (Table 14A-2). There are occasionally other types, as well as mixtures of those listed. Hepatocellular carcinoma (HCC) constitutes about 90% to 95% of primary liver cancers. Cholangiocarcinoma adds approximately 5% to this total. In the western hemisphere, hepatoblastoma represents the most common primary hepatic malignancy of young children.

### HEPATOCELLULAR CARCINOMA

HCC is one of the most prevalent malignant diseases in the world, killing up to 1.25 million persons annually. It constitutes 90% to 95% of primary liver cancers. While HCC is the most common primary malignant liver tumor in adults, hepatoblastoma is the most common primary hepatic cancer of young children. Five different studies demonstrate HCC to have doubled over the past 30 years in the United States. HCC occurs four to nine times more frequently in males than in females, except in the group without preexistent liver disease, in whom the ratio is 1:1. Asians in the United States are approximately eight times at risk for developing the tumor compared with Caucasian populations. HCC makes up a relatively small proportion of the total primary cancers diagnosed on a yearly basis

**TABLE 14A-2.** PRIMARY MALIGNANT NEOPLASMS OF THE LIVER

| *Hepatocellular carcinoma:* | *Others:* |
|---|---|
| Subtype: Fibrolamellar variant | Fibrosarcoma |
| | Leiomyosarcoma |
| *Cholangiocarcinoma:* | Malignant fibrous histocytoma |
| | Primary lymphoma |
| | Familial erythrophagocytic lymphohistiocytosis |
| *Mesenchymal:* | |
| Angiosarcoma | Carcinoid |
| Epithelial hemangioendothelioma | Teratocarcinoma |
| Embryonal rhabdomyosarcoma | Squamous cell carcinoma |
| Undifferentiated sarcoma | |

in the United States. It has an annual incidence in the United States of 1 to 7 per 100,000 population, and it is the 22nd most common type of cancer, with 11,000 to 14,000 new cases per year.

Studies of histocompatibility antigens in South African blacks do not support a genetic basis for the increase of susceptibility of HCC. Rather, emerging data support the role of viral infections or environmental carcinogens. In high-incidence locations, the tumor more often occurs in patients treated for cirrhosis for a long period of time. Chronic liver diseases of any cause probably play an important role in the development of HCC in any part of the world. Epidemiologic and laboratory studies have firmly established a strong and specific association between hepatitis B virus (HBV) and HCC. Other well-documented risk factors include alcoholic cirrhosis blood group B, hepatic adenoma, repeated ingestion of aflatoxin, other types of cirrhosis, or chronic active hepatitis and persistent hepatitis C viral infection. Implicated risk factors for HCC are listed in Table 14A-3.

HBV is the most important etiologic effect identified on a worldwide basis. As accumulated over the past two decades, the evidence of the causal relationship between chronic infection with HBV and the disease is compelling.[7] As many as 98% of indigenous persons are infected with the virus at some time in their lives, and approximately 10% are persistently infected. Studies from both Asia and Africa suggest that HBV is present in as many as 70% to 80%

**TABLE 14A-3.** KNOWN RISK FACTORS FOR HEPATOCELLULAR CARCINOMA

Hepatitis B
Hepatitis C
Alcoholic cirrhosis
Hepatic adenoma
Cirrhosis of any cause
Iron overload
Anabolic steroids
Male sex
Polyvinyl chloride

of patients with HCC. Whether HCC occurs as a consequence of chronic HBV infection or as a result of chronic *liver disease* is not certain. Since HBV vaccine has been available for only a short period of time, it is not known if this will have a significant impact on the incidence of the disease in endemic areas. HBV does not contain an oncochain, but insertional mutagenesis is a potential mechanism. Over expression of *c-myc*, *c-phos*, and *c-herb-a* oncogenes have been demonstrated in tumors, but the relationship to tumorogenesis may be coincidental.

The observations that most strongly support a role for HBV in hepatocellular carcinoma are as follows: (1) The HBV carrier state exists in the same geographic distribution as hepatocellular carcinoma. (2) HCC patients have 100 times greater sensitivity to hepatitis B surface antigen (HBsAg) than population match controls. (3) HBV infections precede the development of carcinoma. (4) In a 5-year study, HBsAg-positive individuals had a 1000 times increased risk of developing malignancy than controls. (5) Progression from chronic states of HBV to cirrhosis and subsequent HCC is well documented. (6) HBV DNA resides in the HCC cell genome. However, genomic integration also occurs in patients without HCC, indicating that this is not the sole explanation for the development of this malignancy.

In contrast to HBV infection, most of the information showing an association between chronic hepatitis C virus (HCV) infection and HCC has been accumulated in western civilizations, where there is relatively little overlap with HBV. HBV and HCV do act as independent risk factors, and the two viruses may have a synergistic effect. HCV is a single strand of RNA that does not become integrated into host DNA. Therefore, it is not certain whether the virus is directly carcinogenic or if its marked propensity to cause chronic necroinflammatory disease is the real culprit. Interaction of either HBV or HCV with the p53 protein might also provide a growth advantage to cells harboring a mutation. Studies in Japan have also implicated HCV as the predominant cause of cirrhosis and HCC. In Japan, HCV infection is present in 51% of the patients with HCC, as opposed to 26% with HBV infection.

Alcoholic cirrhosis appears to be a major predisposing factor for the development of HCC in the United States. About 8% to 10% of patients dying of alcoholic cirrhosis have HCC. In one autopsy study, 55% of alcoholic cirrhotics who had stopped drinking had HCC, which suggests that abstinence from alcohol may allow the alcoholic patient to live long enough to develop a tumor.[8] Implicated, but not proven, risk factors for the development of HCC include aflatoxins, which are potent carcinogens in experimental animals. Aflatoxins are products of the fungus *Aspergillus flavus*, which is found in wheat, soybeans, corn, rice, oats, bread, milk, cheese, and peanuts. The U.S. Food and Drug Administration limits the amounts of aflatoxins allowed in peanut butter to 20 parts per billion.

The risks of HCC developing with the use of oral contraceptives is not clear, although a number of carcinomas have been reported arising within benign adenomas of oral contraceptive users. A type of carcinoma termed fibrolamellar carcinoma characteristically develops in persons younger than the age of 35, and it is possible that some of these tumors are also linked etiologically to oral contraceptives. A number of cases of hepatoma have been reported in males after administration of antigenic or other anabolic steroids for the treatment of aplastic anemia, although it is possible that multiple

**TABLE 14A-4.** HEPATOCELLULAR CARCINOMA COMPARED WITH FIBROLAMELLAR CARCINOMA

| CHARACTERISTIC | HEPATOCELLULAR CARCINOMA | FIBROLAMELLAR CARCINOMA |
| --- | --- | --- |
| Male to female ratio | 4:1–8:1 | 1:1–1:2 |
| Transplantation | Stage I and II (<5 cm) only | Larger lesion acceptable |
| Resectability | Less than 50% | 50–75% |
| Mean survival | 3–4 months | 32–68 months |
| Cirrhosis | 77% | 4% |
| Increased α-fetoprotein | 83% | 7% |
| Hepatitis B positive | 65% | 6% |

transfusions contributed to anemia in these patients. There does appear to be a greater hormone responsiveness in these androgen-related HCCs. Table 14A-4 summarizes available comparative data between HCC and fibrolamellar carcinoma.

**CLINICAL MANIFESTATIONS.** The most common symptoms of HCC are weakness, malaise, upper abdominal or shoulder pain, and weight loss. In one series in the United States, an abdominal mass was the main complaint in 19 of 140 patients (14%) with primary hepatic malignant tumors, and jaundice was present in 34 patients (24%). Approximately 5% of the patients present with a manifestation of metastatic lesions, of which pulmonary metastases are the most common.

A minority of patients initially experience an acute abdominal event such as rupture of the tumor, hemorrhage, or fever of unknown origin. More often, the tumor represents an occult process. The duration of symptoms often is surprisingly short. In one series, over 75% of patients have symptoms for less than 6 weeks.[9] In recent years, the diagnosis has been made preoperatively in the vast majority of patients, primarily because of improved imaging techniques and the increased use of tumor marker α-fetoprotein (AFP).

Physical findings depend on the stage of the disease. Hepatomegaly is the most common sign found in patients. Interestingly, an arterial bruit can be heard in 15% to 20% of patients, which may be diagnostically valuable. Two-thirds of the patients admitted with an obvious cancer exhibit many signs of advanced liver disease (e.g., abdominal pain and tenderness, asthenia, hepatomegaly, splenomegaly, jaundice, ascites, peripheral edema, weight loss, spider angiomas, or evidence of portal hypertension). Ninety percent of these patients have metastatic disease at initial presentation.

The most common perineoplastic manifestation of HCC is probably hypoglycemia. Serum protein abnormalities of globulins, hepatoglobulin, ceruloplasmin, $\alpha_1$-antitrypsin, choriogonadotropins and choriosomatotropins, alkaline phosphatase, and isoferritins can be found. Other abnormalities include hypercholesterolemia, hypertriglyceridemia, porphyria, cystathioninuria, ethanolaminuria, pseudohyperparathyroidism, central changes, hypertrophic pulmonary osteoarthropathy, increased thyroxin binding globulin, and carcinoid syndrome. Increased carcinoembryonic antigen (CEA) occurs in 8% of the cases.

The most sensitive serum marker for the diagnosis of HCC is AFP. This protein has a molecular weight of 64,000 to 74,000 daltons. It is present in large quantities during fetal development but decreases rapidly after birth and thereafter remains at the normal adult level of 10 ng/mL or less. In the United States, 75% of patients with HCC arising in association with HBV cirrhosis had AFP levels above 400 ng/mL. Sixty-five percent of patients with HCC secondary to alcoholic cirrhosis had positive results, whereas only 33% of patients with carcinoma arising in a noncirrhotic liver had positive assays. However, overall AFP has a low specificity, and many cirrhotic patients without HCC have "positive" results (see below). AFP may return to normal after successful surgical resection and is a useful level to follow. Mild elevations of AFP may be found in acute viral hepatitis, chronic liver disease, and some cases of metastatic cancer. Higher levels may be found in adult patients with a fulminant type of HBV infection. Markedly elevated levels may also be found in patients with teratocarcinomas, yolk sac tumors, and, rarely, hepatic metastatic carcinomas from the stomach or pancreas.

Because most tumors that are found asymptomatically are untreatable, screening strategies have been studied. These programs are aimed at evaluating cirrhotic patients for the development of HCC. In HCC, the rationale for screening is based on the concept that tumors usually benign as a single lesion often have a long doubling time, are often encapsulated, and typically have a long asymptomatic stage in the concept that groups at high risk of developing HCC can be identified. The modalities available for screening include AFP, ultrasound, serologic markers, and CT scan and/or ultrasound. Serum AFP values of greater than 20 ng/mL are seen in up to 90% of cases of HCC. Unfortunately AFP has a low specificity. Levels of AFP are elevated in cases of pregnancy, germ cell tumor, and also in acute and chronic hepatitis. In a recent study by Markovic and coworkers,[10] 35.2% of their 131 patients had a normal AFP level. There was insignificant elevation (less than 400 ng/mL) in 65 additional patients (28.4%). In only one-third (36.4%) of the patients ($n = 81$) was the AFP above 400 ng/mL. In other words, two-thirds of patients with cirrhosis may have indeterminate or insignificantly elevated AFP levels.[10] Dr. Morris Sherman[11] conducted a 9-year screening program in Canada. He noted that to be truly effective, screening should result in a decrease in the disease mortality rate. This has not been shown with HCC. Thus, the potential limitations for screening for HCC raise the question as to whether it is ethical to offer screening when the benefits are unknown. The costs of screening for HCC must also be considered. In most studies of HCC screening, the cost per life gained ranged from 16,000 to 55,000 per year. The cost of treating each tumor is $11,000 to $25,000. The cost for each year of life saved is $17,000 and the cost per life saved is greater than $350,000.[11]

DIAGNOSIS. A number of radiologic investigations may be helpful in the diagnosis of HCC. Plain radiographs are not specific and may show an enlarged liver, elevated hemidiaphragm, and, rarely, calcification of the tumor. In conjunction with AFP levels, ultrasonography is frequently used as a "screening test" for HCC. However, the sensitivity of sonography for the detection of HCC in the end-stage cirrhotic liver is only 50%.[12] The majority of small HCCs (<3 cm) are hypoechoic due to their homogenous, purely cellular structure. Larger HCC are typically hypere-

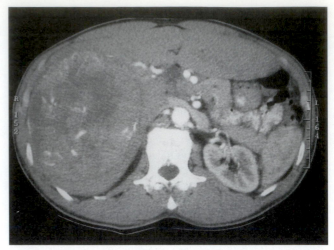

**FIGURE 14A-5.** Helical CT with contrast enhancements demonstrates the presence of a large mass, replacing almost the entire right hepatic lobe. In patients with chronic, active hepatitis B and AFT >16,000, HCC is diagnosed.

choic or of heterogeneous echogenicity due to the presence of one or more of the following: nonliquefactive necrosis, hemorrhage, fatty change, interstitial fibrosis, or sinusoidal dilatation. A hypoechoic halo representing a thin, fibrous capsule is a characteristic finding of HCC.[13]

On enhanced CT scans, the solitary or multinodular form of HCC appears as a solitary mass or multiple masses that are hypodense relative to the normal liver (Fig. 14A-5). However, in a fatty liver, HCC appears denser than the liver parenchyma. Following IV contrast and scanning during the portal venous phase, HCC is generally seen as a hypodense lesion relative to normal liver. For detection of small HCCs, CT scan following intraarterial Lipiodol administration and CT arterial portography (CTAP) are more sensitive studies.[14] CT may also detect lesions as small as 1 cm in diameter and may also differentiate among fatty, cystic, and solid lesions.

In a recent study, Kanematsu and coworkers[15] compared the roles of biphasic, helical CT scans and CTAP on 33 patients with biopsy-proven HCC. They found that biphasic, helical CT scans with both arterial and portal venous enhancement identified 13 more lesions than portal venous phase images in 13 patients. Furthermore, by detecting 23 additional lesions in the same 13 patients, CTAP proved to be even more sensitive than biphasic helical CT.[15] These authors concluded that biphasic, helical CT can be used as an initial screening test for suspicious liver lesions; however, CTAP still seems to be the most sensitive nonsurgical imaging technique for the detection of liver tumor foci.

Hepatic arteriography has been shown to be occasionally helpful in determining the extent of the disease and, in particular, portal or arterial involvement. Although arteriography can also predict the usefulness of direct arterial infusion of chemoembolization for HCC, which may either be hypervascular or hypovascular, currently most of this information can be obtained through the use of biphasic, helical CT scans. However, the disadvantages of these procedures are (1) the degree of invasiveness, and (2) when major hepatic

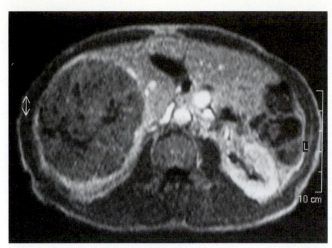

**FIGURE 14A-6.** Dynamic, multiphase, gadolinium-enhanced MR imaging detecting the same tumor as in Fig. 14A-5. As performed to assess the liver for additional nodules, the MRI scan that may not have been appreciated on CT scan.

resection is anticipated, the possibility of thrombosing an artery to the remaining lobe.

Recent developments in MRI techniques have also improved the sensitivity and specificity of HCC detection. Usually HCC is hypodense on T1-weighted images and hyperintense on T2-weighted images. However, the presence of fatty changes, necrosis, or hemorrhage may result in increased signal intensity on T1-weighted images.[16] Dynamic, multiphase, gadolinium-enhanced MR imaging has been shown to improve the detection of HCC and may be superior to dual-phase, spiral CT scan (Fig. 14A-6).[17] In some centers, gadolinium-enchanced MRI is the preferred diagnostic imaging modality used to evaluate patients suspected to have HCC.

Liver-specific contrast agents have developed to improve MRI detection of HCC. On T1-weighted images there is marked signal enhancement of liver parenchyma. Therefore, one can discriminate lesions of hepatocellular origin (HCC, FNA, and regenerative cirrhotic nodules) from other lesions that do not enhance (i.e., liver metastases, cholangiocarcinoma, and lymphoma).[13]

Laparoscopy is emerging as an important tool in the diagnosis and staging of HCC or other suspected liver tumors. Five separate studies demonstrated its usefulness before anticipated resection, particularly in the detection of occult metastases not demonstrated by other modalities. Laparoscopy also offers an opportunity for treatment. Furthermore, the use of laparoscopic ultrasonography has been shown to be a sensitive means of identifying HCC and determining resectability of the tumor.

**HISTOLOGY.** Various classifications confuse the understanding of the pathology of HCC. The traditional classification of Eggel[18] divides the tumor into massive, nodular, or diffuse. The more recent classification by Nagashima[18] has four groups: infiltrative, expansive, mixed infiltrative and expansive, and diffuse. The latter classification also recognizes two special close types of HCC: small (less than 2 cm in diameter) and pedunculated. The classifications are further divided by histopathology. The most common histologic pattern is trabecular, which encompasses the pseudoglandular, pseudofollicular, and mixed trabecular-acinar types. Other histologic adjectives often used with HCC include pseudoglandular, solid, compact, scirrhous, clear cell (replacing), giant cell, pseudocapsular, and sarcomatous. More important than these classifications is the recognition of distinctive variants of HCC in the presence or absence of cirrhosis.

The gross pathologic appearance of HCC varies considerably, depending on the presence or absence of preexisting cirrhosis. In the cirrhotic liver, it is most often multinodular, whereas in the noncirrhotic liver, it is usually a single mass. In an otherwise normal liver, the tumor probably begins as a fairly homogenous mass and then develops satellite lesions. Most satellite lesions occur within the same segment. In the cirrhotic liver, the more diffuse multifocal disease is probably a function of the end-stage disease of the liver.

Percutaneous needle biopsy or fine-needle aspiration for definitive diagnosis generally adds *little* to the evaluation of potentially resectable indeterminate liver masses, and needle biopsy or aspiration carry some hazard for hypervascular masses. Furthermore, rupture and bleeding after biopsy is reported. Needle tract seeding and increased pulmonary metastases have also been reported. Radiologic techniques correlated with serum AFP are useful in diagnosing two-thirds of HCCs, and an indeterminate or negative biopsy aspirate adds little to the decision-making process, except perhaps to establish whether or not the patient has cirrhosis.

**STAGING.** Staging of HCC is largely based on one of two systems. The AJCC staging system defines stage of liver and intrahepatic bile duct cancer by tumor, nodal disease, and metastatic disease. Survivorship based on staging has been correlated. However, unlike other primary malignancies, staging of liver tumor by TNM classification often does not completely analyze the patient's survivorship. This is due to the fact that most patients have accompanying liver failure. The Okuda classification takes into account parameters of liver function.[19] Worsening liver function in spite of small stage of tumor portends a very poor survivorship. Incorporating Child's classification to AJCC/TNM staging is another method of classifying these people. Treatment strategies should incorporate liver function, as well as tumor staging. One such scheme that may be acceptable to these patients is outlined in Fig. 14A-7.

**TREATMENT.** Two common misconceptions about HCC are that it grows rapidly and that it is universally fatal. In general, HCC is actually slower growing than other neoplasms such as colon cancer and bronchogenic carcinoma. Resection has often resulted in cure, particularly in the absence of cirrhosis. Most carcinomas resected in the presence of underlying cirrhosis and chronic hepatitis recur in the liver, although the disease interval may be several years. Usually the "recurrences" are actually new lesions arising in the presence of a cirrhotic liver. Surgical resection is generally accepted as the first choice of treatment for HCC. The indications for surgical treatment are generally consistent. Small, well-defined lesions confined to a single liver lobe are likely to be removed successfully, with a median survival time of greater than 5 years. More recently, in patients with preserved liver function, larger lesions have been resected with acceptable morbidity and mortality rates. Previous studies have shown that larger and less well defined lesions

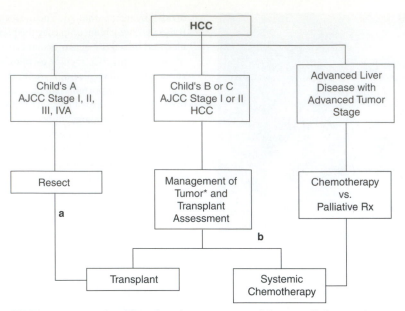

**FIGURE 14A-7.** Algorithm for the treatment of hepatocellular carcinoma (HCC)

*Transarterial chemoembolization, percutaneous ethanol injection, radiofrequency ablation, or cryoablation while waiting on transplant list.

[a]Follow carefully and consider transplant if recurrence with poor liver reserve precludes resection.

[b]Poor prognostic histologic predictors after transplantation or metastatic disease while on waiting list.

---

occupying more than one liver lobe have a much poorer chance of being successfully resected.[20–22] However, patients with T4, any N0, M0 (Stage IVA) tumor, have improved 5-year survival rates with resection. Average survival time after resection is reported to be approximately 3 years. In HCC, nodal metastases are less than 1.6% and routinely are not dissected.[23] Because of improved surgical techniques, the operative mortality rate from major hepatic resection has decreased nearly 20% from 1950 to approximately 2% currently. The mortality rate still relates primarily to postoperative liver failure from accompanying cirrhosis, and in selected patients, a 5-yr survival rate of 35% can be achieved.[24]

Prognostic indices have developed to calculate the risk of hepatectomy in HCC and cirrhosis. Most are based on the modifications of Child's classification, percentage of remaining liver tissue, and patient age. In cirrhosis, wedge resection is as *effective* as more radical procedures in many patients. In addition to resection of occult lesions, intraoperative ultrasonography helps to determine the center of resection and identification of the precise segment of the liver to be removed, which can be done after injection of stain into the portal vein to that segment.

In the 1980s liver transplantation was performed only for otherwise unresectable tumors with only a 20% 2-year survival rate. In contrast, there was an 80% to 90% cure rate with coincidental cancers found in pathologic examinations of the cirrhosis after transplantation. Most deaths after transplantation for tumor are attributable to tumor recurrence. Fibrolamellar HCC had a better prognosis with transplantation, that is, a 30% to 40% 1-year tumor-free survival rate, compared with a 10% survival rate for patients with nonfibrolamellar tumors. Nonprospective studies suggest a doubling of the chance for survival with transplantation compared with resection when resection is an option. This outcome is most evident in patients with cirrhosis and with solitary lesions less than 5 cm in diameter. These data may also support an aggressive combined approach to HCC, including resection or transplantation following another modality such as chemotherapy, chemoembolization, or cryoablation. In the management of HCC, appropriate indications for liver transplantation are currently defined as unresectable stage I or II (where the greatest tumor has a diameter less than 5 cm) HCC and fibrolamellar carcinoma.[25] Transplantation for stage III and IVa tumors is more controversial and cannot be recommended. Despite the shortage of donor livers and the best long-term survival rate of only 20% to 30%, liver transplantation will still remain a therapeutic option for selected patients.

Cryoablation has emerged as a surgical technique in the treatment of HCC and certain other malignancies. The principle of cryotherapy is to use freezing to devitalize neoplastic tissue. Liquid nitrogen at a temperature of −196°C is the most commonly used agent. To achieve tumor ablation, an appropriate margin of at least 1 cm of around apparently normal liver tissue should also be frozen.[26] In HCC, cryotherapy is best performed on tumors less than 3 cm in diameter, although larger tumors have been reported to be effectively treated by multiple probes simultaneously inserted into the tumors.[26] The overall operative morbidity and mortality rates from cryoablation may be less compared with resection, although hepatic failure after cryotherapy is still seen. Therefore, the number of nodules that can be treated may increase or the margin of resection may widen. From Shanghai, Zhou et al.[27] reported treating 87 patients with HCC by cryotherapy. The 1-, 3-, and 5-year survival rates were 60.5%, 32%, and 20.2%, respectively. Among the 30 patients with tumor nodules less than or equal to 5 cm in diameter, the 1-, 3-, and 5-year survival rates were 92.6%, 66.6%, and 50.8%, respectively.[27] However, because some of these patients received other forms of treatment, including hepatic artery ligation and arterial infusion therapy, interpreting the results of cryotherapy was difficult. Complications specific to cryotherapy include cracking the liver with intraoperative hemorrhage, postcryotherapy syndrome with acute renal failure, intrahepatic abscess, and pleural effusion. Long-term data on cryoablation of primary or secondary liver malignancies are not available. Nonetheless, the technique raises a number of interesting possibilities in terms of combined therapy.

More recently, the thermal ablation of liver tumors has been advocated. Radiofrequency ablation (RFA) is a localized thermal treatment technique designed to produce tumor destruction by heating tissue to temperatures in excess of 50°C, temperatures above 50°C being commensurate with cell death. From a surgical standpoint, monopolar or bipolar electrocautery devices used daily in the operating room employ similar technology. The tissue temperature in the tumor to be ablated can be controlled by increasing the radiofrequency power and current delivered. For monopolar tissue ablation, a needle electrode is placed in the tumor via percutaneous or intraoperative approach, and a grounding pad is applied to the patient's skin. A relatively uniform zone of radiant-conductive heat is produced within the first few millimeters of electrode—the tissue interface. The heat emitted from the tissue uniformly radiates out of the electrode; and if the tissue impedance is relatively low, an expanding sphere of ablated tissue is created. The final size of the sphere of heat-ablated tissue is proportional to the square of the radiofrequency current, also known as the radiofrequency power density. Thus, the tissue temperature rapidly falls with increasing distance from the electrode tip, resulting in only a 1-$\mu$ to 1.5-cm sphere of tissue ablation when a single monopolar simple needle is used. Multiple array tips and units with multiple needles have been manufactured, and these have increased the diameter up to 4 cm, across which the radiofrequency current can be passed. Other modifications of the delivery unit involve the use of cooled electrodes and the infusion of saline solution (standard 0.9% or hypertonic 5%), which can be used to increase the radiofrequency current conduction at the needle tip. If the radiofrequency is performed with the application of high power, the tissue heats and is desiccated, resulting in coagulative necrosis; this reduces the propagation of the radiofrequency current and yields a very small zone of coagulative necrosis without radiofrequency ablation. Cooled tips attempt to decrease the desiccation and coagulation by allowing limited heat distribution and more uniform distribution of radiofrequency current and heat. The initial studies for radiofrequency indicate that there may be an apparent advantage of radiofrequency over cryoablation because there may be a lower treatment-related complication rate.[28] The complications just described for cryoablation (cold injury to adjacent organs, coagulopathy, cryoablation syndrome, intrahepatic abscess) have not been seen. Additionally, initial studies suggest that the recurrence rate is lower than with other techniques, but to date, a large clinical experience is lacking. As more experience

is gained, RFA's role as a complement to other ablative techniques, which help to maximize surgical cure in these patients, will be better defined.

Percutaneous ethanol injection (PEI), first advocated by Sugiura and coworkers[29] in 1983, is considered an effective form of direct ablation therapy for HCC. HCC lesions suitable for PEI are those less than 3 cm in size and fewer than three in number. Under local anesthesia, a 22-gauge needle is introduced percutaneously into the tumor through a function probe under ultrasonographic or controlled CT scan guidance. Absolute (99.5%) ethanol is slowly injected into the lesion while the needle position is shifted slowly to achieve uniform and adequate installation and ensure tissue necrosis within and around the tumor. Absolute alcohol induces cellular dehydration, coagulative necrosis, and vascular thrombosis, causing destruction of the tumor cells. The procedure is repeated twice a week for up to four to six sessions.[30] For lesions less than 2 to 5 cm in diameter, PEI has been reported in various series to be satisfactory with 3-year survival rates of 55.7%. Patient survival was also found to be significantly better than for a similar group of patients who had not received treatment.[31]

Percutaneous acetic acid injection has also been shown to be effective therapy for small lesions. In 1996, Ohnishi et al.[32] reported treating 25 patients with solitary HCC lesions of 3 cm or less in diameter by ultrasound-guided percutaneous acetic acid injection. All lesions were smaller after treatment, and there was no evidence of viable HCC in follow-up or biopsy and CT scan. Complete necrosis was seen in two HCCs obtained by means of resection. The 1- and 2-year survival rates were 100% and 92%, respectively, for the 23 patients who did not undergo surgery.[30]

Transcatheter arterial chemoembolization (TACE) has been a popular method for palliation of HCC. TACE is a combination of targeting chemotherapy and arterial embolization. A cytotoxic agent such as cisplatin, doxorubicin, or mitomycin C is first mixed with Lipiodol and then injected into the feeding artery of the tumor by angiographic technique. Lipiodol is a compound that forms a covalent linkage with the chemotherapeutic agent, thus carrying it to the tumor, as well as being an embolizing agent, thus inhibiting neovascularization of the tumor. Small Gelfoam particles are then embolized into the vessel. The technique is contraindicated in cases of poor liver function or when portal hypertension has developed due to tumor thrombosis. Overall survival is not enhanced by TACE, and the toxicity of the approach, combined with the acceleration of underlying liver disease, appears to be a particular problem. It may play a role in control of tumor growth while an HCC patient is waiting for liver transplantation.

SUMMARY OF THERAPEUTIC OPTIONS FOR HCC. Overall, with HCC, staging and degree of liver function are the most important variables affecting the response to treatment and survival. Surgery is highly effective in monofocal HCC with Okuda level 1 and 2 disease without cirrhosis or Child's level A cirrhosis with stage I disease. Liver transplantation is an effective treatment in patients with advanced liver disease (Child's levels B and C) with stage II disease or less (maximal single tumor diameter of 5 cm). Other techniques that are evolving and are important adjuncts in the care of patients with HCC include cryoablation, radiofrequency ablation, acetic acid, or ethanol injection. Prevention is the ideal approach to HCC. Newer studies have shown there to be some benefit to interferon treatment in patients with HCV cirrhosis, with decreased incidence of tumors. Similarly, lamuvidine treatment in HBV cirrhosis may impact the incidence of HCC in this patient group. Because of the heterogeneous nature of HCC, definitive studies to place each treatment in the proper perspective are difficult. Any of these treatments can be accepted as standard in this group, but more rigorous investigation rather than the anecdotal case–reported series will be necessary for a definitive evaluation of each treatment. Until such is achieved and newer treatments are evaluated, only surgical resection should be recommended outside of any clinical research setting.

## INTRAHEPATIC CHOLANGIOCARCINOMA

Another type of primary liver cancer is cholangiocarcinoma, which appears to arise in a peripheral portion of the hepatic parenchyma.[33] This intrahepatic form of bile duct cancer is rare but has some characteristic clinical features. Most commonly, this affects patients in their seventh decade of life. The male-female ratio is 1.7:1. Chronic liver disease is rarely present. Jaundice is slightly more common a clinical presentation compared with HCC, but not nearly as common as with extrahepatic bile duct cancer. Serum AFP levels are occasionally elevated. The radiologic evaluation is similar to that of HCC and usually consists of ultrasound and CT. Biopsy is rarely indicated, and surgical resection with clear margins is the best chance for cure. Liver transplantation may be an appropriate option in those patients with decompensated liver function that precludes resection and who have early stage disease.

## MALIGNANT MESENCHYMAL TUMORS

A number of primary malignant mesenchymal tumors in the liver have been reported. All totaled, these make up less than 2% of primary malignant tumors. Most of the tumors are sarcomas, and the prognosis varies according to cell type and resectability. Most sarcomas are rapidly growing and fatal, but exceptions do occur. True mixtures of sarcomas and carcinomas are extremely rare, but HCC occasionally shows a sarcomatoid (pseudosarcomatous) pattern. The latter behaves like HCC.

Primary hepatic sarcomas have received much attention because of their association with vinyl chloride, or Thorotrast. Angiosarcoma is the principal tumor associated with this agent. It usually occurs as multiple nodules of variable size that rapidly disseminate intravascularly. No single instance of curing angiosarcoma has been reported. The longest reported survivor (5 years) received radiation therapy. Other tumors such as leiomyosarcoma, fibrosarcoma, rhabdomyosarcoma, and mesenchymal sarcoma also rarely appear in the liver. Undifferentiated sarcoma is also generally associated with an extremely poor prognosis, although the authors had a patient who had undergone tumor resection who was a 5-year survivor.

Epithelioid hemangioendotheliomas are considered malignant because of their characteristically diffuse involvement within the liver and the ability to metastasize. Their clinical presentation and course are extremely variable, with most patients dying of liver failure 1 to 10 years after diagnosis. Transplant is indicated in those with evidence of liver failure. Extrahepatic metastases are not neces-

sarily a contraindication since patients can have stable disease after transplantation. Alternatively, in the absence of liver failure, transplant is not necessary. Other malignant tumors reported rarely as primary lesions in the liver include malignant histiocytoma, familial erythrophagocytic lymphohistiocytosis, lymphoma, teratoma, yolk sac tumor, schwannoma, osteosarcoma, and carcinoid.

## REFERENCES

1. Fechner R, Roehm J: Angiographic and pathologic correlations of hepatic focal nodular hyperplasia. Am J Surg Pathol 1:217, 1977.
2. Gordon S et al: Resolution of a contraceptive-steroid-induced hepatic adenoma with subsequent evolution into hepatocellular carcinoma. Ann Intern Med 105:547, 1986.
3. Delbeke D et al: Evaluation of benign vs malignant hepatic lesions with positron emission tomography. Arch Surg 133(5):510, 1998.
4. Kerlin P et al: Hepatic adenoma and focal nodular hyperplasia: Clinical, pathologic, and radiologic features. Gastroenterology 84:994, 1983.
5. Weimann A et al: Benign liver tumors: Differential diagnosis and indications for surgery. W J Surg 21:983, 1997.
6. Brant W et al: The radiological evaluation of cavernous hemangioma. JAMA 257:2471, 1987.
7. Robinson WS: The role of hepatitis B virus in the development of primary hepatocellular carcinoma: I. J Gastroenterol Hepatol 7:622, 1993.
8. Ramming KP et al: Gastrointestinal tract neoplasms, in Cancer Treatment, C Haskel (ed). Philadelphia, Saunders, 1980, pp 231–357.
9. Berman C: Primary carcinoma of the liver. London, HK Lewis, 1951.
10. Markovic S et al: Treatment options in Western hepatocellular carcinoma: a prospective study of 224 patients. J Hepatol 29(4):650, 1988.
11. Sherman M et al: Screening for hepatocellular carcinoma in chronic carriers of hepatitis B virus: Incidence and prevalence of hepatocellular carcinoma in a North American urban population. Hepatology 22(2):432, 1995.
12. Dodd G et al: Detection of malignant tumors in end-stage cirrhotic livers: Efficacy of sonography as a screening technique. Am J Roentgenol 159:727, 1992.
13. Fernandez M, Redvanly R: Primary hepatic malignant neoplasms. Radiol Clin Am 36(2):333, 1998.
14. Takayasu K et al: The diagnosis of small hepatocellular carcinoma: Efficacy of various imaging procedures in 100 patients. Am J Roentgeno 155:49, 1990.
15. Kanematsu M et al: Hepatocellular carcinoma: The role of helical biphasic contrast-enhanced CT versus CT during arterial portography. Radiology 205:75, 1997.
16. Rummeny E et al: Primary liver tumors: Diagnosis by MR imaging. A J Roentgenol 152:63, 1989.
17. Yamashita Y et al: Small hepatocellular carcinoma in patients with chronic liver damage: Prospective comparison of detection with dynamic MR Imaging and helical CT of the whole liver. Radiology 200:79, 1996.
18. Meyers WC: Neoplasms of the liver, in Textbook of Surgery, DC Sabiston Jr (ed). Philadelphia, WB Saunders, 1997, pp 1068–1084.

19. OKUDA K et al: Natural history of hepatocellular carcinoma and prognosis in relation to treatment. Study of 850 patients. Cancer 56(4):918, 1985.

20. INOUE K et al: Surgical treatment of small hepatocellular carcinoma. Gan To Kagaku Ryoho 23:8849, 1996.

21. HU R et al: Surgical resection for recurrent hepatocellular carcinoma: Prognosis and analysis of risk factors. Surgery 120:23, 1996.

22. IKAI I et al: Surgical intervention for patients with stage IVA hepatocellular carcinoma without lymph node metastasis: Proposal as standard therapy. Ann Surg 227(3):433, 1998.

23. LEE C et al: Long-term outcome after surgery for asymptomatic small hepatocellular carcinoma. Br J Surg 83:330, 1996.

24. LAI EC et al: Hepatic resection for hepatocellular carcinoma: An audit of 343 patients. An Surg 221(3):291, 1995.

25. PICHLMAYR R et al: Indications for liver transplantation in hepatobiliary malignancy. Hepatology 20:33S, 1994.

26. CUSCHIERI A et al: Hepatic cryotherapy for liver tumors: Development and clinical evaluation of a high-efficiency insulated multineedle probe system for open and laparoscopic use. Surg Endosc 9:483, 1995.

27. ZHOU X et al: An 18-year study of cryosurgery in the treatment of primary liver cancer. Asian J Surg 15:43, 1992.

28. CURLEY SA et al: Radiofrequency ablation of unresectable primary and metastatic hepatic malignancies: Results in 123 patients. Ann Surg 230:1, 1999.

29. SUGIURA N et al: Treatment of small hepatocellular carcinoma by percutaneous injection of ethanol into tumor with real-time ultrasound monitoring. Acta Hepatol Jpn 24:920, 1983.

30. LIU C, FAN S: Nonresectional therapies for hepatocellular carcinoma. Am J Surg 173:358, 1997.

31. EBARA M et al: Percutaneous ethanol injection for patients with small hepatocellular carcinoma, in *Primary Liver Cancer in Japan*, T Tobe et al (eds). Tokyo, Springer-Verlag, 1992, pp 291–300.

32. OHNISHI K et al: Treatment of hypervascular small hepatocellular carcinoma with ultrasound-guided percutaneous acetic acid injection: comparison with segmental transcatheter arterial embolization. Am J Gastroenterol 91(12):2574, 1996.

33. OKUDA K et al: Clinical aspects of intrahepatic bile duct carcinoma including hilar carcinoma. Cancer 39:232, 1977.

# 14B / NEOPLASMS OF THE EXTRAHEPATIC BILIARY TRACT

*Peter J. Allen and Yuman Fong*

## INTRODUCTION

Tumors of the extrahepatic bile duct occur in approximately 4500 people in the United States each year.[1] The majority of these neoplasms are malignant, and 80% of malignant lesions are adenocarcinomas. Benign lesions will occur in approximately 6% of patients.[2] Tumors from other primary sites may also metastasize to the porta hepatis or the region of the pancreatic head and mimic a bile duct cancer. This pattern of spread has been documented in melanoma, breast carcinoma, renal carcinoma, and colorectal carcinoma.

Tumors of the bile duct may occur anywhere in the biliary tract from within the liver to the ampulla of Vater. These tumors by location have been classified into intrahepatic and extrahepatic categories, with extrahepatic lesions being further subdivided into tumors of the proximal, middle, and distal duct. Since mid bile duct cancers are rare, and the majority of mid bile duct obstructions from cancer result from gallbladder cancer, it is much more useful to separate extrahepatic bile duct cancers into proximal cancers and distal cancers. The proximal lesions are those arising proximal to the cystic duct and include the perihilar tumors, whereas distal lesions are grouped as those distal to the cystic duct and include the periampullary tumors. This latter system of classification will be used in this chapter, since it is practical from a treatment standpoint. Proximal bile duct cancers generally require a combined biliary and liver resection for extirpation, whereas distal tumors require a pancreatic resection. Intrahepatic bile duct tumors are treated in a similar fashion as primary hepatic neoplasms, and the management of these tumors will be addressed in another chapter.

The most common location for malignant tumors of the bile ducts are at the confluence of the hepatic ducts. A recent review from John Hopkins University of 294 patients with cholangiocarcinoma found 196 (67%) to be perihilar in location, 80 (20%) distal, and 18 (6%) within the intrahepatic ducts.[3] This experience is similar to those reported at other institutions.[4–6]

The treatment of malignant bile duct tumors has evolved over the past 30 years. Until recently, liver resection or pancreaticoduodenectomy was associated with a high morbidity and mortality rate, leading to a largely nihilistic attitude toward these tumors. Bile duct cancers, therefore, were considered by most clinicians as incurable and therapy was directed toward palliation. In Klatskin's[7] description of 13 patients with primary proximal bile duct carcinoma in 1965, palliative drainage procedures were the only surgical option employed. All patients in that study died from disease, except for a single patient who died of other causes, and the average survival was 15 months. Another study, performed in 1972, also used palliative procedures, as compared to curative resection, in the majority of patients and similar survival rates were observed.[8] As resections have become increasingly safe, aggressive surgical resection has been shown to improve outcome in patients with cholangiocarcinoma. Several recent studies have documented overall mean survival to be as high as 36 months after curative resection.[9,10]

In this chapter we will summarize the current approach and results of aggressive surgical therapy for bile duct tumors. We will begin with a discussion of bile duct cancer, separating proximal from distal cancers since the curative as well as the palliative approaches are so different. We will then conclude with a short discussion of benign bile duct tumors.

## PROXIMAL BILIARY TRACT CANCERS

### HISTORY

The most common location for malignant tumors of the biliary tract is at the confluence of the hepatic ducts. Approximately 2500 of the 4500 (63%) patients diagnosed annually with cholangiocarcinoma will have their disease occur in this region. In 1965 Dr. Klatskin[7] described 13 patients with cholangiocarcinoma located at hepatic duct bifurcation and this disease has come to be known as Klatskin tumors, though the first resection of a hilar cholangiocarcinoma was reported by Brown and Myers[11] in 1954, and the disease was well described by Altemeier and associates[12] in 1957.

### EPIDEMIOLOGY

The etiology of cholangiocarcinoma remains unknown. Early reports on malignant bile duct tumors postulated a link with cholelithiasis, and several series have reported coincident cholelithiasis in 17% to 37% of patients presenting with malignant bile duct tumors.[13,14]

Carcinoma of the bile duct may also result from an autoimmune or inflammatory etiology such as cases that are associated with ulcerative colitis. In a series of patients from the Mayo Clinic, the risk of intrahepatic cholangiocarcinoma in patients with ulcerative colitis was 75 times higher than that of the general population.[15] Adenocarcinoma of the biliary tract may also develop in patients with longstanding sclerosing cholangitis and series have reported an incidence of cholangiocarcinoma in as many as 20% to 30% of these patients.[16] Finally, choledochal cysts have also been shown to undergo neoplastic change if present for many years.

The biology of cholangiocarcinoma is distinct compared to other tumors of this region. Cholangiocarcinoma tends to grow slowly, and the pattern of spread is most frequently by local extension.[7,17,18] However, nodal metastases may occur in as many as a third of patients at the time of presentation, but blood-borne metastases are distinctly unusual.[19,20]

Approximately 90% of malignant bile duct tumors are adenocarcinomas, and these may be divided into three morphologically distinct variants. These variants include papillary, nodular, and diffuse. Papillary lesions seldom present in the perihilar region, are much more common near the ampulla, and appear as exophytic growths into the duct. They often present with intermittent jaundice and may be multifocal in up to 7% of patients.[18] The nodular variant, on the contrary, occurs more commonly in the upper duct and usually presents as a small, well-localized mass. The diffuse variant presents as a thickening over an extensive area of the duct and may be very difficult to distinguish from sclerosing cholangitis.

Unresected cholangiocarcinoma is rapidly fatal, with mean survival of unresected patients being approximately 3 months.[21,22] The most common causes of death in these patients are liver failure secondary to vascular compromise or cholangitis secondary to biliary obstruction.[23,24]

## PRESENTATION

Biliary tumors may remain clinically silent for long periods of time, and patients with these lesions present with similar nonspecific signs and symptoms as patients who present with benign bile duct tumors. In patients with cholangiocarcinoma, however, these signs and symptoms are often progressive in nature. Jaundice has been reported to occur in as many as 90% of patients, usually occurring within 4 months of diagnosis and becoming progressively more severe.[23] Unilateral biliary obstruction may occur in patients with hilar cholangiocarcinoma, and in these patients serum alkaline phosphatase is the most sensitive indicator of biliary obstruction.[1,25] If unilateral biliary tract obstruction occurs along with portal vein obstruction, ipsilateral hepatic lobar atrophy may occur.[26] Pruritus is often the most distressing symptom associated with obstructive jaundice. Pain is present in approximately 50% of patients, but is more commonly associated with periampullary lesions.[27,28] Anorexia and weight loss are also common findings in patients with advanced disease.

Any patient who presents with obstructive jaundice or with an unexplained elevation in serum alkaline phosphatase level should be evaluated for the possibility of bile duct malignancy.

## EVALUATION

Evaluation of patients should begin as always with a thorough history, physical exam, and routine blood chemistries. Specific attention should be paid to eliciting a history of intermittent jaundice, pruritus, and fever. Family history of ulcerative colitis or sclerosing cholangitis should be addressed. Routine blood tests should include serum liver function tests.

The first imaging test performed is usually sonography. This allows an evaluation for gallstone disease; an evaluation for the presence of biliary or hepatic masses, to distinguish proximal versus distal ductal involvement; and an evaluation of vascular involvement. In addition, sonography may also demonstrate the presence of hepatic lobar atrophy, which is a reliable sign of vascular involvement on the ipsilateral side.[29,30] With expert sonography, often the full extent of local disease can be evaluated at minimal cost (Fig. 14B-1).[31]

Computed tomography (CT) scanning serves as a complementary study to ultrasound and may give more precise assessment of atrophy and of nodal involvement by tumor (Fig. 14B-2). Additional tests to further delineate the extent of local disease include percutaneous transhepatic cholangiography (PTC), and angiography. Often, all of these tests will be performed at considerable costs. Recent developments in MR technology now allow detailed noninvasive imaging of the biliary tree. Such magnetic resonance cholangiopancreatography (MRCP) can often provide equivalent biliary assessment as direct cholangiography while providing equivalent assessment of parenchymal tumor involvement and nodal involvement as CT, and adequate assessment of the vascular involvement (Fig. 14B-3).[32,33]

It is rare that endoscopic retrograde cholangiopancreatography (ERCP) will be useful in the patient with hilar biliary obstruction. This is because of the difficulties of ERCP in visualizing the biliary tree above a high biliary obstruction. ERCP, therefore, provides little information except for the level of obstruction, which is information easily derived from noninvasive imaging. When direct cholangiography is performed, however, biliary drainage should not be routine in patients who are surgical candidates, unless treatment of cholangitis is the goal of the cholangiography. There is no evidence that preoperative biliary drainage of jaundice improves outcome for patients subsequently resected of cholangiocarcinoma.[34,35] On the contrary, in a randomized study of 70 patients with malignant biliary obstruction and jaundice, the group subjected to preoperative drainage had a higher mortality rate than those patients undergoing immediate surgery.[35] Other studies have also shown that preoperative drainage may have an adverse effect on outcome by leading to an increased incidence of postoperative septic complications.[34,36,37] Furthermore, resection after permanent stent placement may be difficult or even impossible because of the extensive inflammatory reaction after placement.

## SURGICAL THERAPY

**SURGICAL RESULTS.** Surgical excision is the only treatment with the potential for cure. However, it was not until recently that surgical excision was routinely feasible and generally accepted as the treatment of choice. Recent improvements in imaging allow for

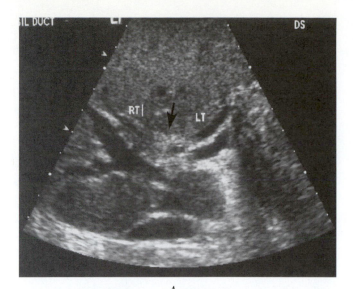
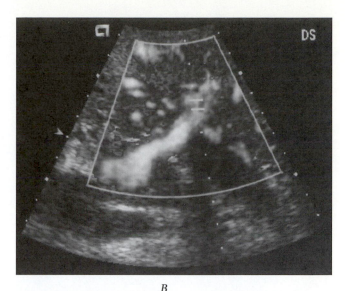

A                                                                 B

**FIGURE 14B-1.** *A.* Sonographic appearance of a cholangiocarcinoma. Note the mass (arrow) at the confluence of the left (LT) and right (RT) hepatic ducts and the dilated left duct. *B.* Doppler ultrasound in the same patient demonstrating patent left and main portal veins, allowing for a right-sided resection of this tumor.

improved diagnosis as well as surgical planning. Furthermore, developments in surgical and anesthetic technique have led to continued improvements in perioperative outcome. Whereas the experience form 1970 to 1989 (Table 14B-1) can be regarded as preliminary, more recent data (Table 14B-2) clearly advocate surgical therapy as safe and effective. In the early years of surgical therapy for hilar cholangiocarcinoma, the experience was uniformly limited, even at major centers (Table 14B-3).[4,37–43] Operative mortality was as high as 33%, and no series had sufficient follow-up to demonstrate clear

benefit from this aggressive approach. More recent data, however, have demonstrated increasing safety of these operations, and have demonstrated favorable long-term outcome.[3,9,36,44–51]

PATIENT SELECTION. Selection of patients is based on three major criteria: medical fitness, no distant metastases, and local resectability. Criteria for medical fitness are as for all major surgical procedures. In addition, because the jaundiced patient is at higher risk for renal failure, assessment should include careful scrutiny of hydration and of renal function. Extraabdominal metastasis is rare. A chest x-ray is used to rule out pulmonary metastases. Abdominal and pelvic CT are used to screen for peritoneal disease and for discontiguous liver metastases.

Our algorithm for evaluating local resectability is outlined in Fig. 14B-4. A quality ultrasound and CT usually secures the diagnosis. If there is no atrophy of the liver, this combination of imaging tests usually suffices as preoperative assessment for exploration. Since portal vein occlusion leads quickly to atrophy, it is unlikely in a patient without atrophy to have lengthy portal vein involvement. In the setting of a tertiary referral center where portal vein reconstructions are routine, we are willing to explore patients to directly assess local structures for resection or for bypass if tumor is not resectable. In institutions where the volume of biliary tumors is lower, it is not unreasonable to obtain further imaging, including MRCP (see Fig. 14B-3), direct cholangiography, and/or angiography before surgery.

In patients with atrophy, the portal vein on that side is usually occluded. In these patients, careful assessment of biliary involvement must be performed. If the tumor involves predominantly the same side as the portal vein occlusion, and there is adequate bile duct on the contralateral side for reconstruction, the tumor is considered

**FIGURE 14B-2.** CT appearance of a cholangiocarcinoma. Note the left lobe atrophy due to left ductal and left portal occlusion. Dilated ducts in the right posterior sector are noted (arrow).

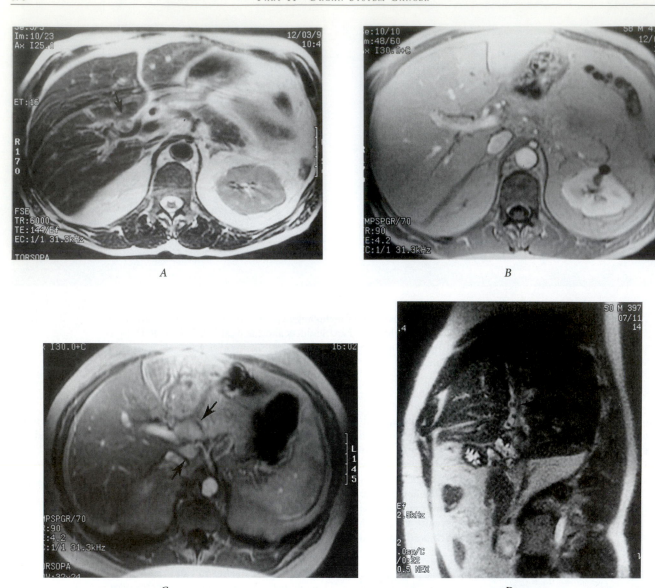

**FIGURE 14B-3.** *A.* MRCP appearance of a cholangiocarcinoma. The tumor (arrow) at the hilum is seen bowing the right hepatic artery behind it. *B.* The portal vein in this same patient is shown not to be involved by tumor. Celiac lymph nodes (arrows) demonstrated to be involved by metastatic cholangiocarcinoma in a different patient. *C.* MRCP can also distinguish other causes of biliary obstruction, such as intrahepatic biliary stones (arrow), as demonstrated on this scan.

"favorable," and exploration is performed for either resection or bypass. Portal involvement on one side with contralateral extensive biliary involvement is considered "unfavorable," and is unlikely to be resectable.[28] These patients are treated palliatively. Additional criteria for unresectable tumors include:

1. Extensive bilateral intrahepatic bile duct spread of tumor
2. Extensive involvement of the main trunk of the portal vein
3. Bilateral involvement of the hepatic arterial or portal venous branches.

Those uncomfortable with portal vein reconstruction should consider referring patients with clear atrophy to a tertiary center for therapy, since reconstruction of the portal vein and the associated temporary ischemia can be particularly hazardous in the jaundiced population.[52–54]

OPERATIVE CONDUCT. For detailed descriptions of the techniques of resection of hilar cholangiocarcinoma, the reader is referred to technical works.[55] The management of bile duct cancer should address two primary objectives: removal of the entire

**TABLE 14B-1.** RESULTS OF STUDIES (1970–1989) EVALUATING SURGICAL RESECTION FOR THE TREATMENT OF DISTAL CHOLANGIOCARCINOMA

| AUTHOR | NO. RESECTED | OPERATIVE MORTALITY | SURVIVAL MONTHS MEAN | MEDIAN |
|--------|--------------|---------------------|------|--------|
| Longmire, 1973[38] | 6 | 15% | NR | — |
| Fortner, 1976[39] | 9 | 33% | 14 | — |
| Launois, 1978[40] | 11 | 18% | 17 | — |
| Akwari, 1979[41] | 4 | 0 | 33 | — |
| Tompkins, 1981[4] | 22 | 23% | — | 10 |
| Cameron, 1982[42] | 10 | 0 | 21* | — |
| Beazley, 1984[37] | 16 | 19% | 17 | — |
| Blumgart, 1984[43] | 18 | 11% | 17 | — |
| Alexander, 1984[5] | 8 | 0 | — | 21 |
| Iwasaki, 1986[91] | 21 | 0 | — | 21* |
| Iida, 1987[92] | 23 | 4% | — | 8* |
| Bengmark, 1988[93] | 22 | 27% | — | 6* |

*Studies reporting 5-year survivors.

**TABLE 14B-2.** RESULTS OF STUDIES (1975–1997) EVALUATING SURGICAL RESECTION FOR THE TREATMENT OF DISTAL CHOLANGIOCARCINOMA

| AUTHOR | RESECTED n | RESECTABILITY, % | OPERATIVE MORTALITY, % | SURVIVAL, % 3 YEAR | 5 YEAR |
|--------|-----------|------------------|------------------------|--------|--------|
| Warren, 1975[72] | 47 | — | 21 | 32 | 25 |
| Nakase, 1977[94] | 161* | 52 | 22 | 8 | 5 |
| Tompkins, 1981[4] | 12 | 67 | 8 | 28 | 28 |
| Alexander, 1984[5] | 14 | 100 | 21 | 20 | 18 |
| Lerut, 1983[73] | 5 | — | — | 0 | 0 |
| Tarazi, 1986[74] | 11 | — | 0 | — | 17 |
| Nagorney, 1993[75] | 22 | 56 | — | 40 | 40 |
| Fong, 1996[76] | 45 | 43 | 4 | 46 | 27 |
| Nakeeb, 1996[3] | — | 91 | 1 | 31 | 28 |

*Collected multiinstitutional series.

**TABLE 14B-3.** RESULTS OF STUDIES (1990–1997) EVALUATING SURGICAL RESECTION FOR THE TREATMENT OF HILAR CHOLANGIOCARCINOMA

| AUTHOR | n | RESECTED n | MORTALITY, % | 5-YR SURVIVAL,% |
|--------|---|-----------|--------------|-----------------|
| Cameron, 1990[44] | 96 | 53(41%) | 2 | 8 |
| Nimura, 1990[45] | NR | 55 | 6 | 40 |
| Hadjis, 1990[46] | 131 | 27(21%) | 7 | 22 |
| Bismuth, 1991[47] | 122 | 22(19%) | 0 | NR |
| Baer, 1993[36] | 48 | 21(44%) | 5 | 45 |
| Guthrie, 1993[48] | 69 | 10(14%) | 10 | 10 |
| Pisters, 1995[49] | 41 | 13(31%) | 8 | 47 |
| Washburn, 1995[9] | 88 | 59(67%) | 10 | 15 |
| Su, 1996[50] | 162 | 49(30%) | 10 | 18 |
| Nakeeb, 1996[3] | 196 | 106(56%) | 4 | 11 |
| Klempnauer, 1997[51] | 339 | 151(55%) | 10 | 28 |

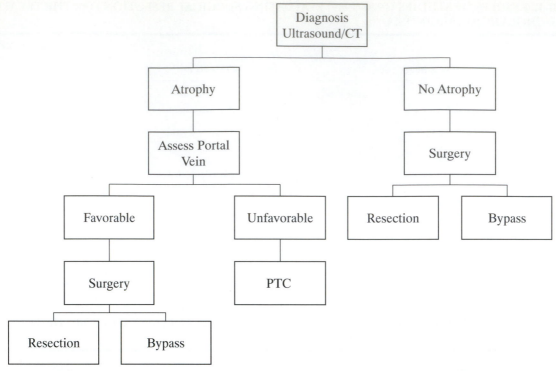

**FIGURE 14B-4.** Algorithm for patient selection for treatment in patients suspected of cholangio-carcinoma.

tumor and relief of jaundice. The only curative treatment is complete surgical resection, yet the resectability rate for all patients with bile duct cancer is approximately 20% to 40%.[56,40] The reason the resectability rate is generally low is because even small tumors at the hepatic hilum often invade many important local structures. In order to obtain adequate exposure of the portal vein for assessment of resectability, we routinely transect the common bile duct just above the duodenum, after an inspection of the abdomen to rule out distant metastases. The bile duct is then reflected superiorly as dissection proceeds to allow safe access to the portal confluence.[1] The distal ductal margin is sent for frozen-section analysis to ensure a negative margin. During dissection, the tumor is mobilized off the underlying vascular structures along with associated lymphatic tissue. Once the back of the confluence of the hepatic duct is reached, dissection proceeds along the right and left hepatic duct to determine extent of ductal involvement proximal to the hilum. If the tumor is small, resection of the hilum along with only a limited portion of the liver at the back of segment IV may suffice for tumor clearance. For the majority of cases, however, one or the other side of the liver will need to be resected for tumor clearance. The hepatic duct is transected after normal-appearing duct is encountered. Stay sutures are placed, and then this margin is sent for frozen section. The accompanying liver resection is then performed after negative margins have been confirmed. Hepatic resection is performed in a standard fashion as an extension of the operation described for local excision.[28,57] Biliary continuity is usually restored by a hepaticojejunostomy using a

70-cm retrocolic Roux-en-Y jejunal limb. It is important to remember that the jaundiced liver does not tolerate ischemia as well as the normal liver, and therefore we attempt to minimize portal occlusion time and avoid arterial ligation when possible.

The importance of the hepatic resection for tumor clearance must be emphasized. The rate of clear surgical margins in the published series to date are clearly related to the aggressiveness with which liver resection is performed (Fig. 14B-5A). It is also not surprising, therefore, that long-term survival is also dependent on rate of liver resection in the respective series (Fig. 14B-5B). Because of the location of the hepatic ducts, direct tumoral extension into the liver most commonly occurs in segment IV; however, anatomic studies have also found that two or three bile ducts drain the caudate lobe directly adjacent to the confluence of the hepatic ducts.[58] Because of the anatomic proximity and reported high incidence of caudate lobe invasion, some surgeons advocate routine resection of the caudate lobe for these lesions.[45,58] We find caudate resections to be necessary in a high percentage of cases but not uniformly indicated. We prefer to judge the need for this resection by direct surgical assessment.

When the biliary tree is entered, bile samples are sent for assessment of bacterial colonization. A positive intraoperative culture prompts a 7-day course of the appropriate antibiotics, since nearly all resected patients will develop a degree of postoperative ascites, and infected ascites is such a morbid complication. All patients with biliary anastomosis are also drained using a closed-suction

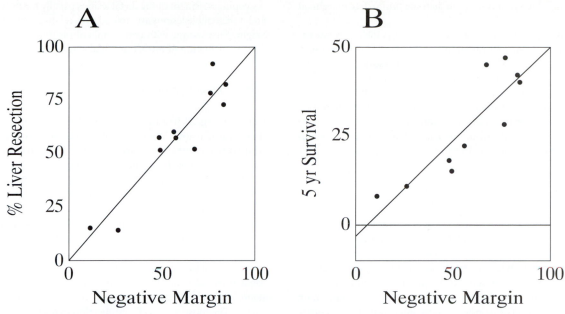

**FIGURE 14B-5.** *A.* Relationship between percentage of liver resected and likelihood of negative surgical margins in various published series. *B.* Relationship of 5-year survival to likelihood of negative surgical margins.

drainage system, although we do not drain routine liver resections otherwise.

Orthotopic liver transplantation has also been employed for hilar tumors that are otherwise unresectable; however, early recurrence and low survival rates have been observed.[59]

## PALLIATIVE THERAPY

When curative resection cannot be performed, a variety of drainage procedures have been described that relieve jaundice. These include operative transtumoral stenting and biliary-enteric bypass, as well as percutaneous and endoscopic endoprostheses.[36,44,60–62] When a patient is found to have disseminated disease, percutaneous stenting is most appropriate. When the disease is locally unresectable, particularly if this is found unresectable at surgery, a surgical bypass at that time is the most appropriate.[63]

## CHEMOTHERAPY AND RADIOTHERAPY

When patients are found to have locally unresectable disease, the use of radiotherapy following decompression has been evaluated with mixed results. Radiation therapy has in some studies been shown to improve survival in unresectable patients who have undergone stenting.[44,64–66] The use of radiotherapy, however, has been associated with measurable morbidity with cholangitis, septicemia, duodenal obstruction, and even death being reported.[44,64] The delivery

of radiotherapy has been by both external beam and intraluminal delivery systems. A recent study from our institution has found the combination of both (external beam radiation and intraluminal iridium 192) to be safe and effective.[67]

The use of chemotherapy in the management of patients with cholangiocarcinoma has also been investigated in both the adjuvant setting and in the treatment of unresectable disease. The most common agents employed have been 5-fluorouracil, doxorubicin, and mitomycin. Both regional administration and systemic treatment have been evaluated.[68,69] Overall partial response rates have been less than 20% in most series, with reports of significant toxicity.[68,70] These response rates, however, have not translated into documented improvements in survival.

## DISTAL BILE DUCT CANCER

### EPIDEMIOLOGY

Distal bile duct cancers are more akin to periampullary tumors in presentation and treatment. It is an uncommon disease, representing only 5% of all cancers in the periampullary region, and occurring only 2000 times each year in the United States. The majority of distal bile duct cancers are adenocarcinomas. Most occur as slow-growing lesions, and although lymphatic metastases occur in approximately one-third of patients, blood-borne metastases are unusual. The tumors spread by local invasion involving neural, perineural, and lymphatic tissues. There is also a well-described subepithelial spread of these cancers, which is important in defining tumor-free margins at resection.

Less common primary distal bile duct tumors include neuroendocrine tumors, cystadenocarcinoma, malignant fibrous histiocytoma, and in infants, rhabdomyosarcoma. These lesions are extremely rare and are mentioned only for completeness.

Surgery represents the only curative option for treatment of distal bile duct cancers.[5,71–75] Patients who are unresectable have a median survival on the order of six to eight months.[5,71–75] Death is usually related to local tumor spread and associated biliary or portal venous obstruction leading to liver failure or biliary sepsis.

## PRESENTATION

The clinical presentation of distal bile duct cancer is very similar to pancreatic adenocarcinoma or higher bile duct tumors, with jaundice, pruritus, and weight loss the predominant presenting symptoms. In our recent review of 104 distal bile duct cancers, jaundice was the most common presenting symptom, occurring in 75% of all patients.[76] Jaundice is usually steadily progressive. However, on occasion presentation of jaundice may be intermittent, particularly if the bile duct cancer is of the papillary variety. Weight loss was also common, occurring in one-third of patients. Pruritus or pain was reported in one-quarter of the patients at presentation.

The differential diagnosis usually includes choledocholithiasis, pancreatitis, as well as other periampullary tumors. Choledocholithiasis as a cause of the biliary obstruction can usually be ruled out by sonography or ERCP. However, distinguishing distal bile duct cancer from other periampullary cancers by preoperative or even operative evaluations is often very difficult.

Evaluation of patients with distal bile duct cancers will usually begin as for all patients, with that of the distal bile duct obstruction. Patients should be questioned for any history consistent with past cholelithiasis, cholecystitis, or pancreatitis, as well as any symptoms of exocrine or endocrine pancreatic insufficiency. Physical examination should include search for distended gallbladder and signs of portal hypertension. The history of jaundice, particularly if it has been intermittent in nature, and the degree of jaundice should be determined.

Imaging usually begins with sonography, to rule out gallstone disease and to determine the level of biliary obstruction. Sonography can also evaluate for mass in the periampullary region, status of the local vasculature, and signs of liver metastases. Usually, a helical CT with thin cuts through the pancreas will be performed to confirm the sonographic findings. If these studies demonstrate extrahepatic bile duct dilation, no signs of biliary stones, and a mass localized to the head of the pancreas, periampullary tumor should be strongly suspected. Barring definitive signs of unresectable tumor, such as encasement of superior mesenteric or portal vessels, plans should be made for surgical intervention. Given the high quality of the helical CT scans, direct angiography is rarely necessary. If no mass is noted, ERCP can be useful in demonstrating a malignant stricture. Cytologic evaluation of specimens obtained by brush biopsy during ERCP may also allow definitive diagnosis prior to therapeutic intervention. In contrast to high biliary obstruction, percutaneous transhepatic cholangiography (PTC) is rarely indicated for distal lesions, since en-

doscopic assessment of the distal lesions usually meets with success, and unresectable lesions are stented with relative ease by endoscopy. Staging laparoscopy with endoscopic ultrasound may also provide further evaluation of intraabdominal spread and resectability.

## SURGICAL RESECTION

Curative surgical treatment for distal bile duct cancer usually requires a pancreaticoduodenectomy. In a minority of cases, patients with truly localized, very early cancers may be treated with wide local duct excision. In the not too distant past, when pancreaticoduodenectomy was associated with an operative mortality of over 20%, some felt that such a morbid procedure was not justified.[77] Over the last two decades, the safety of pancreaticoduodenectomies has steadily improved. In major centers, this operation can now be performed with a perioperative mortality rate of less than 5% (Table 14B-3)[3–5,72,74–76] In our recent series of distal bile duct cancers, the perioperative mortality for 45 resected patients was 4%.[76] Median hospital stay was 17 days (range 1 to 82) for resected patients, and complications occurred in 17 of the resected patients (38%). The most common complications were intraabdominal abscess and pancreatic fistulas.

Not only is surgical therapy being performed with increasing safety, such therapy can result in long-term survival and cure. In the resected patients, median survival can be expected to be between 16 and 33 months, and 5-year survival expected in 17% to 40% of patients (see Table 14B-2). Patients with unresectable disease have a median survival of only 6 to 7 months. Patients palliated by surgical bypass had a longer median survival of 10 months, but were still unlikely to be alive 2 years after diagnosis. Major predictors of long-term outcome were resectability or nodal tumor status. Gender, age, preoperative stenting, preoperative bilirubin level, or tumor grade have not been shown to be influential on outcome. The long-term survival of patients after resection of distal bile duct cancers should be contrasted with patients with other periampullary tumors. It is clear that after curative resection of pancreatic adenocarcinoma, 5-year survival is expected to be less than 15%,[78] whereas 5-year survival for ampullary carcinoma is more likely to approach 50%.[72] The results for distal bile duct cancer resection, therefore, are intermediate, with 5-year survivals of approximately 30% (see Table 14B-2).

## PALLIATION

The two major symptoms occurring in patients with unresectable bile duct cancer requiring palliation are jaundice and gastric outlet obstruction. For the latter, surgical gastrojejunal bypass is indicated, except for patients with far advanced disease who are moribund, where an endoscopically placed gastrostomy may be the best option. For jaundice, decision to pursue surgical or nonsurgical means of relieving the obstruction is based upon the clinical condition of the patient, associated medical problems, and expertise of the particular institution.

Prior to the advent of endoscopic biliary intubation techniques, surgical biliary enteric bypass was the standard of care for obstructive jaundice produced by nonresectable tumors of the periampullary region. The advantages of surgical bypass include complete relief of the obstruction, prolonged patency, and low incidence of cholangitis. These must be weighed, however, against the risks of general anesthesia and the morbidity of a surgical procedure, particularly in the clinical setting of the short survival associated with unresectable malignancies of this region. The absolute indications for surgical bypass are:

1. Failure at endoscopic and percutaneous stenting
2. Gastric outlet obstruction requiring simultaneous gastroenteric bypass
3. Obstructed patients explored for resection of tumor but found to be unresectable.

Recent advances in laparoscopic techniques also allow for laparoscopic biliary bypasses. These have been suggested to have less risk and shorter hospital stays than bypasses performed by the traditional open techniques.

Nonsurgical drainage should be performed for patients with a malignant lesion demonstrated to be clearly unresectable by preoperative imaging, and with no gastric outlet obstruction. Biliary drainage is maintained by either plastic or metallic endoprostheses. The advantages of plastic stents include the ease of placement and exchange of these stents, and the low cost. These stents, however, may migrate and often become occluded by encrustation and therefore require exchange every 2 to 3 months. Metallic expandable stents have a lower risk of migration and have longer patency, but are more expensive, and once deployed are essentially not removable or exchangeable. Our bias is to use plastic stents, accepting the need to replace these stents every 2 to 3 months.

In contrast to high bile duct tumors, where biliary drainage should never be undertaken for jaundice without the presence of pruritus or cholangitis, in the distal duct we feel jaundice alone constitutes adequate indication for drainage. The reason for this more liberal policy regarding the distal duct is the relative risk of life-threatening biliary sepsis at each site. For high bile duct cancers the tumors often grow to involve second- and third-order intrahepatic ducts and excluded segments of liver are not uncommon. Therefore, biliary sepsis after instrumentation insolvable by further instrumentation often occurs. For distal bile duct tumors, drainage is much simpler and infection in the biliary tract can be dealt with in a more straightforward manner. Usually, low bile duct obstruction can be decompressed endoscopically. However, when patients have associated gastric outlet obstruction or other technical factors not allowing access to or cannulation of the papilla, or if a skilled endoscopist is not available, percutaneous drainage may be necessary.

## CHEMOTHERAPY AND RADIOTHERAPY

Because of the rarity of distal bile duct cancers, there are no trials examining chemotherapy or radiotherapy for this disease entity. Clinical practice of these palliative anticancer therapies is based on the little available data for pancreatic cancer extrapolated to distal bile duct cancer. 5-fluorouracil (5-FU) is the chemotherapy most often used in patients with primary, locally unresectable, metastatic, or recurrent low bile duct cancers. There is certainly no study demon-

strating a benefit for postoperative adjuvant chemotherapy after complete resection of tumor. Radiotherapy has also been advocated for patients with locally unresectable, metastatic, or recurrent disease, again based on data extrapolated from pancreatic or high bile duct cancers. Our practice is to use no chemotherapy or radiotherapy in the adjuvant setting. Combined external beam radiation with 5-FU chemotherapy is offered to patients with locally advanced and unresectable disease.

## BENIGN NEOPLASMS OF THE BILIARY TRACT

Benign tumors of the biliary tract are extremely rare. These tumors constitute approximately 2% to 6% of all extrahepatic bile duct neoplasms, and it is estimated that only 200 cases of benign bile duct tumor have been reported in the literature.[2,79-81] The exact incidence of these lesions is difficult to determine accurately, because they are often slow-growing and may remain clinically occult. In autopsy series bile duct hamartoma, an uncommon form of benign bile duct tumor, has been found incidentally in 0.7% of patients.[82]

The most common types of benign bile duct tumor are ones that arise from the epithelium lining the ducts; however, biliary leiomyoma, granular cell myoblastoma, and tumors of neural origin have been reported.[83-86] The most common of the epithelial neoplasms are adenoma and papilloma. Burhans and Meyer[2] reported a review of 84 patients with benign bile duct neoplasms in which 41 (49%) had papilloma, 39 (46%) had adenoma, and the remaining a variety of other histologic subtypes. An additional tumor occasionally found at autopsy, or incidentally at surgery, is the biliary hamartoma. This lesion may also be part of the von Meyenburg complex, which includes a spectrum of fibropolycystic diseases.[82,87] Symptoms or complications from bile duct hamartoma are extremely uncommon.[88,89]

Patients with benign bile duct tumors present with nonspecific symptoms and physical findings. These tumors are often slow-growing, and because of this, the symptoms may develop over long periods of time or be intermittent in nature. The most common presenting symptom for patients with benign tumors of the bile duct is jaundice.[90] Other symptoms described include abdominal pain, nausea, vomiting, or hemobilia. Physical findings are also nonspecific and may include liver enlargement, a palpable gallbladder, abdominal tenderness, and jaundice. Because of the nonspecific presentation of patients with this disease, the diagnostic workup is similar to that described for patients with malignant tumors of the bile duct.

The optimal treatment for these lesions is en bloc surgical resection. The scope of the operation required ranges from local bile duct excisions to extensive liver or pancreatic resections. Dowdy et al reviewed the literature on benign bile duct tumors in 1962 and detailed the operative treatment for 37 patients with these lesions.[95] In that series a total of five patients suffered recurrence of tumor. Four of the five patients who had recurrence, however, had undergone only a local excision of the tumor. Additional studies since 1962 have also shown an increase in tumor recurrence if treatment is less than total surgical excision.[2]

Because of these data we recommend en bloc resection of benign tumors of the bile duct. Procedures such as endoscopic snaring, curettage, and local excision are not recommended unless the patient is otherwise not able to tolerate a larger surgical procedure. Pancreaticoduodenectomy may be necessary for benign tumors in the periampullary region, but in general, the smallest operation that allows complete excision should be performed.

## CONCLUSIONS

In conclusion, cholangiocarcinoma is an uncommon malignancy that most commonly affects the bile duct at its bifurcation. Without treatment this disease results in rapidly progressive jaundice, liver failure, and death. Surgical resection is the only treatment modality that presently can offer a cure, and therefore any patient who presents with obstructive jaundice should be evaluated for malignancy. Surgical resection for distal tumors most often requires pancreaticoduodenectomy, and for proximal tumors bile duct excision with or without hepatic resection. Adjuvant radiotherapy and chemotherapy have not been shown to improve survival after resection. Radiotherapy, however, may improve survival and increase the quality of life in unresectable patients who have undergone palliative procedures. The chemotherapeutic treatment of advanced disease remains of unproven benefit.

## REFERENCES

1. KUVSHINOFF BW et al: Proximal bile duct tumors. Surg Oncol Clin North Am 5:317, 1996.
2. BURHANS R, MEYER RT: Benign neoplasms of the extrahepatic biliary ducts. Am Surg 37:161, 1971.
3. NAKEEB A et al: Cholangiocarcinoma a spectrum of intrahepatic, perihilar, and distal tumors. Ann Surg 224:463, 1996.
4. TOMPKINS RK et al: Prognostic factors in bile duct carcinoma: Analysis of 96 cases. Ann Surg 194:447, 1981.
5. ALEXANDER F et al: Biliary carcinoma: A review of 109 cases. Am J Surg 147:503, 1984.
6. SOREIDE O et al: Clinical spectrum and diagnostic strategies in non-calculous lower bile duct obstruction. Digestive Surg 2:209, 1986.
7. KLATSKIN G: Adenocarcinoma of the hepatic duct at its bifurcation within the porta hepatis. An unusual tumor with distinctive clinical and pathological features. Am J Med 38:241, 1965.
8. TERBLANCHE J et al: Prolonged palliation in carcinoma of the main hepatic duct junction. Surgery 71:720, 1972.
9. WASHBURN WK et al: Aggressive surgical resection for cholangiocarcinoma. Arch Surg 130:270, 1995.
10. WANG YJ et al: Clinical experience in 126 patients with tissue-proved proximal cholangiocarcinoma. J Gastroenterol Hepatol 9:134, 1994.
11. BROWN G, MYERS N: The hepatic ducts. A surgical approach for resection of tumors. Aust NZ J Surg 23:308, 1954.
12. ALTERMEIER WA et al: Sclerosing carcinoma of the major intrahepatic bile ducts. Arch Surg 75:450, 1957.
13. PARKIN DM et al: Cholangiocarcinoma: epidemiology, mechanisms of carcinogenesis and prevention. Cancer epidemiology, biomarkers and prevention. 2:537, 1993.
14. NAKANUMA Y et al: Are hepatolithiasis and cholangiocarcinoma aetiologically related? A morphological study of 12 cases of hepatolithiasis associated with cholangiocarcinoma. Virchows Arch Abt A Pathol Anat 406:45, 1985.
15. AKWARI OE et al: Cancer of the bile ducts associated with ulcerative colitis. Ann Surg 181:303, 1975.
16. CHAPMAN RW: Primary sclerosing cholangitis—A review of its clinical features. Gut 32:1433, 1991.
17. ALTEMEIER WA et al: Sclerosing carcinoma of the intrahepatic (hilar) bile ducts. Surgery 60:191, 1966.
18. WEINBREN K, MUTUM SS: Pathologic aspects of cholangiocarcinoma. J Pathol 139:217, 1983.
19. KIRSCHBAUM JD, KOZOLL DC: Carcinoma of the gallbladder and extrahepatic bile ducts. Surg Gynecol Obstet 73:740, 1941.
20. TSUZUKI T et al: Carcinoma of the bifurcation of the hepatic ducts. Arch Surg 118:1147, 1983.
21. KUWAYTI K et al: Carcinoma of the major intrahepatic and the extrahepatic bile ducts exclusive of the papilla of Vater. Surg Gynecol Obstet 104:357, 1957.
22. FARLEY DR et al: "Natural history" of unresected cholangiocarcinoma: patient outcome after noncurative intervention. Mayo Clin Proc 70:425, 1995.
23. SAKO S et al: Carcinoma of the extrahepatic bile ducts. Review of the literature and report of six cases. Surgery 41:416, 1957.
24. OTTOW RT et al: Treatment of proximal biliary tract carcinoma: an overview of techniques and results. Surgery 97:251, 1985.
25. HADJIS NS et al: Patterns of serum alkaline phosphatase activity in unilateral hepatic duct obstruction: a clinical and experimental study. Surgery 107:193, 1990.
26. HADJIS NS et al: Nonoperative approach to hilar cancer determined by the atrophy-hypertrophy complex. Am J Surg 157:395, 1989.
27. BLUMGART LH, KENNEDY A: Carcinoma of the ampulla of Vater and duodenum: a clinical and pathological study of 31 cases. Br J Surg 60:33, 1973.
28. BENJAMIN IS, BLUMGART LH: Cancer of the bile ducts, in *Surgery of the Liver and Biliary Tract,* 2d ed, LH Blumgart et al (eds). Edinburgh, Churchill Livingstone, 1994, pp 967–995.
29. HANN LE et al: Hepatic lobar atrophy: Association with ipsilateral portal vein obstruction. AJR 167:1017, 1996.
30. LOOSER CH et al: Staging of hilar cholangiocarcinoma by ultrasound and duplex sonography: A comparison with angiography and operative findings. Br J Radiol 65:871, 1992.
31. HANN LE et al: Malignant hepatic hilar tumors: Can ultrasonography be used as an alternative to angiography with CT arterial portography for determination of resectability? J Ultrasound Med 15:37, 1996.
32. SCHWARTZ LH et al: Neoplastic pancreaticobiliary duct obstruction: evaluation with breath-hold MR cholangiopancreatography AJR. 170:1491, 1998.
33. SOTO JA et al: Magnetic resonance cholangiography: Comparison with endoscopic retrograde cholangiopancreatography. Gastroenterology 110:589, 1996.
34. HATFIELD ARW et al: Preoperative external biliary drainage in obstructive jaundice: a prospective controlled clinical trial. Lancet 2:896, 1982.
35. McPHERSON GAD et al: Pre-operative percutaneous transhepatic biliary drainage: The results of a controlled trial. Br J Surg 71:371, 1984.
36. BAER HU et al: Improvements in survival by aggressive resection of hilar cholangiocarcinoma. Ann Surg 217:20, 1993.

37. BEAZLEY RM et al: Clinicopathological aspects of high bile duct cancer. Experience with resection and bypass surgical treatments. Ann Surg 199:623, 1984.

38. LONGMIRE WP et al: Carcinoma of the extrahepatic biliary tract. Ann Surg 178:333, 1973.

39. FORTNER JG et al: Surgical management of carcinoma of the junction of the main hepatic ducts. Ann Surg 184:68, 1976.

40. LAUNOIS B et al: Carcinoma of the hepatic hilum. Ann Surg 190:151, 1979.

41. AKWARI OE, KELLY KA: Surgical treatment of adenocarcinoma. Location: Junction of the right, left, and common hepatic biliary ducts. Arch Surg 114:22, 1979.

42. CAMERON JL et al: Proximal bile duct tumors. Surgical management with silastic transhepatic biliary stents. Ann Surg 196:412, 1982.

43. BLUMGART LH et al: Surgical approaches to cholangiocarcinoma at confluence of hepatic ducts. Lancet 1:66, 1984.

44. CAMERON JL et al: Management of proximal cholangiocarcinomas by surgical resection and radiotherapy. Am J Surg 159:91, 1990.

45. NIMURA Y et al: Hepatic segmentectomy with caudate lobe resection for bile duct carcinoma of the hepatic hilum. World J Surg 14:533, 1990.

46. HADJIS NS et al: Outcome of radical surgery in hilar cholangiocarcinoma. Surgery 107:597, 1990.

47. BISMUTH H et al: Management strategies in resection for hilar cholangiocarcinoma. Ann Surg 215:31, 1992.

48. GUTHRIE CM et al: Changing trends in the management of extrahepatic cholangiocarcinoma. Br J Surg 80:1434, 1993.

49. PISTERS PWT et al: Hilar cholangiocarcinoma—Surgical strategies (abstract). Plenary and Parallel Sessions. Soc Surg Oncol 1996, p 11.

50. SU CH et al: Factors influencing postoperative morbidity, mortality, and survival after resection for hilar cholangiocarcinoma. Ann Surg 223:384, 1996.

51. KLEMPNAUER J et al: Resectional surgery of hilar cholangiocarcinoma: A multivariate analysis of prognostic factors. J Clin Oncol 15:947, 1997.

52. TSUZUKI T, UEKUSA M: Carcinoma of the proximal bile ducts. Surg Gynecol Obstet 146:933, 1978.

53. SAKAGUCHI S, NAKAMURA S: Surgery of the portal vein in resection of cancer of the hepatic hilum. Surgery 99:344, 1986.

54. BLUMGART LH, THOMPSON JN: The management of malignant strictures of the bile duct. Curr Probl Surg 24:69, 1987.

55. FONG Y: Resection for bile duct carcinoma: Technical considerations, in *Hepatobiliary Malignancy—Its Multidisciplinary Management*, J Terblanche (ed). London, Edward Arnold, 1994, pp 571–592.

56. LANGER JC et al: Carcinoma of the extrahepatic bile ducts: Results of an aggressive surgical approach. Surgery 98:752, 1985.

57. BLUMGART LH, BENJAMIN IS: Liver resection for bile duct cancer. Surg Clin North Am 69:323, 1989.

58. MIZUMOTO R et al: Surgical treatment of hilar carcinoma of the bile duct. Surg Gynecol Obstet 162:153, 1986.

59. PICHLMAYR R et al: Radical resection and liver grafting as the two main components of surgical strategy in the treatment of proximal bile duct cancer. World J Surg 12:68, 1988.

60. TERBLANCHE J, LOUW JH: "U"-tube drainage in the palliative therapy of carcinoma of the main hepatic duct junction. Surg Clin North Am 53:1245, 1973.

61. GLATTLI A et al: Unresectable malignant biliary obstruction: treatment by self-expandable biliary endoprostheses. HPB Surg 6:175, 1993.

62. MEN S et al: Palliation of malignant obstructive jaundice. Use of self-expandable metal stents. Acta Radiol 37:259, 1996.

63. JARNAGIN WR et al: Intrahepatic biliary enteric bypass for malignant obstruction at the hepatic duct confluence: effective palliation in selected patients. Am J Surg 175:453, 1998.

64. MEYERS WC, JONES RS: Internal radiation for bile duct cancer. World J Surg 12:99, 1988.

65. ESCHELMAN DJ et al: Malignant biliary duct obstruction: Long-term experience with Gianturco stents and combined-modality radiation therapy. Radiology 200:717, 1996.

66. PITT HA et al: Perihilar cholangiocarcinoma. Postoperative radiotherapy does not improve survival. Ann Surg 221:788, 1995.

67. KUVSHINOFF BW et al: Palliation of irresectable hilar cholangiocarcinoma with biliary drainage and radiotherapy. Br J Surg 82:1522, 1995.

68. OBERFIELD RA, ROSSI RL: The role of chemotherapy in the treatment of bile duct cancer. World J Surg 12:105, 1988.

69. VAUTHEY JN, BLUMGART LH: Recent advances in the management of cholangiocarcinomas. Semin Liver Dis 14:109, 1994.

70. HARVEY JH et al: 5-fluorouracil, mitomycin, and doxorubicin (FAM) in carcinoma of the biliary tract. J Clin Oncol 2:1245, 1984.

71. TOMPKINS RK et al: Prognostic factors in bile duct carcinoma. Analysis of 96 cases. Ann Surg 194:447, 1981.

72. WARREN KW et al: Results of radical resection for periampullary cancer. Ann Surg 181:534, 1975.

73. LERUT JP et al: Pancreaticoduodenal resection. Surgical experience and evaluation of risk factors in 103 patients. Ann Surg 199:432, 1984.

74. TARAZI RY et al: Results of surgical treatment of periampullary tumors: A thirty-five year experience. Surgery 100:716, 1986.

75. NAGORNEY DM et al: Outcomes after curative resections of cholangiocarcinoma. Arch Surg 128:871, 1993.

76. FONG Y et al: Outcome of treatment for distal bile duct cancer. Br J Surg 83:1712, 1996.

77. CRILE G JR: The advantages of bypass operations over radical pancreaticoduodenectomy in the treatment of pancreatic carcinoma. Surg Gynecol Obstet 130:1049, 1970.

78. FONG Y et al: Pancreatic or liver resection for malignancy is safe and effective for the elderly. Ann Surg 222:426, 1995.

79. ISHAK KG, RABIN L: Benign tumors of the liver. Med Clin North Am 59:995, 1975.

80. FOSTER JH: Primary benign solid tumors of the liver. Am J Surg 133:536, 1977.

81. GOLD JH et al: Benign tumors of the liver. Pathologic examination of 45 cases. Am J Clin Pathol 70:6, 1978.

82. CHUNG EB: Multiple bile-duct hamartomas. Cancer 26:287, 1970.

83. DURSI JF et al: Granular cell myoblastoma of the common bile duct: report of a case and review of the literature. Rev Surg 32:305, 1975.

84. CURRY B, GRAY N: Visceral neurofibromatosis. An unusual cause of obstructive jaundice. Br J Surg 59:494, 1972.

85. ARCHAMBAULT H, ARCHAMBAULT R: Leiomyoma of the common bile duct. Arch Surg 64:531, 1952.

86. KUNE GA, POLGAR V: Leiomyoma of the common bile duct causing obstructive jaundice. Med J Aust 1:698, 1976.

87. THOMMESEN N: Biliary hamartomas (von Meyenburg complexes) in liver needle biopsies. Acta Pathol Microbiol Immunol Scand Sect A, Pathol 86:93, 1978.

88. HOMER LW et al: Neoplastic transformation of von Meyenburg complexes of the liver. J Pathol Bacteriol 96:499, 1968.

89. BORNFORS M: The development of cholangiocarcinoma from multiple bile-duct adenomas. Acta Pathol Microbiol Immunol Scand Sect A 92:285, 1984.

90. DAVIES W et al: Extrahepatic biliary cystadenomas and cystadenocarcinoma. Report of seven cases and review of the literature (review). Ann Surg 222:619, 1995.

91. IWASAKI Y: Surgical treatment for carcinoma at the confluence of the major hepatic ducts. Surg Gynecol Obstet 162:457, 1986.

92. IIDA S et al: The long-term survival of patients with carcinoma of the main hepatic duct junction. Cancer 60:1612, 1987.

93. BENGMARK S et al: Major liver resection for hilar cholangiocarcinoma. Ann Surg 207:120, 1988.

94. NAKASE A et al: Surgical treatment of cancer of the pancreas and the periampullary region: cumulative results in 57 institutions in Japan. Ann Surg 185:52, 1977.

95. DOWDY GS et al: Benign tumors of the extrahepatic bile ducts: Report of three cases and a review of the literature. Arch Surg 85:503, 1962.

# CHAPTER 15

# NEOPLASMS OF THE SMALL INTESTINE

*Joshua T. Rubin*

## INTRODUCTION

Primary tumors of the small intestine are great in variety yet limited in frequency. Their clinical significance lies in the complications that they engender, which often require surgical intervention, and their resistance to most forms of therapy when they are malignant. Small-bowel cancer accounts for less than 5% of all gastrointestinal malignancies, even though the small intestine accounts for 75% of the length of the alimentary tract and 90% of its mucosal surface area.[1] The small intestine's relative freedom from neoplasia, in comparison to the stomach proximally and particularly the colon distally, suggests that elucidation of the reasons for this apparent paradox may lead to a better understanding of the more common cancers afflicting western society.

About two-thirds of small-intestinal tumors are malignant.[1] Adenocarcinoma, carcinoid, sarcoma, and lymphoma account for more than 95% of these.[1] Some have a predilection for specific portions of the alimentary tract. Adenocarcinomas tend to cluster in the duodenum, especially near the ampulla of Vater. True ampullary carcinomas are considered extrahepatic biliary tumors rather than small-intestinal tumors. Non-Hodgkin's lymphomas and carcinoid tumors have a predilection for the ileum and particularly its distal extent. Sarcomas occur with even distribution throughout the small intestine.

Primary small-intestinal cancer is sinister because it often presents at an advanced stage, unless incidentally identified in the course of laparotomy or imaging studies performed for unrelated problems. Symptoms, often vague, may be related to obstruction of the small-intestinal lumen due to encroachment by tumor or angulation of the bowel. This is gradual in onset and is often attributed to functional disorders of the gastrointestinal system by unwary physicians and patients. Bleeding, another manifestation of small-bowel neoplasms, may be occult and may only gradually progress to symptomatic anemia. More dramatic complications,

such as intestinal perforation, massive bleeding, intussuception, or complete intestinal obstruction, lead to expeditious diagnosis. Unfortunately, these usually represent late manifestations of advanced disease.

## ANATOMY

The small intestine is arbitrarily divided into three segments based on gross and microscopic anatomic characteristics, which have implications for disease pathogenesis, symptomatology, and therapy. The duodenum is 25 cm in length, extending from the pylorus to the ligament of Treitz. It is unique histologically in that it is the only portion of the small intestine to contain Brunner's glands within the submucosa. Unlike the jejunum and ileum, it is predominantly retroperitoneal. The duodenum is adjacent to and surrounds the pancreatic head, and the pancreaticoduodenal arterial arcades are nestled between these two organs. The pancreas and extrahepatic biliary tree drain into the second portion of the duodenum through the ampulla of Vater. As a result of these anatomic associations, simple segmental resection of invasive duodenal tumors, such as can be easily accomplished with the intraperitoneal small bowel, is often technically impossible or biologically unwise.

The jejunum and ileum are suspended from the retroperitoneum by a mesentery that envelops them and contains their intestinal blood supply and draining lymph nodes. They extend 6 m from the ligament of Treitz to the ileocecal valve. The jejunum contributes about 40% of the length of the small intestine, with the remaining 60% consisting of ileum. The ileum is particularly rich in lymphoid tissue that is arranged into discrete aggregates called Peyer's patches near the ileocecal valve.

The cells that give rise to neoplasms of the small intestine are located within any one of its four histologically discrete layers. The mucosal crypts of Lieberkühn contain multipotent stem cells that give rise to the well-differentiated, columnar epithelial cells of the small-bowel mucosa. Neuroendocrine Kulchitsky cells are also found within these crypts. The underlying lamina propia is rich in lacteals and immunocytes. The submucosal layer contains lymphatic vessels and Meissner's plexus of nerves. The third layer, the muscularis propia, consists of an inner circular and outer longitudinal layer of smooth muscle, within which lie the ganglion cells of Auerbach's plexus and interstitial cells of Cajal. The latter may serve a pacemaker function for coordinated small-intestinal motility.[2,3] These three layers are enveloped in a thin layer of connective tissue referred to as serosa.

An understanding of the lymphatic drainage of the small intestine is important for treating some of its neoplasms. Periduodenal lymph nodes drain into lymph nodes located around the portal vein and the pancreas. Jejunal and ileal lymph nodes drain into adjacent mesenteric lymph nodes. Lymphatic drainage from the jejunum continues to the superior mesenteric artery nodes. The ileal lymphatics drain into the ileocolic lymph nodes. These represent common routes of tumor dissemination. The draining lymph nodes should be removed as part of the curative resection of small-bowel malignancies that are known to disseminate through lymphatic channels. This defines the extent of resection for adenocarcinoma, carcinoid tumors, and some lymphomas.

## EPIDEMIOLOGY AND ETIOLOGY

The incidence of small-bowel cancer is slowly increasing.[1,4,5] There are about 4600 new cases diagnosed every year in the United States.[6] Adenocarcinoma, carcinoid, lymphoma, and sarcoma account for almost all of these. From 1973 to 1982, the incidence of small-bowel carcinoid rose from 2.2 to 3.1 per million Americans.[1,4] The increase in the incidence of carcinoid has been seen more among African Americans than Caucasians.[1,4] From 1983 to 1993, the incidence of small-bowel adenocarcinoma increased from 1.2 to 1.6 per 100,000 among white Americans and from 1.8 to 2.4 per 100,000 among African Americans.[1,4] It has been suggested that environmental factors are responsible, in part, for this trend (Table 15-1). Some studies have found an association between cigarette use, alcohol consumption, and small-bowel cancer.[7,8] There is no apparent association with income, level of education, or socioeconomic level.[1] A weak association with dietary fat, dietary protein, and sugar consumption has been reported.[1,8,9] Age is an independent risk factor. Within subgroups, patients with adenocarcinoma are generally older than patients with lymphoma. Increases in the incidence of small-intestinal lymphoma have been attributed, in part, to the AIDS epidemic.[1]

Several hypotheses have been posited to explain the relatively low incidence of small-intestinal neoplasms (Table 15-2). These focus on either intrinsic mechanisms of defense or vehicles of cell injury that can lead to neoplastic transformation. The IgA-mediated mucosal immune system may protect against the establishment of small-intestinal cancer.[10,11] This is consistent with the observation that patients who are deficient in this immunoglobulin have a higher incidence of small-intestinal cancer than the normal population. Duodenal diamine oxidase purportedly exerts a protective effect against small-intestinal neoplasia,[12,13] and the microsomal enzyme

### TABLE 15-1. RISK FACTORS FOR SMALL-BOWEL CANCER

| RISK FACTOR | STRENGTH OR CONSISTENCY OF ASSOCIATION |
|---|---|
| Crohn's disease | ++++ |
| Adenomas | +++ |
| FAP | +++ |
| Other GI cancers | +++ |
| Cholecystectomy | + |
| Peptic ulcer disease | + |
| Radiation | + |
| Blood type A | + |
| Tobacco use | + |
| Dietary intake of: | |
|    Animal fat | + |
|    Animal protein | + |
|    Sugar | + |
|    Alcohol | + |

benzpyrene hydroxylase may detoxify potential carcinogens in the small intestine.[14] The rapid transit of chyme through the small bowel limits the population of bacteria that can metabolize food to potential carcinogens.[15] Rapid transit also limits exposure of the mucosa to these and other ingested carcinogens. The alkalinity of intestinal chyme may inhibit the generation of carcinogenic nitrosamines.[1] The rapid rate of turnover of the intestinal mucosa and the high rate of programmed cell death may serve a protective effect, because mutated cells are lost before they can become established tumors.[16,17]

Ultimately, alterations in oncogenes and tumor suppressor genes are responsible for neoplasia. This is a multistep process in which a cell accumulates mutations sufficient to release it from the normal genetic control of growth and differentiation. The gross and histologic correlate of this transformation is seen in the adenoma-carcinoma sequence that is a relevant model for small-bowel adenocarcinoma.[18] Like adenomas of the colon, adenomas of the small bowel harbor certain genetic mutations with great frequency, suggesting that they are etiologic. In some series, 50% of evaluated specimens reveal active mutations in cK-ras.[19–22] Forty percent of evaluated tumors display increased expression of cyclin D[17]; p53

### TABLE 15-2. HYPOTHESES TO EXPLAIN THE LOW INCIDENCE OF SMALL-BOWEL MALIGNANCY

Intrinsic mechanisms of mucosal defense:
   IgA
   Diamine oxidase
   Benzpyrene hydroxylase
   Rapid turnover of mucosal epithelium
   Low levels of bcl-2 expression

Limitation of exposure to carcinogens:
   Rapid transit of chyme
   Alkalinity of chyme
   Low numbers of bacteria

mutations have been identified in as many as 73% of specimens.[19,23] A point mutation in the *neu* gene has been identified in small-bowel adenocarcinoma, suggesting that its protein product p185 may play a role in the transformation of small-bowel polyps to carcinoma.[19,23] Finally, expression of the gene bcl-2 is greater in the colonic mucosa than it is in the small-intestinal mucosa of certain murine models.[16] This low level of bcl-2 expression by the small intestine may allow mutated cells to be eliminated by apoptosis before they undergo malignant transformation.

Several heritable defects are known to increase the risk of developing adenocarcinoma of the small intestine. These include germline mutations of the APC gene on chromosome 5 among patients with familial adenomatous polyposis syndrome (FAP).[1,24] Affected patients are prone to develop multiple adenomatous polyps in the small bowel. Small-bowel adenocarcinoma that develops as a result of this mutation is usually located in the periampullary region of the duodenum, just like sporadic adenocarcinoma of the small bowel. Germ-line mutations in the DNA mismatch repair genes hMLH1 and hMSH2 are associated with human nonpolyposis colon carcinoma (HNPCC) or Lynch syndrome.[25–28] Small-bowel adenocarcinoma is less likely to complicate this syndrome than it is to complicate FAP. Patients with Peutz-Jeghers syndrome develop intestinal hamartomatous polyps that may become dysplastic and ultimately progress to adenocarcinoma.[29] The incidence of small-intestinal adenocarcinoma appears to be greater than the risk of colon cancer in these patients.

The observed association of small-intestinal cancer with several chronic intestinal diseases suggests that growth factors may, in part, be etiologic. For example, the risk of small-intestinal cancer is increased among patients with Crohn's disease.[30–32] Unlike sporadic small-intestinal adenocarcinoma, these tumors do not have a predilection for the duodenum and usually develop in propinquity to diseased segments of small intestine. Similarly, adenocarcinoma can develop at anastomotic sites 25 years postoperatively.[33,34] Celiac disease is characterized by intestinal inflammation that presumably is a result of chronic antigenic stimulation. This may be responsible for the increased incidence of adenocarcinoma and lymphoma seen in these patients.[35–39]

## DIAGNOSIS

The diagnosis of benign intestinal tumors is usually made incidentally when x-ray studies are performed for unrelated symptoms or when surgery is performed for unrelated diseases. Benign small-bowel tumors are thought to be symptomatic less frequently than malignant ones. Benign duodenal tumors may be discovered at the time of upper GI endoscopy performed for symptoms of peptic ulcer disease. Malignant tumors of the small intestine are usually diagnosed at an advanced stage as the result of a low level of clinical suspicion.[40–44] The median duration of symptoms before a diagnosis of adenocarcinoma is made approaches 8 months,[45] and as many as one-third of patients have had symptoms for 5 years or more.[45]

No one radiographic procedure has been identified as the most accurate or useful diagnostic test in the setting of small-intestinal tumors. Indeed, many of these investigations complement one another. Enteroclysis may be the most sensitive procedure for identifying small-intestinal tumors, particularly when the diagnosis is suspected beforehand.[46] This study, performed by injecting barium through a nasojejunal tube, can detect partially obstructing tumors that would otherwise be missed by a routine small-bowel follow-through or that are beyond the reach of an enteroscope. The radiographic appearance of the mucosal folds may differentiate small-intestinal adenocarcinoma from submucosal tumors and metastatic lesions. Although CT scans cannot identify small tumors, they may accurately identify tumors associated with high-grade or complete bowel obstruction, and they are much more useful in planning therapy since they help to stage the disease by identifying regional nodal metastases or more distant visceral metastatic lesions.[47] The CT appearance of small-intestinal carcinoid may be pathognomonic due to the dense fibrosis that develops in the adjacent mesentery. Angiography may identify hypervascular tumors that present with intestinal bleeding.

Laboratory tests are useful in the preoperative evaluation of patients with established intestinal tumors. Occult bleeding may lead to the gradual development of anemia. Liver metastases may be associated with an elevation of the hepatic transaminases AST (aspartate aminotransferase) and ALT (alanine aminotransferase). Patients with carcinoid tumor may develop the carcinoid syndrome, which then leads to a characteristic biochemical profile in the urine and blood. Lactate dehydrogenase (LDH) should be determined preoperatively in patients with intestinal lymphoma because of its association with prognosis. Patients with intestinal lymphoma and carcinoid syndrome may develop diarrhea, which can lead to preoperative electrolyte abnormalities. Unfortunately, there are no sensitive or specific serologic tumor markers that allow for early diagnosis or screening for recurrent disease.

## BENIGN INTESTINAL TUMORS

There are a large number of congenital and acquired benign intestinal tumors that must be distinguished from small-intestinal malignancy. These are often discovered incidentally in the course of an evaluation for unrelated symptoms. Their clinical import lies in the need to distinguish them from malignant tumors of the intestinal tract and in their potential for causing significant morbidity.

### HETEROTOPIC TISSUE

Heterotopic pancreas can present as a duodenal excrescence.[48,49] Histologically, it contains ducts and acini, but no islet tissue. The most common location of these benign tumors is near the duodenal ampulla. These tumors occasionally contain smooth muscle, in which case they are labeled adenomyomas. They rarely are the site of a neuroendocrine tumor, adenocarcinoma, or pancreatitis. Heterotopic gastric mucosa can present in a similar fashion.[49] Histologically, these tumors contain fundic mucosa, with both chief and parietal cells.

## HAMARTOMAS

Peutz-Jeghers syndrome is an autosomal dominant trait associated with harmartomatous polyps of the gastrointestinal tract.[50–53] Patients usually have a characteristic pigmentation on the lips or the oral mucosa. Grossly, the intestinal lesions resemble adenomatous polyps. Histologically, however, they contain only smooth muscle, connective tissue, intestinal glands, and mucosal epithelium. These benign lesions can be mistaken for adenocarcinoma of the small intestine, and the incidence of small-intestine adenocarcinoma, as well as the incidence of certain other malignancies, is increased among these patients. Hamartomatous polyps similar to these can appear in patients who are not affected by Peutz-Jeghers syndrome.

Brunner's gland adenomas are unique to the duodenum.[54–56] They represent yet another small-intestinal hamartoma. Histologically, they represent a proliferation of normal duodenal glands. When exuberant, the resulting tumors can be large enough to cause duodenal obstruction or bleeding. Brunner's gland adenomas may be multifocal or diffuse.

## MESENCHYMAL TUMORS

A myriad of benign mesenchymal tumors may also present in the small intestine. They are derived from the vessels, nerves, or smooth muscle of the muscularis mucosa, the submucosa, or the muscularis propria. They present as well-circumscribed submucosal lesions, as opposed to adenocarcinoma, which arises in and destroys the mucosa. Their benign biologic behavior is implied grossly by small size (<5 cm) and microscopically by the near absence of mitoses, absence of necrosis, and low histologic grade.

Leiomyomas are the most common benign mesenchymal tumor.[57–60] Patients are commonly 40 to 50 years old when these tumors are discovered. Duodenal leiomyomas are less common than those occurring in the jejunum and ileum. They may be a manifestation of von Recklinghausen's disease. They occur with equal frequency in men and women. Their clinical significance lies in the inability to easily distinguish them from leiomyosarcomas. They are usually asymptomatic, unless they cause obstruction or bleeding. Perforation is rare. Simple resection with negative margins is adequate therapy.

Lipomas represent the second most common benign tumor of the small intestine.[61–64] At least 60% of these occur in the ileum. Lipomas have a characteristic radiographic appearance. They are usually identified in the course of an evaluation for unrelated symptoms. These tumors may rarely cause ileocolic intussusception or, if pedunculated, may undergo torsion and necrosis. Asymptomatic lipomas can be treated nonoperatively.

Hemangiomas account for about 10% of small-intestinal tumors.[60] At least half of these are cavernous. The remainder are either capillary or mixed.[65,66] These benign vascular tumors are often multiple and are located in the submucosa. They may be a manifestation of systemic vasculopathies such as Osler-Weber-Rendu disease, blue rubber bleb nevus syndrome, Mattucci's syndrome, or Klippel-Trénaunay syndrome. They may rarely cause intussusception. Their most common clinical presentation is bleeding. The most useful diagnostic study for localizing and at times treating these lesions is angiography. Effective angiographic embolization may obviate the need for surgical resection in this setting. Uncomplicated lesions can be observed. Lymphangiomas represent benign malformations of sequestered lymphatic tissue.[60] They are uncommon and may rarely cause protein-losing enteropathy or potassium loss, which can be cured by resection.[66,67] When they attain a large size, they may lead to intestinal obstruction.

There are a plethora of benign tumors of neural origin. Schwannomas (neurilemmomas) are unusual benign neural tumors that can occur in any portion of the small bowel.[60] They are often associated with von Recklinghausen's disease. Women are affected more frequently than men are. Histologically, they consist of schwann cells with myxoid areas (Antoni B) interspersed among cellular areas (Antoni A). Schwannomas do not undergo malignant transformation.

Neurofibromas arise from Auerbach's submucosal plexus of nerves.[60] They are most commonly solitary with a predilection for the jejunum, but they may be multiple in as many as 33% of patients with von Recklinghausen's disease, with which these tumors are often associated.[68] These benign tumors may undergo malignant transformation, with a concomitant increase in size. Growth may also lead to bleeding or intussusception. Treatment for these complications or for suspected malignancy is segmental intestinal resection.

Ganglioneuromas are rare benign tumors that may occur either sporadically or as part of well-described polyposis syndromes, in which setting they are usually multiple. Large lesions can cause intestinal obstruction or bleeding.

Gangliocytic paragangliomas are almost unique to the second portion of the duodenum near the ampulla of Vater.[69,70] These pedunculated, submucosal lesions may ulcerate and bleed, which is the most common clinical presentation. Although these tumors are not endocrinologically active, they are related to somatostatinomas and contain polypeptide hormones. They are almost always benign, yet isolated reports of regional lymph node metastases have been recorded.

## ADENOMAS

Small intestinal adenomas are relatively rare, compared to the frequency with which they develop in the large intestine.[53] They account for about 14% of benign small-intestinal tumors, and they occur with greatest frequency in the duodenum.[57] Like their counterparts in the colon, they may be either tubular, tubulovillous, or villous.[71,72] The latter are thought to be prone to malignant transformation.[73,74] Among duodenal adenomas, 12% were found to harbor carcinoma in situ and 30% had invasive cancer in one study.[75] In contrast to villous adenomas of the colon, size has not been found to invariably correlate with the malignant potential of villous adenomas in the small intestine.[75] They are most often clinically silent, but they may cause either occult or gross bleeding, anemia, intussusception, or jaundice. Their frequency is increased among patients with FAP.

## MALIGNANT INTESTINAL TUMORS

### ADENOCARCINOMA

Adenocarcinoma is the most common malignancy of the small intestine.[1] Its greatest incidence is in the sixth and seventh decades, and it is slightly more common in men than women.[1] It has a propensity to develop in the more proximal small intestine, with 50% of cases located in the duodenum, 40% in the jejunum, and only 10% in the ileum.[1] These rare tumors occur with increased frequency in a variety of clinical settings that include Crohn's disease,[32,76—86] nontropical sprue,[35—39] FAP,[1,24] Lynch syndrome type II,[24—28,87] Peutz-Jeghers syndrome,[29,53] long-standing intestinal anastomoses,[33,34] and cystic fibrosis.[88,89] Villous adenomas of the small bowel are also thought to be premalignant.[73—75,90]

The incidence of adenocarcinoma of the small intestine parallels that of colon carcinoma from country to country.[1] It is more common in the Maori of New Zealand, ethnic Hawaiians, and Swedes than it is in eastern Europeans and Chinese.[1] In the United States, the frequency is greater in men than women, with an average age of onset near 70 years. The incidence of small-intestinal adenocarcinoma increases with age. The frequency of intestinal adenocarcinoma is greater in African Americans than it is in Caucasians.[1]

Adenocarcinoma is usually discovered at a clinically advanced stage.[91] Presenting symptoms may develop as manifestations of intestinal obstruction and include abdominal pain, nausea, and vomiting.[91] Jaundice occurs frequently due to the periampullary location of many of these tumors. Anemia develops commonly as a result of chronic, occult bleeding from the tumor. Anorexia and weight loss are symptoms of advanced disease. At presentation, 67% of patients are found to have lymph node metastases.[40—43] As many as 22% of patients have more distant metastases at that time.[40—43]

Wide segmental resection of the tumor-containing bowel and its adjacent mesentery is the mainstay of therapy. A 5-cm-wide margin of resection on either side of the tumor is advised. For tumors within the first, second, and third portions of the duodenum, a pancreaticoduodenectomy is usually required due to the shared pancreatic and duodenal blood supply, the anatomy of the extrahepatic biliary tree, and the location of the draining lymphatic basin. Extended lymphadenectomy has not been shown to be associated with any survival advantage compared to standard pancreaticoduodenectomy.[92] Segmental resections for tumors in the fourth portion of the duodenum can sometimes be accomplished. Small-intestinal adenocarcinoma affecting the distal ileum should include resection of the right colon and its mesentery in order to accomplish a wide resection of draining lymph nodes. Contraindications to resection include metastatic disease beyond the field of resection or involvement of adjacent structures that cannot be sacrificed. As many as 50% of patients have tumors that are unresectable when diagnosed.[42] Palliation of these patients can sometimes be accomplished by intestinal bypass to allay symptomatic bowel obstruction, limited resection to control bleeding, or urgent operation to manage life-threatening complications.

Prognosis depends on the stage of disease at presentation (Table 15-3).[93] For patients without nodal metastatic disease, the 5-year survival following resection is 70%.[43] The 5-year survival rate for patients with nodal metastatic disease is as low as 13% after attempted curative resection.[43] The overall 5-year survival rate is about 25% in series reported over the past 10 years.[41,94—101] Survival rates for patients with duodenal cancer are a little better than for patients with jejunal or ileal adenocarcinoma.

The role of adjuvant therapy remains undefined. There are no well-designed, prospective, randomized trials evaluating its efficacy. These tumors are thought to be radiotherapy- and chemo-

## TABLE 15-3. AMERICAN JOINT COMMITTEE ON CANCER STAGING OF SMALL-INTESTINAL ADENOCARCINOMA

**Primary tumor (T):**

| | |
|---|---|
| TX | Primary tumor cannot be assessed |
| T0 | No evidence of primary tumor |
| Tis | Carcinoma in situ |
| T1 | Tumor invades lamina propria or submucosa |
| T2 | Tumor invades muscularis propria |
| T3 | Tumor invades into subserosa (peritonealized bowel) |
| | Tumor invades through muscularis propria into surrounding tissue for less than 2 cm (between leaves of mesentery or into retroperitoneum if duodenal) |
| T4 | Tumor invades adjacent organs |
| | Tumor perforates serosa |
| | Tumor extends more than 2 cm into retroperitoneum or between leaves of mesentery |

**Regional lymph nodes (N):**

| | |
|---|---|
| NX | Regional lymph nodes cannot be assessed |
| N0 | No regional lymph node metastases |
| N1 | Regional lymph node metastases present |

**Distant metastases (M):**

| | |
|---|---|
| MX | Presence of distant metastases cannot be assessed |
| M0 | No distant metastases |
| M1 | Distant metastases present |

**Stage:**

| | |
|---|---|
| 0 | Tis, N0, M0 |
| I | T1 or T2, N0, M0 |
| II | T3 or T4, N0, M0 |
| III | Any T, N1, M0 |
| IV | Any T, any N, M1 |

therapy-resistant. Therefore, adjuvant chemoradiation therapy is not generally recommended following resection. For duodenal adenocarcinoma, some clinicians extrapolate from the limited data concerning cancer of the pancreatic head and treat patients with radiation-sensitizing doses of 5-fluorouracil (5-FU) and concomitant radiation therapy. The treatment of metastatic disease is limited to investigational chemotherapy, since response rates to available chemotherapeutics have been exceedingly low. Although for patients with unresectable disease, there are anecdotal reports of long-term survival following treatment using chemotherapy and radiation therapy, most series report survival times that fall well short of 12 months.[40,41,95,102—107]

## SARCOMAS

Mesenchymal tumors of the small intestine do not have a predilection for any subsegment of bowel.[1] They can be broadly categorized as those that belong to a clearly defined cell lineage and those that do not. This has led to their arbitrary division into any one of four major categories based on phenotype.[49,60] The majority of malignant gastrointestinal tumors show clear-cut differentiation toward smooth muscle, as determined by immunohistochemical staining for smooth-muscle actin and desmin. These tumors presumably arise from the muscularis propria, the muscularis mucosa, or vessel-related smooth-muscle cells in the wall of the intestine. Gastrointestinal tumors of smooth-muscle cell lineage are regarded as either benign, borderline, or malignant, based on a constellation of phenotypic characteristics. Those that measure more than 5 cm in diameter, or that are found on light microscopy to have more than five mitotic figures per 10 high-power fields, are hypercellular, and those that have moderate to marked necrosis are considered biologically aggressive and prone to metastasize.

Other small-bowel mesenchymal tumors can clearly be identified as neural in origin.[49,60] Although stains for common neural markers such as chromogranin A and synaptophysin are usually absent, these tumors generally express neuron-specific enolase and S100. In addition, they invariably lack markers of smooth-muscle differentiation. They have been grouped under the rubric of gastrointestinal autonomic nerve tumors (GANTs).

A third category of mesenchymal tumors includes a small number of tumors defined immunohistochemically as expressing both smooth-muscle and neural differentiation markers.[49,60] These are much less common than tumors of singular smooth muscle or neural lineage. A fourth group of tumors lacks evident differentiation toward either smooth-muscle or neural cell lineage. These tumors have been classified as gastrointestinal stromal tumors (GIST) and are thought to develop from the interstitial cells of Cajal.[2] These CD34+ cells form a complex network within the gastrointestinal tract wall, where they may function as a pacemaker system. Like the interstitial cells themselves, GISTs reveal immunoreactivity for the kit receptor and they express CD34. It has been suggested that the term *gastrointestinal pacemaker cell tumor* should replace the previous appellation of *gastrointestinal stromal tumor*. These two groups of tumors are regarded as malignant or potentially malignant.

Leiomyosarcomas are malignant smooth muscle tumors that account for 10% to 20% of small-intestinal malignancies.[60] They usually measure more than 5 cm in diameter and often have invaded surrounding structures at the time of diagnosis. These tumors are distinguished from benign leiomyomas based on a mitotic rate exceeding five figures per high-power field, high cellularity, and presence of necrosis.[49,60] Although they arise in the submucosa, they frequently ulcerate the overlying mucosa and bleed. Leiomyoblastomas are a special variant of malignant smooth-muscle tumors that most commonly develop in the stomach and small intestine. Their histologic diagnosis requires the presence of epithelioid as well as typical spindle-shaped smooth-muscle cells.[108] Determination of the biologic aggressiveness of these tumors is difficult. The long-term prognosis is better for younger patients than it is for older ones. A clinical triad consisting of gastric leiomyoblastoma, pulmonary chondromas, and functional extra-adrenal paragangliomas has been described among young women (Carney's triad). For this reason, radiographic evidence of pulmonary lesions should not be assumed to represent metastatic disease in these patients.[109]

GANTs or plexosarcomas[110] are generally seen in patients close to 60 years of age. Although these tumors frequently metastasize soon after diagnosis, the 5-year survival rate of these patients is reported

to be as high as 60%.[111] Most of these tumors are large, often over 10 cm in diameter, and are locally aggressive. They probably arise from autonomic nerves in the bowel wall.

Intestinal sarcomas most commonly present with bleeding or symptomatic obstruction, or as an abdominal mass. When this diagnosis is suspected, preoperative evaluation should include an abdominopelvic CT scan and a chest radiograph or CT scan to rule out metastatic disease and direct extension to adjacent organs. Visceral angiography is not routinely performed preoperatively, although it may be used to control bleeding in patients whose tumors are not resectable. The role of preoperative biopsy is controversial. Tissue confirmation is advised when nonsurgical disease such as a germ cell tumor or lymphoma must be excluded. Even so, when initial attempts to biopsy these tumors are unsuccessful, aggressive or repetitive attempts must be carefully weighed against the inherent risk associated with these procedures.

The only curative therapy for malignant mesenchymal tumors of the small intestine is wide resection. Simple enucleation of the tumor is inappropriate due to its infiltrative nature. En bloc resection of adjacent organs is not necessary unless they are invaded, in which case organ preservation can usually be achieved without compromising margins of resection. Patients whose tumors invade a kidney and who might require total nephrectomy should undergo preoperative evaluation of their renal function in order to define the likelihood of postoperative chronic renal insufficiency. Patients who for similar reasons may need splenectomy should be treated prophylactically with preoperative vaccination against pneumococcus, meningococcus, and *Hemophilus influenzae* b. Biologically aggressive sarcomas disseminate through vascular channels rather than lymphatics.[112] For this reason, lymph node dissection is not considered a necessary component of curative resection.

The survival rate following complete extirpation of localized intestinal sarcoma approaches 20%.[94,98,113–116] Adjuvant chemotherapy has not been shown to be of survival benefit, but it is unwise to extrapolate from the small number of clinical reports involving limited numbers of patients treated before the availability of ifosfamide. For patients with unresectable and locally advanced tumors, one can make a cogent argument for the use of neoadjuvant ifosfamide and doxorubicin chemotherapy, with or without radiation therapy, followed by resection, if technically feasible following a significant clinical response.

The most common sites of recurrent or metastatic disease are the liver and peritoneum.[117,118] Highly selected patients with isolated hepatic or pulmonary metastases may manifest prolonged survival or even cure as a result of aggressive surgical therapy of their metastatic disease. There is little proven benefit to systemic chemotherapy, however. The most active agents, doxorubicin and ifosfamide, are associated with response rates approaching 30%, but they have not been associated with clear-cut prolongation of survival.

## CARCINOID TUMOR

Carcinoid tumors represent a group of neoplasms arising from endocrine-type cells that constitute the amine precursor uptake and decarboxylation (APUD) system.[119,120] They account for approximately 30% of small-bowel tumors and occur most commonly in the ileum.[121,122] Carcinoid tumors grow as submucosal masses. They may be locally invasive, and, when aggressive, they metastasize via regional lymph nodes. They are often associated with a fibrotic reaction that affects the adjacent small-intestinal mesentery. This may cause kinking of the bowel and obstruction or intestinal ischemia as a result of encasement of mesenteric blood vessels.[123,124] Many of these tumors are found incidentally, either in the course of a radiographic evaluation for related symptoms, during upper gastrointestinal endoscopy, or on evaluation of the appendix following appendectomy.

Symptoms are usually due to local complications, including pain in 27% of patients, nausea and vomiting in 10% of patients, bleeding in 10% of patients, a palpable mass in 10% of patients, and diarrhea in 5% of patients.[125] The median duration of symptoms prior to diagnosis is 21 months.[121,122]

Primary carcinoid tumors are usually of low grade. Benign tumors cannot be differentiated from malignant ones histologically. Only about 30% of small-intestinal carcinoids are biologically aggressive and metastasize.[121] The only curative therapy for carcinoid tumors is wide resection of the involved intestine and its adjacent mesentery in order to eliminate nodal metastatic disease.[126,127] The risk of developing lymph node metastases is directly related to the size of the primary small-bowel tumor.[121,128] Prognosis at the time of diagnosis is related to gender, tumor architecture, tumor size, and the presence or absence of lymph node and distant metastases. Tumors that are less than 1 cm in size rarely metastasize. In one series, 100% of jejunal and ileal carcinoids greater than 2 cm in diameter developed metastatic deposits. Duodenal carcinoids are less likely to metastasize than carcinoids arising in the more distal intestine.[121,122,128] In another series, only 33% of duodenal carcinoids greater than 2 cm in diameter were found to metastasize.

A meticulous search for synchronous intestinal carcinoid tumors should be made during preoperative evaluation and intraoperatively since they are multiple 30% of the time.[129,130] The 5-year survival rate following resection of localized carcinoid tumor is 75%.[131] As many as 65% of patients survive for at least 5 years, even in the presence of nodal metastatic disease.[132] The 5-year survival rate is only 20% for patients who present with metastatic disease.

Carcinoid tumors secrete numerous bioactive amines, including 5-hydroxytryptophan, 5-hydroxytryptamine, synaptophysin, chromogranin A and C, insulin, growth hormone, neurotensin, adrenocorticotropic hormone (ACTH), melanocyte-stimulating hormone (MSH), gastrin, pancreatic polypeptide, calcitonin, substance P, transforming growth factor (TGF) beta, platelet-derived growth factor (PDGF), and beta fibroblast growth factor (FGF).[133–135] These probably contribute to the manifestations of carcinoid syndrome, although the relationship between the syndrome and its mediators has not been fully defined. Manifestations of carcinoid syndrome include diarrhea, crampy abdominal pain, facial flushing, bronchospasm, fibrosis of the right heart valves, and a pellagra-type skin reaction. It is thought that the mediators must gain access to the systemic circulation in order to precipitate the carcinoid syndrome. The ability of the liver to clear these hormones from the portal venous circulation explains why the syndrome is rare among patients with localized small-intestinal carcinoid tumors. The carcinoid syndrome is most commonly seen in patients with liver metastases. Abdominal pain, hypotension, coma, and death characterize carci-

noid crisis, a life-threatening complication precipitated by surgery, stress, anesthesia, chemotherapy, and even fine-needle aspiration biopsy. It is thought to be mediated by bioactive amines secreted by the tumor. For this reason, patients with carcinoid syndrome should be pretreated with octreotide before undergoing biopsy or surgery.

The role of surgery in the treatment of patients with metastatic or unresectable carcinoid tumor is debated. Generally, the goal of therapy in these patients is palliation. For patients who are asymptomatic, observation is usually recommended. Resection or ablation of hepatic metastatic disease and aggressive surgical debulking of extrahepatic metastatic disease have been associated with prolonged regression of symptoms and possibly with prolongation of survival.[122,136–140] This aggressive surgical approach is most appropriate for healthy patients with indolent, metastatic disease. Hepatic arterial chemoembolization has also been associated with palliation.[136,137,141] Systemic chemotherapy is associated with low response rates and short duration of response. 5-FU, streptozotocin, doxorubicin, and dacarbazine (DTIC) are among the more active agents.[142] Some responses have also been seen with interferon α.[143]

Carcinoid syndrome can be confirmed by measuring 24-hour urinary 5-hydroxyindoleacetic acid and serotonin. Borderline cases can be further evaluated by measuring platelet serotonin, serum chromogranin A, substance P, serum serotonin, and urinary 5-hydroxytryptophan. The symptoms of carcinoid syndrome can be controlled by octreotide[144] in as many as 50% to 80% of patients. Responses may often last as long as 2 years.[122] Although tumor regression is rare, as many as 50% of treated patients appear to have stabilization of their disease and their survival may be prolonged.[145,146]

Biochemical responses have also been associated with the use of interferon α; 30% to 60% of treated patients manifest significant decreases in markers of the carcinoid syndrome.[147] Responses may last as long as $1\frac{1}{2}$ years, and clinically significant palliation is often seen in these patients. Only 15% of patients treated with interferon α manifest a decrease in the size of their tumor. However, like octreotide, interferon α has been associated with inhibition of tumor growth and perhaps prolongation of survival.[147]

## LYMPHOMA

Non-Hodgkin's lymphoma accounts for about 20% of small-intestinal cancers and only about 1% to 3% of all gastrointestinal malignancies.[148] The appropriate therapy for small-intestinal lymphoma remains poorly defined due, in part, to the low incidence of this disease in western countries. The ambiguity concerning its classification and the absence of prospective, randomized clinical trials contribute to our poor understanding of the disease.

The classification of small-intestinal lymphomas was improved significantly by the development of a Working Formulation for Clinical Usage by the Non-Hodgkin's Lymphoma Pathologic Classification Project in 1982 (Table 15-4).[149] At that time, six systems of classification were in wide use. Many of them had undergone revision over time. This made the comparison of clinical studies almost impossible. The Working Formulation proposed 10 major types of non-Hodgkin's lymphoma based on morphologic criteria. No immunologic methods were used in developing this system. The 10 groups of non-Hodgkin's lymphoma were generated based on

**TABLE 15-4. WORKING FORMULATION FOR CLASSIFICATION OF NON-HODGKIN'S LYMPHOMA**

I. Low-grade malignant lymphoma
   A. Small lymphocytic
   B. Follicular, predominantly small cleaved cell
   C. Follicular, mixed, small cleaved and large cell
II. Intermediate-grade malignant lymphoma
   D. Follicular, predominantly large cell
   E. Diffuse, small cleaved cell
   F. Diffuse, mixed, small and large cell
   G. Diffuse, large cell, cleaved or noncleaved
III. High-grade malignant lymphoma
   H. Diffuse large cell immunoblastic
   I. Lymphoblastic (convoluted and/or unconvoluted)
   J. Small noncleaved cell (Burkitt's or non-Burkitt's)

clinical correlations such as survival, age, gender, presenting sites, and stage of disease. The Working Formulation was proposed as a means to translate one system to another. Using the Working Formulation, non-Hodgkin's lymphoma is characterized as low grade, intermediate grade, or high grade. There are several subdivisions within each grade, which are easily correlated with those of other existing systems of classification.

Another limitation of the available clinical data is the absence of a consistent definition of primary small-bowel non-Hodgkin's lymphoma. As a result, published clinical series represent a heterogeneous population of patients. Danson and co-workers[150] proposed that patients with superficial lymphadenopathy, mediastinal lymphadenopathy, involvement of the liver and spleen, and abnormal blood counts be excluded from clinical trials evaluating the therapy of primary intestinal non-Hodgkin's lymphoma. Regional lymph node involvement at the time of diagnosis was thought to be consistent with this diagnosis.[150] Some studies have included patients with inguinal lymph node involvement, however. Other clinical series include patients whose lymphoma is not limited to the intestine, but whose clinical picture is dominated by intestinal involvement, or whose tumor bulk is predominantly intestinal. Most patients in these clinical studies are staged using the Ann Arbor system (Table 15-5). Studies using the most strict criteria evaluate patients with disease localized to the small intestine (stage IE) or patients with intestinal

**TABLE 15-5. ANN ARBOR STAGING OF VISCERAL LYMPHOMA**

| | |
|---|---|
| Stage IE | Involvement of a single extralymphatic site |
| Stage IIE | Involvement of a single extralymphatic site and its regional nodes, with or without other lymph node regions on the same side of the diaphragm |
| Stage IIIE | Involvement of a single extralymphatic site and lymph node regions on both sides of the diaphragm |
| Stage IVE | Multifocal involvement of one or more extralymphatic sites, with or without associated lymph node involvement |

tumors and involvement of the adjacent mesenteric lymph nodes only (stage IIE).

The incidence of small-intestinal lymphoma appears to be increasing.[1] It is not clear whether this represents a real increase or statistical aberration due to better identification of patients or better patient registration. There are geographic variations due to genetic differences and endemic diseases. Immunoproliferative small-intestinal disease is an unusual lymphoma in western society but is common in Mediterranean regions and Africa.[1] Patients with celiac disease have a 200-fold increased risk of developing T-cell lymphoma of the small intestine.[151] This may be associated with the human leukocyte antigen DR3.[152] The risk is also increased in the setting of Crohn's disease of the small bowel. Infection with the human immunodeficiency virus (HIV) also seems to increase the risk of developing intestinal lymphoma. The incidence of lymphoma increases as a function of age. The mean and median age of patients at the time of presentation is 60 and 70 years, respectively.

Symptoms at the time of presentation are similar to those seen with other intestinal tumors.[151] Patients with intestinal lymphoma are less likely to bleed than are patients with gastric lymphoma. Diarrhea and visceral perforation are more commonly seen as a complication of small-intestinal lymphoma than they are with gastric lymphoma. Other common manifestations of this disease at diagnosis include abdominal pain, abdominal mass, intestinal obstruction, nausea, vomiting, anorexia, and weight loss.

Once a diagnosis has been made, pretreatment evaluation of these patients should include a complete history with particular attention to the presence of fever, night sweats, and weight loss. These so-called B symptoms have a negative impact on prognosis. The physical examination should evaluate patients for lymphadenopathy and hepatosplenomegaly. It should include an evaluation of Waldeyer's ring, as well. The survey for extra-intestinal disease should also include a bone marrow biopsy and a complete set of chest, abdominal, and pelvic CT scans, looking for involvement of the liver, spleen, or mediastinal, intraabdominal, and retroperitoneal lymph nodes.

A majority of intestinal lymphomas are of high grade. Intermediate and low-grade lymphomas occur with significant frequency, however. Mucosa-associated lymphoid tissue (MALT) lymphomas, common in the stomach, are unusual in the small intestine. Most cases of primary intestinal lymphoma present in the ileum.[1] A significant minority of cases occur in the jejunum, while isolated duodenal lymphoma is much less common.

The role of surgery, radiation therapy, and chemotherapy in the treatment of intestinal non-Hodgkin's lymphoma is controversial. One can make a cogent argument for or against the use of surgical debulking, depending on which of several retrospective reviews one wishes to cite. Although relapse-free survival and overall survival are the most important outcome measures in evaluating therapy, the efficacy of surgery should also be judged in terms of durability of local control, surgical morbidity and mortality, prevention of chemotherapy-associated complications, and impact of the resulting delay of chemotherapy on overall survival. The benefit of surgery may vary, depending on the aggressiveness of the lymphoma. Some investigators have found that the morbidity of chemotherapy is exceedingly high among patients with aggressive intestinal lymphomas, which may bleed or perforate as a result of chemotherapy. They argue that prophylactic resection of the involved intestine permits chemotherapy to be administered more safely.[153] Some clinical series have not found this to be the case, however.[151,154] The purported ability of surgery to prevent chemotherapy-induced complications must be weighed against surgical morbidity, which includes intestinal fistulas, anastomotic breakdown with abscess formation, and postoperative bleeding, all of which serve to further delay the initiation of chemotherapy. There are no studies comparing the mortality directly attributed to surgery with that of chemotherapy. Some series report a 3% risk of postoperative mortality, which approaches the reported risk of intestinal perforation due to chemotherapy in some series.[153]

Three recent studies suggest that surgery should be included in the multimodality therapy of patients with aggressive, high-grade, or intermediate-grade intestinal lymphoma. Over a nine-year period, D'Amore and co-workers[148] evaluated 109 patients with intestinal non-Hodgkin's lymphoma and another 22 patients with combined gastric and intestinal lymphoma. Surgery was associated with an increased risk of early and late complications among patients with gastric lymphoma, and it was therefore suggested that these patients be treated with chemotherapy and radiation rather than resection. However, surgery in combination with chemotherapy was the most effective treatment for small-intestinal lymphoma. This applied to patients with synchronous intestinal and gastric lymphoma, as well. The inclusion of surgery in the primary therapy of intestinal lymphoma was associated with a tenfold reduction in the risk of local recurrence.

List and co-workers[153] evaluated 23 patients with small-intestinal lymphoma. Among patients with intermediate or high-grade lymphomas, surgical resection followed by chemotherapy was associated with a prolongation of disease-free and overall survival, compared to treatment with systemic therapy alone. Patients who underwent complete resection of their tumor also manifested an improvement in local control, compared to patients who were treated with systemic therapy alone or with radiation. Interestingly, tumor-related complications such as bleeding and perforation were only seen among patients whose tumors were not resected.

It is hard to draw clear-cut conclusions concerning surgery from the recent series reported by Ha et al.[155] It is clear that chemotherapy reduced the chances of systemic recurrence after complete response to surgery. Following surgical resection, radiation therapy seems to have enhanced local control, particularly if resection was not histologically complete. Radiation therapy as an adjuvant to surgical resection has also been espoused by Gospadarowicz and co-workers,[156] who found that local control and survival were high among patients with limited, favorable-prognosis disease treated by resection followed by radiation therapy.

Resection of primary intestinal lymphoma has not been consistently demonstrated to be superior to other therapies, however. Salles and co-workers[154] evaluated 91 patients with aggressive lymphoma treated with chemotherapy with or without surgery. There was no apparent benefit to attempted surgical resection of the primary lymphoma. Seventy-eight percent of patients had a complete response following induction chemotherapy. Seventy-five percent of patients who had not previously undergone attempted resection manifested a complete response to chemotherapy administered as the only therapy. None of these patients received adjuvant radiation therapy. Despite this, the local relapse rate was very low. There was

a very low rate of intestinal bleeding and perforation in this series of patients, suggesting that resection of the primary lesion does not necessarily decrease the morbidity associated with chemotherapy. It is possible that the conclusions of this study are skewed by the low rate of complete resection that was achieved in these patients. Since only 31% of these patients were made grossly disease free, the impact of surgery on the final outcome might have been difficult to detect in this small number of patients.

For patients with limited intestinal disease and low-grade lymphoma, surgery and chemotherapy with or without radiation therapy appear to be equally efficacious. The risk of chemotherapy-related complications appears to be low, perhaps because these tumors do not always invade through the full thickness of the bowel. Complete surgical extirpation is more likely to be accomplished for these tumors, which often present with limited disease.

## REFERENCES

1. NEUGUT AI et al: The epidemiology of cancer of the small bowel. Cancer Epidemiol Biomark Prev 7:243, 1998.
2. KINDBLOM LG et al: Gastrointestinal pacemaker cell tumor (GIPACT): Gastrointestinal stromal tumors show phenotypic characteristics of the interstital cells of Cajal. Am J Pathol 152(5):1259, 1998.
3. THUNEBERG L: Interstitial cells of Cajal: Intestinal pacemaker cells? Adv Anat Embryol Cell Biol 71:1, 1982.
4. SEVERSON RK et al: Increasing evidence of adenocarcinoma and carcinoid tumours of the small intestine in adults. Cancer Epidemiol Biomark Prev 5:81, 1996.
5. O'BOYLE CJ et al: Primary small intestinal tumours: Increased incidence of lymphoma and improved survival. Ann R Coll Surg Engl 80:332, 1998.
6. LANDIS SH et al: Cancer Statistics 1998. CA 48:6, 1998.
7. CHEN CC et al: Risk factors for adenocarcinomas and malignant carcinoids of the small intestine: Preliminary findings. Cancer Epidemiol Biomark Prev 3:205, 1994.
8. WU AH et al: Smoking, alcohol use, dietary factors and risk of small intestinal adenocarcinoma. Int J Cancer 70:512, 1997.
9. BROWN I et al: Primary non-Hodgkin's lymphoma in ileal Crohn's disease. Eur J Surg Oncol 18:627, 1992.
10. LOWENFELS AB: Why are small-bowel tumours so rare? Lancet 6:24, 1973.
11. WILLIAMSON RC et al: Adenocarcinoma and lymphoma of the small intestine: Distribution and etiologic associations. Ann Surg 197:172, 1983.
12. ARBONA J, DeCRUICCHI ET: A factor presumably responsible for duodenal resistance to cancer. Curr Ther Res 40:745, 1986.
13. BIEGANSKI T: Biochemical, physiological, and pathophysiological aspects of intestinal diamine oxidase. Acta Physiol Pol 34:139, 1983.
14. WATTENBERG LW: Carcinogen-detoxifying mechanisms in the gastrointestinal tract. Gastroenterology 51(5):932, 1966.
15. HILL MJ et al: Bacteria and aetiology of cancer of large bowel. Lancet 16:95, 1971.
16. POTTEN CS et al: A possible explanation for the differential cancer incidence in the intestine, based on distribution of the cytotoxic effects of carcinogens in the murine large bowel. Carcinogenesis 13:2305, 1992.

17. POTTEN CS: The significance of spontaneous and induced apoptosis in the gastrointestinal tract of mice. Cancer Metastasis Rev 11:179, 1992.

18. SELLNER F: Investigations on the significance of the adenoma-carcinoma sequence in the small bowel. Cancer 66:701, 1990.

19. ARBER N et al: Molecular genetics of small bowel cancer. Cancer Epidemiol Biomark Prev 6:745, 1997.

20. CHO KR, VOGELSTEIN B: Genetic alterations in the adenoma-carcinoma sequence. Cancer Suppl 70:1727, 1992.

21. KIM SH et al: Transgenic mouse models that explore the multi-step hypothesis of intestinal neoplasia. J Cell Biol 123(4):877, 1993.

22. SUTTER T et al: Frequent K-ras mutations in small bowel adenocarcinomas. Dig Dis Sci 41(1):115, 1996.

23. COHEN JA et al: Expression pattern of the neu (NGL gene-encoded growth factor receptor protein [P185$^{neu}$]) in normal and transformed epithelia tissues of the digestive tract. Oncogene 4:81, 1989.

24. O'RIORDAN BG et al: Small bowel tumors: An overview. Dig Dis Sci 14:245, 1996.

25. LYNCH HT, LYNCH JF: 25 Years of HNPCC. Anticancer Res 14:1617, 1994.

26. VASEN HF et al: Cancer risk in families with hereditary non-polyposis colorectal cancer diagnosed by mutation analysis. Gastroenterology 110:1020, 1996.

27. LYNCH HT, LYNCH JF: Clinical implications of advances in the molecular genetics of colorectal cancer. Tumori 81(Suppl 3):19, 1995.

28. PELTOMÄKI P, VASEN HFA: Mutations predisposing to hereditary nonpolyposis colorectal cancer: Database and results of a collaborative study. The International Collaborative Group on Hereditary Nonpolyposis Colorectal Cancer. Gastroenterology 113:1146, 1997.

29. SPIGELMAN AD et al: Polyposis: The Peutz-Jeghers syndrome. Br J Surg 82:1311, 1995.

30. FRESKO D et al: Early presentation of carcinoma of the small bowel in Crohn's disease ("Crohn's carcinoma"): Case reports and review of the literature. Gastroenterology 82:783, 1982.

31. MICHELASSI F et al: Adenocarcinoma complicating Crohn's disease. Dis Colon Rectum 36:654, 1993.

32. RUBIO CA et al: Crohn's disease and adenocarcinoma of the intestinal tract: Report of four cases. Dis Colon Rectum 34:174, 1991.

33. CRUZ DN, HUOT SJ: Metabolic complications of urinary diversions: An overview. Am J Med 102:477, 1997.

34. ATTANOOS R et al: Ileostomy polyps, adenomas and adenocarcinomas. Gut 37:477, 1995.

35. BRUNO CJ et al: Evidence against flat dysplasia as a regional field defect in small bowel adenocarcinoma associated with celiac sprue. Mayo Clin Proc 72:320, 1997.

36. COOPER BT et al: Celiac disease and malignancy. Medicine 59:249, 1980.

37. HOULSTON RS, FORD D: Genetics of coeliac disease. Q J Med 89:737, 1996.

38. STRAKER RJ et al: Adenocarcinoma of the jejunum in association with celiac sprue. J Clin Gastroenterol 11:320, 1989.

39. HOLMES GK et al: Malignancy in coeliac disease: Effect of a gluten free diet. Gut 30:333, 1989.

40. OURIEL K, ADAMS JT: Adenocarcinoma of the small intestine. Am J Surg 147:66, 1984.

41. FROST DB et al: Small bowel cancer: A 30-year review. Ann Surg Oncol 1(4):290, 1994.

42. ROSE MD et al: Primary duodenal adenocarcinoma: A ten-year experience with 79 patients. J Am Coll Surg 183(2):89, 1996.

43. BLACKMAN E, NASH SV: Diagnosis of duodenal and ampullary epithelial neoplasms by endoscopic biopsy: A clinicopathologic and immunohistochemical study. Hum Pathol 16:901, 1985.

44. MAGLINTE DDT et al: The role of the physician in the late diagnosis of primary malignant tumors of the small intestine. Am J Gastroenterol 86:304, 1991.

45. ZOLLINGER RM et al: Primary neoplasms of the small intestine. Am J Surg 151:654, 1986.

46. BESSETTE J et al: Primary malignant tumors in the small bowel: A comparison of the small-bowel enema and conventional follow-through examination. Am J Roentgenol 153:741, 1989.

47. DUDIAK KM et al: Primary tumors of the small intestine: CT evaluation. AJR 152:995, 1989.

48. GAL R et al: Adenomyomas of the small intestine. Histopathology 18:369, 1991.

49. ROSAI J: *Ackerman's Surgical Pathology.* 8th ed, New York, Mosby 1995, pp 645–647.

50. BUCK JL et al: Peutz-Jeghers syndrome. Radiographics 12:365, 1992.

51. CHEN KTK: Female genital tract tumors in Peutz-Jeghers. Hum Pathol 17:858, 1986.

52. CHEN KTK: Benign signet-ring cell aggregates in Peutz-Jeghers polyps: A diagnostic pitfall. Surg Pathol 2:335, 1989.

53. PERGIN KH, BRIDGE MF: Adenomatous and carcinomatous changes in hamartomatous polyps of the small intestine (Peutz-Jeghers syndrome): Report of a case and review of the literature. Cancer 49:971, 1982.

54. MERINO D et al: Hyperplasia of Brunner glands. The spectrum of its radiographic manifestations. Gastrointest Radiol 16:104, 1991.

55. REMINE WH et al: Polypoid hamartomas of Brunner's glands: Report of six surgical cases. Arch Surg 100:313, 1970.

56. RÜFENACHT H et al: "Brunneroma," hamartoma or tumor? Pathol Res Pract 181:107, 1986.

57. WILSON JM et al: Benign small bowel tumor. Ann Surg 181:247, 1975.

58. RIVER L et al: Collective review: Benign neoplasms of the small intestine. A critical comprehensive review with reports of 20 new cases. Inst Abstr Surg 102:1, 1956.

59. EVANS HL: Smooth muscle tumors of the gastrointestinal stromal tumors. Am J Clin Pathol 56:2242, 1985.

60. PASCAL RR et al: Neoplastic diseases of the small and large intestine, in S Silverberg (ed). *Principles and Practice of Sur Path & Cytpath,* 3d ed. New York, Churchill Livingstone, 1997, Chap 39, pp 1801–1866.

61. MAY CW et al: Lipoma of the alimentary tract. Surgery 53:598, 1963.

62. WEISBERG T, FELDMAN M SR: Lipomas of the gastrointestinal tract. Am J Clin Pathol 25:272, 1955.

63. HURWITZ MM et al: Lipomas of the gastrointestinal tract: An analysis of 72 tumors. AJR 99:84, 1967.

64. SMITH FR, MAYO CW: Submucous lipomas of the small intestine. Am J Surg 80:922, 1950.

65. GOOD CA: Tumors of the small intestine. AJR 89:685, 1963.

66. BOYLE L, LACK EE: Solitary cavernous hemangioma of the small intestine. Arch Pathol Lab Med 117:939, 1993.

67. SCHAEFFER JW et al: Colonic lymphangiectasis associated with potassium depletion syndrome. Gastroenterology 55:515, 1968.

68. FULLER CE, WILLIAMS GT: Gastrointestinal manifestations of type 1 neurofibromatosis (von Recklinghausen's disease). Histopathology 19:1, 1991.
69. BURKE AP, HELWIG EB: Gangliocytic paraganglioma. Am J Clin Pathol 92:1, 1989.
70. HASIMOTO S et al: Gangliocytic paraganglioma of the papilla of Vater with regional lymph node metastasis. Am J Gastroenterol 87:1216, 1992.
71. MILLER JH et al: Upper gastrointestinal tract: Villous tumors. AJR 134:933, 1980.
72. KOMOROWSKI RA, COHEN EB: Villous tumors of the duodenum: A clinicopathologic study. Cancer 47:1377, 1981.
73. PERGIN KH, BRIDGE MF: Adenomas of the small intestine. A clinicopathologic review of 5 cases and a study of their relationship to carcinoma. Cancer 48:799, 1981.
74. HAGGITT RC, REID BJ: Hereditary gastrointestinal polyposis syndromes. Am J Surg Pathol 10:871, 1986.
75. WITTEMAN BJM et al: Villous tumors of the duodenum: An analysis of the literature with emphasis on malignant transformation. Neth J Med 42:5, 1993.
76. COLLIER PE et al: Small intestinal adenocarcinoma complicating regional enteritis. Cancer 55:516, 1985.
77. NESBIT RR JR et al: Carcinoma of the small bowel: A complication of regional enteritis. Cancer 37:2948, 1976.
78. SAVAGE RA et al: Carcinoma of the small intestine associated with transmural ileitis (Crohn's disease). Am J Clin Pathol 63:168, 1975.
79. VALDES-DAPENA A et al: Adenocarcinoma of the small bowel in association with regional enteritis: Four new cases. Cancer 37:2938, 1976.
80. RIBIERO MB et al: Adenocarcinoma of the small intestine in Crohn's disease. Surg Gynecol Obstet 173:343, 1991.
81. PEROSIO PM et al: Primary intestinal lymphoma in Crohn's disease: Minute tumor with a fatal outcome. Am J Gastroenterol 87:894, 1992.
82. COLLIER PE et al: Small intestinal adenocarcinoma complicating regional enteritis. Cancer 55:516, 1985.
83. HAWKER PC et al: Adenocarcinoma of the small intestine complicating Crohn's disease. Gut 23:188, 1982.
84. HOCK YL et al: Mixed adenocarcinoma/carcinoid tumour of the large bowel in a patient with Crohn's disease. J Clin Pathol 46:183, 1993.
85. MOHAN IV et al: Crohn's disease presenting as adenocarcinoma of the small bowel. Eur J Gastroenterol Hepatol 10:431, 1998.
86. FRANK JD, SHOREY BA: Adenocarcinoma of the small bowel as a complication of Crohn's disease. Gut 14:120, 1973.
87. LYNCH HT et al: Genetics, natural history, tumor spectrum, and pathology of hereditary nonpolyposis colorectal cancer: An updated review. Gastroenterology 104:1535, 1993.
88. NEGLIA JP et al: The risk of cancer among patients with cystic fibrosis. N Engl J Med 332:494, 1995.
89. SHELDON CD et al: A cohort of cystic fibrosis and malignancy. Br J Cancer 68:1025, 1993.
90. COOPERMAN M et al: Villous adenomas of the duodenum. Gastroenterology 74:1295, 1978.
91. NEUGT AI et al: An overview of adenocarcinoma of the small intestine. Oncology 11:529, 1997.
92. YEO CJ et al: Pancreaticoduodenectomy with or without extended retroperitoneal lymphadenectomy for periampullary adenocarcinoma: Comparison of morbidity and mortality and short-term outcome. Ann Surg 229(5):613, 1999.
93. CONTANT CME et al: Prognostic value of the TNM-classification for small bowel cancer. Hepatogastroenterology 44:430, 1997.
94. DISARIO JA et al: Small bowel cancer: Epidemiological and clinical characteristics from a population based registry. Am J Gastroenterol 89:699, 1994.
95. BAUER RL et al: Adenocarcinoma of the small intestine: 21 year review of diagnosis, treatment, and prognosis. Ann Surg Oncol 1:183, 1994.
96. GARCIA MARCILLA JA et al: Primary small bowel malignant tumors. Eur J Surg Oncol 20:630, 1994.
97. DESA L et al: Primary jejunoileal tumors: A review of 45 cases. W J Surg 15:81, 1991.
98. BROPHY C, CAHOW CE: Primary small bowel malignant tumors. Am Surg 55:408, 1989.
99. DESAI DC et al: Juvenile polyposis. Br J Surg 82:14, 1995.
100. LIOE TF BIGGART JD: Primary adenocarcinoma of the jejunum and ileum: Clinicopathologic review of 25 cases. J Clin Pathol 43:533, 1990.
101. MICHELASSI F et al: Experience with 647 consecutive tumors of the duodenum, ampulla, head of the pancreas, and distal common bile duct. Ann Surg 210:544, 1989.
102. JIGYASU D et al: Chemotherapy for primary adenocarcinoma of the small bowel. Cancer 53:23, 1984.
103. HAQ MM et al: Small bowel adenocarcinoma: A report of three cases and review of literature. Texas Med 81:51, 1985.
104. NIEMIEC TR et al: Adenocarcinoma of the small intestine presenting as an ovarian mass. J Reprod Med 34:917, 1989.
105. GILLEN CD et al: Occult small bowel adenocarcinoma complicating Crohn's disease: A report of three cases. Postgrad Med J 71(833):172, 1995.
106. ZUCCHETTI F et al: Adenocarcinoma of the small intestine. Surgery 76:230, 1991.
107. TEMPLE DF: Adenocarcinoma of small intestine (25 year review—Rosewell Park). J Fla Med Assoc 73:526, 1986.
108. APPELMAN HD, HELWIG EB: Gastric epithelioidleiomyoma and leiomyosarcoma. Cancer 38:708, 1976.
109. CARNEY JA et al: Alimentary tract ganglionemonatosis. N Eng J Med 295:1287, 1976.
110. TORTELLA BJ et al: Gastric astonomic nerve (GAN) tumor and extra adrenal paraganglioma in Carney's triad. Ann Surg 205:221, 1987.
111. PEREZ-ATAYDE AR et al: Neuroectodermal differentiation of gastrointestinal tumors in Carney's triad. Am J Surg Pathol 17:706, 1993.
112. SKANDALAKIS JE, GRAY SW: Smooth muscle tumors of the small intestine, in Smooth Muscle Tumors of the Alimentary Tract: Leiomyomas and Leiomyosarcomas, a Review of 2525 Cases. Springfield, IL, Charles C Thomas, 1962, p 112.
113. DOUGHERTY MJ et al: Sarcoma of the gastrointestinal tract: Separation into favorable and unfavorable prognostic groups by mitotic count. Ann Surg 214:569, 1991.
114. MOROWITZ J et al: An institutional review of sarcomas of the large and small intestine. J Am Coll Surg 180, 1995.
115. CONLON KC et al: Primary gastrointestinal sarcomas: analysis of prognostic variables. Ann Surg Oncol 2(1):26, 1995.
116. KIMURA H et al: Prognostic factors in primary gastrointestinal leiomyosarcoma: A retrospective study. W J Surg 15:771, 1991.
117. NG EH et al: Prognostic implications of patterns of failure for gastrointestinal leiomyosarcomas. Cancer 69:1334, 1992.
118. SALMELA H: Smooth muscle tumors of the stomach: A clinical study of 112 cases. Acta Chir Scand 134:384, 1968.

119. LEWIN KJ: The endocrine cells of the gastrointestinal tract: The normal endocrine cells and their hyperplasias. Pathol Annu 21:1, 1986.

120. SOLCIA E et al: The contribution of immunohistochemistry to the diagnosis of neuroendocrine tumors. Semin Diag Pathol 2:285, 1984.

121. MOERTEL CJ et al: Life history of the carcinoid tumor of the small intestine. Cancer 19:901, 1961.

122. MOERTEL CJ et al: An odyssey in the land of small tumors. J Clin Oncol 5:1503, 1987.

123. ANTHONY PP DRURY RA: Elastic vascular sclerosis of mesenteric blood vessels in argentaffin carcinoma. J Clin Pathol 23:110, 1970.

124. QIZILBASH AH: Carcinoid tumors, vascular elastosis, and ischemic disease of the small intestine. Dis Colon Rectum 20:554, 1977.

125. SAHA S et al: Carcinoid tumors of the gastrointestinal tract: a 44 year experience. South Med J 82:1501, 1989.

126. THOMPSON GB et al: Carcinoid tumors of the gastrointestinal tract: presentation, management and prognosis. Surgery 98:1054, 1985.

127. MAKRIDIS C et al: Surgical treatment of midgut carcinoid tumor. W J Surg 14:377, 1990.

128. BURKE AO et al: Carcinoid tumors of the duodenum. Arch Pathol Lab Med 114:700, 1990.

129. WILSON HW et al: Carcinoid tumors, in *Current Problems in Surgery,* MM Ravich (ed). Chicago, Year Book, 1970.

130. JEFFREE MA, NOLAN DJ: Multiple ileal carcinoid tumors. Br J Radiol 60:402, 1987.

131. GODWIN JD II: Carcinoid tumor: An analysis of 2837 cases. Cancer 36:560, 1975.

132. CARTY S: Endocrine cancer, in *Current Cancer Therapeutics,* J Kirkwood et al (eds). Philadelphia, Churchill Livingstone, 1996, pp 239–249.

133. LANGLEY K: The neuroendrocrine concept today. Ann NY Acad Sci 733:1, 1994.

134. KLOPPEL G, HEITZ PU: Classification of normal and neoplastic neuroendocrine cells. Ann NY Acad Sci 733:18, 1994.

135. CREUTZFELDT W: Historical backround and natural history of carcinoids. Digestion 55:3, 1994.

136. MOERTEL CG: Treatment of the carcinoid tumor and the malignant carcinoid syndrome. J Oncol 1:727, 1983.

137. MARTIN JK JR et al: Surgical treatment of functioning metastatic carcinoid tumors. Arch Surg 118:537, 1983.

138. SOREIDE O et al: Surgical treatment as a principle in patients with advanced abdominal carcinoid tumors. Surgery 111:48, 1992.

139. NAGORNEY DM, QUE FG: Cytoreductive hepatic surgery for metastatic gastrointestinal tumors, in *Endocrine Tumors of the Pancreas: Recent Advances in Research and Management,* M Mignon et al (eds). Basel, Karger, 1995, p 416.

140. COZZI PJ et al: Cryotherapy treatment of patients with hepatic metastases from neuroendocrine tumors. Cancer 76:501, 1995.

141. MOERTEL CG et al: The management of patients with advanced carcinoid tumors and islet cell carcinomas. Ann Intern Med 120:302, 1994.

142. ENGSTROM PF et al: Streptozocin plus fluorouracil versus doxorubicin therapy for metastatic carcinoid tumor. J Clin Oncol 2:1255, 1984.

143. MOERTEL CG et al: Therapy of metastatic carcinoid tumor and the malignant carcinoid syndrome with recombinant leukocyte A interferon. J Clin Oncol 7:865, 1989.

144. KVOLS LK et al: Rapid reversal of carcinoid crisis with somatostatin analogue. N Engl J Med 313:1229, 1985.

145. SALTZ L et al: Octreotide as an antineoplastic agent in the treatment of functional neuroendocrine tumors. Cancer 72:244, 1993.

146. KVOLS LK: Metastatic carcinoid tumors and the malignant carcinoid syndrome. Ann NY Acad Sci 733:464, 1994.

147. OBERG K, ERICKSON B: The role of interferons in the management of carcinoid tumors. Acta Oncol 30:519, 1991.

148. D'AMORE F et al FOR THE DANISH LYMPHOMA STUDY GROUP: Non-Hodgkin's lymphoma of the gastrointestinal tract: A population based analysis of incidence, geographic distribution, clinicopathologic presentation, features and prognosis. J Clin Oncol 12:1673, 1994.

149. ROSENBERG SA: Non-Hodgkin's Lymphoma Pathologic Classification Project: National Cancer Institute sponsored study of classifications of non-Hodgkin's lymphomas: Summary and description of a working formulation for clinical usage. Cancer 49:2112, 1982.

150. DANSON I et al: Primary malignant lymphoid tumors of the intestinal tract. Br J Surg 49:80, 1961.

151. MORTON JE et al: Primary gastrointestinal non-Hodgkin's lymphoma: A review of 175 British national lymphoma investigation cases. Br J Cancer 67:776, 1993.

152. O'DRISCOLL BR et al: HLA type of patients with coeliac disease and malignancy in the west of Ireland. Gut 23:662, 1982.

153. LIST AF et al: Non-Hodgkin's lymphoma of the gastrointestinal tract: An analysis of clinical and pathologic features affecting outcome. J Clin Oncol 6:1125, 1988.

154. SALLES G et al: Aggressive primary gastrointestinal lymphomas: Review of 91 patients treated with the LNH-84 regimen. A study of the group détude des lymphomes agressifs. Am J Med 90:77, 1991.

155. HA CS et al: Primary non-Hodgkin lymphoma of the small bowel. Radiology 211:183, 1999.

156. GOSPADAROWICZ MK et al: Outcome analysis of localized gastrointestinal lymphoma treated with surgery and postoperative irradiation. Int J Rad Oncol Biol Phys 19:1351, 1990.

# CHAPTER 16

# NEOPLASMS OF THE LARGE BOWEL

## 16A / CANCER OF THE COLON

*Leyo Ruo and Jose G. Guillem*

## INTRODUCTION

Malignant neoplasms of the large intestine are among the most common cancers in the general population. Worldwide, colorectal cancer (CRC) accounted for 783,000 new cases in 1990 (9.7%) and caused 437,000 deaths (8.4%).[1] The highest incidence rates occur in developed areas such as Australia and New Zealand, North America, and Europe, whereas, much lower incidence rates are found in Africa and Asia (excluding Japan). The incidence of colon cancer has increased in most regions since 1985, although North America is an exception to this trend. In the United States, CRC is the third most common cancer by incidence and the third most common cause of cancer deaths.[2] The cumulative lifetime risk of developing CRC is estimated at 6%. Overall survival at 5 years is 60% as reported by the Surveillance, Epidemiology, and End Results (SEER) data; 41% by European registries; 42% by Indian registries; and 32% in China.[1] Although geographic differences are thought to represent varying environmental exposures, presumably dietary in nature, CRC occurs more frequently in certain families through genetic predisposition.

## EPIDEMIOLOGY

### PATIENT FACTORS

Colon cancer predominantly affects older patients, with a peak incidence in the sixth decade. However, disease can occur at any age, and may be seen in patients in their twenties and thirties, with 4% of all cases occurring in patients under 45 years of age.[3] Incidence and mortality rates are similar in males and females. Although studies on hormone replacement therapy (HRT) have been inconsistent, most show a lower risk for CRC in women using HRT.[4] The association between physical activity and a reduced risk of colon cancer is a consistent observation in cohort and case-control studies.[5] Epidemiologic studies also suggest that obesity may increase the risk of colon cancer, a more constant finding in men than in women. Black Americans, who once enjoyed a lower incidence of CRC, now experience a higher incidence of disease as well as higher cancer-specific mortality rates.[2] American Indians, Asians, and Hispanics have considerably lower incidence and mortality rates compared with Caucasians or white Americans.

### DIET- AND FOOD-RELATED FACTORS

Caveats regarding the interpretation of dietary data are well known and certainly apply to findings pertaining to CRC. Several cohort and case-control studies indicate a reduced risk of colon cancer with higher consumption of fruits and vegetables, particularly raw, green, and cruciferous vegetables.[4] The beneficial effects of vegetable consumption have been attributed to several micronutrients (carotenoids, ascorbate, folate). However, the data to support these associations are even less compelling.

The role of dietary fiber in colon carcinogenesis was first proposed about 30 years ago with the observation that African natives had a low incidence of CRC. Evidence for an inverse association between dietary fiber and colon cancer risk has been summarized in an analysis of 55 original reports.[6] However, a recent cohort study in over 88,000 women found no association with either colorectal carcinoma or adenoma.[7] The conflicting data on the protective effect of fiber intake on CRC risk may be attributed, in part, to the heterogeneous nature of fiber and the different methods by which it is measured.[8]

Of the studies that have examined meat intake and CRC risk, the results indicate either increased risk or no impact.[4] It is not clear whether the risk observed relates to animal fat, processing, or cooking methods.

Extensive epidemiologic evidence suggests a reduced CRC risk with calcium consumption. Subsequent interventional studies show that calcium not only normalizes the distribution of proliferating cells to the lower 60% of the colonic crypt[9] but also results in a statistically significant reduction in the incidence of metachronous colorectal adenomas in a double-blind, placebo-controlled clinical trial.[10]

## SMOKING AND ALCOHOL

Several studies reveal a higher colon cancer risk among cigarette, cigar, and pipe smokers, especially in those with prolonged smoking histories.[11,12] Tobacco smoke is a major source of carcinogens, including heterocyclic amines, polycyclic hydrocarbons, and nitrosamines. Similarly, excessive alcohol consumption likely increases the risk of CRC, and the association appears to be related to total ethanol intake.[4] Alcohol may exert its effect through acetaldehyde, a product of metabolism that promotes DNA damage or predisposes to nutrient, particularly folate, deficiencies.

## ETIOLOGY AND PATHOGENESIS

CRCs represent a combination of described and probably yet to be described genetic alterations as well as the influence of environmental exposures. This conclusion is partially derived from natural epidemiologic experiments, which show a shift in cancer incidence in successive generations of migrant populations. The current model for colon cancer describes many genetic changes, which are not entirely specific to CRC. In the process of carcinogenesis, environmental factors, such as exposure of the gastrointestinal (GI) tract to intraluminal contents (food, metabolic products, bacteria), modulate the genetic alterations.

## ADENOMA-CARCINOMA SEQUENCE

Most CRCs, if not all, arise through the adenoma-carcinoma sequence.[13] As the cancer grows, it expands on the mucosal surface and replaces previously benign adenomatous tissue.[14] The duration of the polyp-cancer sequence is variable, but on average is about 8 to 10 years.[13,14] Because the prevalence of colonic polyps greatly exceeds the prevalence of carcinoma, few polyps actually progress to carcinoma. The cumulative risk of CRC at the site of the index polyp has been estimated to be 2.5%, 8%, and 24% at 5, 10, and 20 years, respectively.[15] Several observations support the adenoma-carcinoma concept, including the frequent presence of benign adenomatous tissue contiguous with carcinoma in resected specimens;[13,14] a 36% incidence of synchronous polyps in CRC patients;[16] the invariable progression to CRC in familial adenomatous polyposis (FAP) patients;[17] and lastly, the association of genetic abnormalities with adenoma development, growth and progression to malignancy.[18]

## PATHWAYS TO COLORECTAL CANCER

Although some molecular mechanisms are shared, multiple pathways may be responsible for the transformation of a normal colonocyte into CRC (Fig. 16A-1).

SUPPRESSOR PATHWAY. The classic pathway refers to the molecular genetics thought to underlie the adenoma-carcinoma sequence. In order for an adenoma to develop, a mutation in a progenitor colonocyte creates a population of replicating cells with an abnormal phenotype. Allelic loss on chromosome 5q appears to be a critical step in the progression of adenomas to carcinomas.[19,20] It is now clear that mutations of the adenomatous polyposis coli (APC) gene, localized to 5q21, are an integral part of colorectal tumorigenesis.[21,22] Over 60% of sporadic cancers exhibit somatic APC mutations and almost two-thirds have at least one altered allele.[20] APC gene mutations (somatic or germline) produce abnormalities in cell proliferation, migration, and adhesion. As phenotypically abnormal cells accumulate towards the top of the crypt, there is an increased opportunity to sustain further genetic alterations through exposure to luminal promotional agents. Corresponding architectural changes seen on pathology include aberrant crypt foci or microadenomas. However, these premalignant lesions do not commonly develop into cancers.

Within this framework are β-catenin, a cytoskeletal protein that exerts a suppressive effect on cellular proliferation, and Tcf (T-cell factor), a downstream transcriptional activator gene.[23,24] In a normal colonocyte, β-catenin is held by E-cadherin or destroyed, in part, because of wild-type APC. Truncated, inactive APC allows β-catenin accumulation in the nucleus where it can activate transcription and stimulate cellular growth. Evidence suggests that the interaction of β-catenin with APC is important in cellular signaling, and disruption of either of these molecules (as occurs with mutation) can lead to neoplasia via c-*myc*, the target gene of this signaling pathway.[25] These processes characterize the *Wnt* pathway, which plays a role in stimulation of cell growth.[26]

After the activation of the APC–β-catenin–Tcf pathway, a series of specific chromosomal and genetic alterations accumulate in a nonlinear fashion and accompany the transition from normal colonic mucosa to metastatic carcinoma (see Fig. 16A-1).[27] These include K-*ras* (a protooncogene) mutations, changes in methylation patterns, and mutation or loss of p53 (a tumor suppressor gene involved in cell cycle regulation).[28] Other important allelic losses involve the Smad4/DPC4,[29] DCC,[30] and STK (Peutz-Jegher)[31] genes.

MUTATOR PATHWAY. In 1993, replication errors were described in sporadic[31] and familial[32] CRC. Linkage of hereditary nonpolyposis colorectal cancer (HNPCC) to markers on chromosome 2 without increased K-*ras*, p53, and APC mutations suggested that the development of CRC in HNPCC proceeds via a

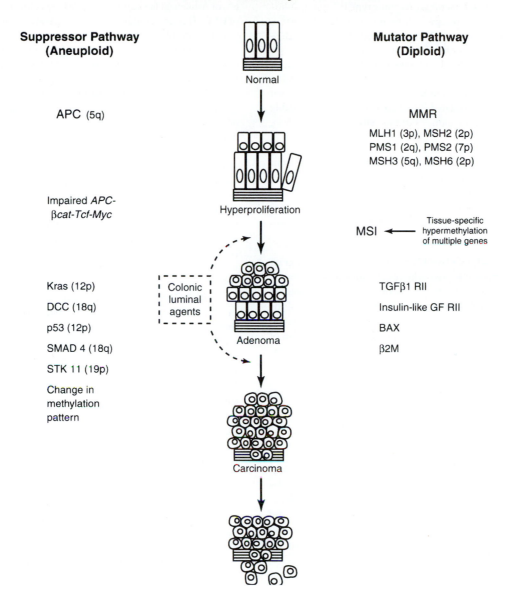

**FIGURE 16A-1.** Pathways to colorectal cancer. Suppressor pathway (left). Mutator pathway (right).

mechanism distinctly different from that mediated by loss of heterozygosity in tumor suppressor genes (APC, p53, DCC) and oncogenes (K-ras). Indeed, the "suppressor pathway" is characterized by gross chromosomal lesions, whereas the "mutator pathway," governed by inactivation of mismatch repair (MMR) genes, is characterized by a more subtle genetic alteration, namely microsatellite instability (MSI). Loss of MMR function may occur through mutation or hypermethylation.[33,34] In the absence of an inherited APC mutation, the likelihood of developing an adenoma in an individual with a MMR defect may not be greatly different from that in

the general population. However, once an adenoma develops, its progression to carcinoma is more rapid.

There are over 100,000 microsatellite sequences scattered throughout the human genome. In CRC, microsatellites containing mononucleotide repeats (particularly $[A]_n$) are most frequently affected by instability. Dinucleotide (particularly $[CA]_n$) and longer repeats are less frequently altered, demonstrating that more simple microsatellite sequences have a higher probability of instability.[35] Genes that are located close to or that contain microsatellites are more susceptible to alteration by a MMR gene mutation. In fact, many MSI-positive tumors accumulate mutations in short mononucleotide sequences close to or contained in genes that play a major role in growth regulation (transforming growth factor β1 receptor type II[36] and insulin-like growth factor type II receptor[37]), in apoptosis (BAX gene[38]), and in immune surveillance (β-2-microglobulin gene[39]). The β-2-microglobulin gene encodes for a subunit of the human leukocyte antigen (HLA) class I molecule, necessary for the presentation of antigens to cytotoxic T cells. In some MSI-positive tumor cells, the inactivation of this gene leads to loss of human leukocyte antigen (HLA) expression, incapacitated T-cell surveillance, and possibly selective growth of a certain clone of tumor cells.

### ESTROGEN RECEPTOR.

ESTROGEN RECEPTOR. Almost all colon cancers arise from cells in which the estrogen receptor (ER) gene has been silenced.[4] The importance of this observation requires further investigation in order to establish why loss of the ER protein is relevant to colonocytes and what hormone response genes may be important downstream.

### CHROMOSOMAL INSTABILITY.

CHROMOSOMAL INSTABILITY. Another recently recognized characteristic of many CRCs is the loss of chromosomal instability, which is consistently associated with loss of a mitotic checkpoint.[40] In some cases, the checkpoint was lost because of mutational inactivation of the human homolog of *BUB1*, a gene important in chromosomal segregation in yeast. Aneuploidy facilitates the loss of other tumor suppressor genes, adding support to genomic hypermutability as a feature of human tumors.

### GENETIC PREDISPOSITION

Individuals with a family history of CRC are at increased risk, not only for belonging to a dominantly inherited syndrome such as FAP or HNPCC, but also when compared to those without a family history. Having one or more first-degree relatives (FDRs) affected by CRC increases that risk three- to six-fold, and the risk is higher with decreasing age of the proband or when additional FDRs are affected.[41–45] To a lesser extent, the risk of developing CRC is also increased in individuals with a second- or third-degree relative diagnosed with CRC.[46]

### FAMILIAL ADENOMATOUS POLYPOSIS.

FAMILIAL ADENOMATOUS POLYPOSIS. Inherited susceptibility for colonic polyps and carcinomas due to a gene passed on in an autosomal dominant fashion was revealed through the analysis of a large pedigree with multiple cases of CRC.[47] Mutations of the APC gene not only represent an early event in sporadic colorectal tumorigenesis but also the genetic basis for FAP. Both copies of the APC gene are generally inactivated in CRC, supporting Knudson's two-hit hypothesis. FAP patients inherit one inactivated allele in all their cells (germline mutation) and, therefore, require only somatic inactivation of the remaining allele to lose APC function.[48] Most affected individuals have mutations that lead to a base substitution, changing an amino acid to a stop codon and resulting in protein truncation.[49] Hypermethylation at 25 CpG sites within the APC gene promoter region may be another mechanism involved in CRC progression.[50] Furthermore, a distinct APC mutation (T to A transversion at nucleotide 3920), which results in a substitution of a lysine for isoleucine at codon 1307, has recently been described in 6% of Ashkenazi Jews and 28% of Ashkenazim with a family history of CRC. This new mutation (I1307K) creates a small hypermutable tract responsible for cancer predisposition.[51]

Individuals with FAP form hundreds of adenomatous polyps, usually in adolescence, and will generally develop CRC by age 40 if a proctocolectomy is not performed.[52] Extracolonic manifestations are common and may include upper GI polyps and cancers, desmoid tumors, epidermoid cysts, mandibular osteomas, dental odontomas, congenital hypertrophy of the retinal pigment epithelium (CHRPE), and a variety of associated benign and malignant tumors (e.g., pancreatic, biliary tree, gastric, small intestinal, thyroid, adrenal, brain).[53] There is a defined risk for transmission of the disease. Thus patients may benefit from molecular techniques to define whether or not FDRs have inherited the genetic predisposition to FAP. Aggressive screening and surveillance is beneficial in this population who may proceed to total proctocolectomy with sphincter preservation, thereby substantially reducing their CRC risk.

### HEREDITARY NONPOLYPOSIS COLORECTAL CANCER.

HEREDITARY NONPOLYPOSIS COLORECTAL CANCER. In the past 20 years, HNPCC has been increasingly recognized through many synonyms, such as cancer family syndrome and Lynch syndromes I and II. The predisposition to cancer in HNPCC arises from germline mutations in MMR genes, which recognize and repair errors from DNA polymerase activity during replication. Mismatched nucleotides in DNA are identified and excised with subsequent resynthesis of the correct sequence. Loss of MMR function results in proofreading errors, subsequent small deletions and insertions, a higher rate of mutations, and eventually CRC. The RER phenotype, also called MSI, refers to unstable short tandem repeat sequences of DNA, which were originally observed in bacteria and yeast[54] and later in human CRC.[32,55] A germline mutation in one allele of an MMR gene along with a somatic mutation in the remaining wild-type allele is necessary to produce MSI. Thus far six human MMR genes have been described: hMLH1, hMSH2, hPMS1, hPMS2, hMSH6, and hMSH3.[56–64] Either mutation[65] or hypermethylation[33,34,66] of MMR genes can potentially lead to CRC.

HNPCC is also a dominantly inherited disease that predisposes to the development of CRC at an early age (average 40 to 45 years).[67] Features of HNPCC include a predominance of right-sided colon cancer, an increased incidence of synchronous and metachronous CRC, and an excess of extracolonic cancers such as endometrial, ovarian, stomach, small bowel, upper urologic tract, hepatobiliary, skin (sebaceous gland), and brain tumors.[67] Currently, low yield and genetic heterogeneity limit the full clinical utility of genetic testing, which should be offered only to select candidates and preferably preceded and followed by genetic counseling. The clinical diagnosis of HNPCC is based on a strong family history of early age-of-onset CRC as specified by the Amsterdam criteria (CRC in at least three first-degree relatives spanning two successive generations of whom one is less than 50 years old at diagnosis).[68] Full colonoscopy with removal of adenomatous polyps is recommended in patients at risk for HNPCC in order to screen for colorectal neoplasms. Because there is a high cumulative risk of metachronous CRC, a total abdominal colectomy with ileorectal anastomosis is recommended for HNPCC patients who develop CRC.[69]

## INFLAMMATORY BOWEL DISEASE

**ULCERATIVE COLITIS.** Patients with ulcerative colitis (UC), especially those with pancolitis (typically defined as disease involvement extending proximal to the splenic flexure) who have been affected greater than 10 years and those with early-onset disease, have an increased risk of CRC.[70,71] This risk increases at a rate of 0.5% to 1.0% per year after 8 to 10 years. Although disease is restricted to the large bowel, screening methods, including surveillance colonoscopy, lack the ability to identify premalignant change accurately. Morphologic markers, such as estimation of dysplasia, are qualitative and suboptimal. In one review, 15% of patients had dysplasia and 20% of these were subsequently found to have colonic cancer.[72] Of note, 10% with cancer did not have dysplasia in any of their biopsies. Thus, the absence of high-grade dysplasia in one part of the bowel does not guarantee that it is absent in the remainder of the colon. The risk for transformation to carcinoma, although increased, is unpredictable and remains based on representative sampling and the qualitative assessment of increased atypia or severity of dysplasia. Unfortunately, molecular changes are also poorly defined. APC mutations are uncommon and p53 mutation appears to be an early genetic event in UC, unlike sporadic CRC.[73]

Considerations for a surveillance program include whether

1. Asymptomatic patients will subject themselves to repeated colonoscopy.
2. Sampling error may miss areas in the bowel with transformation.
3. Active or inactive disease are equally prone to transformation.
4. There is a risk of overlooking early symptoms with a background of inflammatory bowel disease.

As with FAP, sphincter-preserving prophylactic colectomy should be contemplated in select UC patients. Reduction in colon cancer mortality as a result of colonoscopic screening and biopsy for dysplasia has been attributed to prophylactic colectomy for pathologically confirmed dysplasia and detection of carcinoma at an earlier stage.[74] In order for surveillance colonoscopy to be effective, patient education regarding the goal of surveillance and acting upon the discovery of precancerous lesions is essential to receive the full benefit of cancer surveillance.

**CROHN'S DISEASE.** The association between Crohn's disease (CD) and CRC is less well defined, although an excess incidence of colonic cancers has been found from retrospective analyses.[75,76] The relative rarity of inflammatory bowel disease in the general population, selection bias, and potential problems with generalization make it difficult to quantify this risk precisely. The increased risk of cancer is estimated to be equivalent for both CD and UC of similar duration and anatomic extent.[71,76–78] It is not possible to predict which bowel segment will undergo malignant transformation. The recurrent pattern of disease activity makes bowel preservation, rather than prophylaxis against CRC, a priority.

## PREVIOUS COLORECTAL CANCER

Several retrospective studies have attempted to estimate the rate of metachronous neoplasm development after CRC resection. Metachronous adenomatous polyps developed in 24 of 91 (26%) patients at a median interval of 19 months after curative resection for CRC.[79] From two separate reviews, the incidence of metachronous CRC was estimated at 0.35% to 0.61% per year in CRC patients after partial colectomy, excluding those with FAP, HNPCC, and inflammatory bowel disease.[80,81] Early age of onset CRC and HNPCC are risk factors for an increased rate of metachronous neoplasm development.[82–84]

## NONSTEROIDAL ANTI-INFLAMMATORY DRUGS (NSAIDs)

Arachidonic acid (AA), a 20-carbon polyunsaturated fatty acid, is the precursor of prostaglandins (PGs). The first step in PG synthesis is hydrolysis of phospholipids to produce free AA. The next step is catalyzed by cyclooxygenase (COX), which inserts molecular oxygen to produce PGG2, an unstable product. PGG2 is rapidly converted to PGH2, the common precursor for all other prostanoids, by COX peroxidase activity. Cells contain genes encoding at least two isoforms of COX, COX-1, and COX-2. COX-1 is expressed constitutively in most tissues and appears to be responsible for the production of PGs that mediate normal physiologic functions, such as maintaining the integrity of the gastric mucosa and regulating renal blood flow. In contrast, COX-2 is induced by cytokines, growth factors, oncogenes, and tumor promoters, thereby contributing to the synthesis of PGs in inflamed and neoplastic tissues.[85]

PGs accumulate as a consequence of increased COX-2 expression, which in turn is associated with a cancer phenotype.[86,87] Mechanisms by which overexpression of COX-2 contribute to carcinogenesis may involve chronic inflammation, immunosuppression, and angiogenesis as well as modulation of epithelial proliferation, apoptosis, or invasive properties.[88–91] Null mutation of the COX-2 gene reduces the number and size of intestinal polyps in an animal model for FAP.[92] Similarly, inhibition of COX-2 function suppresses polyp formation in mice and azoxymethane-induced colon cancer in rats.[93,94] NSAIDs (aspirin, indomethacin, sulindac, prioxicam) suppress COX-2, inhibit colorectal carcinogenesis in animal studies, and reduce the risk of and mortality from CRC in epidemiologic studies.[4,95] Aspirin reduces the risk of developing adenomatous polyps, especially with prolonged use for longer than 5 years.[96,97] Sulindac causes regression of adenomas in FAP patients.[98] Clinical trials to establish the efficacy of these agents have been initiated and preliminary results show considerable promise.

## PATHOLOGY

Most colonic malignancies are adenocarcinomas, although carcinoid, lymphoma, sarcoma, and squamous cell carcinoma may also originate from the intestine (See Other Malignant Lesions). There are four morphologically distinct types of adenocarcinoma—ulcerative, polypoid, annular, or diffusely infiltrating. A lesion may be well differentiated (20%), moderately differentiated (60%), or poorly differentiated (20%). Differentiation or grade is associated with the presence of lymph node metastases and prognosis. Five-year survival rates are 80%, 60%, and 25% for low-, moderate-, and high-grade carcinomas, respectively, regardless of stage.[99] However, there is no assurance that well-differentiated cancers will not recur or that poorly differentiated cancers will recur.

Colloid or mucinous carcinomas are noted for reported associations with early-onset CRC, involvement of the proximal colon, more advanced stage at diagnosis, and poor prognosis.[100] Mucin is most commonly extracellular. Intracellular mucin, representing a true signet ring cell variety, is relatively rare. Overall, no significant differences characterize mucinous from nonmucinous carcinomas. Although survival is worse in patients with mucinous carcinomas, this has been attributed to presentation with advanced disease.[101]

Several traditional pathologic variables are considered important prognostic factors. These include tumor grade; cell type; depth of bowel wall penetration; lymph node involvement; and lymphatic, venous, or perineural invasion. Other factors identified as independent prognostic factors by multivariate analysis are immune response to tumor, immunologic markers (antigens associated with CRC), oncogenes and molecular markers, nuclear morphology, DNA content (ploidy), proliferating cell nuclear antigen expression, tumor budding, number of mast cells, lymphocytic infiltration, infiltrating border, microacinar growth pattern, autocrine motility factor, sialyl Lewis antigen, sucrase-isomaltase, helix pomatia agglutinin.[102]

## MODES OF SPREAD

Colon cancer may spread by direct local invasion or by transperitoneal, intraluminal, lymphatic, or hematogenous routes. Extension through the bowel wall may result in adherence to intraabdominal viscera, retroperitoneum, or abdominal wall. Transmural penetration also permits transcelomic dissemination throughout the peritoneal cavity, including the omentum.[103] Implantation may also occur through surgical manipulation and resultant deposition on peritoneal surfaces. Intraluminal spread develops through release of tumor cells and distal implantation on raw surfaces, such as hemorrhoidectomy wounds, anal fissures or fistulas, or suture lines.[104] Normal lymphatic flow from the colon is through channels along major arteries. If tumors lie between two major vascular pedicles, lymphatic drainage can proceed via either pedicle. Furthermore, if the central lymph nodes are blocked by tumor, lymphatic flow can be retrograde along the marginal arcades proximally and distally.[102] Hematogenous dissemination, primarily through venous drainage, most commonly progresses to the liver and less often lungs, bone, and brain.

## STAGING

The ultimate purpose of staging is to provide a method of defining disease prognosis for treatment planning and for meaningful comparison of treatments and outcomes analyses. The staging of colon carcinoma is derived from staging systems initially developed for rectal cancer over the past century.

Lockhart-Mummery, the renowned English surgeon, proposed a system that divided rectal tumors into three categories.[105] Favorable cases invading the muscular coat in the absence of gland involvement were classified as stage A. Large, fixed tumors or those with extensive gland involvement were classified as stage C. The definition of stage B rectal cancer was somewhat ambiguous with respect to the phrase, "no extensive involvement of glands." Cuthbert E. Dukes introduced a staging system in 1932 that segregated rectal carcinomas based on "extrarectal" extension and lymph node involvement.[106] Carcinoma limited to the wall of the rectum without spread into the extrarectal tissues or regional lymph nodes represented a stage A cancer. Extension into extrarectal tissues described stage B cancers and tumors with metastases to the regional lymph nodes were classified as stage C. This system was simple and predictive of survival. Subsequent staging systems shared the alphabetized terminology used by Dukes and therefore contributed to the confusion surrounding modifications of Dukes' classification. In 1949, Kirklin, Dockerty, and Waugh[107] proposed a system that described quite different levels of intestinal wall invasion. Stage A tumors were limited to the mucosa. Partial tumor penetration into the muscularis propria was classified as B1 and penetration through the muscularis as B2. Any cancers with lymph node involvement, regardless of the depth of rectal invasion, remained classified as type C lesions. There was no difference in prognosis between lesions above and below the peritoneal reflection, if the depth of invasion was equivalent. Astler and Coller[108] proposed a commonly used modification of Dukes' classification in 1954 that in fact closely paralleled Kirklin's classification.[108] Stage C lesions were subdivided into stage C1, for tumors limited to the intestinal wall with positive lymph nodes, and stage C2, for those with complete penetration of the abdominal wall and associated nodal involvement. The Gunderson and Sosin[109] modification of the Astler Coller staging system subdivided T3 tumors into those with microscopic (B2m or C2m) and gross (B2m+g or C2m+g) tumor penetration. The importance of serosal penetration by tumor was subsequently confirmed in colon cancer, although this was not a significant prognostic factor in rectal cancer.[110,111] Stage D was added by Turnbull et al.[112] to reflect the incurable nature of CRC associated with distant metastases (liver, lung, bone), parietal seeding, or adjacent organ invasion. The Australian system, described by Davis and Newland,[113] included relevant clinical, operative, and pathologic information. Although more complex with a total of nine substages making it cumbersome and less practical, this classification possessed greater prognostic predictive power than either the Dukes or Astler Coller systems.

The American Joint Committee on Cancer (AJCC) and the Union Internationale Contre le Cancer (UICC) have developed a universal staging system for all anatomic sites.[114] The TNM (tumor, node, metastasis) system classified the extent of disease based on clinical and pathologic information. A unified staging system for CRC was formulated in 1988 and has since been updated. The primary advancement in this system was the independent classification within each subcategory (T, N, or M) in greater detail (Table 16A-1)[114] to acknowledge tumor spread that did not progress in an "orderly" fashion as occurs when lymph node metastases are present prior to penetration of the intestinal wall. The number of positive lymph nodes has been included in the TNM classification system because this has been found to be one of the strongest predictors of survival.[115]

**TABLE 16A-1.** TNM CLASSIFICATION (AJCC) FOR CANCER OF THE COLON AND RECTUM

**Primary tumor (T):**

| | |
|---|---|
| TX | Primary tumor cannot be assessed or depth of penetration not specified. |
| T0 | No evidence of primary tumor. |
| Tis | Carcinoma in situ (mucosal): Intraepithelial or invasion of the lamina propria.* |
| T1 | Tumor invades submucosa. |
| T2 | Tumor invades muscularis propria. |
| T3 | Tumor invades through the muscularis propria into the subserosa, or into nonperitonealized pericolic or perirectal tissues. |
| T4 | Tumor perforates the visceral peritoneum, or directly invades other organs or structures.† |

**Regional lymph nodes (N):**

| | |
|---|---|
| NX | Regional lymph nodes cannot be assessed. |
| N0 | No regional lymph node metastasis. |
| N1 | Metastasis in 1 to 3 pericolic or perirectal lymph nodes. |
| N2 | Metastasis in 4 or more pericolic or perirectal lymph nodes. |
| N3 | Metastasis in any lymph node along the course of a named vascular trunk. |

**Distant metastasis (M):**

| | |
|---|---|
| MX | Presence of distant metastasis cannot be assessed. |
| M0 | No distant metastasis. |
| M1 | Distant metastasis. |

* *Note:* Tis includes cancer cells confined within the glandular basement membrane (intraepithelial) or lamina propria (intramucosal) with no extension through the muscularis mucosae into the submucosa.
† *Note:* Direct invasion in T4 includes invasion of other segments of the colorectum by way of the serosa, for example, invasion of the sigmoid colon by a carcinoma of the cecum.

In addition, incorporating the M category included clinical observations of metastatic disease. The stage groupings from 0 to IV paralleled Dukes' classification but avoided the confusion from the numerous modifications of the alphabetically based Dukes' system (Table 16A-2). Prognostically, stages 0 and I were comparable to Dukes' A and stages II and III to Dukes' B and C, respectively. Despite

**TABLE 16A-2.** TNM STAGE GROUPING FOR CANCER OF THE COLON AND RECTUM

| STAGE | T | N | M | DUKES' STAGE |
|---|---|---|---|---|
| 0 | Tis | N0 | M0 | |
| I | T1 | N0 | M0 | A |
| | T2 | N0 | M0 | |
| II | T3 | N0 | M0 | B |
| | T4 | N0 | M0 | |
| III | Any T | N1 | M0 | C |
| | Any T | N2, N3 | M0 | |
| IV | Any T | Any N | M1 | |

the significant advantages of the TNM staging system, the inability to distinguish tumors of different grade, differentiate between $pT_4$ tumors attached to a contiguous organ as opposed to tumor extending to the surface of the specimen, identify potentially resectable $pN_3$ tumors from incurable disease, and acknowledge residual tumor status as microscopic, gross or both (i.e., histologically involved resection margins vs. distant residual tumor) are not yet resolved.

Evaluation of the resected specimen continues to provide the standard for staging with proven prognostic merit. An important consideration of staging systems is that they remain imperfect. Patients with a low probability of recurring (stage I) nevertheless recur, and similarly, patients with high-risk disease (stage III or even some stage IV patients) at presentation may not recur. The inability to predict precise patterns of failure in tumors with "bad biology" continues to drive the identification of markers that will correlate with tumor behavior, particularly at the molecular level (e.g., attachment and invasion of basement membrane, angiogenesis, migration in blood and lymph vessels, and ability to seed and establish growth in target organs). Another significant limitation of the current clinicopathologic staging sytem is the inability to define prognostic categories on the basis of preoperative sampling of the tumor. Thus, the probability or pattern for recurrence cannot be predicted until after surgical resection. This makes it difficult to evaluate preoperative multimodality treatment properly.

## CLINICAL FEATURES

Age at CRC diagnosis is normally distributed. The patients who fall on either end of the spectrum are of particular interest. Survival for younger patients is frequently believed to be lower than the general population of CRC patients, although this is somewhat controversial. Poor prognosis has been attributed to a greater proportion of poorly differentiated tumors; a larger number of mucinous lesions, which are associated with an increased risk of local recurrence; and a lower potential for curative resection because of presentation with advanced stage disease. However, survival rates for young patients with CRC are comparable to those of older patients when stratified by stage.[3] Conflicting reports are found for the prognosis of elderly patients also. A more favorable prognosis is thought to result from less biologically aggressive cancers.

### SYMPTOMS

Typically, patients with colon cancer present with an insidious onset of chronic symptoms. Bleeding is the most common and should be investigated in middle-aged or older individuals, although the most common cause is still likely to be hemorrhoids. Bleeding may be occult, as commonly noted with right-sided lesions, or overt, varying from bright red to dark purple to black, depending on the source in the bowel. A change in bowel habit, either constipation or diarrhea, may be observed with distal lesions because the stool is more formed in consistency and the lumen is narrower. Abdominal pain may be vague and poorly localized, or it may be colicky in nature if the patient is partially obstructed and has associated symptoms of bloating, nausea, or even vomiting. Back pain occurs with invasion of retroperitoneal structures. Nonspecific systemic symptoms of weight loss, deterioration in general health, anemia, and sporadic fever are features of advanced disease. Unusual presentations may consist of acute appendicitis due to a cecal tumor occluding the appendiceal orifice or urinary symptoms (frequency, suprapubic pressure, pneumaturia) secondary to bladder involvement.

Acute symptoms, such as intestinal obstruction, perforation with peritonitis, or hemorrhage, are less common. Approximately 15% of patients present with obstruction, usually due to advanced disease of the left colon where intestinal contents are solid and the configuration of the lesion is more likely to be annular.[116] Perforation associated with colon carcinoma may result in peritonitis, abscess formation, adherence to adjacent structures, or fistulous communication into another viscus. Most commonly, the site of perforation is at the carcinoma itself due to transmural disease. However, patients may first develop obstruction and perforate proximally in the thin-walled cecum. These types of presentations may be confused with inflammatory processes such as diverticulitis, appendicitis, or CD. Typically, a locally confined perforated right colon cancer may produce a large pericecal mass that produces symptoms of chronic iron-deficiency anemia from undiagnosed mucosal bleeding. Although bleeding from colonic carcinoma is very common, massive hemorrhage is not.

### SIGNS

Abdominal examination generally fails to reveal any significant abnormalities, unless the patient presents with complicated disease. A palpable mass usually signifies a large primary tumor or possibly metastases. The liver may be enlarged and irregular. Ascites may be appreciable. Inguinal and left supraclavicular adenopathy occur rarely. A few patients may even be under investigation for fever of unknown origin.

## DIAGNOSIS, SCREENING, AND PREOPERATIVE EVALUATION

### DIAGNOSIS IN SYMPTOMATIC PATIENTS

Digital rectal and sigmoidoscopic examinations are part of the initial workup. The absence of physical signs should not delay additional screening of the large bowel, whether by endoscopy or radiologic studies, if the presenting symptoms implicate a GI origin. There are no prospective randomized data to guide which investigation should be undertaken. However, endoscopy is more accessible, more sensitive and specific, and has the potential to confirm the diagnosis by biopsy. It also provides a means of definitive therapy if the neoplasm is amenable to polypectomy. Colonoscopy is recommended for blood per rectum; other GI symptoms; a polyp found at sigmoidoscopy; a previous history of polyps, CRC, UC, or CD; and a family history of polyps, CRC, or dominantly inherited syndromes (FAP and HNPCC).

### SCREENING ASYMPTOMATIC PATIENTS

Screening of asymptomatic individuals in the general population is directed toward reducing CRC incidence and mortality. Early-stage disease is associated with significantly improved survival, and may be managed by less invasive surgical procedures. Current recommendations developed by the American Cancer Society (Table 16A-3) for an average risk individual (no personal or family history of CRC or adenomatous polyps, no history of inflammatory bowel disease) are annual digital rectal exam with fecal occult blood test (FOBT) beginning at age 40 and flexible sigmoidoscopy beginning at age 50 and every 3 years thereafter.[117] These recommendations are based, in part, on three randomized controlled trials on FOBT that demonstrated a 15% to 33% decrease in mortality from CRC and two case-control studies on screening sigmoidoscopy that reported a 60% to 80% decrease in mortality from cancer of the distal colon or rectum. Although there are no studies to evaluate whether screening colonoscopy can reduce CRC incidence or mortality in average-risk patients, colonoscopy is an effective screening test and endorsed as an alternative modality for screening. Substantial indirect evidence supports the utility of screening average-risk individuals by colonoscopy.[118–120] For many surgeons, the preference is to examine the entire large bowel endoscopically, particularly with the increasing prevalence of more proximal large bowel cancers.

**TABLE 16A-3.** CURRENT RECOMMENDATIONS FOR SCREENING COLON CANCER—AMERICAN CANCER SOCIETY

| RISK CATEGORY | RECOMMENDATION | AGE TO BEGIN | INTERVAL |
|---|---|---|---|
| **AVERAGE RISK (70–80%)**<br>Patients ≥50 yr who do not fit in categories below | FOBT + flexible sigmoidoscopy or TCE | 50 yr | FOBT every 1 yr<br>Flexible sigmoidoscopy every 5 yr<br>Colonoscopy every 10 yr or DCBE every 5–10 yr |
| **MODERATE RISK (15–20%)**<br>Patients with adenomatous polyps | Colonoscopy | At initial polyp diagnosis | Within 3 yr after polyp removal |
| Personal history of CRC s/p curative resection | TCE | Within 1 yr after resection | TCE in 3 yr if normal |
| CRC or adenomatous polyp in FDR <60 yr, or CRC in ≥2 FDR of any age | TCE | Age 40 or 10 yr before the youngest case in the family, whichever is earlier | Every 5 yr |
| **HIGH RISK (5–10%)**<br>Family history of FAP | Early surveillance with endoscopy | 10–12 yr | Every 1–2 yr until colectomy |
| Family history of HNPCC | Colonoscopy | Age 21 yr | Every 2 yr until age 40 then every year |
| Inflammatory bowel disease | Colonoscopy with biopsies for dysplasia | 8 yr after the start of pancolitis; 12–15 yr after the start of left sided colitis | Every 1–2 yr |

NOTE: Digital rectal examination should be performed at the time of each sigmoidoscopy, colonoscopy, or DCBE.
ABBREVIATIONS: TCE = total colorectal examination (includes either colonoscopy or DCBE performed in conjunction with flexible sigmoidoscopy); DCBE = double contrast barium enema; FOBT = fecal occult blood test; yr = years.
SOURCE: Modified from Byers T et al: American Cancer Society guidelines for screening and surveillance for early detection of colorectal polyps and cancer: Update 1997. CA 47(3):154–60, 1997. (By permission.)

## SCREENING HIGH-RISK PATIENTS

Colonoscopy is the preferred examination in patients with a history of adenomatous polyps because of a defined risk for further adenomas and potentially CRC. After removal of colorectal adenomas, repeat colonoscopy can be performed in 3 years for most patients. A shorter interval may be necessary after removal of multiple adenomas, excision of an adenoma with invasive cancer, incomplete or piecemeal removal of a large sessile adenoma, or a suboptimal examination. Longer intervals may be appropriate for patients with a single small tubular adenoma. In fact, if the 3-year follow-up examination is negative, the interval may be, in carefully selected cases, increased to every 5 years.

Individuals with a family cancer history consisting of one or more FDRs affected by CRC or a FDR diagnosed with an adenoma before age 60 are at increased risk for CRC.[41–45,121,122] These patients should undergo screening of their entire colon, beginning at 40 years of age, or 10 years younger than the earliest diagnosed cancer in the family, whichever occurs first.

In patients with FAP, the average age of adenoma detection is 15 years, with approximately 15% of patients manifesting polyps by 10 years, 75% by 20 years, and 90% by 30 years of age.[123] Therefore, FAP registries recommend an annual flexible sigmoidoscopy examination beginning at age 10 to 12 years (Table 16A-3).[53] Because risk decreases with age, the frequency of flexible sigmoidoscopy may be reduced to every 2 years after age 24, every 3 years after age 34, and then every 3 to 5 years after age 44.[124] Once the diagnosis of FAP is made, a full colonoscopy should be performed to evaluate the severity of the phenotype (identify CRC, large polyps, atypical polyps). Genetic counseling and gene testing should also be offered to members of these families. Surveillance for gastric, duodenal, and periampullary adenomas should begin at the time colonic polyposis is diagnosed and continued every 1 to 3 years thereafter. At the time of upper GI endoscopy, a side-viewing endoscope may be advantageous for optimal visualization of the ampulla.

Provisional recommendations for screening have been developed for individuals with MMR gene mutations[69,117,125] who are believed to have an 80% lifetime risk of developing CRC.[126] They may also be appropriate for nontested individuals from a MMR mutation–positive HNPCC family and for individuals belonging to families with an autosomal dominant predisposition to CRC. Full colonoscopy to the cecum with removal of adenomatous polyps is recommended beginning at age 20 to 25 years or 5 years earlier than the age of cancer diagnosis in the youngest affected relative (Table 16A-3).[124,127,128] Full colonoscopy is essential because proximal tumors without associated distal lesions are not uncommon. Examinations are scheduled every 1 to 2 years for the duration of the patient's life. Although there have been no randomized controlled trials to fully substantiate the benefit of colonoscopy in MMR gene mutation carriers, colonoscopic polypectomies of adenomas significantly reduce the incidence of CRC in nontested at-risk individuals of HNPCC kindreds.[129] There was a marked, but not yet significant, reduction in CRC-related mortality. Periodic colorectal examination of HNPCC families also allows the detection of cancer at an earlier stage than in patients not under surveillance.[130] In experimental decision analysis models evaluating cancer prevention strategies in MMR mutation carriers who are 25 years of age, colonoscopic screening increased life expectancy by 7 to 13.5 years and resulted in lower healthcare costs.[131,132] HNPCC families should also be referred for genetic counseling and possible gene testing. Screening for extracolonic malignancies is based on the pattern of disease specific to each family.

Current guidelines for screening in inflammatory bowel disease are the same for both UC and CD because the cancer risk appears to be similar. In patients with pancolitis, colonoscopy should begin after 8 years of symptoms. In patients with left sided colitis, colonoscopy may start after 12–15 years of symptoms. The frequency of examinations should be every 1–2 years. At colonoscopy, mucosal biopsies are taken from any areas of mucosal irregularity or plaque-like lesions as well as grossly normal-appearing mucosa at 10–12 cm intervals throughout the colon. Pathology expertise is essential. If the biopsies are negative or indefinite for dysplasia, surveillance should continue at 1–2 year intervals. Colectomy is indicated for unequivocal low-grade or high-grade dysplasia. Consideration should also be given to patients with medically intractable colitis and those who will not comply with surveillance.

## COLONOSCOPY

Colonoscopy has assumed greater importance in the management of colon cancer, not only in screening patients, but also in the perioperative setting to detect synchronous neoplasms. The standard colonoscope, 160 cm in length, is the most accurate method of detecting lesions less than 1 cm in diameter. It can visualize the entire colon and rectum and portions of the terminal ileum, as well as facilitate a biopsy or polypectomy. Areas adjacent to acute angulations, flexures, and the region behind the ileocecal valve may be difficult to evaluate. When the cecum cannot be reached (5% of patients or fewer[133]), a double-contrast barium enema (DCBE) should be performed. Diagnostic colonoscopy is a safe procedure. Major complications, such as perforation and bleeding, occur in fewer than 0.2% of procedures.[134]

Good bowel preparation and patient compliance are essential for a complete examination. Endoscopic units should be properly equipped for the administration of monitored sedation. The American Society of Colon and Rectal Surgeons has formulated practice parameters for antibiotic prophylaxis to prevent infective endocarditis or infective prosthesis during colon and rectal endoscopy based on recommendations by the American Heart Association (AHA).[135] Potential bacteremia warrants prophylactic antibiotics for high-risk patients, defined by the AHA as those with prosthetic cardiac valves (including bioprosthetic and homograft valves), a history of endocarditis, or a surgically constructed systemic or pulmonary shunt or conduit. Bacterial endocarditis is a moderate risk in patients with most congenital cardiac malformations, rheumatic and other acquired valvular dysfunction, idiopathic hypertrophic subaortic stenosis, and mitral valve prolapse with insufficiency. Broad-spectrum antibiotic coverage is also recommended in patients with prosthetic vascular graft material for at least 1 year after graft implantation and subsequent to this if deemed appropriate.

## DIAGNOSTIC IMAGING

**BARIUM ENEMA.** Well established before the introduction of fiberoptic endoscopy, classical radiologic features of colon carcinomas include the annular "apple-core" appearance with an irregular, jagged outline and overhanging edges or a large filling defect representing a bulky neoplasm projecting into the lumen. Although DCBE is superior for detection of small polyps, constricting lesions are best visualized by single-contrast enema. DCBE is also likely to miss flat lesions and does not allow for diagnostic biopsies or polypectomy. Furthermore, the rectal balloon used in DCBE obscures the distal rectum and limits visualization of this region. Thus, a negative barium enema examination in the setting of clinical suspicion for carcinoma warrants further investigation by colonoscopy.

**COMPUTED TOMOGRAPHY (CT).** When there is suspicion of hepatic metastases or a primary cancer that has invaded adjacent viscera or the abdominal wall, CT of the abdomen may be helpful. Furthermore, CT may identify occult metastases, providing useful information in planning surgical therapy.[136] However, inaccurate staging information is obtained in as many as 50% of patients with known liver metastases.[137] CT underestimated the number of lobes involved in 33% of patients and overestimated involvement in 4%. Extrahepatic disease was found in 12% of patients with a negative preoperative CT. Furthermore, the ability to identify intraabdominal nodal involvement is generally limited to a size threshold of 1 to 1.5 cm.

**CHEST X-RAY.** Routine posteroanterior and lateral chest x-rays are performed before surgery both to evaluate for comorbid disease and identify distant metastases.

## LABORATORY INVESTIGATIONS

A complete blood count and liver function tests are commonly obtained to determine the presence or absence of anemia and whether hepatic metastases may be present. A normal liver profile, however, does not rule out disease.

Carcinoembryonic antigen (CEA) is a glycoprotein secreted onto the luminal surface of the GI tract. Originally thought to be a specific antigen of the fetal digestive tract and adenocarcinoma of the colon, CEA is normally found in feces and pancreaticobiliary secretions, and appears in the plasma in a diverse group of neoplastic and nonneoplastic conditions. Approximately 35% of CRC recurrences do not produce CEA. False-negative results are also common in early stages of carcinoma and poorly differentiated tumors.[138,139] Although CEA has not been advocated as a screening test, a preoperative serum level is determined primarily for surveillance and monitoring response to treatment. An elevated CEA level warrants further investigations to identify and localize asymptomatic recurrences, but does not justify administration of systemic therapy for presumed metastatic disease.[139]

# TREATMENT

Surgery is the primary treatment of potentially curable colon cancers. In most cases, this involves resection of the primary tumor and regional lymph nodes. However, treatment options include endoscopic polypectomy for malignant polyps, laparoscopically assisted colectomy in carefully selected patients, and combined modality therapy for advanced cancers.

## MALIGNANT POLYPS

Approximately 5% to 8% of adenomas may have severe dysplasia and 3% to 5% may have invasive carcinoma at the time of diagnosis.[140,141] Villous adenomas have a 40% risk of containing cancer, whereas tubulovillous and tubular adenomas have a 22% and 5% risk, respectively.[14] The risk of cancer is very low for adenomas under 1 cm in diameter,[142] but increases rapidly to about 50% in polyps over 2 cm.[14]

Colonoscopic polypectomy alone may be appropriate for a malignant polyp with favorable criteria (small, pedunculated polyp with a well-differentiated cancer limited to the head of the polyp), because the risk of residual cancer or nodal metastases under these circumstances is minimal (0.3% to 1.5%).[140,143,144] It is important to mark the area with a submucosal injection of India ink for future endoscopic surveillance or should a resection be indicated.[145] Follow-up colonoscopy and surveillance of the polypectomy site is recommended in 3 to 6 months to assess completeness of excision, and then again at 1 year, before reverting to 3-year follow-up intervals.

Although polypectomy is sufficient treatment for selected malignant polyps, the finding of lymphovascular invasion, poor differentiation, or cancer close to the resection margin (within 2 mm) indicates the need for colonic resection.[143,146] By definition, a sessile polyp has no stalk and the submucosa is immediately adjacent to the muscularis propria. Therefore, sessile polyps with an invasive component generally require a formal colectomy for cure. The decision to proceed with colectomy is based on the risk of residual cancer and regional lymph node metastases as predicted by pathologic determinants balanced against operative morbidity and mortality as well as the life expectancy of the patient.

## CURATIVE RESECTION

**BOWEL PREPARATION.** Preoperative bowel preparation consists of mechanical catharsis and antibiotic prophylaxis. Beyond this general statement, how each is accomplished may vary considerably and is subject to debate. Mechanical cleansing is usually accomplished by ingestion of a hypertonic polyethylene glycol solution such as GoLYTELY or oral sodium phosphate (Fleet PhosphoSoda). Two principles are important when selecting antimicrobial prophylaxis. The administration of antibiotics should be timed to make sure that the tissue concentration of the antibiotic around the wound area is sufficient when bacterial contamination occurs, and coverage should be directed against gram-positive and gram-negative aerobic and anaerobic organisms. The ideal route of administration and selection of specific antibiotics remain controversial. Typical oral regimens consist of neomycin 1 g and erythromycin 1 g given at 1 P.M., 2 P.M., and 11 P.M. the day before surgery. Although oral antibiotics are effective, the surgical wound infection rate may be further lowered by adding parenteral antibiotics just before starting the operation.[147] Single agents administered as a single dose preoperatively are effective in reducing the incidence of surgical wound infections. Elimination of postoperative systemic antibiotics in elective clean-contaminated procedures has resulted in cost savings and reduction in antibiotic-associated morbidity without an apparent increase in surgical wound infections.

**EXPLORATORY LAPAROTOMY.** A Foley catheter is commonly placed into the bladder. An oral gastric tube is placed into the stomach and removed prior to extubation. Access to the peritoneal cavity is generally gained through a vertical midline incision above and below the umbilicus. Some surgeons utilize a transverse incision, which also provides adequate exposure for resections. Paramedian incisions are somewhat antiquated.

A thorough examination by visualization and palpation of the entire peritoneal cavity for metastatic disease is performed with particular attention to the liver, retroperitoneum, ovaries, omentum, small and large bowel mesentery, and serosal surfaces. Intraoperative US of the liver may be helpful to further evaluate hepatic lesions suspicious for metastatic disease. Assessment of the primary tumor at laparotomy is directed toward identification of transmural invasion as well as fixation and/or invasion of adjacent structures. Because the likelihood of lymph node involvement increases with depth of tumor invasion (5.6% for $pT_1$, 10% for $pT_2$, 36.7% for $pT_3$, and 77.7% for $pT_4$ colon carcinoma),[148] invasive adenocarcinomas require ligation and resection of the lymphovascular pedicle draining the intestinal segment containing the tumor. When the lesion is equidistant between two pedicles, then both should be encompassed in the resection. Because intraoperative assessment of T and N status is limited, all invasive colon cancers, small and large alike, should be managed in this manner.

**PRINCIPLES OF RESECTION (FIG. 16A-2).** The extent of resection is defined by ligation of the lymphovascular pedicle. A right hemicolectomy is appropriate for cancers of the cecum to the hepatic flexure. For both oncologic and technical reasons, a right hemicolectomy requires ligation of the ileocolic, right colic, and

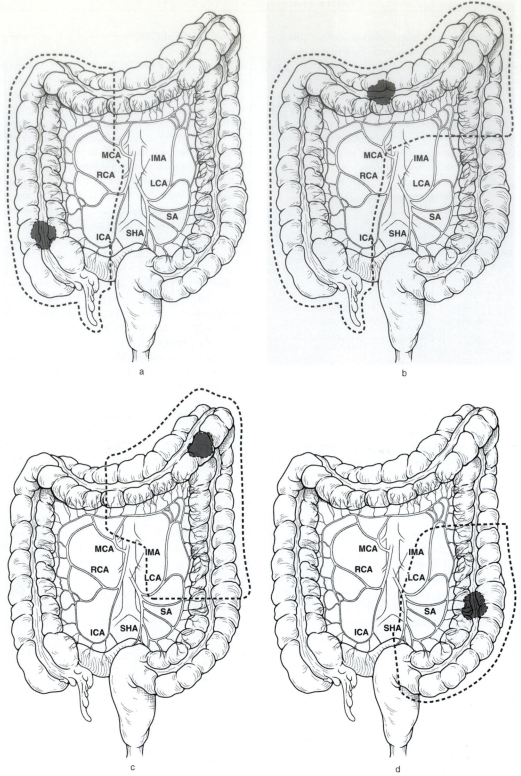

**FIGURE 16A-2.** Extent of surgical resections for colon carcinomas: (a) cecal or ascending colon cancer; (b) transverse colon cancer; (c) splenic flexure colon cancer; (d) descending or sigmoid colon cancer. Abbreviations: ICA = ileocolic artery, RCA = right colic artery, MCA = middle colic artery, IMA = inferior mesenteric artery, LCA = left colic artery, SA = sigmoidal arteries, SHA = superior hemorrhoidal artery.

right branch of the middle colic vessels. Transverse colonic cancers require a transverse colectomy. However, an extended right hemicolectomy, with ligation of the middle colic but preservation of the left colic artery and an ileodescending colon anastomosis, is often preferred because of concerns over tension or inadequate blood supply at the colocolostomy. Adenocarcinomas in the splenic flexure are managed either by an extended right hemicolectomy or by a left hemicolectomy, depending on the blood supply ascertained after a complete splenic flexure mobilization. Cancers in the descending and sigmoid colon should be managed by a left hemicolectomy in which the left branch of the middle colic artery remains intact, but the left colic artery and sigmoidal vessels are ligated. Although resection of primary sigmoid colon cancer does not require high ligation of the inferior mesenteric artery for oncologic reasons, it may facilitate reapproximation of the bowel for reanastomosis without tension. Limited segmental resections may be appropriate for poor-risk patients or patients undergoing a palliative operation.

Although resectability of primary colon cancer is well over 90%, "curative resection" can only be determined after pathologic staging. It is interesting that 19% of patients who presumably had a conventional mesenteric resection as part of their colectomy performed with curative intent had three or fewer lymph nodes examined pathologically.[149] These data suggest that inadequate staging or inadequate surgery may be relevant in a significant proportion of patients undergoing "curative" resection.

Concerns over both hematogenous metastases and implantation of shed malignant cells through manipulation of the tumor have been raised. In an effort to reduce the risk of dissemination, no-touch technique (identification, division, and ligation of mesenteric vessels prior to mobilization of the bowel), occluding the bowel lumen proximal and distal to the primary cancer, and instillation of cytotoxic agents have been suggested. None of these techniques have been shown to improve survival. Interestingly, recent studies utilizing molecular techniques suggest the no-touch technique may decrease cancer cells from being shed into the portal vein during surgical manipulation.[150,151] However, this does not appear to be a consistent observation.[152]

## LAPAROSCOPIC COLECTOMY

As surgeons become more familiar with laparoscopic equipment and techniques, minimal access surgery is being applied to various organs in the peritoneal cavity including the colon. Laparoscopic resection for CRC is controversial. Although decreased hospital costs because of a shorter postoperative stay appear to be the primary benefit, other possible advantages include reduced recuperation time, improvement in quality of life, physiologic and immunologic advantages, and cosmesis. However, these benefits must be balanced against the greater cost of operative equipment and time. There are also potential complications specific to laparoscopic techniques such as unrecognized injuries to the small bowel and ureters, anastomotic leaks, and port site herniations, as well as those arising from the creation of a pneumoperitoneum ($CO_2$ embolization, undesired hemodynamic effects, dysrhythmias). Major oncologic concerns with this technique include inadequate resection for tumor staging, port site recurrences, and altered tumor spread due to pneumoperitoneum.

In a prospective, randomized trial with limited follow-up, laparoscopic techniques were as safe as conventional resection in selected CRC patients.[153] Another early fear was trocar site recurrences, which initially appeared to be greater in laparoscopically assisted CRC resections compared with an open approach. However, subsequent studies report incidences less than 3%.[153,154] Data on laparoscopic colon and rectal procedures have shown that roughly equivalent numbers of nodes draining the cancer are retrieved from the resected specimen when laparoscopic techniques are compared with open resections.[155] Early survival curves for CRC patients treated by laparoscopic resection do not differ from patients treated by conventional surgery.[153,156] Long-term oncologic results are not yet available for laparoscopic-assisted colectomy. If the same principles are applied, current randomized trials comparing open to laparoscopic resection should not lead to major discrepancies in outcome. A trial sponsored by the National Institutes of Health is currently under way and proposes to evaluate diffences between open and laparoscopic colon surgery in 1200 cancer patients with respect to disease-free and overall survival.[154] Additional endpoints include operative morbidity and mortality, as well as quality-of-life issues and cost effectiveness. Further data will also be available from a national laparoscopic-assisted colectomy registry that has been established by the American Society of Colon and Rectal Surgeons in conjunction with the Commission on Cancer of the American College of Surgeons.

The right colon and sigmoid colon appear to be the most accessible to laparoscopic techniques because of their long mesenteries and the relatively straightforward dissection required for mobilization to the midline.

## OBSTRUCTING COLON CANCER

Obstructing or near-obstructing colon cancers present a special challenge. Resection and primary anastomosis are associated with an increased leak rate and poor prognosis.[157] If the patient can be stabilized with resolution of the occlusion, bowel preparation and elective resection is preferred.

When complete obstruction of the colon is secondary to carcinoma, recommended treatment depends on the level of obstruction. Although right or transverse colon lesions are amenable to resection with primary ileocolonic anastomosis, the management of left-sided lesions is more controversial.[158] A three-staged approach, including an initial diversion, a subsequent resection, and ultimately, an anastomosis, is the most conservative option. However, up to 75% of patients may not proceed through to the final stage of restoring GI continuity. Resection with colostomy and either distal mucous fistula or Hartmann's pouch is an alternative. Subtotal colectomy with immediate reanastomosis is a one-stage procedure that avoids a temporary stoma and removes any synchronous lesions,[159,160] but may result in troublesome diarrhea in elderly patients or those requiring postoperative chemotherapy. The ideal circumstances for a subtotal colectomy are an acutely obstructed and resectable carcinoma with a massively distended proximal colon of dubious viability and signs of impending cecal perforation. Intraoperative colonic lavage is another technique that avoids a temporary stoma. Although in carefully selected patients and expert hands this is a safe approach,[161,162] a prospective randomized study documented a morbidity of 17% and an operative mortality of 11%.[163] The most aggressive approach to obstructing colon cancers is to perform a resection with primary anastomosis in the absence of bowel preparation. In a series of 58 patients acutely obstructed by left-sided colonic carcinomas managed by emergency resection and primary anastomosis without intraoperative colonic lavage, only one patient developed a leak at the anastomotic site, requiring pelvic abscess drainage and transverse loop colostomy.[164] One death occurred 12 hours after surgery due to myocardial infarction. In the exceptional case in which the obstructing lesion is deemed unresectable and the distal colon is cleared, a bypass may be considered in lieu of a diverting stoma.

Nonoperative techniques, such as laser recanalization or luminal stenting, may sufficiently relieve bowel obstruction to facilitate a good bowel preparation and allow for resection and primary anastomosis. In 54 patients submitted to recanalization by Nd: YAG laser, two were complicated by perforation, but no further septic sequelae followed an immediate laparotomy.[165] Left hemicolectomy or anterior resection was subsequently performed in 27 of these patients with a leak rate of 26% and mortality rate of 3.7%. Stent placement achieves relief of malignant obstruction in 60% to 92% of patients who are then eligible for a one-stage procedure after routine bowel preparation.[166,167] These novel techniques require special expertise, cautious patient selection, and vigilance for potential complications such as reocclusion and stent migration.

## PERFORATED COLON CANCER

Perforated colon cancer is associated with a high recurrence rate and a poor prognosis.[158] Perforation may lead to diffuse peritonitis or a localized inflammatory process. Each situation is handled individually. In the setting of generalized peritonitis, management includes thorough irrigation of the peritoneal cavity, resection of the perforated segment in order to prevent ongoing contamination, and diversion. Although a Hartmann pouch or mucous fistula is usually necessary, reanastomosis may be feasible in some patients, but should always be protected with a proximal ileostomy or colostomy. Simple closure of the perforation and relief of obstruction by colostomy is less optimal because suture repair in ischemic or inflamed bowel will not hold. Subtotal colectomy with ileorectal or ileosigmoid anastomosis may be necessary in the case of a distal obstructing lesion with perforation of the proximal colon.

## HEMORRHAGE FROM COLON CANCER

Massive hemorrhage from carcinoma is unusual, but when it occurs, an emergent operation is necessary. Because blood in the lumen tends to function as a cathartic, routine mechanical cleansing may not be necessary, and the affected segment may be resected with a primary anastomosis.

## EN BLOC RESECTION

Between 5% and 10% of CRCs without distant metastases have invaded adjacent structures or become attached to the abdominal wall

at the time of resection.[168] Although involvement of the genitourinary system is noted in almost half of all patients who undergo extended resection for locally advanced CRC, other organs frequently involved include small bowel, other segments of large bowel, omentum, stomach, duodenum, spleen, and abdominal wall. The most common extensions of resection in one series involved total hysterectomy (39%), small bowel (21%), urinary bladder (16%), and abdominal wall (4%).[168]

Because extended resections can achieve comparable results in locally advanced CRC as nonextended resections in less advanced cancer, an aggressive surgical approach is warranted, even when multiple adjacent organs or structures are resected.[169,170] Five-year survival rates in 118 patients whose resection of the primary lesion included one or more adjacent secondary organs or structures were 62% and 38% for Dukes' B and C lesions, respectively.[170] In order to perform an adequate curative operation, it becomes necessary to excise en bloc all of the attached tissue. Often these adhesions are inflammatory in nature and not caused by malignant infiltration. However, inadvertent disruption of the tumor capsule during resection should be avoided because negative resection margins are essential for long-term local control and survival.[168] The main objective is en bloc resection, avoiding dissection of adhesions to the CRC, because this potentially leaves disease behind and results in a significant survival disadvantage.

One possible exception to this general recommendation is involvement of the duodenum. Under these circumstances, the morbidity and mortality of radical operation by pancreaticoduodenectomy may exceed the possible benefits. However, in patients carefully selected by experienced surgeons, such radical operations have been safely undertaken.[171]

## OOPHORECTOMY

Recommendation for oophorectomy at the time of primary CRC resection is based on a 3% to 25% incidence (overall approximately 6%) of ovarian involvement, subsequent reoperation in approximately 2% of patients because of symptomatic ovarian metastases, and an apparent five-fold increase in ovarian cancer in women with CRC.[172–175] Oophorectomy removes both microscopic and macroscopic metastases and may diminish morbidity.[176] However, survival is not significantly affected by this procedure, and few patients survive 5 years after operation.[173] In 155 patients randomized to oophorectomy or no oophorectomy during CRC resection, no evidence of ovarian metastases (gross or microscopic disease) was found in 77 patients randomized to oophorectomy.[177] Patients undergoing oophorectomy demonstrated a better recurrence-free survival (80% vs. 65% at 5 years) and a crude survival benefit between 2 and 3 years after surgery that was not statistically significant and did not persist at 5 years. Until mature data become available, the reasons for performing a bilateral oophorectomy are the potential for reducing the risk of primary ovarian carcinoma (particularly in postmenopausal women), the treatment of patients in whom any gross abnormality of the ovaries or involvement by contiguous spread is evident, and reducing the risk of future symptomatic ovarian metastases when peritoneal disease is discovered at CRC resection.

Metachronous ovarian metastases ususally present as a component of diffuse intraabdominal recurrence.[174] Mean survival after operation is 16.6 months. However, if all gross disease can be removed at the time of oophorectomy, mean survival is 48 months compared with 9.6 months for patients with unresectable disease. Furthermore, palliative oophorectomy may be indicated for large symptomatic metastases.

## SYNCHRONOUS COLORECTAL NEOPLASMS

The incidence of synchronous carcinomas reportedly ranges from 2% to 11% of patients and that of adenomatous polyps may be 30% or higher.[178,179] Approximately one-third of patients have synchronous cancers located in a different anatomic segment of the colon, and resection of more colon than anticipated for the index lesion becomes necessary.[178,180] Subtotal colectomy is appropriate for widely separated synchronous carcinomas and for multiple polyps in the colon occurring in the setting of cancer, even if not categorized as hereditary CRC. Although preoperative colonoscopy is prudent to evaluate the entire colon in patients undergoing elective resection, it may not be possible to assess the proximal colon in obstructing cancers or to satisfactorily evaluate the entire colon, and these patients should have postoperative colonoscopy. Surgeons concerned with the fear of implanting malignant cells from exfoliation by preoperative colonoscopy prefer intraoperative palpation to detect synchronous carcinomas and postoperative colonoscopy to clear the residual colon of any missed lesions. However, intraoperative palpation will miss nonpalpable, flat cancers or small lesions that may be excluded from resection.

## PALLIATIVE RESECTION

For patients with metastatic carcinoma from primary colon cancer, resection may be indicated to eliminate the symptoms of local disease and avoid potential complications of obstruction, perforation, bleeding, or local invasion. The role of palliative resection in a patient with limited survival has been questioned, especially if an abdominoperineal resection (APR), which establishes a permanent colostomy, is necessary. In a recent retrospective study of stage IV CRC patients, 66 were resected and compared to 23 with asymptomatic primary colorectal lesions left in situ.[181] In the nonresection group, primary treatment consisted of chemotherapy in 13 patients, external beam radiation therapy in 1, and combination chemoradiation in 9. Only 2 of 23 (8.7%) patients managed without resection eventually developed obstruction at the primary tumor site requiring emergent diversion. For the resection group, the operative morbidity was 30.3%, and the perioperative mortality rate was 4.6%. No survival advantage was gained by resection of asymptomatic primary CRC in the setting of incurable stage IV disease.

In the face of significant comorbid medical illness, extensive hepatic disease, widespread peritoneal seeding, or marked ascites, life expectancy is short and benefits of resection are minimal. However, if the volume of distant metastases is limited, the primary tumor should be evaluated for the possibility of obstruction and palliative resection. As more experience is gained with laser therapy and lu-

minal stenting, an abdominal surgical intervention may be avoided in carefully selected patients.

## RECURRENT DISEASE

Isolated locoregional disease accounts for 5% to 19% of colon recurrences and between 7% and 20% can be resected with curative intent.[182] Surgical resection of local recurrence can result in a mean survival of 33 to 59 months and possibly long-term survival in 30% to 50%, depending on the extent of recurrence and completeness of resection. The use of intraoperative radiation therapy with or without consolidation external beam radiation therapy may increase surgical salvage rates.[183] Endoscopic laser therapy is a palliative modality that may relieve obstruction and control bleeding for unresectable lesions in the distal sigmoid. These symptoms can be controlled in 80% to 90% of patients with minimal morbidity and mortality.[184,185] There is no impact, however, on pain or survival. Treatments can be delivered with little or no sedation, limited hospital stay, and may be repeated as necessary. Complications of laser therapy include bleeding, perforation, abscess, and fistula formation, as well as post-laser stricturing, at an overall rate of 6%.[185]

## METASTATIC DISEASE

Approximately 17% of patients present with synchronous metastases.[149] The liver is the most common site of metastasis followed by the peritoneal surface and the lung.

LIVER. Because the liver is the first major organ draining the intestinal tract, it is the most common site of metastatic disease from colon cancers, and often represents the only site of metastasis. Patients with untreated hepatic metastases have a median survival of 6 to 12 months, which decreases to 4.5 months if metastases are synchronous.[186,187] In this setting, systemic chemotherapy based either on 5-fluorouracil (5-FU) or irinotecan (CPT-11) appears to be palliative, and rarely prolongs survival over 2 years. The lack of therapeutic alternatives has made hepatic resection a potential option for cure. With an increasingly aggressive surgical approach, reported 5-year survival for patients undergoing resection for CRC liver metastases is 25% to 39%, with a median survival of 28 to 40 months and 10-year survival rate in the range of 20%.[188] Morbidity and mortality rates associated with liver resection has improved, and most series report an overall perioperative complication rate of 20% to 50%, and less than 5% mortality rate. A major hepatectomy and colectomy may be overly taxing on most patients. However, in the appropriate setting, concomitant resection of the primary cancer and liver metastases may be safely undertaken in carefully selected patients. Otherwise, a thorough evaluation is performed after colonic resection to assess extent and resectability of synchronous metastatic disease.

A patient who presents with metachronous liver metastases requires an extent of disease workup for both recurrent local disease and other potential sites of metastasis. It is essential to rule out evidence of other metastatic disease because investigation rarely reveals a solitary lesion. A relatively limited group of patients who develop liver metastases will be surgical candidates. A thorough medical evaluation is required to assess comorbid illness. Advanced age alone is not an absolute contraindication to surgery.[189] Preoperative imaging continues to improve, and may incorporate US, CT, CT portography, MRI, and fluorodeoxyglucose positron emission tomography (FDG-PET) in order to identify isolated, well-defined, resectable liver metastases.[188] US is the least invasive and least expensive test and may be useful to define the relationship between the tumor and major vessels. CT is the most widely used because it is readily available. CT portography is a very sensitive method for detection of hepatic metastases and is the gold standard for determining the number of lesions. However, this test is invasive and expensive. Helical CT and MRI compromise sensitivity, but are commonly used instead. FDG-PET is a promising new technology that may be beneficial in preoperative staging, particularly those at high risk for undetected extrahepatic disease. Despite preoperative imaging studies, primarily CT, approximately one-half of patients will be unresectable at laparotomy. Of the unresectable patients, one-third will have unsuspected extrahepatic disease, whereas two-thirds will have more extensive disease in the liver than anticipated.[137] Intraoperative US may further eliminate patients initially thought to have surgically resectable disease.

Currently, there is no firm consensus as to which factors are important in selecting patients for surgical resection of liver metastases and which factors are important for prognosis. Some determinants reported to have a poor prognosis include node-positive primary CRC, short disease-free interval (especially synchronous metastases), resection margin involved by tumor, four or more liver lesions, the presence of satellite nodules, extent of liver involvement greater than 50%, presence of extrahepatic metastases, symptomatic liver metastases, and high preoperative CEA.[188] CRC patients may benefit from metastasectomy if the primary lesion is controlled, there are only one to three preferably unilobar hepatic metastases that can be removed with adequate margins, and there is no evidence of extrahepatic disease. In contrast, the presence of extrahepatic metastases, multiple hepatic metastases replacing more than half of the liver, large lesions encroaching major hepatic veins, contralateral hilar ducts or veins, or lesions that preclude resection with free margins confers an unfavorable prognosis, and resection is unlikely to benefit the patient. Many patients will fall somewhere in between and require individual evaluation by the surgeon in order to make a definitive recommendation. In clinical practice, attempts have been made to formulate a scoring system in order to select patients for surgery and to stratify them based on prognosis. The Memorial Sloan-Kettering Cancer Center scoring system is based on the following: node-positive primary, disease-free interval from primary to metastasis less than 12 months, more than one hepatic tumor, largest hepatic tumor greater than 5 cm, and preoperative CEA level greater than 200 ng/mL.[190] Patients with two or fewer of these criteria can be expected to have a favorable outcome, whereas patients with three or more criteria fare poorly. This system is particularly advantageous because it can be applied to patients prior to surgical resection. Future studies will provide more specific criteria to refine the selection process.

Regional chemotherapy delivered via hepatic artery infusion (HAI) pump has been used for primary treatment of hepatic metastases or in the adjuvant setting following hepatic resection. The rationale for administering chemotherapy by HAI is based on both anatomic and pharmacologic considerations. Liver metastases are perfused almost exclusively by the hepatic artery, whereas the liver parenchyma derives its blood supply predominantly from the portal vein. Some drugs, such as floxuridine (FUDR), are largely extracted by the liver during the first pass through the arterial circulation, so local exposure is substantially increased. The side effects of systemic chemotherapy are almost never observed with HAI. Furthermore, the use of a totally implantable Infusaid pump and a Silastic catheter has resulted in less erosive damage to the intima. The catheter is usually positioned through the gastroduodenal artery such that the tip abuts but does not enter the hepatic artery. After catheter insertion, radionuclide studies are performed to ensure the pump is perfusing the entire liver and to rule out perfusion of extrahepatic tissues. Biliary sclerosis is a dose-limiting toxicity. This complication develops in 6% to 25% of patients, but can be alleviated with the addition of dexamethasone.[191] Other significant complications include arterial thrombosis (9%) and catheter dislodgement (up to 15% prior to use of implantable pumps).

HAI chemotherapy achieves a mean response rate of 44%, approximately three times higher than that noted with systemic chemotherapy.[191] Response rates in previously treated patients with metastatic CRC are somewhat lower. Multi-institutional, prospective, controlled trials comparing intraarterial 5-FU or FUDR with systemic chemotherapy in similarly staged CRC patients with metastatic disease showed significant hepatic tumor response that did not translate into any striking improvement in survival. However, the studies commonly allowed crossover in treatment arms, some were inadequately powered, and some used inadequate systemic chemotherapy. Many patients developed chemical hepatitis and a sclerosing cholangitis-like drug-related effect. In addition to these adverse effects, those patients who were treated by HAI chemotherapy and did not have a tumor response probably had an increased risk of extrahepatic disease, mitigating any obvious potential survival benefit. In a recent randomized, multicenter trial, a subset of patients who have limited disease with an intrahepatic tumor burden of less than 25% were able to gain a survival benefit with an almost two-fold prolonged time to progression.[192] Furthermore, the quality of life on HAI therapy appears to be better, an important consideration if the prospect of cure is low.

The liver is also the most common site of recurrence after resection of hepatic CRC metastases. Initial promising results in retrospective and nonrandomized studies suggested the potential for decreased recurrence and improved survival with HAI after hepatic resection.[193,194] However, randomized trials comparing intrahepatic arterial therapy with either surgery alone or with surgery and adjuvant systemic chemotherapy indicate minimal improvement in survival despite hepatic tumor response.[195,196] Hepatic disease–free survival rate was increased and an increase in 2-year survival rate with HAI plus systemic therapy after liver resection was demonstrated.

Techniques available to ablate liver tumors include cryoablation, alcohol injection, radiofrequency ablation, and embolization.[188] The first three may be used to destroy liver tissue via an open, laparoscopic, or percutaneous approach. There is insufficient evidence to support the use of embolization for metastatic CRC. Ablative modalities may be applied to small lesions in patients with medical contraindications to liver resection, small unresectable recurrences occurring after previous resection, and scattered unresectable cancers. Unfortunately, these techniques are most effective in lesions amenable to resection. However, they may complement current strategies in the treatment of CRC metastases.

It is difficult to establish whether therapy for hepatic metastases has truly resulted in better results because of effective therapy or biologic selection. Nevertheless, in patients with liver-only or liver-preponderant metastatic disease followed to their death, 86% will die of liver failure.[197]

LUNG. Pulmonary metastases usually occur in the setting of generalized recurrence and less than 2% to 4% of CRC patients will develop isolated lung metastases, of which half are potentially resectable.[182] The criteria for determining resectability resemble those applied to hepatic metastases: the primary CRC should be controlled locally, there should be no other evidence of metastases, and the patient's medical condition should allow for pulmonary resection without undue morbidity or mortality. Ideally, pulmonary metastases would be limited to one lung and readily excised. Although video-assisted thoracic surgery may be used as a diagnostic tool, a thoracotomy is required for lung palpation and complete resection, which is essential for long-term survival.[198] There are no uniformly reliable prognostic discriminants in the management of a particular patient. Some factors found to be of favorable prognostic significance include solitary pulmonary metastasis less than 3 cm, normal prethoracotomy CEA level, early-stage primary tumor, complete resection, and prolonged disease-free interval.[182,199–201] An aggressive operative approach toward metastatic disease confined to the lung may result in prolonged disease-free survival and appreciable palliative benefit in very carefully selected patients. Resection of pulmonary metastases is generally associated with little risk and 5-year survival rates as high as 31% to 42% with long-term follow-up.[199,202,203]

LIVER AND LUNG. A very select group of patients with CRC hepatic and pulmonary metastases may benefit from resection. In fact, less than 5% of patients with either pulmonary or hepatic metastases from CRC are eligible for surgical therapy.[200] Thus, operative treatment for patients with both hepatic and pulmonary metastases is rare. In limited series, median survival in the range of 30 months[204] and 5-year survival of approximately 30%[201] is possible.

## ADJUVANT THERAPY

### CHEMOTHERAPY

Adjuvant chemotherapy most likely benefits those patients harboring occult, residual, or disseminated disease. Many agents have been employed singly or in combination in an effort to improve survival rates. The role of 5-FU–based chemotherapy in stage III colon cancer has been firmly established. The precise role for chemotherapy in stage II disease is less clear. In a series of clinical trials, high-risk stage II and stage III colon carcinoma achieved an overall survival benefit with adjuvant chemotherapy.[205–207] 5-FU plus levamisole is well tolerated and accepted as standard surgical adjuvant therapy for patients with stage III colon cancer, but the data in stage II patients suggest a decreased relapse rate without significant improvement in

survival at a median follow-up of 7 years.[207] The combination of 5-FU plus levamisole reduced recurrence by 33% and mortality by 40%, with an absolute improvement of 13% in 5-year survival.[206] Other studies of 5-FU combined with leucovorin suggested that this regimen could be as effective in the adjuvant setting.[206,208,209] Regardless of the specific agents chosen, no significant improvement in patient survival is achieved beyond 6 months of treatment.[208,210] In other studies assessing combination therapy for adjuvant treatment of resected colon cancer, there is no advantage to the addition of levamisole or interferon to a 6-month regimen of 5-FU and leucovorin.[211,212] If extrapolated to the population at large, administration of established adjuvant postoperative combined modality therapy would produce an approximate one-third decrease in the death rate from cancer, which is almost unprecedented in solid tumor adjuvant therapy.

The inability to demonstrate a clear advantage to adjuvant therapy in stage II patients may relate to the low event rate observed in this population, requiring a larger number of patients to detect a significant difference in outcome. Pooled data of B2 colon cancer trials has been reanalyzed and suggests that there is no significant survival benefit, and that chemotherapy should not be considered standard for all patients with stage II colon cancer.[213] Factors associated with increased risk of relapse and worse prognosis in stage II disease include increasing patient age, elevated preoperative CEA level, complete colonic obstruction, perforation, or invasion of the tumor into adjacent organs. Biologic factors also indicative of a poor prognosis in this population are poorly differentiated histology, a high S-phase fraction, loss of DCC protein expression, lack of p27 expression, p53 mutations, and high levels of thymidylate synthase (TS) expression.[212] These potential predictors of outcome are being tested prospectively to determine the efficacy of adjuvant therapy. Another means of identifying stage II patients with worse prognosis is through detection of occult lymph node metastases. Micrometastases were detected in 14 of 26 (54%) patients tested using a CEA-specific nested reverse-transcriptase polymerase chain reaction.[214] The cancer-specific 5-year survival rate was 50% in the group with occult nodal metastases compared with 91% in the 12 patients without micrometastases.

Balanced against the benefits of chemotherapy are the possible toxicities, which may suspend or modify treatment plans because of GI or hematologic complications. Because severe toxic effects (WHO grade 4) occur in fewer than 3% of cases and minimal side effects are experienced with 5-FU–based chemotherapy, compliance with treatment is generally good, with more than 80% of patients completing the planned treatment.[208] Diarrhea is a common side effect. Other toxicities associated with 5-FU include myelosuppression, stomatitis, mild alopecia, and hand-foot syndrome. In combination with other agents, levamisole may increase the severity of myelosuppression and cause hepatic toxicity or cerebral demyelination. When prescribing chemotherapy, consideration should therefore be given to the absolute survival benefit while maintaining optimal quality of life.

Newer agents such as uracil-tegafur, irinotecan (CPT-11), and oxaliplatin have demonstrated activity in treating metastatic colon cancer and hold promise as potentially effective drugs to be tested in the adjuvant setting.[212] Uracil-tegafur (UFT) is an oral fluorinated pyrimidine. These agents are hepatically converted into 5-FU following absorption and expose tissues to 5-FU for a longer duration at lower peak concentrations. In combination with leucovorin, UFT has demonstrated activity in metastatic colon cancer with a favorable toxicity profile. Oxaliplatin is an aminocyclohexane platinum derivative with limited activity as a single agent. However, its ability to synergize with 5-FU has achieved high response rates in metastatic colon cancer patients, including those refractory to 5-FU. The addition of oxaliplatin to current 5-FU regimens may be a promising option for future adjuvant use. The topoisomerase I inhibitor CPT-11 is currently approved for treatment of metastatic colon cancer and will likely find its role in adjuvant therapy. CPT-11 provides a survival advantage over 5-FU infusion in patients with advanced colon cancer for whom bolus 5-FU therapy has failed. Although CPT-11 has both GI and bone marrow side effects, it does not appear to be more toxic than 5-FU even when used in combination with 5-FU. Development of folate-based inhibitors of TS is one approach that attempts to selectively simulate the antitumor activity of 5-FU. Raltitrexed is an example that appears to have efficacy comparable to 5-FU plus leucovorin and is currently used in Europe to treat metastatic colon cancer. In addition to progress in drug development, the future of colon cancer chemotherapy may involve more individualized treatment. Attempts to predict sensitivity to particular agents based on biologic testing of tumors is now under way. High levels of TS or DPD (dihydropyrimidine dehydrogenase) gene expression in colon cancers correlate with a lack of sensitivity to 5-FU. In contrast, low levels of expression predict good response to 5-FU chemotherapy. Other biologic markers being evaluated include p53 status, flow cytometry, allelic deletion of 17p and 18q, expression of the sialosyl-Tn antigen, replication error phenotype (REP), and the presence of the DCC gene product. In the future, it may be possible to formulate specific chemotherapy cocktails for patients based on such biologic tests.

INTRAPERITONEAL CHEMOTHERAPY. Intraperitoneal (IP) delivery of chemotherapy active in the treatment of colon cancer has the potential to increase significantly the exposure of cytotoxic agents to cancer cells present within the peritoneal cavity or liver. It has the greatest therapeutic potential as an adjuvant treatment strategy in colon cancer patients with a high risk for abdominal recurrence. Experience with this technique has primarily utilized IP 5-FU. The agent is administered daily for 4 to 5 days every 3 to 4 weeks.[215] Following IP delivery, 5-FU concentrations are 200- to 400-fold higher in the peritoneal cavity than systemically.[216,217] In a small randomized controlled trial comparing intravenous with intraperitoneal 5-FU delivery, there was a statistically significant decrease in the incidence of recurrences within the peritoneal cavity (documented by second-look procedure), but no differences in disease-free or overall survival.[218] A somewhat larger randomized trial compared IP and systemic 5-FU plus leucovorin with systemic 5-FU plus levamisole in high-risk stage II or stage III resected colon cancer patients.[219] Although there was no survival advantage in stage II patients, an estimated 43% reduction in mortality rate was seen in 196 eligible stage III patients. Trials of IP 5-FU for unresectable hepatic CRC metastases or as an adjuvant strategy after liver resection have not shown any benefit.[215] Although aggressive surgical debulking and IP chemotherapy has been applied to select patients for treatment of peritoneal carcinomatosis from colon cancer, the long-term disease-free survival observed in some patients likely results from biologic factors not directly related to treatment. The major toxicities are abdominal pain and bone marrow suppression. The degree of marrow suppression is increased if patients have undergone aggressive chemotherapy. In an effort to enhance cytotoxic potential, IP 5-FU has been administered in combination, and trials of FUDR as a single agent and in combination have been reported. An interesting pilot study examined IP FUDR and leucovorin given to colon cancer patients at high risk of developing recurrent disease.[220] Three courses of regional therapy were given in conjunction with systemic 5-FU and levamisole. After a median follow-up of 18 months, only four recurrences were observed among 26 patients. The availability of new cytotoxic agents may lead to further exploration of this route of administration.

PORTAL VEIN INFUSION. Regional therapy by portal vein infusion (PVI), which is directed at potential hepatic micrometastases, has also been used in the adjuvant setting for resected colon cancer. In a metaanalysis of 10 clinical trials that randomized patients to 5 to 7 weeks of continuous PVI or to observation, there was a trend toward a survival benefit for patients in the treated group.[221] Although survival with and without PVI appeared to be the same for the first 2 years, it diverged with an absolute survival benefit of 4.7% at 5 years with PVI. Of note, the course of regional chemotherapy is relatively short compared with the 6-month regimen of systemic chemotherapy. Whether the benefit from PVI, modest as it may be, is directly related to the portal route of administration or to systemic exposure of the active agent remains unclear.

## IMMUNOTHERAPY

A potential role for immunotherapy began with bacille Calmette-Guérin (BCG), a nonspecific immunomodulator. However, in National Surgical Adjuvant Breast Project (NSABP) Protocol C-01, the survival advantage in BCG-treated patients was the result of a reduction in deaths not related to carcinoma.[205] A randomized trial of vaccination with BCG and neuramidase-treated autologous carcinoma cells failed to affect disease-free or overall survival.[222] Subsequent efforts, therefore, focused on active specific immunotherapy (ASI) using BCG combined with the patients' irradiated autologous cancer cells to create a tumor vaccine. In recent randomized clinical trials of adjuvant ASI, no significant survival advantage was seen with ASI in surgically resected patients with stage II or III colon cancer.[223,224] However, recurrence-free survival for stage II patients was better for the treated group, and in patients compliant with treatment and exhibiting effective immunity, there was a disease-free and overall survival benefit.

Antibody-based cancer therapy continues to be driven by the prospect of identifying cell-surface antigens with sufficiently restrictive tissue expression to allow specific targeting of antibody to tumor tissue. Recent developments in the therapeutic use of antibodies in colon cancer include unmodified mouse IgG; immune globulin as carrier for targeted delivery of radioisotopes, toxins, and therapeutic molecules; genetically engineered antibody constructs; humanized nonimmunogenic IgG; and novel antigen targets in tumors.[225] Genetically engineered antibody constructs increase the fraction localized to tumors, thereby improving delivery. Because antibodies become activated in the tumor only when bound to antigen, this should minimize nonspecific toxic effects from nonlocalized antibody. Clinical trials are in progress to evaluate the new generation of humanized antibodies. Murine 17-1A monoclonal antibody therapy in 166 patients with resected stage III colon cancer has been shown to reduce recurrence by 23% and mortality by 32% (absolute difference of 20%).[226] Interestingly, therapy was not protective against local recurrence but led to a significant decrease in distant metastases. Another promising approach has been the development of an antiidiotype monoclonal antibody vaccine that mimics CEA, a tumor-associated antigen.[227] Other work has focused on additional immunologic targets such as the blood group–related epitopes Tn and sialylated Tn (sTn).[228]

## RADIATION

Although the major goal of systemic therapy is to impact survival through the prevention of distant recurrence, the addition of adjuvant radiation therapy may be important in patients at particular risk for local failure. In contrast to rectal cancer, the primary failure pattern in colon cancer is abdominal. Local failure does occur, but is less frequent and more difficult to detect. Radiation therapy has been used as adjuvant therapy in cases of incomplete resection. Possible indications for postoperative radiotherapy include residual local disease confirmed by inadequate margins of resection, adherence to retroperitoneal or pelvic (sacrum, pelvic sidewall) structures, macroscopic transmural penetration, extensive microscopic penetration with positive lymph nodes, and tumors associated with abscess or fistula formation. In retrospective and nonrandomized prospective studies, improved local control and survival has been demonstrated in patients with advanced colon cancer.[229–232] A common complication and major concern in patients undergoing radiation is enteritis, which appears to occur more frequently in patients also receiving chemotherapy.

## RESULTS

Five-year survival rate after curative resection depends primarily on the stage of disease, and for node-negative cancers treated by surgery alone, it is 80% to 90%. In node-positive cancers, 5-year survival rate ranges from 69% for one positive node to 27% for six or more positive nodes, with an overall survival rate of 40% to 50%.[233] Although nodal status is the most important prognostic indicator, T stage (depth of tumor invasion) as well as grade (differentiation), lymphatic vessel, blood vessel, and perineural invasion also influence survival.[234] Patients who present with unresectable metastatic disease have an overall 5-year survival of 5% or less.

## SURVEILLANCE

There is no definitive follow-up program for patients after colon cancer resection. The goal of such a program is to identify and char-

acterize asymptomatic resectable local recurrences, liver and lung metastases, metachronous lesions, and symptomatic disease requiring palliation. Because most recurrences are identified when the patient presents with symptoms between scheduled follow-up visits, intensive follow-up regimens are unlikely to be cost effective or improve survival.[235,236] In a prospective randomized study, frequent follow-up diagnosed more recurrences at an earlier and asymptomatic stage, leading to further surgery with curative intent, but did not result in better overall or cancer-related survival.[235] Similarly, patients randomized to follow-up with yearly colonoscopy, CT of the liver, and chest x-ray in addition to clinical review and simple screening tests (CBC, liver profile, CEA, FOBT) did not gain a survival benefit on completion of 5-year follow-up compared with those patients who were followed clinically with simple screening tests alone.[236] Furthermore, the consequences of surveillance may be detrimental, because patients could be informed about an asymptomatic, incurable recurrence.

Proponents of periodic examinations, blood tests and imaging studies aim to detect tumor recurrence early, on the presumption that intervention can affect outcome. In a review of CRC patients monitored by CEA and clinical examinations, 130 developed recurrences.[237] Of the 75 recurrences operated on, 43 were CEA-directed and 32 clinically directed. Recurrent disease was discovered, on the average, 2.5 months earlier in those with a rising CEA level as opposed to new-onset clinical findings, and more patients were able to undergo complete resection (59% vs. 52%). Five-year survival in patients who had second-look surgery was 33%. However, CEA elevation may be unrelated to disease status. Thus, patient selection is important to exclude those with unresectable metastatic disease. A large meta-analysis of 2005 patients comparing clinical follow-up and CEA with no routine follow-up and physician response to symptoms only demonstrated that patients who were in the intensive follow-up group were 2.5 times more likely to have a curative resection and a 3.6-fold higher survival rate after recurrence.[238] Similar findings were reported in a prospective randomized trial for management of local recurrences in CRC.[239] There is no consensus among surgeons as to the ideal duration, intensity, and method of follow-up after CRC resection because of the continuing lack of evidence on which to base patient follow-up.[240] A summary of recommended CRC surveillance guidelines and levels of evidence in support of these guidelines has been formulated by the American Society of Clinical Oncology (Table 16A-4).[139]

Surveillance colonoscopy is recommended because CRC patients have an increased risk of metachronous neoplasms, which occur at a rate of 29% to 60% depending on the interval of follow-up.[140,145,241] A colonoscopy is commonly performed before resection. If this is not possible, colonoscopy is performed after recovering from surgery, usually within a year. If an adenoma with worrisome features is found and removed at colonoscopy, a repeat examination is conducted in 1 year. After a clear colonoscopic examination, the interval may be lengthened to 3 years based on data from the National Polyp Study.[241] A longer interval of up to 5 years between reexaminations is reasonable after a negative colonoscopy.[141] As with all recommendations, management should be individualized, with due consideration for patient-specific factors such as comorbid disease and patient anxiety.

**TABLE 16A-4.** SUMMARY OF COLORECTAL CANCER SURVEILLANCE GUIDELINES—ASCO

| TEST | RECOMMENDATION | LEVEL OF EVIDENCE |
| --- | --- | --- |
| History and physical examination | Every 3–6 mo for the first 3 yr and annually thereafter | V |
| CEA | Every 2–3 mo in patients with stage II or III disease for first 2 yr, then annually thereafter | II |
| CBC | Not recommended | V |
| Liver function tests | Not recommended | II |
| Fecal occult blood test | Not recommended | II |
| CXR | Not recommended (may be considered in symptomatic patients with elevated CEA) | II |
| Colonoscopy | Perioperatively to clear colon, then every 3–5 yr to detect metachronous neoplasms | I |
| CT | Not recommended | II |

## OTHER MALIGNANT LESIONS

### CARCINOID

Carcinoids arise from neuroectodermal cells. These tumors are commonly found in the GI tract, specifically the appendix, small bowel, rectum, stomach, and colon in decreasing order of frequency. Colonic carcinoids make up only 2.8% of all GI carcinoids and represent a very small proportion (0.3%) of all colonic tumors.[242,243] These tumors occur in an older age group with an average age of 64 to 68 (range, 12 to 87) years at the time of diagnosis.[244–246] The most common location is in the cecum.[244,245] Colonic carcinoids present as a simple polyp or as a gross malignancy and may have an apple-core appearance radiologically. Clinical manifestations are difficult to distinguish from those of carcinoma. There is a high incidence of palpable abdominal tumors resulting from a tendency of the tumors to be large (90% over 2 cm).[246] In reported series of colonic carcinoids, 57% to 61% had metastases, 44% to 54% had local spread, and 38% to 42% had distant metastases, primarily involving the liver and lung.[243,246,247] From a population-based study spanning a 25-year period, 64% of the lesions were Dukes D and 22% were Dukes C at diagnosis.[245] Although colonic carcinoids are accompanied by noncarcinoid synchronous and metachronous neoplasms in 10% to 42% of patients, only 4.2% of patients have multiple carcinoids.[242,243]

Carcinoid syndrome refers to a constellation of symptoms associated with the pharmacologic effects of serotonin. Other biochemically active products that may contribute to the carcinoid syndrome are bradykinins, histamine, vasoactive intestinal peptide (VIP), adrenocorticotropic hormone (ACTH), 5-hydroxytrypto-phan, and prostaglandins. Symptoms include flushing (face, neck, anterior chest wall, and hands), diarrhea, and wheezing. Other components are right-sided heart failure (pulmonary stenosis), pulmonary hypertension, edema, pellagra-like skin lesions, peptic ulcers, arthralgia, and weight loss.[248] These findings usually occur in the setting of liver metastases from primary carcinoids of the small bowel. Less than 5% of colonic carcinoids cause the carcinoid syndrome, which correlates with a low detection rate of serotonin by immunohistochemical (66.7%) or laboratory (68.7%) evaluation.[243,246,247]

The macroscopic appearance is variable and may be characterized by a yellowish tinge. Malignancy correlates with lesion size, location, and tissue invasion. Microscopically, carcinoids consist of uniform, small, round, or polygonal cells with prominent round nuclei and eosinophilic cytoplasmic granules. Five histologic patterns are recognized: insular, trabecular, glandular, undifferentiated, and mixed. Tumor stage, histologic pattern, tumor differentiation, nuclear grade, and mitotic rate significantly influence the prognosis.[245,249] Foregut carcinoids are argentaffin-negative, argyrophil-positive, and produce the serotonin precursor 5-hydroxytryptophan. Midgut carcinoids are usually both argentaffin- and argyrophil-positive, multicentric, and associated with carcinoid syndrome. Hindgut carcinoids are rarely argentaffin- or argyrophil-positive, usually unicentric, and not associated with carcinoid syndrome. The most common immunohistochemical pattern of colonic carcinoids is argentaffin-negative, argyrophil-negative, and neuron-specific enolase–positive.[245]

Small polypoid lesions may be adequately treated by polypectomy. Larger lesions require formal resection as for adenocarcinoma.[250] If distant disease is present, resection of the primary tumor is indicated to alleviate symptoms because prolonged survival is possible. For liver metastases, partial hepatectomy should be considered if technically feasible. Patients with unresectable liver metastases may benefit from either operative hepatic dearterialization or hepatic intraarterial embolization with chemotherapy. Aggressive debulking can reduce and occasionally eliminate the manifestations of carcinoid syndrome. Chemotherapeutic agents reportedly effective in carcinoid include systemic 5-FU, doxorubicin, and fluorodeoxyuridine or 5-FU and streptozotocin delivered by hepatic artery or portal vein infusion. Somatostatin analogs have been used to counteract the symptoms of carcinoid syndrome.

Survival after resection of colonic carcinoids without metastatic disease is 41 months.[247] Those with local metastases live an average of 22 months, whereas those with known distant metastases live an average of 15 months. Reported 5-year survival for patients with colonic carcinoids is in the range of 25% to 52%.[242–246] Prognosis for colonic carcinoids appears to be significantly poorer compared with prognosis of appendical and rectal carcinoids.

### LYMPHOMA

Lymphoma may occur as a primary lesion or as part of a generalized malignant process involving the GI tract. Primary colonic lymphomas are rare, as demonstrated by one series over a 20-year period in which these lesions represented 5.8% of all GI lymphomas (15 of 259) and 0.16% of colon cancers (15 of 9193).[251] The cecum is most commonly affected. It occurs twice as often in men at a mean age of 50 (range 3 to 81). The clinical features of colonic lymphomas are nonspecific and indistinguishable from those of carcinoma. Symptoms may include abdominal pain, changes in bowel habit (diarrhea or constipation), blood loss and anemia (especially if ulceration supervenes), weight loss, weakness, and possibly fever. Tender abdominal masses are commonly present. Obstruction occurs in 20% to 25% of patients, but perforation is infrequent. Lymphomas of the colon produce the same radiologic appearance on barium enema (BE) as carcinomas and, similarly, may be indistinguishable from carcinomas at laparotomy. Abdominal CT and endoscopy are the most useful diagnostic tests. A biopsy differentiates the histology but could still be nondiagnostic, especially if superficial in nature. Upon diagnosis, staging is performed with data from history, physical examination, imaging studies, laboratory investigations, and bone marrow aspiration.

Three macroscopic morphologies are seen. The lesion may be annular with plaquelike thickening, bulky and protuberant, or appear as a thickened and aneurysmal dilatation of the bowel wall. The cut surface has an uniform fleshy appearance. Although regional lymph node involvement is common, this is not related to prognosis. Multiple primary foci may be evident and in severe cases, simulate FAP. Criteria for a primary GI lymphoma include

1. No palpable superficial lymphadenopathy
2. Normal roentgenographic findings (specifically, the absence of mediastinal adenopathy on chest x-ray) except at the primary site
3. Normal white blood cell count and differential
4. Predominance of the alimentary tract lesions
5. No involvement of the liver or spleen.[252]

Almost all are non-Hodgkin's B-cell type lymphomas. In order of frequency, they are classified histologically as histiocytic, lymphocytic, mixed, and Hodgkin's disease.

The treatment of primary lymphoma of the colon is complete resection, usually in combination with chemotherapy.[253] Surgery is also performed in the clinical setting of obstruction, bleeding, perforation, or uncertain diagnosis. At laparotomy, staging consists of a thorough exploration and biopsies of all suspicious nodes or organs. Only one-third will be confined to the bowel and regional lymph nodes.[254] Postoperative radiation therapy has been associated with better survival rates. Radiotherapy may also be beneficial for unresectable lesions. Chemotherapy is recommended for systemic disease.

Overall 5-year survival is approximately 40% (range 20% to 55%). For stage I and II disease, overall survival approaches 80%, but decreases to 35% for advanced disease.[255] Prognosis is also affected by tumor size, morphology (intraluminal vs. extramural), and histologic type.

## SARCOMA

Tumors of mesenchymal origin infrequently develop in the colon. These neoplasms are described by their cell type of origin: leiomyosarcoma, liposarcoma, hemangiosarcoma, fibrosarcoma, fibrous his-

tiocytoma, neurofibrosarcoma, lymphangiosarcoma, and Kaposi's sarcoma. The most common type is leiomyosarcoma, with the rest being rare. Symptoms are similar to those of carcinoma and complicated presentations such as bleeding or obstruction can also occur. Although standard radiologic tests with intraluminal contrast may reveal a polypoid or constricting lesion, colonoscopy and biopsy, if performed preoperatively, may be helpful to distinguish the lesion from carcinoma. Macroscopically, the lesion can range from a small nodule to a large mass. In early stages, the overlying mucosa may be intact, but eventually becomes ulcerated with growth. Leiomyosarcomas are usually low-grade malignancies and it is difficult to differentiate histologically benign from malignant variants. As with sarcomas at other sites, regional lymph nodes are rarely involved and hematogenous spread results in metastases, primarily to the liver. Treatment is resection as for carcinoma, and a final diagnosis may only be reached at the time of pathologic examination. Radiation or chemotherapy, alone or in combination, has not been found to be effective.[256] Clinicopathologic factors that adversely affect prognosis are tumor size greater than 5 cm, extraintestinal invasion or perforation, and high histopathologic grade. Patients rarely survive 5 years after operation and there are insufficient data to generate meaningful 5-year survival rates.

## SQUAMOUS CELL CARCINOMA

Squamous cell carcinoma is another exceedingly uncommon neoplasm of the colon, representing 0.1% of colonic carcinomas.[257] The mean age is 53 (range, 33 to 90) and 60 (range, 28 to 91) years for patients with pure squamous cell and mixed adenosquamous cell carcinoma, respectively. Mixed adenosquamous cell carcinoma occurs in men and women with equal frequency, but twice as many men develop squamous cell carcinoma. Synchronous squamous cell carcinoma of the colon occurs in 3.2% of patients, and 10% have either antecedent, synchronous, or metachronous, adenocarcinoma of the colon. These lesions appear to be distributed uniformly throughout the colon.

Criteria to satisfy the diagnosis of primary colonic squamous cell carcinoma are:

1. No evidence of squamous cell carcinoma in any other organ which may have metastasized
2. The affected bowel should not be involved in a fistulous tract lined with squamous epithelium
3. Exclusion of squamous cell carcinoma arising from the anal canal.

Mechanisms proposed for the pathogenesis of this exceedingly uncommon entity include:

1. Proliferation of uncommitted reserve or basal cells after mucosal injury
2. Squamous metaplasia of glandular epithelium, resulting from chronic irritation
3. Embryonal nests of committed or uncommitted ectodermal cells remaining in an ectopic site after embryogenesis

4. Squamous metaplasia of an established colorectal adenocarcinoma
5. Squamous differentiation arising in an adenoma.[257,258]

Clinical presentation, diagnosis, and preoperative assessment are no different from any other colonic neoplasm. Although the gross appearance may not be distinctive, microscopy demonstrates clusters of squamous cells in the stroma. Treatment consists of resection of the affected segment. The 5-year actuarial survival rate after resection of primary squamous cell and adenosquamous cell carcinoma of the colon is 50% for Dukes stage B lesions, 33% for Dukes C lesions, and 0% for Dukes D lesions.[257]

## REFERENCES

1. PARKIN DM et al: Global cancer statistics. CA 49:33, 1999.
2. LANDIS SH et al: Cancer statistics, 1999. CA 49:8, 1999.
3. HEYS SD et al: Colorectal cancer in young patients: A review of the literature. Eur J Surg Oncol 20:225, 1994.
4. POTTER JD: Colorectal cancer: Molecules and populations. J Natl Cancer Inst 91:916, 1999.
5. POTTER JD et al: Colon cancer: A review of the epidemiology. Epidemiol Rev 15:499, 1993.
6. GREENWALD P et al: Dietary fiber in the reduction of colon cancer risk. J Am Diet Assoc 87:1178, 1987.
7. FUCHS CS et al: Dietary fiber and the risk of colorectal cancer and adenoma in women. N Engl J Med 340:169, 1999.
8. POTTER JD: Fiber and colorectal cancer: Where to now? N Engl J Med 340:223, 1999.
9. BOSTICK RM et al: Calcium and colorectal epithelial cell proliferation in sporadic adenoma patients: A randomized, double-blinded, placebo-controlled clinical trial. J Natl Cancer Inst 87:1307, 1995.
10. BARON JA et al: Calcium supplements for the prevention of colorectal adenomas. Calcium Polyp Prevention Study Group. N Engl J Med 340:101, 1999.
11. GIOVANNUCCI E et al: A prospective study of cigarette smoking and risk of colorectal adenoma and colorectal cancer in U.S. men. J Natl Cancer Inst 86:183, 1994.
12. GIOVANNUCCI E et al: A prospective study of cigarette smoking and risk of colorectal adenoma and colorectal cancer in U.S. women. J Natl Cancer Inst 86:192, 1994.
13. MORSON BC: Evolution of cancer of the colon and rectum. Cancer 34(Suppl):845, 1974.
14. MUTO T et al: The evolution of cancer of the colon and rectum Cancer 36:2251, 1975.
15. STRYKER SJ et al: Natural history of untreated colonic polyps. Gastroenterology 93:1009, 1987.
16. CHU DZ et al: The significance of synchronous carcinoma and polyps in the colon and rectum. Cancer 57:445, 1986.
17. BUSSEY HJR: *Familial Polyposis Coli: Family Studies, Histopathology, Differential Diagnosis, and Results of Treatment.* Baltimore, Johns Hopkins University Press, 1975.
18. VOGELSTEIN B et al: Genetic alterations during colorectal-tumor development. N Engl J Med 319:525, 1988.
19. SOLOMON E et al: Chromosome 5 allele loss in human colorectal carcinomas. Nature 328:616, 1987.
20. POWELL SM et al: APC mutations occur early during colorectal tumorigenesis. Nature 359:235, 1992.
21. LEPPERT M et al: The gene for familial polyposis coli maps to the long arm of chromosome 5. Science 238:1411, 1987.
22. BODMER WF et al: Localization of the gene for familial adenomatous polyposis on chromosome 5. Nature 328:614, 1987.
23. MORIN PJ et al: Activation of beta-catenin-Tcf signaling in colon cancer by mutations in beta-catenin or APC. Science 275:1787, 1997.
24. KORINEK V et al: Constitutive transcriptional activation by a beta-catenin-Tcf complex in APC-/-colon carcinoma. Science 275:1784, 1997.
25. HE TC et al: Identification of c-MYC as a target of the APC pathway. Science 281:1509, 1998.
26. PENNISI E: How a growth control path takes a wrong turn to cancer. Science 281:1438, 1441, 1998.
27. FEARON ER, VOGELSTEIN B: A genetic model for colorectal tumorigenesis. Cell 61:759, 1990.
28. BAKER SJ et al: Chromosome 17 deletions and p53 gene mutations in colorectal carcinomas. Science 244:217, 1989.
29. HAHN SA et al: DPC4, a candidate tumor suppressor gene at human chromosome 18q21.1. Science 271:350, 1996.
30. FEARON ER et al: Identification of a chromosome 18q gene that is altered in colorectal cancers. Science 247:49, 1990.
31. HEMMINKI A et al: A serine/threonine kinase gene defective in Peutz-Jeghers syndrome. Nature 391:184, 1998.
32. AALTONEN LA et al: Clues to the pathogenesis of familial colorectal cancer. Science 260:812, 1993.
33. KANE MF et al: Methylation of the hMLH1 promoter correlates with lack of expression of hMLH1 in sporadic colon tumors and mismatch repair-defective human tumor cell lines. Cancer Res 57:808, 1997.
34. HERMAN JG et al: Incidence and functional consequences of hMLH1 promoter hypermethylation in colorectal carcinoma. Proc Natl Acad Sci USA 95:6870, 1998.
35. BOLAND CR et al: A National Cancer Institute Workshop on Microsatellite Instability for cancer detection and familial predisposition: Development of international criteria for the determination of microsatellite instability in colorectal cancer. Cancer Res 58:5248, 1998.
36. MARKOWITZ S et al: Inactivation of the type II TGF-beta receptor in colon cancer cells with microsatellite instability. Science 268:1336, 1995.
37. OUYANG H et al: The insulin-like growth factor II receptor gene is mutated in genetically unstable cancers of the endometrium. stomach, and colorectum. Cancer Res 57:1851, 1997.
38. RAMPINO N et al: Somatic frameshift mutations in the BAX gene in colon cancers of the microsatellite mutator phenotype. Science 275:967, 1997.
39. BICKNELL DC et al: Selection for beta 2-microglobulin mutation in mismatch repair: Defective colorectal carcinomas. Curr Biol 6:1695, 1996.
40. CAHILL DP et al: Mutations of mitotic checkpoint genes in human cancers. Nature 392:300, 1998.
41. LOVETT E: Family studies in cancer of the colon and rectum. Br J Surg 63:13, 1976.
42. BONELLI L et al: Family history of colorectal cancer as a risk factor for benign and malignant tumours of the large bowel. A case-control study. Int J Cancer 41:513, 1988.
43. GUILLEM JG et al: Colonic neoplasms in asymptomatic first-degree relatives of colon cancer patients. Am J Gastroenterol 83:271, 1988.

44. FUCHS CS et al: A prospective study of family history and the risk of colorectal cancer. N Engl J Med 331:1669, 1994.

45. BURT RW et al: Genetics of colon cancer: Impact of inheritance on colon cancer risk. Annu Rev Med 46:371, 1995.

46. SLATTERY ML, KERBER RA: Family history of cancer and colon cancer risk: The Utah Population Database. J Natl Cancer Inst 86:1618, 1994.

47. BURT RW et al: Dominant inheritance of adenomatous colonic polyps and colorectal cancer. N Engl J Med 312:1540, 1985.

48. LEVY DB et al: Inactivation of both APC alleles in human and mouse tumors. Cancer Res 54:5953, 1994.

49. GRODEN J et al: Identification and characterization of the familial adenomatous polyposis coli gene. Cell 66:589, 1991.

50. HILTUNEN MO et al: Hypermethylation of the APC (adenomatous polyposis coli) gene promoter region in human colorectal carcinoma. Int J Cancer 70:644, 1997.

51. LAKEN SJ et al: Familial colorectal cancer in Ashkenazim due to a hypermutable tract in APC. Nat Genet 17:79, 1997.

52. BULOW S: Familial polyposis coli. Dan Med Bull 34:1, 1987.

53. GUILLEM JG et al: Gastrointestinal polyposis syndromes. Curr Probl Surg 36:217, 1999.

54. PELTOMAKI P et al: Microsatellite instability is associated with tumors that characterize the hereditary non-polyposis colorectal carcinoma syndrome. Cancer Res 53:5853, 1993.

55. THIBODEAU SN et al: Microsatellite instability in cancer of the proximal colon. Science 260:816, 1993.

56. LEACH FS et al: Mutations of a mutS homolog in hereditary nonpolyposis colorectal cancer. Cell 75:1215, 1993.

57. FISHEL R et al: The human mutator gene homolog MSH2 and its association with hereditary nonpolyposis colon cancer. Cell 75:1027, 1993.

58. NICOLAIDES NC et al: Mutations of two PMS homologues in hereditary nonpolyposis colon cancer. Nature 371:75, 1994.

59. PAPADOPOULOS N et al: Mutation of a mutL homolog in hereditary colon cancer. Science 263:1625, 1994.

60. BRONNER CE et al: Mutation in the DNA mismatch repair gene homologue hMLH1 is associated with hereditary nonpolyposis colon cancer. Nature 368:258, 1994.

61. DRUMMOND JT et al: Isolation of an hMSH2-p160 heterodimer that restores DNA mismatch repair to tumor cells. Science 268:1909, 1995.

62. PALOMBO F et al: GTBP, a 160-kilodalton protein essential for mismatch-binding activity in human cells. Science 268:1912, 1995.

63. WATANABE A et al: Genomic organization and expression of the human MSH3 gene. Genomics 31:311, 1996.

64. AKIYAMA Y et al: Germ-line mutation of the hMSH6/GTBP gene in an atypical hereditary nonpolyposis colorectal cancer kindred. Cancer Res 57:3920, 1997.

65. THIBODEAU SN et al: Microsatellite instability in colorectal cancer: different mutator phenotypes and the principal involvement of hMLH1. Cancer Res 58:1713, 1998.

66. CUNNINGHAM JM et al: Hypermethylation of the hMLH1 promoter in colon cancer with microsatellite instability. Cancer Res 58:3455, 1998.

67. BABA S: Hereditary nonpolyposis colorectal cancer: An update. Dis Colon Rectum 40(Suppl 10):S86, 1997.

68. VASEN HF et al: The International Collaborative Group on Hereditary Non-Polyposis Colorectal Cancer (ICG-HNPCC). Dis Colon Rectum 34:424, 1991.

69. BURKE W et al: Recommendations for follow-up care of individuals with an inherited predisposition to cancer. I. Hereditary nonpolyposis colon cancer. Cancer Genetics Studies Consortium. JAMA 277:915, 1997.

70. LENNARD-JONES JE et al: Cancer surveillance in ulcerative colitis: Experience over 15 years. Lancet 2:149, 1983.

71. GILLEN CD et al: Ulcerative colitis and Crohn's disease: A comparison of the colorectal cancer risk in extensive colitis. Gut 35:1590, 1994.

72. WAYE JD: Screening for cancer in ulcerative colitis. Front Gastrointest Res 10:243, 1986.

73. BRENTNALL TA et al: Mutations in the p53 gene: An early marker of neoplastic progression in ulcerative colitis. Gastroenterology 107:369, 1994.

74. CHOI PM et al: Colonoscopic surveillance reduces mortality from colorectal cancer in ulcerative colitis. Gastroenterology 105:418, 1993.

75. GILLEN CD et al: Crohn's disease and colorectal cancer. Gut 35:651, 1994.

76. EKBOM A et al: Increased risk of large-bowel cancer in Crohn's disease with colonic involvement. Lancet 336:357, 1990.

77. GREENSTEIN AJ et al: A comparison of cancer risk in Crohn's disease and ulcerative colitis. Cancer 48:2742, 1981.

78. SACHAR DB: Cancer in Crohn's disease: Dispelling the myths. Gut 35:1507, 1994.

79. CARLSSON G et al: The value of colonoscopic surveillance after curative resection for colorectal cancer or synchronous adenomatous polyps. Arch Surg 122:1261, 1987.

80. CALI RL et al: Cumulative incidence of metachronous colorectal cancer. Dis Colon Rectum 36:388, 1993.

81. LEGGETT BA et al: Characteristics of metachronous colorectal carcinoma occurring despite colonoscopic surveillance. Dis Colon Rectum 40:603, 1997.

82. BULOW S et al: Metachronous colorectal carcinoma. Br J Surg 77:502, 1990.

83. SVENDSEN LB et al: Metachronous colorectal cancer in young patients: expression of the hereditary nonpolyposis colorectal cancer syndrome? Dis Colon Rectum 34:790, 1991.

84. MECKIN JP, JARVINEN H: Treatment and follow-up strategies in hereditary nonpolyposis colorectal carcinoma. Dis Colon Rectum 36:927, 1993.

85. HERSCHMAN HR: Prostaglandin synthase 2. Biochim Biophys Acta 1299:125, 1996.

86. EBERHART CE et al: Up-regulation of cyclooxygenase 2 gene expression in human colorectal adenomas and adenocarcinomas. Gastroenterology 107:1183, 1994.

87. KARGMAN SL et al: Expression of prostaglandin G/H synthase-1 and -2 protein in human colon cancer. Cancer Res 55:2556, 1995.

88. TSUJI M, DUBOIS RN: Alterations in cellular adhesion and apoptosis in epithelial cells overexpressing prostaglandin endoperoxide synthase 2. Cell 83:493, 1995.

89. TSUJI M et al: Cyclooxygenase-2 expression in human colon cancer cells increases metastatic potential. Proc Natl Acad Sci USA 94:3336, 1997.

90. ELDER DJ, PARASKEVA C: COX-2 inhibitors for colorectal cancer. Nat Med 4:392, 1998.

91. TSUJI M et al: Cyclooxygenase regulates angiogenesis induced by colon cancer cells. Cell 93:705, 1998.

92. OSHIMA M et al: Suppression of intestinal polyposis in Apc delta

716 knockout mice by inhibition of cyclooxygenase 2 (COX-2). Cell 87:803, 1996.

93. WECHTER WJ et al: R-flurbiprofen chemoprevention and treatment of intestinal adenomas in the APC(Min)/+ mouse model: Implications for prophylaxis and treatment of colon cancer. Cancer Res 57:4316, 1997.

94. KAWAMORI T et al: Chemopreventive activity of celecoxib, a specific cyclooxygenase-2 inhibitor, against colon carcinogenesis. Cancer Res 58:409, 1998.

95. BARNES CJ et al: Non-steroidal anti-inflammatory drug effect on crypt cell proliferation and apoptosis during initiation of rat colon carcinogenesis. Br J Cancer 77:573, 1998.

96. GREENBERG ER et al: Reduced risk of large-bowel adenomas among aspirin users. The Polyp Prevention Study Group. J Natl Cancer Inst 85:912, 1993.

97. LOGAN RF et al: Effect of aspirin and non-steroidal anti-inflammatory drugs on colorectal adenomas: case-control study of subjects participating in the Nottingham faecal occult blood screening programme. BMJ 307:285, 1993.

98. GIARDIELLO FM et al: Treatment of colonic and rectal adenomas with sulindac in familial adenomatous polyposis. N Engl J Med 328:1313, 1993.

99. Morson & Dawson's Gastrointestinal Pathology, 3d ed. Boston, Blackwell Scientific Publications, 1990.

100. UMPLEBY HC et al: Peculiarities of mucinous colorectal carcinoma. Br J Surg 72:715, 1985.

101. GREEN JB et al: Mucinous carcinoma. Just another colon cancer? Dis Colon Rectum 36:49, 1993.

102. COHEN AM et al: Cancer of the colon, in Cancer: Principles and Practice of Oncology, vol 2, VT DeVita et al (eds). Philadelphia, Lippincott, 1997, pp 1144–1196.

103. BRODSKY JT, COHEN AM: Peritoneal seeding following potentially curative resection of colonic carcinoma: Implications for adjuvant therapy. Dis Colon Rectum 34:723, 1991.

104. GORDON PH, NIVATVONGS S: Principles and Practice of Surgery for the Colon, Rectum, and Anus, 2d ed. St Louis, MO, Quality Medical Publishers, 1999.

105. LOCKHART-MUMMERY JP: Two hundred cases of cancer of the rectum treated by perineal excision. Br J Surg 14:110, 1926.

106. DUKES CE: The classification of cancer of the rectum. J Pathol 35:323, 1932.

107. KIRKLIN JW et al: The role of the peritoneal reflection in the prognosis of carcinoma of the rectum and sigmoid colon. Surg Gynecol Obstet 88:326, 1949.

108. ASTLER VB, COLLER FA: The prognostic significance of direct extension of carcinoma of the colon and rectum. Ann Surg 139:846, 1954.

109. GUNDERSON LL, SOSIN H: Areas of failure found at reoperation (second or symptomatic look) following "curative surgery" for adenocarcinoma of the rectum: Clinicopathologic correlation and implications for adjuvant therapy. Cancer 34:1278, 1974.

110. NEWLAND RC et al: The prognostic value of substaging colorectal carcinoma: A prospective study of 1117 cases with standardized pathology. Cancer 60:852, 1987.

111. MINSKY BD et al: Potentially curative surgery of colon cancer: Patterns of failure and survival. J Clin Oncol 6:106, 1988.

112. TURNBULL RB JR et al: Cancer of the colon: the influence of the no-touch isolation technic on survival rates. Ann Surg 166:420, 1967.

113. DAVIS NC, NEWLAND RC: The reporting of colorectal cancer: The Australian clinicopathological staging system. Aust NZ J Surg 52:395, 1982.

114. FLEMING ID, AMERICAN JOINT COMMITTEE ON CANCER, AMERICAN CANCER SOCIETY, AMERICAN COLLEGE OF SURGEONS: AJCC Cancer Staging Manual, 5th ed. Philadelphia, Lippincott-Raven, 1997.

115. WOLMARK N et al: The prognostic value of the modifications of the Dukes' C class of colorectal cancer: An analysis of the NSABP clinical trials. Ann Surg 203:115, 1986.

116. OHMAN U: Prognosis in patients with obstructing colorectal carcinoma. Am J Surg 143:742, 1982.

117. BYERS T et al: American Cancer Society guidelines for screening and surveillance for early detection of colorectal polyps and cancer: Update 1997. American Cancer Society Detection and Treatment Advisory Group on Colorectal Cancer. CA 47:154, 1997.

118. REX DK et al: Screening colonoscopy in asymptomatic average-risk persons with negative fecal occult blood tests. Gastroenterology 100:64, 1991.

119. DISARIO JA et al: Prevalence and malignant potential of colorectal polyps in asymptomatic, average-risk men. Am J Gastroenterol 86:941, 1991.

120. ROGGE JD et al: Low-cost, office-based, screening colonoscopy. Am J Gastroenterol 89:1775, 1994.

121. ST. JOHN DJ et al: Cancer risk in relatives of patients with common colorectal cancer. Ann Intern Med 118:785, 1993.

122. WINAWER SJ et al: Risk of colorectal cancer in the families of patients with adenomatous polyps. National Polyp Study Workgroup. N Engl J Med 334:82, 1996.

123. PETERSEN GM: Genetic testing and counseling in familial adenomatous polyposis. Oncology (Huntington) 10:89; discussion 97, 1996.

124. NATIONAL COMPREHENSIVE CANCER NETWORK: NCCN Colorectal Cancer Screening Practice Guidelines. Oncology (Huntingt) 13:152, 1999.

125. BERTARIO L et al: Clinical aspects and management of hereditary nonpolyposis colorectal cancer (HNPCC). Tumori 82:117, 1996.

126. VASEN HF et al: Cancer risk in families with hereditary nonpolyposis colorectal cancer diagnosed by mutation analysis. Gastroenterology 110:1020, 1996.

127. VASEN HF et al: Surveillance in hereditary nonpolyposis colorectal cancer: An international cooperative study of 165 families. The International Collaborative Group on HNPCC. Dis Colon Rectum 36:1, 1993.

128. AMERICAN SOCIETY FOR GASTROINTESTINAL ENDOSCOPY: Colonoscopy in the screening and surveillance of individuals at increased risk for colorectal cancer. Gastrointest Endosc 48:676, 1998.

129. JARVINEN HJ et al: Screening reduces colorectal cancer rate in families with hereditary nonpolyposis colorectal cancer. Gastroenterology 108:1405, 1995.

130. VASEN HF et al: Hereditary nonpolyposis colorectal cancer: Results of long-term surveillance in 50 families. Eur J Cancer 31A:1145, 1995.

131. SYNGAL S et al: Benefits of colonoscopic surveillance and prophylactic colectomy in patients with hereditary nonpolyposis colorectal cancer mutations. Ann Intern Med 129:787, 1998.

132. VASEN HF et al: A cost-effectiveness analysis of colorectal screening of hereditary nonpolyposis colorectal carcinoma gene carriers. Cancer 82:1632, 1998.

133. WAYE JD, BASHKOFF E: Total colonoscopy: Is it always possible? Gastrointest Endosc 37:152, 1991.

134. HABR-GAMA A, WAYE JD: Complications and hazards of gastrointestinal endoscopy. World J Surg 13:193, 1989.

135. DAJANI AS et al: Prevention of bacterial endocarditis. Recommendations by the American Heart Association. JAMA 277:1794, 1997.

136. GIANOLA FJ et al: Prospective studies of laboratory and radiologic tests in the management of colon and rectal cancer patients: I. Selection of useful preoperative tests through an analysis of surgically occult metastases. Dis Colon Rectum 27:811, 1984.

137. STEELE G JR et al: A prospective evaluation of hepatic resection for colorectal carcinoma metastases to the liver: Gastrointestinal Tumor Study Group Protocol 6584. J Clin Oncol 9:1105, 1991.

138. WOOLFSON K: Tumor markers in cancer of the colon and rectum. Dis Colon Rectum 34:506, 1991.

139. DESCH CE et al: Recommended colorectal cancer surveillance guidelines by the American Society of Clinical Oncology. J Clin Oncol 17:1312, 1999.

140. ECKARDT VF et al: Follow-up of patients with colonic polyps containing severe atypia and invasive carcinoma: Compliance, recurrence, and survival. Cancer 61:2552, 1988.

141. BOND JH: Polyp guideline: diagnosis, treatment, and surveillance for patients with nonfamilial colorectal polyps. The Practice Parameters Committee of the American College of Gastroenterology. Ann Intern Med 119:836, 1993.

142. ROSSINI FP et al: Treatment and follow-up of large bowel adenoma. Tumori 81(Suppl 3):38, 1995.

143. HAGGITT RC et al: Prognostic factors in colorectal carcinomas arising in adenomas: Implications for lesions removed by endoscopic polypectomy. Gastroenterology 89:328, 1985.

144. CRANLEY JP et al: When is endoscopic polypectomy adequate therapy for colonic polyps containing invasive carcinoma? Gastroenterology 91:419, 1986.

145. ZAUBER AG, WINAWER SJ: Initial management and follow-up surveillance of patients with colorectal adenomas. Gastroenterol Clin North Am 26:85, 1997.

146. STEIN BL, COLLER JA: Management of malignant colorectal polyps. Surg Clin North Am 73:47, 1993.

147. SONG F, GLENNY AM: Antimicrobial prophylaxis in colorectal surgery: A systematic review of randomized controlled trials. Br J Surg 85:1232, 1998.

148. HIDA J et al: The extent of lymph node dissection for colon carcinoma: The potential impact on laparoscopic surgery. Cancer 80:188, 1997.

149. BEART RW et al: Management and survival of patients with adenocarcinoma of the colon and rectum: A national survey of the Commission on Cancer. J Am Coll Surg 181:225, 1995.

150. HAYASHI N et al: No-touch isolation technique reduces intraoperative shedding of tumor cells into the portal vein during resection of colorectal cancer. Surgery 125:369, 1999.

151. SALES JP et al: Blood dissemination of colonic epithelial cells during no-touch surgery for rectosigmoid cancer. Lancet 354:392, 1999.

152. GARCIA-OLMO D et al: Experimental evidence does not support use of the "no-touch" isolation technique in colorectal cancer. Dis Colon Rectum 42:1449, discussion 1454, 1999.

153. MILSOM JW et al: A prospective, randomized trial comparing laparoscopic versus conventional techniques in colorectal cancer surgery: A preliminary report. J Am Coll Surg 187:46, discussion 54, 1998.

154. STOCCHI L, NELSON H: Laparoscopic colectomy for colon cancer: trial update. J Surg Oncol 68:255, 1998.

155. FALK PM et al: Laparoscopic colectomy: A critical appraisal. Dis Colon Rectum 36:28, 1993.

156. POULIN EC et al: Laparoscopic resection does not adversely affect early survival curves in patients undergoing surgery for colorectal adenocarcinoma. Ann Surg 229:487, 1999.

157. MULCAHY HE et al: Identifying stage B colorectal cancer patients at high risk of tumor recurrence and death. Dis Colon Rectum 40:326, 1997.

158. MCGREGOR JR, O'DWYER PJ: The surgical management of obstruction and perforation of the left colon. Surg Gynecol Obstet 177:203, 1993.

159. STEPHENSON BM et al: Malignant left-sided large bowel obstruction managed by subtotal/total colectomy. Br J Surg 77:1098, 1990.

160. ARNAUD JP, BERGAMASCHI R: Emergency subtotal/total colectomy with anastomosis for acutely obstructed carcinoma of the left colon. Dis Colon Rectum 37:685, 1994.

161. MEIJER S et al: Intraoperative antegrade irrigation in complicated left-sided colonic cancer. J Surg Oncol 40:88, 1989.

162. MURRAY JJ et al: Intraoperative colonic lavage and primary anastomosis in nonelective colon resection. Dis Colon Rectum 34:527, 1991.

163. THE SCOTIA STUDY GROUP: Single-stage treatment for malignant left-sided colonic obstruction: A prospective randomized clinical trial comparing subtotal colectomy with segmental resection following intraoperative irrigation. Subtotal Colectomy versus on-table irrigation and anastomosis. Br J Surg 82:1622, 1995.

164. NARAYNSINGH V et al: Prospective study of primary anastomosis without colonic lavage for patients with an obstructed left colon. Br J Surg 86:1341, 1999.

165. KIEFHABER P et al: Preoperative neodymium-YAG laser treatment of obstructive colon cancer. Endoscopy 18 (Suppl 1):44, 1986.

166. TEJERO E et al: Initial results of a new procedure for treatment of malignant obstruction of the left colon. Dis Colon Rectum 40:432, 1997.

167. WHOLEY MH et al: Initial clinical experience with colonic stent placement. Am J Surg 175:194, 1998.

168. GALL FP et al: Multivisceral resections in colorectal cancer. Dis Colon Rectum 30:337, 1987.

169. IZBICKI JR et al: Extended resections are beneficial for patients with locally advanced colorectal cancer. Dis Colon Rectum 38:1251, 1995.

170. ROWE VL et al: Extended resection for locally advanced colorectal carcinoma. Ann Surg Oncol 4:131, 1997.

171. KOEA JB et al: Pancreatic and/or duodenal resection for advanced carcinoma of the right colon: Is it justified? Dis Colon Rectum 43:460, 2000.

172. MACKEIGAN JM, FERGUSON JA: Prophylactic oophorectomy and colorectal cancer in premenopausal patients. Dis Colon Rectum 22:401, 1979.

173. O'BRIEN PH et al: Oophorectomy in women with carcinoma of the colon and rectum. Surg Gynecol Obstet 153:827, 1981.

174. MORROW M, ENKER WE: Late ovarian metastases in carcinoma of the colon and rectum. Arch Surg 119:1385, 1984.

175. BIRNKRANT A et al: Ovarian metastasis from colorectal cancer. Dis Colon Rectum 29:767, 1986.

176. GRAFFNER HO et al: Prophylactic oophorectomy in colorectal carcinoma. Am J Surg 146:233, 1983.

177. YOUNG-FADOK TM et al: Prophylactic oophorectomy in colorectal carcinoma: preliminary results of a randomized, prospective trial. Dis Colon Rectum 41:277; discussion, 283, 1998.

178. SLATER G et al: Synchronous carcinoma of the colon and rectum. Surg Gynecol Obstet 171:283, 1990.

179. ARENAS RB et al: Incidence and therapeutic implications of synchronous colonic pathology in colorectal adenocarcinoma. Surgery 122:706, discussion 709, 1997.

180. EVERS BM et al: Multiple adenocarcinomas of the colon and rectum: An analysis of incidences and current trends. Dis Colon Rectum 31:518, 1988.

181. SCOGGINS CR et al: Nonoperative management of primary colorectal cancer in patients with stage IV disease. Ann Surg Oncol 6:651, 1999.

182. TURK PS, WANEBO HJ: Results of surgical treatment of nonhepatic recurrence of colorectal carcinoma. Cancer 71(Suppl 12):4267, 1993.

183. PEZNER RD et al: Resection with external beam and intraoperative radiotherapy for recurrent colon cancer. Arch Surg 134:63, 1999.

184. BOWN SG et al: Endoscopic treatment of inoperable colorectal cancers with the Nd YAG laser. Br J Surg 73:949, 1986.

185. FAINTUCH JS: Endoscopic laser therapy in colorectal carcinoma. Hematol Oncol Clin North Am 3:155, 1989.

186. BENGTSSON G et al: Natural history of patients with untreated liver metastases from colorectal cancer. Am J Surg 141:586, 1981.

187. PALMER M et al: No treatment option for liver metastases from colorectal adenocarcinoma. Dis Colon Rectum 32:698, 1989.

188. FONG Y, SALO J: Surgical therapy of hepatic colorectal metastasis. Semin Oncol 26:514, 1999.

189. FONG Y et al: Pancreatic or liver resection for malignancy is safe and effective for the elderly. Ann Surg 222:426, discussion 434, 1995.

190. FONG Y et al: Clinical score for predicting recurrence after hepatic resection for metastatic colorectal cancer: Analysis of 1001 consecutive cases. Ann Surg 230:309; discussion 318, 1999.

191. KEMENY NE, RON IG: Hepatic arterial chemotherapy in metastatic colorectal patients. Semin Oncol 26:524, 1999.

192. LORENZ M, MULLER HH: Randomized, multicenter trial of fluorouracil plus leucovorin administered either via hepatic arterial or intravenous infusion versus fluorodeoxyuridine administered via hepatic arterial infusion in patients with nonresectable liver metastases from colorectal carcinoma. J Clin Oncol 18:243, 2000.

193. CURLEY SA et al: Adjuvant hepatic arterial infusion chemotherapy after curative resection of colorectal liver metastases. Am J Surg 166:743; discussion 746, 1993.

194. AMBIRU S et al: Adjuvant regional chemotherapy after hepatic resection for colorectal metastases. Br J Surg 86:1025, 1999.

195. LORENZ M et al: Randomized trial of surgery versus surgery followed by adjuvant hepatic arterial infusion with 5-fluorouracil and folinic acid for liver metastases of colorectal cancer. German Cooperative on Liver Metastases (Arbeitsgruppe Lebermetastasen). Ann Surg 228:756, 1998.

196. KEMENY N et al: Hepatic arterial infusion of chemotherapy after resection of hepatic metastases from colorectal cancer. N Engl J Med 341:2039, 1999.

197. GOSLIN R et al: Factors influencing survival in patients with hepatic metastases from adenocarcinoma of the colon or rectum. Dis Colon Rectum 25:749, 1982.

198. MCCORMACK PM et al: Role of video-assisted thoracic surgery in the treatment of pulmonary metastases: results of a prospective trial. Ann Thorac Surg 62:213; discussion 216, 1996.

199. GOYA T et al: Surgical resection of pulmonary metastases from colorectal cancer: 10-year follow-up. Cancer 64:1418, 1989.

200. REGNARD JF et al: Surgical treatment of hepatic and pulmonary metastases from colorectal cancers. Ann Thorac Surg 66:214, discussion 218, 1998.

201. KOBAYASHI K et al: Surgical treatment for both pulmonary and hepatic metastases from colorectal cancer. J Thorac Cardiovasc Surg 118:1090, 1999.

202. MANSEL JK et al: Pulmonary resection of metastatic colorectal adenocarcinoma: A ten year experience. Chest 89:109, 1986.

203. MCAFEE MK et al: Colorectal lung metastases: Results of surgical excision. Ann Thorac Surg 53:780; discussion 785, 1992.

204. MURATA S et al: Resection of both hepatic and pulmonary metastases in patients with colorectal carcinoma. Cancer 83:1086, 1998.

205. WOLMARK N et al: Postoperative adjuvant chemotherapy or BCG for colon cancer: Results from NSABP protocol C-01. J Natl Cancer Inst 80:30, 1988.

206. WOLMARK N et al: The benefit of leucovorin-modulated fluorouracil as postoperative adjuvant therapy for primary colon cancer: Results from National Surgical Adjuvant Breast and Bowel Project protocol C-03. J Clin Oncol 11:1879, 1993.

207. MOERTEL CG et al: Intergroup study of fluorouracil plus levamisole as adjuvant therapy for stage II/Dukes' B2 colon cancer. J Clin Oncol 13:2936, 1995.

208. Efficacy of adjuvant fluorouracil and folinic acid in colon cancer. International Multicentre Pooled Analysis of Colon Cancer Trials (IMPACT) investigators. Lancet 345:939, 1995.

209. O'CONNELL MJ et al: Controlled trial of fluorouracil and low-dose leucovorin given for 6 months as postoperative adjuvant therapy for colon cancer. J Clin Oncol 15:246, 1997.

210. O'CONNELL MJ et al: Prospectively randomized trial of postoperative adjuvant chemotherapy in patients with high-risk colon cancer. J Clin Oncol 16:295, 1998.

211. WOLMARK N et al: Clinical trial to assess the relative efficacy of fluorouracil and leucovorin, fluorouracil and levamisole, and fluorouracil, leucovorin, and levamisole in patients with Dukes' B and C carcinoma of the colon: Results from National Surgical Adjuvant Breast and Bowel Project C-04. J Clin Oncol 17:3553, 1999.

212. MOORE HC, HALLER DG: Adjuvant therapy of colon cancer. Semin Oncol 26:545, 1999.

213. Efficacy of adjuvant fluorouracil and folinic acid in B2 colon cancer. International Multicentre Pooled Analysis of B2 Colon Cancer Trials (IMPACT B2) Investigators. J Clin Oncol 17:1356, 1999.

214. LIEFERS GJ et al: Micrometastases and survival in stage II colorectal cancer. N Engl J Med 339:223, 1998.

215. MARKMAN M: Intraperitoneal chemotherapy in the management of colon cancer. Semin Oncol 26:536, 1999.

216. SPEYER JL et al: Phase I and pharmacological studies of 5-fluorouracil administered intraperitoneally. Cancer Res 40:567, 1980.

217. SPEYER JL et al: Portal levels and hepatic clearance of 5-fluorouracil after intraperitoneal administration in humans. Cancer Res 41:1916, 1981.

218. SUGARBAKER PH et al: Prospective, randomized trial of intravenous versus intraperitoneal 5-fluorouracil in patients with advanced primary colon or rectal cancer. Surgery 98:414, 1985.

219. SCHEITHAUER W et al: Combined intravenous and intraperitoneal chemotherapy with fluorouracil + leucovorin vs fluorouracil + levamisole for adjuvant therapy of resected colon carcinoma. Br J Cancer 77:1349, 1998.

220. KELSEN DP et al: A phase I trial of immediate postoperative intraperitoneal floxuridine and leucovorin plus systemic 5-fluorouracil and levamisole after resection of high risk colon cancer. Cancer 74:2224, 1994.

221. Portal Vein Chemotherapy for Colorectal Cancer: A meta-analysis of 4000 patients in 10 studies. Liver Infusion Meta-analysis Group. J Natl Cancer Inst 89:497, 1997.

222. GRAY BN et al: Melbourne trial of adjuvant immunotherapy in operable large bowel cancer. Aust NZ J Surg 58:43, 1988.

223. VERMORKEN JB et al: Active specific immunotherapy for stage II and stage III human colon cancer: A randomised trial. Lancet 353:345, 1999.

224. HARRIS JE et al: Adjuvant active specific immunotherapy for stage II and III colon cancer with an autologous tumor cell vaccine: Eastern Cooperative Oncology Group Study E5283. J Clin Oncol 18:148, 2000.

225. WELT S, RITTER G: Antibodies in the therapy of colon cancer. Semin Oncol 26:683, 1999.

226. RIETHMULLER G et al: Monoclonal antibody therapy for resected Dukes' C colorectal cancer: Seven-year outcome of a multicenter randomized trial. J Clin Oncol 16:1788, 1998.

227. FOON KA et al: Clinical and immune responses in resected colon cancer patients treated with anti-idiotype monoclonal antibody vaccine that mimics the carcinoembryonic antigen. J Clin Oncol 17:2889, 1999.

228. O'BOYLE KP et al: Immunization of colorectal cancer patients with modified ovine submaxillary gland mucin and adjuvants induces IgM and IgG antibodies to sialylated Tn. Cancer Res 52:5663, 1992.

229. KOPELSON G: Adjuvant postoperative radiation therapy for colorectal carcinoma above the peritoneal reflection. II. Antimesenteric wall ascending and descending colon and cecum. Cancer 52:633, 1983.

230. KOPELSON G: Adjuvant postoperative radiation therapy for colorectal carcinoma above the peritoneal reflection. I. Sigmoid colon. Cancer 51:1593, 1983.

231. DUTTENHAVER JR et al: Adjuvant postoperative radiation therapy in the management of adenocarcinoma of the colon. Cancer 57:955, 1986.

232. WILLETT CG et al: Postoperative radiation therapy for high-risk colon carcinoma. J Clin Oncol 11:1112, 1993.

233. COHEN AM et al: Prognosis of node-positive colon cancer. Cancer 67:1859, 1991.

234. MINSKY BD: Additional pathologic prognostic factors, in *Cancer of the Colon, Rectum, and Anus*, AM Cohen, SJ Winawer (eds). New York, McGraw-Hill, 1995.

235. KJELDSEN BJ et al: A prospective randomized study of follow-up after radical surgery for colorectal cancer. Br J Surg 84:666, 1997.

236. SCHOEMAKER D et al: Yearly colonoscopy, liver CT, and chest radiography do not influence 5-year survival of colorectal cancer patients. Gastroenterology 114:7, 1998.

237. MINTON JP et al: Results of a 400-patient carcinoembryonic antigen second-look colorectal cancer study. Cancer 55:1284, 1985.

238. ROSEN M et al: Follow-up of colorectal cancer: A meta-analysis. Dis Colon Rectum 41:1116, 1998.

239. PIETRA N et al: Role of follow-up in management of local recurrences of colorectal cancer: A prospective, randomized study. Dis Colon Rectum 41:1127, 1998.

240. MELLA J et al: Surgeons' follow-up practice after resection of colorectal cancer. Ann R Coll Surg Engl 79:206, 1997.

241. WINAWER SJ et al: Randomized comparison of surveillance intervals after colonoscopic removal of newly diagnosed adenomatous polyps. The National Polyp Study Workgroup. N Engl J Med 328:901, 1993.

242. GODWIN JD: Carcinoid tumors: An analysis of 2,837 cases. Cancer 36:560, 1975.

243. ROSENBERG JM, WELCH JP: Carcinoid tumors of the colon: A study of 72 patients. Am J Surg 149:775, 1985.

244. BALLANTYNE GH et al: Incidence and mortality of carcinoids of the colon: Data from the Connecticut Tumor Registry. Cancer 69:2400, 1992.

245. SPREAD C et al: Colon carcinoid tumors: A population-based study. Dis Colon Rectum 37:482, 1994.

246. SOGA J: Carcinoids of the colon and ileocecal region: A statistical evaluation of 363 cases collected from the literature. J Exp Clin Cancer Res 17:139, 1998.

247. BERARDI RS: Carcinoid tumors of the colon (exclusive of the rectum): Review of the literature. Dis Colon Rectum 15:383, 1972.

248. WOODS HF et al: Small bowel carcinoid tumors. World J Surg 9:921, 1985.

249. JOHNSON LA et al: Carcinoids: The association of histologic growth pattern and survival. Cancer 51:882, 1983.

250. STINNER B et al: Surgical management for carcinoid tumors of small bowel, appendix, colon, and rectum. World J Surg 20:183, 1996.

251. ZIGHELBOIM J, LARSON MV: Primary colonic lymphoma: Clinical presentation, histopathologic features, and outcome with combination chemotherapy. J Clin Gastroenterol 18:291, 1994.

252. DAWSON IMP et al: Primary malignant lymphoid tumours of the intestinal tract. Br J Surg 49:80, 1961.

253. AMER MH, EL-AKKAD S: Gastrointestinal lymphoma in adults: Clinical features and management of 300 cases. Gastroenterology 106:846, 1994.

254. CONTREARY K et al: Primary lymphoma of the gastrointestinal tract. Ann Surg 191:593, 1980.

255. MIDIS GP, FEIG BW: Cancer of the colon, rectum, and anus, in *The M. D. Anderson Surgical Oncology Handbook*, BW Feig et al (eds). Philadelphia, Lippincott/Williams & Wilkins, 1999, pp. 178–222.

256. NUESSLE WR, MAGILL TR: Leiomyosarcoma of the transverse colon: Report of a case with discussion. Dis Colon Rectum 33:323, 1990.

257. MICHELASSI F et al: Squamous-cell carcinoma of the colon: Experience at the University of Chicago, review of the literature, report of two cases. Dis Colon Rectum 31:228, 1988.

258. VEZERIDIS MP et al: Squamous-cell carcinoma of the colon and retum. Dis Colon Rectum 26:188, 1983.

# 16B / CANCER OF THE RECTUM

*Victor E. Pricolo and Kirby I. Bland*

The management of rectal cancer has undergone significant evolution in the past decade. The overall results of treatment for rectal carcinoma have significantly improved, thanks to several factors: improvement in diagnostic imaging aimed at preoperative staging of the disease, standardization of operative surgical techniques, and demonstrated efficacy of adjuvant radiation therapy and chemotherapy. No other area in the gastrointestinal tract requires such careful planning and individualization of approach to achieve satisfactory oncologic as well as functional results. The desirable goals of preserving anal sphincteric function and avoiding genitourinary complications without compromising the efficacy of a curative resection can now be offered to the vast majority of patients with rectal carcinoma. The diagnostic and therapeutic armamentarium available to the clinician approaching a patient with rectal cancer has never been so rich. The recent literature abounds with information regarding the reliability of new imaging modalities to diagnose primary as well as recurring rectal cancer, the efficacy of adjuvant treatments both in the preoperative and in the postoperative setting, and the feasibility of anal sphincter–saving procedures, ranging from transanal local excisions to coloanal anastomoses. The responsible surgeon must maintain a leading role in the proper planning and coordination of the various management steps in rectal cancer, taking into account patient characteristics as well as tumor variables.

## EPIDEMIOLOGY

Approximately 40% of carcinomas of the large intestine occur in the rectum. The estimated incidence of new cases of rectal cancer in the United States in 2000 is 36,400 (20,200 cases in men, and 16,200 in women). The estimated rectal cancer deaths are 8600 (4700 in men and 3900 in women).[1] Thanks to improved local and systemic control, the mortality figures attributable to rectal cancer have steadily decreased in the past two decades. However, despite efforts in the area of prevention, colorectal cancer remains the second most common malignancy in developed countries and the third most frequent cancer in the world for both genders, after cancer of the lung and stomach in males, and cancer of the breast and cervix in females.[2]

Colorectal cancer is mainly a disease of western industrialized countries. Genetic susceptibility appears to be less relevant than environmental factors, particularly dietary carcinogens, as is evidenced by numerous migrant studies of Asian and eastern European immigrants to the United States and Australia.[3]

Since Burkitt's observation that lack of dietary fiber can play a prominent role, several food items have been associated with an increased risk of colorectal cancer.[4] Generally, a diet high in animal fat (total dietary fat over 20%) from meat and animal protein has been associated with an increased incidence of colorectal cancer. Conversely, large amounts of fiber, especially insoluble (e.g., fresh fruits and vegetables), as well as calcium, β-carotene, vitamin C, and vitamin E may be protective against development of colorectal cancer.[5,6] However, a recent prospective study in nearly 90,000 women failed to show a protective effect of dietary fiber on the risk of colorectal cancer and adenomas.[7] The complex interrelationships among various food components have made the interpretation of some of these studies difficult, since diets high in saturated fats and animal protein tend to be lower in fiber, fruits, and vegetables. The method of food preparation may be important as well, with deep-frying, barbecuing, and smoking being associated with an increased incidence of colorectal cancer.[8]

Alcohol consumption has not been correlated conclusively with the incidence of colon cancer; however, recent cohort studies positively relate alcohol consumption with the incidence of rectal cancer.[9] In addition, recent reports have associated long-term cigarette smoking (at least 35 years) with an increased incidence of colorectal cancer.[10] Pelvic irradiation has also been shown to increase the incidence of rectal carcinoma.[11]

Other risk factors for developing rectal carcinoma are no different from those described for the colon, such as preexisting adenomas, family history of cancer, and inflammatory bowel disease (both ulcerative colitis and Crohn's disease). The occurrence of two-thirds of colorectal malignancies in the rectosigmoid has generally been attributed to stasis in this segment of the large intestine with prolonged exposure of the epithelial lining of the rectosigmoid to environmental carcinogens. Although each specific incidence rate for both colon and rectal carcinoma increases steadily with advancing age, there are no significant gender differences in the incidences of colorectal cancer.[11]

Genetic studies on colorectal carcinoma in the past decade have provided us with crucial information regarding pathogenesis, tumor progression, and prognosis. The observation that the vast majority of colorectal carcinomas arise from premalignant adenomatous polyps that have a monoclonal composition, and the knowledge of several well-known inherited colorectal cancer syndromes, have greatly facilitated the understanding of colorectal carcinogenesis.[12,13]

The identification of genes responsible for familial polyposis coli and its variant, Gardner syndrome, and for Lynch syndromes I and II, has prompted similar investigations of genetic mutations that are involved in sporadic colorectal carcinogenesis.[14] The most frequently studied genes have been the K-*ras*, p53, APC, and the deleted in colorectal carcinoma (DCC) genes.[15,16] The current tumorigenesis model is based on the observation that accumulation of genetic "hits" occurs from aberrant crypt focus, to epithelial hyperplasia, dysplasia, adenoma, and carcinoma.[13] The details of the interactions of environmental factors with the individual genetic background, in order to explain the individual susceptibility to colorectal neoplasms, remain to be better clarified.

On the basis of this knowledge, efforts are under way in the areas of both primary and secondary prevention of colorectal carcinoma. The efficacy of dietary changes in preventing colorectal cancer remains unproven; nonetheless, a diet high in fresh fruits, vegetables, and insoluble fiber and low in meat, fat, and other animal protein, is advisable, particularly for young individuals with first-degree relatives affected by colorectal carcinoma. In several reports, aspirin and other nonsteroidal antiinflammatory medications have been associated with inhibition of carcinogenesis in animal models, as well as with a decreased incidence of colorectal cancer in population-based studies.[17,18] However, conclusive evidence from chemoprevention trials is not available at this time. Presently, the most practical efforts available to the clinician for reducing the incidence of rectal carcinoma are in the areas of secondary prevention: early diagnosis and definitive treatment of premalignant conditions. Digital rectal examination, fecal occult blood testing, and screening proctosigmoidoscopies at regular intervals should allow for detection and endoscopic removal of adenomatous polyps and, therefore, for a reduction in the overall incidence of carcinoma. Several studies have offered conclusive evidence of the impact of screening proctosigmoidoscopy in reducing both colorectal cancer incidence and mortality rates.[19,20]

## PATHOLOGIC STAGING AND PROGNOSIS

The original classification of rectal cancer in stages A, B, and C, as proposed in 1932 by Dr. Cuthbert E. Dukes, pathologist and director of the research laboratory at St. Marks Hospital in London, has been modified over the years to include many other variables that may affect prognosis, such as a more detailed description of depth of invasion, extent of lymph node metastases, and distal metastatic disease.[21] Other classification systems have emphasized histologic features of the neoplasms, such as pattern of tumor growth, tubular configuration, lymphocytic infiltration, neural and vascular invasion, fibrosis, and nuclear polarity.[22] Despite the persistent widespread popularity of Dukes' classification, especially with its Astler-Coller modification, for uniformity's sake it is desirable to use the tumor, node, metastasis (TNM) classification recommended by the American Joint Committee on Cancer and the *Union Internationale Contre le Cancer*. This universal system for staging cancer in all anatomic sites corresponds closely to the modifications of Dukes' classification, and has been endorsed by the American College of Surgeons Commission on Cancer, the Joint Commission on Accreditation of Hospital Organizations, and the American Society of Colon and Rectal Surgeons. (See Chapter 4D by William G. Kraybill and Peter M. Banks, for comprehensive AJCC colorectal carcinoma staging.)

The usefulness of such systems has been evidenced by analyses of clinical trials conducted by the Gastrointestinal Tumor Study Group (GITSG) and the National Surgical Adjuvant Breast and Bowel Project (NSABP), which have emphasized the importance of tumor penetration through the bowel wall and involvement of regional lymph nodes in the prognosis of colorectal cancer.[23,24] TNM staging remains the most accurate predictor of patient outcome and is, therefore, the most important prognostic element in the assessment of patients with rectal carcinoma. The depth of bowel wall penetration closely correlates with the incidence of regional lymph node and metastatic potential (0% with Tis, up to 10% for T1, and as high as 58% for T4 lesions).[25] The presence and number of lymph node metastases in rectal cancer also correlates with prognosis. Survival rate drops from 50% to 55% in patients with one to four positive perirectal lymph nodes, to 22% to 28% in patients with five or more positive regional nodes.[26]

The presence of distal metastases in rectal carcinoma, generally located in the liver and lungs, is associated with a 5-year survival of approximately 1%, which can be significantly improved only by surgical resection or ablation, in appropriately selected patients, with subsequent survivals of 20% to 25% at 5 years. As in other sites in the alimentary canal, tumor size is not a significant prognostic factor in colorectal cancer, and is therefore not included in the TNM classification.

In several studies, tumor obstruction and perforation, as well as extension to adjacent anatomic structures (T4 lesion), have been associated with reduction in disease-free interval as well as with overall survival.[27,28] However, a worse survival rate was not demonstrated in subsequent studies, when the data were corrected for the higher operative mortality in patients with obstructive lesions, and when en bloc resection was performed in patients with direct invasion to adjacent organs.[29] Perforation is associated with a significantly higher risk of free peritoneal and pelvic seeding and is, therefore, associated with a lower 5-year survival rate, limited to 10% to 25%.[30]

There are no significant gender differences in the prognosis of colorectal carcinoma, and the data are somewhat conflicting with regard to the prognosis of colorectal cancer in younger patients. Less than 5% of patients develop colorectal carcinoma before age 40. The assumption, however, that younger patients would carry a worse prognosis has not been proven.[31,32]

Histopathologic variables related to the tumor and assessed by light microscopy have long been associated with prognosis and risk of metastatic spread in rectal cancer. Poor differentiation; mucinous and signet-ring cell type; and neural, lymphatic, and vascular invasion have all been associated with a poorer prognosis.[33–35] More recently, DNA ploidy has been assessed as a parameter that may help predict tumor behavior.[36,37] A significantly elevated preoperative carcinoembryonic antigen (CEA) level is of greater significance in patients with node-positive (stage III) tumors than in patients with node-negative disease.[38]

Molecular genetic analysis of colorectal cancer specimens for the purpose of prognostic evaluation has been investigated in recent years and has yielded very promising data. In view of the fact that the assessment of histopathologic characteristics is quite subjective, semiquantitative, and variable in different areas of the same tumor, the need for more objective prognostic parameters in the preoperative phase of treatment planning has generated a great deal of interest with respect to these molecular biology studies. Several allelic losses,[39] specific deletions on the DCC gene of chromosome 18q,[40] certain K-*ras* mutations,[41] and deletions in the p53 gene on chromosome 17p have been found to be adverse predictors of survival in colorectal carcinoma. Conversely, high-frequency microsatellite instability has been recently associated with a more favorable outcome and a decreased likelihood of metastases.[43]

The feasibility of molecular biology techniques and their applicability in clinical practice may provide important information related not only to the progression of disease during carcinogenesis but also to the clinical behavior of established tumors. It is conceivable that some of these techniques will become part of the standard of care in the prognostic assessment of human neoplasms in the near future.

## DIAGNOSIS: PREOPERATIVE ASSESSMENT AND CLINICAL STAGING

Despite the demonstrated effectiveness of colorectal screening programs, their widespread application is yet to be seen, and most patients still seek medical attention as a result of having observed blood per rectum.[44] Any patient presenting with such symptoms, especially if over 40 years of age, should be promptly evaluated to rule out the possibility of malignant or premalignant conditions of the colon and rectum. Patients can be referred by their primary care physician for either colonoscopy or barium enema examination (Fig. 16B-1). The value of both in rectal cancer is significant, in that they rule out synchronous adenomatous polyps, which occur in up to 50% of patients, as well as synchronous colon carcinomas, which can occur in up to 5% of patients.[45]

It is imperative for the surgeon who will be treating the rectal lesion to conduct a complete evaluation of the patient and the tumor.[46] Patient evaluation includes an assessment of operative risk factors that may play a role in the selection of surgical as well as adjuvant treatment. A complete history and physical examination, as well as laboratory tests; electrocardiogram and chest radiograph; an assessment of cardiovascular diseases, pulmonary function, diabetes, hepatorenal function, and possible disorders of hemostasis, should be performed before a major abdominal operation or administration of a general anesthetic. Age alone should not be considered a contraindication, in the absence of the above-mentioned variables, since it has not been shown to significantly increase morbidity in patients operated on for carcinoma of the colon and rectum.[47]

The clinical assessment of the primary tumor can be conducted by a combination of digital examination and proctoscopy, which remain the most reliable means to determine potential for sphincter preservation. The tumor is assessed for size, location, mobility versus fixation, exophytic versus ulcerative appearance, and for an accurate measurement of the distance of the tumor from the anal verge and/or from the dentate line. As a general rule, tumors measuring less than 3 cm in diameter, preferably with exophytic polypoid growth and located less than 10 cm from the anal verge, may be approachable with local excision.[48] Additional factors to be considered in the choice of operative treatment are patient physique

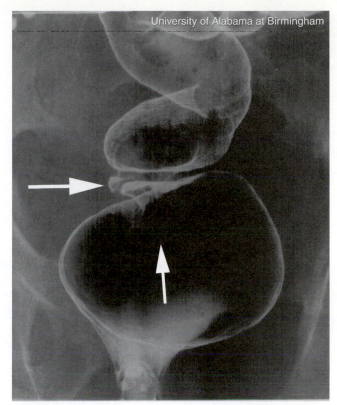

**FIGURE 16B-1.** A 66-year-old man with rectal bleeding. Spot radiograph from double-contrast barium enema reveals a 5-cm annular mass (arrows) in the rectum, approximately 9 cm from anal verge. (*Image courtesy of Cheri L. Canon, M.D.*)

(a morbidly obese male patient with a narrow pelvis may not be suitable for restorative resection), and a weak or incompetent anal sphincter, which may not be worth preserving after a lower anterior resection or coloanal anastomosis.

As stated previously, the colon is evaluated by colonoscopy or barium enema, and biopsies are obtained, confirming the diagnosis of a carcinoma. Once confirmed, the next step in the preoperative assessment is the determination of the extent of the disease, after histopathologic variables of significance have been obtained at the time of biopsy of the rectal tumor. The clinical staging of rectal cancer is aimed at determining three main factors; depth of tumor penetration (T), status of regional lymph nodes (N), and presence of distal metastases (M). Accurate determination of the depth of invasion of the rectal wall can be difficult to define by digital examination alone, although some authors claim up to 80% accuracy.[49] With physical examination alone, there are obvious limitations to the clinical assessment of tumor penetration in the rectal wall. Rectal tumors may not be entirely palpable by rectal examination, and tethering or fixation of the tumor may be due to inflammatory reaction surrounding the tumor, especially after endoscopic biopsy or partial excision. Consequently, in recent years imaging techniques have been utilized in order to improve the overall accuracy of clinical staging in rectal cancer.

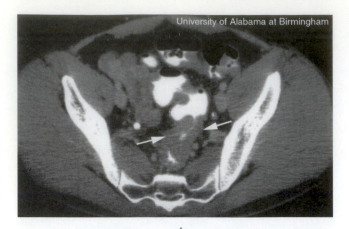
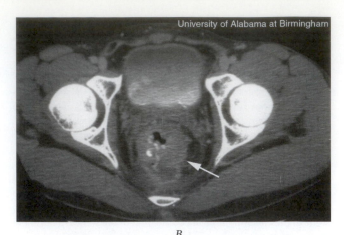

*A*             *B*

**FIGURE 16B-2.** A 34-year-old man with rectal adenocarcinoma. *A.* Intravenous, oral, and rectal contrast-enhanced CT of the pelvis reveals a circumferential mass in the rectosigmoid colon (arrows). *B.* Image through the lower pelvis demonstrates caudal extent of the mass but no regional adenopathy. Pathologically, all lymph nodes were tumor-free. (*Image courtesy of Cheri L. Canon, M.D.*)

## IMAGING TECHNIQUES

### COMPUTED TOMOGRAPHY

Contrast-enhanced CT of the abdomen and pelvis is a valuable test in the preoperative evaluation of rectal tumors (Fig. 16B-2). The determination of liver metastatic disease is generally made by CT in North America (Fig. 16B-3), whereas in several European coun- tries clinicians rely on abdominal ultrasound. The determination of lung metastatic disease is generally assessed with a preoperative chest radiograph, which should be obtained routinely. Chest CT is generally reserved for patients with a chest radiograph suspicious for metastatic disease. The accuracy of pelvic CT in determining the depth of invasion of rectal cancer has generally been reported as ranging between 62% and 79%.[50–53]

The accuracy of CT for determining perirectal lymph node metas- tases is even worse, ranging between 35% and 56%[50–53] (Fig. 16B-4).

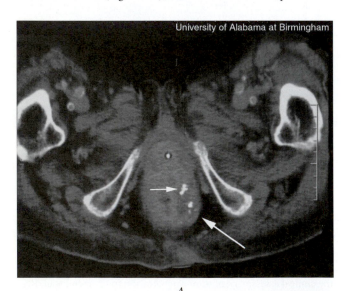
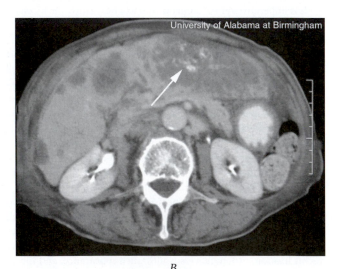

*A*             *B*

**FIGURE 16B-3.** A 70-year-old woman with weight loss, rectal bleeding, hepatosplenomegaly, and el- evated liver function tests. *A.* Intravenous contrast-enhanced CT through the pelvis reveals a low rectal mass (arrow) extending to the anus. Note dense calcifications within the mass (small arrow). *B.* Mul- tiple hepatic metastases are present. Note calcifications in lateral segment lesions (arrow) that have a similar appearance to calcifications in the primary mass. (*Image courtesy of Cheri L. Canon, M.D.*)

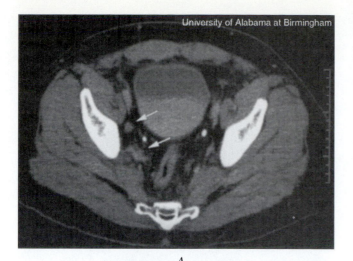

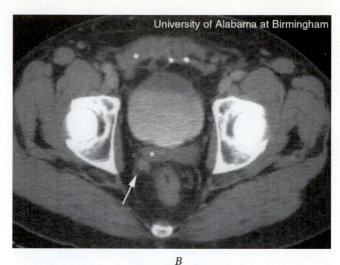

A                                                                                                    B

**FIGURE 16B-4.** A 55-year-old man with rectal carcinoma. *A.* Contrast-enhanced CT through the pelvis reveals mildly enlarged lymph nodes along the right pelvic wall (arrows). *B.* Images that are more caudal demonstrate another enlarged lymph node (arrow) posterior to the right seminal vesicle (asterisk). Although these were thought to represent nodal metastases, all nodes were pathologically negative. (*Image courtesy of Cheri L. Canon, M.D.*)

Isolated reports on relatively small series of patients (40 to 45) have described an overall accuracy in the 90% range for CT in assessing local spread of rectal tumors.[54,55] The need for better imaging techniques has prompted further investigations.

## ENDORECTAL ULTRASOUND

In the past 10 years, endorectal ultrasonography (ERUS) has established itself as a modality proving to be quite accurate in the assessment of both tumor depth and perirectal lymph node metastases. This method should be used whenever possible in the preoperative staging of rectal cancer.[56] The Beynon five-layer model, which is used to define rectal wall anatomy is generally employed.[57] The alternating white and black layers that are visible during endorectal ultrasonography represent mucosal surface, muscularis mucosae, submucosa, muscularis propria, and serosa and/or perirectal fat. The modified ultrasonographic TNM classification has been proposed for the imaging of rectal tumors[56]:

uT1: Tumor confined to mucosa and submucosa
uT2: Tumor penetrating into but not through the muscularis propria
uT3: Extension into perirectal fat
uT4: Extension into adjacent structures

This classification emphasizes the importance of the middle echogenic layer by ultrasonographic imaging (the submucosa). If no invasion of the submucosa is detected, the tumor most likely is not an invasive carcinoma. The accuracy of ERUS in determining depth of rectal wall penetration has ranged between 81% and 94%[58-66] (Fig. 16B-5*A–C*).

In the assessment of wall penetration using ERUS, the interesting limitation is that up to 9% of patients are understaged, but 10% to 21% of patients are overstaged. The relatively high incidence of overstaging should caution the interpretation of downstaging after preoperative chemotherapy and radiation therapy in the treatment of rectal carcinoma. The accuracy of lymph node staging appears to be more limited with ERUS, generally ranging between 58% and 83%.[57,61,64,66,67,68] Generally, lymph nodes can be identified as high hypoechoic areas in the perirectal tissue. Metastatic nodes are generally enlarged and more likely to be round than oval, and most often in close proximity, or just proximal, to the primary neoplasm. The sensitivity and specificity of ERUS aimed at perirectal lymph node staging is on the order of 60% to 80% (Table 16B-1). The availability of ERUS at the time of colonoscopy permits assessment of depth of invasion and presence of metastatic disease, all in one test. The reliability of this technique for colorectal cancer, however, has generally been less than what is achieved with current ERUS probes.[69] The interpretation of ERUS is still operator-dependent. A significant learning curve is required with the technique and the interpretation of imaging, with most errors in interpretation resulting in overstaging of T2 lesions from inflammatory changes, preoperative radiation therapy, and cautery or biopsy artifacts that cause image distortion. Nonetheless, ERUS remains a valuable tool in the overall treatment planning of rectal cancers, especially if local treatment is considered for histologically favorable T1 and T2 lesions. Its use for selected patients may be the most cost-effective method to identify both early cancer for local treatment and more advanced disease for preoperative adjuvant therapy. Ultrasonographic uT3 and uT4 and any N1 lesion should not be considered for local treatment, but should be considered for preoperative adjuvant therapy.

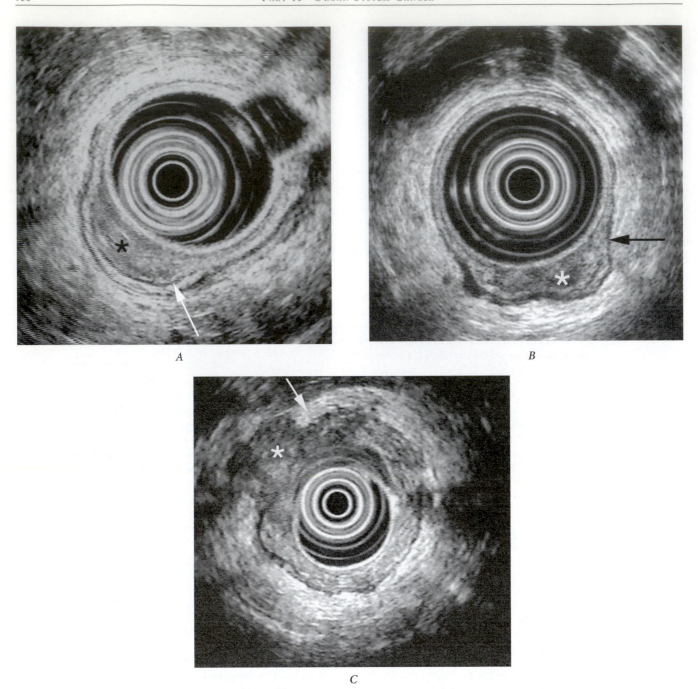

*A*

*B*

*C*

**FIGURE 16B-5.** *A.* Stage uT1: Tumor (*) extends, but not beyond muscularis mucosa (arrow). *B.* Stage uT2: Tumor (*) extends, but not beyond muscularis propria (arrow). *C.* Stage uT3: Tumor (*) extends beyond mucularis propria into perirectal fat (arrow). (*Images courtesy of Craig Philpot, M.D. and Sean C. Fell, M.D.*)

ERUS guided biopsy of suspicious perirectal lymph nodes has yielded an accuracy rate of 77%, with a sensitivity of 71%, a specificity of 89%, a positive predictive value of 92%, and a negative predictive value of 62%.[70] This method may be reserved for patients in whom the ultrasound findings are unclear, and therapeutic decisions then can be based on this information. The extent of tumor spread through the bowel wall (T stage) is most accurately assessed by endoanal ultrasonography, although this technique is less accurate

**TABLE 16B-1.** ACCURACY OF ENDORECTAL ULTRASOUND FOR BOTH DEPTH OF WALL PENETRATION AND LYMPH NODE STATUS

| AUTHOR | YEAR | NO. OF PATIENTS | ACCURACY FOR DEPTH OF WALL PENETRATION, % | ACCURACY FOR LYMPH NODE STAGING, % |
|---|---|---|---|---|
| Boscaini | 1986 | 11 | 91 | |
| Hildebrandt | 1986 | 76 | 88 | |
| Beynon | 1987 | 49 | 90 | |
| Holdsworth | 1988 | 36 | 86 | 61 |
| Yamashita | 1988 | 122 | 78 | |
| Katsura | 1992 | 120 | 92 | |
| Beynon | 1989 | 95 | | 83 |
| Lynmark | 1982 | 63 | 81 | |
| Milsom | 1993 | 67 | 85 | 77 |
| Herzog | 1993 | 118 | 89 | 80 |
| Deen | 1993 | 209 | 82 | |
| Solomon | 1993 | 517 | | 58 |

than both CT and MRI at assessing tumor extension into adjacent organs.[71] Further studies await the comparison of accuracy between ERUS and endorectal MRI.

## MAGNETIC RESONANCE IMAGING

The sensitivity of MRI in detecting rectal wall penetration as well as metastatic perirectal lymph nodes in the pelvis has been limited, and generally comparable with CT scan.[72] More recent MRI techniques (12-mm-thick slices in transverse, coronal, and sagittal planes) did not significantly affect results. The accuracy was about 70% in the determination of rectal wall penetration, and the sen-

sitivity was only 40% in the detection of perirectal lymph node involvement.[73] The use of an endorectal coil for MRI imaging of rectal tumors has received increasing attention in recent years. Endorectal imaging can provide excellent visualization of the layers of the rectal wall in most patients, although it is usually observed over only part of the entire rectal circumference. The overall accuracy rate has been ranging between 60% and 90% in determination of wall invasion and assessment of lymph node status.[74] These data suggest that, at present, endorectal MRI imaging is not superior to ERUS and is certainly far more expensive. At the present time, MRI is generally limited to patients with suspected pelvic recurrences of rectal cancer, where determination of extension into adjacent structures can be better determined than with CT or ultrasound, especially after radiation therapy. MRI is also an option for the evaluation of distant metastases in patients who cannot undergo contrasted CT (e.g., patients with contrast allergy or acute renal failure) (Fig. 16B-6).

## RADIOIMMUNODETECTION

Radioimmunodetection of cancer is generally accomplished by obtaining whole-body gamma scans of patients who have been injected with an antibody labeled or conjugated with a gamma-emitting radionuclide. In colorectal cancer, the most commonly studied antigens have been CEA and TAG-72.[75,76] Although radioimmunodetection is generally used after a negative imaging evaluation in patients with suspected recurrence of colorectal cancer, there have been very few focused studies of radioimmunodetection in the initial staging of colorectal cancer patients. In a study where immunoscintigraphy was performed with [99m]Tc-MoAb BW 431-26, an intact IgG-1 murine monoclonal antibody, the sensitivity for identifying the primary site was 95%, with a specificity of 91%.[77] Other studies have suggested that use of immunoscintigraphy with indium 111 (Oncoscint) may be less useful in identifying liver metastases, but more sensitive than CAT scan in the identification of metastatic extrahepatic disease.[78]

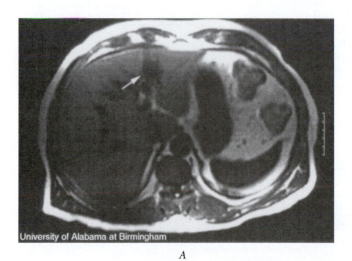
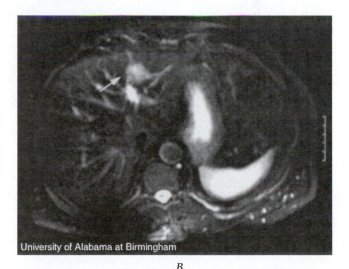

*A*        *B*

**FIGURE 16B-6.** *A.* T1-weighted and *B.* T2-weighted MRI images of rectal carcinoma (*) (*Images courtesy of Ruedi F.L. Thoeni, M.D. and Sean C. Fell, M.D.*)

## POSITRON EMISSION TOMOGRAPHY

PET is an imaging technique that uses a positron-emitting isotope-labeled compound that is incorporated into a biochemical process according to organs and body tissue.[79] In recent years, PET has been applied increasingly by several investigators in evaluation of tumors, including colorectal carcinoma. In small clinical series (14 to 18 patients), PET has been reported as having a sensitivity ranging between 92% and 100% and a specificity ranging between 83% and 100% in the detection of both primary and locally recurring colorectal carcinoma.[80–82]

Despite these encouraging results, there have been a few false-positive reports with PET in patients with malignancy, related to inflammatory changes such as proctitis or abscesses.[83] The use of PET imaging is presently limited to detection of recurrent disease or metastatic disease and is generally not advisable in the preoperative assessment of patients with rectal carcinoma.

## TREATMENT (Fig. 16B-7)

### SURGERY

The ideal curative surgical operation in the treatment of rectal carcinoma should achieve the following goals:

1. It should be curative (i.e., should prevent pelvic recurrence and systemic spread of the disease).
2. It should be associated with acceptable perioperative morbidity.
3. It should be applicable to the majority of patients.
4. It should maintain a satisfactory quality of life (i.e., preservation of enteric continence and genitourinary functions).

More than 90% of patients present with locoregional disease, either limited to the rectal wall or to the perirectal lymph nodes.[84,85]

Rectal carcinoma may spread in five ways:

1. Direct continuity of tissue in and through the bowel wall
2. Extramural lymphatic spread
3. Transperitoneal spread
4. Hematogenous spread
5. Implantation onto raw surfaces or suture lines[84]

The goals of therapy must be clearly defined, after a preoperative assessment of the patient, the tumor, and its stage. In selected cases, curative intent can be achieved with local treatments, although in the majority of patients a curative resection implies a radical pelvic lymphadenectomy (total mesorectal excision with autonomic nerve preservation). If the goals of treatment are limited to palliation of symptoms (patients unfit for major surgery, or in the presence of widespread distant metastatic disease), the goals should be limited

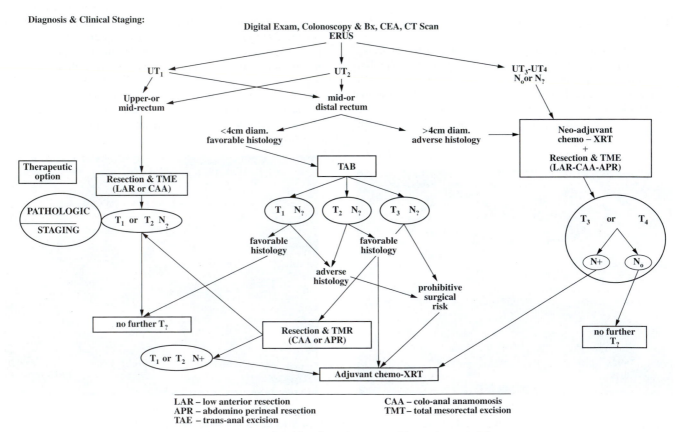

**FIGURE 16B-7.** Management algorithm for primary curable carcinoma of the rectum.

to an operation that would improve patient symptoms with an acceptable morbidity and consequent quality of life. Despite the recent encouraging results of numerous trials emphasizing the effectiveness of radiation therapy and chemotherapy both in the preoperative and the postoperative setting, it is imperative to remember that surgical treatment still remains the mainstay of therapy in rectal carcinoma. The excellent chances of cure of a meticulous, complete pelvic lymphadenectomy should not be compromised by undue reliance on adjuvant treatment modalities.

## SURGICAL TECHNIQUES

ABDOMINOPERINEAL RESECTION. This procedure is generally indicated for lesions of the lower one-third of the rectum or for higher lesions in the presence of an incompetent anal sphincter. W. Ernest Miles[86] reported on 12 such operations in 1908, with a mortality rate of 41.6%. Abdominoperineal resection (APR) remained the standard of treatment for rectal carcinoma for many years, based on the goal of widest possible margins, to prevent the devastating effects of recurrent disease in the pelvis, which at the beginning of the twentieth century was the primary cause of death in the majority of patients. APR includes complete removal of the sigmoid, rectum, and anal sphincteric complex through combined abdominal and perineal approaches, with creation of a permanent colostomy. Until recently, this operation was considered the standard for rectal cancers located less than 5 cm from the dentate line.[87] Nowadays, a sphincter-saving procedure is possible in the majority of rectal cancers. The observation that a 1- to 2-cm distal margin is all that is required to minimize local recurrences, the availability of endoluminal circular stapling devices, and the often significant reduction in size of distal rectal cancer with preoperative radiation therapy have made sphincter preservation the rule rather than the exception for carcinomas of the distal one-third of the rectum. An APR may still be necessary in morbidly obese patients, particularly males with a narrow pelvis, in patients with significant anal sphincter weakness, and with bulky or poorly differentiated lesions located less than 2 cm from the dentate line. In order to minimize postoperative sexual dysfunction and neurogenic bladder dysfunction, it is still desirable to preserve, whenever possible, sympathetic and parasympathetic innervation, during total mesorectal excision. Marking of the stoma site, as well as colostomy counseling by an enterostomal therapy nurse, should be practiced routinely in the preoperative phase.

SPHINCTER-SAVING RESECTIONS. An anal sphincter–preserving resection should attain the goals that have been outlined for an ideal curative operation applicable to most carcinomas of the rectum. Refinement in surgical technique with availability of endoluminal staplers has been the single most important factor in allowing restoration of bowel continuity in the majority of patients with carcinomas located not only in the upper or midrectum, but also in the distal one-third of the rectum. A low anterior resection (LAR) is the procedure most frequently performed for cancers of the upper rectum, whereas a coloanal anastomosis (CAA) may be necessary to achieve adequate mesorectal excision and adequate distal margins for tumors located in the midrectum and distal rectum. The scientific observations that have made APR an ever more infrequent

procedure are related to an appreciation of the adequacy of distal as well as radial margins of resection. The recommended length of distal margins of resection for rectal carcinoma has changed significantly in the past several years. A 5-cm margin had been advocated generally, based on isolated reports from the era of APR, suggesting occasional distal intramural spread of rectal carcinomas.[88,89] Another study, still in the 1950s, recognized that the distal intramural spread of rectal carcinoma is quite uncommon. In this study of 89 patients who underwent a potentially curative resection, only one individual was found to have a distal spread of greater than 1.5 cm. Nonetheless, a distal margin of resection of 2.5 cm in patients with well-differentiated lesions, and a margin of 6 cm in patients with poorly differentiated lesions, was recommended.[90]

In the past 20 years, several reports based on large patient series have demonstrated that distal margins of resections of 2 cm, or slightly less, would not affect adversely local control rates or survival. In a review of 556 patients who underwent low anterior resection for rectal cancer, there was no difference in long-term outcome figures for patients with 2- to 3-cm distal margins when compared with patients with wider margins.[91] In another review of 334 patients treated for carcinoma of the rectum with curative intent, a less than 2-cm margin was found not to adversely affect outcome.[92] The National Surgical Adjuvant Breast and Bowel Project (NSABP) reported no significant difference in disease-free survival when comparing patients with margins of less than 2 cm with those greater than 3 cm.[93] A more recent Japanese study on 610 consecutive rectal cancer patients concluded that a distal margin of resection 1 cm below the lower edge of the tumor is free of cancer cells in most patients. If the tumor had spread distally in the rectum for more than 1 cm, longer resection margins would not necessarily improve overall prognosis. Therefore, a 1-cm distal margin measured on the pathology specimen (accounting for some retraction) may be an appropriate clearance for most rectal cancers.[94] In recent years, greater, and long overdue, attention has been devoted to the need to assess lateral radial margins of resection during radical operations for rectal carcinoma. In a series of 52 patients treated for rectal cancer, the risk of pelvic recurrence was far greater in those with positive radial margins (85%) than in those with negative radial margins of resection (3%).[95]

The pelvic recurrence rate can be greatly reduced by adequate circumferential dissection of the perirectal lymphatics. R.J. Heald and associates[96] deserve credit for attracting the attention of the surgical community to the need for complete excision of the mesorectum during pelvic lymphadenectomy for rectal cancer. The technique of mesorectal excision involves the development of an avascular plane between visceral structures (rectum and mesorectum) and the somatic structures of the autonomic nerve plexuses that can be visualized after division of the superior rectal vessels. Sharp dissection, either with scissors or electrocautery, under direct vision is to be used, completely avoiding any blunt finger dissection that tears into the fragile perirectal tissue planes and may compromise complete clearance of mesorectal lymphatics. The incision on the pelvic peritoneum should be wide, encompassing the entire peritoneal reflection, and division of the middle rectal vessels should be as far from the rectum as possible. Anteriorly, the peritoneum is incised in front of the cul-de-sac in a plane developed between the rectum and the vagina, or the seminal vesicles and the prostate, so that Denonvilliers fascia and the fatty tissue behind it can be excised with the specimen. This dissection can be carried down to the level of the anal sphincteric complex and represents the crucial portion of an adequate curative operation for rectal carcinoma, whether or not the anal sphincters are to be preserved or excised. The mesorectum can be lifted from the levator ani plane posteriorly, drawn up as a "mesorectal tail," and dissected from the distal rectal muscular tube for a distance of approximately 2 to 3 cm.[97] Transection can then be accomplished at the anorectal junction, generally with an angled clamp or a stapling device, with adequate distal margins from the tumor.

In 1992, R.J. Heald and Karanjie[84] reported their results in 192 patients who underwent anterior resection and 21 who underwent APR. Of low anterior resections, 79% were curative and 21% were noncurative. In the 152 specimens from curative LAR, 110 had a resection margin greater than 1 cm and 42 had a resection margin less than 1 cm. The local recurrence rate in the curative resection subgroup was less than 4%. Selection bias notwithstanding (curative versus noncurative procedures), these outstanding results obtained with radical surgery alone in all-stage patients [Dukes' A (22%), B (44%), and C (34%)], emphasize the role of adequate pelvic dissection in rectal carcinoma performed by experienced competent surgeons.[84] A double-stapling technique to restore bowel continuity after low anterior resection is now considered by many surgeons to be the preferred method of reconstruction and has been associated with very acceptable morbidity, as well as favorable oncologic and functional results.[98]

Several other surgeons from Europe and the United States have reported similar results, with low local recurrence rates and very good long-term survival, when surgical treatment alone included total mesorectal excision. W.E. Enker and associates[99] reported on 246 consecutive patients with stage II and stage III primary rectal carcinomas who underwent total mesorectal excision with sphincter preservation and autonomic nerve preservation. The 5-year survival rate was 86.7% for stage II patients and 64% for stage III patients. Pelvic recurrences occurred in 4% of stage II and 8.1% of stage III patients. Statistically significant risk factors for pelvic recurrence were N2 disease and perineural invasion. Adjuvant radiation therapy was of no statistical benefit in preventing local recurrences. The ability of total mesorectal excision to preserve genitourinary function was also retrospectively assessed in 136 patients. Of patients younger than age 60, 86% and patients 60 years and older 67% were able to engage in intercourse; 87% of male patients and 91% of female patients were able to achieve orgasm. Neurogenic bladder was not encountered.[100]

The need for total mesorectal excision, including the distal mesorectal "tail," in order to minimize local recurrence is a concept possibly more relevant than a distal resection margin greater than 1 cm at the mucosal level. Two recent pathologic studies on resected specimens found presence of nodal metastases in the mesorectum, distal to the primary tutor, in approximately 20% of patients.[101,102] These more recent observations confirm Heald's original postulate emphasizing the need for total mesorectal excision, both radially and distally, in order to minimize local recurrences for tumors of the middle and distal one-third of the rectum.

Other factors that have been associated with long-term survival after radical pelvic lymphadenectomy are the level of ligation of the inferior mesenteric artery and the use of periopera-

tive blood products. Ligation of the inferior mesenteric artery, flush with the aorta, should allow for more radical excision of metastatic nodes and possibly an improved prognosis. However, no study has demonstrated a survival advantage, most likely because patients with positive nodal involvement at the base of the inferior mesenteric artery have already developed disseminated disease and would gain no benefit from a high ligation.[103] Several retrospective reviews have indicated a deleterious effect of red blood cell transfusions on survival in cancer patients, most likely as a result of immune suppression.[104] However, other authors have been unable to confirm these findings.[105] Meticulous sharp dissection under direct visualization in the pelvis should greatly reduce the need for perioperative blood transfusions.

The usefulness of total mesorectal excision is particularly apparent in patients with T3 and T4 lesions in the lower rectum and should be extended to at least 5 cm below the tumor for patients with T3 and T4 lesions in the upper rectum. The rectum should be transected at the levator ani plane and an anastomosis can then be performed in the upper surgical anal canal rectum (coloanal anastomosis).[106] Especially if the sigmoid colon is brought down to the distal rectum, patients may experience urgency, frequency of evacuation, and occasional incontinence as a result of the loss of rectal reservoir function. In order to improve functional results after coloanal anastomosis, the construction of a colonic J-shaped pouch was proposed in 1986.[107,108]

A colonic J-shaped pouch, measuring 6 to 8 cm in length, is made by folding the colon and fashioning a side-to-side anastomosis with a linear stapler introduced through the antimesenteric apex of the pouch. The pouch-anal anastomosis is generally performed with a double-stapling technique, or occasionally via a transanal hand sewn technique. The use of a temporary ileostomy is advocated routinely by some surgeons, but is applied selectively by others. In our experience, a diverting ileostomy is used with older patients, with preoperative radiation therapy, and in patients with anemia, malnutrition, immune suppression, or any concern that would affect the integrity of the anastomosis.

Several recent studies have demonstrated superior functional short-term results when comparing colonic J-pouch anal anastomosis with straight coloanal anastomosis.[109–112] Colonic J-pouch anal anastomosis appears to be associated with acceptable morbidity and superior functional results. Patients report decreased frequency of bowel movements during both day and night, ability to defer defecation for more than 30 min, improved continence score, ability to differentiate gas from stool, and decreased need for retarding medications. At 2 months postoperatively, the median frequency of daily bowel movements was 2 for pouch patients versus 6.4 for straight coloanal patients, with a 30% incidence of nocturnal bowel movements in the pouch group versus 62% in the straight coloanal group. At 1 year, the differences were still significant but less marked, with 2 bowel movements per 24 hours in the pouch patients versus 3.5 in the straight group, and a 7% incidence of nocturnal bowel movements versus 24% in the straight coloanal group. A recent study compared 47 patients who underwent colonic J pouch-anal anastomosis with 34 patients who had a low colorectal anastomosis. Functional results were significantly better in the J-pouch group, even when a short rectal segment was present in the straight anastomosis group.[113]

With the advent of sphincter-saving procedures, the operative mortality rate in various series has been in the range of 1% to 3%, with possible complications (anastomotic leak, stricture, bleeding, pelvic sepsis, fecal incontinence, and sexual dysfunction) occurring in 3% to 15% of patients.[114] In 10 series of sphincter-saving resections totaling 1054 patients, the recurrence rate was 12.3%, which is virtually identical to the 12.8% recurrence rate in a cumulative series of 2210 patients treated by APR.[115]

The availability of laparoscopic technology has prompted some surgeons to perform anterior resection by laparoscopy-assisted methods in patients with upper rectal cancers. A prospective nonrandomized comparison of laparoscopic and conventional techniques revealed comparable numbers of resected lymph nodes, but generally shorter distal margins.[116] However, to our knowledge, there is no description of a meticulous total mesorectal excision performed by laparoscopic technique. A cooperative trial from the Cancer and Leukemia Group B (CALGB), comparing randomized patients with colon cancers treated laparoscopically versus conventional technique, has shown no significant difference in outcome at 3 years; however, most patients entered in this study had right colon tumors.

Another technical option in the treatment of cancers of the middle and distal rectum has been abdominotranssacral resection, which involves abdominal mobilization of the left and sigmoid colon with pelvic lymphadenectomy, followed by transsacral rectosigmoid resection and colorectal anastomosis. Although in morbidity and mortality the recurrence rates are comparable with LAR and APR, peculiar to this operation are sacral fecal fistula complications and an approximately 10% incidence of anastomotic complications.[117] In recent years, this technique has been virtually abandoned in favor of low anterior resections and coloanal anastomoses.

A Hartmann's procedure, which involves removal of the rectosigmoid with an end colostomy and closure of the rectal stump, finds its indications in patients with obstructed or perforated rectosigmoid carcinoma, palliative resections, and in patients in whom immediate colorectal anastomosis is not generally advisable.[118] The morbidity rate of a second major operation, required for reestablishment of intestinal continuity, can be assessed on the basis of the chance of cure and patient-related variables.[119]

Adjacent organ resection in the treatment of T4 rectal carcinoma may be required in approximately 5% of patients with rectal cancer.[120] In the absence of metastatic disease, concomitant resection of adjacent organs such as ovaries, uterus, bladder, small intestine, colon, and ureter is advised, since the 5-year survival is based on the stage of the disease.[121]

The advocates of prophylactic oophorectomy during resection for colorectal cancer have cited a 3% to 25% incidence of ovarian metastases and possible prevention of ovarian carcinoma.[122] However, a survival benefit achieved by removal of the ovaries is yet to be demonstrated.

**LOCAL EXCISION.** Nowadays, local excision of early tumors of the distal and middle third of the rectum is generally performed via transanal technique. Posterior surgical approaches to the rectum via a transsacral (Kraske) or a transsphincteric (Mason) approach have been largely abandoned. The major advantage of a transanal local excision of a rectal tumor lies in its low morbidity, lower anesthetic requirement, and faster recovery. Patient selection is crucial, since approximately only 5% of all patients with rectal cancer are good candidates for this procedure. Ideally, all patients considered for local excision should be evaluated by preoperative ERUS. An ideal candidate is a patient with an exophytic, mobile tumor, measuring less than 4 cm in diameter, located within 10 cm of the anal verge, with well- or moderately well-differentiated tumor, confined to the submucosa (T1) or muscularis propria (T2).[123] The key factor in choosing this technique is the prediction of perirectal lymph node involvement, which cannot be removed adequately by this method. A 0% incidence of lymph node metastases in the perirectal tissue has been reported in several studies in patients with well-differentiated sessile exophytic T1 rectal tumors. T1 tumors with unfavorable histology (poor differentiation, lymphovascular invasion, and colloid features) carry a risk of perirectal lymph node metastases of approximately 10%, whereas the risk of lymph node metastases ranges between 22% and 28% for T2 lesions. The incidence of lymph node metastases correlates with tumor grade (0% for grade 1 tumors, 22% for grade 2 tumors, and 50% for grade 3 tumors) and presence of lymphovascular invasion (31% if present, and 19% if absent).[124,125]

Endoscopic local excision of early rectal carcinomas with the snare cautery technique may be adequate therapy for pedunculated lesions with well- or moderately well-differentiated histology and a greater than 2 mm free margin.[126,127]

In order to obtain satisfactory results in transanal excision of rectal tumors, close attention to meticulous surgical technique is paramount. The procedure can be performed under either general or spinal anesthesia and, in high-risk patients, with locoregional pudendal nerve block anesthesia. My preference is to place the patient in the Buie prone jack-knife position for lesions located in the anterior and lateral walls, and in the lithotomy position for lesions located in the posterior wall. The exposure is achieved by using a Pratt rectal bivalve retractor along with a Lone-Star TM retractor in order to obtain adequate visualization during the procedure. It is essential not to disrupt the integrity of the lesion, in order to minimize the risk of implantation of tumor fragments on the suture line. The normal rectal mucosa surrounding the tumor is outlined with a needle-tipped cautery at a margin of greater than 1 cm circumferentially, after traction sutures are placed. A full-thickness excision of all layers of the rectal wall is performed and hemostasis is achieved with the cautery or with suture ligatures, as needed. The specimen is properly oriented for pathologic evaluation and the rectal wall defect is closed, whenever possible, in a transverse fashion to avoid luminal narrowing. An incomplete local excision is considered palliative.[128]

Several studies have proven the effectiveness of this method for curative intent. Local excision alone achieved a 5-year actuarial recurrence-free survival of 87%, and local control of 96%, in 28 patients with favorable histology who were undergoing local excision; although the results were 57% and 68%, respectively, for 28 patients with unfavorable histology (e.g., poor differentiation and lymphovascular invasion).[129] In a review of 10 published series in which local excision alone was used, the cancer-specific survival rate was 89%, with a local recurrence rate of 19%, and a 50% chance of cure after salvage surgery and adjuvant therapy.[130] In a more recent study of 48 patients prospectively evaluated after local excision,

21 patients with favorable histology received local excision alone, whereas patients with T2 or T3 lesions received adjuvant chemoradiation therapy. The overall local or distal recurrence rate was 8%, with recurrence primarily related to the presence of positive margins or aggressive histology.[131]

There is general agreement that positive margins, poor differentiation, or lymphovascular invasion should be an indication for further therapy, even in T1 lesions, and certainly for T2 lesions, since the risk of perirectal adenopathy is on the order of 10% to 30%. These findings have prompted authors to use adjuvant chemoradiation for T2 lesions and selected T3 cancers. Locoregional failure after local excision with radiation therapy, with or without concurring chemotherapy, was evaluated in a review of 11 studies.[132] Local failure was 0% in most studies for T1 lesions (with isolated reports of failure in histologically unfavorable tumors), between 0% and 25% for T2 lesions, and between 20% and 33% in most studies with an adequate number of T3 lesions. On the basis of these findings, most authors would agree that histologically favorable T1 lesions can be treated by local excision alone. In the treatment of T2 lesions, the addition of chemoradiation therapy can significantly decrease the local recurrence rate.[133] Most pathologic T3 lesions benefit from further surgery if patients can tolerate it. Preoperative radiation therapy followed by local excision is less commonly used and makes transanal excision technically more difficult.[134]

A technical variation on transanal excision has been proposed by using a sophisticated operating proctoscope with magnified vision and a variety of instruments for grasping, cutting, coagulating, and suturing.[135] This method of transanal endoscopic microsurgery (TEM), introduced in Germany in 1983, is rather expensive and is presently used in a limited number of centers with special interest in the technique.

Local excision of rectal tumors can also be used for palliative purposes in patients unfit for a major abdominal operation. My experience suggests that survival and symptomatic control can be surprisingly acceptable in older patients.

Other methods for local control include electrocoagulation, endocavitary irradiation, and laser ablation. Electrocoagulation can be used in a limited group of patients who meet selection criteria for cure or palliation, as mentioned. The procedure requires general anesthesia, a formal bowel preparation, and a 1- to 3-day postoperative hospital stay. The overall complication rate (bleeding, stricture, urinary retention, electrical burns, perianal sepsis, perforation, and rectovaginal fistulas in women) is as high as 21%, with a mortality rate of 2.7%.[136] Five-year survival in patients with small exophytic cancers is greater than 70%. However, the recurrence rate is as high as 40%. This method is generally limited to treatment of small lesions in older patients. In similar cases, European centers have reported encouraging results with the use of cryosurgery.[137]

Endocavitary irradiation of early rectal cancer for cure was championed by Jean Papillon.[138] The procedure can be performed in an outpatient setting, and consists of endorectal applications of low-voltage irradiation (20 to 30 Gy during a 6-week period). In a series of 312 patients, the 5-year disease-free survival rate was 74%.[139] This method can also be utilized for palliation, in cases with advanced local disease.[140] The major disadvantage of endocavitary irradiation alone is the inability to obtain a pathologic specimen for adequate staging purposes.

Other methods that have been used in recent years for palliation or preoperative recanalization of the obstructive rectal carcinomas have included use of metallic self-expandable stents and Nd:YAG laser photoablation.[141–143]

In general, if the goals of therapy are limited to palliation to alleviate or significantly reduce the patient's symptoms caused by primary or recurring rectal disease not thought to be resectable for cure, nonresectional, transanal, or endoscopic methods offer the advantage of less morbidity.

## ADJUVANT THERAPY

The impetus to consider adjuvant radiation therapy and chemotherapy in the treatment of adenocarcinoma of the rectum came from the observation of treatment failures as high as 70%, with overall survival averaging 70% for stage II patients, and 40% for stage III patients, 5 years postoperatively.[144] The most common pattern of treatment failure is characterized by locoregional recurrence in the overwhelming majority of patients [70% to 80% of patients have pelvic recurrences alone or in combination with distant metastases], whereas 20% to 30% of treatment failure is characterized by distant metastases alone.[145] If one compares these data with the outstanding results that have been achieved with the technique of total mesorectal excision, leading to local recurrence rates generally ranging between 4% and 10%, it becomes apparent that these exceedingly high local treatment failure rates were due to inadequate technique of resection. It is also clear from the results of studies that have used total mesorectal excision alone in the treatment of patients in stages II and III, that excellent local control will lead to higher overall survival rates as well. Nonetheless, adenocarcinoma of the rectum, the cancer considered fraught with an exceedingly high local recurrence rate and overall worse survival than carcinoma of the colon, was also considered relatively radioresistant and chemoresistant, until a few years ago. A striking comparison can be drawn between adequacy of surgical treatment and of adjuvant treatment in carcinoma of the rectum. In fact, inadequate dosages of radiation therapy and chemotherapy had yielded disappointing results in both the preoperative and postoperative settings, much like inadequate surgery did.[146] Once doses greater than 45 Gy in the preoperative phase were utilized in European studies, a reduction in local recurrence was finally achieved, although a survival benefit could not be demonstrated.[147,148]

What drew the attention of American surgeons to the importance of the combination of chemotherapy plus radiation therapy in the adjuvant treatment of carcinoma of the rectum were clinical studies conducted by the Gastrointestinal Tumor Study Group (GTSG),[149] and by the North Central Cancer Treatment Group (NCCTG).[150] Subsequently, a National Institutes of Health Consensus Development Conference concluded that a combination of postoperative chemotherapy and radiation therapy improved local control, as well as survival, in stages II and III carcinoma of the rectum and recommended that these measures be followed in clinical practice.[151]

The GTSG study revealed a suggestion of improvements in recurrence and survival evident with combination chemoradiation, although this trial failed to achieve statistical significance. The NCCTG study did show an improvement in survival with chemoradiation at 7 years (54% vs. 38%, $p < 0.043$) and this finding was supported by the NSABP R-01 trial, which showed statistically improved disease-free and overall survival in postoperative chemotherapy versus radiotherapy in advanced rectal cancer—although radiotherapy did decrease local recurrence it did not improve survival.[152] From this, the consensus NIH statement from 1990 recommended a postoperative course of chemoradiation to optimize the improvement in survival afforded by postoperative chemotherapy, and the decrease in local recurrence by postoperative radiotherapy. Additional trials followed by verifying that radiotherapy did decrease local recurrence, but did not improve survival among those patients. The NSABP R-02 trial has recently confirmed these earlier findings, revealing that combination chemoradiation does not have an improvement in survival over chemotherapy alone, thus further defining only a local impact from radiotherapy.[153]

The NSABP R-03 trial, designed to evaluate the advantage(s) of preoperative versus postoperative irradiation using chemotherapy-based adjuvant approaches was closed due to poor patient accrual. Nonetheless, additional prospective analyses are essential to evaluate the advantages of preoperative chemoirradiation over those using postoperative therapies. Unfortunately, the early observations from these studies led most American surgeons to focus on the postoperative phase in considering adjuvant therapy in rectal carcinoma, after the tumor could be accurately staged by pathologic methods, whereas our European colleagues, especially those in Scandinavian countries, were focusing on the preoperative assessment and consideration of preoperative radiation therapy.

The theoretical advantages of administering preoperative radiotherapy are several: "sterilization" of circumferential margins around the primary tumor with enhanced radiotherapy effect, since the tumor blood supply has not been disrupted; "sterilization" of pelvic lymphatics to minimize seeding during surgical resection; reduction in size of the primary tumor, which may increase the chances of analsphincter preservation.[154] Chemotherapy agents such as 5-fluorouracil (5-FU) may also have a radiosensitizing effect, and thus enhance the potential for locoregional control.[155] The greatest caveat in the use of any neoadjuvant therapy comes from the limitations inherent in the accuracy of preoperative staging methods, which were discussed in the section on diagnosis. With ERUS, there is up to a 10% chance of understaging the disease, and up to a 20% chance of overstaging the disease, which may lead to erroneously attributing a "downstaging" effect to the neoadjuvant therapy. Nonetheless, several studies have recently claimed a downstaging effect in advanced rectal cancer with the use of preoperative chemoradiation. In a study of 31 patients (24 with fixed, 3 with partially fixed, and 4 with advanced fixed tumors), 23 (74%) were clinically downstaged, and surgical resection could be completed with negative margins in 29 patients (94%).[156] Another study achieved downstaging with preoperative chemoradiation in 14 of 20 patients staged with ERUS. A complete oncologic response (no tumor detected in the rectal wall) was achieved in 7 of 20 patients.[157] Enhanced local control and decreased metastases, in addition to tumor downstaging, were also demonstrated in another study of 23 patients who underwent chemoradiation in the preoperative stage and were compared with T2 and T3 lesions to assess survival, disease-free interval, and pelvic recurrence rate. Treatment included fluorouracil, cisplatin, and 4500 cGy administered preoperatively in a 5-week period. Rectal wall involvement was assessed by CT scan. A sterile pathologic specimen was achieved in 27% of patients and local recurrence rate at short-term follow-up (ranging between 3 and 15 months) was seen in less than 5% of patients. Increased survival, disease-free survival, and decreased pelvic recurrence rates were observed when compared with control patients.[158]

The use of adjuvant therapy in the postoperative setting for stages II and III rectal cancer patients after curative surgery has undergone further modifications with the introduction of protracted infusion of fluorouracil in combination with radiation therapy. In a study of 660 patients, groups were assigned intermittent bolus injections versus protracted venous infusion, as well as systemic chemotherapy with semustin plus fluorouracil, or fluorouracil alone in a higher dose, both before and after the pelvic irradiation. With a median follow-up of 46 months in surviving patients, the group receiving protracted infusion of fluorouracil had a significantly increased time before relapse and improved survival, although there was no evidence of a beneficial effect in patients who received semustin plus fluorouracil.[159]

In addition to the oncologic results, another consideration in choosing whether to use adjuvant therapy in the preoperative or in the postoperative setting pertains to the long-term functional results. In a study of 100 patients with Astler-Coller stage B2 or C tumors, 41 received postoperative chemotherapy and 59 did not. The patients who had chemoradiotherapy had significantly more frequent bowel movements, more "clustering" of bowel movements, more nighttime bowel movements, more frequent incontinence, more need to wear a perineal pad, and were more often unable to defer defecation for more than 15 minutes. Patients who received postoperative chemoradiotherapy also experienced more liquid stools, perianal skin irritation, inability to differentiate stool from gas, and the need to use antidiarrheal medication significantly more often. These effects lasted for the entire duration of follow-up, ranging between 2 and 5 years.[160,161]

On the other hand, when high-dose preoperative radiation therapy (40 + 20 Gy) was delivered in the preoperative setting in 21 patients who then underwent coloanal anastomosis with colonic J-pouch, functional results were quite acceptable. Continence, frequency of bowel movements, and urgency were not significantly different than those reported by surgeons who performed colonic J-pouch anal anastomoses without any adjuvant therapy.[157] However, every effort should be made not to use radiation therapy indiscriminately, and to assess the predictive factors for local recurrence. In fact, a recent randomized study on 203 patients in the Swedish Rectal Cancer Trial showed significantly better functional results in the surgery alone group than in the preoperatively irradiated group.[162]

On the basis of these data, it appears that patients in stages II or III at the time of the preoperative assessment should be considered strongly for preoperative adjuvant therapy. An ongoing controversy is whether or not chemotherapy should be used in addition to radiation therapy in the preoperative phase, since several studies have shown significant beneficial effects in terms of local control if radiation therapy alone is used in the preoperative setting. In a study of 71 patients with clinically resectable adenocarcinoma of the rectum who were treated with preoperative radiation therapy and compared with patients treated with surgery alone, there were similar incidences of postoperative morbidity in their occurrences and severity. With a minimum follow-up of 3 years, the locoregional recurrence rate was 7.8%, and the combined incidence of locoregional recurrence and/or distant metastases was 28%. The 5-year disease-free survival of 71% for the preoperative radiation group compared with 41% for the historical control group of patients treated with surgery alone.[163] As previously mentioned, the dose of radiation plays a crucial role in determining the effectiveness of therapy. A large prospective randomized trial from the Veterans Administration on 361 male patients compared surgery alone [abdominoperineal resection (APR)] with 3150 cGy of preoperative radiotherapy. Five-year survival was 50% for both treated and control patients, and the incidence of positive lymph nodes in the resected specimens was 35% in the preoperative radiation group and 41% in the APR alone controls.[164] Higher doses of preoperative radiation therapy were necessary to achieve results. A group of 161 patients with cancer of the rectum was treated with a total of 5500 to 6000 cGy, then underwent sphincter-preserving surgery for cancer of the rectum 4 to 8 weeks after completion of radiation. They were then followed for a median of 5 years. The overall 5-year Kaplan-Meier survival rate was 79%, with a disease-free survival rate of 73%, and a local recurrence rate of 12.4%.[165] In another study of 90 patients treated with 4500 cGy of preoperative radiation over a 5-week period, followed by a 6-week waiting period before surgery for Dukes' stage A, B, and C rectal adenocarcinoma, an overall 5-year survival rate of 86% with a local recurrence rate of only 1.8% was achieved.[166] A recent retrospective study on 1423 patients from the Mayo Clinic also concluded that surgery alone could only achieve 60% 5-year disease-free survival in stage III.[167]

Although these studies achieved excellent local control and satisfactory 5-year survival, they did not receive the attention they deserved, most likely as a result of the fact that they did not use a control group, were nonrandomized, and included patients with stage I disease who are not likely to benefit from adjuvant therapy. Consequently, most clinicians practicing in the United States were familiar only with the NIH consensus statement of 1990, advocating postoperative adjuvant chemoradiation in patients with stages II and III rectal carcinoma as a treatment with proven effectiveness, both in terms of local control and improvement in survival. A very important and much-awaited contribution came from the Swedish Rectal Cancer Trial data published in April of 1997; 1168 patients with resectable rectal cancer were randomly assigned to undergo preoperative irradiation (25 Gy delivered in five fractions in 1 week, followed by surgery within 1 week) or surgery alone. The radiation treatment did not increase postoperative mortality rates, and at 5 years' follow-up the local recurrence rate was 11% in the group receiving radiotherapy and 27% in the group treated with surgery alone. The overall 5-year survival rate was 68% in the radiotherapy plus surgery group and 48% in the surgery alone group. The cancer-specific survival rates after 9 years were 74% and 65%, respectively. Although the treatment dosage, fractionation of doses, and "rest" before surgery are different from what most American radiation oncologists use, this study deserves credit for demonstrating improved survival as well as local control in a large prospective randomized group of patients with rectal cancer.[168]

Of the 10 randomized trials of preoperative radiation therapy for resectable rectal cancer, 5 have reported a significant decrease in the rate of local recurrence, some found survival improvement in subgroup analysis, but none had shown a significant advantage for the whole group of treated patients.[169] A recently published trial

has analyzed clinically resectable T3 rectal cancer in a total of 32 patients. They received 5-FU, low-dose leucovorin, and concurrent radiation therapy, using doses and techniques of administration that are considered more conventional in the United States, with surgery delayed until 4 to 6 weeks after completion of radiation therapy. 5-FU and leucovorin were administered preoperatively by daily bolus five times and radiation therapy was begun concurrently on day 1 for a total dose of 5040 cGy. Postoperatively, the patients received a median of two monthly cycles of 5-FU leucovorin (range, 0 to 10). There was a complete response rate of 22% (9% pathologic and 13% clinical). Total grade 3 plus acute toxicity was 25%. Of the 20 patients who were thought initially to require an APR, 17 (85%) were able to undergo sphincter-preserving surgery. At a median follow-up of 22 months (range, 3 to 59 months), there was no local failure and the 3-year actuarial disease-free survival rate was 60%.[170] In addition, there are three randomized trials comparing preoperative with postoperative combination therapy for clinically resectable stage III rectal cancer. There are presently two active trials in the United States (the Radiation Therapy Oncology Group, RTOG Study 94-01, and the National Surgical Adjuvant Breast and Bowel Project (NSABP) Protocol RO3) and one in Germany (CAO/ARO/AIO 94). All three studies are using conventional doses and techniques for delivering radiation therapy and concurrent fluorouracil-based chemotherapy but, unfortunately, low accrual has resulted in recent closure of RTOG 94-01 and may jeopardize NSABP RO3 as well.[171]

The combination of hyperthermia with chemoradiation in a preoperative phase has also been advocated in order to improve surgical results. In a group of 84 patients with carcinoma of the rectum, the 5-year survival rate in the hyperthermic chemoradiation therapy (HCRT) plus surgery patients was 91.3% as compared with 64% in patients undergoing surgery only. However, no significant difference was observed in postoperative prognosis in cases without lymph node metastases or with tumors limited to the muscularis propria.[172] Similarly encouraging results for T3 and T4 rectal cancers have been observed in a more recent series of 37 patients with a 38-month survival rate of 86%.[173]

Other ongoing trials are addressing the question of the relative value of preoperative chemoradiotherapy sequencing in patients with T3 rectal cancer, from the Eastern Cooperative Oncology Group (ECOG), the South West Oncology Group (SWOG), the Cancer and Leukemia Group B (CALGB) and North Central Cancer Treatment Group (NCCTG). Other phase I and II trials are addressing the effectiveness of newer chemotherapeutic agents and preoperative radiation in patients with locally advanced or recurrent rectal cancer. The clinicians who will bear the greatest responsibility in meeting accrual targets are surgeons, since we are usually the first treatment consultants. It is imperative that surgical technique be standardized just as precisely as dosage and delivery intervals of radiation therapy and chemotherapy. Total mesorectal excision with autonomic nerve preservation should be documented carefully in a registry of operative procedures following the examples of our Swedish and Norwegian colleagues.

## TREATMENT OF LOCALLY RECURRENT RECTAL CANCER

Local recurrence in the pelvis after curative treatment for rectal carcinoma poses a significant challenge to the oncologic surgeon. As discussed in the previous sections of this chapter, there is a great variability in the incidence of this event, generally related to the extent of surgery as well as the utilization of adjuvant treatment modalities. There is general agreement in the literature that the recurrence rate of APR and sphincter-saving resection are virtually identical.[174]

Local recurrence can be of five types[175]:

1. Anastomotic, when it arises from within the bowel, generally as a result of inadequate distal margins.
2. Perianastomotic, when it occurs in proximity to anastomosis, by extrinsic disease with an inward growth pattern, generally from inadequate mesorectal excision.
3. Perineal, in the scar following APR, generally from direct tumor implantation at the time of surgery.
4. Pelvic wall, posterolateral, often fixed to bone and major neurovascular structures.
5. Anterior genitourinary, in the proximity of prostate, seminal vesicles, urinary bladder, uterus, or ovaries.

Pelvic recurrence is generally suspected in the presence of pelvic pain or pressure, or new onset of rectal bleeding, vaginal bleeding or discharge, or dysuria. A complete physical examination including rectal and pelvic exam, will generally detect the problem. Endoscopic evaluation of the neorectum, for sphincter-saving resections, is necessary to obtain visualization and biopsies. Imaging tests rely on the use of CT to assess the pelvic extent of the disease as well as the presence of distant metastatic deposits, and rectal or vaginal ultrasonography.

In recent years, magnetic resonance imaging (MRI) as well as positron emission tomography (PET) imaging have shown significant accuracy in detecting locally recurring colorectal carcinoma.[176,177]

Another imaging modality that may be particularly useful in the overall treatment planning in this setting (determination of recurrent disease as well as exclusion of distant metastatic disease) is radioimmunoscintigraphy with the use of monoclonal antibodies.[178] A pelvic recurrence is often suspected on the basis of an elevated carcinoembryonic antigen (CEA) level, and the use of radiolabeled antibodies to CEA has been a logical step toward precise recognition and direction of treatment for the recurrent disease. A more accurate prognostic assessment along with the improvements in diagnostic imaging in recent years have replaced the "second-look" procedures for cancer of the rectum.[179] After completion of a diagnostic evaluation, an assessment of the goals of treatment has to be considered. If distant extrapelvic disease is present, the goals of therapy are going to be palliative, and the potential morbidity and mortality of extensive pelvic surgery must be weighed against the likely inability to achieve a cure. In this setting, symptomatic control and maintenance of the patient's quality of life must be the essential goals of palliation. Palliative efforts directed at prevention of large bowel obstruction may require the use of a sigmoid colostomy. Alternatively, reestablishment of intestinal luminal patency can be achieved by electrofulguration, laser ablation, or placement of self-expandable metallic stents. Maintenance of nutritional status can be achieved by gastrostomy or jejunostomy tube placement by surgical or endoscopic method. Palliation of pain may be required in a large number of these patients. Radiation therapy alone or in combination with chemotherapy may be used for palliation of both bleeding and pain. Narcotic analgesics

are generally necessary, and the use of neurosurgical procedures such as cordotomy or rhizotomy are rarely necessary.

If salvage therapy is considered for a curative effort, an assessment of resectability of the pelvic recurrence is essential, since surgery is the only treatment that can provide any hope for a cure. It has been estimated that up to 50% of local recurrences of rectal cancer represent failure of adequate locoregional treatment.[170] In these patients, an aggressive surgical approach, often with concomitant use of radiation and chemotherapy, may achieve a potential cure. The technique of abdominosacral resection, with or without pelvic exenteration, to remove pelvic recurrence and its musculoskeletal extension was used in 63 patients with recurrent rectal cancer with curative intent in 47 and for palliation in 6. Long-term survival for 4 years was achieved in 14 of 43 patients (33%), with significant mortality rate (88.5%) in the curative group.[180] In another study of 43 consecutive patients with pelvic recurrence of colorectal adenocarcinoma, a multimodality treatment protocol was reported, with 5 weeks of pelvic external-beam radiation therapy (45 Gy) and continuous intravenous infusion of 5-FU and/or cisplatin. This was followed by surgery that included intraoperative radiation therapy boost (10 to 20 Gy) for 21 patients and brachytherapy for 4 patients. In 77% of patients, resection could be achieved with curative intent, and 88% of patients had margin-negative resection, with 48% undergoing sphincter-preserving operation. At a median follow-up of 26 months, the local recurrence rate was 67% with a median survival for resected patients of 34 months, actuarial 5-year disease-free survival of 37%, and an overall survival of 58%.[181]

Intraoperative radiation therapy has been advocated as an adjunct to palliative surgery for locally recurrent rectal carcinoma in a series of 42 patients to improve local control and possibly improve survival.[182] Although the exact role of chemotherapy and radiation therapy in the treatment of pelvic recurrences is yet to be clearly defined, it would appear that an aggressive regimen of preoperative chemoradiation may facilitate subsequent extended surgical resection with negative margins and curative intent in this unfortunate group of patients.

## Acknowledgments

*The authors appreciate the assistance of Cheri L. Canon, M.D., Sean Fell, M.D., Ruedi F.L. Thoeni, M.D. and Craig Philpot, M.D., of the Department of Radiology, University of Alabama in Birmingham; and Robert O. Santaella, M.D., Chief Resident in Surgery, University of Alabama in Birmingham.*

## REFERENCES

1. GREENLEE RT et al: Cancer statistics. CA: Cancer J Clin 50:7, 2000.
2. COLEMAN M et al: Trends in cancer incidence and mortality. International Agency for Research on Cancer 1993; 121:1–806.
3. WHITTEMORE AS et al: Diet, physical activity, and colorectal cancer among Chinese in North America and China. J Natl Cancer Inst 82:915, 1990.
4. BURKITT DP: Epidemiology of cancer of the colon and rectum. Cancer 28:3, 1971.
5. WILMINK AB: Overview of the epidemiology of colorectal cancer. Dis Colon Rectum 40:483, 1997.

6. Potter JD: Nutrition and colorectal cancer. Cancer Causes Control 7:127, 1996.

7. Fuchs CS et al: Dietary fiber and the risk of colorectal cancer and adenoma in women. N Engl J Med 340:169, 1999.

8. Gerhardsson de Verdier M et al: Meat, cooking methods, and colorectal cancer: A case reference study in Stockholm. Intl J Cancer 49:520, 1991.

9. McMichael A, Giles G: Colorectal cancer, in Trends in Cancer Incidence and Mortality, R Doll et al (eds). Cold Spring Harbor, NY, Cold Spring Harbor Laboratory Press, 1994, pp 77–98.

10. Giovannucci E et al: The prospective study of cigarette smoking and risk of colorectal adenoma and colorectal cancer in US men and women. J Natl Cancer Inst 86:192, 1994.

11. Levitt MD et al: Rectal cancer after pelvic irradiation. J Roy Soc Med 83:153, 1990.

12. Wilmink AB: Overview of the epidemiology of colorectal cancer. Dis Colon Rectum 40:483, 1997.

13. Fearon E, Vogelstein B: A genetic model for colorectal tumorigenesis. Cell 61:759, 1990.

14. Vogelstein B et al: Genetic alterations during colorectal tumor development. N Engl J Med 319:525, 1988.

15. Pricolo VE et al: Topographic genotyping of colorectal carcinoma: from a molecular carcinogenesis model to clinical relevance. Ann Surg Oncol 4:269, 1997.

16. Reymond MA et al: DCC protein as a predictor of distant metastases after curative resection for rectal cancer. Dis Colon Rectum 41:755, 1998.

17. Marnett L: Aspirin and the potential role of prostaglandins in colon cancer. Cancer Res 52:5575, 1992.

18. Paganini HA: Aspirin and the prevention of colorectal cancer: A review of the evidence. Semin Surg Oncol 10:158, 1994.

19. Newcomb P et al: Screening sigmoidoscopy and colorectal cancer mortality. J Natl Cancer Inst 84:1572, 1992.

20. Selby J et al: A case control study of screening sigmoidoscopy and mortality from colorectal cancer. N Engl J Med 326:6537, 1992.

21. Schubert W: Dukes' classification: American chaos versus British order. Can J Surg 33:8, 1990.

22. Jass JR et al: The grading of rectal cancer: histological perspective in a multivariate analysis of 444 cases. Histopathology 10:437, 1986.

23. Gastrointestinal Tumor Study Group. Prolongation of the disease-free survival in surgically treated rectal carcinoma. N Engl J Med 312:1465, 1985.

24. Wolmark N et al: The prognostic value of the modification of the Dukes' C class of colorectal cancer: An analysis of the NSABP clinical trials. Ann Surg 203:115, 1986.

25. Abel ME et al: Practice parameters for the treatment of rectal carcinoma. Dis Colon Rectum 36:989, 1993.

26. Hojo K et al: Lymphatic spread and its prognostic value in patients with rectal cancer. Am J Surg 144:350, 1982.

27. Freedman LS et al: Multivariate analysis of prognostic factors for operable rectal cancer. Lancet 2:733, 1984.

28. Phillips RKS et al: Large bowel cancer: Surgical pathology and its relationship to survival. Br J Surg 71:604, 1984.

29. Orkin BA et al: Extended resection for locally advanced primary adenocarcinoma of the rectum. Dis Colon Rectum 32:286, 1989.

30. Bear HD et al: Colon and rectal carcinoma in the west of Scotland: Symptoms, histologic characteristics, and outcome. Am J Surg 147:441, 1984.

31. Taylor MC et al: Prognostic factors in colon and rectal carcinoma of young adults. Can J Surg 31:150, 1988.

32. Enblad G et al: Relationship between age and survival in cancer of the colon and rectum with special reference to patients less than 40 years of age. Br J Surg 77:611, 1990.

33. Lockhart-Mummery HF, Dukes CE: The surgical treatment of malignant rectal polyps. Lancet 269:751, 1952.

34. Morson BC: Factors influencing the prognosis of early cancer of the rectum. Proc Roy Soc Med 59:607, 1966.

35. Horn A et al: Venous and neural invasion as predictors of recurrence in rectal adenocarcinoma. Dis Colon Rectum 34:798, 1991.

36. Wahlstrom B et al: Association of ploidy and cell proliferation, Dukes' classification and histopathologic differentiation in adenocarcinomas of colon and rectum. Eur J Surg 158:237, 1992.

37. Moran MR et al: Multifactorial analysis of local recurrences in rectal cancer, including DNA ploidy studies: A predictive model. World J Surg 17:801, 1993.

38. Moertel CG et al: The preoperative carcinoembryonic antigen test in the diagnosis, staging and prognosis of colorectal cancer. Cancer 58:603, 1986.

39. Laurent-Puig P et al: Survival and acquired genetic alterations in colorectal cancer. Gastroenterology 102:1136, 1992.

40. Jen J et al: Allelic loss of chromosome 18q and prognosis in colorectal cancer. N Engl J Med 331:213, 1994.

41. Pricolo VE et al: Prognostic value of TP53 and K-ras 2 mutational analysis in stage III carcinoma of the colon. Am J Surg 171:41, 1996.

42. Pricolo et al: Mutated p53 gene as an independent adverse predictor of survival in colon carcinoma. Arch Surg 132:371, 1997.

43. Gryfe R et al: Tumor microsatellite instability and clinical outcome in young patients with colorectal cancer. N Engl J Med 342:69, 2000.

44. Soderberg CH et al: Changing trends in the overall management of rectal cancer. RI Med 78:167, 1995.

45. Pricolo VE: Gastrointestinal endoscopy, in Care of the Surgical Patient. Surgical Technique Supplement American College of Surgeons, 2:1, 1993.

46. Durdey P, Williams NS: Preoperative evaluation of patients with lower rectal carcinoma. World J Surg 16:430, 1992.

47. Coburn MC et al: Factors affecting prognosis and management of carcinoma of the colon and rectum in patients more than eighty years of age. J Am Coll Surg 179:65, 1994.

48. Morson BC et al: Policy of local excision for early carcinoma of the colorectum. Gut 18:1045, 1977.

49. Nicholls RJ et al: The clinical staging of rectal cancer. Br J Surg 69:404, 1992.

50. Freeny PC et al: Colorectal carcinoma evaluation with CT: Preoperative staging and detection of postoperative recurrence. Radiology 158:347, 1986.

51. Grabbe E et al: The perirectal fascia: Morphology and staging of rectal carcinoma. Radiology 149:241, 1983.

52. Dixon AK et al: Preoperative computer tomography of carcinoma of the rectum. Br J Radiol 54:655, 1981.

53. Thompson WM et al: Preoperative and postoperative CT staging of rectosigmoid carcinoma. AJR 146:703, 1986.

54. Thoeni RF et al: Detection and staging of rectal and rectosigmoid cancer by computed tomography. Radiology 141:135, 1981.

55. Williams NS et al: Preoperative staging of rectal neoplasms

and its impact on clinical management. Br J Surg 72:868, 1985.

56. Orrum WJ et al: Endorectal ultrasound in the preoperative staging of rectal tumors. Dis Colon Rectum 33:654, 1990.

57. Beynon J et al: Preoperative staging of local invasion in rectal cancer using endoluminal ultrasound. J Roy Soc Med 80:23, 1987.

58. Hildebrandt U, Feifel G: Preoperative staging of rectal cancer by endorectal ultrasound. Dis Colon Rectum 28:42, 1995.

59. Boscaini M et al: Transrectal ultrasonography: Three years experience. Intl J Colorectal Dis 1:208, 1986.

60. Danon J: An evaluation of the role of rectal endosonography in rectal cancer. Ann Roy Coll Surgeons [England] 71:131, 1989.

61. Holdsworth PJ et al: Endoluminal ultrasound and computed tomography in the staging of rectal cancer. Br J Surg 75:1019, 1988.

62. Katsura Y et al: Endorectal ultrasonography for the assessment of wall invasion and lymph node metastases and rectal cancer. Dis Colon Rectum 35:362, 1992.

63. Lindmark G et al: The value of endosonography in preoperative staging of rectal cancer. Intl J Colorectal Dis 7:162, 1992.

64. Milsom JW, Graffner H: Intrarectal ultrasonography in rectal cancer staging and in evaluation of pelvic disease. Clinical uses of intrarectal ultrasound. Ann Surg 212:602, 1990.

65. Herzog U et al: How accurate is endorectal ultrasound in the preoperative staging of rectal cancer? Dis Colon Rectum 36:127, 1993.

66. Deen KI et al: Preoperative staging of rectal neoplasms with endorectal ultrasonography. Semin Colon Rectal Surg 6:78, 1985.

67. Yamashita Y et al: Evaluation of endorectal ultrasound for the assessment of wall invasion of rectal cancer. Dis Colon Rectum 31:617, 1988.

68. Solomon MJ et al: Reliability and validity studies of endoluminal ultrasonography for anorectal disorders. Dis Colon Rectum 37:546, 1994.

69. Yoshida M et al: Endoscopic assessment of invasion of colorectal tumors with the new high frequency ultrasound probe. Gastrointest Endosc 41:587, 1995.

70. Milsom JW et al: Preoperative biopsy of perirectal lymph nodes in rectal cancer using endoluminal ultrasonography. Dis Colon Rectum 37:364, 1994.

71. Heriot AG et al: Preoperative staging of rectal carcinoma. Br J Surg 86:17, 1999.

72. Hodgman CG et al: Preoperative staging of rectal carcinoma by computed tomography and 0.15T magnetic resonance imaging. Dis Colon Rectum 29:446, 1986.

73. Kusonoki M et al: Preoperative detection of local extension of carcinoma of the rectum using magnetic resonance imaging. J Am Coll Surg 179:653, 1994.

74. Schnall MD et al: Rectal tumor stage: Correlation of endorectal MR imaging and pathologic findings. Radiology 190:709, 1994.

75. Goldenberg DM et al: Clinical studies of cancer radioimmunodetection with carcinoembryonic antigen monoclonal antibody fragments labeled with indium 123 [$^{123}$In] or $^{99m}$Tc. Cancer Res 50:909, 1990.

76. Gero EJ et al: The CA 72-4 radioimmunoassay for detection of the TAG-72 carcinoma associated antigen in serum of patients. J Clin Lab Anal 3:363, 1989.

77. Lind T et al: Anticarcinoembryonic antigen immunoscintigraphy and serum CA levels in patients with suspected primary and recurring colorectal carcinoma. J Nucl Med 32:3213, 1991.

78. Beatty JD et al: Preoperative imaging of colorectal carcinoma with 111In-labeled anticarcinoembryonic antigen monoclonal antibody. Cancer Res 46:6494, 1986.

79. Tempero M et al: New imaging techniques in colorectal cancer. Semin Oncol 22:448, 1995.

80. Ito M et al: Recurrent rectal cancer in scar: Differentiation with PET and MR imaging. Radiology 182:549, 1992.

81. Schlag P et al: Scar or recurrent rectal cancer. Positron emission tomography is more helpful for diagnosis than immunoscintigraphy. Arch Surg 124:197, 1989.

82. Gupta NC et al: PET-FDG imaging for follow-up evaluation of treated colorectal cancer. Radiology 199:181, 1991.

83. Tahara T et al: High [18F] fluorodeoxyglucose uptake in abdominal abscesses: A PET study. J Comput Assist Tomogr 13:829, 1989.

84. Heald RJ, Karanjie ND: Results of radical surgery for rectal cancer. World J Surg 16:848, 1992.

85. Enker WE: Designing the optimal surgery for rectal carcinoma. Cancer 78:1847, 1996.

86. Miles WE: A method of performing abdominoperineal excision for carcinoma of the rectum and of the terminal portion of the pelvic colon. Lancet 2:1812, 1908.

87. Kirwan W et al: Declining indications for abdominoperineal resection. Br J Surg 76:1061, 1989.

88. Cole PP: The intramural spread of rectal carcinoma. Br Med J 1:431, 1913.

89. Grinnell RS: Distal intramural spread of carcinoma of the rectum and rectosigmoid. Surg Gynecol Obstet 99:421, 1954.

90. Quer EA et al: Retrograde intramural spread of carcinoma of the rectum and rectosigmoid. Surg Gynecol Obstet 96:24, 1953.

91. Wilson SM, Beahrs OH: The curative treatment of carcinoma of the sigmoid, rectosigmoid and rectum. Ann Surg 183:556, 1976.

92. Pollett WG, Nicholls RJ: The relationship between the extent of distal clearance and survival in local recurrence rates after anterior resection for carcinoma of the rectum. Ann Surg 198:159, 1983.

93. Wolmark N, Fisher B: An analysis of survival and treatment failures following abdominal perineal and sphincter-saving resection in Dukes' B and C rectal carcinoma. Ann Surg 204:480, 1986.

94. Shirouzu K et al: Distal spread of rectal cancer and optimal distal margin of resection for sphincter-preserving surgery. Cancer 76:388, 1995.

95. Quirk EP et al: Local recurrence of rectal adenocarcinoma due to inadequate surgical resection. Histologic study of lateral tumor spread in surgical excision. Lancet 2:996, 1986.

96. Heald RJ et al: The mesorectum and rectal cancer—The clue to pelvic resection? Br J Surg 69:613, 1982.

97. Heald RJ, Rya RD: Recurrence and survival after mesorectal excision for rectal cancer. Lancet 1:1476, 1986.

98. Laxamana A et al: Long-term results of anterior resection using the double-stapling technique. Dis Colon Rectum 38:1246, 1995.

99. Enker WE et al: Total mesorectal excision in the operative treatment of carcinoma of the rectum. J Am Coll Surg 181:335, 1995.

100. Havenga K et al: Male and female sexual and urinary function after total mesorectal excision with autonomic nerve preservation for carcinoma of the rectum. J Am Coll Surg 182:495, 1996.

101. Scott N et al: Total mesorectal excision and local recurrence: a study of tumour spread in the mesorectum distal to rectal cancer. Br J Surg 82:1031, 1995.

102. HIDA J et al: Lymph node metastases detected in the mesorectum distal to carcinoma of the rectum by the clearing method: justification of total mesorectal excision. J Am Coll Surg 84:584, 1997.

103. GRINNELL RS: Results of ligation of inferior mesenteric artery of the aorta and resection of carcinoma of the descending and sigmoid colon and rectum. Surg Gynecol Obstet 121:1031, 1965.

104. STEPHENSON KR et al: Perioperative blood transfusion associated with decreased times recurrence and decreased survival after resection of colon and rectal metastases. Ann Surg 208:679, 1988.

105. WEIDEN PL et al: Perioperative blood transfusion does not increase the risk of colon and rectal recurrence in cancer. Cancer 60:870, 1987.

106. MACFARLANE JK et al: Mesorectal excision for rectal cancer. Lancet 341:457, 1993.

107. LAZORTHES F et al: Resection of the rectum with construction of a colonic reservoir in coloanal anastomosis for carcinoma of the rectum. Br J Surg 73:136, 1986.

108. PARC R et al: Resection in coloanal anastomosis with colonic reservoir for rectal carcinoma. Br J Surg 73:139, 1986.

109. CAVALIERE F et al: Coloanal anastomosis for rectal cancer: long-term results at the Mayo and Cleveland Clinics. Dis Colon Rectum 38:807, 1995.

110. SEOW-CHOEN F, GOH HS: Prospective randomized trial comparing J colonic pouch anal anastomosis and straight coloanal reconstruction. Br J Surg 82:608, 1995.

111. WANG JY et al: Staple colonic J pouch anal anastomosis without a diverting colostomy for rectal carcinoma. Dis Colon Rectum 40:30, 1997.

112. HALLBOOK O et al: Randomized comparison of straight and colonic J pouch anastomosis after low anterior resection. Ann Surg 224:58, 1996.

113. DEHNI N et al: Long term functional outcome after low anterior resection. Dis Colon Rectum 41:817, 1998.

114. CORMAN ML: *Colon and Rectal Surgery,* 2d ed. Philadelphia, JB Lippincott, 1989, pp 534–539.

115. HACKFORD AW: The extent of major resection for rectal cancer. Semin Colon Rectal Surg 1:16, 1990.

116. TATE JJT et al: Prospective comparison of laparoscopic and conventional anterior resection. Br J Surg 80:1396, 1993.

117. LOCALIO SA, ENG K: *Abdominosacral Resection in Colorectal Tumors.* Philadelphia, JB Lippincott, 1986, pp 185–190.

118. DIXON AR, HOLMES JT: Hartmann's procedure for carcinoma of the rectum and distal sigmoid colon: five-year audit. J Roy Coll Surg [Edinb] 35:166, 1990.

119. GHORRA S et al: Colostomy closure: Impact of preoperative risk factors on morbidity. Am J Surg 65(3):266, 1999.

120. HORTON BA et al: Extended resection for locally advanced primary carcinoma of the rectum. Dis Colon Rectum 32:286, 1989.

121. BOEY J et al: Pelvic extenteration for locally advanced colorectal carcinomas. Ann Surg 195:513, 1982.

122. O'BRIEN P et al: Oophorectomy in women with carcinoma of the colon and rectum. Surg Gynecol Obstet 163:827, 1981.

123. BIGGERS OR et al: Local excision of rectal cancer. Dis Colon Rectum 29:374, 1986.

124. MINSKY BD et al: Selection criteria for local excision with or without adjuvant radiation therapy for rectal cancer. Cancer 63:1421, 1989.

125. BRODSKY J et al: Variables correlated with the risk of lymph node metastases in early rectal cancer. Cancer 69:322, 1992.

126. NIVATVONGS S et al: The risk of lymph node metastases in colorectal polyps with invasive adenocarcinoma. Dis Colon Rectum 34:323, 1991.

127. TANAKA S et al: Clinical pathologic features of early rectal carcinoma and indications for endoscopic treatment. Dis Colon Rectum 39:959, 1995.

128. MORSON BC et al: Policy of local excision for early cancer of the colorectum. Gut 18:1045, 1977.

129. WILLETT CJ et al: Selection factors for local excision or abdominoperineal resection of early stage rectal cancer. Cancer 73:2716, 1994.

130. GRAHAM RA et al: Local excision of rectal carcinoma. Am J Surg 160:306, 1990.

131. BLEDAY R et al: Prospective evaluation of local excision for small rectal cancers. Dis Colon Rectum 40:388, 1997.

132. NG AK et al: Sphincter preservation therapy for distal rectal carcinoma. A review. Cancer 79:671, 1996.

133. BLEDAY R, STEELE G JR: Adjuvant therapy after local excision for rectal cancer. Semin Colon Rectal Surg 7:55, 1986.

134. DESPRETZ J et al: Conservative management of tumors of the rectum by radiotherapy and local excision. Dis Colon Rectum 33:113, 1990.

135. BUESS G: Review: Transanal endoscopic microsurgery (TEM). J Roy Coll Surg (Edinb) 38:239, 1993.

136. EISENSTADT TE, OLIVER GC: Electrocoagulation for adenocarcinoma of the lower rectum. World J Surg 16:458, 1992.

137. HEBLER G et al: Local procedures in the management of rectal cancer. World J Surg 11:499, 1987.

138. PAPILLON J: Intracavitary irradiation of early rectal cancer for cure: a series of 186 cases. Cancer 36:696, 1975.

139. PAPILLON J, BERARD PH: Endocavitary irradiation in the conservative treatment of adenocarcinoma of the lower rectum. World J Surg 16:451, 1992.

140. SISCHY B et al: Treatment of rectal carcinoma by means of endocavitary irradiation: a progress report. Cancer 46:1957, 1980.

141. ECKHAUSER ML et al: The role of preresectional laser regionalization for obstructive carcinoma of the colon and rectum. Surgery 106:710, 1989.

142. ITABASHI M et al: Self-expanding stainless steel stent application in rectosigmoid stricture. Dis Colon Rectum 36:508, 1993.

143. BANEKER GW et al: Endoscopic laser recanalization is effective for prevention and treatment of obstruction in sigmoid and rectal cancer. Arch Surg 126:1348, 1991.

144. BLEDAY R, WONG WD: Recent advances in surgery for colon and rectal cancer. Curr Probl Cancer 17:1, 1993.

145. SHINGLETON WW, PROSNITZ LI: Adjuvant therapy for colorectal cancer. Curr Probl Cancer 9:1, 1985.

146. GALLOWAY DJ et al: Adjuvant multimodality treatment of rectal cancer. Br J Surg 36:440, 1989.

147. GERARD A et al: Preoperative radiation as adjuvant treatment in rectal cancer. Ann Surg 208:606, 1988.

148. WILKING N: Preoperative short-term radiation therapy in operable rectal carcinoma. Cancer 66:49, 1990.

149. KROOK JE et al: Effective surgical adjuvant therapy for high risk rectal carcinoma. N Engl J Med 324:709, 1991.

150. KROOK JE et al: Radiation versus sequential radiation-chemotherapy-radiation: A study of the North Central Cancer Treatment Group, Duke University and the Mayo Clinic (abstract). Proc Am Soc Clin Oncol 5:82, 1986.

151. NIH CONSENSUS STATEMENT: Adjuvant therapy for patients with colon and rectal cancer. 264:1444, 1990.

152. FISHER B et al: Postoperative adjuvant chemotherapy or radiation therapy for rectal cancer: Results from NSABP Protocol R-01. J Natl Cancer Inst 80:21, 1988.

153. WOLMARK N et al: Randomized trial of postoperative adjuvant chemotherapy with or without radiotherapy for carcinoma of the rectum: NSABP Protocol R-02. J Natl Cancer Inst 92:388, 2000.

154. OTA DM: Preoperative radiation for rectal cancer: benefits and controversies. Ann Surg Oncol 3:419, 1996.

155. BYFIELD JE et al: Pharmacologic requirements for obtaining sensitization of human tumor cells in vitro to combined 5-fluorouracil or Ftorafur and x-rays. Int J Rad Oncol Biol Phys 8:1923, 1982.

156. CHEN CT et al: Downstaging of advanced rectal cancer following combined preoperative chemotherapy and high dose radiation. Intl J Rad Oncol Biol Phys 30:169, 1994.

157. MEADE PG et al: Preoperative chemoradiation downstages locally advanced ultrasound staged rectal cancer. Am J Surg 170:609, 1995.

158. CHARI RL et al: Preoperative radiation and chemotherapy in the treatment of adenocarcinoma of the rectum. Ann Surg 221:778, 1995.

159. O'CONNELL MJ et al: Improving adjuvant therapy for rectal cancer by combining protracted infusion of fluorouracil with radiation therapy after curative surgery. N Engl J Med 331:502, 1994.

160. KOLLMORGEN CS et al: The long-term effect of adjuvant postoperative chemoradiotherapy for rectal carcinoma and bowel function. Ann Surg 220:676, 1994.

161. ROUANET P et al: Conservative surgery for low rectal carcinoma after high-dose radiation: functional and oncologic results. Ann Surg 221:67, 1995.

162. DAHLBERG M et al: Preoperative irradiation affects functional results after surgery for rectal cancer. Dis Colon Rectum 41:543, 1998.

163. MENDENHALL WM et al: Preoperative irradiation for clinically resectable rectal adenocarcinoma. Semin Radiat Oncol 3:48, 1993.

164. HIGGINS GA et al: Preoperative radiation and surgery for cancer of the rectum. Veterans Administration Surgical Oncology Group Trial II. Cancer 68:352, 1986.

165. MOHIUDDIN M, MARKS G: Patterns of recurrence following high-dose preoperative radiation and sphincter-preserving surgery for cancer of the rectum. Dis Colon Rectum 36:117, 1993.

166. KODNER IJ et al: Preoperative irradiation for rectal cancer improves local control and long-term survival. Ann Surg 209:194, 1989.

167. ZAHEER S et al: Surgical treatment of adenocarcinoma of the rectum. Ann Surg 227:800, 1998.

168. SWEDISH RECTAL CANCER TRIAL: Improved survival with preoperative radiotherapy in resectable rectal cancer. N Engl J Med 336:980, 1997.

169. COHEN AM et al: Cancer of the rectum, in *Cancer: Principles and Practice of Oncology,* 5th ed. VT DeVita et al (eds). Philadelphia, Lippincott-Raven, 1997, pp 1197–1234.

170. GRANN A et al: Preliminary results of preoperative 5-fluorouracil, low-dose leucovorin, and concurrent radiation-therapy for clinically resectable T3 rectal cancer. Dis Colon Rectum 40:515, 1997.

171. MINSKY BD: Adjuvant therapy for rectal cancer—A good first step. N Engl J Med 336:1016, 1997.

172. OHNO S et al: Improved surgical results after combining preoperative hyperthermia with chemotherapy and radiotherapy for patients with carcinoma of the rectum. Dis Colon Rectum 40:401, 1997.

173. RAU B et al: Preoperative hyperthermia combined with radiochemotherapy in locally advanced rectal cancer: a phase II clinical trial. Ann Surg 227:380, 1998.

174. SAGAR PN, PEMBERTON JH: Surgical management of locally recurrent rectal cancer. Br J Surg 83:293, 1996.

175. PILIPSHEN SJ: Cancer of the rectum: Local recurrence, in *Current Therapy in Colon and Rectal Surgery,* VW Fazio (ed). Hamilton, Ontario, BC Decker, 1990, pp 137–149.

176. KRESTIN GP: Is magnetic resonance imaging the method of choice in the diagnosis of recurring rectal carcinoma. Abdom Imaging 22:343, 1997.

177. KEOGAN NT et al: Local recurrence of rectal cancer: Evaluation with F18 fluorodeoxyglucose PET imaging. Abdom Imaging 22:332, 1997.

178. SCHULTE WJ: Use of monoclonal antibodies in colorectal cancer: A review. World J Surg 22:38, 1996.

179. WANGENSTEEN OH et al: An interim report on the "second look" procedure for cancer of the stomach, colon and rectum and for limited intraperitoneal carcinosis. Surg Gynecol Obstet 99:257, 1954.

180. WANEBO HJ et al: Pelvic resection of recurrent rectal cancer. Ann Surg 220:586, 1994.

181. LOWY AM et al: Preoperative infusional chemoradiation, selective intraoperative radiation and resection for locally advanced pelvic recurrence of colorectal carcinoma. Ann Surg 223:177, 1996.

182. SUZUKI K et al: Intraoperative irradiation after palliative surgery for locally recurrent rectal cancer. Cancer 75:939, 1995.

# 16C / ANAL CANCER

*John H. Scholefield and John MA Northover*

## INTRODUCTION

Anal cancer is a rare tumor, accounting for only 3% to 5% of all large-bowel malignancies. Over 80% of anal cancers are of squamous origin (the largest group of the epidermoid anal tumors). Squamous cancers may arise from the squamous epithelium of the anal canal and perianal area; 10% are adenocarcinomas arising from the glandular mucosa of the upper anal canal, the anal glands, and ducts. A very rare and particularly malignant tumor is anal melanoma. Lymphomas and sarcomas of the anus are even less common, but they have increased in incidence in recent years, particularly among patients with human immunodeficiency virus (HIV) infection. There has also been a rise in the incidence of other anal epidermoid tumors among patients with HIV.

Traditionally the anal region is divided into the anal canal and the anal margin or verge. The natural history, demography, and surgical management differ among these areas. There has been controversy regarding the exact definition of the anal canal. Anatomists see it as lying between the dentate line and the anal verge, whereas surgically it is defined as lying between the anorectal ring and the anal verge. For pathologists, the anal canal has been defined as corresponding to the longitudinal extent of the internal anal sphincter.[1] The canal above the dentate line is lined by rectal mucosa, except for a small zone immediately above the line called the transitional or junctional zone.[2] Inferiorly, the canal is covered by stratified squamous epithelium. Further confusion relates to the definition of the anal canal and anal margin as sites for cancer. The anal margin is variously described as the visible area external to the anal verge, or as the area below the dentate line. This argument has become less important as surgery plays a decreased role in treatment, but reports of surgical results from past decades are confused by this variation in definition.

## EPIDERMOID TUMORS

### ETIOLOGY AND PATHOGENESIS

Anal squamous cell carcinomas are relatively uncommon tumors; there are between 250 and 300 new cases per year in England and Wales. Based on these figures, each consultant general surgeon might expect to see one anal carcinoma every 3 to 4 years. However, anal cancers are probably underreported, since some anal canal tumors are misclassified as rectal tumors and some perianal tumors as squamous carcinomas of skin.

The Office of Population Censuses and Surveys' Cancer Statistics for England and Wales[3] recorded 289 cases of anal cancer in 1988. The average age at presentation is 57 years for both sexes, but canal tumors are more common in women, whereas margin tumors are more common in men. However, these figures must be interpreted with caution since the distinction between anal canal and anal margin is poorly defined.

There is wide geographic variation in the incidence of anal cancers around the world,[4] but again these figures must be interpreted with caution for reasons given above. Nevertheless, a low incidence (2 cases per 100,000 of population) is reported by Rizal in the Philippines, and the highest incidence (36 cases per 100,000 of population) is reported in Geneva, Switzerland. Other areas of high incidence are Poland (Warsaw) and Brazil (Recife).[4] It is notable that these areas also have a high incidence of cervical, vulval, and penile tumors (possibly reflecting increased incidence of infection with the common proposed etiological agent—papillomaviruses). The United Kingdom's incidence of anal cancer lies between these extremes.

The increasing incidence of HIV infection in the United States has resulted in an increase in the incidence of anal cancer.[5] Areas such as San Francisco, with a large homosexual population, have reportedly seen a dramatic increase in the prevalence of anal cancers. A recent study from Denmark has reported a doubling in the incidence of anal cancer, particularly in women, over the last 10 years.[6] No other countries have reported similar increases to date, but the Cancer Registry data in Denmark are renowned for their remarkable accuracy and completeness.

Recent epidemiologic evidence has suggested that anal cancer may be associated with anal sexual activity; Cooper[7] observed four cases of anal cancer arising in homosexual men with long histories of anoreceptive intercourse. The occurrence of a disproportionately high incidence of anal cancer among male homosexual communities was reported from San Francisco and Los Angeles. Daling et al.[8] identified risk factors for the development of squamous cell carcinoma of the anus. A history of receptive anal intercourse in males increased the relative risk of developing anal cancer by 33 times compared with controls with colon cancer. A history of genital warts also increased the relative risk of developing anal cancer (27-fold in men and 22-fold in women). These studies suggest that a sexually transmissible agent may be an etiological factor in the development of anal squamous cell carcinoma.

Similarly, epidemiologic data and molecular biologic data have shown an association between a sexually transmissible agent and female genital cancer. Using nucleic acid hybridization techniques, human papillomavirus (HPV) type 16 DNA, and less commonly types 18, 31, and 33 DNA, was consistently found to be integrated into the genome in genital squamous cell carcinomas.[9] Recently, the same HPV DNA types have also been identified in a similar proportion of anal squamous cell carcinomas.[10] HPVs are DNA viruses, of which there are more than 60 types capable of causing a wide variety of lesions on squamous epithelium. Common warts can be found on the hands and feet of children and young adults and are caused by the relatively infectious HPV types 1 and 2. Anogenital papillomaviruses are less infective than types 1 and 2 and are exclusively sexually transmitted. The epidemiology of genital papillomavirus infection is poorly understood, largely due to the social and moral taboos surrounding sexually transmissible infections. Anogenital papillomavirus-associated lesions range from condyloma through intraepithelial neoplasia to invasive carcinoma. The most common HPV types causing genital warts are types 6 and 11. HPV types 6 and 11 may also be isolated from low-grade intraepithelial neoplasia. HPV types 16, 18, 31, and 33 are much less commonly associated with genital condylomas, but are more commonly found in high-grade intraepithelial neoplasias and invasive carcinomas. Once one area of the anogenital epithelium is infected, spread of papillomavirus infection throughout the rest of the anogenital area probably follows, but remains occult in the majority of individuals.[11] Therefore, the commonly held belief that anal cancer only occurs in individuals who practice anal intercourse is probably unfounded.

## PREMALIGNANT LESIONS

Anal and genital papillomavirus-associated lesions may be identified clinically either by naked eye inspection or more usually with an operating microscope (colposcope) and the application of acetic acid to the epithelium, resulting in an "aceto-white" lesion. Colposcopic examination may suggest the degree of dysplasia and permits targeted biopsy of a lesion, but histologic examination remains the diagnostic standard. Although the natural history of cervical papillomavirus infection and intraepithelial neoplasia are reasonably well understood, the same is not true for anal lesions, probably because they have only been diagnosed over the last 5 to 10 years. Consequently, the natural history and malignant potential of anal intraepithelial neoplasia are both uncertain.

Anogenital intraepithelial neoplasia of the cervix (CIN), vulva (VIN), vagina (VAIN), and anus (AIN) are graded from I to III, according to the number of thirds of epithelial depth that appear dysplastic on histologic section. Thus in grade III the cells of the whole thickness of the epithelium appear dysplastic, being synonymous with carcinoma in situ.

High-grade AIN lesions may be characterized by hyperkeratosis or changes in the pigmentation of the epithelium. Thus carcinoma in situ may appear white, red, or brown, and however pigmented, the pigmentation is commonly irregular. These lesions may be flat or raised; ulceration, however, is suggestive of invasive disease. It is important that any suspicious area be biopsied and examined

histologically. The terms Bowen's disease of the anus and leukoplakia are best avoided because they are confusing and convey no specific information. The malignant potential of both Bowen's disease and leukoplakia is also uncertain.

At the present time multifocal genital intraepithelial neoplasia represents a difficult clinical problem, which may be further complicated by the occurrence of synchronous or metachronous AIN.[12] The management of these patients is controversial because the natural history of these lesions remains poorly understood.

## COCARCINOGENS

Carcinogenesis is a multistep process, papillomavirus infection probably being only one of a number of factors in the pathogenesis of these tumors. Other potential cocarcinogens are being investigated, such as the effect of cigarette smoking and other infective agents such as chlamydia and HIV.

There are few published data on the prevalence of HPV infection among HIV-infected patients, but it appears that anogenital HPV infection is particularly common in this group. There has been a dramatic increase in the incidence of anal cancer in areas where HIV infection is prevalent. This supports the hypothesis that suppression of cell-mediated responses to HPV infection are involved in the pathogenesis of anal cancer. This is further supported by the increased prevalence of squamous carcinomas in patients receiving systemic immunosuppression following organ transplantation.

## HISTOLOGIC TYPES

Included within the category of epidermoid tumors are squamous cell carcinomas, basaloid (or cloacogenic) carcinomas, and mucoepidermoid cancers. The different morphological types of anal cancer do not appear to have different prognoses.[13] Tumors arising at the anal margin tend to be well differentiated and keratinizing, whereas those arising in the canal are more commonly poorly differentiated. Basaloid tumors arise in the transitional zone around the dentate line and form 30% to 50% of all anal canal tumors.

## PATTERNS OF SPREAD

Anal canal cancer spreads locally, mainly in a cephalad direction, so that the tumor may appear to have arisen in the rectum. The tumor also spreads outward into the anal sphincters and into the rectovaginal septum, perineal body, and the vagina in more advanced cases. Lymph node metastases occur frequently, especially in tumors of the anal canal.[14] Spread initially occurs to the perirectal group of nodes and thereafter to inguinal, hemorrhoidal, and lateral pelvic lymph nodes. The frequency of nodal involvement is related to the size of the primary tumor together with its depth of penetration.[15] Approximately 14% of patients will present with inguinal lymph node involvement, but this rises to approximately 30% when the primary tumor is greater than 5 cm in diameter.[16,17] Only 50% of patients with enlarged nodes at presentation will subsequently be shown to contain tumor. Synchronously involved nodes carry a particularly poor prognosis, whereas the salvage rate is much higher when metachronous spread develops.

Hematogenous spread tends to occur late and is usually associated with advanced local disease. The principal sites of metastases are the liver, lung, and bones.[18] However, metastases have been described in the kidneys, adrenals, and brain.

## CLINICAL PRESENTATION

Since anal cancer is rare but anal and rectal bleeding are common symptoms, it is not surprising that 75% of anal cancers are misdiagnosed initially as benign conditions.[19] The predominant symptoms of epidermoid anal cancer are pain and bleeding, which are present in about 50% of patients.[20] The presence of a mass is noted by a minority of patients, around 25%. Pruritus and discharge occur in a similar proportion. Advanced tumors may involve the sphincter mechanism, causing fecal incontinence. Invasion of the posterior vaginal wall may cause a discharging fistula through the vagina.

Cancer of the anal margin usually has the appearance of a malignant ulcer, with a raised, everted, indurated edge. Lesions within the canal may not be visible, although extensive lesions spread to the anal verge, or can extend via the ischiorectal fossa to the skin of the buttock.[21] Digital examination of the anal canal is usually painful, and may reveal the distortion produced by the tumor. Since the anal cancer tends to spread upward, there may be involvement of the distal rectum, perhaps giving the impression that the lesion has arisen there. Involvement of the perirectal lymph nodes may be palpable on digital examination, rather more than may be apparent in disseminating rectal cancer. If the tumor has extended into the sphincter muscles, the characteristic induration of a spreading malignancy may be felt around the anal canal.

Although up to one-third of patients will have inguinal lymph nodes that are enlarged, biopsy will confirm metastatic spread in only 50% of these; the rest are due to secondary infection.[20] Biopsy or fine-needle aspiration is recommended by many to confirm involvement of the groin nodes if radical block dissection is contemplated. Distant spread is unusual in anal cancer, so hepatomegaly, although it must be looked for, is very uncommon. Frequently other benign perianal conditions will exist in association with anal cancer, such as fistulas, condylomas, or leukoplakia.

## INVESTIGATION

The most important investigation in the management of anal cancer is examination under anesthesia. Ideally this should be carried out jointly by the surgeon and radiotherapist. Examination under anesthesia permits optimum assessment of the tumor in terms of size, involvement of adjacent structures, nodal involvement, and also provides the best opportunity to obtain a biopsy for histologic confirmation. Sigmoidoscopic examination is probably best performed at this examination.

## CLINICAL STAGING

No one system of staging for anal tumors has been adopted universally. However, that of the Union Internationale Contre le Cancer (UICC)[22] is the one most widely used.

This system has been criticized for its application to anal canal lesions because it requires assessment of involvement of the external sphincter. To overcome this, a system has been suggested by Papillon[23] as follows:

T1    <2 cm
T2    2–4 cm
T3    >4 cm, mobile
T4a   invading vaginal mucosa
T4b   extension into structures other than skin or rectal or vaginal mucosa

Although insertion of the probe may be difficult or impossible due to discomfort, ultrasound scanning can provide accurate information regarding sphincter involvement.[24] Computed tomography and magnetic resonance scanning may provide information on spread beyond the anal canal.

Measurement of levels of serum tumor markers and other measures of biologic activity such as DNA ploidy are generally unhelpful because they do not provide reliable information.

## TREATMENT

### HISTORICAL

Traditionally, anal cancer has been seen as a "surgical" disease. Anal canal tumors were treated by radical abdominoperineal excision and colostomy, whereas anal margin lesions were treated generally by local excision. Over the past decade, nonsurgical radical treatments—radiotherapy with or without chemotherapy—have taken over as primary treatments of choice in most cases.

Overall the results of surgery for anal cancer are disappointing for what is essentially a locoregional disease. For decades radical abdominoperineal excision of the rectum and anus was the preferred method of treatment at most centers around the world. Abdominoperineal excision for anal canal cancer differs little from the procedure used for rectal cancer, but particular care is taken to clear the space below the pelvic floor. Although extended pelvic lymphadenectomy in addition to abdominoperineal excision has been practiced, such extensive operations did not appear to improve 5-year survival rates.[25] Compared to margin cancer, anal canal cancer is more likely to be locally advanced at presentation and to be associated with subsequent metastasis,[26] perhaps explaining the general preference for radical surgery. Around 20% are found to be surgically incurable at presentation. Results published since the mid-1980s reporting series collected over the previous several decades, have varied widely in their survival outcome; on average, the 5-year survival rate has been around 55% to 60%.[14,20,27] Most postsurgical relapses occur locoregionally.

Around 75% of cancers at the anal margin have been treated in the past by local excision.[20,28] The rationale for this was based on the perception that margin lesions rarely metastasize, although this has not always been confirmed by prolonged follow-up. It may be postulated that disappointing 5-year survival rates of around 50% to 70% might have been better if radical surgery had been applied more frequently, but this must remain a matter for speculation.

## CURRENT TREATMENT

Radiotherapists have been treating anal tumors for many years, achieving equivalent survival rates but with the advantage of stoma avoidance in the majority of patients who might otherwise have required radical surgery. Ironically it was a surgeon, Norman Nigro, reporting the use of combined chemotherapy and radiotherapy to try to turn patients with inoperable disease into candidates for surgical salvage, who began to turn surgeons away from operation as first-choice therapy.[29]

## RADIATION-ALONE THERAPY

The initial treatment for anal cancer was radiotherapy because the mortality and morbidity rates of surgical treatment of anal carcinoma were unacceptable. By the 1930s, however, it was recognized that the low-voltage radiotherapy used frequently produced severe radionecrosis. As surgery became safer, abdominoperineal excision for invading lesions, and local excision for small growths, became the standard treatment for the next four decades.

More recently, the development in the 1950s of equipment that could deliver high-energy irradiation by the cobalt source generator or more recently by linear accelerators, enabled radiotherapists to deliver higher penetrating doses to more deeply placed structures with less superficial expenditure of energy. Radiation damage to surrounding tissues was consequently reduced while simultaneously delivering an enhanced tumoricidal effect. Interstitial irradiation alone may produce local tumor control rates of 47%.[30] Improved results have been described using a technique of external beam irradiation, combined with interstitial therapy[31]—two-thirds of patients survived for 5 years, the majority maintaining adequate sphincter function. An alternative is high-dose external beam radiotherapy alone, for which 5-year survival rates of 75% at 3 years have been described.[32]

## CHEMOIRRADIATION THERAPY (COMBINED MODALITY THERAPY)

Combined modality therapy for anal cancer was championed by Norman Nigro.[29] Nigro chose to use 5-fluorouracil (5-FU) and mitomycin C empirically as a preoperative regimen aimed at improving the results of radical surgery. The radiotherapy then consisted of 30 Gy of external beam irradiation delivered over a period of 3 weeks. A bolus of mitomycin C was given on day 1 of treatment, and 5-FU was delivered in a synchronous continuous 4-day infusion during the first week of radiotherapy. After the completion of radiotherapy, a further infusion of 5-FU was administered and patients later proceeded to abdominoperineal excision. It was evident to Nigro that the majority had quite dramatic tumor shrinkage; in

this 1974 publication, the tumor was reported to have disappeared completely in all three patients. No tumor was found in the surgical specimen in both the patients who underwent abdominoperineal excision; the third refused surgery. Nigro's experience over the ensuing 10 years bore out his early enthusiasm. As he became more confident, he no longer routinely pressed his patients to undergo radical surgery, initially confining himself to excising the site of the primary tumor after combined modality therapy. Later he dropped even this relatively minor surgical step if the primary site looked and felt normal after treatment.[33]

A variety of similar techniques have subsequently been described. With wider experience, it became clear that higher doses of radiotherapy (45 to 60 Gy) could be applied, usually split into two courses to minimize morbidity. Chemotherapy comprised intravenous infusion of 5-FU at the beginning and end of the first radiotherapy course, and a single bolus of mitomycin C given on the first day of treatment. Modifications of chemotherapy dosage and prophylactic antibiotic therapy were necessary in elderly or frail patients, and those with extensive ulcerated tumors.

All the reported series describe excellent results, but it has yet to be determined whether similar levels of local tumor control and survival can be achieved without chemotherapy, perhaps thereby avoiding some morbidity. The only analysis comparing patients who have been treated with the combined regimen and those receiving radiotherapy alone has suggested that initial local tumor control may be achieved in about 90% of patients receiving various combined treatment protocols compared with 56% with radiotherapy alone.[34] This retrospective review compared patients who had received a combined treatment program with historical controls treated by radiotherapy alone in the same institution. The overall uncorrected 5-year survival rate of the two groups of patients was similar at 58%. This group also looked at the role of mitomycin C in the treatment regimen and concluded from noncontrol data that this contributes to optimum local tumor control.[35]

The most recent data on combined modality therapy from the United Kingdom Co-ordinating Committee on Cancer Research compared chemoirradiation with radiotherapy alone in a randomized multicenter study.[36] This study randomized 585 patients, making it the largest single trial in anal cancer research. The trial showed that combined modality therapy gave superior local control of disease compared with radiotherapy alone. Only 36% of patients receiving combined therapy had "local failure," whereas 59% of patients receiving radiotherapy alone had local failure. Although there was no significant overall survival advantage for either treatment regime, the risk of death from anal cancer was significantly less in the combined modality therapy group. As a result of this trial, it seems that the standard treatment for anal squamous carcinoma should be a combination of radiotherapy, and intravenous 5-FU with mitomycin. Surgery may then be reserved for those in whom combined modality therapy fails.[36]

## THE ROLE OF SURGERY TODAY

Although surgeons no longer play the central therapeutic role, they nevertheless have important contributions to make.

**INITIAL DIAGNOSIS.** Most patients present to surgeons, and surgeons are best suited to perform examination under anesthesia to confirm diagnosis and assess local extent.

**LESIONS AT THE ANAL MARGIN.** Small lesions at the anal margin may still best be treated by local excision alone, obviating the need for protracted courses of nonsurgical therapy. There is some evidence that the risk of regional lymph node metastasis is not related to primary tumor size. This may explain the disappointing results sometimes reported after local excision, but it conflicts with the view that tumor size is related to stage, which is said to account for the excellent results of local excision in small tumors.[14]

**TREATMENT COMPLICATIONS AND DISEASE RELAPSE.** Surgeons retain an important role in treatment of anal cancer after failure of primary nonsurgical treatment, either early or late.[37] Four situations may require surgery after primary nonsurgical treatment:

1. Residual tumor
2. Complications of treatment
3. Incontinence or fistula after tumor resolution
4. Subsequent tumor recurrence

The appearance of the primary site is often misleading after radiotherapy. In most patients complete remission is indicated by the tumor disappearing completely. In some, however, a lump may remain, occasionally looking like an unchanged primary tumor. Only generous biopsy will reveal whether the residual lump contains tumor or consists merely of inflammatory tissue.[38] Thus histologic proof of residual disease is mandatory before radical surgery is recommended to the patient.

Complications of nonsurgical treatment for anal cancer do occur in a proportion of patients, and may range from radionecrosis, fistula, or incontinence. Severe anal pain due to radionecrosis of the anal lining may necessitate either a colostomy, in the hope that the lesion may heal after fecal diversion, or radical anorectal excision.

Occasionally, a tumor is so locally extensive that the patient will be rendered incontinent as a consequence of primary tumor shrinkage. Although rectovaginal fistula may be amenable to repair, sphincter damage is unlikely to improve with local surgery, therefore necessitating abdominoperineal excision of the anorectum.

Should clinical evidence of recurrent disease develop after initial resolution, biopsy is again mandatory prior to surgical intervention. If high-dose radiotherapy was used for primary treatment, further nonsurgical therapy for recurrence is usually contraindicated, therefore making radical surgical removal necessary.

**INGUINAL METASTASES.** Inguinal lymph nodes are enlarged in 10% to 25% of patients with anal cancers. Although inguinal lymph node involvement may be treated by radiotherapy, some argue that this should be treated surgically. Histologic confirmation is advisable before radical groin dissection because up to 50% of cases of inguinal lymphadenopathy may be due to inflammation alone.[20] Enlargement of groin nodes some time after primary therapy is most likely to be due to recurrent tumor; radical groin dissection is indicated in this situation, with up to 50% 5-year survival.[18]

**TREATMENT OF INTRAEPITHELIAL NEOPLASIA.** HPV infection of the anogenital area is very common. It has been reported that over 70% of sexually active adults have at some time had occult or overt genital HPV infection.[39] In most individuals the infection remains occult, but in a minority, for reasons which are currently uncertain, the infection may manifest itself as either condylomas or as intraepithelial neoplasia. As with other viral infections, it is impossible to eradicate HPV infection by surgical excision, and for this reason surgical excision of condylomas is effectively performed more for relief of symptoms and cosmesis than to eradicate infection. Similarly, the natural history of low-grade AIN (AIN I and II) seems to be relatively benign, and therefore a policy of observation alone is probably adequate. This is likely to be particularly advisable when large areas of the anogenital epithelium are affected. However, for high-grade AIN (AIN III), the advice is more circumspect because we do not know the natural history of this condition. If the area of AIN III is small, it is probably prudent to excise it locally and then to observe the patient. If the area of AIN III is too large for local excision to be possible without risk of anal stenosis, then a careful observational policy with 6-month review may be an option. Aggressive surgical excision of the whole perianal skin and anal canal and resurfacing with split skin has been performed in some patients, but this requires the use of a defunctioning colostomy to permit the grafts to take. This sort of surgery requires multiple procedures and carries significant morbidity, which for a condition of uncertain malignant potential may make the treatment worse than the disease.

## RARER TUMORS

### BUSCHKE LOWENSTEIN TUMORS

These rare tumors occur in several genital sites, including the anal margin. They are notable for their encephaloid appearance and rapid growth. They are caused by papillomavirus infection, but their rapid growth and typically condylomatous appearance distinguish them from other anal squamous cancers.

Although these tumors may appear like florid condylomas, they usually contain a squamous carcinoma and may invade locally into surrounding tissues. These tumors are difficult to assess clinically; examination under anesthesia usually reveals that they extend up the anal canal to the dentate line.

Treatment by surgical excision is recommended for these lesions. However, such excision may lead to significant anal stenosis because the whole of the anal circumference is involved. Alternatives are the use of perianal rotation flaps or the use of split skin grafts (and a defunctioning colostomy).

### ADENOCARCINOMA

Adenocarcinoma in the anal canal is usually simply a very low rectal cancer that has spread downward to involve the canal, but true adenocarcinoma of the anal canal does occur, probably arising from the anal glands, which arise around the dentate line and pass radially outward into the sphincter muscles. This is a very rare tumor, quite radiosensitive, but usually still treated by radical surgery.

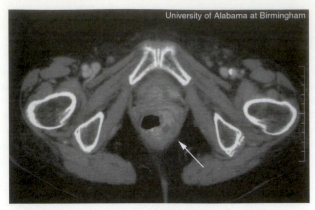

*A*

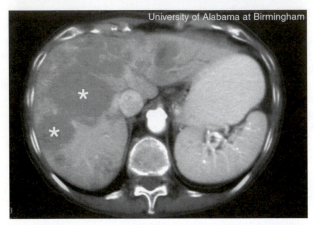

*B*

**FIGURE 16C-1.** 86-year-old woman with rectal bleeding. *A.* Intravenous, oral, and rectal contrast-enhanced CT of the pelvis demonstrates a mass at the anorectal junction (arrow). *B.* Image through the liver demonstrates multiple metastases (asterisks). Although this is a typical appearance for metastatic adenocarcinoma, malignant melanoma was diagnosed at rectal biopsy. (*Courtesy of C. Canon, MD.*)

## MALIGNANT MELANOMA

This tumor is very rare, accounting for just 1% of anal canal malignant tumors. The lesion may mimic a thrombosed external pile due to its color, although amelanotic tumors also occur. It has an even worse prognosis when occurring in the anal canal than at other sites. Because the chances of cure are minimal, radical surgery as primary treatment has been all but abandoned at some centers.[40] (See Fig. 16C-1.)

## REFERENCES

1. MORSON B et al: Morson and Dawson's Gastrointestinal Pathology. Oxford, Blackwell, 1990.

2. FENGER C: The anal transitional zone. Location and extent. Acta Pathol Microbiol Immunol Scand 87:379, 1979.

3. OFFICE OF POPULATION CENSUSES AND SURVEYS: *Cancer Statistics Registrations.* HMSO, 1988.

4. MUIR C, WATERHOUSE J: *Cancer in Five Continents (V).* Lyon, IARC Scientific Publications, 1987.

5. WEXNER S et al: The demographics of anal cancers are changing. Identification of a high risk population. Dis Colon Rectum 30:942, 1987.

6. FRISCHE M, MELBYE M: Trends in the incidence of anal carcinoma in Denmark. Br Med J 306:419, 1993.

7. COOPER H et al: Cloacogenic carcinoma of the anorectum in homosexual men: an observation of four cases. Dis Colon Rectum 22:557, 1979.

8. DALING J et al: Sexual practices, sexually transmitted diseases and the incidence of anal cancer. N Engl J Med 317:973, 1987.

9. ZUR HAUSEN H: Papilloma viruses in human cancers. Mol Carcinogen 1:147, 1989.

10. PALMER JG et al: Anal cancer and human papillomaviruses. Dis Colon Rectum 32:1016, 1989.

11. SYRJANEN et al: Anal condylomas in homosexual/bisexual and heterosexual males II. Histopathological and virological assessment. VIIth International Papillomavirus Workshop, 1988, p 127.

12. SCHOLEFIELD J et al: Anal intraepithelial neoplasia: Part of a multifocal disease process. Lancet 340:1271, 1992.

13. MORSON B: The pathology and results of treatment of squamous cell carcinoma of the anal canal and anal margin. Proc R Soc Med 53:22, 1960.

14. BOMAN B et al: Carcinoma of the anal canal. A clinical and pathologic study of 188 cases. Cancer 54:114, 1984.

15. LOYGUE J, LAUGIER A: Cancer epidermoide de l'anus. Chirurgie 6:710, 1980.

16. KLOTZ R et al: Transitional cell cloagenic carcinoma of the anal canal. Cancer 20:1724, 1967.

17. STEARNS M et al: Cancer of the anal canal. Curr Probl Cancer 4:1, 1980.

18. GREENALL M et al: Recurrent epidermoid cancer of the anus. Cancer 57:1437, 1986.

19. EDWARDS A et al: Anal cancer: The case for earlier diagnosis. J R Soc Med 84:395, 1991.

20. PINTOR MP et al: Squamous cell carcinoma of the anus at one hospital from 1948 to 1984. Br J Surg 76:806, 1989.

21. NELSON R et al: Anal carcinoma presenting as a perirectal abscess or fistula. Arch Surg 120:632, 1985.

22. UICC: *TNM Classification of Malignant Tumors,* 4th ed. Heidelberg, Springer-Verlag, 1985.

23. PAPILLON J et al: A new approach to the management of epidermoid carcinoma of the anal canal. Cancer 51:1830, 1987.

24. GOLDMAN S et al: Transanorectal ultrasonography in the staging of anal epidermoid carcinoma. Int J Colorectal Dis 6:152, 1991.

25. PARADIS P et al: The clinical implications of a staging system for carcinoma of the anus. Surg Gynecol Obstet 141:411, 1975.

26. JENSEN S et al: Long term prognosis after radical treatment for squamous call carcinoma of the anal canal and anal margin. Dis Colon Rectum 31:273, 1988.

27. GREENALL M et al: Epidermoid cancer of the anal margin. Pathologic features, treatment and clinical results. Am J Surg 149:95, 1985.

28. GREENALL M et al: Treatment of epidermoid carcinoma of the anal canal. Surg Gynecol Obstet 161:509, 1985.

29. NIGRO N et al: Combined therapy for cancer of the anal canal. A preliminary report. Dis Colon Rectum 27:354, 1974.

30. JAMES R et al: Local radio-therapy in the management of squamous carcinoma of the anus. Br J Surg 72:282, 1985.

31. PAPILLON J: *Rectal and Anal Cancers.* Berlin, Springer-Verlag, 1982.

32. GREEN J et al: Anal carcinoma: Therapeutic concepts. Am J Surg 140:151, 1980.

33. NIGRO N: Treatment of squamous cell cancer of the anus. Cancer Treat Res 18:221, 1984.

34. CUMMINGS B et al: Epidermoid anal cancer: treatment by radiation alone or by 5-fluorouracil with or without mitomycin C. Radiat Oncol 21:1115, 1991.

35. CUMMINGS B et al: Mitomycin in anal canal carcinoma. Oncology 50(Suppl 1):63, 1993.

36. UKCCCR ANAL CANCER TRIAL WORKING PARTY: Epidermoid anal cancer: results from the UKCCCR randomised trial of radiotherapy alone versus radiotherapy, 5 fluorouracil, and mitomycin. Lancet 348:1049, 1996.

37. SALMON R et al: Prognosis of cloacogenic and squamous cancers of the anal canal. Dis Colon Rectum 29:336, 1986.

38. NORTHOVER J: The non-surgical management of anal cancer. Br J Radiol 61:755, 1988.

39. SYRJANEN K: Anogenital human papilloma virus and the problem of persistence. Eur J Dermatol 8:5, 1998.

40. QUAN S: Anal cancers. Squamous and melanoma. Cancer 70(Suppl 5):1384, 1992.

# CHAPTER 17

# UROLOGIC NEOPLASMS

## 17A / CANCER OF THE KIDNEY AND URETER

*Inoel Rivera and Zev Wajsman*

### RENAL CELL CARCINOMA

Renal cell carcinoma accounts for approximately 85% of all primary renal neoplasms and 3% of all adult malignancies. About 23,000 cases are expected to be diagnosed every year, and an estimated 11,000 patients[1] will succumb to this disease. Men are affected about two times more commonly than women, and the disease generally occurs at a median age of 65. Renal cell carcinoma occurs bilaterally in 2% to 4% of patients, either synchronously or at a later time after diagnosis. Heredity has a role in renal cell carcinoma. Approximately 30% of patients with Hippel-Lindau disease develop renal cell carcinoma, which is metastatic in half of the cases at diagnosis. These tumors are often bilateral and multifocal with an equal male-to-female ratio. Renal cell carcinoma is also associated with other genetic diseases, including adult polycystic disease, horseshoe kidney, tuberous sclerosis, and acquired renal cystic disease. After an average interval of 5 or 6 years, secondary primary tumors develop in 7% of patients successfully treated for renal cell carcinoma.[2,3] The incidence of acquired renal cystic disease in patients on long-term dialysis is approximately 35% to 95%, and the reported incidence of renal cell carcinoma in this group of patients is 4% to 7%.

#### CLINICAL PRESENTATION

Many patients who harbor renal cell carcinoma are asymptomatic. About 25% of patients with newly diagnosed renal cell cancer have evidence of distant metastasis. The classic triad of flank pain, hematuria, and palpaple mass is present in approximately 5% of patients and usually is a manifestation of advanced disease. Hematuria, gross or microscopic, is found in 59% of patients, flank or abdominal pain in 50%, palpable mass in 40%, and weight loss in 28% of patients.[4–7]

Because of its protean manifestations, renal cancer can present with a myriad of systemic symptoms. In 10% to 40% of patients, the presentation will include a paraneoplastic syndrome not always associated with metastatic disease.[8–9] These paraneoplastic manifestations may be due to tumor cells secreting specific hormones, which can include insulin, gonadotropins, an ACTH-like substance, a PTH-like hormone, erythropoietin, human chorionic gonadotropin, glucagon, renin, and prostaglandins. An example of a paraneoplastic syndrome without evidence of metastatic disease is Stauffer's syndrome. This syndrome is characterized by abnormal liver function test, leukopenia, fever, and areas of hepatic necrosis. However, in many patients, after the kidney is removed, function returns to normal. Nevertheless Stauffer's syndrome is still a poor prognostic factor. Return of abnormal liver function tests is usually a sign of recurrent disease. The sudden appearance of a scrotal varicocele that does not subside in the supine position has been the presenting sign in 2% to 11% of patients with renal cancer. Usually on the left side, this is caused by obstruction of the left gonadal vein by tumor thrombus in the left renal vein. In rare instances, tumor thrombus in the inferior vena cava can obstruct the right gonadal vein.

Renal cell carcinoma was known as the "internist's tumor" because of its systemic manifestations. However, now, with the frequent incidental findings of these tumors on radiologic evaluations, a more appropriate name would be the radiologist's tumor.

#### HISTOPATHOLOGY AND CYTOGENETICS

Renal cell carcinomas seem to arise from the proximal convoluted tubule cells. Electron microscopy studies have revealed a striking similarity of the microvilli forming a brush border appearance in the cells of renal cell carcinomas and the proximal convoluted tubule cells.[10] This origin of renal cell carcinoma was also confirmed by a number of investigators using monoclonal antibody probes.[11] These tumors are usually round, varying from several centimeters in diameter to a size almost filling the whole abdominal cavity. Some authors consider tumors less than 3 cm in diameter to be renal adenomas because they rarely metastasize. Nevertheless, there are multiple reports of small renal cell carcinomas that presented with early metastatic disease.[12,13] Microscopically, renal cell carcinomas can be divided into four histologic groups: clear cell, granular cell, chromophobe, and sarcomatoid. The most common type is clear cell, accounting for 80% of these neoplasms. Microscopically, they are characterized by sheets of large, clear cells separated by fibrous septae. These cells are clear because of the abundance of glycogen, lipids, and cholesterol in their cytoplasm. Less frequently, cells with a granular and eosinophilic cytoplasm are found in these tumors. Both of these cell types may be present in different foci of this tumor, but usually one of them is predominant. The chromophobe cell type, which represents approximately 4% of renal tumors, is characterized by transparent cytoplasm with fine reticular appearance. The sarcomatoid type is found infrequently, is characterized by spindle cells, and usually has a poor prognosis.[14]

The most common chromosomal alterations in renal cell carcinoma are deletions and translocations in the short arm of chromosome 3 (3p). Balanced reciprocal translocations between chromosomes 3 and 8, and 3 and 6, have been found in patients in each member of two families with renal cell carcinoma.[15,16] In this group, patients developed multiple or bilateral cancers at an earlier age. In patients with Hippel-Lindau and renal tumors, a gene on the short arm of chromosome 3 has also been identified. Metastatic disease and poor outcome have also been associated with mutations on the tumor suppressor gene p53.[17]

Renal oncocytoma is a solid tumor of the kidney with the histologic pattern of large eosinophilic cells with granular cytoplasm and almost invariably benign clinical behavior. However, the current radiologic modalities are not reliable for differentiating between pure oncocytoma and renal cell carcinoma, and oncocytomas may have foci of renal cell carcinoma. For these reasons, most oncocytomas require an aggressive surgical approach.

## STAGING

It has been shown that tumor thrombus extending to the renal vein or inferior vena cava without lymph node involvement does not significantly affect survival. On the other hand, overall 5-year survival rates for patients with positive lymph nodes are similar to those for patients with distant metastasis (less than 20%). The tumor-node-metastasis (TNM) system separates nodal involvement from vascular invasion. The 5-year survival rates for TNM stages T1, T2, T3a, T3b, T3c, and T4 are 100%, 91%, 72%, 56%, 30%, and 25%, respectively.[18]

### TNM CLASSIFICATION OF PRIMARY RENAL CELL CARCINOMA

#### PRIMARY TUMOR

TN    Primary tumor cannot be assessed.
TO    No evidence of primary tumor.
T1    Tumor 2.5 cm or less in greatest dimension limited to the kidney.
T2    Tumor more than 2.5 cm in greatest dimension limited to the kidney.
T3a   Tumor extends into major veins or invades adrenal gland or perinephric tissues but not beyond Gerota's fascia.
T3b   Tumor invades adrenal gland or perinephric tissues but not beyond Gerota's fascia.
T3c   Tumor grossly extends into renal vein(s) or vena cava.
T4    Tumor invades beyond Gerota's fascia.

#### REGIONAL LYMPH NODES (N)

NX   Regional lymph nodes cannot be assessed.
NO   No regional lymph node metastasis.
N1    Metastasis in a single lymph node, 2 cm or less in greatest dimension.
N2    Metastasis in a single lymph node, more than 2 cm but not more than 5 cm in greatest dimension; or multiple lymph nodes, none more than 5 cm in greatest dimension.
N3    Metastasis in a lymph node more than 5 cm in greatest dimension.

#### DISTANT METASTASIS (M)

MX   Presence of distant metastasis cannot be assessed.
MO   No distant metastasis.
M1    Distant metastasis.

## RADIOGRAPHIC IMAGING

Traditionally, a renal mass has been diagnosed on intravenous pyelography with infusion nephrotomography. However, many more renal masses are being demonstrated with ultrasound and CT scans than with urography. Currently, it is estimated that two-thirds of all locally confined renal tumors are found serendipitously.[19] The differential diagnosis of a renal mass includes the following: tumor, simple or complex cyst, angiomyolipoma, xanthogranulomatosis, pyelonephritis, oncocytoma, or hamartoma. Renal ultrasound can distinguish a cystic mass from a solid mass with a sensitivity of 97% and specificity of 97%. The sonographic criteria for a simple cyst include the following: absence of internal echoes, smooth wall, round or oval shape, sound transmission, and an acoustic shadow arising from the edges of the cyst. Any lesion that does not meet these criteria must be evaluated with a CT scan. Cyst aspirations for diagnostic purposes are rarely indicated today. Patients with no severe medical conditions and any doubtful radiologic appearance of renal masses require surgical exploration.

CT scan is now the single most useful test for the diagnosis and staging of renal cancer.[20–22] Several studies have shown that CT scan allows the correct diagnosis of renal vein involvement, vena cava extension, perirenal extension, lymph node metastasis, and extension to adjacent organs.[20–22] Limitations of the CT scan include the tendency to overestimate the local extension of the disease. This is particularly significant in upper renal masses, where CT scanning infrequently demonstrates false local extension to the liver. CT also gives inadequate insight into the extent of cava involvement. It will not detect limited node involvement unless the node is of an adequate size. CT scan also does not distinguish between reactive and metastatic nodes; thus, in selected patients, these findings should be confirmed with needle biopsy or at the time of surgery.

MRI provides the most useful information about invasion of the renal vein or inferior vena cava without the need for invasive venacavography. MRI can detect the level of the vena cava thrombus with 100% sensitivity, as can cavography. MRI can image the tumor in multiple planes and seems to be more accurate in staging the renal lesion, especially if the mass is less than 3 cm in diameter.[23,24] MRI has better resolution of tissue planes, thus reducing the false-positive interpretations of perirenal involvement by CT scan. Selective renal angiography is rarely used anymore in the evaluation of renal tumors. Angiography is reserved for patients in whom nephron-sparing surgery is anticipated, or in selected cases for renal artery embolization before resection. In renal carcinoma, the classic angiographic findings are neovascularity, microaneurysms, arteriovenous fistulae, contrast media pooling, capsular vessel accentuation, and tumor blush with epinephrine. Cystic adenocarcinoma and hypovascular renal cell carcinomas fail to demostrate these classic angiographic findings.

Further metastatic workup includes complete blood count (CBC), liver function tests with alkaline phosphatase, and chest x-ray. Bone scan is reserved for patients with elevated alkaline phosphatase or bone pain.

## SURGICAL TREATMENT OF RENAL CELL CARCINOMA

Radical nephrectomy is the procedure of choice for localized renal cell carcinoma. This encompasses en bloc resection of the kidney, perinephric fat, Gerota's fascia, and ipsilateral adrenal gland. In 45% of patients with renal cell carcinoma, there is extension to perirenal tissues, making radical nephrectomy the logical surgical procedure.[25] Presently, there is no curative chemotherapy, radiotherapy, or immunotherapy available, thus making radical or partial nephrectomy the only available curative option.

Preoperative renal artery embolization is advocated as a procedure to diminish blood loss in patients with large or locally advanced renal tumors.[26] In our experience, the use of alcohol for angioinfarction of large tumors or tumors with extension to the renal hilum decreases blood loss from parasitic vessels and allows early renal vein ligation. The use of regional lymph node dissection along with radical nephrectomy is controversial. As mentioned previously, patients with evidence of positive lymph nodes on pathologic specimens have poor survival rates similar to those for patients with distant metastasis. At present, our approach is to perform hilar lymph node removal with the specimen, primarily for staging purposes. Renal-sparing surgery is usually performed in patients with bilateral renal tumors or renal carcinoma in a solitary kidney for whom a radical nephrectomy would render the patient anephric. Patients with unilateral renal cancer and a compromised contralateral kidney (for example, patients with calculus disease, diabetes, renal artery stenosis, ureteral reflux, or pyelonephritis) are also candidates for nephron-sparing surgery. Caval thrombus is found in approximately 10% of patients, more commonly on the right side and directly related to the size of the primary tumor. Many authors have shown that if the tumor can be completely removed, survival for patients with renal vein and vena cava tumor thrombus approaches that for patients with stage T2 disease.[27,28] The recent increase in the availability and improved resolution of ultrasonography and CT as diagnostic modalities has resulted in a progressive rise in the diagnosis of the incidentally discovered renal mass. Currently, 30% of the surgically amenable renal tumors are discovered incidentally.[29] This accounts for a number of important issues regarding the evaluation and treatment of the incidental renal mass. The 5-year survival rate for partial nephrectomy in masses of 4 cm or less is 87% to 90%, similar to that for radical nephrectomy. These excellent results have stimulated extending the use of partial nephrectomy to patients with a normal contralateral kidney. In some series, long-term follow-up of patients with masses of less than 3 cm revealed a low incidence of metastatic disease and a slow progression rate, introducing the issue of observation for poor-surgical-risk and elderly patients.[30] Survival rates for metastatic renal cell carcinoma are quite poor, with a 5-year survival rate of 0% to 8%. Nevertheless, there is evidence of improved survival in patients with solitary metastasis after surgical removal of all cancer. This advantage has not been seen in patients with multiple metastases. The 3-year survival rate for patients with solitary metastasis is 19%, compared with 4.3% for patients with multiple metastases after complete surgical resection. It has been suggested that the best results are obtained in patients with solitary metastasis to the lung.[31]

RADICAL NEPHRECTOMY.   The incision selected to perform a radical nephrectomy is dictated by the size of the tumor, previous surgical procedures, body habitus of the patient, extrarenal pathology that requires another operation to be done simultaneously, need for bilateral renal procedures, and experience of the surgeon. The general principles of radical nephrectomy include excision of the kidney with early ligation of the renal artery and vein, excision of perinephric tissue within Gerota's fascia, ipsilateral adrenalectomy, and regional lymph node dissection.

For most of our nephrectomies, including for large tumors, we use a generous extraperitoneal flank approach. In obese patients, this incision provides excellent exposure and can be extended to the chest or peritoneal cavity, if needed. For large upper-pole tumors or very bulky disease, we prefer the intrapleural-intraperitoneal thoracoabdominal approach. Exposure is a key factor in performing cancer surgery. The incision extension and selection need to provide the surgeon with an adequate field to remove the tumors, with limited complications.

The bed of the 11th or 12th rib is most commonly used for the flank approach. The selection of the rib depends on the position of the kidney and the location of the lesion. The patient is placed in the lateral position with the back close to the edge of the table. The brake of the table is placed just above the iliac crest. The table is flexed and the kidney rest is elevated. This maneuver increases the space between the 12th rib and the iliac crest, creating tension on the skin and flank muscles (Fig. 17A-1). The incision is made directly over the selected rib from the posterior axillary line to the lateral border of the rectus muscle. The external oblique, latissimus dorsi, and serratus posterior inferior muscles are divided with electrocautery, and the rib is exposed. After the periostium of the rib is mobilized, the proximal end of the rib is transsected as far back as possible with the rib cutter. If the 11th rib is resected, care must be taken to avoid the pleural reflection. The pleura may be reflected upward by sharply dividing the fascial attachments to the diaphragm. Sharply, the bed of the rib is incised and Gerota's fascia is exposed. The peritoneum is mobilized off the posterior aspect of the transversalis muscle and fascia. Gerota's fascia is mobilized from the inner side of the diaphragm and off the quadratus and psoas muscles. At this time a retractor is placed. However, entering the peritoneal cavity at this stage may add markedly to the

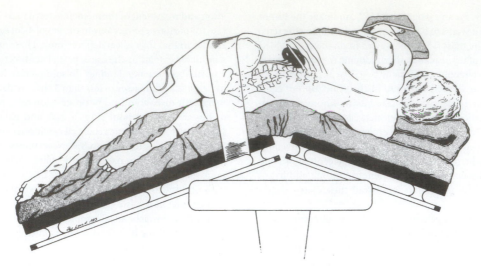

**FIGURE 17A-1.** Position of the patient for flank incision. (With permission from AC Novick and SB Streem: *Campbell's Urology.* Philadelphia, Saunders, 7th ed, 1996, p 3012.)

exposure, especially on the right side, allowing a safe mobilization of the duodenum and good exposure of the vena cava and renal vein. Retracting the colon superiorly, a plane between the mesocolon and Gerota's fascia can be identified (Fig. 17A-2). Dissecting

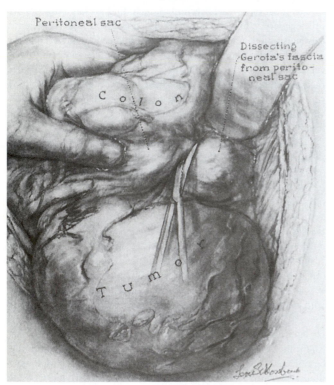

**FIGURE 17A-2.** Mobilization of colon from Gerota's fascia. (With permission from FF Marshall: *Textbook of Operative Urology.* Philadelphia, Saunders, 1996, vol 27, p 254.)

between this plane, Gerota's fascia can be mobilized laterally and the colon can be mobilized medially. The renal artery can be identified posteriorly, ligated, and divided. When identification of the renal artery is difficult, the aorta can be approached medially and the renal artery can be ligated from an anterior approach (Fig. 17A-3). A posterior access to the renal hilum is very helpful in bulky disease. The anterior approach may be associated with inadvertent injury to other organs such as duodenum, ligation of iliac vessels, or, as reported previously, ligation of the superior mesenteric artery. After ligation of the renal artery, the renal vein is ligated and divided to avoid venous hypertension and to decrease bleeding. Nevertheless, if access to the renal artery is obstructed by the renal vein, early ligation of the vein is warranted. Ligation and division of the ureter and gonadal vessels are performed at the time of dissection of the lower pole of the kidney (Fig. 17A-4). Care must be taken during dissection of the upper Gerota's fascia to identify and ligate the vascular branches to the adrenal gland. En bloc resection of the kidney inside Gerota's fascia accompanies perihilar lymph node dissection (Fig. 17A-5). Recent data demonstrate a low incidence of adrenal metastasis after radical nephrectomy. These data suggest that ipsilateral adrenalectomy may be reserved for patients with large tumors or tumors at the upper pole of the kidney.

**PARTIAL NEPHRECTOMY.** The indications for partial nephrectomy for renal carcinoma were defined earlier in this chapter. Patients with solitary kidneys or compromised contralateral kidneys are the usual candidates for nephron-sparing surgery. In 1995, Nissenkorn et al.[32] reported an incidence of 0% to 3.7% for satellite malignant nodules in patients with renal cell carcinoma 3 cm or smaller, and they claimed that patients with this tumor size are overtreated if they have a nephrectomy 96% to 100% of the time.

A flank, extraperitoneal approach is usually preferred. This approach allows excellent exposure of the kidney near the surgeon's hands and, if renal cooling is required, provides isolation from the peritoneal cavity and chest. The peritoneum is mobilized away

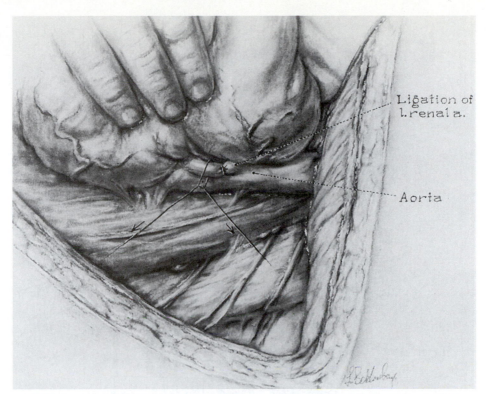

**FIGURE 17A-3.** Posterior approach for renal artery. (With permission from FF Marshall: *Textbook of Operative Urology*. Philadelphia, Saunders, 1996, vol 27, p 253.)

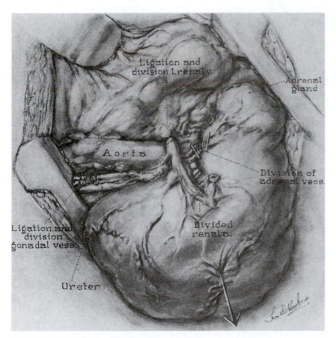

**FIGURE 17A-4.** Arterior exposure of renal vein, ureter, gonadal vessels, and adrenal vessels are ligated. (With permission from FF Marshall: *Textbook of Operative Urology*. Philadelphia, Saunders, 1996, vol 27, p 254.)

from Gerota's fascia. The renal vasculature is identified, and before any manipulation, 12.5 mg of mannitol is given to provide diuresis. If fluids and mannitol are not successful in producing diuresis, furosemide could be added to increase urine output. Cross clamping the renal vessels provides the surgeon with a bloodless field for approximately 30 min of warm ischemia without major damage to renal function. Nevertheless, if a more complex resection is contemplated, in situ cooling of the kidney protects the renal parenchyma from damage for as long as 3 h. Cooling of the kidney should always be used when partial resection cannot be performed in less than 30 min of vascular occlusion. Before resection, the whole kidney must be inspected and palpitated to rule out multifocal disease. Intraoperative ultrasound may prove useful in this matter.

An intestinal bag is placed around the kidney and the renal artery is occluded; if the tumor is near the renal hilum, occlusion of the renal vein is also recomended to avoid major bleeding. Ringer's lactate ice slush is placed around the kidney for 10 to 15 min for cooling before resection. Care is taken to replace the ice slush as needed, and to aspirate the melted ice to avoid hypothermia. The renal capsule is incised sharply with 1 cm of normal renal tissue surrounding the tumor (Fig. 17A-6A). The renal parenchyma is divided bluntly, and any intraparenchymal vessels are identified and ligated individually (Fig. 17A-6B). Perinephric fat is left intact over the tumor. If the collecting system is entered, it must be closed with absorbable sutures. If extensive reconstruction of the collecting system is anticipated,

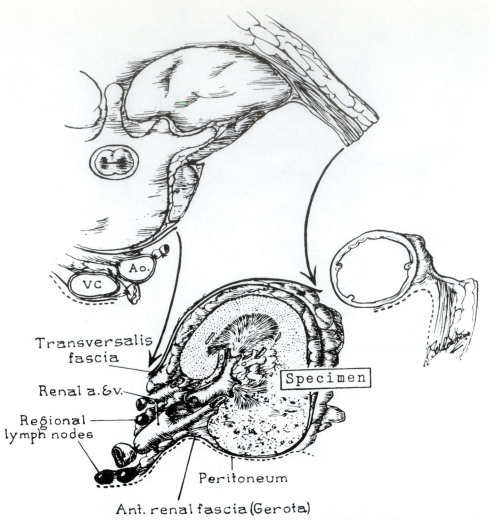

Transversalis fascia

Renal a. & v.

Regional lymph nodes

Specimen

Peritoneum

Ant. renal fascia (Gerota)

Ao.

VC

**FIGURE 17A-5.** En bloc resection of the kidney through a flank incision. (With permission from FF Marshall: *Textbook of Operative Urology.* Philadelphia, Saunders, 1996, vol 27, p 249.)

a ureteral stent can be placed preoperatively to inject methylene blue into the collecting system to facilitate reconstruction. Intermittent renal artery occlusion must be avoided. Nevertheless, the renal vascular clamp can be opened briefly to identify major bleeding vessels. Avitene (collagen) and an argon beam coagulator are helpful in maintaining homeostasis. Before the vascular clamps are removed, the renal parenchyma can be approximated with interrupted mattress sutures of absorbable material (Fig. 17A-6*D*). The remodeling of the kidney is easier at this time because of the malleability of the renal parenchyma during ischemia. Perinephric fat can be incorporated into the closure (Fig. 17A-6*C*). A closed drainage is left inside Gerota's fascia in most cases. In older patients with solitary kidneys or in patients with solitary kidneys and renal insufficiency, we prefer to start the patient on renal doses of dopamine after the vessels are unclamped to improve renal blood perfusion. Temporary or permanent hemodialysis is rarely required with such an approach;

nevertheless, the patient and the surgeon must be prepared for this event.

Angiography is helpful in identifying blood supply for renal masses, especially in large tumors or when nephron-sparing surgery is contemplated. Intraoperative ultrasound is an excellent tool to use to perform partial nephrectomies on patients with tumors located deep in the renal parenchyma. Ultrasound will clarify tumor extension and help to achieve good surgical margins. Complications of partial nephrectomy include hemorrhage, urinary fistula formation, ureteral obstruction, renal insufficiency, and infection. Retroperitoneal postoperative hemorrhage is usually self-limiting and can be treated conservatively. If bleeding persists, arteriography with angioinfarction may be required. Open surgery is seldom used. Urinary fistula usually presents with persistent output through the drain. This can be confirmed by creatinine analysis of the fluid. An intravenous pyelogram or ultrasound must be performed to rule

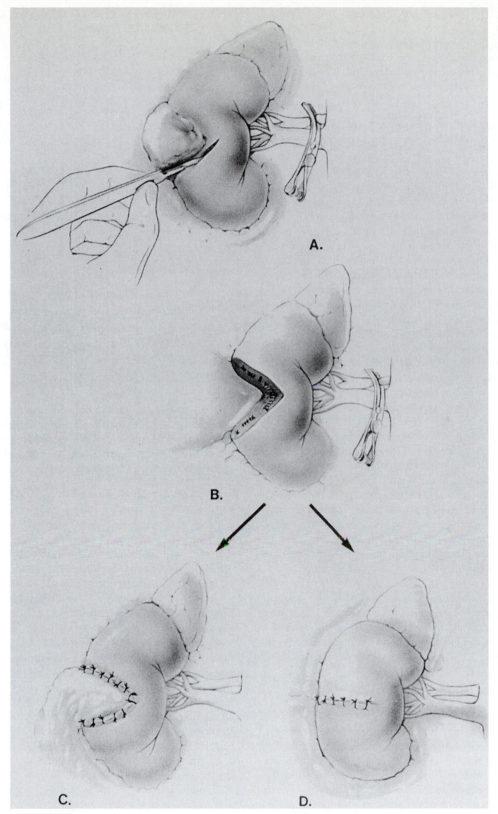

**FIGURE 17A-6.** Technique of wedge resection for a peripheral tumor on the surface of the kidney (*A* and *B*). The renal defect may be closed on itself (*D*) or covered with perirenal fat (*C*). (With permission from AC Novick and SB Streem: *Campbell's Urology*. Philadelphia, Saunders, 7th ed, 1996, p 3012.)

out obstruction. In the absence of obstruction, most of these fistulas resolve spontaneously and surgery is rarely necessary. Ureteral obstruction is usually related to blood clots, and drainage can be improved with a ureteral stent while the clots dissolve.

## MANAGEMENT OF RENAL TUMOR WITH EXTENSIVE INVOLVEMENT OF THE VENA CAVA

Diagnostic procedures today have achieved a high degree of accuracy in defining the extent of a vena caval thrombus. Our experience with magnetic resonance imaging (MRI) is such that it has become the single test we use in evaluating the extent of renal tumors. Intraoperative transesophageal echocardiography aids significantly in the management of patients with inferior vena caval and atrial involvement. The complex surgical situation in the management of extensive renal cell tumors requires a team approach with a urologic surgeon, a cardiovascular surgeon, and, often, a cardiac anesthesiologist to be able to manage difficult situations during this type of surgery.

Renal cell carcinoma invading the vena cava can be divided into three types: (1) that located in the infrahepatic cava, (2) that located in the retrohepatic cava, or (3) that extending into the right atrium above the diaphragm. Recognition of extension of the tumor into the vena cava is important because it determines what approach can be used to resect the tumor (Fig. 17A-7). An infrahepatic caval tumor can be resected by simply cross clamping the vena cava above the level of the tumor, without danger of embolization into the heart. Depending on the level of involvement, a retrohepatic caval tumor can be treated with or without cardiopulmonary bypass. At the time of surgery, if the end of the tumor is palpable in the retrohepatic cava and a number of short hepatic veins can be taken down to get a safe cross clamp above the tumor, then cardiopulmonary bypass will not be necessary. If the tumor extends up to or near the diaphragm, above the point at which the inferior vena cava can be safely clamped, or if the tumor extends into the right atrium, then cardiopulmonary bypass should be used to resect the tumor.

The diagnostic tests used to indicate the extent of the tumor thrombus include CT scanning with contrast, MRI, and preoperative transesophageal echocardiography. Our preference is MRI imaging to determine the extent of an inferior vena caval thrombus and transesophageal echocardiography to determine the extent of right atrial involvement.

## TECHNIQUE

In most patients with an inferior vena cava thrombus, the tumor is bulky and extends toward the renal hilum, which is often surrounded by a large collateral venous circulation. In addition, an extensive fibrotic and desmoplastic reaction is frequently seen, affecting the renal hilum and the retroperitoneum and encasing the vena cava. In such situations, radical nephrectomy becomes a formidable procedure, in which routine isolation of the renal hilum and typing of the renal artery are difficult and often result in blood loss. Preoperative alcohol embolization has been used in our institution for the last 8 years. This allows the complete mobilization of the kidney, mak-

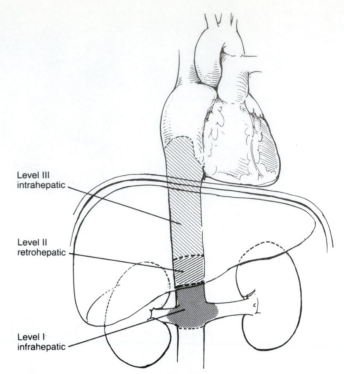

**FIGURE 17A-7.** Level I: Tumor in the vena cava within 1 cm of the renal vein. Level II: Tumor thrombus located in the vena cava behind the liver. Level III: Tumor thrombus located in the intrahepatic vena cava. (With permission from WR Mayfield and Z Wajsman: *Atlas of Surgical Oncology.* Philadelphia, Saunders, 1995, vol 21, p 591.)

ing dissection of the renal hilum safer and reducing blood loss to a minimum. It is especially important to prevent significant hemodynamic instability before the various bypass procedures required during vena cava thrombectomy. Intraoperative blood loss is also relieved by using intraoperative autotransfusion.

When a bypass technique is considered and systemic heparinization is planned, meticulous dissection and hemostasis of the retroperitoneal space are mandatory to reduce further intraoperative and postoperative hemorrhaging. First, the abdomen is explored through a transverse abdominal incision extending between the costal margins. The right colon is completely mobilized, and the parietal peritoneum is incised well above the hepatic flexure, over the kidney toward the inferior vena cava. This is done before any pedicle manipulation, and it is facilitated by prior alcohol embolization. In patients with large upper-pole tumors, the sternum is opened early during exploration, allowing an additional incision into the diaphragm. Additional exposure, if needed, can be obtained by opening the pericardial sac at this time. Hepatic ligaments are incised, allowing mobilization of the liver and its retraction into the chest and medially to expose the retrohepatic vena cava. The porta hepatis is identified and mobilized. Short hepatic veins can be ligated at this time or clipped. The kidney is mobilized and dissected so that it is approached from the posterior aspect, with the kidney displaced medially. In large tumors, the posterior approach to the renal artery avoids difficult dissection anteriorly and decreases the chance of vascular injury or inadvertent ligation of the mesenteric or celiac axis. Here again, previous alcohol embolization is helpful.

After ligation and transsection of the renal arterial pedicle, the inferior vena cava is dissected distally and proximally to the renal vein insertion. The kidney is completely mobilized to the point of transsection of the renal vein. The left renal vein is isolated and surrounded with umbilical tape and pseudo-Rummel. The inferior vena cava also is mobilized distally toward the iliac veins, and an umbilical tape is placed around it, well below the renal vein insertion. In addition, tape is placed around the inferior vena cava above the renal veins and above the planned incision into the inferior vena cava to allow exclusion of hepatic flow during the resuturing of the opening in the vena cava without additional backflow. The hilum of the liver is identified, and the hepatic artery, portal vein, and common bile duct are identified and surrounded by an umbilical tape so that a Pringle maneuver can be performed. At this stage, the cardiovascular team is called in (Fig. 17A-8). As previously described by Mayfield and co-workers,[33] there are three basic bypass techniques that can be used for the resection of caval and atrial tumors. They are venovenous bypass, moderate hypothermic cardiopulmonary bypass, and deep hypothermic circulatory arrest. In all cases, intraoperative transesophageal echocardiography is used. Transesophageal echocardiography is invaluable for the detection of intraoperative embolization of a tumor thrombus into the heart. This occurred once in the authors' experience when simple caval clamping was performed; on removal of the clamp, a large tumor embolus to the right atrium was immediately demonstrated. Fortunately, inflow occlusion could be performed immediately, and the tumor was extracted before embolization into the pulmonary arteries occurred.

A venovenous bypass can be used in a fashion similar to that used for liver transplantation. This technique is restricted to use in the removal of caval tumors that do not invade the right atrium (Fig. 17A-9). Cannulation of the inferior vena cava or a femoral vein and cannulation of the axillary internal jugular vein or right atrium are performed. These cannulas are connected by a heparinized circuit through a centrifugal pump. The vena cava is clamped at the diaphragm, a venous bypass is instituted, and the tumor is extracted from below. Even in this setting, tumor embolization into the right side of the heart can occur, and we believe that cardiopulmonary bypass helps avoid this complication.

Deep hypothermic circulatory arrest or moderate hypothermic cardiopulmonary bypass is used for intrahepatic and intracardiac thrombectomy. A sternotomy is performed (if not done earlier for exposure), the pericardium is opened, and the patient is heparinized with 300 units/kg of heparin. The ascending aorta and superior vena cava are cannulated. The latter can be cannulated either through the right atrial appendage or directly. The superior vena cava and cannula are surrounded by an umbilical tape and pseudo-Rummel below the level of the azygous vein to allow azygous return to be directed toward the heart-lung machine.

To perform the thrombectomy, the inferior vena cava is clamped below the level of the renal veins. A Pringle maneuver is performed. Simultaneously, the patient undergoes cardiopulmonary bypass and the temperature is allowed to drift to 32°C. The superior vena caval tape is tightened. The renal vein is incised in a circular fashion around

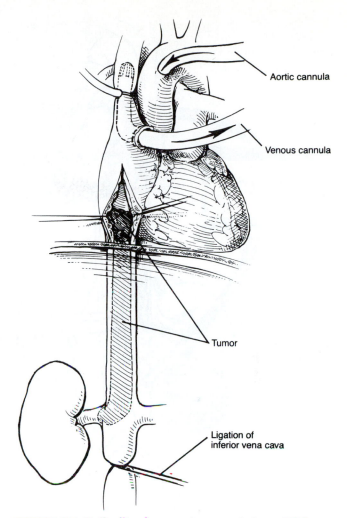

**FIGURE 17A-8.** Cardiopulmonary bypass technique. (With permission from WR Mayfield and Z Wajsman: *Atlas of Surgical Oncology.* Philadelphia, Saunders, 1995, vol 21, p 593.)

the inferior vena cava insertion, and the incision into the inferior vena cava then can be extended cephalad when needed. The renal vein is divided, and traction is placed on the tumor thrombus. Simultaneously, the heart is fibrillated, the right atrium is opened, and the tumor is identified. Pressure is placed on the tumor in an attempt to deliver it through the renal vein. There may be moderate adherence of the thrombus to the wall of the vena cava. The thrombus can be taken down bluntly using an endarterectomy instrument, a tonsil clamp, or sometimes, a finger in the correct plane. In the majority of cases, the tumor is easily endarterectomized and slips out through the renal vein. Pump suction should be used in the coronary sinus and at the level of the hepatic veins to improve visualization during this part of the procedure. A third vent or pump suction can be used in the abdomen to control hepatic and renal venous return into the vena cava.

Rewarming is begun as the right atrial closure is beginning. The heart is defibrillated. The superior vena caval tape is loosened, and the right atrial and vena caval closures are completed. Often,

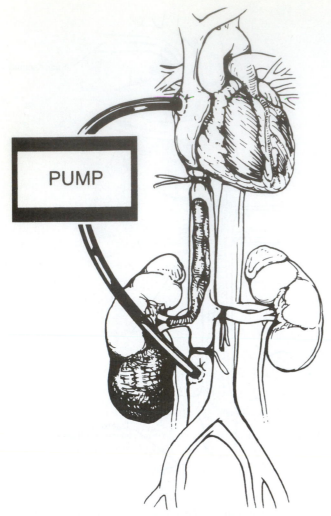

**FIGURE 17A-9.** Venous bypass technique. (With permission from AC Novick: Surgery of renal cell carcinoma, in AC Novick and SB Streem: *Campbell's Urology*. Philadelphia, Saunders, 7th ed, 1996, p 3008.)

a thrombus is seen extending into the left renal vein; usually it is pulled out only during removal of the inferior vena caval tumor. Extension of the tumor thrombus below the renal veins toward the iliac veins is rare. Frozen section of the infrarenal thrombus should be performed, and if present, a tumor should be extracted. Usually, however, as a result of the tumor occlusion above it, the inferior vena cava is filled with a well-organized thrombus. In most of our cases, below the renal vein, we transected or ligated the inferior vena cava with heavy silk ligation or umbilical tape to reduce any possibility of pulmonary embolization in these high-risk patients.

The patient is weaned from the cardiopulmonary bypass. Intraoperative echocardiography is continued to ensure that any tumor embolus is detected.

Deep hypothermic circulatory arrest can be performed as a simple extension of this cannulation technique. This allows a bloodless

field for inspection of the vena cava if it is deemed necessary or when resection of the vena cava is needed.

The average time on bypass is 20 to 25 min. Visualization is adequate for complete tumor thrombectomy.

## CONTRAINDICATIONS

Contraindications to the use of cardiopulmonary bypass include a recent cerebral infarction, any source of acute bleeding (such as peptic ulcer disease), an allergy to heparin, and/or a tumor stage that would preclude surgical care.[33]

## TRANSITIONAL CELL CARCINOMA OF THE RENAL PELVIS AND URETER

Transitional cell carcinoma of the renal pelvis and ureter is a relatively uncommon tumor, accounting for only 5% to 7% of all primary tumors of the kidney. Renal pelvic tumors are three to four times as common as ureteral tumors.[34,35] These neoplasma occur more frequently in the sixth and seventh decades and appear two and a half times more often in men than in women. Upper-tract transitional cell carcinoma occurs in 2% to 4% of patients with bladder cancers; approximately 45% of patients with upper-tract lesions will have tumors in the bladder either synchronously or metachronously. Cystoscopy must be performed as part of the workup and long-term follow-up of these patients.

### ETIOLOGY

The most important etiologic factor in the development of transitional cell carcinoma is tobacco smoke. Environmental factors such as exposure to industrial chemicals, for example, those used in the rubber and textile industries, are particularly important in the development of these tumors. Long-term, high-dose exposure to phenacetin, an anti-inflammatory agent, produces a nephropathy, as well as upper-tract urothelial cancers.[36,37] Upper-tract urothelial tumors have also been associated with a history of cyclophosphamide therapy. Chronic infection or chronic inflammation from stone disease has been associated with the development of squamous cell carcinomas.[38,39] Studies of familial cancer syndromes in which chromosomal abnormalities have been found in some patients have implicated hereditary factors.[40–45]

### PATHOLOGY AND GRADE

Transitional cell carcinoma accounts for more than 90% of upper-tract urothelial tumors. Most upper-tract tumors are papillary.[1,46] Squamous cell carcinoma accounts for 0.7% to 7% of upper-tract tumors.[47] Typically, these are moderately to poorly differentiated tumors, and they characteristically present with advanced disease.[48,49] Adenocarcinoma of the renal pelvis is an extremely rare tumor, representing less than 1% of all renal pelvis tumors. As with squamous cell carcinoma, adenocarcinoma is associated with calculi, long-term obstruction, and inflammation.[50,51] The most commonly used grading system for transitional cell carcinomas is based on the degree of cellular anaplasia. This system groups tumors into three grades corresponding to well (G1, 20%), moderately (G2, 60%), and poorly (G3, 20%) differentiated. Grades 1 and 2 are usually papillary, whereas grade 3 tumors are solid or infiltrating in 50% of cases. After radical surgical treatment, the 5-year survival rate for patients with grade 1 tumors approaches 100%; for grade 2 tumors, it is 80%, and for grade 3 tumors, it is 29%.[52,53]

## STAGING

Tumor grade and stage were found to be the most clinically useful parameters for predicting the prognosis of upper-tract urothelial tumors. The 5-year survival rates for patients with tumors of the renal pelvis and ureter treated with radical surgery according to pathologic stage are as follows: Tis—75%; Ta—54% to 100%; T1—90%; T2—54% to 80%; T3—0% to 54%; T4—0% to 54%; and with nodal involvement, less than 5%.[54] A criticism of the TNM system has been that stage T3 understages ureteral cancer and overstages renal pelvic cancer. Better prognoses have been reported in patients with pelvic tumors invading the renal parenchyma than in patients with ureteral tumors invading periureteral tissues.

### STAGING TRANSITIONAL CELL CARCINOMA OF THE RENAL PELVIS AND URETER

#### *T OR PT (PRIMARY TUMOR)*

TX    Primary tumor is occult and cannot be assessed; for example, positive cytology findings in ureteral urine without (or prior to) demonstration of tumor.

TO    No evidence of primary tumor.

Tis    Carcinoma in situ (flat or nonpapillary carcinoma in situ).

Ta    Noninvasive papillary carcinoma.

T1    Carcinoma involves subepithelial connective tissue.

T2    Carcinoma invades muscularis.

T3    Carcinoma invades beyond muscularis into periureteric or peripelvic fat; carcinoma invades into renal parenchyma.

T4    Carcinoma invades adjacent organs or extends through kidney into perinephric fat.

#### *N OR PN (REGIONAL LYMPH NODES)*

NX    Regional lymph nodes cannot be assessed.

NO    No regional lymph node metastasis.

N1    Metastasis in a single lymph node 2 cm or less in diameter.

N2    Metastasis in a single lymph node 2 to 5 cm in diameter or metastases to multiple lymph nodes, none more than 5 cm in diameter.

N3    Metastasis in a lymph node more than 5 cm in diameter.

#### *M (DISTANT METASTASIS)*

MX    Presence of distant metastasis cannot be assessed.

MO    No distant metastasis.

M1    Distant metastasis.

## DIAGNOSIS

The most common presenting symptom or sign of upper urothelial tumors is gross or microscopic hematuria, occurring in more than 75% of patients.[55] Flank pain occurs in up to 30% of patients and usually is dull because of gradual obstruction and distention of the collecting system. However, acute colic occurs from passage of blood clots, which obstruct the collecting system. Approximately 10% to 15% of patients are asymptomatic, with tumor diagnosed as an incidental finding on an imaging study obtained for other reasons. The diagnosis of upper-tract urothelial tumors relies on the well-performed intravenous urogram, which reveals an abnormality in 50% to 75% of cases.[56] Careful examination of the contralateral collecting system must be performed because of the 2% to 4% incidence of bilateral lesions.

Characteristically, a filling defect that is irregular and in continuity with the wall of the collecting system is found. Obstruction of varying degrees and occasional nonvisualization may occur in 30% of patients.[39] The differential diagnosis of urinary filling defects includes kidney stone, fungus ball, external compression, blood clots, air bubble, and sloughed papilla. Retrograde pyelography is particularly helpful in patients with high-grade obstructions or with poor visualization or nonvisualization on excretory urography. Retrograde pyelography establishes the diagnosis of urothelial cancer with greater than 75% accuracy.[56] Ultrasonography is useful for distinguishing renal stones from soft-tissue masses and hydronephrosis. CT scan provides the same information as ultrasonography in many instances, but its main role is detecting local and distant extension of the disease. Cytology from a voided sample has a very low sensitivity for the diagnosis of upper-tract urothelial cancers. Barbotage specimens from the renal pelvis provide more accurate results but are still associated with a high incidence of false-negative (22% to 35%) and false-positive results.[57–59] However, positive cytology from the upper tract, in addition to a filling defect on intravenous urography, may be regarded as sufficient evidence of upper tract malignancy. The development of rigid and flexible ureteroscopes has increased the accuracy of upper-tract tumor diagnosis and has decreased dramatically the incidence of nephroureterectomy performed for otherwise benign lesions. Streem and co-workers[60] reported that ureteropyeloscopy increased the percentage of definitive diagnosis from 58% to 83%.

## MANAGEMENT

The treatment options for localized upper-tract tumors include nephroureterectomy, distal ureterectomy, and endoscopic resection with topical chemotherapy. Patients with low-grade, low-stage tumors do well with either conservative or radical surgery. Patients with intermediate-grade tumors do better with radical surgery. Patients with high-grade, high-stage tumors do poorly with either treatment. Nephroureterectomy is the standard treatment for upper-tract urothelial tumors. This procedure includes en bloc resection of the kidney, ureter, and a cuff of bladder. Use of this procedure is based on many studies that have demonstrated a 30% to 75% incidence of tumor recurrence in the ureteral stump or around the ipsilateral ureteral orifice if not removed at nephroureterectomy.[61–63]

The reported 5-year survival rates for total ureterectomy are for stages Tis, Ta, and T1, 91%; stage T2, 43%; stage T3 or T4 or NI or N2, 23%; and for stage N3 or M1, 0%.[64] Conservative surgery is indicated in a select group of patients with low-grade tumors, low-stage tumors, bilateral tumors, or renal dysfunction. Retrograde ureteropyeloscopy and percutaneous ureteropyeloscopy are used in the resection or ablation of upper-tract urothial tumors with a reported recurrence rate of 25% to 40%.[65,66] The only true indications for topical chemotherapy are the treatment of carcinoma in situ or recurrent superficial tumors in a solitary kidney.

NEPHROURETERECTOMY. Removal of the kidney, ipsilateral ureter, and a cuff of bladder surrounding the ureteral orifice is the most common surgical treatment for transitional cell carcinoma of the upper urinary tract. Nephroureterectomy may be performed either through a single incision or two separate ones. The decision is based on the preference of the surgeon, as well as the body habitus of the patient. In both, en bloc removal of the surgical specimen is performed. In the one-incision technique, the patient is positioned with the side of the tumor elevated about 30 to 45° . A sand bag under the patient's shoulder and flank can be used for this purpose. The pelvis remains nearly in the supine position. Usually the incision is made from the tip of the 12th rib, with or without rib resection, although occasionally higher intercostal incisions are required and continued as a paramedian incision down to the pubis (Fig. 17A-10). A complete extraperitoneal approach is used. The peritoneal envelope is mobilized across the midline, providing excellent exposure to the entire ureter and bladder. In the two-incision technique, the patient is placed in a lateral decubitus position, and the nephrectomy is performed through a flank incision. To avoid ureteral transsection, the kidney is pushed down to the pelvis and the incision is closed. Then the patient is placed in the supine position, and the kidney, ureter, and bladder cuff are removed through a Pfannenstiel incision. Careful mobilization of the ipsilateral side of the bladder with ligation of vesical branches of the hypogastric artery greatly facilitates exposure as well as lymph node dissection. In both techniques, the bladder is opened and an intravesical or extravesical removal of the ureter is performed. The cystotomy is closed with two layers of absorbable sutures, a cystostomy tube is placed, and a closed drain is located at the pelvic area before closure.

DISTAL URETERECTOMY. The indications for distal ureterectomy include the following: bilateral tumors, solitary kidney, and renal insufficiency. Relative indications are low-grade, low-stage tumor and distal ureteral tumor. The contraindications include the following: multiple tumors, presence of carcinoma in situ, and muscle-invasive disease. The patient is placed in the supine position and the table is flexed. A number of incisions, including the Pfannensteil, Gibson, midline, or paramedian, can be used to gain access to the distal ureter and bladder. The lower midline incision offers good exposure to the distal ureter, bladder, and lymph nodes, with the advantage that any urologist is familiar with this approach. The perivesical space is dissected and the peritoneum is mobilized cranially and medially. The ureter is identified as it crosses the iliac vessels, and a vessel loop is passed around it. Then the ureter is dissected down to its entry into the intramural tunnel. A midline cystotomy is made, and the ureteral orifice is identified. A no. 5F

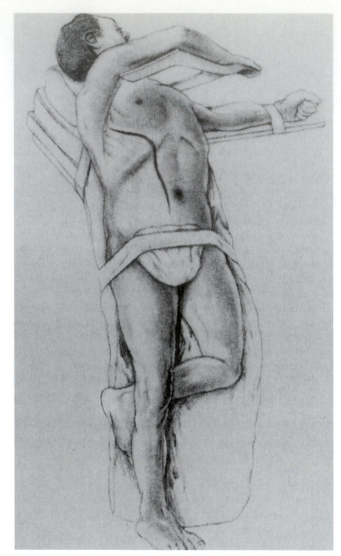

**FIGURE 17A-10.** Position of patient for extraperitoneal nephroureterectomy. (With permission from FF Marshall: *Textbook of Operative Urology.* Philadelphia, Saunders, 1996, vol 31, p 279.)

feeding tube is placed inside the ureter and a figure-of-eight suture is used to close the ureter (Fig. 17A-11). To facilitate traction, this stitch includes the stent. A circumferential incision is made around the ureteral orifice and, using sharp dissection, the ureter is freed up (Fig. 17A-12). The ureter is brought outside the bladder, and ligated and transsected proximal to the tumor. A circumferential piece of the ureter proximal to the ligature is sent for frozen section analysis to assure a tumor-free margin. A tension-free reimplantation of the remaining ureter is performed. In cases where a long portion of distal ureter is removed, a psoas hitch or Boari flap is very helpful to close the gap between the ureter and bladder. A transureteroureterostomy is contraindicated because of the possibility of tumor seeding on the unaffected side. The ureteral hiatus and the cystotomy are closed with two layers of absorbable sutures. A cystotomy tube and a Foley catheter are used for drainage. In patients with minimal bleeding

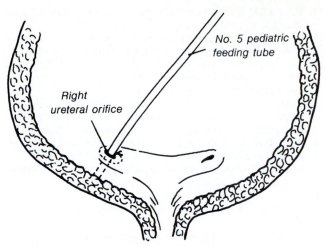

**FIGURE 17A-11.** The trigone is exposed, and a no. 5F pediatric feeding tube is passed up the orifice to be resected and sutured in place. Incision into the bladder mucosa is started in the inferomedial aspect of the bladder mucosa, allowing an appropriate cuff to be circumcised. (With permission from R Donohue: *Current Genitourinary Cancer Surgery.* Philadelphia, Williams & Wilkins, 1997, vol 10, p 113.)

during the procedure, we leave a Foley catheter for drainage only. Also, a closed drain is left in the perivesical space.

**CONSERVATIVE SURGERY.** Endoscopic management may benefit patients with tumors in a solitary kidney; patients with bilateral tumors; renal insufficiency; multiple low-grade, low-stage lesions; and those unable to undergo major open surgery. For patients with these condition, ureteroscopy can be used for the treatment

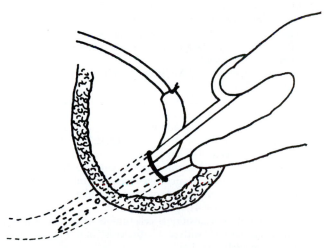

**FIGURE 17A-12.** After adequate ureteral mobilization, scissors are used to complete the tunnel to the extravesical pelvis. (With permission from DE Crawford: *Current Genitourinary Cancer Surgery.* Baltimore, Waverly, 1997, vol 10, p 114.)

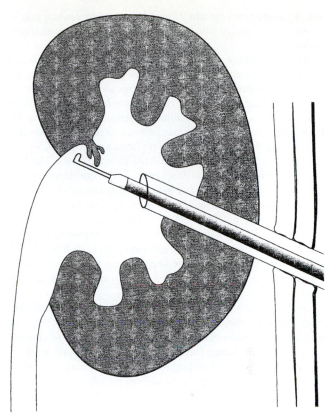

**FIGURE 17A-13.** Percutaneous access for removal of upper trace urothelial tumor. (With permission from DE Crawford: *Current Genitourinary Cancer Surgery.* Baltimore, Waverly, 1997, vol 12, p 131.)

of upper urothelial tumors. The patient is placed in the lithotomy position, and cystoscopy with retrograde pyelography is performed to identify the lesion and plan the procedure. The location of the tumor and the anatomy of the ureter dictate the type of ureteroscopic instrument to be used during the procedure. Rigid ureteroscopes provide the best optics and control for managing upper-tract tumors, but they may be difficult to advance into segments of the ureter proximal to the iliac vessels. In this situation, a flexible ureteroscope is preferable. A 0.038-inch guidewire is advanced into the renal pelvis and used as a safety access. The ureteroscope is advanced to the renal pelvis with or without dilation of the distal ureter and the ureter is carefully examined. The entire collecting system is inspected. The visual appearance of the tumor is important. Low-grade, low-stage tumors appear papillary with a narrow base. Histologic confirmation is preferable, but for purposes of staging, it is often difficult to obtain adequate samples from the tumor base. Tumor resection can be accomplished using a rigid resectoscope, or tumor ablation can be achieved using a bugbee electrode or neodymium:yttrium-aluminum-garnet (Nd:YAG) laser. To prevent perforations, caution must be taken to perform the procedure under constant direct vision. A double-pigtail ureteral catheter is placed after the procedure to avoid obstruction due to tissue edema. The patient must have close follow-up with intravenous urograms and cytology every 3 months. Ureteroscopy may be used for follow-up every 6 months, or when there is any abnormality on urograms and/or cytology.

Percutaneous surgery of the upper collecting system is usually reserved for patients with urothelial tumors in a solitary kidney, for those with compromised contralateral renal units, or when uretero-scopic treatment is not feasible. Nephroscopes are of larger caliber than ureteroscopes, which facilitates access and visualization. Tumors with considerable bulk may be resected using this approach. A percutaneous nephrostomy tube is placed several days before the procedure to allow the tract around the tube to mature. The tract is dilated to no. 30F and an Amplatz sheath is introduced into the renal pelvis. Rigid and flexible nephroscopes are used to visualize the collecting system. Bladder resectoscopes may be used for tumor resection (Fig. 17A-13). After completion of the resection, a nephroureteral stent and nephrostomy tube are placed. On post-operative day 3, an antegrade nephrostogram is performed, and, if there is no extravasation, the nephrostomy tube is removed. At this time, a second look can be performed to eradicate any residual tumor.

With a percutaneous approach, there is concern about the potential for implantation of tumor cells along the nephrostomy tract or perinephric tissues. Smith[67] reported on 25 patients with urothelial tumors of the kidney treated percutaneously with no incidence of tumor cell implantation along the nephrostomy tract. The follow-up in this group of patients is the same as the follow-up previously described for endoscopic treatment.

## REFERENCES

1. BORING CC et al: Cancer statistics, 1994. CA 44:7, 1994.
2. KANTOR AF: Current concepts in the epidemiology and etiology of primary renal cell carcinoma. J Urol 117:415, 1977.
3. WYNDER EL et al: Epidemiology of adenocarcinoma of the kidney. J Natl Cancer Inst 53:1619, 1974.
4. SKINNER DG et al: Diagnosis and management of renal cell carcinoma: A clinical and pathologic study of 309 cases. Cancer 28:1165, 1971.
5. PATEL NP, LAVENGOOD RW: Renal cell carcinoma: Natural history and results of treatment. J Urol 119:722, 1978.
6. WATERS WB, RICHI JP: Aggressive surgical approach to renal cell carcinoma: Review of 130 cases. J Urol 122:306, 1979.
7. RICHES CW et al: New growths of the kidney and ureter. Br J Urol 23:297, 1971.
8. LASKI ME: Paraneoplastic syndromes in hypernephroma. Abst AUA 89:25, 1994.
9. RUBIN AL et al: Symposium on endocrine functions of the kidney: Foreword. Am J Med 58:1, 1975.
10. OBERLING C et al: Ultrastructure of the clear cells in renal carci-nomas and its importance for the demonstration of their renal origin. Nature 186:402, 1960.
11. BANDER NH et at: Analysis of mouse monoclonal antibody that reacts with a specific region of the human proximal tubule and subsets of renal cell carcinomas. Cancer Res 49:6774, 1989.
12. BELL ET: *Renal Diseases*, 2d ed. Philadelphia, Lea & Febiger, 1950.
13. HICKS WK: Benign tubular adenoma with malignant transfor-mation. J Urol 71:162, 1954.
14. TOMERA KM et al: Sarcomatoid renal carcinoma. J Urol 130:657, 1983.
15. COHEN AJ et al: Hereditary renal cell carcinoma associated with a chromosomal translocation. N Engl J Med 301:592, 1979.
16. KOVACS G et al: Tissue-specific expression of a constitutional 3;6 translocation: Development of multiple bilateral renal cell carcinomas. Int J Cancer 43:422, 1989.
17. UHLMAN DO et al: Association of immunohistochemical staining for p53 with metastatic progression and poor survival in patients with renal cell carcinoma. J Natl Cancer Inst 86:1470, 1994.
18. BASSIL B et al: Validation of the tumor, nodes, and metastases classification of renal cell carcinoma. J Urol 134:450, 1985.
19. KONNAK JW, GROSSMAN HB: Renal cell carcinoma as an incidental finding. J Urol 134:1094, 1985.
20. JASCHKE W et al: Accuracy of computed tomography in stag-ing of kidney tumors. Acta Radiol (Diagn) (Stockh) 23:593, 1982.
21. RICHIE JP et al: Computerized tomography scan for diagnosis and staging of renal cell carcinoma. J Urol 129:1114, 1983.
22. LANG EK: Comparison of dynamic and conventional computed tomography, angiography and ultrasonography in the staging of renal cell carcinoma. Cancer 54:2205, 1984.
23. HORAN J et al: The detection of renal carcinoma extension into the renal vein and inferior vena cava: A prospective com-parison of venacavography and magnetic resonance imaging. J Urol 142:943, 1989.
24. STEWART BH, DUNNICK NR: Imaging renal neoplasms. Prob Urol 4:175, 1990.
25. ROBSON CJ et al: The results of radical nephrectomy for renal cell carcinoma. Trans Am Assoc Genitourin Surg 60:122, 1968.
26. RICHIE JP: Renal Cell Carcinoma. Harvard Medical School Uro-logic Cancer 1992.
27. CHERRIE RJ et al: Prognostic implications of vena caval extension of renal cell carcinoma. J Urol 128:910, 1982.
28. SKINNER DG et al: Extension of renal cell carcinoma into the vena cava: The rationale for aggressive surgical management. J Urol 107:711, 1972.
29. RODRIGUEZ R et al: Differential diagnosis and evaluation of the incidentally discovered renal mass. Semin Urol Oncol 13:246, 1995.
30. MORGAN WR, ZINCKE H: Progression and survival after renal conserving surgery of renal cell carcinoma: Experience in 104 patients and extended follow-up. J Urol 144:852, 1990.
31. MALDAZYS JD et al: Prognostic factors in renal cell carcinoma. J Urol 136:376, 1986.
32. NISSENKORN I, BERNHEIM J: Multicentricity in renal cell carcinoma. J Urol 153:620, 1995.
33. MAYFIELD W, WAJSMAN Z: Surgical management of renal cell car-cinoma. Atlas Surg Oncol 591, 1995.
34. HUBEN RP et al: Tumor grade and stage as prognostic variables in upper tract urothelial tumors. Cancer 62:2016, 1988.
35. WALLACE DMA et al: The late results of conservative surgery for upper tract urothelial carcinomas. Br J Urol 53:537, 1981.
36. JENSEN OM et al: The Copenhagen case-control study of renal pelvis and ureter cancer: Role of smoking and occupational ex-posures. Int J Cancer 41:557, 1988.
37. PALVIO DH et al: Transitional cell tumors of the renal pelvis and ureter associated with capillarosclerosis indicating analgesic abuse. Cancer 41:557, 1987.
38. STEIN A et al: Adenocarcinoma of the renal pelvis: Report of two cases, one with simultaneous transitional cell carcinoma of the bladder. Urol Int 43:299, 1988.

39. BABAIAN RJ, JOHNSON DE: Primary carcinoma of the ureter. J Urol 123:357, 1980.

40. FRISCHER Z et al: Bilateral transitional cell carcinoma of the renal pelvis in the cancer family syndrome. J Urol 134:1197, 1985.

41. ORPHALI SI et al: Familial transitional cell carcinoma of renal pelvis and upper ureter. Urology 27:394, 1986.

42. LYNCH HT et al: The Lynch syndrome II and urological malignancies. J Urol 143:24, 1990.

43. HECHT F et al: Nonreciprocal chromosome translocation t(5;14) in cancers of the kidney: Adenocarcinoma of the renal parenchyma and transitional cell carcinoma of the kidney pelvis. Cancer Genet Cytogenet 14:197, 1985.

44. SANDBERG AA et al: Chromosome change in transitional cell carcinoma of the ureter. Cancer Genet Cytogenet 19:335, 1986.

45. GIBAS Z et al: Trisomy 7 AMD o(5p) in a transitional cell carcinoma of the ureter. Cancer Genet Cytogenet 25:369, 1987.

46. SAY CS, JORI JM: Transitional cell carcinoma of the renal pelvis: Experience from 1940 to 1972 and literature review. J Urol 112:438, 1974.

47. BABAIAN RJ et al: Metastases from transitional cell carcinoma of the urinary bladder. Urology 16:142, 1980.

48. LI MK, CHEUNG WL: Squamous cell carcinoma of the renal pelvis. J Urol 138:269, 1987.

49. PETERSON RO: Urologic Pathology. Philadelphia, Lippincott, 1986, p 762.

50. SPIRES SE et al: Adenocarcinoma of renal pelvis. Arch Pathol Lab Med 117:1156, 1993.

51. STEIN A et al: Adenocarcinoma of the renal pelvis: Report of two cases, one with simultaneous transitional cell carcinoma of the bladder. Urol Int 43:299, 1988.

52. MOSTOFI FK et al: Histological Typing of Urinary Bladder Tumors (International Histological Classification of Tumors No. 10). Geneva, World Health Organization, 1973.

53. HENEY NM et al: Prognostic factors in carcinoma of the ureter. J Urol 125:632, 1981.

54. MELAMED MR, RUETER VE: Pathology and staging of urothelial tumors of the kidney and ureter. Urol Clin North Am 20:333, 1993.

55. MURPHY DM et al: Primary grade 1 transitional cell carcinoma of the renal pelvis and ureter. J Urol 123:629, 1980.

56. MURPHY DM et al: Management of high grade transitional cell cancer of the upper urinary tract. J Urol 125:25, 1981.

57. HAUTREY CE: Fifty-two cases of primary ureteral carcinoma: A clinical-pathologic study. J Urol 105:188, 1971.

58. SARNACKI CT et al: Urinary cytology and the clinical diagnosis of urinary tract malignancy: A clinicopathologic study of 1,400 patients. J Urol 106:761, 1971.

59. ZINCKE H et al: Significance of urinary cytology in the early detection of transitional cell cancer of the upper urinary tract. J Urol 116:781, 1976.

60. STREEM SB et al: Ureteropyeloscopy in the evaluation of upper tract filling defects. J Urol 136:383, 1986.

61. BLOOM NA et al: Primary carcinoma of the ureter: A report of 102 new cases. J Urol 103:590, 1970.

62. KAKIZOE T et al: Transitional cell carcinoma of the bladder in patients with renal, pelvic and ureteral cancer. J Urol 124:17, 1980.

63. MULLEN JB, KOVACS K: Primary carcinoma of the ureteral stump: A case report and a review of the literature. J Urol 123:113, 1980.

64. BATATA MA et al: Primary carcinoma of the ureter: A prognostic study. Cancer 35:1626, 1975.

65. GHAZI MR et al: Primary carcinoma of the ureter. Report of 27 new cases. Urology 14:18, 1979.

66. HATCH TR et al: Time related recurrence rates in patients with upper tract transitional cell carcinoma. J Urol 140:40, 1988.

67. SMITH AD et al: Percutaneous management of renal pelvic tumors: A treatment option in selected cases. J Urol 137:852, 1987.

# 17B / CANCER OF THE BLADDER

*Sherri Machele Donat and William R. Fair*

## INTRODUCTION

### INCIDENCE

The bladder is one of the more common sites for appearance of cancer in the genitourinary tract, accounting for 7% of all cancers in males and 4% of all cancers in females.[1,2] Overall, the incidence of bladder cancer has been relatively stable and continues to occur at a rate of about 17 per 100,000. It is estimated that there will be 54,200 new patients with bladder cancer and 12,100 related deaths in 1999,[55] making it the fourth leading site of cancer in men after prostate, lung, and colorectal cancers, and the eighth leading site of cancer in females. This translates into a 260% higher incidence in men than women, and 70% higher in whites than blacks. Although bladder cancer is uncommon in some ethnic groups (American Indians, Filipinos, Asians, Hispanics), the incidence continues to be greater in males regardless of ethnicity as shown by the Surveillance, Epidemiology, and End Results (SEER) data (Fig. 17B-1).[2] The lifetime risk for developing bladder cancer is estimated to be 2.8% and 0.9% for white and black men, respectively, and 1% and 0.6% for white and black women, respectively.[2,3]

Due to advances in chemotherapy, radiation, and surgical management, mortality rates have decreased to about 3 per 100,000 since 1993,[1] but the majority of patients continue to die of metastatic disease. About 74% of bladder cancers are diagnosed early while the disease is still localized, and in this instance 5-year relative survival rates are correspondingly good at 93%. Survival rate declines dramatically when patients are diagnosed with advanced disease, with 5-year relative survival rates of around 49% for patients with regional disease at diagnosis, and only 6% for patients with distant disease at the time of diagnosis.[1] Beyond 5 years, survival rate continues to fall for all patients, with 71% of patients surviving 10 years after diagnosis and 65% surviving 15 years. When examining 5-year survival rates, it appears that survival is poorer in blacks than whites. Mortality rates, however, are identical between the two groups at 3.9 per 100,000 in whites and 3.8 per 100,000 in blacks, with only the incidence of bladder cancer being significantly greater in whites at 15.4 per 100,000 versus 8.6 per 100,000 in blacks.[1–3] This would indicate the detection of a greater number of lower-stage or biologically less aggressive tumors in whites, thereby increasing the incidence of cancer but not affecting the mortality rates.

## ETIOLOGY

Most bladder cancers are thought to be induced by environmental carcinogen exposure superimposed on a genetic predisposition, although rare cases of familial bladder cancers have been reported. It is considered a field change disease and, therefore, may affect the entire urothelium from the renal pelvis to the urethra. Of these, the bladder is the most common site of malignant transformation. Although the probability of developing upper tract tumors in patients with bladder cancer is only 2% to 4%, the risk of developing bladder cancer subsequent to an upper tract tumor is 15% to 50%.[4] Following radical cystectomy for bladder cancer, patients have a 1% to 9% risk of developing an upper tract tumor over the ensuing 10 years, the majority arising within the first 3 years, with a reported range of 8 months to 20 years.[4,5]

Several environmental and occupational factors have been identified as etiologic agents or risk factors associated with the development of transitional cell carcinoma of the urinary tract. This allows the unique opportunity, not yet present with most malignancies, of patient counseling to reduce the risk of tumor recurrence or even prevention of tumors in patients known to be at high risk for their development. In general, countries with higher degrees of industrialization have a higher incidence of tumors. The first reported link between an environmental agent and bladder cancer came in 1895 when Rehn identified an association between the development of bladder tumors and aniline dye exposure in factory workers.[3] This association was further supported in 1938 when Hueper was able to demonstrate a relationship between upper tract tumors and B-naphthylamine, an intermediate compound of dyes. These original associations were difficult to make secondary to an average delay of 15 to 20 years from the time of the initial exposure to the actual manifestation of tumor.[4] This latency period also accounts to some degree for the greater association of bladder cancer and advancing age, with the most common onset in the sixth and seventh decades of life. Since 1938, several other chemicals and their derivatives have been elucidated, including the aromatic amines, benzidine, α- and β-naphthylamine, 4-aminobiphenyl, polycyclic aromatic hydrocarbons (PAHs), and nitropyrenes. In addition, associations have been noted between dye, rubber, paint, and organic chemicals, and a higher incidence of tumors in patients working in occupations involving exposure to these agents.[4] It is estimated that occupational exposure to these agents accounts for 1% to 6% of all female bladder cancers and 18% to 35% of male bladder cancers.[6]

| RACIAL GROUP | FEMALE INCIDENCE | MALE INCIDENCE |
|---|---|---|
| American Indian | 0.4 | 3.5 |
| Filipino | 3 | 5.9 |
| Hispanic | 3.3 | 11.3 |
| Chinese | 3.9 | 13.9 |
| African American | 5.6 | 15.1 |
| White | 7.6 | 29.6 |

**FIGURE 17B-1.** Bladder cancer incidence by racial group and sex according to the Surveillance, Epidemiology, End Results (SEER) Program. (*Derived from Fadet Y: Epidemiology of bladder cancer, in* Comprehensive Textbook of Genitourinary Oncology, *Vogelzang NJ et al (eds). Baltimore, Williams & Wilkins, 1996, chap 17.*)

Cigarette smoking is by far the most significant risk factor for the development of bladder cancer and is estimated to account for 31% of the bladder cancers in women and at least 50% of the bladder cancers in men.[3,4] Smokers have up to a fourfold higher incidence of bladder cancer than nonsmokers. This finding has been consistent in almost every country studied, as demonstrated in Table 17B-1, where the relative risk of developing bladder cancer in smokers is shown to range from 1.6 to 4.2.[6] The risk is further supported by the finding of a dose-response relationship, showing a linear increase in the risk of developing a bladder cancer associated with increasing exposure (i.e., pack-years) to cigarette smoking. Patients who have smoked greater than 25 years have been found to have a relative risk ($p < 0.0001$) of developing tumors 4.5 times greater than nonsmokers.[3,7] In addition, there appears to be a strong relationship between the amount smoked per day, the number of years smoked, and the pack-year history of use with the development of both bladder and upper tract tumors. Smokers can reduce their risk by as much as 60% to 70% by quitting, but it may take several years before their risk declines to that of nonsmokers.[2–4,6] Again, the causative agents found in the urine of smokers include

## TABLE 17B-1. CIGARETTE SMOKING AND BLADDER CANCER

| | | RELATIVE RISK | | |
|---|---|---|---|---|
| AUTHOR | COUNTRY | MALE | FEMALE | TOTAL |
| Glashan | England | 1.8 | 1.6 | |
| Gonzalez | Spain | | | 2.3 |
| Mommsen | Denmark | 3.5 | 3.2 | 2.7 |
| Ohno | Japan | 1.87 | 3.53 | |
| Hartge | United States | 2.2 | | |
| Vineis | Italy | | 2.1 | |
| Morrison | United States | 1.9 | 4.2 | |
| Miller | Canada | 3.9 | 2.6 | |

SOURCE: Taken with permission from Thompson IM, Fair WF: The epidemiology of bladder cancer. AUA Update Series 8:213, 1989.

β-naphthylamine, 3,4-benzpyrene, pyrene, anthracene, and other polycyclic aromatic hydrocarbons. Others have suggested that although cigarette smoking has not been shown to alter significantly the kinds of mutations sustained in the p53 gene, it may act to increase the extent of DNA damage per mutagenic event.[2,8] Cigar and pipe smoking also increase the risk of developing bladder cancer, but not significantly.

Two pharmaceutical agents that have been associated with transitional cell carcinoma (TCC) are phenacetin, an analgesic agent whose chronic use translates into a relative risk of developing tumors similar to that of smoking, and cyclophosphamide, an alkylating agent used in the treatment of malignant neoplasms. Phenacetin-related tumors seem to be associated with chronic use of the drug and are more common in the upper tract than the bladder. About six cases of upper tract TCC have been reported in patients following cyclophosphamide therapy as well, with an average induction time of 5 years.[9] Cyclophosphamide is an alkylating agent widely used in the treatment of carcinomas of B-cell origin such as lymphoma and multiple myeloma. Its urinary metabolite, acrolein, is thought to be the primary carcinogen, with a latency period ranging from 6 to 13 years.[10] Most urologic oncologists are familiar with the more immediate complications of the therapy, including hemorrhagic cystitis and bladder fibrosis. The use of 2-mercaptoethanesulfonic acid (MESNA) before the start of and during cyclophosphamide therapy not only helps reduce the incidence of hemorrhagic cystitis, but may also help reduce the risk of a subsequent bladder cancer.

Radiation exposure has been reported to portend a two- to fourfold increased risk of developing bladder cancer, and has been seen in patients receiving radiation to the pelvic area for cervical and prostate cancer and in women treated with radiation for dysfunctional uterine bleeding. It has also been reported in patients receiving radioactive iodine for thyroid disease and in survivors of atomic bomb exposure in Japan.[10] Radiation-associated cancers often are high-grade and locally advanced at the time of diagnosis, probably due to a delay in diagnosis. This delay in diagnosis may be related to the similarity in presentation between the irritative voiding symptoms and hematuria frequently seen with a benign radiation cystitis and those seen with a bladder cancer.

Chronic irritative stimulants known to be associated with the development of bladder cancer are recurrent urinary tract infections, long-term indwelling catheters, infections with *Schistosoma haematobium,* and lesser associations with viral infections, including retroviruses and papilloma, herpes, and adenoviruses.[10]

On rare occasions an autosomal dominant hereditary pattern can be identified; however, the majority of hereditary bladder cancers appear to be inherited in a polygenetic pattern involving both a genetic predisposition and environmental interactions. Chromosomal aberrations occur frequently, with loss of 9q, 17p, 5q, and 3p having been reported. Overexpression of protooncogenes and/or inactivation of tumor suppressor genes are also felt to play a role in the transformation of cells to malignancy. Associations have been reported with overexpression of p53, retinoblastoma gene product (Rb), and c-*erb* B-2/neu and bladder cancer.[8,10] In addition, smokers seem to have a higher frequency of multiple mutations, which indicates that smoking may increase the extent of DNA damage.[11]

Dietary factors such as coffee, artificial sweeteners, chlorinated water, fatty foods, and foodstuffs with high sodium content have been suggested as possible risks for the development of bladder cancer, but none have been substantiated by case control studies. Because no clear link between these dietary factors and bladder cancer has been demonstrated, recommendations for avoidance of these foodstuffs cannot be made at this time.

## PREVENTIVE MEASURES

Bladder cancer is a unique cancer in that several environmental and occupational carcinogens placing patients at higher risk for developing the cancer have been identified. Avoidance of known risk factors may be beneficial in both preventing the occurrence of the cancer as well as subsequent recurrences. This allows for the possibility of preventing or decreasing the risk of developing bladder cancer in some patients by simply avoiding environmental and occupational exposure to the known carcinogens. In addition, patients identified as being at increased risk for the development of bladder cancer are perhaps the best group for which to consider periodic screening. Detection of the cancer in its earliest stages can translate into better survival rates. High-risk groups in the population for whom to consider periodic screening or chemoprevention are all patients with known occupational or environmetal exposure, those with known genetic predisposition by family history, those with previous history of a bladder tumor or upper tract tumor, those with iatrogenic exposure to cyclophosphamide or pelvic radiation, those with exposure to chronic irritation of the bladder (i.e., catheters, recurrent infections), those with a history of heavy smoking, and men above age 60 because of the greater association of bladder cancer with advancing age.

Chemoprevention is another area of interest in clinical research because of the ability to identify people at an increased risk for the development of bladder cancer. Agents under current study include retinoids, difluoromethylornithine (DFMO), and megadoses of vitamins A, $B_6$, C, E, and zinc. To date, no oral agent has demonstrated the ability to reduce the recurrence of bladder cancer or prevent its progression to muscle-invasive disease.

## CLINICAL MANIFESTATIONS

### CLINICAL SIGNS AND SYMPTOMS

The diagnosis of bladder cancer is often delayed because of the intermittent nature of symptoms and their commonality with other benign disorders such as urinary tract infections, interstitial cystitis, prostatitis, and the passage of renal calculi.

*Intermittent gross painless hematuria* is the most common presenting symptom of bladder cancer, although up to 12.5% of patients with asymptomatic microscopic hematuria will also be found to have a bladder carcinoma.[12] The degree of blood in the urine is not predictive of the probability of cancer being present. Microhematuria, most of which is attributed to benign causes, is estimated to be present in 13% of the general population. Benign causes for hematuria can include urinary tract infection, urinary calculi, sickle cell

**TABLE 17B-2.** THE MOST COMMON CAUSES OF HEMATURIA BY AGE AND SEX

0–20 years
 Acute glomerulonephritis
 Acute urinary tract infection
 Congenital urinary tract anomalies with obstruction

20–40 years
 Acute urinary tract infection
 Stones
 Bladder tumor

40–60 years (males)
 Bladder tumor
 Stones
 Acute urinary tract infection

40–60 years (females)
 Acute urinary tract infection
 Stones
 Bladder tumor

60 years (males)
 Benign prostatic hyperplasia
 Bladder tumor
 Acute urinary tract infection

60 years (females)
 Bladder tumor
 Acute urinary tract infection

SOURCE: Taken with permission from Gillenwater JY, Duckett JW et al (eds). *Adult and Pediatric Urology.* St. Louis, Mosby-Year Book, 1996, p 67.

anemia, vasculitis, renal vein thrombosis, renal infarction, nephritis, renal cysts, renal contusion or trauma, heavy exercise, benign prostatic hyperplasia, and unknown causes. The most likely cause for hematuria varies according to the patient's age and sex (Table 17B-2). Any patient with the finding of microhematuria on repetitive occasions or a single episode of gross hematuria, whether in association with no other symptoms, urinary symptoms, or with risk factors for bladder cancer, should have a workup, including a thorough physical examination, a cystoscopy, a urine specimen for cytology, and an intravenous pyelogram. About 75% of patients will be diagnosed with this initial workup. Additional studies such as utereroscopy, retrograde pyelograms, renal ultrasound, or CT scanning may be required to diagnose the remaining cases; however, no cause may be found for hematuria in approximately 5% to 10% of patients.[13]

The point at which gross hematuria is noted in the urine can be helpful in localizing where it may be originating from and thus the cause.

*Initial hematuria* occurs primarily at the beginning of the stream and usually is predictive of a urethral source. When blood is only noticed as a discharge between voidings or as a stain on undergarments while the urine itself appears clear on voidings indicates disease at the urethral meatus or the anterior urethra.

*Terminal hematuria* occurs primarily at the end of voiding and indicates disease at the bladder neck or prostatic urethral area. Total gross hematuria occurring throughout the entire voiding can occur with disease in the bladder, ureters, or kidneys.

*Irritative voiding symptoms* occur in approximately one-third of patients with bladder cancer and are most common in patients with carcinoma in situ or invasive carcinoma. They may consist of any one or a combination of the following: daytime and/or nocturnal frequency, urgency, dysuria, or urge incontinence.

*Obstructive voiding symptoms* are less common and may be due to tumor location at the bladder neck or prostatic urethra. Symptoms are usually straining, intermittency, nocturia, decreased force of stream, and a feeling of incomplete voiding.

Flank pain, suprapubic or abdominal pain, perineal pain, lower-extremity edema, pelvic mass, weight loss, fatigue, and bone pain usually indicate an advanced local tumor and/or metastatic disease.[14]

## DIAGNOSIS

### HISTORY AND PHYSICAL

In addition to a routine history, questions should include occupational and environmental exposures, smoking history, bleeding tendencies, family history of cancer or genetic syndromes, past genitourinary conditions or surgery, voiding symptoms, previous history of hematuria, and past or present conditions or medications with potential impact on the genitourinary system such as diabetes mellitus, tuberculosis, or bleeding disorders. Since 75% to 85% of bladder cancers are superficial at first presentation, the *physical examination* is usually normal. Patients with locally advanced or metastatic disease may have a palpable pelvic mass on bimanual or rectal exam, a palpable vaginal mass, adenopathy, lower-extremity edema, flank tenderness, bone pain, neurologic changes, prostatic enlargement or mass, or a palpable urethral mass or induration. Although adenopathy is more commonly seen in the pelvis or retroperitoneum, any palpable node should be considered for fine-needle or excisional biopsy if suspicious.

The *bimanual exam* is best performed under anesthesia before attempting resection of the tumor to assess tumor stage, mobility, and separability of the bladder from the iliac vessels. In a male, one or two fingers are placed in the rectum and the other hand is placed on the abdomen over the suprapubic area so that the bladder can be balloted between the two. In a female, two fingers are placed in the vagina and the bladder is balloted between the vagina and the abdominal wall. Induration, a palpable mass, or fixation in a patient that has not received previous radiation therapy to the pelvis are indications of the presence of an invasive tumor and perivesical disease. When a patient has received pelvic radiation in the past, it is difficult to differentiate between fixation due to radiation effect and tumor invasion. Any concerns of rectal wall involvement or a second primary tumor of the colon should be investigated by a barium enema and a flexible sigmoidoscopy or colonoscopy prior to planning surgery. The urethra should be palpated as well for induration, masses, fixation, and bloody discharge. Findings and interpretation of the bimanual exam may be affected by the size of the tumor, body habitus of the patient, previous pelvic surgery or radiation, the degree of relaxation of the abdominal wall, as well as the experience of the examiner.

**LABORATORY FINDINGS.** The *urinalysis* should include both a microscopic and gross examination and a dipstick chemical test. To avoid any distortion in readings, the urine should be examined within 30 min of collection or it should be refrigerated. The color of the urine can be affected by its concentration, ingestion of certain foods or medications, and bacteria. Urinary pigments that may mimic hematuria are anthocyanins such as beets or berries, phenolphthalein, phenazopyridine, vegetable dyes, urates, myoglobin, and *Serratia marcescens*. In these instances the microscopic exam will show no red blood cells (RBCs), but the dipstick analysis will be positive for blood. The specific gravity of a specimen is important to note because of its ability to influence the stability of white blood cells (WBCs) or RBCs. For example, when the urinary flow rate is high and the specific gravity is hypotonic at a gravity of less than 1.007, RBCs are lysed and therefore will not be present on microscopic examination even in the presence of pathology. The average individual excretes about 30,000 RBCs per hour, which on microscopic examination would appear as 1 RBC per high-power field (HPF). Microhematuria, however, is not considered significant unless it is greater than 3 RBCs per HPF. The morphology of the RBCs may also indicate the etiology of the hematuria in that cells of glomerular origin will often be dysmorphic or formed in casts.[13]

*Urine cytology* is frequently used to follow patients with TCC of both the lower and upper tracts. A positive cytology in a patient with no evidence of disease in the bladder should prompt a thorough evaluation of the upper tracts and the prostatic urethra. Lesions in these areas may not produce symptoms and, therefore, are easily missed early in the disease course. The greatest value of urine cytology is in the diagnosis of carcinoma in situ, where it has a sensitivity of about 90%. Unfortunately, urine cytologies have an overall false-negative rate of 65% in diagnosing upper tract TCC, and as high as 96% in low-grade upper tract tumors, and therefore are of limited value for the diagnosis of these tumors.[4,15] In fact, urine cytologies are negative in up to 80% of patients with low-grade tumors regardless of the tumor location.[16] This is thought to be due to the fact that lower-grade tumors have fewer morphological alterations that lead to the loss of intercellular attachments and adhesiveness, thus making them identifiable on cytologic analysis. When they are exfoliated, low-grade tumors are therefore shed in large papillary fragments with uniform size, minimal changes in nuclear-to-cytoplasmic ratios, and small or absent nucleoli. High-grade tumors, on the other hand, tend to have greater morphological changes leading to exfoliation and discovery on cytologic examination. High-grade tumor cells tend to be more isolated in loose clusters and elongated with marked pleomorphism, to have increased nuclear-to-cytoplasmic ratios, and to have variable nucleoli size.

If the cytology is positive and there is no discernible upper tract lesion, selective ureteral and renal pelvis washings may be performed. The diagnostic accuracy of these washings is still debated because of possible contamination from the bladder. However, some investigators report an accuracy rate of up to 80% in detecting carcinoma in situ of the upper tract with appropriate barbotage methods.[17]

To maintain a high level of diagnostic accuracy, it is important that the urine cytology specimens be collected and stored in the proper manner. Catheterized specimens can denude normal surface epithelial cells, which can coalesce in papillary groups and be misinterpreted as low-grade TCC. Voided specimens with prolonged exposure to concentrated urine or specimens from female patients contaminated with vaginal, cervical, endometrial, or epithelial cells can also be misinterpreted.[17] Chronic urinary tract infections, inflammatory conditions, and stone disease can also result in degenerative changes and cellular atypia. Recent instrumentation or intravesical therapy create well-described changes in cells that can be misinterpreted as well, and finally, the ability of the cytopathologist to interpret the specimen plays some role.

*DNA ploidy analysis* has been used to evaluate the DNA content of transitional cell tumors, and currently may be measured by flow cytometry or quantitative fluorescence image analysis. Flow cytometry allows for the analysis of up to 1000 cells per second, but it is not possible to assign DNA content to the morphology of a specific cell. Image analysis, on the other hand, is a slower method, but it permits the DNA measurement of cells already diagnosed visually as tumor cells.[1] The identification of abnormal DNA content in bladder cancer is being studied to determine if there may be any prognostic value to the individual patient in terms of survival and progression of disease. Tumor heterogeneity, individual cell cycle phases of tumors, morphology, and DNA content may all be determined by these methods.

Several *biochemical and immunologic markers* have been studied, but none have demonstrated reliable diagnostic results to date. Urinary enzyme tests for lactate dehydrogenase and alkaline phosphatase do not appear to be specific, and the levels of these enzymes do not appear to be reliably increased in patients with TCC. Carcinoembryonic antigen (CEA) is detectable in urine and serum, and its levels can be elevated in proportion to the mass and surface area of the tumor. However, elevated CEA levels may also simply reflect tissue breakdown secondary to infection or other tissue-destructive lesions, and therefore are also nonspecific and unreliable. Levels of tumor-specific or tumor-associated antigens in the serum or urine have not been found to be specifically or reliably increased either. There are several *molecular markers* under study as well, with the hope of identifying reliable associations between the pathologic features of a tumor, its molecular expression, and prognosis. Chromosomal aberrations (loss of 9q, 17p, 5q, and 3p), overexpression of protooncogene (p53, retinoblastoma gene product and c-*erb* B-2/neu), and/or inactivation of tumor suppressor genes are felt to play a role in the transformation of cells to malignancy, and associations have been reported with bladder cancer.

## RADIOGRAPHIC FINDINGS

An *intravenous pyelogram* (IVP) is recommended for all patients with a suspected urothelial carcinoma. It allows visualization of the entire urinary tract for localization of gross disease in both the bladder and upper tracts. More importantly, it is more sensitive in detecting small lesions of the ureter or renal pelvis, whereas CT scan or renal ultrasound are much better tests for the evaluation of renal parenchymal disease. However, IVP use may be limited in patients with renal insufficiency, diabetes mellitus, or contrast agent allergies. In these instances, retrograde pyelograms at the time of cystoscopy may be performed. Patients with known prior allergic reactions may also be prophylactically treated with steroids (prednisone, 50 mg orally 12, 7, and 1 hr before contrast administration) and an antihistamine (diphenhydramine, 50 mg orally 1 hr before contrast administration) prior to the scan. Baseline and periodic visualizations of the upper tracts by pyelograms are recommended in all patients with known superficial or invasive bladder cancer.

The *scout film* (before contrast) is rarely helpful in the detection of a TCC of the bladder, although some tumors (up to 6.7%) may develop a stippled or mottled calcification secondary to tumor necrosis, hemorrhage, or cystic degeneration.[18] The bony structures visible on the scout film should also be reviewed for evidence of bony metastases, which are usually lytic in appearance. The *cystogram phase* of the IVP detects 60% to 85% of large bladder tumors; however, smaller tumors may be missed and will only be seen with cystoscopy. Both the cystogram phase (Fig. 17B-2A) and the postvoid film (Fig. 17B-2B) should be examined for filling defects, which are usually irregular frondlike or nodular defects that are persistent from film to film. Invasive tumors of the bladder may cause a distal ureteral obstruction and secondary hydronephrosis by obstructing the ureteral orifice and/or the intramural tunnel (Fig. 17B-3A–C). The lack of this finding does not rule out invasive disease; however, its presence is associated with invasive disease in about 92% of patients.[18] Ideally, the IVP should be obtained prior to the transurethral resection of the tumor to avoid misinterpretation of postoperative changes.

The classic urographic findings for upper tract TCC are a meniscus-shaped ureteral filling defect known as the "goblet" or "Bergmann" sign, and the "stipple sign" produced by contrast medium being trapped in the fronds of a papillary tumor. Filling defects may be the result of the parietal implantation of tumor, the uneven jagged contours of papillary fronds, or obstruction of a ureter with proximal dilatation. This is diagnostic in 47% to 98% of patients with upper tract tumors, although fewer than 10% of patients with bladder cancer will have simultaneous upper tract involvement. About 50% of patients with a filling defect either in the renal pelvis or ureter will have an associated hydronephrosis, hydroureter, or nonvisualization of the kidney secondary to obstruction.[4] Nonvisualization is usually a symptom of advanced disease, and is frequently associated with invasion of tumor into the renal parenchyma, indicating a poorer prognosis. Stenosis is also a specific sign of infiltrating disease and is more commonly seen in the renal pelvis than the ureter. In contrast, if no abnormalities are found on IVP and a tumor is present on other studies, it will be low grade in 85% of patients.[17] As alluded to previously, *retrograde pyelograms* are often used to evaluate the ureters and renal pelvis in patients who either cannot receive intravenous contrast due to allergy or renal insufficiency, or in patients in whom the ureters and renal pelvis were poorly visualized on an IVP. Retrograde pyelograms are performed at the time of cystoscopy by using a ureteral catheter to inject contrast medium directly up the ureters in a retrograde fashion. This is usually performed under fluoroscopy to ensure optimal visualization of all parts of the upper tracts.

*Ultrasound* is not very useful in the diagnosis or staging of bladder cancer. It can confirm a soft tissue mass, but it is unable to

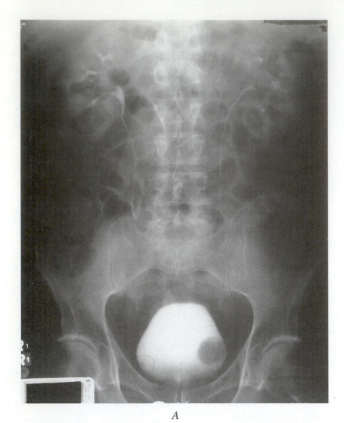
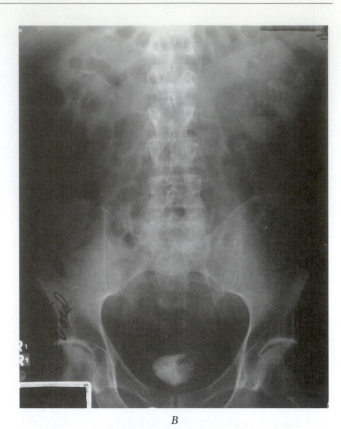

*A*
*B*

**FIGURE 17B-2.** Cystogram and postvoid phases of the intravenous pyelogram demonstrating a filling defect in the bladder.

differentiate depth of invasion, extravesical disease, or nodal status, and will miss small lesions. It is useful in evaluating the upper tracts for renal parenchymal disease and to differentiate a nonradiopaque stone from a soft tissue mass by differences in echogenicity.

*Computed tomography* (CT) is routinely used in clinical staging of patients with invasive or locally advanced bladder carcinomas. It can demonstrate extravesical extension; nodal involvement in the pelvis or retroperitoneum; visceral, pulmonary, or osseous metastasis; and upper tract function, involvement, or obstruction. In addition, it is useful for comparison examinations in patients receiving chemotherapy for advanced disease to evaluate response. Although CT provides better visualization of tumors than ultrasound, it may also miss tumors less than 1 cm in size, and cannot differentiate depth of bladder wall invasion (i.e., mucosal vs. lamina propria vs. muscularis propria invasion). Alternatively, CT scanning is about 80% accurate in differentiating locally advanced tumors involving extravesical adipose tissue (Fig. 17B-4) or surrounding structures from less invasive tumors.[18] Unfortunately, most patients are not scanned until after a transurethral resection and bimanual exam of the tumor have been performed for tissue diagnosis and clinical staging, making it difficult to distinguish inflammatory or traumatic edematous changes from true extravesical extension of tumor. Bladder muscle wall thickening on CT can only suggest the presence

of a muscle-invasive tumor and requires tissue for diagnosis. Nodal involvement can only be implied (Fig. 17B-5) because its sensitivity in detecting nodal metastasis is relatively low (false-negative rate 68%; false-positive rate 16%), and requires a needle or excisional biopsy for confirmation.[19]

*Magnetic resonance imaging* (MRI) is used in a similar fashion to CT for staging of invasive or locally advanced disease. MRI may be used in patients allergic to the contrast agents required for CT scanning, but it is difficult to tolerate by claustrophobic patients and cannot be used in patients with pacemakers or other metallic foreign bodies such as vascular clips, implants, or projectiles. Open MRI imaging is available for claustrophobic patients, but the trade-off is poorer image resolution due to the smaller magnet.

*Nuclear bone scanning* is used to evaluate the presence of osseous metastasis and is recommended only in patients with invasive or locally advanced tumors and skeletal symptoms or elevated alkaline phosphatase levels. Increased uptake is a nonspecific finding and may represent areas of degenerative change, trauma, previous fracture sites, or metastatic disease. Plain films, bone windows on CT, or MRI of areas of concern are necessary to confirm a metastasis. If the added studies are not confirmatory, a bone biopsy may be performed. Occasionally, ureteral obstruction may be noted on a bone scan (see Fig 17B-3*A*).

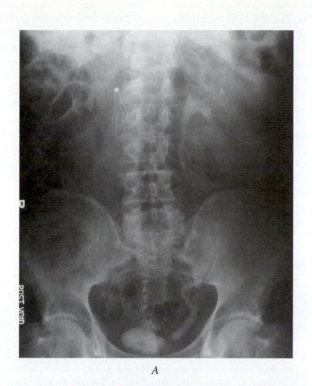

*A*

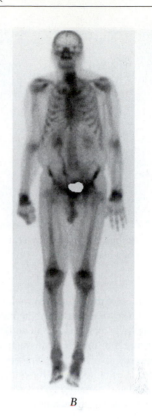

*B*

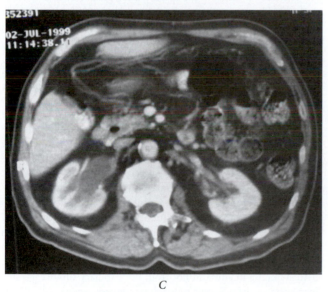

*C*

**FIGURE 17B-3.** Invasive tumor causing hydronephrosis by obstructing the distal ureter as demonstrated by *A.* Intravenous pyelogram *B.* Bone scan, and *C.* Computed tomography.

*Chest radiographs* are used as an initial screening tool and for periodic monitoring in patients at risk for pulmonary metastases, although it will be unable to detect lesions less than 1 cm in diameter. Metastatic lesions are characteristically noncalcified soft tissue densities. If the chest film is suspicious for metastatic disease, a CT scan of the chest will give optimal visualization of any lesions less than 1 cm and an assessment of mediastinal and paratracheal nodes for enlargement. The CT can also be used to direct needle biopsy of pulmonary lesions to confirm the diagnosis. If old films are available for comparison, they are useful to help differentiate benign lesions that usually do not progress with time from metastasis.

## ENDOSCOPIC FINDINGS

*Cystoscopy* with a bimanual exam and tumor biopsy is the most accurate method for establishing the diagnosis and clinical stage of a bladder cancer. It is best performed under anesthesia to allow

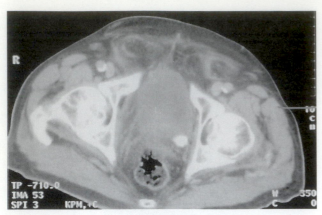

**FIGURE 17B-4.** Computed tomography scan demonstrating extravesical extension of a bladder tumor.

for complete relaxation of the abdominal wall. A bimanual exam is performed as previously described after the induction of anesthesia and the size, mobility, pelvic side wall and anterior abdominal wall involvement, urethral involvement, vaginal wall or prostatic involvement, and rectal involvement are recorded. Once the endoscope is introduced, a urine specimen for cytology is obtained and the bladder is inspected systematically, recording the size, location, architecture (papillary, sessile, flat), and number of all tumors on a bladder map (Fig. 17B-6). In addition, the status of the intervening mucosa; ureteral orifices (patency and character of the efflux); presence of trabeculation, cellules, or diverticuli; and involvement of the bladder neck or urethra should be noted. Patients with positive urine cytologies and no visible tumor in the bladder should have random bladder and prostatic urethral biopsies, as well as retrograde studies and selective ureteral washes for cytology to try to determine the source of the positive cytology.

If possible, each bladder tumor should be resected completely, including the muscle layer below to delineate the histologic type and depth of invasion of the tumor. Selected biopsies of the grossly normal-appearing intervening mucosa should also be performed to determine if carcinoma in situ or dysplasia exists, which may affect

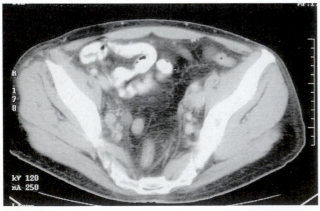

**FIGURE 17B-5.** Nodal enlargement on computed tomography implying metastatic disease that must be confirmed by biopsy.

treatment options (i.e., bladder sparing or continent diversion). The findings of the endoscopic exam coupled with the cytology or pathology results, radiologic evaluation, and bimanual exam determine the clinical stage of the patient. The true pathologic stage can only be determined at the time of cystectomy. The understaging error of clinical staging is estimated to be 40% to 50%.[20] This is essentially due to the inability to detect microscopic extension of disease and the inability to differentiate inflammation and tumor fibrosis or necrosis from viable tumor by radiologic evaluation. Despite the inadequacies, the restaging transurethral biopsy and bimanual exam performed under anesthesia are increasingly used to help determine the need for neoadjuvant therapy, response to radiation or chemotherapy, and to direct the need for further therapy or the feasibility of bladder preservation.

## HISTOLOGY

### CELL TYPES

Primary carcinoma of the bladder includes, in descending order of frequency, TCC, squamous cell carcinoma, adenocarcinoma, and undifferentiated carcinoma (Table 17B-3). The predominant (90% to 95%) urothelial carcinoma in the United States is TCC, which can occur anywhere in the lining of the urinary tract from the renal pelvis to the distal two-thirds of the urethra. Although a tumor can occur anywhere in the lining of the urinary tract, greater than 90% occur in the bladder, 8% in the renal pelvis, and only 2% in the ureter or urethra. TCCs may occur as solitary or multifocal lesions exhibiting several growth patterns, the most common being papillary (70%), and the remaining nodular (10%), and sessile or mixed (20%).[21] Transitional epithelium has a high metaplastic potential; thus mixed histologic patterns, including squamous, adenocarcinomatous, and spindle cells are seen in up to one-third of TCCs.

Tumors with mixed histology tend to be more invasive, but the presence of these elements does not change the primary classification of the tumor. Reuter et al., in an unpublished paper, have described a sequence in tumor development progressing from mucosal hyperplasia to an invasive papillary carcinoma (Fig. 17B-7). This sequence is supported by the common finding of areas of carcinoma in an otherwise benign-appearing papilloma, described as papilloma with carcinoma in situ. This suggests that the pathogenesis of papillary carcinoma may be through the transformation of a preexisting papilloma, although it is also possible for some patients to develop an invasive carcinoma from the accompanying flat carcinoma in situ and not from the papillary tumor.[22] Transformation of the adjacent mucosa may grossly appear as a flat or micropapillary carcinoma in situ and is found in 7% to 25% of patients undergoing cystectomy for invasive carcinoma of the bladder. It is more commonly found in patients with multiple recurrences over time or multifocal disease where involvement of the distal ureter may represent an extension of the bladder cancer into the distal ureter. The panurothelial nature of carcinoma in situ is further supported by the finding of increased risk (20%, 26/128 patients) of the development of upper tract tumors over time in patients whose bladders have been preserved by successful intravesical bacillus Calmette-Guérin (BCG) therapy.[23,24] Such tumors have been detected as late as 15 years or more after treatment of

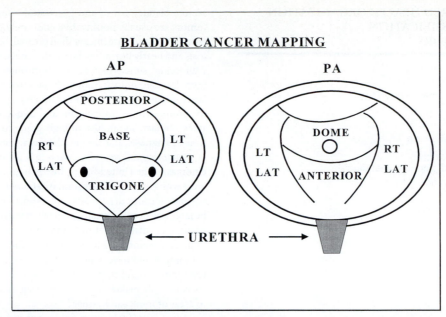

**FIGURE 17B-6.** Bladder map used to record size, location, and architecture of all tumors at cystoscopy. (*Adapted from Scher HI, et al: Cancer of the bladder, in* Cancer Principles and Practice of Oncology, *5th ed, DeVita VT et al (eds). Philadelphia, Lippincott-Raven, 1997, chap 33.3.*)

the initial bladder tumor, mandating surveillance of the upper tracts probably for the lifetime of the patient. Flat carcinoma in situ may also develop in the ureter or renal pelvis unrelated to the condition of the bladder and is usually asymptomatic and found incidentally on workup of a positive urine cytology. Flat carcinoma in situ is

Mucosal Hyperplasia

⇓

Papilloma

⇓

Atypical Papilloma

⇓

Papilloma with Focal CIS

⇓

Non-invasive Papillary Carcinoma

⇓

Papillary Carcinoma with Invasion

**FIGURE 17B-7.** Proposed transformation of urothelium from hyperplasia to invasive papillary carcinoma. (*Taken with permission from Melamed MR, Reuter VE: Pathology and staging of urothelial tumors of the kidney and ureter. Urol Clin North Am 20:333, 1993.*)

difficult to define grossly because the mucosal appearance may vary from being slightly thickened and pale white when epithelial hyperplasia is present to an erythemic congested appearance when there is an increase in subepithelial vascularity.

It is unclear whether the development of new tumors represents multifocality in a carcinoma-prone urothelium or dissemination of cells from the initial tumor.[4,22] Two arguments favoring the multifocal origin of tumors are the occurrence of bilateral upper tract tumors and the common finding of separate areas of carcinoma and carcinoma in situ in cystectomy series. Conversely, the theory of tumor dissemination can be supported through the high incidence of the subsequent development of bladder cancer in patients presenting with upper tract tumors as opposed to the very low incidence of the reverse, the decreasing incidence of developing subsequent tumor in the bladder over time after a nephroureterectomy, the reported cases of percutaneous tract and retroperitoneal seeding after pyelotomies for renal pelvis tumors, the recent demonstration of common genetic markers in what appear to be separate urinary tract tumors,[25] the increased risk (15 to 20 times) of bladder cancer patients with vesicoureteral reflux developing upper tract tumors, and the experimental animal evidence that tumor has the potential to spread by dissemination.[4]

Grading systems for TCC are based on histologic parameters that categorize tumors based on the degree of the cellular organization, cytoplasmic features, nuclear features, and their degree of resemblance to normal urothelium. Only the TCCs are graded, and one of the more commonly used systems is the World Health Organization (WHO) grading system, which categorizes tumors into low-grade (G1), intermediate grade (G2), or high grade (G3). Normal urothelium is composed of 3- to 7-cell-layer thick epithelium resting on

## TABLE 17B-3. WORLD HEALTH ORGANIZATION HISTOLOGIC CLASSIFICATION OF BLADDER TUMORS

Epithelial tumors
  Transitional cell papilloma
  Transitional cell papilloma, inverted type
  Squamous cell papilloma
  Transitional cell carcinoma
    With squamous metaplasia
    With glandular metaplasia
    With squamous and glandular metaplasia
  Squamous cell carcinoma
  Adenocarcinoma
  Undifferentiated carcinoma

Nonepithelial tumors
  Benign
  Malignant
  Rhabdomyosarcoma
  Other

Miscellaneous tumors
  Pheochromocytoma
  Lymphomas
  Carcinosarcomas
  Malignant melanoma
  Others

Metastatic tumors and secondary extensions

Unclassified tumors

Epithelial abnormalities
  Papillary (polypoid) "cystitis"
  Brunn's nests
  Cystitis cystica
  Glandular metaplasia
  "Nephrogenic adenoma"
  Squamous metaplasia

Tumorlike lesions
  Follicular cystitis
  Malakoplakia
  Amyloidosis
  Fibrous (fibroepithelial) polyp
  Endometriosis
  Hamartomas
  Cysts

Source: Taken with permission from Hudson HA, Catalona WJ: Urothelial tumors of the bladder, upper tracts, and prostate. In *Adult and Pediatric Urology*, Gillenwater JY et al (eds). St Louis, Mosby-Year Book, 1996, chap. 29.

a basement membrane, with the most superficial layer composed of large, flat umbrella cells. Below the basement membrane is a loose connective tissue layer called the lamina propria with scattered smooth muscle fibers (muscularis mucosae). Below the lamina propria is a smooth muscle layer, the muscularis propria, beyond which

are the bladder serosa and perivesical fat. Grade 1, or low-grade, tumors are usually noninvasive and rarely progress to higher-stage lesions. Cell layers are thicker than normal, but uniform with rare mitosis and nearly normal polarity, thickness, and polarization. Grade 2 tumors are similar to grade 1 tumors but with a thicker epithelium, more frequent mitosis, more cellular crowding, and a preserved polarity. Grade 3 tumors are considered high grade, with a loss of polarity, prominent pleomorphism, and frequent progression to higher stages. In fact, about 50% of high-grade tumors are invasive at the time of diagnosis, and almost all invasive tumors are high-grade.[10,21]

*Squamous cell carcinoma* accounts for only 5% of bladder carcinomas in the United States, but as high as 75% of carcinomas in areas with endemic schistosomiasis. Growth patterns vary from sessile and ulcerated to papillary, polypoid, or nodular, and they tend to be large and deeply invasive even when well differentiated. They also occur in the distal one-third of the urethra where squamous epithelium predominates. Microscopically, they are usually abundantly keratinized and have a similar histologic pattern as squamous cell carcinomas found elsewhere in the body. Tumors often have an associated leukoplakia or keratinizing squamous metaplasia adjacent to areas of frank carcinoma.[21]

*Adenocarcinoma* is even more uncommon and accounts for only 0.5% to 2% of bladder carcinomas. They most commonly occur spontaneously (66%), but may be associated with exstrophy of the bladder, endometriosis, or may be of urachal origin (33%). The nonurachal tumors tend to occur in clinical settings of chronic irritation such as exstrophy (85%) and neurogenic bladders (15%). Microscopically, the tumors have a glandular growth pattern predominantly and may be subclassified into mucinous (23%), enteric (19.4%), signet-ring cell (16.7%), mixed (12.5%), and adenocarcinoma unspecified (27.8%). Grossly, they may be nodular, papillary, ulcerative, or sessile, and are often mucoid. Tumors with a predominantly signet cell subtype have a poorer prognosis than those with other components.

*Undifferentiated carcinomas* of the bladder are rare and may demonstrate histologic features of small cell carcinoma, undifferentiated large cell carcinoma, and lymphoepithelioma. The small cell subtype can be confused with lymphoma, often necessitating the use of immunohistochemical stains for lymphoid or epithelial markers to differentiate the two. Grossly, the tumors tend to be large and either polypoid or ulcerated. Histologically, depending on the subtype, they may appear as sheets of small oat-shaped cells (small cell), or large pleomorphic cells with components of malignant giant cells (undifferentiated large cell).

Metastatic cancers to the bladder are rare and have included pheochromocytoma, melanoma, lymphoma, and small cell carcinoma.

## PROGNOSTIC FACTORS

The identification of factors that influence the outcome of a patient's disease is important not only in predicting the clinical course for the patient, but to help in treatment selection. For instance, a more aggressive treatment might be selected for patients identified to be at high risk for progression of disease or local and/or distant recurrence than would be chosen for a patient judged to have a tumor with minimal biologic risk. This can be especially important when

**TABLE 17B-4.** SURVIVAL BASED ON PATHOLOGIC STAGE

| SERIES | YEAR | PATIENTS | 5-YEAR SURVIVAL RATE, % | | |
| --- | --- | --- | --- | --- | --- |
| | | | P2 | P3 | P4 |
| Richie | 1975 | 134 | 39 | 40 | — |
| Whitmore | 1980 | 174 | 50 | 25 | 18 |
| Mather | 1981 | 58 | 70 | 33 | 29 |
| Skinner | 1982 | 130 | 47 | 39 | 25 |
| Skinner | 1984 | 197 | 69 | 29 | 22 |
| Montie | 1984 | 99 | 63 | 57 | — |
| Giuliani | 1991 | 202 | 56 | 19 | — |
| Roehrborn | 1991 | 280 | 61 | 36 | 27 |
| Pagano | 1991 | 261 | 50 | 15 | 21 |
| Wishnow | 1992 | 71 | 75 | 48 | — |
| Waehre | 1997 | 227 | 60 | 31 | 29 |
| Herr | 1999 | 686 | 58 | 22 | 15 |
| Totals | | 2519 | 57 | 31 | 24 |

considering bladder preservation. Radiation, chemotherapy, and surgery can all have serious toxicities, including death. In addition, all treatments affect quality of life. Therefore, the morbidity of a treatment, both in terms of physical side effects and quality-of-life changes, must always be weighed against its potential for benefit or cure in the individual patient. Reliable prognostic factors can be of great benefit to this end. Many factors have been examined concerning their ability to predict prognosis and treatment outcome including age, sex, race, tumor grade, tumor size, depth of invasion, vascular or lymphatic invasion, clinical and pathologic stage, involvement of vonn Brun's nests, tumor multifocality and frequency of recurrence, associated carcinoma in situ, ploidy and molecular markers (p53, Rb), nodal involvement, positive margins, ureteral involvement, prostatic duct or stromal involvement, and cell type (squamous, adenomatous, undifferentiated, etc.) and degree of differentiation. The most reliable prognostic variables among the factors studied by multivariate analysis are tumor grade, stage, and presence of carcinoma in situ.[10] In addition, several laboratory parameters, including the expression of Thompson-Friedenreich (T) antigen, lectin-binding carbohydrate structures, ABH blood group antigens, Lewis x antigen, oncofetal protein expression, epidermal growth factor receptor content, and chromosomal abnormalities have been evaluated for their prognostic significance, and some significant correlations with tumor progression have been shown, although none of these have been adopted yet to the degree that they are used to make treatment decisions.[26] It is hoped that some of these markers or a combination of markers will help stratify patients into good-risk versus poor-risk categories prior to treatment selection. For superficial tumors, the presence of Tis (carcinoma in situ) has been identified as the most significant ($p = 0.0001$) variable in predicting progression, followed by multifocality ($p = 0.006$), lamina propria invasion (T1; $p = 0.02$), and tumor grade ($p = 0.04$).[27] By definition, carcinoma in situ is composed of grade 3 cells. Patients with low-grade Ta tumors seldom progress, develop metastasis, or die from their tumors, accounting for a 20% to 30% difference in survival when compared with patients with superficial tumors with lamina propria invasion (T1), which are predominantly high grade by nature.[28]

**TABLE 17B-5.** SURVIVAL OF PATIENTS WITH NODE-POSITIVE BLADDER CANCER

| SERIES | YEAR | PATIENTS | 5-YEAR SURVIVAL RATE, % |
| --- | --- | --- | --- |
| Whitmore | 1981 | 134 | 7 |
| Smith | 1983 | 230 | 4 |
| Skinner | 1984 | 36 | 35 |
| Vieweg | 1991 | 229 | 19 |
| Pagano | 1991 | 26 | 4 |
| Herr | 1999 | 193 | 22 |

The most significant prognostic factor in treatment outcome with invasive cancers appears to be the pathologic stage of disease and more specifically, whether the tumor is organ-confined (T3a or less) or non-organ-confined (T3b or greater or node-positive any T stage). Several series have consistently demonstrated the relationship of pathologic stage of the tumor and nodal status to survival (Table 17B-4). In the event of node-positive disease, the 5-year survival rate is dismal (4% to 35%) without any systemic therapy (Table 17B-5). Distant metastatic disease to bone, lung, viscera, brain, or soft tissue portends an even graver prognosis, with median survivals of less than 1 year (6 to 9 months) and an almost 0% 5-year survival rate.[14]

## STAGING OF DISEASE

The staging systems for bladder cancer were originally derived from pathologic studies of cystectomy specimens, which were then correlated with patient outcome, including risk of metastasis and survival. This is where the first associations of depth of invasion of a tumor and treatment outcomes were made. It has been through the pathologic analysis of radical cystectomy specimens that our current staging system arose (see Table 17B-6) as well as the realization that there is a significant clinical staging error rate.[14] It is estimated that 35% to 50% of patients are understaged, whereas 23% of patients are overstaged. Many systems have been devised over the years, with the most common two being the Jewett and

**TABLE 17B-6.** TNM VERSUS PATHOLOGIC STAGING FOR RADICAL CYSTECTOMY PATIENTS

| T STAGE | NO. OF PATIENTS* | PATIENTS FOR WHOM T < P, % | PATIENTS FOR WHOM T > P, % |
| --- | --- | --- | --- |
| T1/Tis | 124 | 23 (19) | 18 (15) |
| T2 | 181 | 71 (39) | 45 (25) |
| T3a | 104 | 37 (36) | 19 (18) |
| T3b | 56 | 32 (57) | 23 (45) |
| Total | 465 | 163 (35) | 105 (23) |

* Combined series from Whitmore, Prout, Richie, and Skinner.
SOURCE: Taken with permission from Fair FW et al: Cancer of the bladder, in *Cancer Principles and Practice of Oncology*, 4th ed, DeVita VT et al (eds). Philadelphia, Lippincott-Raven, 1993, chap 34.

**TABLE 17B-7.** BLADDER CANCER: CLINICAL STAGING CLASSIFICATION

| | MARSHALL-JEWETT | TNM | DESCRIPTION |
|---|---|---|---|
| | | T0 | No evidence of tumor |
| Superficial | CIS | Tis | Flat tumor: carcinoma in situ |
| | O | Ta | Noninvasive papillary carcinoma |
| | A | T1 | Invades lamina propria |
| Infiltrating | B1 | T2a | Invades superfical half of muscle |
| | B2 | T2b | Invades deep half of muscle |
| | C | T3a (microscopic) | Invades perivesical fat |
| | | T3b (macroscopic) | Invades perivesical fat |
| Invasion of adjacent structures | D1 | T4a | Invades prostate, uterus, vagina |
| | | T4b | Invades abdominal wall, pelvic wall |
| Lymph node involvement | D2 | N1–3 | Dependent on number and size of nodes involved |
| | D3 | | |
| Distant disease | D4 | M1 | Distant metastasis |

Strong and the TNM (tumor, node, metastasis) systems. The Jewett and Strong system was originally proposed in 1946 and later modified by Marshall by adding findings of the bimanual exam and microscopic findings of tissue removed at biopsy. Since then the International Union Against Cancer (IUAC) and the American Joint Commission for Cancer (AJCC) have adopted the TNM system, which provides a means of differentiating the two patterns of growth and clinical behavior of superficial tumors and more clearly defines the extent of extravesical spread as depicted in Fig. 17B-8 and Table 17B-7. In addition, the TNM system has two classifications, allowing for the distinction between pretreatment clinical staging and postsurgical histopathologic staging. Treatment options for bladder

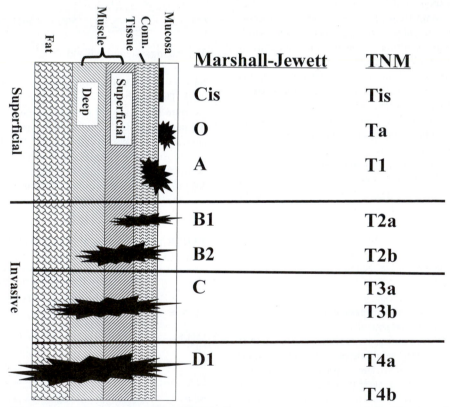

**FIGURE 17B-8.** Comparison of the Marshall-Jewett and TNM systems of classification of bladder cancer. (Abbreviation: conn. = connective.)

**TABLE 17B-8.** SENSITIVITY AND SPECIFICITY (%) OF CT AND MRI FOR DETERMINING NODAL STATUS IN BLADDER CANCER

| SERIES | NO. | % SENSITIVITY | % SPECIFICITY | % UNDERSTAGING | % OVERSTAGING |
|---|---|---|---|---|---|
| CT | | | | | |
| Voges et al | 164 | 10 | 95 | 90 | 5 |
| Koss et al | 25 | 60 | 100 | 40 | 0 |
| Vock et al | 44 | 94 | 85 | 6 | 15 |
| Weinerman et al | 36 | 57 | 100 | 43 | 0 |
| Sawczuk et al | 8 | 0 | 83 | 100 | 17 |
| Giri et al | 17 | 37 | 89 | 63 | 11 |
| All series | 294 | 48 | 94 | 52 | 6 |
| | | | | | |
| MRI | | | | | |
| Buy et al | 40 | 83 | 100 | 17 | 0 |
| Tavares et al | 22 | 50 | 100 | 50 | 0 |
| Johnson et al | 9 | 100 | 100 | 0 | 0 |
| All series | 71 | 74 | 100 | 26 | 0 |

SOURCE: Taken with permission from See WA, Fuller JR: Staging of advanced bladder cancer. Urol Clin North Am 19:663, 1992.

cancer are based on the stage of the disease; therefore, it is imperative that the staging be as accurate as possible. Today, most patients are staged by a combination of pathologic and clinical (exam, laboratory, and radiographic findings) procedures; however, the most accurate staging appears to come at the time of cystectomy and lymph node dissection (pathologic staging).[14] This is due to our inability by radiograph, endoscopic biopsy, bimanual exam, and physical exam to identify microscopic extension of disease, or to differentiate postsurgical changes or trauma or postchemotherapy or radiation fibrosis or necrosis from viable tumor. Staging by transurethral resection is thought to underestimate the pathologic extent of disease in 30% to 50% of patients.[29] About 50% of all patients with invasive cancer will have metastatic disease.[30] Due to the increasing frequency of metastases with increasing depth of invasion of the bladder wall, any patient thought to have muscle invasion (T2–4) will go on to have testing to evaluate the possibility of regional spread prior to choosing a definitive therapy. However, the accuracy of defining regional lymph node involvement by MRI or CT is less than desirable, as seen in multiple series addressing this issue (Table 17B-8).[19,31] Despite the inaccuracies, most practitioners continue to use these modalities for lack of better alternatives. If the patient is felt to be at significant risk for distant disease, then a staging evaluation for the most common sites of distant metastases, including lymph nodes, bone, liver, lungs, and adrenals, is usually performed. The lungs can be evaluated by a chest radiograph or CT. Although a chest CT is more sensitive, it also has a higher false-positive rate, and most investigators agree that it should be reserved for evaluating patients at high risk or in patients who demonstrate a suspicious abnormality on a chest radiograph.[31] A CT-guided needle biopsy, thoracoscopic wedge biopsy, or open thoracotomy may be used to obtain a pathologic confirmation of suspected lung disease. Liver disease is less common (30% of patients dying of bladder cancer are found to have liver disease), and usually evaluated at the time of the regional evaluation by CT or MRI of the abdomen. The bone is evaluated with a radionuclide bone scan and plain films, if necessary. Bone disease is only seen in about 5% of early-stage invasive disease (T1–2) and in about 15%

of patients with locally advanced disease. However, the impact its presence has on treatment decisions warrants the investigation in patients at high risk or suspicion due to bone symptoms and/or elevated alkaline phosphatase levels. Areas of increased uptake suspicious for disease can then be further evaluated by plain films, bone windows on CT, MRI, or biopsy as clinically indicated. Brain metastasis can occur, but it is rare and usually seen as a site of relapse in patients who have failed aggressive chemotherapy as a neoadjuvant complement to their primary definitive therapy (radiation or surgery) or for metastasis to other sites.[30] Brain scans are not usually performed as part of a standard systemic workup, but are reserved for patients with clinical suspicion of disease based on symptoms or as part of a protocol requirement.

## TREATMENT BY STAGE OF DISEASE

The clinical behavior, primary management, and prognosis of bladder cancer are determined by its depth of invasion and stage. There is a range of disease from superficial to invasive to metastatic. Accordingly, treatments range from the endoscopic removal of a tumor, to partial or complete removal of the bladder, to systemic chemotherapy. It is exceedingly important that the cancer be staged as accurately as possible prior to making a treatment decision. Therefore, it is our practice at Memorial Sloan-Kettering Cancer Center (MSKCC) to perform a restaging or second transurethral resection (TUR) of the tumor site prior to deciding on a treatment course due to the high reported incidence (20% to 40%) of local recurrence, a 43% reported incidence of understaging secondary to inadequate first resections, and the low likelihood that intravesical therapy will have an effect on residual invasive tumor cells.[32,34] In our experience, a restaging TUR decreases the uncertainty of the depth of tumor invasion, improves control of the primary tumor by ensuring the most complete resection possible, and provides additional material for pathologic analysis that may help in selecting the appropriate therapy. The extent of disease and age and comorbidities of the patient also dictate the type of treatment and whether a single treatment modality will be sufficient or if the patient might benefit from a combined-modality approach. In the case of invasive disease, although radical cystectomy may afford the best chance for cure, a subset of patients who either desire not to have their bladder removed or medically are too high risk for a major surgery have the options of radiation therapy or a combined-modality approach that may include any combination of the following: radiation therapy, aggressive transurethral resection, or partial cystectomy and chemotherapy. The goals of a treatment approach may range from the prevention or delay of a local recurrence, to organ sparing, to the prevention of distant metastasis, to palliation. In general, systemic therapy is used in three disease scenarios: known metastatic disease, locally advanced disease as neoadjuvant or adjuvant therapy, or in bladder-sparing protocols.

## SUPERFICIAL DISEASE

Of bladder cancers, 80% are superficial, meaning that they are confined to the epithelium (Ta, Cis) or submucosa (T1). The treatment intent for superficial tumors is to prevent recurrences or progression to more invasive or incurable disease. The conventional treatment modality to manage superficial tumors in the bladder is *endoscopic transurethral resection* (TURBT). Very small, low-grade recurrent papillary Ta (confined to the mucosa) tumors are often fulgurated in the office setting using cystoscopy with either a Bugby electrode or laser. This does not provide any tumor for pathologic analysis, however, and is usually reserved for patients with documented superficial low-grade disease who on surveillance cystoscopy grossly appear to have a similar low-grade recurrence. Approximately 65% to 85% of patients with Ta tumors will experience a recurrence, but the overall 5-year survival rate is 95%.[10] At the time of initial staging, it is very important to include muscularis propria in the staging resection of bladder tumors and to resect the tumor as completely as possible to ensure the most accurate clinical staging and assessment of depth of invasion. As a matter of routine, the pathologist should indicate whether muscularis propria is or is not present in the specimen and whether it is involved by tumor or not.

Most patients will develop new tumors over time, with about 30% progressing to a higher stage at recurrence. The risk of progression or recurrence is related to the depth of invasion (Ta, T1, Tis), tumor grade, and differentiation. This risk necessitates a diligent surveillance program with cystoscopy, urine cytology, and repeat TURs as needed at 3-month intervals. Patients at high risk for recurrence or progression may be considered for adjuvant or prophylactic *intravesical instillation therapy* with chemotherapeutic agents, immunologic agents, or cytokines. The indications for these agents vary from institution to institution, but in general, intravesical therapy is rarely advocated for an initial low-grade superficial Ta tumor. It is, however, frequently used as an adjuvant therapy following the endoscopic resection of an initial T1 (lamina propria invasion) tumor, or for superficial tumors with an associated carcinoma in situ.[33] At MSKCC, the use of prophylactic intravesical therapy is restricted to the treatment of patients in high-risk categories, which include four or more tumor recurrences in a year, greater than 40% involvement of the bladder surface by tumor, the presence of diffuse carcinoma

in situ (Tis), or the presence of T1 disease.[23,29] Beneficial effects seen with BCG in these settings have been a delay in progression to a higher stage, a decreased need for cystectomy, and improved survival.[23,29]

The therapeutic effects of intravesical instillation agents are thought to be secondary to both a direct toxic effect on tumor cells (topical) and an associated immune or nonspecific inflammatory response. Local and systemic toxicities are related to the degree of absorption of the agent, which is dependent on the size of the molecule given, urine pH, and the time of the instillation relative to the last bladder biopsy or resection. In general, most of the intravesical agents can cause irritative voiding symptoms such as frequency, dysuria, nocturia and bladder spasms, intermittent hematuria or passage of debris, fever, myelosuppression, or contact dermatitis. Although rare, deaths have also resulted from the systemic absorption of intravesical instillation agents when administered too close to the time of resection.

## HIGH-RISK SUPERFICIAL DISEASE

By definition, T1 disease is superficially invasive into the lamina propria. It does not involve the muscularis propria and therefore is considered superficial disease; however, it is clear in observing the natural history of these tumors that their propensity for progression to invasive disease is much greater. About 50% of T1 tumors will recur within 1 year and 90% within 5 years if managed by transurethral resection alone. In addition, one-third will progress to muscle-invasive disease within 5 years of diagnosis and 39% to 53% within 10 years when treated with transurethral resection alone (Table 17B-9).[32,34] The size, grade, associated carcinoma in situ, and number of tumors also play a role in risk of progression as outlined in the previous section. None of these factors alone should be relied upon independently to decide in favor of a cystectomy versus an organ-sparing approach. Attempts have been made to distinguish between involvement of the muscularis mucosae (T1b) and no involvement (T1a) as a prognostic factor for risk of progression, but due to the problems in the orientation (i.e., tangential cuts) and quality (i.e., cautery artifact, inadequate material, inadequate depth of resection) of transurethral resection specimens, this method of classification has been difficult to evaluate for reliability.

Treatment options considered after the initial diagnosis of a T1 tumor are surveillance, intravesical therapy, repeat transurethral resection, chemotherapy, radiation, and cystectomy.[35] The decision is based on the individual characteristics of each patient's disease, including grade, multifocality, degree of associated carcinoma in situ, number of recurrences, and to some degree now, the biologic marker status of the tumor.[26] Despite this, there is no reliable method for predicting who will fail intravesical therapy or who will progress to muscle-invasive or metastatic disease, and therefore early radical cystectomy for T1 disease remains controversial. External beam radiation appears to be of little value in low-stage (Ta, Cis, T1) bladder cancer.[36,37] The dilemma, therefore, is in balancing a bladder-sparing approach against the risk of progression versus immediate cystectomy in a patient who might not have progressed (50%) and the impact of the surgery on quality of life. The decision between

**TABLE 17B-9.** T1 BLADDER TUMORS: CURE AND TUMOR PROGRESSION RATES AFTER TUR ALONE

| SERIES | NO. OF PATIENTS | NO. OF PATIENTS (%) WITH | | FOLLOW-UP, MONTHS |
|---|---|---|---|---|
| | | NO RECURRENCE | PROGRESSION | |
| England et al | 192 | 57 (30%) | 53 (28%) | 5 |
| Heney et al | 63 | 21 (33%) | 19 (30%) | 5 |
| Malmstrom et al | 28 | 10 (35%) | 8 (29%) | 5 |
| Torti et al | 51 | 21 (41%) | 14 (27%) | 5 |
| Wolf et al | 77 | 20 (26%) | 32 (42%) | 10 |
| Sarkis et al | 43 | 5 (11%) | 22 (51%) | 10 |
| Holmang et al | 99 | 13 (13%) | 39 (39%) | 20 |
| Herr | 47 | 2 (4%) | 25 (53%) | 15 |
| Totals | 600 | 149 (25%) | 212 (35%) | |

SOURCE: Taken with permission from Herr HW: High-risk superficial bladder cancer: Transurethral resection alone in selected patients with T1 tumor. Semin Urol Oncol 15:142, 1997.

bladder-sparing and immediate radical cystectomy is especially significant when one considers the decreasing survival with increasing stage of disease. Five-year survival rates for disease pathologically confined to the lamina propria (pT1) is 80% versus 58% for muscle-invasive disease (pT2, pT3a), versus 36% for patients with nodal metastases.[38] Therefore, when considering a bladder-sparing approach, survival must be considered the primary goal. With this in mind, bladder sparing should only be attempted in selected cases where there is a high likelihood of eradicating the primary tumor in the bladder, the risk of recurrence is low, and bladder function is not compromised. In addition, the refinement of nerve-sparing and continent urinary diversion techniques certainly have improved the quality-of-life issues associated with radical cystectomy. All of these issues should be discussed with the patient so that an informed decision can be made.

## MUSCLE-INVASIVE DISEASE (ORGAN-CONFINED OR EXTRAVESICAL EXTENSION)

Certainly, the most common therapy for muscle-invasive disease of the bladder in the United States and much of western Europe is a *radical cystectomy with a bilateral pelvic lymph node dissection,* which consists of taking the bladder, perivesical fat and visceral peritoneum, prostate, and seminal vesicles en bloc with or without the urethra in a male, and the bladder, perivesical fat and visceral peritoneum, anterior vaginal wall, urethra, uterus, cervix, fallopian tubes, and ovaries en bloc in a female (Fig. 17B-9). The pelvic node dissection is considered a standard portion of the procedure because it improves the staging accuracy, and it may be of therapeutic benefit in those with minimal nodal involvement while adding little time or morbidity to the surgery. With improvements in surgical technique, significant operative complications and mortality rates have declined from around 14% in the 1950s to less than 2% by the 1980s.[14] The type of urinary diversion chosen should take into consideration patient preference, patient physical and mental capabilities to manage a diversion, body habitus and anatomy, tumor stage and location, renal function, likelihood of local or distant recurrence necessitat-

ing local and/or systemic therapy, the history of prior therapy or surgery (i.e., pelvic radiation, previous bowel resections), and past medical history (i.e., colitis, Crohn's disease, malabsorption syndromes, history of other malignancies, renal insufficiency, diabetes, heart disease, or other comorbidities.).[39–41] There are two types of urinary diversion reservoirs: an ileal conduit noncontinent stomal diversion or a continent urinary reservoir that may either have a catheterizable cutaneous stoma or internal anastomosis to the urethra. The ileal conduit is the oldest diversion, originally described by Bricker in 1950. It consists of a small segment of isolated small bowel (usually ileum) brought out the anterior abdominal wall, usually in the right lower quadrant. The left ureter is brought under the sigmoid mesocolon to the right side and then both ureters attached to the blind end of the loop. The urine drains spontaneously into an external collection device worn over the stoma. It is a well-tolerated diversion with few complications.[41]

Attempts to improve quality of life in patients requiring the total removal of their bladder have led to the development of several continent urinary diversions. The continent diversions come in a variety of forms, but may be divided into continent catheterizable cutaneous stomas versus internalized orthotopic pouches attached to the proximal urethra that may or may not require catheterization. These diversions may be constructed out of small bowel entirely, colon, or a combination of the two. Metabolic abnormalities are more common than with the ileal loops secondary to the longer lengths of bowel used for the construction and the absorptive properties of the bowel segment used. Surgical complications requiring reoperation and continence rates have improved over the past few years with improvements in surgical technique and experience. However, the continent reservoir requires a more active role by the patient, some manual dexterity, reliability, some intellectual capacity, and the willingness to catheterize their pouch. There are both relative and absolute contraindications for each type of diversion as outlined in Table 17B-10.

An alternative therapy to radical cystectomy that is widely used in Great Britain and Canada, but not in the United States, is *definitive external beam radiation,* which can be followed by a salvage radical cystectomy in patients who demonstrate persistent disease. Several studies comparing radical cystectomy alone to *preoperative*

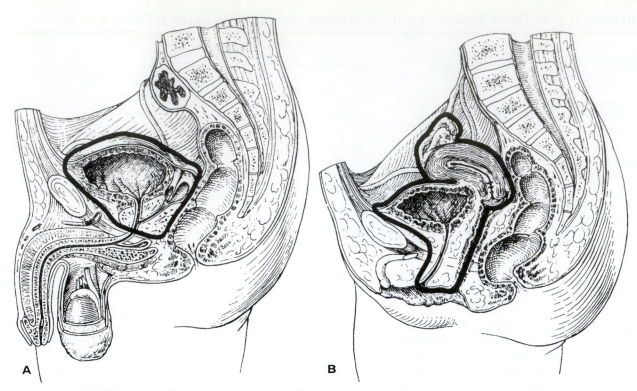

**FIGURE 17B-9.** Illustration of the limits of the pelvic surgical dissection in *A.* a male, and *B.* a female undergoing radical cystectomy for bladder cancer. (*Taken with permission from Fair WF et al: Cancer of the bladder, in Cancer Principles and Practice of Oncology, 4th ed, DeVita VT et al (eds). Philadelphia, Lippincott-Raven, 1993, chap 34.*)

*radiation therapy* plus cystectomy have failed to demonstrate a significant survival advantage (0% to 10%); therefore, it is no longer routinely performed in the United States.[14,37,42] In fact, significant toxicities have been reported when radiation has been administered for documented local recurrences, including a 30% incidence of small bowel obstruction. Radiation therapy has demonstrated the ability to eradicate some bladder tumors; however, the level of tumoricidal radiation dose has not been clearly defined. Most contemporary series have recommended a dose of 65 Gy at daily single doses of 1.8 to 2 Gy to the primary tumor. The dose to the whole bladder and surrounding perivesical tissue is usually restricted to 47.5 to 55 Gy.[14] Toxicities may be acute or chronic and may include irritative bowel and/or bladder symptoms, persistent proctitis, rectal bleeding, hematuria, rectal mucous secretion, impotence, decreased bladder capacity, bowel obstruction, inflammation of the overlying skin, general fatigue, and the occurrence of secondary tumors in the bladder or surrounding tissues (late). The probability for cure is dependent on the ability to achieve local control or complete eradication of the primary tumor. Unfortunately, only 23% to 41% of patients with invasive tumors achieve a durable local control with radiation alone, and when restaged with cystoscopy and bladder biopsy following completion of radiation, only 40% to 52% of patients achieve a complete response (Table 17B-11).[14,29] This is reflected in the overall 5-year survival results using radiotherapy

as a lone treatment for invasive bladder cancer, which have been a disappointing 30% to 45% (Table 17B-12).[14,32] Since the bladder is still in situ, the incidence of local failure is much higher than in patients who undergo cystectomy for the same stage of disease (59% to 67% vs. 10%). Davidson et al.[44] reported that of patients who succumb to their disease following definitive radiation therapy, 46% die with both a local recurrence and distant metastasis, 13% die with distant metastasis only, and about 13% die of other causes. A retrospective review from the Massachusetts General Hospital showed that the 5-year survival rate was 79% in patients with T2 or T3 disease if local control was achieved, but only 11% in patients who developed a local recurrence.[44] As with radical cystectomy, the degree of local control appears to be affected by T stage and grade, tumor morphology, and the amount of residual tumor after transurethral resection. Ureteral obstruction and anemia are also poor prognostic factors and are usually indicators of advanced stage of disease. Due to the poor prognosis of a local recurrence following definitive radiation therapy, *salvage radical cystectomy* has become an option in patients whose comorbidities will allow major surgical intervention.

Five-year survival rates after salvage cystectomy have been reported to be 40% to 45% as opposed to 11% when the bladder cannot be removed.[14] One must keep in mind when comparing mortality rates from radiation data with those of surgery, that in many

## TABLE 17B-10. CONTRAINDICATIONS TO CONTINENT URINARY DIVERSION AND NEOBLADDER

| ALL CONTINENT DIVERSIONS "STOMAL" | NEOBLADDER DIVERSION "ORTHOTOPIC" |
|---|---|
| Relative | Relative |
| Advanced age | Recurrent urethral strictures |
| Advanced stage disease | Tumor at the bladder neck (in males) |
| Need for adjuvant chemotherapy | Prostatic dual involvement |
| Poor medical health | Multifocal bladder CIS (controversial) |
| Prior radiation therapy | |
| Morbid obesity | |
| | |
| Absolute | Absolute |
| Mental or physical inability to catheterize | Advanced local disease |
| Poor renal function | Prostatic stroma invasion |
| Chronic inflammatory bowel disease | Tumor at the bladder neck (in females) |
| Advanced local disease | Prostatic urethra (controversial) |
| | Poor renal function |
| | Chronic inflammatory bowel disease |

SOURCE: Taken with permission from Cespedes RD et al: Bladder preservation and continent urinary diversion in T3b transitional cell carcinoma of the bladder. Semin Urol Oncol 14:103, 1996.

radiation series most of the patients treated with radiation alone were regarded as poor candidates for cystectomy in the first place due to advanced age or intercurrent medical problems contraindicating surgery. Trials looking at radical cystectomy in the salvage setting suggest that deferring the cystectomy to the time of a documented local recurrence does not appear to compromise survival or adversely affect the incidence of distant progression of disease.[29] A recent M.D.

Anderson Cancer Center trial including 133 patients with clinical stage T3b disease looking at the possible benefits of preoperative radiation followed by immediate cystectomy versus no preoperative radiation and adjuvant multiagent chemotherapy, demonstrated a significant decrease in the incidence of local recurrences (9% vs. 28%) in a subset of patients with true pathologic stage T3b. This advantage was not seen in patients with T2 or T3a pathologic disease and did not translate into a survival advantage for any patient at 5 years.[45] The majority of patients relapse systemically and are not routinely restaged locally, making it difficult to know the true rate of pelvic recurrence in the surgical patients in most series. In addition, preoperative radiation has the potential drawback of increasing surgical complications related to irradiated bowel and distal ureters in patients who may otherwise be candidates for a continent internal diversion.

A *partial cystectomy* is considered only in selected patients ideally meeting all of the following criteria: small muscle-invasive tumors in an area of the bladder that allows complete resection (posterior wall or dome) with adequate margins (2 cm), no concomitant carcinoma in situ, negative random bladder biopsies, and negative prostatic urethral biopsies. Tumor at the bladder neck or trigone remain relative contraindications to partial cystectomy. Its clinical use remains controversial, but in selected patients it may provide adequate local control while allowing for bladder preservation in a patient who either has an intercurrent medical condition precluding surgical intervention or does not wish to have his or her entire bladder removed.[29,39,40] Currently, about 5% to 10% of patients with invasive bladder cancer may be candidates for a partial cystectomy. However, with the recent improvements in continent diversions, the number of partial cystectomies may actually decline. The use of preoperative methotrexate, vinblastine, doxorubicin and cisplatin (M-VAC) treatment has been shown to increase the proportion of tumors that could be removed by partial cystectomy from 10% to about 27%.[29,47] Low-dose preoperative external beam radiation of 9 to 12 Gy may be used to minimize the risk of tumor seeding. Preoperative radiation, however, will not alter the biologic potential of the remaining mucosa to develop recurrent invasive or superficial tumor over time, or the metastatic potential that each of the new recurrences may bring. At least 50% of patients will experience an invasive or superficial recurrence following a partial cystectomy.[14,29] Table 17B-13 demonstrates the modern experience in bladder sparing using various combined-modality therapies.

## TABLE 17B-11. LOCAL CONTROL BASED ON CLINICAL STAGING USING RADIOTHERAPY ALONE

| SERIES | NO. OF PATIENTS | STAGE | 5-YEAR SURVIVAL RATE, % | 5-YEAR RATE OF LOCAL CONTROL IN THE BLADDER, % |
|---|---|---|---|---|
| London Hospital | 182 | T2–T3 | 40 | 41 |
| UK Cooperative Group | 157 | T3 | 23 | 45 |
| Princess Margaret Hospital | 121 | T2–T4a | 40 | 35 |
| Sydney, Prince of Wales | 342 | T1–T4b | — | 45 |
| Belgium/Netherlands Group | 147 | T2, T3 | 31 | 35 |

SOURCE: Taken with permission from Fair WF et al: Cancer of the bladder, in *Cancer Principles and Practice of Oncology*, 4th ed, DeVita VT et al (eds). Philadelphia, Lippincott-Raven, 1993, chap 34.

**TABLE 17B-12.** FIVE-YEAR SURVIVAL AND LOCAL CONTROL RATES FOR PATIENTS WITH INVASIVE CARCINOMA OF THE URINARY BLADDER TREATED WITH RADICAL RADIATION THERAPY

| INVESTIGATIONS | NO. OF PATIENTS | LOCAL CONTROL, % | OVERALL 5-YEAR SURVIVAL, % | FIVE-YEAR SURVIVAL (%) BY STAGE | | | |
|---|---|---|---|---|---|---|---|
| | | | | T1 | T2 | T3 (T3a/T3b) | T4 (T4a/T4b) |
| Goffinet, 1975 | 384 | 24 | 40 | | 46 | 35 | |
| Rider, 1976 | 554 | | | 56 | 50 | 18 | 20 |
| Blandy, 1980 | 704 | 30 | 29 | 70 | 27 | 38 | 9 |
| Yu, 1985 | 356 | 36 | | 66 | 42 | 35/23 | 23 |
| Duncan, 1986 | 917 | 23 | 36 | 61 | 40 | 26 | 12 |
| Jenkins, 1988 | 182 | 41 | 40 | | 46 | 35 | |
| Gospodarowicz, 1989 | 121 | 35 | 45 | | 59 | 52/29 | 50/16 |
| Davidson, 1990 | 709 | | 31 | 87 | 49 | 28 | 2 |
| Greven, 1990 | 116 | 27 | 34 | 39 | 59 | 10 | 0 |

Source: Taken with permission from Fair WF et al: Cancer of the bladder, in *Cancer Principles and Practice of Oncology*, 4th ed, DeVita VT et al (eds). Philadelphia, Lippincott-Raven, 1993, chap 34.

The major cause of death in patients with invasive bladder cancer is metastatic disease.[48] Experience with *systemic multidrug chemotherapy regimens* in patients with metastatic disease has given insight to other possible uses in patients with clinically localized disease in an attempt to improve cure rates, preserve bladder function, or both.

In patients thought to have clinically localized invasive bladder cancer, chemotherapy can be used in either an adjuvant setting following radiation or surgery (definitive or bladder sparing) or in a neoadjuvant setting before a definitive therapy is given. Chemotherapy alone for treatment of invasive bladder cancers has not been adequate. Analysis of cumulative data shows that the proportion of bladders rendered tumor free by chemotherapy alone is inversely proportional to the T stage, with pathologic complete response rates being less than 10% in patients with T3b or greater disease or a palpable mass at presentation.[29] Nontransitional, mixed histology, and carcinoma in situ present an added challenge due to their decreased sensitivity to chemotherapy.[14] Half of patients with muscle-invasive disease will succumb to their disease within 5 years, usually from distant metastasis not apparent at the time of cystectomy.[29] The incidence of both distant and local failure increases with advancing stage of disease, with a distinct increased risk once the disease involves extravesical tissues (T3b+) or pelvic lymph nodes. These observations, along with clinical patterns of progression of disease, support the concept that patients with invasive disease are at increased risk for harboring undetected micrometastatic disease at the time of their initial therapy, which later accounts for treatment failure.

*Neoadjuvant therapy* is directed at treating presumed micrometastasis as the primary cause of treatment failure. The advantage to neoadjuvant therapy is that the response in the primary tumor can be used as a marker for treatment efficacy outside the bladder.[49] This allows treatment to be given to the point of maximal clinical response rather than an arbitrarily preselected number of courses, and may prevent some patients from receiving unnecessary therapy. Previous experience at MSKCC with M-VAC for operable invasive bladder

**TABLE 17B-13.** RESULTS OF COMBINED MODALITY THERAPIES FOR SURVIVAL AND SURVIVAL WITH BLADDER PRESERVED*

| SERIES | THERAPY | NO. PATIENTS | 5-YEAR SURVIVAL RATE, % | 5-YEAR SURVIVAL RATE WITH BLADDER PRESERVED, % |
|---|---|---|---|---|
| Dunst | TUR-CP+RT | 79 | 52 | 41 |
| Tester | MCV-CP+RT | 91 | 62 | 44 |
| Kachnic | TUR-MCV-CP+RT | 106 | 52 | 43 |
| Shipley | TUR-MCV-CP+RT | 123 | 49 | 38 |
| Housett | TUR-5-FU−CP+RT | 120 | 63 | – |
| Given | TUR-MCV-CP+RT | 93 | 51 | 18 |
| Srougi | MVAC+PC | 30 | 53 | 20 |
| Sternberg | TUR+MVAC | 64 | 50 | 33 |
| Cervek | TUR-MCV+RT | 105 | 58 | 45 |
| MSKCC | TUR+MVAC+TUR/PC | 111 | 48 | 30 |

* Bladder preservation selected by complete tumor response to induction therapy.

cancer (T2–T4a, N0, M0) has shown an improved survival rate for patients with resectable extravesical disease (T3b–T4). Despite apparent complete response (T0) in the bladder following completion of chemotherapy, this cannot be relied on alone as a replacement for definitive local therapy in most patients. This is illustrated in the cumulative data Scher et al. reported on 444 patients with residual disease in the bladder before chemotherapy. The data showed a complete response or pathologic response (Po) in only 30% of patients at cystectomy. In addition, our ability to detect clinically residual invasive tumor is limited, with most series showing 50% of patients thought to be Po endoscopically in fact harbored residual tumor at the time of cystectomy.[29,50] The MSKCC experience looking at patient outcomes (5-year follow-up) following a delay to definitive surgery secondary to neoadjuvant M-VAC chemotherapy is similar to the previously reported radiation experience and delayed salvage cystectomy, in that there appears to be no adverse effect on multivariate analysis secondary to the delay of definitive surgical therapy.[49,51] Our M-VAC experience in patients with resectable extravesical disease led to recent attempts to improve local control and survival of patients who present with unresectable bladder cancer by downstaging the tumor with neoadjuvant chemotherapy prior to complete resection of residual pelvic tumor and regional nodes.[52] Results indicate that an aggressive approach to unresectable bladder cancer, including chemotherapy and radical surgery, may translate into a survival advantage for patients who achieve a complete response (T0), but may be of little advantage in palliation or survival in patients who achieve only a partial response or no response to neoadjuvant chemotherapy.

## METASTATIC DISEASE

Prior to the development of effective chemotherapy, median survival times rarely exceeded 3 to 6 months.[48] Several single agents have shown activity in bladder cancer, but experience has shown that better and more durable response rates can be achieved with multidrug regimens, and the combined experience of several contemporary trials is seen in Table 17B-14. Combination therapy with three to four agents is currently considered first-line therapy. Response usually occurs quickly and can be assessed after one to two cycles of therapy. The primary limitations of therapy have been the inability to deliver adequate doses due to compromised renal function and/or the inability to maintain hydration in patients with cardiac compromise. Common toxicities with these multidrug regimens may include neutropenic fever in 20% to 30%, mucositis in 10% to 20%, renal insufficiency, decreased auditory acuity, peripheral neuropathy, and a 3% to 4% mortality rate. Most treatment-related deaths are seen in patients with adverse prognostic features (i.e., lower performance status, weight loss, or hypercalcemia). Complete clinical response rates are reported in the 10% to 20% range.[29]

## FOLLOW-UP AND FREQUENCY

Although the incidence of bladder cancer has increased 36% over the past decade, mortality rates have declined by 20%. This decline is attributed to better detection of carcinoma in situ and improved treatment.[32] The aims of surveillance are to discern the clinical pattern or natural history of an individual patient's disease, to detect recurrent tumors at risk for progression of disease early enough for cure, and to monitor for progression of disease outside the bladder so that treatment may be instituted while the volume of disease is low. The interval of follow-up and type of tests used are predicated on past clinical observations of the behavior of the disease in the majority of cases, and then tailored to the patient's clinical history and disease.

## SUPERFICIAL DISEASE

Even though 80% of bladder cancers are superficial at presentation, 10% to 30% will progress over time to muscle-invasive disease, which has a poorer prognosis in terms of local or distant progression and ultimately death. Progression can be defined as either the development of muscle-invasive disease or metastasis. For surveillance to be effective, it must identify disease early enough in its course when there are effective therapies. The grim prognosis of muscle-invasive disease has led to a strategy of vigilant follow-up and repeat

**TABLE 17B-14.** COMBINATION CHEMOTHERAPY PROGRAMS

| REGIMEN | DRUGS | NO. OF TRIALS | EVALUABLE PATIENTS | COMPLETE RESPONSES, % | COMPLETE AND PARTIAL RESPONSES, % | 95% CONFIDENCE INTERVAL, % |
|---------|-------|---------------|---------------------|------------------------|------------------------------------|-----------------------------|
| MTX/DDP | Methotrexate, cisplatin | 9 | 293 | 41 (14) | 135 (46) | (17–34) |
| CMV | Cisplatin, methotrexate, vinblastine | 4 | 157 | 35 (22) | 82 (52) | (29–39) |
| CAP/CISCA | Cyclophosphamide, doxorubicin, cisplatin | 10 | 293 | 65 (22) | 166 (57) | (13–31) |
| MVAC | Methotrexate, vinblastine, doxorubicin, cisplatin | 12 | 526 | 106 (20) | 281 (53) | (22–34) |

SOURCE: Scher HI, Norton L: Chemotherapy for urothelial tract malignancies. Semin Surg Oncol 8:316, 1992.

**TABLE 17B-15. FOLLOW-UP OF PATIENTS WITH URINARY BLADDER CANCER (SUPERFICIAL BLADDER TUMORS): MEMORIAL SLOAN-KETTERING CANCER CENTER**

| | YEAR | | | | |
| --- | --- | --- | --- | --- | --- |
| | 1 | 2 | 3 | 4 | 5 |
| Office visit* | 4 | 4 | 3 | 3 | 2 |
| Cystoscopy[†] | 4 | 4 | 3 | 3 | 2 |
| Urine cytology | 4 | 4 | 3 | 3 | 2 |
| Intravenous pyelography | 1 | 1 | 1 | 1 | 1 |

* Symptoms assessed at each visit are hematuria, dysuria, and frequency.

[†] For patients with papilloma TaG1, cystoscopy is performed every 6 months for the first 3 years and annually thereafter. For patients with TaG2 focal tissue Tis, it is performed every 3 months for the first 2 years, every 6 months for years 3 and 4, and annually thereafter. For patients with T1G2,3 diffuse Tis, cystoscopy is performed every 3 months for the first 2 years, every 4 months for years 3 and 4, every 6 months for year 5, and annually thereafter. Follow-up intervals may shift according to changes in patterns of recurrence. With every recurrence patients return to cystoscopy every 3 months for at least the following year.

SOURCE: Taken with permission from Herr HW: Urinary bladder carcinoma, in *Cancer Patient Follow-up*, Johnson FE, Virgo KS (eds). St. Louis, Mosby-Year Book, 1997.

transurethral endoscopic resection of recurrent superficial tumors. The type and interval of follow-up is based on prognostic factors of the presenting and recurrent tumors, such as focality, grade, and depth of invasion, which are predictive of recurrence patterns and progression rates. For instance, low-grade tumors such as papillomas or Ta grade 1 tumors tend to recur only every 1 to 3 years, have long disease-free intervals, and have little risk of progression. The follow-up interval may therefore be less frequent than for a patient with carcinoma in situ or a T1 tumor who may be at greater risk for recurrence or progression of disease.[24] The incidence of developing upper tract tumors (renal pelvis or ureters) is small, but appears to increase over time, with about a 15% incidence at 3 years, 20% at 5 years, and up to 30% between 5 and 10 years.[4] Table 17B-15 illustrates the routine follow-up schedule at MSKCC for patients with superficial bladder tumors.[32–34]

## MUSCLE-INVASIVE DISEASE

In patients with invasive disease who have undergone radical cystectomy with or without chemotherapy or radiation, follow-up studies are aimed at the detection of local or distant recurrences, monitoring the long-term effects of urinary diversions (i.e., renal insufficiency, malabsorption syndromes, metabolic disorders, and urinary tract infections [UTIs]), the detection of new urothelial tumors of the upper tracts, urethral recurrences, or, in the case of bladder-sparing techniques, the development of local recurrences. Again surveillance is aimed at identifying recurrent disease or problems for which effective treatments are available. Most urethral recurrences occur within the first 2 to 3 years following cystectomy, and are highly curable if

caught early. Relapse occurs in 3% to 10% of patients, but if caught early by urethral washings, the results of therapeutic urethrectomy are excellent.[32,34,54] A bloody discharge or a palpable urethral mass are often signs of more advanced recurrence, which has a poorer prognosis. Patients at high risk for relapse have multifocal disease involving the bladder neck and extending into the prostatic urethra or ducts. Urethral washes are obtained 4 to 8 weeks postoperatively, then every 3 to 4 months for 3 years, then every 6 months for 2 years. If there are no symptoms and no evidence of disease after 5 years, recurrence is unlikely and no further exam is necessary.

Following cystectomy the incidence of upper tract disease in all patients is about 2% to 4%. Most occur in the first 3 to 5 years; however, patients remain at risk for life.[4] The presence of diffuse carcinoma in situ in the bladder and distal ureters increases the lifetime risk up to as much as a 20%.[23] Most local or distant recurrences after cystectomy for muscle-invasive disease occur within the first 2 years (70%), followed by a 20% incidence the third year, and 10% in the fourth and fifth years. Pelvic recurrences occur in 10% to 20% of patients with organ-confined tumors, 30% to 40% of patients with extravesical extension, and up to 50% of patients with node-positive disease. Of patients, 10% succumb to local regional disease only, although distant metastases are present in 90% as well.[32,34]

The sites of distant metastatic disease most often seen, in descending order of frequency, are the lung, nodes, bone, and liver. Patients with limited visceral metastasis, pelvic recurrences, or isolated retroperitoneal nodes respond well to cisplatin-based chemotherapy regimens (M-VAC), with 18% remaining alive and disease-free beyond 5 years.[23] Although unusual, the brain has become a more common site of relapse in patients after salvage chemotherapy in the past few years.[30] Taking all of this into consideration, Table 17B-16 shows the follow-up recommendations for invasive tumor following cystectomy.

## SUMMARY

The incidence of bladder cancer is relatively stable at about 17 patients per 100,000 population, with the overall incidence greater in males than females. More than 54,200 patients were newly diagnosed in 1999, but advances in treatment have led to declines in mortality rates. Several environmental and occupational factors have been identified as carcinogens, creating the unique opportunity of prevention through patient education. Tobacco smoking is perhaps the greatest offender and presents the greatest risk for development of carcinoma of the bladder. An understanding of the pathogenesis of the disease through the study of mutations of genes and clonal origin of tumors are evolving and may have some prognostic benefit in the future. Careful observation of the natural history of the disease and its behavior relative to the stage of disease and tumor characteristics have led to stage-specific treatment, multiple-modality therapy, bladder preservation when possible, and better survival rates. Appropriate initial staging of the disease is imperative. Understaging can lead to undertreatment, with subsequent progression of disease and death, and overstaging can lead to unnecessary local or systemic treatments with their associated toxicities. Cystectomy is no

**TABLE 17B-16.** FOLLOW-UP OF PATIENTS WITH URINARY BLADDER CANCER (AFTER CYSTECTOMY): MEMORIAL SLOAN-KETTERING CANCER CENTER

| | YEAR | | | | |
|---|---|---|---|---|---|
| | 1 | 2 | 3 | 4 | 5 |
| Office visit* | 5 | 3 | 2 | 2 | 2 |
| Complete blood count | 5 | 3 | 2 | 2 | 2 |
| Electrolytes | 5 | 3 | 2 | 2 | 2 |
| Multichannel blood tests† | 5 | 3 | 2 | 2 | 2 |
| Liver function tests | 5 | 3 | 2 | 2 | 2 |
| Voided urine or ileal conduit cytology‡ | 5 | 3 | 2 | 2 | 2 |
| Urethral washings§ | 4–5 | 3–4 | 3–4 | 2 | 2 |
| Abdominal computed tomography¶ | 3 | 2 | 1 | 1 | 1 |
| Pelvic computed tomography¶ | 3 | 2 | 1 | 1 | 1 |
| Chest x-ray | 2 | 2 | 1 | 1 | 1 |
| Intravenous pyelography or renal ultrasound | 2 | 1 | 1 | 1 | 1 |

\* Symptoms assessed at each visit are urinary, stoma, and hematuria, sexual, abdominal pain, weight loss, and back pain. Office visit should include physical examination of the abdomen, groin, lymph nodes, stoma, urethra, penis, and perirectal lymph nodes and digital rectal examination.
† Consists of blood urea nitrogen and creatinine.
‡ For patients receiving an orthotopic internal reservoir to the urethra.
§ The first urethral wash should be obtained 4 to 8 weeks after cystectomy.
¶ The first computed tomographic scan should be obtained at 3 months.
SOURCE: Taken with permission from Herr HW: Urinary bladder carcinoma, in *Cancer Patient Follow-up*, St. Louis, Mosby-Year Book, 1997.

longer the gold standard for treatment of all invasive disease, but is the standard to which all alternative treatments must be compared for survival. Surgical advancements and refinements in urinary diversion techniques have improved overall quality of life in patients who must undergo a radical cystectomy. Metastatic disease portends a poor prognosis. Some advances have been made with multidrug chemotherapy regimens, but work continues to find a more effective systemic therapy.

## REFERENCES

1. AL-ABADI H, NAGEL R: Transitional cell carcinoma of the renal pelvis and ureter: Prognostic relevance of nuclear deoxyribonucleic acid ploidy studied by slide cytometry: an eight year survival time study. J Urol 148:31, 1992.
2. FRADET Y: Epidemiology of bladder cancer, in *Comprehensive Textbook of Genitourinary Oncology*, NJ Vogelzang et al (eds). Baltimore, Williams & Wilkins, 1996, pp 298–303.
3. SILVERMAN DT et al: Epidemiology of bladder cancer. Hematol Oncol Clin North Am 6:1, 1992.
4. DONAT MD, HERR HW: Transitional cell carcinoma of the renal pelvis and ureter: diagnosis, staging, management, and prognosis, in *Urologic Oncology*, JE Osterling, JP Richie (eds). Philadelphia, WB Saunders, 1997, pp 215–234.
5. MALKOWICZ SB, SKINNER DG: Development of upper tract carcinoma after cystectomy for bladder cancer. Urology 36:20, 1990.
6. THOMPSON IM, FAIR WF: The epidemiology of bladder cancer. AUA Update Series, 8:210, 1989.
7. ROSS RK et al: Analgesics, cigarette smoking, and other risk factors for cancer of the renal pelvis and ureter. Cancer Res 49:1045, 1989.
8. DALBAGNI G et al: Molecular genetic alterations of chromosome 17 and p53 nuclear overexpression in human bladder cancer. Diagn Molec Pathol 2:4, 1993.
9. LEVINE E: Transitional cell carcinoma of the renal pelvis associated with cyclophosphamide therapy. AJR 159:1027, 1992.
10. HUDSON MA, CATALONA WJ: Urothelial tumors of the bladder, upper tracts, and prostate, in *Adult and Pediatric Urology*, 3d ed. JY Gillenwater et al (eds). St. Louis, Mosby-Year Book, 1996, pp 1379–1464.
11. SHIRAI T et al: The etiology of bladder cancer—Are there any new clues or predictors of behavior? Int J Urol 2:64, 1995.
12. CARSON CC III et al: Clinical importance of microhematuria. JAMA 241:149, 1979.
13. BUSHMAN W, WYKER AW: Standard diagnostic considerations, in *Adult and Pediatric Urology*, JY Gillenwater et al (eds). St. Louis, Mosby-Year Book, 1996, pp 63–77.
14. FAIR WF et al: Cancer of the bladder, in *Principles and Practice of Oncology*, 4th ed, VT DeVita et al (eds). Philadelphia, JB Lippincott, 1993, pp 1052–1072.
15. SARNACKI CT et al: Urinary cytology and the clinical diagnosis of urinary tract malignancy: a clinicopathologic study of 1400 patients. J Urol 106:761, 1971.
16. VICENTE J et al: Transitional cell carcinoma in the upper urinary tract: diagnosis and management. Urol Int 2:7, 1995.
17. KLEER E, OSTERLING JE: Transitional cell carcinoma of the upper tracts. Prob Urol 6:531, 1992.
18. BADALAMENT RA et al: Imaging, in *Comprehensive Textbook of Genitourinary Oncology*, NJ Vogelzang et al (eds). Baltimore, Williams & Wilkins, 1996, pp 371–385.
19. HERR HW, HILTON S: Routine CT scan in cystectomy patients: Does it change management? Urology 47:324, 1996.
20. WHITMORE WF: Management of invasive bladder neoplasms. Semin Urol 1:34, 1983.
21. YOUNG RH: Pathology of bladder cancer, in *Comprehensive Textbook of Genitourinary Oncology*, NJ Vogelzang et al (eds). Baltimore, Williams & Wilkins, 1996, pp 326–337.
22. MELAMED MR, REUTER VE: Pathology and staging of urothelial tumors of the kidney and ureter. Urol Clin North Am 20:333, 1993.
23. HERR HW et al: Bacillus Calmette-Guerin therapy for superficial bladder cancer: A 10 year follow-up. J Urol 147:1020, 1992.
24. HERR HW, WHITMORE WF: Ureteral carcinoma in situ after successful intravesical therapy for superficial bladder tumors: incidence, pathogenesis and management. J Urol 138:292, 1987.
25. SIDRANSKI D et al: Clonal origin of bladder cancer. N Engl J Med 326:737, 1992.
26. DALBAGNI G et al: Markers of progression in bladder tumor. Crit Rev Oncol Hematol 16:33, 1994.
27. BOSL GM et al: Bladder cancer: Advances in biology and treatment. Crit Rev Oncol Hematol 16:33, 1994.

28. PAULSON D et al: Optimal staging procedures, including imaging, to define prognosis of bladder cancer. Int J Urol 2:1, 1995.

29. SCHER HI et al: Cancer of the bladder, in *Cancer: Principles and Practice of Oncology: Cancers of the Genitourinary System*, 5th ed, VT DeVita et al (eds). Philadelphia, Lippincott-Raven, 1997, pp 1300–1322.

30. ROSENSTEIN M et al: Treatment of brain metastases from bladder cancer. J Urol 149:480, 1993.

31. SEE WA, FULLER JR: Staging of advanced bladder cancer. Urol Clin North Am 19:663, 1992.

32. HERR HW: High-risk superficial bladder cancer: Transurethral resection alone in selected patients with T1 tumor. Semin Urol Oncol 15:142, 1997.

33. PHAM HT, SOLOWAY MS: High-risk superficial bladder cancer: intravesical therapy for T1 G3 transitional cell carcinoma of the urinary bladder. Semin Urol Oncol 15:147, 1997.

34. HERR HW: Urinary bladder carcinoma, in *Cancer Patient Follow-up*, FE Johnson, KS Virgo (eds). St Louis, Mosby -Year Book, 1997, pp 432–35.

35. MONTIE JE, KLEIN EA: High-risk superficial bladder cancer. Semin Urol Oncol 15:141, 1997.

36. WHITMORE WF, PROUT GR: Discouraging results for high dose external beam radiation therapy in low stage (O and A) bladder cancer. J Urol 127:902, 1982.

37. ZEITMAN AL et al: The case for radiotherapy with or without chemotherapy in high risk superficial and muscle-invading bladder cancer. Semin Urol Oncol 15:161, 1997.

38. ESRIG D et al: Early cystectomy for clinical stage T1 transitional cell carcinoma of the bladder. Semin Urol Oncol 15:154, 1997.

39. CESPEDES RD et al: Bladder preservation and continent urinary diversion in T3b transitional cell carcinoma of the bladder. Semin Urol Oncol 14:103, 1996.

40. ROWLAND RG: Continent cutaneous diversion. Semin Urol Oncol 15:179, 1997.

41. CARLIN BI et al: Comparison of the ileal conduit to the continent cutaneous diversion and orthotopic neobladder in patients undergoing cystectomy: a critical analysis and review of the literature. Semin Urol Oncol 15:189, 1997.

42. MONTIE JE et al: Radical cystectomy without radiation therapy for carcinoma of the bladder. J Urol 131:477, 1984.

43. DAVIDSON SE et al: Assessment of factors influencing the outcome of radiotherapy for bladder cancer. Br J Urol 66:288, 1990.

44. SHIPLEY WU et al: Full dose irradiation for patients with invasive bladder carcinoma: Clinical and histologic factors prognostic of improved survival. J Urol 134:679, 1985.

45. COLE CJ et al: Local control of muscle-invasive bladder cancer: preoperative radiation therapy and cystectomy versus cystectomy alone. Int J Radiat Oncol Biol Phys 32:331, 1995.

46. SWEENEY P et al: Partial cystectomy. Urol Clin North Am 19:701, 1992.

47. STEMBERG CN et al: Neoadjuvant m-vac (methotrexate, vinblastine, adriamycin, and cisplatin) chemotherapy and bladder preservation for muscle-infiltrating transitional cell carcinoma of the bladder. Urol Oncol 1:127, 1995.

48. YAGODA A: Chemotherapy for advanced urothelial cancer. Semin Urol 1:60, 1983.

49. SCHULTZ PK et al: Neoadjuvant chemotherapy for invasive bladder cancer: Prognostic factors for survival of patients treated with m-vac with 5 year follow-up. J Clin Oncol 12:1394, 1994.

50. SCHER HI: Chemotherapy for invasive bladder cancer: Neoadjuvant versus adjuvant. Semin Oncol 17:555, 1990.

51. SCHER HI et al: Neo-adjuvant chemotherapy for invasive bladder cancer: Experience with the m-vac regimen. Br J Urol 64:250, 1989.

52. DONAT SM et al: Methotrexate, vinblastine, doxorubicin, and cisplatin chemotherapy and cystectomy for unresectable bladder cancer. J Urol 156:368, 1996.

53. HERR HW et al: An overview of intravesical therapy for superficial bladder tumors. J Urol 138:1363, 1987.

54. HARDEMAN SW, SOLOWAY MS: Urethral recurrence following radical cystectomy. J Urol 144:666, 1990.

55. LANDIS SH, MURRAY T, BOLDEN S, WINGO PA: Cancer statistics. CA Cancer J Clin 49:8, 1999.

# 17C / CANCER OF THE PENIS AND URETHRA

*David A. Corral and Curtis A. Pettaway*

## INTRODUCTION

Malignant tumors of the penis and urethra are uncommon lesions in North America. Their treatment outcome is largely dependent upon the initial stage of disease at presentation. In this chapter, we discuss the diagnosis, staging, and therapy of penile cancer, including surgical techniques for treating local and regional disease, minimally invasive approaches to the treatment of low-stage disease, and propose a practical treatment algorithm based on the initial stage. Management of cancer of the male and female urethra is also addressed.

## PENILE CANCER

Squamous cell carcinoma (SCC) is by far the most common type of penile cancer, accounting for 95% of such malignancies.[1] In western countries the incidence of this disease is approximately 1 in 100,000 males, comprising less than 0.5% of all male malignancies.[2] However, in developing areas of the world, particularly in Central and South America, Central Africa, India, and China, the incidence of penile SCC is much higher, accounting for approximately 10% of malignancies in males.[2–5] The increased incidence of penile SCC is clearly influenced by cultural and religious practices and standards of hygiene. It has long been noted that the incidence of penile cancer correlates inversely with the practice of neonatal circumcision and that this disease is virtually nonexistent in cultures in which it is universally performed.[6] It has been suggested that factors present in smegma and recurrent balanitis predispose to the development of penile SCC. Phimosis has also been strongly correlated with penile cancer, occurring in up to 50% of patients.[2,7] The presence of a foreskin may predispose to sexually transmitted diseases, including infection by the human papillomavirus (HPV), which has been associated with benign, premalignant, and malignant lesions of the penis. Condylomae caused by HPV are commonly located on the glans, corona, meatus, fossa navicularis, and penile, scrotal, and perineal skin. These nondysplastic genital warts are most frequently associated with viral subtypes HPV-6 and HPV-11. In contrast, other viral subtypes, predominantly HPV-16 and HPV-18, have been associated with dysplastic and malignant transformation in both cervical and penile lesions. Previously, epidemiologic data have demonstrated that men whose sexual partners have HPV-related cervical lesions are at increased risk for the development of penile intraepithelial neoplasia.[8] The recent development of advanced molecular biologic techniques, including polymerase chain reaction and in situ hybridization, has provided increased evidence for an etiologic role for HPV by identifying specific DNA sequences from HPV-16, -18, -30, -6, and -11 in primary penile SCC, but not in normal foreskins.[9,10] HPV-16 DNA was also detected in a lymph node metastasis, the same viral subtype found in the primary tumor,[10] and has been demonstrated in Bowenoid carcinoma in situ.[11] It has also been noted that the HPV genome encodes oncoprotein E6, which complexes with the tumor suppressor protein p53,[12] and oncoprotein E7, which binds the retinoblastoma protein, pRB.[13]

Although a substantial body of evidence indicates that HPV plays an etiologic role in the development of invasive penile cancer, its prevalence of only 31% to 63%[14] indicates that it is not the exclusive causative agent. Other factors such as smoking and chronic dermatitis have also been associated with penile SCC.[15] In fact, the single common factor underlying the association of penile cancer with lack of circumcision, smegma, poor hygiene, balanitis, and HPV infection is chronic inflammation and its attendant cell turnover. Although neonatal circumcision clearly minimizes the risk of penile SCC, perhaps by minimizing the risk of HPV infection, it has been suggested that diligent penile hygiene in uncircumcised men may be sufficient to prevent its occurrence.[16] Because cultural and religious practices are difficult to change, preventive strategies may best be directed at minimization of risk through proper hygiene and avoidance of infection by HPV.

### CLINICAL MANIFESTATIONS

In its early stages, penile cancer often follows an indolent course, beginning as a small lesion producing local symptoms (mass, ulceration, bleeding, pain, and discharge) of varying duration prior to presentation and histologic confirmation. For multiple reasons, including denial, ignorance, and embarrassment, delayed presentation is common. More than half of all patients with penile cancer will delay seeking medical attention for at least 6 months after the appearance of symptoms, with one-third of patients waiting more than a year.[17] For this reason, it is not uncommon for tumors to have metastasized beyond the primary site at the time of presentation. Tumor spread occurs via regional lymphatic vessels that act as conduits for tumor emboli.[18] Metastatic deposits enlarge in the inguinal nodal areas, eventually producing ulceration and infection.

Death often results from sepsis or, less commonly, hemorrhage following erosion of the tumor into the femoral vessels.[7] Although fewer than 10% of patients have distant metastasis at presentation, advanced regional disease is often a harbinger of its development, which can occur in several organs including lung, liver, bone, and brain.[7,19]

## DIAGNOSIS

Because the gross appearance of the primary lesion in penile cancer varies widely, from an exophytic papillary mass to an ulcerative lesion, it can be confused with benign conditions involving the penis. Nonmalignant lesions of the penis are relatively rare, with the exception of condyloma acuminatum. Condylomas are caused by HPV and grossly appear as either painless sessile or papillary exophytic lesions in the locations described earlier. Although HPV viral subtypes 16 and 18 are frequently associated with dysplastic condylomas and have been implicated in the etiology of penile SCC as discussed above, the majority of these lesions are nondysplastic, caused by the nontransforming HPV viral subtypes 6 and 11. These lesions are treated with topical podophylin, freezing, or laser ablation. Other benign lesions of the penis include herpes genitalis, caused by herpes simplex virus type 2, and appear as a small, painful ulcerated lesion, and balanitis xerotica obliterans (lichen sclerosis et atrophicus) characterized by white epidermal plaques often involving the glans or prepuce. Distinction of these benign lesions from penile cancer can only be definitively made by histologic examination of a biopsy specimen. When malignancy is suspected, small lesions are best managed by excisional biopsy rather than incisional or punch dermatologic biopsy. Lesions involving the prepuce are most often treated by circumcision. No disfiguring procedure should be considered without first establishing a histologic diagnosis of cancer.

## HISTOLOGY

Preinvasive lesions of the penis include erythroplasia of Queyrat and Bowen's disease. Erythroplasia of Queyrat appears as a shiny, red, velvety elevated plaque involving the prepuce or glans, most commonly occurring in uncircumcised men in the fifth or sixth decade of life. Bowen's disease appears as a scaly plaque on the shaft of the penis without erythematous discoloration and typically arises one decade earlier than erythroplasia of Queyrat. Although originally described separately due to these slightly differing clinical presentations, these two entities are best classified together as penile carcinoma in situ.[20,21] These intraepithelial neoplasms progress to invasive SCC in approximately 10% of patients.[22] Histologically, these lesions demonstrate proliferation of large atypical cells, multinucleated cells, loss of polarity, and numerous mitoses, but these findings are restricted to the epithelium (Fig. 17C-1B). In contrast, Bowenoid papulosis is a term describing a similar condition that occurs in younger men, but may be multicentric, follows an indolent course, and does not progress to invasive carcinoma.

SCC of the penis is histologically identical to that in other areas of the body and is most often graded by degree of differentiation according to the Broder's system used for cutaneous SCC.[23] Well-differentiated penile SCC consists of hyperkeratotic epidermis giving rise to fingerlike projections of atypical squamous cells with associated keratin pearls (Fig. 17C-1D). With progression to higher grades, keratin pearls are lost and nuclear pleomorphism and mitotic figures are more prominent (Fig. 17C-E, F).

Verrucous carcinoma, also known as giant condyloma of Buschke-Lowenstein, is a variant of penile SCC that presents as a large fungating, often ulcerated mass, arising most commonly from the coronal sulcus. Histologically, this lesion is a well-differentiated SCC with an exophytic papillary growth pattern and may represent malignant degeneration of HPV condyloma (Fig. 17C-1C). Clinically, these tumors extend locally by burrowing into normal tissue, but do not metastasize.

Nonsquamous malignancies account for only 5% of penile cancers. These tumors include a variety of sarcomas, basal cell carcinoma, and melanoma.[22] The incidence of Kaposi's sarcoma of the penis has dramatically increased secondary to the rise in incidence of acquired immunodeficiency syndrome (AIDS) and is the presenting sign in up to 3% of AIDS patients.[22] These lesions can be managed by local excision or radiotherapy.

## STAGING

Two staging systems currently used to evaluate the extent of disease in patients with penile cancer are the Jackson staging system (Table 17C-1)[24] and the American Joint Committee on Cancer (AJCC) tumor-node-metastasis (TNM) staging system (Table 17C-2).[25] The Jackson system is simple to use, correlates with survival, and had been widely accepted by many physicians. However, it has largely been replaced by the TNM system, which provides improved stratification of the depth of invasion of the primary tumor and nodal involvement. Because prognosis and therapeutic decisions are largely dependent upon the stage at presentation, particularly the depth of invasion in low-stage disease, an accurate assessment of the extent of disease is mandatory.

Staging studies begin with a physical examination of the primary lesion and the inguinal region, tumor biopsy, chest x-ray, and computed tomography (CT) of the abdomen and pelvis. Unfortunately, noninvasive staging of regional disease has long been considered highly inaccurate because only 35% to 60% of palpable adenopathy is actually caused by nodal metastasis, with the remainder

**TABLE 17C-1.** THE JACKSON SYSTEM OF STAGING OF PENILE SQUAMOUS CARCINOMA

| STAGE | DEFINITION |
| --- | --- |
| I | Lesions confined to the glans and/or prepuce |
| II | Lesions extending onto the shaft of the penis |
| III | Lesions associated with operable malignant inguinal lymph nodes |
| IV | Lesions extending off the shaft of the penis and/or inoperable inguinal metastases or distant metastasis |

Source: Data from Jackson SM.[24]

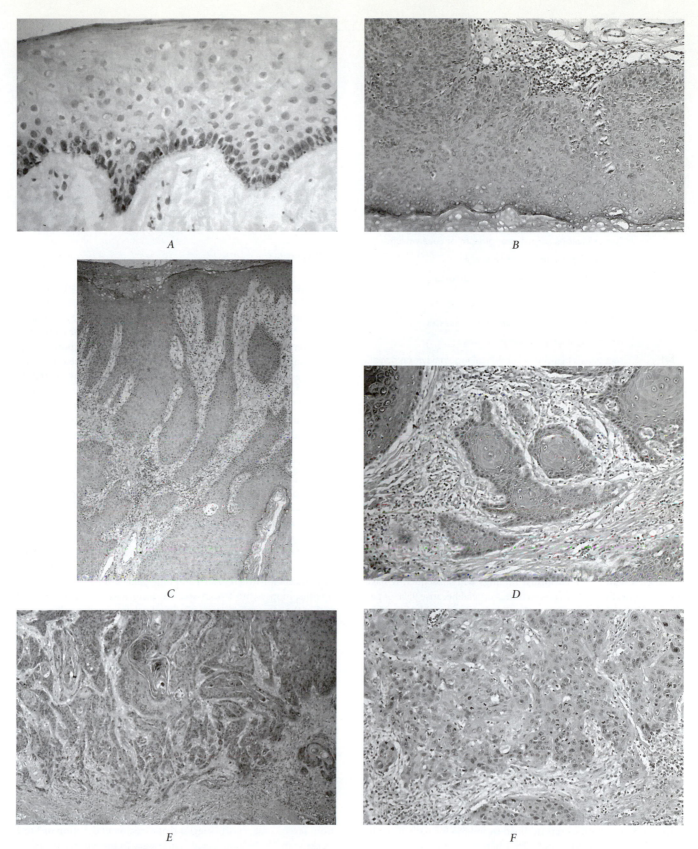

**FIGURE 17C-1.** Histologic sections of squamous cell carcinoma (SCC) of the penis. *A*. Normal penile skin. *B*. Carcinoma in situ. *C*. Verrucous carcinoma. *D*. Well-differentiated SCC. *E*. Moderately differentiated SCC. *F*. Poorly differentiated penile SCC.

**TABLE 17C-2.** AMERICAN JOINT COMMITTEE ON CANCER TNM SYSTEM OF STAGING PENILE SQUAMOUS CANCER

| STAGE | DEFINITION |
|---|---|
| **Primary tumor (T)** | |
| Tx | Primary tumor cannot be assessed |
| T0 | No evidence of primary tumor |
| Tis | Carcinoma in situ |
| Ta | Noninvasive verrucous carcinoma |
| T1 | Tumor invades subepithelial connective tissue |
| T2 | Tumor invades corpus spongiosum or cavernosum |
| T3 | Tumor invades urethra or prostate |
| T4 | Tumor invades other adjacent structures |
| **Regional lymph nodes (N)** | |
| Nx | Regional lymph nodes cannot be assessed |
| N0 | No regional lymph node metastasis |
| N1 | Metastasis in a single superficial inguinal lymph node |
| N2 | Metastasis in multiple superficial inguinal lymph nodes unilateral or bilateral |
| N3 | Metastasis in deep inguinal or pelvic lymph node(s), unilateral or bilateral |
| **Distant metastasis (M)** | |
| Mx | Presence of distant metastasis cannot be assessed |
| M0 | No distant metastasis |
| M1 | Distant metastasis |

SOURCE: Data from American Joint Committee of Cancer: Penis.[25]

resulting from inflammation or infection. Conversely, up to 66% of patients with palpably normal findings will subsequently have nodal metastasis.[26,27] This distinction is crucial because 95% of patients with proven nodal metastasis treated conservatively die within 3 years of diagnosis, compared with a 77% 5-year survival rate for patients with nonmetastatic disease.[27,28] Depth of invasion of the primary lesion is the most prognostically useful indicator of lymph node involvement. Tumors limited to the prepuce and subepithelium of the glans (AJCC stage T1) are associated with nodal metastasis in only 5% to 11% of patients.[29] In contrast, in patients with corporal invasion (Jackson stage II and AJCC stages T2, T3, and T4), the incidence of nodal involvement rises to 47% to 68%.[30]

The prognosis of patients with penile carcinoma is greatly dependent on stage, particularly regional nodal involvement. The 5-year survival rate falls sharply from 66% to 90% for patients with Jackson stage I disease to 20% to 24% and 0% to 5% for patients with Jackson stages III and IV, respectively.[2,29] Furthermore, the extent of nodal involvement adversely impacts survival. In a study of 201 patients by Ravi, the 5-year survival rate declined from 95% for patients without nodal disease to 81% and 50% when 1 to 3 or greater than 3 inguinal lymph nodes were positive, respectively. No patient with pelvic nodal disease survived to 5 years.[31]

Ilioinguinal lymphadenectomy, a surgical procedure with both therapeutic and diagnostic advantages, remains the most reliable technique to assess regional nodal status. However, because of its invasive nature and attendant morbidity,[32] less invasive techniques are often employed, such as superficial node dissection with intraoperative lymphatic mapping, which is discussed later in this chapter. Other less invasive strategies for the evaluation of regional node status include needle aspiration (with or without lymphangiography)[33] and sentinel lymph node biopsy.[34] Understandably, the reliability of either of these techniques depends on minimizing the sampling error. DNA flow cytometric studies of the penile tumor have not proved useful in predicting lymph node metastases.[35]

## TREATMENT

The consideration of treatment options begins with an adequate assessment of the primary lesion. Superficial lesions limited to the prepuce with a normal-appearing rim of skin may be managed conservatively by circumcision. Cancer-free margins should be confirmed by frozen section. In the past, high recurrence rates reported after circumcision appear to be related more to poor patient selection and lack of adequate negative margins than to failure of the procedure itself.[36] Lesions also commonly appear on the glans, coronal sulcus, or both. Definitive therapy of lesions in these locations may require a therapeutic approach that permanently disfigures the patient, such as partial or total penectomy. When less invasive therapy is being considered to maintain a functionally and cosmetically intact penis, adequate histologic confirmation of malignancy and precise determination of the depth of invasion is essential. With small localized lesions of the glans, tissue confirmation may be accomplished by simple wedge excision. However, the surgeon must remember that this procedure may not be curative and has been associated with a 40% local recurrence rate when used alone.[37] Large primary lesions or diffuse glanular lesions should be assessed by incisional biopsy with a scalpel or a dermatologic punch. In the case of large obvious cancers for which partial and total penectomy are the only two options, biopsy with frozen-section confirmation can be obtained within the same anesthetic period as the definitive procedure.

## TREATMENT OPTIONS FOR LOW TUMOR BURDEN (JACKSON STAGE I OR AJCC STAGE TIS, TA, OR T1)

In the past, surgery was the mainstay of therapy for penile cancer. However, it has been recognized that less invasive techniques are suitable for the treatment of patients with low-stage disease. When considering therapeutic options for these patients, the urologic surgeon weighs the benefit of functional organ preservation using minimally invasive therapy, such as topical chemotherapy, radiation therapy, circumcision, laser ablation, or Mohs micrographic surgery, against the risk of recurrent or persistent disease. Topical chemotherapy is an effective alternative for the treatment of carcinoma in situ. Data from several case reports suggest that a treatment duration of 3 to 7 weeks with 5% 5-fluorouracil is necessary to prevent recurrence.[38] Potential drawbacks include inadequate treatment because of poor patient compliance or severe local skin irritation.

Radiotherapy may be delivered as external beam therapy, brachytherapy, or iridium 192 wire-impregnated mold. These techniques may effectively treat selected patients with distal penile lesions (Jackson stage I or AJCC stage T1) with control rates in several series ranging from 78% to 90%.[39–42] However, complications are common and include stricture, fistula formation, and distal penile or skin necrosis in 17% to 40% of treated patients. Approximately 20% of patients with low-stage lesions require subsequent amputation after radiation therapy as a result of recurrent disease or iatrogenic complications.[40] For these reasons radiotherapy should be reserved for patients with low-stage lesions who refuse surgical therapy.

More recently, microscopically controlled tumor excision (Mohs micrographic surgery)[43,44] and laser tumor ablation[45] have become popular therapeutic options for low-stage disease. Mohs micrographic surgery involves fixation of the tumor with a topical solution followed by layer-by-layer tumor excision until a negative frozen-section surgical margin is obtained. In one series, local tumor control in 35 patients was 94% at 5 years with a survival rate of 86% and 62% for clinical stage I and II disease, respectively.[44] A potential drawback of the Mohs technique is that it may require multiple treatment sessions and specialized equipment and personnel that may not be readily available at all centers. Furthermore, those lesions that are amenable to treatment with Mohs micrographic surgery are also likely to be successfully treated more rapidly by laser ablation.

When organ preservation is appropriate, laser ablation of small-volume penile cancer has become a popular technique. Overall, local control in four early series of patients (AJCC stages Tis, T1, and T2) using the neodymium:yttrium-aluminum garnet (Nd:YAG) laser ranged from 68% to 100% with a mean follow-up of 17 to 60 months.[45–48] Local failure commonly occurs when invasive lesions (AJCC stage T2 or greater) are treated with this modality.[49] Laser ablation is usually accomplished in one outpatient session and is without the morbid complications of radiation therapy. In general, healing takes approximately 6 weeks, with excellent cosmesis and sexual function at 3 months.[46] At The University of Texas M. D. Anderson Cancer Center, we routinely offer laser ablation to sexually active patients with small, superficial lesions (AJCC stages Tis and Ta).

## TREATMENT OF LOCALLY ADVANCED LESIONS (JACKSON STAGE II OR AJCC STAGE T2, T3, T4, OR BULKY TA)

Verrucous carcinoma, although classically noninvasive, may present as a bulky mass replacing the glans penis.[50] These lesions, as well as invasive SCC, require either partial or total penectomy. Partial penectomy is the option of choice when the primary tumor can be removed with a 2-cm disease-free margin and the remaining corpus is sufficient to allow the patient to stand and direct the urine stream during voiding. If these requirements cannot be met, a total penectomy with creation of a perineal urethrostomy is the only remaining option. In either case, a confirmation of negative surgical margins by frozen section is imperative. Local recurrence rates after partial and total penectomy are similarly low, ranging from 0% to 6%.[3,27]

It is our practice to prescribe antibiotics for patients at the time of diagnosis because lesions requiring partial or total penectomy are often associated with ulceration and infection. In anticipation of regional surgical staging procedures, antibiotics are continued postoperatively for an extended period. Penile amputation is most conveniently performed in the dorsal lithotomy position so that if unexpected intraoperative findings are noted, partial penectomy can be readily converted to total penectomy.

During surgery, the lesion is covered with a plastic drape, condom, or glove held in place with a suture. The entire penis, scrotum, perineum, and suprapubic region are included in the surgical preparation. Standard dorsal lithotomy drapes are used, including an adhesive drape or towel to exclude the rectum from the field.

TECHNIQUE OF PARTIAL PENECTOMY. A tourniquet is applied around the base of the penis to control bleeding during the procedure. Prior to beginning, it is beneficial to use a skin marker to define the incision. An oblique circumferential skin incision is made beginning over the dorsal penile surface 2 to 3 cm proximal to the lesion (Fig. 17C-2A). It is necessary to leave sufficient ventral skin to create the urethrocutaneous anastomosis. The proximal skin margin is mobilized free from the underlying fascia toward the base of the penis in a circumferential fashion.

The urethra is mobilized proximally beginning 2 cm proximal to the lesion (Fig. 17C-2B). The dorsal neurovascular bundle is isolated and ligated with a 3-0 absorbable suture proximal to the site of corporal transection. The urethra is next retracted ventrally away from the corporal bodies, and the corpora are transected 2 cm proximal to the lesion. Following this, the urethra is divided 1 cm distal to the level of corporal transection (Fig. 17C-3A). The specimen is sent for frozen-section confirmation of negative corporal and urethral margins. The corporal bodies are closed in unison with interrupted 0-Vicryl horizontal mattress sutures (Fig. 17C-3B), the tourniquet is removed, and hemostasis is assured. If necessary, the urethra may be further mobilized from the corporal bodies proximally to gain sufficient length to allow a tension-free urethrocutaneous anastomosis.

The urethra is next spatulated over its dorsal surface, and skin closure is begun in a dorsal-to-ventral direction with 3-0 Vicryl suture (Fig. 17C-4). The new urethrocutaneous anastomosis is created in the ventral aspect of the wound with interrupted 4-0 Vicryl suture. A Foley catheter is placed, and the penis is wrapped with a loose compression dressing and taped superiorly to the abdomen. After 24 hours, the dressing is removed and the catheter is left indwelling for an additional 2 to 4 days.

TECHNIQUE OF TOTAL (RADICAL) PENECTOMY. Because the corporal bodies are rarely completely removed, this procedure is, in fact, a subtotal penectomy. The level at which the corpora will be transected and the need to create a perineal urethrostomy are the main considerations during radical penectomy.

The patient's position and surgical draping are identical to those for the partial penectomy. A circumferential skin incision is made around the penile base from its dorsal aspect and extending onto the upper scrotum. After the plane is entered deep to Scarpa's fascia, the subcutaneous tissues and the scrotal contents are bluntly dissected away from the corporal bodies (Fig. 17C-5A). The penis

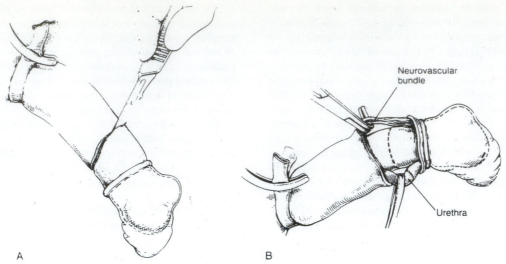

A                                                        B

**FIGURE 17C-2.** Partial penectomy. *A*. Tourniquet is placed proximally and lesion is excluded from the surgical field by a condom. *B*. Exposure of the urethra and neurovascular bundle. (*Reproduced with permission from CA Pettaway, AC von Eschenbach: Surgery of penile carcinoma, in Atlas of Surgical Oncology, KI Bland et al (eds). Philadelphia, WB Saunders, 1995.*)

is now retracted upward, and Buck's fascia is incised over the corpus spongiosum. The spongiosum is mobilized proximally, incising the musculi bulbospongiosus that cover the pendulous and bulbous portions of the urethra (Fig. 17C-5*B*). Distally, the dissection is limited to allow at least a 2-cm margin proximal to the lesion. The

corpus spongiosum is ligated distally and sharply transected at this level. A Foley catheter is passed into the bladder through the proximal urethral stump.

Downward traction is next placed on the penile shaft (Fig. 17C-6*A*), and the suspensory ligament is identified in the dorsal

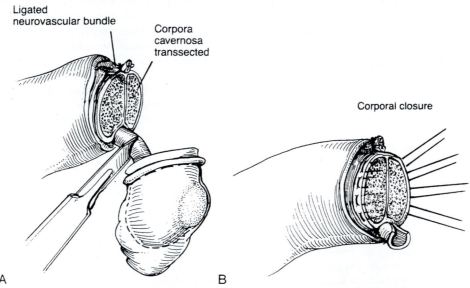

A                                                        B

**FIGURE 17C-3.** Partial penectomy. *A*. The neurovascular bundle is ligated and the corpora are transected. The urethra is transected 1 cm distal to the level of corporal transection. *B*. Corpora are closed with horizontal mattress sutures and the urethra is spatulated dorsally (*Reproduced with permission from CA Pettaway, AC von Eschenbach: Surgery of penile carcinoma, in Atlas of Surgical Oncology, KI Bland et al (eds). Philadelphia, WB Saunders, 1995.*)

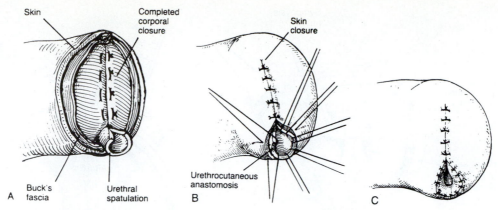

**FIGURE 17C-4.** Partial penectomy. *A*. Completed corporal closure. *B*. Skin closure and completed urethrocutaneous anastomosis. *C*. Completed partial penectomy. (*Reproduced with permission, from CA Pettaway, AC von Eschenbach: Surgery of penile carcinoma,* in Atlas of Surgical Oncology, *KI Bland et al (eds). Philadelphia, WB Saunders, 1995.*)

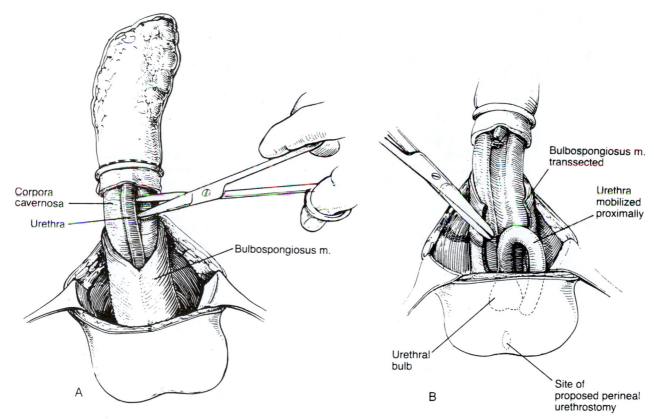

**FIGURE 17C-5.** Radical penectomy. *A*. Urethral dissection. *B*. Transection of the distal urethra and mobilization of the proximal segment. (*Reproduced with permission from CA Pettaway, AC von Eschenbach: Surgery of penile carcinoma,* in Atlas of Surgical Oncology, *KI Bland et al (eds). Philadelphia, WB Saunders, 1995.*)

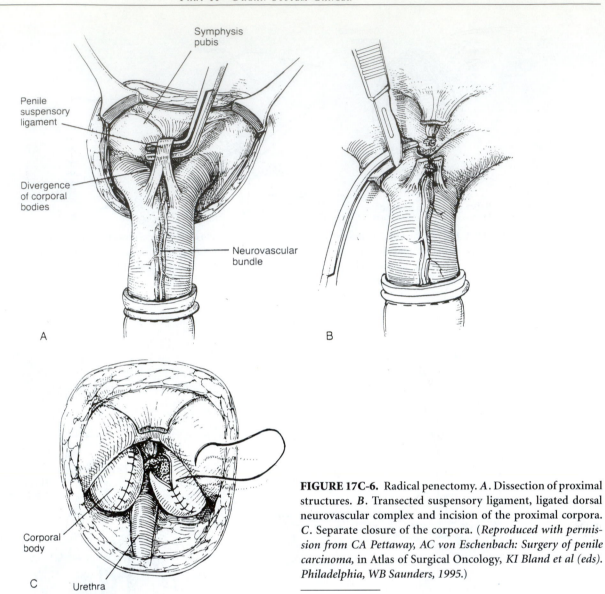

**FIGURE 17C-6.** Radical penectomy. *A*. Dissection of proximal structures. *B*. Transected suspensory ligament, ligated dorsal neurovascular complex and incision of the proximal corpora. *C*. Separate closure of the corpora. (*Reproduced with permission from CA Pettaway, AC von Eschenbach: Surgery of penile carcinoma,* in Atlas of Surgical Oncology, *KI Bland et al (eds). Philadelphia, WB Saunders, 1995.*)

midline. This ligament is then elevated with a right-angle clamp and transected with electrocautery, with care taken not to injure the dorsal vessels prematurely. Next, the dorsal neurovascular bundle is ligated with a 2-0 or 3-0 absorbable suture as close to the symphysis pubis as is possible and transected. At this level, the corporal bodies diverge. The urethra is retracted downward, and the corpora are encircled with a large curved clamp. Depending on the proximal extent of the penile lesion, the corporal bodies may be divided separately at this level (Fig. 17C-6*B*), or may require further mobilization from the pubic ramus prior to transection. Corporal closure is performed separately (Fig. 17C-6*C*) (with a running Vicryl suture) and the surgical specimen is sent for frozen section to assess the surgical margins.

To construct a perineal urethrostomy, a space is developed by blunt dissection in the scrotal midline toward the base of the scrotum. After the appropriate position is determined, the scrotum is elevated, and a small ellipse of perineal skin is removed. The urethra is next transposed to the perineum (Fig. 17C-7*A*), and the excess urethral length is removed. The urethra is spatulated and the urethrocutaneous anastomosis is created with 4-0 Vicryl suture (Fig. 17C-7*B*). The scrotum is reconstructed over Penrose drains in a layered fashion with absorbable suture. The skin is closed in a transverse fashion by approximating scrotal skin to prepubic skin with permanent suture or wound clips (Fig. 17C-8), which serves to elevate the scrotal contents away from the perineal urethrostomy site. The drains are brought out through the lateral aspect of the wound. A Foley catheter and perineal pressure dressings are left at the conclusion of the procedure. The Foley catheter is left for approximately 4 to 6 days to protect the anastomosis and to allow perineal edema to resolve. The perineal dressings and Penrose drains are removed after 24 to 48 hours, depending on the amount of drainage.

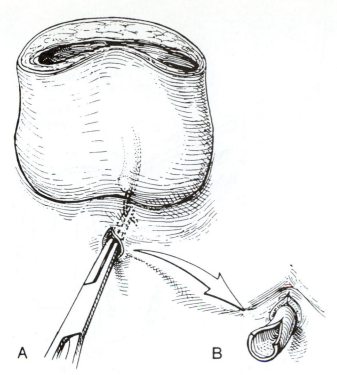

**FIGURE 17C-7.** Radical penectomy. *A*. Transposition of the urethra to the perineum. *B*. Urethral spatulation after removal of excess length. (*Reproduced with permission from CA Pettaway, AC von Eschenbach: Surgery of penile carcinoma, in Atlas of Surgical Oncology, KI Bland et al (eds). Philadelphia, WB Saunders, 1995.*)

**FIGURE 17C-8.** Radical penectomy. Spatulated urethrocutaneous anastomosis, scrotal flap elevation, and wound closure with placement of Penrose drains. (*Reproduced with permission from CA Pettaway, AC von Eschenbach: Surgery of penile carcinoma, in Atlas of Surgical Oncology, KI Bland et al (eds). Philadelphia, WB Saunders, 1995.*)

At the conclusion of radical or partial penectomy, if infection in the primary lesion has been well controlled, we proceed directly with inguinal staging procedures under the same anesthetic.

**FOLLOW-UP.** Patients should be followed carefully to detect urethral stricture occurring at the penile stump or at the perineal urethrostomy site. Urethral stricture may respond to periodic dilation or, in more severe cases, may require lysis or revision. With adequate surgical margins, local tumor recurrence is rare. For those patients who have undergone a prior partial penectomy and have developed a recurrence in the penile stump, a radical penectomy is indicated.

In patients free of disease for 1 to 2 years who desire the return of sexual function, reconstruction following penectomy may be indicated. The goals and considerations of phallic reconstruction include: (1) a one-stage microsurgical procedure, (2) creation of a competent urethra to achieve normal voiding, (3) restoration of phallic tactile and erogenous sensibility, (4) ability of soft tissue to tolerate a prosthetic device, and (5) aesthetic acceptance by the patient. To achieve this, collaboration between the urologist and plastic surgeon is of paramount importance. A discussion of current reconstructive surgical techniques is reviewed by Schellhammer[51] and others.[52]

## ASSESSMENT AND MANAGEMENT OF REGIONAL DISEASE

The rarity of inguinal metastasis in patients with carcinoma in situ and verrucous carcinoma[53] suggests that these patients can be safely observed without initial groin dissection or biopsy. Also, patients with well-differentiated (grade 1, G1) tumors appear to be at a lower risk for nodal involvement than those with higher-grade lesions. Solsona et al.[30] found that 0 of 19 patients with T1, G1 disease had nodal involvement and Theodorescu et al.[26] found a 45% long-term actuarial relapse-free survival rate in patients with G1 tumors managed initially by surveillance. These studies suggest that patients with T1, G1 lesions may be offered either prophylactic lymphadenectomy or careful surveillance. The latter option should be restricted to those individuals considered reliable with regard to follow-up examinations who also have no palpable inguinal adenopathy.

Palpable inguinal adenopathy at presentation may be secondary to regional metastasis or to the chronic infection that commonly accompanies these lesions. Therefore, for those patients who present with minimal, shotty inguinal adenopathy, it may be acceptable to give a 4-week course of oral antibiotic therapy prior to reexamining and proceeding with surgical staging if the adenopathy persists.

The survival rate of patients with penile cancer correlates not only with the presence or absence of nodal disease but also the extent of regional nodal involvement.[54–55] In contrast to earlier reports, a survival advantage has been shown in patients with positive nodes who undergo an early, rather than a delayed, node dissection.[27,54] All of these findings argue for routine lymphadenectomy in patients with penile cancer. However, a clinical dilemma surrounds the fact that only one-third of patients ultimately benefit from ilioinguinal node dissection, although the procedure is associated with significant morbidity in up to 50% of patients.[32] Several efforts have been made to minimize morbidity while identifying metastases at the earliest stage by limiting the scope of dissection to target only the first echelon of lymphatic drainage. The original concept and rationale for this approach were described by Cabanas,[34] who noted that contrast medium injected into the dorsal penile lymphatic vessels drained into a lymph node radiographically projected over the femoral head. Upon anatomic dissection, this node was found to reside superomedially to the superficial epigastric vein near the epigastric saphenous junction. In patients with positive results from sentinel lymph node biopsies who subsequently underwent ilioinguinal node dissection, it was often the only involved node. Furthermore, there were no cases in which other nodes were positive and the sentinel node was negative. The 5-year survival rate in the presence of a negative sentinel lymph node biopsy was 90%. More recently, however, a few cases have been reported in which, despite what the surgeons thought was an adequate negative sentinel lymph node biopsy, patients relapsed with unresectable disease, calling into question the concept that removal of only the sentinel node provides adequate staging.[56–57]

To avoid false-negative biopsy results caused by either sampling error or variations in lymphatic drainage, a bilateral extended sentinel lymph node dissection (ESLND) has been proposed. This modification removes all superficial lymph node tissue clustered around the superficial epigastric vein in the superomedial lymph node quadrant (Fig. 17C-9). The procedure is converted to a standard ilioinguinal dissection on the affected side if a grossly positive node is encountered, or a modified dissection that spares the saphenous vein, as described by Catalona[58] for microscopic disease. However, in our experience at the M. D. Anderson Cancer Center, we found that of 20 consecutive patients who underwent extended sentinel lymph node dissection, all with negative pathology, 5 (25%) developed inguinal metastasis at a median of 10 months.[59] Therefore, we have abandoned this approach and now perform complete superficial dissection with intraoperative lymphatic mapping for patients with stage T1 or greater disease and clinically negative inguinal lymphatics. This experimental technique involves intradermal injection of isosulfan blue (a vital blue dye) at the junction of the tumor and normal skin[60] with the goal of identifying the first echelon of drainage, and ultimately sparing these patients the morbidity of further dissection. Intraoperative lymphatic mapping may become an important staging tool in the future, however, at present, its use is investigational. In general practice for this group of patients we recommend complete bilateral superficial dissection with progression to deep inguinal and pelvic node dissection if frozen-section analysis is positive. If the superficial lymph nodes are negative by frozen section, the procedure is concluded. Because data from Cabanas[34] and Srinivas[55] refute the occurrence of pelvic metastasis without prior inguinal metastasis, a pelvic lymph node dissection is not performed.

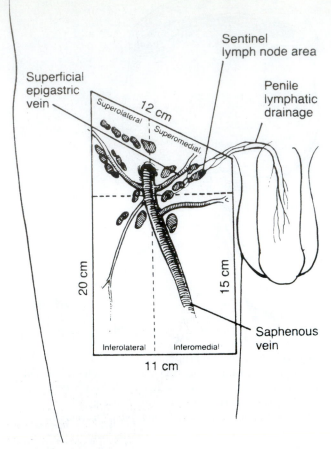

**FIGURE 17C-9.** Anatomy of inguinal lymphatics. The boundaries of the inguinal lymph node dissection (*solid border*) are shown. The superficial inguinal nodes are divided into four quadrants by lines intersecting the saphenofemoral junction (*dotted lines.*) (*Reproduced with permission from CA Pettaway, AC von Eschenbach: Surgery of penile carcinoma,* in Atlas of Surgical Oncology. *KI Bland et al (eds). Philadelphia, WB Saunders, 1995.*)

Patients with persistent unilateral palpable adenopathy (no response following a 4-week course of antibiotics) undergo standard ilioinguinal dissection on the affected side. Because of possible occult contralateral disease, we perform complete superficial dissection with frozen-section analysis on the contralateral side. Those with bilaterally persistent adenopathy should be considered for neoadjuvant or adjuvant chemotherapy and complete bilateral inguinal and pelvic dissection.

The preoperative preparation of patients undergoing regional staging (inguinal dissection, or ilioinguinal dissection) includes those studies required for any major surgery: chest x-ray, electrocardiography, complete blood count, coagulation profile, serum electrolytes, urinalysis and blood type and screen.

Because patients are kept at bedrest several days postoperatively, bowel movements can be problematic. For bowel evacuation, we use enemas or laxatives preoperatively in patients scheduled for inguinal procedures. Occasionally, if an extensive pelvic and inguinal dissection is anticipated, whole-bowel lavage is performed by having the patient drink a colonic lavage solution (GoLYTELY), 1 gallon during a period of 3 to 4 hours. Intestinal antisepsis with oral agents is generally not required.

Preoperative intravenous antibiotics are given at least 1 hr prior to surgery for patients undergoing inguinal staging procedures. Patients with ulcerated inguinal masses are admitted several days prior to surgery for optimization of wound care by intravenous antibiotics, dressing changes, whirlpool baths, and local antisepsis. Plans for wound closure (skin graft or flap coverage) are anticipated in patients requiring wide resection of the skin. If necessary, plastic surgery consultation is obtained preoperatively.

### ANATOMIC CONSIDERATIONS.

Lymphatic drainage of the penis has been studied extensively.[53,61,62] Briefly, the lymphatic vessels run along the dorsum of the penis toward the penile base. During transit, lymphatics from the right and left sides freely communicate. Cutaneous lymphatic vessels of the shaft skin form right and left trunks that drain into the superficial inguinal nodes, primarily of the superomedial group (see Fig. 17C-9). Lymphatic drainage from the glans with tributaries from the urethra and cutaneous lymphatic vessels unite to form one to four collecting trunks on the dorsal penile surface. These trunks run under the fascia in association with the deep dorsal vein. In the area of the penile suspensory ligament, the lymphatic trunks anastomose to form a presymphyseal plexus, which then sends lymphatic trunks bilaterally to terminate in the superomedial inguinal nodes. The penile corporal lymphatic trunks also follow the deep dorsal vein to the symphysis pubis and either divide into discrete right or left trunks or anastomose with the presymphyseal lymphatic plexus, which then divides into lateral trunks.[53] The superomedial inguinal nodes also receive drainage from the corpora.

Daseler et al.[62] previously reported the location and zonal distribution of the inguinal and iliac lymph node chains based on 450 anatomic dissections. The inguinal lymph nodes (see Fig. 17C-9) were found within a quadrilateral area bounded as follows: superiorly by a line 12 cm long and 1 cm above the inguinal ligament to the pubic tubercle, medially by a line dropped vertically 15 cm from the pubic tubercle, laterally by a line dropped vertically 20 cm from the superior lateral margin, and inferiorly by a line 11 cm in length, connecting the lower aspects of the medial and lateral margins. The superficial inguinal lymph nodes are located above the fascia lata of the thigh and are separated into four quadrants and a central zone, divided by horizontal and vertical lines crossing at the saphenofemoral junction. According to Rouviere,[61] lymph nodes primarily from the medial quadrants and the central zone receive penile afferent lymphatic vessels. Only occasionally do penile afferent lymphatic vessels drain into the superolateral quadrant and, rarely, into the inferolateral quadrant. The deep inguinal nodes lie beneath the fascia lata clustered about the femoral vessels within the femoral sheath. They also receive lymph drainage from the superficial inguinal nodes.

Communication with the pelvic nodes occurs via the node of Cloquet, which lies within the femoral canal. The pelvic nodal field is familiar to most urologic surgeons and includes the lymph nodes associated with the iliac vessels from the aortic bifurcation to the inguinal ligament, including the hypogastric and obturator lymph node chains.

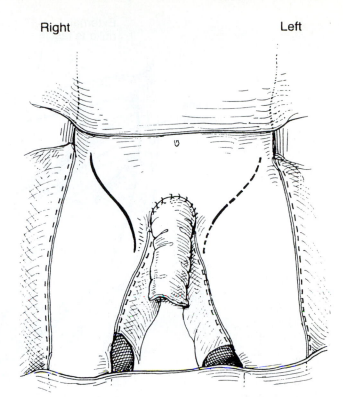

**Right**                                        **Left**

**FIGURE 17C-10.** Regional staging procedures. A superficial inguinal lymph node dissection incision (*left*), which can be extended as necessary for an ilioinguinal lymphadenectomy (*right*). (*Reproduced with permission from CA Pettaway, AC von Eschenbach: Surgery of penile carcinoma*, in Atlas of Surgical Oncology, *KI Bland et al (eds). Philadelphia, WB Saunders, 1995.*)

### INGUINAL LYMPH NODE DISSECTION.

Patients are positioned supine on the operating table with their legs flexed at the knee in a "frog-leg" position. Padding is placed to support the knees and the heels. A Foley catheter is placed, and the abdomen, scrotum, perineum, and thighs are shaved, prepared, and draped (Fig. 17C-10).

### ILIOINGUINAL NODE DISSECTION.

At The University of Texas M. D. Anderson Cancer Center, we perform a modified S-shaped incision (Fig. 17C-10, right). It begins 2 cm medial to the anterior superior iliac spine, curving gently downward to run parallel to and below the inguinal ligament. The final portion of the incision curves downward over the medial thigh. If an inguinal mass appears to involve the skin, an ellipse of skin is resected as part of the incision. Skin flaps are next raised, starting with the superior margin. It is important to remember that the flaps must be developed deep to Scarpa's fascia and handled gently throughout the procedure with skin hooks or sutures placed in the dermis to preserve adequate blood supply and avoid postoperative skin flap necrosis. The superior flap is raised cephalad at least 2 cm above the inguinal ligament. The medial margin of this same flap is developed to expose the spermatic cord and is then carried medially and inferiorly to expose the

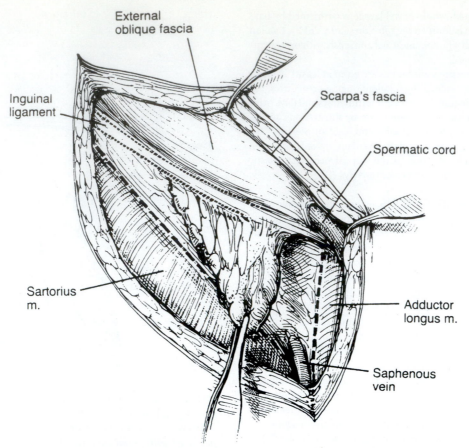

**FIGURE 17C-11.** Ilioinguinal node dissection. Elevation of the superior flap to expose the external oblique fascia. The superomedial aspect of the nodal specimen is ligated and divided near the midline. Dotted lines represent the inguinal ligament and the sites of the fascial incisions over the sartorius and adductor longus muscles. (*Reproduced with permission from CA Pettaway, AC von Eschenbach: Surgery of penile carcinoma,* in Atlas of Surgical Oncology. *KI Bland et al (eds). Philadelphia, WB Saunders, 1995.*)

midpoint of the adductor longus muscle (Fig. 17C-11). The inferior flap is undermined in an inferolateral direction to expose the mid-plane of the sartorius muscle laterally and the apex of the femoral triangle inferiorly.

Once the flaps have been developed, the superficial inguinal dissection begins superiorly over the lower abdominal wall. The lymphatic and adipose tissues are sharply dissected off the external oblique muscle superiorly and are then retracted inferiorly. The specimen is tethered superomedially by lymphatic vessels coursing to the prepubic area. This pedicle is ligated as close to the midline as possible and is retracted laterally (Fig. 17C-11). To define the medial limits of the dissection, the fascia over the lateral edge of the adductor longus is incised. The specimen, including the muscular fascia, is next sharply mobilized in an inferolateral direction off the adductor and pectineus muscles toward the femoral sheath. Venous branches, including the superficial epigastric and external pudendal vessels, are ligated as they are encountered. This procedure is best

performed with the surgeon standing opposite the side of dissection so that the specimen can be rotated toward the surgeon. The saphenous vein is encountered at the apex of the femoral triangle and may be divided between ligatures (Fig. 17C-12).

The lateral limit of dissection is defined by incising the muscular fascia over the sartorius muscle from below the iliac spine to the apex of the femoral triangle. The lymphatic specimen is mobilized medially toward the femoral sheath. At this point in the procedure, it is helpful to retract superiorly the inferior aspect of the specimen containing the ligated saphenous vein. The femoral sheath is incised along the midpoint of the lateral aspect of the distal femoral artery and vein. The femoral sheath and lymphatic specimen are then sharply dissected off the femoral vessels in a superior direction (Fig. 17C-13A), securing any sizable vessels with clips or ligatures. While mobilizing the lateral aspect of the lymphatic specimen, it is important to avoid injury to the femoral nerve as a result of dissection under the sartorius muscle.

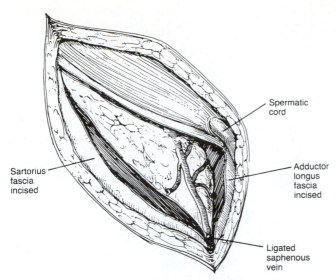

Sartorius
fascia
incised

Spermatic
cord

Adductor
longus
fascia
incised

Ligated
saphenous
vein

**FIGURE 17C-12.** Ilioinguinal node dissection. The specimen is mobilized inferiorly exposing the inguinal ligament. The fascia over the edge of the adductor longus muscle and the medial border of the sartorius muscle are incised. The saphenous vein is ligated at the apex of the femoral triangle. (*Reproduced with permission from CA Pettaway, AC von Eschenbach: Surgery of penile carcinoma,* in Atlas of Surgical Oncology. *KI Bland et al (eds). Philadelphia, WB Saunders, 1995.*)

The specimen is freed from the proximal femoral artery by dividing the superficial circumflex iliac artery and other branches at their origin (Fig. 17C-13*B*). The nodal specimen is next retracted superomedially and unwrapped from the femoral vein by incising the femoral sheath and adventitia over the vein. The saphenofemoral junction is delineated, and if the saphenous vein is to be sacrificed, it is ligated or oversewn at its junction. The specimen is now held by attachments at the femoral canal (Fig. 17C-13*B*). At this point, the specimen can be divided beneath the inguinal ligament prior to performing a pelvic lymphadenectomy, or it can be delivered subsequently en bloc. If a pelvic lymphadenectomy will not be performed, the inguinal ligament is retracted upward. Cloquet's node is identified lying within the femoral canal. The specimen is ligated, divided above Cloquet's node, and removed. The wound is then thoroughly irrigated, and meticulous hemostasis is obtained.

If a pelvic lymphadenectomy is to be performed, it can be accomplished prior to or at the conclusion of the inguinal procedure. In patients with CT scan evidence of pelvic adenopathy, the pelvic procedure is performed initially to assess the operability of the lesion and the likelihood of cure prior to consideration of an inguinal node dissection. If it is desirable to avoid an open surgical procedure, or if neoadjuvant chemotherapy is being considered, fine-needle aspiration of the pelvic nodes under CT guidance can be used to confirm tumor involvement.

Pelvic lymphadenectomy is accomplished through the incision used for ilioinguinal dissection or through a separate midline infraumbilical incision. After the external oblique fascia is exposed,

it is incised 2 cm medial to the anterosuperior iliac spine, traveling obliquely toward the pubic tubercle. The retroperitoneal space is entered in a standard fashion by dividing the abdominal wall muscles, being careful to mobilize the peritoneal contents medially. Exposure for the pelvic dissection is illustrated in Fig. 17C-14. The surgical technique of pelvic lymphadenectomy is further described in Chap. 17D, Cancer of the Prostate, and will not be discussed further here. In certain cases in which an inguinal mass is present, it is desirable to perform an en bloc ilioinguinal lymphadenectomy. Elevation of the inguinal ligament allows mobilization of the lymphatic contents within the femoral canal so that the specimen can be delivered. If it is necessary to divide or resect the inguinal ligament or a portion of the lower abdominal wall, plastic reconstruction with Marlex mesh grafting and myocutaneous flap rotation gives excellent results.

If a standard inguinal dissection is performed, we routinely transpose the sartorius muscle. This is accomplished by mobilizing the sartorius from its origin at the anterior superior iliac spine, then rotating the sartorius anteriorly and medially over the femoral vessels and suturing it to the inguinal ligament using horizontal mattress sutures (Fig. 17C-15*A*). The abdominal wall musculature is closed in several layers, and a closed-suction drain is placed in the wound through a stab wound placed well away from the undermined skin flaps (Fig. 17C-15*B*). The skin is inspected, and any areas appearing "dusky" are excised to bleeding edges. Injection of fluorescein dye and inspection with a Wood's lamp can be beneficial if the integrity of the skin edges is in question. Finally, the subcutaneous tissue is closed over the abdominal and inguinal areas with absorbable suture, and the skin is closed with staples.

To decrease lymphatic flow from the distal extremity, it is imperative that the patient be maintained at bedrest. During this period, leg elevation is maintained, and fitted elastic stockings or elastic bandages are wrapped in a snug fashion. A functioning closed-suction drain prevents accumulation of lymphatic fluid under the groin flaps. The patient receives antibiotics for several days postoperatively to prevent wound infection, and administration of subcutaneous heparin 5000 units twice daily should be considered for deep venous thrombosis (DVT) prophylaxis until the patient ambulates. A Foley catheter is kept in place until lymph drainage decreases dramatically and ambulation is possible. The period of bedrest varies, but it ranges from 3 to 7 days. When drainage becomes minimal during the preceding 24 hr, the patient may attempt ambulation. If drainage does not increase during the next 24 hr, the inguinal drains can be removed, usually at approximately 7 days postoperatively. While ambulating, the patient should wear either a fitted elastic stocking or elastic bandages wrapped well around the legs. It is important to monitor the wound daily for evidence of seroma formation, skin necrosis, or infection. When ambulatory and when the wound appears to be healing satisfactorily, the patient may be discharged. Fitted stockings are used for the first 3 to 6 months if an inguinal or combined ilioinguinal dissection has been performed. After this time, a trial period of ambulation without stockings begins. If edema reappears, the patient will probably require continued use of fitted stockings.

Skin flap necrosis is the most common postoperative complication in up to 50% of patients.[32] Risk of this complication is minimized

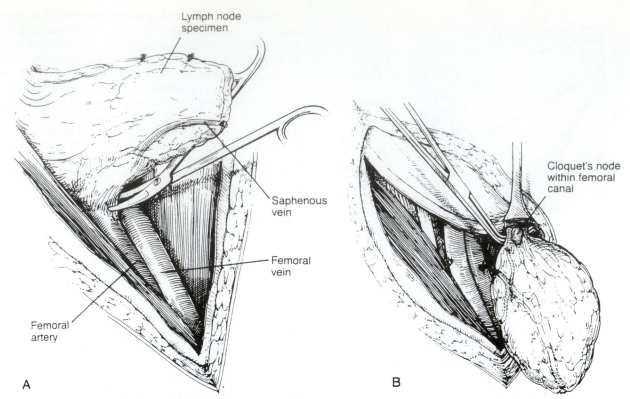

Lymph node
specimen

Saphenous
vein

Femoral
vein

Femoral
artery

A

Cloquet's node
within femoral
canal

B

**FIGURE 17C-13.** Ilioinguinal node dissection. *A.* Femoral sheath is incised and the specimen is mobilized superiorly toward the saphenofemoral junction. *B.* Femoral arterial and venous tributaries including the saphenofemoral junction are ligated at their origins. The specimen is divided above the node of Cloquet. (*Reproduced with permission from CA Pettaway, AC von Eschenbach: Surgery of penile carcinoma, in Atlas of Surgical Oncology. KI Bland et al (eds). Philadelphia, WB Saunders, 1995.*)

by careful attention to the handling of the skin flaps during dissection and by excision of all marginal-appearing skin edges before closure. Provided the wound is clean, excision of necrotic tissue can take place after the area of slough is fully demarcated. Small areas of skin necrosis will usually heal after excision by secondary intention. Occasionally, when larger areas of skin are lost, a skin graft will be required. If necessary, undrained collections of fluid under skin flaps can be aspirated using sterile technique with a needle and syringe. If the fluid is purulent or reaccumulates rapidly, an additional percutaneous drain is placed or incision and drainage is performed with wound packing. Soft tissue infection, presenting as wound cellulitis or a drain tract infection, may occur in 10% of patients.

Cellulitis is treated aggressively with intravenous antibiotics to prevent progressive lymphatic obstruction with resultant edema and possible progressive skin loss. Extremity edema has been noted to occur in up to 50% of patients and ranges in severity from minimal to severe with or without associated skin changes. Careful intraoperative ligation of all lymphatic vessels, along with postoperative leg elevation and the use of compression stockings, helps to minimize risk of this complication. Furthermore, careful selection of appropriate patients for saphenous vein preservation is recommended.

## ADJUVANT OR NEOADJUVANT MODALITIES

Radiation therapy plays a limited role in the management of regional disease. When given as prophylaxis in the setting of clinically negative regional lymphatics, the rate of subsequent development of symptomatic nodal metastasis approaches 25%, similar to that of untreated patients.[63] As monotherapy for clinically involved lymph nodes, radiation therapy is inferior to surgery.[64,65] External beam therapy may be most useful as palliation of inoperable fungating nodal metastases.

Chemotherapy may play a role in the treatment of patients with advanced disease. Cisplatin, bleomycin, and methotrexate have been used as monotherapy with response rates between 25% and 50%,[66] but these are mostly partial and of short duration. Combination chemotherapy regimens have had modest success in controlling advanced disease. A prospective phase II study of combination methotrexate, cisplatin, and bleomycin for advanced genitourinary SCC at our institution achieved an objective response rate of 55% with a median survival of 17 months for responders.[67] Future studies will emphasize the integration of chemotherapy and surgical management to achieve greater duration of disease-free status.

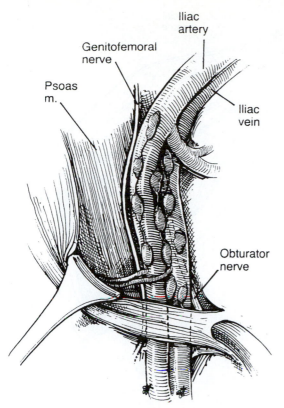

**FIGURE 17C-14.** Relationship of the pelvic lymph nodes to the iliac artery, vein and obturator nerve. (*Reproduced with permission from CA Pettaway, AC von Eschenbach: Surgery of penile carcinoma, in Atlas of Surgical Oncology. KI Bland et al (eds). Philadelphia, WB Saunders, 1995.*)

## SUMMARY OF THERAPEUTIC OPTIONS FOR PENILE CANCER

The options for management of penile cancer discussed in this chapter are driven mainly by clinical stage, and each has its own attendant morbidity. The goal of therapy is to maximize the potential for cure while preserving as much function as possible. We propose the treatment algorithms shown in Fig. 17C-16, with the caveat that individual therapeutic strategies must be patterned around individual patient needs.

## URETHRAL CANCER

Carcinoma of the urethra is exceedingly rare, with only approximately 1200 female and 600 male urethral cancers reported.[68] It is the only urologic malignancy with a higher incidence in women than men. As in penile cancer, development of urethral cancer has been associated with chronic inflammation and HPV infection,[69] and is frequently noted at a site of previous stricture formation in men. In distinction to penile cancer, where the battle for cure is won or lost

at the level of the regional lymphatics, death from urethral cancer results from failure of local control of the primary tumor.

## ANATOMY AND HISTOLOGY

The histologic composition of the urethral epithelium changes with anatomic location in both the female and male urethra, and these variations are reflected in tumor histology. The male urethra can be divided into three anatomic segments: prostatic, membranous, and penile. The prostatic urethra is lined by transitional epithelium, whereas stratified and pseudostratified columnar epithelium line the membranous and penile urethra up to the fossa navicularis, where the epithelium changes to stratified squamous. Anatomically, the bulbar urethra makes up the proximal one-third of the penile urethra. However, carcinomas arising in this urethral segment have similar presentation, prognosis, and management to those arising more proximally, and therefore should be classified with carcinomas of the membranous and prostatic urethra.

In the female, the urethra can be divided anatomically into the proximal third, which is lined by transitional epithelium, and the distal two-thirds, lined mostly by stratified squamous epithelium with smaller areas of pseudostratified and stratified columnar epithelium.

Carcinoma of the urethra may originate from any of the lining epithelial cell types or from associated glands. In males, the bulbomembranous urethra is the most common site of occurrence, with 56% to 59% arising in this segment. The penile urethra is the site of origin in one-third of patients, whereas 10% urethral cancers arise in the prostatic urethra.[68] Accordingly, SCC accounts for 70% to 80% of male urethral cancer, whereas 20% are transitional cell carcinoma and 5% are adenocarcinoma. In females, half of the urethral cancers arise in the distal two-thirds of the urethra. Approximately 70% of female urethral cancers are SCC and 15% each are adenocarcinoma and transitional cell carcinoma. A small percentage of urethral cancers in both sexes are classified as undifferentiated, and rarely sarcomas and melanomas are encountered.

As with histology, lymphatic drainage varies along the length of the urethra. In the male the lymphatic drainage of the penile urethra accompanies that of the glans penis, emptying into the presymphyseal plexus and then to the superficial and deep inguinal and external iliac chains. Lymphatics draining the bulbar, membranous, and prostatic urethra follow a complex course culminating in the presacral, external, and internal iliac chains. Similarly, in the female, lymphatics of the proximal urethra drain into the obturator, external, and internal iliac chains, whereas those of the distal urethra drain to the superficial and deep inguinal nodes. Due to these anatomic differences, tumors arising in the distal urethra spread regionally to the inguinal nodes, whereas those originating in the proximal urethra will metastasize directly to pelvic lymphatics.

## PRESENTATION, DIAGNOSIS, AND STAGING

As with penile cancer, there is a significant delay of 6 months to 3 years from the onset of symptoms to presentation and diagnosis.[68,70] Because of this, patients often present with locally or regionally

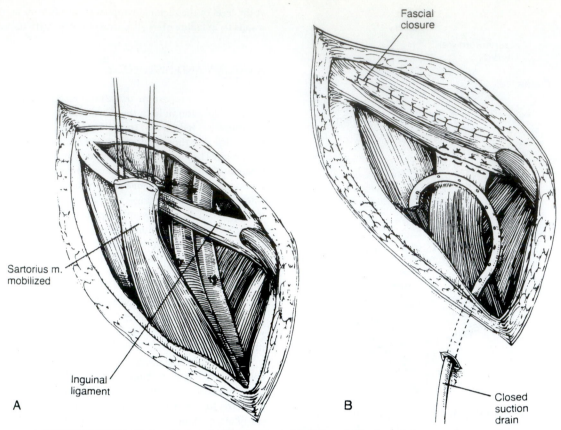

**FIGURE 17C-15.** Ilioinguinal node dissection. *A.* Medial mobilization of the sartorius muscle to cover the femoral vessels. *B.* The sartorius is sutured to the inguinal ligament and a closed-suction drain is brought out through the skin away from the incision. (*Reproduced with permission from CA Pettaway, AC von Eschenbach: Surgery of penile carcinoma,* in Atlas of Surgical Oncology, *KI Bland et al (eds). Philadelphia, WB Saunders, 1995.*)

advanced disease. The presenting signs and symptoms in the male vary with the anatomic location of the lesion. Tumors in the penile urethra commonly present with irritative or obstructive voiding difficulty. These tumors often arise at the site of a urethral stricture, and therefore should be suspected when a "benign" stricture becomes more difficult to manage. These lesions may produce a palpable ventral mass, whereas those arising from the bulbomembranous urethra may give rise to a solid or fluctuant perineal mass.[70] Lesions in the prostatic urethra bulbomembranous urethra, and advanced lesions of the penile urethra often present with decreased force and caliber of stream, obstruction, or overflow incontinence, and may produce a filling defect on retrograde urethrogram. Hematuria or purulent discharge may be noted with lesions at any level. In the female, urethral or vaginal bleeding is the most common presenting symptom, and may be associated with a mass or ulceration on physical examination that requires histologic examination to be distinguished from benign lesions such as urethral caruncle, condyloma, or diverticulum.

The diagnosis is made by urethroscopic biopsy, although very distal lesions may be amenable to direct visual biopsy, especially in the female patient. Several staging systems have been proposed for defining the extent of disease in male and female patients with urethral carcinoma. The Grabstald staging system[71] for female urethral cancer and the Ray staging system[72] for male urethral cancer are given in Table 17C-3. Although these clinical staging systems are simple, the TNM staging system of the International Union Against Cancer,[73] shown in Table 17C-4, emphasizes tumor invasion, extent of regional node involvement, and distant metastasis. A thorough bimanual exam under anesthesia with attention to the anus, rectum, urogenital diaphragm, and vagina (female patients) defines the local extent of disease and is conveniently performed at the time of urethroscopy and biopsy. Simultaneously, a careful inguinal examination is performed to detect the presence of inguinal adenopathy. Because as patients with urethral carcinoma often present with advanced disease, a routine chest x-ray and serum chemistries are indicated for staging purposes. A CT scan of the abdomen and pelvis should also be performed to assess the status of pelvic and retroperitoneal lymph nodes and abdominal viscera. Fine-needle aspiration of suspicious lymph nodes detected by palpation or CT scan should be performed if clinically indicated. MRI of the pelvis may be of value in defining the extent of soft tissue or bony involvement by extensive perineal lesions.

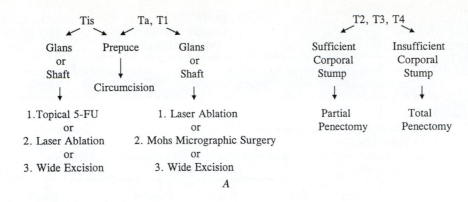

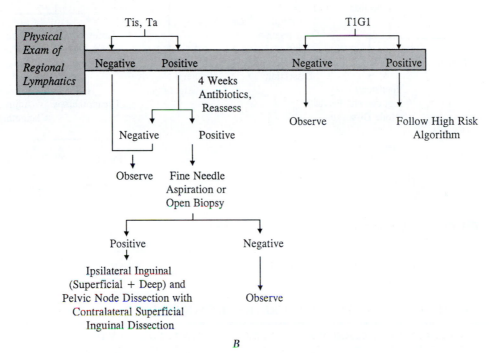

**FIGURE 17C-16.** Proposed algorithm for the treatment of SCC of the penis (5-FU-5-fluorouracil). *A.* Management of the primary tumor. *B.* Management of regional disease in low-risk patients. *C.* Management of regional disease in high-risk patients. (*C* is on page 808.)

## TREATMENT

The rarity of urethral cancer makes the establishment of a uniform treatment strategy difficult. In general, the specific histologic type of a tumor does not markedly affect prognosis. Tumor stage and anatomic location within the urethra are the most important determinants of local control and survival in both males and females and, therefore, treatment options are strongly dictated by these factors.

### FEMALE URETHRAL CARCINOMA

***ANTERIOR URETHRA.*** In the female, small, well-defined lesions confined to the mucosa of the anterior urethra can be effectively treated by transurethral resection or distal urethrectomy. Stage Tis, T1, and T2 anterior urethral tumors are amenable to distal urethrectomy if negative margins can be confirmed by frozen section. Urinary continence should be maintained in patients undergoing distal urethrectomy. Low-stage anterior urethral cancer in the female can also be treated with radiation therapy delivered as brachytherapy,[74,75] brachytherapy combined with external beam radiation,[76,77] or in combination with surgery, with an expected survival of 40% to 100% at 5 years.[78] However, complications, including incontinence, fistula, and stricture, are not uncommon.[74,78] A common theme for distal-only urethral carcinomas is that local control via surgical excision and interstitial brachytherapy with or without external beam radiotherapy are facilitated by the favorable location. This translates into

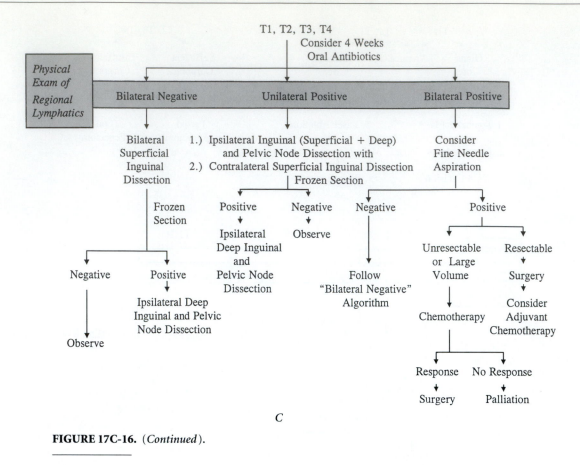

*C*

**FIGURE 17C-16.** (*Continued*).

**TABLE 17C-3.** CLINICAL STAGING SYSTEMS FOR URETHRAL CANCER

| STAGE | FEMALE: GRABSTALD SYSTEM DESCRIPTION | STAGE | MALE: RAY SYSTEM DESCRIPTION |
|---|---|---|---|
| 0 | Carcinoma in situ | 0 | Confined to mucosa |
| A | Submucosal extension | A | Invasion into but not beyond the lamina propria |
| B | Invasion of periurethral muscle | B | Invasion into but not beyond the corpus spongiosum |
| C | Periurethral extension:<br>  C1 Invasion of muscular wall of vagina<br>  C2 Invasion of muscular wall of vagina with invasion of vaginal mucosa<br>  C3 Invasion of adjacent structures (bladder, labia, clitoris) | C | Direct extension into tissues beyond the corpus spongiosum (corpus cavernosa, muscle, fat, fascia, skin, bone) or beyond the prostatic capsule |
| D | Metastasis:<br>  D1 Inguinal lymphatics<br>  D2 Pelvic lymphatics below the aortic bifurcation<br>  D3 Pelvic lymphatics above the aortic bifurcation<br>  D4 Distant metastasis | D | Metastasis:<br>  D1 Regional, including inguinal or pelvic lymph nodes<br>  D2 Lymph nodes above the aortic bifurcation or distant metastasis |

## TABLE 17C-4. INTERNATIONAL UNION AGAINST CANCER TNM STAGING SYSTEM FOR URETHRAL CANCER

| STAGE | DEFINITION |
| --- | --- |
| **PRIMARY TUMOR (T)** | |
| Tx | Primary tumor cannot be assessed |
| T0 | No evidence of primary tumor |
| Tis | Carcinoma in situ |
| Ta | Noninvasive papillary, polypoid, or verrucous carcinoma |
| T1 | Tumor invades subepithelial connective tissue |
| T2 | Tumor invades periurethral musculature (corpus spongiosum or prostate) |
| T3 | Tumor invades anterior vagina or bladder neck (corpus cavernosum or beyond prostate or bladder neck) |
| T4 | Tumor invades other adjacent structures |
| **REGIONAL LYMPH NODES (N)** | |
| Nx | Regional lymph nodes cannot be assessed |
| N0 | No regional lymph node metastasis |
| N1 | Metastasis in a single superficial inguinal lymph node, 2 cm or less in greatest dimension |
| N2 | Metastasis to a single lymph node, >2 cm but <5 cm in greatest dimension, or multiple nodes involved, none >5 cm |
| N3 | Metastasis to a lymph node >5 cm in greatest dimension |
| **DISTANT METASTASIS (M)** | |
| Mx | Presence of distant metastasis cannot be assessed |
| M0 | No distant metastasis |
| M1 | Distant metastasis |

5-year survival of greater than 50% in most series.[75] Inguinal lymphadenectomy is recommended for palpably involved nodes and will be histologically positive for tumor in approximately 80% of cases. Conversely, prophylactic lymphadenectomy has not proved to be of therapeutic benefit in the face of clinically negative inguinal nodes.[79]

**POSTERIOR URETHRA.** Tumors of the posterior urethra in the female that invade beyond the mucosa in the absence of gross pelvic nodal involvement are best managed by anterior exenteration, including resection of a cuff of vagina. These tumors have a poorer prognosis than tumors of the anterior urethra due to higher stage at presentation, with a historic 5-year survival rate between 10% and 17%.[79] The addition of radiation therapy may be beneficial.[76] Grigsby and Herr[80] recently described four evaluable female pa-

tients with invasive proximal urethral cancer treated with preoperative radiotherapy combined with anterior exenteration, resection of the genitourinary diaphragm, partial symphysectomy, and lymphadenectomy. Two were cured and two died subsequent to local and distant failure within 5 months of surgery.[80] Narayan et al.[79] reviewed the results of four small series of 34 patients treated with preoperative radiotherapy and surgery and noted an average 5-year survival rate of 55%.[79] Thus, an incremental improvement in local control and survival with neoadjuvant radiotherapy in selected patients may be achieved.

### MALE URETHRAL CARCINOMA

**ANTERIOR URETHRA (FOSSA NAVICULARIS, PENILE URETHRA).** In the male, the treatment of carcinoma of the distal urethra is also determined by stage. Stage Tis, Ta, and T1 tumors are treated with aggressive transurethral resection, whereas stage T2 or greater tumors are resected by partial penectomy if a 2-cm negative margin can be achieved while preserving a sufficient length of the penile stump, or by total penectomy if these criteria cannot be met. In a series of 23 male patients with anterior urethral cancer treated at the M. D. Anderson Cancer Center, all four patients with tumors located in the fossa navicularis were disease-free at a mean follow-up of 93 months and 6 of 11 patients with penile urethral tumors were disease-free at a mean of 48 months.[81] No local recurrences were noted in four patients with fossa navicularis primaries. Further, eight of nine patients with penile urethral tumors (in whom local control was attempted) were free of local recurrence. Adjuvant chemotherapy in combination with partial or total penectomy may have aided in local control.

**POSTERIOR URETHRA (BULBOUS, MEMBRANOUS, AND PROSTATIC URETHRA).** Occasionally, superficial lesions (Ta, Tis, T1) occuring within the posterior urethra can be managed with transurethral resection (TUR). The vast majority consist of squamous cell or papillary (or in situ) transitional cell carcinomas of the bulbous or prostatic urethra.[82] Aggressive TUR can assist in staging and have therapeutic benefit in some cases. Invasion into and beyond the periurethral smooth muscle, prostatic ducts, and, most importantly, the prostatic stroma is more ominous and requires extensive surgical resection for local control to maximize the possibility of long-term survival. Such procedures include radical en bloc excision of the penis, scrotum, prostate, and bladder with pelvic lymphadenectomy and excision of the pubic ramus for suspected invasion. Even with these extensive surgical procedures, the 5-year survival rate has been poor (20%) due to a failure of local control and distant metastases. Two small series suggest that an incremental benefit in local control and survival may be achieved by the integration of chemotherapy or radiotherapy with surgery [6 of 14 patients or 43% (combined series) with disease-free survival more than 16 months] over historical series.[80,81]

**MANAGEMENT OF INGUINAL LYMPH NODES.** As with female urethral carcinoma, there remains no proven benefit to prophylactic inguinal dissection in males with urethral carcinoma. Due to the morbidity of lymphadenectomy, standard management consists of close observation by physical examination every 2 months for patients with no palpable adenopathy. However, several series attest to the therapeutic value of lymphadenectomy in patients with palpably positive nodes.[82] In an attempt to decrease morbidity, Dinney et al.[81] have described the use of a limited sentinel lymph node dissection in nine patients with urethral carcinoma, two of whom had a normal physical examination. In both patients, with a normal physical examination, the sentinel lymph node was the only node positive, and both patients were treated with radical groin dissection and subsequent chemotherapy. Both patients achieved durable long-term survival, although one patient had a subsequent recurrence with distant metastasis at 46 months. This prophylactic approach may prove useful in patients with invasive anterior or distal urethral lesions where the lymphatic drainage is directed to the inguinal lymph nodes. Potentially, patients found to have early metastatic dissemination could be stratified for adjuvant systemic therapy. We are continuing to gain experience with this technique prior to its routine implementation.

## NOVEL COMBINATION REGIMENS FOR LOCALLY ADVANCED URETHRAL CARCINOMA OF THE MALE AND FEMALE URETHRA.

It is clear that failure to obtain local control or the subsequent development of distant metastasis in patients with invasive urethral carcinomas results in dismal survival rates. Aggressive surgical procedures alone have failed to impact the natural history of the disease. The suggestion that incremental improvements in local control and survival could be achieved with the addition of chemotherapy and/or radiation with surgery have led to attempts to integrate these modalities.[79–81]

At Memorial Sloan-Kettering Cancer Center, 11 patients with stage T2–4, N0, M0 tumors of the posterior urethra were treated with neoadjuvant methotrexate vinblastin adriomycin and cisplatin (M-VAC) chemotherapy.[80] Of 10 evaluable patients, 4 were downstaged to T0. Of five patients with transitional cell carcinoma, 3 achieved a complete remission. Complete remissions were not achieved in patients with mixed or nontransitional histology with this regimen. In responding patients, conservative surgical procedures led to dissappointing local recurrences that were incurable with subsequent aggressive procedures.[80] Thus, optimal treatment requires systemic therapy directed by histology combined with an aggressive surgical resection from the outset.

At the University of Texas M. D. Anderson Cancer Center, we have initiated several combination regimens for patients with locally advanced urethral carcinoma (T2–4, N0 or T1–4, N1–3, M0) that combine aggressive systemic and local therapy stratified by the primary tumor histology. For patients with primarily transitional cell carcinoma of the urethra, five cycles of neoadjuvant M-VAC chemotherapy are followed by stage-directed surgical resection to achieve wide negative margins. SCCs are sensitive to cisplatin-containing chemotherapeutic regimens and are also radiosensitive.[83] Thus, patients exhibiting this histology will receive neoadjuvant radiotherapy (50 Gy) and concomitant cisplatin–5-fluorouracil chemotherapy followed by aggressive surgical resection.

Adenocarcinoma is relatively radioresistant and responds poorly to standard chemotherapy. Accumulating experience suggests that the combination of taxol and cisplatin (or carboplatin) is active in a variety of cancers, including breast, prostate, lung, bladder, gastrointestinal, ovarian, and endometrial.[84–88] Patients with primary adenocarcinoma of the urethra will receive five cycles of taxol and cisplatin and subsequently undergo surgical consolidation to assess response to therapy, local and distant control, and survival. The goal of our studies is to gain a significant experience with patients treated in a standard aggressive fashion. This will allow a more definitive assessment of the results of therapy so that future refinements can be tested.

## Acknowledgments

*The authors wish to thank Dr. Nora Morganstern for providing photomicrographs used in this chapter.*

## REFERENCES

1. JOHNSON DE et al: Carcinoma of the penis: Experience with 153 cases. Urology 1:404, 1973.
2. SUFRIN G, HUBEN R: Benign and malignant lesions of the penis, in *Adult and Pediatric Urology*, 2d ed. JY Gillenwater et al (eds). St Louis, Mosby-Year Book, 1987, pp 1643–1681.
3. PERSKY L, deKERNION J: Carcinoma of the penis. CA Cancer J Clin 6:258, 1986.
4. DODGE OG, LINSELL CA: Carcinoma of the penis in Uganda and Kenya Africans. Cancer 16:1255, 1963.
5. RIVEROS M, LEBRON R: Geographic pathology of cancer of the penis. Cancer 16:798, 1963.
6. WOLBARST AL: Circumcision and penile cancer. Lancet 1:150, 1932.
7. SCHELLHAMMER PF et al: Tumors of the penis, in *Campbell's Urology*, 6th ed. PC Walsh et al (eds). Philadelphia, WB Saunders, 1992, pp 1264–1295.
8. BARRASSO R et al: High prevalence of papillomavirus-associated penile intraepithelial neoplasia in sexual partners of women with cervical intraepithelial neoplasia. N Engl J Med 317:916, 1987.
9. VARMA VA et al: Association of human papillomavirus with penile carcinoma: A study using polymerase chain reaction and in situ hybridization. Hum Pathol 22:908, 1991.
10. IWASAWA A et al: Detection of human papillomavirus deoxyribonucleic acid in penile carcinoma by polymerase chain reaction and in situ hybridization. J Urol 149:59, 1993.
11. SARKAR FH et al: Detection of human papillomavirus in squamous neoplasm of the penis. J Urol 147:389, 1992.
12. WERNESS BA: Cervical cancer: Search for an infectious etiology. Contemp Oncol 45, 1994.
13. MUNGER K et al: The E6 and E7 genes of the human papillomavirus type 16 together are necessary and sufficient for transformation of primary human keratinocytes. J Virol 63:4417, 1989.
14. WEINER JS, WALTHER PJ: The association of oncogenic human papillomaviruses with urologic malignancy. Surg Oncol Clin North Am 4:257, 1995.
15. MADEN C et al: History of circumcision, medical conditions and sexual activity and risk of penile cancer. J Natl Cancer Inst 85:19, 1993.
16. THOMPSON HC et al: Report of the ad hoc task force on circumcision. Pediatrics 56:610, 1975.

17. NARAYANA AS et al: Carcinoma of the penis: Analysis of 219 cases. Cancer 49:2185, 1982.
18. EKSTROM T, EDSMYR F: Cancer of the penis: A clinical study of 229 cases. Acta Chir Scand 115:25, 1958.
19. STAUBITZ WJ et al: Carcinoma of the penis. Cancer 8:371, 1955.
20. GERBER GS: Carcinoma in situ of the penis. J Urol 151:829, 1994.
21. KAYE V et al: Carcinoma in situ of penis: Is distinction between erythroplasia of Queyrat and Bowen's disease relevant? Urology 36:479, 1990.
22. AYALA AG, RO JT: Pathology of penile cancer, in *Principles and Practice of Genitourinary Oncology.* D Raghavan et al (eds). Philadelphia, Lippincott-Raven, 1997, pp 927–936.
23. BRODERS A: Squamous cell epithelioma of the skin. Ann Surg 73:141, 1928.
24. JACKSON SM: The treatment of carcinoma of the penis. Br J Surg 53:33, 1966.
25. AMERICAN JOINT COMMITTEE of CANCER (eds): Penis, in *Manual for Staging Cancer,* 3d ed. JB Lippincott (ed). Philadelphia, 1998, pp 189–191.
26. THEODORESCU D et al: Outcomes of initial surveillance of node negative invasive squamous cell carcinoma of the penis. J Urol 155:1626, 1996.
27. McDOUGAL WS et al: Treatment of carcinoma of the penis: The case for primary lymphadenectomy. J Urol 136:38, 1986.
28. FRALEY EE et al: Cancer of the penis: Prognosis and treatment plans. Cancer 55:1618, 1985.
29. MUKAMEL E, DEKERNION JB: Early versus delayed lymph node dissection versus no lymph node dissection in carcinoma of the penis. Urol Clin North Am 14:707, 1987.
30. SOLSONA E et al: Corpus cavernosum invasion and tumor grade in the prediction of lymph node condition in penile carcinoma. Eur Urol 22:115, 1992.
31. RAVI, R: Correlation between the extent of nodal involvement and survival following groin dissection for carcinoma of the penis. Br J Urol 72:817, 1993.
32. JOHNSON DE, LO RK: Complications of groin dissection in penile cancer: Experience with 101 lymphadenectomies. Urology 14:312, 1984.
33. SCAPPINI P et al: Penile cancer. Aspiration biopsy cytology for staging. Cancer 58:1526, 1986.
34. CABANAS RM: An approach for the treatment of penile carcinoma. Cancer 39:456, 1977.
35. HALL MC et al: Deoxyribonucleic acid flow cytometry and traditional pathologic variables in invasive penile carcinoma: Assessment of prognostic significance. Urology 52:111, 1998.
36. HARDNER GJ et al: Carcinoma of the penis: Analysis of therapy in 100 consecutive cases. J Urol 108:428, 1972.
37. HANASH KA et al: Carcinoma of the penis: A clinicopathologic study. J Urol 104:291, 1970.
38. GOETTE DK, CANON TE: Erythroplasia of Queyrat: Treatment with topical 5-fluorouracil. Cancer 38:1498, 1976.
39. EL-DEMIRY MI et al: Reappraisal of the role of radiotherapy and surgery in the management of carcinoma of the penis. Br J Urol 56:724, 1984.
40. HAILE K, DELCLOS L: The place of radiation therapy in the treatment of carcinoma of the distal end of the penis. Cancer 45:1980, 1980.
41. GRABSTALD H, KELLEY CD: Radiation therapy of penile cancer. Six to ten year follow-up. Urology 15:575, 1980.
42. DUNCAN W, JACKSON SM: The treatment of early cancer of the penis with megavoltage x-rays. Clin Radiol 23:246, 1972.
43. MOHS FE et al: Microscopically controlled surgery in the treatment of carcinoma of the penis. J Urol 133:961, 1985.
44. MOHS FE et al: Mohs micrographic surgery for penile tumors. Urol Clin North Am 19:291, 1992.
45. MALLOY TR et al: External genital lesions, in *Lasers in Urological Surgery,* 2d ed, JA Smith Jr et al (eds). Chicago: Year Book, 1989, pp 23–34.
46. VON ESCHENBACH AC et al: Results of laser therapy for carcinoma of the penis. Organ preservation. Prog Clin Biol Res 370:407, 1991.
47. BOON TA: Sapphire probe laser surgery for localized carcinoma of the penis. Eur J Surg Oncol 14:193, 1988.
48. ROTHENBERGER KH: Value of the neodymium: YAG laser in the therapy of penile carcinoma. Eur Urol 12:34, 1986.
49. MALEK RS: Laser treatment of premalignant and malignant squamous cell lesions of the penis. Lasers Surg Med 12:246, 1992.
50. JOHNSON DE et al: Verrucous carcinoma of the penis. J Urol 133:216, 1985.
51. Schellhammer PF: A concise plan for managing carcinoma of the penis. Contemp Urol 4:13, 1992.
52. BISSADA NK: Penile reconstuction after total penectomy or urethra-sparing total penectomy. J Urol 137:1173, 1987.
53. JOHNSON DE: Cancer of the penis: Overview, in *Genitourinary Tumors: Fundamental Principles and Surgical Techniques.* DE Johnson, MA Boileau (eds). New York: Grune & Stratton, p 189, 1982.
54. JOHNSON DE, LO RK: Management of regional lymph nodes in penile carcinoma: Five year results following therapeutic groin dissections. Urology 14:308, 1984.
55. SRINIVAS V et al: Penile cancer. Relation of extent of nodal metastasis to survival. J Urol 137:880, 1987.
56. PERINETTI E et al: Unreliability of sentinel lymph node biopsy for staging penile carcinoma. J Urol 124:734, 1980.
57. WESPES E et al: Cabanas approach: Is sentinel node biopsy reliable for staging penile carcinoma? Urology 28:278, 1986.
58. CATALONA WJ: Modified groin lymphadenectomy for carcinoma of the penis, in *Urologic Surgery,* presented by Bristol Laboratories and Mead Johnson Pharmaceuticals. New Scotland, NY, Learning Technologies, 1988.
59. PETTAWAY CA et al: Sentinel lymph node dissection for penile carcinoma: The M. D. Anderson Cancer Center Experience. J Urol 1544:1999, 1995.
60. LEVENBACK C et al: Intraoperative lymphatic mapping for vulvar cancer. Obstet Gynecol 84:163, 1994.
61. ROUVIERE H: The lymphatics of the male genital organs, in *Anatomy of the Human Lymphatic System,* MJ Tobias (ed). Ann Arbor, Edwards Brothers, 1938, pp 218–226.
62. DASELER EH et al: Radical excision of the inguinal and iliac lymph glands. Surg Gynecol Obstet 87:679, 1948.
63. JONES WG, EIWELL CM: Radiation therapy for penile cancer, in *Comprehensive Textbook of Genitourinary Oncology,* NJ Vogelzang et al (eds). Baltimore, Williams & Wilkins, 1996, pp 1109–1114.
64. HORENBLAS S et al: Squamous cell carcinoma of the penis. II. Treatment of the primary tumor. J Urol 147:1533, 1992.
65. NEWAISHY GA, DEELEY TJ: Radiotherapy in the treatment of carcinoma of the penis. Br J Radiol 41:519, 1968.
66. STADLER W: Chemotherapy for penile cancer, in *Comprehensive Textbook of Genitourinary Oncology.* NJ Vogelzang et al (eds). Baltimore, Williams & Wilkins, 1996, pp 1114–1116.
67. CORRAL DA et al: Combination chemotherapy for metastatic

or locally advanced genitourinary squamous cell carcinoma: A phase II study of methotrexate, cisplatin and bleomycin (MPB). J Urol 160:1770, 1998.

68. Terry PJ et al: Carcinoma of the urethra and scrotum, in *Principles and Practice of Genitourinary Oncology,* D Raghavan et al (eds): Philadelphia: Lippincott-Raven, 1997, pp 347–354.

69. Weiner JS et al: Oncogenic human papillomavirus type 16 is associated with squamous cell cancer of the male urethra. Cancer Res 52:5018, 1992.

70. Mostofi FK et al: Carcinoma of the male and female urethra. Urol Clin North Am 19:347, 1992.

71. Grabstald H et al: Cancer of the female urethra. JAMA 197:835, 1966.

72. Ray B et al: Experience with primary carcinoma of the male urethra. J Urol 117:591, 1977.

73. Beahrs OH et al (eds): *Manual for Staging of Cancer,* 3d ed, Philadelphia, JP Lippincott (ed). 1988, p 210.

74. Garden AS et al: Primary carcinoma of the female urethra: Results of radiation therapy. Cancer 71:3102, 1993.

75. Sailer SL et al: Carcinoma of the female urethra: A review of results with radiation therapy. J Urol 140:1, 1988.

76. Weghaupt K et al: Radiation therapy for primary carcinoma of the female urethra: A survey over 25 years. Gynecol Oncol 17:58, 1984.

77. Forman JD, Lichter AS: The role of radiation therapy in the management of carcinoma of the male and female urethra. Urol Clin North Am 19:383, 1992.

78. Bracken RB et al: Primary carcinoma of the female urethra. J Urol 116:188, 1976.

79. Narayan P, Konety B: Surgical techniques of female urethral cancer. Urol Clin North Am 19:373, 1992.

80. Grigsby PW, Herr HW: Urethral tumors, in *Comprehensive Textbook of Genitourinary Oncology,* N Vogelzang (eds). Baltimore, Williams & Wilkins, 1996, pp. 1117–1123.

81. Dinney CPN et al: Therapy and prognosis for male anterior urethral carcinoma: An update. Urology 43:506, 1994.

82. Zeidman EJ et al: Surgical treatment of carcinoma of the male urethra. Urol Clin North Am 19:359, 1992.

83. Hussein AM et al: Chemotherapy with cisplatin and 5-fluorouracil for penile and urethral squamous cell carcinomas. Cancer 65:433, 1990.

84. Ajani JA et al: Paclitaxel in the treatment of patients with upper gastrointestinal carcinomas. Semin Oncol 23:55, 1996.

85. Pienta KJ, Smith DC: Paclitaxel, estramustine and etoposide in the treatment of hormone-refractory prostate cancer. Semin Oncol 24:72, 1997.

86. Price FV et al: A trial of outpatient paclitaxel and carboplatin for advanced recurrent, and histologic high-risk endometrial carcinoma: preliminary report. Semin Oncol 24:78, 1997.

87. Roth BJ: Preliminary experience with paclitaxel in advanced bladder cancer. Semin Oncol 22:1, 1995.

88. Abu-Rustum NR et al: Salvage weekly paclitaxel in recurrent ovarian cancer. Semin Oncol 24:62, 1997.

# 17D / CANCER OF THE PROSTATE

*Peter N. Schlegel, Sarah K. Girardi, and E. Darracott Vaughan, Jr.*

## INTRODUCTION

Prostate cancer is the most common nonskin malignancy in men, and is the second leading cause of cancer death after lung cancer. It is estimated that in 1998 approximately 184,000 men were diagnosed with prostate cancer and 39,200 died of the disease.[1] Despite a decade of aggressive efforts at early detection and treatment, the mortality rate from prostate cancer has decreased slowly. The most significant risk factors for developing prostate cancer are age, race, and family history.

The disease exists in two forms. One is the indolent variety, referred to as latent or histologic prostate cancer, which remains silent throughout life and is only discovered incidentally, such as during a transurethral resection for benign prostatic enlargement or at autopsy. The other is the clinically aggressive variety that can be detected because of an abnormal digital rectal examination (DRE) or after investigation of an elevated prostate-specific antigen (PSA) level and eventually progresses inexorably to osseous metastases and death. Significant confusion has existed between these two clinically very different but histologically similar diseases.

## EPIDEMIOLOGY

Prostate cancer presents many challenges to the epidemiologist. Because prostate cancer is a disease of aging; men who are affected may not present until late in life, or their disease may remain silent throughout life and they ultimately succumb to other causes. Prior to the discovery of PSA, prostate cancer was only detected when tumors grew large enough to be noticed on DRE or when the cancer was metastatic. Early diagnosis was only possible after transurethral resection (TUR) of the prostate, but many of these tumors were latent. This is reflected in the former staging system, which classified tumors as stage A1 or stage A2 depending on the amount of cancer found in a transurethrally resected specimen (Table 17D-1). With the advent of PSA measurement and the concomitant decrease in the number of TURs being performed, more prostate cancers are being diagnosed at an early stage with clinically significant volume of disease, whereas latent tumors (found on TUR) are rarely detected. This has led to both lead-time and length-of-time bias in evaluating the efficacy of treatment strategies. In addition, since the natural history of prostate cancer differs depending on the method of detection, studies that do not control for detection method can be misleading.

With the introduction of PSA measurement and its subsequent widespread use came an apparent epidemic of cases. The age-adjusted incidence of prostate cancer reported by the Surveillance, Epidemiology, and End Results (SEER) program in the United States rose rapidly from 84.4 per 100,000 in 1984 to 163 per 100,000 in 1991. Stephenson et al.[2] tracked age-adjusted prostate cancer incidence

in trends from the population-based Utah Cancer Registry and compared them with the SEER data. A rapid rise in incidence was seen in the Utah registry between 1988 and 1991, reflecting the widespread use of PSA measurement. The incidence of prostate cancer in Utah peaked at 236.2 per 100,000 in 1992, and subsequently fell to 195.0 and 164.0 per 100,000 in 1993 and 1994, respectively. This rise and fall in prostate cancer incidence demonstrates another basic epidemiologic principle. As is true of any new detection test, especially when it is applied to a disease of long duration, initial screening is really a prevalence screen. It will detect disease that is ongoing as well as new cases. Once the test has been used for several years and the prevalence is established, the screening test will begin to yield true incidence values. This principle is illustrated in Fig. 17D-1.

Despite all the challenges prostate cancer presents to the epidemiologist, careful studies of affected populations and individual families have resulted in a much better understanding of disease prevalence, incidence, and epigenetic factors that may play a role in the development of prostate cancer. There are now compelling data to support a significant role for age, race, family history, and dietary factors in the development of prostate cancer.

## AGE

The single greatest risk factor for prostate cancer is age. It is estimated that 30% to 40% of men over age 50 harbor foci of prostate cancer.[3] The probability of developing prostate cancer is less that 1 in 10,000 for men under age 39, 1 in 103 for men between ages 40 and 50, and 1 in 8 for men between ages 60 and 79.[4] Approximately 50% of men diagnosed with prostate cancer will develop metastatic and

**TABLE 17D-1. JEWETT CLASSIFICATION OF PROSTATE CANCER STAGES**

| STAGE | DESCRIPTION |
|---|---|
| A1 | Cancer found incidentally in TURP specimen, <5% resected specimen involved, Gleason <6 |
| A2 | Cancer found incidentally in TURP specimen, ≥5% specimen with cancer and/or Gleason ≥7 |
| BIN | Nodule ≤1 cm in size |
| B1 | Palpable abnormality of prostate on one side only |
| B2 | Palpable abnormality of prostate on both sides |
| C | Palphable extracapsular extension of cancer |
| D0 | Biochemical (acid phosphaten) evidence of extracapsular prostate cancer; includes elevated PSA after local therapy |
| D1 | Lymph node metastasis |
| D2 | Bouj metastasis |

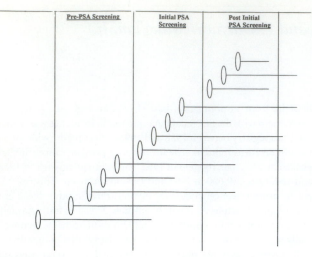

**FIGURE 17D-1.** The initial increase and subsequent decrease yield of PSA screening. With the introduction of PSA, cases of longstanding duration and new cases are detected as incident cases. After several years, when prevalence is established, the screening test becomes a more accurate reflection of true incidence.

therefore incurable disease. Therefore, efforts have been aimed at cancer prevention and early detection in individuals at increased risk for developing prostate cancer.

## RACE

There are significant racial differences in prostate cancer incidence. Rates of incidence are low in Japanese men, high in American whites, and highest in black American men.[5] The frequency of histologic prostate cancer in Japan and the United States is similar, whereas clinical prostate cancer rates are much higher in the United States. When Japanese men migrate to the United States, they develop clinical prostate cancer at a rate that approaches that of American men.[6] American black men develop clinical prostate cancer at a younger age, higher grade and stage, and progress more rapidly to advanced disease than their white counterparts,[7,8] even when controls for access to medical care and socioeconomic factors are used.[9] Higher intake of dietary fats,[10] higher levels of circulating testosterone,[11] and reduced ability to produce vitamin D in response to sunlight exposure[12] have all been implicated as potential explanations for the increased prostate cancer risk in black Americans.

## FAMILY HISTORY

Prostate cancer may be inherited as a hereditary disease with an autosomal dominant pattern and 85% penetrance.[13] Men with a first-degree relative with prostate cancer are two times as likely to develop prostate cancer as their age-matched counterparts. Men with two or three affected first-degree relatives are 5 and 11 times as likely to develop prostate cancer as their age-matched counterparts, respectively (Table 17D-2). The age of the affected relative is important. An individual with a father or brother diagnosed with

**TABLE 17D-2.** PROSTATE CANCER RISK BASED ON FAMILY HISTORY

| NUMBER OF FIRST-DEGREE RELATIVES AFFECTED | RELATIVE RISK OF DEVELOPING PROSTATE CANCER |
| --- | --- |
| 1 | 2 |
| 2 | 5 |
| 3 | 11 |

Source: Adapted from Carter et al.[14]

prostate cancer at age 70 and with no other relatives affected is at no increased risk for developing prostate cancer, whereas a man with one or more affected first-degree relatives and a father or brother diagnosed at age 50 is seven times as likely to develop prostate cancer as his age-matched counterpart (Table 17D-3).[14]

Prostate cancer families have been classified at Johns Hopkins University as hereditary, familial, or sporadic. Hereditary prostate cancer is defined as having three consecutive generations affected in either the paternal or maternal lineage, at least two affected brothers age 55 or less, or three first-degree relatives affected. Although hereditary prostate cancer accounts for approximately 43% of men who are diagnosed at age 55 or less, it accounts for only 9% of prostate cancer cases over all.[14] There is evidence that men in families with female members with breast and ovarian cancer who are carriers for the *BRCA1* and *BRCA2* genes may also be at increased risk for developing prostate cancer.[15]

## DIETARY FACTORS

There is increasing evidence to support a role for dietary factors in the development of prostate cancer. Epidemiologic studies have shown that although the incidence of histologic prostate cancer is relatively consistent among diverse populations, clinical prostate cancer rates are highly variable. This supports the concept that endogenous factors may be responsible for the initiation of prostate cancer, but environmental factors such as diet may be responsible for the development of clinical disease. Perhaps the most compelling data are those for dietary fats.

Fair et al.[16] showed that when nude mice injected with human prostate cancer cell line (LnCaP) are fed a high-fat diet, tumor growth is increased. Furthermore, when their diets are fat-restricted, tumor growth slows. Giovannucci et al.[17] collected dietary histories of men participating in the Health Professionals Follow-up Study, a prospective cohort of 51,529 United States' men who had completed food-frequency questionnaires in 1986. Follow-up questionnaires

**TABLE 17D-3.** PROSTATE CANCER RISK BASED ON FAMILY HISTORY AND AGE AT DIAGNOSIS

| AGE AT ONSET, YEARS | ADDITIONAL RELATIVES | RELATIVE RISK |
| --- | --- | --- |
| 70 | 1 or more | 1.0 |
| 60 | 1 or more | 5.0 |
| 50 | 1 or more | 7.0 |

Source: Adapted from Carter et al.[14]

were sent in 1988 and 1990 aimed at documenting new disease histories and updated exposure histories. They found that total fat consumption was directly related to risk of advanced prostate cancer. They concluded that animal fat, especially from red meat, was associated with an increased risk of developing prostate cancer.

Several mechanisms have been proposed to account for the association between dietary fat and prostate cancer, including increases in sex hormone levels from excess fat intake or alterations in 5α-reductase activity by unsaturated fatty acids. Linolenic acid specifically has been postulated to damage cell membranes and DNA through the formation of free radicals.[18]

## VITAMINS

The role of retinol (vitamin A) and β-carotene (provitamin A) in the development of prostate cancer has been debated. Giovannucci et al.[19] assessed dietary intake over a 1-year period in a cohort of 47,894 subjects and found no relationship between risk of prostate cancer detection and overall intake of vegetables and fruits.[19] Intake of the carotenoids β-carotene, carotene, lutein, and β-crytoxanthin were not risk factors for prostate cancer. Lycopene intake alone was related to a lower risk (age- and energy-adjusted RR = 0.79; 95% confidence interval = 0.64–0.99).

Several laboratory studies have shown that in addition to its role in calcium homeostasis, vitamin D plays a role in the regulation of cell growth and differentiation. In vitro studies of prostate cancer cell lines have shown that vitamin D can significantly reduce the growth of prostate cancer cells.[20] Based on a report that a series of common polymorphisms in the vitamin D receptor gene were associated with osteoporosis, Taylor et al.[21] set out to determine whether these vitamin D receptor polymorphisms might also be associated with increased prostate cancer risk. In a case-control study of 108 men undergoing radical prostatectomy and 170 controls, men who were homozygous for the T allele (which was shown to be associated with higher serum levels of the active metabolite of vitamin D) had one-third the risk of developing prostate cancer than men who were heterozygous or homozygous for the T allele. Other studies, however, have failed to show an association. Gann et al.[22] conducted a case-control study of men in which vitamin D metabolite and vitamin D–binding protein assays were measured in 232 prostate cancer patients and age-matched controls. Median levels of 25-D, 1,25-D, and vitamin D–binding protein were indistinguishable between cases and controls. Isaacs et al.[23] studied specific vitamin D receptor genotypes for an association between specific genotypes and advanced prostate cancer and found no association. Cofactors important in vitamin D activity may partially explain these conflicting reports.

## HORMONES

The role of hormones in the development of prostate cancer is poorly understood. African-American men have been shown to have circulating testosterone levels that are 15% higher than their white counterparts.[24] This difference has been postulated to account for the increased risk of prostate cancer in black American men. Elevated levels of circulating testosterone have not been consistently observed in men with prostate cancer, however. In a study comparing 5α-reductase activity in white and black American men and Japanese men, different levels of androgen metabolites were seen in white and black Americans when compared to Japanese men, suggesting an association between low 5α-reductase activity and low risk for prostate cancer.[25]

## VASECTOMY

In 1993 Giovannucci et al.[25] reported an association between vasectomy and prostate cancer risk. A total of 10,055 men who were part of the Health Professionals Follow-up Study between the ages of 40 and 75 had undergone a vasectomy at the time of study entry in 1986 compared to 37,800 who had not. Three hundred new cases of prostate cancer were diagnosed in participants who were initially free of cancer. Vasectomy was associated with an elevated risk of prostate cancer after controlling for diet, physical activity, smoking, alcohol consumption, educational level, body mass index, and geographic area of residence. The authors concluded that based on the elevated risk and lack of confounding factors, the association was causal. The findings have been vigorously debated.[25,26] No biologic explanation has been found, and the epidemiologic method has been seriously questioned. Extension of this study obviated any association between vasectomy and subsequent development of prostate cancer. In a study by John et al.[27] in 1995, of 1642 patients with prostate cancer and 1636 controls, no association between increased prostate cancer risk and vasectomy was found.

## SUMMARY

Over the past decade, significant progress has been made in our understanding of the epidemiology of prostate cancer. Studies of diverse populations suggest that prostate cancer develops as the result of both genetic and environmental influences. Individuals with a family history of prostate cancer are clearly at increased risk, as are black American men. Dietary fats likely play an important role in prostate cancer development and may explain some of the variability in prostate cancer incidence across populations. Vitamin A is reported by some to be protective; however, the supporting data currently are lacking. The early data on vitamin D are intriguing and may indeed lead to an important role for vitamin D in prostate cancer prevention. Continued laboratory and population-based studies will be needed to design effective strategies for chemoprevention of prostate cancer.

# HISTOLOGY

Almost all prostate cancers are adenocarcinomas. They tend to arise from the peripheral zone of the prostate in 85% of patients. Adenocarcinoma of the prostate is multifocal in more than 85% of patients. Even if it appears to be unilateral on rectal examination, these lesions are bilateral in approximately 70% of surgical specimens that are examined pathologically. Although prostatic adenocarcinoma can be found in up to 50% of men in autopsy series, these lesions are small, low-grade, and clinically insignificant. These tumors are very rarely detected during clinical screening with PSA blood tests, rectal examination, and transrectal ultrasound-guided biopsy of the prostate.[28]

## PRECURSOR LESIONS

High-grade prostatic intraepithelial neoplasia (PIN) is a clinically significant finding on prostate biopsies that is associated with the presence of invasive carcinoma. PIN consists of architecturally benign prostatic acini or ducts lined with cytologically atypical cells (Fig 17D-2). Low-grade PIN, previously referred to as mild dysplasia or PIN-1, is of no prognostic significance. Patients with low-grade PIN are at no measurable risk of having an invasive carcinoma found on repeat biopsy. When high-grade PIN is found on needle biopsy, there is a 30% to 50% risk of finding carcinoma on subsequent biopsies.[29] By itself, PIN does not give rise to elevated serum PSA levels. The finding of high-grade PIN without invasive carcinoma on needle biopsy should result in subsequent additional prostatic biopsies. Biopsies should be performed both in the region where PIN was seen as well as other areas of the prostate, in the typical sextant pattern. Although high-grade PIN appears to be a precursor lesion to many peripheral intermediate-grade and high-grade adenocarcinomas, PIN is not a required precursor for carcinomas to arise within the prostate.[30]

## GRADING, CYTOLOGIC, AND NUCLEAR FEATURES

Numerous grading systems have existed for evaluation and diagnosis of prostate cancer. By far, the Gleason grading system is the most widely accepted. The Gleason system of prostate cancer grading is based on the glandular pattern of the tumor as evaluated at relatively low magnification. Cytologic features are not important in grading of the tumor. The Gleason grading system combines the two most common (primary and secondary) architectural patterns of cancer within the sampled specimen. Each of the two most common patterns is assigned a grade from 1 to 5, with 1 being the most

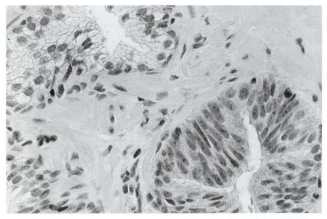

**FIGURE 17D-2.** High-grade prostatic intraepithelial neoplasia.

differentiated and 5 the least differentiated or anaplastic pattern (Fig. 17D-3). The value of the Gleason grading system is its ability to predict survival rates. Importantly, Gleason grading may provide prognostic information that is to some degree independent of the extent of local tumor. The Gleason sum score is reported as the two scores added together. For example, if the most common pattern of grading was a 3 pattern and the second most common pattern was a 4, the Gleason grade would be reported as Gleason $3 + 4 = 7$ (Fig. 17D-4).[31]

## TUMOR VOLUME

In general, the size of a prostate cancer correlates with its risk of metastatic spread. Capsular penetration is uncommon in tumors that are less than 0.5 $cm^3$ in volume. However, tumors that have grown greater than 4 $cm^3$ in volume have an increased risk of lymph node metastases or seminal vesicle invasion. Almost by definition, prostate cancer volumes of less than 0.2 $cm^3$ with no Gleason 4 pattern present are almost certainly insignificant tumors. These insignificant or "latent" tumors are found in autopsy series that are rarely if ever detected with transrectal ultrasound-guided biopsies that are performed because of elevated PSA levels.

## SURGICAL SPECIMENS

Pathologic evaluation of radical prostatectomy specimens should include several important points. Whole-mount sectioning of the prostate is easier to evaluate; however, these pleasing sections are usually not performed, and routine sectioning allows accurate identification of important pathologic features. Detection of seminal vesicle invasion and lymph node metastasis are important prognostic factors for radical prostatectomy. Only 25% of men with seminal vesicle invasion and virtually no men with lymph node metastases are free of progression at 10 years following radical prostatectomy. Although the prostatic capsule is incomplete in many areas around the prostate, evaluation of penetration of tumor into the capsule or extension outside of the prostate into periprostatic soft tissue is of prognostic significance. In addition, evaluation of margins to detect focal or extensive tumor at the margin is of value. Even in the face of positive margins, only approximately 50% of men will demonstrate cancer progression and recurrence after radical prostatectomy. In general, tumor volume correlates well with pathologic stage and Gleason grade in clinical T2 cancers. However, tumor volume is not an independent prognostic variable after radical prostatectomy. Evaluation of DNA ploidy is also of limited independent value.[30]

## OTHER CARCINOMAS

Mucinous adenocarcinomas are a subtype of tumor that have very aggressive biologic behavior. As with standard adenocarcinomas, they have a propensity to develop bone metastases and produce PSA and acid phosphatase with advanced disease.[32] Approximately 0.5% of prostatic cancers arise from the prostatic ducts and are referred to as prostatic duct adenocarcinomas. These tumors are often clinically underestimated because they produce limited amounts of

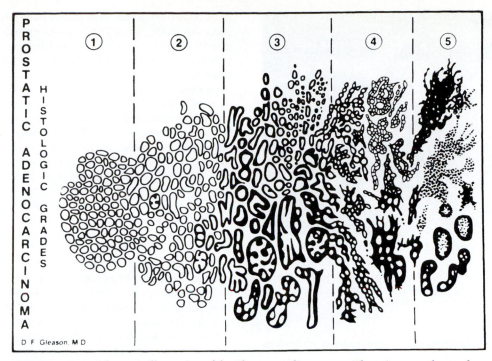

**FIGURE 17D-3.** Schematic illustration of the Gleason grading system. The primary and secondary patterns of prostate cancer cell architecture are identified and added together to obtain the Gleason sum score.

PSA. Most prostatic duct adenocarcinomas have an advanced stage at presentation with a subsequent aggressive clinical course.[33]

Transitional cell carcinomas of the prostate are rarely primary, and usually present as T4 transitional cell carcinomas of the bladder. Their behavior and management is considered in Chap. 17B, Cancer of the Bladder. Other unusual lesions include pure primary squamous carcinoma of the prostate, sarcomas of the prostate, and primary prostatic lymphoma.[34]

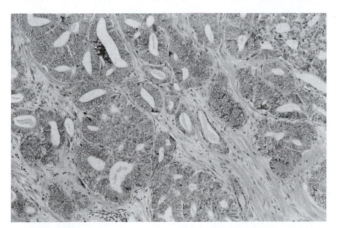

**FIGURE 17D-4.** Invasive prostate cancer with areas of cribiform growth pattern (Gleason score 3).

## SUMMARY

In summary, complete Gleason scoring, evaluation of the local specimen as having organ-confined tumor, focal capsular penetration, or extracapsular extension as well as margin, seminal vesicle, and lymph node status are important in evaluation of radical prostatectomy specimens.

## DIAGNOSIS

Unfortunately, the location of most carcinomas of the prostate in the peripheral zone region of the gland results in a paucity of symptoms for patients with early localized prostate cancer. Similarly, except for the uncommon prostatic nodule,[35] the DRE is normal in most patients with potentially curable T1 disease and an abnormal DRE is often not due to prostatic carcinoma.[36]

In contrast to the limitations of the history and physical exam, there have been a series of increasingly more precise serum markers to diagnose prostate cancer. The initial marker utilized to identify prostate carcinoma was the enzymatic determination of serum acid phophatase.[37] A level above 0.8 U/L almost always signified metastatic disease. The test is not utilized routinely today because of the advent of prostatic-specific antigen (PSA) and methodologic difficulties in standardizing enzymatic assays. However, if performed

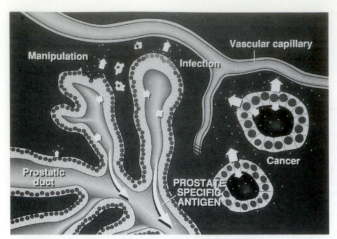

**FIGURE 17D-5.** Physiology of PSA showing normal secretion through the prostatic ducts. Mechanisms for increased serum PSA level is through manipulation, infection, or cancer, where there is direct secretion into the bloodstream.

properly, enzymatic acid phosphatase evaluations are a useful indices of metastatic disease.

The enzymatic acid phosphatase assay was followed by the radioimmunoassay method. This test today has no clinical utility and should not be applied because of an unacceptable frequency of false-positive and false-negative results.

## PROSTATE-SPECIFIC ANTIGEN

PSA is a member of the kallikrein gene family. It is a serine protease produced by the prostate epithelium and periurethral glands in the male. PSA is secreted into seminal fluid in high concentration and is involved in the liquefaction of the ejaculate. As shown in Fig. 17D-5, PSA is primarily secreted outside of the body and only backs up into the bloodstream to significant degrees when the prostate is affected by infection or has been manipulated, such as after a biopsy has been performed. Because prostate cancer glands do not secrete PSA out of the body, PSA may also be detectable in blood if a prostate cancer is present. whether it is in the prostate gland or has spread into other areas of the body. As a prostate cancer grows. PSA levels in blood tend to increase as well. This finding allows the response to

prostate cancer treatment to be followed with serial measurement of PSA levels. Production of PSA by normal prostate function as well as prostate cancer is dependent on male hormones (androgens) being present in the body at normal levels. For example, patients who are taking the 5α-reductase inhibitor finasteride to limit symptoms of benign enlargement of the prostate (BPH) will typically see a 50% decrease in serum levels of PSA due to marked suppression of the potent androgen dihydrotestosterone. Patients who are on complete hormonal ablation (usually with a gonadotropin-releasing hormone (GnRH) agonist and an antiandrogen) have dramatic decreases in the PSA level because of the low hormone levels in the body. Because PSA is normally secreted outside of the body, the presence of an elevated PSA level suggests either that the prostate is enlarged or an abnormal condition exists within the prostate, whether it is caused by BPH, inflammation, infection, or prostatic cancer. However, the presence of an elevated PSA level in blood does not confirm the presence of prostate cancer.

The Tandem assay (Hybritech, San Diego, California), with a normal range up to 3.99 mg/mL, has been utilized in the majority of studies evaluating PSA and prostatic cancer detection. It is now clear in numerous studies that the routine use of PSA increases the early detection of prostate cancer[38] over that of DRE alone. With further refinements of the definition of a "normal" use of PSA, there is an increase in the detection of localized organ-confined prostatic cancer.

Thus it is now recommended that men at age 50 should begin annual PSA measurements and DRE. Annual PSA assays and DRE should begin at age 40 in men with a family history of prostate cancer and men of African descent (Table 17D-4, 17D-5).

PSA testing has led to a dramatic increase in the detection of potentially curable localized cancer. Studies utilizing frozen sera collected before clinical detection of prostate cancer have found that with appropriate PSA testing, the tumor could have been detected as much as 5 years earlier (Fig. 17D-6), presumably at an earlier stage.[18,39,40]

The prostate enlarges with age in men with normal testicular function at a rate of 0.2 to 1.2 g/yr. Thus it is logical to expect a progressive rise in PSA for an individual over time. Thus a fixed definition of a "normal" PSA value may not be appropriate for all subpopulations of men. Several refinements of the PSA test have been offered.

**PSA VELOCITY.** A more accurate way to evaluate the significance of a PSA blood test is to measure the change in PSA levels over time.[39] This measurement is referred to as PSA velocity, and is usually represented as an increase in PSA level in nanograms per

**TABLE 17D-4.** CHANCE OF CANCER AS A FUNCTION OF SERUM PSA LEVEL AND DRE FINDINGS

| STUDY | CHANCE OF CANCER ON BIOPSY, %: PSA <4.0 ng/mL | | CHANCE OF CANCER ON BIOPSY, %: PSA >4.0 ng/mL | |
| --- | --- | --- | --- | --- |
| | NEGATIVE DRE | POSITIVE DRE | NEGATIVE DRE | POSITIVE DRE |
| Cooner et al, 1990 | 9 | 17 | 25 | 62 |
| Hammerer and Huland, 1994 | 4 | 21 | 12 | 72 |
| Ellis et al, 1994 | 6 | 13 | 24 | 42 |
| Catalona et al, 1994b | — | 10 | 32 | 49 |

ABBREVIATIONS: PSA = prostate-specific antigen; DRE = digital rectal examination.
SOURCE: Adapted from *Campbell's Urology*, Walsh PC et al (eds), Philadelphia, WB Saunders, 1994.

## TABLE 17D-5. CANCER DETECTION WITH SERUM PSA AND DRE

| METHOD OF DETECTION | CANCER DETECTION RATE, %, AMONG 6630 MEN | NO. OF CANCERS DETECTED, %, $n = 264$ |
|---|---|---|
| DRE | 3.2 | 48(18) |
| PSA | 4.6 | 118(45) |
| DRE/PSA | 5.8 | 98(37) |

ABBREVIATIONS: DRE = digital rectal examination; PSA = prostate-specific antigen.
SOURCE: Adapted from Catalona WI J Urol 151:1283, 1994.

milliliter per year. To obtain valid measurements of PSA velocity, a series of at least three PSA blood tests must be obtained over 1.5 years. If the PSA level increase is greater than 0.75 ng/mL per year, then there is increased suspicion that prostate cancer is causing this PSA level to rise. The relative increase in PSA levels over time for men with benign enlargement of the prostate or prostate cancer is demonstrated in Fig. 17D-6.

PSA DENSITY. The calculation of PSA density (serum PSA level divided by prostate volume [cm³]) is an approach to enhance the specificity of serum PSA measurement.[41] In the PSA range of 4 to 10 mg/mL, many patients who undergo a biopsy are not found to have cancer, and it is believed that the elevation of PSA level is caused by BPH component. Because the enlarged prostate has additional BPH tissue, and BPH tissue is known to produce PSA, this calculation was designed to remove the contribution to the serum PSA

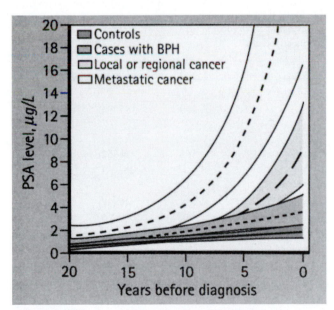

**FIGURE 17D-6.** Changes in PSA level over time before diagnosis of prostate cancer, which is the basis for PSA velocity. Patients eventually diagnosed with prostate cancer have a logarithmic change in PSA as opposed to patients with benign prostatic hyperplasia. (*From HB Carter et al.[39] Reproduced with permission.*) (See also Plate 27.)

level by the BPH tissue. This removal is done by determining the quotient of the serum PSA divided by the volume of the prostate. This calculation gained acceptance in the mid-1990s when it was determined that prostate cancer caused a tenfold greater increase in PSA compared with BPH. For patients with a PSA density greater than 0.15, an increased risk of detection of prostate cancer was reported in some studies. If a patient had a previous negative biopsy, an elevated PSA density suggested the need for a repeat biopsy. Although there is not complete agreement in the literature as to the benefit of PSA density measurement, for clinical management of the man with a PSA level of 4 to 10 ng/mL, the determination of PSA density for many urologists remains a helpful concept in determining the need for prostate biopsy. The PSA density calculation requires an ultrasound-determined prostate volume measurement.

AGE-SPECIFIC PSA LEVEL. As previously stated, it is now well documented that in the aging male with normal testicular function, there is an increase in the size of the prostate (ranging from 0.4 to 1.2 g/yr). A logical extension is that serum PSA levels should also increase with age.[42] This concept has led to community-based determinations of age-specific normal PSA levels (Tables 17D-6 and 17D-7). Thus, rather than accepting a single "normal" PSA level, the PSA level in a younger patient is expected to be lower and in an older patient, higher. One should be suspicious of prostatic cancer if the patient's age-specific PSA level is abnormal. The use of the age-specific PSA level is believed to enhance the specificity and sensitivity of the test and also to avoid unnecessary biopsies.

However, this concept has recently been challenged by the fear that using higher PSA cutoffs for older men with nonpalpable prostate cancer may make it less likely to diagnose the disease at an earlier age, when it is most likely to be curable. Further studies are necessary, but an important concept is that in the younger patient, the PSA level is significantly lower than the commonly used cutoff range of PSA in most laboratories.

FREE AND TOTAL PSA. In addition to evaluating the total amount of PSA protein that is present in blood, evaluation of the type of PSA may also be helpful in considering the significance of an abnormal PSA level for an individual patient. PSA may exist in either free form or bound to proteins in blood.[43] When it is bound to proteins, PSA normally binds to the proteins $\alpha_2$-macroglobulin or $\alpha_1$-antichymotrypsin. Regardless of what the PSA is bound to, the proportion of free to total PSA (total PSA = free PSA + bound PSA) may be evaluated as percent free PSA. For any given PSA value in men with PSA levels between 4 and 10 ng/mL, the chance of prostate cancer being present may be further evaluated based on

## TABLE 17D-6. SERUM PSA LEVEL AND PATIENT AGE

| AGE RANGE, YEARS | MEDIAN VALUE, ng/mL | INTERQUARTILE RANGE, ng/mL | REFERENCE RANGE, ng/mL |
|---|---|---|---|
| 40–49 | 0.7 | 0.5–1.1 | 0–2.5 |
| 50–59 | 1.0 | 0.6–1.4 | 0–3.5 |
| 60–69 | 1.4 | 0.9–3.0 | 0–4.5 |
| 70–79 | 2.0 | 0.9–3.2 | 0–6.5 |

SOURCE: From Oesterling et al.[92] Reproduced with permission.

## TABLE 17D-7. AGE-SPECIFIC REFERENCE RANGE FOR SERUM PSA LEVEL ACCORDING TO INDIVIDUAL YEAR OF LIFE

| AGE, YR | PSA RANGE, ng/mL | AGE, YR | PSA RANGE, ng/mL |
|---------|------------------|---------|------------------|
| 40 | 2.0 | 60 | 3.8 |
| 41 | 2.1 | 61 | 4.0 |
| 42 | 2.2 | 62 | 4.1 |
| 43 | 2.3 | 63 | 4.2 |
| 44 | 2.3 | 64 | 4.4 |
| 45 | 2.4 | 65 | 4.5 |
| 46 | 2.5 | 66 | 4.6 |
| 47 | 2.6 | 67 | 4.7 |
| 48 | 2.6 | 68 | 4.9 |
| 49 | 2.7 | 69 | 5.1 |
| 50 | 2.8 | 70 | 5.3 |
| 51 | 2.9 | 71 | 5.4 |
| 52 | 3.0 | 72 | 5.6 |
| 53 | 3.1 | 73 | 5.8 |
| 54 | 3.2 | 74 | 6.0 |
| 55 | 3.3 | 75 | 6.2 |
| 56 | 3.4 | 76 | 6.4 |
| 57 | 3.5 | 77 | 6.6 |
| 58 | 3.6 | 78 | 6.8 |
| 59 | 3.7 | 79 | 7.0 |

Source: From Oesterling et al.[92]

percent free PSA (Table 17D-8). For example, although the overall possibility of finding cancer on biopsy for men with a PSA level of 4 to 10 ng/mL is 25%, when one subdivides these men based on the percent free PSA, the probability of cancer being present on biopsies may be as low as 8% or as high as 56%. The value of the percent free PSA measurement is further demonstrated in Fig. 17D-7, where the probability of finding cancer is subdivided based on patient age. For men between 50 and 64 years of age, the risk of finding prostate cancer is rather similar, given an individual percent free PSA value relative to what is seen in men with a much higher prevalence of prostate cancer (men 65 to 75 years of age). In general, the clinical decision to perform an initial prostate biopsy is usually made based on evaluation of a single age-adjusted "cutoff value." Percent free PSA is then used to modify the risk of cancer being present and the potential need for subsequent biopsies. For men with percent free PSA values greater than 25%, the risk of prostate cancer being present may be so low that subsequent prostate biopsy may be avoided or deferred even if the absolute PSA value is abnormal. In summary, the fact that prostate cancers usually release a form of PSA that is bound to proteins into blood (which is different from the PSA released by prostate glands with benign enlargement) provides the basis for using percent free PSA measurement to further refine the sensitivity and specificity of the PSA blood test.

**PSA EVALUATION AFTER THERAPY FOR PROSTATE CANCER.** PSA has its greatest clinical value in detection of recurrent disease after local therapy, especially radical prostatectomy. With the prostate gland removed, PSA levels should be undetectable (≤0.1 ng/mL). Detectable PSA, with subsequent increases on serial

## TABLE 17D-8. COMPARISON OF CLINICAL AND PATHOLOGIC STAGES IN RADICAL PROSTATECTOMY SERIES

| REFERENCE | NO. OF PATIENTS | ORGAN-CONFINED NO. (%) | NON-ORGAN-CONFINED NO. (%) |
|-----------|-----------------|------------------------|----------------------------|
| **T1a** | | | |
| Partin et al, 1993c; Johns Hopkins University | 31 | 31 (100) | — |
| Catalona and Bigg, 1990; Washington University | 13 | 13 (100) | — |
| Zincke et al, 1994; Mayo Clinic | 49 | 44 (90) | 5 (10) |
| Total | 93 | 88 (94) | 5 (6) |
| **T1b** | | | |
| Partin et al, 1993c; Johns Hopkins University | 71 | 50 (70) | 21 (30) |
| Catalona and Bigg, 1990; Washington University | 40 | 26 (65) | 14 (35) |
| Zincke et al, 1994; Mayo Clinic | 177 | 120 (68) | 57 (32) |
| Total | 288 | 196 (68) | 92 (32) |
| **T1c (nonpalpable)** | | | |
| Epstein et al, 1994a; Johns Hopkins University | 157 | 80 (51) | 77 (49) |
| Paulson, 1994; Duke University | 142 | 81 (57) | 61 (43) |
| Total | 299 | 161 (54) | 138 (46) |
| **T2** | | | |
| Partin et al, 1993c; Johns Hopkins University | 565 | 294 (52) | 271 (48) |
| Paulson, 1994; Duke University | 131 | 49 (37) | 64 (63) |
| Zincke et al, 1994; Mayo Clinic | 2944 | 1333 (45) | 1289 (55) |
| Catalona and Bigg, 1990; Washington University | 197 | 103 (52) | 94 (48) |
| Total | 3837 | 1779 (46) | 1718 (54) |
| **T3a** | | | |
| Partin et al, 1993c; Johns Hopkins University | 36 | 7 (19) | 26 (81) |

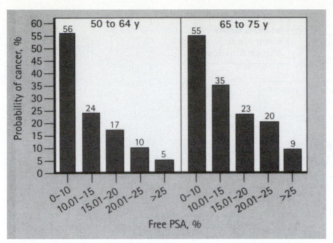

**FIGURE 17D-7. A.** Probability of cancer as calculated by % free PSA and age for patients with PSA levels between 4 and 10 ng/mL. (*From WJ Catalona et al.*[43] *Reproduced with permission.*) (See also Plate 28.)

| PSA | Probability of cancer, % | | Percent Free PSA | Probability of cancer, % |
|---|---|---|---|---|
| 0–2 ng/mL | 1 | | 0–10 | 56 |
| 2–4 ng/mL | 15 | | 10–15 | 28 |
| 4–10 ng/mL | 25 | | 15–20 | 20 |
| >10 ng/mL | >50 | | 20–25 | 16 |
| | | | >25 | 8 |

**FIGURE 17D-7. (Continued.) B.** Probability of prostate cancer based on prostate-specific antigen (PSA) and percent free PSA results (for men with nonsuspicious digital rectal examination results, regardless of patient age). Adapted from WJ Catalonia et al.[43] (See also Plate 29.)

testing, reflects evidence of local or distant prostate cancer recurrence. After radiation, nadir levels of PSA may take 18 to 24 months to be achieved. The best prognosis is obtained when men have a PSA level less than 0.5 ng/mL that does not subsequently increase. PSA may also be used to follow patients after hormonal or other systemic therapy as a rough guide of disease status. Since PSA production is androgen-dependent, androgen status must be considered when evaluating men treated for prostate cancer.

**HYPERSENSITIVE PSA MEASUREMENT.** PSA may also be measured using a series of hypersensitive assays that allow detection of very low levels of PSA in the bloodstream. The hypersensitive assays may be helpful in the early detection of recurrent prostate cancer after effective local treatment such as local prostatectomy. The use of this test may allow detection of recurrent cancer 1 to 2 years before what would be possible with standard PSA assays. Unfortunately, very low levels of PSA are also found in nonprostate tissues such as the urethral glands. Therefore, a significant frequency of false-positive results may occur with widespread use of the hypersensitive PSA for detection of prostate cancer recurrences. Even women will have detectable hypersensitive PSA levels, although women have no prostate tissue. The use of hypersensitive PSA analysis is limited to patients who have had treatment for localized prostate cancer. A hypersensitive PSA does not provide additional information over that provided by total and percent free PSA for initial detection of prostate cancer.

**POLYMERASE CHAIN REACTION TECHNOLOGY.** New techniques have allowed identification of circulating blood cells that produce PSA, as well as the previously described tests that measure the amount of PSA protein present in the blood. These procedures involve taking a sample of blood, usually from a peripheral vein, and analyzing it with detailed molecular techniques, including reverse transcriptase polymerase chain reaction (RT-PCR), to amplify very small amounts of RNA to determine if there are PSA-producing cells in blood. Normally, PSA-producing cells are not present in blood; they are only present in the prostate. However, in the presence of prostate cancer, circulating blood cells, presumably prostate cancer cells, that produce PSA may exist. With PCR techniques, as few as one cell in one million can be detected. The presence of PSA-producing cells in blood does correlate with the stage and aggressiveness of prostate cancer. However, all tumors, including localized tumors, will occasionally release prostate cancer cells into the bloodstream, and their presence on a blood test does not determine whether cancer has spread to other areas of the body. In addition, most men with established extensive spread of prostate cancer to other areas of the body will have "negative" PSA-PCR blood tests. Technical problems with degradation of RNA in blood samples and interlaboratory differences in performing RT-PCR have been problematic for this test. The role of RT-PCR technology in detecting circulating prostate cancer cells is limited at present in the management of men with prostate cancer.

## SUMMARY

Men over 50 should have an annual measurement of PSA level and a DRE. Earlier screening is appropriate for patients at high risk of developing prostate cancer, including African-American men and those with a family history of prostate cancer. All patients with an abnormal DRE should have a transrectal ultrasound (TRUS) and biopsy. The precise use of age-specific PSA and free and total ratio remains to be validated. However, if the age-specific PSA level is elevated and/ or the free PSA is less than 20% (total PSA range 3 to 10 ng/mL), then a TRUS and biopsy of the prostate gland are indicated (Fig. 17D-8).

## TRANSRECTAL ULTRASOUND

The development of TRUS has been a dramatic advance in our ability to image the prostate. Prior to TRUS, perineal prostatic biopsy or transrectal aspiration of the prostate were blind procedures directed toward abnormalities found on DRE. The evolution of PSA identifies patients with possible T1c localized prostate cancer with a normal DRE. Without TRUS to direct systematic biopsy of the prostate, appropriate utilization of PSA data would have been

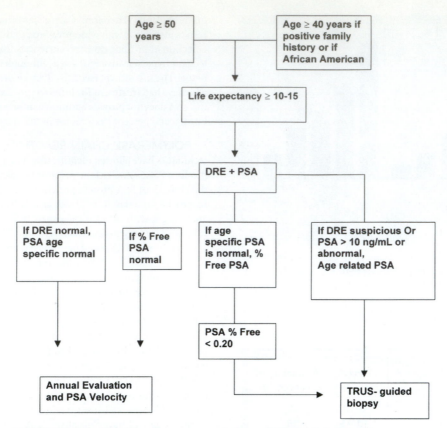

**FIGURE 17D-8.** Algorithm for recommended use of PSA in clinical practice.

difficult. Thus TRUS is now most commonly utilized in conjunction with transrectal prostatic biopsy. The biopsy is rapid, easily performed by a trained urologist, well tolerated by the patient, and is performed in an outpatient setting.

The transrectal approach for prostatic ultrasonography gives more accurate images than the transabdominal approach. Thus the size, symmetry, consistency of the prostate; the relationship to the bladder; and evaluation of the seminal vesicles can be obtained. However, it is apparent that there is not a single characteristic ultrasound appearance of prostate cancer. Indeed, many prostate cancers are too small and diffuse to detect by ultrasound. Prostate cancer is often described as hypoechoic, but it may also be isoechoic and can be hyperechoic. Therefore the TRUS findings have poor specificity and TRUS is never utilized in isolation to rule out the diagnosis of prostatic cancer. The role of color doppler imaging with TRUS is under investigation. TRUS may be utilized to estimate prostatic volume using the prostate ellipsoid formula: (anterior-posterior diameter) × (transverse diameter) × (sagittal diameter/2). There is more variability in this method than with planimetric methods, but planimetric methods are more time consuming and so are rarely performed. Newer machines allow three-dimensional imaging, which may estimate prostate volume more accurately. Prostate size determinations are utilized to determine PSA density, to select patients with BPH for treatment with alpha blockade (<35 g) or finasteride (>35 g), to estimate response to therapy, and at times as a guide for brachytherapy.

## TRUS-GUIDED PROSTATIC BIOPSY

Prostate biopsy is usually performed with ultrasound guidance. This is an office procedure and does not require anesthesia. The prostate is visualized using ultrasound, and an 18-gauge biopsy needle is used. Patients routinely receive antibiotic prophylaxis for prostate biopsy, and the complications of bleeding or infection are rare. A series of at least six biopsies is mapped throughout the prostate to allow sampling of the entire gland. At the time of biopsy, the ultrasound allows determination of the prostate size and the detection of any anatomic abnormalities (Fig.17D-9).

Although TRUS does not have adequate specificity to detect prostate cancer, abnormal areas seen on ultrasound are sampled with needle biopsy in addition to the sextant pattern. In the ultrasound image shown in Fig. 17D-10, a prostate cancer is seen in the lower left as a discrete, hypoechoic area.

Because prostate cancer cannot usually be seen as a discrete lesion on ultrasound, biopsies are performed in a predetermined pattern to sample the peripheral zone adequately. TRUS permits biopsy planning by providing complete visualization of all zones of the prostate. To detect any cancer of 1 cm or larger, biopsies are performed at 1.0-cm spacing in the peripheral zone (PZ). In the most common prostate sizes (40 g), this represents three biopsy cores in the right and left PZ for a total of six biopsy specimens. Hence the name "sextant pattern" is applied to this method of ultrasound-guided prostate biopsy (Fig. 17D-11).

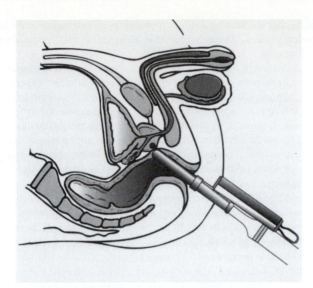

**FIGURE 17D-9.** TRUS-guided prostatic biopsy, using an automated biopsy gun. (See also Plate 30.)

The relationship of prostate size to the identification of cancer during biopsy also demonstrates the importance of prostate size in determining the number of biopsy cores to be performed. Using the standard sextant pattern in the 40-g prostate, a 1-cm cancer should be detected. However, in the larger prostate, the pattern may miss the cancer; therefore, additional biopsy cores are needed in the larger prostate[45] (see Fig. 17D-11).

Patients with abnormal serum PSA levels but a single negative biopsy represent a clinical dilemma. Most urologists suggest at least one additional TRUS biopsy, since at least 12% of repeat biopsies will reveal prostate carcinoma.[36]

Repeat prostatic biopsy should include sampling of the transition zone,[46] which may reveal carcinoma in as many as 30% of patients. An additional indication for repeat biopsy is the presence of high-grade PIN on initial biopsy (see Fig. 17D-2).

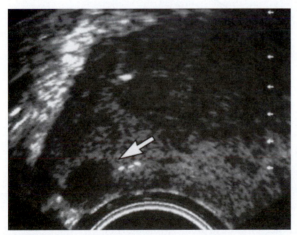

**FIGURE 17D-10.** TRUS image of prostate cancer. The lesion can be seen in the lower left, as it is in the hypoechoic area.

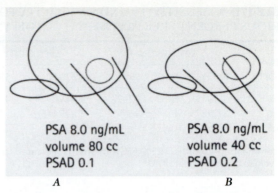

| PSA 8.0 ng/mL volume 80 cc PSAD 0.1 | PSA 8.0 ng/mL volume 40 cc PSAD 0.2 |
| --- | --- |
| *A* | *B* |

**FIGURE 17D-11.** In the larger prostate, the pattern shown in panel A misses the cancer. Therefore, additional biopsy cores are needed in the larger prostate. (*From RG Uzzo et al.[45] Reproduced with permission.*)

TRUS does not accurately stage prostatic cancer. However, if the prostatic biopsies are at the base and high grade (Gleason 7 to 10), some investigators have recommended TRUS biopsy of the seminal vesicles to identify T3c disease.

## STAGING

Precise staging following the diagnosis of prostate cancer is critical. The extent of disease directs the therapy to be utilized and directly correlates with prognosis. Treatment is directed to eradicate localized disease with the hope of cure, whereas treatment of metastatic disease is only palliative at the present time. Staging techniques are directed to the evaluation of local extension of disease first, and secondly the presence of metastatic disease.

### TNM CLASSIFICATION

It is now acceptable to use the TNM classification in lieu of the older Jewett-Whitmore (A to D) staging. An important addition to the classification is the T1c category for patients identified by PSA abnormalities alone with a normal DRE. In fact, at the present time this is the most common initial presentation.

Clinical pathologic T1a to T2c patients are candidates for total prostatectomy, whereas T3 to T4 patients are more commonly recommended to have radiotherapy, often with neoadjuvant hormonal treatment. A continuing problem in staging is the inability to accurately distinguish between T2 and T3 disease. Thus there is significant understaging by DRE and TRUS in the diagnosis of prostate cancer. This understaging is evident upon pathologic staging showing the presence of pathologic extracapsular extension disease in patients with clinically localized disease (Table 17D-9).

It suffices to say that at this time there are no imaging studies, TRUS, pelvic computerized axial tomography (CT), or pelvic or transectal magnetic resonance (MRI), that accurately delineate T2 and T3 disease. Neither pelvic CT nor MRI is recommended to stage patients with clinically localized disease.

**TABLE 17D-9.** SENSITIVITY AND SPECIFICITY FOR VARIOUS PERCENT FREE PSA (%FPSA) CUTOFFS*

| % FPSA CUTOFFS | SENSITIVITY | | SPECIFICITY | |
|---|---|---|---|---|
| | n/n (%) | 95% CI | n/n (%) | 95% CI |
| <25% | 358/379 (95) | 92–97 | 80/394 (20) | 16–24 |
| <32% | 373/379 (98) | 96–99 | 25/394 (6) | 4–9 |
| <55% | 379/379 (100) | | 0/394 (0) | |

*Recommended cutoff is >25% FPSA (biopsy is indicated in men with values below this cutoff ).

## EVALUATION FOR METASTATIC DISEASE

The most common sites for the appearance of early metastatic disease are the pelvic lymph nodes and bone. Recently, based upon retrospective analysis of a large number of operative specimens and postoperative clinical data, a predictor of pathologic stage from clinical data has been reported (Fig. 17D-12).[47] Taken together, these and other studies reveal a low probability of metastatic disease in patients with a PSA level of less than 10 ng/mL and a Gleason score below 7.

Accordingly, the routine use of bone scans and pelvic or abdominal CT preoperatively in such patients is not cost-effective. However, the radionuclide bone scan is the most sensitive method for detecting metastatic disease, and nonspecific findings can be documented prior to treatment. In patients at higher risk for metastatic disease, PSA above 20 ng/mL or Gleason score of 7 to 10, on biopsy, bone scan and pelvic CT scanning is more reasonable. If suspicious pelvic lymph nodes are demonstrated, then percutaneous or laparoscopic node biopsy can be performed.

Additional staging techniques under study include monoclonal imaging positive emission tomography (PET) and detection of circulating prostatic cells by (RT-PCR), as previously discussed. None of these techniques has been validated. Monoclonal imaging is limited by both false-positive and false-negative studies, and the relationship of RT-PCR–detected cells with eventual development of metastatic disease is unknown. Both studies should be considered experimental at this time and not utilized routinely.

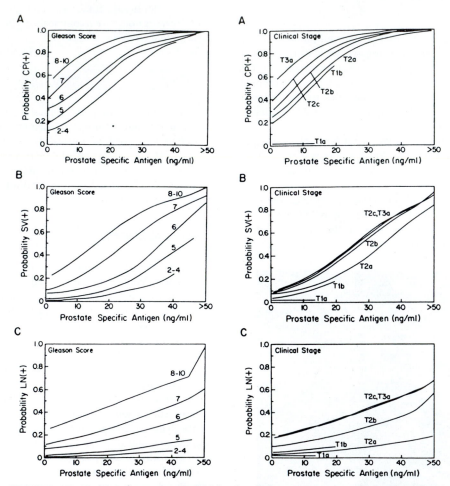

**FIGURE 17D-12.** Use of preoperative PSA level and Gleason score to predict probability of capsular penetration (CP), seminal vesicle involvement (SV), and lymph node involvement (LN). At right, similar curves are developed depending on clinical stage. (*From CP Partin et al.[47] Reproduced with permission.*)

## MANAGEMENT OF PROSTATE CANCER

Prostate cancer may be divided, based on its clinical presentation, into localized or advanced disease. For men with clinical T1–2,NX, M0 prostate cancer, curative therapy or observation are options. For men with advanced disease (T3, N+ or M+), hormonal therapy and other palliative treatments are the primary approaches for consideration. In men who have a less than 10-year life expectancy with localized disease, as well as men with less than 5-year life expectancy and asymptomatic advanced disease, expectant management is the optimal initial treatment.

Management of localized prostate cancer is a controversial issue, in part because the natural history of localized prostate cancer has been only segmentally elucidated. At present, prostate cancer is the most common cancer diagnosed in men in the United States and the second most common cause of cancer death. The ratio of death rate to incidence suggests that between 20% and 50% of men with a clinical diagnosis of prostate cancer will die of the disease. In considering the management of localized prostate cancer, it is important to remember that men with latent, incidental microscopic tumors can only rarely have these cancers detected using today's screening tests of PSA level and TRUS-guided biopsies.[48] Preliminary studies that have evaluated a program of observation or watchful waiting rather than screening with a PSA-based approach suggest that the death rate from prostate cancer will decrease with screening. In addition, the small decrease in prostate cancer death rates associated with the increased screening by PSA measurement (with a 5- to 7-year lag period) suggests that earlier screening, detection, and treatment of men with prostate cancer may result in saving lives. Since prostate cancer screening has only been available for a little over a decade and the lag time between detection of localized disease and death may be 10 to 15 years or more, it is understandable that proof of the benefit of early screening in decreasing death rates does not yet exist. In distinction, there is widespread acceptance that breast cancer is an important cause of death in women and early detection (introduced more than 20 years ago) decreases the death rate from breast cancer.[29]

Studies of the natural history of localized prostate cancer have suffered from selection biases, but they allow us some insight into what would occur if patients with localized disease were not treated with curative intention. Almost all of these studies indicate that men with metastatic disease had unrecognized advanced disease at least 10 years prior to diagnosis. This is supported by the studies of Carter et al.,[13] where serum PSA levels were followed serially in a number of patients in the Baltimore Longitudinal Study of Aging. Therefore, patients who are candidates for curative local therapy should have a 10-year life expectancy.

## OBSERVATION

Patients with prostate cancer who are followed expectantly should have regular physical examinations and serial PSA levels obtained. Progressive increases in PSA level, development of local cancer growth as suggested by physical examination, or evidence of metastatic disease should be evaluated. For men with localized disease who demonstrate progression, repeat prostatic biopsies or treatment may be indicated. It is unclear how many patients can still be treated with curative intent after a period of observation and subsequent disease progression. Four major series have reported long-term results following deferred therapy. Whitmore and colleagues reported on 75 men who were selected out of a pool of 4000 patients seen at Memorial Hospital during his career. Johansson and co-workers reported on 223 of 306 eligible men from Sweden.[49] Aus in 1994 performed a retrospective analysis of 536 patients with known diagnoses of prostate cancer who died in Goteborg, Sweden, between 1988 and 1990.[49A] Although Whitmore and Johansson reported cancer-specific survival of 84% and 87% at 10 years, the Aus analysis indicates that for patients who had no metastases at the time of diagnosis and survived more than 10 years, 63% eventually died of prostate cancer. Aus further concluded that 15 years was the earliest time when cancer-specific mortality analysis had any significance. In men less than 65 years of age with nonmetastatic cancer at the time of diagnosis, 75% died of prostate cancer when managed with noncurative intent. Using the Connecticut Cancer Registry, Albertson et al.[50] found that men with a Gleason score of 5 to 7 tumors had a potential lost life expectancy of 4 to 5 years, based on a series of patients who were followed without treatment. For men with a Gleason score of 8 to 10 tumors, 6 to 8 years of life expectancy was lost. Taken together, these series suggest that with localized prostate cancer and moderately well differentiated tumors, approximately 50% of men who live 15 years or more after diagnosis will die of prostate cancer if no treatment is provided.

Adolfsson and colleagues[51] as well as Chodak et al.[52] performed a pooled analysis of 823 case records from six nonrandomized studies done since 1985. They reported that the metastatic rates at 10 and 15 years were substantial. For men with histologic-grade tumors, 42% developed metastatic disease within 10 years, and 70% developed metastatic disease within 15 years. These studies are somewhat flawed by the fact that many patients received hormonal therapy at the time of progression, which may have delayed the appearance of metastatic disease. Additional studies, such as that of Fleming et al.,[53] have attempted to use a Markov model to analyze the potential therapeutic benefit from early intervention and treatment. A quality-of-life analysis was used to evaluate the potential benefit of curative therapy. This study is somewhat flawed by the low rates of progression used in the Markov model analysis. The rates of progression were clearly lower than that reported by Chodak et al.[52] Beck et al.[54] reevaluated these data based on the results of Chodak et al. and found a significant benefit from treatment of well-differentiated lesions as well as moderately and poorly differentiated lesions when quality-of-life adjustments were taken into account. Results following radical prostatectomy suggest that the 10-year actuarial progression-free survival likelihood of 69% as reported from Johns-Hopkins[29] is clearly better than the 53% for untreated patients in Johannson's series of 44% treated with interstitial iodine125.[55] Therefore, a potential benefit of treatment is suggested.

Further studies by Labrie et al.[56] suggest that screening with PSA followed by treatment will result in a decreased death rate from prostate cancer. Subsequent randomized studies by this author have provided early evidence for a survival benefit with PSA screening for prostate cancer. In addition, the decrease in prostate cancer deaths observed in the SEER database from 1992 to 1995 suggests that death rates may be being affected both by therapy and earlier diagnosis (NCI, 1998). Further, a well-controlled randomized series may be necessary to document the potential benefits of treatment.

Men who have a limited life expectancy (less than 10 years) either due to advanced age at diagnosis (typically greater than age 75) or significant comorbidity are therefore not candidates for treatment of localized prostate cancer with intent to cure. For patients who have mild comorbidities and life expectancy greater than 10 years, the risks and benefits of treatment should be balanced and the patient informed of his options, including watchful waiting, radiation, and surgery. For men who have no significant comorbidities, are young, and have a greater than 10- to 15-year life expectancy, all available data suggest that local treatment is important and likely to be effective. Watchful waiting to determine if a cancer will progress is limited by the sensitivity of DRE to detect cancer growth and the uncertain nature of PSA changes for patients who have local cancer progression.

Despite its epidemic incidence, prostate cancer treatment still generates controversy. Prostate cancer treatment is associated with some degree of morbidity, may be applied to patients who have micrometastatic disease, and many patients at the time of diagnosis will have local disease that cannot be cured. Until 10- to 15-year data are available from early detection (PLCO) or treatment (PIVOT) studies for localized cancer, we will not have definitive information as to whether aggressive or conservative treatment should be provided for men with localized prostate cancer. However, the vast majority of prostate cancers that are detected as localized disease at this point are clinically important.[48] Slow but inevitable progression of clinically detected localized cancer occurs without treatment. Surgical treatment appears to be quite effective if cancers are detected early.

## CLINICAL IMPORTANCE OF CANCERS DETECTED WITH PSA AND DRE

One concern with earlier detection of prostate cancers is that PSA and DRE alone may detect latent or clinically insignificant carcinomas. These findings have not been supported by studies to date. In fact, evaluation of prostate cancer volume in radical prostatectomy specimens detected by PSA and DRE in the contemporary era indicates that more than 95% of cancers are clinically significant. Even for men with a normal rectal examination who have cancers detected by PSA level elevation alone and who have microscopic solitary tumors seen on TRUS-guided needle biopsies, over 90% of these tumors are clinically significant.[48]

## RADICAL PROSTATECTOMY

Radical prostatectomy is an effective treatment for localized prostate cancer that may be performed by either a retropubic or perineal approach. Most surgeons currently prefer the retropubic approach, because it allows access to the pelvic lymph nodes and simultaneous performance of a lymph node dissection. In addition, contemporary techniques for urethral anastomosis have very low complication rates with good continence, and wider excision or preservation of the neurovascular bundles may be more easily effected by the retropubic approach. Although perineal prostatectomy has the potential advantages of lower blood loss and more direct urethral anastomosis, these advantages may be outweighed by the inability to remove periprostatic fascias with the prostate using a perineal ap-

proach. During perineal prostatectomy, the dissection is performed essentially along the prostatic gland, whereas the primary dissection during retropubic prostatectomy is performed outside of the prostatic fascias.

Since its introduction by Millen in 1947, the retropubic approach to prostatectomy has been a standard treatment. However, the popularity of this procedure was low until the last 20 years because of the frequent complications of bleeding, incontinence, and impotence. More recently, a series of anatomic discoveries have improved surgeons' ability to remove all tumor and substantially decrease associated morbidity. Delineation of the periprostatic vascular anatomy, the relationship of the neurovascular bundles to the prostate, and subsequent elucidation of the urethral sphincter mechanism inferior to the prostate have allowed a decrease in perioperative blood loss. In addition, improved rates of postoperative potency and urinary continence have been achieved. Many of these advances are based on anatomic work that was described by Walsh et al.[58,59] and others[56,57] at the James Buchanan Brady Urological Institute of the Johns Hopkins Hospital.

One major source of potential bleeding during prostatectomy is the dorsal vein complex that passes over the prostate gland. The dorsal vein complex enters the pelvis under the public bone. It is located just above the urethral sphincter muscles and below the periprostatic fascias. During division of the fascias and urethral sphincter, the dorsal vein complex is opened. Control of this vascular structure is usually performed with sutures. It must be performed carefully to avoid compromising urethral sphincter function. The dorsal vein complex from the penis then fans out over the prostate, and it must be further secured on the lateral and superior portions of the prostate during completion of the prostatectomy.[56]

The autonomic innervation of the penis travels in the cavernous nerves that are located just posterolateral to the prostate in close association with the lateral prostatic fascia and rectum. These nerves are derived from branches of the pelvic plexus that lie in a fenestrated plate along the lateral sidewall of the rectum between 5 and 11 cm from the anal verge. The pelvic plexus is derived from hypogastric nerves that travel lateral to the sigmoid colon as well as sacral roots 2, 3, and 4, which provide parasympathetic efferent preganglionic fibers. For patients in whom it is clinically appropriate to preserve the cavernous nerves, their location can be identified because they travel with the capsular veins of the prostate in a group posterolateral to the prostate. This neurovascular bundle complex is located outside of the prostate.[60] Preservation of the neurovascular bundle does not result in any compromise to removal of the entire prostate with its capsule (Fig. 17D-13.)

During radical prostatectomy, the neurovascular bundle can be isolated and preserved by incising the lateral prostatic fascia just anterior to the neurovascular bundle. After small branches of the neurovascular bundle to the prostate are clipped and divided, the neurovascular bundle then stays on the rectal surface in close association with the lateral prostatic fascia as the prostate is removed. The striated urethral sphincter surrounds the urethra and attaches to the prostate. Preservation of this urethral sphincter complex is critical to the early and effective restoration of continence for men after radical prostatectomy. Again, the striated urethral sphincter is outside of the prostate. Division of the striated urethral sphincter may be carried out under direct vision during apical dissection of the

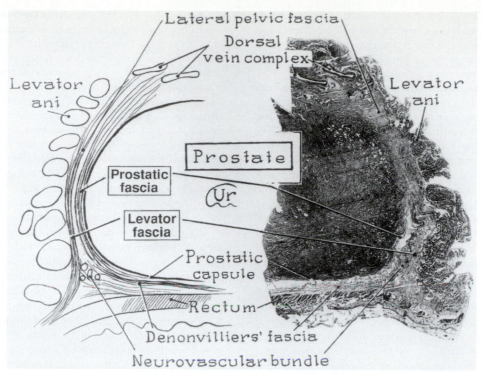

**FIGURE 17D-13.** Cross-sectional anatomy of the adult human prostate. The relationship of the prostate to lateral prostatic fascias, endopelvic fascia, Denonvilliers' fascia, and the neurovascular bundle is shown (*From Walsh, 1998.*[59] © *1996 Brady Urological Institute.*)

prostate. Direct incision of this region may be effected after dorsal vein complex control is obtained. Maintenance of an optimal length of urethral sphincter (striated) muscle is important. During all portions of the apical dissection, the surgeon must be certain that the entire prostate is removed and only urethral muscle is preserved. Reestablishment of the striated urethral sphincter muscle relationship to the puboprostatic ligaments and periurethral fascias around the dorsal vein complex is important to provide normal anatomic relationship between the urethra and the pubis postoperatively.

## PREOPERATIVE PREPARATION

Surgery is often deferred for 6 to 8 weeks after needle biopsy of a prostate, and 12 weeks after transrectal resection, to allow resolution of any inflammatory reaction that may occur from these biopsies. With the newer 18-gauge needle biopsies of the prostate, periurethral and periprostatic inflammation is typically minor. Some patients will choose to have autologous blood stored preoperatively or to receive recombinant erythropoietin preoperatively to decrease their risk of receiving heterologous blood transfusion. Patients may receive a limited bowel preparation with magnesium citrate and should have an enema on the morning prior to surgery.

Many surgeons prefer a regional or a spinal anesthetic for this operation. Regional anesthesia is associated with lower blood loss and a decreased risk of deep venous thrombosis and pulmonary emboli.

Since pulmonary emboli are the most common cause of perioperative mortality, use of epidural anesthesia is supported.[61,62] The patient is placed supine on the table, which is flexed to extend the distance between the umbilicus and the pubis. Position of table flexion is initially located at the level of the umbilicus. The patient is prepped and draped with the phallus available for manipulation during the procedure. A 16- to 18-French Foley catheter is placed per urethra with 40 to 50 mL of water in the Foley catheter balloon. A standard lower abdominal midline incision is fashioned and the retroperitoneal space is opened. Direct care should be taken to open the transversalis fascia sharply, since preservation of this structure may be important to prevent postoperative hernia formation. The peritoneum is then mobilized superiorly on both sides up to the level of the iliac vessels and psoas muscle if lymph node dissection is planned.

## SURGICAL PROCEDURE

Sampling lymph node dissection is performed in the obturator space with the lateral margin of dissection being the pelvic wall and external iliac vein, the distal margin being the node of Cloquet, and the proximal margin being the hypogastric vessels. The posterior margin is the obturator nerve within the pelvis. Removal of the obturator vessels is neither helpful nor beneficial. In occasional patients, the obturator artery provides blood supply to the phallus and removal of the obturator artery may compromise penile blood flow.

A self-retaining retractor, such as the Balfour retractor, is used during the procedure. A retracting arm with a notched blade, such as the Yu-Holtgrewe blade, can then be used to retract the Foley catheter within the bladder superiorly. This provides optimal access to the prostate and its attachments to the pubis.

The endopelvic fascia is then defined by removing any fat from this structure, and an incision is fashioned sharply in the endopelvic fascia just lateral to the capsular veins of the prostate. Care should be taken during this time to incise only the fascia. This incision allows separation of the endopelvic muscles from the prostate. Small veins in this region may be controlled with electrocautery. After incision in the endopelvic fascia on both sides, the prostate can now be moved laterally to allow better access to the apex. At this point, a running suture of 0 or 2-0 chronic can be placed into the fascia overlying the prostate from the midportion of the prostate laterally on each side over its anterior surface. This allows the dorsal vein vessels to be trapped between the fascia and the prostate itself. This maneuver decreases back bleeding through the dorsal venous complex over the prostate. The fascia covering the prostate is then divided sharply, which includes division of the puboprostatic ligaments. Separation of the puboprostatic ligaments from the public symphysis is discouraged, because this prevents reestablishment of the normal urethral sphincter relationship to the pubic bone through its reattachment to the periurethral fascias. The dorsal vein complex is then entered and oversewn with 2-0 or 3-0 absorbable sutures (Fig. 17D-14). As noted above, care must be taken to avoid extending these sutures into the urethral sphincter complex, because this may limit its function postoperatively.

The striated urethral sphincter and anterior urethra are then divided just distal to the apex of the prostate (Fig. 17D-15). Removal of an excess length of urethral sphincter muscle does not improve cancer control, and can increase the risk of postoperative incontinence. Care should be taken to divide the urethral muscle around the Foley catheter. The posterior portion of the urethra is not directly visualized at this point and is not divided. The urethral sphincter sutures can then be placed for the subsequent urethrovesicle anastomosis. Viewed from the patient's head, sutures are placed at 6, 8, 10, 12, 2, and 4 o'clock. Placement of the sutures at this time is easy to effect by pushing the prostate inferiorly; sutures are placed in an inside-out fashion only for the 12 o'clock suture, and other sutures are placed in an outside-in fashion. For the anterior sutures, the urethral mucosa and a small cross-segment of urethral muscle is included in the suture as well as the anterior segment of fascia that was previously above the urethral sphincter. This allows restoration of the normal urethral angle postoperatively. After five of these six sutures have been placed, the catheter is then brought up through the incision in the urethra and retracted cephalad. The 6 o'clock suture can then be placed in the posterior urethra. A right-angle clamp is placed behind the urethra and the posterior segment of urethra is divided sharply. Attention may then be turned to the lateral prostatic fascias.

The prostate is rolled laterally without excessive traction on the urethral catheter. The lateral prostatic fascia alone is divided just above the neurovascular bundle complex at the posterolateral level of the prostate. Small vessels that come off the neurovascular bundle are identified and clipped. The prostate should then be released from the neurovascular bundle starting at the apical level (Fig. 17D-16). The Denonvilliers' fascia can then be easily identified, and a right-angle clamp is placed behind Denonvilliers' fascia and behind the posterior portion of the urethral sphincter muscle at the level of the apical prostate. Care must be taken at this point to avoid an incision into the posterior portion of the prostate. Blunt dissection on the rectum should be avoided to prevent tearing or neuropraxia to the neurovascular bundles. Although neurovascular bundles are still attached to the prostate, they are highly susceptible to traction injury. The Denonvilliers' fascia is then incised just medial to the neurovascular bundle, freeing the bundle from the prostate.

In cases where it is appropriate to unilaterally or bilaterally perform wide excision of the neurovascular bundle, the neurovascular bundle is isolated at the level at the apex of the prostate and absorbable sutures are used to tie this neurovascular bundle

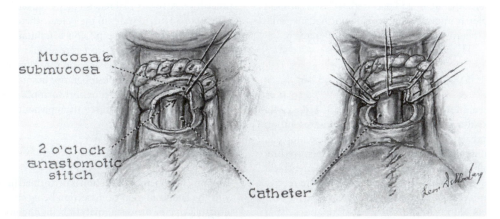

**FIGURE 17D-14.** A hemostatic running suture has been placed around the dorsal vein and anterior fascia of the prostate with care taken not to entrap the striated urethral muscle. The correct placement of urethral sutures without compression or shortening of the urethral muscle is demonstrated. (*From Walsh, 1998.*[59] © *1996 Brady Urological Institute.*)

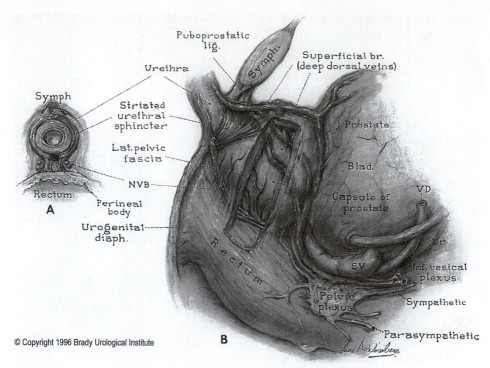

**FIGURE 17D-15.** The anatomic relationships of the urethral muscles to the neurovascular bundle is seen in the inset. A lateral view of pelvic neuroanatomy, its relationship to the fascias around the prostate, bladder, rectum and urethra are demonstrated. (*From Walsh, 1998.*[59] © *1996 Brady Urological Institute.*)

complex. A right angle should be placed completely around the neurovascular bundle with care taken to avoid entry into the rectum at this point. Incision in the lateral prostatic fascia for wide excision of the neurovascular bundle is performed posterior to the bundle itself.

After the urethral sphincter is divided posterior to Denonvilliers' fascia, the prostate may then be mobilized up to the level of the posterolateral base of the prostate near its junction with the bladder. Major vessels and branches of the inferior vesicle artery entering the prostate should be secured at this level with clips or ligatures. After the prostate is mobilized laterally, Denonvilliers' fascia is then incised over the level of the seminal vesicles. This allows dissection to be performed along the seminal vesicles up laterally over the bladder. An arterial complex is typically found just anterior to the seminal vesicle on each side, between the seminal vesicle and the bladder. This arterial complex should be specifically ligated before its division. Attention may then be turned to the anterior surface of the junction of the bladder and the prostate. The bladder is entered, with care taken to avoid entry into the prostate. The best maneuver to avoid entry into the prostate is to maintain dissection on the bladder muscle itself. Once the bladder has been widely opened, the Foley catheter balloon may be deflated and both ends of the Foley catheter used to retract the prostate inferiorly.

After intravenous infusion of indigo carmine, blue efflux from the ureteral orifices may be directly identified. This can be used to avoid incision into the ureteral orifices. The bladder muscle is then divided posteriorly, leaving the prostate specimen attached only by the seminal vesicles and vas deferens. Midline dissection is then performed to isolate the vas deferens that is separated off the seminal vesicle along its entire length. Separation of the vas from the seminal vesicle allows identification of the vessels at the superior tip of the seminal vesicles. The vas deferens and its associated vessels are clipped and divided. Attention is then turned to the seminal vesicles. Care must be taken to avoid avulsion of the seminal vesicle and its associated blood supply. Seminal vesicle blood supply is clipped and divided, and the prostate specimen can be removed. An initial review for bleeding within the pelvis should then be performed.

The bladder neck can then be narrowed in a tennis-racquet fashion. Initial sutures of 2-0 chronic are placed at the level of the ureteral orifices to reapproximate the bladder muscle. The bladder is closed along its length. An approximately 30-French opening is left at the anterior portion of the bladder neck closure. The urethral mucosa can be everted with 4-0 sutures to improve the opportunity for mucosa-to-mucosa anastomotic connection postoperatively (Fig. 17D-17). The sutures that were previously placed into the urethra can then be placed in a corresponding fashion at 12, 2, 4, 6, and 10 o'clock. These sutures are placed after a new urethral catheter has been brought out anteriorly within the pelvis. The Foley catheter is placed into the bladder prior to placement of the 12 o'clock suture, but after placement of all other sutures.

The urethrovesical anastomosis is then completed by tying each of the sutures circumferentially around the urethra; 2-0 or 3-0 Monocryl sutures are used for the anastomosis, because they tie

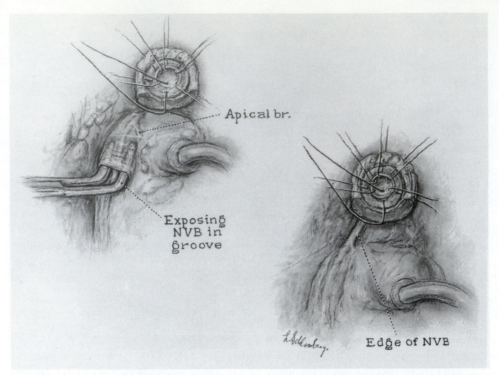

**FIGURE 17D-16.** Sutures have been placed in the urethra at 12, 2, 4, 6, 8, and 10 o'clock. Release of the lateral prostatic fascia is demonstrated in one illustration, and dissection of the prostate off of the neurovascular bundle in its groove posterolateral to the prostate is shown. (*From Walsh, 1998.*[59] © *1996 Brady Urological Institute.*)

easily, are fairly rapidly absorbed after healing of the anastomosis, and are durable. There should be no gaps in the anastomosis and the bladder should come down easily. If there is difficulty in bringing the bladder down to the urethra, the obliterated umbilical artery should be divided, the flexion should be decreased on the operating table, and the peritoneal reflection should be freed up laterally to allow the bladder to more easily reach the urethra without tension.

Pelvic drains may then be placed into the lower abdomen to collect any urethral leakage that may occur from the anastomosis perioperatively as well as lymphatic fluid. If clinically detectable hernias are present, these may be repaired at this time. Simultaneous preperitoneal repair of hernias in men who are undergoing radical prostatectomy may be effectively accomplished with polypropylene mesh with low morbidity and excellent results.[63]

## PERINEAL PROSTATECTOMY

A perineal prostatectomy is performed with the patient in the exaggerated lithotomy position. The perineum is opened, and dissection is performed anterior to the external rectal sphincter fibers. The rectourethralis muscle is divided, and Denonvilliers' fascia is left on the prostate (Fig. 17D-18). The vascular pedicles to the prostate are ligated at the prostate base. The seminal vesicles and vasa deferentia are isolated and removed, and the prostate is separated from the bladder. Anastomosis is carried out to the urethral stump after removal of the prostate.

## RESULTS AFTER PROSTATECTOMY

After radical prostatectomy patients should have an undetectable PSA level. Systemic PSA detection ($\geq$0.2 ng/mL) is indicative of recurrent local or systemic disease. The risk of biochemical recurrence is dependent on the local extent of tumor (organ confined vs. extracapsular penetration), invasion of seminal vesicles or lymph nodes, and Gleason sum score. Long-term overall results from Johns Hopkins Hospital are presented in Fig. 17D-19. Gleason sum score and extent of local disease in the prostatic specimen provide a means of estimating the risk of disease recurrence.[64]

Results for return of urinary control after prostatectomy vary greatly from surgeon to surgeon in different series. Urinary continence returns for 75% to 98% of patients postoperatively. Return of erectile function may take as much as 12 to 18 months, and achievement of erections adequate for vaginal penetration and climax occur in 40% to 80% of men in selected series, based on whether one or both neurovascular bundles are preserved, the age of the patient, preoperative erectile function, and extent of tumor.

## RADIOTHERAPY

Radiotherapy, the use of ionizing radiation to destroy cancer cells, has been proven effective in the treatment of many cancers. Its role in the treatment of prostate cancer is somewhat limited by the relative

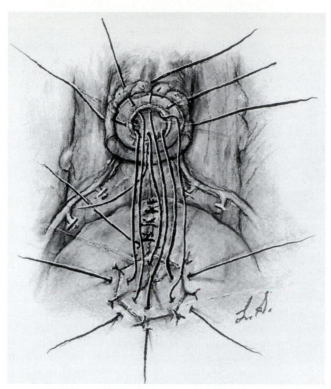

**FIGURE 17D-17.** Anastomosis of the urethra to the reconstructed bladder neck is demonstrated. Note the tennis racquet type closure of the posterior bladder, with eversion of bladder mucosa at the anterior bladder neck. (*From Walsh, 1998.*[59] © *1996 Brady Urological Institute.*)

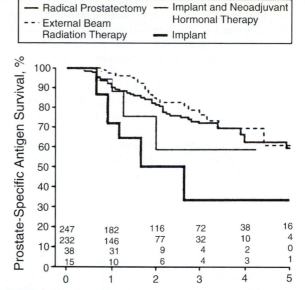

**FIGURE 17D-19.** Proportion of patients remaining biochemically free of disease by PSA criteria after radical prostatectomy (RP), external beam radiation therapy (RT), brachytherapy (implant) or neoadjuvant hormonal therapy followed by brachytherapy (neoadjuvant/implant). (*From AV D'Amico et al.*[66] *Reproduced with permission.*)

radiation insensitivity of prostate cancer.[65] Radiation can be delivered either as external-beam radiotherapy, which is usually produced using a linear accelerator, or as interstitial tissue seeds. A linear accelerator is essentially a tube into which electrons are injected and

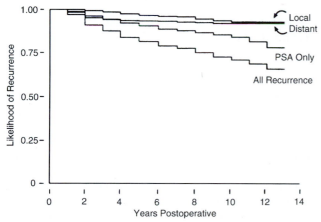

**FIGURE 17D-18.** Survival curve demonstrating the risk of recurrence after radical retropubic prostatectomy for 1,623 patients operated at Johns Hopkins Hospital (*From CR Pound et al.*[64] *Reproduced with permission.*)

allowed to accelerate on a radiofrequency carrier wave. A focused beam of radiation therapy is then forced to impact on a target, which converts this energy into x-rays or photons. The energy produced by a linear accelerator is variable and can be much higher than the energy used in the past by cobalt 60 machines. Energy levels are important in radiation therapy because higher energy levels allow deeper penetration into tissue. This is important for the treatment of tumors that are present deep within the body, such as prostate cancers.[66]

A second approach to the treatment of localized prostate cancer is the administration of permanent implants such as iodine 125 or palladium 103. Brachytherapy with iodine 125 has the potential advantage of delivering very high doses of local radiation therapy with a minimum of scatter and subsequent injury to surrounding structures such as bowel, bladder, and urethral sphincter and urethra. However, accurate placement of the implants is critical to delivery of radiation therapy. Since localized prostate cancers tend to be multifocal, treatment of the entire prostate gland is required. In addition, since most prostate cancers are peripheral in location, loading of radiation dose to the posterior part of the prostate, and therefore the rectum, is required during radiation therapy.

Combinations of external-beam radiation therapy and brachytherapy have also been applied. Both external-beam radiation as well as brachytherapy have been enhanced in their effectiveness by the use of imaging modalities such as CT scans and TRUS. Optimal contemporary external-beam radiation therapy includes planning with three-dimensional CT-guided treatment planning (three-dimensional conformal therapy). With this approach, dose enhancement is possible with a minimization of radiation energy delivered to, and therefore complications from, surrounding structures such as rectum and bladder. The importance of dose escalation is reflected by data from Zelefsky et al.[65] at Memorial Hospital in New York. These authors have demonstrated that prostate biopsies after external-beam radiation therapy are commonly positive unless a dose of 81 cGy is delivered. It should be remembered that postradiation biopsies detect only gross tumors. A negative biopsy, especially in the face of a rising PSA level, may well reflect persistent tumor in the prostate or elsewhere that has not responded to or been treated by radiation.

Rapid evolution of prostate radiation therapy techniques has occurred over the past several years. Given the very long natural history and follow-up that is required to evaluate patients with localized prostate cancer for treatment effectiveness, very few patients have been treated with contemporary radiation techniques and had adequate follow-up to evaluate its effectiveness. Perhaps the best study that has evaluated patients with clinically localized prostate cancer treated with external-beam radiation, interstitial radiotherapy, or radical prostatectomy was recently published by D'Amico.[66] In this study of 1872 men treated between January of 1989 and October of 1997, actuarial freedom from PSA failure (defined as three increases in PSA level after reaching a PSA nadir) was evaluated. Patients were categorized based on Gleason score and PSA values as being in low-risk, intermediate-risk, and high-risk groups. There was no difference in 5-year PSA-based failure rate for low-risk patients who were treated with radical prostatectomy, external radiation therapy, or brachytherapy with or without neoadjuvant deprivation. Intermediate- and high-risk patients treated with radical prostatectomy or radiation therapy did better than those treated with brachytherapy.

A second study attempted to compare the results of interstitial radiation therapy published by Ragde et al.[67] with radical prostatectomy at John's Hopkins Hospital in a comparable series of patients who were matched by PSA level and Gleason score. Patients after radical prostatectomy had a 98% likelihood of being free from biochemical progression, measured as PSA less than 0.2 ng/mL, whereas patients treated with interstitial [125]I had only a 79% chance of being disease-free.[68] Overall series comparing the effectiveness of radiation and radical prostatectomy have shown little difference in 5-year disease-free survival rates, with a 10% to 20% disease-free survival benefit to surgery at 10 years of follow-up. Many of these studies are limited by the fact that PSA evaluations postoperatively have not been used. In addition, none of these series represent randomized controlled studies comparing the two attempted treatment modalities for localized prostate cancer.

## HORMONAL THERAPY WITH RADIATION

One approach to optimizing the effectiveness of radiation therapy is to decrease the amount of tumor present using neoadjuvant hormone therapy for 3 to 6 months prior to radiation treatment. RTOG86-10, a study of patients with stage C (T3) prostate cancer involved two arms. Patients were randomized to either receive the gonadotropin releasing hormone (GnRH) agonist goserelin with flutamide, the antiandrogen, for 3 months and then radiation ther-

apy of 65 Gy versus radiation therapy alone. A 3-year interim analysis with 255 evaluated patients demonstrated significant improvement in digitally evaluated local control for the patients receiving cytoreduction (84% versus 71%) $p = 0.003$). The disease-free survival rate using PSA level over 4.0 ng/mL as evidence of disease progression was 46% versus 26% ( $p = 0.0001$), with an advantage to the group that was treated with hormonal therapy prior to radiation.[69] Unfortunately, many patients have been continuously treated with hormonal therapy after radiation, which confounds the results of PSA evaluation, because early hormonal therapy is known to delay disease progression without necessarily affecting survival.

## EVALUATION OF TREATMENT EFFECT

After radical prostatectomy, PSA levels should decrease to undetectable ($\leq 0.1$ ng/mL), as PSA production from other glands in the body such as periurethral glands is minimal, and this PSA can generally not be detected in a serum blood test. PSA is normally produced at detectable levels only by benign prostate tissue, localized prostate cancer, and prostate cancer elsewhere in the body. Therefore, with the prostate gland and localized cancer removed, a detectable PSA ($\geq 0.2$ ng/mL) represents biochemical evidence of prostate cancer recurrence, either locally or systemically. Unfortunately, it is more difficult to evaluate PSA levels after radiation therapy. First of all, radiation therapy may take 18 to 24 months to effect complete cancer cell destruction. In addition, small amounts of PSA may be produced by benign prostatic tissue after effective localized radiation. Several studies have demonstrated that clinical progression of prostate cancer after radiation occurs more commonly when patients have a nadir PSA level post treatment greater than 4.0 ng/mL or even greater than 1.0 ng/mL (ASTRO consensus panel, 1997). The lowest rates of development of clinical prostate cancer occur when patients have nadir PSA levels of less than 0.5 ng/mL with no progressive increase in PSA after radiation therapy, whether delivered by external-beam or interstitial therapy.

## TREATMENT FOR ADVANCED DISEASE AFTER ATTEMPTED LOCAL THERAPY

Patients who have been treated with curative intent for localized prostate cancer who have positive biopsies or progressively increasing serum PSA levels should be considered to have progressive prostate cancer. Since the interval from PSA detection in serum after radical prostatectomy to clinical progression with bone metastases has a median interval of 8 years, significant uncertainty may exist as to the location of disease recurrence at the time of its biochemical detection with elevated PSA level alone. The presence of a positive biopsy in the pelvis, either after surgery or radiation therapy, provides information only regarding the presence of local disease. The curative success of additional local treatment is dependent on the presence or absence of metastatic disease. Since CT scan, bone scan, and Prostascint evaluation are limited in their ability to detect microscopic metastatic disease, significant uncertainty may exist as to whether patients with prostate cancer recurrence after attempted local treatment have local or systemic disease or both.

In general, most patients with local recurrences alone will have delayed detection of PSA recurrence (greater than 3 years after prostatectomy) with a slow PSA increase (PSA doubling time of 1 year or more).[70] These patients are the most suitable candidates for additional local treatment. Patients who have initially undetectable PSA levels after radical prostatectomy with a rapid increase in PSA are far more likely to have metastatic disease.[71]

## RADIATION AFTER PROSTATECTOMY

Patients receiving postprostatectomy irradiation have not been adequately studied to have well-defined standardization for treatment delivery. Patients may be treated who have adverse prognostic factors found at the time of prostatectomy, such as gross positive surgical margins, or they may be treated at the time of PSA recurrence. Typically, patients with pathologic T3 disease who are being treated adjuvantly in the absence of pelvic node irradiation are given 60 to 64 Gy to the prostatic bed. Although early treatment may appear to have significant benefit, approximately 50% of patients with "positive surgical margins" will never have detectable PSA recurrences without adjuvant treatment.[31] These results must be compared to the 50% to 60% disease-free survival rates for patients who receive localized pelvic irradiation for adverse prognostic findings in the adjuvant setting after radical prostatectomy.[72] In distinction, patients who are treated at the time of PSA reappearance after radical prostatectomy will have an approximately 20% chance of long-term PSA-measured response to localized radiation therapy.[73] These observations may reflect that: (1) most patients who fail after radical prostatectomy have systemic disease alone, (2) radiation therapy is ineffective at managing local disease after radical prostatectomy, and (3) most patients with positive surgical margins at the time of radical prostatectomy are cured by radical prostatectomy alone. If radiation is elected as an adjuvant treatment after surgical prostatectomy, treatment should be delayed at least 5 to 8 weeks until urinary continence is achieved. An increased rate of urethral stricture formation and incontinence as well as impotence is expected when radiation is delivered after radical prostatectomy.[74]

## SALVAGE PROSTATECTOMY AFTER RADIATION

Surgical (salvage) prostatectomy for presumed localized disease is a treatment option for men who have defined localized persistence of prostate cancer after radiation therapy. In the absence of demonstrable metastatic disease, one option is to perform salvage prostatectomy. When PSA levels have been used to detect recurrence after salvage prostatectomy, actuarial nonprogression rates at 5 and 8 years were 55% and 33%, respectively.[75] Rectal injuries occur intraoperatively for approximately 15% of patients, 27% develop urethrovesical anastomtic strictures, and urinary incontinence persisted in 58%. Many patients will have advanced disease with seminal vesicle invasion, lymph node metastases, or both despite negative imaging evaluations preoperatively. Salvage prostatectomy is technically challenging and has the potential to provide excellent local control of radiopersistent cancer. If cancer is confined to the prostate or in the immediate periprostatic tissue, a high proportion of patients can be effectively treated. To consider salvage prostatectomy, patients should be in good health with a life expectancy of greater than 10 years, have a local tumor demonstrated on biopsy, and no evidence of metastatic disease. Salvage prostatectomy should be performed before the PSA level rises above 10 ng/mL. Patients should be advised of the high risk of preoperative complications prior to salvage prostatectomy.

## HORMONAL THERAPY IN THE MANAGEMENT OF PROSTATE CANCER

The traditional treatment of patients with metastatic prostate cancer has been directed against testicular androgen production since the classic work of Huggins et al.[76] Huggins and associates were the first to show that orchiectomy or treatment with diethylstilbesterol (DES) improved symptoms in patients with prostate cancer. Interestingly, although this work was honored by the Nobel Prize and hormonal treatment remains the mainstay of treatment today, there is no evidence that endocrine treatment cures prostate cancer, and the overall effect on patient survival in symptomatic patients is marginal. Undoubtedly symptoms are relieved, although at the price of impaired libido and impotence.

Endocrine treatment can be expected to result in objective and subjective responses in about 80% of patients. In patients with demonstrable metastases, the median time to clinical progression on hormonal therapy is 18 to 24 months and death is 30 to 36 months. The availability of PSA testing now allows early detection of patients who have escaped primary treatment. The response of these patients to hormonal ablation is longer than the response in symptomatic patients, due primarily to a lead-time bias of detection of metastatic disease. The optimal timing for initiation of therapy remains controversial. Some asymptomatic patients prefer nonconventional treatment including low-fat diet, vitamin E, selenium, and high soy intake prior to beginning endocrine therapy.[77,78]

## METHODS OF ENDOCRINE TREATMENT

Surgical castration remains the gold standard of endocrine therapy. It is easily performed on an outpatient basis, is well-tolerated, inexpensive, and completely eliminates testicular testosterone production. However, today there is great reluctance by patients to undergo this treatment, since there are medical alternatives that are potentially reversible. A recently published prospective study has shown that the addition of an androgen receptor blocker does not add to the efficacy of orchiectomy alone.[79] The major side effects of orchiectomy are loss of libido and potency.

DIETHYLSTILBESTEROL (DES). Although other estrogens have been utilized to inhibit testosterone, the major clinical studies have used DES. A series of Veterans' Administration studies published in the 1960s showed an unexpectedly high death rate due to cardiovascular events in patients treated with 5 mg of DES a day. Later studies showed cardiovascular side effects at a dose of 3 mg/day.[80] The effect is minimal at a dose of 1 mg/day, but this dosage does not completely suppress testosterone.[81] However, the effectiveness in preventing prostate cancer deaths appears to be similar. DES at 1 to 3 mg/day in conjunction with aspirin to avoid cardiovascular complications may be as effective as more expensive luteinizing hormone–releasing hormone (LH-RH) analogs. Further studies are warranted but not contemplated at this time.

LUTEINIZING HORMONE–RELEASING HORMONE. Schally and co-workers[82] described the structure of GnRH, which stimulates the release of follicle-stimulating hormone (FSH) and LH. Subsequently numerous LH-RH synthetic analogs, which have both agonist and antagonist activity, have been produced. Depo LH-RH agonists have now been developed that have a 1-, 3-, or 4-month duration of action after intramuscular or subcutaneous administration. The effects on testosterone are similar to castration and the side effects are the same, allowing the term *medical castration* to be applied to this treatment. One critical difference is the initial stimulation of LH and testosterone for the first 1 to 2 weeks after GnRH analog treatment.

This phenomenon has been termed the flare effect and may result in increased symptoms. An androgen receptor blocker should be co-administered during the initial month of LH-RH analog therapy and is begun prior to administration of the LH-RH drug.

ANDROGEN RECEPTOR BLOCKER. These drugs are steroidal and nonsteroidal compounds that bind to the androgen receptor in a competitive fashion. Some steroid antiandrogens have additional mechanisms of action including suppression of gonadotrophins. However, compounds commonly utilized in this country— flutamide, bicolutamide, and nilutamide—are pure "antiandrogens." Androgen receptor blockers clinically abolish the flare effect of testosterone on prostate cancer and may block the effect of adrenal analogues when administered together with an LHRH drug as complete androgen blockade.[83] To date, trials of androgen receptor blockers as monotherapy have failed to show the efficacy of medical or surgical castration.[84] The advantage is preservation of potency but at the expense of painful gynecomastia due to increases in serum testosterone with subsequent elevation of circulating estrogens.

COMPLETE ANDROGEN BLOCKADE. The concept of maximal androgen blockade was introduced by Labrie and co-workers[85] to describe the concept of complete blockade of both testicular and adrenal androgens. Subsequently, there have been numerous prospective randomized studies utilizing a variety of combinations of LH-RH analogs or orchiectomy in combination with different androgen receptor blockers. Pivotal studies by Labrie and associates[86] showed that administration of leuprolide acetate with the antiandrogen flutamide showed a significant benefit in time to progression and overall survival compared to leuprolide acetate alone. The mean time to progression and survival differed by 2.1 and

7.3 months, respectively. One criticism of this study is that the flare effect may account for the differences in progression and survival, not continued use of the antiandrogen throughout the duration of LHRH treatment. In addition, the benefit of improved survival was seen for only 3% of patients treated. This single study has led to the widespread use of total endocrine ablation in this country. However, a comprehensive review of data from 21 studies[87] and a recent additional review by Eisenberger,[88] concluded that there is no advantage of complete androgen blockade over orchiectomy or medical castration alone. The observation of clinical remission after antiandrogen withdrawal is described below under "Management of Advanced Prostate Cancer."[89]

INTERMITTENT ENDOCRINE THERAPY. The continuous use of androgen withdrawal is accompanied by loss of libido and potency, weight gain, bone demineralization, loss of muscle mass, and hot flashes. Moreover, a population of hormone-resistant cells refractory to androgen ablation inevitably arise.

The notion of intermittent hormonal ablation was offered to give a period of freedom from side effects and perhaps to prolong hormone dependency.[82] Most protocols provide treatment to reduce the PSA level below 4 ng/mL and then to withhold treatment until a predetermined PSA-level rise occurs (10 to 20 ng/mL). Reinstitution of androgen deprivation treatment is then provided.[82] Prospective studies are currently in progress, but definitive results are not yet available.

## MANAGEMENT OF ADVANCED PROSTATE CANCER

For patients who have hormone-resistant prostate cancer growth, several options, including investigational treatments, are available. Most patients who are treated with hormone-resistant prostate cancer have symptomatic disease and the goal of the treatment is palliation. This is true because there are no treatment options available with high effectiveness to cure patients in this situation. Palliative therapy may involve management of pain from bony metastases, or urinary diversion for obstructive uropathy, either from local prostate cancer growth into the bladder base obstructing the ureters or retroperitoneal lymph node enlargement from metastatic disease.

### SPINAL CORD COMPRESSION

Spinal cord compression is a serious emergency for patients with advanced metastatic prostate cancer. For patients with evidence of spinal cord compression, immediate hormonal therapy should be instituted, preferably with ketoconazole 400 mg orally every 8 hr. Immediate orchiectomy is an alternative treatment. Patients who have previously received hormonal therapy should be treated with high-dose steroids and subsequently receive neurosurgical consultation and consideration of emergent radiation therapy. Spinal cord compression may occur secondary to vertebral collapse from metastatic prostate cancer or epidural metastases. These can be effectively evaluated with MRI scans.

## PALLIATIVE RADIATION THERAPY

Patients with isolated bony metastases that are symptomatic typically present with unrelenting, continuous localized pain. They may be effectively treated with localized radiation therapy of 30 Gy in 10 divided fractions.[66] Patients should also be evaluated by an orthopedic surgeon. If a pathologic fracture has occurred in a weight-bearing region, surgical fixation is required for pain control and to allow healing. Postoperative irradiation may then be provided.

## SYSTEMIC RADIONUCLIDE THERAPY

For patients with extensive bony metastases that are symptomatic, systemic radionuclide therapy may be administered with good results. Strontium 89 is quickly taken up in the mineral matrix of bone. The proportion of strontium 89 retained is directly related to the metastatic tumor burden and varies from 20% to 80% of the administered dose. Preferential accumulation occurs in and around metastatic bone deposits, where strontium 89 releases beta energy directly to the tumor. Elimination occurs through the kidneys, so careful disposal of urine is required for 7 to 10 days after treatment. Patients who receive strontium 89 typically have myelosuppression, with platelet counts decreasing 20% to 50% starting approximately 3 weeks after treatment. Strontium 89 significantly delays the appearance of new, painful bony sites and also prolongs the time until additional radiotherapy is required, compared with patients who received control treatments.[66] Treatment may be repeated after 3 months. Buchali[90] suggested a median survival advantage of more than 8 months in patients who are treated with strontium 89. Mertens et al.[91] noted an 8-month improvement in survival for patients treated with strontium 89 and low-dose cisplatin. However, a survival advantage for strontium-treated patients has not been definitively demonstrated. Controlled trials are required to determine whether systemic radionuclide therapy provides any survival advantage over supportive care alone.

## MEDICAL MANAGEMENT OF HORMONE-REFRACTORY DISEASE

Management of hormone-refractory prostate cancer involves a difficult problem for the patient with advanced prostate cancer. Unfortunately, almost 40,000 men will die of prostate cancer per year, the second leading cause of cancer death in men in the United States. Previous trials for treatment of men with hormone-refractory prostate cancer have been limited in their ability to demonstrate benefits. One problem is that 80% to 90% of patients do not have bidimensionally measurable disease, making standard phase II criteria of tumor response difficult. Use of PSA level alone may be limited by variations in PSA levels in individual patients without therapy. The strongest evidence to support a role for PSA as a marker of response is a correlation between magnitude of PSA decline and survival.[92] For patients with greater than 50% decline in PSA levels after treatment, median survival was 21 months, versus only 8 months in those patients who had a less than a 50% decline in PSA level after treatment

($p = 0.0002$). Palliative end points may also be important for evaluating response to treatment of hormone-refractory prostate cancer, because pain and debility are significant problems for patients with this condition. Validated quality-of-life instruments have been used for men with hormone-refractory prostate cancer and can be used to follow patients after treatment.[94]

Four steps may be considered in the management of hormone-refractory prostate to decrease tumor growth. First, the maintenance of testicular androgen suppression should be confirmed. Castrate levels of testosterone should be reliably less than 50 ng/mL. Unfortunately, many patients who are on long-term GnRH-agonist therapy may have "acute on chronic" effects of GnRH agonist, leading to subtle biochemical flare of testosterone and PSA levels with recurrent treatment. If symptomatic disease is demonstrated in patients, or biochemical evidence of disease progression occurs related to repeat GnRH-depot treatments, then steps should be taken such as orchiectomy or shortening the interval of depot injections to confirm adequate androgen suppression.

Secondly, antiandrogen therapy should be discontinued if it is in place. Antiandrogen withdrawal may result in clinical and PSA responses in up to 21% of men previously treated with the antiandrogens flutamide, bicalutamide, and megesterol acetate.[95] The phenomenon occurs within days of stopping flutamide, but may take up to 6 weeks after cessation of treatment with bicalutamide. The apparent agonist activity of flutamide has been suggested to occur as an activation of certain mutant androgen receptors present in prostate cancer cells.[96,97] Thirdly, second-line hormonal therapy should be considered. For patients who have not previously received antiandrogens, antiandrogen therapy may be provided. Androgen-independent prostate cancer may respond to 150 to 200 mg of bicalutamide per day for about 25% of patients, after previously receiving flutamide therapy. Megesterol acetate has progestational activity that results in objective response rates of 0% to 9% and significant PSA declines in 12% to 14% of patients. Side effects may include thrombophlebitis and fluid retention.

Adrenal androgen synthesis inhibitors such as aminoglutethamide or ketoconazole may also be used in patients with a low, partial response rate. Patients who are maintained on ketoconazole or aminoglutethamide should also receive hydrocortisone to prevent symptomatic systemic adrenal insufficiency. Estrogens and antiestrogens have also been applied to patients with hormone-refractory prostate cancer. Up to three-quarters of patients treated with high-dose estrogen had effective pain relief, and approximately one-third had PSA level declines of greater than 50%. This may be related to a direct mitotic arrest or cytotoxic effects on prostate cancer cells.[97]

An additional step is to consider chemotherapy for patients with hormone-refractory prostate cancer. Unfortunately, even recent chemotherapy trials in hormone-refractory prostate cancer have not resulted in dramatic measurable responses for most patients. However, subjective responses can be seen. Apparently active agents include estramustine, cyclophosphamide, etoposide, platinum, paclitaxel or adriamycin or vinblastine. The results of recent trials are summarized in Table 17D-10.[97] Adjunctive therapies with the use of systemic radiation have been previously discussed. In addition, investigational targets for therapy include growth-factor inhibitors, differentiation agents, cdk inhibitors, activators of apoptosis,

**TABLE 17D-10.** RECENT CHEMOTHERAPY TRIALS IN HORMONE REFRACTORY PROSTATE CANCER

| REFERENCES | THERAPY | NO. OF PATIENTS | % PSA DECLINE GREATER THAN 50% (95% CI) | % MEASURABLE RESPONSE (95% CI) | SUBJECTIVE RESPONSE |
|---|---|---|---|---|---|
| Tannock et al | Mitoxantrone + steroids | 80 | 33 (21–47) | Not reported | Yes |
| Kantoff et al | | 119 | 33 (24–42) | Not reported | Yes |
| Amato et al | Estramustine + vinblastine | 22 | 50 (28–72) | 14 (0–58) | Yes |
| Seidman et al | | 25 | 54 (31–72) | 43 (10–82) | Yes |
| Hudes et al | | 36 | 31 (16–48) | 40 (5–85) | Yes |
| Hudes et al | Estramustine + paclitaxel | 23 | 65 (43–84) | 57 (18–90) | Not reported |
| Petrylak et al | Estramustine + docetaxel | 21 | 62 (38–81) | 43 (10–82) | Yes |
| Pienta et al | Estramustine + | 42 | 52 (36–68) | 50 (26–74) | Not reported |
| Raghavan et al | Oral cyclophosphamide | 50 | 30 (12–54) | 20 (8–39) | Yes |
| Maulard-Durdux et al | Oral cyclophosphamide + oral etoposide | 20 | 35 (15–59) | Not reported | Yes |
| Frank et al | Estramustine + etoposide + platinum | 18 | Not reported | 61 (36–83) | Not reported |
| Smith et al | Estramustine + etoposide + paclitaxel | 23 | 53 (31–73) | 40 (5–85) | Not reported |
| Sella et al | Adriamycin + ketoconazole | 39 | 55 (38–71) | 58 (28–85) | Not reported |
| Ellerhorst et al | Adiamycin + ketoconazole/vinblastine-estramustine | 46 | 67 (52–80) | 75 (47–92) | Yes |

antiangiogenesis agents, monoclonal antibodies directed against tumor epitopes and immunotherapy including vaccines.[97]

## SUMMARY

The challenge of the future for treatment of prostate cancer will involve development and application of effective treatments for systemic disease. It is fortunate that prostate cancer is so hormonally sensitive in its growth pattern, because this allows effective palliation for advanced disease. Chemotherapy currently offers palliative benefits to a small subset of patients; however, multidrug combinations may offer some potential for curative treatment in the future. Despite the promise of local therapies in decreasing the death rate from prostate cancer, management of advanced hormone-refractory prostate cancer will remain an important issue for treatment of patients with this genitourinary disease.

## REFERENCES

1. LANDIS SH et al: Cancer statistics, 1998. CA Cancer J Clin 48:6, 1998.
2. STEPHENSON RA et al: The fall in incidence of prostate carcinoma. On the down side of a prostate specific antigen induced peak in incidence—Data from the Utah Cancer Registry. Cancer 77: 1342, 1996.
3. SCARDINO PT et al: Early detection of prostate cancer. Hum Pathol 23:211, 1992.
4. WINGO PA et al: Cancer statistics, 1995. CA Cancer J Clin 45:8, 1995.
5. PIENTA KJ, ESPER PE: Risk factors for prostate cancer. Ann Intern Med 118:793, 1993.
6. SHIMIZU H et al: Cancers of the prostate and breast among Japanese and white immigrants in Los Angels County. Br J cancer 63:963, 1991.
7. MEBANE C et al: Current status of prostate cancer in North American black males. J Natl Med Assoc 82:782, 1990.
8. DENMARK-WAHNEFRIED W et al: Knowledge, beliefs, and prior screening behavior among blacks and whites reporting for prostate cancer screening. Urology 46:346, 1995.
9. BAQUET CR et al: Socioeconomic factors and cancer incidence among blacks and whites. J Natl Cancer Inst 83:551, 1991.
10. WHITTEMORE AS et al: Prostate cancer in relation to diet, physical activity, and body size in blacks, whites, and Asians in the United States and Canada. J Natl Cancer Inst 87:652, 1995.
11. ROSS RK et al: Serum testosterone levels in healthy young black and white men. J Natl Cancer Inst 76:45, 1986.
12. MORTON RA: Racial differences in adenocarcinoma of the prostate in North American Men. Urology 44:637, 1994.
13. CARTER BS et al: Mendelian inheritance of familial prostate cancer. Proc Natl Acad Sci USA 89:3367, 1992.
14. CARTER BS et al: Hereditary prostate cancer: epidemiologic and clinical features. J Urol 150:797, 1993.
15. FORD D et al: Risks of cancer in BRCA-1 mutation carriers. Lancet 343:692, 1994.
16. WANG Y et al: Decreased growth of established human LnCaP tumors in nude mice fed a low fat diet. J Natl Cancer Inst 87:1456, 1995.
17. GIOVANNUCCI E et al: A prospective study of dietary fat and risk of prostate cancer. J Natl Cancer Inst 85:1571, 1993.
18. GANN PH et al: Prospective study of plasma fatty acids and risk of prostate cancer. J Natl Cancer Inst 86:281, 1994.
19. GIOVANNUCCI E et al: Intake of carotenoids and retinol in relation to risk of prostate cancer. J Natl Cancer Inst 87:1767, 1995.
20. WANG X et al: The in vitro effect of vitamin D3 analogue EB-1089 on a human prostate cancer cell line (PC-3). Br J Urol 80:260, 1997.
21. TAYLOR JA et al: Association of prostate cancer with vitamin D receptor gene polymorphism. Cancer Res 56:4108, 1996.
22. GANN PH et al: Circulating vitamin D metabolites in relation to subsequent development of prostate cancer. Cancer Epidemiol Biomarkers Prev (United States) 5:121, 1996.

23. KIBEL AS et al: Vitamin D receptor polymorphisms and lethal prostate cancer. J Urol 160:1405, 1998.

24. ROSS RK et al: 5-alpha-reductase activity and risk of prostate cancer among Japanese and US white and black males. Lancet 339:887, 1992.

25. GIOVANNUCCI E et al: A retrospective cohort study of vasectomy and prostate cancer in US men. *JAMA* 269:878, 1993.

26. DERSIMONIAN R et al: Vasectomy and prostate cancer risk: Methodological review of the evidence. J Clin Epidemiol 46:163, 1993.

27. JOHN EM et al: Vasectomy and prostate cancer: results from a multiethnic case-control study. J Natl Cancer Inst 87:662, 1995.

28. WALSH PC, PARTIN AW: Treatment of early stage prostate cancer: Radical prostatectomy, in *Important Advances in Oncology,* De Vita VT Jr et al (eds). Philadelphia, J B Lippincott, 1994, pp 211–223.

29. KEETCH D et al: Morphometric analysis and clinical follow up of isolated prostatic intraepithelial neoplasia in needle biopsy of the prostate. J Urol 154:347, 1995.

30. EPSTEIN JI: Pathologic evaluation of prostatic c carcinoma: Critical information for the oncologist. Oncology 10:527, 1996.

31. EPSTEIN JI et al: Prediction of progression following radical prostatectomy. A multivariate analysis of 721 men with long tern follow-up. Am J Surg Pathol 20:286, 1996.

32. EPSTEIN JI, LIEBERMAN P: Mucinous adenocarcinomas of the prostate gland. Am J Surg Pathol 9:299, 1985.

33. EPSTEIN JI, LIEBERMAN P, WOODRUFF J: Prostatic carcinomas with endometroid features: A light microscopic and immunohisto-chemical study of ten cases. Cancer 57:111, 1986.

34. RANDOLPH TL et al: Histologic variants of adenocarcimona and other carcinomas of prostate: Pathologic criteria and clinical significance. Mod Pathol 10:612, 1997.

35. JEWETT HJ: Significance of the palpable prostatic nodule. JAMA 160:8, 1956.

36. BRAWER MK et al: Screening for prostate carcinoma with PSA. J Urol 147:841, 1992.

37. GUTMAN AB, GUTMAN EB: Acid phosphatase occurring in serum of patients with metastasizing prostate gland. J Clin Invest 17:473, 1938.

38. COONER WH et al: Prostate cancer detection in a clinical urologic practice with ultra sonography, digital rectal examination and prostate specific antigen. J Urol 143:11, 1990.

39. CARTER HB et al: Longitudinal evaluation of prostate specific antigen levels in men with and without prostate disease. JAMA 267:2215, 1992.

40. TIBBLIN G et al: The value of prostatic specific antigen in early diagnosis of prostate cancer: The study of men born in 1913. J Urol 154:1386, 1995.

41. BENSON MC et al: Prostatic specific antigen density; a means of distinguishing benign prostatic hypertrophy from prostate cancer. J Urol 147:815, 1992.

42. OSTERLING JE et al: Serum prostatic specific antigen in a community based population of healthy men: Establishment of age specific reference ranges. JAMA 150:110, 1993.

43. CATALONA WJ et al: Evaluation of percentage of free serum prostatic specific antigen to improve specificity of prostate cancer screening. JAMA 274:1214, 1995.

44. KATZ AE et al: Molecular staging of prostate cancer with the use of enhanced reversed transcriptase-PCR assay. Urology 43:765, 1994.

45. UZZO RG et al: The influence of prostate size on cancer detection. Urology 46:831, 1995.

46. STAMEY TA et al: Large, organ confined, impalpable transition zone cancer: Association with metastatic levels of prostatic specific antigen. J Urol 149:510, 1993.

47. PARTIN AW et al: The use of prostatic specific antigen, clinical stage and Gleason score to predict pathological stage in patients with localized prostate cancer. J Urol 150:110, 1993.

48. GARDNER TA et al: Microfocal prostate cancer: Biopsy cancer volume does not predict actual tumor volume. Br J Urol 81:839, 1998.

48A. WARNER J, WHITMORE WF JR: Expectant management of clinically localized prostatic cancer. J Urol 152(2):1761, 1994.

49. JOHANSSON JE et al: High 10 year survival rate in patients with early, untreated prostatic cancer. JAMA 267:2191, 1992.

49A. AUS G: Prostate cancer. Mortality and morbidity after non-curative treatment with aspects on diagnosis and treatment. Scand J Urol Nephrol Suppl 167:1, 1994.

50. ALBERTSON PC et al: Long term survival among men with conservatively treated localized prostate cancer. JAMA 274, 1995.

51. ADOLFSSON J et al: Recent results of management of palpable clinically localized prostate cancer. Cancer 72:310, 1993.

52. CHODAK GW et al: Results of conservative management of clinically localized prostate cancer. N Engl J Med 330:242, 1994.

53. FLEMING C et al: A decision analysis of alternative treatment strategies for clinically localized prostate cancer. JAMA 269:2650, 1993.

54. BECK JR et al: A critique of the decision analysis for clinically localized prostate cancer. J Urol 152:1894, 1994.

55. FUKS Z et al: The effect of local control of metastatic dissemination in carcinoma of the prostate: Long-term results in patients treated with iodine implantation. Int J Radiat Oncol Biol Phys 21:537, 1991.

56. LABRIE F et al: Diagnosis of advanced or noncurable prostate cancer can be practically eliminated by prostate specific antigen. Urology 47:212, 1996.

56A. BRAWLEY OW, FIGUEROA-VALLES N: Prostate cancer research and the National Cancer Institute. Semin Urol Oncol 16(4):235, 1998.

56B. MILLIN T: Retropubic urinary surgery. London, Livingstone, 1947.

57. REINER WG, WALSH PC: An anatomical approach to the surgical management of the dorsal vein and Santorini's plexus during radical retropublic surgery. J Urol 121:198, 1979.

58. WALSH PC et al: Radical prostatectomy with preservation of sexual function: anatomical and pathological considerations. Prostate 4:473, 1983.

59. WALSH PC: Radical retropubic prostatectomy, in *Campbell's Urology,* Walsh PC et al (eds). Philadelphia, WB Saunders, 1998.

60. SCHLEGEL PN, WALSH PC: Neuroanatomical approach to radical cystoprostatectomy with preservation of sexual function. J Urol 138:1402, 1987.

61. PETERS C, WALSH PC: Blood transfusion and anesthetic practices in radical retropubic prostatectomy. J Urol 434:81, 1985.

62. MAHOLTRA V et al: Comparison of epidural anesthesia, general anesthesia and combined epidural general anesthesia for radical prostatectomy. [Abstract.] Presented at the Annual Meeting of American Society of Anesthesiologists, Oct. 17, 1994.

63. CHOI BB et al: Preperitoneal prosthetic mesh hernioplasty during radical retropubic prostatectomy. J Urol 161:840, 1999.

64. POUND CR et al: Prostate specific antigen after anatomic radical retropubic prostatectomy. Urol Clin North Am 24:395, 1997.

65. ZELFESKY MJ, WHITMORE WF JR: Long-term results of retropubic permanent Iodine implantation of prostate for clinically localized prostatic cancer. J Urol 158:23, 1997.

66. D'AMICO AV et al: Biochemical outcome after radical prostatectomy, external beam radiation therapy, or interstitial radiation therapy for clinically localized prostate cancer. JAMA 280:969, 1998.

67. RAGDE H et al: Interstitial iodine 125 without adjuvant therapy in the treatment of clinically localized prostate carcinoma. Cancer 80:442, 1997.

68. POLASCIK TJ et al: Comparison of radical prostatectomy and Iodine 125 interstitial radiotherapy for the treatment of clinically localized prostate cancer: A 7 year biochemical (PSA) progression analysis. Urology 51:88, 1998.

69. PORTER AT, FORMAN JD: Prostate brachytherapy. An overview. Cancer 71(Suppl):953, 1993.

70. POUND CR et al: Natural history of progression after PSA elevation following radical prostatectomy. JAMA 281:1591, 1999.

71. PATEL A et al: Recurrence patterns after radical retropubic prostatectomy: Clinical usefulness of prostate specific antigen doubling times and log slope prostate specific antigen doubling times and long slope prostate specific antigen. J Urol 158:1441, 1997.

72. SCHILD SE et al: The use of radiotherapy for patients with isolated elevation of serum prostate specific antigen following radical prostatectomy. J Urol 156:1725, 1996.

73. CADEDDU JA et al: Long term results of radiation therapy for prostate cancer recurrence following radical prostatectomy. J Urol 159:173, 1998.

74. PETROVICH Z et al: Radiotherapy following radical prostatectomy in patients with adenocarcinoma of the prostate. Int J Radiat Oncol Biol Phys 21:940, 1991.

75. ROGERS E et al: Salvage radical prostatectomy: Outcome measured by serum prostate specific antigen levels. J Urol 153:104, 1995.

76. HUGGINS C et al: Studies on prostate cancer: The effect of castration on advanced carcinoma of the prostate gland. Arch Surg 49:209, 1941.

77. NELSON MA et al: Selenium and prostate cancer prevention. Semin Urol Oncol 17:91, 1999.

78. MOYAD M: Soy, disease prevention and prostate cancer. Semin Urol Oncol 17:97, 1999.

79. EISENBERGER MA et al: Bilateral orchiectomy with or without flutamide for metastatic prostate cancer. N Engl J Med 339:1936, 1998.

80. DE VOUGHT HJ et al: Members of the all EORTC_GU: Cardiovascular side effects of diethylstilbesterol, cyproterones, acetate, mederoxyprogesterone, acetate and estramustin, phosphate used for the treatment of advanced prostate cancer: Results from European organization for research on treatment of cancer trials. J Urol 135:30761, 1986.

81. KENT JR et al: Estrogen dosage and suppression of testosterone levels in patients with prostate carcinoma. J Urol 109:858, 1973.

82. SCHALLY EV et al: Isolation and properties of the FSH and LH-Releasing hormone. Bioch

83. LABRIE F et al: New approaches in the treatment of prostate cancer: Complete instead of partial withdrawl of androgens. Prostate 4:579, 1983.

84. KAISAY Y et al: Comparison to LH-RH analog (Zoladex) with orchiectomy in patients with metastatic prostate carcinoma. Br J Urol 67:502, 1971.

85. LABRIE F et al: Diagnosis of advanced or noncurable prostate cancer can be practically eliminated by prostate specific antigen. Urology 47:212, 1996.

86. LABRIE F et al: The controlled trial of Leuprolide with and without flutamide in prostate cancer. N Engl J Med 321, 1989.

87. DALESIO O et al: Maximum androgen ablation in advanced prostate cancer: An overview of 22 randomized trials with 3,289 deaths in 5,710 patients. Lancet 46:346, 1995.

88. EISENBERGER, 1999 AUA update in press.

89. SCHER HI, KELLY WK: The flutamide withdrawal syndrome: Its impact on clinical trials and hormonal refractory prostate cancer. J Clin Oncol 11:66, 1993.

90. BUCHALI K et al: Results of a double blind study of 89-strontium therapy of skeletal metastases of prostatic carcinoma. Eur J Nucl Med 14:349, 1988.

91. MERTENS WC et al: Strontium-89 and low dose infusion cisplatin for patients with hormone refractory prostate carcinoma metastatic to bone: A preliminary report. J Nucl Med 33:1437, 1992.

92. KELLY WK et al: Prostate specific antigen as a measure of disease outcome in metastatic hormone refractory prostate cancer. J Clin Oncol 11:607, 1993.

93. KELLY WK, SCHER HI: Prostate specific antigen decline after antiandrogen withdrawal: The flutamide withdrawal syndrome. J Urol 149:607, 1993.

94. FENTON MA et al: Functional characterization of mutant androgen receptors from androgen independent prostate cancer. Clin Cancer Res 3:1383, 1997.

95. CULIG Z et al: Androgen receptor gene mutations in prostate cancer. Implications for disease progression and therapy. Drugs Aging 10:50, 1997.

96. ROBERTSON CN et al: Induction of apoptosis by diethylstilbestrol in hormone insensitive prostate cancer cells. J Natl Cancer Inst 88:908, 1996.

97. OH WK, KANTOFF PW: Management of hormone refractory prostate cancer: Current standards and future prospects. J Urol 160:1220, 1998.

# 17E / CANCER OF THE TESTIS

*Steve W. Waxman and E. David Crawford*

## INTRODUCTION

Testicular carcinoma accounts for only 1% of all cancer in males; however, it is the most common solid tumor malignancy in men between the ages of 15 and 35. Approximately 2 to 3 new patients per 100,000 males is reported in the United States each year. This accounts for approximately 6500 new patients with testicular carcinoma diagnosed each year in the United States.[1] In the 1960s, survival rates for testicular cancer were poor (in the 65% range); however, with advances in surgical treatment and chemotherapy, overall cure rates now are greater than 95%. All phases of testicular carcinoma management have improved. These advances include more sensitive diagnostic equipment, reliable tumor markers, a thorough understanding of the surgical anatomy from both a cancer and fertility standpoint, and finally more effective and safer chemotherapeutic regimens. It is this multimodality approach that has made testicular cancer one of the most curable malignancies and serves as a model for the treatment of other solid tumors.

## ETIOLOGY

Greater than 90% of all primary testicular cancer has a germ cell origin (seminoma and nonseminoma). Non–germ cell tumors (gonadoblastoma, Sertoli cell, Leydig cell) are rare and will not be covered in this chapter. Germ cell tumors of the testes are the most common solid tumor malignancy in men ages 20 through 34. This also corresponds to the maximum sexual activity period in males, giving rise to hypotheses that these tumors may be at least in part hormonally dependent. There is also some evidence to support germinal epithelium damage as a risk factor for the development of testicular germ cell tumors by the observation of poor semen quality in patients at the time of diagnosis. Another theory regarding hormonal environment in the development of testicular carcinoma is the finding of elevated gonadotroping levels [particularly follicle-stimulating hormone (FSH)] in a large percentage of these patients.

Cryptorchidism has the strongest association with the development of testicular carcinoma. The risk of cancer developing in cryptorchid testes has been estimated to be 48 per 100,000 (a 22-fold increased risk over that of the general population).[2] Intraabdominal testes have a sixfold higher incidence of testicular carcinoma when compared to other cryptorchid locations. The incidence of testicular cancer is higher on the right side, which parallels the increased incidence of right-sided cryptorchidism. Orchidopexy facilitates the examination of the testis; however, whether it alters its malignant potential remains controversial.

Exogenous estrogen during pregnancy has also been implicated as a possible risk factor for testicular cancer, with an increased incidence of 2% to 5% over that of the general population. Other factors such as viral infection, mumps, trauma, and atrophy have all been studied as possible risk factors for development of germ cell tumors; however, a direct causal relationship is not established at this time.

## CLINICAL MANIFESTATIONS

The majority of patients present with a nodule in or painless enlargement of one testicle. Sometimes the patient may only complain of heaviness or fullness in the scrotum. Other presentations include acute pain in the scrotum, either spontaneous or following minor trauma. Rarely, a patient may notice growth in a previously atrophic testis. The enlargement is usually gradual and delays in seeking medical attention are not uncommon. Delays in diagnosis may occur due to patient unawareness, reluctance, or fear to seek medical attention. Misdiagnosis may also hamper prompt evaluation and treatment of testicular neoplasms. Patients treated with antibiotics for suspected epididymitis or epididymoorchitis must be reexamined after several weeks to assess improvement. If the testis is not better or if more enlarged, then further evaluation (i.e., scrotal ultrasound) is indicated.[3] Although up to half of patients may have evidence of metastatic disease at the time of diagnosis, only 10% present with signs and symptoms related to metastatic disease. This may present as an enlarged supraclavicular lymph node or systemic complaints such as respiratory (cough or dyspnea), gastrointestinal (vomiting or hemoptysis), central nervous system symptoms (CNS metastasis), lower-extremity swelling (iliac or vena caval obstruction), flank or back pain (bulky retroperitoneal disease). Gynecomastia may be seen in approximately 5% of patients due to either excessive estrogen secretion or deficient androgen production associated with the testicular germ cell tumor.

## DIAGNOSIS

A thorough history and physical are crucial in the diagnosis and treatment of testicular cancer. As stated before, there is often a significant delay (3 to 6 months) between the first onset of signs and symptoms and the patient seeking medical care. Added to this is the fact that an incorrect diagnosis is made at the time of initial examination by the physician in up to 25% of patients. These facts, combined with the rapid doubling time of testicular neoplasms, accounts for the finding of metastatic disease in up to 50% of patients at the time of diagnosis. Many investigators have looked at the prognostic implications of rapid doubling time as evidenced by cellular proliferation markers. Some embryonal cell carinomas may have doubling times as rapid as 3 days.[4] Patient education and instruction in self-examination are crucial to promoting earlier detection and treatment in this disease.

Patients who have undergone orchidopexy for undescended testes should be especially careful to perform monthly testicular self-examination because they are at siginificantly increased risk of developing testicular cancer. Other diagnoses that are frequently mistaken for an early testicular neoplasm include epididymitis, epididymoorchitis, hydrocele, spermatocele, and epidermoid cysts.

Scrotal evaluation begins with a thorough examination of the contralateral testis to evaluate the size, shape, consistency, and associated paratesticular structures. The testis is carefully palpated between the thumb and first two fingertips. Upon examining the suspect testicle, any firm nodular or fixed areas within the substance of the testis or tunica albuginea should be considered a germ cell tumor until proven otherwise. If a hydrocele is present, a thorough examination may be compromised. Hydroceles and spermatoceles easily transilluminate, and this may be helpful in defining solid versus fluid-filled masses. If a mass is felt to be truly involving the testicular parenchyma, then the patient should undergo inguinal exploration with biopsy and/or orchiectomy. Scrotal ultrasound has proved to be very helpful in distinguishing solid versus cystic and testicular versus paratesticular masses. It is more than 90% sensitive and specific in the diagnosis of a solid testicular mass.[5] Scrotal ultrasounds are noninvasive and inexpensive, and one should not hesitate to use them if scrotal examination is suboptimal secondary to either a large hydrocele or if there is any suspicion as to the possibility of a testicular parenchymal lesion. MRI scanning, while providing excellent images of the testicle parenchyma, is expensive and not necessary in the diagnosis of testicular tumors.

## PREOPERATIVE EVALUATION

Although most patients are relatively young and healthy, preoperative testing prior to inguinal exploration with possible biopsy or orchiectomy is related mainly to the possibility that the patient may have a testicular neoplasm. The biochemical markers α-fetoprotein (AFP), human chorionic gonadotropin—beta subunit (β-HCG), and lactate dehydrogenase (LDH) are all clinically useful in the diagnosis, staging, and monitoring of treatment response in testicular germ cell tumors. Therefore, patients suspected of having a testicular tumor must have these markers drawn prior to inguinal exploration on the possibility that there may be a germ cell tumor. AFP is a glycoprotein with a half-life of 4 to 6 days, and it is detected usually only in trace amounts in adults. AFP is not seen in pure seminoma or choriocarcinoma. Embryonal cell carcinoma and yolk sac tumors both produce AFP, causing elevated levels in the serum. β-HCG is a

glycoprotein with a half-life of 24 hr. Its level is found to be elevated in all patients with choriocarcinoma as well as half of those with embryonal cell carcinoma. It is also interesting to note that up to 25% of patients with pure seminoma may have elevated levels of β-HCG.

LDH is not specific for any histologic type of testicular cancer; however, its degree of elevation in the serum does correlate with the bulk of disease. It is crucial to obtain these serum markers prior to orchiectomy because the monitoring of postorchiectomy marker levels will be aided by knowing preoperative levels. If AFP and β-HCG levels decline with the appropriate kinetics after orchiectomy, this may be indicative of disease confined to the testis. It is possible, however, to have levels of tumor markers that were preoperatively elevated fall to zero and still have residual disease. It is also important to realize that many seminomas and some nonseminomas may not have any elevation in these tumor marker levels prior to orchiectomy. Prior to inguinal exploration and possible biopsy or orchiectomy, patients may also need a chest x-ray if they have any symptoms or physical findings of pulmonary disease possibly related to metastases.

## RADICAL INGUINAL ORCHIECTOMY

Percutaneous biopsy, scrotal exploration, and/or biopsy can all potentially change the normal metastatic pathway of testicular tumors, and therefore should never be performed in any patient suspected of having a testicular tumor. In patients who have undergone scrotal exploration with the unexpected finding of a testicular germ cell tumor, scrotal or inguinal lymphatic cancer recurrence is seen in as many as 24% of patients. Overall survival rates in these patients, however, has not been shown to suffer due to effective and aggressive adjuvant treatment.[6] Once a patient is suspected of having a parenchymal tumor, he should undergo an inguinal exploration with possible testicular biopsy and/or orchiectomy.

### TECHNIQUE

The patient is prepped and draped in a supine position. The abdomen and groin, including the entire scrotum, are prepped into the field. A curvilinear inguinal incision is then performed along the skin lines and the incision carried down through the subcutaneous tissues. The aponeurosis of the external oblique muscle is then incised down through the external inguinal ring.

The ilioinguinal nerve is identified and preserved. The entire spermatic cord structures are then isolated at the level of the public tubercle. A noncrushing clamp can then be placed across the spermatic cord at this time or the spermatic cord can be compressed with a Penrose drain utilizing a Potts tie so as to isolate the vascular and lymphatic drainage from the involved testicle.

The testicle is then manipulated from the scrotum into the operative field using the Penrose drain for traction on the cord. Care is taken not to violate the fascial tunic covering the testicle. The gubernaculum is divided between clamps and ligated. After the testicle has been freed from the scrotum, it is brought up into the operative field. The testicle and spermatic cord are draped and isolated from the surrounding operative field. At this point, the testicle is examined thoroughly while still attached to its tunics. If the mass is felt to be truly within the substance of the testicle, then the inguinal orchiectomy should be performed. If the mass is felt to possibly be outside of the tunica albuginea, then a biopsy may be indicated.

If one is to perform a biopsy, the tunica vaginalis is incised, care being taken to wall off the field around the testicle and spermatic cord with extra towels and laparotomy pads to prevent any possible tumor spillage. Once the tunica vaginalis is incised, the testicle and epididymis are inspected. If the diagnosis is in doubt, one may perform wedge biopsy and frozen-section analysis on the testis.

If the mass is benign, then the tunica albuginea can be closed with an absorbable suture and the testis returned to the scrotum. As stated before, upon delivery of the testicle into the inguinal incision, if a mass is felt to be within the body of the testicle, one should proceed ahead with inguinal orchiectomy.

To complete the orchiectomy, the spermatic cord structures should be ligated at the level of the internal inguinal ring. The vas deferens should be ligated separately with nonabsorbable sutures. The remainder of the spermatic cord should be ligated with large, permanent sutures so as to allow easy identification of the spermatic cord stump at the time of retroperitoneal lymph node dissection (RPLND). The incision and hemiscrotum are then thoroughly irrigated. The scrotal skin is invaginated up so that the inside of the scrotum can be inspected for hemostasis. If a large defect is seen at the level of the internal inguinal ring, this can be closed with sutures. The aponeurosis of the external oblique is then closed with a 2-0 polyglycolic acid (PGA) suture. Scarpa's fascia is closed with 3-0 chromic suture. The skin is closed with a 4-0 PGA subcuticular suture or skin clips. Complications of inguinal exploration and radical inguinal orchiectomy are uncommon and similar to that of inguinal herniorrhaphy. The principal complication, hemorrhage and/or hematoma, can be minimized by careful attention to hemostasis in the dissection of the testicle from the hemiscrotum.

The procedure is easily performed on an outpatient basis using a general, regional, or even local anesthetic. Inguinal exploration with radical inguinal orchiectomy provides not only the histologic diagnosis, but also the definitive treatment in patients whose testicular cancer is confined to the gonad (Figs. 17E-1 and 17E-2).

## HISTOLOGY

Of all testicular tumors, 90% to 95% are of germ cell origin. Testicular germ cell tumors are divided into seminoma and nonseminoma types. Seminoma is the most common germ cell type, found in 35% to 70% of testicular neoplasms. Although classically divided into typical, anaplastic, and spermatocytic, prognostic differences between typical and anaplastic are debatable. The spermatocytic subtype is usually associated with an older age and is unlikely to metastasize. The seminomas as a group are most often found in the fourth and fifth decades of life. Pure seminoma may be associated with an elevated β-HCG level in up to 30% of patients. AFP level, however, is never elevated in cases of pure seminoma, and an elevation in the level of this marker in cases where only seminoma is found in the orchiectomy specimen should prompt further reevaluation by the pathologist. Nonseminomas are composed of embryonal cell carcinoma, yolk sac carcinoma, choriocarcinoma, and teratoma. Multiple cell types are found in up to 25% of nonseminomas.

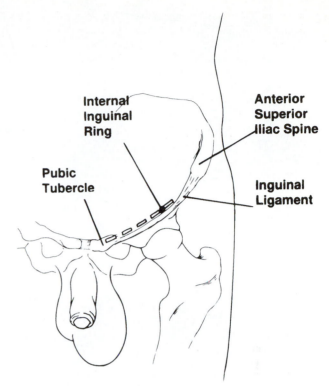

**FIGURE 17E-1.** Anatomic landmarks and proposed incision for radical inguinal orchiectomy. (*From Crawford ED, Das S (eds): Current Genitourinary Surgery, 2d ed. Baltimore, Williams & Wilkins, 1997, Fig. 35-2, p 455.*)

Germ cell tumors that are composed of both seminomatous and nonseminomatous elements are considered nonseminomas and are treated accordingly, as will be discussed later in this chapter. The most common combination of nonseminomatous elements is that of embryonal cell carcinoma and teratoma. This combination of cell types is designated teratocarcinoma. Elevations in β-HCG levels are seen in 40% to 60% of nonseminomas. In nonseminomas containing embryonal cell or yolk sac elements, the AFP level will be elevated in up to 70% of patients.

## STAGING

Clinical staging begins once an intratesticular lesion is suspected as serum is drawn for tumor markers and a radical orchiectomy performed. Pathologic analysis of the specimen then establishes the cell type (seminoma, nonseminoma, etc.). Repeat serum samples are then drawn to evaluate the rate of decay in these markers as compared with their half-lives. The pathologic evaluation of the orchiectomy specimen should not only provide the histologic cell type or types if more than one is present, but also the relative percentage in cases of nonseminoma. Also, the presence of vascular or lymphatic invasion should be noted, along with any involvement of the spermatic cord, epididymis, or cord margin.

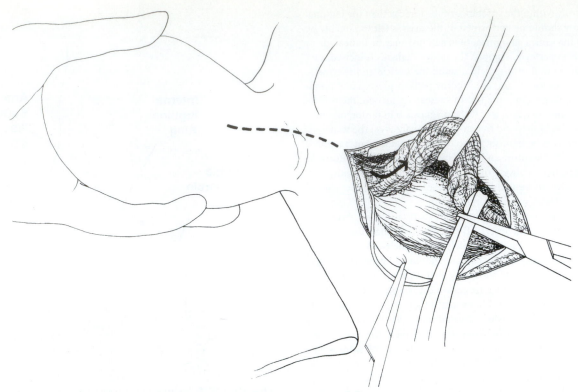

**FIGURE 17E-2.** Gentle external pressure is placed on the testicle as it is delivered from the scrotum into the wound. (*From Crawford ED, Das S (eds):* Current Genitourinary Surgery, *2d ed. Baltimore, Williams & Wilkins, 1997, Fig. 35-6, p 457.*)

Primary testicular lesions that invade adjacent structures, show vascular invasion, contain embryonal or undifferentiated cells, or lack yolk sac cells, are considered to be at increased risk of metastatic disease. The TNM staging system for testicular cancer is listed in Table 17E-1.

## TABLE 17E-1. CLINCAL STAGES OF TESTICULAR CANCER

| STAGE | DESCRIPTION |
|---|---|
| A or I | Tumor limited to the testis alone |
| B1 or IIA | Tumor of the testis and retroperitoneal lymph nodes |
| B2 or IIB | Tumor of retroperitoneal lymph nodes 2–6 cm in greatest dimension by computed tomography (CT) |
| B3 or IIC | Tumor of retroperitoneal lymph nodes >6 cm in greatest dimension by CT |
| C or III | Tumor above the diaphragm or involving abdominal solid organs |

SOURCE: From Gillenwater J et al (eds): *Adult and Pediatric Urology*, 3d ed. St Louis, Mosby-Yearbook, 1996, Table 39-3, p 1926.

Once the histopathologic diagnosis of a germ cell neoplasm has been made, initial staging involves the imaging of the retroperitoneal lymph nodes and chest. Although lymphangiography was previously used to evaluate the retroperitoneal lymph nodes, CT scanning has replaced this modality in the evaluation and staging of the abdomen and retroperitoneum. Although CT scanning is the most sensitive method for evaluating the lungs and mediastinum, a standard posteroanterior (PA) and lateral chest x-ray are the initial method for staging the chest. Any questionable areas can then be followed up with a CT scan. Serum marker levels, CT scan of the abdomen, and chest x-ray provide the initial staging following orchiectomy and thus allow one to clinically stage the patient (Table 17E-2).

Numerous staging systems have been developed over the years, with differences mainly related to the extent of the retroperitoneal nodal disease. The size and extent of retroperitoneal lymph node involvement is important because it guides initial treatment and has prognostic significance. CT scanning of the retroperitoneal lymph nodes has improved markedly over the years; however, there is still a false-positive and -negative rate of 25% and 33% respectively.[7,8]

False-positive and false-negative results by CT scanning are inevitable, because this modality cannot pick up micrometastases, and lymphadenopathy does not always represent metastatic disease. The sensitivity and specificity of imaging modalities, serum marker

**TABLE 17E-2.** TNM STAGING SYSTEM FOR
TESTICULAR CANCER

| | |
|---|---|
| T$_0$ | No apparent primary |
| T$_1$ | Testis only (excludes rete testis) |
| T$_2$ | Beyond the tunica albuginea |
| T$_3$ | Rete testis or epididymal involvement |
| T$_4$ | Spermatic cord |
| | a: Spermatic cord |
| | b: Scrotum |
| N$_0$ | No nodal involvement |
| N$_1$ | Ipsilateral regional nodal involvement |
| N$_2$ | Contralateral or bilateral abdominal or groin nodes |
| N$_3$ | Palpable abdominal nodes or fixed groin nodes |
| N$_4$ | Juxtaregional nodes |
| M$_0$ | No distant metastases |
| M$_1$ | Distant metastases present |

SOURCE: From Gillenwater J et al (eds): *Adult and Pediatric Urology*, 3d ed. St Louis, Mosby-Yearbook, 1996, Table 39-5, p 1926.

levels, and the histologic cell types are important not only to the initial clinical staging, but also to the treatment options that are possible and finally in following patients on surveillance or status after surgery, chemotherapy, or radiation therapy. RPLND is the gold standard for the pathologic staging of the retroperitoneum, with the advantage of not only detecting micrometastases but also in providing surgical cure in a large number of patients. The indications, risks, benefits, complications, and technique of RPLND will be discussed later in the chapter.

## SEMINOMA

### TREATMENT

The treatment options for low-stage seminoma and nonseminoma differ greatly, and therefore will be discussed separately. Low-stage seminoma traditionally has been treated with radical orchiectomy followed by external-beam radiation therapy to the regional lymph nodes. The distribution of lymph node metastases from testicular neoplasms was mapped out in 1970s and 1980s.[9,10] Although the location of retroperitoneal lymph node metastases was mapped out for nonseminomatous tumors based on RPLND, this route of metastatic spread also holds true for seminoma (Fig. 17E-3).

Testicular neoplasms spread from the parenchyma to the lymphatics at the mediastinum testis. With the exception of choriocarcinoma, testicular neoplasms typically spread in a predictable stepwise manner. The first echelon of lymph node drainage from the right testicle is to the interaortocaval nodes at the level of the second vertebral body. The first echelon of nodal drainage from the left testis is to the paraaortic lymph nodes. From the retroperitoneal lymph nodes, spread may occur to the suprahilar region or via the cisterna chyli or thoracic duct to the supraclavicular nodes. Although the initial landing sites for testicular tumors are fairly constant, cross metastases can occur (more often with right-sided tumors). Inguinal lymph

nodes are typically not involved in the spread of testicular germ cell tumors, because these lymph node chains drain the legs, penis, and scrotum. Inguinal lymph node involvement can occur when there has been scrotal violation due to unrecognized testicular tumor during an exploration for a presumably nonmalignant process and/or a biopsy. It is crucial to perform all testicular explorations through an inguinal incision when testicular tumor is a possibility because the lymphatic drainage of the testicle remains relatively constant. Distant metastases are primarily to the lung with subsequent spread possible to the liver, brain, and bone.

### LOW-STAGE SEMINOMA

Traditionally, the treatment for low-stage seminoma is radical orchiectomy followed by radiotherapy to the regional lymph nodes. Low-stage seminoma is extremely sensitive to external-beam radiation therapy. In patients with stage I disease (no retroperitoneal lymphadenopathy), the retroperitoneal lymph nodes are treated with 20 to 35 Gy; this has a less than 5% relapse rate. Concern for overtreatment in up to 80% of patients with clinical stage I seminoma has led to the option of surveillance in some of these patients. Patients who may be candidates for surveillance must have no lymphadenopathy and must also be very reliable and willing to undergo close follow-up with frequent office visits and periodic imaging studies with chest x-ray and CT scanning. Surveillance is a viable option because it is known that patients who do relapse (most in the retroperitoneal area; some in the pelvic or inguinal nodes) can be salvaged with radiotherapy and/or cisplatin based chemotherapy. However, it is the authors' opinion that irradiation therapy is the gold standard.

Another concern regarding external-beam radiation therapy to the retroperitoneum is the small, but not insignificant, risk of secondary primary cancers in the gastrointestinal tract, urinary tract, and leukemia. The risk of developing a secondary cancer following radiation has been calculated to be 10% after 20 years.[11]

### STAGE II SEMINOMA

Stage II seminoma has traditionally been treated with radical orchiectomy followed by external-beam radiation to the regional lymph nodes. The radiation dose and technique are tailored to the location and extent of disease. The most common presentation of stage II disease is that of IIa (lymph node mass 2 cm or less in greatest dimension). Stage IIb disease is a lymph node mass greater than 2 cm but not more than 5 cm in the greatest dimension or multiple nodes with none greater than 5 cm in the greatest dimension. The failure rates for radiation therapy in stage IIa and IIb disease are 10% to 20%.[12]

Stage IIc (bulky retroperitoneal disease) denotes a lymph node mass more than 5 cm in its greatest dimension. When treated with external-beam radiation therapy, results are poor, with a 20% to 50% failure rate. These poor results led investigators to apply chemotherapy (previously only used in nonseminoma), with results equal to that for equivalent-stage nonseminoma. Retroperitoneal lymphadenectomy is reserved for special cases where radiotherapy or

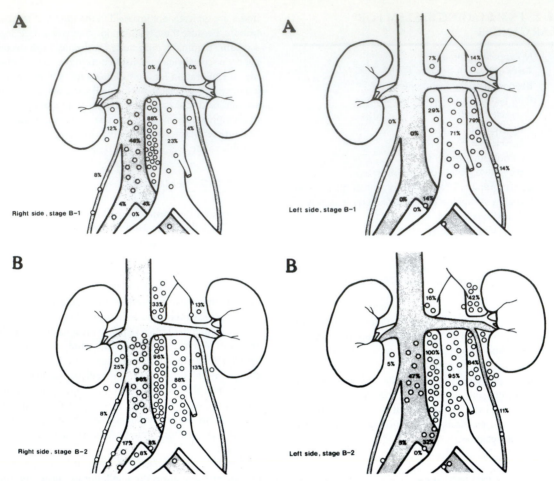

**FIGURE 17E-3.** Distribution of retroperitoneal lymph node metastases in early-stage nonseminomatous testicular cancer based on the appearance of the nodes during operation. Stages are shown for each testicle: *A.* Grossly negative (stage B1). *B.* Grossly positive (stage B2). (*From Donohue JP, Zachary JM, Maynard BR. Distribution of nodal metastases in nonseminomatous testis cancer. J Urol 128:315–320, 1982.*)

chemotherapy is contraindicated (i.e., inflammatory bowel disease or contralateral seminoma following prior irradiation).

## STAGE III SEMINOMA

Metastatic seminoma has been shown to be remarkably sensitive to cisplatin-based chemotherapy, with response rates of greater than 85%.[13] Four cycles of the combination of cisplatin and etoposide has been shown to be very effective in the treatment of advanced seminoma (stage II and III). Residual retroperitoneal masses may persist after radiation or chemotherapy. A persistent mass following chemotherapy will rarely have teratoma cells, and a retroperitoneal lymphadenectomy following chemotherapy for seminoma is technically very difficult when compared with nonseminoma. Perioperative morbidity rate for salvage RPLND is high, and one may

consider adjuvant radiotherapy in patients with residual mass following chemotherapy. Complications of chemotherapy will be discussed in the section under nonseminoma.

## NONSEMINOMA

The marked decline in morbidity and mortality rates in nonseminoma is primarily due to advances in the technique of RPLND and combination chemotherapy. The inability to detect micrometastases by current imaging modalities results in up to 30% of patients having occult metastatic (lymph node) disease. This finding becomes important when deciding which patients are cured following radical orchiectomy and thus possibly candidates for surveillance versus those patients who harbor occult metastatic disease and thus require subsequent RPLND. To help improve the odds of finding those

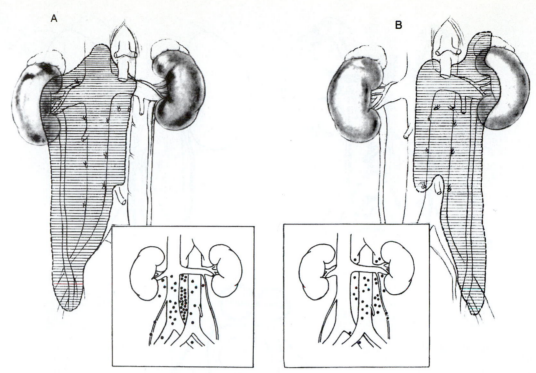

**FIGURE 17E-4.** Limits of modified nerve-sparing RPLND, *A.* on the right side, and *B.* left side for patients with grossly negative nodes. The dissection is complete within the anatomic area and is designed to remove all nodes likely to contain metastases yet preserve the contralateral sympathetic chain and hypogastric plexus. The postganglionic sympathetic nerves (L1 to L3) can be identified prospectively and preserved within the field of dissection. Insets: Margins of dissection overlaid on distribution of nodes in stage B1. (*From Crawford ED, Das S (eds):* Current Genitourinary Surgery, *2d ed. Baltimore, Williams & Wilkins, 1997, Fig. 36-2, p 463.*)

patients who at are high risk of having micrometastases at the time of radical orchiectomy, several investigators have determined risk factors that can predict either recurrence on surveillance or occult nodal disease following radical orchiectomy. The most widely agreed upon risk factors that increase the possibility of relapse or occult nodal disease are the presence of vascular or lymphatic invasion or a high percentage of embryonal cell carcinoma in the primary tumor. The presence of yolk sac tumor in a clinical stage I nonseminoma may have a favorable impact on the chance for relapse or in predicting occult nodal disease.

## CLINICAL STAGE I NONSEMINOMA

Patients with clinical stage I nonseminoma have tumor confined to the testis with no spread through the capsule or into the spermatic cord, and no evidence of lymphadenopathy and normal levels of post orchiectomy tumor markers. As stated before, approximately 25% to 30% of patients with clinical stage I nonseminoma are understaged with current imaging modalities. Reliable patients who have low risk factors for relapse or occult metastatic disease may be candidates for surveillance. Those patients who do relapse may be treated with either RPLND and/or combination chemotherapy with no apparent adverse impact on the overall cure and survival rates. Concerns over fertility and morbidity following RPLND in patients with clinical stage I nonseminoma have been lessened with the development and improved understanding of the anatomy and techniques of performing the operation. Patients with clinical stage I nonseminoma who are either unreliable, unwilling to undergo frequent surveillance, or have elevated risk factors should undergo RPLND. RPLND has been shown to be less expensive than surveillance over a 5-year period by cost-and-benefit risk analysis. Also, from a morbidity standpoint concerning fertility, toxicity, and late relapse, RPLND is the favored option.[14]

**RPLND IN CLINICAL STAGE I NONSEMINOMA.** The modifications in RPLND have resulted in the preservation of ejaculation in 90% to 100% of patients depending on the method used and the proficiency of the surgeon. Popularization of retroperitoneal lymphadenectomy came about with the realization that the primary

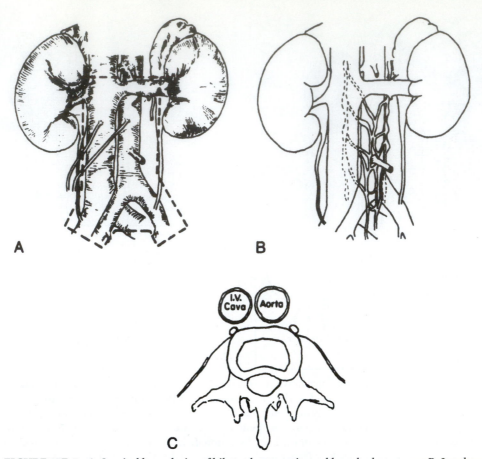

**FIGURE 17E-5.** *A*. Surgical boundaries of bilateral retroperitoneal lymphadenectomy. *B*. Lumbar sympathetic chain and postganglionic fibers forming the superior hypogastric plexus. *C*. Cross section of the sympathetic trunks in relation to the psoas muscles, vertebral bodies, and great vessels. (*From Crawford ED, Das S (eds):* Current Genitourinary Surgery, *2d ed. Baltimore, Williams & Wilkins, 1997, Fig. 37-1, p 484.*)

spread of testicular germ cell tumors was to the retroperitoneal lymph nodes. Up until the 1980s, RPLND for testicular carcinoma meant a full bilateral RPLND with removal of all obvious lymphatic tissue between the ureters from above the renal hilum down to the iliac vessels. This resulted in the loss of emission and ejaculation because the postganglionic sympathetic fibers were also removed along with the lymphatic tissue. Mapping studies by Donahue and associates[9,15] refined our knowledge of the primary landing sites for left-sided and right-sided testicular tumors, thus making it possible to modify the RPLND in clinical stage I nonseminomas and thus preserve fertility. This was even further elucidated so that the individual postganglionic sympathetic fibers could be preserved and thus allow the preservation of ejaculation in up to 100% of patients. It is well known that up to 50% of patients with germ cell tumors are hypofertile at the time of diagnosis. Following nerve-sparing RPLND, approximately 75% of patients have normal semen parameters and overall, 75% of patients are successful in impregnating their sexual partner. Whether one uses a modified template or a nerve-sparing

RPLND, studies have shown no compromise in the diagnostic or therapeutic value of the procedure.[16,17]

In patients with pathologically confirmed stage I nonseminoma treated with radical orchiectomy followed by modified RPLND, 99.6% are cured of their disease. It should be noted that a very small percentage of patients may have primary spread of their tumor to sites other than the retroperitoneal lymph nodes who, therefore, relapse at these metastatic sites and thus require salvage chemotherapy (Figs. 17E-4, 17E-5).

**MODIFIED-TEMPLATE RPLND.** Using the mapping studies of Donahue and associates,[9,15] Narayan and associates[17] described their modified RPLND with the preservation of ejaculation in half their patients. Subsequent investigators showed the modified-template RPLND to be effective in both the diagnostic and therapeutic management of low-stage nonseminoma while preserving fertility in up to 90% of patients.[18]

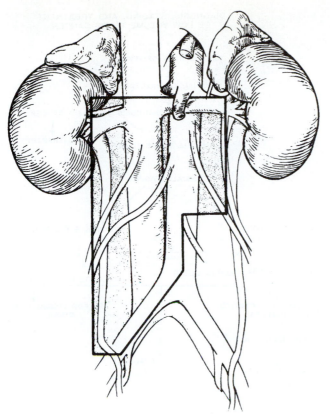

**FIGURE 17E-6.** Modified right-sided retroperitoneal lymph node dissection template. The dissection is complete above the level of the inferior mesenteric artery but limited to the unilateral/ipsilateral side below the level of the inferior mesenteric artery. (*From Osterling J, Richie J: Urologic Oncology. Philadelphia, Saunders, 1997, Fig. 34-3, p 487.*)

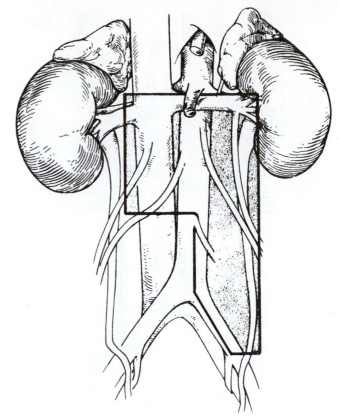

**FIGURE 17E-7.** Template for modified left-sided retroperitoneal lymph node dissection. The right-sided border is near the right margin of the inferior vena cava. (*From Osterling J, Richie, J: Urologic Oncology. Philadelphia, Saunders, 1997, Fig. 34-4, p 487.*)

The technique can be performed either through a thoracoabdominal or midline transabdominal incision. This limited dissection is from the renal hilum bilaterally, then extending down to the inferior mesenteric artery with bilateral dissection to the ureters laterally. The dissection then carries unilaterally inferior to the inferior mesenteric artery on the site of the primary tumor, care being taken not to disrupt the hypogastric plexus overlying the bifurcation of the aorta. The inferior limit of dissection laterally is where the ureter crosses the iliac vessels. The ipsilateral spermatic vessels are removed along with the specimen. Utilizing a spit and roll technique, lymphatic tissue is removed in packets around and in between the great vessels as indicated in Figs. 17E-6 and 17E-7.

## CLINICAL STAGE II NONSEMINOMA

Clinical stage II nonseminoma can be divided into micrometastatic, small-volume, and bulky retroperitoneal disease. Patients who have elevated tumor markers following radical orchiectomy for clinical stage I disease are presumed to harbor micrometastases. Small-volume RPLND can be divided into IIA or IIB. Patients with clinical stage II nonseminoma (retroperitoneal lymphadenopathy) should undergo a RPLND if on gross examination they have small-volume disease (lymph nodes less than 2 to 3 cm in diameter).

These patients should undergo a full bilateral lymph node dissection. Patients with pathologic stage N1 or N2a disease may be cured by the RPLND alone, and then may be observed closely. Patients with stage N2b (larger-volume retroperitoneal disease) should undergo two cycles of combination chemotherapy with bleomycin, etoposide, and cisplatin after the RPLND. Because the retroperitoneal lymph nodes may be the first and only site of metastatic deposits in patients with micrometastatic or minimal nodal disease, RPLND may be truly curative, thus sparing the patient potentially unnecessary combination chemotherapy (Fig. 17E-8).

## CHEMOTHERAPY FOR STAGE II NONSEMINOMA

As stated earlier, patients with micrometastatic lymph node disease following RPLND are typically observed closely because their relapse rate is as low as 10% but may be up as high as 20% to 30%. When looking at low-stage II disease (N1 and N2a), relapse rates are less

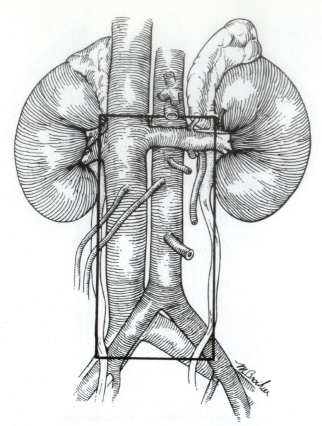

**FIGURE 17E-8.** Margins of dissection of full bilateral retroperitoneal lymph node dissection, including right and left suprahilar areas. (*From Gillenwater J et al (eds):* Adult and Pediatric Urology, *3d ed. St Louis, Mosby-Yearbook, 1996, Fig. 39-14, p 1928.*)

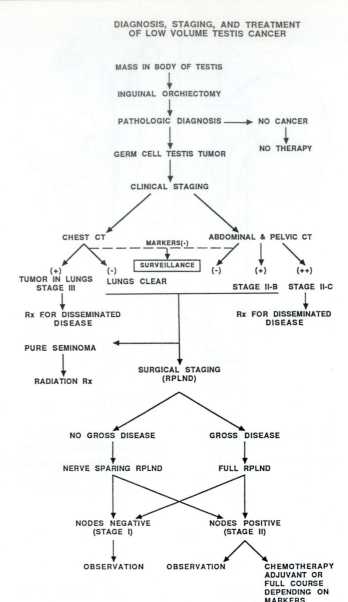

**FIGURE 17E-9.** Algorithm for the diagnosis of testicular cancer and for the treatment of low-stage disease. Note that the treatment of high-stage tumors (B3 and C) is shown in Figure 17E-10. Stage I indicates stage A; stage II, stage B; stage III, stage C. RPLND = retroperitoneal lymph node dissection. (*From Gillenwater J et al (eds):* Adult and Pediatric Urology, *3d ed. St Louis, Mosby-Yearbook, 1996, Fig. 39-19, p 1934.*)

likely following RPLND, and those who do relapse can be salvaged with four cycles of combination chemotherapy. Studies have been performed regarding the adjuvant use of chemotherapy in patients with low-stage II nonseminoma following RPLND. When analyzing all positive lymph node disease following RPLND, the relapse rate is up to 48%.[19] This high relapse rate for all stage II disease following RPLND was compared to a very low relapse rate of 2% for all stage II patients treated with two cycles of adjuvant chemotherapy postoperatively. An effective strategy for stage II disease, therefore, is primary RPLND for minimal stage II disease (N1 and N2a) followed by observation with salvage chemotherapy should the patient relapse. Patients with bulkier stage II disease (stage N2b) are at higher risk of relapse and should undergo two courses of adjuvant chemotherapy. This selective approach to adjuvant chemotherapy will spare those patients less likely to undergo relapse from the potentially toxic effects of combination chemotherapy. Those patients at higher risk of relapse will undergo two rather than four cycles of combination chemotherapy and achieve nearly complete freedom from relapse with a lower overall dose of chemotherapy than would have been necessary in a salvage situation (Fig. 17E-9).

## BULKY RETROPERITONEAL DISEASE

Patients with large-volume retroperitoneal disease (N3) but without distant metastases should undergo combination chemotherapy initially with three to four cycles followed by restaging. Patients who have achieved a complete response judged by a completely normal

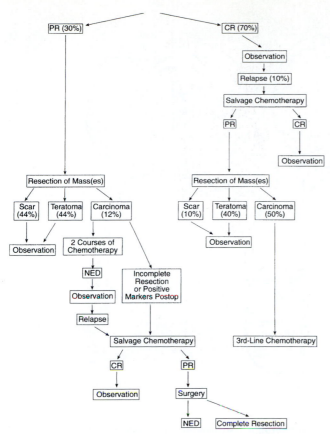

**FIGURE 17E-10.** Algorithm for the treatment of high-stage disease. CR = complete clinical remission; PR = partial clinical remission; NED = no evidence of disease. (*From Gillenwater J et al (eds):* Adult and Pediatric Urology, *3d ed. St Louis, Mosby-Yearbook, 1996, Fig. 39-20, p 1937.*)

CT scan along with normal levels of tumor markers may potentially be observed, but more than likely should undergo a RPLND. Those patients who achieve a partial response should then undergo a full bilateral RPLND. Following initial combination chemotherapy with a partial response, a RPLND will yield either scar tissue, teratoma, or residual carcinoma. The finding of residual carcinoma will require that the patient undergo further chemotherapy. In patients who have either scar tissue or teratoma found at the time of RPLND following chemotherapy, close follow up with no further chemotherapy is advisable (Fig. 17E-10).

Currently, the combination of bleomycin, etoposide, and cisplatin (BEP) is given in three cycles for patients with advanced testicular carcinoma. This combination has a cure rate of approximately 70% in patients with advanced testicular carcinoma. In patients whose tumor marker levels do not normalize after three cycles of BEP, salvage chemotherapy is indicated. RPLND following combination chemotherapy with BEP has a potential for complications related mainly to bleomycin. Patients who have received bleomycin need to undergo pulmonary function testing preopera-

tively, and care should be taken to avoid overhydration and to limit inspired oxygen to room air concentrations in the perioperative period. Patients whose tumor marker levels do not normalize after three cycles of combination chemotherapy should undergo salvage chemotherapy with vinblastine, ifosfamide, and cisplatin (VIP); this combination has an approximate 30% salvage rate. Patients who are salvaged with the second-line chemotherapy should then undergo a full bilateral RPLND with the possible finding of scar tissue, teratoma, or a residual carcinoma. Patients who fail first- and second-line combination chemotherapy may potentially be salvaged with an autologous bone marrow transplant.

## RPLND FOLLOWING CHEMOTHERAPY

RPLND following combination chemotherapy can be technically challenging and may be associated with a higher morbidity and even mortality rates if one does not pay close attention to operative and perioperative details. Patients who have undergone chemotherapy with bleomycin should be treated carefully, as stated earlier. Patients with a large retroperitoneal mass following chemotherapy require a full bilateral RPLND. A thoracoabdominal or transabdominal approach may be used. Large masses extending into the suprahilar region are best exposed with a thoracoabdominal incision. As described before, the small bowel and ascending colon are mobilized completely and placed in a bowel bag on the patient's chest. The aorta and vena cava are identified and dissected free of surrounding tissues below and above the tumor mass. The ureters are identified and vessel loops placed around them so as to prevent injury. The renal veins are likewise identified and preserved. Care is then taken to dissect the retroperitoneal mass free of all surrounding structures and up into the retrocrural space. The desmoplastic reaction that occurs at edges of the tumor mass make it occasionally difficult to dissect the tumor free of the aorta and inferior vena cava, potentially leading to inadvertent entry into the vessels with significant blood loss. Most perioperative complications whether gastrointestinal, lymphatic, or renal are temporary and usually treated conservatively[20] (Fig. 17E-11).

## WIDELY METASTATIC NONSEMINOMA

Patients who present with widely metastatic disease initially undergo two cycles of combination chemotherapy with BEP. If the patient's markers do not normalize and/or there is obvious widespread residual disease or the disease progresses while on treatment, then salvage chemotherapy should be undertaken with VIP. Patients who receive ifosfamide should also be treated with Mesna to avoid the potential complication of hemorrhagic cystitis. Patients not responding to salvage chemotherapy may be candidates for autologous bone marrow transplantation with high-dose chemotherapy.[21]

## MODIFICATIONS IN RPLND

A number of factors come into play when deciding on the type of RPLND most appropriate for each individual patient. Mapping

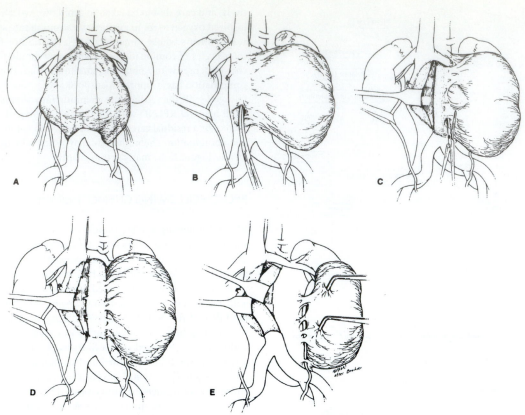

**FIGURE 17E-11.** A–E. Technique for removing bulky tumor during a postchemotherapy retroperitoneal lymph node dissection (RPLND). The mass is removed by separating it into a bundle anterior to each of the great vessels and the ureters. Once the bulky mass has been resected, a standard full bilateral RPLND can be performed. (*From Gillenwater J et al (eds):* Adult and Pediatric Urology, *3d ed. St Louis, Mosby-Yearbook, 1996, Fig. 39-21, p 1939.*)

studies and large series have shown which techniques and limits of dissection are most appropriate with each stage of disease. In patients with no retroperitoneal lymphadenopathy, either a modified template or nerve-sparing technique is indicated. Although the template method is familiar to most urologists, a nerve-sparing dissection is an excellent procedure with a moderate learning curve. Patients with low-volume retroperitoneal disease (N2a) who undergo initial RPLND should have slightly wider surgical boundaries extending bilaterally above the inferior mesenteric artery and below, as well with preservation of the sympathetic nerves and hypogastric plexus, thus preserving ejaculation in up to 90% of patients.[22] Finally, the type of RPLND performed following combination chemotherapy should be a full bilateral lymph node dissection with nerve preservation in only highly selected patients.[23]

## SUMMARY

Testicular carcinoma has become one of the most curable solid tumors in men due to improvements and discoveries both surgically and chemotherapeutically. Patients with low to medium-volume disease now achieve a greater than 90% cure rate overall. Cisplatin-based chemotherapeutic regimens have led the way in treating patients with advanced nonseminoma and seminoma although effective salvage chemotherapeutic regimens have also been developed. An understanding of the natural history of metastatic spread in testicular carcinoma along with the sympathetic innervation for emission and ejaculation have allowed surgical techniques to achieve excellent diagnostic and therapeutic cure while preserving fertility. Research continues to lower the toxicity of chemotherapeutic regimens while increasing their efficacy so as to improve disease-free survival and overall survival rates in patients presenting with widely metastatic disease.

## REFERENCES

1. BORING CC et al: Cancer statistics, 1994. CA Cancer J Clin 44:7, 1994.
2. CROMIE WJ: Cryptorchidism and malignant testicular disease, in *Cryptorchidism, Management and Implications.* F Hadziselimovic (ed). New York, Springer-Verlag, 1983.

3. PRESTI JC JR: Testicular cancer, an overview, in *Current Genitourinary Cancer Surgery*, 2d ed, ED Crawford, S Das (eds). Baltimore, Williams & Wilkins, 1997, pp 445–453.

4. MOUL JW, HEIDENREICH A: Prognostic factors in low-stage nonseminomatous testicular cancer. Oncology 10:1359, 1996.

5. BENSON CJ: The role of ultrasound in diagnosis and staging of testicular cancer. Semin Urol 6:189, 1988.

6. GIGUERE JK et al: The clinical significance of unconventional orchiectomy approaches in testicular cancer: A report from the testicular intergroup study. J Urol 139:1225, 1988.

7. DONOHUE JP et al: The role of retroperitoneal lymphadenectomy in clinical stage B testis cancer; the Indiana University experience (1965–1989). J Urol 153:85, 1995.

8. FERNANDEZ EB et al: Retroperitoneal imaging with third and fourth generation computed axial tomography in clinical stage I nonseminomatous germ cell tumors. Urology 44:548, 1994.

9. DONOHUE JP et al: Distribution of nodal metastases in nonseminomatous testicular cancer. J Urol 128:315, 1982.

10. RAY B et al: Distribution of retroperitoneal lymph node metastases in testicular germinal tumors. Cancer 33:340, 1974.

11. STEIN ME et al: Second primary cancer in irradiated stage I testicular seminoma. Strahlenther Onkol 11:1672, 1993.

12. EVENSEN J et al: Testicular seminoma: Histological findings and their prognostic significance for stage II disease. J Surg Oncol 36:166, 1987.

13. MENCEL PJ et al: Advance seminoma: Treatment results, survival and prognostic factors in 142 patients. J Clin Oncol 12:120, 1994.

14. BANIEL J, DONOHUE JP: Cost and risk benefit considerations in low stage (I and II) nonseminomatous testicular tumors. AUA Update Series Lesson 7, 16: 50, 1977.

15. DONOHUE JP et al: Nerve-sparing retroperitoneal lymphadenectomy with preservation of ejaculation. J Urol 144:287, 1990.

16. FOSTER RS et al: The fertility of patients with clinical stage I testis cancer managed by nerve sparing retroperitoneal lymph node dissection. J Urol 152:1139, 1994.

17. NARAYAN P et al: Ejaculation and fertility after extended retroperitoneal lymph node dissection for testicular cancer. J Urol 127:685, 1982.

18. RICHIE JP: Clinical stage I testicular cancer: The role of modified retroperitoneal lymph adenectomy. J Urol 144:1160, 1990.

19. WILLIAMS SD et al: Immediate adjuvant chemotherapy versus observation with treatment at relapse in pathologic stage II testicular cancer. N Engl J Med 317:1433, 1987.

20. BANIEL J et al: Testis cancer: Complications of post chemotherapy retroperitoneal lymph node dissection. J Urol 153:976, 1995.

21. SIEGERT W et al: High-dose treatment with carboplatin, etoposide, and ifosfamide followed by autologous stem cell transplantation in relapsed or refractory germ cell cancer: A phase I/II study. J Clin Oncol 12:1223, 1994.

22. STEELE GS, RICHIE JP: Current role of retroperitoneal lymph node dissection in testicular cancer. Oncology 5:717, 1997.

23. WAHLE GR et al: Nerve sparing retroperitoneal lymphadenectomy after primary chemotherapy for metastatic testicular carcinoma. J Urol 152:428, 1994.

# CHAPTER 18

# GYNECOLOGIC NEOPLASMS

## 18A / CANCER OF THE VULVA AND VAGINA

*Dennis S. Chi, Borys Mychalczak, and William J. Hoskins*

### CANCER OF THE VULVA

Cancer of the vulva is a relatively rare neoplasm accounting for approximately 4% of all gynecologic malignancies and fewer than 1% of all cancers in women.[1] Since the vulva is covered by squamous epithelium, about 80% to 90% of primary vulvar malignancies are squamous cell carcinomas. Consequently, the data regarding patterns of spread, prognostic factors, and survival for vulvar cancer are based predominantly on studies of squamous cell neoplasms. However, a wide variety of other malignancies are found on the vulva, including malignant melanoma, carcinoma arising from the Bartholin's gland, basal cell carcinoma, and soft-tissue sarcoma.

Surgery is the mainstay of treatment for vulvar cancer, and during the past 60 years, surgical management has come full circle.[2] In the early part of the century, conservative procedures such as simple vulvectomy were frequently performed. However, the 5-year survival rate was only 20% to 25%.[3,4] Due to these poor results, Basset[5] advocated a more radical en bloc dissection of the vulva and regional lymph nodes. Using Basset's approach, Taussig[6] and Way[7] reported 5-year survival rates of 60% to 70%. However, this radical surgery resulted in significant physical and psychologic morbidity, and in recent years a more conservative surgical approach with integration of radiation therapy has been advocated. With careful patient selection, survival does not seem to be compromised.

### EPIDEMIOLOGY

In the United States, invasive vulvar cancer occurs with an average annual age-adjusted incidence rate of 1.2 per 100,000 woman-years.[8] The median age of patients diagnosed with vulvar carcinoma in situ is approximately 45 to 50 years. The median age for invasive vulvar cancer is about 65 to 70 years, with a peak incidence of 20 per 100,000 in women over age 75. The incidence of invasive vulvar cancer has not changed over the past 20 years. However, recent studies have reported that the incidence of vulvar carcinoma in situ between 1973 and 1987 nearly doubled from 1.1 to 2.1 per 100,000 woman-years.[8,9] The increased incidence was most notable in women under 55 years of age. The relatively stable incidence of invasive disease despite a steady increase in carcinoma in situ suggests that more effective treatment of in situ disease has prevented an increase in invasive cancers or that invasive and in situ disease have different etiologic factors.[8,9]

Several infectious agents have been proposed as possible etiologic factors in vulvar cancer, including granulomatous infections, herpes simplex virus, and human papillomaviruses (HPV). Most recently, areas of investigation have focused on the neoplastic potential of vulvar HPV infections. Strong associations between HPV infection and the later development of vulvar carcinoma have been identified.[10] The postulated mechanism of HPV-induced carcinogenesis is thought to involve inactivation of the p53 tumor-suppressor gene via mutation or interaction of the p53 protein with the protein encoded for by the HPV E6 oncogene.[11,12] However, although 80% to 90% of all vulvar intraepithelial neoplasias (VINs) contain HPV DNA, only 30% to 50% of invasive lesions contain evidence of HPV infection.[13–17]

An analysis of the differences in HPV DNA content between intraepithelial and invasive vulvar cancers in conjunction with data from other epidemiologic, histopathologic, and molecular studies has led several authors to suggest that patients with invasive squamous cell carcinomas of the vulva can be divided into two groups whose cancers may have different etiologies.[18–21] Younger patients (35 to 55 years) tend to have carcinomas associated with HPV infection and VIN (Table 18A-1). Their tumors are frequently multifocal and appear histologically as poorly differentiated, nonkeratinizing, and "basaloid" or "warty."[18–20] The risk factors for these patients are

**TABLE 18A-1.** TWO PROPOSED SUBSETS OF PATIENTS WITH SQUAMOUS CELL CARCINOMA OF THE VULVA

|  | I | II |
|---|---|---|
| Age | 35–55 years | 55–85 years |
| Associated with human papillomavirus (HPV) infection | Yes | No |
| Preexisting lesion | Vulvar epithelial neoplasia (VIN) | Vulvar inflammation, lichen sclerosis |
| Multifocal lesions | Yes | No |
| Histopathology of tumor | Poorly differentiated, nonkeratinizing, basaloid or warty | Well-differentiated, keratinizing |
| Similar risk factors or cervical carcinoma | Yes | No |

similar to those for squamous cell carcinoma of the cervix (smoking, young age at first sexual intercourse, history of multiple sexual partners, history of sexually transmitted disease). Older patients (55 to 85 years) generally have a history of vulvar inflammation or lichen sclerosis and rarely demonstrate evidence of HPV infection or VIN. Their tumors are usually unifocal, well-differentiated, and exhibit exuberant keratin formation.

## ANATOMY

The vulva includes the mons pubis, labia majora and minora, clitoris, vaginal vestibule, perineal body, and their supporting subcutaneous tissues (Fig. 18A-1). The mons pubis is a fatty prominence anterior to the public symphysis that becomes covered with coarse public hair at the time of puberty. The labia majora are two elongated skin folds that course posteriorly from the mons pubis and blend into the perineal body. The skin of the labia majora is pigmented, with hair follicles on the lateral surface and sebaceous glands medially. The labia minora are a second, smaller set of skin folds that lie between the labia majora. Posteriorly, they meet to form the margin of the vaginal vestibule; anteriorly, they split to enclose the clitoris, forming the prepuce anteriorly and the frenulum posteriorly. The skin of the labia minora contains numerous sebaceous glands but no hair follicles.[22]

The clitoris is located about 2 to 3 cm anterior to the urethral meatus. It is composed of erectile tissue and consists of a glans, body, and two crura. Only the glans is visible externally. The body is composed of a pair of fused corpora cavernosa that extend superiorly beneath the labia before dividing into the two crura. The crura are attached to the ischial rami and are covered by the corresponding ischiocavernosus muscle.

The vaginal vestibule is situated in the center of the vulva and is demarcated circumferentially by the labia minora and posteriorly by the perineal body. In the virgin, the vaginal orifice is guarded by a thin mucosal fold, the hymen, which tears at first coitus. After rupture, the fragments of hymen that persist as small rounded

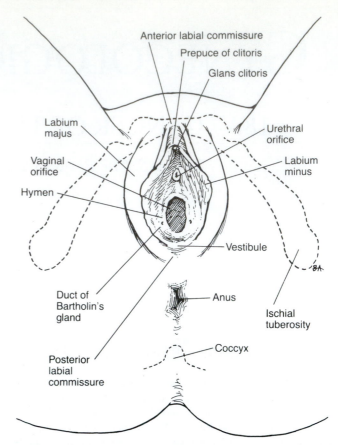

**FIGURE 18A-1.** Female external genitalia. (Reprinted from Hacker NF. Surgery for malignant tumors of the vulva. In: Gershenson DM, DeCherney AH, Curry SL, eds. *Operative Gynecology*. Philadelphia, PA: W. B. Saunders Company; 1993:174, with permission.)

tags are known as hymenal caruncles. The Bartholin's glands are a pair of pea-sized mucus-secreting glands located in the subcutaneous tissue of the posterior labia majora. Each gland drains via a simple duct that opens onto the posterolateral portion of the vestibule. The glands are normally impalpable but become readily palpable if malignant transformation of the gland or its duct occurs.

The perineal body is a 3- to 4-cm band of skin that forms the posterior margin of the vagina and separates the vaginal vestibule from the anus.

The blood supply to the vulva is derived primarily from the internal pudendal artery, which is a terminal branch of the anterior division of the hypogastric artery. The internal pudendal artery emerges from the pelvis around the ischial spine to reach the posterolateral vulva, where it divides into branches that supply the various vulvar structures. These branches also anastomose freely with branches from the superficial and deep external pudendal arteries, which arise from the femoral artery and travel medially to supply the labia majora and their deep structures.

Lymphatics from the vulva course anteriorly through the labia majora, turn laterally at the mons pubis, and drain primarily into the superficial inguinal lymph nodes (Fig. 18A-2). Approximately

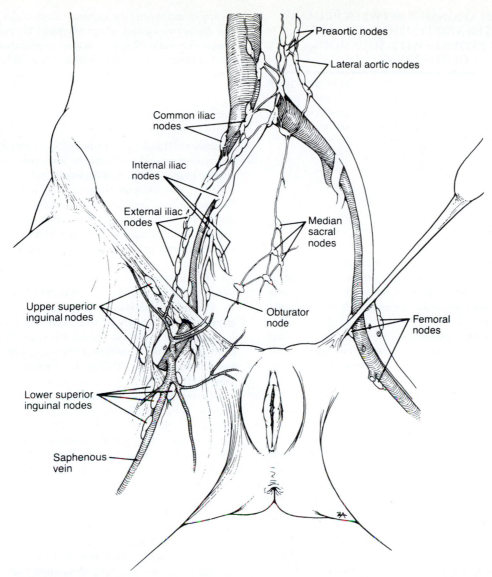

**FIGURE 18A-2.** Inguinofemoral lymph nodes. (Reprinted from Hacker NF. Surgery for malignant tumors of the vulva. In: Gershenson DM, DeCherney AH, Curry SL, eds. *Operative Gynecology.* Philadelphia, PA: W.B. Saunders Company; 1993:175, with permission.)

10 to 12 superficial inguinal lymph nodes lie along the saphenous vein, which branches between Camper's fascia and the cribriform fascia overlying the femoral vessels. These superficial nodes are located in the femoral triangle formed by the inguinal ligament superiorly, the border of the sartorius muscle laterally, and the border of the adductor longus muscle medially. Dye studies by Parry-Jones[23] have demonstrated that the vulvar lymphatics are confined within the labiocrural folds and do not spread laterally onto the thigh. The lymphatic drainage generally does not cross the midline, unless the site of dye injection is at the clitoris or perineal body, where bilateral lymphatic flow may occur.[24]

Lymphatic drainage proceeds from the superficial to the deep inguinal (or femoral) lymph nodes located beneath the cribriform fascia medial to the femoral vein. There are usually three to five deep nodes, with the most cephalad node of the group, known as Cloquet's node, located under the inguinal ligament. The deep inguinal nodes drain into the external iliac nodes and up to the para-aortic chains. Although direct lymphatic pathways have been described from the clitoris to the pelvic nodes, these channels seem to be of minimal clinical significance.[25,26]

## NATURAL HISTORY AND PATTERNS OF SPREAD

About 70% of vulvar squamous carcinomas involve the labia majora or minora. Labial lesions occur three times more frequently on the

**TABLE 18A-2.** RELATIONSHIP BETWEEN PRIMARY TUMOR DIAMETER AND LYMPH NODE METASTASES IN PATIENTS WITH SQUAMOUS CELL CARCINOMA OF THE VULVA

| TUMOR DIAMETER | NUMBER OF PATIENTS | PATIENTS WITH LYMPH NODE METASTASES | PERCENTAGE OF PATIENTS WITH LYMPH NODE METASTASES |
|---|---|---|---|
| ≤1 cm | 101 | 13 | 13 |
| 1.1–2.0 cm | 210 | 38 | 18 |
| 2.1–4.0 cm | 289 | 110 | 38 |
| >4.0 cm | 148 | 71 | 48 |
| Total | 748 | 232 | 31 |

labia majora than on the labia minora. Approximately 15% to 20% of cases involve the clitoris, and a similar proportion involve the perineal body. In about 10% of patients, the lesion is too extensive to determine the original site, and in approximately 5% of patients, the lesions are multifocal.[27–29]

Vulvar cancers have three modes of spread: (1) direct extension into adjacent organs such as the vagina, urethra, and anus; (2) embolization to regional lymph nodes; and (3) hematogenous dissemination to distant organs such as the liver, lungs, and bone.

The overall incidence of lymph node metastases in vulvar cancer is about 30% to 45%.[2,27] Initial lymph node metastases are usually to the superficial inguinal nodes. Although lymphatic spread generally proceeds in a stepwise fashion from the superficial inguinal to the deep inguinal and then to the pelvic nodes, patients with metastases to the deep inguinal nodes without involvement of the superficial nodes have been reported.[30–32] The incidence of lymph node metastasis increases with the size of the primary tumor and its depth of stromal invasion. Table 18A-2 demonstrates the incidence of nodal metastases in relation to the diameter of the primary tumor.[31,33,34] Table 18A-3 shows the incidence of lymph node metastasis for patients with vulvar carcinomas measuring less than 2 cm in relation to the depth of stromal invasion by the primary tumor.[29,30,35–44]

**TABLE 18A-3.** RELATIONSHIP BETWEEN DEPTH OF STROMAL INVASION AND LYMPH NODE METASTASES IN PATIENTS WITH SQUAMOUS CELL CARCINOMA OF THE VULVA

| DEPTH OF STROMAL INVASION | NUMBER OF PATIENTS | PATIENTS WITH LYMPH NODE METASTASES | PERCENTAGE OF PATIENTS WITH LYMPH NODE METASTASES |
|---|---|---|---|
| ≤ 1 mm | 178 | 0 | 0 |
| 1.1–2.0 mm | 181 | 12 | 7 |
| 2.1–3.0 mm | 157 | 17 | 11 |
| 3.1–5.0 mm | 158 | 38 | 24 |
| >5.0 mm | 126 | 47 | 37 |
| Total | 800 | 114 | 14 |

Any spread beyond the inguinal lymph nodes is considered distant metastasis. Distant site involvement is uncommon at initial presentation but is often seen in women with recurrent vulvar cancer. The lungs are the most common site of distant hematogenous metastasis.

## HISTOLOGY

Squamous VIN and extramammary Paget's disease of the vulva (adenocarcinoma in situ) are the two preinvasive lesions of the vulva recognized by the International Society for the Study of Vulvar Disease (ISSVD).[45] Previously used terms such as "erythroplasia of Queyrat," "Bowen's disease," and "carcinoma in situ simplex" have been reclassified as squamous carcinoma in situ, or VIN 3.

Histologic findings in VIN include disruption of the normal vulvar epithelial architecture with crowded, disorganized cells demonstrating nuclear atypia, high mitotic activity, and high nuclear-cytoplasmic ratios. When the cellular changes are confined to the lower third of the epithelium, VIN 1 (mild dysplasia) is the diagnosis. A lesion is classified as VIN 2 (moderate dysplasia) if the cellular changes extend through approximately one-third to two-thirds of the epithelium. When the cellular atypia involves more than two-thirds of the full thickness of the epithelium (disregarding the keratin layer), the diagnosis is VIN 3 (severe dysplasia) or carcinoma in situ (also designated as VIN 3), if the change is essentially full thickness.

Microscopically, vulvar Paget's disease is characterized by the presence of Paget's cells, which are large cells with pale, vacuolated cytoplasm and prominent nuclei. These cells are generally found in higher concentration near the basement membrane but are also seen throughout the epithelium. Paget's cells may appear singly or may be clustered together, occasionally having an acinar or glandlike arrangement.[22]

Approximately 80% to 90% of invasive vulvar cancers are squamous cell carcinomas. Most squamous cell carcinomas of the vulva can be categorized into one of three main histologic subtypes: basaloid, warty (condylomatous), or keratinizing. Basaloid carcinomas are characterized by variable-sized nests of immature squamous cells showing little, if any, squamous maturation. Warty (condylomatous) carcinomas have multiple papillary projections with keratinized epithelial surfaces and fibrovascular cores.[45] Basaloid and warty carcinomas are usually poorly differentiated. Keratinizing carcinomas are generally well differentiated and demonstrate whorls and nests of keratin. About 5% of vulvar carcinomas are anaplastic and may consist of large immature cells, spindle sarcomatoid cells, or small cells. The latter may simulate small-cell anaplastic carcinomas of the lung or Merkel-cell tumors, and have demonstrated an aggressive biologic behavior in the few reported cases.[9,46,47]

Malignant melanoma is the second most common vulvar malignancy, accounting for 2% to 9% of cases.[2,9,45] There are three distinct histopathologic types of vulvar melanomas: (1) superficial spreading melanoma; (2) acral lentiginous melanoma; and (3) nodular melanoma. They are differentiated from one another based on the appearance and growth patterns of their atypical melanocytic cells. Superficial spreading melanoma, as its name implies, rarely invades deeply early in its development. Acral lentiginous melanoma, which also tends to remain superficial during early development, can later

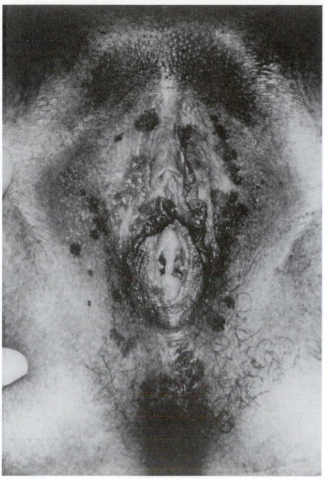

**FIGURE 18A-3.** Hyperpigmented lesions of vulvar carcinoma in situ. (Reprinted from DiSaia PJ, Creasman WT. Preinvasive disease of the vagina and vulva. In: DiSaia PJ, Creasman WT, eds. *Clinical Gynecologic Oncology.* 4th ed. St. Louis, MO: Mosby-Year Book, Inc; 1993:50, with permission.)

appear as a flat freckle that can become quite extensive. Nodular melanoma, the most aggressive of the three types, is a raised lesion that penetrates deeply and may widely metastasize.

Primary carcinoma of the Bartholin's gland accounts for about 5% of vulvar malignancies. Bartholin's carcinomas are termed *squamous* if they originate near the orifice of the duct, *papillary* if they arise from the transitional epithelium of the duct, and *adenocarcinoma* if they arise from the gland itself. Although primary adenocarcinomas of the vulva arise within the Bartholin's gland, adenocarcinomas may also arise from the periurethral Skene's glands or from vulvar adnexal structures associated with Paget's disease.

Although basal cell carcinomas of the skin are extremely common, they represent only about 2% of vulvar cancers. The histologic pattern of vulvar basal cell carcinoma resembles that of basal cell carcinoma found elsewhere on the skin. Small, elongated cells with deeply basophilic nuclei characteristically show palisading at the pe-

riphery of the involved rete ridges. Although metastases to regional lymph nodes do occur, the overall prognosis for these tumors is excellent, and no patients have died as a result of the disease.[45]

Although they account for only 1% to 2% of primary vulvar malignancies, sarcomas can arise from any of the supporting mesenchymal tissues of the vulva. Soft-tissue sarcomas of the vulva include leiomyosarcoma, rhabdomyosarcoma, malignant fibrous histiocytoma, angiosarcoma, liposarcoma, and others. The most common vulvar sarcoma, leiomyosarcoma, is composed of interlacing smooth-muscle cells that have a perinuclear area, or halo, when sectioned on long axis.[45]

## CLINICAL PRESENTATION

Patients with VIN may experience vulvar pruritus, irritation, or a mass, but up to 50% are asymptomatic at the time of diagnosis.[48,49] Typically, the lesions of VIN have a raised surface and about one-quarter are hyperpigmented (Fig. 18A-3). The remainder may be pink, gray, red, or white in color.[45] The lesions may be macular or papular, as well as single or multiple (Fig. 18A-4).

Patients with vulvar Paget's disease typically present with an eczematoid, red, weeping, pruritic area on the vulva (Fig. 18A-5). This disease typically occurs in older, postmenopausal Caucasian women. Because of its eczematoid appearance, it is not unusual for vulvar Paget's disease to be misdiagnosed as eczema or contact dermatitis. Unlike its counterpart in the breast, which is invariably associated with an underlying ductal carcinoma, approximately 15% to 20% of women with vulvar Paget's disease have an underlying adenocarcinoma. These adenocarcinomas usually arise within apocrine glands or the underlying Bartholin's gland and are more often clinically apparent than microscopic or occult. In addition, 30% of patients will have, or will later develop, an adenocarcinoma at another location.[50] The most commonly observed sites are breast, colon, rectum, and upper female genital tract.

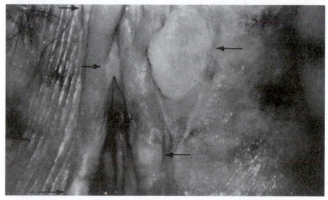

**FIGURE 18A-4.** Multiple white lesions of VIN. (Reprinted from DiSaia PJ, Creasman WT. Preinvasive disease of the vagina and vulva. In DiSaia PJ, Creasman WT, eds. *Clinical Gynecologic Oncology.* 4th ed. St. Louis, MO: Mosby-Year Book, Inc; 1993:49, with permission.)

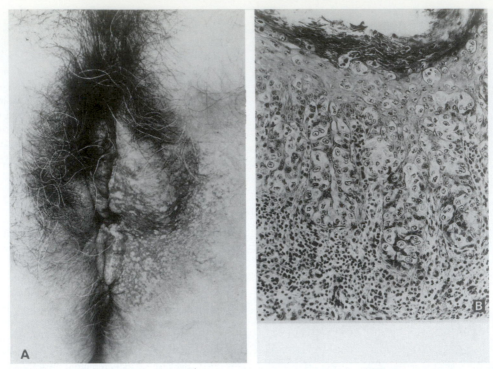

**FIGURE 18A-5.** Paget's disease of the vulva. (Reprinted from Woodruff JD, Buscema J. Surgical conditions of the vulva. In: Thompson JD, Rock JA, eds. *Te Linde's Operative Gynecology.* 7th ed. Philadelphia, PA: J. B. Lippincott Co; 1992:1086, with permission.)

Most women with invasive squamous cell carcinoma present with vulvar pruritus and a recognizable lesion. The lesion may occur as an exophytic or papillomatous mass or an endophytic ulcer (Fig. 18A-6). Unfortunately, some women ignore or deny obvious symptoms and lesions for long periods of time and present with advanced disease (Fig. 18A-7). The presentation in such cases is generally dominated by local pain, bleeding, and surface drainage from the tumor.[22] Metastatic disease in the inguinal lymph nodes or at distant sites may also be symptomatic. Verrucous carcinoma is a rare variant of squamous cell carcinoma. It is a slow-growing, nonaggressive tumor that resembles (and is frequently misdiagnosed as) extensive condyloma acuminata. Even with extensive local invasion, metastases are rare.[51]

Vulvar melanomas occur predominantly in postmenopausal Caucasian women, most commonly on the labia minora or the clitoris. The tumor may arise from preexisting pigmented lesions or from normal-appearing skin. Typical presentations include an asymptomatic pigmented lesion or an identified mass that may be painful or bleeding (Fig. 18A-8).

Primary carcinoma of the Bartholin's gland generally occurs in older women and is rare in patients under the age of 50. Patients usually present with an enlargement in the gland that may be mistaken for a cyst. These tumors are typically solid, deeply infiltrative, and difficult to detect in their early growth. They range in size from 1 to 7 cm in diameter, and pain and ulceration occur with increasing local growth. Approximately 20% of patients have lymph node metastases at the time of diagnosis.[45]

Vulvar basal cell carcinomas are found primarily in elderly Caucasian women who present with pruritus or a firm mass that generally measures less than 2 cm and is confined to the labia majora. The lesion may have an area of central ulceration surrounded by an elevated, "rolled up" margin.[52]

Most vulvar sarcomas arise in the labia majora, and a wide age range (6 to 64 years) is noted.[45] Leiomyosarcoma is the most common sarcoma involving the vulva. Local pain and an enlarging mass are typical presenting symptoms.[53] The tumors are frequently 5 cm or larger when first detected. Lymphatic metastases are uncommon.

## DIAGNOSIS

Since there are no pathognomonic features of vulvar diseases, early diagnosis of vulvar cancer requires maintenance of a high index of suspicion and biopsy of any vulvar abnormality. A wedge biopsy with a knife or a circular biopsy with a Keye's or Baker's dermal punch under local infiltration anesthesia provides an excellent specimen. The biopsy specimen should include some surrounding skin, underlying dermis, and connective tissue so the pathologist can adequately evaluate the depth and nature of stromal invasion. Excisional biopsy is preferred for lesions smaller than 1 cm in diameter.

Initial evaluation should include a detailed physical examination that includes measurements of the vulvar lesion, assessment of extension to adjacent structures, bimanual pelvic examination, and

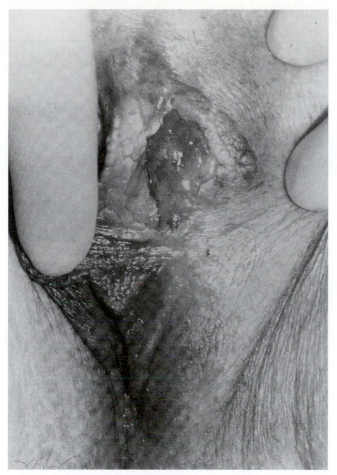

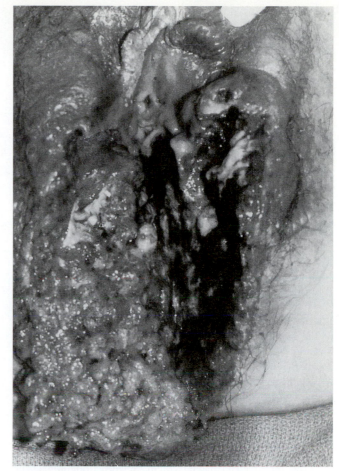

**FIGURE 18A-6.** This T2 lesion arises on the left labium majus and demonstrates the typical irregular surface features and superficial ulceration of a squamous cell carcinoma. (Reprinted from Burke TW, Eifel P, McGuire W, Wilkinson EJ. Vulva. In: Hoskins WJ, Perez CA, Young RC, eds. *Principles and Practice of Gynecologic Oncology.* 2nd ed. Philadelphia, PA: Lippincott-Raven Publishers; 1997:721, with permission.)

**FIGURE 18A-7.** This patient ignored symptoms and an obvious tumor for more than a year. (Reprinted from Burke TW, Eifel P, McGuire W, Wilkinson EJ. Vulva. In Hoskins WJ, Perez CA, Young RC, eds. *Principles and Practice of Gynecologic Oncology.* 2nd ed. Philadelphia, PA: Lippincott-Raven Publishers; 1997:722, with permission.)

assessment of inguinal lymph node involvement. Because neoplasia of the female genital tract is often multifocal, the vagina and cervix should be carefully inspected, and a Papanicolaou (Pap) smear of the cervix must be obtained.

Women with small cancers and clinically negative inguinal lymph nodes require few diagnostic studies other than those needed for surgical clearance. Additional studies should be considered for those patients with large primary tumors or suspected metastases. Cystoscopy and proctoscopy may be performed in women with advanced lesions or with tumors that are near the urethra or anus, respectively. Patients who complain of bone pain or who have tumor fixed to pelvic bones should have appropriate skeletal radiographs. Computed tomography (CT) or magnetic resonance imaging (MRI) may be helpful in outlining the extent of tumor and in evaluating the deep inguinal, pelvic, and para-aortic lymph nodes. Fine-needle aspiration biopsy from sites of suspected metastases may eliminate

the need for surgical exploration in some patients with advanced tumors.

## STAGING OF THE DISEASE

In 1983, the International Federation of Gynecology and Obstetrics (FIGO) adopted a clinical TNM staging system for vulvar carcinoma. Staging was based on a clinical assessment of the primary tumor and the regional lymph nodes. Although this system provided reliable information regarding the primary lesion, it rendered an inaccurate assessment of inguinal lymph node status in 20% to 30% of cases. Due to the relatively large magnitude of these staging errors, FIGO changed to a modified surgical staging system in 1989. Nodal status is determined by the surgical evaluation of the groin, and the presence or absence of distant metastases is based on an unspecified diagnostic workup tailored to the patient's clinical presentation. The staging

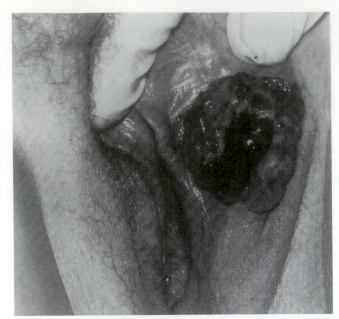

**FIGURE 18A-8.** Nodular, darkly pigmented malignant melanoma of the left labium majus. (Reprinted from Burke TW, Eifel P, McGuire W, Wilkinson EJ. Vulva. In: Hoskins WJ, Perez CA, Young RC, eds. *Principles and Practice of Gynecologic Oncology.* 2nd ed. Philadelphia, PA: Lippincott-Raven Publishers; 1997:746, with permission.)

system was further revised in 1995, dividing stage I into stages IA and IB based on the depth of stromal invasion.[54] Table 18A-4 shows the most recent FIGO staging system for vulvar carcinoma. The American Joint Commission on Cancer (AJCC) has published a TNM classification scheme that is correlated with the FIGO staging system (Table 18A-4).[55]

The FIGO staging system used for vulvar carcinoma is not applicable for vulvar melanoma because these lesions are usually much smaller and the prognosis is related to the depth of penetration rather than to the diameter of the lesion. Three microstaging systems have been described which determine the stage of melanoma based on either its depth of local invasion or tumor thickness.[56–58] A comparison of the three systems is shown in Table 18A-5. Of these three systems, the Breslow system of levels, which is based on tumor thickness as multiples of 0.75 mm, appears to have the most prognostic significance for vulvar melanoma.[59] No formal staging system exists for vulvar sarcomas, although the FIGO system for vulvar carcinomas is occasionally applied.

## PROGNOSTIC FACTORS

For patients with vulvar squamous cell carcinomas, lymph node metastasis is the single most important prognostic factor. In a study of 588 patients treated on two Gynecologic Oncology Group (GOG) trials, Homesley and co-workers[60] reported a 5-year survival rate of 91% in patients with negative inguinal lymph nodes, which

## TABLE 18A-4. STAGING OF VULVAR CARCINOMA

**Primary tumor (T):**

TX   Primary tumor cannot be assessed.

T0   No evidence of primary tumor.

Tis  Carcinoma in situ.

T1   Tumor confined to the vulva or perineum; 2 cm or less in greatest dimension.

T2   Tumor confined to the vulva or perineum; more than 2 cm in greatest dimension.

T3   Tumor of any size with adjacent spread to the lower urethra, vagina, or anus.

T4   Tumor invades the upper urethra, bladder mucosa, rectal mucosa, or pelvic bone.

**Regional lymph nodes (N):**

NX   Regional lymph nodes cannot be assessed.

N0   No regional lymph node metastasis.

N1   Unilateral regional lymph node metastasis.

N2   Bilateral regional lymph node metastasis.

**Distant metastasis (M):**

MX   Presence of distant metastasis cannot be assessed.

M0   No distant metastasis.

M1   Distant metastasis.

**STAGE GROUPINGS**

| FIGO | AJCC | CLINICAL/PATHOLOGIC FINDING |
|---|---|---|
| 0 | Tis N0 M0 | Carcinoma in situ; intraepithelial carcinoma. |
| I | T1 N0 M0 | Tumor confined to the vulva or perineum; 2 cm or less in greatest dimension; no nodal metastases. |
| IA | | Stromal invasion ≤ 1 mm. |
| IB | | Stromal invasion > 1 mm. |
| II | T2 N0 M0 | Tumor confined to the vulva or perineum; more than 2 cm in greatest dimension; no nodal metastases. |
| III | T1 N1 M0<br>T2 N1 M0<br>T3 N0 M0<br>T3 N1 M0 | Tumor of any size with adjacent spread to the lower urethra, vagina, or anus; and/or unilateral lymph node metastasis. |
| IVA | T1 N2 M0<br>T2 N2 M0<br>T3 N2 M0<br>T4 Any N M0 | Tumor invades the upper urethra, bladder mucosa, rectal mucosa, or pelvic bone; and/or bilateral regional lymph node metastasis. |
| IVB | Any T Any N M1 | Any distant metastasis including pelvic lymph nodes. |

SOURCE: Modified from Beahrs OH et al: Gynecologic tumors, in *Manual for Staging of Cancer*, 4th ed, OH Beahrs et al (eds). Philadelphia, Lippincott, 1992, pp 155–180. Used with permission.

**TABLE 18A-5. MICROSTAGING SYSTEMS FOR VULVAR MELANOMAS**

| LEVEL | CLARK ET AL[56] | CHUNG ET AL[57] | BRESLOW[58] |
|---|---|---|---|
| I | Intraepithelial | Intraepithelial | <0.76 mm |
| II | Into papillary dermis | ≤1 mm from granular layer | 0.76–1.50 mm |
| III | Filling dermal papillae | 1.1–2.0 mm from granular layer | 1.51–2.25 mm |
| IV | Into reticular dermis | >2 mm from granular layer | 2.26–3.0 mm |
| V | Into subcutaneous | Into subcutaneous fat | >3.0 |

decreased to 75%, 36%, 24%, and 0% in patients with one or two, three or four, five or six, or seven or more positive lymph nodes, respectively. Patients with bilateral lymph node involvement had a survival rate of 25%, compared to 71% for those with unilateral involvement.

Other major prognostic factors include FIGO stage, tumor size, depth of invasion, tumor grade, and the presence of lymph vascular space invasion.[34,60–62] These features tend to be correlated with one another and all are predictive of lymph node metastasis.

Van der Velden and colleagues'[63] recent review of 71 patients with vulvar squamous cell carcinoma and positive lymph nodes demonstrated that extracapsular growth of lymph node metastases in the groin is also an important predictor of poor survival. Twenty-eight of 44 patients (64%) with extranodal spread died of disease, compared to 3 of 22 patients (14%) without this finding.

Studying the relationship between surgical resection margins and tumor recurrence, Heaps and co-workers[64] demonstrated a sharp rise in the incidence of local recurrence based on the width of the tumor-free margins. In the 91 patients with a tumor-free margin of greater than 8 mm, none had a local recurrence, compared to a 48% (21 out of 44 patients) local recurrence rate in patients with a margin of less than 8 mm. Since their analysis was performed on formalin-fixed specimens, they suggested that the 8-mm margin would correspond to 1-cm margins in fresh, unfixed tissue.

The data on prognostic factors for nonsquamous cell vulvar malignancies is much less extensive. For patients with vulvar melanoma, both the thickness of the melanoma and its depth of invasion have been shown to correlate with its pattern of spread and prognosis.[56–59] As with squamous carcinomas, lymph node status is highly prognostic for patients with Bartholin's carinomas. The prognosis of patients with vulvar leiomyosarcoma appears to depend on three main factors: lesion size, tumor contour, and mitotic activity. Lesions larger than 5 cm in diameter with infiltrating margins and more than five mitotic figures per 10 high-power fields have the worst prognosis.[53,65,66]

## TREATMENT

Due to the pioneering work of Taussig[6] and Way[7] during the 1940s and 50s, en bloc radical vulvectomy with bilateral inguinofemoral (superficial and deep inguinal) lymphadenectomy became the standard treatment for most patients with operable vulvar cancer. Although this operative approach achieved gratifying 5-year survival rates of 60% to 70%, the surgery caused significant physical and psychologic morbidity.[67] Numerous subsequent studies demonstrated that operating through separate vulvar and groin incisions achieves comparable cure rates with less morbidity than traditional radical vulvectomy. Based on these study results, the management of vulvar carcinoma has evolved over the past two decades from a one-disease, one-operation approach to a philosophy of maximum individualization, conservation, and restoration.[68] Modern optimal management requires careful consideration of less radical surgery for early-stage disease, the use of plastic reconstructive techniques for large surgical defects, and the incorporation of radiation therapy into the treatment regimen of locoregionally advanced disease.

## PREINVASIVE DISEASE

*VULVAR INTRAEPITHELIAL NEOPLASIA (VIN).* Several studies have reported that approximately 4% of patients with VIN will progress to invasive vulvar cancer.[69,70] However, what is generally not emphasized in these follow-up studies is that most of the patients were treated for their VIN. In one of the few studies of untreated VIN followed prospectively, seven of eight women with VIN 3 who received no treatment went on to develop invasive vulvar carcinoma.[71] Although several cases of spontaneous remission of VIN have been reported, due to its clear potential for progression to invasive carcinoma, the recommended treatment for VIN is surgical excision.

After invasive carcinoma has been excluded by performing a sufficient number of excisional biopsies, the surgical excision of VIN should be as conservative as possible. Wide local excision with removal of the full thickness of skin or mucosa followed by primary closure can be performed in most patients. Although surgical excision margins of only 2 to 3 mm are required, skin flaps or skin grafts may occasionally be necessary to restore normal anatomy in patients with large surgical defects. Patients with extensive or diffuse VIN may require superficial (skinning) vulvectomy in which full or partial thickness of the vulva skin or mucosa are removed, preserving the subcutaneous and other deeper tissues.[68] Some authors use the carbon dioxide ($CO_2$) laser to vaporize multifocal lesions. However, this method does not provide a specimen for histologic review. Therefore, most authorities recommend the restriction of the $CO_2$ laser to physicians experienced in vulvar disease to avoid vaporizing unrecognized invasive carcinoma.[68,72]

VIN often recurs at or near the margins of resection, even when the histologic analysis demonstrates that the initial lesions were completely resected. This phenomenon most likely represents the multifocal nature of the disease, as VIN has even been reported to recur within the donor skin from a skin graft.[73] Most patients with recurrent disease can be managed by repeat wide local excision.

*VULVAR PAGET'S DISEASE.* In the absence of clinical or biopsy evidence of invasive carcinoma, wide local excision is the standard treatment for vulvar Paget's disease. Although underlying adenocarcinomas are usually clinically apparent, this is not invariable. Thus, the underlying dermis should be removed for adequate histologic evaluation. For this same reason, laser therapy is unsatisfactory for primary disease. Unlike VIN, where the histologic extent of disease usually correlates closely with the macroscopic lesion, vulvar Paget's disease usually extends subepithelially well beyond the gross lesion.[74] While in the operating room, frozen section diagnosis of surgical margin status is recommended to ensure complete removal.

Local recurrence rates of approximately 30% have been reported, but most of these recurrences may be attributable to positive margins at the time of resection.[68] Recurrent lesions are almost always in situ. Due to the low risk of invasion, it is reasonable to treat recurrent disease with either repeat local excision or laser ablation. However, if a primary or recurrent lesion is associated with an invasive adenocarcinoma, the patient should be managed according to the extent of invasion, as outlined for squamous cell carcinoma.[72]

## T1 SQUAMOUS CELL CARCINOMA

*MANAGEMENT OF THE PRIMARY LESION.* Traditionally, invasive squamous cell carcinoma was considered a "diffuse disease involving the entire vulva."[75] Anything less than radical vulvectomy was considered inadequate treatment with a high likelihood of local recurrence. In addition, there was concern that without an en bloc resection, intervening tissue left between the primary tumor and the inguinal lymph nodes would contain residual microscopic tumor foci in the draining lymphatics. However, it has been shown that squamous carcinomas spread by lymphatic embolization rather than permeation, and experience with a separate incision technique for inguinal lymph node dissection has confirmed that metastases rarely occur in the intervening skin bridge in patients without clinically suspicious inguinal nodes.[72,76–79] Moreover, in a recent literature review of patients with T1 vulvar carcinomas, Hacker and van der Velden[80] reported a similar, locally invasive recurrence rate of 7% in 165 patients treated conservatively by radical local excision, compared to 6% in 365 patients treated with traditional radical vulvectomy.

Most authorities agree that aggressive but local resection of T1 vulvar carcinoma is safe and effective treatment. Various terms have been used to describe the procedure, including the following: "radical local excision," "radical wide excision," "wide deep excision," "modified vulvectomy," and "radical hemivulvectomy." The procedure requires a wide and deep excision of the primary tumor; the surgical margins should be at least 1 to 2 cm, with the dissection carried down to the inferior fascia of the urogenital diaphragm.[22,64] Most excision sites for small tumors can be closed primarily.

*MANAGEMENT OF THE INGUINAL LYMPH NODES.* Patients who have T1 tumors with stromal invasion of less than 1 mm have minimal risk of lymph node metastases (see Table 18A-3). Due to the negligible risk of lymphatic dissemination (provided that the groin nodes are clinically negative), these patients can be managed with radical local excision alone. However, patients with T1 tumors and stromal invasion of greater than 1 mm have a significant risk of inguinal lymph node metastases (see Table 18A-3). The optimal management of the inguinal lymph nodes in these patients has been addressed in two recent GOG studies.

In the first study,[81] patients with clinically negative groins who had their T1 to T3 tumors totally removed by radical vulvectomy were randomized to receive either bilateral superficial and deep inguinal dissection or bilateral inguinal irradiation. Those patients who underwent groin dissections and were found to have positive lymph nodes received postoperative irradiation to the inguinal and pelvic nodes on the involved side. After only 58 of the planned 300 patients were enrolled in the study, it was closed prematurely when interim monitoring revealed an excessive number of groin relapses on the radiation regimen. There were 5 inguinal relapses among the 27 patients (18.5%) on the groin irradiation regimen and none on the groin dissection regimen. Although the technique and dosage used in the irradiation arm of the study have been criticized, the significantly superior progression-free and overall survival for the patients treated with groin dissection confirmed the benefit of inguinal dissection as part of the standard management approach for this group of patients.

In the second GOG study,[82] patients with T1 vulvar carcinoma and clinically negative inguinal lymph nodes were treated with modified radical hemivulvectomy and ipsilateral superficial inguinal lymphadenectomy. Patients who, after having a frozen section removed during the operation, were found to have metastasis to the superficial inguinal nodes underwent radical vulvectomy and bilateral superficial and deep inguinal lymphadenectomy. These patients were then excluded from further analysis. The resultant study group was composed of 121 patients with T1 tumors less than 5 mm thick and surgically documented negative superficial inguinal lymph nodes. This study group was compared to a similar group of patients from a prior GOG study. Patients in the historic control group had all been treated with radical vulvectomy and bilateral superficial and deep inguinal lymphadenectomy. There was no difference in the overall survival rates between the two groups, while the acute and long-term morbidity rates were less in the patients treated with more conservative surgery. However, 6 of the 121 study patients (5%) had recurrence in the operated (ipsilateral) node-negative groin, compared to no groin recurrences in the 96 historic control patients. Moreover, five of the seven deaths due to cancer in the study group occurred among patients whose first recurrence was in the groin. The authors concluded that the recurrence rate in the operated groin was troubling and may have been attributable to the decision to leave the deep inguinal lymph nodes intact.

The data from these two GOG studies and others in the literature demonstrate that patients with lateral T1 vulvar carcinomas that invade greater than 1 mm may be safely managed with radical local excision and unilateral groin dissection. However, for more centrally located T1 tumors within 2 cm of the clitoris or perineal body, a bilateral groin dissection should be performed, due to the potential for bilateral lymphatic flow. In order to avoid the high mortality rate associated with groin recurrence, most authors recommend that groin dissections routinely include a thorough superficial and deep inguinal lymphadenectomy.[68,72]

*TECHNIQUE FOR INGUINOFEMORAL LYMPHADENECTOMY.* The incisions used for radical local excision and bilateral groin dissection are shown in Fig. 18A-9. The operation is usually done with the patient in the low lithotomy position. In performing the groin dissection, the incision is continued down directly to the inguinal ligament. The superficial subcutaneous fat is left attached to the skin to provide blood supply, but is separated from

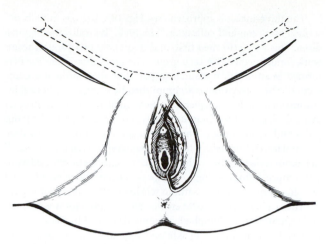

**FIGURE 18A-9.** Radical hemivulvectomy (radical local excision) with bilateral groin dissection through three separate incisions. Separate groin incisions begin at the anterior superior iliac spine, 2 cm below the inguinal ligament, and extend to the public tubercle. (Reprinted from Woodruff JD, Buscema J. Surgical conditions of the vulva. In: Thompson JD, Rock JA, eds. *Te Linde's Operative Gynecology.* 7th ed. Philadelphia, PA: J.B. Lippincott Co; 1992:1109, with permission.)

the underlying nodal tissue by dissecting inferiorly at the level of Camper's fascia. The specimen is developed by continuing the inferior dissection along the borders of the sartorius muscle laterally and the adductor longus muscle medially. The cribriform fascia is then opened along the sartorius muscle and mobilized medially as part of the specimen. This helps identify the femoral vessels, which are dissected free so that the deep nodes can be removed in continuity with the superficial nodes. The saphenous vein is generally tied off at its point of entry into the femoral vein and again at the lower margin of the dissection at the apex of the femoral triangle.

Many surgeons protect the femoral vessels by dividing the sartorius muscle at its origin from the anterior superior iliac spine and then suturing its free edge to the inguinal ligament medially, thus transposing the muscle over the vessels. A recent review of 101 patients undergoing inguinofemoral lymphadenectomy demonstrated a 25% decrease in significant groin morbidity in patients who had sartorius muscle transposition, compared to those who did not.[83] At the conclusion of the dissection, a closed suction drain is placed to prevent lymphocyst formation and the incision is closed in layers.

*ADDITIONAL TREATMENT.* Most authors recommend no additional treatment for patients managed in the above fashion who are found to have zero or one microscopically involved lymph nodes.[84–86] Even if one microscopically involved lymph node is found in a patient who has undergone a unilateral groin dissection, the risk of metastases to the contralateral groin or pelvic lymph nodes is low—provided that the groin does not contain clinically suspicious nodes.[26,84,85] The prognosis for this group of patients is excellent, and only careful observation is required.[60,85,86]

Patients who have two or more positive inguinal lymph nodes are at increased risk for metastases to the contralateral groin and pelvic

lymph nodes.[84,85] In a prospective trial performed by the GOG,[85] 114 patients with positive inguinal lymph nodes after radical vulvectomy and bilateral inguinofemoral lymphadenectomy were randomized to receive either pelvic node dissection on the involved side(s) or bilateral pelvic and inguinal irradiation. The study was closed early due to a clear-cut superiority in the 2-year survival rate of the pelvic irradiation treatment arm (68% versus 54%). The survival advantage was limited to patients with clinically evident groin nodes or more than one positive inguinal lymph node. These data indicate that patients with two or more positive groin nodes are best treated with bilateral pelvic and inguinal irradiation consisting of 4500 to 5000 cGy delivered over 5 to 6 weeks.[85]

Patients who have a single positive lymph node with either macroscopic involvement or extracapsular tumor growth are at high risk for recurrent disease and therefore should also receive postoperative irradiation.[63,86] In patients with tumor-free surgical resection margins measuring less than 1 cm, the central vulva area should be included in the radiation field due to their high risk of local recurrence.[64]

Management becomes somewhat controversial for patients who have undergone a unilateral groin dissection and are found to have a single high-risk positive node or two or more positive nodes. Some authors recommend inguinofemoral lymphadenectomy of the undissected groin prior to radiation therapy,[68,86] while others recommend radiotherapy alone because of the high morbidity rate associated with inguinofemoral lymphadenectomy combined with groin irradiation.[72,87,88]

*POSTOPERATIVE MORBIDITY.* Although the more limited surgical approach to women with small vulvar cancers has substantially decreased postoperative morbidity, the incidence of groin complications and lower-extremity lymphedema is still significant. With the use of separate incisions, the incidence of inguinal wound breakdown has decreased from over 80% to between 40% and 50%, while the incidence of chronic lower-extremity lymphedema has decreased from approximately 30% to 15%.[9,68,76] The risk of lymphedema and chronic groin complications is related to the extent of inguinal dissection. Patients who undergo superficial and deep inguinal lymphadenectomy followed by irradiation have the greatest likelihood of morbidity.[22]

In an effort to further reduce the postoperative morbidity associated with groin dissection, Levenback and colleagues[89] are currently investigating the use of intraoperative lymphatic mapping to identify the sentinel inguinal lymph node. If this method proves to be a reliable and accurate means of predicting nodal metastases, certain subsets of patients may be able to avoid extensive inguinal lymphadenectomy and its associated morbidity.

### T2 SQUAMOUS CELL CARCINOMA

*CONSERVATIVE MANAGEMENT.* During the past decade, the role of radical local excision for vulvar carcinoma has expanded to encompass select patients with T2 tumors. Although the reported experience is less extensive than that for T1 lesions, recent studies have demonstrated that as long as surgical margins of at least 1 cm are obtained, the local recurrence rate for patients with T2 tumors treated with radical local excision is identical to that for similarly treated patients with T1 carcinomas.[85,89] As with T1 tumors, as long as the inguinal lymph nodes are clinically negative and the T2 lesion is located greater than 2 cm from the midline structures, unilateral groin dissection may be performed.[68] However, regardless of the type of resection used for the primary tumor, any and all enlarged, fixed, or ulcerating inguinal lymph nodes should be removed. Nodes with these features are highly suggestive of metastatic disease,[34,61] and their resection will improve local control and probably enhance the curative potential of postoperative irradiation.[22,72,85] As with T1 tumors, due to the potential for bilateral lymphatic flow, bilateral inguinofemoral lymphadenectomy is required for T2 lesions where the tumor is less than 2 cm away from the clitoris or perineal body.

*RADICAL VULVECTOMY AND INGUINOFEMORAL LYM-PHADENECTOMY.* Radical vulvectomy is indicated for cancers that are so extensive that a more conservative resection would leave the patient with a vulva that has no functional or cosmetic benefit. The operation has two main variants: (1) vulvectomy and inguinofemoral lymphadenectomy using separate incisions (Fig. 18A-10); and (2) vulvectomy and inguinofemoral lymphadenectomy using a single incision (Fig. 18A-11). Although separate incisions are preferred because of the associated reduction in morbidity,[76,79,90] leaving all or most of the mons pubis in the treatment of locally extensive disease carries an increasing risk of local failure as the tumor size increases and approaches the retained tissue. Therefore, the size and geographic distribution of the carcinoma must be the deciding factors in designing the resection.[68]

The three-incision approach (see Fig. 18A-10) was initially described by Byron and colleagues[91] in 1962. Typically, the inguinal dissections are performed first, and frequently two surgical teams work simultaneously on each groin. The groin dissections are performed in an identical manner to that described in the preceding section. The vulvectomy is accomplished by using two elliptical incisions: an inner incision placed at the vaginal introitus and an outer incision placed at the labiocrural folds and brought across the mons pubis and perineal body. The incision is carried down to the deep perineal fascia, from which the ring-shaped specimen is detached. If the tumor is close to the urethra, the distal 2 cm may be resected without compromising continence. Primary closure is often possible, but this should be performed without tension on the urethra or vagina.

The original technique for en bloc radical vulvectomy with bilateral inguinofemoral lymphadenectomy described by Stanley Way[7] removed a large amount of skin and subcutaneous tissue over the mons pubis and femoral triangles, making closure always under tension, if achievable at all. Consequently, delayed healing because of granulation of open wounds and prolonged hospitalization were the norm. Over the past two decades, the skin incision has been modified (Fig. 18A-11) to minimize the skin resected, thereby improving primary healing.[92] With the modified skin-sparing incision, the superior portion extends from the lateral margins of the groin dissections across the mons pubis. The lateral vulvar incisions are placed along the labiocrural folds. These incisions are taken down to the level of the deep inguinal and perineal fascia to permit en bloc removal of the superficial and deep inguinal lymph nodes, the entire vulva, and an intervening skin bridge (Fig. 18A-12). Following removal of

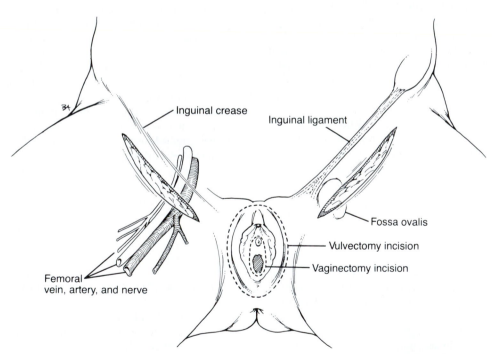

**FIGURE 18A-10.** Vulvectomy and bilateral groin dissection through three separate incisions. (Reprinted from Hacker NF. Surgery for malignant tumors of the vulva. In: Gershenson DM, DeCherney AH, Curry SL, eds. *Operative Gynecology.* Philadelphia, PA: W.B. Saunders Company; 1993:181, with permission.)

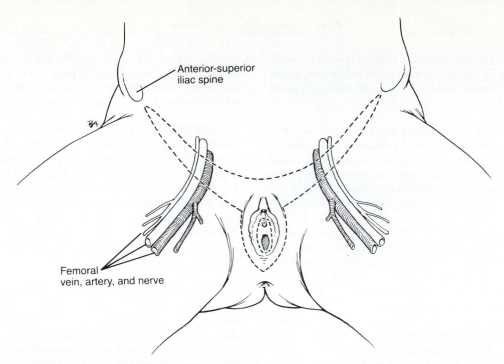

**FIGURE 18A-11.** Modified, skin-sparing incision for en bloc radical vulvectomy and bilateral groin dissection. (Reprinted from Hacker NF. Surgery for malignant tumors of the vulva. In: Gershenson DM, DeCherney AH, Curry SL, eds. *Operative Gynecology*. Philadelphia, PA: W.B. Saunders Company; 1993:184, with permission.)

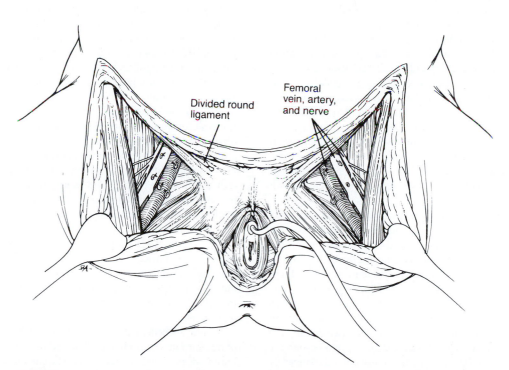

**FIGURE 18A-12.** Femoral triangle after dissection of the inguinal and femoral lymph nodes. (Reprinted from Hacker NF. Surgery for malignant tumors of the vulva. In: Gershenson DM, DeCherney AH, Curry SL, eds. *Operative Gynecology*. Philadelphia, PA: W.B. Saunders Company; 1993:182, with permission.)

the specimen, closed suction drains are usually placed in the groin sites. By undermining and mobilizing the skin and mucosal edges, primary closure of the vulvar incision can usually be accomplished without tension.

*CLOSURE OF LARGE SURGICAL DEFECTS.* Although it is usually possible to close vulvar defects primarily, occasionally extensive resections and/or poor tissue mobility make primary closure without tension impossible. In these cases, the main surgical options available for repair of the defect involve covering the defect with a full-thickness skin flap or reconstructing the area with a myocutaneous flap.

The rhomboid flap is a full-thickness skin flap that has proved to be an excellent option for the repair of vulvar defects not amenable to primary closure.[93,94] It is a local tissue advancement flap that draws its blood supply from the subcutaneous vascular network. These flaps can be developed at any level of the vulva. Single or combination flaps can be made to cover a wide variety of defects. The maximum practical flap size for the vulva is about 4 cm × 4 cm. Larger flaps require extensive local tissue dissection and can be difficult to rotate into the desired position because of poor mobility.

The rhomboid flap is created by making a V-shaped incision adjacent to the tissue defect needing coverage (Fig. 18A-13). The flap size should be slightly larger than the measured surgical defect to allow for flexibility in trimming the flap edge to accommodate the shape of the defect. The incision is carried down approximately 1 to 1.5 cm into the subcutaneous tissue, and the flap is then mobilized by undermining the tissue adjacent to the flap. The flap can then be rotated over the defect and sutured into place.

Myocutaneous flaps contain skin, subcutaneous tissue, and a segment of muscle. They receive their blood supply and innervation through a clearly defined neurovascular pedicle. Because these flaps bring in a new blood supply to the area, they are particularly helpful if the vulva is poorly vascularized due to prior surgery or irradiation. And since these flaps are large, thick tissue sources, they are capable of reconstructing substantial tissue defects. Various types of myocutaneous flaps have been used to repair large vulvar and groin defects, including rectus abdominis flaps, gluteus maximus flaps, tensor fascia lata flaps, and gracilis flaps. While each of these flaps has its own unique advantages, the most reported experience is with the gracilis flap.

The gracilis muscle is a broad, flat muscle located in the superficial portion of the medial thigh. It is a weak adductor, whose absence produces little perceptible deficit. The flap design is initiated by drawing a guideline from the pubic tubercle to the medial femoral condyle.[95] The muscle lies directly beneath this line. An elliptically shaped skin paddle is then outlined adjacent to the guideline (Fig. 18A-14). The dimensions of the paddle should be no greater than 10 to 12 cm × 6 to 8 cm, because larger flaps have a higher incidence of necrosis and wound separation.[96] The skin-paddle incision is carried down to the gracilis fascia, and the muscle is transected about 3 cm beyond the distal margin of the paddle. The myocutaneous unit is developed by continuing the dissection proximally. The main vascular bundle is usually encountered approximately 7 cm below the pubic tubercle. This pedicle should be preserved; however, if additional mobility is necessary, it can be sacrificed. Flap viability is thought to be retained through blood supply derived from the more proximal obturator branches.[22] Once fully developed, the flap is mobilized through a subcutaneous tunnel to reach the perineum or groin. The flap can be trimmed and sutured into position and the thigh donor site closed with interrupted fascial sutures and skin staples.

*ADDITIONAL TREATMENT.* Postoperatively, the recommended management for these patients is similar to patients with T1 tumors: observation for patients with zero or one microscopically positive lymph node and bilateral inguinal and pelvic irradiation for those with a single high-risk (macroscopic involvement or extracapsular tumor growth) node or two or more positive nodes.[84–86] There is no general consensus as to whether patients who undergo unilateral groin dissection and have a single high-risk node or two or more positive nodes should have their contralateral groins dissected prior to the radiation therapy.

T3 AND T4 SQUAMOUS CELL CARCINOMA. For patients with small T3 tumors that invade the vagina or lower urethra, partial vaginectomy or urethrectomy may be combined with radical vulvectomy to obtain adequate surgical margins. If the margins are inadequate, postoperative radiation therapy can be delivered to prevent local recurrence.[9] However, for larger tumors or those that involve the anus, rectum, or proximal urethra, extended radical vulvectomy will not remove all of the disease. In these cases, adequate surgical clearance of the primary tumor is possible only by partial or total pelvic exenteration combined with radical vulvectomy and bilateral groin dissection.

In a cumulative literature review, Cavanagh and Hoffman[97] reported a 46% 5-year disease-free survival rate for 184 patients who underwent exenteration for vulvar cancer from 1970 to 1995. However, the substantial risks of postoperative mortality (up to 20%)[97] and acute and long-term complications (over 50%)[98,99] associated with this ultraradical procedure have led investigators to search for less morbid treatment options.

Boronow and colleagues[100] have used preoperative radiation therapy to shrink locally advanced vulvovaginal carcinoma to the point where a more limited resection could be performed. With this approach, the authors report improved resection margins, spared organ function, and improved quality of life for most patients. Forty-eight patients with primary and recurrent disease were treated with this method. Bladder and rectal resection were required in only two and three patients, respectively. Seventeen of the 40 vulvectomy specimens (42.5%) contained no evidence of residual cancer. The 5-year survival rate for the 37 primary cases was 75.6%. Several other investigators have reported excellent responses and high local control rates for locally advanced vulvar carcinomas treated with preoperative radiation therapy.[22] The irradiation generally involves external-beam therapy of moderately high doses (4500 to 5000 cGy) delivered over 5 to 6 weeks.

In 1993, Benedetti-Panici and co-workers[101] reported on the use of neoadjuvant chemotherapy followed by surgery in patients with locally advanced vulvar carcinoma. The chemotherapeutic regimen consisted of cisplatin, bleomycin, and methotrexate given for two or three cycles. Two of the 21 patients (10%) had partial responses in the primary tumor, and 14 (67%) had partial responses in their nodal disease. Local control was achieved in 12 patients (57%) and the 3-year survival rate was only 24%.

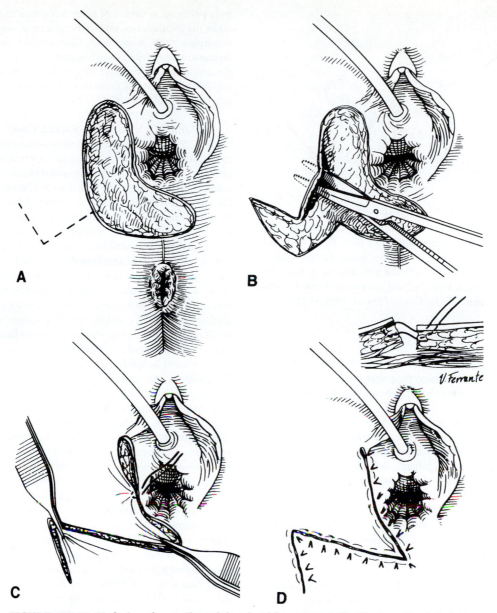

V. Ferrante

**FIGURE 18A-13.** Technique for a unilateral rhomboid flap repair. *A.* The flap is outlined. *B.* A 1-cm-thick flap of skin and subcutaneous tissue is raised. The area is undermined. *C.* The flap is rotated, and stay sutures are placed. *D.* Completed repair. (Reprinted from Burke TW, Eifel P, McGuire W, Wilkinson EJ. Vulva. In: Hoskins WJ, Perez CA, Young RC, eds. *Principles and Practice of Gynecologic Oncology.* 2nd ed. Philadelphia, PA: Lippincott-Raven Publishers; 1997:739, with permission.)

Thomas and colleagues[102] added concurrent 5-fluorouracil (5-FU) chemotherapy with or without mitomycin C to radiation therapy in the treatment of 33 patients with vulvar cancer. There were six complete vulvar responses in the nine patients treated with primary chemoradiation alone. However, three of the six subsequently had a local recurrence, suggesting the need to combine the chemoradiation with excision of the primary tumor bed. Berek and co-workers[103] treated 12 patients with advanced vulvar carcinoma with preoper-

ative chemoradiation using cisplatin and 5-FU. The 3-year survival rate was 83%.

With the experience now accrued, preoperative radiation, with or without concurrent chemotherapy, should be regarded as the treatment of first choice for patients with advanced vulvar carcinoma who would otherwise require some type of pelvic exenteration.[72] Although the data at this time are insufficient to determine whether concurrent chemotherapy adds to the efficacy of preoperative

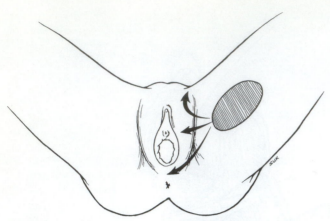

**FIGURE 18A-14.** Diagrammatic representation of possible external placements for a gracilis myocutaneous flap. These flaps can be used to reconstruct large defects of the groin, labium majus, or perineal body. (Reprinted from Burke TW, Morris M, Roh MS, Levenback C, Gershenson DM. Perineal reconstruction using single gracilis myocutaneous flaps. *Gynecol Oncol.* 1995;57:223, with permission.)

radiation therapy, impressive responses have been described for some very advanced lesions, suggesting that the results of preoperative chemoradiation may prove to be better than those attainable with radiation alone.

The GOG[104] is currently evaluating the role of preoperative concurrent radiation and chemotherapy in the treatment of advanced vulvar cancers not amenable to radical vulvectomy. Preliminary results are promising, as 34 of 71 patients (48%) had no visible tumor following preoperative treatment with cisplatin, 5-FU, and irradiation. Moreover, among the 50 patients who presented with vulvar cancers that would have otherwise required exenteration, only two (4%) required exenterative surgery to resect residual disease after chemoradiation. The final analysis of these data will help determine the optimum treatment regimen for this group of patients.

### DISTANT METASTATIC (M1) SQUAMOUS CELL CARCINOMA.

The incidence of pelvic node metastases in vulvar carcinoma is less than 10%. Due to the documented efficacy of inguinal and pelvic irradiation for patients with positive groin nodes, the routine use of pelvic lymphadenectomy in these patients has largely been abandoned. However, in the GOG study reported by Homesley,[84] the incidence of pelvic recurrence was higher in the group of patients receiving pelvic irradiation, possibly because of the inability of external beam radiotherapy to sterilize bulky positive pelvic lymph nodes. Furthermore, collated results from the literature suggest that approximately 20% of patients with involved pelvic lymph nodes may be rendered disease-free by pelvic lymphadenectomy.[86] For these reasons, some authorities recommend resection of all enlarged pelvic lymph nodes detected by radiologic imaging techniques, followed by radiation therapy or chemoradiation therapy to the groin and pelvis.[72,105]

Although occasional apparent cures have been described for various combinations of surgery, irradiation, and chemotherapy, the treatment of patients with other distant metastases is essen-

tially palliative. A variety of drugs have been tested in Phase II trials in the treatment of metastatic recurrent vulvar squamous cell carcinoma. Only doxorubicin (Adriamycin) and bleomycin have demonstrated activity as single agents.[106,107] Combination regimens containing bleomycin have shown significant responses, but the number of patients in these series is too small to make any definite recommendations.[108,109]

### RECURRENT SQUAMOUS CELL CARCINOMA.

Approximately 15% to 40% of patients with squamous cell carcinoma of the vulva will develop recurrence following treatment.[97] Recurrence correlates most closely with the number of positive inguinal lymph nodes.[84] Patients with fewer than three positive nodes, particularly if the nodes are only microscopically involved, have a low incidence of recurrence at any site. Patients with three or more positive nodes have a high incidence of local, regional, and systemic recurrences.[84,85]

Isolated vulvar recurrences account for about half of all recurrences. Many occur at sites remote from the primary tumor site or many years after apparently successful treatment, suggesting that some of these local recurrences represent the development of new disease. Up to 75% to 80% of these patients can be salvaged by further radical local excision.[97,110,111] If further surgical excision is not feasible, combination external-beam irradiation with interstitial brachytherapy has been used to treat isolated recurrences. Although this treatment is highly effective, the associated morbidity rate is high, with up to a 60% incidence of severe radionecrosis.[112,113]

Curative resection may still be possible when vulvar recurrence extends to the urethra or anus. Selected patients have achieved long-term survival after partial or total pelvic exenteration.[98,99] The surgical approach in these cases should be individualized to the size and location of the recurrent tumor. Due to their universally dismal prognosis, patients with recurrent nodal disease should not undergo exenterative surgery. Patients who develop regional groin recurrence are rarely curable,[38,110,114] because they have a high likelihood of also having pelvic and systemic disease. A small percentage of patients with recurrence in a previously unirradiated groin may be salvaged with resection followed by radiotherapy. However, surgical resection in a previously irradiated groin is unlikely to be curative and is associated with a substantial risk of wound breakdown. The debility caused by a combination of unresolved recurrence and surgical wound breakdown is worse than that of progressive recurrence alone.[22] Since no effective chemotherapy exists at this time for patients with recurrence in a previously irradiated groin, management of these patients should therefore be considered palliative in nature.

As for patients who have distant metastases at presentation, patients who develop systemic recurrence have a dismal prognosis, and all therapy is essentially palliative.

### TREATMENT OF NONSQUAMOUS CELL MALIGNANCIES.

Due to their infrequent occurrence, there is relatively little definitive information regarding the treatment of nonsquamous cell vulvar malignancies. Most available data are derived from small case series spanning long periods of time.

*MELANOMA.* The major treatment modality for vulvar melanoma is surgical. As with squamous cell carcinoma, the recent trend has been away from radical vulvectomy and toward a more conservative resection. The current recommendation for treatment is radical local excision of the primary lesion with a surgical margin of at least 2 cm.[105,115] Trimble and co-workers[116] and others have shown that survival with more conservative resection is similar to that achieved with radical vulvectomy.[115,117] Inguinal lymph node metastases are rare in patients with Breslow or Clark's Level I or II melanoma.[57,59] Therefore, lymphadenectomy can be avoided in these patients, and they may be treated with radical local excision alone. Furthermore, although regional lymph node dissection in vulvar melanoma probably serves more of a prognostic value than a therapeutic one,[59,118] most authorities recommend inguinofemoral lymphadenectomy for melanomas that are deeper than Level II.[72,105,116]

Radiation therapy may be useful in enhancing local and regional control for some high-risk patients[22]; doses in the range of 4000 cGy to 5000 cGy have been used effectively.[119] Systemic chemotherapy is generally ineffective in vulvar melanoma. Biologic and immunologic approaches are currently being investigated.[120]

Overall, the 5-year survival rate for women with vulvar melanoma is about 50%.[121,122] Patients with superficial lesions (Levels I and II) have an excellent chance for cure following surgical resection. However, patients with deeper invasion or metastases at the time of diagnosis have a poor prognosis.[57,59] These patients should be considered for investigational trials.

*BARTHOLIN'S GLAND CARCINOMA.* Bartholin's gland carcinoma traditionally has been treated by radical vulvectomy with bilateral inguinal and pelvic node dissection. The decision to perform a pelvic node dissection or administer pelvic irradiation should be based on the same criteria as used for squamous cell carcinoma.[105] Similarly, radical local excision may be as effective as radical vulvectomy.[123] Since the incidence of inguinal metastases is about 30%,[124] ipsilateral inguinofemoral lymphadenectomy should be included with the primary resection. Postoperative irradiation may reduce the incidence of vulvar and regional recurrence.[123] Because of the deep location of the Bartholin's glands, these cases tend to be more advanced at the time of diagnosis than squamous cell carcinomas. However, stage for stage, the prognosis is similar.

*BASAL CELL CARCINOMA.* Basal cell carcinomas are managed by radical local excision with a minimum surgical margin of 1 cm.[125] Although metastases to regional lymph nodes have been reported,[126] this is an exceedingly rare event and routine inguinal dissection is not indicated. The local recurrence rate is about 20%.[127] However, no patients have died as a result of this disease.

*SARCOMAS.* Leiomyosarcoma is the most common vulvar sarcoma. Occasional cures have been obtained with aggressive resection of either primary or locally recurrent disease. Radiation therapy may help to enhance local control. However, the natural history of vulvar leiomyosarcoma is characterized by a protracted course of frequent local recurrence, followed by distant fatal metastases. Chemotherapy is used chiefly for palliation rather than for cure.[105]

## FOLLOW-UP AND SURVIVAL

After completing treatment, patients should be examined every 3 to 4 months for 2 years and then every 6 months for the next 3 years.

Thereafter, visits should be made annually. In a GOG study[114] on sites and times to failure in 143 conservatively treated patients, all 12 cases of groin recurrence were diagnosed within the first 2 years of follow-up. Vulvar recurrences were found up to 89 months after initial treatment.

In addition to examination of the vulva and groins, a pelvic examination, Pap smear of the cervix and/or vagina, and a rectal examination should be performed at each visit, because these patients are also at high risk for the development of cancers of the cervix, vagina, and anus.[128]

The 5-year survival rate for all stages of vulvar squamous cell carcinoma combined is about 70%.[60] Approximately two-thirds of patients present with FIGO Stage I and II tumors, where 5-year survival rates of 80% to 90% are routinely reported.[60,62,85] However, 5-year survival rates fall to 60% and 15% for Stage III and IV patients, respectively.[62]

## SUMMARY

Cancer of the vulva is a relatively rare neoplasm, accounting for approximately 4% of all gynecologic malignancies and fewer than 1% of all cancers in women. The most common histologic type is squamous cell carcinoma, which represents 80% to 90% of all vulvar cancers. Most women present with vulvar pruritus and a recognizable lesion.

Modern optimal management of squamous cell carcinoma of the vulva includes careful consideration of less radical surgery for early-stage disease, the use of plastic reconstructive techniques for large surgical defects, and the incorporation of radiation therapy into the treatment regimen of locoregionally advanced disease. By taking a more individualized treatment approach, physical and psychologic morbidity has been significantly decreased without compromising overall survival.

The single most important factor influencing survival is lymph node status. Overall, the 5-year survival rate for patients with positive lymph nodes is 30% to 40% less than for patients with negative nodes. Better treatment options are needed for patients with nodal metastases. Multimodality therapy that incorporates radiation therapy, chemotherapy, and surgery has demonstrated encouraging results in the treatment of locally advanced vulvar cancer and appears to be the most promising area of investigation in the management of node-positive patients.

The prognosis for patients with distant metastases is dismal and points to the need for the development of effective systemic therapy.

## CANCER OF THE VAGINA

Cancer of the vagina that involves the vulva or the cervix is classified as primary vulvar or cervical cancer with vaginal extension. Similarly, cancer occurring in the vagina within 5 years of therapy for vulvar or cervical cancer is considered recurrent disease rather than a new primary vaginal malignancy. Partially due to this classification system, primary vaginal cancer is an uncommon entity, accounting for only 1% to 2% of all gynecologic malignancies.[129,130] The majority (80% to 90%) of vaginal malignancies are metastatic, involving the vagina by direct extension or via lymphatic or hematogenous routes.[130]

Since the vagina is lined by squamous epithelium, about 80% to 90% of primary vaginal malignancies are squamous cell carcinomas. Consequently, as with vulvar cancer, the data regarding patterns of spread, prognostic factors, and survival for vaginal cancer are based predominantly on studies of squamous cell malignancies. Other primary neoplasms found on the vagina include adenocarcinomas, soft-tissue sarcomas, and malignant melanomas.

Radiation therapy has been the standard treatment for vaginal cancer since the early years of this century. Initial results were extremely poor, with overall 5-year survival rates of less than 25%.[129,131] However, due to the increased sophistication of modern radiotherapy techniques, along with a more individualized approach to treatment, more recent series have reported overall 5-year survival rates of approximately 50%.[132-134] And although radiation therapy remains the treatment of choice for most patients with vaginal malignancies, in properly selected cases surgery can be equally effective.[134-136]

## EPIDEMIOLOGY

In the United States, invasive vaginal cancer occurs with an average annual incidence rate of approximately 0.5 per 100,000 women-years.[137] It is a disease primarily of postmenopausal women. The median age of patients diagnosed with vaginal carcinoma in situ is approximately 50 to 55 years, while the median age for invasive vaginal cancer is about 60 to 65 years.

The etiology of vaginal squamous cell carcinoma is unknown. However, up to 30% of women with primary vaginal squamous cell carcinoma have a history of in situ or invasive squamous cell carcinoma of the cervix.[132,136,138] This phenomenon has given rise to the "field effect" theory, which postulates that the entire lower female genital tract is at risk for the development of a squamous cell abnormality once an initial malignancy has occurred.[139,140] Recent studies have focused on HPV infection as the cause of this field effect.[141,142] Numerous reports have documented the strong association of HPV infection with in situ and invasive cervical and vulvar lesions, and HPV DNA has been found in over 50% of patients with vaginal cancer and in about 70% of vaginal intraepithelial neoplasias (VAIN).[142,143] Since the vagina does not have a transformation zone of immature epithelial cells susceptible to HPV infection, HPV-induced vaginal lesions are thought to arise in areas of squamous metaplasia that develop during healing of mucosal abrasions caused by coitus or tampon use.[144]

In a case-control study of 138 patients, Brinton and colleagues[145] identified a history of HPV infection, a previous abnormal Pap smear, early hysterectomy, and low socioeconomic level as potential risk factors for vaginal carcinoma in situ or invasive carcinoma. A history of vaginal trauma had less significance as a risk factor.

Prior pelvic irradiation has been suggested as a possible cause of primary squamous cell carcinoma of the vagina.[146,147] However, an analysis of 1200 patients treated over a period of 20 years at Washington University failed to demonstrate an increase in the incidence of second pelvic neoplasias following radiation therapy.[148]

In 1971, Herbst and colleagues[149] first reported a highly significant association between clear-cell adenocarcinoma of the vagina and maternal ingestion of diethylstilbestrol (DES) during pregnancy.

From 1943 to 1971, DES was given to women to maintain high-risk pregnancies. The findings of Herbst and colleagues led to the establishment of a registry to gather information about cases of clear-cell adenocarcinoma in the United States. More than 500 cases of clear-cell carcinoma of the vagina or cervix have been reported to the registry.[150] Sixty percent of the registered patients had been exposed to DES or similar synthetic estrogens in utero. The tumors were primary vaginal carcinomas in 60% of cases and primary cervical cancers in 40%. The age at diagnosis ranged from 7 to 34 years, with a median of 19 years. The risk of developing adenocarcinoma of the cervix or vagina in the exposed female population from birth to 34 years of age was approximately one case per 1000 women. The risk is greatest for those patients who were exposed to DES during the first 16 weeks in utero and declines for those whose exposure began in the 17th week or later.

Although the risk of clear-cell adenocarcinoma of the vagina is small in DES-exposed women, 45% of these patients have areas of vaginal adenosis (a condition in which glandular epithelium is present in the vagina after its development is complete) and 25% have structural abnormalities of the uterus, cervix, or vagina. It has also been reported that the incidence of cervical and vaginal intraepithelial neoplasia in DES-exposed women is twice as high as in unexposed women.[151] The reason for this increased risk is not clear.

## ANATOMY

The vagina is a muscular, dilatable tube averaging 7.5 cm in length that extends from the uterus to the vulva.[152] It is situated anterior to the rectum and posterior to the base of the bladder and urethra. At its uppermost extent, the vaginal wall meets the uterine cervix. The circular groove formed at the juncture of the vagina and the cervix is called the fornix.

The vaginal wall is composed of three layers: the mucosa, the muscularis, and the adventitia. The inner mucosal layer is formed by a thick, nonkeratinizing, stratified, squamous epithelium. This epithelium normally contains no glands but is lubricated by mucous secretions originating from the cervix. The muscularis contains an inner, circular, smooth-muscle layer and an outer, longitudinal, thicker muscular portion. Skeletal muscle at the introitus creates a vaginal sphincter. The adventitial layer is a thin, outer connective-tissue layer that merges with that of adjacent organs.

The blood supply to the upper vagina is derived from branches of the descending division of the uterine artery and the internal pudendal artery.[153] The vaginal artery usually arises from one of these two arteries but may also come from other components of the hypogastric system. The lower vagina is supplied by the inferior rectal artery and other branches of the internal pudendal artery.

The lymphatic drainage of the vagina consists of an extensive anastomotic network that combines laterally into larger drainage trunks. The lymphatics in the upper portion of the vagina drain primarily via the lymphatics of the cervix, while those in the lower portion drain either cephalad to cervical lymphatics or follow the drainage patterns of the vulva into the inguinal and femoral nodes (see Fig. 18A-2).

## NATURAL HISTORY AND PATTERNS OF SPREAD

Approximately 50% of vaginal carcinomas arise in the upper one-third of the vagina.[129,133,134,138] Although Plentl and Friedman[129] found that tumors most commonly arose on the posterior vaginal wall, recent reviews have reported a more even distribution of lesions on the anterior, posterior, and lateral walls.[133,134,138]

Vaginal cancers have three modes of spread: (1) direct extension into adjacent organs such as the urethra, bladder, and rectum; (2) embolization to regional lymph nodes; and (3) hematogenous dissemination to distant organs such as the lungs, liver, and bone.

There are limited data on the incidence of lymph node metastasis from vaginal cancer. In a review of early reports, Plentl and Friedman[129] found an overall incidence of 20.8% in 679 patients with vaginal cancer. Rubin and colleagues[136] reported that 16 of 38 patients (42%) with all stages of disease had abnormal lymphangiograms, but the lymphangiograms were performed in select patients only, and many of these abnormalities were not confirmed histologically. Al-Kurdi and Monaghan[154] performed lymph-node dissections on 35 patients and reported positive pelvic nodes in 10 (28.6%). Positive inguinal nodes were found in 6 of 19 patients (31.6%) who had disease involving the lower vagina. Generally, inguinal node metastases occur only in patients whose tumors involve the lower one-third of the vagina.[133,134,138,155] However, regardless of the tumor location, the pelvic lymph nodes (particularly the external iliac group) are at risk for metastases, emphasizing the importance of regional treatment for the majority of patients.[138]

Hematogenous metastases usually occur late in the natural history of the disease, when the local tumor is quite advanced. The most frequent site of distant metastasis is the lung.

## HISTOLOGY

In contrast to the high prevalence of intraepithelial lesions of the cervix and vulva, vaginal intraepithelial neoplasia (VAIN) is relatively rare. VAIN is characterized histologically by the presence of nuclear atypia and disordered squamous maturation with increased mitotic activity, abnormal mitotic figures, and dyskeratosis.[130] Lesions are graded from VAIN 1 to 3, corresponding to mild, moderate, and severe dysplasia. VAIN 3 also includes carcinoma in situ. As with VIN, the grade for VAIN corresponds to the level of cellular abnormalities within the epithelium.

Squamous cell carcinoma represents about 80% to 90% of primary vaginal malignancies. Histologically, squamous cell carcinomas of the vagina are similar to squamous tumors in other sites. Generally, these tumors contain pleomorphic squamous cells that display a lack of organization and a loss of cellular cohesion. They may exhibit keratinization manifested by squamous pearls and intercellular bridges.[152]

Approximately 4% to 9% of primary vaginal neoplasms are adenocarcinomas.[129,156] Adenocarcinoma of the vagina not associated with in utero DES exposure microscopically resembles adenocarcinoma arising in other areas. DES-related clear-cell adenocarcinomas exhibit three basic histologic patterns: tubulocystic (which is the most common), papillary, and solid. The tumor cells are cuboidal or columnar, with clear cytoplasm and a distinct cell membrane; or

they are hobnail type, with large atypical, protruding nuclei surrounded by a small rim of cytoplasm.[152]

About 3% of primary vaginal cancers are soft-tissue sarcomas.[156] Primary vaginal sarcomas that have been reported include leiomyosarcoma, rhabdomyosarcoma, endometrial stromal sarcoma, malignant fibrous histiocytoma, angiosarcoma, and hemangiopericytoma. Leiomyosarcoma is the most common vaginal sarcoma in adults and histologically is composed of interlacing bundles of spindle-shaped cells with blunt-ended nuclei and fibrillar cytoplasm. Embryonal rhabdomyosarcoma is characterized microscopically by a continuous zone of condensed round or spindle cells (the cambium layer) seen immediately beneath the intact vaginal epithelium. Elsewhere, the tumor is composed of small, dark cells sparsely distributed in a myxoid stroma.[152]

Malignant melanomas account for approximately 2% to 3% of primary vaginal cancers.[156] Fewer than 200 cases have been reported.[157] Histologically, vaginal melanomas are similar to those in other sites. The tumor may be composed of spindle-shaped, epithelioid, or small lymphocyte-like cells. The cells may or may not be pigmented. Poorly differentiated lesions that are difficult to distinguish from sarcomas or squamous cell carcinomas can be identified by their distinctive ultrastructural features or immunoperoxidase staining pattern.[158]

## CLINICAL PRESENTATION

Patients with VAIN are usually asymptomatic, and in most instances there is no grossly identifiable lesion in the vagina. Occasionally, the epithelium appears raised, roughened, and white or pink. More often, the diagnosis is made by a colposcopically directed biopsy performed during investigation of an abnormal Pap smear. The process is multifocal or diffuse in almost half of the cases and is usually located in the upper third of the vagina.[130]

Between 50% and 60% of patients with invasive squamous cell carcinoma of the vagina present with abnormal vaginal bleeding.[159–161] The bleeding is often postmenopausal, since that is the population most likely to develop the disease (Fig. 18A-15). However, in younger patients, the abnormal bleeding may be postcoital or intermenstrual. Patients may also complain of vaginal discharge or a palpable mass. The mass may exhibit an exophytic or ulcerative, infiltrating pattern of growth. Pain or symptoms referable to the bladder or rectum usually occur with more advanced disease. Ten to twenty percent of patients are asymptomatic at the time of diagnosis. Verrucous carcinoma is an uncommon variant of well-differentiated squamous cell carcinoma. The tumor appears as a relatively large, well-circumscribed, soft, cauliflower-like mass. Verrucous carcinoma may extensively infiltrate surrounding tissues but rarely metastasizes.[152]

Adenocarcinomas not associated with in utero DES exposure occur primarily in postmenopausal women. The presentation is similar to that of vaginal squamous cell carcinomas, but patients with vaginal adenocarcinomas tend to present with more advanced disease. These tumors often pose difficult diagnostic problems and must be distinguished from metastatic tumors originating in other sites. Occasionally, cancer arising in the kidney, breast, colon, or pancreas first becomes manifest as a vaginal lesion.

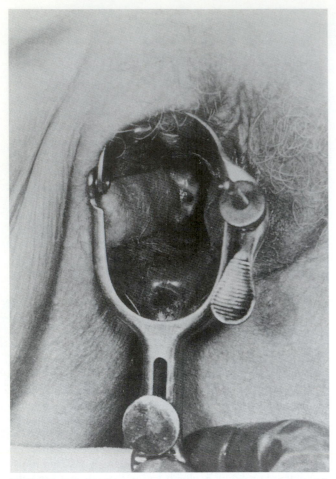

**FIGURE 18A-15.** Stage I squamous cell carcinoma of the middle third of the vagina presented as postmenopausal bleeding. (Reprinted from Morrow CP, Curtin JP, Townsend DE. Tumors of the vagina. In: Morrow CP, Curtin JP, Townsend DE, eds. *Synopsis of Gynecologic Oncology.* 4th ed. New York, NY: Churchill Livingstone; 1993:94, with permission.)

Clear-cell adenocarcinomas associated with in utero DES exposure occur in young women, with a median age at diagnosis of 19 years. Small tumors are usually asymptomatic and are detected by palpation or Pap smear. Larger tumors generally cause symptoms such as abnormal vaginal bleeding or discharge. Clear-cell carcinomas may involve any portion of the vagina; however, most arise on the anterior wall, usually in the upper third of the vagina (Fig. 18A-16). The tumors vary greatly in size (1 to 30 cm), with most being exophytic and superficially invasive.[162] Adenosis is associated with 97% of vaginal clear-cell adenocarcinomas. The classic gross appearance of adenosis is red, velvety, grapelike clusters in the vagina. The process may involve the surface epithelium and/or glands in the superficial stroma.[152]

Leiomyosarcoma is the most common vaginal sarcoma in adults. The age range extends from 25 to 86 years. Abnormal vaginal bleed-

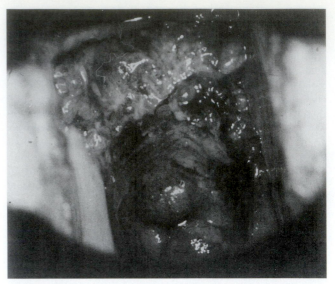

**FIGURE 18A-16.** Clear-cell adenocarcinoma of the vagina in a 20-year-old DES-exposed woman. The lesion is typically exophytic and is located in the anterior vaginal fornix. (Reprinted from Morrow CP, Curtin JP, Townsend DE. Tumors of the vagina. In: Morrow CP, Curtin JP, Townsend DE, eds. *Synopsis of Gynecologic Oncology.* 4th ed. New York, NY: Churchill Livingstone; 1993:105, with permission.)

ing is the most common presenting symptom. The tumors are usually bulky masses that occur most commonly in the upper vagina. For frankly malignant lesions, lymphatic and hematogenous dissemination is common. Embryonal rhabdomyosarcoma (sarcoma botryoides) is the most common malignant neoplasm of the vagina in infants and children. The average age at diagnosis is 2 years, with nearly 90% of cases diagnosed before 5 years of age.[130] Most children present with symptoms of a vaginal mass or bleeding. The tumor is usually located along the anterior wall of the vagina and appears as a polypoid mass resembling a bunch of grapes, hence the term *botryoides.* Frequently, the tumor fills and protrudes from the vagina (Fig. 18A-17).

The average age at diagnosis for primary vaginal melanomas is 55 years, with a range of 22 to 83. Typically, patients present with vaginal bleeding, vaginal discharge, or a vaginal mass. Malignant melanoma may arise anywhere in the vagina, but it most commonly arises on the anterior wall of the distal third.[163] The tumor is generally exophytic, deeply invasive, and brownish to black in color; however, a variety of colors may be seen, such as red and yellow. Approximately 5% are amelanotic.

## DIAGNOSIS

The diagnosis of vaginal cancer is often missed on first examination, particularly if the lesion is small and situated in the lower two-thirds of the vagina, where it may be covered by the blades of the speculum.

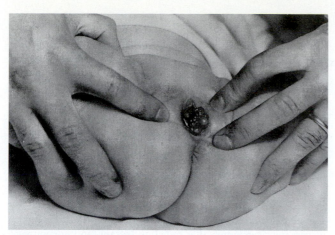

**FIGURE 18A-17.** Sarcoma botryoides. Typical mass resembling a cluster of grapes protruding from the vagina. (Reprinted from Hilgers RD, Malkasian GD, Soule EH. Embronal rhabdomyosarcoma (botryoid type) of the vagina: a clinicopathological review. *Am J Obstet Gynecol.* 1970;107:484, with permission.)

Frick and co-workers[164] reported that at least 10 of 52 (19%) cases in their series were missed on initial examination. The speculum should be rotated as it is withdrawn so that anterior or posterior wall lesions will not be overlooked. Pap smears may detect early squamous cell lesions, but may not detect adenocarcinomas, which often grow in submucosal locations.[165] For this reason, bimanual pelvic and rectal examinations are integral elements in the clinical evaluation of these patients.

Definitive diagnosis is usually made by biopsy of a gross lesion. In patients with an abnormal Pap smear and no gross abnormality, careful vaginal colposcopy and the liberal use of Lugol's iodine to stain the vagina will be necessary.

All patients with pathologically confirmed invasive vaginal cancer should have a complete blood count, biochemical profile, chest radiograph, cystoscopy, and proctoscopy. A barium enema or skeletal radiographs may also be needed in select cases. CT and MRI are being increasingly used as part of the metastatic evaluation.[152]

## STAGING OF THE DISEASE

Vaginal carcinoma is staged using the FIGO staging system (Table 18A-6). It is a clinical staging system based on the findings of physical examination, chest radiographs, cystoscopy, proctoscopy, and skeletal radiographs (if the latter are indicated to rule out bone involvement). Information obtained from lymphangiography, CT, MRI, or surgical staging cannot change the clinical stage. The AJCC has suggested a TNM staging system; however, this system is rarely used (see Table 18A-6).[55]

The distribution of patients with vaginal carcinoma by FIGO stage from seven recent series is shown in Table 18A-7.[132–134,160,166–168] The staging system does not take into account the size or location of

## TABLE 18A-6. STAGING OF VAGINAL CARCINOMA

**Primary tumor (T):**

TX   Primary tumor cannot be assessed.

T0   No evidence of primary tumor.

Tis   Carcinoma in situ.

T1   Tumor confined to the vagina.

T2   Tumor invades paravaginal tissues but not to the pelvic wall.

T3   Tumor extends to the pelvic wall.

T4   Tumor invades the mucosa of the bladder or rectum and/or extends beyond the true pelvis.

**Regional lymph nodes (N):**

NX   Regional lymph nodes cannot be assessed.

N0   No regional lymph node metastasis.

**Upper two-thirds of the vagina:**

N1   Pelvic lymph node metastasis.

**Lower one-third of the vagina:**

N1   Unilateral inguinal lymph node metastasis.

N2   Bilateral inguinal lymph node metastasis.

**Distant metastasis (M):**

MX   Presence of distant metastasis cannot be assessed.

M0   No distant metastasis.

M1   Distant metastasis.

### STAGE GROUPINGS

| FIGO | AJCC | CLINICAL FINDINGS |
|------|------|-------------------|
| 0 | Tis N0 M0 | Carcinoma in situ; intraepithelial carcinoma. |
| I | T1 N0 M0 | Tumor is limited to the vaginal wall. |
| II | T2 N0 M0 | Tumor involves the subvaginal tissues but not to the pelvic wall. |
| III | T1 N1 M0 T2 N1 M0 T3 N0 M0 T3 N1 M0 | Tumor extends to the pelvic wall. |
| IV | | Tumor extends beyond the true pelvis or has involved the mucosa of the bladder or rectum. |
| IVA | T1 N2 M0 T2 N2 M0 T3 N2 M0 T4 Any N M0 | Tumor has spread to adjacent organs. |
| IVB | Any T Any N M1 | Tumor has spread to distant organs. |

SOURCE: Modified from Beahrs OH et al: Gynecologic tumors, in *Manual for Staging of Cancer*, 4th ed, OH Beahrs et al (eds). Philadelphia, Lippincott, 1992, pp 155–180. Used with permission.

**TABLE 18A-7.** DISTRIBUTION OF PRIMARY VAGINAL CARCINOMA BY FIGO STAGE

| STAGE | NUMBER OF PATIENTS | PERCENT |
| --- | --- | --- |
| I | 246 | 24 |
| II | 322 | 31 |
| III | 303 | 30 |
| IV | 153 | 15 |
| Total | 1024 | 100 |

the tumor, and in many cases it is difficult if not impossible to distinguish on clinical grounds a tumor that is "limited to the vaginal wall" versus one that has "involved the subvaginal tissue." This in part may explain the wide variation in stage distribution and survival rates reported in the literature.[136]

Although there are rather limited data on staging patients with vaginal melanoma, the use of the microstaging system described by Breslow is remommended by most authors.[58,163,169,170] No formal staging system exists for vaginal sarcomas; however, the FIGO system for vaginal carcinomas is occasionally applied.

## PROGNOSTIC FACTORS

In vaginal squamous cell carcinoma, the most significant factor influencing prognosis is the clinical stage of disease.[132–135,138,160] Tumor size also appears to be an important predictor of outcome. In a review of 271 patients with primary squamous cell carcinoma of the vagina, Chyle and colleagues[138] found a higher rate of local and distant failure for tumors larger than 5 cm in diameter. Other investigators have reported poorer survival rates for patients who are symptomatic or have tumors that involve more than one-third of the vaginal canal[132,134,160,174]; generally, both of these factors are a function of tumor size or bulk.

There is no general consensus as to whether patient age, tumor grade, or tumor location are significant, independent prognostic factors. In a review of 434 patients with primary carcinoma of the vagina treated at the University of Vienna, Kucera and Vavra[160] reported that factors in addition to early stage of disease that were associated with improved prognosis were as follows: (1) patient age under 60; (2) well-differentiated tumors; and (3) tumors located in the upper third of the vagina. However, other authors have not found these factors to be of significance.[132–134,172] Similarly, Chyle and colleagues[138] reported significantly poorer survival for patients with vaginal adenocarcinoma versus squamous cell carcinoma. However, other investigators have found no difference in their outcomes.[132–135,172]

In a review of the literature on vaginal melanoma, Reid and colleagues[163] found that tumor thickness and tumor size were significant prognostic factors for disease-free interval and survival, respectively. The prognosis of patients with vaginal sarcomas appears to depend on three main factors: lesion size, cytologic atypia, and mitotic activity. Lesions larger than 3 cm in diameter with marked cytologic atypia and more than five mitotic figures per 10 high-power fields suggest a poor prognosis.[173]

## TREATMENT

The treatment of vaginal cancer must be individualized, taking into consideration the age and overall medical status of the patient, her desire to maintain a functional vagina, and the stage, size, and location of the tumor. Radiation therapy is the preferred treatment modality for most vaginal malignancies. This treatment preference is based on the fact that the close proximity of the vagina to the bladder and rectum makes radical resection with adequate surgical margins and organ preservation technically quite difficult in most cases and virtually impossible in others. Furthermore, most of these patients are elderly and not good candidates for radical surgery. For these reasons, along with the excellent tumor control and functional results obtained with radiation therapy, the role of surgery is reserved for select cases of early-stage disease, centrally recurrent or persistent carcinoma after radiation therapy, and nonepithelial tumors.

**PREINVASIVE DISEASE (VAIN).** Patients with only HPV infection or VAIN 1 do not require treatment. These lesions often regress spontaneously, are frequently multifocal, and recur quickly after attempts at ablative therapy. VAIN 2 is usually treated by laser ablation.[9]

However, with VAIN 3, there is a significant risk that the patient may be harboring an undiagnosed invasive lesion. Hoffman and co-workers[174] found occult invasion in the surgical specimens from 9 of 32 (28%) patients who underwent upper vaginectomy for VAIN 3. Furthermore, although the malignant potential of VAIN is probably quite low, future progression to invasion does occur. In a review of 136 patients with vaginal carcinoma in situ, Benedet and Saunders[175] reported that four cases (3%) progressed to invasive vaginal carcinoma in spite of various treatment methods. Moreover, Aho and co-workers[176] followed 23 patients with biopsy-confirmed VAIN without treatment for at least 3 years; two cases (9%) progressed to invasive cancer. Due to the possibility of harboring or progressing to an invasive cancer, VAIN 3 requires definitive treatment. If the lesions have been adequately sampled to rule out invasion, they may be treated conservatively. The two most commonly employed conservative approaches are $CO_2$-laser ablation and topical 5-fluorouracil (5-FU). Krebs[177] reported treatment failure rates of 27% and 19%, respectively.

Local excision with a margin of 3 to 5 mm of normal mucosa is frequently used for small, single VAIN 3 lesions or for multiple lesions located in a single portion of the vagina. Rarely, total vaginectomy is required for extensive lesions or for those patients who fail conservative therapy. A total vaginectomy starts at the hymenal ring and progresses to the vaginal apex (Fig. 18A-18). Great care must be taken not to enter the bladder or the rectum while the dissection is being performed. During the dissection, it is critical that the vesicovaginal and rectovaginal septums are identified with certainty to avoid injury to the bladder and rectum (Fig. 18A-19). A uterine sound placed through the urethra into the bladder and the operator's finger placed in the rectum can greatly assist in this dissection.[178] Vaginal reconstruction with a split-thickness skin graft is then recommended. The overall treatment failure rate for surgical excision is approximately 12%.[179]

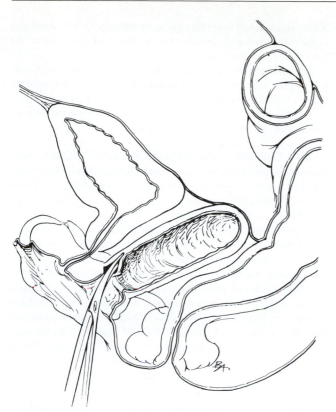

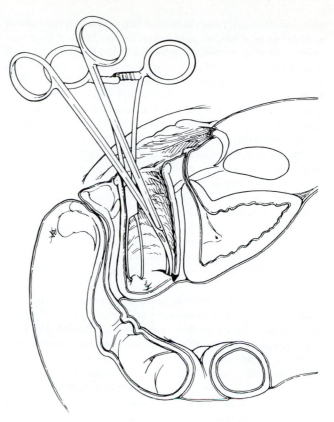

**FIGURE 18A-18.** Dissection begins at the hymenal ring for total vaginectomy. The vaginal mucosa is dissected from the underlying tissue. (Reprinted from Hopkins MP. Surgery for cancer of the vagina. In: Gershenson DM, DeCherney AH, Curry SL, eds. *Operative Gynecology.* Philadelphia: Saunders; 1993:205, with permission.)

**FIGURE 18A-19.** In the upper vagina, the bladder and rectum are in close proximity. It is important to identify the vesicovaginal and rectovaginal septa to avoid injury. (From Hopkins MP. Surgery for cancer of the vagina. In: Gershenson DM, DeCherney AH, Curry SL, eds. *Operative Gynecology.* Philadelphia: Saunders; 1993:205, with permission.)

## STAGE I SQUAMOUS CELL CARCINOMA

*RADIATION THERAPY.* Patients with Stage I squamous cell carcinoma of the vagina are usually treated with radiation therapy. Many authors recommend that patients with small superficial tumors be treated with brachytherapy alone.[155,160,161] Perez and colleagues[155] achieved similar tumor control and survival in 22 select Stage I patients treated with brachytherapy alone, compared to 27 other Stage I patients treated with a combination of external beam irradiation and brachytherapy. Tumors less than 2 cm in diameter and less than 0.5 cm thick can be treated with an intracavitary cylinder delivering 6000 to 7000 cGy to the entire vaginal mucosa with an additional dose of 2000 to 3000 cGy to the tumor area. If the lesion is thicker and localized to one wall, a single plane interstitial implant may be added to increase the depth dose and limit excessive irradiation to the vaginal mucosa. A dose of 6000 to 6500 cGy is delivered to the entire vaginal mucosa with an additional 1500 to 2000 cGy (calculated 0.5 cm beyond the plane of the implant) given to the tumor. This delivers an estimated total dose of 8000 to 10,000 cGy to the involved vaginal mucosa.[152]

Larger Stage I tumors should be treated with a combination of external beam irradiation and brachytherapy. The external beam field must include the primary tumor and the regional lymph nodes. When tumors involve the lower one-third of the vagina, the field should be enlarged to include the medial inguinal lymph nodes. The whole pelvis is initially treated with 1000 to 2000 cGy. An additional parametrial dose is then delivered with a midline block to give a total of 5000 cGy to the parametria. Brachytherapy follows, aiming to deliver a total of 7000 to 7500 cGy to the tumor.[9] Lee and colleagues[180] treated 15 Stage I vaginal carcinoma patients with external beam irradiation and brachytherapy, and none developed recurrent disease. In their series, which included a total of 65 patients, they found that the overall treatment time was a significant predictor of pelvic control: if the entire course of radiotherapy was completed within 9 weeks, the pelvic control rate was 97%, compared to 54% if the treatment time extended beyond 9 weeks.

*SURGERY.* In the treatment of Stage I vaginal carcinoma, there are no large studies comparing the efficacy of surgery versus radiation. However, from the limited data available, it appears that surgery can be as effective as radiation therapy in select Stage I patients. In four recent studies that included a total of 51 patients with Stage I vaginal carcinoma, the overall survival rate achieved with surgery was similar to that achieved with radiation therapy.[134–136,181] In the study that included the most Stage I patients, Davis and co-workers[135] reported a 5-year survival rate of 85% in 25 patients treated by surgery alone, compared to 65% in 14 patients treated with radiation therapy alone.

The patients with Stage I vaginal carcinoma who can be treated surgically are those whose tumors are located in the upper third of the vagina. Patients whose uterus is still in situ can be managed by radical hysterectomy, pelvic lymphadenectomy, and radical upper vaginectomy. Patients who have already had a hysterectomy may be treated with a radical upper vaginectomy and pelvic lymphadenectomy. Upper posterior lesions are more amenable to a surgical approach because the rectum reflects away from the posterior vagina but the bladder stays in close proximity to the anterior vagina for its entire length.

Radical vaginectomy usually requires an abdominoperineal approach. The abdominal procedure is performed first to evaluate the nodal areas and confirm that surgery should proceed. The para-aortic lymph nodes should be sampled and sent for frozen section diagnosis. If metastatic disease is present in the para-aortic lymph nodes, then the procedure should not be performed. If the para-aortic nodes are negative, bilateral pelvic lymphadenectomy and radical hysterectomy may be performed as described for cervical cancer in the next section of this chapter.

When the dissection has neared the perineum, attention is turned to the perineal phase. An incision is made around the circumference of the vaginal vault at a level at least 2 cm distal to the tumor. The incision is carried down to the pubocervical fascia beneath the urethra and the perirectal fascia overlying the rectum. Laterally, the vaginal branches of the pudendal artery are identified and divided. The dissection is continued beneath the urethra, over the rectum, and laterally to join the abdominal dissection. This allows the entire specimen to be removed from above. A split-thickness skin graft can be used to reconstruct the vagina.[152]

### STAGE II SQUAMOUS CELL CARCINOMA.

Patients with Stage II vaginal carcinoma require a comprehensive approach to treatment that should include external-beam irradiation and brachytherapy. In a study of 165 patients with a mean follow-up of 7.6 years, Perez and colleagues[152] reported a pelvic control rate of 66% in 62 Stage II patients treated with a combination of external beam irradiation and brachytherapy, compared to 31% in 13 Stage II patients treated with either mode of therapy alone. The data also demonstrated the importance of adequate radiation dosage for tumor control. Only 1 of the 10 (10%) Stage II patients who received a tumor dose of greater than 7500 cGy had a pelvic recurrence, compared to 7 of the 20 (35%) Stage II patients whose tumor dose was less than 7500 cGy. Other authors have also stressed the importance of delivering at least 7000 to 7500 cGy to the primary tumor.[133,172]

In general, the irradiation for patients with Stage II vaginal carcinoma consists of 2000 cGy to the whole pelvis, followed by a supplemental dose of 3000 cGy to the parametria using a midline shielding block. This external beam therapy is combined with interstitial and intracavitary radiation to deliver a minimum of 7500 cGy to the tumor.

Selected patients with Stage II disease may be cured with radical surgical treatment.[134–136] However, an exenterative procedure is often required to remove the tumor. Therefore, primary surgical treatment of Stage II carcinoma is generally reserved for patients with a previous history of pelvic irradiation.

### STAGE III AND IV SQUAMOUS CELL CARCINOMA.

Stages III and IVA tumors are usually bulky, highly infiltrative lesions involving most or all of the vagina as well as the pelvic wall, bladder, or rectum. The standard treatment is radiation therapy, which has produced less than satisfactory results. Pelvic tumor control has been achieved in fewer than half of the patients at this stage of disease.

All patients require treatment with external beam irradiation, and most authors advocate the addition of brachytherapy, whenever possible. Perez and colleagues[152] recommend a total of 5500 to 6000 cGy of external-beam therapy in combination with interstitial and intracavitary insertions to deliver a total tumor dose of 7500 to 8000 cGy.[152] However, Chyle and colleagues[138] reported a relatively high 10-year relapse-free rate of 47% in 55 Stage III patients, even though 40 (73%) of these patients were treated with external beam radiation alone. Patients treated with only external irradiation received doses up to 8000 cGy using a shrinking field technique after 4500 to 5000 cGy. Although brachytherapy is an important part of disease management in most patients, a greater emphasis is placed on treatment with external beam irradiation in patients with very large tumors, since it is difficult to implant large areas while limiting the dose to intimately associated critical normal structures.[9,151]

The treatment of patients with Stage IVB vaginal carcinoma is essentially palliative. A variety of drugs have been tested in Phase II trials in the treatment of vaginal squamous cell carcinoma. Only doxorubicin (Adriamycin) has demonstrated significant activity as a single agent,[182] and while combination regimens containing cisplatin have shown significant responses, the number of patients in these series is too small to make any definite recommendations.[172,183,184]

### COMPLICATIONS OF THERAPY.

Major complications of therapy are usually reported in 10% to 20% of patients treated for primary vaginal carcinoma, whether the treatment is by surgery or radiation.[133,134,138,155] The complication rates are generally higher than those reported for the treatment of carcinoma of the cervix, primarily because the close proximity of the urethra, bladder, and rectum to the vagina predisposes these structures to injury. The most frequently reported complications are fistulae, cystitis, urethral strictures, rectal strictures or ulceration, and vaginal necrosis, ulceration, or stenosis. There have been no comprehensive studies of posttreatment vaginal function in these patients.

### RECURRENT SQUAMOUS CELL CARCINOMA.

Recurrent vaginal squamous cell carcinoma after radiation therapy should be approached with pelvic exenteration as the primary mode of therapy, provided there is no evidence of metastatic disease. If the recurrence is located on the anterior or posterior vaginal wall, an anterior or posterior exenteration can be performed. When the recurrence is located at the vaginal apex after a previous hysterectomy, a total exenteration should be performed because the bladder and rectum will be contiguous with the upper vagina.[178]

Eddy and colleagues[132] reported a 5-year disease-free survival in three of six patients who underwent exenterative surgery because of persistent vaginal carcinoma after radiation therapy. Stock and colleagues[134] salvaged 5 of 50 patients with local or pelvic recurrence: 3 underwent exenteration, 1 had a radical vulvectomy and partial vaginectomy, and 1 had 5000 cGy of interstitial radiation given to a suburethral nodule.

### TREATMENT OF NONSQUAMOUS CELL MALIGNANCIES. 
Due to their infrequent occurrence, there is relatively little definitive information regarding the treatment of nonsquamous cell vaginal malignancies. As with vulvar malignancies, most available data are derived from small case series spanning long periods of time.

*ADENOCARCINOMA.* The treatment of vaginal adenocarcinomas is similar to that of vaginal squamous cell carcinomas. However, women with DES-related clear cell adenocarcinomas are very young, with a median age at diagnosis of 19 years, so every effort should be made to preserve vaginal and ovarian function. A combination of wide local excision, retroperitoneal lymphadenectomy, and local irradiation can be effective therapy for small Stage I tumors.[185] Local excision alone is not recommended, since about 17% of patients with Stage I disease have positive pelvic nodes and even very small clear cell adenocarcinomas have been reported to metastasize to the pelvic lymph nodes.[162,186] Furthermore, Senekjian and colleagues[185] reported a recurrence rate of over 40% at 10 years in 17 patients with Stage I disease treated by local excision alone, compared to 0% in 11 Stage I patients treated with local excision and local irradiation (5 of these patients also had a retroperitoneal node dissection).

A high percentage of patients with larger DES-related Stage I tumors of the upper vagina have been successfully treated with radical hysterectomy, pelvic lymphadenectomy, radical vaginectomy, and vaginal reconstruction with a split-thickness skin graft. Jones and colleagues[187] reported no recurrences in 9 Stage I patients treated in this manner, with a follow-up of up to 10 years. Since the tumor often spreads subepithelially, it is important to obtain frozen-section biopsies of the distal margins whenever surgical resection is performed.

When more advanced lesions are treated with whole-pelvic irradiation, ovarian transposition to preserve ovarian function should be considered before the initiation of the radiotherapy.

Most recurrences occur within 3 years of initial therapy. However, recurrences have been reported to occur up to 20 years after treatment.[188,189] About one-third of relapses are first detected at distant sites, most commonly in the lungs of extrapelvic lymph nodes.[9] To date, no effective chemotherapeutic regimen has been reported.[188,189]

The overall actuarial 10-year survival rate of patients treated for vaginal clear-cell adenocarcinoma is 79%. The 10-year survival rates are excellent for patients with Stage I and II tumors, approximately 90% and 80%, respectively.[185,190] However, fewer than 30% of patients with Stage III and IV disease are long-term survivors.[179]

*SARCOMA.* For adult patients with vaginal sarcomas, surgical excision is the mainstay of treatment. Although 5-year survival rates of approximately 30% have been reported, Curtin and colleagues[65] recently reported a relatively high 70% overall 5-year survival rate for 24 patients with sarcoma of the vagina and vulva. Fifteen of the 24 patients (63%) had vaginal sarcomas that were treated initially with surgery, ranging from wide-local excision to posterior exenteration. Based on the data regarding management of soft-tissue sarcomas of the extremities, patients with high-grade tumors, or recurrent low-grade tumors that were successfully resected received brachytherapy to the tumor site. Some patients also received external beam radiation to provide an additional dose to the tumor bed. Although 6 of the 15 patients (40%) with vaginal sarcomas experienced disease recurrence, only 2 (13%) recurred locally. Reid and colleagues[191] also reported favorable survival when patients with leiomyosarcomas localized to the vagina were treated by exenteration.

Exenterative surgery no longer plays a role in the primary management of children with vaginal embryonal rhabdomyosarcoma. Excellent results have been achieved by the Intergroup Rhabdomyosarcoma Study Group using a regimen of preoperative vincristine, actinomycin D, and cyclophosphamide (VAC) chemotherapy and conservative surgery, followed by radiation therapy in select cases.[192,193]

*MELANOMA.* Limited data are available on which to base recommendations for the management of patients with primary vaginal melanoma. Reid and colleagues[163] pooled their data on 15 patients with 115 patients reported in the literature. They noted four different treatment strategies: (1) surgery only; (2) radiation therapy only; (3) surgery plus radiation therapy; and (4) chemotherapy plus surgery or radiation therapy. There were no significant differences in survival among these treatment regimens. The 55 patients who underwent surgery only were then divided into two groups based on the extent of their surgical procedures. There was no difference in survival or disease-free interval between the 24 patients who had undergone conservative procedures (wide local excision, partial vaginectomy) versus the 31 patients who underwent radical procedures (radical hysterectomy, radical vaginectomy, exenteration).

Van Nostrand and colleagues[157] subsequently pooled the data on 8 of their patients with 111 patients reported in the literature. They found that 2-year survival rates were 48% for the 50 patients treated with radical surgery compared to 20% for the 69 patients treated with conservative surgery. The authors concluded that radical surgery for patients with primary vaginal melanoma should be performed for lesions less than 10 cm$^2$.

Because these two reviews are based largely on the same cases, it is difficult to understand how they could have reached such contradictory conclusions. In the absence of more definitive data, it seems reasonable to offer patients with vaginal melanoma surgery tailored to achieve adequate deep and lateral margins consistent with the management of cutaneous melanoma.[170] Radiation therapy may be added to improve locoregional control, with exenterative procedures reserved for persistent or recurrent disease.[194] Adjuvant chemotherapy and immunotherapy (including vaccines) have not yet been proved to be of any benefit in patients with vaginal melanoma.

The overall prognosis for patients with vaginal melanoma is poor. In the review by Reid and colleagues,[163] the mean disease-free interval was 15 months. Once a recurrence was noted, the mean survival time was 8.5 months. The overall 5-year survival rate in collected series is 15% to 20%.[121,122,157,163]

## FOLLOW-UP AND SURVIVAL

After completing their treatment for vaginal squamous cell carcinoma, patients should be examined every 3 to 4 months for 2 years and then every 6 months for the next 3 years. Thereafter, visits should be made annually. In addition to an examination and Pap smear of the vagina, examination of the vulva and groins, Pap smear of the cervix, and a rectal examination should be performed at each visit, because these patients are also at high risk for the development of cancers of the vulva, cervix, and anus.[128,139,140]

The 5-year survival rate for all stages of vaginal squamous cell carcinoma combined is about 50%.[132–134,160] Survival from different series is difficult to accurately compare or pool because of the varied ways that the survival rates have been reported (crude, disease-free, actuarial, corrected, uncorrected, and so on). However, the 5-year survival rate by stage for patients with vaginal carcinoma can be approximated as follows: Stage 1, 75%; Stage II, 50%; Stage III, 35%; Stage IVA, 20%; and Stage IVB, 0%.[179]

## SUMMARY

Vaginal cancer is a rare entity accounting for fewer than 1% to 2% of all gynecologic malignancies. The most common histologic type is squamous cell carcinoma, which represents 80% to 90% of all vaginal cancers. Patients generally present with abnormal vaginal bleeding or a mass, although 10% to 20% of patients are asymptomatic at the time of diagnosis. Prognosis depends on the stage of the disease, and therapy should be individualized for each patient based on her age, the histologic cell type, and the stage of the tumor. Radiation therapy is the standard treatment for the majority of patients. However, in select patients, surgery can be equally effective.

The prognosis of patients with advanced disease is poor. The use of hypoxic sensitizers to enhance the effects of irradiation in large tumors is currently under investigation.[152] The development of effective chemotherapeutic agents is necessary to treat the high percentage of patients who develop distant metastases.

## REFERENCES

1. PARKER SL et al: Cancer statistics, 1997. CA 47:5, 1997.
2. HACKER NF: Surgery for malignant tumors of the vulva, in *Operative Gynecology,* DM Gershenson et al (eds). Philadelphia, Saunders, 1993, pp 173–200.
3. BLAIR-BELL W, DATNOW MM: Primary malignant diseases of the vulva, with special reference to treatment by operation. J Obstet Gynaecol Br Emp 43:755, 1996.
4. WAY S: The anatomy of the lymphatic drainage of the vulva and its influence on the radical operation for carcinoma. Ann R Coll Surg Engl 3:187, 1948.
5. BASSET A: Traitement chirurgical operatoire de l'epithelioma primifif du clitoris. Indications-technique-results. Rev Chir 46:546, 1912.
6. TAUSSIG FJ: Cancer of the vulva: An analysis of 155 cases. Am J Obstet Gynecol 40:764, 1940.
7. WAY S: Carcinoma of the vulva. Am J Obstet Gynecol 79:692, 1960.
8. STURGEON SR et al: In situ and invasive vulvar cancer incidence trends (1973–1987). Am J Obstet Gynecol 166:1482, 1992.
9. EIFEL PJ et al: Cancer of the cervix, vagina, and vulva, in *Cancer: Principles and Practice of Oncology,* 5th ed, VT Devita et al (eds). Philadelphia, Lippincott-Raven, 1997, pp 1433–1478.
10. BRINTON LA et al: Case-control study of cancer of the vulva. Obstet Gynecol 75:859, 1990.
11. LEE YY et al: Carcinoma of the vulva: HPV and p53 mutations. Oncogene 9:1655, 1994.
12. KIM YT et al: p53 mutations and clonality in vulvar carcinomas and squamous hyperplasias: Evidence suggesting that squamous hyperplasias do not serve as direct precursors of human papillomavirus-negative vulvar carcinomas. Hum Pathol 27:389, 1996.
13. ANSINK AC et al: Human papillomavirus, lichen sclerosis, and squamous cell carcinoma of the vulva: Detection and prognostic significance. Gynecol Oncol 52:180, 1994.
14. BLOSS JD et al: Clinical and histologic features of vulvar carcinomas analyzed for human papillomavirus status: Evidence that squamous cell carcinoma of the vulva has more than one etiology. Hum Pathol 22:711, 1991.
15. CRUM CP: Carcinoma of the vulva: Epidemiology and pathogenesis. Obstet Gynecol 79:448, 1992.
16. HORDING U et al: Vulvar squamous cell carcinoma and papillomaviruses: Indications for two different etiologies. Gynecol Oncol 52:241, 1994.
17. MONK BJ et al: Prognostic significance of human papillomavirus (HPV) DNA in primary invasive vulvar cancer. Obstet Gynecol 85:709, 1995.
18. TOKI T et al: Probable nonpapillomavirus etiology of squamous cell carcinoma of the vulva in older women: A clinicopathologic study using in situ hybridization and polymerase chain reaction. Int J Gynecol Pathol 10:107, 1991.
19. ANDERSEN WA et al: Vulvar squamous cell carcinoma and papillomaviruses: Two separate entities. Am J Obstet Gynecol 165:329, 1991.
20. KURMAN RJ et al: Basaloid and warty carcinoma of the vulva. Am J Surg Pathol 17:133, 1993.
21. TRIMBLE CL et al: Heterogeneous etiology of squamous carcinoma of the vulva. Obstet Gynecol 87:59, 1996.
22. BURKE TW et al: Vulva, in *Principles and Practice of Gynecologic Oncology,* 2d ed, WJ Hoskins et al (eds). Philadelphia, Lippincott-Raven, 1997, pp 717–751.
23. PARRY-JONES E: Lymphatics of the vulva. J Obstet Gynecol Br Empire 70:751, 1963.
24. IVERSEN T, AAS M: Lymph drainage from the vulva. Gynecol Oncol 16:179, 1983.
25. PIVER MS, XYNOS FP: Pelvic lymphadenectomy in women with carcinoma of the clitoris. Obstet Gynecol 49:592, 1977.
26. CURRY SL et al: Positive lymph nodes in vulvar squamous carcinoma. Gynecol Oncol 9:63, 1980.
27. PLENTL AA, FRIEDMAN EA: Clinical significance of vulvar lymphatics, in *Lymphatic System of the Female Genitalia,* AA Plentl and EA Friedman (eds). Philadelphia, Saunders, 1971, pp 27–50.

28. SHIMM DS et al: Prognostic variables in the treatment of squamous cell carcinoma of the vulva. Gynecol Oncol 24:343, 1986.

29. ANDREASSON B, NYBOE J: Predictive factors with reference to low-risk of metastases in squamous cell carcinoma in the vulvar region. Gynecol Oncol 21:196, 1985.

30. PARKER RT et al: Operative management of early invasive epidermoid carcinoma of the vulva. Am J Obstet Gynecol 123:349, 1975.

31. HACKER NF et al: Superficially invasive vulvar cancer with nodal metastases. Gynecol Oncol 15:65, 1983.

32. CHU J et al: Femoral node metastases with negative superficial inguinal nodes in early vulvar cancer. Am J Obstet Gynecol 140:337, 1981.

33. RUTLEDGE F et al: Carcinoma of the vulva. Am J Obstet Gynecol 196:1117, 1970.

34. HOMESLEY HD et al: Prognostic factors for groin node metastasis in squamous cell carcinoma of the vulva (a Gynecologic Oncology Group study). Gynecol Oncol 49:279, 1993.

35. BINDER SW et al: Risk factors for the development of lymph node metastasis in vulvar squamous carcinoma. Gynecol Oncol 37:9, 1990.

36. ROSS MJ, EHRMANN RL: Histologic prognosticators in stage I squamous cell carcinoma of the vulva. Obstet Gynecol 70:774, 1987.

37. HOFFMAN JS et al: Microinvasive squamous carcinoma of the vulva: Search for a definition. Obstet Gynecol 61:615, 1983.

38. HACKER NF et al: Individualization of treatment for stage I squamous cell vulvar carcinoma. Obstet Gynecol 63:155, 1984.

39. MAGRINA JF et al: Stage I squamous cell cancer of the vulva. Am J Obstet Gynecol 134:453, 1979.

40. IVERSEN T et al: Individualized treatment of stage I carcinoma of the vulva. Obstet Gynecol 57:85, 1981.

41. WILKINSON EJ et al: Microinvasive carcinoma of the vulva. Int J Gynecol Pathol 1:29, 1982.

42. BOICE CR et al: Microinvasive squamous carcinoma of the vulva: Present status and reassessment. Gynecol Oncol 18:71, 1984.

43. ROWLEY K et al: Prognostic factors in early vulvar cancer. Gynecol Oncol 31:43, 1988.

44. STRUYK APHB et al: Early stage cancer of the vulva: A pilot investigation on cancer of the vulva in gynecologic oncology centers in the Netherlands. Proc Int Gynecol Cancer Soc 2:303, 1989.

45. WILKINSON EJ: Premalignant and malignant tumors of the vulva, in Blaustein's Pathology of the Female Genital Tract, 4th ed. RJ Kurman (ed). New York, Springer-Verlag, 1994, pp 87–129.

46. CHEN KT: Merkel's cell (neuroendocrine carcinoma of the vulva). Cancer 73:2186, 1994.

47. LORET DE MOLA JR et al: Merkel cell carcinoma of the vulva. Gynecol Oncol 151:272, 1993.

48. FRIEDRICH EG et al: Carcinoma in situ of the vulva: A continuing challenge. Am J Obstet Gynecol 136:830, 1980.

49. BERNSTEIN SG et al: Vulvar carcinoma in situ. Obstet Gynecol 61:304, 1983.

50. HART WR, MILLMAN RB: Progression of intraepithelial Paget's disease of the vulva to invasive carcinoma. Cancer 40:2333, 1977.

51. LUCAS WE et al: Verrucous carcinoma of the female genital tract. Am J Obstet Gynecol 119:435, 1974.

52. PALLADINO VS et al: Basal cell carcinoma of the vulva. Cancer 24:460, 1969.

53. TAVASSOLI FA, NORRIS HJ: Smooth muscle tumors of the vulva. Obstet Gynecol 53:213, 1979.

54. CREASMAN WT: New gynecologic cancer staging. Gynecol Oncol 58:157, 1995.

55. BEAHRS OH et al: Gynecologic tumors, in Manual for Staging of Cancer, 4th ed, OH Beahrs et al (eds). Philadelphia, Lippincott, 1992, pp 155–180.

56. CLARK WH et al: The histogenesis and biologic behavior of primary human malignant melanomas of the skin. Cancer Res 29:705, 1969.

57. CHUNG AF et al: Malignant melanoma of the vulva: A report of 44 cases. Obstet Gynecol 45:638, 1975.

58. BRESLOW A: Thickness, cross-sectional area and depth of invasion in the prognosis of cutaneous melanoma. Ann Surg 172:902, 1970.

59. PHILLIPS GL et al: Malignant melanoma of the vulva treated by radical hemivulvectomy: A prospective study of the Gynecologic Oncology Group. Cancer 73:2626, 1994.

60. HOMESLEY HD et al: Assessment of current International Federation of Gynecology and Obstetrics staging of vulvar carcinoma relative to prognostic factors for survival (a Gynecologic Oncology Group study). Am J Obstet Gynecol 164:997, 1991.

61. SEDLIS A et al: Positive groin lymph nodes in superficial squamous cell vulvar cancer (a Gynecologic Oncology Group study). Am J Obstet Gynecol 156:1159, 1987.

62. RUTLEDGE FN et al: Prognostic indicators for invasive carcinoma of the vulva. Gynecol Oncol 42:239, 1991.

63. VAN DER VELDEN J et al: Extracapsular growth of lymph node metastases in squamous cell carcinoma of the vulva: The impact on recurrence and survival. Cancer 75:2885, 1995.

64. HEAPS JM et al: Surgical-pathologic variables predictive of local recurrence in squamous cell carcinoma of the vulva. Gynecol Oncol 38:309, 1990.

65. CURTIN JP et al: Soft-tissue sarcoma of the vagina and vulva: A clinicopathologic study. Obstet Gynecol 86:269, 1995.

66. NIRENBERG A et al: Primary vulvar sarcomas. Int J Gynecol Pathol 14:55, 1995.

67. ANDERSEN BL, HACKER NF: Psychological adjustment after vulvar surgery. Obstet Gynecol 63:155, 1984.

68. MORROW CP, CURTIN JP: Surgery for vulvar neoplasia, in Gynecologic Cancer Surgery, CP Morrow, JP Curtin (eds). New York, Churchill Livingstone, 1996, pp 381–450.

69. BUCEMA J, WOODRUFF JD: Progressive histobiologic alterations in the development of vulvar cancer. Am J Obstet Gynecol 138:146, 1980.

70. HORDING U et al: Vulvar intraepithelial neoplasia III: A viral disease of undetermined progressive potential. Gynecol Oncol 56:276, 1995.

71. JONES RW, ROWAN DM: Vulvar intraepithelial neoplasia III: A clinical study of the outcome in 113 cases with relation to the later development of invasive vulvar carcinoma. Obstet Gynecol 84:741, 1994.

72. HACKER NF: Vulvar cancer, in Practical Gynecologic Oncology, JS Berek and NF Hacker (eds). Baltimore, Williams & Wilkins, 1994, pp 403–439.

73. COX SM et al: Recurrent carcinoma in situ of the vulva in a skin graft. Am J Obstet Gynecol 155:177, 1986.

74. GUNN RA, GALLAGER HS: Vulvar Paget's disease: A topographic study. Cancer 46:590, 1980.

75. GREEN TH JR et al: Epidermoid carcinoma of the vulva: An analysis of 238 cases, parts I and II. Am J Obstet Gynecol 73:834, 1958.

76. HACKER NF et al: Radical vulvectomy and bilateral inguinal lymphadenectomy through separate groin incisions. Obstet Gynecol 58:574, 1981.

77. CHRISTOPHERSEN W et al: Radical vulvectomy and bilateral groin lymphadenectomy utilizing separate groin incisions: Report of a case with recurrence in the intervening skin bridge. Gynecol Oncol 21:247, 1985.

78. SCHULZ MJ, PENALVER M: Recurrent vulvar carcinoma in the intervening tissue bridge in early invasive stage I disease treated by radical vulvectomy and bilateral groin dissection through separate incisions. Gynecol Oncol 35:383, 1989.

79. GRIMSHAW RN et al: Radical vulvectomy and bilateral inguinofemoral lymphadenectomy through separate incisions—experience with 100 cases. Int J Gynecol Cancer 3:18, 1993.

80. HACKER NF, VAN DER VELDEN J: Conservative management of early vulvar cancer. Cancer 71:1673, 1993.

81. STEHMAN FB et al: Groin dissection versus groin radiation in carcinoma of the vulva: A Gynecologic Oncology Group study. Int J Radiat Oncol Biol Phys 24:39, 1992.

82. STEHMAN FB et al: Early stage I carcinoma of the vulva treated with ipsilateral superficial inguinal lymphadenectomy and modified radical hemivulvectomy: A prospective study of the Gynecologic Oncology Group. Obstet Gynecol 79:490, 1992.

83. PALEY PJ et al: The effect of sartorious muscle transposition on wound morbidity following inguinal-femoral lymphadenectomy. Gynecol Oncol 64:237, 1997.

84. HOMESLY HD et al: Radiation therapy versus pelvic node resection for carcinoma of the vulva with positive groin nodes. Obstet Gynecol 68:733, 1986.

85. HACKER NF et al: Management of regional lymph nodes and their prognostic influence in vulvar cancer. Obstet Gynecol 61:408, 1983.

86. THOMAS GM et al: Changing concepts in the management of vulvar cancer. Gynecol Oncol 42:9, 1991.

87. PETEREIT DG et al: Inguinofemoral radiation of N0, N1 vulvar cancer may be equivalent to lymphadenectomy if proper radiation technique is used. Int J Radiat Oncol Biol Phys 27:963, 1993.

88. BURKE TW et al: Surgical therapy of T1 and T2 vulvar carcinoma: Further experience with radical wide excision and selective inguinal lymphadenectomy. Gynecol Oncol 57:215, 1995.

89. LEVENBACK C et al: Potential applications of intraoperative mapping in vulvar cancer. Gynecol Oncol 59:216, 1995.

90. FARIAS-EISNER R et al: Conservative and individualized surgery for early squamous cell carcinoma of the vulva: The treatment of choice for stages I and II (T1-2, N0-1, M0) disease. Gynecol Oncol 53:55, 1994.

91. BYRON RL et al: The surgical treatment of invasive carcinoma of the vulva. Surg Gynecol Obstet 121:1243, 1965.

92. ABITBOL MM: Carcinoma of the vulva: Improvements in the surgical approach. Am J Obstet Gynecol 117:483, 1973.

93. LISTER GD, GIBSON T: Closure of rhomboid skin defects: The flaps of Limberg and Dufourmentel. Br J Plast Surg 25:300, 1972.

94. BURKE TW et al: Closure of complex vulvar defects using local rhomboid flaps. Obstet Gynecol 84:1043, 1994.

95. BURKE TW et al: Perineal reconstruction using single gracilis myocutaneous flaps. Gynecol Oncol 57:221, 1995.

96. SOPER JT et al: Short gracilis flaps for vulvovaginal reconstruction after radical pelvic surgery. Obstet Gynecol 74:185, 1989.

97. CAVANAGH D, HOFFMAN MS: Controversies in the management of vulvar carcinoma. Br J Obstet Gynaecol 103:293, 1996.

98. HOPKINS MP, MORLEY GW: Pelvic exenteration for the treatment of vulvar cancer. Cancer 70:2835, 1992.

99. MILLER B et al: Pelvic exenteration for primary and recurrent vulvar cancer. Gynecol Oncol 58:202, 1995.

100. BORONOW RC et al: Combined therapy as an alternative to exenteration for locally advanced vulvovaginal cancer. II. Results, complications and dosimetric and surgical considerations. Am J Clin Oncol 10:171, 1987.

101. BENEDETTI-PANICI P et al: Cisplatin (P), bleomycin (B), and methotrexate (M) preoperative chemotherapy in locally advanced vulvar carcinoma. Gynecol Oncol 50:49, 1993.

102. THOMAS G et al: Concurrent radiation and chemotherapy in vulvar carcinoma. Gynecol Oncol 34:263, 1989.

103. BEREK JS et al: Concurrent cisplatin and 5-fluorouracil chemotherapy and radiotherapy for advanced stage squamous carcinoma of the vulva. Gynecol Oncol 42:197, 1991.

104. MOORE DH et al: Preoperative chemoradiation for advanced vulvar cancer: A phase II study of the Gynecologic Oncology Group. 27th Ann Proc SGO, 1996.

105. HOMESLEY H: Management of vulvar cancer. Cancer 76:2159, 1995.

106. DEPPE G et al: Adriamycin treatment of advanced vulvar carcinoma. Obstet Gynecol 50:13, 1977.

107. TROPE C et al: Bleomycin alone or combined with mitomycin C in treatment of advanced or recurrent squamous cell carcinoma of the vulva. Cancer Treat Rep 64:639, 1980.

108. BELINSON JL et al: Bleomycin, vincristine, mitomycin C, and cisplatin in the management of gynecologic squamous cell cancer. Gynecol Oncol 20:387, 1985.

109. DURRANT KR et al: Bleomycin, methotrexate, and CCNU in advanced inoperable squamous cell carcinoma of the vulva: A phase II study of the EORTC Gynaecological Cancer Cooperative Group (GCCG). Gynecol Oncol 37:359, 1990.

110. HOPKINS MP et al: The surgical management of recurrent squamous cell carcinoma of the vulva. Obstet Gynecol 75:1001, 1990.

111. PIURA B et al: Recurrent squamous cell carcinoma of the vulva: A study of 73 cases. Gynecol Oncol 48:189, 1993.

112. PREMPREE T, AMORNMARN R: Radiation treatment of recurrent carcinoma of the vulva. Cancer 54:1943, 1984.

113. HOFFMAN M et al: Interstitial radiotherapy for the treatment of advanced or recurrent vulvar and distal vaginal malignancy. Am J Obstet Gynecol 162:1278, 1990.

114. STEHMAN FB et al: Sites of failure and times to failure in carcinoma of the vulva treated conservatively: A Gynecologic Oncology Group study. Am J Obstet Gynecol 174:1128, 1996.

115. ROSE PG et al: Conservative therapy for melanoma of the vulva. Am J Obstet Gynecol 159:52, 1988.

116. TRIMBLE EL et al: Management of vulvar melanoma. Gynecol Oncol 45:254, 1992.

117. DAVIDSON T et al: Vulvovaginal melanoma: Should radical surgery be abandoned? Br J Obstet Gynaecol 94:473, 1987.

118. BALCH CM: The role of elective lymph node dissection in melanoma: Rationale, results and controversies. J Clin Oncol 6:163, 1988.

119. HABERMALZ HJ, FISCHER JJ: Radiation therapy of malignant melanoma: Experience with high individual treatment doses. Cancer 38:2258, 1976.

120. Kirkwood JM et al: Interferon alfa-2b adjuvant therapy of high-risk cutaneous melanoma: The Eastern Cooperative Oncology Group Trial EST 1684. J Clin Oncol 14:7, 1996.

121. Ragnarsson-Olding B et al: Malignant melanoma of the vulva and vagina: Trends in incidence, age distribution, and long-term survival among 245 consecutive cases in Sweden 1960–1984. Cancer 71:1893, 1993.

122. Weinstock MA: Malignant melanoma of the vulva and vagina in the United States: Patterns of incidence and population-based estimates of survival. Am J Obstet Gynecol 171:1225, 1994.

123. Copeland LJ et al: Bartholin gland carcinoma. Obstet Gynecol 67:794, 1986.

124. Leuchter RS et al: Primary carcinoma of the Bartholin gland: A report of 14 cases and a review of the literature. Obstet Gynecol 60:361, 1982.

125. Breen JL et al: Basal cell carcinoma of the vulva. Obstet Gynecol 46:122, 1975.

126. Hoffman JS et al: Basal cell carcinoma of the vulva with inguinal node metastases. Gynecol Oncol 29:113, 1988.

127. Palladino VS et al: Basal cell carcinoma of the vulva. Cancer 24:460, 1969.

128. Sturgeon SR et al: Second primary cancers after vulvar and vaginal cancers. Am J Obstet Gynecol 174:929, 1996.

129. Plentl AA, Friedman EA: Clinical significance of the vaginal lymphatics, in Lymphatic System of the Female Genitalia, AA Plentl and EA Friedman (eds). Philadelphia, Saunders, 1971, pp 57–74.

130. Zaino RJ et al: Diseases of the vagina, in Blaustein's Pathology of the Female Genital Tract, 4th ed, RJ Kurman (ed). New York, Springer-Verlag, 1994, pp 131–183.

131. Palmer JP, Biback SM: Primary cancer of the vagina. Am J Obstet Gynecol 67:377, 1954.

132. Eddy GL et al: Primary invasive vaginal carcinoma. Am J Obstet Gynecol 165:292, 1991.

133. Kirkbride P et al: Carcinoma of the vagina: Experience at the Princess Margaret Hospital (1974–1989). Gynecol Oncol 56:435, 1995.

134. Stock RG et al: A 30-year experience in the management of primary carcinoma of the vagina: Analysis of prognostic factors and treatment modalities. Gynecol Oncol 56:45, 1995.

135. Davis KP et al: Invasive vaginal carcinoma: Analysis of early-stage disease. Gynecol Oncol 42:131, 1991.

136. Rubin SC et al: Squamous carcinoma of the vagina: Treatment, complications, and long-term follow-up. Gynecol Oncol 20:346, 1985.

137. Cramer DW, Cutler SJ: Incidence and histopathology of malignancies of the female genital organs in the United States. Am J Obstet Gynecol 118:443, 1974.

138. Chyle V et al: Definitive radiotherapy for carcinoma of the vagina: Outcome and prognostic factors. Int J Radiat Oncol Biol Phys 35:891, 1996.

139. Newman W, Cromer JK: The multicentric origin of carcinoma of the female anogenital tract. Surg Gynecol Obstet 108:273, 1959.

140. Marcus S: Multiple squamous cell carcinomas involving the cervix, vagina, and vulva: The theory of multicentric origin. Am J Obstet Gynecol 80:802, 1960.

141. Weed JC et al: Human papilloma virus in multifocal, invasive female genital tract malignancy. Obstet Gynecol 62:832, 1983.

142. McCance DJ et al: Human papillomavirus types 6 and 16 in multifocal intraepithelial neoplasia of the female lower genital tract. Br J Obstet Gynecol 82:1101, 1985.

143. Ikenberg H et al: Human papillomavirus DNA in invasive carcinoma of the vagina. Obstet Gynecol 76:432, 1990.

144. Hoffman MS et al: Upper vaginectomy for in situ and occult, superficially invasive carcinoma of the vagina. Am J Obstet Gynecol 166:30, 1992.

145. Brinton LA et al: Case-control study of in situ and invasive carcinoma of the vagina. Gynecol Oncol 38:49, 1990.

146. Pride GL et al: Primary invasive squamous carcinoma of the vagina. Obstet Gynecol 53:218, 1979.

147. Boice JD et al: Radiation dose and second cancer risk in patients treated for cancer of the cervix. Radiat Res 116:3, 1988.

148. Lee JY et al: The risk of second primaries subsequent to irradiation for cervix cancer. Int J Radiat Oncol Biol Phys 8:207, 1982.

149. Herbst AL et al: Adenocarcinoma of the vagina: Association with maternal stilbestrol therapy with tumor appearance in young women. N Engl J Med 284:878, 1971.

150. Hicks ML, Piver MS: Conservative surgery plus adjuvant therapy for vulvovaginal rhabdomyosarcoma, diethylstilbestrol clear cell adenocarcinoma of the vagina, and unilateral germ cell tumors of the ovary. Obstet Gynecol Clin North Am 19:219, 1992.

151. Bornstein J et al: Development of cervical and vaginal squamous cell neoplasia as a late consequence of in utero exposure to diethylstilbestrol. Obstet Gynecol Surv 43:15, 1988.

152. Perez CA et al: Vagina, in Principles and Practice of Gynecologic Oncology, 2nd ed, WJ Hoskins et al (eds). Philadelphia, Lippincott-Raven, 1997, pp 753–783.

153. Morrow CP, Curtin JP: Surgical anatomy, in Gynecologic Cancer Surgery, CP Morrow and JP Curtin (eds). New York, Churchill Livingstone, 1996, pp 67–139.

154. Al-Kurdi M, Monaghan JM: Thirty-two years experience in management of primary tumors of the vagina. Br J Obstet Gynaecol 88:1145, 1981.

155. Perez CA et al: Definitive irradiation in carcinoma of the vagina: long-term evaluation of results. Int J Radiat Oncol Biol Phys 15:1283, 1988.

156. Hacker NF: Vaginal cancer, in Practical Gynecologic Oncology, JS Berek and NF Hacker (eds). Baltimore, Williams & Wilkins 1994 pp 441–456.

157. Van Nostrand KM, Lucci JA, Schell M et al: Primary vaginal melanoma: Improved survival with radical pelvic surgery. Gynecol Oncol 55:234, 1994.

158. Berman ML et al: Primary malignant melanoma of the vagina: Clinical, light, and electron microscopic observations. Am J Obstet Gynecol 139:963, 1981.

159. Nori D et al: Radiation therapy of primary vaginal carcinoma. Int J Radiat Oncol Biol Phys 9:1471, 1983.

160. Kucera H, Vavra N: Radiation management of primary carcinoma of the vagina: Clinical and histopathological variables associated with survival. Gynecol Oncol 40:12, 1991.

161. Stock RG et al: The importance of brachytherapy technique in the management of primary carcinoma of the vagina. Int J Radiat Oncol Biol Phys 24:747, 1992.

162. Herbst AL et al: Clear-cell adenocarcinoma of the vagina and cervix in girls: analysis of 170 Registry cases. Am J Obstet Gynecol 119:713, 1974.

163. REID GC et al: Primary melanoma of the vagina: A clinicopathologic analysis. Obstet Gynecol 74:190, 1989.

164. FRICK HC et al: Primary carcinoma of the vagina. Am J Obstet Gynecol 101:695, 1968.

165. BARBER HRK, SOMMERS SC: Vaginal adenosis, dysplasia, and clear cell adenocarcinoma after diethylstilbestrol treatment in pregnancy. Obstet Gynecol 43:645, 1974.

166. PREMPREE T: Role of radiation therapy in the management of primary carcinoma of the vagina. Acta Radiol Oncol 21:195, 1982.

167. BENEDET JL et al: Primary invasive carcinoma of the vagina. Obstet Gynecol 62:715, 1983.

168. LEUNG S, SEXTON M: Radical radiation therapy for carcinoma of the vagina—impact of treatment modalities on outcome: Peter MacCallum Cancer Institute experience 1970–1990. Int J Radiat Oncol Biol Phys 25:413, 1993.

169. LEVITAN Z et al: Primary malignant melanoma of the vagina: Report of four cases and review of the literature. Gynecol Oncol 33:85, 1989.

170. TRIMBLE EL: Melanomas of the vulva and vagina. Oncology 10:1017, 1996.

171. CHU AM, BEECHINOR R: Survival and recurrence patterns in the radiation treatment of carcinoma of the vagina. Gynecol Oncol 19:298, 1984.

172. PETERS WA et al: Carcinoma of the vagina: Factors influencing treatment outcome. Cancer 55:892, 1985.

173. TAVASSOLI FA, NORRIS HJ: Smooth muscle tumors of the vagina. Obstet Gynecol 53:689, 1979.

174. HOFFMAN MS et al: Upper vaginectomy for in situ and occult, superficially invasive carcinoma of the vagina. Am J Obstet Gynecol 166:30, 1992.

175. BENEDET JL, SAUNDERS BH: Carcinoma in situ of the vagina. Am J Obstet Gynecol 148:695, 1984.

176. AHO M et al: Natural history of vaginal intraepithelial neoplasia Cancer 68:195, 1991.

177. KREBS HB: Treatment of vaginal intraepithelial neoplasia with laser and topical 5-fluorouracil. Obstet Gynecol 73:657, 1989.

178. HOPKINS MP: Surgery for cancer of the vagina, in Operative Gynecology, DM Gershenson et al (eds). Philadelphia, Saunders, 1993, pp 201–211.

179. MORROW CP, CURTIN JP: Tumors of the vagina, broad ligament, and fallopian tube, in Gynecologic Cancer Surgery, CP Morrow and JP Curtin (eds). New York, Churchill Livingstone, 1996, pp 717–743.

180. LEE WR et al: Radiotherapy alone for carcinoma of the vagina: The importance of overall treatment time. Int J Radiat Oncol Biol Phys 29:983, 1994.

181. MANETTA A et al: Primary invasive carcinoma of the vagina. Obstet Gynecol 76:639, 1990.

182. PIVER MS et al: Adriamycin alone or in combination in 100 patients with carcinoma of the cervix or vagina. Am J Obstet Gynecol 131:311, 1978.

183. BELINSON JL et al: Bleomycin, vincristine, mitomycin-C, and cisplatin in the management of gynecological squamous cell cancer. Gynecol Oncol 20:387, 1985.

184. KATIB S et al: The effectiveness of multidrug treatment by bleomycin, methotrexate, and cisplatin in advanced vaginal carcinoma. Gynecol Oncol 21:101, 1985.

185. SENEKJIAN EK et al: Local therapy in stage I clear cell adenocarcinoma of the vagina. Cancer 60:1319, 1987.

186. CHAMBERS J et al: Minute clear cell carcinoma of the vagina with early metastasis to pelvic lymph nodes. Am J Obstet Gynecol 131:223, 1978.

187. JONES WB et al: Clear-cell adenocarcinoma of the lower genital tract: Memorial Hospital 1974–1984. Obstet Gynecol 70:573, 1987.

188. JONES WB et al: Late recurrence of clear cell adenocarcinoma of the vagina and cervix: A report of three cases. Gynecol Oncol 51:266, 1993.

189. FISHMAN DA et al: Late recurrences of vaginal clear cell adenocarcinoma. Gynecol Oncol 62:128, 1996.

190. SENEKJIAN E et al: An evaluation of stage II vaginal clear cell adenocarcinoma according to substages. Gynecol Oncol 31:56, 1988.

191. REID GC et al: The role of pelvic exenteration for sarcomatous malignancies. Obstet Gynecol 74:80, 1989.

192. HAYS DM et al: Clinical staging and treatment results in rhabdomyosarcoma of the female genital tract among children and adolescents. Cancer 61:1893, 1988.

193. ANDRASSY RJ et al: Conservative surgical management of vaginal and vulvar pediatric rhabdomyosarcoma: A report from the Intergroup Rhabdomyosarcoma Study III. J Pediatr Surg 30:1034, 1995.

194. BONNER JA et al: The management of vaginal melanoma. Cancer 62:2066, 1988.

# 18B / CANCER OF THE CERVIX AND UTERINE FUNDUS

*Thomas W. Burke and Charles Levenback*

The uterus is a complex reproductive organ capable of dramatic transformation during pregnancy. It contains three distinct epithelia, smooth-muscle components, and generalized and specialized stromal elements. Consequently, a wide variety of benign and malignant tumors can originate from this organ. The uterus is divided into two major portions—the fundus and the cervix—on the basis of anatomic and functional criteria. Because each portion of the uterus has its own distinct histology, each produces a group of malignant tumors derived from the elements native to that part of the organ. Thus, cervix and fundal malignancies are generally considered as discrete entities with differing cell-type profiles, prognostic features, diagnostic evaluations, staging criteria, and treatment. This chapter has been divided into two sections in order to provide an overview of the clinical aspects of both categories of tumors.

## CERVICAL CANCER

### INCIDENCE

The incidence of cervical cancer varies widely throughout the world, with the highest incidences in the countries of Central and South America and the lowest in Mediterranean countries such as Italy, Greece, and Spain.[1] In the United States the incidence of cervical cancer is 2.5 per 100,000, and the lifetime risk of acquiring the disease is less than 1%. In 2000, the estimated number of new cases in the United States was 12,800, with 4600 deaths from the disease predicted. The incidence among Vietnamese American women, 43 per 100,000, is the highest of any racial or ethnic group in the United States; the next highest incidence, 16.2 per 100,000, is among Hispanic American women; and third highest, 13.2 per 100,000, is among African American women.[2]

The incidence of cervical cancer has dropped since the Papanicolaou (Pap) test of exfoliative cervical cytology was introduced for screening purposes in the 1940s. In one population that has had ready access to screening and treatment, women from the Canadian province of British Columbia, the incidence of invasive cervical cancer dropped over a 20-year period from more than 30 per 100,000 in 1955 to fewer than 5 per 100,000 in 1985.[3] The mortality from this type of cancer in the United States has dropped 70% over the past 40 years.[4] However, the incidence of cervical cancer remained stable during the 1980s and 1990s. Several explanations for this

stability have been proposed, including the persistence of under-screened populations. Even in 2000, 50% of patients with cervical cancer had never had Pap-smear screening.

### PATHOGENESIS AND RISK FACTORS

One of the unique aspects of cervical cancer is its resemblance to sexually transmitted diseases (STDs). A variety of STDs, including gonorrhea and herpes, have previously been associated with cervical cancer; however, human papillomavirus (HPV) now seems to be the most likely causative agent.[5] HPV DNA has been found in more than 90% of squamous cell cancers of the cervix. Certain subtypes of HPV are thought to produce proteins that disrupt the normal mechanisms that regulate cell growth; moreover, incorporation of HPV genes E6 and E7 into the host genetic material results in malignant transformation. Although HPV infection has been closely linked with the development of cervical cancer, many women infected with HPV never develop cervical cancer. However, HPV has several subtypes, and the lower-risk subtypes are associated with benign condyloma and low-grade intraepithelial neoplasia. In addition to HPV infection, additional host immune factors probably must be present to result in a malignancy.

Major risk factors for cervical cancer are listed in Table 18B-1. Cervical cancer is rare in women under the age of 20 years. Its incidence peaks between the ages of 45 and 60 years, although the incidence in African American women seems to continue increasing into the seventh and eighth decades of life. The presence of cervical cancer in young women should always raise the suspicion of immunosuppression from HIV infection or other causes.

The incidence of cervical cancer is usually higher in women in lower socioeconomic groups, presumably because women in these groups are screened less frequently and have less access to health care.

Other risk factors for cervical cancer include age at first intercourse (coitarche), number of sexual partners, and sexual history of those partners. The significance of age at coitarche, specifically the period between menarche and coitarche, may be related to the vulnerability of the metaplastic epithelium of the cervical transformation zone, which develops after menarche, to HPV infection. In one study, an interval of less than 5 years between menarche and coitarche was associated with a significant increase in the risk of

**TABLE 18B-1.** RISK FACTORS FOR CERVICAL CANCER

| FACTOR | RELATIVE RISK INCREASE (X) |
|---|---|
| Age | 2 |
| HPV infection | 40–60 |
| Age of first intercourse | 2–4 |
| Multiple sexual partners | 2–5 |
| Male partners' sexual behavior | 1.5–2 |
| Low socioeconomic status | 2.3 |
| Long-term smoking | 2.5 |
| Long-term oral contraceptive use | 1.5–2 |
| Nutritional deficiency | 2.3 |

developing cervical cancer.[6] The number of sexual partners and the sexual history of male partners are other important risk factors; women with partners who have had multiple sexual partners are at increased risk for invasive cervical cancer.[7]

The influence of contraceptive methods on the risk of developing cervical cancer has been studied extensively. Use of oral contraceptives for more than 5 years seems to increase the risk factor, although a plausible explanation for this increase has yet to be found. One hypothesis is that women who use oral contraceptives do not use barrier methods, which may physically prevent HPV infection.

Although well documented, the increased risk of cervical cancer associated with smoking is not fully understood. High nicotine levels in the cervical mucus found in women who smoke may play a role in the development of cervical cancer.[8] Women who are immunosuppressed, through infection with HIV or through immunosuppressive therapy for organ transplantation, are at increased risk for both cervical dysplasia and invasive cervical cancer.[9,10]

## SCREENING AND EARLY DETECTION

Of the estimated 50 million Pap smears performed each year in the United States, 4 million are abnormal. A variety of factors can cause false-negative or false-positive results, including patient factors such as recent douching and provider factors such as poor sampling or fixing techniques, laboratory errors in processing, and interpretative errors by cytopathologists and clinicians. False-negative rates reportedly range between 5% and 50%, with the most common being 20%.[11]

The Bethesda system for classifying cervical cytologic samples was introduced in 1988 to clarify the evaluation of abnormal Pap smears; however, this system led to additional confusion regarding classification of "atypical squamous cells of undetermined significance" (ASCUS). Since 20% to 30% of women with ASCUS have cervical dysplasia, patients with ASCUS on a Pap smear require further evaluation.[12]

With regard to screening frequency, most providers in the United States follow the 1996 American Cancer Society guidelines, which have been endorsed by the American College of Obstetricians and Gynecologists and the American Academy of Family Practitioners.

The American Cancer Society recommends annual Pap smears beginning with the onset of sexual activity, or at age 18 years; after 3 normal consecutive smears, the screening frequency can be reduced at the physician's discretion, for low-risk patients. Risk assessment is difficult in most clinical settings, since the sexual behavior of the patient and male partners can be awkward to obtain. For this reason, many clinicians continue to recommend an annual Pap smear. Finally, there are several commercially available HPV subtyping cervical cytology tests; however, there are no standard recommendations for their use. No recommendations have been established for HPV screening, either for the general population or for patients with abnormal Pap smears.

The primary purpose of colposcopy after an abnormal Pap smear is to identify the presence of occult invasive disease. Premalignant lesions can be treated with a variety of methods. A recent study conducted at the University of Texas M. D. Anderson Cancer Center found that cryotherapy, laser vaporization, and loop electrosurgical excision treatments for squamous intraepithelial lesions were equally effective in terms of complications, persistence, and recurrence of disease.[13]

## MICROINVASIVE CERVICAL CANCER

Some very small invasive cervical cancers behave similarly to high-grade squamous intraepithelial lesions; thus, subjecting women to radical surgery for these microinvasive lesions exposes them to unnecessary risks. In 1974, the Society of Gynecologic Oncologists (SGO) introduced a definition for microinvasion that was embraced by practitioners in the United States.[14] The SGO defined microinvasion as invasion of 3 mm or less, negative cone margins, and no lymphatic space invasion. This definition was quickly embraced by the gynecology community, even though it was not reflected in International Federation of Gynecology and Obstetrics (FIGO) staging for cervical cancer at the time. A few years later, this definition was expanded to include estimates of tumor volume, since tumors with a volume of less than 400 $mm^2$ had minimal chances of metastasis or recurrence.[15] In 1995, the most recent staging system for cervical cancer was adopted by FIGO (Table 18B-2). This system includes a category of microscopic tumors (stage IA), with two subcategories based on the depth of invasion and lateral spread. Lateral spread is not commonly reported by pathologists in the United States; clinicians must either ask for this measurement or, more often, recommend treatment on the basis of depth rather than volume.

Microinvasive cervical cancer, as defined by the SGO, is treated by extrafascial hysterectomy. Some patients who wish to preserve their reproductive options can be treated adequately by cone biopsy with negative margins.[16]

## CLINICAL MANIFESTATIONS OF INVASIVE CERVICAL CANCER

The most common initial symptom of invasive cervical cancer is abnormal vaginal bleeding. Cervical cancer arises at the squamocolumnar junction. In premenopausal women, this junction is located on the ectocervix; after menopause, this junction migrates toward the

**TABLE 18B-2. INTERNATIONAL FEDERATION OF GYNECOLOGY AND OBSTETRICS STAGING SYSTEM FOR CARCINOMA OF THE CERVIX UTERI**

| STAGE | DESCRIPTION | COMMENTS |
|---|---|---|
| Stage 0 | Carcinoma in situ, intraepithelial carcinoma. | Notes about the staging: |
| Stage I | The carcinoma is strictly confined to the cervix. | |
| Stage IA | Invasive cancer identified only microscopically. All gross lesions even with superficial invasion are stage IB cancers. Invasion is limited to measured stromal invasion with maximum depth of 5 mm and no wider than 7 mm. | Stage IA carcinoma should include minimally microscopically evident stromal invasion, as well as small cancerous tumors of measurable size. Stage IA should be divided into those lesions with minute foci of invasion visible only microscopically as stage IA1 and macroscopically measurable microcarcinoma as stage IA2, in order to gain further knowledge of the clinical behavior of these lesions. The term "IB occult" should be omitted. |
| Stage IA1 | Measured invasion of stroma no greater than 3 mm in depth and no wider than 7 mm. | The diagnosis of both stage IA1 and IA2 cases should be based on microscopic examination of removed tissue, preferably a cone, which must include the entire lesion. The lower limit of stage IA2 should be measurable macroscopically (even if dots need to be placed on the slide prior to measurement), and the upper limit of stage IA2 is given by measurement of the two largest dimensions in any given section. |
| Stage IA2 | Measured invasion of stroma greater than 3 mm and no greater than 5 mm in depth, and no wider than 7 mm. | |
| Stage IB | Clinical lesions confined to the cervix or preclinical lesions greater than stage IA. | The depth of invasion should not be more than 5 mm taken from the base of the epithelium, either surface or glandular, from which it originates. The second dimension, the horizontal spread, must not exceed 7 mm. Vascular space involvement, either venous or lymphatic, should not alter the staging but should be specifically recorded, as it may affect treatment decisions in the future. |
| Stage IB1 | Clinical lesions no greater than 4 cm in size. | The depth of invasion should not be more than 5 mm taken from the base of the epithelium, either surface or glandular, from which it originates. The second dimension, the horizontal spread, must not exceed 7 mm. Vascular space involvement, either venous or lymphatic, should not alter the staging but should be specifically recorded, as it may affect treatment decisions in the future. Lesions of greater size should be classified as stage IB. |
| Stage IB2 | Clinical lesions greater than 4 cm in size. | |
| Stage II | The carcinoma extends beyond the cervix but has not extended to the pelvic wall. The carcinoma involves the vagina but not as far as the lower third. | |
| Stage IIA | No obvious parametrial involvement. | As a rule, it is impossible to estimate clinically whether a cancer of the cervix has extended to the corpus or not. Extension to the corpus should therefore be disregarded. |
| Stage IIB | Obvious parametrial involvement. | |
| Stage III | The carcinoma has extended to the pelvic wall. On rectal examination, there is no cancer-free space between the tumor and the pelvic wall. The tumor involves the lower third of the vagina. All cases with a hydronephrosis or nonfunctioning kidney are included unless they are known to be due to other causes. | A patient with a growth fixed to the pelvic wall by a short and indurated but not nodular parametrium should be allotted to stage IIB. It is impossible, at clinical examination, to decide whether a smooth and indurated parametrium is truly cancerous or only inflammatory, therefore, the case should be placed in stage III only if the parametrium is nodular on the pelvic wall or if the growth itself extends to the pelvic wall. |
| Stage IIIA | No extension to the pelvic wall. | The presence of hydronephrosis or nonfunctioning kidney due to stenosis of the ureter by cancer permits a case to be allotted to stage III even if, according to the other findings, the case should be allotted to stage I or stage II. |
| Stage IIIB | Extension to the pelvic wall and/or hydronephrosis or nonfunctioning kidney. | |
| Stage IV | The carcinoma has extended beyond the true pelvis or has clinically involved the mucosa of the bladder or rectum. A bullous edema as such does not permit a case to be allotted to stage IV. | The presence of bullous edema, as such, should not permit a case to be allotted to stage IV. Ridges and furrows in the bladder wall should be interpreted as signs of submucous involvement of the bladder if they remain fixed to the growth during palpation. (i.e., examination from the vagina or the rectum during cystoscopy). A finding of malignant cells in cytologic washings from the urinary bladder requires further examination and biopsy from the wall of the bladder. |
| Stage IVA | Spread of the growth to adjacent organs. | |
| Stage IVB | Spread to distant organs. | |

SOURCE: Adapted from Shepard JH, Staging announcement: FIGO staging of gynecologic cancers: Cervical and vulva. *Int J Gynecol Cancer* 5:319, 1995.

endocervix. Cervical cancers usually infiltrate locally. Tumors that arise on the ectocervix are easily visible on gynecologic examination and often cause postcoital bleeding. By contrast, tumors that arise from the endocervix can cause expansion of the cervix but are generally less visible, and bleeding may be less prominent. As cervical tumors continue to expand and infiltrate locally, additional symptoms, usually pain, develop. Hip, buttock, flank, and sciatic pain all indicate that the tumor has reached the pelvic sidewall. Direct extension of the tumor into the bladder or rectum is rare and must be confirmed by bladder or rectal biopsy. However, ureteral obstruction can occur at the pelvic sidewall. Because this condition is frequently asymptomatic, with only minimal changes in serum creatinine present, intravenous pyelography is the standard staging test.

Lymphatic metastases are the most common form of regional spread, and the status of the lymph nodes has great prognostic significance. The lymphatic spread generally follows a predictable sequence from the pelvic nodes to the para-aortic nodes and then typically along the path of the thoracic duct to the left supraclavicular nodes. Therefore, physical examination of a patient with cervical cancer should always include careful palpation of the supraclavicular area.

## EVALUATION OF PATIENTS WITH STAGE IB THROUGH STAGE IV DISEASE

In contrast to other major gynecologic cancers, cervical cancer is staged with clinical methods because most patients are treated with radiotherapy rather than with surgery. Clinical staging begins with a careful digital examination of the vagina and rectum, with documentation of the findings in an annotated drawing, in the medical record. When the clinical findings are unclear, pelvic examination under anesthesia is an option. If there is any doubt as to parametrial or pelvic sidewall extension, the lower stage should be assigned.

In addition to physical examination, the minimum staging procedures for all patients are a chest x-ray, liver and renal function laboratory tests, and an intravenous pyelogram. Barium enema is useful in patients with suspected rectal involvement or other colorectal disease that might influence radiotherapy. Flexible sigmoidoscopy offers the possibility of biopsy, as well. Flexible sigmoidoscopy and cystoscopy are necessary only for patients with advanced disease whose physical examination or symptoms suggest bladder or rectal invasion.

Imaging the pelvic and para-aortic lymph nodes is a vital component of the modern evaluation of patients with cervical cancer. Although none of the available modalities is ideal (Table 18B-3), lymphangiography remains the diagnostic mode of choice for evaluating lymph nodes.[17,18] Surgical staging can detect micrometastases to lymph nodes and confirm palpation findings in the pelvis.[19] In addition, some evidence suggests that "debulking" the metastatic nodes improves long-term outcome.[20,21] Retroperitoneal staging clearly reduces the risk of complications compared to transperitoneal staging if patients are treated with radiotherapy.

**TABLE 18B-3.** TECHNIQUE FOR IMAGING LYMPH NODES

| TECHNIQUE | ADVANTAGES | DISADVANTAGES |
|---|---|---|
| Lymphangiography | Images internal structure of nodes; high sensitivity | Labor intensive; high potential for complications; poor availability |
| Computed tomography | Images all structures of abdomen and pelvis; replaces intravenous pyelography; widely available | Increased risk of false positives due to inflammatory changes |
| Magnetic resonance imaging | Best images of primary tumor; safe in pregnancy | Expensive |
| Ultrasonography | Least risk | Lowest sensitivity |

## TREATMENT OF INVASIVE CERVICAL CANCER

Consensus holds that patients with stage IB1 squamous carcinoma of the cervix with negative preoperative lymph node imaging findings can be treated with radical hysterectomy and pelvic lymphadenectomy or pelvic radiation. The choice of treatment depends on factors such as the desire for ovarian preservation, the presence of co-morbid conditions, the risk of side effects, and the availability of subspecialists in the treatment of cervical cancer.

Controversy remains regarding the merits of radical hysterectomy for patients with stage IB2 cervical cancers. In one study, more than 70% of patients with stage IB2 cervical cancer received postoperative radiotherapy for a variety of high-risk histologic findings, and the 5-year survival rate for this group was 72.8%.[22] In another study, the disease-specific 5-year survival rate was similar for patients with 5-cm tumors that had been treated with radiation only. The similarity in these results has been interpreted as a caution against combining therapies when one will suffice.[23] Curtin[24] argues that surgery remains the treatment of choice, noting that complications associated with high-dose intracavitary radiation are complex and difficult to manage and that adherence to nationally accepted standards for radiotherapy of cervical cancer by radiation oncologists is poor.[25] In general, we believe that radical hysterectomy should be avoided for patients whose preoperative evaluation indicates that postoperative radiation would be needed should the radical hysterectomy be performed. Such indications would include bulky (greater than 4-cm) tumors, extensive lymphovascular involvement, high-grade adenocarcinoma, and pelvic lymph node metastases.

The debate over radiation versus surgery may be resolved by the recently announced results of several multi-institutional phase III trials. Between 1990 and 1997, the Radiation Therapy Oncology Group randomly assigned 403 patients who had tumors of 5 cm or larger and disease confined to the pelvis to receive either extended field radiation or a combination of 5-fluorouracil, cisplatin, and pelvic radiation. Patients who received chemoradiation had an estimated 5-year survival rate of 73% compared with 58% for the other group. In another trial, patients with locally advanced disease were assigned to receive radiation in combination with hydroxyurea, or hydroxyurea, cisplatin, and 5-fluorouracil or weekly cisplatin. The treatments that included cisplatin significantly increased the progression-free survival rate, and the cisplatin-only group had the best toxicity profile. These results suggest that patients whose tumors are 5 cm or larger (stage IB2) may be best treated with radiation and chemotherapy as opposed to surgery and radiation (Fig. 18B-1). Based on the results of five studies,[26–30] the National Cancer Institute took the unusual step of releasing a clinical announcement on February 22, 1999: "Results from each of 5 randomized phase III trials shows overall survival advantage for cisplatin-based chemotherapy given concurrently with radiation therapy. Although trials vary somewhat in terms of stage of disease, dose of radiation, and schedule of cisplatin and radiation, they all demonstrate significant sur-

vival benefit for this combined approach. The risk of death from cervical cancer was decreased by 30 percent to 50 percent by concurrent chemoradiation. Based on these results, strong consideration should be given to the incorporation of concurrent cisplatin-based chemotherapy with radiation therapy in women who require radiation therapy for treatment of cervical cancer."

Standard pelvic radiation is given in two phases and involves the use of an external beam with megavoltage energies in two anterior-posterior opposed fields. This approach treats the pelvic nodes and shrinks the primary tumor. Brachytherapy techniques and the relative radioresistance of the cervix, uterus, and vagina allow the use of very high local doses. Low-dose-rate brachytherapy is given in two applications usually 2 weeks apart. Each requires general anesthesia and a 2- to 3-day hospitalization. High-dose-rate brachytherapy is an alternative to low-dose-rate in some centers. High-dose-rate brachytherapy may be given on an outpatient basis, although it requires up to five applications.

**Treatment Algorithm**

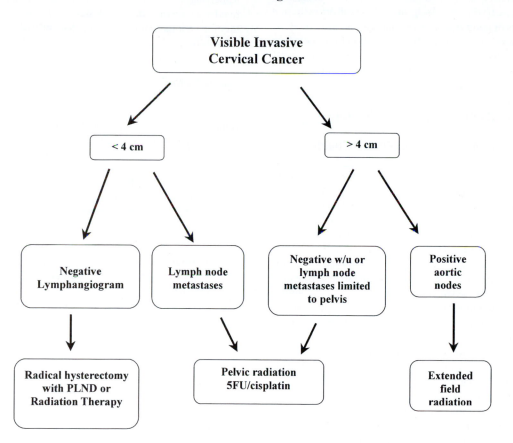

PLND = pelvic lymph node dissection.

**FIGURE 18B-1.** Algorithm for management of patients with invasive cervical cancer. This strategy emphasizes chemoradiation for patients with advanced disease, defined as large volume or pelvic metastases.

A recent innovation in the surgical management of patients with invasive cervical cancer who wish to retain their fertility is radical vaginal trachelectomy.[31] Several successful pregnancies have been reported after this operation.[32]

## TREATMENT OF RECURRENT CERVICAL CANCER

Recurrent cervical cancer presents a complex treatment problem with little likelihood of success. Small recurrences in the vagina and pelvis after radical hysterectomy can be cured with radiotherapy. However, survival rates for patients in this group range from 50%, if tumor is limited to the vagina, to less than 20%, if the pelvic sidewall is involved. Pelvic exenteration provides the only significant possibility of cure when disease recurs after radiation therapy—but only if that recurrence manifests as central pelvic tumors that can be extirpated in this way. Survival rates of up to 50% have been reported in well-selected patients treated with pelvic exenteration after pelvic radiotherapy.

Patients whose disease cannot be cured by surgery or radiotherapy are usually treated with chemotherapy. Numerous drugs have been tested in phase II trials. Single-agent cisplatin still offers the best regimen in terms of good response and manageable toxicity. However, tumors in a previously irradiated area respond very poorly to chemotherapy, with only about 15% of patients having a complete or partial response and another 30% having stabilization of disease.

## UTERINE FUNDAL CANCERS

### INCIDENCE, EPIDEMIOLOGY, AND RISK FACTORS

Most tumors of the fundal portion of the uterus arise within the epithelial glandular lining and can be categorized as endometrial adenocarcinomas. Endometrial adenocarcinomas constitute the most common gynecologic malignancy and will be diagnosed in about 36,000 U.S. women this year.[2] Histologic subtypes include typical endometrial adenocarcinoma (90%), papillary adenocarcinoma (3%), papillary serous carcinoma (3%), clear-cell carcinoma (2%), and mucinous carcinoma (2%)[33,34] Malignant tumors arising from mesenchymal elements of the uterus are much less common, accounting for about 3500 cases annually. The major histologic categories include leiomyosarcoma (LMS), endometrial stromal sarcoma (ESS), and malignant mixed müllerian tumors (MMMT).

Uterine fundal malignancies of all types are typically tumors of postmenopausal women, with about three-quarters of cases diagnosed in women over the age of 50 years.[33–35] These cancers are more common in developed countries and tend to occur more often in the higher socioeconomic social groups. This profile is similar to that observed in women with breast and ovarian cancers and would seem to suggest that a high-fat diet may play some role in predisposing individuals to these cancers. Although the majority of endometrial adenocarcinomas appear as sporadic cases, a genetic syndrome has been identified in some families with breast, ovary, or colon cancers.[36,37] In addition, women with a previous diagnosis of breast, ovarian, or colon cancer are at higher risk for developing endometrial cancer—as are those with a family history

of these malignancies.[38] Some retrospective reviews have identified prior pelvic irradiation as a potential predisposing factor in the development of uterine sarcomas.[39–41]

Several medical conditions have been associated with an increased risk of developing endometrial adenocarcinomas. These include obesity, hypertension, diabetes mellitus, and gallbladder disease. While some authors have argued that these medical conditions are routinely seen in the obese postmenopausal woman and are not cancer risk factors, careful epidemiologic reviews employing multivariate analysis have identified these conditions as independent risk factors.[42–45]

The normal endometrial glands undergo intense proliferation in response to estrogenic stimulation. During the reproductive years, this estrogenic stimulation of the proliferative phase of the ovarian cycle is normally counterbalanced by the equally strong maturational effects of progesterone secreted by the corpus luteum after ovulation. Clinical conditions causing chronic unopposed exposure of the endometrium to estrogenic stimulation have all been associated with an increased risk of endometrial cancer.[46–50] Obesity also represents a chronic estrogenic stimulation state in that peripheral fat cells are capable of converting adrenal androstenedione to estrone, a weak estrogen. A summary of epidemiologic risk factors for endometrial cancer and their relative risks is outlined in Table 18B-4.

### CLINICAL MANIFESTATIONS

Most endometrial malignancies occur in postmenopausal women. Initial tumor growth is centered within the uterine cavity, where friable polypoid portions of tumor frequently produce bleeding or

**TABLE 18B-4. RISK FACTORS FOR ENDOMETRIAL ADENOCARCINOMA**

| FACTOR | RELATIVE RISK INCREASE (X) |
|---|---|
| Epidemiologic features: | |
| Postmenopausal reproductive status | 5–7 |
| Caucasian race | 2 |
| Home in Europe or North America | 2.5 |
| Higher economic status | 1.5 |
| Associated medical conditions: | |
| Obesity | 2–4 |
| Hypertension | 1.5 |
| Diabetes mellitus | 3 |
| Gallbladder disease | 4 |
| Family history (breast, colon, endometrial cancer) | 2 |
| Continuous estrogen exposure: | |
| Exogenous estrogens (unopposed) | 2–12 |
| Early menarche/late menopause | 1.5–4 |
| Nulliparity | 2–3 |
| Anovulation | 2–5 |
| Estrogen-secreting tumors | 10–15 |

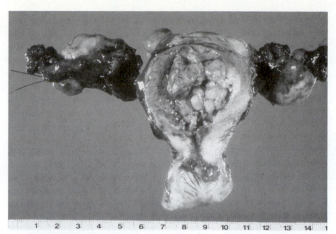

**FIGURE 18B-2.** Hysterectomy specimen opened to demonstrate the extensive polypoid growth pattern of an endometrial carcinoma. The tumor fills the entire endometrial cavity and presents a readily accessible target for outpatient biopsy.

spotting from the vagina (Fig. 18B-2). Because normal menstruation has usually ceased, women easily recognize the presence of any bleeding. Furthermore, postmenopausal bleeding is a widely publicized and identified symptom of cancer. Consequently, most women with this symptom seek prompt medical evaluation. Tumors that occur in premenopausal or perimenopausal women frequently produce a bleeding pattern that is substantially different from normal menstruation. These women also tend to seek medical evaluation because they view their abnormal bleeding as an annoying problem that interferes with their daily function.

Both primary-care physicians and gynecologists have been trained to identify abnormal bleeding patterns and seek a rapid diagnosis. As a result, about 75% of all cases of endometrial cancer are diagnosed while the tumor is still confined to the uterus.[51,52] In such cases, the woman tends to have no symptoms other than abnormal vaginal bleeding. The mechanisms of tumor spread beyond the uterus include direct local extension, intraperitoneal implantation, retroperitoneal lymphatic metastasis, and distant hematogenous dissemination. Fortunately, relatively few patients present with clinically advanced endometrial cancer. The clinical presentation for these cases will be dictated by the mechanism and route of spread. Direct local growth produces a large bulky tumor that usually extends to involve the cervix first and then the adjacent organs such as ovary, bladder, and rectosigmoid. Pain, bleeding, and a palpable mass are the hallmarks of this presentation. In very advanced tumors, fistulae to the bladder or rectum may occur. Intraperitoneal implantation can occur if the primary tumor penetrates the uterine serosa and releases microfragments of tumor into the peritoneal cavity or if malignant cells traverse the fallopian tubes to reach the peritoneum. Intraperitoneal tumors tend to produce multiple surface nodules, an omental "cake," and ascites. This presentation may resemble that commonly seen in women with advanced ovarian cancers. In fact, papillary serous tumors of the uterus (histologically identical to those seen in the ovary) often present in this fashion. Retroperi-

toneal lymphatic spread is usually clinically silent and only detected at the time of staging laparotomy. Enlarged nodes may be detected by preoperative imaging studies such as computed tomography (CT) or magnetic resonance imaging (MRI) or may cause identifiable symptoms if they compress or entrap nerve roots. Unusual, but well-described, lymphatic presentations for endometrial cancer include palpable groin metastasis caused by tumor embolization through lymphatic channels that parallel the round ligament; suburethral metastases, thought to result from retrograde flow of lymph through the vaginal plexus; and left scalene adenopathy, resulting from direct tumor embolization via the thoracic duct. Hematogenous dissemination produces metastases to the lung, liver, bone, or brain. The clinical presentations of such patients will obviously depend upon the site and extent of their distant disease.

## DIAGNOSIS AND EVALUATION

The traditional diagnostic approach to the woman with postmenopausal bleeding consisted of an examination under anesthesia, dilatation of the cervix, and fractional curettage to obtain separate specimens from the endocervix and the endometrium. This approach has largely been replaced by office sampling procedures that are simpler and less risky and provide equivalent diagnostic specimens.[53-55] A variety of outpatient biopsy instruments are available; all of them provide adequate tissue samples for histologic diagnosis. About 10% of cases present diagnostic dilemmas in which a more invasive diagnostic approach is necessary. These include situations in which the cervix is stenotic and cannot be dilated in the clinic, the patient cannot tolerate the discomfort of outpatient biopsy, previously obtained diagnostic material is inadequate, or a large tumor distorts anatomy so as to make the site of origin uncertain. In such settings, examination under anesthesia with dilatation and hysteroscopically directed biopsy is the current diagnostic method of choice. The hysterscope permits direct visualization of both the endocervical and endometrial linings and facilitates targeted biopsy of gross abnormalities.

Pelvic ultrasound may be a useful diagnostic tool in some high-risk asymptomatic women. Ultrasonic measurement of "endometrial stripe" thicknesses greater than 8 mm has been correlated with an increased risk of benign and malignant endometrial neoplasms in long-term tamoxifen users.[56-59] However, routine application of ultrasound as a screening technique for the entire population of postmenopausal women is not warranted because of its relatively high expense and low yield.

Endometrial carcinoma is a surgically staged disease. In addition, most women have tumors that are clinically confined to the uterus at the time of diagnosis. Consequently, once the diagnosis has been established, most of the clinical evaluation is directed toward an assessment of the patient's operative risk rather than an assessment of disease spread. This preoperative evaluation should include a complete history and physical examination, a chest radiograph, an electrocardiogram, and laboratory studies to evaluate hematopoietic, renal and hepatic functions. When abnormal organ function that may influence surgical therapy is detected, a more complete evaluation is indicated. A serum CA-125 level, if elevated, may be a useful predictor of occult extrauterine disease.[60,61] More sophisticated imaging studies such as CT, MRI, ultrasound, and intravenous pyelography should be reserved for patients with large pelvic tumors or symptoms suggestive of metastatic disease.

## STAGING

Prior to 1988, uterine fundal cancers were clinically staged according to guidelines published by FIGO. This schema relied upon a fractional biopsy procedure and a detailed pelvic examination. A number of large surgical staging experiences undertaken and published in the late 1970s and 1980s identified the major weaknesses of the clinical staging system: extrauterine disease was rarely detected, biopsy of the endocervix was frequently a contaminated specimen that inaccurately predicted the presence of tumor, and there were significant discrepancies in assessing histologic grade and cell type between preoperative and postoperative specimens.[62–64] For all of these reasons, FIGO adopted and published a surgical staging system for uterine fundal cancers in 1988 (Table 18B-5). This schema accounts for histologic grade; depth of myometrial penetration; extension to the cervix; and spread to adnexal structures, peritoneal surfaces, or retroperitoneal nodes as major prognostic factors.[65] Features not included that might have prognostic importance are presence of lymph-vascular space invasion, extent of uterine cavity involvement by tumor, presence of certain molecular markers (p53, ras, etc.), and variant cell type.[66–79]

The surgical staging schema provides a detailed framework for categorizing major histopathologic risk factors. However, it fails to specify a precise surgical approach required for adequate staging. Furthermore, there is no current evidence that complete surgical staging results in a survival advantage for patients. Because most women with endometrial cancer have low-grade and low-risk tumors with survival rates above 95%, we have used a stratified approach to staging. Women with superficially invasive grade 1 cancers undergo total hysterectomy with bilateral salpingo-oophorectomy

**TABLE 18B-5.** SURGICAL STAGING OF UTERINE CANCERS, 1998 INTERNATIONAL FEDERATION OF GYNECOLOGY AND OBSTETRICS CRITERIA

| | |
|---|---|
| Stage I. | Cancer is confined to the fundus. |
| A. | Tumor involves only endometrium. |
| B. | Tumor invades <1/2 of myometrium. |
| C. | Tumor invades >1/2 of myometrium. |
| Stage II. | Cancer involves the cervix. |
| A. | Tumor limited to endocervical glands. |
| B. | Tumor invades cervical stroma. |
| Stage III. | There is regional spread of cancer. |
| A. | Tumor invades uterine serosa, tube, ovary, or positive peritoneal cytology. |
| B. | Tumor metastasis to vagina. |
| C. | Tumor metastasis to pelvic or para-aortic lymph nodes. |
| Stage IV. | Bulky pelvic cancer or distant spread is present. |
| A. | Tumor invasion of bladder or rectal mucosa. |
| B. | Distant metastatic disease. |

only. Intraoperative evaluation of the uterine specimen is routinely performed in order to detect the 5% to 10% of stage 1 tumors with deep myometrial invasion or cervical extension. All others have an extended staging operation in addition to their hysterectomy. This surgical strategy is highlighted in the treatment algorithm shown in Fig. 18B-3.

There are a number of surgical approaches to staging. Most of the controversies surrounding them are focused on the extent of the sampling technique and the clinical impact of the information obtained. Our approach is to begin with an exploratory laparotomy through a midline lower abdominal incision. Careful exploration is followed by the collection of pelvic washings for cytologic analysis. We then proceed immediately with the hysterectomy because this is the therapeutic portion of the procedure. The staging portion of the operation can be divided into peritoneal and retroperitoneal phases. Intraperitoneal evaluation includes the cytologic specimen collected at the time of abdominal entry, biopsy of all palpable visual abnormalities, and an omental biopsy.[80] Random sampling of peritoneal surfaces that are grossly normal has an exceedingly low yield for detecting occult disease. Retroperitoneal assessment is aimed at the detection of lymph node metastases. We remove an identifiable lymph node from each of four pelvic nodal groups: external iliac, hypogastric, obturator, and common iliac. These sampling biopsies are performed bilaterally. Additional nodal biopsies are taken from the right and left para-aortic nodal chains at a level near the origin of the ovarian arteries, because lymphatic drainage of the uterine fundus appears to bypass the lower para-aortic lymph nodes. This systematic and selective approach to lymph node sampling appears to provide accurate prognostic information regarding the presence of lymphatic metastases.[81,82] Although most surgeons perform some type of lymphatic sampling, some have advocated complete pelvic and para-aortic lymphadenectomy as both a staging and a therapeutic procedure.[83–85] Recent retrospective review has suggested that women undergoing lymphadenectomy do have a slight survival advantage.[86] These observations require additional confirmation. Postoperatively, all surgical and cytologic specimens are reviewed so that the patient can be assigned to a stage grouping.

FIGO's surgical staging scheme was defined by and developed for women with adenocarcinomas of the endometrial lining. It is unclear whether or not women with uterine sarcomas should be operatively managed in the same fashion. Pure mesenchymal tumors have a greater tendency for lymphatic and hematogenous dissemination (LMS and ESS), while the mixed müllerian tumors (MMMT) have features of both epithelial and mesenchymal lesions. Because all forms of uterine sarcoma are rare, we have tended to perform an extended staging operation whenever possible as a means of learning more about their spread patterns and natural history.

## TREATMENT

Hysterectomy with bilateral salpingo-oophorectomy is the primary treatment modality for women with endometrial cancers that are clinically confined to the uterus. Surgical removal of the uterus is curative for most patients. An abdominal approach through a midline incision is usually employed to allow adequate access for

**Treatment Algorithm**

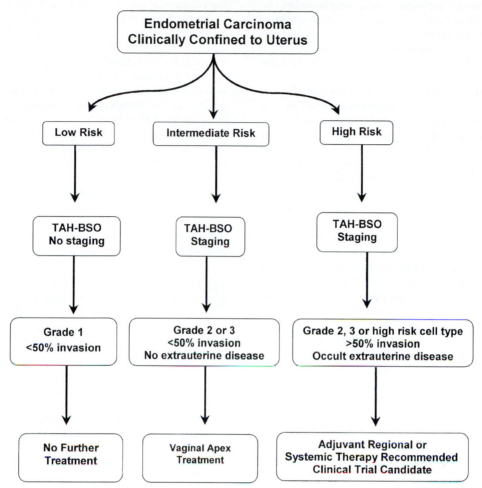

**FIGURE 18B-3.** Treatment algorithm for staging and treatment of endometrial carcinomas confined to the uterus. The outlined strategy limits extended staging operations and potentially morbid adjuvant therapy to those patients at greatest risk for development of recurrent tumor, while eliminating these risks in the large subset of low-risk patients who are likely to be cured by surgical resection alone.

extended staging procedures in high-risk cases. Laparoscopically assisted vaginal hysterectomy with or without additional staging biopsies has been used as an alternative by some surgeons skilled in these techniques.[87] Current evidence suggests that laparoscopic procedures can provide histopathologic material equivalent to that obtained at open laparotomy. Total vaginal hysterectomy has also been used as a potentially less morbid approach for massively obese women with low-grade tumors.[88–90] This technique avoids an abdominal incision but precludes a staging assessment of the peritoneal cavity and retroperitoneal lymph nodes. In our experience, the vaginal approach is as technically difficult as an abdominal one in the obese woman and offers no distinct advantage.

Several centers have successfully treated subsets of endometrial carcinoma patients with radiation alone.[91–94] Typically, irradiation-only therapy has been reserved for patients thought to have exorbitant operative risks because of obesity or medical illness. The best treatment results appear to be achieved when therapy is weighted toward the brachytherapy component rather than external-beam treatment of the whole pelvis. Techniques that use uterine packing sources, such as Heyman or Simon capsules, seem to be more effective than an intrauterine tandem and ovoid apparatus. Virtually all of the experience reported for radiation-only treatment describes a disease-free survival rate that is 15% to 20% less than that reported for surgical therapy. Since few medically compromised patients have an operative mortality risk this high, we have reserved radiotherapy as sole treatment of only the most severely ill women.

Tumors that grossly expand the cervix (stage IIB) may present a diagnostic and treatment dilemma. It is often impossible to determine the precise site of origin in these cases. To address the potential risk of incomplete resection by extrafascial hysterectomy, a more aggressive therapeutic approach is usually recommended. Options include surgical removal by radical hysterectomy as employed for cervical carcinomas and combined treatment using preoperative external-beam irradiation and a single brachytherapy application followed by extrafascial hysterectomy. Reported outcomes for either approach appear comparable.[95–99]

Fortunately, the number of patients who present with advanced unresectable pelvic disease or distant metastases is small. In these cases, curative treatment is usually not possible and must be individualized to disease location and volume as well as patient condition.

A large selection of postoperative adjuvant and adjunctive treatment options have been added to hysterectomy in an attempt to reduce the incidence of recurrent disease. Additional therapy is usually not recommended for women with superficially invasive low-grade cancers, because their chance for cure following surgery alone is greater than 90%. Adjuvant therapy can be considered for stage I and II cases with high-risk features such as grade 3 histology or deep myometrial invasion. Although external-beam irradiation to the whole pelvis with or without vaginal cuff brachytherapy is probably the most frequently employed adjuvant treatment, systemic treatment with a variety of chemotherapeutic or hormonal agents has also been used in this setting.[100,101] Postoperative irradiation can reduce the risk of isolated vaginal apex failure by about 50%.[102–104] However, isolated vaginal recurrence is a relatively uncommon event. Several large trials have failed to demonstrate a survival advantage for either adjuvant external beam pelvic irradiation or progestational therapy.[105–110] Reported experience with adjuvant chemotherapy suggests an advantage but has not yet been tested in large randomized trials.[111,112]

For patients who have documented extrauterine disease, postoperative adjunctive therapy is recommended, because recurrence risk is extremely high in stage III and IV cases.[113–115] External-beam irradiation to the pelvis, extended fields to the para-aortic nodal regions, or whole abdominal fields can be selected based on disease extent and location. Residual disease volume is an important predictor of survival, especially for locations outside of the pelvis where less intensive therapy can be safely delivered. Systemic chemotherapy may be effective in some cases. Combined modality therapy is currently under investigation.[116]

Most women who develop tumor recurrence die of their disease. The rare patient who presents with central pelvic failure can be salvaged by irradiation (if not previously used) or by exenterative resection.[117,118] However, most recurrences are not amenable to local or regional approaches. Systemic therapy should be considered palliative. Occasional long-term responses to hormonal therapy with progestational agents have been reported, but are uncommon.[119–122] There is a perception that low-grade lesions metastatic to the lung may be particularly sensitive to progestational therapy. The majority of metastases do not respond to hormonal agents and must be treated with cytotoxic chemotherapy. Agents with demonstrated activity include cisplatin, carboplatin, doxorubicin, and paclitaxel (Taxol).[123–130] Although response rates for single-agent therapy approach 30% to 35%, response duration is generally short and long-term survival is unusual.

## UTERINE SARCOMAS

The treatment of uterine sarcomas parallels that of endometrial carcinomas with a few minor differences. Surgical resection by hysterectomy remains the primary treatment of choice. We perform extended staging in all cases because of the higher potential for extrauterine disease. Reported recurrence incidence for women with tumors confined to the uterus is as high as 50%.[131–133] Uterine sarcomas have a predilection for distant dissemination via lymphatic or hematogenous routes.[134] Although postoperative external-beam irradiation is often employed, there is no documented advantage to any adjuvant therapeutic modality in women with uterine sarcoma.[135–136] Our approach is to reserve treatment for women who develop recurrent disease, even though such treatment is not likely to be curative. Radiotherapy can be used for local or regional palliation of pelvic or nodal recurrence. Systemic agents with some activity include doxorubicin, cisplatin, ifosfamide, and dacarbazine.[137–142] Anecdotal responses to hormonal agents have been reported but are very unusual, with the exception of low-grade endometrial stromal sarcomas, which are exquisitely sensitive to progestational agents.[143,144]

## REFERENCES

1. WINGO PA et al: Cancer statistics, 1995. CA 45(1):8, 1995.
2. LANDIS SH et al: Cancer statistics, 1998. CA 48:6, 1998.
3. ANDERSON GH et al: Organisation and results of the cervical cytology screening programme in British Columbia, 1955–85. Br Med J Clin Res Ed 296(6672):975, 1988.
4. KOSS LG: The Papanicolaou test for cervical cancer detection: A triumph and a tragedy. JAMA 261(5):737, 1989.
5. MUNOZ N et al: The role of HPV in the etiology of cervical cancer. Mutat Res 305(2):293, 1994.
6. PETERS RK et al: Risk factors for invasive cervical cancer among Latinas and non-Latinas in Los Angeles Country. J Natl Cancer Inst 77(5):1063, 1986.
7. ZUNZUNEQUI MV et al: Male influences on cervical cancer risk. Am J Epidemiol 123(2):302, 1986.
8. SCHIFFMAN MH et al: Biochemical epidemiology of cervical neoplasia: measuring cigarette smoke constituents in the cervix. Cancer Res 47(14):3886, 1987.
9. HALPERT R et al: Human papillomavirus and lower genital neoplasia in renal transplant patients. Obstet Gynecol 68(2):251, 1986.
10. MAIMAN M et al: Prevalence, risk factors, and accuracy of cytologic screening for cervical intraepithelial neoplasia in women with the human immunodeficiency virus. Gynecol Oncol 68(3):233, 1998.
11. Screening, in *Cancer of the Cervix,* HM Shingleton and JW Orr Jr (eds). Philadelphia, Lippincott, 1995, pp 17ff.
12. MONTZ FJ et al: Natural history of minimally abnormal Papanicolaou smear. Obstet Gynecol 80(3 Pt 1):385, 1992.
13. MITCHELL MF et al: A randomized clinical trial of cryotherapy, laser vaporization, and loop electrosurgical excision for treatment of squamous intraepithelial lesions of the cervix. Obstet Gynecol 92(5):737, 1998.
14. SESKI JC et al: Microinvasive squamous carcinoma of the cervix: Definition, histologic analysis, late results of treatment. Obstet Gynecol 50(4):410, 1977.

15. Burghardt E et al: Objective results of the operative treatment of cervical cancer. Bailieres Clin Obstet Gynecol 2(4):987, 1988.

16. Morris M et al: Cervical conization as definitive therapy for early invasive squamous carcinoma of the cervix. Gynecol Oncol 51(2):193, 1993.

17. Heller PB et al: Clinical-pathologic study of stage IIB, III and IVA carcinoma of the cervix: extended diagnostic evaluation for paraaortic node metastasis—A Gynecologic Oncology Group study. Gynecol Oncol 38(3):425, 1990.

18. Wallace S et al: Is lymphangiography worthwhile? Int J Radiat Oncol Biol Phys 5:1873, 1979.

19. Nordqvist SR et al: Selective therapy for early cancer of the cervix. I. Surgically explored nonresected cases. Gynecol Oncol 7(2):248, 1979.

20. Hacker NF et al: Resection of bulky positive lymph nodes in patients with cervical carcinoma. Int J Gynecol Cancer 5:250, 1995.

21. Potish RA et al: The role of surgical debulking in cancer of the uterine cervix. Int J Radiat Oncol Biol Phys 17(5):979, 1989.

22. Finan MA et al: Radical hysterectomy for stage IB1 vs IB2 carcinoma of the cervix: Does the new staging system predict morbidity and survival? Gynecol Oncol 62(2):139, 1996.

23. Grigsby PW: Stage IB1 vs IB2 carcinoma of the cervix: Should the new FIGO staging system define therapy? (editorial) Gynecol Oncol 62(2):135, 1996.

24. Curtin JP: Radical hysterectomy—The treatment of choice for early-stage cervical carcinoma. (editorial) Gynecol Oncol 62(2):137, 1996.

25. Montana GS et al: Carcinoma of the cervix: Patterns in care studies: Review of 1978, 1983, and 1988–1989 surveys. Int J Radiat Oncol Biol Phys 32(5):1481, 1995.

26. Morris M et al: Pelvic radiation with concurrent chemotherapy versus pelvic and para-aortic radiation for high-risk cervical cancer: A randomized Radiation Therapy Oncology Group clinical trial. NEJM 340:1137, 1999.

27. Rose PG et al: Concurrent cisplatin-based chemoradiation improves progression-free and overall survival in advanced cervical cancer: Results of a randomized Gynecologic Oncology Group study. NEJM 340:1144, 1999.

28. Whitney CW et al: A randomized comparison of fluorouracil plus cisplatin versus hydroxyurea as an adjunct to radiation therapy in stages IIB–IVA carcinoma of the cervix with negative para-aortic lymph nodes. A Gynecologic Oncology and Southwest Oncology Group Study. J Clin Oncol 17:1339, 1999.

29. Peters WA III et al: Cisplatin and 5-fluorouracil plus radiation therapy are superior to radiation therapy as adjunctive in high-risk early-stage carcinoma of the cervix after radical hysterectomy and pelvic lymphadenectomy: Report of a phase III intergroup study. Gynecol Oncol 72:443 (abstract), 1999.

30. Keys HM et al: Cisplatin, radiation, and adjuvant hysterectomy compared with radiation and adjuvant hysterectomy for bulky stage IB cervical carcinoma. NEJM 340:1154, 1999.

31. D'Argent D, Mathevet P: Schauta's vaginal hysterectomy combined with laparoscopic lymphadenectomy. Bailieres Clin Obstet Gynecol 9(4):691, 1995.

32. Roy M, Plante M: Pregnancies after radical vaginal trachelectomy for early-stage cervical cancer. Am J Obstet Gynecol 179(6 Pt 1):1491, 1998.

33. Burke TW et al: Treatment failure in endometrial carcinoma. Obstet Gynecol 75:96, 1990.

34. Connelly PJ et al: Carcinoma of the endometrium III: Analysis of 865 cases of adenocarcinoma and adenoacanthoma. Obstet Gynecol 59:569, 1982.

35. Morrow CP et al: Relationship between surgical-pathological risk factors and outcome in clinical stage I and II carcinoma of the endometrium: A Gynecologic Oncology Group Study. Gynecol Oncol 40:55, 1991.

36. Lynch HT et al: Endometrial carcinoma: Multiple primary malignancies constitutional factors and heredity. Am J Med Sci 252:381, 1966.

37. Lynch HT et al: Cancer family syndrome, in *Cancer Genetics*, HT Lynch (ed). Springfield, IL, Charles C Thomas, 1976, pp 355–388.

38. Mitchell MF et al: Patients with both breast and endometrial cancer. Proc Soc Gynecol Oncol (Abstr) 49:143, 1993.

39. Peters III WA et al: The selective use of vaginal hysterectomy in the management of adenocarcinoma of the endometrium. Am J Obstet Gynecol 146:285, 1983.

40. Hannigan EV, Gomez LG: Uterine leiomyosarcoma: A review of prognostic clinical and pathological features. Am J Obstet Gynecol 134:557, 1979.

41. Larson B et al: Prognostic factors in uterine leiomyosarcoma. Acta Oncol 29:185, 1990.

42. Wynder EL et al: An epidemiological investigation of cancer of the endometrium. Cancer 19:489, 1966.

43. MacMahon B: Risk factors for endometrial cancer. Gynecol Oncol 2:122, 1974.

44. Davies JL et al: A review of the risk factors for endometrial carcinoma. Obstet Gynecol Surv 36:107, 1981.

45. Parazzina F et al: Review: The epidemiology of endometrial cancer. Gynecol Oncol 41:1, 1991.

46. Smith DC et al: Association of exogenous estrogen and endometrial carcinoma. N Engl J Med 293:1164, 1975.

47. Ziel HK, Finkle WD: Increased risk of endometrial carcinoma among users of conjugated estrogens. N Engl J Med 293:1167, 1975.

48. Gray LA et al: Estrogens and endometrial cancer. Obstet Gynecol 49(4):385, 1977.

49. Antunes CMF et al: Endometrial cancer and estrogen use: Report of a large case-control study. N Engl J Med 300:9, 1979.

50. Ernster VL et al: Benefits and risks of menopausal estrogen and/or progestin hormone use. Prev Med 17:201, 1988.

51. Hendrickson M et al: Uterine papillary serous carcinoma: A highly malignant form of endometrial adenocarcinoma. Am J Surg Pathol 6:93, 1982.

52. Christopherson WM et al: Carcinoma of the endometrium V: An analysis of prognosticators in patients with favorable subtypes and stage I disease. Cancer 51:1705, 1983.

53. Greenwood SM, Wright DJ: Evaluation of the office endometrial biopsy in the detection of endometrial carcinoma and atypical hyperplasia. Cancer 43:1474, 1979.

54. Koss LG et al: Endometrial carcinoma and its precursors: Detection and screening. Clin Obstet Gynecol 25:49, 1982.

55. Grimes DA: Diagnostic office curettage—Heresy no longer. Contemp Obstet Gynecol 28:96, 1986.

56. Hann LE et al: Endometrial thickness in tamoxifen-treated patients: Correction with clinical and pathologic findings. Am J Roentgenol 168:657, 1997.

57. Fisher B et al: Five versus more than five years of tamoxifen therapy for breast cancer patients with negative lymph nodes and estrogen receptor-positive tumors. J Natl Cancer Inst 88:1529, 1996.

58. FISHER B et al: Endometrial cancer in tamoxifen-treated breast cancer patients: Findings from the National Surgical Adjuvant Breast and Bowel Project (NSABP) B-14. J Natl Cancer Inst 86:527, 1994.

59. KILLACKEY MA et al: Endometrial adenocarcinoma in breast cancer patients receiving antiestrogens. Cancer Treat Rep 69:237, 1985.

60. PATSNER B et al: Predictive value of preoperative serum CA 125 levels in clinically localized and advanced endometrial carcinoma. Am J Obstet Gynecol 158:399, 1988.

61. ROSE PG et al: Serial CA-125 measurements for evaluation of recurrence in patients with endometrial carcinoma. Obstet Gynecol 84:12, 1994.

62. COWLES TA et al: Comparison of clinical and surgical staging in patients with endometrial carcinoma. Obstet Gynecol 66:413, 1985.

63. BORONOW RC et al: Surgical staging in endometrial cancer: Clinical-pathologic findings of a prospective study. Obstet Gynecol 63:825, 1984.

64. DISAIA PJ et al: Risk factors and recurrence patterns in stage I endometrial cancer. Am J Obstet Gynecol 151:1009, 1985.

65. CREASMAN WT: New gynecologic cancer staging. Obstet Gynecol 75:287, 1990.

66. SCHINK JC et al: Tumor size in endometrial cancer: A prognostic factor for lymph node metastasis. Obstet Gynecol 70:216, 1987.

67. HANSON MB et al: The prognostic significance of lymph-vascular space invasion in stage I endometrial cancer. Cancer 55:1753, 1985.

68. INOUE Y et al: The prognostic significance of vascular invasion by endometrial carcinoma. Cancer 78:1447, 1996.

69. HENDRICKSON M et al: Adenocarcinoma of the endometrium: Analysis of 256 cases with carcinoma limited to the uterine corpus. Gynecol Oncol 13:373, 1982.

70. JEFFREY JF et al: Papillary serous adenocarcinoma of the endometrium. Obstet Gynecol 67:670, 1986.

71. SILVERBERG SG, DE GIORGI LS: Clear cell carcinoma of the endometrium: Clinical pathologic and ultrasonic findings. Cancer 31:1127, 1973.

72. KURMAN RJ, SCULLY RE: Clear cell carcinoma of the endometrium: An analysis of 21 cases. Cancer 37:872, 1976.

73. SUTTON GP et al: Malignant papillary lesions of the endometrium. Gynecol Oncol 27:294, 1987.

74. SALAZAR OM et al: Adenosquamous carcinoma of the endometrium: An entity with an inherent poor prognosis? Cancer 40:119, 1977.

75. ENOMOTO T et al: K-ras activation in premalignant and malignant epithelial lesions of the human uterus. Cancer Res 51:5308, 1991.

76. HETZEL DJ et al: HER-2/neu expression: A major prognostic factor in endometrial cancer. Gynecol Oncol 47:179, 1992.

77. LUKES AS et al: Multivariable analysis of DNA ploidy, p53, and HER-2/neu as prognostic factors in endometrial cancer. Cancer 73:2380, 1994.

78. MILLER B et al: Nucleolar organizer regions: A potential prognostic factor in adenocarcinoma of the endometrium. Gynecol Oncol 54:137, 1994.

79. PISANI AL et al: HER-2/neu, p53, and DNA analyses as prognosticators for survival in endometrial carcinoma. Obstet Gynecol 85:729, 1995.

80. MARINO BD et al: Staging laparotomy for endometrial carcinoma: Assessment of peritoneal spread. Gynecol Oncol 56:34, 1995.

81. CHUANG L et al: Staging laparotomy for endometrial carcinoma: Assessment of retroperitoneal lymph nodes. Gynecol Oncol 58:189, 1995.

82. CLARKE-PEARSON D et al: Morbidity and mortality of selective lymphadenectomy in early stage endometrial cancer (Abstract). Proc Soc Gynecol Oncol 32:14, 1991.

83. ORR JW JR et al: Surgical staging of uterine cancer: An analysis of perioperative morbidity. Gynecol Oncol 42:209, 1991.

84. LARSON DM et al: Pelvic and para-aortic lymphadenectomy for surgical staging of endometrial cancer: Morbidity and mortality. Obstet Gynecol 79:998, 1992.

85. GIRARDI F et al: Pelvic lymphadenectomy in surgical treatment of endometrial cancer. Gynecol Oncol 49:177, 1993.

86. KILGORE LC et al: Adenocarcinoma of the endometrium: Survival comparisons of patients with and without pelvic node sampling. Gynecol Oncol 56:29, 1995.

87. CHILDERS JN et al: Laparoscopic assisted surgical staging (LASS) of endometrial carcinoma. Gynecol Oncol 51:33, 1993.

88. PRATT JH et al: Vaginal hysterectomy for carcinoma of the fundus. Am J Obstet Gynecol 88:1063, 1964.

89. PETERS III WA et al: Prognostic features of sarcomas and mixed tumors of the endometrium. Obstet Gynecol 63:550, 1984.

90. BLOSS JD et al: Use of vaginal hysterectomy for the management of stage I endometrial cancer in the medically compromised patient. Gynecol Oncol 40:74, 1991.

91. KUPELIAN PA et al: Treatment of endometrial carcinoma with radiation therapy alone. Int J Radiat Oncol Biol Phys 27:817, 1993.

92. LANDGREN RC et al: Irradiation of endometrial cancer in patients with medical contraindication to surgery or with unresectable lesions. Am J Roentgenol 26:148, 1976.

93. ANDERSEN WA et al: Radiotherapeutic alternatives to standard management of adenocarcinoma of the endometrium. Gynecol Oncol 16:383, 1983.

94. FISHMAN DA et al: Radiation therapy as exclusive treatment for medically inoperable patients with stage I and II endometrioid carcinoma of the endometrium. Gynecol Oncol 61:189, 1996.

95. RUTLEDGE F: The role of radical hysterectomy in adenocarcinoma of the endometrium. Gynecol Oncol 2:331, 1974.

96. PARK RC et al: Treatment of adenocarcinoma of the endometrium. Gynecol Oncol 2:60, 1974.

97. HERNANDEZ W et al: Stage II endometrial carcinoma: Two modalities of treatment. Am J Obstet Gynecol 131:171, 1978.

98. KINSELLA TJ et al: Stage II endometrial carcinoma: 10-year follow-up of combined radiation and surgical treatment. Gynecol Oncol 10:290, 1980.

99. ONSRUD M et al: Endometrial carcinoma with cervical involvement (stage II): Prognostic factors and value of combined radiological-surgical treatment. Gynecol Oncol 13:76, 1982.

100. CHUNG CK et al: The role of adjunctive radiotherapy for stage I endometrial carcinoma: Preoperative vs postoperative irradiation. Int J Radiat Oncol Biol Phys 7:1429, 1989.

101. MEERWALDT JH et al: Endometrial adenocarcinoma adjuvant radiotherapy tailored to prognostic factors. Int J Radiat Biol Phys 18:299, 1990.

102. MORROW CP, TOWNSEND DE: Synopsis of Gynecologic Oncology. New York, Churchill Livingstone, 1987.

103. BROWN JM et al: Vaginal recurrence of endometrial carcinoma. Am J Obstet Gynecol 100:544, 1968.

104. Phillips GL et al: Vaginal recurrence of adenocarcinoma of the endometrium. Gynecol Oncol 13:323, 1982.

105. Onsrud M et al: Postoperative external pelvic irradiation in carcinoma of the corpus stage I: A controlled clinical trial. Gynecol Oncol 4:222, 1976.

106. Aalders J et al: Postoperative external irradiation and prognostic parameters in stage I endometrial carcinoma. Obstet Gynecol 56:419, 1980.

107. Lewis GC et al: Adjuvant progestogen therapy in primary definitive treatment of endometrial cancer. Gynecol Oncol 2:368, 1974.

108. Kauppila A et al: Adjuvant progestin therapy in endometrial carcinoma. Prog Cancer Res Ther 25:219, 1983.

109. DePalo G et al: A controlled clinical study of adjuvant medroxyprogesterone acetate (MPA) therapy in pathologic stage I endometrial carcinoma with myometrial invasion (Abstract). Proc Ann Meet Am Soc Clin Oncol 4:121, 1985.

110. MacDonald RR et al: A randomized trial of progestogens in the primary treatment of endometrial carcinoma. Br J Obstet Gynaecol 95:166, 1988.

111. Stringer CA et al: Adjuvant chemotherapy with cisplatin, doxorubicin, and cyclophosphamide (PAC) for early-stage high-risk endometrial cancer: A preliminary analysis. Gynecol Oncol 38:305, 1990.

112. Burke TW et al: Postoperative adjuvant cisplatin, doxorubicin, and cyclophosphamide (PAC) chemotherapy in women with high-risk endometrial carcinoma. Gynecol Oncol 55:47, 1994.

113. Potish RA et al: Paraaortic lymph node radiotherapy in cancer of the uterine corpus. Obstet Gynecol 65:251, 1985.

114. Potish RA et al: Role of whole abdominal radiation therapy in the management of endometrial cancer: Prognostic importance of factors indicating peritoneal metastases. Gynecol Oncol 21:80, 1985.

115. Greer BE, Hamberger AD: Treatment of intraperitoneal metastatic adenocarcinoma of the endometrium by the whole-abdomen moving-strip technique and pelvic boost irradiation. Gynecol Oncol 16:365, 1983.

116. Reisinger SA et al: A phase I study of weekly cisplatin and whole abdominal radiation for the treatment of stage III and IV endometrial carcinoma: A gynecologic oncology group pilot study. Gynecol Oncol 63:299, 1996.

117. Morris M et al: Treatment of recurrent adenocarcinoma of the endometrium with pelvic exenteration. Gynecol Oncol 60:288, 1996.

118. Barber HRK, Brunschwig A: Treatment and results of recurrent cancer of corpus uteri in patients receiving anterior and total pelvic exenteration 1974–1963. Cancer 22:949, 1968.

119. Kelley RM, Baker WH: Progestational agents in the treatment of carcinoma of the endometrium. N Engl J Med 264:216, 1961.

120. Reifenstein EC: Hydroxyprogesterone caproate therapy in advanced endometrial cancer. Cancer 27:485, 1971.

121. Podratz KC et al: Effects of progestational agents in treatment of endometrial carcinoma. Obstet Gynecol 66:106, 1985.

122. Lenz SA et al: High dose megestrol acetate in advanced or recurrent endometrial cancer: A Gynecologic Oncology Group study. J Clin Oncol 14:357, 1996.

123. Thigpen JT et al: Phase II trial of Adriamycin in the treatment of advanced or recurrent endometrial carcinoma: A Gynecologic Oncology Group study. Cancer Treat Rep 63:21, 1979.

124. Trope C et al: A phase II study of cisplatinum for recurrent corpus cancer. Eur J Cancer 16:1025, 1980.

125. Seski JC et al: Cisplatin chemotherapy for disseminated endometrial cancer. Obstet Gynecol 59:225, 1982.

126. Thigpen JT et al: Phase II trial of cisplatin as first-line chemotherapy in patients with advanced and recurrent endometrial carcinoma: A Gynecologic Oncology Group study. Gynecol Oncol 33:68, 1989.

127. Long HJ et al: Phase II evaluation of carboplatin in advanced endometrial carcinoma. J Natl Cancer Inst 80:276, 1988.

128. Green JB et al: Carboplatin therapy in advanced endometrial cancer. Obstet Gynecol 75:696, 1990.

129. Burke TW et al: Treatment of advanced or recurrent endometrial carcinoma with single-agent carboplatin. Gynecol Oncol 51:397, 1993.

130. Ball HG et al: A phase II trial of taxol in advanced and recurrent adenocarcinoma of the endometrium: A Gynecologic Oncology Group study (Abstract). Gynecol Oncol 62:278, 1996.

131. Spanos WJ Jr et al: Patterns of recurrence in malignant mixed müllerian tumor of the uterus. Cancer 57:155, 1986.

132. George M et al: Uterine sarcomas: Prognostic factors and treatment modalities—study on 209 patients. Gynecol Oncol 24:58, 1986.

133. Major FJ et al: Prognostic factors in early-stage uterine sarcoma. Cancer 71:1702, 1993.

134. Moskovic E et al: Survival patterns of spread and prognostic factors in uterine sarcoma: A study of 76 patients. Br J Radiol 66:1009, 1993.

135. Hornback NB et al: Observations on the use of adjuvant radiation therapy in patients with stage I and II uterine sarcoma. Int J Radiat Oncol Biol Phys 12:2127, 1986.

136. Sorbe B: Radiotherapy and/or chemotherapy as adjuvant treatment of uterine sarcomas. Gynecol Oncol 20:281, 1985.

137. Piver MS, Barlow JJ: Adriamycin in localized and metastatic uterine sarcomas. J Surg Oncol 12:263, 1979.

138. Hannigan EV et al: Treatment of advanced uterine sarcoma with Adriamycin. Gynecol Oncol 16:101, 1983.

139. Omura GA et al: A randomized study of Adriamycin with and without dimethyl triazenoimidazole carboxamide in advanced uterine sarcomas. Cancer 52:626, 1983.

140. Currie JL et al: Combination chemotherapy with hydroxyurea, dacarbazine (DTIC), and etoposide in treatment of uterine leiomyosarcoma: A Gynecologic Oncology Group study. Gynecol Oncol 61:27, 1996.

141. Sutton GP et al: Phase II trial of ifosfamide and mesna in leiomyosarcoma of the uterus: A Gynecologic Oncology Group study. Am J Obstet Gynecol 166:556, 1992.

142. Sutton GP et al: A phase II trial of ifosfamide and mesna in patients with advanced or recurrent mixed mesodermal tumors of the ovary previously treated with platinum-based chemotherapy: A Gynecologic Oncology Group study. Gynecol Oncol 53:24, 1994.

143. Styron SL et al: Low-grade endometrial stromal sarcoma recurring over three decades. Gynecol Oncol 35:275, 1989.

144. Katz L et al: Endometrial stromal sarcoma: A clinicopathologic study of 11 cases with determination of estrogen and progestin receptor levels in three tumors. Gynecol Oncol 26:87, 1987.

# 18C / CANCER OF THE FALLOPIAN TUBE

*Cheung Wong and M. Steven Piver*

## INTRODUCTION

Primary carcinoma of the fallopian tube is the least common malignancy of the female genital tract and is estimated to account for less than 1.0% of all gynecologic malignancies.[1,2] Worldwide, the incidence of fallopian tube carcinoma ranges from 2.9 to 3.6 cases per million women.[3] The mean age at diagnosis of fallopian tube carcinoma ranges from 54 to 63 years; however, cases of primary carcinoma of the fallopian tubes have been reported in women as young as 17 to 19 years of age.[4,5] Similar to epithelial ovarian cancer, the majority of patients are white (87%) and postmenopausal (66%).[1] Despite being diagnosed at an earlier stage, the overall 5-year survival rate for all stages ranges from 14% to 36.5%; the 5-year survival rate in stages I and II ranges from 17% to 50.8% compared to 0% to 51% in stages III and IV.[6–8]

Although the etiology of fallopian tube carcinoma remains unknown, pelvic inflammatory disease and infertility have been suggested as possible causal factors.[2,6,9] In a study of 71 patients with primary fallopian tube cancer, Eddy et al.[1] reported chronic salpingitis in 11% of patients; likewise, Ayhan et al.[2] identified pelvic inflammatory disease among 25% of patients. Recently, there is doubt whether pelvic inflammatory disease is related to carcinoma of the fallopian tubes since the rate of pelvic inflammatory disease in patients with fallopian tube cancer is no higher than that in the general population. In a retrospective study of 40 patients with fallopian tube cancer, Mei-Liu et al.[5] reported a history of sterility among 42.5% of patients; furthermore, among infertile patients, there was a 5-fold higher incidence of bilateral invasive fallopian tube carcinoma than in fertile patients.

## CLINICAL MANIFESTATIONS

Unlike primary epithelial ovarian cancer, which is often described as a "silent" disease, primary fallopian tube cancer is characterized with a relative abundance of nonspecific symptoms. Abdominal pain, vaginal bleeding, and watery vaginal discharge are the most common presenting symptoms (Table 18C-1).[1,9] In 1916, Latzko[10] described the "hydrops tubae profluens" phenomenon, which is considered to be pathognomonic for fallopian tubal cancer: colicky lower abdominal pain, adnexal mass, and pain that is relieved after profuse serous discharge from the vagina; this triad of symptoms has

been reported in only 8% to 20% of patients.[11] Among 71 patients, Eddy and colleagues[1] reported 50% to be symptomatic for less than 2 months, 71% to be symptomatic for less than 6 months, 87% to be symptomatic for less than 12 months, and 13% are symptomatic for more than 1 year. The most frequently described physical findings are pelvic mass (61%), abdominal mass (23%), and ascites (5%).[1]

## DIAGNOSIS

The preoperative diagnosis of fallopian tube carcinoma is usually delayed because up to 20% of the patients may be asymptomatic at presentation, whereas the remainder of the patients have inconsistent, nonspecific symptoms[12]; in fact, less than 3% of patients are correctly diagnosed preoperatively.[1,11] Currently, there are no preoperative screening examinations for fallopian tube carcinoma; however, cytology, serology, and radiographic studies may be helpful in diagnosing this rare malignancy.

Based on its natural history, malignant cells from the fallopian tubes are suspected to be expelled into the uterus and ultimately into the vagina, resulting in abnormal cervical and vaginal cytology. The incidence of abnormal Pap smears ranges from 11% to 60%.[16–19] The low sensitivities of Pap smears prohibit them from being a reliable diagnostic tool for the diagnosis of fallopian tube cancer. A discrepancy between Pap smears, colposcopy, cervical biopsy, and endometrial curettage should raise the suspicion of fallopian tube cancer.

Serum CA 125 levels may be elevated in 59% to 100% of patients; however, its value as a diagnostic test is limited, since serum CA 125 levels may be elevated in other malignant conditions (ovarian cancer, uterine cancer) and benign conditions (pelvic inflammatory disease, endometriosis, fibroids).[17–19] Serum CA 125 may perhaps be most useful in the management and follow-up of patients with fallopian tube cancer. In a small study of five patients with fallopian tube cancer, Tokunaga et al.[19] reported that all patients demonstrated a rapid decrease in CA 125 levels as they responded to treatment; among the three patients who remained free of disease, CA 125 levels continued to be less than 5 U/mL, but the two patients who developed recurrence demonstrated elevated levels of CA 125.

Radiologic imaging has been proposed as a possible tool for diagnosing fallopian tube carcinoma. Martzloff,[20] in 1940, proposed the use of hysterosalpingography in diagnosing this rare malignancy; however, this technique has not been widely accepted because of the theoretical potential of initiating or potentiating intraperitoneal

**TABLE 18C-1.** PRESENTING SYMPTOMS
OF FALLOPIAN TUBE CARCINOMA

Abdominal pain
Vaginal bleeding
Vaginal discharge
Asymptomatic

**TABLE 18C-2.** FINN AND JAVERT'S CRITERIA FOR
DIAGNOSING FALLOPIAN TUBE CANCER

FINN AND JAVERT'S GROSS CRITERIA
1. The fallopian tubes, at least in the distal portion, are
   abnormal. The fimbrated end may be dilated and occluded.
2. Papillary growth is found in the endosalpinx.
3. Uterus and ovaries are grossly normal or affected by
   lesions other than cancer.

FINN AND JAVERT'S MICROSCOPIC CRITERIA
1. The epithelium of the endosalpinx is replaced in whole or
   in part by adenocarcinoma; histologically, the cells resemble
   the epithelium of the endosalpinx.
2. The endometrium and ovaries are normal or contain
   malignant lesions which are secondary to the tubal primary
   tumor.
3. Tuberculosis is excluded.

spread of malignant cells from the fallopian tube. Images of cystic, solid, or complex adnexal masses with free fluid in the cul-de-sac are often seen on CT scan, MRI, or sonography; consequently, these images are often misinterpreted for the more common ovarian tumors, tuboovarian abscess, or ectopic pregnancies. Recent advances in color and pulsed transvaginal doppler have aided in accurately diagnosing fallopian tube malignancies.[21] Currently, there is no ideal screening test for fallopian tube cancer; instead, a constellation of signs; symptoms; and serologic, cytologic, and radiographic data should raise the suspicion of this rare malignancy in the preoperative state.

## HISTOLOGY

The histopathologic similarities between primary ovarian cancer and primary fallopian tube cancer often make it difficult to differentiate between the two entities. In 1949, Finn and Javert[22] proposed criteria, both gross and microscopic, for the diagnosis of primary fallopian tube cancer (Table 18C-2). Subsequently, additional diagnositic criteria, first proposed by Hu et al.[23] in 1950, then modified by Sedlis[11] in 1978, used in the diagnosis of primary fallopian tube cancer are:

1. The histological pattern reproduces the epithelium of the tubal mucosa
2. The tumor arises from the endosalpinx
3. Transition from benign to malignant epithelium is found
4. Ovaries and endometrium are normal or with tumor smaller than tumor in the tube

The gross appearance of the fallopian tubes is variable. Bilateral fallopian tube carcinoma has been reported in 13% to 26% of patients.[11,12] The tubes vary from being moderately enlarged (2 cm in diameter) to large sausagelike tubes (17 cm in diameter) (Fig. 18C-1). In 55% a patients, a friable tumor is noted to be extruding from the fimbriated end of the affected tube, although examination of the fallopian tube mucosa usually demonstrates the tumor to be in the distal third of the tube.[23] Salpingitis is present in approximately 37% of patients.[24] Dissection of the tube often demonstrates bloody or purulent fluid, making the diagnosis of fallopian tube carcinoma difficult to differentiate from hydrosalpinx or pyosalpinx.[23]

Preinvasive (in situ) carcinoma of the fallopian tubes has been described by several investigators.[25–27] To accurately diagnose carcinoma in situ of the fallopian tubes, the epithelial cells lining the endosalpinx must form papillae with mitotically active malignant nuclei.[28] Invasive fallopian tube carcinoma is classified as either

epithelial, mixed epithelial-mesenchymal, or mesenchymal (Table 18C-3). The majority of the tumors are histologically similar to serous adenocarcinomas; the tumors are composed of branching papillae with one or more layers of epithelial cells consisting of hyperchromatic nuclei and abnormal mitoses[28] (Fig. 18C-2). An abrupt transition from normal to malignant epithelium may be seen. Less common histologic subtypes of the fallopian tubes are mucinous carcinomas, endometrioid carcinoma, leiomyosarcomas, mixed mesodermal tumors,[29,30] clear cell carcinoma,[31] and squamous cell carcinoma.[32]

## STAGING

The staging system for ovarian cancer has been adopted and modified for the staging of fallopian tube cancer because of the clinical, therapeutic, and prognostic similarities between the two disease entities. In 1991, International Federation of Gynecology

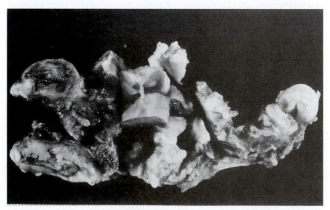

**FIGURE 18C-1.** Fallopian tube carcinoma: gross specimen. Note the papillary growths in the mucosa.

## TABLE 18C-3. CLASSIFICATION OF FALLOPIAN TUBE CARCINOMA

**Malignant Epithelial Tumors**
Carcinoma in situ
Serous carcinoma
Mucinous carcinoma
Endometriod carcinoma
Clear cell carcinoma
Squamous cell carcinoma

**Mixed Epithelial-Mesenchymal Tumors**
Mesodermal (mullerian) mixed tumors
Homologous (carcinosarcoma)
Heterologous

**Mesenchymal Tumors**
Leiomyosarcoma

and Obstetrics (FIGO) accepted an official staging system for fallopian tube cancer[33] (Table 18C-4).

## PATTERNS OF SPREAD

Fallopian tube carcinoma tends to spread intraabdominally in a manner similar to epithelial ovarian cancer. Sedlis[34] reported that peritoneal involvement was the most common site of metastasis, followed by the ovaries and uterus (Table 18C-5). In a study of 15 patients, none of which underwent pelvic lymphadenectomy, Tamimi et al.[35] reported an overall lymph node metastases of 53%: 5 patients with paraaortic lymph node involvement, 1 patient with groin lymph node involvement, 1 patient with groin and supraclavicular lymph node involvement, and 1 patient with mediastinal lymph node involvement. Similarly, in a study of 33 patients with primary fallopian tube carcinoma (27% and 72% of the patients underwent systematic pelvic or paraaortic lymphadenectomy and selective lymph node sampling, respectively), Cormio et al.[36]

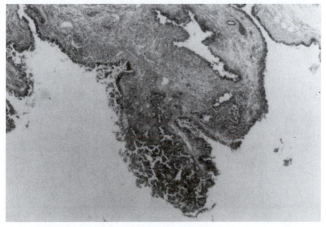

**FIGURE 18C-2.** Fallopian tube carcinoma: Microscopic specimen.

## TABLE 18C-4. FIGO FALLOPIAN TUBE CARCINOMA STAGING

| Stage 0 | Carcinoma in situ (limited to tubal mucosa). |
|---|---|
| Stage I | Growth limited to the fallopian tubes. |
| Stage IA | Growth is limited to one tube with extension into the submucosa and/or muscularis but not penetrating the serosal surface; no ascites. |
| Stage IB | Growth is limited to both tubes with extension into the submucosa and/or muscularis but not penetrating the serosal surface; no ascites. |
| Stage IC | Tumor either stage IA or IB with tumor extension through or onto the tubal serosa; or with ascites present containing malignant cells or with positive peritonel washings. |
| Stage II | Growth involving one or both fallopian tubes with pelvic extension. |
| Stage IIA | Extension and/or metastasis to the uterus and/or ovaries. |
| Stage IIB | Extension to other pelvic tissues. |
| Stage IIC | Tumor either stage IIA or IIB and ascites present containing malignant cells or positive peritoneal washings. |
| Stage III | Tumor involves one or both fallopian tubes with peritoneal implants outside of the pelvis and/or positive retroperitoneal or inguinal nodes. Superficial liver metastases equals stage III. |
| Stage IIIA | Tumor is limited to the true pelvis with negative nodes but histologically confirmed seeding of the abdominal peritoneal surfaces. |
| Stage IIIB | Tumor involving one or both tubes with histologically confirmed implants of abdominal peritoneal surfaces, none exceeding 2 cm in diameter. Lymph nodes are negative. |
| Stage IIIC | Abdominal implants greater than 2 cm in diameter and/or positive retroperitoneal or inguinal nodes. |
| Stage IV | Growth involving one or both fallopian tubes with distant metastases. If pleural effusion is present, there must be positive cytology. Parenchymal liver metastases equals stage IV. |

## TABLE 18C-5. METASTATIC SITES OF FALLOPIAN TUBE CARCINOMA, IN ORDER OF MOST COMMON FREQUENCY

Peritoneum
Ovaries
Uterus
Intestine
Vagina
Lymph nodes
Liver

reported an overall 45% lymph node involvement: 40% with only paraaortic lymph node involvement, 33% with only pelvic lymph node involvement, and 28% demonstrated both pelvic and paraaortic lymph node involvement.

## TREATMENT

### SURGERY

Surgery remains to be the initial treatment for patients with fallopian tube carcinoma. Careful surgical staging should be performed for patients with early-stage disease, which includes total abdominal hysterectomy, bilateral salpingoophorectomy, peritoneal washings, systematic inspection and biopsy of the peritoneal cavity, omentectomy, and bilateral pelvic and paraaortic lymphadenectomy. Among those with advanced stage disease, optimal cytoreductive surgery (<1 cm residual disease) demonstrates a significant survival advantage over those with suboptimal cytoreductive surgery. Eddy et al.[1] reported an overall 5-year survival rate of 29% among patients with no gross residual disease: 5-year survival among those with less than 2 cm residual disease versus those with more than 2 cm residual disease was 15% and 7%, respectively. In addition, Podratz et al.[13] reported a survival rate of 80% at 2 years among patients with residual tumor less than 1 cm to be significantly superior to the 30% survival rate among patients with more than 1 cm residual disease.

### RADIOTHERAPY

External beam radiotherapy, intraperitoneal isotopes, and vaginal and uterine radioactive implants have been proposed as treatment options for patients with fallopian tube carcinoma. Phelbs and Chapman[37] reported that 89% of stage I and II patients treated with postoperative radiotherapy survived 18 months to 16 years, whereas all patients with stage III disease treated with postoperative radiation died for a minimum follow-up of one year. Likewise, Schray et al.[38] reported that 52% of patients with primary fallopian tube cancer (stage I to IV) remain free of disease after being treated with postoperative radiotherapy. Survival data from postoperative radiotherapy should be viewed with caution because of the lack of uniformity among radiotherapy regimens in most clinical trials.

### CHEMOTHERAPY

The natural history of fallopian tube cancer remains poorly defined. Because of its metastatic pattern, the biology of fallopian tube cancer has been assumed to be similiar to that of ovarian cancer. Of patients with fallopian tube cancer, 35% to 43% have intraperitoneal involvement, and over 30% of patients are reported to have paraaortic lymph node involvement.[34,35] Consequently, cisplatin-based chemotherapy regimens, similar to those used in treating ovarian cancer, have been adapted in the treatment of fallopian tube cancer. Due to the rarity of this disease and the small number of clinical trials, the efficacy of chemotherapy in the treatment

**TABLE 18C-6. RESPONSE RATE OF FALLOPIAN TUBE CANCER TO CISPLATIN-BASED CHEMOTHERAPY**

| AUTHOR | NO. OF PATIENTS | CHEMOTHERAPY REGIMEN* | OVERALL RESPONSE |
|---|---|---|---|
| Maxson[39] | 12 | PC ± A | 92% |
| Peters[40] | 16 | PC ± A | 81% |
| Muntz[41] | 12 | PC ± A | 71% |
| Morris[42] | 15 | PAC | 53% |
| Jacobs[43] | 9 | PAC | 44% |

* P = cisplatin; C = cyclophosphamide; A = Adriamycin.

of fallopian tube cancer is limited but promising. Overall, in advanced cases, the response rate to chemotherapy of fallopian tube cancer ranges from 50% to 90% (Table 18C-6). In a study of 23 patients with fallopian tube cancer (12 with measurable disease) treated with cisplatin and cyclophosphamide with or without doxorubicin, Maxson and colleagues[39] reported an overall response rate of 92% with a 2-year survival rate among stage I and II and stage III and IV patients 92% and 43%, respectively. In a study comparing single-agent therapy, multiagent treatment without cisplatin, and cisplatin-based combination therapy, Peters et al.[40] reported a significant survival advantage in treating advanced-stage patients with cisplatin-based chemotherapy: patients treated with cisplatin-based chemotherapy had an overall response rate of 81%, which was significantly higher than the response rate of 29% and 9% for patients treated with multiagent therapy without cisplatin or single-agent therapy, respectively; furthermore, Peters et al.[40] demonstrated a significant improvement in the 5-year survival rate among those patients treated with a cisplatin-based multiagent chemotherapy regimen versus those treated with other forms of chemotherapeutic regimens, 40% versus 10%, respectively. In the study by Peters et al.,[40] an important difference between the study groups should be noted: only 19% of patients in the cisplatin-based chemotherapy arm developed recurrent disease, whereas almost 60% of patients in the two other treatment arms developed recurrent disease. In a study from Memorial Sloan-Kettering Cancer Center, Barakat et al.[8] reported an overall 5-year survival rate of 51% among 38 patients treated with cisplatin-based combination chemotherapy following primary surgery; in addition, those patients with no residual disease following surgery had a significantly higher 5-year survival rate than those with gross residual disease, 83% versus 28%, respectively.

### Acknowledgment

*Pathologic figures are courtesy of Tamara Kalir, MD, PhD, The Mount Sinai School of Medicine, New York, New York.*

## REFERENCES

1. EDDY GL et al: Fallopian tube carcinoma. Obstet Gynecol 64:546, 1984.
2. AYHAN A et al: Primary carcinoma of the fallopian tube: A study of 8 cases. Eur J Gynaec Oncol 15:2, 1994.

3. NORDIN AJ: Primary carcinoma of the fallopian tube: A 20 year literature review. Obstet Gynecol Survey 49:349, 1994.

4. BLAUSTEIN A: Tubal adenocarcinoma coexistent with other genital neoplasms. Obstet Gynecol 21:62, 1963.

5. LIU MM et al: Diagnosis of primary adenocarcinoma of fallopian tube. J Cancer Res Clin Oncol 110:136, 1985.

6. ROSEN A et al: Primary carcinoma of the fallopian tube—A retrospective analysis of 115 patients. Br J Cancer 68:605, 1993.

7. ROSE PG et al: Fallopian tube cancer. The Roswell Park experience. Cancer 66:2661, 1990.

8. BARAKAT RR et al: Cisplatin-based combination chemotherapy in carcinoma of the fallopian tube. Gynecol Oncol 42:156, 1991.

9. BAEKELANDT M et al: Primary adenocarcinoma of the fallopian tube. Review of the literature. Int J Gynecol Cancer 3:65, 1993.

10. LATZKO W: Linseitiges Tubenkarizinom rechtsietige karzinomatose tubo-ovarian cyste. Zentralbl Gynakol 40:599, 1916.

11. SEDLIS A: Carcinoma of the fallopian tube. Surg Clin North Am 58:121, 1978.

12. DODSON MG et al: Clinical aspects of fallopian tube carcinoma. Obstet Gynecol 36:935, 1970.

13. PODRATZ KC et al: Primary carcinoma of the fallopian tube. Am J Obstet Gynecol 154:1319, 1986.

14. BOUTSELIS JG, THOMPSON JN: Clinical aspects of primary carcinoma of the fallopian tube. A clinical study of 14 cases. Am J Obstet Gynecol 111:98, 1971.

15. FIDLER HK, LOCK DR: Carcinoma of the fallopian tube detected by cervical smear. Am J Obstet Gynecol 67:1103, 1954.

16. CORMIO G et al: Primary carcinoma of the fallopian tube. A retrospective analysis of 47 patients. Ann Oncol 7:271, 1996.

17. KOL S et al: Preoperative diagnosis of fallopian tube carcinoma by transvaginal sonography and CA-125. Gynecol Oncol 37:129, 1990.

18. NILOFF JM et al: Evaluation of serum CA 125 in carcinomas of the fallopian tube, endometrium, and endocervix. Am J Obstet Gynecol 148:1057, 1984.

19. TOKUNAGA T et al: Serial measurement of CA 125 in patients with primary carcinoma of the fallopian tube. Gynecol Oncol 36:335, 1990.

20. MARTZLOFF KH: Primary carcinoma of the fallopian tube. Am J Obstet Gynecol 40:804, 1940.

21. KURJAK A et al: Preoperative diagnosis of primary fallopian tube carcinoma. Gynecol Oncol 68:29, 1998.

22. FINN WJ, JAVERT CT: Primary and metastatic cancer of the fallopian tube. Cancer 2:803, 1949.

23. HU CY et al: Primary carcinoma of the fallopian tube. Am J Obstet Gynecol 59:58, 1950.

24. PETERS WA et al: Prognostic features of carcinoma of the fallopian tube. Obstet Gynecol 71:757, 1988.

25. GREENE TH, SCULLY RE: Tumors of the fallopian tube. Clin Obstet Gynecol 886, 1962.

26. HAYDEN GE, POTTER EL: Primary carcinoma of the fallopian tube. With report of 12 new cases. Am J Obstet Gynecol 79:24, 1960.

27. RYAN GM: Carcinoma in situ of the fallopian tube. Am J Obstet Gynecol 84:198, 1962.

28. WHEELER JE: Diseases of the fallopian tube, in *Blaustein's Pathology of Female Genital Tract*, 4th ed, RJ Kurman (ed). New York, Springer-Verlag, 1994, pp 529–562.

29. MUNTZ HG et al: Carcinosarcoma and mixed mullerian tumors of the fallopian tube. Gynecol Oncol 34:109, 1989.

30. CARLSON JA et al: Malignant mixed mullerian tumor of the fallopian tube. Cancer 71:87, 1993.

31. VOET RL, LIFSHITZ S: Primary clear cell adenocarcinoma of fallopian tube: Light microscopic and ultrastructural findings. Int J Gynecol Pathol 1:292, 1982.

32. MALINAK LJ et al: Primary squamous cell carcinoma of the fallopian tube. Am J Obstet Gynecol 95:1167, 1966.

33. PETTERSSON F: Staging rules for gestational trophoblastic tumors and fallopian tube cancer. Acta Obstet Gynecol Scand 71:224, 1992.

34. SEDLIS A: Primary carcinoma of the fallopian tube. Obstet Gynecol Surv 16:209, 1961.

35. TAMIMI HK, FIGGE DC: Adenocarcinoma of the uterine tube: Potential for lymph node metastases. Am J Obstet Gynecol 141:132, 1981.

36. CORMIO G et al: Lymph node involvement in primary carcinoma of the fallopian tube. Int J Gynecol Cancer 6:405, 1996.

37. PHELPS HM, CHAPMAN KE: Role of radiation therapy in treatment of primary carcinoma of the uterine tube. Obstet Gynecol 43:669, 1974.

38. SCHRAY MF et al: Fallopian tube cancer: The role of radiation therapy. Radiother Oncol 10:267, 1987.

39. MAXSON WZ et al: Primary carcinoma of the fallopian tube: Evidence for activity of cisplatin combination therapy. Gynecol Oncol 26:305, 1987.

40. PETERS WA et al: Results of chemotherapy in advanced carcinoma of the fallopian tube. Cancer 63:836, 1989.

41. MUNTZ HG et al: Combination chemotherapy in advanced adenocarcinoma of the fallopian tube. Gynecol Oncol 40:268, 1991.

42. MORRIS M et al: Treatment of fallopian tube carcinoma with cisplatin, doxorubicin, and cyclophosphamide. Obstet Gynecol 76:1020, 1990.

43. JACOBS AJ et al: Treatment of carcinoma of the fallopian tube using cisplatin, doxorubicin, and cyclophosphamide. Am J Clin Oncol 9:436, 1986.

# 18D / GESTATIONAL TROPHOBLASTIC TUMORS

*Cheung Wong and M. Steven Piver*

## INTRODUCTION

Gestational trophoblastic disease encompasses a spectrum of inter-related diseases that arises from tumor growths of the human trophoblasts; these disease entities include complete and partial molar pregnancies, gestational choriocarcinoma, and placental site trophoblastic disease. The malignant potential of each of these disease entities depends on the extent of trophoblastic hyperplasia.

The incidence of hydatidiform moles varies in different parts of the world. In North America or Europe the incidence ranges from 0.6 to 1.1 per 1000 pregnancies, whereas in Japan there is an apparent twofold increase in the incidence of hydatidiform moles (2.0 per 1000 pregnancies).[1] The high incidence of hydatidiform moles in certain parts of the world may be attributed to racial, socioeconomic, and dietary factors. In a study from Hawaii, Matsuura et al.[2] reported an increased incidence of developing hydatidiform moles among Filipinos and other Oriental groups in comparison to whites and native Hawaiians, 1 in 571 pregnancies versus 1 in 1300 pregnancies, respectively. Women at extreme ends of their reproductive life also have an increased risk of developing molar pregnancies. Women over the age of 50 reportedly have a 300- to 400-fold increased risk of developing hydatidiform moles, whereas women under the age of 15 have a sixfold increased risk over women between the ages of 25 and 29.[2,3] Interestingly, Parazzini and colleagues[4] reported that paternal age over 45 years is associated with a 2.9 times increased relative risk for the development of complete molar pregnancies. Risk of developing molar pregnancies is independent of paternal race.[2]

Worldwide studies have consistently found that diet is an important risk factor for the development of hydatidiform moles. In a case control study of 140 patients from Italy, Parazzini et al.[5] reported that patients with gestational trophoblastic disease have a significantly decreased consumption of vitamin A, β-carotene, and animal protein. Likewise, in the United States, Berkowitz et al.[6] observed a 50% decrease in the risk of gestational trophoblastic disease among women with increased animal fat and β-carotene consumption.

Several case control studies have found an increased risk for hydatidiform moles among women with a previous history of gestational trophoblastic disease or spontaneous or therapeutic abortions. Among patients with a history of prior molar pregnancies, Palmer et al.[1] reported a tenfold increase in subsequent risk for molar pregnancies. In a case control study of 331 cases and 662 controls, Briton and colleagues[7] reported a significantly decreased risk of molar pregnancies among patients with prior term pregnancies (odds ratio 0.5), but a significantly increased risk (odds ratio 2.8) among those who underwent prior therapeutic abortions. Women with two consecutive spontaneous abortions have been reported to have a significantly increased risk of developing molar pregnancies.[8]

The incidence of gestational choriocarcinoma has been reported to be one case per 19,920 live births.[9] Risk factors for the development of gestational choriocarcinoma are similar to those for the development of hydatidiform moles. Previous history of hydatidiform moles, maternal age greater than 45, and history of spontaneous abortions are important risk factors in the development of gestational choriocarcinoma.

## CLINICAL MANIFESTATIONS

The clinical presentations of patients with gestational trophoblastic disease are the result of trophoblastic hyperplasia and the concurrent elevation in β human chorionic gonadotropin (β-HCG). Vaginal bleeding and abnormal uterine enlargement (uterus larger than the expected gestational age) are the two most common presenting symptoms (Table 18D-1). Of patients with molar pregnancies, 25% may present with hypertension (preeclampsia), typically occurring prior to 24 weeks' gestation. Hyperthyroidism and hyperemesis are also frequently seen in patients with molar pregnancies, 25% and 10%, respectively. Of patients with hydatidiform moles, 25% to 35% will present with theca lutein cysts of the ovary.[10,11]

Gestational trophoblastic disease has been reported to metastasize to all organ systems, with the lung being the most common site of metastasis (Table 18D-2). Patients with metastatic disease to the lungs may present with dyspnea, coughing, hematoptysis, or pleuritic chest pain. Likewise, patients with cerebral metastases may present with convulsions, focal neurologic signs, or increased intracranial pressure.[12]

## DIAGNOSIS

Patients with molar pregnancies and choriocarcinomas have varying quantities of cytotrophoblast and syncytiotrophoblast; consequently, the β-HCG levels in these patients may be markedly elevated above normal pregnancy levels. Conversely, patients with placental site trophoblastic tumor have a small population of

**TABLE 18D-1.** COMMON PRESENTING SYMPTOMS

Bleeding
Nausea, vomiting
Preeclampsia
Abdominal pain
Hyperthyroidism
Enlarged uterus

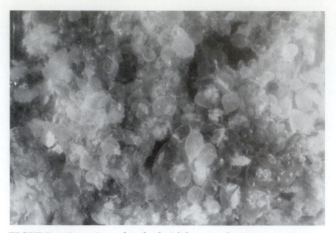

**FIGURE 18D-1.** Complete hydatidiform mole: Gross specimen.

syncytiotrophoblastic elements but a greater population of intermediate cytotrophoblast; therefore, human placental lactogen (HPL) is a more reliable tumor marker than β-HCG among these patients.[13]

Ultrasonography has widely been used to help make the diagnosis of gestational trophoblastic tumors. Sonographic images of gestational trophoblastic disease often demonstrate multiple endometrial hypoechoic channels and spaces.[14] With the addition of transvaginal color Doppler ultrasonography, abundant vascularization with low resistance index are helpful in differentiating gestational trophoblastic tumors from other pathologic entities such as incomplete pregnancies.[15,16] Pelvic magnetic resonance imaging (MRI) has been used in gestational trophoblastic diseases to identify areas of myometrial invasion; however, its role as a diagnostic tool for identifying gestational trophoblastic disease has not yet been fully defined.[17] In a study of 39 patients with abnormally elevated serum β-HCG level with a tentative diagnosis of gestational trophoblastic disease, incomplete pregnancies, or ectopic pregnancies, Barton and colleagues[18] reported overlapping MRI findings, such as increased uterine volume, increased endometrial distension, increased myometrial disruption, and increased myometrial mass in all 39 patients, whereas only 26 of these patients were subsequently pathologically confirmed to have gestational trophoblastic disease. In this study, Barton et al.[18] failed to identify the classic "snowstorm" or "cluster of grapes" images in all 26 patients with documented gestational trophoblastic disease.

## PATHOLOGY

### COMPLETE HYDATIDIFORM MOLE

The chromosomes of all complete molar pregnancies are diploid and paternal in origin.[19] In over 90% of the patients, an anuclear ovum is fertilized by a haploid (23,X) sperm, which duplicates and produces a complete molar pregnancy with 46,XX; however, in 10% of patients, 46,XY may be found when an anuclear ovum is fertilized by two sperms.[20,21] Classically, complete molar pregnancies have been described to have a triad of histologic features:

**TABLE 18D-2.** COMMON SITES OF METASTASES

| | |
|---|---|
| Lungs | Spleen |
| Liver | Kidney |
| Brain | Cecum |
| Vagina | Gastrointestinal tract |

diffuse hydropic swelling of the chorionic villi, diffuse hyperplasia of both syncytiotrophoblast and cytotrophoblast, and lack of identifiable fetal tissue (Figs. 18D-1, 18D-2, 18D-3).[22,23] Because fetal death occurs before the development of the fetal circulation, nucleated fetal erythrocytes are not seen in the villous capillaries (Table 18D-3).[24]

### PARTIAL MOLAR PREGNANCY

Partial molar pregnancies have a triploidy genotype, which is the result of dispermic fertilization of a normal ovum.[25] The ratio of 69,XXX to 69,XXY is approximately 2:3; interestingly, 69,XYY partial moles are very rare.[22] Histologic features of partial moles demonstrate focal hydropic villi, focal trophoblastic hyperplasia, scalloping of the villi, and evidence of fetal tissue (Fig. 18D-4). Since the embryo usually survives for a period of 8 weeks, there is evidence of fetal tissue in partial moles and evidence of nucleated fetal erythrocytes.[26]

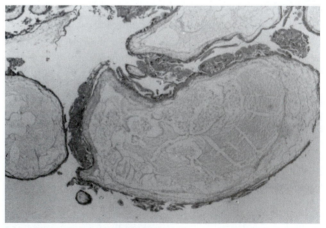

**FIGURE 18D-2.** Complete hydatidiform mole: Microscopic specimen. Note the hydropic chorionic villi.

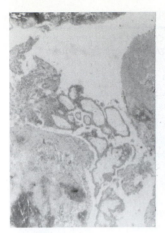
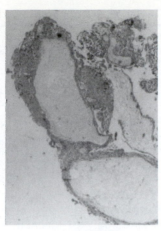

**FIGURE 18D-3.** Comparison of normal chorionic villi versus complete hydatidiform mole (both taken at same magnification). Note the hydropic chorionic villi in the complete mole (left side).

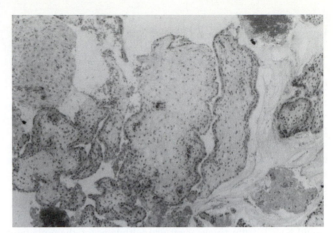

**FIGURE 18D-4.** Partial hydatidiform mole: Microscopic specimen.

## GESTATIONAL CHORIOCARCINOMA

Gestational choriocarcinoma is the result of malignant transformation of molar tissue or from normal pregnancies. Grossly, choriocarcinomas are yellow-white tumors with large areas of necrosis and extensive hemorrhage. Microscopically, choriocarcinomas demonstrate cytotrophoblast and syncytiotrophoblast without any evidence of chorionic villi. Gestational choriocarcinoma readily invades into the blood vessels resulting in myometrial invasion and intravascular tumor emboli.[12,13]

## PLACENTAL SITE TROPHOBLASTIC TUMOR

Placental site trophoblastic tumors are the rarest of gestational trophoblastic tumors. Grossly, placental site trophoblastic tumors have a yellow cut surface with necrotic foci. Microscopically, placental

**TABLE 18D-3. COMPARISON OF COMPLETE VERSUS PARTIAL HYDATIDIFORM MOLES**

| | COMPLETE MOLE | PARTIAL MOLE |
|---|---|---|
| Cytogenetic analysis | 46,XX (most common) Diploidy Paternal origin | 69,XXX (most common) Triploidy Paternal and maternal origin |
| Pathology: Hydropic villi | Diffuse | Focal |
| Trophoblastic proliferation | Diffuse | Focal |
| Scalloping of chorionic villi | Absent | Present |
| Fetus & fetal RBCs | Absent | Present |

site trophoblastic tumors lack the biphasic morphologic pattern of cytotrophoblasts and syncytiotrophoblasts that are characteristic of choriocarcinoma. Placental site trophoblastic tumors metastasize primarily by the hematogenous route, thus demonstrating metastases in the liver, lungs, brain, kidney, and stomach. Aggressive placental site trophoblastic tumors tend to demonstrate 7 or more mitoses per 10 high-power fields, large areas of necrosis, and the presence of many cells with clear cytoplasm.[27,28]

## TREATMENT

### MANAGEMENT OF COMPLETE AND PARTIAL MOLAR PREGNANCIES

Initial treatment of molar pregnancies consists of surgical evacuation and close monitoring of postevacuation β-HCG levels. For women who wish to maintain fertility, suction curettage is the treatment of choice. Oxytocin is usually given before the initiation of the curettage in order to help control bleeding; also, in order to avoid uterine perforations in those uteri that are distended and soft, the uterus should not be sounded prior to curettage. After the suction curettage, the uterine lining is gently curetted with a sharp curette to ensure complete evacuation of molar tissue. Oxytocin infusion should be continued at least 24 h after evacuation. If fertility is no longer desired, hysterectomy is a reasonable option for patients with molar pregnancies. The use of oxytocin or prostaglandins to induce labor is not recommended for the evacuation of molar pregnancies because of the potential risk of disseminating trophoblastic tissue into the systemic circulation. Surgical evacuation is curative in 80% to 90% of the patients. Of patients, 10% may subsequently develop into invasive moles and 2.5% may develop into choriocarcinoma.[29] Close monitoring of postevacuation β-HCG is imperative. Quantitative serum HCG levels should be followed every 1 to 2 weeks until negative for three consecutive weeks then followed up every 3 months for 1 year. Contraception should be used during the follow-up period.

## MANAGEMENT OF LOW-RISK AND HIGH-RISK METASTATIC GESTATIONAL TROPHOBLASTIC DISEASE

### STAGING

Three classification systems have been used for the staging of gestational trophoblastic disease: the Federation of Gynecology and Obstetrics (FIGO) staging system, National Institute of Health (NIH) classification, and the World Health Organization (WHO) scoring system (Table 18D-4). In a retrospective study comparing the three prognostic classification systems, Dubuc-Lissoir et al.[30] reported that none of the scoring systems is clearly superior to the others. The prognostic scoring systems are helpful in identifying which patients would benefit from single-agent or multiple-agent chemotherapy and the scoring systems are more predictive of the clinical outcome. Patients with a prognostic score of 8 or greater are considered to be at high risk and are more likely to require combination chemotherapy to achieve complete remission. Conversely, patients with prognostic scores less than 8 are considered to be at low risk and would benefit from single-agent chemotherapy.[30,31]

## THERAPY FOR NONMETASTATIC GESTATIONAL TROPHOBLASTIC DISEASE

The introduction of an effective single chemotherapeutic agent, namely methotrexate, has significantly improved the cure rates of patients with nonmetastatic gestational trophoblastic disease. In a study of 58 patients with nonmetastatic gestational trophoblastic disease, Hammond et al.[33] reported an overall response rate of 98%; 93% of the patients remained in complete remission after being treated with single-agent methotrexate; of the four patients resistant to methotrexate, three patients entered remission after being treated with hysterectomy or actinomycin D chemotherapy. With better understanding of methotrexate's mechanism of action, folinic acid has been added to rescue normal cells from the inhibition of dihydrofolate reductase induced by methotrexate. In 1985, Berkowitz and colleagues[34] reported that methotrexate and folinic acid achieved excellent outcomes with limited systemic toxicities among patients with nonmetastatic gestational trophoblastic disease; methotrexate and folinic acid induced complete remission in 90.2% of patients with nonmetastatic disease and 82.3% sustained complete remission after only one course of chemotherapy. The combination of methotrexate and folinic acid was associated with granulocytopenia, thrombocytopenia, and hepatotoxicity in 5.9%, 1.6%, and 14.1% of the patients, respectively. Similarly, multiple studies have demonstrated cure rates ranging from 76% to 93% among patients with nonmetastatic gestational trophoblastic disease initially treated with methotrexate; furthermore, in these studies, most patients resistant to methotrexate were subsequently treated with actinomycin D or combination chemotherapy with excellent response[33–37] (Table 18D-5). Alternative single chemotherapeutic agents used in the treatment of nonmetastatic gestational trophoblastic disease are actinomycin D, 5-fluorouracil and etoposide, all of which have a reported remission rate ranging from 84% to 98%.[38–40]

## TABLE 18D-4. CLASSIFICATION SYSTEMS

FEDERATION OF INTERNATIONAL GYNECOLOGIC ONCOLOGY (FIGO) STAGING SYSTEM FOR GESTATIONAL TROPHOBLASTIC TUMORS

| STAGE | DESCRIPTION |
|---|---|
| I | Limited to the uterine corpus |
| II | Extends to the adnexae, outside the uterus, but limited to the genital structures |
| III | Extends to the lungs with or without genital tract involvement |
| IV | All other metastatic sites |

NATIONAL INSTITUTE OF HEALTH (NIH) CLASSIFICATION OF GESTATIONAL TROPHOBLASTIC TUMORS

| GROUP | DESCRIPTION |
|---|---|
| I | Nonmetastatic disease: No evidence of disease outside the uterus |
| II | Metastatic disease: Any disease outside the uterus<br>A. Good-prognosis metastatic disease<br>  1. Short duration (last pregnancy <4 months)<br>  2. Low pretreatment HCG titers: <100,000 IU/24 h in urine or <40,000 mIU/mL of serum<br>  3. No metastasis to brain or liver<br>  4. No significant prior chemotherapy<br><br>B. Poor-prognosis metastatic disease<br>  1. Long duration (last pregnancy >4 months)<br>  2. High pretreatment HCG titer: >100,000 IU/24 h in urine or >40,000 mIU/mL of serum<br>  3. Brain or liver metastasis<br>  4. Significant prior chemotherapy<br>  5. Term pregnancy |

WORLD HEALTH ORGANIZATION (WHO) SCORING SYSTEM FOR GESTATIONAL TROPHOBLASTIC TUMORS

| SCORE | PROGNOSTIC FACTOR | | | |
|---|---|---|---|---|
| | 0 | 1 | 2 | 4 |
| Age, years | <39 | >39 | | |
| Antecedent pregnancy | Mole | Abortion | Term | |
| Interval between end of antecedent pregnancy and start of chemo, months | <4 | 4–6 | 7–12 | >12 |
| HCG, mIU/mL | <$10^3$ | $10^3$–$10^4$ | $10^4$–$10^5$ | >$10^5$ |
| ABO group (female × male) | | O × A<br>A × O | B<br>AB | |
| Largest tumor, cm, including uterus | <3 | 3–5 | >5 | |
| Site of metastases | | Spleen, kidney | GI, liver | Brain |
| Number of metastases | | 1–4 | 4–8 | >8 |
| Prior chemotherapy | | | Single agent | Two or more drugs |

**TABLE 18D-5.** RESPONSE RATE OF NONMETASTATIC GESTATIONAL TROPHOBLASTIC DISEASE TO METHOTREXATE

| AUTHOR | NO. OF PATIENTS | CHEMOTHERAPY | RESPONSE RATE |
|---|---|---|---|
| Hammond[33] | 54 | MTX | 93% |
| Berkowitz[34] | 185 | MTX/FAR | 87.6% |
| Wong[35] | 33 | MTX | 75.8% |
| Barter[36] | 15 | MTX | 87% |

Abbreviations: MTX = methotrexate; FAR = folinic acid rescue.

## THERAPY FOR LOW-RISK, GOOD-PROGNOSIS METASTATIC GESTATIONAL TROPHOBLASTIC DISEASE

Single-agent chemotherapy with methotrexate or actinomycin D is considered treatment of choice for patients with low-risk metastatic gestational trophoblastic disease. In 1965, the National Cancer Institute treated 36 patients with metastatic gestational trophoblastic disease with methotrexate or actinomycin D; in this prospective study, Ross and colleagues[41] reported comparable response rates with methotrexate and actinomycin D, 72% and 79%, respectively. Side effects from methotrexate and actinomycin D were acceptable with no cases of chemotherapy-related mortality. A retrospective study of 52 patients with low-risk metastatic gestational trophoblastic disease from the Southeastern Trophoblastic Disease Center reported 60% of patients achieving complete remission with a median of three cycles of single chemotherapeutic regimen of methotrexate.[42] In a study of 80 patients with low-risk and 5 patients with intermediate-risk gestational trophoblastic disease treated with single-agent high-dose methotrexate with folinic acid rescue, Elit and associates[43] reported an 84% (71 of 85 patients) response rate; the remaining 14 patients who failed to achieve remission with methotrexate were successfully salvaged with second-line chemotherapy. Besides methotrexate, single-agent 5-fluorouracil and etoposide have been demonstrated to be active chemotherapeutic agents in the treatment of low-risk gestational trophoblastic disease. In a study of 173 cases of invasive moles and 139 cases of choriocarcinoma treated initially with 5-fluorouracil, Sung et al.[39] reported a complete remission rate of 84.9% and 59.3% for invasive moles and choriocarcinoma, respectively. Likewise, Wong et al.[38] reported that 59 of 60 patients with persistent or metastatic gestational trophoblastic disease achieved remission after being initially treated with oral etoposide therapy.

## THERAPY FOR HIGH-RISK, POOR-PROGNOSIS GESTATIONAL TROPHOBLASTIC DISEASE

The use of combination chemotherapy for the treatment of high-risk gestational trophoblastic disease has improved the prognosis of these patients in the past two decades. Hammond et al.[44] from 1966

to 1971, reported an overall cure rate of 47% after treating 17 patients with poor-prognosis metastatic trophoblastic disease with two treatment protocols; the first protocol treated patients primarily with combination chemotherapy and the second protocol used combination chemotherapy after failing initial single-agent chemotherapy. Ten patients initially treated with combination triple chemotherapy consisting of methotrexate, actinomycin D, and chlorambucil (MAC) demonstrated a cure rate of 70%. A cure rate of 14% was reported among the seven patients who demonstrated resistance to conventional single-agent methotrexate or actinomycin D and were secondarily treated with MAC chemotherapy. Subsequent trials have commonly substituted cyclophosphamide for chlorambucil in the MAC regimen. Lurain and Brewer[45] reported an overall cure rate of 51% among 73 patients with metastatic poor-prognosis gestational trophoblastic disease who were treated with MAC. A cure rate of 63% was reported among patients treated primarily with MAC and a cure rate of 30% was reported among patients treated secondarily with MAC. In a report that reviewed the results of patients with metastatic gestational trophoblastic tumor treated at the New England Trophoblastic Disease Center, DuBeshter et al.[46] reported that survival was markedly improved in the past two decades with the use of combination chemotherapy (MAC) in comparison to those treated with single-agent chemotherapy (methotrexate, methotrexate with folinic acid, or actinomycin D) for patients with high-risk metastatic disease (Table 18D-6).

In 1976, Bagshawe[47,48] reported a seven-drug combination consisting of hydroxyurea, vincristine, methotrexate, folinic acid, actinomycin D, cyclosphosphamide, and doxorubicin (Adriamycin) (CHAMOMA) to be highly effective in the treatment of high-risk gestational trophoblastic disease. Subsequent studies have also demonstrated that CHAMOMA is effective in the treatment of high-risk gestational trophoblastic disease. Data from the Southeastern Regional Trophoblastic Disease Center reported a 56% remission rate among patients with poor prognosis; commonly reported toxicities were myelosuppression and severe thrombocytopenia, 78% and 39%, respectively.[49] Likewise, Wong et al.[50] reported that CHAMOMA was highly effective in treating patients with high-risk gestational trophoblastic disease (cure rate of 82%), but the CHAMOMA regimen had notable side effects: 34% developed moderate leukopenia, 18% developed severe leukopenia, 10% developed

**TABLE 18D-6.** HIGH-RISK METASTATIC GESTATIONAL TROPHOBLASTIC TUMORS: RESULTS OF THERAPY BY DECADES*

| THERAPY | REMISSION RATE PER PERIOD | | |
|---|---|---|---|
| | 1965–1975 | 1976–1985 | 1980–1985 |
| Primary single-agent chemotherapy | 48% | 17% | 0% |
| Primary combination chemotherapy | 33% | 73% | 92% |
| Secondary combination chemotherapy | 25% | 80% | 90% |

* Adapted from Dubeshter et al.[46]

**TABLE 18D-7.** MAC VERSUS CHAMOMA: RESPONSE RATE

| REGIMEN | REMISSION WITH PRIMARY TREATMENT | REMISSION WITH SECONDARY TREATMENT |
|---|---|---|
| MAC | 73% | 23% |
| CHAMOMA | 65% | 5% |

ABBREVIATIONS: MAC = methotrexate, dactinomycin, chlorambucil; CHAMOMA = methotrexate, dactinomycin, cyclophosphamide, doxorubicin, melphalan, hydroxyurea, and vincristine.

moderate thrombocytopenia, and 6% developed severe thrombocytopenia. In a randomized prospective study comparing MAC versus CHAMOMA, the Gynecologic Oncology Group reported that MAC appeared to be as effective but much less toxic than the CHAMOMA regimen[51] (Table 18D-7).

Because etoposide has been reported to be effective in the treatment of gestational trophoblastic disease, it has been included in the multichemotherapeutic regimen in the treatment of high-risk gestational trophoblastic disease.[38,52] The combination of etoposide, methotrexate, actinomycin D, cyclophosphamide, and vincristine (EMA/CO) has been used to treat patients with poor-prognosis gestational trophoblastic disease, with an overall response rate ranging from 80% to 86% (Table 18D-8). In a study of 36 patients with high-risk gestational trophoblastic disease treated with the EMA/CO regimen, 22 as first-line therapy and 14 as second-line therapy, Bolis and colleagues[53] documented an overall response rate of 86%. The overall relapse rate after complete response was 19% at 5.5 months (median time). Toxicity was acceptable, with 40.9% developing neutropenia and 22.7% developing thrombocytopenia. In a nonrandomized study of 148 patients with high-risk gestational trophoblastic tumors (76 patients had received no prior chemotherapy and 72 had received prior chemotherapy), Newlands et al.[54] reported an 82% remission rate among patients who had received no prior chemotherapy, and 89% remission rate among those who received prior chemotherapy. Among the patients who demonstrated resistance to EMA/CO, the addition of cisplatin salvaged 82% of these patients. In 1997, Bower et al.[55] reported the results of 272 patients, of which 121 patients had previously received chemotherapy, with high-risk gestational trophoblastic disease who were treated with weekly EMA/CO. The overall 5-year survival rate was 86.2%, with 78% of patients achieving complete remission. Multivariate analysis demonstrated that liver metastases, brain metastases, and antecedent term pregnancies were independent adverse prognostic factors. Forty-seven patients developed resistance to EMACO, but 70% of these patients were salvaged with further cisplatin-based chemotherapy and surgery. Alopecia, nausea, reversible neurotoxicity, and myelosuppression are common reported toxicities of EMA/CO.

## ROLE OF SURGERY IN THE TREATMENT OF GESTATIONAL TROPHOBLASTIC DISEASE

Surgery has a limited role in the treatment of patients with gestational trophoblastic disease because of the introduction of effective chemotherapy regimens. However, surgery may be useful in removing the only known focus of disease (either during primary or secondary chemotherapy treatments), in controlling hemorrhage, in relieving obstructions, or in treating other complications that may otherwise interfere with the potential cure of chemotherapy. Surgical procedures used in the treatment of gestational trophoblastic disease include hysterectomy, bowel resection, craniotomy, thoracotomy, and nephrectomy.[57,58] In a comprehensive review of their experience from the Southeastern Regional Center for Trophoblastic Disease, Hammond et al.[58] reported that hysterectomies performed during the administration of systemic chemotherapy significantly reduce the duration of hospitalization and the amount of chemotherapy required to achieve complete remission (Table 18D-9). Chemotherapy did not delay wound healing or increased the risk of any other postoperative complications.[58]

**TABLE 18D-8.** HIGH-RISK GESTATIONAL TROPHOBLASTIC TUMORS: RESPONSE RATES TO EMA/CO

| AUTHOR | OVERALL RESPONSE RATE |
|---|---|
| Bolis[53] | 86% |
| Newlands[54] | 85% |
| Bower[55] | 86% |
| Soper[56] | 87.5% |

**TABLE 18D-9.** RESULTS OF THERAPY AND THE ROLE OF OPERATION IN THE TREATMENT OF GESTATIONAL TROPHOBLASTIC DISEASES (GTD)

| | NONMETASTATIC GTD | |
|---|---|---|
| | DAYS HOSPITALIZED | NO. OF COURSES OF CHEMOTHERAPY |
| Chemotherapy & hysterectomy | 32.8 | 2.2 |
| Chemotherapy alone | 50.8 | 4.0 |
| | GOOD-PROGNOSIS METATSTATIC GTD | |
| Chemotherapy & hysterectomy | 56.6 | 3.8 |
| Chemotherapy alone | 76.6 | 5.9 |
| | POOR-PROGNOSIS METASTATIC GTD | |
| Chemotherapy & hysterectomy | 86.7 | 5.6 |
| Chemotherapy & other operation | 107 | 8.2 |
| Chemotherapy alone | 91.5 | 6.9 |

**Acknowledgment**

*Pathologic figures courtesy of Tamara Kalir, MD, PhD, The Mount Sinai School of Medicine, New York, New York.*

# REFERENCES

1. PALMER JR: Advances in the epidemiology of gestational trophoblastic disease. J Reprod Med 39:155, 1994.
2. MATSUURA J et al: Complete hydatidiform mole in Hawaii: An epidemiological study. Gene Epidem 1:271, 1984.
3. BAGSHAWE KD et al: Hydatidiform mole in England and Wales 1973–83. Lancet 1:673, 1986.
4. PARAZZINI F et al: Parental age and risk of complete and partial hydatidiform mole. Br J Obstet Gynecol 93:582, 1986.
5. PARAZZINI F et al: Dietary factors and risk of trophoblastic disease. Am J Obstet Gynecol 158:93, 1988.
6. BERKOWITZ RS et al: Risk factors for complete molar pregnancy from a case-control study. Am J Obstet Gynecol 152:1016, 1985.
7. BRINTON LA et al: Gestational trophoblastic disease: A case-control study from the People's Republic of China. Am J Obstet Gynecol 161:121, 1989.
8. ACAIA B et al: Increased frequency of complete hydatidiform mole in women with repeated abortion. Gynecol Oncol 31:310, 1988.
9. BRINTON LA et al: Choriocarcinoma incidence in the United States. Am J Epidemiol 123:1094, 1986.
10. CURRY SL et al: Hydatidiform mole. Diagnosis, management, and long-term followup of 347 patients. Obstet Gynecol 45:1, 1975.
11. MONTZ FJ et al: The natural history of theca lutein cysts. Obstet Gynecol 72:247, 1988.
12. FISHER PM, HANCOCK BW: Gestational trophoblastic diseases and their treatment. Cancer Treat Reviews 23:1, 1997.
13. MAZUR MT, KURMAN RJ: Choriocarcinoma and placental site tumor, in *Gestational Trophoblastic Disease*, AE Szulman, HJ Buchsbaum (eds). New York, Springer-Verlag, 1987, p 45.
14. MANGILI G et al: Transvaginal ultrasonography in persistent trophoblastic tumor. Am J Obstet Gynecol 169:1218, 1993.
15. HUANG SC, CHOU CY: The role of transvaginal ultrasonography in the management of gestational trophoblastic tumor. Am J Obstet Gynecol 172:1063, 1995.
16. YAHATA T et al: Primary choriocarcinoma of the uterine cervix: Clinical, MRI, and color Doppler ultrasonographic study. Gynecol Oncol 64:274, 1997.
17. HRICAK H et al: Gestational trophoblastic neoplasm of the uterus: MR assessment. Radiology 161:11, 1986.
18. BARTON JW et al: Pelvic MR imaging findings in gestational trophoblastic disease, incomplete abortion, and ectopic pregnancy: Are they specific? Radiology 186:163, 1993.
19. KAJII T, OHAMA K: Androgenic origin of hydatidiform mole. Nature 268:633, 1977.
20. SURTI U et al: Complete (classic) hydatidiform mole with 46,XY karyotype of paternal origin. Hum Genet 51:153, 1979.
21. PATTILLO RA et al: Genesis of 46,XY hydatidiform mole. Am J Obstet Gynecol 141:104, 1981.
22. SZULMAN AE, SURTI U: The syndromes of hydatidiform mole. 1. Cytogenetic and morphologic correlations. Am J Obstet Gynecol 131:665, 1978.
23. SZULMAN AE: Trophoblastic disease: Clinical pathology of hydatidiform moles. Obstet Gynecol Clin North Am 15:433, 1988.
24. SZULMAN AE, SURTI U: The syndromes of hydatidiform mole. 2. Morphologic evolution of the complete and partial mole. Am J Obstet Gynecol 132:20, 1978.
25. JACOBS PA et al: Human triploidy: Relationship between paternal origin of additional haploid complement and development of partial hydatidiform mole. Ann Hum Genet 46:223, 1982.
26. SZULMAN AE, SURTI U: The clinicopathologic profile of the partial hydatidiform mole. Obstet Gynecol 59:597, 1982.
27. HOPKINS M et al: Malignant placental site trophoblastic tumor. Obstet Gynecol 66:95S, 1985.
28. YOUNG RH, SCULLY RE: Placental site trophoblastic tumor: Current status. Clin Obstet Gynecol 27:248, 1984.
29. LURAIN JR et al: Natural history of hydatidiform mole after primary evacuation. Am J Obstet Gynecol 145:591, 1983.
30. DUBUC-LISSOIR J et al: Metastatic gestational trophoblastic disease: A comparsion of prognostic classification systems. Gynecol Oncol 45:40, 1992.
31. LURAIN JR et al: Prognostic factors in gestational trophoblastic tumors: A proposed new scoring system based on multivariate analysis. Am J Obstet Gynecol 164:611, 1991.
32. BREWER JI et al: Choriocarcinoma: Absolute survival rates of 122 patients treated by hysterectomy. Am J Obstet Gynecol 85:84, 1963.
33. HAMMOND CB et al: Primary chemotherapy for nonmetastatic gestational trophoblastic neoplasms. Am J Obstet Gynecol 98:71, 1967.
34. BERKOWITZ RS et al: Ten years' experience with methotrexate and folinic acid as primary therapy for gestational trophoblastic disease. Gynecol Oncol 23:111, 1986.
35. WONG LC et al: Methotrexate with cirtrovorum factor rescue in gestational trophoblastic disease. Am J Obstet Gynecol 152:59, 1985.
36. BARTER JF et al: Treatment of nonmetastatic gestational trophoblastic disease with oral methotrexate. Am J Obstet Gynecol 157:1166, 1987.
37. BAGSHAWE KD: Risk and prognostic factors in trophoblastic neoplasia. Cancer 38:1373, 1976.
38. WONG LC et al: Primary oral etoposide therapy in gestational trophoblastic disease. Cancer 58:14, 1986.
39. SUNG HC et al: Reevaluation of 5-fluorouracil as a single therapeutic agent for gestational trophoblastic neoplasms. Am J Obstet Gynecol 150:69, 1984.
40. GOLDSTEIN DP et al: Actinomycin D as initial therapy of gestational trophoblastic disease: A re-evaluation. Obstet Gynecol 45:341, 1975.
41. ROSS GT et al: Sequential use of methotrexate and actinomycin D in the treatment of metastatic choriocarcinoma and related trophoblastic diseases in women. Am J Obstet Gynecol 93:225, 1965.
42. SOPER JT et al: 5-day methotrexate for women with metastatic gestational trophoblastic disease. Gynecol Oncol 54:76, 1994.
43. ELIT L et al: High dose methotrexate for gestational trophoblastic disease. Gynecol Oncol 54:282, 1994.
44. HAMMOND CB et al: Treatment of metastatic trophoblastic disease: Good and poor prognosis. Am J Obstet Gynecol 115:453, 1973.
45. LURAIN JR, BREWER JI: Treatment of high-risk gestational trophoblastic disease with methotrexate, actinomycin D, and cyclophosphamide chemotherapy. Obstet Gynecol 65:830, 1985.
46. DUBESHTER B et al: Metastatic gestational trophoblastic disease: Experience at the New England Trophoblastic Disease Center, 1965 to 1985. Obstet Gynecol 69:390, 1987.

47. BAGSHAWE KD: Treatment of trophoblastic tumours. Ann Acad Med 5:273, 1976.

48. BAGSHAWE KD, BEGENT RHJ: Trophoblastic tumors, clinical features and management, in *Gynecologic Oncology: Fundamental Principles and Clinical Practice,* M Coppleson (ed). Edinburgh & New York, Churchill Livingstone, 1981, pp 757–772.

49. WEED JC et al: Chemotherapy with the modified Bagshawe protocol for poor prognosis metastatic trophoblastic disease. Obstet Gynecol 59:377, 1982.

50. WONG LC et al: Modified Bagshawe's regimen in high-risk gestational trophoblastic disease. Gynecol Oncol 23:87, 1986.

51. CURRY SL et al: A prospective randomized comparison of methotrexate, dactinomycin, and chlorambucil versus methotrexate, dactinomycin, melphalan, hydroxyurea, and vincristine in "poor prognosis" metastatic gestational trophoblastic disease: A gynecologic oncology study. Obstet Gynecol 73:357, 1989.

52. NEWLANDS ES, BAGSHAWE KD: Epipodophyllin derivative (VP 16-213) in malignant teratomas and choriocarcinomas. Lancet 2:87, 1977.

53. BOLIS G et al: EMA/CO regimen in high-risk gestational trophoblastic tumor (GTT). Gynecol Oncol 31:439, 1988.

54. NEWLANDS ES et al: Results with the EMA/CO (etoposide, methotrexate, actinomycin D, cyclophosphamide, vincristine) regimen in high risk gestational trophoblastic tumours, 1979 to 1989. Br J Obstet Gynaecol 98:550, 1991.

55. BOWER M et al: EMA/CO for high risk gestational trophoblastic tumors: Results from a cohort of 272 patients. J Clin Oncol 15:2636, 1997.

56. SOPER JT et al: Alternating weekly chemotherapy with etoposide-methotrexate-dactinomycin/cyclophosphamide-vincristine for high-risk gestational trophoblastic disease. Obstet Gynecol 83:113, 1994.

57. HAMMOND CB et al: The role of operation in the current therapy of gestational trophoblastic disease. Am J Obstet Gynecol 136:844, 1980.

58. LEWIS JL et al: Surgical intervention during chemotherapy of gestational trophoblastic neoplasms. Cancer 19:1517, 1966.

# 18E / CANCER OF THE OVARY

*Elizabeth A. Poynor and William J. Hoskins*

## EPIDEMIOLOGY

Ovarian cancer is the fourth leading cause of cancer death in women in North America and accounts for approximately 5% of all cancer deaths in women. It is the leading cause of death from gynecologic malignancies. Approximately 25,200 cases are expected to be diagnosed in 2000, leading to 14,500 deaths.[1] The incidence of ovarian cancer in the United States is lower for African American women than for Caucasian women: 10.3 per 100,000 African American women, compared to 15.6 per 100,000 Caucasian women.[2] The median age at diagnosis of epithelial ovarian cancer is 63; this type of cancer is rare in women under the age of 40. The incidence increases from 15 to 16 per 100,000 women in the 40 to 44 years age group to 57 per 100,000 women in the 70 to 74 years age group.[3] After the age of 75 years, the rates begin to decline. Germ cell tumors are far more common in young women, with a median age at diagnosis of 16 to 20 years. The etiology of ovarian cancer is poorly understood; genetic, environmental, and reproductive factors are associated with the risk for the development of epithelial ovarian cancer.

Reproductive risk factors associated with an elevated risk for the development of ovarian cancer include those associated with an increased number of ovulations in a woman's lifetime. Menstrual factors have been inconsistently associated with a risk for the development of epithelial ovarian cancer; an early age of menarche and late menopause have been associated with a twofold increase in the risk of developing ovarian cancer.[4] Conversely, factors that decrease the number of ovulatory cycles, such as oral contraceptive use and pregnancy, are associated with a decreased risk for the development of ovarian cancer. Oral contraceptive use may be associated with up to an 80% reduction in the risk for the development of the disease. The relative risk (RR) decreases to 0.75 for women who have ever used oral contraceptives, and although oral contraceptives begin to be protective after a few months of use, the risk decreases with longer duration of use.[5-8] The strongest reproductive factor associated with a lower risk for ovarian cancer is the number of full-term pregnancies. Women who have ever been pregnant have 30% to 60% less risk of developing ovarian cancer when compared to women who have never been pregnant.[9] Women who have had more than three pregnancies have RR of up to 0.35 compared to women who have never been pregnant.

To date, the strongest risk factor for the development of ovarian cancer is a family history of the disease. If a woman has a first-degree relative with epithelial ovarian cancer, her lifetime risk is elevated to 4% to 5%,[10] compared to a 1.6% risk in a woman without a family history. If she has two affected family members, her risk is elevated to 7%. Approximately 7% of all women diagnosed with ovarian cancer will report a relative with ovarian cancer.[11] Ovarian cancer is a component of three hereditary cancer syndromes: hereditary breast and ovarian cancer syndrome, hereditary site-specific ovarian cancer, and the Lynch II syndrome; however, true hereditary ovarian cancers account for only 5% to 10% of all epithelial ovarian cancers. If a woman is a member of a hereditary breast and ovarian cancer family or a hereditary ovarian cancer family, her lifetime risk of developing ovarian cancer may be as high as 50%.[12] If she is a member of a Lynch II family, her lifetime risk of developing ovarian cancer is 10%. A personal history of cancer also affects a woman's risk of developing ovarian cancer; if she has a diagnosis of breast cancer, her risk of ovarian cancer may be doubled; however, if she has a diagnosis of premenopausal breast cancer, her risk may be elevated by fourfold.[13]

Few data exist to associate specific environmental factors with the development of ovarian cancer. However, one environmental risk factor that has been consistently associated with an increased risk for the disease is the exposure to talc powder on the perineal area. Surgical interventions that decrease a woman's exposure to environmental agents have been associated with a lower rate of development of the disease. Hysterectomy and tubal ligation both decrease the risk of ovarian cancer; however, the reason for this is uncertain but may be due to ablating a potential entry of environmental agents into the peritoneal cavity.[14] Higher levels of dietary fat have been suggested to be associated with an elevated risk for the disease, but case-controlled studies have failed to demonstrate this association.[15] Use of hormone replacement therapy, coffee and alcohol consumption, and tobacco use have not been found to affect a woman's risk for the development of ovarian cancer. No definitive associations with environmental carcinogens or radiation have been established.

Fertility drugs have been a controversial topic when considering whether they are related to an increased incidence of developing ovarian cancer. One study has demonstrated that the use of clomiphene, a drug commonly used to induce ovulation in women, for greater than 12 months is associated with a twofold to threefold increase in the risk of developing ovarian cancer.[16] The lifetime risk of developing an ovarian tumor for a woman exposed to prolonged fertility medications is estimated to be 4% to 5%. This may, however, be related to her infertility alone, because women who do not conceive are at an increased risk of developing ovarian cancer; the issue as to whether fertility drugs actually play a causal role in the development of ovarian cancer requires further evaluation in a prospective fashion.[17-20]

Germ cell tumors account for only approximately 25% of all ovarian neoplasms; however, only 3% of these tumors are malignant.[21] In the first two decades of life, 70% of tumors are of germ cell origin and approximately 30% of these are malignant.[21,22] Epithelial tumors and stromal tumors are rare in this age group, so that germ cell tumors account for approximately two-thirds of all malignancies in this age group. Germ cell tumors account for fewer than 5% of all ovarian malignancies in North America, but account for a higher proportion of malignant ovarian neoplasms in African American and Asian communities, due to the fact that epithelial tumors are less common in these groups. Sex cord–stromal tumors account for 5% to 8% of all ovarian malignancies.[21-23]

## GENETICS AND OVARIAN CANCER

The genetic etiology of sporadic ovarian cancer, or that which occurs in the absence of a family history of the disease, is poorly understood. However, the genetic etiology of hereditary ovarian cancer is well understood. Epithelial ovarian cancer is a component of three hereditary cancer family syndromes: hereditary breast and ovarian cancer, hereditary site-specific ovarian cancer, and the Lynch II syndrome. Table 18E-1 outlines the major cancer predisposition syndromes associated with ovarian cancer. By far the most common form of hereditary ovarian cancer is the hereditary breast and ovarian

cancer syndrome. This is characterized by the autosomal dominant transmission of breast and ovarian cancer within a family. Approximately 5% to 10% of all ovarian cancers are thought to be hereditary in etiology. The median age at diagnosis in families with hereditary ovarian cancer is approximately 10 years younger than that in the general population, with the median age at diagnosis being 49 years among these women.[24]

Mutations in the tumor-suppressor BRCA1 gene account for the vast majority of hereditary ovarian cancers, and the remainder are accounted for by mutations in a second tumor-suppressor gene, the BRCA2 gene. The BRCA1 gene, which is located on chromosome 17q21, was cloned in 1994.[25] The gene consists of 100 kilobases (kb), and encodes for a protein of 1863 amino acids. Originally, the gene was identified by linkage analysis from hereditary breast and ovarian cancer families. Therefore, the penetrance was estimated to be quite high, at up to 26% to 85% for a woman's chance of developing ovarian cancer in her lifetime and up to 90% for a woman's chance for developing breast cancer in her lifetime.[26] If a woman carries a BRCA1 mutation, once she has breast cancer diagnosed, she has a 44% chance of developing ovarian cancer.[27] As the gene has been studied, estimates for the penetrance estimates for mutations in the BRCA1 gene have been decreased. Mutations have been found throughout the coding region for the BRCA1 gene, and no single "hotspot" for mutations exists, making the study of the gene very difficult. Certain "founder" mutations have been identified in populations. For example, the 185delAG and the 5382insC mutations are found in 1% and 0.2% of Ashkenazi Jewish women,

**TABLE 18E-1.** SUMMARY OF MAJOR HEREDITARY CANCER PREDISPOSITION SYNDROMES ASSOCIATED WITH THE DEVELOPMENT OF OVARIAN CANCER

| GENE(S) | LOCATION | HEREDITARY CANCER SYNDROME | CHARACTERISTICS OF SYNDROME | RISK OF MALIGNANCY |
|---------|----------|----------------------------|-----------------------------|---------------------|
| BRCA1 | 17q | Hereditary breast and ovarian cancer | Autosomal dominant transmission of breast and/or ovarian cancer | 80–90% lifetime risk of breast cancer* 40–50% lifetime risk of ovarian cancer* Fourfold increase of colorectal cancer Threefold increased risk of prostate cancer |
| BRCA2 | 13q | Hereditary breast and ovarian cancer | Autosomal dominant transmission of breast and/or ovarian cancer | 80–90% lifetime risk of breast cancer <25% lifetime risk of ovarian cancer Increased risk of male breast cancer Increased risk of pancreatic cancer |
| HNPCC-associated genes | | HNPCC syndrome | Autosomal dominant transmission of colon cancer | 68–75% lifetime risk of colon cancer 30–39% risk of endometrial cancer 10% lifetime risk of ovarian cancer |
| hMSH2 | 2p | | | |
| hMLH1 | 3p | | | |
| PMS1 | 2q | | Autosomal dominant transmission of colon cancer with associated adenocarcinomas of endometrium, lung, pancreas, ovary | 68–75% lifetime risk of colon cancer 30–39% risk of endometrial cancer 10% lifetime risk of ovarian cancer |
| PMS2 | 7p | Lynch II syndrome | | |

* The penetrance estimates for the BRCA1 and BRCA2 genes have been primarily evaluated in families with multiple cancer cases. It is suspected that as these genes are studied further, the penetrance estimates would drop.

respectively.[28,29] Mutations in the *BRCA1* gene are also associated with an increased risk for the development of colorectal and prostate cancers, with lifetime risks of 6% and 8%, respectively.[30] To date, the function of the *BRCA1* protein is unknown. It has been postulated to be a transcription factor and may play a role in DNA repair pathways. Mutations in this gene are uncommon in sporadic ovarian cancers.

The *BRCA2* gene is located in 13q and was also recently cloned.[31] Mutations in this gene account for most of the remainder of hereditary ovarian cancer; however, this gene is associated with a greater proportion of hereditary breast cancer. Similar to the *BRCA1* gene, *BRCA2* is a large gene, with mutations identified throughout the coding region. Mutations in this gene are associated with a RR to develop ovarian cancer of tenfold, for a lifetime risk of less than 10%.[32] Male breast cancer and pancreatic cancer are also associated with *BRCA2* mutations. Similar to *BRCA1* mutations, founder mutations have also been identified in specific populations; for example, the 6174delT is found in 1% of Ashkenazi Jewish women.[28] The function of the BRCA2 protein is unknown and, like the *BRCA1* gene, is thought to play a role in DNA repair.

Although the vast majority of hereditary ovarian cancer is linked to mutations in the *BRCA1* and *BRCA2* genes (discussed above), a small percentage cannot be accounted for by these genes. The Lynch II syndrome is characterized by an autosomal dominant transmission of colorectal cancer in families, along with other adenocarcinomas such as endometrial, ovarian, gastrointestinal, and urinary tract cancers. Mutations in the mismatch repair genes, *hMLH1*, *hMSH2*, *PMS1*, and *PMS2*, account for this syndrome. Endometrial cancer is the most common component of the syndrome; however, women who are members of these families have an associated risk of 10% to develop ovarian cancer.[33]

The genetic origins of sporadic ovarian cancer are poorly understood. There have been a variety of gene mutations discovered in known tumor-suppressor genes and oncogenes; however, there has been no one gene mutation identified in a majority of ovarian tumors. Mutations in the tumor-suppressor gene *p53* are by far the most common gene mutations in epithelial ovarian cancers.[34,35] The frequency of mutations in this gene increases as the tumor stage and grade increase, and mutations in this gene are found in approximately 50% of advanced-stage tumors. Mutations in the oncogenes *c-myc, h-ras, k-ras,* and *erb*B2 have also been identified.[36]

Ovarian tumors are also associated with other genetic disorders. Peutz-Jeghers syndrome, characterized by mucocutaneous pigmentation and intestinal polyposis, is associated with sex cord–stromal tumors with annular tubules, and in rare cases, with mucinous tumors.[37] Individuals with mixed gonadal dysgenesis are at elevated risk to develop gonadoblastomas.[38] Germ cell tumors of the ovary may be a component of the Li-Fraumeni family cancer syndrome.[39] Individuals with the multiple nevoid basal cell carcinomas are at increased risk for ovarian fibromas.[40]

## SCREENING AND PREVENTION

The poor overall 5-year survival rate in women with epithelial ovarian cancer is due to the fact that a majority of patients present with advanced-stage disease, where the 5-year survival rate is only 5% to 20%. The 5-year survival rate in women with disease confined to the ovary is 90%, compared to 20% and 5% for stage III and IV tumors, respectively.[41] Since surviving ovarian cancer is influenced heavily by the stage at which the disease is diagnosed, early detection through screening has the potential to reduce disease-related morbidity and mortality. It has been estimated that if the proportion of ovarian cancer detected at stage I disease could be increased to 75%, the number of deaths from ovarian cancer could be cut in half;[42] however, the role of screening for ovarian cancer remains controversial. A recent National Institutes of Health Consensus Statement (1994)[43] did not endorse screening for ovarian cancer outside of research protocols and recommended that further prospective research be done to evaluate its potential impact on the reduction of related morbidity and mortality. However, the demand for ovarian cancer screening from the general public appears to be high, and practitioners are providing screening with ultrasound and cancer antigen 125 (CA-125) in the general setting.

Screening methods for epithelial ovarian cancer consist of physical examination, measuring CA-125 level, and performing a transvaginal ultrasound. The major problems with these forms of detection for ovarian cancer are as follows: the CA-125 level has only a 50% sensitivity for detection of stage I ovarian cancer, the transvaginal ultrasound has a very high false-positive rate, and the combined positive predictive value of these tests is low. Overall, 16,563 women have been screened for ovarian cancer and reported on in the literature; 17 ovarian cancers have been detected (10 invasive and 7 borderline) along with 3 granulosa cell tumors.[44,45] Of the 20 ovarian cancers detected, 17 were stage I, 1 was stage II, and 2 were stage III. In order to improve on the low positive predictive value, investigators have sought to screen only women who are at elevated risk for ovarian cancer based on personal cancer history or family history; the positive predictive value of ultrasound (USG) is the highest for this group of women, at 9.8%.[45]

Other methods that have been employed to improve on ovarian cancer screening techniques are the use of morphology indices and Doppler flow of the ovary and cysts. One group has reported a positive predictive value of 47% for ovarian cancer utilizing the morphology of the cyst, including the tumor volume, wall structure, and septal structure.[46] There has, however, been no agreement on a standard "morphology index," and there has been no long-term testing of these indices. Doppler flow evaluation of vessels that supply ovarian masses has also been utilized to predict whether a cyst is malignant. The initial studies demonstrated a positive predictive value for ovarian cancer of 98%;[47] however, these early, very promising results have not been reproduced. (In one screening study, two patients with stage I ovarian cancers had normal Doppler flow indices.[48]) As with the morphology index, there have been no large-scale studies of stage I ovarian cancers designed to determine the actual efficacy of these methods for screening purposes. One group has reported that if an ovarian mass was to have a morphology index and Doppler flow both suggestive of malignancy, two of five ovarian cancers found would have been missed.[48] These methods require further investigation.

Investigators have also tried to combine multiple tumor markers in order to improve on screening methods. Others have attempted to use CA-125 levels monitored over time, instead of using a cutoff level for a normal value. The sensitivity of the CA-125 value for ovarian cancer detection can be increased by evaluating levels below the standard threshold of 35 U/dL, and the specificity can be increased by evaluating these levels over time.[49] These methods are currently under investigation.

Preventing ovarian cancer has also been difficult due to the fact that there is little known about the etiology of ovarian cancer. Using oral contraceptives to prevent ovarian cancer is the most well proven. The risk of ovarian cancer can be decreased by up to 60% to 80% by the use of this medication, and this risk-reducing effect appears to be translated over to other high-risk populations, such as those with a family history of the disease and those with BRCA1 or BRCA2 mutations.[50] The use of oral contraceptives should also be balanced by the potential increase in breast cancer; there are few data concerning this in women who have a BRCA1 or BRCA2 mutation. In women with a family history of breast cancer, however, there appears to be little effect on breast cancer risk with the use of oral contraceptive.[51] Studies have also demonstrated that any increased risk in breast cancer with the use of oral contraceptives appears to be short-term.[52] Other risk-reducing strategies include the use of prophylactic oophorectomy in patients who are determined to be at the highest risk for ovarian cancer, based on a known mutation in the BRCA1 or BRCA2 gene, or a member of a family with a hereditary ovarian cancer syndrome. A recent National Institutes of Health consensus conference recommended a prophylactic oophorectomy for women with two or more first-degree relatives with epithelial ovarian cancer after completion of childbearing or at age 35 years.[52,53] This is based on the finding that the majority of hereditary ovarian cancers occur in patients in their mid to late 40s, with 17% diagnosed before the age of 40 in one series.[54] The failure of prophylactic oophorectomy is reported to be between 2% to 11%.[54–56] This is due to the fact that these women remain susceptible to the development of primary peritoneal cancer. Proponents of prophylactic oophorectomy have cited the lack of proven efficacy of ovarian cancer screening, combined with the high mortality of this disease, as strong justification for prophylactic surgery. This must, however, be balanced by the fact that these women will be subjected to an early surgical menopause, with the side effects of vasomotor symptoms, vaginal dryness, osteoporosis, and potential cardiovascular complications. There are few data concerning the impact on breast cancer of the use of estrogen replacement therapy in women who carry a mutation in BRCA1 or BRCA2 genes. Risk associated with postmenopausal hormone replacement therapy and breast cancer has been reported to be both unaffected and increased by a family history of breast cancer.[57–59]

In summary, screening the general population for ovarian cancer with currently employed methods has little value outside of a research setting; however, high-risk populations of women may benefit from ovarian cancer screening. The women at highest risk, based on a personal history of a mutation in a cancer-predisposition gene, may benefit from prophylactic surgery. However, these women should be counseled that the procedure is not 100% effective, and the risks and benefits of hormone replacement therapy should be discussed prior to surgery. Prevention with oral contraceptive use should also be discussed.

## CLINICAL PRESENTATION OF OVARIAN MALIGNANCIES

Symptoms of an adnexal mass in a woman include pelvic pain, urinary frequency, dysuria, constipation, and dyspareunia. Unfortunately, because there are no signs and symptoms associated with early-stage ovarian cancer, the majority of epithelial ovarian cancers are advanced at the time of diagnosis. Abdominal distension due to ascites is one of the most common symptoms of epithelial ovarian cancer; pleural effusions may also be present with ascites. Other symptoms include vague abdominal bloating, nausea, early satiety, heartburn, and abnormal vaginal bleeding. It is important to note that most of these symptoms may be associated with a variety of other intra-abdominal and gastrointestinal conditions. Women may also present with shortness of breath due to a pleural effusion. Hypercalcemia may be associated with small-cell tumors of the ovary. Benign etiologies of a pelvic mass, ascites, and pleural effusion include benign ovarian fibromas, the so-called Meigs syndrome, along with tuberculous peritonitis with genital tract tuberculosis. In the differential diagnosis of the above conditions, liver disease and metastatic tumors from other sources must also be considered.

Germ cell tumors are most commonly found in young women, with a peak incidence occurring in women in their 20s. Abdominal pain and a pelvic mass are present in 85% of cases,[60] and 10% of women present with an acute abdomen due to rupture, torsion, or hemorrhage into the tumor. This is due to the fast-growing nature of these tumors (in contrast to slow-growing epithelial tumors). Abdominal distension presents in 35% of cases. Feminization (in the form of isosexual precocious puberty) and vaginal bleeding are also present in 10% of cases.

Steroid hormone production is found in a majority of the sex cord–stromal tumors, with the exception of the ovarian fibroma. These tumors may present as an adnexal mass with abdominal pain and other symptoms related to an adnexal mass. Notable for their production of androgens and estrogens, these tumors may be associated with androgenic symptoms such as voice deepening, hirsutism, breast atrophy, clitoromegaly, loss of female contour, and temporal hair recession. Patients with virilization have an elevated testosterone level; typically, tumors associated with androgen production result in serum testosterone levels greater than 200 ng/dL, and the androstenedione may also be increased. Typically, the 17-ketosteroids are normal. Symptoms of estrogen excess include isosexual precocious puberty, menorrhagia, intermenstrual bleeding, and postmenopausal bleeding. Associated conditions include endometrial hyperplasia and endometrial carcinoma.

## PATTERNS OF SPREAD AND STAGING

Epithelial ovarian cancer may arise from inclusion cysts of the surface epithelium of the ovary. Little is known about the natural history of ovarian cancer, and it is usually diagnosed at an advanced stage, due to the intra-abdominal location of the ovaries. Ovarian cancer may spread by three routes: (1) surface shedding of tumor cells transperitoneally, (2) lymphatic spread, and (3) hematogenous spread. By far the most common spread pattern is transperitoneal, so that at the time of laparotomy, one will typically find the following: large unilateral or bilateral pelvic masses and tumor implants on the peritoneal surfaces of intra-abdominal organs, the omentum, the undersurface of the diaphragm, the mesentery of the bowel, and the sigmoid colon. The tumor spreads via the flow of peritoneal fluid: up the right paracolic gutter, to the right hemidiaphragm, to the omentum, so that the majority of diaphragmatic tumor implants may be on the right side.

The second location in which tumor is commonly found in the lymph nodes, and the pelvic, paraaortic, and inguinal lymph nodes may contain metastatic tumor. The tumor spreads via the infundibulopelvic ligament to the para-aortic lymph nodes to the level of the renal vessels, via the broad ligament to the external and internal iliac and obturator lymph nodes, and via the round ligament to the inguinal lymph nodes. Nodal disease may also involve the supraclavicular nodes. This lymph node disease may not be clinically apparent at the time of laparotomy, and the presence of metastatic disease in the lymph nodes has important treatment, as well as prognostic, implications. It is estimated that in apparent stage I disease, the paraaortic lymph nodes will be positive 18% of the time and 20% in stage II disease.[61]

The third and less common form of spread is via the bloodstream. This is extremely uncommon, however; the most common form of distant disease is as a right pleural effusion. Distant spread to other organs such as bone, brain, subcutaneous tissues, and pericardium may also occur. It usually does so in the form of recurrent disease, after the initial diagnosis of intraperitoneal disease has been diagnosed and treated. It has been reported that 38% of patients will go on to develop some form of distant disease.[62]

The staging of ovarian cancer is surgical in nature and reflects the spread patterns discussed above. Therefore, careful attention must be paid to these areas. Table 18E-2 outlines the surgical staging of ovarian cancer.

## PROGNOSTIC FACTORS

Survival is dependent on many factors. For epithelial ovarian cancer, the stage of the disease is the greatest prognostic factor. Other factors that may be important include grade of the tumor, histopathologic subtype, performance status and age of patient, volume of disease prior to surgery, volume of disease remaining after primary surgery, and presence of ascites. For advanced-stage tumors, the volume of disease remaining at the completion of surgery is the greatest prognostic factor. Individuals with stage I disease enjoy a 95% to 99% 5-year survival rate, while the survival rates of patients with stage III and IV disease are 20% and 5%, respectively.[63,64] For patients with stage I disease, the grade of the tumor is quite important, as well as the histopathologic subtype. Patients with grade 1 tumors have a 5-year survival rate greater than 90% without adjuvant treatment with chemotherapy; however, individuals with grade 3 or clear-cell tumors require adjuvant therapy.[65] Patients with clear-cell tumors of the ovary may also have a worse prognosis on a stage-for-stage basis; overall survival is 60% for

**TABLE 18E-2.** FIGO STAGING OF OVARIAN CANCER

| Stage I | Growth limited to the ovaries. |
| --- | --- |
| | Stage IA | Growth limited to one ovary, no ascites, no tumor on the external surfaces and capsule intact. |
| | Stage IB | Growth limited to both ovaries, no ascites, no tumor on the external surfaces and capsule intact. |
| | Stage IC | Tumor is either stage IA or IB, but with tumor on the surface of one or both ovaries, or with capsule ruptured; or with ascites present containing malignant cells as peritoneal wash positive for malignant cells. |
| **Stage II** | Growth involving one or both ovaries with pelvic extension. |
| | Stage IIA | Extension or metastases involving the uterus or the tubes. |
| | Stage IIB | Extension to other pelvic tissues. |
| | Stage IIC | Tumor is either stage IIA or IIB, but with tumor on the surface of one or both ovaries, or with capsule ruptured; or with ascites present containing malignant cells or a peritoneal wash positive for malignant cells. |
| **Stage III** | Tumor involving one or both ovaries with peritoneal implants outside the pelvis and/or positive retroperitoneal or inguinal lymph nodes. Tumor is limited to the true pelvis with histologically proven malignant extension to the small bowel or omentum. Superificial liver metastases are stage III disease. |
| | Stage IIIA | Tumor is grossly limited to the true pelvis with negative lymph nodes but with histologically confirmed disease of the abdominal peritoneal surfaces. |
| | Stage IIIB | Tumor involving one or both ovaries with histologically confirmed implants of abdominal peritoneal surfaces, none exceeding 2 cm in diameter. Nodes are negative. |
| | Stage IIIC | Abdominal implants greater than 2 cm in diameter or positive retroperitoneal or inguinal lymph nodes. |
| **Stage IV** | Growth involving one or both ovaries with distant metastases. If pleural effusion is present, there must be positive cytology. Parenchymal liver metastases are Stage IV disease. |

individuals with stage I tumors and 12% for those with tumors of all other stages.[66] No other histopathologic subtype carries any prognostic value for epithelial ovarian cancers. Tumor grade has not been demonstrated to be of value in the prognosis of advanced-stage patients, and this is most likely due to interobserver variation. For early-stage disease, the presence of malignant ascites, capsular penetration, and dense adhesions to the pelvic peritoneum are all poor-prognosis features.[67] Although tumor rupture and spillage of cyst fluid contents at surgery has generally warranted treatment with adjuvant therapy, it has not reliably been found to be a poor-prognosis feature.[68–71]

Investigators have also evaluated DNA ploidy as a prognostic feature of ovarian tumors. Aneuploidy increases as the tumor stage and grade increase.[72] Ploidy analysis has been correlated with stage in early-stage disease. The 5-year survival rate of patients with diploid tumors approaches 100%, compared to 58% in aneuploid tumors.[73] Mutations in the *p53* gene have been associated with a worse prognosis in early-stage disease.[74] The association with amplification or overexpression of *erbB*2 and poor prognosis has been noted by some, but not by others.[75,76] Some investigators have found the presence of a *BRCA1* mutation associated with a good prognosis with a prolonged median survival of 77 months, compared to 29 months in advanced-stage patients without a *BRCA1* mutation.[77] This has not been confirmed by others.

The absolute value of CA-125 has not been found to be an independent prognostic factor, but the postoperative decline has been found to be important.[78] If patients had a CA-125 level greater than 100 after 3 cycles of chemotherapy, their median survival was 7 months, compared to a 50% survival in patients with a CA-125 level of less than 10.[79]

Survival is also dependent on the age of a patient at diagnosis. The overall 5-year survival rate is 70% for women below the age of 45 at diagnosis, compared to 20% for women age 75 or older at the time of diagnosis. Women with advanced-stage disease who are below the age of 45 at diagnosis have a 45% 5-year survival rate, compared to 13% for women ages 65 to 74.[80]

## TUMOR MARKERS

### EPITHELIAL TUMORS

Epithelial ovarian cancers are associated with an elevation in CA-125. The CA-125 tumor antigen is recognized by the mouse monoclonal antibody, OC-125. This antibody was developed by immunizing mice with the ascites from a patient with a papillary serous ovarian cancer.[81] The CA-125 molecule is a high-molecular-weight glycoprotein. It is present on the fetal tissues of the müllerian tract and coelomic epithelium.[82] It is also present on the adult derivatives of the coelomic epithelium, including the pleura, pericardium, and peritoneum. This marker is elevated in malignant and nonmalignant conditions, and its use has primarily been applied to determine a patient's response to therapy for ovarian malignancies, and not for diagnosis. It is elevated in 80% of clinically apparent ovarian cancers, but in only 50% of stage I ovarian cancers.[83] Elevated CA-125 levels may also be found in germ cell tumors and Sertoli-Leydig

**TABLE 18E-3. MALIGNANT AND NONMALIGNANT ETIOLOGIES OF AN ELEVATED CA-125**

| MALIGNANT | NONMALIGNANT |
|---|---|
| Ovarian carcinoma | Endometriosis |
| Fallopian-tube carcinoma | Pregnancy |
| Uterine carcinoma | Leiomyomas |
| Endocervical carcinoma | Adenomyosis |
|  | Menses |
| Breast carcinoma | Pelvic inflammatory disease |
| Colon carcinoma |  |
| Pancreatic carcinoma | Laparotomy |
| Lung carcinoma | Pancreatitis |
|  | Peritonitis |
|  | Cirrhosis |
|  | Thoracotomy |

cell tumors, along with adenocarcinomas of the fallopian tube, endometrium, and endocervix.

Nongynecologic malignancies are also associated with elevations in CA-125; these include pancreatic carcinoma (59%), lung (32%), breast (12%), and colon (22%) cancers. Therefore, CA-125 cannot be used in determining the origin of a malignancy. CA-125 elevations are typically the highest for women with ovarian carcinomas (in the thousands of units per milliliter range); the levels in other carcinomas are usually in the several hundreds of units per milliliter range. The CA-125 level can also be elevated in a variety of benign conditions, including endometriosis, adenomyosis, leiomyomas, pregnancy, pelvic inflammatory disease, and menses. Other benign nongynecologic conditions associated with elevated CA-125 values include cirrhosis, pancreatitis, recent laparotomy or thoracotomy, peritonitis, and peritoneal tuberculosis. Table 18E-3 outlines the malignant and nonmalignant etiologies of an elevated CA-125.

The clinical use of CA-125 has been primarily employed in the management of patients with an established epithelial ovarian cancer diagnosis. There is a close correlation of progression or regression of disease.[84–86] The CA-125 is also utilized to follow patients in order to detect recurrent disease. In 90% of cases of ovarian cancer recurrence, the CA-125 began to rise before signs and symptoms developed. The CA-125 is also clinically applied to evaluation before second-look surgery. In virtually all patients with an elevated CA-125 prior to second-look evaluation, disease will be found if the CA-125 is elevated.[87] The role of CA-125 levels in screening for ovarian cancer should be investigational only, or with certain high-risk women, based on family history and personal cancer history. The marker does not reach the appropriate sensitivity of specificity when a single value is used; however, investigation is currently under way to employ the marker in a more valuable way.

### GERM CELL TUMORS

Germ cell tumors also produce tumor markers. These tumors may be composed of a single cell type or may be mixed, and the components that make up the tumor will determine the markers produced. α-Fetoprotein (AFP) is an oncofetal antigen that is elevated in germ cell tumors and hepatocellular carcinomas. The endodermal sinus tumor produces AFP, along with the embryonal carcinoma. β-Human chorionic gonadotropin (βhCG) is produced by the choriocarcinoma and the embryonal carcinoma. Dysgerminomas are classically devoid of AFP; they may produce βhCG due to small numbers of syncytiotrophoblast, which may be present in this tumor. Dysgerminomas may also be associated with the production of lactate dehydrogenase (LDH) and CA-125. In all patients undergoing surgery for an adnexal mass, a serum sample should be obtained and diagnosed preoperatively and subsequently monitored. If a germ cell tumor is found, assays for AFP, βhCG, LDH, and CA-125 should be performed. If an individual with a diagnosis of a dysgerminoma is found to have an elevated AFP, a search for other components to the tumor should be conducted, because it may have implications for treatment. Immature teratomas usually do not produce markers but may produce AFP.

## SEX CORD–STROMAL TUMORS

Sex cord–stromal tumors are most often associated with hormone production. Granulosa cell and theca cell tumors produce estrogens and occasionally progesterone. Sertoli-Leydig cell tumors produce testosterone, dehydroepiandrosterone (DHEA), and also occasionally estradiol and progesterone. Granulosa cell tumors are also associated with the production of inhibin, which is a normal secretory product of the granulosa cell tumors in the follicular phase of the menstrual cycle.[88] CA-125 may also be elevated in some sex cord–stromal tumors, and AFP may also be produced by Sertoli-Leydig cell tumors.[89]

## MANAGEMENT OF THE ADNEXAL MASS

It is not uncommon for an adnexal mass to be detected either preoperatively or during the time of a laparotomy or laparoscopy being performed for other reasons. Preoperatively, time is available for an appropriate evaluation in order to determine how to manage the mass. At the time of surgery for other causes, however, this is not possible, and decisions will need to be based on the available information such as patient's age, menstrual status, underlying disease, and size and appearance of the ovary. Approximately two-thirds of tumors of the ovary of patients between the ages of 20 and 44 are benign, and the chance that a tumor is malignant in a patient less than 45 years is less than 7%.[90] Adnexal masses may be placed in the following categories: functional cysts, neoplastic masses, inflammatory masses, ectopic pregnancy, and tubal masses.

Preoperatively, the assessment of an adnexal mass should include an ultrasound (with or without Doppler studies) and a βhCG in the premenopausal woman, an ultrasound, and a CA-125 level in the postmenopausal woman. Attention to the ovarian cyst's characteristics is important: internal septations, solid areas, wall thickness, and the cyst's fluid must be noted. In the premenopausal woman, cysts can be divided into functional and neoplastic. The most common functional cyst is the follicular cyst, and most are less than 8 cm in

size and resolve in 1 to 2 months. Other forms of the functional cyst include the corpus luteum cyst (>2 cm in size) and the theca lutein cyst. Theca lutein cysts are associated with pregnancy and are most common in molar pregnancies. Ultrasound characteristics of these cysts include a smooth-walled, unilocular structure, and they are characterized by an absence of blood flow to the cyst on Doppler USG. Theca lutein cysts are usually multilocular.

It should also be noted that a patient on oral contraceptives may produce functional cysts. Of the neoplastic masses in the premenopausal women, the benign cystic teratoma (or the dermoid cyst) is the most common. On USG, the most common characteristics of the dermoid cyst include calcification, layering of fat, and presence of fluid. However, these may also be simple cysts with smooth walls. Benign mucinous and serous cysts tend to be simple cysts, without septation or solid areas and with normal blood flow. Malignant epithelial carcinomas of the ovary are characterized by thick septations (>2 mm), solid areas, and abnormal blood flow on Doppler USG. Malignant masses are characterized by vascular flow, and because the vessels that supply the tumor tend to have less smooth muscle, the blood faces less impedance through normal vessels. The lower resistance to blood flow is expressed generally as a pulsatility index, as follows:

$$\frac{\text{Peak systolic flow–end diastolic velocity}}{\text{Mean systolic velocity}}$$

A malignant tumor tends to have a lower pulsatility index than a benign mass. If there is no blood flow in the mass, the likelihood of malignancy is significantly reduced. If a constant blood flow with a continuing diastolic blood flow is present, the diagnosis of a malignant lesion should be entertained. Inflammatory masses tend to be complex in nature, with a combination of cystic and solid components. These tend to be quite irregular in shape and are characteristically tender. These masses tend to be associated with fevers and systemic signs of infection in the patient. Ectopic pregnancy may also present as an adnexal mass in a woman of reproductive age, and the most common location for an ectopic pregnancy is in the fallopian tube. These are characterized by a positive pregnancy test, hemorrhage into the tube, and adnexal pain. Figure 18E-1 outlines the management scheme for an adnexal mass in a premenopausal woman.

In the postmenopausal woman, functional cysts will not be present, and all adnexal masses must be considered potentially neoplastic. The risk for a mass being malignant is also increased in the age group. Criteria similar to those used in premenopausal women are used to evaluate an adnexal mass in the postmenopausal women. However, the CA-125 value enters into the management scheme. In this age group, any adnexal mass associated with an elevated CA-125 requires removal, as well as any complex mass that contains septation or solid areas. A particular problem in this age group has been the asymptomatic, simple ovarian cyst. With the advent of improved imaging studies and the more frequent use of ultrasound and CT scans, these are detected with increasing frequency. The issue in this situation is whether these cysts require removal. In one prevalence study, 6.6% of asymptomatic postmenopausal women were found to have a simple ovarian cyst 5 cm or less in size.[91] On follow-up, 24% of the cysts resolved, 50% persisted, and 17% were lost to follow-up. Numerous studies have demonstrated that these are most always

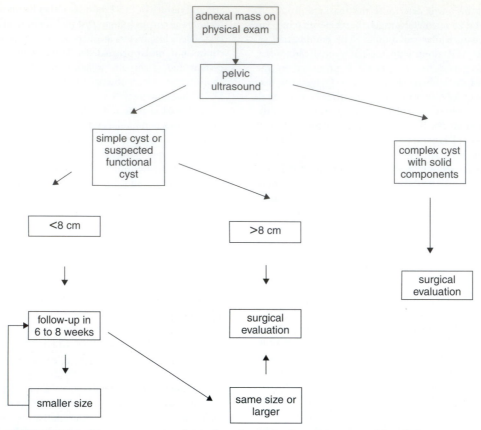

**FIGURE 18E-1.** The management of the adnexal mass in the premenopausal female.

benign. Of 43 postmenopausal women with simple cysts undergoing surgical evaluation, none were found to be malignant.[92] In a study that included larger simple cysts, 3 of 144 (2%) were found to be malignant; the mean sizes of the malignant simple cysts were 7, 11, and 18 cm.[93] For a woman in this age group to have a cyst managed conservatively, she must have a normal CA-125. An algorithm for managing the adnexal mass in the postmenopausal woman is outlined in Fig. 18E-2.

After it is decided that a mass requires surgical removal, the next question that must be answered is whether it can be safely removed via laparoscopy. As a general rule, any mass that is highly suspicious for malignancy should be removed via laparotomy, and any mass in a postmenopausal woman should be removed intact, or aspirated without spillage of fluid contents into the peritoneal cavity. Requirements for a mass to be removed through the laparoscope in a postmenopausal woman include a normal CA-125, a simple cyst by USG, and a size less than 10 cm. The requirements for premenopausal women are somewhat more relaxed, due to the low incidence of malignancy in this age group. A number of studies have demonstrated the efficacy of the use of the laparoscope to evaluate and remove an adnexal mass that is not suspected to be malignant.[94–96] The management of the adnexal mass in a woman with a history of nongynecologic malignancies has also been evaluated. In one study,

30 patients with a previously diagnosed nongynecologic malignancy who underwent a laparoscopy for the diagnosis of an adnexal mass were evaluated.[97] The mean age of the patients was 57; 24 of the patients had benign disease and 6 had metastatic disease. In this population of patients, it was concluded that laparoscopy could be safely used to manage an adnexal mass, and it should be considered in the initial method of surgical evaluation in this population of patients.

All patients who sign a consent for laparosopic management of an adnexal mass should also sign a consent for a laparotomy. This is done for two reasons: (1) if it is not technically feasible to remove the mass via the laparoscope, and (2) if the mass is found to have characteristics of a malignancy. Characteristics of a malignant mass include excrescences on the surface of the ovary, peritoneal implants, and ascites.

## PATHOLOGY

The ovary is composed of three cell types: germ cells, stromal cells, and epithelial cells derived from the coelomic epithelium. Cancers of the ovary can originate from any of these three cell types. By far the most common type of ovarian tumor is derived from the

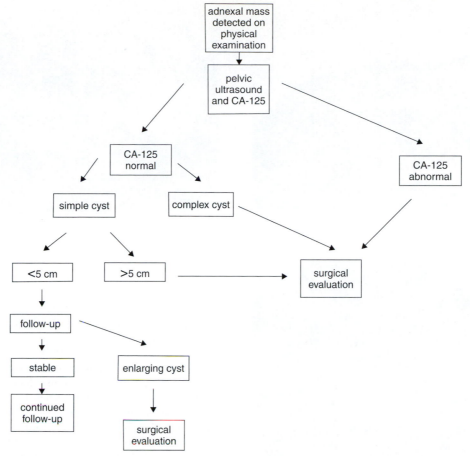

**FIGURE 18E-2.** The management of the adnexal mass in the postmenopausal female.

epithelial covering of the ovary; 70% of ovarian tumors are epithelial in derivation, 20% are germ cell–derived, 10% are stromal, and 5% are metastatic. Germ cell tumors are found most commonly in young women.

Epithelial tumors account for 90% of all malignancies. These are predominantly glandular in nature, and the histology resembles müllerian-derived epithelium of the genital tract. Epithelial tumors are divided into histologic subtypes; within each of these various histologic subtypes, there are three types of tumors: benign, borderline, and invasive. The most common form of ovarian cancer is of the serous histopathologic subtype. Two-thirds of epithelial cancers are invasive, and one-third are borderline. Grossly, most ovarian tumors are cystic in nature. This is due to the repair process that occurs when a woman ovulates. The repair process to the disrupted epithelium results in inclusion cyst formation, and these inclusion cysts may then become neoplastic. Gross characteristics of malignant ovarian tumors include solid areas inside the cyst wall and excrescences on the surface of the ovary. However, not all solid tumors are malignant in nature; ovarian fibromas are a benign form of a solid ovarian tumor. Figure 18E-3 shows a benign tumor of the ovary.

The nomenclature of ovarian tumors reflects the cell type of the tumor and the degree of biologic malignancy. The neoplastic

epithelium may resemble any one of the forms of epithelium of the genital tract, and these are categorized into subtypes based on this histologic resemblance: cells that compose serous ovarian tumors

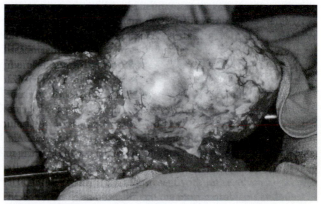

**FIGURE 18E-3.** A malignant ovarian cyst, characterized by solid areas within the cyst.

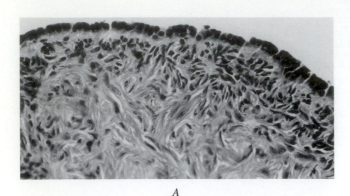

*A*

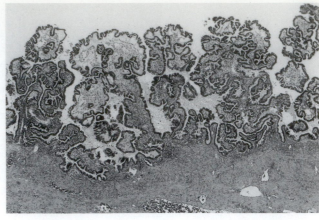

*B*

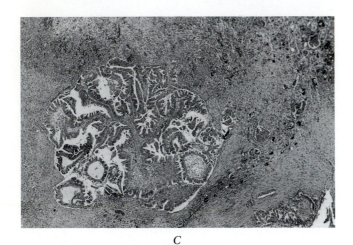

*C*

**FIGURE 18E-4.** The pathologic spectrum of serous ovarian neoplasm: (*a*) A benign serous ovarian tumor. These neoplasms are characterized by being lined by a single layer of serous cells. (*b*) A borderline serous ovarian tumor. Epithelial cells covering fibrovascular cores and an absence of invasion into the ovarian stroma characterizes these. (*c*) A serous invasive ovarian carcinoma. Sheets of proliferating cells invading into and replacing the ovarian stroma characterize these. (See also Plate 31.)

resemble the cells of the fallopian tube; mucinous tumors resemble the cells of the endocervix; endometrioid neoplasms resemble the endometrium; clear-cell tumors resemble the endometrial glands of pregnancy; and transitional-cell tumors resemble cells of urothelial differentiation. Specimen examination by pathology requires careful inspection of the tumor and attention to solid areas within the cyst and excrescences on the surface of the tumor. These areas should be well sampled at the time of pathologic examination. Serous tumors are notable for having a uniform histology, while mucinous tumors may demonstrate a great variation in histopathology in one specimen, ranging from areas of benign, borderline, and malignant tumor cells within one specimen. Thus, careful sectioning of these tumors must be performed so as not to overlook a malignant component of the tumor. This has implications for a frozen-section diagnosis.

## EPITHELIAL OVARIAN TUMORS

**SEROUS EPITHELIAL OVARIAN TUMORS.** These are the most common form of epithelial neoplasms and account for 46% of all epithelial tumors. Fifty percent of these are benign, 30% are malignant, and 20% are borderline. Figure 18E-4 demonstrates the pathologic spectrum of these tumors. Benign epithelial tumors, which are characterized by a single layer of cells lining a cyst, are usually unilocular. They may also have a few papillary excrescences involving the cyst wall. Approximately 20% of serous tumors are adenofibromas, consisting of a firm, white fibroma component containing multiple neoplastic cysts. Psammoma bodies, which are calcium deposits, may also be present in these tumors. They may vary in size from 1 cm to very large (>30 cm in size), and approximately 20% are bilateral. The median age at diagnosis is 45 years. The premalignant potential of the benign, serous epithelial tumors is unknown, but pathologic sections have revealed a transition from benign to malignant epithelium in 20% of cases, suggesting that they may have a premalignant potential; however, this remains controversial.[98]

Borderline epithelial ovarian tumors (see Fig. 18E-4*B*) are characterized by moderate to marked cellular proliferation. The cysts are lined by multiple layers of cells, but the cells do not invade into the stroma of the ovary. The cytology of the cells resembles that of a well-differentiated serous adenocarcinoma. The borderline tumor is characterized by tufts of epithelial cells growing on fibrovascular

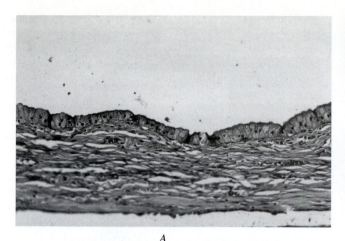
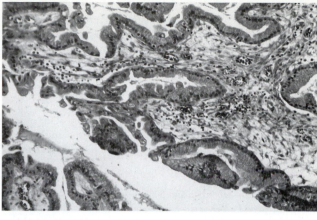

A                                                                 B

**FIGURE 18E-5.** (*a*) A benign tumor consisting of a single layer of cells. (*b*) A malignant mucinous tumor, consisting of sheets of cells. (See also Plate 32.)

cores, and approximately 30% are bilateral. The median age at diagnosis is 48 years. These tumors are generally considered malignant tumors with an indolent course and are not thought to progress into invasive ovarian cancer. They do have the potential to metastasize, but the majority present at an early stage.

Invasive serous tumors (see Fig. 18E-4*C*), which are the most common form of epithelial ovarian cancer, are usually quite large by the time they are diagnosed and are characterized by solid areas. They may also undergo hemorrhage and necrosis. Invasive serous tumors are graded based on their cytology and architecture[99]: grade 1 tumors are characterized by fine papillae throughout; grade 2 tumors demonstrate more cellular atypia; and grade 3 tumors consist of large sheets of undifferentiated cells. There is a close correlation between stage and grade of these tumors: 90% of advanced-stage tumors are grades 2 or 3, and 70% of early-stage tumors are grade 1.[100] Psammoma bodies are more commonly found in well-differentiated tumors. Approximately 30% of stage I tumors are bilateral. The mean age at diagnosis of serous epithelial ovarian cancer is 56 years.

MUCINOUS EPITHELIAL TUMORS. The cells of mucinous tumors predominantly resemble the cells of the endocervix but may also resemble the cells of the colon. These tumors comprise 34% of all epithelial neoplasms and the vast majority are benign: 81% are benign, 14% are borderline, and 5% are malignant. These tumors commonly reach very large sizes, are multilocular, and are filled with a mucinous material. Benign mucinous tumors (Fig. 18E-5*A*) are lined by a single layer of cells that resembles the endocervix, or less commonly, the colon. Only 2% are bilateral, and the median age at diagnosis is 44 years.

Borderline mucinous epithelial ovarian tumors are also composed of cells resembling the endocervix or the colon; however, the intestinal form is far more common and is present in approximately 83% of these tumors.[101] The cyst wall lining of this tumor is one to three cell layers' thick and is characterized by mild to moderate cel-

lular atypia. Six percent are bilateral, and the median age at diagnosis is 49 years.

Malignant mucinous tumors (Fig. 18E-5*B*) are relatively rare and are characterized by sheets of cells or as tumor invading into the stroma of the ovary. Because these tumors become less well differentiated, they may lose their mucinous component and may be difficult to distinguish from other epithelial carcinomas. Forty-seven percent are bilateral, and the median age at diagnosis is 52 years.

ENDOMETRIOID OVARIAN TUMORS. The cells comprising endometrioid tumors (Fig. 18E-6) resemble the cells of the endometrium. Endometrioid ovarian tumors comprise 8% of all common epithelial tumors and most are malignant: 77% are malignant, 19% are borderline, and 4% are benign. Approximately 10% of these tumors are associated with endometriosis, suggesting that

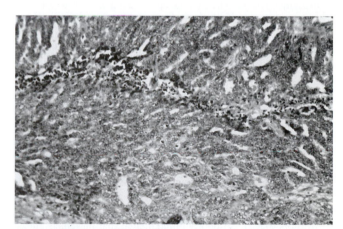

**FIGURE 18E-6.** Endometrioid cancers of the ovary resemble cells of the endometrium.

some of these tumors may arise from a neoplastic transformation of the endometriosis.[102] Similar to other epithelial tumors, the median ages for diagnosis of benign, borderline, and malignant tumors are 40, 48, and 57 years, respectively. Endometrioid carcinomas may contain squamous metaplasia, termed *adenoacanthomas,* and also may contain a poorly differentiated squamous component, termed *adenosquamous carcinoma.* Poorly differentiated endometrioid carcinomas may be difficult to distinguish from serous tumors. Very importantly, approximately 25% of endometrioid tumors of the ovary are associated with an underlying cancer of the uterus, so that any surgery for an endometrioid adenocarcinoma requires an investigation of the uterus.

### CLEAR-CELL TUMORS OF THE OVARY.

Clear-cell tumors account for 3% of all ovarian epithelial tumors, and the vast majority are malignant. These tumors are bilateral 13% of the time and grossly resemble serous tumors. Borderline clear-cell tumors are exceedingly rare but exist and may be difficult to distinguish from an invasive tumor.[103] The cells comprising the clear-cell tumor are characterized by clear cells and "hobnail" cells. Microscopically, they may resemble the steroid-cell tumors and the endodermal sinus tumor. This tumor should not be confused with a metastatic clear-cell tumor from the kidney, which may be evident only after the diagnosis of an ovarian mass.[104]

### TRANSITIONAL-CELL TUMORS (BRENNER TUMORS).

Brenner tumors are ovarian tumors containing cells that resemble the urothelium. They are almost always benign, with only 1% borderline and an additional 1% malignant. These tumors comprise 2% of all epithelial neoplasms. They are typically solid in appearance, and 7% are bilateral. As with other ovarian tumors, they may reach a large size. A transitional-cell carcinoma of the ovary differs from a malignant Brenner tumor of the ovary in that no benign Brenner areas are evident. In addition, this tumor tends to be more aggressive than a malignant Brenner tumor.

### CARCINOSARCOMAS.

Commonly referred to as mixed müllerian tumors, carcinosarcomas are the most common form of ovarian sarcoma. The average age of women with this tumor is 60 years. Carcinosarcomas are composed of a malignant sarcomatous component and a malignant carcinomatous component, and are classified as homologous or heterologous. The homologous tumor components resemble those found in the müllerian tract, and the heterologous tumor elements resemble tissue found outside of the genital tract. These tumors tend to be highly aggressive, with only a 30% survival rate in patients with stage I disease.[105]

### OTHER CARCINOMAS OF THE OVARY.

Approximately 3% of all ovarian tumors are of the mixed variety. The most common form of a mixed tumor is that of the clear-cell and endometrioid carcinoma, which may arise in endometriosis.[106] A tumor is considered "mixed" if greater than 10% of the tumor consists of one of the components.

Tumors that are so poorly differentiated that placement into a distinct histopathologic subtype is impossible, are referred to as undifferentiated carcinomas, comprising approximately 2% of all ovarian tumors. The small cell carcinoma is a form of the undifferentiated carcinoma. Two types of small cell carcinoma exist: the

hypercalcemic and the pulmonary. The hypercalcemic type is found in young women, with a median age at diagnosis of 28 years. Sixty percent will have an elevated serum calcium, and once the tumor is resected, the calcium decreases.[107] These are highly aggressive tumors, with an extremely poor prognosis. The pulmonary type resembles the small cell ("oat cell") carcinoma of the lung.[108] Neuron-specific enolase is commonly elevated in women with these tumors. Like the hypercalcemic small tumor, these are highly aggressive tumors, with a median time from diagnosis to death of just 8 months.

## GERM CELL TUMORS

These tumors typically occur in young women. Childhood ovarian tumors are rare, but when they occur, they are invariably of germ cell origin. The median age at diagnosis of germ cell tumors of the ovary is 20 years. Table 18E-4 outlines the World Health Organization (WHO) classification of germ cell tumors of the ovary. These tumors

### TABLE 18E-4. THE WHO CLASSIFICATION OF GERM CELL TUMORS

Primitive germ cell tumors:

Dysgerminoma:
  Variant: with syncytiotrophoblast cells

Yolk sac tumor (endodermal sinus tumor):
  Variants:
    Polyvesicular vitelline tumor
    Hepatoid
    Glandular

Embryonal carcinoma

Polyembryoma

Choriocarcinoma

Teratoma:
  Immature:

  Mature:
    Solid
    Cystic:
      Dermoid cyst
        With secondary tumor formation
        Retiform

  Monodermal:
    Struma ovarii:
      With thyroid tumor
    Carcinoid:
      Insular
      Trabecular
    Strumal carcinoid
  Micunbous carcinoid:
    Neuroectodermal tumors
    Sebaceous tumors
    Other

Mixed

may be malignant or benign. The benign dermoid cyst, otherwise known as a mature teratoma, accounts for virtually all of the benign germ cell tumors of the ovary. Malignant germ cell tumors may derive from two sources: as a malignant component of an otherwise benign dermoid or directly from the germ cells of the ovary, referred to as primitive germ cell tumors. These tumors typically recapitulate normal embryonic and extraembryonic structures.

DERMOID CYST. The dermoid cyst accounts for approximately 25% to 30% of all ovarian tumors. These tumors are most common in women of the reproductive age group, but they may also be encountered in women in older age groups and in children. This tumor is bilateral in 12% of cases and usually consists of epidermoid components, with skin being the most prominent feature of this teratoma. It also typically contains sebum, hair, and teeth and may contain derivatives of any of the three germ layers. Any component of these tumors may undergo malignant degeneration. Malignant degeneration occurs in approximately 1% of these tumors, and squamous cell carcinoma is the most commonly found malignant component. Other types of malignant tumors that may be found in dermoid are melanoma, basal cell carcinoma, adenocarcinomas, and neuroendocrine tumors. Malignant changes found within germ cell tumors account for 2% to 3% of all ovarian cancers, and the age incidence is similar to that of epithelial ovarian cancers. Struma ovarii refers to a specialized type of dermoid consisting of thyroid tissue. These tumors are rarely functional at a clinical level and are malignant in only approximately 5% of cases. In contrast, carcinoid tumors of the dermoid cyst are functional and may produce carcinoid syndrome in approximately 30% of cases.

PRIMITIVE GERM CELL TUMORS. These tumors account for 20% of all ovarian tumors but a far smaller proportion of malignancies, and are most common in young women, with a peak incidence in the third decade of life.

DYSGERMINOMA. Dysgerminomas (Fig. 18E-7) are composed of a monotonous group of cells resembling the primordial germ cells of the embryo. They are the most common of the primitive germ cell tumors, of which they account for 50%. Usually a solid tumor, they are grossly bilateral in 10% of cases. In an additional 10% of cases, a microscopic focus will be found in a grossly normal contralateral ovary. Approximately 5% of dysgerminomas contain syncytiotrophoblasts, and are therefore associated with βhCG production. These tumors may also have estrogenic and androgenic manifestations.

IMMATURE TERATOMA. These tumors account for 20% of primitive germ cell tumors. They consist of a mix of cells from all three germ layers, some of which will be immature in appearance. Immature neural tissue comprises the largest immature component of these tumors. Characteristically, they will have a solid, white appearance due to the neural component of the tumor. Less than 5% of these tumors are bilateral, and a mature teratoma will occupy the contralateral ovary in approximately 10% of cases. The tumors are graded based on the amount of immature neural tissue present in the tumor. These tumors, along with benign dermoid, may also

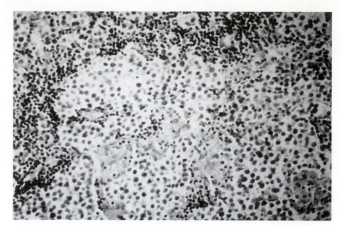

**FIGURE 18E-7.** A dysgerminoma of the ovary characterized by a monotonous group of cells resembling the primordial germ cells of the embryo.

be associated with deposits of mature neural tissue throughout the peritoneal cavity. This tissue does not alter stage of the tumor nor prognosis. It may, however, occasionally require surgical removal, because it can grow, although usually quite slowly.

YOLK SAC TUMOR (ENDODERMAL SINUS TUMOR). These tumors comprise approximately 20% of primitive germ cell tumors and usually consist of a solid mass. The most common form of these tumors is the reticular form, consisting of cells that form irregular anastomosing spaces, which resemble extra-embryonic differentiation. Schiller-Duval bodies (Fig. 18E-8) are characteristic of these tumors. They consist of a single papilla lined by tumor cells, containing a central vessel projecting into the space. These tumors may also recapitulate normal embryonic structures derived from the yolk sac. The cells of the yolk sac tumor stain positive for AFP.

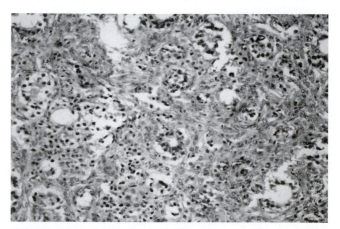

**FIGURE 18E-8.** Schiller-Duval bodies, characteristic of the endodermal sinus tumor.

**TABLE 18E-5. GERM CELL TUMOR COMPONENTS AND THEIR SECRETED SUBSTANCES**

| TUMOR | ASSOCIATED MARKER SUBSTANCES |
|---|---|
| Dysgerminoma | LDH |
| | CA-125 |
| Immature teratoma | AFP |
| Embryonal carcinoma | AFP |
| | βhCG |
| Endodermal sinus tumor | AFP |
| Choriocarcinoma | βhCG |

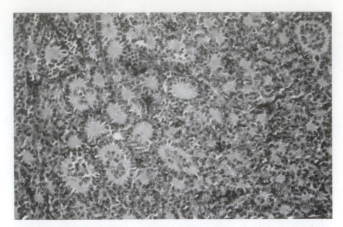

**FIGURE 18E-9.** Cal Exner bodies characteristic of the granulosa-cell tumor.

**OTHER GERM CELL TUMORS.** Embryonal carcinomas and choriocarcinomas of the ovary rarely occur by themselves but may occur as components of other tumors. Embryonal carcinomas are similar to testicular carcinomas. Choriocarcinomas are composed of syncytiotrophoblasts, cytotrophoblasts, and intermediate trophoblasts. Both of the above tumors produce βhCG and are therefore associated with endocrine changes such as isosexual precocious puberty and abnormal vaginal bleeding. Mixed primitive germ cell tumors account for 10% of primitive germ cell tumors of the ovary. The most common form of mixed germ cell tumor is composed of dysgerminoma and yolk sac components. The degree of bilaterality depends on the presence or absence of dysgerminomatous components. Because a small portion of one component may change postoperative treatment, it is important to recognize mixed forms. Table 18E-5 outlines the germ cell components and associated secreted substances.

### SEX CORD–STROMAL TUMORS

This large and heterogenous group of ovarian tumors arises from the ovarian matrix, which consists of sex cords and mesenchyme. The granulosa cells of the ovary are responsible for estrogen production and are derived from the sex cords. The mesenchymal cells are the precursors of the stromal and theca cells of the ovary. Theca cells of the ovary are responsible for androgen production. Sex cord–stromal tumors are rare in childhood and adolescence, occurring most frequently in postmenopausal women, with the peak age range from 50 to 70 years. They comprise 7% of all malignant neoplasms, and the vast majority are of an indolent nature. Classically, these tumors may also produce estrogen and androgens and, many times, may present with endocrinologic manifestations such as isosexual precocious puberty, excessive amounts of vaginal bleeding in the menstruating female, or postmenopausal bleeding. Androgenic effects seen as virilization may also be found.

**GRANULOSA CELL TUMOR.** These tumors are those derived from the sex cord. They comprise 5% of all ovarian malignancies and 70% of all malignant sex cord–stromal tumors. The average age at diagnosis of these tumors is 52 years. Two forms of the granulosa tumor exist: the adult form and the juvenile form. The adult type comprises 95% of all granulosa cell tumors. Due to the estrogen production of these tumors, one of the most common manifestations is abnormal vaginal bleeding; they are associated with atypical endometrial hyperplasia 42% of the time, and with invasive endometrial cancer 22% of the time.[109] Virilizing symptoms may also present with granulosa cell tumors.[110]

In most cases, these tumors are large at the time of discovery; however, they may be microscopic.[111] They may be solid or cystic in gross characteristics. The cells of this tumor consist predominantly of granulosa cells along with a minor component of theca cells and/or fibroblasts. The most common growth form of this tumor is microfollicular, characterized by Call-Exner bodies, which are small cavities containing eosinophilic fluid, degenerating nuclei, and a hyalinized basement membrane (Fig. 18E-9). Other growth patterns such as trabecular also exist.

Juvenile granulosa cell tumors present primarily in prepubertal girls and women under the age of 30. Due to estrogen production by the tumor, prepubertal patients will present with isosexual pseudo-precocious puberty.[112,113] Some individuals will present with virilization due to elevated levels of androgens.[113–115] Approximately 5% of these tumors are bilateral,[115] and the vast majority (88%) are stage IA at the time of diagnosis. Juvenile granulosa cell tumors are found as a component of Ollier's disease and Marfucci's syndrome. Similar to the adult form of the tumor, they may be solid or cystic. The classic Call-Exner bodies are rarely found in the juvenile tumors. Cytology distinguishes the juvenile form of this tumor from the adult type, as does the mitotic rate, which is significantly higher in these tumors when compared to the adult form.

**FIBROMAS AND THECOMAS.** Fibromas and thecomas are derived from the mesenchymal cells of the ovary, and the vast majority of these tumors are benign. They may be composed of theca cells, smooth-muscle cells, or both. The thecoma consists of lipid-rich theca cells. They comprise 10% of all ovarian neoplasms and primarily occur in postmenopausal women. The tumors may reach sizes of up to 40 cm, and ascites may be present.[116–118] These tumors are the most hormonally active of the sex cord–stromal tumors, and 60% of patients will have abnormal vaginal bleeding due to estrogen production.[117,118] As with any tumor that produces excess estrogen for the body, endometrial hyperplasia and invasive cancer may also be present. These tumors may also be associated with androgen production.

The ovarian fibroma, the most common tumor in the sex cord–stromal category, accounts for 4% of all ovarian neoplasms. It is composed of a collection of bland smooth-muscle cells, is most commonly present in postmenopausal women, and does not produce active sex hormones. The tumor is typically a solid tumor, which may reach quite large proportions. Ascites may also be produced by this benign tumor, arising from stromal edema of the tumor, and occurs in approximately 10% of fibromas greater than 10 cm in size.[119] Meigs' syndrome is a classic syndrome associated with ovarian fibromas and is characterized by pleural effusion and ascites.[120] Gorlin's syndrome is characterized by an inherited predisposition of ovarian fibromas and basal cell nevi at an early age.[121] A low malignant potential form of the ovarian fibroma exists, characterized by increased cellular density of the tumor, nuclear atypia, and three or fewer mitotic figures per 10 high-power fields.[122] A malignant form of the fibroma, the fibrosarcoma, also exists—but it is extremely rare. These tumors are highly malignant and are characterized by nuclear pleomorphism and more than four mitotic figures per 10 high-power fields.

**SERTOLI-LEYDIG CELL TUMORS.** These tumors are extremely rare, with an average size of 16 cm and an average age of diagnosis of 25 years. The tumors may be composed of Sertoli cells or Sertoli and Leydig cells. Sertoli-Leydig cell tumors tend to be well differentiated and manifest a primarily tubular pattern,[123] but they may also be moderately or poorly differentiated. The Sertoli cells are estrogen producing, and the Leydig cells are androgen producing. These tumors typically produce androgens, and thus they are associated with virilization and menstrual disorders such as amenorrhea and oligomenorrhea. The peripheral conversion of androgens into estrogen may also lead to postmenopausal bleeding in older women. Excessive renin production may occur with Sertoli cell tumors, so that hypertension and hypokalemia may also occur.[124–126] Only 2% to 3% have spread by the time of diagnosis, and 18% of these tumors are malignant.[127] Inhibin and AFP may be produced by these tumors.[128]

**OVARIAN SEX CORD TUMOR WITH ANNULAR TUBULES (SCTAT).** This tumor has features that are intermediate between the histopathology of the Sertoli cell tumor and the granulosa cell tumor. The cells of this tumor form simple or complex ring-shaped tubules.[129] Approximately 30% of these tumors occur in women with Peutz-Jeghers syndrome,[130] where they tend to be small, bilateral, and multifocal. Fifteen percent of women with Peutz-Jeghers syndrome and SCTAT will have an associated cervical neoplasm, termed *adenoma malignum,* which tends to be highly aggressive.[130,131] These tumors are estrogen producing, and the presenting signs and symptoms are related to this hyperestrogenic state.

**STEROID CELL TUMORS.** Steroid cell tumors are rare, accounting for just 0.1% of all ovarian neoplasms. These tumors are composed of steroid hormone–producing cells, including lutein cells, Leydig cells, and adrenocortical cells, and are divided into three classes: (1) the stromal luteoma, (2) the Leydig cell tumor, and (3) the steroid tumor not otherwise specified. The large, round cells that compose these tumors contain large lipid vacuoles. Crystals of Reineke are characteristic of the Leydig cell tumors,[132] which are thought to arise from the Leydig cells of the epithelium of the ovary. The stromal luteoma and the Leydig cell tumor are usually benign. The stromal luteoma may present with postmenopausal bleeding. Leydig cell tumors are small (their average size is 2.7 cm) and the average age at diagnosis is 58 years.[132,133] The initial manifestation of these tumors is a hyperandrogenic state; however, a hyperestrogenic state may also be present.

The steroid tumor not otherwise specified lacks the characteristic cells of the stromal luteoma or the Leydig cell tumor. The signs and symptoms of androgen excess may be seen years prior to the diagnosis. Estrogen excess, as in the other sex cord–stromal tumors, may also be seen. In contrast to the stromal luteoma and the Leydig cell tumor, these tumors are associated with a high risk of malignancy, and 43% of women with these tumors will have extra-ovarian disease diagnosed either at initial presentation or at follow-up.[134]

## OVARIAN SARCOMAS

Ovarian sarcomas are exceedingly rare. The most common form of sarcoma that occurs in the ovary is the carcinosarcoma (referenced under epithelial tumors). Other sarcomas of the ovary that have been reported include leiomyosarcomas and angiosarcomas.

## METASTATIC TUMORS TO THE OVARY

Approximately 5% of all ovarian tumors are metastatic. A hallmark of metastatic disease to the ovary is bilaterality. Both gynecologic and nongynecologic tumors may metastasize to the ovary. The most common gynecologic tumor to metastasize to the ovary is from the fallopian tubes, which will involve the ovary, due to its close proximity, in approximately 13% of cases.[135] Other sites of gynecologic malignancies that may involve the ovary include tumors of the cervix, in fewer than 1% of cases, and tumors of the endometrium, in approximately 5% of cases.[136] The endometrioid carcinoma of the ovary existing with an adenocarcinoma of the uterus is not always metastatic disease, however, since they may be dual primaries.

Nongynecologic sites of cancer metastasizing to the ovary include breast, colon, biliary, and stomach. In a study of 121 women with a new adnexal mass and a history of breast cancer, 50% had a benign neoplasm and 50% had a malignant tumor, with a ratio of 3:1 of a primary ovarian cancer to metastatic breast cancer.[137] The classic Krukenberg tumor of the ovary accounts for 40% of all metastatic tumors to the ovary.[138] It is characterized by mucin-filled signet-ring cells located in the ovarian stroma. The most common site of origin of this tumor is the stomach, but it may also originate from the colon, breast, or the biliary tract. Other gastrointestinal tumors may also metastasize to the ovary and may not have the characteristics of a Krukenberg tumor. Metastatic mucinous carcinoma from the colon can resemble a primary mucinous carcinoma of the ovary.[139,140] In an evaluation of 35 women with a history of colon cancer and a newly diagnosed mass, 57% had metastatic colon cancer, 26% had a benign ovarian neoplasm, and 17% had a primary epithelial ovarian cancer.[141] Carcinoid tumors may metastasize to the ovary; however,

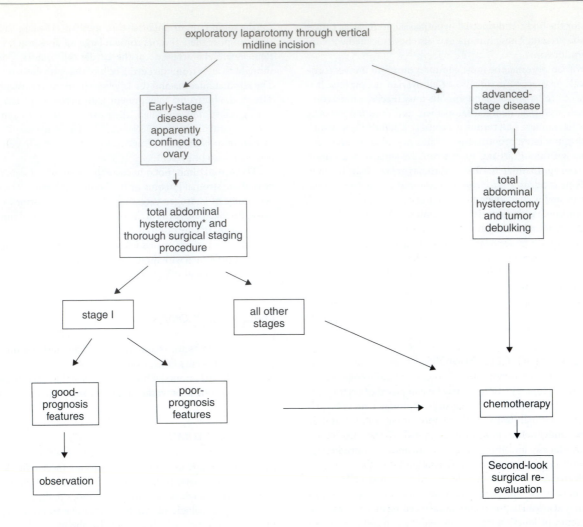

* In selected young patients who desire to maintain future fertility, the contralateral ovary and uterus may be left in place.

**FIGURE 18E-10.** The general management scheme for epithelial ovarian cancer.

these are very rare and occur in fewer than 2% of carcinoids, and account for only 2% of metastatic tumors to the ovary.[136,142] Any diagnosis on frozen section of an ovarian carcinoid should lead to an aggressive search for a primary tumor.[143] Lymphomas and leukemias may also involve the ovary. Hodgkin's disease involves the ovary in approximately 15% of cases, and Burkitt lymphomas involve the ovary quite commonly.[144]

## PRINCIPALS OF TREATMENT OF OVARIAN CANCER

The treatment of ovarian cancer remains a combination of surgery and chemotherapy. The treatment of early-stage ovarian cancer consists of a thorough surgical staging and, in selected cases, no treat-

ment with chemotherapy. In patients with high-grade or clear-cell tumors of the ovary, treatment with chemotherapy is recommended. In advanced-stage ovarian cancer, the treatment consists of tumor cytoreductive surgery and chemotherapy. Figure 18E-10 outlines the general management scheme for early-stage and advanced-stage ovarian cancers.

## SURGICAL MANAGEMENT

**PREOPERATIVE EVALUATION.** Ovarian cancer is a surgically diagnosed and staged disease, and it usually presents with an adnexal mass, with or without ascites. One of the initial evaluations will be by pelvic ultrasound or CT scan of the pelvis. Once a decision has been made that a patient has a possible ovarian malignancy, preoperative evaluation should include chest x-ray, electrocardiogram, urinalysis, and bloodwork, including a complete blood count, chemistries, a CA-125 measurement, and a CEA. In the young patient with a suspected ovarian malignancy, tumor markers for germ cell tumors (LDH, βhCG, AFP) should be drawn either preoperatively or intraoperatively. Any pleural effusion on a chest x-ray (CXR) should be tapped, if possible, and sent for cytology. A CT scan may be ordered in order to alert a surgeon to possible metastatic sites, such as intraparenchymal liver metastases, and it also allows evaluation of the pancreas and gallbladder. Mammograms should also be ordered preoperatively due to the fact that metastatic breast cancer may resemble ovarian cancer in its presentation. If a patient has bowel symptoms, an upper endoscopy, colonoscopy, or barium enema should be performed. Metastatic gastric and colon cancer can resemble ovarian cancer in its presentation. Patients with ovarian cancer may have symptoms of rectosigmoid obstruction. All patients with a suspected diagnosis of advanced-stage ovarian cancer will need a careful discussion of the potential surgical procedures that may be required to cytoreduce tumor, including sterilization, bowel resection with possible colostomy, splenectomy, possible blood transfusion, and intensive care unit postoperative care, along with complete mechanical bowel prep with antibiotics. Prophylactic intravenous antibiotics should be given preoperatively.

## SURGICAL MANAGEMENT OF EARLY-STAGE OVARIAN CANCER.

Approximately 10% to 15% of patients will present with early-stage ovarian cancer, and it is of utmost importance that a woman with a diagnosis of ovarian cancer is properly staged. In selected well-staged, early-stage ovarian cancers, treatment with chemotherapy will not be necessary. The surgical staging procedure is based on the patterns of spread of ovarian cancer and includes a thorough visual inspection of all peritoneal surfaces along with biopsies and a thorough evaluation of pelvic and para-aortic lymph nodes. Table 18E-6 outlines the components of a thorough surgical staging procedure for ovarian cancer patients. In a postmenopausal woman, or a woman desiring no future fertility, a total abdominal hysterectomy and bilateral salpingo-oophorectomy are performed. In selected women, a normal ovary and the uterus may be left in place for future fertility. If the uterus is left in place, an evaluation of the endometrium with a dilatation and curettage should be performed.

The abdominal incision should be vertical in a woman suspected of having a possible ovarian cancer. This is necessary to gain access to the upper abdomen and to the diaphragmatic surfaces. If a transverse incision has been made and an ovarian malignancy has been encountered, the incision can be extended at its lateral aspect vertically, along the lateral aspect of the rectus muscle. Upon opening the abdominal cavity, a thorough palpation of the abdominal cavity is undertaken with particular attention directed to the diaphragmatic surfaces, omentum, retroperitoneal lymph node areas, liver, stomach, spleen, pancreas, kidneys, and pelvis. All surfaces of the bowel should be inspected, and the small bowel should be run from the ligament of Treitz to the distalmost portion of the ileum. If peritoneal fluid or ascites is present, it should be aspirated and sent for cytology. Washings of the pelvis are then taken. In a woman of reproductive age, a cystectomy should be performed, with careful

**TABLE 18E-6. COMPONENTS OF THE SURGICAL STAGING PROCEDURE FOR OVARIAN CANCER**

Vertical midline incision

Aspiration and cytologic evaluation of any free pelvic fluid

Systematic inspection of all peritoneal surfaces and of the small and large bowel

Total abdominal hysterectomy and bilateral salpingo-oophorectomy*

Peritoneal washes:
  Pelvis
  Right and left paracolic gutters
  Right and left hemidiaphragms

Peritoneal biopsies:
  Anterior and posterior cul de sac
  Right and left paracolic gutters
  Right and left hemidiaphragms
  Intestinal mesentery
  Any suspicious areas

Omentectomy

Lymph-node sampling:
  Right and left para-aortics
  Common iliac lymph nodes
  External iliac
  Internal iliac
  Obturator

*In selected young patients who desire to maintain future fertility, the contralateral ovary and uterus may be left in place.

attention not to rupture the cyst. In a postmenopausal woman, the ovary with the cyst should be removed. After the frozen section has returned positive for an epithelial malignancy, attention is directed to performing the remainder of the surgical staging procedure. In a postmenopausal woman, the remaining ovary should be removed, and hysterectomy should be performed. In a young woman, conservative surgery may be performed, and sterilizing procedures should not be performed on the basis of a frozen section. After the removal of the primary tumor and the remaining ovary and uterus, attention is directed to peritoneal biopsies and an omentectomy. Biopsies of adequate size should be taken; 2- to 3-cm strips of peritoneum can be removed by grasping the peritoneum with an Allis clamp and removing with cautery. Sites for sampling include bladder peritoneum, posterior cul de sac, right and left pelvic sidewalls, right and left paracolic gutters, and the right and left diaphragm peritoneum. Saline washings are obtained from the left and right paracolic gutters and the left and right hemidiaphragms. These can be placed with the prior pelvic wash and sent as one sample. Attention should be directed to any adhesions, and these should be sampled and sent for permanent section. Attention is then directed to performing pelvic lymph node sampling. Lymph nodes are sampled in the obturator space, external iliac, and hypogastric regions. Careful attention should also be directed to a palpation of the inguinal lymph node regions, because it is possible for these areas to also be involved with tumor via spread down the round ligament of the uterus. If any

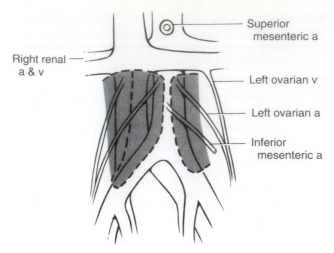

**FIGURE 18E-11.** Aortic node dissection for ovarian cancer staging, frontal view. The shaded areas indicate the tissue zones to be removed for staging. The broken lines indicate the initial incision lines used to mobilize the tissue zones for this dissection. The aortocaval nodes are removed along with the precaval and right paracaval nodes and the left para-aortic and adjacent preaortic nodes are removed. The ipsilateral common iliac nodes are excised.

suspicious lymph nodes are palpated in the inguinal region, they should be removed. Para-aortic lymph nodes and common iliac lymph nodes are also sampled. Careful attention should be directed to the para-aortic nodes due to the fact that it is possible for direct extension to these nodal areas to occur without involvement of pelvic lymph nodes. High aortic nodes must be thoroughly sampled where the gonadal vessels enter the inferior vena cava and the renal vein on the left side. The nodal areas that should be sampled are the precaval, periaortic, aortocaval, right caval, and left para-aortic. The boundaries for this important lymph node dissection include the common iliac nodes, inferiorly, and the renal veins, superiorly. Figure 18E-11 diagrams the aortic nodal dissection for early-stage ovarian cancer.

Table 18E-7 outlines the locations in which occult tumor may be found in women with apparent early-stage ovarian cancer. Approximately 33% of patients who have an apparent stage I tumor will be upstaged by the above procedure, and of those patients who

**TABLE 18E-7.** LOCATIONS OF OCCULT TUMOR IN WOMEN WITH APPARENT EARLY-STAGE (STAGES I AND II) EPITHELIAL OVARIAN CANCER

| DIAPHRAGM | AORTIC LYMPH NODES | PELVIC NODES | OMENTUM | POSITIVE CYTOLOGY |
|---|---|---|---|---|
| 13/177 | 17/114 | 3/51 | 14/162 | 32/121 |
| 7.3% | 18.1% | 5.9% | 8.6% | 26.4% |

SOURCE: Modified from JS Berek: Epithelial ovarian cancer, in *Practical Gynecologic Oncology*, in *Practical Gynecologic Oncology*, JS Berek, NF Hacker (eds). Williams and Wilkins, 1994, p 338. Reprinted with permission from *Ovarian Malignancies*, MS Piver (ed). Endinburgh, Churchill Livingstone, 1987, p 112.

are upstaged, 77% will have advanced-stage disease.[145] It is also important to note that visually negative areas do not correlate with being pathologically negative. In a series of patients with omental and diaphragmatic metastases, approximately 50% in each group had normal surfaces by visualization and palpation.[146] Palpably and visually abnormal lymph nodes contain tumor 88% of the time, and microscopic metastases are present in 33% of grossly normal lymph nodes.[147]

Many times, a tumor will be adherent to the pelvis in the absence of direct tumor extension, and the question arises as to whether these patients should be categorized as stage I or stage II patients. When the adherence is dense, these patients should be placed at stage II, due to the fact that these patients will experience a relapse rate similar to stage II patients.[148,149] Dense adherence is defined as follows: (1) cyst rupture at the time of dissection, (2) sharp dissection is required, or (3) raw areas remain in the area of the dissection.

Complications occur a significant proportion of the time with comprehensive surgical staging procedures. In one series reporting on 86 women undergoing surgical staging, intraoperative complications occurred 15% of the time.[150] Reported intraoperative complications include damage to the vena cava, ureter, and intestine. In addition to bowel obstruction, postoperative complications also include lymphocyst formation, which may occur after pelvic and para-aortic lymph node sampling.

**SURGICAL MANAGEMENT OF ADVANCED-STAGE OVARIAN CANCER.** The primary goal for surgical management of advanced-stage epithelial ovarian cancer is the removal of as much tumor as possible at the time of initial surgery. Survival is correlated to the amount of surgical debulking that can be performed, so that an aggressive approach to this disease is necessary. However, the radicalness of the procedure must be balanced with the potential morbidity to the patient. Thus, there is no one standard or "formula" operation, and the extent of surgery will be determined by the extent of disease, the pattern of tumor spread, and the medical condition of the patient. The theory supporting the principle of maximal surgical cytoreduction is that epithelial ovarian cancer is a chemosensitive tumor and that, by removing a large proportion of the tumor, the remaining cells will be thrown into active division and will therefore be more sensitive to chemotherapy.

Tumors have an exponential growth rate, but the growth slows as the tumor gets quite large and outgrows its blood supply (and thus its nutrients). This flattening of the portion of the growth curve is referred to as the Gompertzian phenomenon.[151] The concept of surgical debulking of chemosensitive ovarian tumors is based on the following hypothesis: by decreasing the tumor burden, more cells are actively proliferating and are thus more sensitive to chemotherapeutic agents. Other hypotheses that have also been proposed include the following: (1) cytoreduction leads to a lower tumor burden and thus fewer cell kills are needed in order to achieve eradication of the tumor based on first-order kinetics; and (2) a smaller number of cells results in fewer opportunities for the cells to develop drug-resistance mutations.

The concept of maximal surgical effort was first introduced in 1968 in a study demonstrating that women who had a "definitive operation" did better than those who had biopsy only.[152] Table 18E-8[152–160] reviews the existing literature on the effects of

**TABLE 18E-8.** SUMMARY OF THE DATA DEMONSTRATING THE EFFECTIVENESS OF TUMOR CYTOREDUCTION OF EPITHELIAL OVARIAN CANCER

| AUTHOR | DATE | RESIDUAL DISEASE, CM | MEDIAN SURVIVAL, MONTHS |
|---|---|---|---|
| Griffiths[152] | 1975 | 0 | 39 |
| | | 0–0.5 | 29 |
| | | 0.6–1.5 | 18 |
| | | >1.5 | |
| | | | 11 |
| Hacker et al.[153] | 1983 | <0.5 | 40 |
| | | 0.6–1.5 | 18 |
| | | >1.5 | 6 |
| Vogl et al.[154] | 1983 | <2 | 40 |
| | | ≥2 | 16 |
| Pohl et al.[155] | 1984 | <2 | 45 |
| | | ≥2 | 16 |
| Delgado et al.[156] | 1984 | <2 | 45 |
| | | ≥2 | 16 |
| Redman et al.[157] | 1986 | <3 | 38 |
| | | ≥3 | 26 |
| Conte et al.[158] | 1986 | <2 | 40 |
| | | ≥2 | 16 |
| Nejit et al.[159] | 1987 | <1 | 40 |
| | | ≥1 | 21 |
| Piver et al.[160] | 1988 | <2 | 48 |
| | | ≥2 | 21 |
| *Total* | | *Optimal** | *36* |
| | | *Suboptimal* | *16* |

* Optimal and suboptimal are as defined by the author of the study comprising this summary.
SOURCE: Modified from WJ Hoskins: Primary surgical management of epithelial ovarian cancer, in *Ovarian Cancer*, SC Rubin, GP Sutton (eds). New York, McGraw-Hill, 1993, p 248.

surgical debulking on the disease outcome in women. This table demonstrates that "optimal" surgical debulking has an impact on overall survival as well as on the disease-free interval in women with ovarian cancer and thus provides the surgical basis for the treatment of epithelial ovarian cancer. All reports on the effects of surgical debulking use the largest remaining tumor nodule as the measurement of residual disease. As discussed above, the definition of "optimal" may vary from study to study. A summary of these data demonstrates that women who are "optimal" at the end of cytoreduction have an improved median progression-free interval (31 versus 13 months) and a better median survival (36 versus 16 months). The findings at the time of second-look surgery, a surrogate endpoint, also demonstrate the advantages of optimal surgical cytoreduction. In a summary of the data concerning second-look surgery, those patients who are optimally cytoreduced have a much better chance of having no disease found at the time of second-look surgery. Women who have no disease left at the end of pri-

mary cytoreductive surgery have a 76% chance of having no disease found at the time of second-look surgery. Women who have optimal cytoreduction have a 46% chance of negative second-look findings. Women who have suboptimal disease left have a 23% chance of a negative second look.[161] The overall response rate was not significantly different for the two groups (61% versus 59%). This is to be expected and further supports tumor debulking as the surgical treatment for ovarian cancer, because it demonstrates the chemosensitivity of ovarian cancer that renders a person with a lower tumor burden in a more advantageous position for successful treatment.

One debate that has been raised in the discussion of the benefits of tumor cytoreduction concerns the biology of the tumor versus the actual benefits of surgical cytoreduction. It has been questioned whether the surgery itself is the factor that improves the disease-free survival of these patients, or whether this is instead a result of tumor biology. Those tumors that are able to be "effectively" cytoreduced may be less aggressive than those in which debulking cannot take place, and therefore it is the tumor biology that actually has the impact on the survival of the patient. As mentioned above, this question will not be answered in a prospective, randomized manner due to the fact that it would be considered unethical not to attempt cytoreductive surgery. One study has addressed this issue in a retrospective fashion. It reported patients who required extensive surgery for cytoreduction and found that they did not have as good a rate of survival as those who did not require extensive operations to achieve optimal cytoreduction.[162] Investigators have also addressed the outcome if patients require bowel surgery, such as sigmoid or low anterior resections, in order to achieve optimal cytoreduction. Patients appear to achieve a survival benefit, even if bowel resections are required for cytoreduction.[163] A few retrospective studies have also addressed the benefit of tumor cytoreductive surgery in stage IV disease and have shown it to be of benefit.[164,165]

The spread patterns of epithelial ovarian cancer include transperitoneal, lymphatic, and hematogenous spread. Transperitoneal spread of the tumor is the most common form of spread, and the entire abdomen is at risk for tumor spread. Figure 18E-12A and B show the typical presentation of advanced-stage ovarian cancer. The typical finding in the abdomen of a woman with stage III or IV epithelial ovarian cancer is involvement of the omentum with a large tumor "cake," involvement of the peritoneal surfaces of the diaphragm, involvement of the surfaces of the small and large bowel, peritoneal involvement of the surfaces of the paracolic gutters, and dense involvement of the pelvis with tumor spreading directly from the ovaries. This pelvic disease will also commonly involve the rectosigmoid colon. The tumor tends to involve the peritoneal surfaces of intraabdominal organs and usually does not invade these structures; it tends to grow in a manner such that surgical debulking usually involves the removal of tumor from the surfaces of these organs. Exceptions to this may be the involvement of the rectosigmoid colon and intraparenchymal liver disease. The tumor usually does not involve the retroperitoneal surfaces, such as the ureter.

If, on physical examination, fixed disease is palpated in the posterior cul de sac and it is anticipated that a rectosigmoid resection will be a possibility, the patient is placed in the low lithotomy position, and pneumatic compression stockings are placed on the patient. If the abdomen is distended by ascites, a small incision is made near

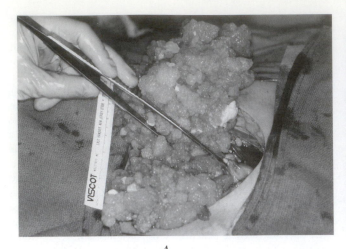

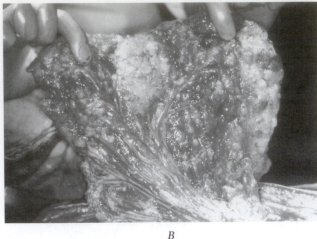

A                                                      B

**FIGURE 18E-12.** (*a*) The typical presentation of advanced-stage ovarian cancer. Pictured is the ovary. (*b*) Pictured is the omentum involved with tumor.

the umbilicus, the ascites drained and sent for cytology. Upon opening the abdomen, in order to plan the operation, the surgeon must make a thorough evaluation as to whether optimal debulking is feasible. The pelvic disease is usually amenable to debulking; however, a bowel resection may be required. It is usually possible to "clear" the tumor in the pelvis. The disease in the upper abdomen, therefore, determines the resectability of the tumor. Upper abdominal disease that will limit the extent of debulking includes the following: extensive disease on the diaphragmatic surfaces that is invasive into the muscle, extensive disease in the bowel mesentery, extensive intraparenchymal liver disease, celiac nodal metastases, and metastases to the porta hepatis. The patient's medical status must also be taken into account before performing an extensive surgical resection.

After a thorough assessment through a large vertical midline incision has been made, attention is directed to performing the tumor resection. The omentum is the second most common site of tumor involvement, and thus it is usually involved in advanced ovarian cancer. A frozen-section biopsy may also be sent at this point. The disease on the omentum is usually removed first in order to facilitate packing the bowel out of the pelvis to obtain exposure. In some cases, the omental cake can be removed from the transverse colon, and an infracolic omentectomy is performed. If the tumor involves the entire omentum, it is also removed from the stomach. When performing the omentectomy, care must be taken not to avulse tumor from the spleen because it is not uncommon for tumor to track up into the upper abdomen and involve the omentum in the left upper quadrant. It may be of benefit to remove as much of this omental tumor as possible. Patients may achieve symptomatic relief with its resection; therefore, regardless of whether the patient can be optimally debulked, it should be resected.

After the omentectomy is performed, attention is directed to the pelvis, and the bowel is packed away. Attention is first directed to securing the blood supply to the pelvic organs by ligating the infundibulopelvic ligaments (IP ligaments—the gonadal vessels) and

the uterine arteries. The round ligaments of the uterus are ligated, and the retroperitoneal space is first entered laterally to the IP ligaments and the external iliac vessels. The ureter is then identified; it lies on the medial leaf of the peritoneal incision. The IP ligaments are then secured at the pelvic brim. The uterine arteries are also secured after the paravesical and pararectal spaces are entered, and the ureter is dissected away from the pelvic peritoneum at the level of the uterine artery. Attention is then directed to dissecting the bladder away from the tumor and cervix. The tumor is then swept medially, and attention is directed to removing the ovaries, uterus, and cervix. If the cul de sac is filled with tumor, a retrograde hysterectomy may be performed in order to dissect the tumor away from the colon. In this technique, the ureters are dissected out of the parametria of the uterus, mobilized, and retracted laterally. The bladder is dissected off the lower uterus and cervix, and the vagina is then entered anteriorly. This incision is carried to the posterior aspect of the vagina in a circumferential fashion, and the uterus, cervix, ovaries, and tumor are removed without entering the posterior cul de sac. The cardinal and uterosacral ligaments are clamped in a retrograde fashion, similar to that in a vaginal hysterectomy. If the tumor invades the rectal wall, the rectum may be removed with the specimen. Bowel resections potentially requiring a colostomy should only be undertaken if (1) the patient can be optimally debulked, or (2) for palliative purposes, if the patient has an impending obstruction. The majority of the time, the rectum can be anastomosed with a transanal stapling device, but a patient should always be counseled preoperatively that a colostomy may be necessary. Rectosigmoid resection in the setting of tumor cytoreduction is associated with major morbidity in about 25% of cases, with the most common major complications being infection in about 13% of cases.[166]

Resection of other intraabdominal disease can then be undertaken. Many times, as mentioned above, the tumor only involves the surface of organs, and thus an attempt can be made to remove tumor from the surfaces. It may, however, be necessary to remove intraabdominal organs in order to remove tumor. A general rule is that an organ or resection should not be performed unless it has the potential to render the patient optimal at the end of the procedure. Other sites of tumor include the spleen, liver, diaphragmatic surfaces, and small and large intestine.

Splenectomy is commonly performed in order to achieve optimal cytoreduction. Small-volume intraparenchymal liver metastases may be resected if they render the patient optimal at the end of the procedure, as well as small and large bowel resections. Many times, diaphragmatic disease may be resected with proper exposure. Diffuse miliary disease may require "diaphragmatic stripping of the peritoneum." This may require mobilizing the liver by transecting the falciform, triangular, and coronary ligaments as necessary. The dissection starts laterally at the costal margin and extends medially and posteriorly to where the anterior leaf of the coronary ligament and the right triangular ligament reflect onto the anterior surface of the liver. If the tumor has not penetrated throughout the diaphragm, it will usually strip quite easily from this area. In this dissection, care must be taken to clip perforating vessels from the branches of the inferior phrenic vessels. The integrity of the diaphragm should be checked after this procedure. Other methods to address with this disease include using the Cavitron Ultrasonic Suction Aspirator (CUSA) and the argon beam coagulator. Transdiaphragmatic involvement of the pleura will limit the resectability of extensive disease; however, limited resections of penetrating lesions may be performed.

Other sites that may be involved with tumor include retroperitoneal lymph nodes. Approximately 75% of women with bulky intraabdominal disease will have nodal involvement.[167] If bulky lymph nodes are encountered, they should be removed if possible. Nodal areas that may be involved with tumor include the obturator, hypogastric, external iliac, common iliac, and the para-aortic areas. The infrahilar high para-aortic lymph nodes have potential for involvement, but the suprahilar nodal area may also be involved, and these areas should be thoroughly inspected. Many times it is the case that this is feasible; however, these nodes may be densely adherent to the wall of the vessels, limiting the ability to resect them. Occasionally, it may be necessary to resect a portion of a vein or an artery. The benefit achieved by complete lymphadenectomy at the time of surgical cytoreduction remains controversial. It has been argued by some that a complete lymphadenectomy can improve the prognosis of women with advanced-stage cancers, and thus they advocate the use of complete pelvic and para-aortic lymphadenectomy at the time of cytoreduction. A complete systematic lymphadenectomy for ovarian cancer should include the periaortic nodes (from above the origin of the inferior mesenteric artery (IMA) to the insertion of the gonadal vessels into the vena cava and the left renal vein); the common, external, and internal iliac arteries and veins should be skeletonized and the nodes removed. The inferior boundary for this dissection is the crossing of the circumflex iliac vein over the external iliac artery. Nodes are also removed from the obturator and presacral spaces after identification of the obturator and the sciatic nerves. One case-control study, in which women were divided into two groups based on the performance of a systematic lymphadenectomy at the time of cytoreductive surgery, demonstrated that in the group in which the lymphadenectomy was performed, a survival advantage was achieved

in patients who were optimally cytoreduced.[168] In a retrospective study, women who underwent a lymphadenectomy achieved a better survival rate than those who did not.[167] Other studies have also demonstrated similar findings.[169,170] It is, however, not standard in the United States to perform a systematic lymphadenectomy in women with advanced ovarian cancer, and the issue of whether this significantly impacts survival requires a prospective, randomized study.

Numerous studies have reported on the morbidity of cytoreductive surgery; however, they are of limited value. Each operative procedure is based on the tumor that the patient presents with, and therefore the radicalness of each cytoreductive procedure will vary; approximately 25% of all patients undergoing cytoreductive surgery will experience complications other than prolonged ileus, the most common being wound infection.

## PRIMARY CHEMOTHERAPY

Surgery is rarely curative for advanced-stage ovarian cancer. For selected patients with early ovarian cancer, there appears to be no benefit to adjuvant chemotherapy. In a Gynecologic Oncology Group (GOG) trial, patients with favorable prognostic criteria were randomized to receive either oral melphalan (0.2 mg/kg daily for 5 days; repeat cycles every 4 to 6 weeks for 12 courses or 18 months of therapy, whichever came first) or no chemotherapy.[171] Favorable prognostic criteria were defined as stage IA or IB disease, grade 1 or 2 tumors. Unfavorable prognostic criteria were defined as stage IA or IB, grade 3 tumors, tumor on the external surface of the ovary, ruptured capsule, ascites or positive washings, and all stage II tumors. After a complete staging laparotomy was performed, 81 patients were available for comparison. The 5-year disease-free survival rates for the two groups of favorable-prognosis patients were 91% in the untreated group and 98% in the treated group. In the group of 812 patients, there was one death due to aplastic anemia. Based on this study, for patients with early-stage ovarian cancers and good-prognosis factors, the overall survival rate is greater than 90%, and these patients can be spared treatment with cytotoxic chemotherapy.

Numerous regimens have been utilized in the treatment of ovarian cancer; however, the two most active agents against this tumor are platinum and paclitaxel (Taxol). In a study published in 1986, platinum was demonstrated to be a superior agent in the treatment of epithelial ovarian cancer.[172] This GOG study compared a regimen consisting of platinum doxorubicin (Adriamycin) and cyclophosphamide (Cytoxan) (PAC) to one containing Adriamycin and Cytoxan alone, and found a response rate of 51% in the platinum-containing regimen, compared with 26% in the two-drug regimen. This study, along with two others,[159,173] laid the foundation for treating patients with epithelial ovarian cancer with a platinum-based regimen. After these initial studies, PAC became the standard of treatment for epithelial ovarian cancer. Next, the role of Adriamycin was studied and was demonstrated to be expendable. In a randomized study, the GOG compared PAC to platinum and Cytoxan in 349 patients with advanced-stage disease.[174] This study demonstrated similar response rates and overall survival rates. However, a large

Italian clinical trial has demonstrated a higher complete remission rate for the PAC regimen.[158] In a meta-analysis of these studies and two others, it appears that there may be a 5% to 7% survival rate at 2 years and at 6 years.[175] These studies are limited, however, due to the fact that in some of these regimens the dose of cisplatin was not increased in the two-drug regimen, as it was in the GOG study.

Cisplatin is the drug most thoroughly evaluated in the treatment of ovarian cancer. It is thought that the primary action of cisplatin is its binding to DNA and the production of intrastructural cross-links and formation of DNA adducts.[176] These cross-links affect DNA replication by inducing changes in conformation. Potential side effects of cisplatin administration include anaphylactic reactions, delayed nausea and vomiting; dose-limiting nephrotoxicity, ototoxicity, and neurotoxicity may occur. Adequate hydration and mannitol diuresis are important in order to prevent nephrotoxicity and ototoxicity. Carboplatin is the second platinum compound that is utilized in the treatment of ovarian cancer. The toxicities of this drug differ significantly from those of cisplatin. This drug demonstrates little nephrotoxicity, but its dose-limiting toxicity is myelosuppression with thrombocytopenia and leukopenia. Aggressive hydration is not required for this medication, and thus it is well suited for outpatient treatments. In a long-term study of previously untreated patients with advanced ovarian cancer, there was no statistically significant difference in patients treated with cisplatin compared with those treated with carboplatin.[177]

Generally, patients are treated with 6 cycles of a platinum-containing regimen. In a prospective study comparing 5 cycles versus 10 cycles, or 6 versus 12 cycles, of treatment with PAC in patients with stage III and IV disease, the survival rate was not improved in patients treated with the prolonged regimens.[178,179] Prior to the demonstrated effectiveness of platinum, the standard postoperative treatment for epithelial ovarian cancer consisted of either cisplatin (75 mg/m²) or carboplatin (350 mg/m², or dosed to an AUC of 6–7 combined with cyclophosphamide (750 mg/m² when combined with cisplatin, and 600 mg/m² when combined with carboplatin).

Combination chemotherapy that includes a platinum compound and paclitaxel is now the standard primary treatment for ovarian cancer. Paclitaxel was first isolated from a crude extract of the bark of the Pacific yew, *Taxus brevifolia*, and was first reported to have significant activity in ovarian cancer in 1989.[180] Paclitaxel is a member of a class of drugs called taxanes. These drugs exert their effects by binding to the microtubules of the cells. This results in the stabilization of the structure and shifts the equilibrium to microtubule assembly, so that the cell is arrested at G2/M. Side effects of paclitaxel include hypersensitivity reactions, and patients should be premedicated with steroids, diphenhydramine, and cimetidine. These reactions may be severe and occur within 10 minutes of drug infusion. Myelosuppression (primarily neutropenia) is the major dose-limiting toxicity. Neurotoxicity, primarily peripheral neuropathy, is the second most common dose-limiting toxicity.

The GOG performed the prospective, randomized study that has established paclitaxel as a component in first-line therapy of epithelial ovarian cancer.[181,182] In this study, 385 patients with suboptimal stage III or IV disease were randomized to be treated with cyclophosphamide and cisplatin versus paclitaxel (135 mg/m², 24-hr infusion) and cisplatin (75 mg/m²). In this study there was an

**TABLE 18E-9. STANDARD INTRAVENOUS CHEMOTHERAPY REGIMENS IN THE TREATMENT OF EPITHELIAL OVARIAN CANCER AFTER INITIAL LAPAROTOMY FOR THE DISEASE**

| | |
|---|---|
| Cisplatin | 75–100 mg/m² |
| Taxol | 135–175 mg/m² |
| | |
| Carboplatin | AUC of 7.5 |
| Taxol | 135–175 mg/m² |

improvement in the median survival of 1 year in the group treated with the paclitaxel combination: 37.5 months in the paclitaxel group, compared with 24 months in the Cytoxan-treated group. The clinical response rate was 67% for the Cytoxan group, compared with 77% for the paclitaxel group. Subsequent studies have demonstrated the safety and efficacy of a 3-hour infusion of paclitaxel, at a higher dose of 175 mg/m², combined with carboplatin, dosed to an AUC of 7.5.[183,184] This regimen was based on a European-Canadian trial that demonstrated the safety of the 3-hr infusion, with decreased neutropenia and an increase in time to progression in the 3-hr infusion group. In this trial, a complete response rate of 67% was observed with the 3-hr paclitaxel infusion.[98] Table 18E-9 outlines standard chemotherapy regimens for the treatment of advanced-stage epithelial ovarian cancer.

Most recently, a large cooperative group has demonstrated a possible survival benefit to women who are optimally cytoreduced and treated with intraperitoneal chemotherapy.[185] In this study, 539 patients with advanced-stage disease who were optimally cytoreduced were randomized to receive either IP or IV cisplatin at 100 mg/m² along with Cytoxan at 600 mg/m² IV. The estimated median survival was superior at 49 months in the IP group versus 41 months in the IV group ($p < 0.05$). No clinical trials have been published to date comparing IP platinum in combination with paclitaxel to the standard regimens of IV platinum and IV paclitaxel.

Future investigations in the treatment of epithelial ovarial cancer with platinum and paclitaxel-based regimens include the following: clinical trials evaluating the dose, schedule, and duration of therapy of paclitaxel-based regimens; comparisons of cisplatin and paclitaxel with carboplatin and paclitaxel; appropriate dose intensity of these regimens; and the role of IP therapy combined with paclitaxel.

## SECOND-LOOK SURGERY

Second-look surgery refers to the reassessment of an individual with ovarian cancer who is in a complete clinical remission and who has had a staging laparotomy and has completed first-line chemotherapy. This procedure is performed because up to 50% of women in a complete clinical remission, as determined by CA-125 level, physical examination, and CT scan, will have disease detectable by surgical evaluation only. This reevaluation allows one to determine which patients (1) need further treatment, (2) require observation only, and (3) may be eligible for consolidation chemotherapy. In addition, this second reassessment allows the surgeon to determine a patient's response to the initial chemotherapy and to perform additional tumor debulking. Second-look surgery should not be performed on women who will not undergo further therapy based on the results of the surgery. There has been much debate surrounding the use of second-look surgical reassessment. At present, there has been no study to demonstrate a survival benefit associated with the procedure, and it has lost favor in the community. Recent studies suggest, however, that patients treated with consolidation chemotherapy after a negative second look may have a better survival rate than those who do not undergo further treatment. The procedure also offers the surgeon a second opportunity at cytoreduction if the patient is responding to chemotherapy. Thus, some institutions actively pursue this course of management for ovarian cancer patients.

### OUTLINE OF THE SURGICAL PROCEDURE.

A thorough second-look procedure should be done by a surgeon experienced in the management of epithelial ovarian cancer. This procedure will typically yield 20 to 30 pathologic specimens. Laparotomy has been the traditional method used to reassess a patient's status; however, laparoscopy may also be utilized. Regardless of the method of reassessment, the principles of the procedure remain the same. A pelvic examination under anesthesia is initially performed. If a laparotomy is performed, a generous vertical incision should be utilized so that entrance to the upper abdomen may be gained. If tumor is initially obvious, a frozen-section diagnosis should be obtained. Surgical debulking of persistent disease is also attempted, in order to enhance the response to salvage chemotherapy.

If no tumor is identified at the time of surgery, a systematic exploration of the peritoneal cavity and retroperitoneal spaces must be pursued. Saline washings are obtained from the pelvis, right and left paracolic gutters, and left and right hemidiaphragms. The residual omentum should be closely examined and removed. The small bowel should be run, and special attention paid to small implants on the peritoneal surfaces of the intestine and its mesentery. The remainder of the infundibulopelvic ligaments should be re-excised and sent for permanent section. The operative note from the initial surgery should be carefully reviewed prior to surgery so that special attention can be paid to areas of residual tumor remaining at the end of the initial surgery. Adhesions must be carefully lysed, and multiple biopsies should be sent from these areas. Multiple peritoneal biopsies should also be taken in the anterior and posterior cul de sacs, the left and right pericolic gutters, and the left and right hemidiaphragms. Any residual omentum should be excised, along with the uterus and adnexal structures (if they remained at the end of the initial surgery). If the pelvic and para-aortic lymph nodes were not sampled at the initial laparotomy, this should be done at the time of the second-look reassessment. If there was disease present in the lymph nodes at the initial surgery, careful attention should be paid to these areas at the time of this surgery.

One study has evaluated the use of laparoscopy in second-look surgery[186] and found it to be feasible. This study consisted of 31 patients who underwent a laparoscopy, 70 patients who underwent a laparotomy, and 8 patients who underwent both procedures. At a median follow-up time of 22 months, recurrences were noted in 14% of both groups.

### PATIENT SELECTION FOR SECOND-LOOK SURGERY.

The first criterion for the patient to be eligible for second-look evaluation is that she be willing to undergo further treatment based on the surgical findings. If a woman will not undergo further treatment based on the findings, the surgical-pathologic results have no implications for patient management. Individuals who are considered eligible to undergo second-look evaluation usually have been diagnosed with advanced-stage disease; women with comprehensively staged stage I disease will have a low yield of positive findings. Ninety-five percent of these women will have a negative second-look evaluation.[187] However, women who have been diagnosed with clinical stage I disease and who have undergone first-line treatment but have not undergone comprehensive surgical staging are eligible. These individuals will have disease found approximately 20% of the time.[187] To be eligible for second-look reassessment, a woman must also have a normal CA-125 and CT scan. Virtually all women with an elevated CA-125 will have persistent disease at the time of surgery.[188] Surgery will document disease in approximately 50% of women with a normal CA-125.[188–190] Patients with negative imaging by a CT scan will also not necessarily be without evidence of disease at the time of surgery; CT scanning cannot detect disease less than 1 to 2 cm.[191,192] Newer methods of disease evaluation include positron emission scanning (PET); however, there are no data currently available to evaluate its sensitivity.

### SECOND-LOOK SURGICAL FINDINGS.

Surgical reexploration will reveal tumor in about 55% of advanced-stage patients.[193] This will be microscopic disease about 30% of the time.[194] The two most important variables related to second-look findings include tumor stage and amount of residual disease at the initial laparotomy. Table 18E-10 demonstrates the findings based on initial stage of disease. Patients who have only microscopic disease at the end of their initial surgery will have a negative second look 76% of the time, patients who were optimally debulked will have a negative second look 46% of the time, and patients who were suboptimally debulked will have a negative second look 23% of the time[193] (Table 18E-11).

Due to the fact that 95% of comprehensively staged stage I patients will have a negative second look, these patients are not

**TABLE 18E-10.** FINDINGS AT THE TIME OF SECOND-LOOK SURGICAL REASSESSMENT BASED ON THE INITIAL SURGICAL STAGE

| STAGE | % NEGATIVE |
| --- | --- |
| Comprehensively staged, stage I | 95 |
| I | 82 |
| II | 71 |
| III | 33.6 |
| IV | 32.8 |

SOURCE: Modified from Ozols RF: Epithelial ovarian cancer. In: Hoskins WJ, Perez CA, Young RC (eds). *Principles and Practice of Gynecologic Oncology*, 1st ed. Philadelphia, JB Lippincott Co., 1992, p 760.

**TABLE 18E-11.** FINDINGS AT THE TIME OF SECOND-LOOK SURGICAL REASSESSMENT BASED ON THE RESIDUAL DISEASE AT THE COMPLETION OF INITIAL LAPAROTOMY

| RESIDUAL | % NEGATIVE |
| --- | --- |
| None | 72 |
| Optimal | 50 |
| Suboptimal | 23 |

SOURCE: Modified from Ozols RF. Epithelial ovarian cancer. In: Howkins WJ, Perez CA, Young RC (eds). *Principles and Practice of Gynecologic Oncology*, 2nd ed. Philadelphia, Lippincott-Raven Publishers, 1997, p 960.

routinely recommended to undergo the procedure. However, patients who were inadequately staged at their initial laparotomy will have positive findings approximately 20% of the time; therefore, if these patients are not restaged immediately before adjuvant chemotherapy treatment, they should undergo a second-look procedure.

Patients with a negative second-look assessment will have a much better prognosis.[195] Podratz and his colleagues[196] reported an 83% 5-year survival rate for patients with no tumor at second-look surgery, compared to a 43% 5-year survival rate for those patients with microscopic disease. Patients in this series with gross residual disease had the worse prognosis, with 5-year survival of less than 30%. One group has reported that 80% of patients will die from their disease within 3 years if gross residual disease is found. Actuarial survival rates have been reported to be 96% for 2 years and 71% at 5 years in a group of patients with either microscopic or no residual disease.[197]

Despite negative second-look surgical findings, patients with advanced-stage disease remain at significant risk for relapse. Patients with stage II, III, or IV disease will have relapse rates of 50%.[198] The mean time to recurrence is 24 months. This recurrence rate is also dependent on the amount of tumor remaining at the end of the initial laparotomy. Patients with small-volume disease have a relapse rate of 32%, compared to 61% in patients with large-volume residual disease.

**SECONDARY SURGICAL DEBULKING.** Second-look surgery is primarily a diagnostic procedure, but it may confer a therapeutic benefit when significant tumor debulking is achieved. It is calculated that approximately 40% of patients undergoing a second-look operation will be eligible for debulking, and the procedure is technically feasible in up to 80% of cases. However, the benefit of cytoreduction at the time of second-look surgery remains controversial. Many studies have demonstrated no benefit to surgical cytoreduction at the time of second-look surgery; however, other studies have demonstrated a survival benefit to secondary surgical debulking at the time of second-look surgery.[199–201] In one study, patients who were cytoreduced to microscopic disease had a 5-year survival rate of 51%, which was similar to that of patients who were found to have microscopic disease at the time of second look, and significantly better than that of women left with gross residual disease (who had a 5-year survival rate of 14%).[199] Another study has

also demonstrated a very similar result.[200] In this study, patients whose disease was rendered microscopic at second look had a 5-year survival rate of 51%, compared to 62% in a group of patients who were found to have microscopic disease. In patients with gross residual disease, the 5-year survival rate was less than 10%. The data must be analyzed in reference to those patients who are responsive to chemotherapy; intuitively, however, these would be the patients who would benefit from further surgical cytoreduction. This appears to be the case; in a study of 33 patients who were nonresponders to chemotherapy, it was demonstrated that such patients fare poorly regardless of whether secondary surgical debulking is possible or not, and the authors concluded that it is of little benefit in patients whose tumors are not chemosensitive.[202] At present, there is no proven, highly effective drug for second-line therapy, and thus, this is the case.

**MANAGEMENT OF PATIENTS BASED ON SECOND-LOOK FINDINGS.** Figure 18E-13 outlines possible treatment options after second-look surgery. In the subset of patients with negative findings, these patients may be observed, but 50% of advanced-stage patients will ultimately have a recurrence. Thus, the concept of consolidation chemotherapy has been applied to ovarian cancer. Studies have evaluated IP P32, IV, and IP chemotherapy as consolidation treatments. Preliminary results suggest that IP platinum may decrease recurrences and prolong the disease-free interval. One group has reported a 5-year survival rate of 80% in patients who had an additional three courses of IP cisplatin.[203] In a study comparing 40 patients with negative second look undergoing treatment with IP cisplatin (110 mg/m$^2$) and etoposide (200 mg/m$^2$) to those who underwent observation only after surgery, the treated group had a recurrence rate of 39%, compared to 54% in the observation group.[204] The median disease-free survival time was 28.5 months in the observation group, and was not reached in the treatment group.

For patients with gross residual disease that has responded to chemotherapy, an attempt should be made at cytoreduction of the tumor. These patients should be offered salvage chemotherapy, and, optimally, most will participate in research protocols. Patients who have had a dramatic response to their initial systemic chemotherapy can be continued on this regimen. Patients with small-volume disease may be treated with IP chemotherapy.[205] IP P32 and whole abdominal radiation (WAR) do not appear to be as safe or effective as chemotherapy.[203,206–208]

## FOLLOW-UP AFTER PRIMARY TREATMENT

Patients who recur after second-look surgery will usually do so within 2 years of the procedure. After a patient has stopped treatment, she should be examined at 3-month intervals for 2 years. This should consist of a complete physical examination, with pelvic examination and a measure of CA-125 level. The symptoms of recurrent disease are similar to the initial presentation of ovarian cancer, and any rise in the CA-125 should be considered recurrent disease until proven otherwise. If the patient has either one of the two, she should undergo a CT scan of the abdomen and pelvis. Generally, disease will not be detected on a CT scan until the CA-125 is greater than

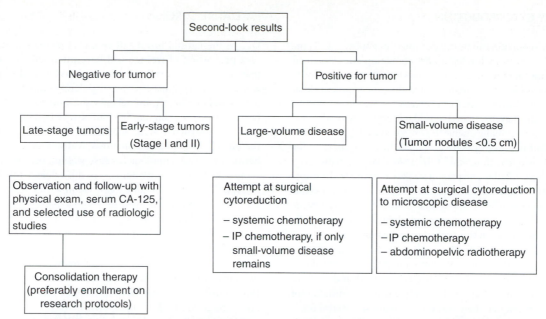

**FIGURE 18E-13.** Treatment options based on second-look surgery findings. Used with permission from Poyner EA, Hoskins WJ. The role of second-look surgery in the management of epithelial ovarian cancer. Contemp Oncol 1995. [Special Report on Ovarian Cancer: State of the Art Diagnosis and Management, JR Lurain (ed.)]

100 units/dL. If the CA-125 is elevated and there is no disease on CT scan, consideration should be given to performing a laparoscopy to evaluate disease status. Women should also have a Pap smear every year, along with a mammogram. After 2 years, the patient is examined at 6-month intervals. Further treatment options for patients with recurrent disease will depend on the disease-free interval and response to platinum-based chemotherapy. Patients who have a greater than 1-year disease-free interval may benefit from additional cytoreductive surgery and reinduction chemotherapy.[209,210] Patients who recur more than 6 months after treatment with platinum-based therapy should also be retreated with one of these agents.

## SALVAGE CHEMOTHERAPY

Salvage chemotherapy refers to that which is given to patients who develop recurrent disease or to patients who have persistent disease at the end of their initial surgery. Because ovarian cancer is a chemosensitive tumor, a variety of agents have been utilized to treat patients in the salvage setting. The choice of agents is guided by the disease-free interval and prior response to platinum-based regimens.

Women who recur more than 6 months after treatment with cisplatin should be treated with carboplatin in this situation because this will produce a response rate of approximately 30%.[211,212] In this situation, carboplatin is chosen due to its better toxicity profile. Patients who recur more than 6 months after treatment with carboplatin can be treated with carboplatin or cisplatin.[213] Patients who

are resistant to a platinum-paclitaxel regimen should undergo treatment with nonplatinum compounds. IP paclitaxel has also been applied in the salvage situation, after prior treatment with IV paclitaxel.

Patients with recurrent disease who are asymptomatic may be good candidates to use hormonal agents as treatment. Response rates of 15% have been reported with the use of progestational agents[214] and of up to 18% with tamoxifen.[215,216] These agents provide a good alternative to cytotoxic chemotherapy in patients who are asymptomatic or in patients who cannot tolerate the side effects of cytotoxic chemotherapy.

Newer agents that are being utilized in the salvage setting for epithelial ovarian cancer include topotecan, gemcitabine, and liposomal doxorubicin. Topotecan is an analogue of camptothecin and is a topoisomerase I inhibitor. Response rates of 12% have been reported in platinum-resistant patients, and 20% in platinum-sensitive patients.[217] Major toxicities are hematologic, with a grade 4 neutropenia occurring in 82% of these patients at a dose of 1.5 mg/m$^2$ per day for 5 consecutive days. Gemcitabine is a pyrimidine antimetabolite with a structure that closely resembles cytosine arabinoside. The drug is generally given in doses of 800 mg/m$^2$ once a week for 3 weeks, with 1 week of rest. Patients with platinum-resistant disease have an approximately 20% response rate to this drug.[218] Major toxicities include leukopenia and thrombocytopenia. Due to the differences in mechanism of actions and toxicity profiles, gemcitabine has also been combined with cisplatin and found to be synergistic.[219] Liposomal doxorubicin has also been recently employed in the treatment of recurrent-persistent ovarian cancer, and response rates of up to 26% have been reported.[220]

## SECONDARY CYTOREDUCTION

Secondary cytoreduction can be divided into three subtypes: (1) interval cytoreduction, which refers to cytoreduction after a defined course of chemotherapy in a patient in whom initial cytoreduction was not possible; (2) cytoreduction at the time of second-look surgery; and (3) cytoreduction for recurrent disease.

Multiple studies have evaluated secondary surgical cytoreduction in women who were initially unable to be cytoreduced. These studies have proved that the surgery is feasible, and thus reexploration for this indication is not without merit. In a summary of eight series from the literature, totaling 286 patients, 56% were rendered optimal by various criteria, and more recent studies have demonstrated this to be the case in 60% to 80% of the time. Thus, the surgery is technically feasible, but the question remains whether women actually gain a survival benefit from this type of management. In a prospective study of 22 patients with advanced-stage ovarian cancer, one group of patients underwent treatment with chemotherapy after a laparotomy in which biopsy only had been performed, and a second group underwent surgical cytoreduction prior to the initiation of chemotherapy.[221] Overall, there was no difference in survival times between the two groups, and those who had interval optimal surgical cytoreduction demonstrated a survival benefit. A Danish group has demonstrated a similar finding.[222] When compared to initial cytoreduction, women who underwent interval optimal cytoreduction demonstrated a similar 50% 3-year survival. A large prospective, randomized trial has demonstrated the effectiveness of this strategy.[223] In this study, patients who were suboptimally debulked at the time of initial laparotomy were treated with three cycles of cisplatin and Cytoxan. Patients who were not progressing on therapy were subsequently randomized to undergo interval debulking or further treatment with chemotherapy. There were 150 patients in each arm. Patients who underwent interval surgical debulking demonstrated a significant improvement in median survival and disease-free interval compared to those patients who did not undergo interval cytoreduction. A second endpoint of quality of life has been suggested as measuring the benefit of interval, and other forms of secondary surgical debulkings. Quality of life has been studied after initial surgical debulking.[224] In a study of 34 patients, 19 optimally debulked and 15 suboptimally debulked, women who underwent optimal surgical cytoreduction were more likely to enjoy a better quality of life. Eighty-two percent of the women who underwent optimal surgical debulking could continue normal activities, compared to only 46% of the suboptimally debulked patients. The second scenario has been discussed under the second-look surgery section.

The third scenario in which secondary cytoreduction is employed involves the patient who has recurrent disease but who has had a significant disease-free interval from the time of initial treatment. Among patients who are reexplored for recurrent or persistent disease, those who are able to be cytoreduced to optimal disease have a significant improvement in median survival compared to those who were unable to be cytoreduced.[225] One study, reported on in the form of an abstract, prospectively randomized patients into debulking or no debulking.[226] A significant survival advantage was found in the debulking group. Surgery for recurrent disease is usually reserved for individuals who are responsive to chemotherapy, defined as a complete response to initial therapy and a disease-free interval of greater than 12 months.

## PALLIATIVE SURGERY

Due to the natural history of epithelial ovarian cancer, a significant proportion of women will have intestinal tract involvement that arises from obstructive complications late in the disease. These women are usually at a relatively high level of functioning when this occurs and may be in minimal pain; thus, surgical intervention may be warranted. Women may have an obstruction based on a discrete mass, or obstructive symptoms based on a global dysfunction of the intestine due to carcinomatosis. A distinction should be made between the two situations because women who have obstructive symptoms based on carcinomatosis will achieve little benefit from a surgical intervention, and a gastrostomy tube may be placed for symptomatic relief. For those in whom a discrete point of obstruction exists, palliation may be gained from a bypass procedure. Other options for these patients include intravenous hydration and gastric decompression.

When considering a surgical intervention in an advanced-stage ovarian cancer patient, general medical status, future treatment options, and patient desires should be kept in mind. The patient should always be given a trial of conservative management. Total parenteral nutrition may be started in order to prepare patients for surgery; it should not be used in a patient for whom no surgical intervention is planned. The site of obstruction is most commonly the small bowel. In a report on 54 patients undergoing a palliative operative procedure for advanced-stage ovarian cancer, the small bowel was the site of obstruction 44% of the time, the large bowel was obstructed 33% of the time, and both were involved 22% of the time.[227] It was possible to perform a definitive procedure for relief of obstruction 70% of the time. Of those patients, 80% were discharged from the hospital with intestinal function, and the mean postsurgical survival time was 6.8 months. Thus, these patients should be offered a palliative procedure because it may improve the quality of their remaining months of life.

Some studies have attempted to determine which patients will benefit most from such a procedure. One group has identified factors such as advanced age, poor nutritional status, and presence of palpable tumor masses[228−230] as predictors of rate of success of surgery and survival. Other studies have found no preoperative predictors of operability or survival postoperatively.[227] Therefore, it seems reasonable to offer intestinal surgery for women who are in appropriate medical condition to tolerate the procedure.

The other condition that may be a chronic problem for advanced-stage patients is ascites. In the absence of a response to a chemotherapeutic agent, there is little that can be done for this condition. Intermittent removal of the ascites will provide temporary relief, but it will always reaccumulate when the patient is not being treated or is not responding to treatment. The experience with peritoneal-venous shunts has been poor in this situation[231,232] and they are not generally utilized.

## RADIATION THERAPY

The role of radiation therapy in the treatment of ovarian cancer is primarily in the palliative situation. Radiation therapy for the treatment of ovarian cancer must encompass the entire abdominal cavity. This may be accomplished by the moving-strip technique and the open-field technique. Today, the latter form is the most commonly employed. Whole abdominal radiation therapy (WAR) is reserved for patients with small-volume disease (<2 cm largest residual). Treatment with radiation therapy for patients whose disease is optimally debulked to less than 2 cm results in a survival rate of 30% to 35%, compared to 35% in platinum-based therapy.[233,234] The standard adjuvant treatment for ovarian cancer remains chemotherapy; however, radiation therapy may be effective in treating small-volume disease. Some investigators have advocated its use in combination with chemotherapy.[235] Others have proposed WAR in the treatment of microscopic disease remaining after treatment with chemotherapy.[236,237]

Radiation in the palliative setting for ovarian cancer is probably underutilized, but may be very successful in patients who have one area of disease that may be encompassed in a radiation field. The most common situation in which this arises is a pelvic mass causing bowel or bladder symptoms, or bleeding. Radiation may also be employed for isolated retroperitoneal nodal areas. Investigators have reported a response rate of up to 71% in a palliative setting.[238] Other studies have reported similar response rates,[239,240] with median survivals of 19.5 months after palliative radiation therapy.

## INTRAPERITONEAL CHEMOTHERAPY

The theoretical advantage to drugs delivered directly to the surface of the tumor is that the tumor will be exposed to higher concentrations of the drugs for more prolonged periods of time. Table 18E-12 shows drugs that are commonly employed in the intraperitoneal treatment of epithelial ovarian cancer. This treatment has been applied in the initial treatment of ovarian cancer, salvage, and consolidation treatments. Its role continues to be investigated. The prerequisites for the treatment of a patient with intraperitoneal therapy are that the patient has small-volume disease, less than 1 cm residual, and that there are no adhesions limiting the distribution of the drug throughout the abdominal cavity. One study has addressed the topic of whether retroperitoneal nodal disease is a contraindication to IP therapy, and this does not appear to be the case.[241]

IP therapy is delivered via an implantable, permanent port-a-catheter device. This can be placed at the time of initial debulking surgery or during second-look surgery. In a review of 249 catheters placed in ovarian cancer patients, 17% of patients had major catheter complications. These included catheter blockage (9%), infection (8.8%), and catheter erosion into the bowel in eight patients.[242] In order to decrease the risk of erosion and infection, it has been recommended that the catheter not be placed at the time of bowel surgery. Since a higher proportion of catheters are now being placed at the time of laparoscopy instead of laparotomy, the complication rate may be reduced.

## SPECIAL CONSIDERATIONS

**REPRODUCTIVE CONSERVATION.** It is now acceptable to manage the woman who desires future childbearing and who has an early-stage cancer with conservative surgery consisting of an

**TABLE 18E-12.** DRUGS COMMONLY EMPLOYED IN THE INTRAPERITONEAL TREATMENT OF EPITHELIAL OVARIAN CANCER AND THEIR ASSOCIATED PHARMACOKINETIC ADVANTAGE (EXPRESSED AS PEAK PERITONEAL CAVITY CONCENTRATION/PEAK PLASMA CONCENTRATION)

| DRUG | PHARMACOKINETIC ADVANTAGE |
|------|---------------------------|
| Cisplatin | 20 |
| Carboplatin | 18 |
| Melphalan | 93 |
| Mitoxantrone | 620 |
| Doxorubicin | 474 |
| 5-FU | 298 |
| Mitomycin | 71 |

SOURCE: Modified from Markman, M. Intraperitoneal chemotherapy, In Rubin SC, Sutton GP (eds). *Ovarian Cancer.* New York: McGraw-Hill 1993, p 325.

oophorectomy and a staging procedure. Survival does not appear to be compromised in this situation.[243,244] It is not recommended that the contralateral ovary be biopsied if it appears normal, due to the possible risk of adhesions and resulting infertility and ovarian failure. The risk of disease in a contralateral ovary of normal appearance is quite low. These patients may require adjuvant chemotherapy, and pregnancies have been reported after this form of management.[245] These patients may be placed on oral contraceptives postoperatively until childbearing is desired. However, there are no data regarding the use of oral contraceptives in this patient population diagnosed with ovarian cancer. The retained ovary should also be followed with ultrasound imaging on a periodic basis. In patients with advanced-stage tumors, surgical treatment should consist of a hysterectomy and bilateral salpingo-oophoretomy.

**THE INADEQUATELY STAGED OVARIAN CANCER PATIENT.** It is not unusual for a patient to be operated on in a community where a staging procedure is not completed. For patients with well-differentiated tumors who apparently have early-stage disease, it is important that they undergo a staging laparotomy. Approximately 30% of the time, more advanced-stage disease will be found, which will require further treatment with chemotherapy. If the staging laparotomy confirms stage IA or IB disease, these patients will not need any further treatment. In the apparent early-stage patient with poor-prognosis features, such as high-grade tumors or stage IC or II disease, further treatment with chemotherapy will be required. The question thus becomes whether to perform a staging laparotomy immediately or after treatment with chemotherapy. A CT scan should be obtained, and if there is any evidence of bulky disease in the nodal areas or upper abdomen, immediate surgery should be performed. In a small percentage of cases, immediate surgery may be necessary, even in the setting of a normal CT scan, because bulky intraabdominal or retroperitoneal disease may be missed on a CT scan.

## BORDERLINE TUMORS

The first report on a borderline tumor of the ovary occurred in 1929, when Taylor[246] reported on an epithelial tumor of the ovary that had the histologic features of an ovarian cancer but behaved in a benign fashion. In 1961, the borderline tumor was recognized as an entity, and the World Health Organization created a category for these tumors, "carcinoma of low malignant potential."[246] These tumors possess the cytology of a malignant cell, including nuclear atypia and mitoses along with epithelial hyperplasia and stratification; however, the tumor demonstrates no invasion into the ovarian stroma. These tumors may metastasize, but they grow in an indolent fashion. Borderline tumors may occur in any histopathologic subtype; however, the serous and mucinous histopathologic subtypes are the most common. The distinction between borderline tumors of the ovary and well-differentiated invasive carcinoma may be a difficult one to make, and therefore, a consultation with a pathologist skilled in the differential diagnoses of epithelial ovarian tumors is often required. It is generally accepted by most clinicians that these tumors do not represent a transition from benign to malignant neoplasms, but instead are thought to represent a unique disease entity. This is demonstrated by the fact that they rarely recur as invasive malignancies, although scattered reports of this phenomenon do exist.

### EPIDEMIOLOGY

Borderline tumors of the ovary may represent up to 20% of serous and mucinous ovarian tumors.[247] The frequency of these tumors will reflect the population being studied: borderline tumors of the ovary will account for a higher proportion of early-stage tumors, with up to 30% of stage I tumors being borderline,[248] compared to advanced-stage tumors, in which only 7% of patients with stage IIIA and IIIB tumors are borderline tumors.[247] The mean age of patients with borderline tumors is lower than that of women with invasive ovarian tumors: 45.7 versus 52.5 years.[249] The majority of patients with borderline tumors of the ovary are less than 50 years of age. Nulliparity and nulligravidity have been reported in up to 43% and 39% of patients, respectively.[250,251] These tumors may be a component of the hereditary breast and ovarian cancer; however, Jewish women who carry one of the common *BRCA1* mutations, 185 del AG, are not at elevated risk to develop borderline tumors.[252]

### PROGNOSTIC FACTORS

As in other types of ovarian cancer, stage of disease is an important prognostic factor; however, even women with advanced-stage disease enjoy a good prognosis. Usually, unlike invasive epithelial ovarian cancers, borderline tumors of the ovary are diagnosed at an early stage; only 20% will be stage III or IV. In a thoroughly staged patient with a borderline tumor, disease will be found in up to 30% of cases.[253] The 5-year survival rate for stage I patients is 95% to 100%. The 5-year survival rate in women with advanced-stage disease ranges from 64% to 96%;[254,255] however, the rate steadily declines after 5 years, with a mortality rate of 30%.[256] DNA ploidy has

also been identified as a prognostic factor; in a Norwegian study, patients over the age of 60 with advanced-stage tumors that were diploid had a 15-year survival rate of 75%, compared to 20% for patients with tumors that were aneuploid.[257] Other investigators have also identified aneuploidy as an independent prognostic factor.[258,259] Some investigators have divided peritoneal implants of borderline tumors into invasive and noninvasive types. Invasive implants are characterized as such based on the findings of infiltration into the underlying tissue, and they are associated with a poorer prognosis.[260] These tumors are placed into the borderline category, based on the primary ovarian tumor; however, they should be treated as an invasive epithelial ovarian cancer, with adjuvant chemotherapy.

### SURGICAL TREATMENT

The mainstay of treatment for borderline tumors of the ovary is surgery. The patterns of spread of borderline tumors are similar to those of invasive ovarian tumors, and the principles of surgical management of borderline tumors are also similar to those for invasive tumors. Common types of disease involvement include intraperitoneal disease; involvement in the contralateral ovary (in 10% to 30% of cases);[247,261,262] lymph node metastases (in 20% of cases);[263] and involvement of the omentum (in 15% of patients with apparent stage I disease and in 40% of patients with stage III tumors).[262,264,265] Approximately 7% of women who have stage I disease will have positive washings.[265] Stage IV borderline tumors are very rare, but they do occur.

Surgical staging plays a role in the treatment of borderline tumors of the ovary, but not to the same extent as in treatment of its invasive counterpart, since chemotherapy decisions are not typically based on staging findings. The surgery for a woman who has completed her childbearing includes a total abdominal hysterectomy, omentectomy, and a thorough staging as outlined above. It is not uncommon for a woman to be referred for a borderline tumor of the ovary that is diagnosed postoperatively. It may be of value to reexplore a woman who desires no future fertility and has not had a hysterectomy and bilateral salpingo-oophorectomy, or a woman in whom the upper abdomen has not been thoroughly explored.

Since many of the women with borderline tumors of the ovary are in their childbearing years at the time of diagnosis, conservative surgical therapy plays an important role in management. This may consist of a unilateral salpingo-oophorectomy, unilateral salpingo-oophorectomy and cystectomy of the contralateral ovary, and bilateral ovarian cystectomies—all with conservation of the uterus. Multiple studies evaluating the survival of women with early-stage tumors that were treated conservatively reveal no difference from that of women who were treated with bilateral salpingo-oophorectomy.[266–270] Generally, it is not recommended that a grossly normal contralateral ovary be biopsied, due to the fact that this may lead to adhesions and fertility problems in the future, although an abnormal area on an ovary destined for retention should be biopsied. These studies reveal that for early-stage borderline tumors, survival approaches 100%, regardless of treatment with bilateral salpingo-oophorectomy versus unilateral salpingo-oophorectomy. For a woman with bilateral involvement, the situation becomes more complex. An acceptable treatment for these women includes unilateral salpingo-oophorectomy and cystectomy or bilateral cystectomies. In two studies evaluating cystectomies as treatment, it was shown that recurrence can be expected in up to 15% of cases.[251,271,272] None of the patients died of disease, however, and all were salvaged with subsequent surgery. Factors associated with recurrence included positive margins on cystectomy specimen and multiple cystectomies in the same ovary. Eight pregnancies were achieved in 16 patients. In the series from Chambers,[255] one of the patients developed a recurrence that was invasive. This is an exceedingly rare situation; however, one must be aware that it may occur.

Only 20% of borderline tumors are advanced at the time of diagnosis. The treatment of these tumors is also surgically based. An attempt should be made to remove all gross tumor at the time of laparotomy. This is done because the tumor is slowly growing and is considered to be resistant to chemotherapy. Therefore, the treatment even for advanced-stage tumors is attempted at complete surgical resection.

## ADJUVANT THERAPY

Borderline tumors are generally considered to be resistant to chemotherapy, presumably because they grow so slowly. Multiple studies have demonstrated that adjuvant therapy adds nothing to the already excellent prognosis of these tumors.[273–276] In the past, these patients were typically treated with alkylating agents, which have been demonstrated to cause leukemia, and the literature contains numerous reports of these patients going on to develop leukemia. Radiation therapy has also been employed in the adjuvant treatment of borderline tumors. In one prospective study, a group employed the use of whole pelvic radiation therapy with or without radioactive gold.[248] There were more deaths from the treatment in this study than from the disease. In conclusion, women with completely resected stage I disease enjoy an excellent prognosis, and the risk of therapy generally outweighs the risk of death from disease.

As with early-stage tumors, there are few data to support the treatment of advanced-stage borderline tumors with chemotherapy. In a summary of eight series involving 58 patients with stages II and III borderline tumors treated with surgery alone, 24% of the patients recurred and 8.6% died of disease.[256] In a summary of 10 series involving 134 patients with stages II and III borderline tumors, 16.5% of the patients recurred and 10.5% died of disease.[256] Similar findings have also been demonstrated with adjuvant radiation therapy; in a summary of 28 patients, 14% recurred and 11% died.[256] Thus, even though after adjuvant treatment the recurrence rate may be slightly higher, the proportion of women who will die from disease is the same. Some investigators have utilized second-look surgery in order to assess the response to chemotherapy. In a study of alkylating agents in the treatment of advanced-stage tumors, 10 of 13 women had persistent tumor after treatment.[277] Similar results have been found by others.[278,279] Other studies, however, have reported higher response rates.[280,281] In one study of 20 patients with advanced-stage tumors with macroscopic residual disease at the end of the initial laparotomy, there was a partial response rate of 40% and a complete response rate of 40%, for an overall response rate of 80%.[282] A GOG study[265] of adjuvant combination chemotherapy demonstrated a complete response rate of 25%. In conclusion, there has been no clear, established benefit of adjuvant therapy for advanced-stage borderline tumors. The policy at our institution regarding management of these tumors is not to treat women with completely resected advanced-stage borderline tumors. However, for those patients with gross residual disease left at the time of laparotomy, treatment with platinum-based combination chemotherapy is instituted.

Two groups may benefit from adjuvant chemotherapy treatment: (1) those with aneuploid tumors and (2) those with invasive implants. Although aneuploidy is a strong prognostic factor, there have been no prospective studies that demonstrate a benefit to adjuvant treatment in this group of patients. As mentioned above, those patients with invasive implants should be treated as if they have an invasive epithelial ovarian cancer, because they have a poorer prognosis compared to those patients with noninvasive implants.

## RECURRENT DISEASE

The important aspect of borderline tumors that must be kept in mind after the initial diagnosis and surgical treatment is that since these are indolent tumors, they have a propensity to occur late (up to 5 years after diagnosis). Thus, continued surveillance of these women by a qualified physician is important. The median time to recurrence is 5 years.[247,283]

## PSEUDOMYXOMA PERITONEI

The entity known as pseudomyxoma peritonei was first described in 1842, and the term was first applied in 1844, when the entity was associated with a ruptured ovarian cyst.[284] It was found in association with a mucocele of the appendix and described in 1901.[285] This entity is characterized by the accumulation of gelatinous material in large amounts in the abdominal cavity. The tumor is most often related to neoplasms of the ovary and the appendix, but it may also originate from mucinous neoplasms of the endometrium, colon, common bile duct, ovarian teratoma, fallopian tube tumors, and umbilical and urachal lesions. It is typically slow growing and refractory to therapy. The entity has been associated with 1.7% of benign mucinous tumors of the ovary,[286,287] 15.4% of borderline mucinous tumors of the ovary,[288] and 30% of frankly malignant mucinous tumors of the ovary.[289] The etiology is poorly understood and various hypotheses have been proposed to account for the phenomenon. Some of these hypotheses include rupture of a tumor, leading to spread of cellular debris, metaplasia of the peritoneum, mucin leaks leading to a type of foreign-body reaction, and colonic differentiation of peritoneal mesothelium.

The mean age range at diagnosis of this tumor is from 49 to 63 years.[290] Patients usually present with abdominal distension, an abdominal mass, pain, or hernia. Radiographic studies will demonstrate multiloculated cystic masses in the abdomen and pelvis. Treatment remains a combination of surgery and chemotherapy, although these tumors are poorly responsive to chemotherapy. Because the tumor is exceedingly rare, no prospective studies exist, and consensus concerning the proper treatment is lacking.

In one study in which patients were treated with no adjuvant therapy, all developed recurrences at a median time of 18 months.[291] Adjuvant therapies have included radiation therapy, chemotherapy, immunotherapy, and instillation of mucolytic agents. Fernandez and Daly[292] have reported a 75% 5-year survival rate in patients receiving radiation therapy, compared to 44% in these patients receiving melphalan. One group has reported a 56% response rate to PAC chemotherapy[293] Sugarbaker and his colleagues[294] have advocated aggressive surgical management with peritoneal stripping, combined with IP 5-FU and mitomycin C. Mucolytic agents that have been employed include glucose and dextran solutions.[295]

## GERM CELL TUMORS OF THE OVARY

### SURGICAL MANAGEMENT

Since the majority of germ cell tumors occur in women of young age, reproductive preservation is an important component in the management of germ cell tumors of the ovary. Standard management of germ cell tumors consists of a unilateral salpingo-oophorectomy and staging procedure for early-stage malignancies, and surgical cytoreduction and unilateral salpingo-oophorectomy for advanced-stage malignancies. All of the germ cell malignancies will require adjuvant chemotherapy, with the exception of stage IA dysgerminomas and grade 1 immature teratomas. In order to determine the most appropriate treatment, it is important to check tumor markers in patients with germ cell tumors of the ovary. For example, in women with a dysgerminoma and an elevated AFP, mixed germ cell tumors may occur and tumor markers may intensify the search for the mixed elements. A search should be made for other elements within the tumor.

The dysgerminoma is the only germ cell tumor that is associated with a significant rate of bilateral involvement, and these tumors involve the contralateral ovary in approximately 15% of cases. Staging of germ cell malignancies is the same as that outlined for epithelial ovarian cancer. This consists of a thorough examination of the peritoneal surfaces, along with multiple biopsies and a thorough lymph node sampling (see Table 18E-6). Dysgerminomas are the most common germ cell tumor of the ovary and are stage I in 75% of cases.[296,297] This tumor primarily spreads through the lymphatic system so that a thorough lymph node sampling is warranted. If disease is found outside of the ovary, the contralateral ovary and uterus may be left in place due to the chemosensitivity of this tumor. A small focus on the contralateral ovary may be resected in order to preserve fertility, with the use of adjuvant chemotherapy. Dysgerminomas that develop in dysgenic gonads require the removal of both ovaries; however, the uterus may be left in place for future embryo transfer. The treatment for immature teratomas is similar to that of the dysgerminoma; however, this tumor has a greater predilection for transperitoneal spread. The endodermal sinus tumor and the embryonal carcinoma are treated in a similar fashion, but extensive surgical staging may not be necessary due to the fact that all of these patients will receive postoperative chemotherapy.

**TABLE 18E-13. CHEMOTHERAPY REGIMENS EMPLOYED IN THE TREATMENT OF GERM CELL TUMORS OF THE OVARY.**

| REGIMEN | DOSE | SCHEDULE |
|---|---|---|
| *BEP* | | |
| Bleomycin | 15 units/m$^2$/week | Weekly |
| Etoposide | 100 mg/m$^2$/day | Days 1–5 every 3 weeks |
| Cisplatin | 20 mg/m$^2$/day | Days 1–5 every 3 weeks |
| *VHP* | | |
| Vinblastine | 0.15 mg/kg days 1 and 2 | Every 3 weeks |
| Bleomycin | 15 units/m$^2$/week | Weekly |
| Cisplatin | 100 mg/m$^2$ on day 1 | Every 3 weeks |
| *VAC* | | |
| Vincristine | 1–1.5 mg/m$^2$ on day 1 | Every 4 weeks |
| Actinomycin-D | 0.5 mg/day | Days 1–5 every 4 weeks |
| Cytoxan | 150 mg/m$^2$/day | Days 1–5 every 4 weeks |

### ADJUVANT CHEMOTHERAPY

Patients who have the diagnosis of a well-staged stage IA dysgerminoma of the ovary do not require treatment with adjuvant chemotherapy. The relapse rate in this population is 5% to 10%; however, at the time of recurrence, most can be treated successfully with chemotherapy. Treatment options for women with advanced-stage tumors include chemotherapy and radiation therapy. Chemotherapy is generally employed because radiation therapy is associated with the loss of reproductive potential. Germ-cell tumors have been treated with vinblastine, actinomycin and cisplatin (VAC); bleomycin, etoposide, and cisplatin (BEP); and cisplatin, vinblastine, and bleomycin (PVB) (Table 18E-13). The standard treatment of germ-cell malignancies of the ovary was VAC, but experience with testicular tumor has demonstrated the superiority of BEP. BEP results in a shorter treatment time and lower relapse rate.[298,299] The standard therapy for ovarian germ cell malignancies has now become three or four cycles of BEP in the adjuvant setting.

Patients with a stage IA, grade 1 immature teratoma do not require adjuvant therapy. All other patients with immature teratomas are treated with adjuvant therapy. All patients with embryonal carcinomas and endodermal sinus tumors are treated with adjuvant therapy. For patients with early-stage disease and completely resected advanced-stage disease, three cycles of BEP may be utilized. For patients with incompletely resected disease, treatment with two cycles past negative tumor markers should be administered.

### SECOND-LOOK SURGERY

Second-look surgery is generally not warranted in early-stage germ cell tumors or completely resected advanced-stage tumors.[300–302] When performing a second-look surgery in advanced-stage patients with immature teratomas, one may find mature teratomatous elements throughout the peritoneal cavity. This should be resected if possible, and chemotherapy should be discontinued. The value of second-look surgery for endodermal sinus tumors is not determined. One can assume, however, that if the AFP remains elevated, the patient has persistent tumor and alternative chemotherapy should be instituted.

## RECURRENT DISEASE

Women with stage IA dysgerminomas of the ovary have a 95% disease-free survival; however, 5% to 10% of women with a retained gonad will develop recurrent disease. Approximately 75% of recurrences will occur in the first year,[300] and these women can be salvaged with treatment with BEP. The prognosis of women with immature teratomas of the ovary is dependent on grade and stage of the tumor.[303] The amount of residual disease at the end of laparotomy is also an important prognostic factor; the 5-year survival rate for women with incompletely resected disease is 50% and rises to 95% if the disease is completely resected.

In patients with germ cell tumors who fail treatment with platinum-based regimens, durable responses may be attained with VAC or ifosfamide-cisplatin combinations.[304] Autologous marrow rescue may also be an option for some of these patients. The role of secondary cytoreduction has not been determined but may be of some benefit in women with immature teratomas of the ovary.

## SEX CORD–STROMAL TUMORS

The vast majority of stromal tumors are indolent, and therefore surgery remains the mainstay of treatment. In the woman who desires future fertility, a unilateral salpingo-oophorectomy may be performed. In the postmenopausal female, a hysterectomy with bilateral salpingo-oophorectomy is usually performed.

The treatment for a granulosa cell tumor in young women is a unilateral salpingo-oophorectomy; these tumors are bilateral in only 2% of cases. For the woman who desires no future fertility, treatment with a bilateral salpingo-oophorectomy is the standard, along with a staging procedure. These tumors are estrogen producing and are thus associated with endometrial hyperplasia or a uterine malignancy in up to 25% to 50% of cases.[305] Thus, a thorough endometrial sampling with a dilation and curettage (D&C) is warranted in patients who retain their uterus. These patients enjoy a good prognosis because this tends to be an indolent tumor. Surgical resection alone is treatment. However, 15% to 20% of patients with granulosa cell tumors will recur, with the median interval to recurrence being 6 years. Recurrences at 10 to 20 years are also not uncommon.[306] Aggressive surgical management of recurrent disease is warranted, and exenteration procedures with en bloc removal of the bowel or bladder may be indicated. In patients in whom surgical resection is not possible, chemotherapy and radiation therapy may be employed. These tumors may also spread hematogenously, so that metastases may be found in the liver, brain, and lung.

Treatment for Sertoli-Leydig cell tumors of the ovary is surgery; however, chemotherapy may be given in the adjuvant setting in the treatment of poorly differentiated tumors or of advanced-stage disease. These tumors are rarely bilateral (<1% of the time).

## PRIMARY PERITONEAL CARCINOMA

Primary peritoneal cancer pathologically resembles epithelial ovarian cancer in its presentation, treatment, and response to treatment. It arises from the "secondary müllerian system," which is comprised of the pelvic and lower abdominal mesothelial lining and subjacent mesenchyme. The entity was first described by Swerdlow in 1959.[307] The tumor is characterized by involvement of the peritoneal cavity with tumor and may also involve the surface of the ovaries. This tumor is indistinguishable from ovarian cancer, and may also occur after the removal of the ovaries for benign conditions. Other terms applied to primary peritoneal carcinomas are peritoneal serous papillary carcinoma and serous surface papillary carcinoma. The majority of these tumors are of the serous type, but may be of any histologic subtype resembling epithelial ovarian carcinomas. They may be of low malignant potential or malignant. The tumor may be difficult to distinguish from a peritoneal mesothelioma; electron microscopy and immunohistochemistry may be utilized to help make the proper diagnosis.[308] The tumors present as similar to epithelial ovarian cancers. They are characterized by surface growths of tumors on the peritoneal surfaces and involve the omentum, intestinal serosa, and the surface of other intraabdominal organs. The ovaries in these patients are absent or are involved with surface growths of tumor, usually with little stromal invasion. Studies involving primary peritoneal carcinomas usually limit the size of the ovaries from 3 to 4 cm in size at the time of assessment. The tumors are thought to account for up to 15% of advanced-stage ovarian carcinoma tumors.[309] The epidemiologic characteristics of epithelial ovarian cancers and primary peritoneal cancers are similar, except the women with primary peritoneal cancers may be older at the time of diagnosis (mean age of 63.8 versus 55 years for women with ovarian cancer.)[310] The genetics of primary peritoneal cancer and their relationship to BRCA1 and BRCA2 mutations is not yet elucidated. One study has evaluated BRCA1 gene mutations in 17 women with primary peritoneal cancer and found that 11% (2/17) had mutations in the BRCA1 gene.[311] Women who have undergone a prophylactic oophorectomy for a family history of ovarian cancer have up to 11% chance of developing a primary peritoneal cancer after a prophylactic oophorectomy. More genetic and prospective studies are required to determine the exact risks for women with a family history of breast and ovarian cancer.

The treatment of primary peritoneal cancer consists of a combination of cytoreductive surgery and chemotherapy. The same surgical principals that attempt to complete cytoreduction of epithelial ovarian cancer apply to these tumors. Treatment with cisplatin and paclitaxel combination chemotherapy for six cycles along with the possibility of second-look reassessment are also employed as treatments, identical to epithelial ovarian cancer. Numerous authors have reported 5-year survival rates similar to those in advanced-stage epithelial ovarian cancer.[312–315] At least one study has suggested a better prognosis for papillary serous peritoneal cancers when compared to ovarian cancer,[316] and at least one study has suggested a worse prognosis.[317]

## OVARIAN MALIGNANCIES IN CHILDREN AND ADOLESCENTS

Symptoms of these tumors may be related to the mass itself and include abdominal-pelvic pain, urinary frequency, rectal pressure, hormone production, menstrual irregularities, or vaginal bleeding in premenarchal girls. Preoperative evaluation for any ovarian mass in a girl or young woman should include an USG or CAT scan of the abdomen and pelvis tumor markers, including AFP, LDH, hCG, and CXR. Germ cell malignancies represent two-thirds of malignancies in women less than the age of 20. In this age group, approximately 70% of ovarian tumors are germ cell, and 30% of these are malignant. In women less than 10 years of age, 80% of the germ cell tumors are malignant. Although germ cell tumors are the most common malignancies in children and adolescents, stromal and epithelial tumors may also occur. Juvenile granulosa cell tumors (JGCT) of the ovary are a distinct entity from adult granulosa cell tumors. The mean age of diagnosis of these tumors is 6 years. Signs of these tumors arise from estrogen production. These consist of isosexual pseudopuberty. Precocious puberty is found in 80% of girls with granulosa cell tumors, and postmenarchal girls may have signs such as menstrual irregularities. Treatment consists of unilateral oophorectomy, surgical staging and tumor debulking. Small cell carcinoma of the ovary is a rare epithelial neoplasm. The average age of diagnosis of this tumor is 20 years, and 70% of these patients present with hypercalcemia.

Of the germ cell tumors, the dysgerminoma is the most common. These tumors are not typically associated with an elevation in tumor markers; however, approximately 5% will contain syncytiotrophoblast and produce βhCG. These may cause symptoms of isosexual precocious puberty.[318] The vast majority are stage I at diagnosis.

A karyotype is recommended for premenarchal girls (those without secondary sexual characteristics) who have been diagnosed with germ-cell tumors. This is because treatment for germ cell tumors is a unilateral salpingo-oophorectomy, except in cases of girls with gonadal dysgenesis; in such cases, both ovaries should be removed. Gonadal dysgenesis is characterized by primary amenorrhea, virilization, and other abnormalities of secondary sexual characteristics. Prepubertal females may have no outward signs, and therefore a karyotype is recommended for these patients. This is important because 25% to 30% of patients with gonadal dysgenesis will develop germ cell malignancies, frequently in association with gonadoblastomas. Fifty percent of gonadoblastomas are associated with dysgerminomas, and 10% are associated with other malignant germ cell tumors.[319]

## FALLOPIAN TUBE CANCER

Fallopian tube cancer is an extremely rare malignancy, and it accounts for 0.3% of gynecologic malignancies. The hallmarks of fallopian tube cancer are (1) a profuse, watery vaginal discharge, (2) pelvic pain, and (3) a pelvic mass. The histologic features of fallopian tube cancers, along with the surgical treatment, are the same as those for epithelial ovarian cancer. This tumor may also be associated with ascites and transperitoneal spread of the tumor, thus closely resembling ovarian cancer. A dense lymphatic network surrounds the fallopian tube; therefore, retroperitoneal lymph node disease is common. Staging procedures are the same as those for ovarian cancer, and tumor debulking is performed in a similar manner. These patients are generally treated with adjuvant chemotherapy—even patients with stage I disease with low-grade tumors. The data for observation alone after surgical treatment are not present to support this type of management, and therefore platinum-based therapy with paclitaxel is employed.

## REFERENCES

1. Landis SH et al: Cancer statistics, 1999. CA 49:8, 1999.
2. Wingo PA et al: Cancer statistics, 1995. CA 45:8, 1995.
3. Yanick R: Ovarian Cancer. Age contrasts in incidence, histology, disease stage at diagnosis, and mortality. Cancer 71:517, 1993.
4. Casagrande JT et al: "Incessant ovulation" and ovarian cancer. Lancet 2:170, 1979.
5. The reduction in risk of ovarian cancer associated with oral-contraceptive use. The Cancer and Steroid Hormone Study of the Centers for Disease Control and the National Institute of Child Health and Human Development. N Engl J Med 316:650, 1987.
6. Booth M et al: Risk factors for ovarian cancer: A case-control study. Br J Cancer 60:592, 1989.
7. Risch HA et al: Parity, contraception, infertility, and the risk of epithelial ovarian cancer. Am J Epidemiol 140:585, 1994.
8. Rosenberg L et al: Epithelial ovarian cancer and combination oral contraceptives. JAMA 247:3210, 1982.
9. Greene MH et al: The epidemiology of ovarian cancer. Semin Oncol 11:209, 1984.
10. Schildkraut JM, Thompson WD: Familial ovarian cancer: A population-based case-control study. Am J Epidemiol 128:45, 1988.
11. Whittemore AS: Characteristics relating to ovarian cancer risk: Implications for prevention and detection. Gynecol Oncol 55:S15, 1994.
12. Lynch HT et al: Hereditary carcinoma of the ovary and associated cancers: A study of two families. Gynecol Oncol 36:48, 1990.
13. Thompson WD, Schildkraut JM: Family history of gynaecological cancers: Relationships to the incidence of breast cancer prior to age 55. Int J Epidemiol 20:595, 1991.
14. Whittemore AS et al: Characteristics relating to ovarian cancer risk: Collaborative analysis of 12 US case-control studies. II. Invasive epithelial ovarian cancers in white women. Collaborative Ovarian Cancer Group. Am J Epidemiol 136:1184, 1992.
15. Byers T et al: A case-control study of dietary and nondietary factors in ovarian cancer. J Natl Cancer Inst 71:681, 1983.
16. Rossing MA et al: Ovarian tumors in a cohort of infertile women. N Engl J Med 331:771, 1994.
17. Whittemore AS: The risk of ovarian cancer after treatment for infertility. N Engl J Med 331:805, 1994.

18. PARAZZINI F et al: Treatment for infertility and risk of invasive epithelial ovarian cancer. Hum Reprod 12:2159, 1997.

19. MOSGAARD BJ et al: Infertility, fertility drugs, and invasive ovarian cancer: A case-control study. Fertil Steril 67:1005, 1997.

20. BRISTOW RE, KARLAN BY: Ovulation induction, infertility, and ovarian cancer risk. Fertil Steril 66:499, 1996.

21. SCULLY RE: Tumors of the ovary and maldeveloped gonads, in *Atlas of Tumor Pathology,* Fascicle 16. Washington, DC, Armed Forces Institute of Pathology, 1979.

22. BEREK JS, HACKER NF: Ovarian and fallopian tubes, in *Cancer Treatment,* 3rd ed, Haskell M (ed). Philadelphia, PA, Saunders, 1990, p 295.

23. SLAYTON RE: Management of germ cell and stromal tumors of the ovary. Semin Oncol 11:299, 1984.

24. BEWTRA C et al: Hereditary ovarian cancer: A clinicopathological study. Int J Gynecol Pathol 11:180, 1992.

25. MIKI Y et al: A strong candidate for the breast and ovarian cancer susceptibility gene BRCA1. Science 266:66, 1994.

26. EASTON DF et al AND THE BREAST CANCER LINKAGE CONSORTIUM: Breast and ovarian cancer in BRCA1 mutation carriers. Am J Hum Genet 56:265, 1995.

27. FORD D et al: Risks of cancer in BRCA1-mutation carriers. Breast Cancer Linkage Consortium. Lancet 343:692, 1994.

28. ODDOUX C et al: The carrier frequency of the BRCA2 6174delT mutation among Ashekenazi Jewish individuals is approximately 1%. Nat Genet 14:188, 1996.

29. STRUEWING JP et al: The carrier frequency of the BRCA1 185delAG mutation is approximately 1 percent in Ashkenazi Jewish individuals. Nat Genet 11:198, 1995.

30. FORD D et al AND THE BREAST CANCER LINKAGE CONSORTIUM: Risks of cancer in BRCA1 mutation carriers. Lancet 343:692, 1994.

31. WOOSTER R et al: Localization of a breast cancer susceptibility gene BRCA2 to chromosome 13q 12-13. Science 265:2088, 1994.

32. FORD D, EASTON DF: The genetics of breast and ovarian cancer. Br J Cancer 72:805, 1995.

33. WATSON P, LYNCH HT: Extracolonic cancers in hereditary non-polyposis colorectal cancer. Cancer 71:677, 1993.

34. KOHLER MF et al: Spectrum of mutation and frequency of allelic deletion of the p53 gene in ovarian cancer. J Natl Cancer Inst 85:1513, 1993.

35. MARKS JR et al: Overexpression and mutations of the p53 in epithelial ovarian cancer. Cancer Res 51:2979, 1991.

36. PEREZ RP et al: Ovarian cancer biology. Semin Oncol 18:186, 1991.

37. SCULLY RE: Sex cord tumors with annular tubules: A distinctive ovarian tumor of the Peutz Jeghers syndrome. Cancer 25:1107, 1970.

38. BARAKAT B et al: 46 XY gonadal dysgenesis with secondary amenorrhea, virilization and bilateral gonadoblastoma. S Med J 72:1163, 1979.

39. HARTLEY AC et al: Are germ cell tumors part of the Li Fraumeni cancer family syndrome. Cancer Genet Cytogent 42:221, 1989.

40. CLENDENNING WE et al: Ovarian fibromas and mesenteric cysts: Their association with hereditary basal cell cancer of the skin. Am J Obstet Gynecol 87:1008, 1963.

41. YANCIK R: Ovarian cancer. Age contrasts in incidence, histology, disease stage at diagnosis, and mortality. Cancer 71(2 Suppl 2):517, 1993.

42. VAN NAGELL JR JR et al: Ovarian cancer screening in asymptomatic postmenopausal women by transvaginal sonography. Cancer 68:458, 1991.

43. MARWICK C: Consensus panel says benefits of screening women for ovarian cancer currently unproven. JAMA 271:1305, 1994.

44. CAMPBELL S et al: Transabdominal ultrasound screening for early ovarian cancer. BMJ 299:1363, 1989.

45. BOURNE TH et al: Screening for early familial ovarian cancer with transvaginal ultrasonography and colour blood flow imaging. BMJ 306:1025, 1993.

46. DEPRIEST PD et al: The efficacy of a sonographic morphology index in indentifying ovarian cancer: A multi-institutional investigation. Gynecol Oncol 55:174, 1994.

47. KURJAK A, PREDANIC M: New scoring system for prediction of ovarian malignancy based on transvaginal color Doppler sonography. J Ultrasound Med 11:631, 1992.

48. VAN NAGELL JR JR et al: Ovarian cancer screening. Cancer 76(Suppl 10):2086, 1995.

49. SKATES SJ et al: Toward an optimal algorithm for ovarian cancer screening with longitudinal tumor markers. Cancer 76:2004, 1995.

50. NAROD SA et al: Oral contraceptives and the risk of hereditary ovarian cancer. Hereditary Ovarian Cancer Clinical Study Group. N Engl J Med 339:424, 1998.

51. PAUL C et al: Oral contraceptives and risk of breast cancer. Int J Cancer 46:366, 1990.

52. HARRIS RE et al: Oral contraceptives and breast cancer risk: A case-control study. Int J Epidemiol 19:240, 1990.

53. NIH CONSENSUS CONFERENCE: Ovarian cancer: Screening, treatment, and follow-up. NIH consensus development panel on ovarian cancer. JAMA 273:491, 1995.

54. BURKE W et al: Recommendations for follow-up care of individuals with an inherited predisposition to cancer. II. BRCA1 and BRCA2. Cancer Genetics Studies Consortium. JAMA 277:997, 1997.

55. TOBACMAN JK et al: Intra-abdominal carcinomatosis after prophylactic oophorectomy in ovarian-cancer-prone families. Lancet 2:795, 1982.

56. PIVER MS et al: Primary peritoneal carcinoma after prophylactic oophorectomy in women with a family history of ovarian cancer: A report of the Gilda Radner Familial Ovarian Cancer Registry. Cancer 71:2751, 1993.

57. COLDITZ GA et al: Hormone replacement therapy and risk of breast cancer: Results from epidemiologic studies. Am J Obstet Gynecol 168:1473, 1993.

58. STANFORD JL et al: Combined estrogen and progestin hormone replacement therapy in relation to risk of breast cancer in middle-aged women. JAMA 274:137, 1995.

59. SCHUURMAN AG et al: Exogenous hormone use and the risk of postmenopausal breast cancer: Results from the Netherlands Cohort Study. Cancer Causes Control 6:416, 1995.

60. WILLIAMS SD et al: Ovarian germ-cell tumors, in *Principles and Practice of Gynecologic Oncology,* 2nd ed, Hoskins WJ et al (eds). Philadelphia, Lippincott-Raven, 1997, pp 987–999.

61. BURGHARDT E et al: Pelvic lymphadenectomy in operative treatment of ovarian cancer. Am J Obstet Gynecol 155:315, 1986.

62. DAUPLAT J et al: Distant metastases in epithelial ovarian carcinoma. Cancer 60:1561, 1987.

63. YOUNG RC et al: Adjuvant therapy in stage I and II epithelial ovarian cancer: Results of two prospective randomized trials. N Engl J Med 322:1021, 1990.

64. YANCIK R: Ovarian cancer: Age contrasts in incidence, histology, disease stage at diagnosis, and mortality. Cancer 71:517, 1993.

65. YOUNG RC: The treatment of early stage ovarian cancers. Semin Oncol 22:76, 1995.

66. VERGOTE IB et al: Analysis of prognostic factors in stage I epithelial ovarian carcinoma: Importance of degree of differentiation and deoxyribonucleic acid ploidy in predicting relapse. Am J Obstet Gynecol 157:88, 1987.

67. DEMBO AJ et al: Prognostic factors in patients with stage I epithelial ovarian cancer. Obstet Gynecol 75:263, 1990.

68. KODAMA S et al: Multivariate analysis of prognostic factors in patients with ovarian cancer stage I and II. Int J Gynaecol Obstet 56:147, 1997.

69. SAINZ DE LA CUESTA R et al: Prognostic importance of intraoperative rupture of malignant ovarian epithelial neoplasms. Obstet Gynecol 84:1, 1994.

70. DEMBO AJ et al: Prognostic factors in patients with stage I epithelial ovarian cancer. Obstet Gynecol 75:263, 1990.

71. SEVELDA P et al: Prognostic value of the rupture of the capsule in stage I epithelial ovarian carcinoma. Gynecol Oncol 35:321, 1989.

72. PUNNONEN R et al: Prognostic assessment in stage I ovarian cancer using a discriminant analysis with clinicopathological and DNA flow cytometric data. Gynecol Obstet Invest 27:213, 1989.

73. GAJEWSKI WH et al: Prognostic significance of DNA content in epithelial ovarian cancer. Gynecol Oncol 53:5, 1994.

74. HARTMANN LC et al: Prognostic significance of p53 immunostaining in epithelial ovarian cancer. J Clin Oncol 12:64, 1994.

75. SLAMON DJ et al: Studies of the HER-2/neu proto-oncogene in human breast and ovarian cancer. Science 244:707, 1989.

76. RUBIN SC et al: Prognostic significance of HER-2/neu expression in advanced epithelial ovarian cancer: A multivariate analysis. Am J Obstet Gynecol 168:162, 1993.

77. RUBIN SC et al: Clinical and pathological features of ovarian cancer in women with germ-line mutations of BRCA1. N Engl J Med 335:1413, 1996.

78. RUSTIN GJ et al: Use of CA-125 to predict survival of patients with ovarian carcinoma. North Thames Cooperative Group. J Clin Oncol 7:1667, 1989.

79. MOGENSEN O: Prognostic value of CA 125 in advanced ovarian cancer. Gynecol Oncol 44:207, 1992.

80. VOEST EE et al: A meta-analysis of prognostic factors in advanced ovarian cancer with median survival and overall survival (measured with the log (relative risk] as main objectives. Eur J Cancer Clin Oncol 25:711, 1989.

81. BAST RC JR et al: Reactivity of a monoclonal antibody with human ovarian carcinoma. J Clin Invest 68:1331, 1981.

82. KABAWAT SE et al: Tissue distribution of a coelomic-epithelium-related antigen recognized by the monoclonal antibody OC125. Int J Gynecol Pathol 2:275, 1983.

83. JACOBS I, BAST RC JR: The CA 125 tumour-associated antigen: A review of the literature. Human Reprod 4:1, 1989.

84. ALTARAS MM et al: The role of cancer antigen 125 (CA 125) in the management of ovarian epithelial carcinomas. Gynecol Oncol 30:26, 1988.

85. ZYGMUNT A et al: Estimation of the usefulness of neoplastic markers TPS and CA 125 in diagnosis and monitoring of ovarian cancer. Eur J Gynaecol Oncol 20:298, 1999.

86. PODCZASKI E et al: Use of CA 125 to monitor patients with ovarian epithelial carcinomas. Gynecol Oncol 33:193, 1989.

87. BEREK JS et al: CA 125 serum levels correlated with second-look operations among ovarian cancer patients. Obstet Gynecol 67:685, 1986.

88. LAPPOHN RE et al: Inhibin as a marker for granulosa-cell tumors. N Engl J Med 321:790, 1989.

89. MANN WJ et al: Elevated serum alpha fetoprotein associated with Sertoli-Leydig cell tumors of the ovary. Obstet Gynecol 67:141, 1986.

90. SCULLY RE: Tumors of the Ovary and Maldeveloped Gonads. Armed Forces Institute of Pathology, Fascicle 16. Washington, DC, 1979.

91. CONWAY C et al: Simple cyst in the postmenopausal patient: Detection and management. J Ultrasound Med 17:369, 1998.

92. KROON E, ANDOLF E: Diagnosis and follow-up of simple ovarian cysts detected by ultrasound in postmenopausal women. Obstet Gynecol 85:211, 1995.

93. OBWEGESER R et al: The risk of malignancy with an apparently simple adnexal cyst on ultrasound. Arch Gynecol Obstet 253:117, 1993.

94. PARKER WH et al: A multicenter study of laparoscopic management of selected cystic adnexal masses in postmenopausal women. J Am Coll Surg 179:733, 1994.

95. DOTTINO PR et al: Laparoscopic management of adnexal masses in premenopausal and postmenopausal women. Obstet Gynecol 93:223, 1999.

96. YUEN PM et al: A randomized prospective study of laparoscopy and laparotomy in the management of benign ovarian masses. Am J Obstet Gynecol 177:109, 1997.

97. CHI DS et al: Laparoscopic management of adnexal masses in women with a history of nongynecologic malignancy. Obstet Gynecol 86:964, 1995.

98. PULS LE et al: Transition from benign to malignant epithelium in mucinous and serous ovarian cystadenocarcinoma. Gynecol Oncol 47:53, 1992.

99. SCULLY RE: Tumors of the ovary and maldeveloped gonads. Atlas of Tumor Pathology, 3rd ed. Washington, DC, in press.

100. RUSSELL P, BALLANTYNE P: Surgical Pathology of the Ovaries. New York, Churchill Livingstone, 1989, p 539.

101. BELL DA et al: Ovarian epithelial tumors of borderline malignancy. Prog Reprod Urinary Tract Pathol 1:1, 1989.

102. HEAPS JM et al: Malignant neoplasms arising in endometriosis. Obstet Gynecol 75:1023, 1990.

103. OZOLS RF et al: Epithelial ovarian cancer, in Principles and Practice of Gynecologic Oncology, 2nd ed, Hoskins WJ et al (eds). Philadelphia, Lippincott-Raven, 1997, pp 919–986.

104. WEBB M et al: Factors influencing survival in stage I ovarian cancer. Am J Obstet Gynecol 116:222, 1973.

105. CHANG J et al: Carcinosarcoma of the ovary: Incidence, prognosis, treatment and survival of patients. Ann Oncol 6:755, 1995.

106. LAGRENADE A, SILVERGERG SG: Ovarian tumors associated with atypical endometriosis. Hum Pathol 19:108, 1988.

107. YOUNG RH et al: Small cell carcinoma of the ovary hypercalcemic type: A clinicopathologic analysis of 150 cases. Am J Surg Pathol 18:1102, 1994.

108. EINCHHORN JH et al: Primary ovarian small cell carcinoma of pulmonary type: A clinicopathologic, immunohistologic, and flow cytometric analysis of 11 cases. Am J Surg Pathol 16:926, 1992.

109. GUSBERG SB, KARDON P: Proliferative endometrial response to theca-granulosa-cell tumors. Am J Obstet Gynecol 111:633, 1971.

110. NAKASHIMA N et al: Androgenic granulosa-cell tumors of the ovary: A clinicopathologic analysis of 17 cases and review of the literature. Arch Pathol Lab Med 108:786, 1984.

111. FATHALLA MF: The occurrence of granulosa and theca tumours in clinically normal ovaries. J Obstet Br Cwlth 74:279, 1967.

112. LACK EE et al: Granulosa theca cell tumors in premenarchal girls: clinical and pathologic study of 10 cases. Cancer 48:1846, 1981.

113. PLANTAZ D et al: Tumeurs de la granulosa de l'ovaire chez l'enfant et l'adolescente. Arch Fr Pediatr 49:793, 1992.

114. VASSAL G et al: Juvenile granulosa cell tumor of the ovary in children: A clinical study of 15 cases. J Clin Oncol 6:990, 1988.

115. YOUNG RH et al: Juvenile granulosa cell tumor of the ovary: A clinicopathological analysis of 125 cases. Am J Surg Pathol 8:575, 1984.

116. BARRENETXEA G et al: Pure theca cell tumors: A clinicopathologic study of 29 cases. Eur J Gynecol Oncol 11:429, 1990.

117. BJORKHOLM E, SILFVERSWARD C: Prognostic factors in granulosa-cell tumors. Gynecol Oncol 11:261, 1981.

118. NORRIS HJ, TAYLOR HB: Prognosis of granulosa-theca tumors of the ovary. Cancer 21:225, 1968.

119. SAMANTH KK, BLACK WC: Benign ovarian stromal tumors associated with free peritonial fluid. Am J Obstet Gynecol 107:538, 1970.

120. MEIGS JV: Fibroma of the ovary with ascites and hydrothorax Meigs' syndrome. Am J Gynecol 22:697, 1931.

121. RAGGIO M et al: Recurrent ovarian fibromas with basal cell nevus syndrome (Gorlin syndrome). Obstet Gynecol 61:95, 1983.

122. PRAT J, SCULLY RE: Cellular fibromas and fibrosarcomas of the ovary: A comparative clinicopathic analysis of 17 cases. Cancer 47:2663, 1981.

123. YOUNG RH, SCULLY RE: Well-differentiated ovarian Sertoli-Leydig cell tumors: A clinicopathological analysis of 23 cases. Int J Gynecol Pathol 3:277, 1984.

124. AIBA M et al: Spironolactone bodylike structure in renin-producing Sertoli-cell tumors of the ovary. Surg Pathol 3:143, 1990.

125. EHRLICH EN et al: Aldosteronism and precocious puberty due to an ovarian androblastoma (Sertoli-cell tumor). J Clin Endocrinol Metab 23:358, 1963.

126. KORSETS A et al: Resistant hypertension associated with a renin-producing ovarian Sertoli-cell tumor. Am J Clin Pathol 85:242, 1986.

127. YOUNG RH, SCULLY RE: Ovarian Sertoli-Leydig cell tumors: A clinicopathological analysis of 207 cases. Am J Surg Pathol 9:543, 1985.

128. GAGNON S et al: Frequency of alpha-fetoprotein production of Sertoli-Leydig cell tumors of the ovary: An immunohistochemical study of 8 cases. Mod Pathol 2:63, 1989.

129. SCULLY RE: Sex cord tumor with annular tubules a distinctive ovarian tumor of the Peutz-Jeghers syndrome. Cancer 25:1107, 1970.

130. YOUNG RH et al: Ovarian sex cord tumor with annular tubules: Review of 74 cases including 27 with Peutz-Jeghers syndrome and four with adenoma malignum of the cervix. Cancer 50:1384, 1982.

131. NOMURA K et al: Ovarian sex cord tumor with annular tubules. Acta Pathol Jpn 41:701, 1991.

132. PARASKEVAS M, SCULLY RE: Hilus cell tumor of the ovary. Int J Gynecol Pathol 8:299, 1989.

133. DUNNIHOO DR et al: Hilar-cell tumors of the ovary. Obstet Gynecol 27:703, 1966.

134. HAYES MC, SCULLY RE: Stromal luteoma of the ovary: A clinicopathological analysis of 63 cases. Am J Surg Pathol 11:835, 1987.

135. SEDLIS A: Carcinoma of the fallopian tube. Surg Clin North Am 58:121, 1978.

136. WOODRUFF JD et al: Metastatic ovarian tumors. Am J Obstet Gynecol 107:202, 1970.

137. CURTIN JP et al: Ovarian disease in women with breast cancer. Obstet Gynecol 84:449, 1994.

138. WOODRUFF JD, NOVAK ER: The Krukenberg tumor: Analysis of 48 cases from the Emil Novak Ovarian Tumor Registry. Obstet Gynecol 15:351, 1960.

139. WEBB MJ et al: Cancer metastatic to the ovary: Factors influencing survival. Obstet Gynecol 45:391, 1975.

140. KIKKAWA F et al: Mucinous carcinoma of the ovary. Clinicopathologic analysis. Oncology 53:303, 1996.

141. ABU-RUSTUM N et al: Ovarian and uterine disease in women with colorectal cancer. Obstet Gynecol 89:85, 1997.

142. YOUNG RH et al: Metastatic ovarian tumors in children: A report of 14 cases and review of the literature. Int J Gynecol Pathol 12:8, 1993.

143. ROBBOY SJ et al: Carcinoid metastatic to the ovary: A clinocopathologic analysis of 35 cases. Cancer 33:798, 1974.

144. ARSENEAU JC et al: American Burkitt's lymphoma: A clinicopathologic study of 30 cases. I. Clinical factors relating to prolonged survival. Am J Med 58:314, 1975.

145. YOUNG RC et al: Decker staging laparotomy in early ovarian cancer. JAMA 250:3072, 1983.

146. BUCHSBAUM HJ et al: Surgical staging of carcinoma of the ovaries. Surg Gynecol Obstet 169:226, 1989.

147. WU PL et al: Lymph node metastasis of ovarian cancer: A preliminary survey of 74 cases of lymphadenectomy. Am J Obstet Gynecol 155:1103, 1986.

148. DEMBO AJ et al: Prognostic factors in patients with stage I epithelial ovarian cancer. Obstet Gynecol 75:263, 1990.

149. SEVELDA P et al: Prognostic factors for survival in stage I epithelial ovarian carcinoma. Cancer 65:2349, 1990.

150. TRIMBOS JB et al: Reasons for incomplete surgical staging in early ovarian carcinoma. Gynecol Oncol 37:374, 1990.

151. GOLDIE JH, COLDMAN JA: A mathematical model for relating the drug sensitivity of tumors of their spontaneous mutation rate. Cancer Treat Rep 63:1727, 1979.

152. GRIFFITHS CT: Surgical resection of tumor bulk in the primary treatment of ovarian cancer. Nat Cancer Inst Monogr 42:101, 1975.

153. HACKER NF et al: Primary cytoreductive surgery for epithelial ovarian cancer. Obstet Gynecol 61:413, 1983.

154. VOGL SE et al: Cis-platin based combination chemotherapy for advanced ovarian cancer: High overall response rate with curative potential only in women with small tumor burdens. Cancer 51:2024, 1983.

155. POHL R et al: Prognostic parameters in patients with advanced ovarian malignant tumors. Eur J Gynaecol Oncol 5:160, 1984.

156. DELGADO G et al: Stage III epithelial ovarian cancer: The role of maximal surgical reduction. Gynecol Oncol 18:293, 1984.

157. REDMAN JR et al: Prognostic factors in advanced ovarian carcinoma. J Clin Oncol 4:515, 1986.

158. CONTE PF et al: A randomized trial comparing cisplatin plus cyclophosphamide versus cisplatin, doxorubicin, and cyclophosphamide in advanced ovarian cancer. J Clin Oncol 4(6):965, 1986.

159. NEJIT JP et al: Randomized trial comparing combination chemotherapy regimens (Hexa-CAF vs CHAP-5) in advanced ovarian carcinoma. J Clin Oncol 5:1157, 1987.

160. PIVER MS et al: The impact of aggressive debulking surgery and

cisplatin-based chemotherapy on progression-free survival in stage III and IV ovarian carcinoma. J Clin Oncol 6:983, 1988.

161. BARNHILL DR et al: The second-look surgical reassessment for epithelial ovarian carcinoma. Gynecol Oncol 19:148, 1984.

162. POTTER ME et al: Primary surgical therapy of ovarian cancer: How much and when. Gynecol Oncol 40:195, 1991.

163. WEBER AM, KENNEDY AW: The role of bowel resection in the primary surgical debulking of carcinoma of the ovary. J Ann Coll Surg 179:465, 1994.

164. BRISTOW RE et al: Survival impact of surgical cytoreduction in stage IV epithelial ovarian cancer. Gynecol Oncol 72:278, 1999.

165. CURTIN JP et al: Stage IV ovarian cancer: Impact of surgical debulking. Gynecol Oncol 64:9, 1997.

166. SOPER JT et al: The role of partial sigmoid colectomy for debulking epithelial ovarian carcinoma. Gynecol Oncol 41:239, 1991.

167. KIGAWA J et al: Evaluation of cytoreductive surgery with lymphadenectomy including para-aortic nodes for advanced ovarian cancer. Eur J Surg Oncol 19:273, 1993.

168. SCARABELLI C et al: Systematic pelvic and para-aortic lymphadenectomy during cytoreductive surgery in advanced ovarian cancer: Potential benefit on survival. Gynecol Oncol 56:328, 1995.

169. KIKKAWA F et al: Prognostic evaluation of lymphadenectomy for epithelial ovarian cancer. J Surg Oncol 60:227, 1995.

170. DI RE F et al: Systemic pelvic and paraaortic lymphadenectomy for advanced ovarian cancer: Prognostic significance of node metastases. Gynecol Oncol 62:360, 1996.

171. YOUNG RL et al: Adjuvant therapy in stage I and stage II epithelial ovarian cancer: Results of two prospective randomized trials. N Engl J Med 322:1021, 1990.

172. OMURA G et al: A randomized trial of cyclophosphamide and doxorubicin with or without cisplatin in advanced ovarian carcinoma. A Gynecologic Oncology Group Study. Cancer 57:1725, 1986.

173. DECKER DG et al: Cyclophosphamide plus cis-platinum in combination: Treatment program for stage III or IV ovarian carcinoma. Obstet Gynecol 60:481, 1982.

174. OMURA GA et al: Randomized trial of cyclophosphamide plus cisplatin with or without doxorubicin in ovarian carcinoma: A Gynecologic Oncology Group Study. J Clin Oncol 7:457, 1989.

175. OMURA GA et al: CP versus CAP chemotherapy of ovarian carcinoma: A meta-analysis. J Clin Oncol 9:1668, 1991.

176. REED E et al: Platinum-DNA adducts in leukocyte DNA correlate with disease response in ovarian cancer patients receiving platinum-based chemotherapy. Proc Natl Acad Sci USA 84:5024, 1987.

177. ROZENZWEIG M et al: Randomized trial of carboplatin versus cisplatin in advanced ovarian cancer, in Carboplatin: Current Perspectives and Future Directions, Bunn PA et al (eds). Philadelphia, Saunders, 1990, p 95.

178. HAKES T et al: Randomized prospective trial of 5 versus 10 cycles of cyclophosphamide, doxorubicin and cisplatin (CAP) in stage III and IV ovarian cancer. Proc ASCO 9:156, 1990.

179. BERTELSEN K et al: A prospective randomized comparison of 6 and 12 cycles of cyclophosphamide, adriamycin, and cisplatin in advanced epithelial ovarian cancer: A Danish Ovarian Study Group trial (DACOVA). Gynecol Oncol 49:30, 1993.

180. MENCZER J et al: Abdominopelvic irradiation for stage II–IV ovarian carcinoma patients with limited or no residual disease at second-look laparotomy after completion of cisplatinum-

based combination chemotherapy. Gynecol Oncol 24:149, 1986.

181. MCGUIRE WP et al: A phase III trial comparing cisplatin/cytoxan (PC) and cisplatin/taxol (PI) in advanced ovarian cancer (AOC) (Abstr 808). Proc ASCO 12:255, 1993.

182. MCGUIRE WP et al: Taxol and cisplatin (TP) improves outcome in advanced ovarian cancer (AOC) as compared to cytoxan and cisplatin (CP) (Abstr 771). Proc ASCO 14:275, 1995.

183. OZOLS RF et al: Phase I and pharmacokinetic study of taxol (T) and carboplatin C in previously untreated patients (PTS) with advanced epithelial ovarian cancer (OC): A pilot study of the Gynecologic Oncology Group (Abstr 824). Proc ASCO 12:259, 1993.

184. BOOKMAN MA et al: Carboplatin and paclitaxel in ovarian carcinoma: A phase I study of the Gynecologic Oncology Group. J Clin Oncol 14:1895, 1996.

185. ALBERTS DS et al: Intraperitoneal cisplatin plus intravenous cyclophosphamide versus intravenous cisplatin plus intravenous cyclophosphamide for stage III ovarian cancer. N Engl J Med 335:1950, 1996.

186. ABU-RUSTUM NR et al: Second-look operation for epithelial ovarian cancer: Laparoscopy or laparotomy? Obstet Gynecol 88:549, 1996.

187. WALTON L et al: Results of second-look laparotomy in patients with early-stage ovarian carcinoma. Obstet Gynecol 70:770, 1987.

188. NILOFF JM et al: Predictive value of CA 125 antigen levels in second-look procedures for ovarian cancer. Am J Obstet Gynecol 151:981, 1985.

189. RUBIN SC et al: Serum CA 125 levels and surgical findings in patients undergoing secondary operations for epithelial ovarian cancer. Am J Obstet Gynecol 160:667, 1989.

190. BEREK JS et al: CA 125 serum levels correlated with second-look operations among ovarian cancer patients. Obstet Gynecol 67:685, 1986.

191. LUND B et al: Correlation of abdominal ultrasound and computed tomography scans with second- or third-look laparotomy in patients with ovarian carcinoma. Gynecol Oncol 37:279, 1990.

192. BRENNER DE et al: Abdominopelvic computed tomography: Evaluation in patients undergoing second-look laparotomy for ovarian carcinoma. Obstet Gynecol 65:715, 1985.

193. OZOLS RF et al: Epithelial ovarian cancer, in Principles and Practice of Gynecologic Oncology, WJ Hoskins et al (eds). Philadelphia, Lippincott, 1992, p 731.

194. BEREK JS et al: Second-look laparotomy in stage III epithelial ovarian cancer: Clinical variables associated with disease status. Obstet Gynecol 64:207, 1984.

195. SCHWARTZ PS, SMITH JP: Second look operation in ovarian cancer. Am J Obstet Gynecol 138:1124, 1980.

196. PODRATZ KC et al: Second-look laparotomy in ovarian cancer: Evaluation of pathologic variables. Am J Obstet Gynecol 152:230, 1985.

197. COPELAND LJ et al: Microscopic disease at second-look laparotomy in advanced ovarian cancer. Cancer 55:472, 1985.

198. RUBIN SC et al: Prognostic factors for recurrence following negative second-look laparotomy in ovarian cancer patients treated with platinum-based chemotherapy. Gynecol Oncol 42:137, 1991.

199. HOSKINS WJ et al: Influence of secondary cytoreduction at the time of second look laparotomy on the survival of patients with epithelial ovarian cancer. Gynecol Oncol 34:365, 1989.

200. LIPPMAN SM et al: Second look laparotomy in epithelial ovarian cancer: Prognostic factors associated with survival duration. Cancer 61:2571, 1988.

201. PODRATZ KC et al: Evaluation of treatment and survival after positive second look laparotomy. Gynecol Oncol 31:9, 1988.

202. MORRIS M et al: Secondary cytoreductive surgery in epithelial ovarian cancer: Nonresponders to first line-therapy. Gynecol Oncol 33:1, 1989.

203. BRUZZONE M et al: Chemotherapy versus radiotherapy in the management of ovarian cancer patients with pathological complete response or minimal residual disease at second look. Gynecol Oncol 38:392, 1990.

204. BARAKAT RR et al: A phase II trial of intraperitoneal cisplatin and etoposide as consolidation therapy in patients with Stage II–IV epithelial ovarian cancer following negative surgical assessment. Gynecol Oncol 69:17, 1998.

205. MARKMAN M: Intraperitoneal therapy of ovarian cancer. Semin Oncol 25:356, 1998.

206. HACKER NF et al: Whole abdominal radiation as salvage therapy for epithelial ovarian cancer. Obstet Gynecol 65:60, 1985.

207. PETERS WA 3d et al: Salvage therapy with whole-abdominal irradiation in patients with advanced carcinoma of the ovary previously treated by combination chemotherapy. Cancer 58:880, 1986.

208. SMITH JP et al: Postoperative treatment of early cancer of the ovary: A random trial between postoperative irradiation and chemotherapy. Natl Cancer Inst Monogr 42:149, 1975.

209. GERSHENSON DM et al: Re-treatment of patients with recurrent epithelial ovarian cancer with cisplatin-based chemotherapy. Obstet Gynecol 73:798, 1989.

210. REICHMAN B et al: Intraperitoneal cisplatin and etoposide in the treatment of refractory/recurrent ovarian carcinoma. J Clin Oncol 7:1327, 1989.

211. CANETTA R et al: Carboplatin: Current status and future prospects. Cancer Treat Rev 15(Suppl B):17, 1988.

212. OZOLS RF et al: High dose carboplatin in refractory ovarian cancer patients. J Clin Oncol 5:197, 1987.

213. GORE ME et al: Treatment of relapsed carcinoma of the ovary with cisplatin or carboplatin following initial treatment with these compounds. Gynecol Oncol 36:207, 1990.

214. THIGPEN JT et al: New drugs and experimental approaches in ovarian cancer treatment. Semin Oncol 11:314, 1984.

215. MYERS AM et al: Advanced ovarian carcinoma: Response to antiestrogen therapy. Cancer 48:2368, 1981.

216. SCHWARTZ PE et al: Tamoxifen therapy for advanced ovarian cancer. Obstet Gynecol 59:583, 1982.

217. BOOKMAN MA et al: Topotecan for the treatment of advanced epithelial ovarian cancer: An open-label phase II study in patients treated after prior chemotherapy that contained cisplatin or carboplatin and paclitaxel. J Clin Oncol 16:3345, 1998.

218. LUND B et al: Phase II study of gemcitabine in previously platinum-treated ovarian cancer patients. Anticancer Drugs 6(Suppl):61, 1996.

219. PETERS GJ et al: Interaction between cisplatin and gemcitabine in vitro and in vivo. Semin Oncol 22(Suppl 11):72, 1995.

220. MUGGIA FM: Clinical efficacy and prospects for use of pegylated liposomal doxorubicin in the treatment of ovarian and breast cancers. Drugs 54(Suppl 4):22, 1997.

221. JACOB JH et al: Neoadjuvant chemotherapy and interval de-

222. WILS J et al: Primary or delayed debulking surgery and chemotherapy consisting of cisplatin, doxorubicin, and cyclophosphamide in stage III and IV epithelial ovarian carcinoma. J Clin Oncol 4:1068, 1986.

223. VANDER BURG MEL et al: The effect of debulking surgery after induction chemotherapy on the prognosis of advanced epithelial ovarian cancer. N Engl J Med 332:669, 1995.

224. BLYTHE JG, WAHL TP: Debulking surgery: Does it increase the quality of survival? Gynecol Oncol 14:396, 1982.

225. SEGNA RA et al: Secondary cytoreduction for ovarian cancer following cisplatin therapy. J Clin Oncol 11:434, 1993.

226. FIORENTINO MV et al: Randomized study of redebulking in epithelial ovarian cancer (abstr). Proc ASCO 12:A854, 1993.

227. RUBIN SC et al: Palliative surgery for intestinal obstruction in advanced ovarian cancer. Gynecol Oncol 34:16, 1989.

228. KREBS HB, GOPLERUD DR: Surgical management of bowel obstruction in advanced ovarian carcinoma. Obstet Gynecol 61:327, 1983.

229. CLARKE-PEARSON DL et al: Intestinal obstruction in patients with ovarian cancer: Variables associated with surgical complications and survival. Arch Surg 123:42, 1988.

230. FERNANDES JR et al: Bowel obstruction in patients with ovarian cancer: A search for prognostic factors. Am J Obstet Gynecol 158(2):244, 1988.

231. CAREY M et al: Testing the validity of a prognostic classification in patients with surgically optimal ovarian carcinoma: A 15 year review. Int J Gynecol Cancer 3:24, 1993.

232. SOUTER RG et al: Surgical and pathologic complications associated with peritoneovenous shunts in management of malignant ascites. Cancer 55:1973, 1985.

233. DEMBO AJ: Abdominopelvic radiotherapy in ovarian cancer: A 1-year experience. Cancer 55:2285, 1985.

234. OMURA G et al: Randomized trial of cyclophosphamide plus cisplatin with or without doxorubicin in ovarian carcinoma: A Gynecologic Oncology Group study. J Clin Oncol 7:457, 1989.

235. FUKS Z et al: The multimodal approach to the treatment of stage III ovarian carcinoma. J Clin Oncol 5:897, 1987.

236. LEDERMANN JA et al: Outcome of patients with unfavorable optimally cytoreduced ovarian cancer treated with chemotherapy and whole abdominal radiation. Gynecol Oncol 41:30, 1991.

237. MORTON G, THOMAS GM: Role of radiotherapy in the treatment of cancer of the ovary. Semin Surg Oncol 10:305, 1994.

238. ADELSON MD et al: Palliative radiotherapy for ovarian cancer. Int J Radiat Oncol Biol Phys 13:17, 1986.

239. MAY LF et al: Palliative benefit of radiation therapy in advanced ovarian cancer. Gynecol Oncol 37:408, 1990.

240. CORN BW et al: Recurrent ovarian cancer: Effective radiotherapeutic palliation after chemotherapy failure. Cancer 74:2979, 1994.

241. BARAKAT RR et al: Salvage intraperitoneal therapy of advanced epithelial ovarian cancer: Impact of retroperitoneal nodal disease. Eur J Gynaecol Oncol 18:161, 1997.

242. WOODRUFF JD et al: Metastatic ovarian tumors. Am J Obstet Gynecol 107:202, 1970.

243. MARCHETTI M et al: Malignant ovarian tumors: Conservative surgery and quality of life in young patients. Eur J Gynaecol Oncol 19:297, 1998.

244. ZANETTA G et al: Conservative surgery for stage I ovarian carcinoma in women of childbearing age. Br J Obstet Gynaecol 104:1030, 1997.

245. SHIBAHARA H et al: A case of a patient diagnosed with malignant mixed Mullerian tumor of the ovary who concieved after conservative surgery and adjuvant chemotherapy. Gynecol Oncol 65:363, 1997.

246. TAYLOR HC: Malignant and semimalignant tumor of the ovary. Surg Gynecol Obstet 48:702, 1929.

247. Hopkins MP et al: An assessment of pathologic features and treatments modalities in ovarian tumors of low malignant potential. Obstet Gynecol 70:923, 1987.

248. KOLSTAD P et al: Individualized treatment of ovarian cancer. Am J Obstet Gynecol 128:617, 1977.

249. AURE JC et al: Clinical and histologic studies of ovarian carcinoma. Obstet Gynecol 37:1, 1971.

250. KLIMAN L et al: Low malignant potential tumors of the ovary. A study of 76 cases. Obstet Gynecol 68:338, 1986.

251. CHAMBERS JT et al: Borderline ovarian tumors. Am J Obstet Gynecol 159:1088, 1988.

252. GOTLIEB WH et al: Rates of Jewish ancestral mutations in BRCA1 and BRCA2 in borderline ovarian tumors. J Natl Cancer Inst 90:995, 1998.

253. YOUNG RC et al: Staging laparotomy in early ovarian cancer. JAMA 250:3072, 1983.

254. CREASMAN WT et al: Stage I borderline ovarian tumors. Obstet Gynecol 59:93, 1982.

255. CHAMBERS JT: Borderline ovarian tumors: A review of treatment. Yale J Biol Med 62:351, 1989.

256. SUTTON GP: Ovarian tumors of low malignant potential in ovarian cancer, in *Ovarian Cancer,* Rubin SC, Sutton GP (eds). New York, NY, McGraw-Hill, 1993, pp 425–449.

257. KAERN J et al: Cellular DNA content as a new prognostic tool in patients with borderline tumors of the ovary. Gynecol Oncol 38:452, 1990.

258. DRESCHER CW et al: Prognostic significance of DNA content and nuclear morphology in borderline ovarian tumors. Gynecol Oncol 48:242, 1993.

259. PADBERG B-C et al: DNA cytophotometry and prognosis in ovarian tumors of borderline malignacy. Cancer 69:2510, 1992.

260. SEIDMAN JD, KURMAN RJ: Subclassification of serous borderline tumors of the ovary into benign and malignant types. A clinicopathologic study of 65 advanced stage cases. Am J Surg Pathol 20:1331, 1996.

261. BELL DA, SCULLY RE: Clinical perspective on borderine tumors of the ovary, in *Current Topics in Obstetrics and Gynecology,* Hale RW (ed). New York, NY, Elsevier, 1991, 119–134.

262. YAZIGI R et al: Primary staging in ovarian tumors of low malignant potential. Gynecol Oncol 31:402, 1988.

263. LEAKE JF et al: Retroperitoneal lymphatic involvement with epithelial ovarian tumors of low malignant potential. Gynecol Oncol 42:124, 1991.

264. NATION JG, KREPART GV: Ovarian carcinoma of low malignant potential: Staging and treatment. Am J Obstet Gynecol 154:290, 1986.

265. SUTTON GP et al: Stage III ovarian tumors of low malignant potential treated with cisplatin combination therapy (a Gynecologic Oncology Group study). Gynecol Oncol 41:230, 1991.

266. BOSTWICK DG et al: Ovarian epithelial tumors of borderline malignancy. Cancer 58:2052, 1986.

267. TAZELAAR HD et al: Conservative treatment of borderline ovarian tumors. Obstet Gynecol 66:417, 1985.

268. MUNNELL EW: Is conservative therapy ever justified in stage I (IA) cancer of the ovary? Am J Obstet Gynecol 103:641, 1969.

269. HART WR, NORRIS HJ: Borderline and malignant mucinous tumors of the ovary: Histologic criteria and clinical behavior. Cancer 31:1031, 1973.

270. RUSSELL P, MERKUR H: Proliferative ovarian "epithelial" tumors: A clinicopatholigical analysis of 144 cases. Aust NZJ Obstet Gynaecol 19:45, 1979.

271. LIM-TAN SK et al: Ovarian cysectomy for seous borderline tumors: A follow-up study for 35 cases. Obstet Gynecol 72:775, 1988.

272. TROPE C, KAERN J: Management of borderline tumors of the ovary: State of the art. Semin Oncol 25:372, 1998.

273. MASSAD LS JR et al: Epithelial ovarian tumors of low malignant potential. Obstet Gynecol 78:1027, 1991.

274. CREASMAN WT et al: Stage I borderline ovarian tumors. Obstet Gynecol 59:93, 1982.

275. BARNHILL D et al: Epithelial ovarian carcinoma of low malignant potential. Obstet Gynecol 65:53, 1985.

276. BOSTWICK DG et al: Ovarian epithelial tumors of borderline malignancy. Cancer 58:2052, 1986.

277. O'QUINN AG, HANNIGAN EV: Epithelial ovarian neoplasms of low malignant potential. Gynecol Oncol 21:177, 1985.

278. MANCHUL LA et al: Borderline epithelial ovarian tumors: A review of 81 cases with an assessment of the impact of treatment. Int J Radiat Oncol Biol Phys 22:867, 1992.

279. TAMAKOSHI K et al: Clinical behavior of borderline ovarian tumors: A study of 150 cases. J Surg Oncol 64:147, 1997.

280. FORT MG et al: Evidence for the efficacy of adjuvant therapy in epithelial ovarian tumors of low malignant potential. Gynecol Oncol 32:269, 1989.

281. GERSHENSON DM, SILVA EG: Serous ovarian tumors of low malignant potential with peritoneal implants. Cancer 65:578, 1990.

282. BARAKAT RR et al: Platinum-based chemotherapy for advanced-stage serous ovarian carcinoma of low malignant potential. Gynecol Oncol 59:390, 1995.

283. NIKRUI N: Survey of clinical behavior of patients with borderline epithelial tumors of the ovary. Gynecol Oncol 12:107, 1981.

284. WERTH R: Pseudomyxoma peritonei. Arch Gynecol Obstet 24:100, 1984.

285. FRAENKEL E: Uber das sogennante pseudomyxoma peritonei. Munch Med Wschr 48:965, 1901.

286. MASSON JC, HAMRICK RA: Pseudomyxoma peritonei of ovarian origin: An analysis of thirty cases. Surg Clin North Am 10:61, 1930.

287. RUSSELL P: The pathological assessment of ovarian neoplasms. I. Introduction to the common "epithelial" tumors and analysis of benign "epithelial" tumors. Pathology 11:5, 1979.

288. RUSSELL P: The pathological assessment of ovarian neoplasms. II. The proliferating "epithelial" tumors. Pathology 11:251, 1979.

289. RUSSELL O: The pathological assessment of ovarian neoplasms. III. The malignant "epithelial" tumors. Pathology 11:493, 1979.

290. MICHAEL H et al: Ovarian carcinoma with extracellular mucin production: Reassessment of "pseudomyxoma ovarii et peritonei." Int J Gynecol Pathol 6:298, 1987.

291. LIMBER GK et al: Pseudomyxoma peritonei: A report of ten cases. Ann Surg 178:587, 1973.

292. FERNANDEZ RN, DALY JM: Pseudomyxoma peritonei. Arch Surg 115:409, 1980.

293. JONES CM, HOMESLEY HD: Successful treatment of pseudomyxoma peritonei of ovarian origin with cisplatin, doxorubicin, and cyclophosphamide. Gynecol Oncol 22:257, 1985.

294. Sugarbaker PH et al: Malignant pseudomyxoma peritonei of colonic origin: Natural history and presentation of a curative approach to treatment. Dis Colon Rectum 30:772, 1987.

295. Green N et al: Pseudomyxoma peritonei of appendiceal origin: Clinicopathologic aspects. Am J Surg 109:235, 1965.

296. Freel JH et al: Dysgerminoma of the ovary. Cancer 43:798, 1979.

297. Gordon A et al: Dysgerminoma: A review of 158 cases from the Emil Novak Ovarian Tumor Registry. Obstet Gynecol 58:497, 1981.

298. Williams SD et al: Adjuvant therapy of ovarian germ cell tumors with cisplatin, etoposide, and bleomycin: A trial of the Gynecologic Oncology Group. J Clin Oncol 12:701, 1994.

299. Gershenson DM et al: Treatment of malignant germ cell tumors of the ovary with bleomycin, etoposide, and cisplatin. J Clin Oncol 8:715, 1990.

300. Slayton RE: Management of germ cell and stromal tumors of the ovary. Semin Oncol 11:299, 1984.

301. Gershenson DM et al: Second-look laparotomy in the management of malignant germ cell tumors of the ovary. Obstet Gynecol 67:789, 1986.

302. Thomas GM et al: Current therapy for dysgerminoma of the ovary. Obstet Gynecol 70:268, 1987.

303. Curry SL et al: Malignant teratoma of the ovary: prognostic factors and treatment. Am J Obstet Gynecol 131:845, 1978.

304. Loehrer P et al: Salvage therapy in recurrent germ cell cancer: Salvage therapy in recurrent germ cell cancer: Ifosfamide and cisplatin plus either vinblastine or etoposide. Ann Intern Med 109:540, 1988.

305. Bjorkholm E, Pettersson F: Granulosa-cell and theca cell tumors: The clinical picture and long-term outcome for the Radiumhemmet series. Acta Obstet Gynecol Scand 59:361, 1980.

306. Fox H et al: A clinicopathologic study of 92 cases of granulosa cell tumor of the ovary with special reference to the factors influencing prognosis. Cancer 35:231, 1975.

307. Swerdlow M: Mesothelioma of the pelvic peritoneum resembling papillary cystodeoncarcinoma of the ovary. Am J Obstet Gynecol 77:197, 1959.

308. Ordonez NG: Role of the immunohistochemosatry in distinguishing epithelial peritoneal mesotheliomas from peritoneal and ovarian serous carcinomas. Am J Surg Pathol 22:1203, 1998.

309. Dalrymple JC et al: Extraovarian peritoneal serous papillary carcinoma: A cliniopathologic study of 31 cases. Cancer 64:110, 1989.

310. Eltabbakh GH et al: Epidemiologic differences between women with borderline ovarian tumors and women with epithelial ovarian cancer. Gynecol Oncol 74:103, 1991.

311. Badera CA et al: BRCA1 gene mutations in women with papillary serous carcinoma of the peritoneum. Obstet Gynecol 92:596, 1998.

312. Altaras MM et al: Primary peritoneal papillary serous adenocarcinoma: clinical and management aspects. Gynecol Oncol 40:230, 1991.

313. Bloss JD et al: Extraovarian peritoneal serous papillary carcinoma: A case-control retrospective comparison to papillary adenocarcinoma of the ovary. Gynecol Oncol 50:347, 1993.

314. Taus P et al: Primary serous papillary carcinoma of the peritoneum: A report of 18 patients. Eur J Gynaecol Oncol 18:171, 1997.

315. Ben-Barouch G et al: Primary peritoneal serous papillary carcinoma: A study of 25 cases and comparison with stage III-IV ovarian papillary serous carcinoma. Gynecol Oncol 60:393, 1996.

316. Piura B et al: Peritoneal papillary serous carcinoma: Study of 15 cases and comparison with stage III-IV ovarian papillary serous carcinoma. J Surg Oncol 68:173, 1998.

317. Killackey MA, Davis AR: Papillary serous carcinoma of the peritoneal surface: Matched-case comparison with papillary serous ovarian carcinoma. Gynecol Oncol 51:171, 1993.

318. Gershenson D: Malignant germ cell tumors of the ovary: Clinical features and management, in Gynecologic Oncology, M Coppleson (ed). London, Churchill Livingstone, 1992, p 936.

319. Tlaerman A: Germ cell tumors of the ovary, in Blaustein's Pathology of the Female Genital Tract, RJ Kurman (ed). New York, Springer-Verlag, 1987, p 659.

# CHAPTER 19

# NEOPLASMS OF THE BREAST

*Maureen A. Chung and Kirby I. Bland*

Breast cancer is a prevalent and devastating disease. Worldwide, it is the most frequent cancer in women,[1] accounting for 16% and 11%, respectively, of all cancer deaths of women in developed and developing countries.[2] In the United States, one woman in eight will develop breast cancer during her lifetime.[3] This chapter presents an overview of the diagnosis and treatment of breast cancer, including discussions on the controversy of screening mammography, treatment of minimally invasive breast cancer, and optimal management of the clinically negative axilla. The final section reviews the management of special cases of breast cancer, including the clinically occult breast cancer, phyllodes tumors, male breast cancer, Paget's disease of the nipple, and pregnancy-associated breast cancer.

## RISK FACTORS

Sex and age are the two most important risk factors for breast cancer, which is predominantly a malignancy of postmenopausal women. In North America, the incidence of breast cancer is 1 in 217 for women under the age of 39, and rapidly increases to 1 in 14 for women aged 60 to 79 years. This risk is further modified by age at menarche and menopause, as well as age at first pregnancy. Since it is known that breast cancers have estrogen receptors and antiestrogen therapy has been used in the treatment of this malignancy, it has been suggested that endogenous and exogenous estrogen exposure is an important factor in breast cancer carcinogenesis. The relative risk in women who receive estrogen replacement after menopause has been evaluated extensively. In a recent meta-analysis of 51 studies involving more than 150,000 subjects,[4] the risk of breast cancer was found to be 1.14, as compared to women who had never received hormonal replacement therapy. This risk was increased with prolonged estrogen use; 5 years of replacement therapy being associated with 1 extra breast cancer for 1000 users. After 13 years of hormonal replacement, there was 1 extra breast cancer case for every 100 users. There is also a small increase for women who use birth control pills for more than 10 years.[5] However, exposure to environmental estrogens in the form of 1,1-dichloro-2,2-bis( *p*-chlorophenyl)ethylene

(DDE) and polychlorinated biphenyls (PCBs) does not appear to increase breast cancer risk.[6]

Carcinogenesis is an interplay between the genetic make-up of the individual and his or her environment, with genetic factors thought to contribute to 30% of cases diagnosed before the age of 30. If a first-degree relative has breast cancer, the relative risk is 1.7, and this risk increases threefold if there was premenopausal onset of this malignancy. If the breast cancer was bilateral, the relative risk increases fivefold.[7] Aside from this genetic influence on carcinogenesis in sporadic breast cancer, there are true hereditary breast cancers and breast cancer syndromes. Hereditary breast cancers constitute approximately 5% to 10% of all breast cancers and can be suspected if onset is at an earlier age when compared to the general population, multiple family members are affected, and the cancer is multifocal with an increased incidence of bilateral involvement. Table 19-1 outlines the hereditary breast cancer syndromes that are currently known. Some of the difficulty in studying these syndromes and distinguishing hereditary breast cancers from sporadic cancers with a strong family history results from the degree of phenotypic variation that is present in hereditary breast cancers.[8]

Much of the recent focus on hereditary breast cancer has involved two genes, *BRCA1* and *BRCA2. BRCA1,* a large gene with more than 100 identified mutations, influences susceptibility to breast and ovarian cancer and is located on chromosome 17.[9] *BRCA1* is a tumor suppressor gene and is inherited in an autosomal dominant manner. The coding region for *BRCA1* measures over 7.8 kilobase (kB). Because of its size, sequencing the entire gene is time-consuming, and, therefore, diagnostic tests to identify *BRCA1* mutations have focused on mutations most frequently identified in hereditary breast cancer. This has created some difficulty in understanding a negative result from commercially available kits designed to identify patients with *BRCA1* mutations. Furthermore, the coding sequence of *BRCA1* contains many genetic polymorphisms that have no detrimental effect on function.[10] Therefore, even if the gene is sequenced in its entirety and an abnormality is identified, unless the mutation has been previously reported, the "abnormality" may represent a genetic polymorphism. *BRCA1* has been reported to be involved with

**TABLE 19-1.** HEREDITARY BREAST CANCERS AND CANCER SYNDROMES: OUTLINE OF GENETIC MUTATIONS IN HEREDITARY CANCERS AND THE PROPOSED FUNCTION OF THE INVOLVED GENES

| MUTATION | POSITION | ACTION | CANCER |
|---|---|---|---|
| p53 | ch17p13 | Apoptosis, transcription factor, cell cycle | Li-Fraumeni syndrome: Colorectal and breast carcinomas, sarcomas |
| BRCA1 | ch17q21 | Transcription activation | Breast and ovarian cancer |
| BRCA2 | ch13q12-13 | Transcription activation | Breast cancer (male and female) |
| MSH2 | 2p22 | DNA repair | HNPCC: Syndrome with predominance of colon cancer, but also associated with endometrial, breast, urinary tract, and ovarian cancers |
| hMLH1 | 3p21-23 | DNA repair | HNPCC |
| HPMS1 | 2q31-33 | DNA repair | HNPCC |
| HPMS2 | 7q22 | DNA repair | HNPCC |
| PTEN (MMAC1) | ch10q23 | Tumor suppressor | Cowden disease: Syndrome with elevated risk for breast, thyroid, skin neoplasms |

cell cycle regulation through its association with the cyclin independent kinase inhibitor, p21.[11] BRCA1 may also be involved with DNA repair mechanisms.[12]

BRCA2, the second gene known to cause a breast cancer predisposition, has been mapped to chromosome 13.[13] Different from BRCA1, BRCA2 mutations are associated with breast cancer alone, but also lead to a predisposition of male breast cancer. Ashkenazi Jews are predisposed to having BRCA2 mutations. Studies of this population have concluded that approximately 2% are carriers of the mutation, and carriers have a 56% chance of developing breast cancer through the age of 70.[14] The coding region for BRCA2 is twice as long as that for BRCA1, making it less amenable for genetic testing. BRCA2 has also been reported to be important for DNA repair and integrity.[15]

The prevalence of BRCA1 and BRCA2 mutations in the general population is not known. It has been estimated that 16% of patients with a strong family history or an early age at onset of breast cancer will have a BRCA1 mutation.[16] BRCA2 mutations have been found at a lower frequency.[17] The cumulative risk of breast cancer in women with a germline mutation of one of these genes has been estimated to range from 40% to 85%.

Unlike other genetic mutations, BRCA1 and BRCA2 mutations have been rarely identified in sporadic breast cancers. This discrepancy may partially be explained by the "caretaker, gatekeeper" hypothesis. As cells proliferate, mutations in the DNA are constantly occurring. The majority of these mutations are recognized by "caretaker genes" and the DNA errors repaired. BRCA1 and BRCA2 are examples of gatekeeper genes. Their role is to maintain DNA integrity by identifying and repairing errors in the DNA. If these genes are mutated, errors in the DNA may accumulate, including mutations in "caretaker" genes. It is the accumulation of mutations in the caretaker genes that results in carcinogenesis.

Less frequent hereditary syndromes involving breast cancer are the Li-Fraumeni syndrome, Cowden disease, ataxia-telangectasia, and hereditary nonpolyposis colon cancer (HNPCC). The Li-Fraumeni syndrome is due to an inherited mutation in p53, a tumor suppressor gene that has been widely implicated in sporadic human cancers. Patients who have an inherited mutation in this gene are predisposed to the development of soft tissue sarcomas and osteosarcomas, breast cancer, adrenocortical cancer, brain tumors, and leukemias. Li-Fraumeni syndrome accounts for about 1% of breast cancers diagnosed before the age of 40.[18] Cowden syndrome is a rare genetic disorder that includes breast cancer predisposition.[19] It is transmitted in an autosomal fashion. The candidate gene responsible for Cowden disease is PTEN. PTEN, also known as MMAC1,[20] behaves like a tumor suppressor gene and maps to chromosome 10q23.[21] Ataxia-telangectasia results from a genetic defect in DNA repair. It is unclear if patients with this disease are at an increased risk for breast cancer.[22,23] HNPCC is also a genetic disease resulting from a mutation in genes important for the recognition and repair of DNA damage. It is associated predominantly with an increased incidence of colon cancer. However, this syndrome is also associated with an increase in endometrial, ovarian, urinary tract, and breast cancers.[24]

Despite advances in molecular biology and the continual identification of genes implicated in carcinogenesis, it is probable that there are other genes, not yet identified, which play an important role in hereditary breast cancer. In a recent study of 100 breast and breast-ovarian families in Finland, only 21% of these breast cancer families had identifiable mutations or linkage to BRCA1 or BRCA2.[25] These data indicate that other genes are likely to be important in hereditary breast cancer.

Because breast cancer is found predominantly in developed countries, a high-fat, low-fiber diet, alcohol use, and sedentary lifestyle have been implicated as risk factors for this malignancy. In 1976, the Nurses Health Study was initiated in the United States and data collected prospectively on more than 100,000 nurses living in 11 states. Through questionnaires, follow-up has been collected every 2 years. Data from this study indicate that there was no relationship between fat intake and breast cancer.[26] However, an increase in body mass index to 31 kg/m$^2$ resulted in a 1.59 relative risk of breast cancer.[27] This increased risk was limited to postmenopausal women, indicating that weight gain alone does not cause breast cancer. While vegetable and fruit consumption have suggested an inverse relationship to breast cancer risk, indicating the potential importance of micronutrient composition in this disease,[28] alcohol consumption equivalent to two drinks per day has been associated with a 25% increase in risk.[29]

The risk of breast cancer after a benign breast biopsy depends on the histological characteristics of the breast tissue. Nonproliferative breast biopsies are not associated with a subsequently increased incidence of breast cancer. Proliferative changes on a breast biopsy, however, such as moderate or florid hyperplasia, papilloma with fibrovascular core or atypical ductal or lobular hyperplasia, are associated with an increased cancer risk.[30] Data from the Nurses' Health Study[31] indicate that a benign breast biopsy for atypical hyperplasia is associated with a relative risk of breast cancer of 3.7. When stratified according to menopausal status, premenopausal women with atypical hyperplasia of the breast had a relative risk for breast cancer of 5.9; the risk for postmenopausal women was 2.3. A personal history of breast cancer is an important risk factor for the development of a subsequent breast malignancy, estimated to be as high as 1% per year from the time of diagnosis of the initial cancer. The interrelationship between known risk factors is summarized in Table 19-2. For example, the relative breast cancer risk with atypical hyperplasia is 3.7. For atypical hyperplasia, in the presence of a family history positive for breast cancer, the relative breast cancer risk increases to 7.3. The ability to identify women with increased relative risk for breast cancer is important not only because these women need to be followed closely with mammography and clinical examinations, but also because they become candidates for breast cancer prevention treatments (see later section on breast cancer prevention in this chapter).

Another known risk factor for breast cancer is previous radiation exposure (e.g., for Hodgkin's disease). In a retrospective multicenter analysis of women treated with radiotherapy plus or minus

chemotherapy for Hodgkin's disease, 63 women developed breast cancer.[32] Breast cancer occurred after a median interval of 16 years, and 13 women had bilateral breast cancer. The breast cancers fell into two groups: lesions detected at an earlier stage with a slow tumor doubling time, and other cancers diagnosed at a later stage that were highly aggressive. Therefore, women who have a history of Hodgkin's disease, and who have been treated with mantle radiation, should be considered at an increased risk for breast cancer development. These women should have yearly mammography starting approximately 8 years after irradiation.[33]

Breast cancer is a multifactorial disease. Since the contribution and interaction of the known risk factors to cancer causation and progression are unknown, it is difficult to interpret the contribution of each respective risk factor. With the exception of the hereditary breast cancers, it is difficult to assess an individual woman's breast cancer risk. It would, however, seem prudent to eliminate lifestyle risk factors as a possible aid in decreasing this risk.[34]

## DIAGNOSIS

A diagnosis of breast cancer is usually suspected by finding a suspicious lump during breast examination or by abnormalities present on a mammogram. In the past, the majority of breast cancers were detected by breast examination, done either by the patient or by the physician as part of a physical examination. With the increased availability of mammography, there has been an increase in the detection of breast cancers before they can be palpated on breast examination. The importance of breast self-examination should not be minimized, however, since when done correctly, risk of death from breast cancer may be reduced.[35]

Since tumor size is an important prognostic indicator of outcome in breast cancer, and detection of breast cancer at a nonpalpable stage usually denotes a smaller tumor size or an in situ lesion, mammographic screening of breast cancer has become more widespread. Breast cancer screening has resulted in a decreased mortality rate from this disease in women over 50 years of age.[36] Current recommendations for women in this age group include monthly self breast examinations and an annual physical examination by a physician coupled with screening mammography. However, screening mammography is more controversial for women under the age of 50 with no known risk factors for breast cancer. This controversy became apparent in the early 1990s when the National Cancer Institute changed its guidelines to not recommend routine screening for women aged 40 to 49 years of age.[37] The change in recommendation was partly a result of the Canadian National Breast Screening Study (CNBSS),[38] which concluded that there was no benefit for routine breast cancer screening in women aged 40 to 49 years. This issue was further addressed at the National Institutes of Health (NIH) Consensus Development Conference in early 1997, where an update of the eight randomized trials addressing this issue was presented.[39] Five of these trials were conducted in Sweden[40] (Kopparberg, Ostergotland, Malmo, Stockholm, and Gothenburg), and one each in England (Edinburgh[41]), Canada (CNBSS), and the United States of America (Health Insurance Plan of Greater New York[42]). In this meta-analysis of eight randomized trials of screening mammography involving

**TABLE 19-2. BREAST CANCER RISK AFTER A BREAST BIOPSY FOR BENIGN DISEASE: INTERPLAY BETWEEN AGE, MENOPAUSAL STATUS, AND FAMILY HISTORY**

| RISK FACTOR | RELATIVE RISK |
|---|---|
| LCIS with no family history for breast cancer | 5.4 |
| LCIS with history of fibrocystic disease and positive family history for breast cancer | 7.2 |
| Proliferative disease with atypia | 13.2 |
| Atypical hyperplasia | 3.7 |
| Atypical hyperplasia in a premenopausal woman | 5.9 |
| Atypical hyperplasia in a postmenopausal woman | 2.3 |
| Atypical hyperplasia with a positive family history for breast cancer | 7.3 |

SOURCE: Compiled from data obtained in: AJ London et al: A prospective study of benign breast disease and risk of breast cancer. JAMA 267:941–944, 1992.

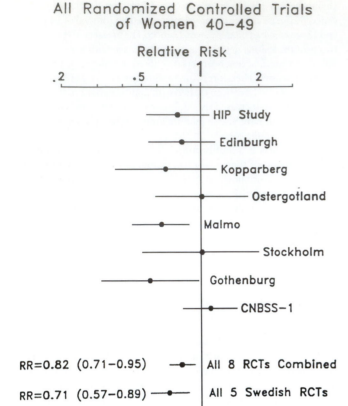

## All Randomized Controlled Trials of Women 40–49

Relative Risk

RR=0.82 (0.71–0.95)    All 8 RCTs Combined

RR=0.71 (0.57–0.89)    All 5 Swedish RCTs

**FIGURE 19-1.** In women aged 40 to 49 at entry, outcome of screening mammography expressed as relative risk of dying from breast cancer. (*From Hendrick RE et al: Benefit of screening mammography in women aged 40–49: A new meta-analysis of randomized controlled trials.* J Natl Cancer Inst Monogr 22:87–92, 1998.)

women aged 40 to 49 at time of entry, there was an 18% mortality rate reduction (95% CI = 0.71–0.95) with an average follow-up period of 12.7 years (Fig. 19-1). It is important to note that the benefit of screening in women 40 to 49 years of age did not become apparent until at least 8 years after the initiation of screening and continues to increase as the follow-up period becomes more prolonged.[43]

The approach to the work-up of a breast mass or mammographic abnormalities is depicted in Fig. 19-2. Excisional biopsy after needle localization has been the usual approach for nonpalpable solid lesions suspicious for a malignancy. Stereotactic needle biopsy has proved to be a viable alternative to surgical biopsy of mammographic abnormalities.[44] Although all surgical biopsies should be approached as if the lesion were malignant, one benefit of stereotactic core needle biopsy is that subsequent surgical excision of the abnormality results in a lower incidence of a positive or close surgical margin.[45,46] If a breast carcinoma is diagnosed by stereotactic needle biopsy, surgical excision of the biopsy site and needle tract should be part of the definitive treatment.

## STAGING

Since stage is based on the extent of disease, staging of tumors is one of the most important prognostic indicators of outcome. A uniform system for classification of breast cancers has been developed by the American Joint Committee on Cancer (AJCC) and the Union Internationale contre le Cancer (UICC).[47] The AJCC-UICC staging system is based on the premise that as tumor size increases, the risk of nodal metastases increases until finally, distant metastases occur. The TNM staging system is outlined in Table 19-3. In lesions with a mixed in situ and invasive cancer, the tumor size is based on the size of the invasive component. Microinvasive breast cancer refers to breast cancers where the invasive component is less than 2 mm in size.[48] Minimally invasive breast cancer usually refers to lesions less than 1 cm in size (T1a,b) while early breast cancer refers to stage I and II lesions. Survival is inversely related to stage: patients with stage I breast cancer have a survival of approximately 90%, while few patients with stage IV disease survive 5 years after diagnosis.

## PROGNOSTIC FACTORS

Prognostic factors depend on both intrinsic tumor characteristics and host environment. Tumor size and nodal status (clinical stage), the most important prognostic determinants of outcome in breast cancer, act independently but in an additive manner.[49] However, it is clear that other factors must also play a role in cancer progression and survival, since some patients with small, node-negative breast cancer still die from this disease, while others with advanced disease have a more favorable outcome than would be predicted solely by clinical stage.

Histologic grade is a measurement of the intrinsic malignant potential of the neoplasm. The most common grading system used in breast cancer is the Scarff-Bloom-Richardson classification, which classifies this disease into three grades based on architecture, nuclear pleomorphism, and number of mitoses. Worsening histologic grade (grade 3) has been shown to be associated with a worse survival within a clinical stage.[50] However, since tumor size and lymph node involvement are associated with increasing grade, it is not clear if histologic grade is, in fact, an independent prognostic factor in breast cancer.[51] Furthermore, interobserver variation and lack of a universally accepted grading system have hampered its use in the design of clinical trials.[52] Other histologic features that affect prognosis are vascular invasion and neural invasion. Lymphatic permeation, associated with an increased rate of lymph node involvement and local recurrence after breast conservation, has been shown to be a prognostic indicator independent of clinical stage.[53] Expression of estrogen (ER) and progesterone (PR) receptors has been associated with a more favorable outcome in breast cancer. Using the data obtained from the National Surgical Adjuvant Breast and Bowel Project Protocol B-06 (NSABP B-06) trial, it was found that in node-negative patients, there were 8% and 10% differences in disease-free and overall survival rates, respectively, in women with ER-positive tumors.[54] A similar positive result in survival rates was obtained for PR-positive tumors.

# TABLE 19-3. DEFINITION OF TNM

*Primary tumor (T):*

TX  Primary tumor cannot be assessed.

T0  No evidence of primary tumor.

Tis  Carcinoma in situ: Intraductal carcinoma, lobular carcinoma in situ, or Paget's disease[1] of the nipple with no tumor.

T1  Tumor 2 cm or less in greatest dimension.

    T1mic  Microinvasion 0.1 cm or less in greatest dimension.

    T1a  Tumor more than 0.1 cm, but not more than 0.5 cm, in greatest dimension.

    T1b  Tumor more than 0.5 cm, but not more than 1 cm, in greatest dimension.

    T1c  Tumor more than 1 cm but not more than 2 cm, in greatest dimension.

T2  Tumor more than 2 cm, but not more than 5 cm, in greatest dimension.

T3  Tumor more than 5 cm in greatest dimension.

T4  Tumor of any size with direct extension to (a) chest wall or (b) skin, only as described below:

    T4a  Extension to chest wall.

    T4b  Edema (including *peau d'orange*) or ulceration of the skin of the breast or satellite skin nodules confined to the same breast.

    T4c  Both (T4a and T4b).

    T4d  Inflammatory carcinoma (see definition of inflammatory carcinoma in the introduction).

*Regional lymph nodes (N):*

NX  Regional lymph nodes cannot be assessed (e.g., previously removed).

N0  No regional lymph node metastasis.

N1  Metastasis to movable ipsilateral axillary lymph node(s).

N2  Metastasis to ipsilateral axillary lymph node(s) fixed to one another or to other structures.

N3  Metastasis to ipsilateral internal mammary lymph node(s).

*Pathologic classification (pN):*

pNX  Regional lymph nodes cannot be assessed (e.g., previously removed, or not removed, for pathologic study).

pN0  No regional lymph node metastasis.

pN1  Metastasis to movable ipsilateral axillary lymph node(s).

    pN1a  Only micrometastasis (none larger than 0.2 cm).

    pN1b  Metastasis to lymph node(s), any larger than 0.2 cm.

    pN1bi  Metastasis in 1 to 3 lymph nodes, any more than 0.2 cm and all less than 2 cm in greatest dimension.

    pN1bii  Metastasis to 4 or more lymph nodes, any more than 0.2 cm and all less than 2 cm in greatest dimension.

    pN1biii  Extension of tumor beyond the capsule of a lymph node metastasis less than 2 cm in greatest dimension.

    pN1biv  Metastasis to a lymph node 2 cm or more in greatest dimension.

pN2  Metastasis to ipsilateral axillary lymph nodes that are fixed to one another or to other structures.

pN3  Metastasis to ipsilateral internal mammary lymph node(s).

*Distant metastasis (M):*

MX  Distant metastasis cannot be assessed.

M0  No distant metastasis.

M1  Distant metastasis (includes metastasis to ipsilateral supraclavicular lymph node[s]).

*Stage grouping:*

| | | | |
|---|---|---|---|
| Stage 0 | Tis | N0 | M0 |
| Stage I | T1 | N0 | M0 |
| Stage IIA | T0 | N1 | M0 |
| | T1[2] | N1[3] | M0 |
| | T2 | N0 | M0 |
| Stage IIB | T2 | N1 | M0 |
| | T3 | N0 | M0 |
| Stage IIIA | T0 | N2 | M0 |
| | T1[2] | N2 | M0 |
| | T2 | N2 | M0 |
| | T3 | N1 | M0 |
| | T3 | N2 | M0 |
| Stage IIIB | T4 | Any N | M0 |
| | Any T | N3 | M0 |
| Stage IV | Any T | Any N | M1 |

[1] Paget's disease associated with a tumor is classified according to the size of the tumor.

[2] T1 includes T1 mic.

[3] The prognosis of patients with N1a is similar to that of patients with pN0.

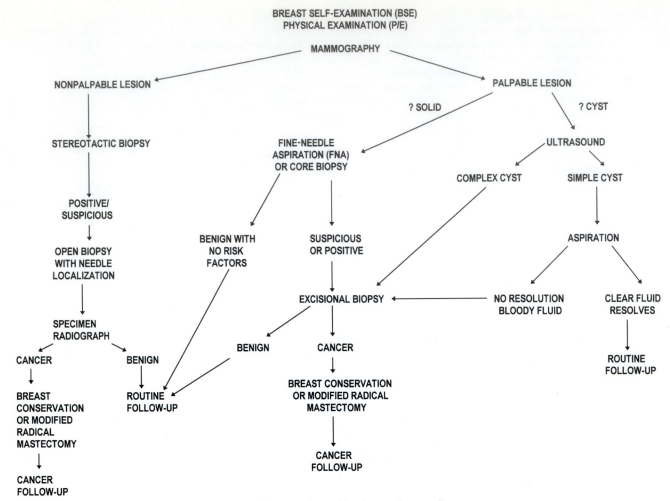

**FIGURE 19-2.** Approach to a patient with a breast abnormality.

With the advent of newer molecular techniques and the identification of oncogenes and tumor suppressor genes involved in carcinogenesis, there has been an attempt to link oncogene expression with respect to breast cancer prognosis. The two most frequent molecular abnormalities in breast cancer are overexpression of erbB-2,[55] a cell surface protein in the epidermal growth factor family, and mutation of p53, a tumor suppressor gene important in transcription and apoptosis.[56] Approximately 21% of primary invasive breast cancers are positive for erbB-2 overexpression. By using paraffin tissue blocks obtained from patients enrolled in NSABP B-06, it was found that erbB-2 overexpression correlated with an increase in the mortality rate (twofold increase), particularly in tumors of good nuclear grade, where there was an approximate fivefold increase in the mortality rate.[57] Overexpression of p53 in breast tissue has been shown to correlate with tumor size, stage, and steroid receptor status, and in multivariate analysis, both p53 and erb B-2 overexpression are independent prognostic variables of disease-free and overall survival.[58] The number of molecular markers that are known to be aberrantly expressed in breast cancer is increasing rapidly,[59] and although the specific abnormality may be important, the total number of defects may play a role in prognosis. Bland and co-workers[60] evaluated the role of individual and co-expression of oncogenes in breast cancer recurrence. Utilizing Ha-ras, c-myc, c-fos, and p53 overexpression as potential prognostic indicators, the authors found that increased oncogene expression correlated inversely with breast cancer survival. While the recurrence rate for one oncogene was 17.2%, the recurrence rate increased to 56.3% when two oncogenes were overexpressed and to 100% when more than three were involved.

Tumor growth is a result of both intrinsic tumor characteristics and the environment. An important prognostic indicator of survival is a woman's age at breast cancer diagnosis. Chung and co-workers[61] analyzed breast cancer survival according to age and found that women 40 years old and younger at the time of breast cancer diagnosis had a worse 5-year survival prognosis than did other age groups. This difference in survival was not a reflection of difficulty in diagnosing cancer among younger age groups, since the younger women still had an inferior survival rate when survival was analyzed according to stage. Initial results from NSABP B-06 suggested that race may be an important prognostic factor for survival. In the evaluation of 22 pathologic and 5 clinical factors for a 10-year survival rate, better survival was noted for Caucasians as compared with African Americans.[62] However, it was not clear if this disparity in survival rate was a reflection of differences in mean stage of disease with each racial group. A follow-up study from the NSABP reported that information obtained from two randomized clinical trials indicated comparable survival rates for Caucasians and African Americans with lymph node–negative breast cancer.[63] This study did confirm that African-American women with breast cancer tended to have less favorable baseline characteristics, which may explain the differences in survival rate that were noted earlier. The host immune response is also an important prognostic factor. Patients with early breast cancer, or those with advanced breast cancer, who are alive and have no residual disease have been found to have an increased number of tumor-infiltrating lymphocytes as compared with patients with advanced disease who have had a recurrence or died.[64]

Despite an increase in the number of prognostic factors associated with breast cancer, tumor size and lymph node status remain the most important and clinically useful. Other factors such as grade, hormone receptor status, and oncogene expression may identify subcategories at risk for recurrence within each stage. The use of computerized prognostic models in the future may overcome the difficulty of integrating the effect of each prognostic indicator.[65]

## GENERAL PRINCIPLES OF MASTECTOMY

Surgery remains the mainstay for the local and regional treatment of breast cancer. The type of operation is governed by the size and the position of the lesion, the primary tumor characteristics, and whether the lesion is close to the skin or fixed to underlying structures. The predominant operations for breast cancer include the following: (1) the removal of the entire breast and axillary contents (MRM), and (2) breast conservation procedures, which include removal of the lesion with a margin of normal tissue (tumorectomy, lumpectomy, tylectomy, quadrantectomy) and a noncontiguous axillary nodal dissection.

A pathologic diagnosis of breast cancer can be made on the basis of a fine-needle aspiration biopsy, a core biopsy, or an excisional biopsy. Since no architectural information is contained in an aspiration cytology biopsy, an invasive carcinoma cannot be differentiated from an intraductal cancer. Although it is possible to distinguish invasiveness on a needle core biopsy, it may be difficult to distinguish between pathologic lesions that are similar such as atypical ductal hyperplasia and low-grade ductal carcinoma in situ.

When performing an excisional biopsy, care should be taken in deciding where to place the incision. The incision should be designed in a manner such that if a mastectomy is required, the mastectomy incision will easily incorporate the biopsy scar. Incisions for breast biopsies are usually placed along the lines of Langer, which provide an acceptable scar once the incision has healed (Fig. 19-3). Some surgeons prefer a radial incision for lesions in the lower half of the breast, particularly if skin is to be included in the biopsy, because removal of skin in this area may alter the inframammary fold and affect the cosmetic result. It is not necessary to remove skin unless the lesion is superficial or a previous biopsy scar is present. In any event, the skin incision should be placed over the lesion; tunneling from a circumareolar incision to a peripheral lesion should be avoided.

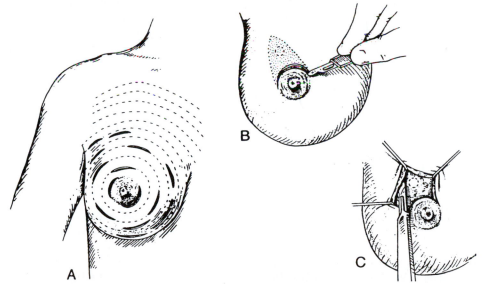

**FIGURE 19-3.** The recommended locations of incisions for performing breast biopsy. *A.* The most cosmetically acceptable scars result from circumareolar incisions that follow the contour of Langer's lines. *B* and *C.* The technique for dissection of breast masses within 2 cm of the areolar margin. Thick skin flaps are advised to ensure cosmetically contoured and viable tissues about the aerola. (*From Bland KI, Copeland EM III (eds): The Breast: Comprehensive Management of Benign and Malignant Diseases.* Philadelphia, WB Saunders, 1998, p. 812.)

An excisional biopsy can be the definitive breast operation if the primary tumor characteristics indicate that the lesion can be treated by breast conservation and the tumor margins are adequate. If breast conservation is desirable and the excisional biopsy specimen is inadequate, i.e., positive or close tumor margins, the entire biopsy site, including the biopsy scar should be re-excised. If a mastectomy is required, the mastectomy incision should incorporate the biopsy scar with a 1- to 2-cm margin of skin. The preferred mastectomy incision is usually performed slightly oblique from the transverse line and extended cephalad towards the axilla (modified Orr incision) (Fig. 19-4). This type of incision removes the nipple-areola complex, the mammary parenchyma, allows access to the axilla, and provides an acceptable cosmetic result. If a previously placed biopsy scar makes fashioning of the mastectomy incision difficult, the oncologic aspect of the operation should not be sacrificed. For all mastectomy procedures, radical excision of the skin is not deemed essential for local tumor control.

Lesions of the inner lower and upper outer quadrants can be easily removed by the modified Orr incision. This incision allows for easy reconstruction of the breast using myocutaneous or subpectoral

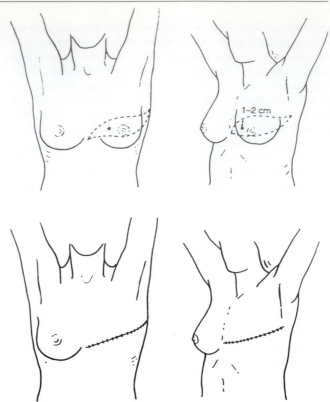

**FIGURE 19-5.** Design of the obliquely placed modified Stewart incision for cancer of the inner quadrant of the breast. The medial extent of the incision often must incorporate skin to the midsternum to allow 1- to 2-cm margin in all directions from the edge of the tumor. Lateral extent of the incision ends at the anterior margin of the latissimus dorsi muscle. (*From Bland KI, Copeland EM III (eds): The Breast: Comprehensive Management of Benign and Malignant Diseases.* Philadelphia, WB Saunders, 1998, p. 826.)

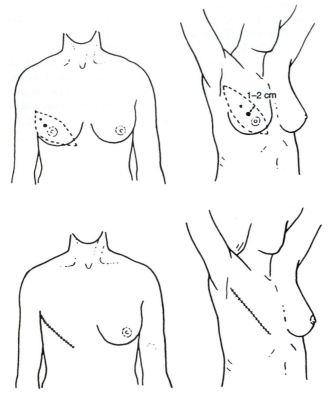

**FIGURE 19-4.** Design of the classic Orr incision for carcinoma of the upper outer quadrants of the breast. The skin incision is placed 1 to 2 cm from the margin of the tumor in an oblique plane that is directed cephalad toward the ipsilateral axilla. This incision is a variant of the original Greenough, Kocher, and Rodman techniques for flap development. (*From Bland KI, Copeland EM III (eds): The Breast: Comprehensive Management of Benign and Malignant Diseases.* Philadelphia, WB Saunders, 1998, p. 827.)

augmentation breast implants. Lesions of the upper inner quadrant are usually the most difficult to manage because of their anatomic position. These lesions, as well as lesions in the lower outer quadrant and central subareolar primaries, should be removed by a modified Stewart incision (Fig. 19-5). None of these mastectomy incisions requires the removal of more than 1 to 2 cm of skin around the previous biopsy scar.

Mastectomy, either simple or modified radical, with the excision of a minimum amount of overlying skin is referred to as a skin-sparing mastectomy (SSM). Since the inframammary fold is left in place and native breast skin gives the best possible color match, a SSM can be cosmetically superior for breast reconstruction after a standard MRM. A SSM must include the nipple-areola complex (and not just the nipple because the areola also contains mammary ducts[66]) and all previous biopsy sites with a margin of intact skin, and provide access to the axilla.[67] SSM may be considered in patients with multicentric disease, invasive carcinoma with an extensive intraductal component greater than 25% of tumor volume, T2 lesions with features that are difficult to detect either clinically or mammographically, and a central lesion that would require excision of the nipple-areola complex. If patients are carefully selected for SSMs, the risk of local recurrence is quite low. When compared to conventional mastectomy, the local recurrence rate after SSM has been found to be equivalent (SSM = 4.8%, non-SSM = 9.5%), with no difference in native skin flap necrosis.[68] Kroll and colleagues[69] reported the MD Anderson experience with 104 patients who had a SSM and found a local recurrence rate of 6.7% with a minimum follow-up period of 5 years. These results indicate that in the carefully selected patient, a SSM can be a safe oncologic procedure.

As is discussed later in this chapter, an axillary dissection is usually included as part of the surgical treatment of invasive breast cancer. The majority of breast primaries drain preferentially to the axilla. The exceptions to this rule are primary tumors that arise medially. These lesions may drain preferentially to the internal mammary lymph nodes, in which case axillary sampling may be an inadequate staging procedure. Morrow and Foster[70] evaluated 7070 patients with breast cancer who had sampling of both axillary and internal mammary lymph nodes and found that only 5% to 10% of patients had internal mammary nodes involved in the absence of axillary metastases. For patients at risk for internal mammary lymph node metastases, irradiation of these nodes is justified.

The axillary dissection can be done as part of the breast operation (MRM) or, if breast conservation is chosen, through a separate incision in the axilla. The lymph nodes within the axilla can be divided into groups based on their anatomic position: external mammary, subscapular, axillary vein, central nodal, and subclavicular (apical) lymph nodes. Lymph nodes in the external mammary, subscapular, and axillary vein groups are considered level I lymph nodes, while those in the central nodal and apical groups are considered level II and III lymph nodes, respectively. An axillary dissection should include level I and II nodes, with an average number of nodes to be removed greater than 10. A routine level III axillary dissection is not required since this procedure increases the risk of arm lymphedema.

## NONINVASIVE BREAST CANCER

With the advent of screening mammography, there has been an increase in literature dedicated to in situ or noninvasive breast cancers. In situ cancers have cells that are cytotypically similar to invasive cancers but are confined to the ductal structure. The predominant forms of in situ breast cancers are lobular carcinoma in situ (LCIS) and ductal carcinoma in situ (DCIS), and their names depict the anatomic site from which they are felt to arise. However, these two noninvasive cancers are vastly different in their pathology, with LCIS considered a risk factor for the subsequent development of breast cancer and DCIS considered a premalignant breast neoplasm.

### LOBULAR CARCINOMA IN SITU

The term *lobular carcinoma in situ* (LCIS) was first coined by Foote and Stewart[71] to describe a noninfiltrating, proliferative lobular lesion of the breast. LCIS is characterized by the distention and distortion of the lobular unit with characteristic cells; the natural history and optimal treatment of this pathologic entity have been controversial. LCIS tends to occur in premenopausal women and regresses

to some degree after menopause. LCIS has no clinical manifestations nor does it produce mammographic abnormalities. This pathologic entity is usually multicentric and bilateral. The risk for developing a breast cancer persists for up to 20 years after a biopsy positive for LCIS, with approximately 75% of the subsequent breast cancers having predominantly a ductal histology.[72] As the natural history of this pathologic entity is better understood, the treatment of LCIS has gone through an evolutionary change.[73] Initially treated as an invasive cancer with MRM, breast conservation became more popular in the 1980s.[74] Haagensen and co-workers[75] retrospectively evaluated the Columbia experience with LCIS, which involved 211 women, the majority of whom did not undergo mastectomy. The mean follow-up in this study was 14 years. Overall, 17.1% of the women developed an invasive breast carcinoma; approximately one-half involved the breast initially diagnosed with lobular neoplasia. Examination of the subsequent carcinomas revealed that the majority were of ductal origin. Haagensen further examined the relative risk of carcinoma in women with lobular neoplasia and a family history of breast cancer. Overall, the relative risk for breast cancer in women with a breast biopsy positive for lobular neoplasia was 7.2. This number increased to 13.8 if the patient had family history of breast cancer in a first-degree relative.

More conservative figures for the development of a breast cancer after diagnosis with LCIS have been obtained from NSABP B-17.[76] This randomized prospective study was designed in order to determine the optimal treatment for DCIS. However, 182 women with LCIS only were enrolled in this study; these women were treated with lumpectomy alone. At a mean follow-up of 5 years, there were 11 breast tumor recurrences (incidence of subsequent breast cancer was 6%); 7 in the ipsilateral breast and 4 in the contralateral breast. Half of the breast cancers diagnosed in this group were invasive lobular carcinomas. The long-term results of this study will help address the true incidence of breast cancer after a biopsy of LCIS.

There are two dramatically different choices in the management of LCIS: bilateral prophylactic mastectomy or lifelong observation. Prophylactic mastectomy is the only means of preventing breast cancer. However, since some skin overlying the breast remains after mastectomy, and since it is difficult to remove all breast tissue from this skin, the risk of developing breast cancer after a prophylactic mastectomy is not an absolute zero. Furthermore, since the cancer risk with LCIS involves both breasts, bilateral mastectomy is the treatment option. This option, however, should only be recommended to the patient with other known risk factors for breast cancer, such as a family history that is suggestive of hereditary breast cancer, and only after extensive discussion of the available options. Since LCIS is a marker of breast cancer risk in both breasts, the preferable alternative is lifelong surveillance with mammography and clinical examination.[77] The use of chemopreventive breast cancer agents such as tamoxifen may have a role in the management of women with LCIS.[78]

### DUCTAL CARCINOMA IN SITU

DCIS presents a spectrum of diseases, from a nonpalpable lesion detected by microcalcifications to a palpable mass with a high incidence of an associated invasive component. Beginning in the 1980s with the implementation of mammographic screening, the incidence of DCIS has increased. Data from the National Cancer Institute's Surveillance, Epidemiology, and End Results (SEER) program indicate that the incidence of DCIS had increased 200% from 1983 to 1992.[79] It is possible that in the future, a large proportion of breast cancer cases will involve DCIS.

Unlike LCIS, DCIS is a true premalignant lesion. Histologically, the malignant cells in DCIS are confined to the natural ductal boundaries with no evidence of stromal invasion. Architecturally, the cells can be organized into a papillary pattern (the earliest type), followed by a cribriform growth pattern, and finally comedonecrosis occurs when the proliferating cells have outstripped their blood supply. Calcium deposition occurs in the area of necrosis, and these deposits can be seen on a mammogram as microcalcification. There are several classification schemes for DCIS based on architectural morphology, nuclear characteristics, and presence or absence of necrosis. DCIS can be classified into well, moderately, and poorly differentiated lesions based on cytonuclear and architectural differentiation.[80] Monomorphic nuclei, few mitoses, and inconspicuous nucleoli are characteristic of well-differentiated DCIS. Architectural differentiation is present in these lesions and necrosis is usually absent. At the other end of the spectrum are poorly differentiated lesions that have pleomorphic nuclei, frequent mitoses, prominent nucleoli, and are usually accompanied by necrosis. Moderately differentiated lesions have characteristics between these two extremes. However, there are other published classifications for DCIS that are based primarily on nuclear grade and the presence or absence of necrosis.[81] To overcome some of the confusion associated with the differing classification systems, a Consensus Conference on the Classification of Ductal Carcinoma in Situ was held in Philadelphia in April 1997. Although the panel could not endorse any specific classification system, the panel agreed that DCIS should be stratified predominantly by nuclear grade into low (NG1), intermediate (NG2), and high-grade (NG3) lesions that partially correlate with prognosis.[82] Other factors that were found useful in the classification of DCIS were presence and quantification of necrosis, cell polarization, and architectural pattern. This panel also recommended that documentation of margins, extent and distribution of disease, association of microcalcifications with DCIS, and correlation of tissue specimen with the mammographic abnormalities be included in the final pathology report since this information may be useful in the prognosis and the design of a treatment plan.

Before the advent of screening mammography, DCIS was infrequently diagnosed as the predominant lesion. During the premammographic era, DCIS tended to be a large lesion and was treated predominantly by mastectomy. In addition to the large size, it was unclear whether DCIS was a multicentric lesion and therefore required a mastectomy for complete removal. Using Egan's serial subgross method,[82] Holland and colleagues[83] evaluated mastectomy specimens removed for DCIS. All but one of these DCIS specimens had a localized lesion. However, using a similar technique, Faverly and co-workers[84] showed that 63% of DCIS lesions studied at mastectomy extended beyond 5 cm. Regardless of whether DCIS is more likely to be more extensive or multicentric than IDC, the local recurrence rate after mastectomy for DCIS ranges from 0% to 4% and this treatment method remains the gold standard.[85] However, the advent of breast conservation as a treatment option for invasive carcinoma raised the possibility of this treatment approach for DCIS. The treatment options evaluated for management of DCIS included lumpectomy with and without radiation, and the need for axillary nodal dissection.

In the mid-1980s to 1990s, several centers reported their results of DCIS treated with excisional breast biopsy and breast irradiation[86-94] (Table 19-4). The earlier reports came from the Institut Curie[86] and Fox Chase Cancer Center.[87] The series from the Institut Curie had 54 patients, all with tumors of less than 5 cm. There were 3 recurrences after a median follow-up of 55 months: one recurrence had an invasive carcinoma and this patient later died of systemic disease. The Fox Chase study had a similar recurrence rate of 10% (4/40) and half of the recurrences were of invasive cancers. All patients with recurrences were salvaged by a mastectomy. Subsequent to these reports, several groups reported their experience with DCIS treated with breast conservation and radiotherapy. A majority of the studies had fewer than 100 patients. Follow-up ranged from

**TABLE 19-4.** RETROSPECTIVE STUDIES EVALUATING LOCAL RECURRENCE FOR DCIS TREATED WITH BREAST-CONSERVING SURGERY AND ADJUVANT IRRADIATION[93]

| SERIES | TIME | NUMBER (% NONPALPABLE) | FOLLOW-UP PERIOD (MEDIAN) | LOCAL RECURRENCE RATE | MEDIAN TIME TO FAILURE | % INVASIVE |
|---|---|---|---|---|---|---|
| Zafrani et al.[86] | 1967–83 | 54 | 55 mo | 5.5% | | 33% |
| Recht et al.[87] | 1976–83 | 40 | 44 mo | 10% | | 50% |
| McCormick et al.[88] | 1977–88 | 55 (67%) | 36 mo | 18% (3 yr) 25% (6 yr) | | |
| Ray et al.[89] | 1976–90 | 56 | 60 mo | 11% (8 yr) | 34 mo | |
| Solin et al.[90] | 1978–85 | 51 | 68 mo | 6% (5 yr) | 58.4 mo | |
| Solin et al.[91] | 10 centers | 270 | 124 mo | 19% (15 yr) | 52 mo | |
| Haffty et al.[92] | 1974–87 | 60 | 36 mo | 5% (5 yr) | | |
| Solin et al.[93] | 10 centers | 110 (100%) | 112 mo | 7% (5 yr) 14% (10 yr) | 5 yr | 40% |
| Hiramatsu et al.[94] | 1976–90 | 76 (71%) | 74 mo | 4% (5 yr) 15% (10 yr) | 47 mo | 57% |

**TABLE 19-5.** STUDIES EVALUATING LOCAL RECURRENCE FOR DCIS TREATED WITH BREAST-CONSERVING SURGERY ONLY

| SERIES | TIME | NUMBER (% NONPALPABLE) | FOLLOW-UP PERIOD (MEDIAN) | LOCAL RECURRENCE RATE | % INVASIVE |
|---|---|---|---|---|---|
| Page et al.[95] | 1952–68 | 28 (0%) | 24 yr | 25% (10 yr) 32% (24 yr) | 100 |
| Eusebi et al.[96] | 1964–76 | 80 | 17.5 yr | 20% | 70 |
| Fisher et al.[97]* | 1976–84 | 21 | 8 yr | 43% | 56 |
| Arnesson et al.[98] | 1982–84 | 38 (100%) | 5 yr | 13% | 40 |
| Schwartz et al.[99] | 1978–90 | 70 (100%) | 49 mo | 15.3% | |
| Lagios et al.[100] | 1975–87 | 79 (100%) | 48 mo | 10.1% | 50 |

*These results were obtained from women who were enrolled in the NSABP B-06 study on invasive breast cancer, but who, on pathologic review, were found to have intraductal breast cancer only.

3 to 10 years, and the local recurrence rate was 5% to 25%. Solin and co-workers[90] reported the results of 10 institutions and found a local recurrence rate of 19% at 15 years; the median time to failure was 52 months.

The range in local recurrence rates for DCIS is a reflection not only of treatment differences but also of patient selection. In an evaluation of 110 nonpalpable lesions,[93] the local recurrence rate at 10 years was only 14%, a rate much lower than in other series. Regardless of the local recurrence rate, most authors agree that approximately one-half of the recurrences after breast conservation surgery and radiotherapy for DCIS will be invasive cancers.

DCIS has also been treated by lumpectomy alone, i.e., without adjuvant radiotherapy [95–100] (Table 19-5). Earlier studies included only DCIS that had been detected clinically; later studies evaluated mammographically detected DCIS. In the earlier studies,[95–97] the local recurrence rate for DCIS treated with lumpectomy alone was up to 43%; greater than 50% were invasive cancers. In the later studies that included only mammographically detected DCIS, the local recurrence rate had decreased to 15%. For example, Lagios and co-workers[100] reported the UCSF experience of a 10% local recurrence rate after lumpectomy alone for DCIS, with the recurrence rate increasing to 19.1% for DCIS associated with high-grade nuclear morphology and comedo-type necrosis. Half of the recurrent lesions were invasive carcinomas. Half of the DCIS leisons greater than 56 mm had an associated occult invasive carcinoma.

The results of these retrospective studies stimulated the NSABP to design Protocol B-17,[101] which prospectively and randomly compared lumpectomy with and without radiation for the treatment of DCIS. In this trial of 818 women and after a mean follow-up of 90 months, the section treated with lumpectomy and breast irradiation had a lower recurrence rate of 12.1% as compared with the section treated by lumpectomy alone (recurrence rate of 26.8%). In the arm of the study treated by lumpectomy alone, half the recurrences were invasive cancers. For the group treated with lumpectomy and irradiation, only one third of the recurrences were invasive cancers. Extended follow-up is needed to determine the long-term recurrence rate with lumpectomy and radiation.

One of the criticisms of the NSABP trial is that DCIS was treated as one disease entity. The recurrence rate after lumpectomy alone for the NSABP trial was twice that seen in the UCSF experience, where only lesions less than 2.5 cm in size were treated with lumpectomy.

This has raised the issue of whether DCIS, when associated with good prognostic features, can be treated with lumpectomy alone, especially when the lesion is nonpalpable. Tumor size has been found to be an important prognostic factor for DCIS, with larger tumors being more likely to recur after breast-conservation surgery. The majority of DCIS detected today are nonpalpable, and tumor size is estimated from the mammogram and the extent of microcalcifications that are present. However, when estimating tumor size from a mammogram, care must be taken because mammography tends to underestimate the size of DCIS involvement present in the breast.[102] Paradoxically, this discrepancy is more likely with micropapillary and cribriform lesions than with more advanced DCIS.

Nuclear grade has been found to be one of the most important prognostic indicators for DCIS. When tumor recurrence after lumpectomy was evaluated by Lagios and colleagues,[100] it was found that DCIS with high nuclear grade was associated with a 19% local recurrence rate. Conversely, none of the low-grade lesions in this series recurred during the same time period. Aside from nuclear grade and tumor size, the presence of comedonecrosis and involvement of the margins with tumor are other prognostic markers associated with an increased likelihood of recurrence.[103] In an effort to consolidate the known prognostic features for DCIS, Silverstein and colleagues[104] evaluated the outcome of their patients with DCIS according to these characteristics and developed the Van Nuys Prognostic Index (VNPI). The VNPI combines three prognostic features—tumor size, tumor margin, and grade—to give an overall score that can be used to guide therapy (Table 19-6). Silverstein and associates[104] have reported that the recurrence rate approaches 0% for those women with VNPI scores of 3 or 4 who were treated with lumpectomy alone or lumpectomy and breast irradiation. Women with VNPI scores of 5 to 7 had a lower recurrence rate when radiation was added to lumpectomy, while those with high VNPI scores had an extremely high rate of recurrence (80%), whether or not the breast had been irradiated. Mastectomy may be the best option in these high-risk patients.

Although the recurrence rate for DCIS is around 10% after radiation, the majority of series report that one-third to one-half of the recurrences are invasive carcinomas. Either breast conservation or mastectomy can be used to treat these recurrences. Close observation after breast conservation suggests that detection of these recurrences at an early stage (minimally invasive breast cancer) should afford these women a high rate of cure.

**TABLE 19-6.** THE VAN NUYS PROGNOSTIC INDEX (VNPI) SCORING SYSTEM FOR DCIS

| SCORE | 1 | 2 | 3 |
|---|---|---|---|
| Size tumor, mm | ≤15 | 16–40 | ≥41 |
| Margin width, mm | ≥10 | 1–9 | <1 |
| Pathologic classification | Non-high-grade without necrosis | Non-high-grade with necrosis | High-grade with or without necrosis |

One to three points are awarded for each predictor of local breast recurrence. The total score is the Van Nuys Prognostic Index (ranging from 3–9) and treatment recommendations are based on this score (VNPI).

| VNPI | LOCAL RECURRENCE RATE | TREATMENT RECOMMENDATION |
|---|---|---|
| 3 or 4 | 2/101 | Wide local excision alone |
| 5, 6, 7 | 40/209 | Lumpectomy and breast irradiation |
| 8 or 9 | 13/23 | Mastectomy |

SOURCE: Adapted from information in Silverstein MJ et al: A prognostic index for ductal carcinoma in situ of the breast. Cancer 77:2267–74, 1996.

Although DCIS is an intraductal tumor, lymph node metastases should not occur unless there is a missed invasive component. When axillary lymph node dissections have been performed for DCIS, the incidence of lymph node metastases approaches 0%.[105] Therefore, the current recommendation is that axillary node dissections should not be performed routinely for DCIS. Treatment options of DCIS have undergone an evolution from radical therapy with MRM to conservative therapy with lumpectomy alone. DCIS is a heterogeneous disease. The challenge is to identify subgroups within this disease so as to design optimal treatment guidelines for each subgroup.

## INVASIVE DISEASE

Breast tissue is composed of lobules and ducts, and malignancies can arise in either of these two components. The majority of breast carcinomas have an infiltrating ductal histology and are classified as ductal carcinomas, no special type (NST) or not otherwise specified (NOS). Approximately 10% of breast carcinomas arise from the lobular breast tissue and are classified as lobular carcinomas. Some ductal carcinomas have recognizable histologic features that allow for their special histologic classification into subtypes which includes medullary, tubular, and mucinous carcinomas. The presence of these special subtypes is usually associated with a more favorable outcome as compared to that observed with ductal carcinomas, NOS.[106] Less common subtypes of breast carcinomas include solid papillary and signet ring carcinomas.

Infiltrating lobular carcinoma (ILC) of the breast is the second most frequent type of invasive breast cancer. It accounts for 5% to 10% of all breast carcinomas and is characterized by a high incidence of multicentricity and bilateral breast involvement. In the past there was some reluctance to treat these lesions with breast conservation because of the fear that the recurrence rate would be unacceptably high. The incidence of ipsilateral breast recurrence for ILC treated by breast conservation is summarized in Table 19-7.[107] The majority of series report an equivalent rate of local recurrence for both IDC and ILC treated with breast conservation indicating that this histologic entity can be treated by lumpectomy and breast irradiation instead of mastectomy. Furthermore, the rate of bilateral breast cancer is not increased as compared with IDC. ILC is unique in its pattern of systemic metastases in that visceral metastases and meningeal metastases occur more frequently than that seen with IDC.

Tubular carcinoma of the breast is a rare subtype of invasive carcinoma with a distinct histologic pattern characterized by irregular tubular formation. It accounts for 1% to 2% of all breast carcinomas and has a more favorable prognosis than other infiltrating ductal carcinomas. This lesion tends to be small at diagnosis, with a mean size of around 1 cm.[108] The incidence of lymph node metastases is low, which may be a reflection of the associated small tumor size or the low tendency of this histologic lesion to metastasize. Because of their excellent prognosis and low propensity to metastasize, it has been suggested that tubular carcinomas may be treated by lumpectomy alone, without adjuvant radiation or axillary dissection.[109]

Mucinous (colloid) carcinomas can be subcategorized into either pure or mixed lesions. Pure mucinous carcinoma consists of small aggregates of tumor cells floating in abundant extracellular mucin. Mixed mucinous carcinomas contain areas of abundant extracellular mucin but also have areas of malignant cells that are devoid of mucin. These subtypes appear differently on mammography, with pure lesions appearing as circumscribed, lobular lesions and mixed mucinous cancers having an irregular contour.[110] Clinically pure and mixed carcinomas behave differently as well, with pure mucinous lesions having a low propensity to metastasize and a better survival rate.[111]

Generally, subtypes of breast carcinomas are well-differentiated lesions with a low histologic grade. Medullary carcinoma is the exception. Although characterized by histologic features of a high-grade malignancy such as lack of tubular formation, a high mitotic rate, and nuclear pleomorphism with medullary carcinoma,[112] patients with medullary carcinoma have a good prognosis.[113] In a recent review of 52 women with medullary carcinoma,[114] it was observed that 11% of patients had tumors larger than 4 cm and 33% of patients had axillary metastases. Despite these poor prognostic factors, the 10-year survival rate in this group of patients was 85%.

**TABLE 19-7.** 5-YR LOCAL RECURRENCE AND OVERALL SURVIVAL ACCORDING TO HISTOLOGY[107]

| AUTHOR | TIME PERIOD | STUDY GROUP | | NUMBER | LOCAL RECURRENCE | p | OVERALL SURVIVAL | p |
|---|---|---|---|---|---|---|---|---|
| Schnitt et al.[270] | | Stage I/II with breast conservation | ILC | 49 | 14% | NS | | |
| | | | IDC | 561 | 12% | | | |
| Kurtz et al.[271] | 1977–1985 | Stage I/II with breast conservation | ILC | 67 | 13.5% | NS | 92% | |
| | | | IDC | 709 | 9% | | 88% | |
| duToit et al.[272] | 1973–1987 | T < 5 cm matched controls | ILC | 71 | 42.1% | <0.05 | | |
| | | | IDC | 342 | 16.7% | | | |
| Poen et al.[273] | 1981–1987 | All treated with breast conservation | ILC | 60 | 2% | | 91% | |
| Weiss et al.[274] | 1977–1986 | Stage I/II with breast conservation | ILC | 41 | 9% | NS | 91% | NS |
| | | | IDC | 386 | 7% | | 87% | |
| White et al.[275] | 1980–1987 | Stage I/II with breast conservation | ILC | 30 | 3.3% | NS | 100% | 0.05 |
| | | | IDC | 346 | 4.2% | | 84.5% | |
| Veronesi et al.[276] | | All treated with breast conservation | ILC | 431 | 4.6% | a | | |
| | | | IDC | 1987 | 3.5% | | | |
| | | | IDC + EIC | 150 | 11.3% | | | |
| Sastre-Garau et al.[277] | 1981–1991 | All patients | ILC | 726 | 9% | NS | 87% | NS |
| | | | IDC | 10,061 | 11% | | 89% | |
| Salvadori et al.[278] | 1973–1989 | All treated with QUART | ILC | 286 | 8.0% | NS | | |
| | | | IDC | 1,903 | 8.2% | | | |
| Chung et al.[107] | 1984–1994 | All patients | ILC | 316 | 2.8%–4.3% | NS | 68% | NS |
| | | | IDC | 4,570 | 2.1%–2.5% | | 71% | |

ABBREVIATIONS: EIC = extensive intraductal component; IDC = infiltrating ductal carcinoma; ILC = infiltrating lobular carcinoma; NS = not statistically significant; QUART = quadrantectomy plus adjuvant radiotherapy.
NOTE: No statistically significant difference in LRR between ILC and IDC; $p < 0.05$ when IDC with EIC compared to IDC or ILC.[107]
SOURCE: Reprinted with permission from Chung MA et al: Optimal surgical treatment of invasive lobular carcinoma of the breast. Ann Surg Oncol 4:545, 1997.

## TREATMENT OF EARLY BREAST CANCER

Treatment of early breast cancer can be divided into MRM or breast conservation, with or without breast irradiation, and with or without a concomitant axillary nodal dissection. Known as the "gold standard" for breast cancer, MRM is the treatment against which all other treatment modalities are compared. Treatment objectives are cure of the disease, local control, adequate staging, and acceptable cosmetic result. There have been several prospective randomized trials addressing the issue of breast conservation in the management of early breast cancer (Table 19-8). Six of these trials compared the gold standard with lumpectomy, axillary nodal dissection, and breast irradiation. Since the trials comparing MRM to breast conservation surgery and radiotherapy were conducted in the 1970s and 1980s, these trials have had a longer follow-up period than the trials comparing lumpectomy, with and without breast irradiation.

One of the first trials to compare less radical surgery with a more conservative approach for breast cancer was conducted at Guy's Hospital.[115] This trial, which was conducted between 1961 and 1971, compared the outcome of women treated by Halsted radical mastectomy versus wide local excision of the tumor with a 3-cm margin of normal tissue. Both groups received adjuvant radiotherapy. As expected, the local recurrence rate for patients treated with the more conservative surgery was higher than for those treated with mastectomy. There was no difference in the 10-year overall survival rate

for patients with stage I breast cancer. However, the 10-year overall survival rate was decreased in women with stage II disease in the tumorectomy group (30% for those treated with tumorectomy; 43% for those treated with Halsted mastectomy). This is the only randomized trial that has shown an adverse effect in survival rates for women treated with the more conservative surgery. This discrepancy may be a reflection of the radiotherapy techniques used during this study, which would not be acceptable by today's standards.

The earliest randomized trial that showed no decrease in survival rate when breast cancer was treated with breast conservation surgery and adjuvant radiotherapy was conducted at the Institut Gustave-Roussy (IGR).[116] To be eligible, patients had to have a tumor smaller than 2 cm on gross examination; lumpectomy patients had a 2-cm margin of normal tissue excised with the surgical specimen. A lower axillary dissection was performed on all patients; complete axillary dissection was only performed if, on frozen section, there was lymph node involvement. All patients who had undergone breast conservation surgery received adjuvant breast irradiation. Node-positive patients were further randomized to receive axillary nodal irradiation. No chemotherapy or hormonal treatment was administered. With a follow-up period of 15 years, women treated with breast conservation surgery and radiation had an increase in the local recurrence rate to 18%, but no decrease in overall survival.

The National Cancer Institute Trial[117] was a single-institution trial and had the broadest eligibility criteria. Women who had stage I or II breast cancer were randomized to MRM or lumpectomy,

**TABLE 19-8.** SUMMARY OF THE RANDOMIZED TRIALS THAT EVALUATED THE INCIDENCE OF LOCAL RECURRENCE AND SURVIVAL RATES FOR BREAST CANCER TREATED BY MODIFIED RADICAL MASTECTOMY OR BREAST CONSERVATION WITH BREAST IRRADIATION

| SERIES | T | INCLUSION | F/U | TREATMENT | N | LRR | OS | DFS |
|---|---|---|---|---|---|---|---|---|
| Guy's Hospital[115] | 1961–1971 | Stage I/II | 10 yr | LAND + RT | 182 | 37%/57% | 52%/30% | NS |
| | | | | RM + RT | 188 | 15%/35% | 58%/43% | |
| IGR[116] | 1972–1979 | T < 2 cm | 15 yr | LAND + RT | 88 | 13% | 73% | NA |
| | | | | MRM | 91 | 18% | 65% | NA |
| NCI[117] | 1979–1987 | Stage I/II | 10 yr | LAND + RT | 121 | 5% | 77% | 72% |
| | | | | MRM | 116 | 10% | 75% | 69% |
| Milan I[118] | 1973–1980 | T < 2 cm | 13 yr | MRM | 349 | 2.0% | 69% | NS |
| | | | | QUART | 352 | 3.1% | 71% | |
| EORTC[119] | 1980–1986 | Stage I/II | 8 yr | MRM | 425 | 9% | 73% | NS |
| | | | | LAND + RT | 456 | 15% | 71% | |
| Danish (DBCG)[120] | 1983–1989 | | 6 yr | LAND + RT | | | 79% | 70% |
| | | | | MRM | | | 82% | 66% |

ABBREVIATIONS: F/U = Follow-up expressed in years; N = number of women in study; LRR = local recurrence rate; OS = overall survival rate; DFS = disease-free survival; LAND + RT = lumpectomy, axillary node dissection, and breast irradiation; MRM = modified radical mastectomy; NS = not significant; NA = not available.

axillary dissection, and breast irradiation. If the axillary lymph nodes were positive for disease, then patients in the breast conservation arm also received irradiation of the internal mammary and supraclavicular lymph nodes. For lumpectomy patients, the tumor had to be grossly excised; microscopic negative tumor margins were not necessary. All patients with positive lymph nodes received adjuvant chemotherapy. In this trial, which included 247 women with a median follow-up of 10.1 years, the local recurrence rate was twofold greater in women treated with breast conservation and radiation. The overall survival rates did not differ between these two arms.

The Milan I trial[118] was limited to women with tumors less than 2 cm in diameter. The randomization was to Halsted mastectomy or quadrantectomy, axillary dissection, and radiotherapy (QUART). A quadrantectomy was defined as removal of the primary tumor with a 2- to 3-cm margin of normal breast tissue, overlying skin, and pectoral fascia. As with the other trials, the overall survival rate did not differ between the two treatment arms. Although there was an increase in the local recurrence rate in the women treated by QUART, the local recurrence rate was only 3.1%. This low local recurrence rate may be a reflection of the use of a quadrantectomy instead of a lumpectomy for removal of the primary tumor.

Although the EORTC trial[119] included women with stage I and II breast cancer, the specific aim of this trial was to evaluate MRM or breast conservation surgery and irradiation in women with stage II disease. In this trial of 902 patients, 81% had stage II disease. As with the other trials, the survival rates did not differ between the two treatment arms. The 8-year local recurrence rate was one and a half times greater in the group treated with lumpectomy, axillary dissection, and radiotherapy. When the women were stratified according to tumor size, the local recurrence rate in the lumpectomy group was 7% for TI lesions and 16% for TII tumors. Tumor size did not influence the likelihood of local recurrence in the mastectomy group. The Danish Breast Cancer Cooperative Group trial also compared breast conservation therapy with mastectomy.[120] In this

study of 905 patients, the 6-year overall survival rate was similar in the two treatment groups.

With the exception of the Guy's Hospital trial, the results of these trials concluded that despite the increase in local recurrence for women treated with breast conservation surgery and adjuvant irradiation, there was no difference in overall survival rate. Furthermore, breast conservation surgery with adjuvant radiotherapy could be offered, not only to women with small tumors, but also to women with tumors up to 5 cm in size.

Once it had been established that stage I and II breast cancers could be treated with breast conservation surgery and adjuvant radiotherapy, without a decrement in survival, the next set of trials evaluated the need for radiotherapy after lumpectomy. The Milan II[121] and Milan III,[122] Uppsala,[123,124] and Toronto[125] trials compared breast conservation surgery, with and without breast irradiation (Table 19-9).

The Milan II and Milan III trials evaluated the extent of local surgery and adjuvant therapy in the management of small breast cancers. Both of these trials were limited to women with tumors smaller than 2.5 cm. The Milan II trial compared QUART with tumorectomy, axillary dissection, and radiotherapy (TART). The definition of QUART was the same as in the first Milan trial. TART was defined as excision of the tumor with 2 cm of normal tissue, axillary dissection and radiotherapy; minimal skin was excised. The local recurrence rate was 2.3% with QUART and 7.0% with TART. There was no difference in the overall survival. When margins were evaluated, despite the appearance of normal tissue at the margin, 16% of the TART specimens and 3% of the QUART specimens had microscopic positive margins. Milan III evaluated the need for adjuvant radiotherapy; the two arms were QUART and quandrantectomy and axillary dissection (QUAD). After a median follow-up of 39 months, the local recurrence rate was 0.3% and 8.8% in the QUART and QUAD treatment arms, respectively. Again, there was no difference in survival rates. The results of the three Milan trials have been

**TABLE 19-9.** LOCAL RECURRENCE RATES, OVERALL SURVIVAL AND DISEASE-FREE SURVIVAL RATES IN WOMEN TREATED WITH BREAST CONSERVATION SURGERY, WITH AND WITHOUT ADJUVANT RADIOTHERAPY

| SERIES | T | INCLUSION | F/U | TREATMENT | N | LRR | OS | DFS |
|---|---|---|---|---|---|---|---|---|
| Milan II[121] | 1985–1987 | T < 2.5 cm | 4 yr | QUART | 360 | 2.3% | NS | NS |
| | | | | TART | 345 | 7.0% | | |
| Milan III[122] | 1987–1989 | T < 2.5 cm | 39 mo | QUART | 294 | 0.3% | NS | NS |
| | | | | QUAD | 273 | 8.8% | | |
| Uppsala-Orebro[123,124] | 1981–1988 | T < 2 cm | 5 yr | LAND + RT | 187 | 2.3% | 91% | 90% |
| | | | | LAND | 194 | 18.4% | 90% | 87% |
| Toronto (PMH)[125] | 1984–1989 | T < 4 cm | 7.6 yr | LAND + RT | 416 | 11% | 79% | |
| | | | | LAND | 421 | 35% | 76% | |
| NSABP B-06[126] | 1976–1984 | T < 4 cm | 12 yr | MRM | 494 | — | 59% | 49% |
| | | | | LAND + RT | 515 | 10% | 63% | 50% |
| | | | | LAND | 520 | 35% | 58% | 45% |

ABBREVIATIONS: T = Tumor size; F/U = follow-up period (yr); N = number of patients in study; LRR = local recurrence rate; OS = overall survival rate; DFS = disease-free survival rate; QUART = quadrantectomy and breast radiotherapy; TART = tumorectomy and breast radiotherapy; LAND + RT = lumpectomy, axillary node dissection, and breast radiotherapy; LAND = lumpectomy and axillary node dissection; MRM = modified radical mastectomy; NS = not significant; NA = not available.

updated and pooled (Table 19-10).[126] There was no difference in the survival rate according to treatment modality. The local recurrence rates were highest in the TART and QUAD treatment arms. Similar local recurrence rates were obtained for women treated with Halsted mastectomy or QUART.

The Uppsala-Orebro Breast Cancer Study Group randomized 381 women with conditions ranging from stage I breast cancer to lumpectomy with or without adjuvant radiotherapy. The lumpectomy specimen had to include the underlying fascia; multifocal lesions were excluded. After a 3-year follow-up period, the local recurrence rates were 2.3% and 18.4% in women treated with or without radiotherapy, respectively. The Toronto study, run by the Ontario Clinical Oncology Group, also only included women with node-negative disease but increased the tumor size to 4 cm. There was a fourfold increase in local recurrences in the group treated with lumpectomy alone as compared to those women treated with

**TABLE 19-10.** LONG-TERM FOLLOW-UP OF THE THREE MILAN TRIALS (MILAN I, II, AND III) WITH THE DATA POOLED INTO THE FOUR TREATMENT ARMS; HALSTED MASTECTOMY, QUART, TART, AND QUAD

| TREATMENT | NUMBER | LOCAL RECURRENCE RATE |
|---|---|---|
| Halsted mastectomy | 349 | 2.3% |
| QUART | 1006 | 3.3% |
| TART | 345 | 12.8% |
| QUAD | 273 | 11.7% |

SOURCE: Compiled from data obtained in Veronesi U et al: Breast conservation is a safe method in patients with small cancer of the breast: Long-term results of three randomized trials on 1,973 patients. Eur J Cancer 31A:1574–1579, 1995.

lumpectomy and radiotherapy. In both of these trials, there were no differences in overall survival rate, irrespective of the treatment modality.

NSABP B-06[127] was a three-armed trial that compared MRM and lumpectomy, with and without breast irradiation. Again, the local recurrence rate was significantly greater when breast irradiation was omitted after breast conservation surgery. At 12 years of follow-up, the overall survival rates and disease-free survival rates were similar for all three arms of this study.

Despite the increase in local recurrence in women treated by lumpectomy alone, it is assumed that the majority of local recurrences can be salvaged by a mastectomy, with no decrease in overall survival. In the Milan, Toronto, and Uppsala trials, the survival rate was comparable with or without breast irradiation. However, a recent report reanalyzing the data suggested that breast irradiation with lumpectomy may offer a survival benefit as compared with lumpectomy alone. Using a Bayesian analysis, Levitt and collegues[128] have reported that there is a 10% relative reduction in cancer mortality in favor of irradiated patients, and this benefit increases to 17.5% at 10 years. From these randomized trials, it can be summarized that women with breast cancer treated with lumpectomy, breast irradiation, and axillary nodal dissection have a comparable disease-free and overall survival rate as compared with those treated by MRM. Treatment of early breast cancer by lumpectomy alone results in approximately a threefold increase in local disease recurrence, which may or may not have an adverse effect on survival.

Although the majority of early breast cancers are amenable to breast conservation, there are certain prognostic factors that are associated with an increased likelihood of local tumor recurrence. Approximately 10% of patients treated by breast conservation and adjuvant radiation will have local disease recurrence.[129] Eighty percent of local recurrences occur within the first 5 years. Although the studies cited previously indicate that a local tumor recurrence does not affect survival, patients who have a local recurrence have an eightfold relative risk for a distant recurrence.[130] A consistent prognostic factor for local recurrence is presence of tumor at the surgical margin. An excision with a microscopically positive margin for tumor cells is associated with an increased risk of local recurrence. In an analysis of 143 patients who had recurrence of their breast cancer, Noguchi and colleagues[131] found that a positive surgical margin increased the likelihood of a local recurrence to 16.7 times that when the surgical margin was negative. When margin status is subdivided into negative (tumor present greater than 1 mm from excision margin), close (tumor present within 1 mm but not at margin), and positive (carcinoma at inked margin), the 5-year local recurrence rates are 3%, 2%, and 16%, respectively.[132] Therefore, if a positive surgical margin is present after excision, re-excision of the biopsy should be performed since attempts to sterilize positive margins with radiotherapy will still result in a high rate of local recurrence.[133]

Tumor characteristics can predict which patients are more likely to have a local recurrence after local therapy. Extensive intraductal component (EIC) is defined as the presence of intraductal carcinoma in more than 25% of the specimen. The presence of an extensive intraductal component[134] or comedocarcinoma[135] is associated with an increased risk for local recurrence. Increasing tumor size is another prognostic risk factor for locoregional recurrence after both mastectomy[136] and breast conservation surgery with tumors larger than 2 cm having a twofold increase in local recurrence.[137] It is debatable whether lymph node status is a prognostic indicator of local tumor recurrence. Some groups have shown that the presence of positive lymph nodes or tumor emboli within the lymphatics increases the relative risk for a local recurrence.[135] However, multivariate analysis of results, obtained from NSABP B-06, suggests that nodal status alone is not a prognostic factor for local recurrence.[138] Breast cancers with lymphatic vessel invasion[139] or poor nuclear grade[140] are more likely to recur as compared to similar cancers without these histologic features. Mammographic findings suggestive of multifocal disease such as diffuse microcalcifications or a stellate lesion with microcalcifications within the lesion are associated with more local recurrences.[141,142] With the increasing analysis of cancers with molecular markers, there is early evidence that some of these markers such as the percentage of tumor cells actively dividing (S-phase fraction) and p53 overexpression will be important prognostic factors for local recurrence.[131]

In terms of host factors, age less than 45[143] or 50[144,145] years was associated with more local recurrences. Factors that are associated with an increased local recurrence are summarized in Table 19-11.

Not all women are candidates for breast conservation. Although large tumor size is not a contraindication to breast conservation, the surgeon has to be able to remove the lesion with a contiguous rim of normal breast tissue. There should be an acceptable cosmetic result in the remaining breast tissue. The appearance of multiple, scattered-appearing calcifications or factors suggestive of multicentricity that cannot be adequately excised are indications for a mastectomy. The present use of breast conservation in early breast cancer includes adjuvant radiation to the remaining breast tissue. Contraindications to adjuvant breast irradiation include first and second trimester pregnancy, a history of prior therapeutic radiation to the breast region (e.g., mantle radiation for Hodgkin's disease), and some collagen vascular disorders.

**TABLE 19-11.** RISK OF LOCAL RECURRENCE AFTER BREAST CONSERVATION SURGERY AND ADJUVANT RADIOTHERAPY

| PROGNOSTIC FACTOR | RR OF LOCAL RECURRENCE* |
|---|---|
| Age <45 | 4.09 |
| Age <50 | 1.2–2.0 |
| Mammogram suggestive of multicentricity | 2.3 |
| Diffuse microcalcifications | 3.8 |
| Presence of EIC | 2.2–9.0 |
| Presence of comedocarcinoma | 3.5 |
| Histology (lobular versus ductal) | 2.8 |
| Positive surgical margin | 2.6–16.7 |
| Tumor size (>2 cm) | 2.0 |
| Positive lymph nodes | 2.5 |
| p53 overexpression | 9.28 |

* Relative risk (RR) expressed as a multiple if prognostic factor is absent or age is greater than 65.

The optimal time interval between surgery and the initiation of adjuvant radiotherapy remains to be resolved. Hartsell and colleagues[146] reported that in a retrospective review of 474 patients treated with breast conservation, a delay in the initiation of breast irradiation beyond 120 days resulted in an increase in local recurrence in patients who had node-positive disease. However, other groups have reported that a delay in initiating breast radiotherapy of up to 16 weeks did not result in an increased risk of a local recurrence in patients with node-negative breast cancer.[147] The Steering Committee on Clinical Practice Guidelines for the Care and Treatment of Breast Cancer recently concluded that although the optimal interval between surgery and breast irradiation was not known, local breast irradiation should be initiated as soon as possible after surgery, and preferably not later than 12 weeks.[148] The optimal timing of breast irradiation in patients who are to receive adjuvant chemotherapy is even more complicated. Some groups have suggested that a delay in the initiation of radiotherapy so that chemotherapy can be completed resulted in an increased local recurrence rate of 41%; patients who received radiotherapy earlier in their treatment had a local failure rate of 4% to 6%.[149] However, utilizing data obtained from two randomized trials evaluating adjuvant chemotherapy in node-positive women, the International Breast Cancer Study Group concluded that the likelihood of local recurrence was equivalent in premenopausal, perimenopausal, and postmenopausal women who had radiation therapy 4 or 7, or 2 or 4 months, respectively, after surgery.[150]

Two recent controversies regarding the management of early breast cancer include the optimal management of the axilla (i.e., whether an axillary nodal dissection is a diagnostic or therapeutic tool) and the need for adjuvant breast irradiation in patients with minimally invasive breast cancers (tumors less than 1 cm in size).

In 1985, NSABP reported the results of trial B-04,[151] which had two distinct objectives. One part of the trial addressed the management of patients with clinically negative nodes and randomized patients to receive MRM, mastectomy, and axillary radiotherapy or mastectomy alone followed by delayed axillary dissection for a clinically positive axilla. At 10 years of follow-up, there was no difference in disease free or overall survival for any of the three arms. The conclusion from this part of the study was that there is no therapeutic benefit for axillary dissection in the patient with clinically negative nodes. Since clinical evaluation of the axilla is inaccurate in up to 40% of patients and lymph node metastases is one of the most important prognostic factors, an immediate axillary dissection was beneficial because it identified which patients would be good candidates for adjuvant chemotherapy.

The second objective of this study addressed management of the patient with clinically positive nodes. These women were randomized to receive MRM or axillary radiation; they did not receive adjuvant hormonal or chemotherapy. At 10 years of follow-up, 25% of the women had no recurrence of disease, indicating that treatment of the axilla may prevent distant metastases. Furthermore, recurrence in the axilla was 1% for women treated with surgery versus 11% treated with axillary radiation. Since these results have been published, there has been great controversy as to whether an axillary dissection is solely a diagnostic tool or whether it has some therapeutic benefit as well.[152] The Breast Carcinoma Collaborative Group of the Institut Curie found that the 5-year survival rate for women who received an axillary nodal dissection was significantly better than for those who had no dissection (96.6% versus 92.6%, p < 0.05). However, patients who had nodal metastases had received adjuvant therapy, which may account for their survival advantage.[153]

Until recently, radiotherapy has been used to control local and regional disease; it was thought that its use had no impact on overall survival. This dogma has been challenged with the publication of the results of two randomized trials that compared the outcomes of patients who did, or did not, receive axillary irradiation after surgical dissection. Both of these studies were limited to premenopausal females. The larger of the two studies was conducted by the Danish Breast Cancer Cooperative Group, which randomly selected among 1708 high-risk, premenopausal women to receive cyclophosphamide, methotrexate, and fluorouracil (CMF) plus or minus axillary irradiation.[154] Factors considered "high risk" were positive axillary lymph nodes, tumor size greater than 5 cm, and tumor extension to the skin or pectoral muscles. In this study, the addition of axillary irradiation resulted in a 10-year survival rate of 54%; patients who received CMF alone had a 10-year survival rate of 45% (p < 0.001). Multivariate analysis revealed that the benefit of axillary irradiation was independent of the number of positive lymph nodes or tumor size. A similar trial was conducted in Canada with 318 premenopausal women with positive lymph nodes randomized to CMF plus or minus chest wall and axillary radiotherapy; all women had undergone MRM.[155] Not surprisingly, the 5-, 10-, and 15-year local recurrence rates were lower in the group randomized to the CMF and radiotherapy arm (Table 19-12). This decrease in locoregional recurrence was statistically significant in women who had four or more positive lymph nodes. However, as with the Danish study, there was also an improvement in the overall survival rate, with the CMF and radiotherapy group having a 29% reduction in breast cancer mortality. One of the criticisms of the Danish study is that half of the patients had fewer than 10 lymph nodes removed during the axillary dissection. These studies were conducted 15 years ago, and today, different chemotherapeutic regimens are being used

**TABLE 19-12.** LOCOREGIONAL RECURRENCE, OVERALL SURVIVAL RATE, AND BREAST CANCER–SPECIFIC SURVIVAL RATE IN PREMENOPAUSAL NODE-POSITIVE WOMEN RANDOMIZED TO RECEIVE CMF PLUS OR MINUS CHEST WALL AND AXILLARY RADIOTHERAPY

LOCOREGIONAL RECURRENCE RATE

|  | 5 yr | 10 yr | 15 yr |
| --- | --- | --- | --- |
| CMF alone | 79% | 75% | 67% |
| CMF plus RT | 90% | 87% | 87% |
| p = 0.003 |  |  |  |

OVERALL SURVIVAL RATE

|  | 5 yr | 10 yr | 15 yr |
| --- | --- | --- | --- |
| CMF alone | 70% | 54% | 46% |
| CMF plus RT | 76% | 64% | 54% |
| p = 0.07 |  |  |  |

BREAST CANCER–SPECIFIC SURVIVAL RATE

|  | 5 yr | 10 yr | 15 yr |
| --- | --- | --- | --- |
| CMF alone | 70% | 56% | 47% |
| CMF plus RT | 76% | 65% | 57% |
| p = 0.05 |  |  |  |

ABBREVIATIONS: CMF = Cytoxan, methotrexate, 5-fluorouracil; RT = chest wall and axillary radiotherapy, see text for chemotherapy regimen.
SOURCE: Results from the British Columbia Cancer Agency (compiled from data in Ragaz J et al: Adjuvant radiotherapy and chemotherapy in node-positive premenopausal women with breast cancer. N Engl J Med 337:956–962, 1997.

and breast cancer is being diagnosed at an earlier stage. Despite this, the results of these two trials have challenged the notion that locoregional control has little impact on overall survival rate and that axillary metastases may be able to metastasize.

An axillary dissection has some morbidity, with a loss of cutaneous sensation and a decrease in shoulder mobility, and carries the long-term risk of arm lymphedema. To help resolve the above controversy, sentinel lymph node mapping has been popularized. In breast cancer, the sentinel lymph node is the first lymph node or nodes into which the lymphatics from the breast cancer area drain. Using a blue dye and/or radioactive colloid, the sentinel lymph node (SLN) can be identified. Since only one to three nodes are removed in the axilla, these sentinel lymph nodes can be examined not only by standard histologic examination, but also by immunohistochemistry, which increases the detection of micrometastases.[156] It has been hypothesized that since the SLN is the first lymph node draining the cancer, if it is free of tumor, then the rest of the axilla should also be disease-free.

The John Wayne Cancer Institute[157] was one of the first groups to systematically study the feasibility of SLN mapping in breast cancer. Using a blue dye to identify the SLN, Giuliano and colleagues[157] were able to perform a SLN biopsy in 174 patients with breast cancer. In this initial series, 65.5% of patients had a SLN identified. Completion axillary dissections were performed on all patients in this study, and only 4.4% of the patients had a nonsentinel axillary lymph node positive for metastatic disease with a SLN negative for metastases (i.e., false-negative rate). Overall 30% of the patients had metastases in their SLN; of these, only 43% had metastases in the SLN only. After his seminal paper, Giuliano then conducted extensive analysis of sentinel and nonsentinel axillary lymph nodes to determine if the sentinel node was able to accurately predict the presence or absence of regional disease. In 70 breast cancer patients with a negative SLN, completion axillary dissections were performed and all lymph nodes examined by standard histology, followed by immunohistochemistry.[158] Out of 1078 lymph nodes examined, by hematoxylin and eosin staining, all were negative and by immunohistochemistry, only one was positive. This study concluded that the SLN is a true predictor of axillary lymph node status.

Since these initial results have been reported, Giuliano has updated his results and other groups have reported their observations (Table 19-13).[157–164] The tracers used to identify the SLN have included technetium sulfur colloid, technetium albumin, technetium-labeled dextran, patent blue V dye, and isosulfan blue dye. Overall, the ability to identify the SLN ranges from 60% to 70% when only a dye is used, to over 90% when both a dye and radiocolloid are combined. In most reported series, there have been some patients in whom it was not possible to localize the SLN ("failed sentinel lymph node"). The factors responsible for a failed SLN are not clear. A report from Free University in Amsterdam[163] has suggested that the presence of a previous biopsy cavity influences the ability to identify the SLN. In this study of 130 patients, the failure

rate was significantly higher for patients who had had a previous biopsy (36%) than for those who had a palpable tumor in situ (4%). However, the results from the H. Lee Moffitt Cancer Center do not support this conclusion.[160]

Most series on sentinel node biopsy for breast cancer that have more than 100 patients and that have included axillary dissections as part of their protocol have had false-negative results. A falsely negative SLN occurs when the SLN is free of disease, but there are metastases in other axillary lymph nodes. False-negative SLNs may be more likely with increasing tumor size,[164] multicentric lesions,[53] or if the SLN has been completely replaced by tumor.[162] Using careful technique, fewer than 5% of cases have involved a false-negative SLN. Some groups no longer perform a completion axillary dissection if the SLN is free of metastatic disease.

One of the advantages of SLN biopsy is that careful pathologic examination of the SLN can be performed. Previously, the standard mode for examining lymph nodes involved single sections through the lymph node. With the advent of SLN biopsy, the SLN can be carefully examined with multiple, thin hematoxylin and eosin stained sections, immunohistochemistry, and even reverse transcriptase polymerase chain reaction (RT-PCR) to identify the presence of epithelial-derived mRNA in the lymph node. The overall result is that the proportion of breast cancer patients in whom lymph nodes are determined to be positive for regional disease has increased to 40% to 50%. Many of these lymph nodes have had micrometastases only. The significance of lymph node micrometastases in breast cancer is controversial, and it is unclear whether patients with lymph node micrometastases only have a decreased survival rate and should be treated with adjuvant systemic therapy.[156]

In an effort to resolve some of the controversy associated with SLN biopsy, four large multicenter studies have been designed to

**TABLE 19-13.** THE ACCURACY OF SENTINEL LYMPHADENECTOMY TO PREDICT AXILLARY STATUS IN BREAST CANCER

| SERIES | NUMBER OF PATIENTS | SLN IDENTIFIED | % WITH POSITIVE SLN | FALSE NEGATIVE |
|---|---|---|---|---|
| John Wayne Cancer Institute[157] | 174 | 114/174 (65.5%) | 37/114 (29.8%) | 5/114 (4.4%) |
| John Wayne Cancer Institute[159] | 107 | 100/107 (93.4%) | 42/100 (42%) | 0/100 (0%) |
| H. Lee Moffitt Cancer Center[160] | 466 | 440/466 (94/4%) | 105/440 (23.8%) | 1/440 (0.21%) |
| European Institute of Oncology[53] | 163 | 160/163 (985) | 81/160 (47.9%) | 4/160 (2.5%) |
| Mercer University School of Medicine[161] | 20 | 14/20 (66%) | 5/14 (35.7%) | 0/14 (0%) |
| Kaiser Permanente[162] | 145 | 103/145 (71.0%) | 28/103 (21.5%) | 3/103 (2.9%) |
| Academisch Ziekenhuis van de Vrije Universitet[163] | 130 | 122/130 (94%) | 44/104* (42%) | 1.104* (1%) |
| Memorial Sloan-Kettering Cancer Center[164] | 60 | 55/59 (93%) | 20/55 (36%) | 3/55 (5.5%) |

* Only 104 of the patients underwent a completion axillary dissection. These 130 patients form the denominator for determination of false-negative SLN biopsy rate.

**TABLE 19-14. INCIDENCE OF POSITIVE LYMPH NODE METASTASIS IN PATIENTS WITH T1 BREAST CANCERS**

| SERIES | TIME PERIOD | SIZE, % |
|---|---|---|
| Deaconess[137] | 1979–1988 | T1a,b = 13% |
| North Carolina[166] | 1987–1994 | T1a = 4% |
| Van Nuys, CA[168] | 1979–1995 | T1 = 23% |
| | | T1a = 4% |
| | | T1b = 17% |
| | | T1c = 28% |
| Rhode Island and Massachusetts[167] | 1984–1995 | T1a = 11.3% |
| | | T1b = 17.3% |
| BI/Albert Einstein (NYC)[170] | 1990–1991 | T1a,b = 5% |
| | | T1c = 35% |

address the pros and cons of SLN biopsy.[165] The American College of Surgeons Oncology Group (ACoSOG) will study the impact of positive SLN and no axillary dissection on regional recurrence and survival and the significance of micrometastases. The Bay Area Sentinel Lymph Node Study will evaluate the techniques used to identify the SLNs and try to determine which patients are most appropriate for SLN biopsy. The Moffit Center/Department of Defense Study is similar to the ACoSOG and will study regional recurrence and survival rates in patients who are SLN-positive, who have an axillary dissection, and patients who are SLN-negative, who have no further dissection. Finally, the University of Vermont/NSABP will compare survival and morbidity rates in patients who have a standard axillary dissection or a SLN biopsy. These studies have been designed to start accruing patients in 1998; it will be some time before the results are available.

Another approach to the controversy of a routine axillary dissection for breast cancer is to determine which patients are least likely to benefit from an axillary dissection (either from a diagnostic or a therapeutic approach) and to not treat the axilla in these patients. Since the risk of nodal metastases is proportional to tumor size, the smallest tumors are the ones least likely to have regional disease. The incidence of lymph node metastases in patients with T1 lesions ranges from 4% to 35% (Table 19-14). The lower percentages are found in the studies where the pathologic material has been carefully reviewed[166]; higher percentages are more likely with data derived solely from cancer registries. Lymph node metastases with T1 lesions are most often found in young women under 40 years of age,[167] higher nuclear grade,[168] lesions that were palpable at diagnosis,[169] and lesions with lymphovascular invasion.[170] In an analysis of T1 breast lesions identified in a mammographically screened population, increasing grade was found to correlate with the incidence of axillary metastases, with only 5% of grade I lesions having lymph node involvement as compared to 18% with grade III lesions.[171] Since older women with small (T1a), well-differentiated, nonpalpable breast cancers are the least likely to have nodal metastases, these women may be candidates for local treatment only.

The role of using axillary irradiation after an axillary dissection remains controversial. The addition of axillary irradiation to surgical dissection has often been used for patients considered at high risk for tumor recurrence in the axilla. This includes patients with large tumor size, four or more lymph nodes positive for tumor, and extracapsular disease. However, recent retrospective reports analyzing the benefit of nodal irradiation have challenged this practice. Although extranodal disease has been shown to be associated with the likelihood of extensive nodal involvement and overall decreased survival rate, it has not resulted in an increase in axillary failure when the axilla was not irradiated.[172–174] Similar results have been reported for patients with more than four lymph nodes involved with tumor who have not had axillary irradiation after surgical dissection.[175,176]

## CHEMOTHERAPY

There is little doubt that the introduction of adjuvant chemotherapy to the management of women at risk for systemic breast cancer has resulted in an increased survival benefit. The current status of adjuvant chemotherapy for breast cancer was reviewed recently,[177] and some of the present controversies surrounding its use are outlined in Table 19-15.

The literature on adjuvant chemotherapy in breast cancer is overwhelming, with each published study being unique. In an effort to consolidate the available data, the Early Breast Cancer Trialists' Collaborative Group[178] pooled the information of all randomized trials on adjuvant chemotherapy begun before 1985 in order to determine the benefit of hormonal, cytotoxic, and immune therapy in early breast cancer. This study included 30,000 women on tamoxifen trials; 30,000 women who underwent ovarian ablation; 11,000 who received polychemotherapy; 15,000 who received other forms of chemotherapy; and 6000 women who received immunotherapy.

The Early Breast Cancer Trialists' Collaborative Group validated the use of adjuvant chemotherapy in the management of breast cancer, finding that the combination of more than one chemotherapeutic agent was superior to single-agent therapy. For women who received an adjuvant polychemotherapy regimen, there was a 28% reduction in disease recurrence and a 16% reduction in cancer death at 10 years of follow-up. Six months appears to be the optimal duration of therapy, however, since additional cycles have shown little survival benefit. These results included women with and without nodal disease after 20 years of follow-up.[179] The benefit of adjuvant chemotherapy in node-positive breast cancer remains consistent.

With respect to tamoxifen, the Early Breast Cancer Trialists' Collaborative Group concluded that there was a 25% reduction in the recurrence rate and a 17% decrease in the mortality rate from

**TABLE 19-15. CONTROVERSIES IN ADJUVANT CHEMOTHERAPY**

*Candidates suitable for adjuvant chemotherapy:*
- Optimal chemotherapy regimen
- Number of chemotherapy cycles
- Timing of adjuvant chemotherapy: Preoperative, perioperative, postoperative
- Sequencing of adjuvant radiotherapy and chemotherapy
- Duration of adjuvant hormonal therapy

breast cancer. The results were better for women with nodes positive for disease as compared with those with local disease only. However, the benefit of adding chemotherapy to tamoxifen was debatable in women older than 50 years of age who had node-positive disease. A meta-analysis of 3920 postmenopausal women with node-positive disease found that although the addition of adjuvant chemotherapy increased disease-free and overall survival rates, the increase was small and the benefit diminished by the morbidity of the chemotherapy regimens.[180] These results differ from those obtained from NSABP B-16, which found that at 3 years of follow-up, the addition of chemotherapy to tamoxifen increased the survival rates in a similar group of women from 73% to 83%.[181]

In an effort to resolve some of the issues associated with tamoxifen use in the adjuvant treatment of breast cancer, the Early Breast Cancer Trialists' Collaborative Group reviewed the data obtained from the randomized trials of adjuvant tamoxifen among women with early breast cancer.[182] This study included all randomized trials that began before 1990 and included results up to 1995. With a database of 38,000 women (8000 with estrogen receptor [ER]-negative tumors, 18,000 with ER-positive tumors, and 12,000 with tumors of an unknown ER status), it was concluded that tamoxifen use for 5 years decreased the local recurrence of breast cancer by 47% in women with ER-positive tumors. Tamoxifen use for 5 years also decreased the mortality rate by 25% in these women. The decrease in the local recurrence rate was present in the first 5 years; the mortality rate decrease persisted for up to 10 years. Tamoxifen use also resulted in a decrease in the rate of a contralateral breast cancer (26 cases out of 1000 versus 47 cases out of 1000 for women who took and did not take tamoxifen for 5 years, respectively). There was a fourfold increased rate of endometrial cancer associated with tamoxifen use (11/1000 and 3/1000 for tamoxifen and no-tamoxifen use, respectively). The beneficial effects of tamoxifen on breast cancer were present in both premenopausal and postmenopausal women and were independent of lymph node status. However, there appeared to be little benefit associated with tamoxifen use in women who had ER-negative tumors.

The optimal length of adjuvant tamoxifen therapy remains debatable, with the length of adjuvant treatment ranging from 2 years to indeterminate. In the Swedish Breast Cancer Cooperative Group Trial, women with early breast cancer were randomized to 2 versus 5 years of adjuvant tamoxifen.[183] In this study of 3887 women, there was a significant increase in disease-free and overall survival rates with the longer period of tamoxifen use, with an 18% reduction in recurrence rate and mortality rate. However, results from the Eastern Cooperative Oncology Group suggest that there seems to be no benefit in extending tamoxifen use beyond 5 years.[184] Therefore, it would appear from these studies that the use of tamoxifen in the adjuvant setting should be extended to 5 years, with little benefit thought likely beyond this time period.

Since many breast cancers have estrogen receptors, the role of ovarian ablation was investigated in the Early Breast Cancer Trialists' Collaborative Group study. While little benefit was found for women older than 50, in younger women ovarian ablation resulted in a 26% decrease in disease recurrence and a 25% decrease in breast cancer deaths. However, the benefit in young women was statistically significant for those with node-positive disease; for those with node-negative disease, the benefit is less clear.

It remains unclear as to when adjuvant chemotherapy should be given. Chemotherapy for early breast cancer is usually administered in the postoperative setting, since this allows accurate pathologic staging of the tumor. However, with the advent of breast conservation and the need for adjuvant radiotherapy, the sequencing of the adjuvant therapies is less clear. In those patients at high risk for systemic disease, it appears that a sandwich therapeutic regimen (three cycles of chemotherapy, radiotherapy, followed by three cycles of chemotherapy) would be most beneficial.[185] Preoperative chemotherapy in women with operable breast cancer has been shown to decrease tumor size and the number of lymph nodes involved, as well as to increase the likelihood of breast conservation.[186] However, a meta-analysis including 6093 women has shown that although there is an increase in disease-free survival, the use of perioperative chemotherapy in operable breast cancer does not translate into an increase in survival benefit.[187]

Because it was noted that tamoxifen can decrease the risk for the development of a contralateral breast cancer, some authors have suggested that this drug be used as a chemopreventive breast cancer drug. To test whether tamoxifen can prevent breast cancer, the NSABP Protocol P1 was designed. This study, which was initiated in 1992, randomized high-risk women to receive either tamoxifen or placebo. Women considered at high risk for developing breast cancer included any women over the age of 65 (age was the risk factor), significant family history of breast cancer, and previous breast biopsy for lobular carcinoma in situ. After 4 years, the study was closed and preliminary results released through the media in the spring of 1998. The preliminary results showed that the use of tamoxifen decreased the risk of breast cancer by one-half in all women, irrespective of age. However, there was an associated increase in thrombotic events and endometrial carcinoma in the tamoxifen arm, particularly in women older than 65. It was concluded by the investigators involved with the study that the benefit of tamoxifen, in terms of cancer development, outweighed the side effects, especially in women under the age of 65. To date, the results have not been formally published and scrutinized. Therefore, it remains controversial whether women at high risk for breast cancer should receive tamoxifen as a breast cancer preventive agent.

## LOCALLY ADVANCED BREAST CANCER

Locally advanced breast cancer (LABC) includes patients with stage III or inflammatory breast cancer. Usually defined pathologically by the presence of tumor emboli in the dermal lymphatics (true IBC), inflammatory breast cancer (IBC) accounts for 2% of all breast cancers and is associated with a clinical presentation of skin inflammation with erythema and "peau d'orange" changes.[188] A subtype of IBC (pseudo-IBC) has the same clinical appearance but lacks the extensive lymph node involvement and permeation of the dermal lymphatics. Although pseudo-IBC appears clinically similar to true IBC, the distinction is important in that treatment may differ.

Historically, LABC has had a dismal prognosis. Initially treated by surgery and/or radiation, the 5-year survival rate with this disease was less than 5%, with patients often succumbing to metastatic disease. The advent of chemotherapy in the 1970s allowed the use of multimodality treatment for IBC, consisting of induction chemotherapy followed by local treatment and further chemotherapy, if a clinical response had been obtained. The overall survival rate for LABC after multimodality treatment ranges from a low of 29% (6-year survival rate)[189] to 45%[190] to 50%[191] (5-year survival rate). Attia-Sobol and colleagues[192] reported their results on 109 patients treated with an adriamycin-based induction chemotherapy, followed by radiotherapy (if complete or near complete response) or surgery, and then more chemotherapy. With a median follow-up period of 120 months, the median survival length was 70 months and the median disease-free survival length was 45 months. MD Anderson recently reported their results for 178 women with IBC treated between 1974 and 1993 with doxorubicin-based combination chemotherapy.[193] After a mean follow-up period of 89 months, 5- and 10-year survival rates for the group were 36% and 24%, respectively. Twenty six percent of their patients had a local recurrence, with 98% of these patients dying of their disease. Factors associated with a local recurrence included treatment by radiotherapy alone and a poor response to induction chemotherapy.[194] These authors concluded that the addition of mastectomy to combination chemotherapy and radiotherapy in patients with IBC who responded to induction chemotherapy improved local control and resulted in a more favorable outcome in overall survival.

However, the benefit of mastectomy in the management of IBC is not clear. Touboul and colleagues[195] reported their results of stage II breast cancers greater than 3 cm or locally advanced breast cancers treated by induction chemotherapy, preoperative radiation, and further chemotherapy. Locoregional disease was treated by either MRM, lumpectomy, axillary dissection and adjuvant radiation, or radiotherapy alone. The 10-year overall survival rate was 66% and did not differ in the three treatment arms. The local recurrence rate was lowest for patients treated by mastectomy (6%) and similar for those treated by wide excision and radiotherapy or radiotherapy alone (23% and 20%, respectively). As with the MD Anderson study, these authors observed that local failure was associated with a decreased survival rate. Schwartz and associates[196] have reported the Jefferson experience with LABC treated by breast conservation. This study began in 1979 with induction chemotherapy, followed by MRM and further chemotherapy. Since 1990, patients who were candidates for breast conservation surgery had wide excision of the tumor with radiation as local treatment. In 108 stage III patients, the 5-year survival rate was 68% and 63% for responders treated by mastectomy and breast conservation, respectively. In the Jefferson study, there were an inadequate number of patients with IBC to draw any conclusion about IBC treated by breast conservation. The largest series of patients with LABC who were treated with breast conservation has been reported by Bonadonna and colleagues.[197] In the Milan experience, the 3-year local relapse rate was 3.5% for 220 women with LABC treated by induction chemotherapy, breast conservation and radiation and followed by chemotherapy. The difficulty in comparing survival outcomes based on local therapy is an inherent selection bias in all the studies, since those patients most likely to have breast conservation are usually those whose tumors responded to the induction chemotherapy. It is accepted that chemotherapy responders have a better prognosis as compared with nonresponders; therefore, patients having breast conservation may, as a group, be different from those patients undergoing mastectomy or radiotherapy alone. With the introduction of induction chemotherapy, the controversy

in LABC is the optimal management of the breast and axilla. Although the majority of LABC patients die from metastatic disease, those patients who do recur locally have a worse outcome than those patients with good local control. It is not clear if treating the breast by mastectomy, breast-conserving surgery, or radiotherapy alters survival. It is feasible, however, that patients whose tumors respond to induction chemotherapy may be candidates for breast conservation.

Because of the increase in survival seen with induction chemotherapy, it is not surprising that more aggressive chemotherapeutic agents are being used in the management of locally advanced breast cancer, including the use of high-dose chemotherapy and stem cell rescue.[198,199] It is hoped that these more aggressive regimens will result in an increased survival rate for this once dismal disease.

## SURVIVAL RATES FOR BREAST CANCER

The most important predictor of survival for breast cancer is the clinical stage. Approximately 24% of women diagnosed with breast cancer will die of their disease. However, there is a positive trend in breast cancer survival for women diagnosed with this disease in the United States. From 1960 to 1992, there has been an increase in breast cancer survival: from 63% to 85% for caucasian women, and 46% to 70% for African American women.[3] This improvement in survival may be a reflection of the increased use of mammographic screening and diagnosing breast cancer at an earlier clinical stage.

The overall survival of women with breast cancer is summarized in Fig. 19-6. Clearly, it can be seen that women with early breast cancer have a significantly better survival rate than those with more advanced disease. It is rare for a women with DCIS (stage 0) to die of breast cancer. Women with tumors less than 2 cm in size and no nodal metastases (stage I) have a survival rate of 90%, with a step-off decrease in survival for larger tumors and positive nodal metastases. As mentioned, tumor size and nodal metastases are two of the most important prognostic factors of outcome in breast cancer, with factors such as age and histologic and molecular features of the cancer playing a secondary role in survival. These features are important for deciding which women, within each clinical stage, are most likely to have a recurrence, locally or distally, and who should be candidates for more aggressive treatment.

## FOLLOW-UP

The follow-up of women with breast cancer has two primary functions: the identification of recurrent disease and the diagnosis of a new primary breast cancer. Practice guidelines provide a guide for clinical practice and do not replace clinical judgment. Table 19-16 summarizes the American Society of Clinical Oncology guidelines for breast cancer surveillance.[200] These guidelines were recommended on the basis of clinical trial results, meta-analyses of retrospective studies, and potential benefit to the patient. These guidelines emphasize the importance of clinical examination at frequent intervals. With the advent of tumor markers for breast cancer screening and detection of recurrent disease,[201] these guidelines underscore the concept that radiologic and serologic testing, in the absence of symptoms, is rerely beneficial to the patient. The exception to this is

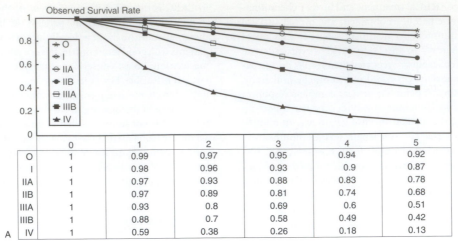

| | 0 | 1 | 2 | 3 | 4 | 5 |
|---|---|---|---|---|---|---|
| O | 1 | 0.99 | 0.97 | 0.95 | 0.94 | 0.92 |
| I | 1 | 0.98 | 0.96 | 0.93 | 0.9 | 0.87 |
| IIA | 1 | 0.97 | 0.93 | 0.88 | 0.83 | 0.78 |
| IIB | 1 | 0.97 | 0.89 | 0.81 | 0.74 | 0.68 |
| IIIA | 1 | 0.93 | 0.8 | 0.69 | 0.6 | 0.51 |
| IIIB | 1 | 0.88 | 0.7 | 0.58 | 0.49 | 0.42 |
| IV | 1 | 0.59 | 0.38 | 0.26 | 0.18 | 0.13 |

A

Years After Diagnosis

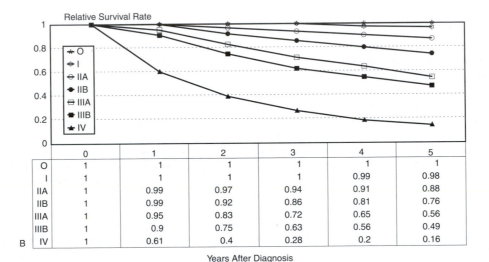

| | 0 | 1 | 2 | 3 | 4 | 5 |
|---|---|---|---|---|---|---|
| O | 1 | 1 | 1 | 1 | 1 | 1 |
| I | 1 | 1 | 1 | 1 | 0.99 | 0.98 |
| IIA | 1 | 0.99 | 0.97 | 0.94 | 0.91 | 0.88 |
| IIB | 1 | 0.99 | 0.92 | 0.86 | 0.81 | 0.76 |
| IIIA | 1 | 0.95 | 0.83 | 0.72 | 0.65 | 0.56 |
| IIIB | 1 | 0.9 | 0.75 | 0.63 | 0.56 | 0.49 |
| IV | 1 | 0.61 | 0.4 | 0.28 | 0.2 | 0.16 |

B

Years After Diagnosis

**FIGURE 19-6.** Breast cancer survival according to stage. (*From Fleming ID et al. (eds): Breast, in AJCC Cancer Staging Manual.* Philadelphia, Lippincott-Raven, 1997, p. 175.)

the use of routine mammography to detect recurrent and new breast disease. The incidence of a contralateral breast cancer in a patient with a previous breast cancer is 1% per year, and mammography allows the detection of nonpalpable and early breast lesions.[202] The need for mammographic survillance of both the ipsilateral breast for recurrent disease and the contralateral breast for a new primary breast cancer is important, since up to 50% of women with a history of breast cancer, who also have mammographic abnormalities in the contralateral breast, will have a new malignancy.[203]

## CONTRALATERAL BREAST CANCER

A previous history of breast cancer is one of the risk factors for development of a secondary breast cancer. A contralateral breast cancer occurs in approximately 2.5%[204] of women who have breast cancer, underscoring the need for close surveillance. In women with a history of this disease, the risk for a metachronous breast cancer at 5 and 10 years after initial diagnosis is 4%[205] and 7%,[206] respectively. Risk factors for the development of a contralateral breast cancer are as follows: young age at the time of the primary breast cancer diagnosis, a family history of breast cancer,[207] and infiltrating lobular carcinoma as the initial cancer.[208] Adjuvant chemotherapy and tamoxifen are thought to decrease the risk of a contralateral breast cancer in women with a previous history of this disease.

Contralateral breast cancer can be managed in a similar manner to that of unilateral breast cancer with breast conservation.[209] Survival after the development of a contralateral breast cancer is dependent on stage of disease with a similar survival rate to that of unilateral breast cancer.[210]

**TABLE 19-16.** ASCO RECOMMENDATIONS FOR BREAST CANCER FOLLOW-UP CARE

| TEST | FREQUENCY | LEVEL OF EVIDENCE | GRADE OF RECOMMENDATION |
|---|---|---|---|
| *Recommended* | | | |
| History/eliciting of symptoms and physical examination | Every 3–6 mo × 3 yr; every 6–12 mo × 2 yr; then annually | III, expert consensus | B |
| Breast self-examination | Monthly | III, expert consensus | D |
| Mammography, contralateral | Annually | I | A |
| Ipsilateral | Annually | IV | C |
| Pelvic examination | Annually | III, expert consensus | B |
| Patient education regarding symptoms of reoccurrence | N/A | V, expert consensus | D |
| Coordination of care | N/A | V, expert consensus | D |
| *Not Recommended* | | | |
| Complete blood count | | | |
| Automated chemistry studies | | I | A |
| Chest roentgenography | | I | A |
| Bone scan | | I | A |
| Ultrasound of the liver | | I | A |
| Computed tomography of chest, abdomen, and pelvis | | V, expert consensus | D |
| Tumor marker CA 15-3 | | III, expert consensus | NG |
| Tumor marker CEA | | III, expert consensus | NG |

SOURCE: American Society of Clinical Oncology: Recommended breast cancer surveillance guidelines. J Clin Oncol 15:2149–2156, p. 2150, 1997.

## RECURRENT BREAST CANCER

One reason for following breast cancer patients who have had potentially curative therapy is to identify those women who will develop recurrent disease. Breast cancer can recur locally, distally, or both locally and distally. Approximately one-third of recurrences will occur locally, one-third distally, and one-third will occur locally and distally. As such, patients who appear to have only local recurrent disease should undergo a metastatic survey to determine if they have disseminated disease.

For patients who have only local recurrence, management will depend on whether breast conservation or mastectomy was the initial procedure. The prognosis is worse for patients who relapse after mastectomy than for those who recur after breast conservation. The local relapse rate after breast conservation (i.e., lesions treated with lumpectomy and adjuvant radiotherapy) is approximately 5% at 5 years and increases to 8% at 10 years.[211] The majority of these patients will be salvaged with a completion mastectomy, although, in select patients, repeat lumpectomy and radiation can be used.[212] The prognosis after salvage mastectomy is dependent on several factors, including the time from primary cancer diagnosis to diagnosis of the second breast cancer, method of detection of recurrent disease (mammographic changes versus clinical suspicion), the extent of the recurrence and the histology of the recurrent lesion.[213] Pa-

tients who have a recurrence soon after the initial diagnosis not only have a poorer prognosis after salvage mastectomy, but also are more likely to develop systemic disease. Up to half of those who have a recurrence within 4 years of initial diagnosis develop disseminated disease.[214]

## TREATMENT OF METASTATIC DISEASE

Approximately 10% of women with breast cancer will present with metastatic disease, while another 50% with initially localized breast cancer will relapse with systemic breast cancer. The treatment goal in women with metastatic breast cancer is palliative, i.e., primarily to alleviate symptoms, preserve health-related quality of life, and, if possible, to prolong life without undue toxicity.[215] Patient selection is paramount in the management of these patients.[216] The modalities used to treat metastatic breast cancer include surgery, radiotherapy, hormonal antagonists, and chemotherapy.

Patients with locally advanced disease can undergo "toilet" mastectomies, although it may be necessary to resect the chest wall with appropriate reconstruction.[217] The role of surgery in resecting metastatic disease is less clear. If it is unclear whether the lesion is metastatic breast cancer or a new primary, then a diagnostic surgical procedure may be indicated. The use of surgery to perform

**TABLE 19-17.** SURVIVAL OUTCOME FOR PATIENTS WITH CLINICALLY OCCULT BREAST CANCER AND AXILLARY METASTASIS TREATED WITH SURGERY AND/OR RADIOTHERAPY

| SERIES | PERIOD | NO. OF PATIENTS | TREATMENT | OCCULT CA | SURVIVAL |
|---|---|---|---|---|---|
| MSKCC[224] | 1975–1988 | 35 | Surgery, 33 | 67% | 5 yr = 75% |
| | | | | | 10 yr = 55% |
| Dutch study[225] | 1980–1991 | 15 | Observation, 14 | NA | 7.5 yr = 73% |
| Milan Institute[222] | 1945–1987 | 60 | Breast surgery, 33 | 81.8% | 5 yr = 76.6% |
| | | | Breast RT, 6 | | 10 yr = 58.3% |
| | | | Observation, 17 | | Breast surgery or RT = 10 yr, 68% |
| | | | | | Observation = 10 yr, 45% |
| MD Anderson[226] | 1944–1987 | 42 | Breast surgery, 18 | 11% | 5 yr, 71.8% |
| | | | Breast RT, 16 | | 10 yr, 65% |
| | | | Observation, 13 | | |

NOTES: Breast surgery = patients treated with breast surgery and axillary dissection. Breast RT = patients treated with breast irradiation and axillary dissection. Observation = 5 patients who had an axillary dissection and had treatment of the breast only when the lesion became clinically apparent.

metastectomies is discouraged. Radiotherapy can be used to control local disease or to provide pain relief, and in the case of bone metastases, decrease the risk of pathologic fracture.[218]

For patients with hormone receptor–positive tumors, hormonal manipulation with aminoglutethemide and tamoxifen remain viable options. Approximately 30% of all patients will respond to tamoxifen therapy. In a phase III study comparing tamoxifen with aminoglutethemide, the response rate for the latter was 45%, while that for tamoxifen was 27%.[219] Aminoglutethemide was associated with greater toxicity. Despite these differences, the overall survival rates were similar for these two drugs, underscoring the need to measure quality-of-life issues.

Patients with hormone receptor–negative tumors, rapidly progressive disease or visceral metastases may benefit from chemotherapy. Systemic treatment of metastatic breast cancer can increase the median survival rate of women with breast cancer, and in the rare case, prolong survival. Chemotherapy in this setting usually consists of cyclophosphamide and fluorouracil in conjunction with methotrexate or adriamycin.[220] Treatment with these combinations in excess of 9 months, however, has not been shown to increase survival.[221] Patients whose disease progresses after receiving these drug combinations can be switched to a taxol-based regimen or newer drug regimens including other taxenes, topoisomerase inhibitors, Navelbine, or immunologic modulators. The role of high-dose chemotherapy and autologous bone marrow transplant in patients with metastatic breast cancer is not clear.

## SPECIAL CASES

### CLINICALLY OCCULT BREAST CANCER WITH AXILLARY METASTASES

Axillary metastases in women with both normal mammography and clinical examination usually arise from a breast primary. These clinically occult breast cancers are rare and account for fewer than 1% of all breast cancers. Axillary sampling of patients usually re-

veals extensive nodal involvement with half of the patients having more than four nodes positive for metastatic disease, and a tendency for extranodal involvement.[222] Treatment of the breast is controversial. If it is surgically removed, the primary tumor will be found up to 70% of the time (clinically occult) and the tumor will tend to have poor prognostic indicators, such as poor differentiation, high nuclear grade, and lymphatic invasion.[223] However, there is no difference in overall survival if a wait-and-see approach is taken, with a mastectomy performed if the primary tumor becomes apparent (Table 19-17).[224–226] Despite the poor prognostic features associated with this disease, the associated 5- and 10-year survival rates are better than those seen with similar staged breast cancers.

## PHYLLODES TUMORS AND OTHER HISTOLOGIES

Phyllodes tumors, rare lesions, have an incidence of 2 cases per 1 million women. The peak age at diagnosis is 45 to 49 years of age, with a slight increase in incidence found in Latina women.[227] Phyllodes tumors can be categorized as benign, borderline, and malignant, based on growth at tumor margins, cellularity, and composition of connective tissue component, cellular atypia and number of mitoses per high-power field.[228] These neoplasms can be treated with wide local excision, particularly if less than 5 cm and of benign or borderline histotype.[229] Although there is local recurrence in up to 50% of patients, some of these patients can be treated by wide excision (less than mastectomy) with no adverse effect on survival.[230,231] Grade[232] and histologic classification are the most important prognostic factors, with a 5-year disease-free survival rate of 95% for benign lesions, 73% for borderline lesions, and 66% for the malignant histotype.[233]

Sarcomas of the breast are primary malignancies of breast connective tissue, half being angiosarcomas or stromal sarcomas. In the MD Anderson series of 60 cases,[234] patients who had lesions locally excised with tumor-free margins did equally as well as those who had mastectomy. As with soft-tissue sarcomas, local control may be improved with radiation. Axillary dissection did not affect outcome since lesions metastasized preferentially to the lung. The median overall survival period in this series was 67 months, with a median disease-free survival period of 18 months. The most important prognostic marker was a tumor size less than 5 cm.

Primary squamous carcinomas of the breast are rare lesions that most likely arise from either myoepithelial cell or luminal epithelial cells. These lesions are usually diagnosed at a late stage. Because of the rarity of this neoplasm, optimal management is unknown, but the conventional treatment for this tumor has been MRM.[235]

## MALE BREAST CANCER

Although breast cancer is most common among women, men can and do develop this disease. The incidence of female to male breast cancer is approximatley 125:1. Breast cancer in males tends to be diagnosed at later stages than in women because of a lower index of suspicion and less breast tissue in males.[236] The risk factors for male breast cancer include a positive family history (particularly if a *BRCA2* mutation is involved), gynecomastia, and previous chest wall irradiation. On physical examination, 95% of the patients will present with a lump that is usually central in location[237] and mammography will reveal an uncalcified, subareolar mass.[238] Occasionally, microcalcifications will be present, suggesting the presence of a malignancy.

Treatment of male breast cancer is usually by mastectomy. On histologic examination, the neoplasm tends to stain strongly positive for estrogen receptors and more than 50% of the lesions will have lymphatic invasion.[239] The presence of estrogen receptors on these cancers suggests the possibility of using tamoxifen as an adjuvant treatment.[240]

Survival rates for male breast cancer tend to be worse than for females, which may be a reflection of the more advanced clinical stage at diagnosis in men. Overall, the 5-year survival rates with male breast cancer is 57% to 76% and at 10 years, drops to 31% to 66%.[241–243] Nodal status is an important predictor of outcome.[244] In the MD Anderson study of 335 men with breast cancer, 5-year survival rates were 90%, 73%, and 55%, respectively, for men without nodal disease, one to three positive lymph nodes, and more than four positive lymph nodes.[245]

## PAGET'S DISEASE OF THE NIPPLE

Paget's disease of the nipple (nipple eczema containing Paget cells without a palpable lump) is a rare disease that is often mistreated as a benign skin condition because of its difficulty in diagnosis. There is much controversy as to whether the cells arise in situ or migrate from the skin into the breast parenchyma.[246] Regardless of its origin, the clinician should remain suspicious of eczematous changes around the nipple, since temporary healing of Paget's disease has been reported.[247] This disease is difficult to diagnose clinically because often the mammogram is normal and there is no associated underlying mass.[248] In a review of 34 patients with typical skin changes associated with Paget's disease, 50% of the patients had a normal mammogram, 30% had nipple, areolar, or subareolar abnormalities, and 20% had a mass or calcifications on mammography.[249]

Scrape cytology of the skin along with fine-needle aspiration cytology may aid in making the diagnosis.[250]

The majority of patients with Paget's disease will have an underlying carcinoma, DCIS, or invasive ductal carcinoma.[251] This carcinoma is often multifocal and if a palpable mass is present, more likely it is an invasive malignancy. Up to 50% of patients with an invasive carcinoma will have axillary metastases.[252] Treatment of this disease has ranged from radiotherapy to breast conservation and mastectomy, with or without axillary node dissection. Axillary node status is the most important predictor of outcome[253] since women with Paget's disease and an associated invasive cancer have a similar survival as women with an invasive cancer and no skin abnormalities.[254] Although there have been reports of Paget's disease of the nipple being treated by radiotherapy alone,[255] the current therapy for this disease includes a mastectomy with or without an axillary dissection.[256] Since the likelihood of an invasive cancer with associated axillary involvement is high for lesions presenting with a palpable mass, MRM is recommended for these patients.[257] Further studies evaluating the use of breast conservation surgery in this disease are warranted.[258]

## BREAST CANCER DURING PREGNANCY OR LACTATION

Approximately 1% to 3% of women will develop breast cancer while pregnant or lactating,[259] and the number of women who develop breast cancer during pregnancy will probably increase as women postpone having children into their thirties and forties.[260] The physiologic changes that occur in the breast during this time period make the diagnosis of breast cancer a challenge. Despite this difficulty, mammography coupled with ultrasonography will often show abnormalities consistent with a breast malignancy.[261]

The clinical stage of the disease and the trimester during which the cancer is diagnosed governs the manner in which the cancer should be treated. Carcinoma of the breast associated with pregnancy is usually diagnosed at an advanced stage, with up to 75% of patients having nodal metastases.[262] In the first trimester, breast irradiation is contraindicated, and these women may not be candidates for breast conservation therapy. If the cancer is advanced and chemotherapy is required, termination of the pregnancy would be recommended. In the second and third trimesters, breast conservation and adjuvant irradiation may be used. Chemotherapy, if needed, can be delayed until after delivery. In the event that the lesion is a locally advanced breast cancer, induction chemotherapy may be required. If the breast cancer is diagnosed during the lactational period, lactation should be suppressed and the cancer treated either with breast conservation or MRM.[262] Women diagnosed with breast cancer while pregnant or lactating should wait at least 1 year, and preferably 2, before becoming pregnant again.[263,264]

Whether or not women who develop breast cancer while pregnant or lactating have a worse prognosis as compared to similarly aged women with this malignancy is controversial. It is clear, however, that these pregnant women are more likely to be diagnosed at an advanced stage and therefore have an overall worse prognosis.[265–268] Particularly in women under the age of 30, even after accounting for disease stage, there appears to be a worse prognosis for breast cancer associated with pregnancy.[269]

## CONCLUSION

Breast cancer is a common disease, and the number of women who will be diagnosed with this malignancy will increase as the "baby boomer" generation enters menopause. With better surveillance mechanisms, the proportion of breast cancers that are diagnosed at an earlier stage will increase, resulting in better survival rates for women with this neoplasm. However, breast cancer is a heterogeneous disease, and surgeons who treat this disease have to be aware of which women can be treated with breast conservation and which women should be treated more aggressively with MRM and chemotherapy. Furthermore, as women live longer, the issues of hormone replacement, secondary breast cancers, and follow-up after breast cancer will become more important. As we begin to unravel the prognostic factors important in breast cancer recurrence and survival, we will be able to determine the answers to these questions. These improvements should result in generally less morbidity for women with breast cancer and a continual increase in the proportion of women who have been cured of this malignancy.

## REFERENCES

1. PARKIN DM et al: Estimates of the worldwide incidence of eighteen major cancers in 1985. Int J Cancer 54:594, 1993.
2. PISANI P et al: Estimates of the worldwide mortality from eighteen major cancers in 1985: Implications for prevention and projections of future burden. Int J Cancer 55:891, 1993.
3. PARKER SL et al: Cancer statistics, 1997. CA 47:5, 1997.
4. COLLABORATIVE GROUP ON HORMONAL FACTORS IN BREAST CANCER: Breast cancer and hormone replacement therapy: Collaborative reanalysis of data from 51 epidemiological studies of 52,705 women with breast cancer and 108,411 women without breast cancer. Lancet 350:1047, 1997.
5. HELZLSOUER KJ, COUZI R: Hormones and breast cancer. Cancer 76:2059, 1995.
6. HUNTER DJ et al: Plasma organochlorine levels and the risk of breast cancer. N Engl J Med 337:1253, 1997.
7. HILL AD et al: Hereditary breast cancer. Br J Surg 84:1334, 1997.
8. LYNCH HT et al: Phenotypic variation in hereditary breast cancer: Cancer control implications. Arch Surg 129:806, 1994.
9. MIKI Y et al: A strong candidate for the breast and ovarian cancer susceptibility gene BRCA1. Science 266:66, 1994.
10. SHATTUCK-EIDENS D et al: BRCA1 sequence analysis in women at high risk for susceptibility mutations: Risk factor analysis and implications for genetic testing. JAMA 278:1242, 1997.
11. SOMASUNDARAM K et al: Arrest of the cell cycle by the tumour suppressor BRCA1 requires the CDK-inhibitor p21 WAF1/CiP1. Nature 389:187, 1997.
12. SCULLY R et al: Association of BRCA1 with Rad51 in mitotic and meiotic cells. Cell 88:265, 1997.
13. WOOSTER R et al: Localization of a breast cancer susceptibility gene, BRCA2, to chromosome 13q12-13. Science 265:2088, 1994.
14. STRUEWING JP et al: The risk of cancer associated with specific mutations of BRCA1 and BRCA2 among Ashkenazi Jews. N Engl J Med 336:1401, 1997.
15. SHARAN S et al: Embryonic lethality and radiation hypersensitivity mediated by Rad51 in mice lacking BRCA2. Nature 386:804, 1997.
16. VOUCH FJ et al: BRCA1 mutations in women attending clinics that evaluate the risk of breast cancer. N Engl J Med 336:1409, 1997.
17. KRAINER M et al: Differential contributions of BRCA1 and BRCA2 to early-onset breast cancer. N Engl J Med 336:1414, 1997.
18. SIDRANSKY D et al: Inherited p53 gene mutations in breast cancer. Cancer Res 52:2984, 1992.
19. BROWNSTEIN MH et al: Cowdens disease: A cutaneous marker of breast cancer. Cancer 41:2393, 1978.
20. TSOU HC et al: The role of MMAC1 mutations in early-onset breast cancer: Causative in association with Cowden syndrome and excluded in BRCA1-negative cases. Am J Hum Genet 61:1036, 1997.
21. LIAW D et al: Gremlin mutations of the PTEN gene in Cowden's disease, an inherited breast and thyroid cancer syndrome. Nat Genet 16:64, 1997.
22. CORTESSIS V et al: Linkage analysis of DRD2, a marker linked to the ataxia-telangectasia gene, in 64 families with premenopausal bilateral breast cancer. Cancer Res 53:5083, 1993.
23. FITZGERALD MG et al: Heterozygous ATM mutations do not contribute to early onset of breast cancer. Nat Genet 15:307, 1997.
24. RISINGER J et al: Molecular genetic evidence of the occurrence of breast cancer as an integral tumor in patients with the hereditary nonpolyposis colorectal carcinoma syndrome. Cancer 77:1836, 1996.
25. VEHMANEN P et al: Low proportion of BRCA1 and BRCA2 mutations in Finnish breast cancer families: Evidence for additional susceptibility genes. Hum Mol Genet 6:2309, 1997.
26. WILLETT WC et al: Dietary fat and fiber in relation to risk of breast cancer: An eight year follow-up. JAMA 268:2037, 1992.
27. HUANG Z et al: Dual effects of weight and weight gain on breast cancer risk. JAMA 278:1407, 1997.
28. TRICHOPOULOU A et al: Consumption of olive oil and specific food groups in relation to breast cancer risk in Greece. J Natl Cancer Inst 87:110, 1995.
29. LONGNECKER MP: Alcoholic beverage consumption in relation to risk of breast cancer: meta-analysis and review. Cancer Causes Control 5:73, 1994.
30. DUPONT WD, PAGE DL: Risk factors for breast cancer in women with proliferative breast disease. N Engl J Med 312:146, 1985.
31. LONDON SJ et al: A prospective study of benign breast disease and the risk of breast cancer. JAMA 267:941, 1992.
32. CUTULI B et al: Breast cancer in patients treated for Hodgkin's disease: Clinical and pathological analysis of 76 cases in 63 patients. Eur J Cancer 33:2315, 1997.
33. GOSS PE, SIERREA S: Current perspectives on radiation-induced breast cancer. J Clin Oncol 16:338, 1998.
34. HUNTER DJ, WILLETT WC: Nutrition and breast cancer. Cancer Causes Control 7:56, 1996.
35. HARVEY BJ et al: Effect of breast self-examination techniques on the risk of death from breast cancer. Can Med Assoc J 157:1205, 1997.
36. FLETCHER SW et al: Report of the International Workshop on screening for breast cancer. J Natl Cancer Inst 85:1644, 1993.
37. METTLIN C, SMART CR: Breast cancer detection guidelines for women aged 40 to 49 years: Rationale for the American Cancer Society reaffirmation of recommendations. CA 44:248, 1994.

38. MILLER AB et al: Canadian National Breast Screening Study: 1. Breast cancer detection and death rates among women aged 40 to 49 years. Can Med Assoc J 147:1459, 1992.

39. HENDRICK RE et al: Benefit of screening mammography in women aged 40–49: A new meta-analysis of randomized controlled trials. J Natl Cancer Inst Monogr 22:87, 1998.

40. NYSTROM L et al: Breast cancer screening with mammography: Overview of Swedish randomised trials. Lancet 341:973, 1993.

41. ALEXANDER FE: The Edinburgh Randomized Trials of breast cancer screening, in NIH Consensus Development Conference, Breast Cancer Screening for Women Ages 40–49, Program and Abstracts Bethesda (MD). National Institutes of Health, 1997, p 49.

42. SHAPIRO S: Periodic screening for breast cancer: The Health Insurance Plan of Greater New York Randomized Controlled Trial, in NIH Consensus Development Conference, Breast Cancer Screening for Women Ages 40–49, Program and Abstracts Bethesda (MD). National Institutes of Health, 1997, pp 41–48.

43. FLETCHER SW: Breast cancer screening among women in their forties: An overview of the Issues, in NIH Consensus Development Conference, Breast Cancer Screening for Women Ages 40–49, Program and Abstracts Bethesda (MD). National Institutes of Health, 1997, pp 5–9.

44. MIKHAIL RA et al: Stereotactic core needle biopsy of mammographic breast lesions as a viable alternative to surgical biopsy. Ann Surg Oncol 1:363, 1994.

45. YIM JH et al: Mammographically detected breast cancer: Benefits of stereotactic core versus wire localization biopsy. Ann Surg 223:688, 1996.

46. SMITH DN et al: Large core needle biopsy of non-palpable breast cancers. The impact on subsequent surgical excisions. Arch Surg 132:256, 1997.

47. FLEMING ID et al (eds). Breast, in AJCC Cancer Staging Manual. Philadelphia, Lippincott-Raven, 1997, pp 171–180.

48. SILVER SA, TAVASSOLI FA: Mammary ductal carcinoma in situ with microinvasion. Cancer 82:2382, 1998.

49. CARTER CL et al: Relation of tumor size, lymph node status, and survival in 24,740 breast cancer cases. Cancer 63:181, 1989.

50. HENSON DE et al: Relationship among outcome, stage of disease, and histologic grade for 22,616 cases of breast cancer: The basis for a prognostic index. Cancer 68:2142, 1991.

51. BURKE HB, HENSON DE: Histologic grade as a prognostic factor in breast carcinoma: Counterpoint. Cancer 80:1703, 1997.

52. ROBERTI NE: The role of histologic grading in the prognosis of patients with carcinoma of the breast: Is this a neglected opportunity? Cancer 80:1708, 1997.

53. FISHER B et al: Relative worth of estrogen or progesterone receptor and pathologic characteristics of differentiation as indicators of prognosis in node negative breast cancer patients: Findings from National Surgical Adjuvant Breast and Bowel Project Protocol B-06. J Clin Oncol 6:1076, 1988.

54. VERONESI U et al: Sentinel-node biopsy to avoid axillary dissection in breast cancer with clinically negative lymph-nodes. Lancet 349:1864, 1997.

55. MITTRA I et al: Prognosis of breast cancer: Evidence for interaction between c-erbB-2 overexpression and number of involved axillary lymph nodes. J Surg Oncol 60:106, 1995.

56. ALEXIEV BA et al: Expression of c-erbB-2 oncogene and p53 tumor suppressor gene in benign and malignant breast tissue: Correlation with proliferative activity and prognostic index. Gen Diagn Pathol 142:271, 1997.

57. PAIK S et al: Pathologic findings from the National Surgical Adjuvant Breast and Bowel Project: Prognostic significance of erbB-2 protein overexpression in primary breast cancer. J Clin Oncol 8:103, 1990.

58. MARKS JR et al: Overexpression of p53 and HER-2/neu proteins as prognostic markers in early stage breast cancer. Ann Surg 219:332, 1994.

59. JIANG M et al: P21/waf1/cip1 and mdm-2 expression in breast carcinoma patients as related to prognosis. Int J Cancer 74:529, 1997.

60. BLAND KI et al: Oncogene protein coexpression: Value of Ha-ras, c-myc, c-fos, and p53 as prognostic determinants for breast carcinoma. Ann Surg 221:706, 1995.

61. CHUNG M et al: Younger women with breast carcinoma have a poorer prognosis than older women. Cancer 77:97, 1996.

62. FISHER ER et al: Pathologic findings from the National Surgical Adjuvant Breast Project protocol B-06: 10 year pathologic and clinical prognostic determinants. Cancer 71:2507, 1993.

63. DIGNAM JJ et al: Prognosis among African-American women and white women with lymph node negative breast carcinoma: Findings from two randomized clinical trials of the National Surgical Adjuvant Breast and Bowel Project (NSABP). Cancer 80:80, 1997.

64. MARROGI AJ et al: Study of tumor infiltrating lymphocytes and transforming growth factor-beta as prognostic factors in breast carcinoma. Int J Cancer 74:492, 1997.

65. BURKE HB et al: Artificial neural networks improve the accuracy of cancer survival prediction. Cancer 79:857, 1996.

66. SCHNITT SJ et al: Mammary ducts in the areola: Implications for patients undergoing reconstructive surgery of the breast. Plast Reconstr Surg 92:1290, 1993.

67. TOTH BA, LAPPERT P: Modified skin incisions for mastectomy: The need for plastic surgical input in preoperative setting. Plast Reconstr Surg 87:1048, 1991.

68. CARLSON GW et al: Skin-sparing mastectomy: Oncologic and reconstructive considerations. Ann Surg 225:570, 1997.

69. KROLL SS et al: Risk of recurrence after treatment of early breast cancer with skin-sparing mastectomy. Ann Surg Oncol 4:193, 1997.

70. MORROW M, FOSTER RS Jr: Staging of breast cancer: A new rationale for internal mammary node biopsy. Arch Surg 116:748, 1981.

71. FOOTE FW, STEWART FW: Lobular carcinoma in situ: A rare form of mammary cancer. Am J Pathol 17:491, 1941.

72. BODIAN CA et al: Lobular neoplasia: Long term risk of breast cancer and relation to other factors. Cancer 78:1024, 1996.

73. ROSEN PP et al: Lobular carcinoma in situ of the breast: Preliminary results of treatment by ipsilateral mastectomy and contralateral breast biopsy. Cancer 47:813, 1981.

74. WALT AJ et al: The continuing dilemma of lobular carcinoma in situ. Arch Surg 127:904, 1992.

75. HAAGENSEN CD et al: Lobular neoplasia (so-called lobular carcinoma in situ) of the breast. Cancer 42:737, 1978.

76. FISHER ER et al: Pathologic findings from the National Surgical Adjuvant Breast Project (NSABP) Protocol 17: Five year observations concerning lobular carcinoma in situ. Cancer 78:1403, 1996.

77. OSBORNE MP, HODA SA: Current management of lobular carcinoma in situ of the breast. Oncology 8:45, 1994.

78. OSBORNE MP, BORGEN PI: Atypical ductal and lobular hyperplasia and breast cancer risk. Surg Clin North Am 2:1, 1993.

79. ERNSTER VL et al: Incidence of and treatment for ductal carcinoma in situ of the breast. JAMA 275:913, 1996.

80. HOLLAND R et al: Ductal carcinoma in situ: A proposal for a new classification. Semin Diagn Pathol 11:167, 1994.

81. DOUGLAS-JONES AG et al: A critical appraisal of six modern classifications of ductal carcinoma in situ of the breast (DCIS): Correlation with grade of associated invasive carcinoma. Histopathology 29:397, 1996.

82. The Consensus Conference Committee: Consensus Conference on the classification of ductal carcinoma in situ. Cancer 80:1798, 1997.

83. HOLLAND R et al: Extent, distribution, and mammographic/histologic correlations of breast ductal cacinoma in situ. Lancet 335–519, 1990.

84. FAVERLY DRG et al: Three dimensional imaging of mammary ductal carcinoma in situ: Clinical implications. Semin Diagn Pathol 11:193, 1994.

85. FRYKBERG ER et al: Ductal carcinoma in situ of the breast. Surg Gynecol Obstet 117:425, 1993.

86. ZAFRANI B et al: Conservative management of intraductal breast carcinoma with tumorectomy and radiation therapy. Cancer 57:1299, 1986.

87. RECHT A et al: Intraductal carcinoma of the breast: Results of treatment with excisional biopsy and irradiation. J Clin Oncol 3:1339, 1985.

88. MCCORMICK B et al: Duct carcinoma in situ of the breast: An analysis of local control after conservation surgery and radiotherapy. Int J Radiat Oncol Biol Phys 21:289, 1991.

89. RAY GR et al: Ductal carcinoma in situ of the breast: Results of treatment by conservative surgery and definitive irradiation. Int J Radiat Oncol Biol Phys 28:105, 1994.

90. SOLIN LJ et al: Definitive irradiation for intraductal carcinoma of the breast. Int J Radiat Oncol Biol Phys 19:843, 1990.

91. SOLIN LJ et al: Fifteen-year results of breast-conserving surgery and definitive breast irradiation for the treatment of ductal carcinoma in situ of the breast. J Clin Oncol 14:754, 1996.

92. HAFFTY BG et al: Radiation therapy for ductal carcinoma in situ of the breast. Conn Med 54:482, 1990.

93. SOLIN LJ et al: Mammographically detected, clinically occult ductal carcinoma in situ treated with breast-conserving surgery and definitive breast irradiation. Cancer J Sci Am 2:158, 1996.

94. HIRAMATSU H et al: Local recurrence after conservative surgery and radiation therapy for ductal carcinoma in situ: Possible importance of family history. Cancer J Sci Am 1:55, 1995.

95. PAGE DL et al: Continued local recurrence of carcinoma 15–25 years after a diagnosis of low grade ductal carcinoma in situ of the breast treated only by biopsy. Cancer 76:1197, 1995.

96. EUSEBI V et al: Long term follow-up of in situ carcinoma of the breast. Semin Diagn Pathol 11:223, 1994.

97. FISHER ER et al: Conservative management of intraductal carcinoma (DCIS) of the breast. J Surg Oncol 47:139, 1991.

98. ARNESSON LG et al: Follow-up of two treatment modalities for ductal cancer in situ of the breast. Br J Surg 76:672, 1989.

99. SCHWARTZ GF et al: Subclinical ductal carcinoma in situ of the breast. Treatment by local excision and surveillance alone. Cancer 70:2468, 1992.

100. LAGIOS MD et al: Mammographically detected duct carcinoma in situ: Frequency of local recurrence following tylectomy and prognostic effect of nuclear grade on local recurrence. Cancer 63:618, 1989.

101. FISHER B et al: Lumpectomy and radiation therapy for the treatment of intraductal breast cancer: Findings from National Surgical Adjuvant Breast and Bowel Project B-17. J Clin Oncol 16:441, 1998.

102. HOLLAND R et al: Extent, distribution, and mammographic/histological correlations of breast ductal carcinoma in situ. Lancet 335:519, 1990.

103. FISHER ER et al: Pathologic findings from the National Surgical Adjuvant Breast Project (NSABP) Protocol B-17. Intraductal carcinoma (ductal carcinoma in situ). The National Surgical Adjuvant Breast and Bowel Project Collaborating Investigators. Cancer 75:1310, 1995.

104. SILVERSTEIN MJ et al: A prognostic index for ductal carcinoma in situ of the breast. Cancer 77:2267, 1996.

105. SILVERSTEIN MJ et al: Axillary lymph node dissection for intraductal breast carcinoma—Is it indicated? Cancer 59:1819, 1987.

106. GAMEL JW et al: The impact of stage and histology on the long-term clinical course of 163,808 patients with breast carcinoma. Cancer 77:1459, 1996.

107. CHUNG MA et al: Optimal surgical treatment of invasive lobular carcinoma of the breast. Ann Surg Oncol 4:545, 1997.

108. MCBOYLE MF et al: Tubular carcinoma of the breast: An institutional review. Am Surg 63:639, 1997.

109. BAKER RR: Unusual lesions and their management. Surg Clin North AM 70:963, 1990.

110. WILSON TE et al: Pure and mixed mucinous carcinoma of the breast: pathologic basis for differences in mammographic appearance. Am J Roentgenol 165:285, 1995.

111. RASMUSSEN BB et al: Prognostic factors in primary mucinous breast carcinomas. Am J Clin Pathol 87:155, 1987.

112. SIMPSON JF, PAGE DL: Prognostic value of histopathology in the breast. Semin Oncol 19:254, 1992.

113. PEDERSEN L et al: Medullary carcinoma of the breast: Prevalence and prognostic importance of classical risk factors in breast cancer. Eur J Cancer 31A:2289, 1995.

114. REINFUSS M et al: Typical medullary carcinoma of the breast: a clinical and pathological analysis of 52 cases. J Surg Oncol 60:89, 1995.

115. HAYWARD JL: The Guy's trial of treatments of "early" breast cancer. World J Surg 1:314, 1977.

116. ARRIAGADA R et al: Conservative treatment versus mastectomy in early breast cancer: Patterns of failure with 15 years of follow-up data. Institut Gustave-Roussy Breast Cancer Group. J Clin Oncol 14:1558, 1996.

117. JACOBSON JA et al: Ten year results of a comparison of conservation with mastectomy in the treatment of stage I and II breast cancer. N Engl J Med 332:907, 1995.

118. VERONESI U et al: Breast conservation is the treatment of choice in small breast cancer: Long term results of a randomized trial. Eur J Cancer 26:668, 1990.

119. VAN DONGEN JA et al: Factors influencing local relapse and survival and results of salvage treatment after breast-conserving therapy in operable breast cancer: EORTC trial 10801, breast conservation compared with mastectomy in TNM stage I and II breast cancer. Eur J Cancer 28A:801, 1992.

120. BLICHERT-TOFT M et al: Danish randomized trial comparing breast conservation therapy with mastectomy: Six years of life-table analysis. Danish Breast Cancer Cooperative Group. J Natl Cancer Inst Monogr 11:19, 1992.

121. VERONESI U et al: Quadrantectomy versus lumpectomy for small size breast cancer. Eur J Cancer 26:671, 1990.

122. VERONESI U et al: Radiotherapy after breast-preserving surgery in women with localized cancer of the breast. N Engl J Med 328:1587, 1993.

123. The Uppsala-Orebro Breast Cancer Study Group: Sector resection with or without postoperative radiotherapy for stage I breast cancer: A randomized trial. J Natl Cancer Inst 82:277, 1990.

124. LILJEGREN G et al: Sector resection with or without postoperative radiotherapy for stage I breast cancer: Five year results of a randomized trial. Uppsala-Orebro Breast Cancer Study Group. J Natl Cancer Inst 86:717, 1994.

125. CLARK RM et al: Randomized clinical trial of breast irradiation following lumpectomy and axillary dissection for node-negative breast cancer: An update. Ontario Clinical Oncology Group. J Natl Cancer Inst 88:1659, 1996.

126. VERONESI U et al: Breast conservation is a safe method in patients with small cancer of the breast: Long-term results of three randomised trials on 1,973 patients. Eur J Cancer 31A:1574, 1995.

127. FISHER B et al: Reanalysis and results after 12 years of follow-up in a randomized clinical trial comparing total mastectomy with lumpectomy with or without irradiation in the treatment of breast cancer. N Engl J Med 333:1456, 1995.

128. LEVITT SH et al: The impact of radiation on early breast carcinoma survival: A Bayesian analysis. Cancer 78:1035, 1996.

129. Early Breast Cancer Trialists' Collaborative Group: Effects of radiotherapy and surgery in early breast cancer: An overview of the randomized trials. N Engl J Med 333:1444, 1995.

130. KEMPERMAN H et al: Prognostic factors for survival after breast conserving therapy for stage I and II breast cancer: The role of local recurrence. Eur J Cancer 31A:690, 1995.

131. NOGUCHI S et al: A case-control study on risk factors for local recurrences or distant metastases in breast cancer patients treated with breast-conserving therapy. Oncology 54:468, 1997.

132. GAGE I et al: Pathologic margin involvement and the risk of recurrence in patients treated with breast-conserving therapy. Cancer 78:1921, 1996.

133. RENTON SC et al: The importance of the resection margin in conservative therapy for breast cancer. Eur J Surg Oncol 22:17, 1996.

134. SCHNITT SJ et al: Pathologic predictors of early local recurrence in stage I and II breast cancer treated by primary radiation therapy. Cancer 53:1049, 1984.

135. McCRADY DR et al: Factors associated with local breast cancer recurrence after lumpectomy alone. Ann Surg Oncol 3:358, 1996.

136. CROWE JP et al and PARTICIPATING INVESTIGATORS: Local-regional breast cancer recurrence following mastectomy. Arch Surg 126:429, 1991.

137. CADY B et al: New therapeutic possibilities in primary invasive cancer. Ann Surg 218:338, 1993.

138. FISHER B et al: Significance of ipsilateral breast tumor recurrence after lumpectomy. Lancet 338:327, 1991.

139. LEITNER SP et al: Predictors of recurrence for patients with small (one centimeter or less) localized breast cancer (T1a,bN0M0). Cancer 76:2266, 1995.

140. STIERER M et al: Long term analysis of factors influencing the outcome in carcinoma of the breast smaller than one centimeter. Surg Gynecol Obstet 175:151, 1992.

141. DALBERG K et al: Mammographic features, predictors of early ipsilateral breast tumour recurrences? Eur J Surg Oncol 22:483, 1996.

142. LILJEGREN G et al: Risk factors for local recurrence after conservative treatment in stage I breast cancer: Definition of a subgroup not requiring radiotherapy. Ann Oncol 8:235, 1997.

143. ELKHUIZEN PH et al: Local recurrence after breast-conserving therapy for invasive breast cancer: High incidence in young patients and association with poor survival. Int J Radiat Oncol Biol Phys 40:850, 1998.

144. DALBERG K et al: Breast conserving surgery for invasive breast cancer: Risk factors for ipsilateral breast tumor recurrences. Breast Cancer Res Treat 43:73, 1997.

145. HAFFTY BG et al: Prognostic factors for local recurrence in the conservatively treated breast cancer patient: A cautious interpretation of the data. J Clin Oncol 9:997, 1991.

146. HARTSELL WF et al: Delaying the initiation of intact breast irradiation for patients with lymph node positive breast cancer increases the risk of local recurrence. Cancer 76:2497, 1995.

147. VUJOVIC O et al: Does delay in breast irradiation following conservative breast surgery in node-negative breast cancer patients have an impact on risk of recurrence? Int J Radiat Oncol Biol Phys 40:869, 1998.

148. THE STEERING COMMITTEE ON CLINICAL PRACTICE GUIDELINES FOR THE CARE AND TREATMENT OF BREAST CANCER: Breast radiotherapy after breast-conserving surgery. CMAJ 158(Suppl 3): S35, 1998.

149. RECHT A et al: Integration of conservative surgery, radiotherapy, and chemotherapy for the treatment of early-stage, node positive breast cancer: Sequencing, timing, and outcome. J Clin Oncol 9:1662, 1991.

150. WALLGREN A et al: Timing of radiotherapy and chemotherapy following breast-conserving surgery for patients with node-positive breast cancer. International Breast Cancer Study Group. Int J Radiat Oncol Biol Phys 35:649, 1996.

151. FISHER B et al: Ten-year results of a randomized clinical trial comparing radical mastectomy and total mastectomy with or without radiation. N Engl J Med 312:674, 1985.

152. LIN PP et al: Impact of axillary lymph node dissection on the therapy of breast cancer patients. J Clin Oncol 11:1536, 1993.

153. CABANES PA et al: Value of axillary dissection in addition to lumpectomy and radiation in early breast cancer. The Breast Carcinoma Collaborative Group of the Institut Curie. Lancet 339:1245, 1992.

154. OVERGAARD M et al: Postoperative radiotherapy is high-risk premenopausal women with breast cancer who receive adjuvant chemotherapy. N Engl J Med 337:949, 1997.

155. RAGAZ J et al: Adjuvant radiotherapy and chemotherapy in node-positive premenopausal women with breast cancer. N Engl J Med 337:956, 1997.

156. DOWLATSHAHI K et al: Lymph node micrometastases from breast carcinoma. Reviewing the dilemma. Cancer 80:1188, 1997.

157. GIULIANO E et al: Lymphatic mapping and sentinel lymphadenectomy for breast cancer. Ann Surg 220:391, 1994.

158. TURNER RR et al: Histopathologic validation of the sentinel lymph node hypothesis for breast carcinoma. Ann Surg 226:271, 1997.

159. GUILIANO AE et al: Sentinel lymphadenectomy in breast cancer. J Clin Oncol 15:2345, 1997.

160. COX CE et al: Guidelines for sentinel node biopsy and lymphatic mapping of patients with breast cancer. Ann Surg 227:645, 1998.

161. DALE PS, WILLIAMS JT 4TH: Axillary staging utilizing selective sentinel lymphadenectomy for patients with invasive breast carcinoma. Am Surg 64:28, 1998.

162. Guenther JM et al: Sentinel lymphadenectomy for breast cancer in a community managed care setting. Cancer J Sci Am 3:336, 1997.

163. Borgstein PJ et al: Sentinel lymph node biopsy in breast cancer: Guidelines and pitfalls of lymphoscintigraphy and gamma probe detection. J Am Coll Surg 186:275, 1998.

164. O'Hea BJ et al: Sentinel lymph node biopsy in breast cancer: Initial experience at memorial Sloan-Kettering Cancer Center. J Am Coll Surg 186:423, 1998.

165. McNeil C: Sentinel node biopsy: Studies should bring needed data. J Nat Can Instit 90:728, 1998.

166. Whitten TM et al: Axillary lymph node metastases in stage T1a breast cancer: A pathologic review of 82 patients. Am Surgeon 63:144, 1997.

167. Mustafa IA et al: The impact of histopathology on nodal metastases in minimal breast cancer. Arch Surg 132:384, 1997.

168. Barth A et al: Predictors of axillary lymph node metastases in patients with T1 breast carcinoma. Cancer 79:1918, 1997.

169. Silverstein MJ et al: Predicting axillary node positivity in patients with invasive carcinoma of the breast by using a combination of T category and palpability. J Am Coll Surg 180:700, 1995.

170. Chadha M et al: Predictors of axillary lymph node metastases in patients with T1 breast cancer: A multivariate analysis. Cancer 73:350, 1994.

171. Arnesson LG et al: Histopathology grading in small breast cancer < or = 10 mm: Results from an area with mammography screening. Breast Cancer Res Treat 44:39, 1997.

172. Pierce LJ et al: Microscopic extracapsular extension in the axilla: Is this an indication for axillary radiotherapy? Int J Radiat Oncol Biol Phys 33:253, 1995.

173. Leonard C et al: Are axillary recurrence and overall survival affected by axillary extranodal tumor extension in breast cancer? Implications for radiation therapy. J Clin Oncol 13:47, 1995.

174. Fisher BJ et al: Extracapsular axillary node extension in patients receiving adjuvant systemic therapy: An indication for radiotherapy? Int J Radiat Biol Phy 38:551, 1997.

175. Mehta K, Haffty BG: Long-term outcome in patients with four or more positive lymph nodes treated with conservative surgery and radiation therapy. Int J Radiat Oncol Biol Phys 35:679, 1996.

176. Vicini FA et al: The role of regional nodal irradiation in the management of patients with early-stage breast cancer treated with breast-conserving therapy. Int J Radiat Oncol Biol Phys 39:1069, 1997.

177. Hortobagyi GN, Buazdar AU: Current status of adjuvant systemic therapy for primary breast cancer: Progress and controversy. CA 45:199, 1995.

178. Early Breast Cancer Trialists' Collaborative Group: Systemic treatment of early breast cancer by hormonal, cytotoxic, or immune therapy: 133 randomized trials involving 31,000 recurrences and 24,000 deaths among 75,000 women. Lancet 339:1, 71, 1992.

179. Bonadonna G et al: Adjuvant cyclophosphamide, methotrexate, and fluorouracil in node positive breast cancer: The results of 20 years of follow-up. N Engl J Med 332:901, 1995.

180. Gelber RD et al: Adjuvant chemotherapy plus tamoxifen compared with tamoxifen alone for post-menopausal breast cancer: Meta-analysis of quality adjusted survival. Lancet 347:1066, 1996.

181. Fisher B et al: Postoperative chemotherapy and tamoxifen compared with tamoxifen alone in the treatment of positive-node breast cancer patients aged 50 years and older with tumors responsive to tamoxifen: Results from the National Surgical Adjuvant Breast and Bowel Project B-16. J Clin Oncol 8:1005, 1990.

182. Early Breast Cancer Trialists' Collaborative Group: Tamoxifen for early breast cancer: An overview of the randomised trials. Lancet 351:1451, 1998.

183. Swedish Breast Cancer Cooperative Group: Randomized trial of two versus five years of adjuvant tamoxifen for postmenopausal early stage breast cancer. J Natl Cancer Inst 88:1543, 1996.

184. Tormeay DC et al: Postchemotherapy adjuvant tamoxifen therapy beyond five years in patients with lymph node-positive breast cancer. Eastern Cooperative Oncology Group. J Natl Cancer Inst 88:1828, 1996.

185. Recht A et al: The sequencing of chemotherapy and radiation therapy after conservative surgery for early-stage breast cancer. N Engl J Med 334:1356, 1996.

186. Fisher B et al: Effect of preoperative chemotherapy on local-regional disease in women with operable breast cancer: Findings from the National Adjuvant Breast and Bowel Project B-18. J Clin Oncol 15:2483, 1997.

187. Clahsen PC et al: Overview of randomized perioperative polychemotherapy trials in women with early stage breast cancer. J Clin Oncol 15:2526, 1997.

188. Bonnier P et al: Inflammatory carcinomas of the breast: A clinical, pathological, or a clinical and pathological definition? Int J Cancer 62:382, 1995.

189. Colozza M et al: Induction chemotherapy with cisplatin, doxorubicin, and cyclophosphamide (CAP) in a combined modality approach for locally advanced and inflammatory breast cancer. Long-term results. Am J Clin Oncol 19:10, 1996.

190. Fein DA et al: Results of multimodality therapy for inflammatory breast cancer: An analysis of clinical and treatment factors affecting outcome. Am Surg 60:220, 1994.

191. Thomas F et al: Pattern of failure in patients with inflammatory breast cancer treated by alternating radiotherapy and chemotherapy. Cancer 76:2286, 1995.

192. Attia-Sobol J et al: Treatment results, survival and prognostic factors in 109 inflammatory breast cancers: Univariate and multivariate analysis. Eur J Cancer 29A:1081, 1993.

193. Fleming RY et al: Effectiveness of mastectomy by response to induction chemotherapy for control in inflammatory breast cancer. Ann Surg Oncol 4:452, 1997.

194. Ueno NT et al: Combined-modality treatment of inflammatory breast carcinoma: Twenty years of experience at M.D. Anderson Cancer Center. Cancer Chemother Pharmacol 40:321, 1997.

195. Touboul E et al: Primary chemotherapy and preoperative irradiation for patients with stage II larger than 3 cm or locally advanced non-inflammatory breast cancer. Radiother Oncol 42:219, 1997.

196. Schwartz GF et al: Breast conservation following induction chemotherapy for locally advanced carcinoma of the breast (stages IIB and III): A surgical perspective. Surg Oncol Clin N Am 4:657, 1995.

197. Bonadonna G et al: Preoperative chemotherapy in operable breast cancer (Lett). Lancet 341:1485, 1993.

198. Safah H, Weiner RS: The role of bone marrow transplantation in the management of advanced local disease. Surg Oncol Clin N Am 4:735, 1995.

199. Somlo G et al: High-dose chemotherapy and stem-cell rescue in the treatment of high-risk breast cancer: Prognostic indicators

of progression-free and overall survival. J Clin Oncol 15:2882, 1997.

200. AMERICAN SOCIETY OF CLINICAL ONCOLOGY: Recommended breast cancer surveillance guidelines. J Clin Oncol 15:2149, 1997.

201. PECTASIDES D et al: Clinical value of CA 15-3, mucin-like carcinoma associated antigen, tumor polypeptide antigen, and carcinoembryonic antigen in monitoring early breast cancer patients. Am J Clin Oncol 19:459, 1996.

202. MORROW M et al: Breast cancer surgical practice guidelines. Society of Surgical Oncology Practice Guidelines: Breast cancer. Oncology 11:877, 1997.

203. ROUBIDOUX MA et al: Women with breast cancer: Histologic findings in the contralateral breast. Radiology 203:691, 1997.

204. ROBINSON E et al: Survival of first and second primary breast cancer. Cancer 71:172, 1993.

205. BROET P et al: Contralateral breast cancer: Annual incidence and risk parameters. J Clin Oncol 13:1578, 1995.

206. HEALEY EA et al: Contralateral breast cancer: Clinical characteristics and impact on prognosis. J Clin Oncol 11:1545, 1993.

207. GOGAS J et al: Bilateral breast cancer. Am Surg 59:733, 1993.

208. COOK LS et al: A population-based study of contralateral breast cancer following a first primary breast cancer. Cancer Causes Control 7:382, 1996.

209. GOLLAMUDI SV et al: Breast-conserving therapy for stage I-II synchronous bilateral breast carcinoma. Cancer 79:1362, 1997.

210. SINGLETARY SE et al: Occurrence and prognosis of contralateral carcinoma of the breast. J Am Coll Surg 178:390, 1994.

211. DEWAR JA et al: Local relapse and contralateral tumor rates in patients with conservative surgery and radiotherapy (Institut Gustave Roussy 1970–1982). IGR Breast Cancer Group. Cancer 76:2260, 1995.

212. MULLEN EE et al: Salvage radiotherapy for local failures of lumpectomy and breast irradiation. Radiother Oncol 42:25, 1997.

213. OSBORNE MP, SIMMONS RM: Salvage surgery for recurrence after breast conservation. World J Surg 18:93, 1994.

214. HAFFTY BG et al: Ipsilateral breast tumor recurrence as a predictor of distant disease: Implications for systemic therapy at the time of local relapse. J Clin Oncol 14:52, 1996.

215. OSOBA D: Health-related quality of life as a treatment endpoint in metastatic breast cancer. Can J Oncol 5(Suppl 1):47, 1995.

216. HENDERSON IC et al: Comprehensive management of disseminated breast cancer. Cancer 66(Suppl 6):1439, 1990.

217. SWEETLAND HM et al: Radical surgery for advanced and recurrent breast cancer. J R Coll Surg Edinb 40:88, 1995.

218. THERIAULT RL, HORTOBAGYI GN: Bone metastasis in breast cancer. Anticancer Drugs 3:455, 1992.

219. GALE KE et al: Hormonal treatment for metastatic breast cancer: An Eastern Cooperative Oncology Group Phase III trial comparing aminoglutethimide to tamoxifen. Cancer 73:354, 1994.

220. OVERMOYER BA: Chemotherapeutic palliative approaches in the treatment of breast cancer. Semin Oncol 2(Suppl 3):2, 1995.

221. WONG K, HENDERSON IC: Management of metastatic breast cancer. World J Surg 18:98, 1994.

222. MERSON M et al: Breast carcinoma presenting as axillary metastases without evidence of a primary tumor. Cancer 70:504, 1992.

223. ROSEN PP, KIMMEL M: Occult breast carcinoma presenting with axillary lymph node metastases: A follow-up study of 48 patients. Hum Pathol 21:518, 1990.

224. BARON PL et al: Occult breast cancer presenting with axillary metastases: Updated management. Arch Surg 125:210, 1990.

225. VAN OOIJEN B et al: Axillary nodal metastases from an occult primary consistent with breast carcinoma. Br J Surg 80:1299, 1993.

226. ELLERBROEK N et al: Treatment of patients with isolated axillary nodal metastases from an occult primary carcinoma consistent with breast origin. Cancer 66:1461, 1990.

227. BERNSTEIN L et al: The descriptive epidemiology of malignant cystosarcoma phyllodes tumors of the breast. Cancer 71:3020, 1993.

228. SALVADORI B et al: Surgical treatment of phyllodes tumors of the breast. Cancer 63:2532, 1989.

229. ROWELL MD et al: Phyllodes tumors. Am J Surg 165:376, 1993.

230. ZURRIDA S et al: Which therapy for unexpected phyllode tumor of the breast? Eur J Cancer 28:654, 1992.

231. COHN-CEDERMARK G et al: Prognostic factors in cystosarcoma phyllodes: A clinicopathologic study of 77 patients. Cancer 68:2017, 1991.

232. REINFUSS M et al: Malignant phyllodes tumours of the breast: A clinical and pathological analysis of 55 cases. Eur J Cancer 29A:1252, 1993.

233. REINFUSS M et al: The treatment and prognosis of patients with phyllodes tumor of the breast: An analysis of 170 cases. Cancer 77:910, 1996.

234. GUTMAN H et al: Sarcoma of the breast: Implications for extent of therapy. The M.D. Anderson experience. Surgery 116:505, 1994.

235. BAUER RL, BUSCH ER: Primary sqamous cell carcinoma of the breast. Surg Rounds 10:325, 1997.

236. CHUNG HC et al: Male breast cancer: A 20 year review of 16 cases at Yonsei University. Yonsei Med J 31:242, 1990.

237. JAIYESIMI IA et al: Carcinoma of the male breast. Ann Intern Med 117:771, 1992.

238. TUKEL S, OZCAN H: Mammography in men with breast cancer: review of the mammographic findings in five cases. Australas Radiol 40:387, 1996.

239. CUTULI B et al: Male breast cancer: Results of the treatments and prognostic factors in 397 cases. Eur J Cancer 31A:1960, 1995.

240. MCLACHLAN SA et al: Male breast cancer: An 11 year review of 66 patients. Breast Cancer Res Treat 40:225, 1996.

241. GOUGH DB et al: A 50-year experience of male breast cancer: Is outcome changing? Surg Oncol 2:325, 1993.

242. JOSHI MG et al: Male breast carcinoma: An evaluation of prognostic factors contributing to a poorer outcome. Cancer 77:490, 1996.

243. SALVADORI B et al: Prognosis of breast cancer in males: An analysis of 170 cases. Eur J Cancer 30A:930, 1994.

244. SULYOK Z, KOVES I: Male breast tumours. Eur J Surg Oncol 19:581, 1993.

245. GUINEE VF et al: The prognosis of breast cancer in males: A report of 335 cases. Cancer 71:154, 1993.

246. LAGIOS MD et al: Paget's disease of the nipple: Alternative management in cases without or with minimal extent of underlying breast carcinoma. Cancer 54:545, 1984.

247. DIXON AR et al: Paget's disease of the nipple. Br J Surg 78:722, 1991.

248. SAWYER RH, ASBURY DL: Mammographic appearances in Paget's disease of the breast. Clin Radiol 49:185, 1994.

249. IKEDA DM et al: Paget disease of the nipple: Radiologic-pathologic correlation. Radiology 189:89, 1993.

250. GUPTA RK et al: The role of cytology in the diagnosis of Paget's disease of the nipple. Pathology 28:248, 1996.

251. YIM JH et al: Underlying pathology in mammary Paget's disease. Ann Surg Oncol 4:287, 1997.

252. CHAUDARY MA et al: Paget's disease of the nipple: A ten year review including clinical, pathological, and immunohistochemical findings. Breast Cancer Res Treat 8:139, 1986.

253. PAONE JF, BAKER RR: Pathogenesis and treatment of Paget's disease of the breast. Cancer 48:825, 1981.

254. FREUND H et al: Paget's disease of the breast. J Surg Oncol 9:93, 1977.

255. BULENS P et al: Breast conserving treatment of Paget's disease. Radiother Oncol 17:305, 1990.

256. JAMALI FR et al: Paget's disease of the nipple-areola complex. Surg Clin North Am 76:365, 1996.

257. SALVADORI B et al: Analysis of 100 cases of Paget's disease of the breast. Tumori 62:529, 1976.

258. PIERCE LJ et al: The conservative management of Paget's disease of the breast with radiotherapy. Cancer 80:1065, 1997.

259. TITCOMB CL: Breast cancer and pregnancy. Hawaii Med J 49:18, 1990.

260. KUERER HM et al: Breast carcinoma associated with pregnancy and lactation. Surg Oncol 6:93, 1997.

261. LIBERMAN L et al: Imaging of pregnancy-associated breast cancer. Radiology 191:245, 1994.

262. RIBEIRO G et al: Carcinoma of the breast associated with pregnancy. Br J Surg 73:607, 1986.

263. HORNSTEIN E et al: The management of breast carcinoma in pregnancy and lactation. J Surg Oncol 21:179, 1982.

264. CLARK RM, CHUA T: Breast cancer and pregnancy: The ultimate challenge. Clin Oncol (R Coll Radiol) 1:11, 1989.

265. DIFRONZO LA, O'CONNELL TX: Breast cancer in pregnancy and lactation. Surg Clin North Am 76:267, 1996.

266. LETHABY AE et al: Overall survival from breast cancer in women pregnant or lactating at or after diagnosis. Auckland Breast Cancer Study Group. Int J Cancer 67:751, 1996.

267. PETREK JA et al: Prognosis of pregnancy-associated breast cancer. Cancer 67:869, 1991.

268. HOOVER HC JR: Breast cancer during pregnancy and lactation. Surg Clin North Am 70:1151, 1990.

269. GUINEE VF et al: Effect of pregnancy on prognosis for young women with breast cancer. Lancet 343:1587, 1994.

270. SHNITT SJ et al: Influence of infiltrating lobular histology on local tumor control in breast cancer patients treated with conservative surgery and radiotherapy. Cancer 64:448, 1989.

271. KURTZ JM et al: Conservation therapy for breast cancers other than infiltrating ductal carcinoma. Cancer 63:1630, 1989.

272. DU TOIT RS et al: An evaluation of differences in prognosis, recurrence patterns and receptor status between invasive lobular and other invasive carcinomas of the breast. Eur J Surg Oncol 17:251, 1991.

273. POEN JC et al: Conservation therapy for invasive lobular carcinoma of the breast. Cancer 69:2789, 1992.

274. WEISS MC et al: Outcome of conservative therapy for invasive breast cancer by histologic type. Int J Radiat Oncol Biol Phys 23:941, 1992.

275. WHITE JR et al: Conservative surgery and radiation therapy for infiltrating lobular carcinoma of the breast. The role of preoperative mammograms in guiding treatment. Cancer 74:640, 1994.

276. VERONESI U et al: Local recurrences and distant metastases after conservative breast cancer treatments: Partly independent events. J Natl Can Inst 87:19, 1995.

277. SASTRE-GARAU X et al: Infiltrating lobular carcinoma of the breast. Clinicopathologic analysis of 975 cases with reference to data on conservative therapy and metastatic patterns. Cancer 77:113, 1996.

278. SALVADORI B et al: Conservative surgery for infiltrating breast carcinoma. Br J Surg 84:106, 1997.

# CHAPTER 20

# SARCOMAS

## 20A / SARCOMAS OF THE SOFT TISSUES

*Constantine P. Karakousis*

## INCIDENCE

Soft tissue sarcomas arise in tissues that include the organs of locomotion, e.g., muscles, tendons, supportive tissues, fibrous tissue, adipose tissue, and synovial tissue. The muscles in the human body compose about 40% of the adult body weight. Supportive tissues of viscera may also give rise to soft tissue sarcoma. The word *sarkoma* is of Greek origin and means "fleshy growth." Soft tissues constitute over 50% of the weight of the body.[1] They arise from tissues derivative of the primitive mesenchyme. An exception to this rule is the neurogenic sarcoma, which, although arising from an ectodermal structure, is categorized along with other soft tissue sarcomas due to similarities in behavior and treatment.

There are about 8100 new cases of soft tissue sarcoma (including heart) and 4600 deaths from this disease in the United States per year.[2] Soft tissue sarcomas comprise about 1% of all cancers[1] other than skin cancers in adults, but their relative frequency is higher in children. There is little information regarding epidemiologic or etiologic factors for patients with soft tissue sarcoma. The Li-Fraumeni syndrome[3] is associated with an increased incidence of soft tissue sarcoma, as well as other tumors. Lymphangiosarcoma may occur in the arm of women after mastectomy and axillary node dissection (Stewart-Treves syndrome),[4] arising from prolonged, advanced lymphedema of the extremity. Soft tissue sarcomas have a slightly increased incidence in a variety of genetically transmitted diseases such as Werner's syndrome, intestinal polyposis, and Gardner's syndrome.[1] In multiple neurofibromatosis (von Recklinghausen's disease), there is a 5% to 10% chance of development of a neurofibrosarcoma over the lifetime of a patient.[5] Many patients tend to refer to a history of trauma as an initiating factor for the development of a sarcoma, but an unequivocal etiologic association has not been established. In experimental animals, 3-methylcholanthrene and viruses can cause a soft tissue sarcoma. In humans, there are conflicting reports that environmental exposure to phenoxyacetics (in some herbicides) and chlorophenols (wood preservatives) may be associated with an increased risk of development of soft tissue sarcoma. Thorotrast, a radiologic contrast agent used in the past; vinyl chloride; and arsenic have an established role in the development of sarcomas of the liver.[6] Sarcomas may occur in areas previously exposed to radiation,[6] following a long latency period of 10 to 15 years on average.

## PATHOLOGIC CLASSIFICATION

Each of the soft tissues can give rise to benign or malignant growth, the latter usually arising de novo, transformation of a benign growth into a malignant sarcoma being rare. The pathologic classification is usually based upon the recognition of the tissue of origin for each tumor. Occasionally, this may not be possible and the pathologic classification tends to be merely descriptive, e.g., round cell or spindle cell sarcoma, when the predominant cell in the lesion may be identified. Without recognizable tissue of origin or a predominant cell type, the diagnosis of poorly differentiated or undifferentiated sarcoma is made. Various histologic subtypes are shown in Table 20A-1.[7] The most common of these are liposarcoma and malignant fibrous histiocytoma. There has been an evolution in the pathologic criteria defining some soft tissue sarcomas. The entity of malignant fibrous histiocytoma was defined in the mid-1960s, but the classification did not become popular until the 1980s and now is one of the most common histologic subtypes.

There are tumors that occupy an intermediate position between benign varieties and sarcomas. Desmoid tumors exhibit a locally invasive behavior and have a tendency for local recurrence if inadequate resection has been performed, but practically never metastasize. Dermatofibrosarcoma protuberans also shows a locally invasive pattern, with a tendency for local recurrence if inadequately treated, but metastases rarely occur.

**TABLE 20A-1. FREQUENCY OF HISTOLOGIC SUBTYPES IN PRIMARY SOFT TISSUE SARCOMAS**

| HISTOLOGIC SUBTYPE | PERCENT |
| --- | --- |
| Liposarcoma | 30 |
| Malignant fibrous histiocytoma | 27 |
| Leimyosarcoma | 11 |
| Synovial sarcoma | 8 |
| Unclassified | 5 |
| Fibrosarcoma | 5 |
| Spindle cell sarcoma | 3 |
| Rhabdomyosarcoma | 3 |
| Hemangiosarcoma | 3 |
| Clear cell sarcoma | 2 |
| Epitheloid sarcoma | 1 |
| Malignant schwannoma | 1 |
| Other | 3 |

## SITES OF SOFT TISSUE SARCOMAS

The sites in which soft tissue sarcomas occur are cited in Table 20A-2, as reported by Memorial Sloan Kettering Cancer Center (1982–1995) for 2678 patients.[8] In a 1987 survey by the American College of Surgeons of 4500 cases of soft tissue sarcomas, these tumors most commonly occurred in the lower extremities (46%), followed by the trunk (19%), retroperitoneum (13%), upper extremities (13%), and the head and neck area (9%).[9]

## PRESENTATION AND INITIAL WORKUP

Soft tissue sarcomas present often as asymptomatic soft tissue masses associated with little or no pain. In deep-seated tissues, particularly in areas with a large amount of tissues or cavities, these tumors may become 10 to 15 cm in size or larger, before they are appreciated by the patient. In the peripheral portions of the extremities, they are usually detected when they are much smaller. Occasionally, soft tissue sarcomas occur near the course of peripheral nerves such as the femoral or sciatic nerve, and they may compress the trunk or roots of this nerve and thereby produce symptoms in the nerve distribution. In these cases, plain x-rays may not reveal any soft tissue density,

**TABLE 20A-2. DISTRIBUTION BY SITE OF SOFT TISSUE SARCOMAS**

| SITE | DISTRIBUTION, % |
| --- | --- |
| Lower extremity | 35 |
| Upper extremity | 15 |
| Retroperitoneum | 14 |
| Trunk | 10 |
| Visceral | 15 |
| Other | 11 |

and the cause of pain at the distribution of the nerve may be attributed to benign causes such as osteoarthritis, resulting in a delay in diagnosis. A plain x-ray of the affected area may first be obtained because even this will often reveal a soft tissue density and also provide evidence as to the existence or not of any bone involvement. Although plain radiographs are useful as a diagnostic tool, computed tomography (CT) scan provides further information, and magnetic resonance imaging (MRI) can provide additional information in delineating a soft tissue tumor as, in addition to the cross sections of the area, it provides coronal and sagittal views. MRI scans provide a clear outline of the extent of the tumor and its possible relationship with major vessels, muscles, or underlying bones. Arteriography may occasionally be required in order to further demonstrate the relationship of the tumor mass to adjacent major vessels, as well as to demonstrate the major arterial feeding branches of the tumor, and on the venous site of the study provide evidence on the venous return. Bone scan may occasionally be helpful in delineating the extent of any bone involvement, although with the use of MRI, both angiography and bone scans are rarely required today.

## PROGNOSTIC FACTORS AND STAGING

The single most important prognostic factor in soft tissue sarcomas is the histologic grade of the tumor. The grade of the tumor is based on factors such as the histologic subtype, the number of mitoses, degree of necrosis, presence or absence of pleomorphism, cellularity, vascularity, or lymphatic invasion and characteristics of the primary lesion. Various grading systems have been developed over the years, with the most common based on the distinction between well differentiated and poorly differentiated sarcomas in a three-grade system: grade I—well differentiated; grade II—intermediately differentiated, and grade III—poorly differentiated. There is also a four-grade system, with grade I—well-differentiated lesions, grade II and grade III—various degrees of intermediate differentiation, and grade IV—undifferentiated lesions. Finally, due to the difficulty in recognizing and quantitating an intermediate grade, some pathologists have advanced the notion of a two-grade system, i.e., of well and poorly differentiated sarcomas.

The staging system is based on the most important prognostic parameter of the primary tumor, which is the grade of the tumor, followed in prognostic significance by the size. With regards to the latter, tumor masses are distinguished into T1 or ≤5 cm and T2 >5 cm. Recently, the location of the primary tumor has been found to be of prognostic importance, with masses superficial to the investing fascia in the extremities having better prognosis, other factors being equal, than masses deep to or invading the deep fascia. Sarcomas arising in cavities are by definition deep lesions. Until recently, the accepted staging system was based primarily on the grade of the tumor, with stage I, stage II, and stage III being tumor masses with grade I, II, or III tumors, respectively. Each of these first three stages was subdivided into A and B depending upon the size of the tumor, i.e., ≤5 cm or >5 cm. Stage IV was further distinguished into IVA, presenting with lymph node metastases in addition to the primary tumor, and IVB, characterized by distant (hematogenous) disease. The most recent staging system, which incorporates the location of the primary sarcoma as a prognostic parameter, is depicted

**TABLE 20A-3.** STAGE GROUPING

| | | | | |
|---|---|---|---|---|
| *Stage I* | | | | |
| A. Low-grade, small, superficial, and deep | G1–2, | T1a–1b, | N0, | M0 |
| B. Low-grade, large, superficial | G1–2, | T2a, | N0, | M0 |
| *Stage II* | | | | |
| A. Low grade, large, deep | G1–2, | T2b, | N0, | M0 |
| B. High-grade, small, superficial, deep | G3–4, | T1a–1b, | N0, | M0 |
| C. High-grade, large, superficial | G3–4, | T2a, | N0, | M0 |
| *Stage III* High-grade, large, deep | G3–4, | T2b, | N0, | M0 |
| *Stage IV* any metastasis | any G, | any T, | N1, | M0 |
| | any G, | any T, | N0, | M1 |

ABBREVIATIONS: G1, well differentiated; G2, moderately differentiated; G3, poorly differentiated; G4, undifferentiated; T1, tumor ≤ 5 cm; T1a, superficial tumor; T1b, deep tumor; T2, tumor > 5 cm; T2a, superficial tumor; T2b, deep tumor; N0, no regional lymph node metastases; N1, regional lymph node metastases; M0, no distant metastases; M1, distant metastases.

in Table 20A-3.[10] There is good correlation in the new staging system between the various stages and 5-year disease-free survival, the latter being 78% for stage 1, 64% for stage 2, and 36% for stage 3.[6] The Enneking system of classification adopted in the orthopedic literature for soft tissue sarcomas of the extremities is based on the two-grade system and the extent of the tumor, i.e., whether confined within a muscular compartment of the extremity or extending beyond the compartment.

## INDIVIDUAL FEATURES OF THE VARIOUS HISTOLOGIC SUBTYPES

There is a commonality in biologic behavior as well as treatment for soft tissue sarcomas. However, there are also individual features that distinguish one histologic subtype from another.

Fibrosarcoma was the most common histologic subtype in the years before 1970, but has become a rare diagnosis as the refinement of pathologic criteria and diagnosis has permitted detection and definition of other histologic subtypes (particularly malignant fibrous histiocytoma).

Rhabdomyosarcoma, arising in striated muscle, is further distinguished into pleomorphic, alveolar, embryonal, and botryoid subtypes. The latter three subtypes usually occur in childhood. For childhood rhabdomyosarcoma, the efficacy of adjuvant chemotherapy is considered proven. Pleomorphic rhabdomyosarcoma affects patients over 30 years of age, usually occurring in the extremities of males.

Leiomyosarcomas derive from smooth muscle and as such can arise from the wall of blood vessels or from the wall of the viscera. They are common sarcomas in the retroperitoneal area. Desmin and smooth muscle actin are the most common immunohistochemical stains. Mitotic activity appears to be the best indicator of prognosis.

Liposarcomas derive from adipose tissue and occur anywhere in the body but more commonly in the thigh and retroperitoneum. Well-differentiated liposarcomas rarely metastasize but tend to recur locally if inadequately treated. After repeat failure of local control, they may dedifferentiate and become more apt to metastasize. Myxoid liposarcoma accounts for 40% to 50% of all liposarcomas and is a low- to intermediate-grade lesion. There is a typical translocation in myxoid liposarcoma t(12;16) (q13–14;p11). Round cell sarcoma has the same translocation. Fibroblastic liposarcoma, composed of fibroblastlike cells, is of higher grade than myxoid liposarcoma. Pleomorphic liposarcoma is a highly malignant lesion.

Synovial sarcomas arise from tendon synovial tissue and occur most frequently in the extremities near joints involving the capsule (knee, ankles, foot, hand). They are distinguished into monophasic and biphasic types. The biphasic type includes epithelial cells surrounded by spindle or fibrous cells. They are generally considered to be high-grade sarcoma. Calcified areas appear in 20% of these tumors and, according to some authors, this is a favorable prognostic sign.

Neurofibrosarcomas arise from the nerve sheath of peripheral nerves and are also reported as neurogenic sarcomas, malignant schwannomas, or malignant peripheral nerve sheath tumors (MPNSTs). They are frequently associated with von Recklinghausen's disease, which carries a 5% chance of development of a neurofibrosarcoma,[6] but higher rates have also been reported in the literature. Any rapid change in size of one of the known neurofibromas or the development of symptoms from a previously existing neurofibroma, is an indication for resection.

Angiosarcomas, i.e., hemangiosarcomas and lymphangiosarcomas, arise from blood and lymphatic vessels, respectively. They are often high-grade lesions and have a poor prognosis. The lymphangiosarcomas, some arising in the lymphedematous arm of women following radical mastectomy, often require radical amputation due to their diffuse nature and involvement of the extremity.

Malignant hemangiopericytomas consist of cells resembling pericytes, cells arranged along capillaries and veins. In adults, they occur in the lower extremities and pelvis. There are indolent varieties but often these tumors behave like high-grade sarcomas. Malignant hemangiopericytomas should be treated as sarcomas.

Malignant fibrohistiocytomas are sarcomas containing both fibroblastlike and histiocytelike cells. Although this entity was first described in 1964,[11] this diagnosis did not become popular until the mid-1970s, and many cases previously diagnosed as pleomorphic rhabdomyosarcoma or undifferentiated fibrosarcoma are now considered to be malignant fibrohistiocytomas. They usually occur in adults. There are four recognized variants: (1) storiform pleomorphic, (2) myxoid, (3) malignant giant cell tumor of the soft parts, and (4) inflammatory malignant fibrous histiocytoma. Prognosis is related to histologic grade and size of tumor.

Alveolar soft part, epithelioid, and clear cell sarcomas are other histologic subtypes.

Overall, the incidence of metastasis to regional lymph nodes of soft tissue sarcoma is only about 5%.[6] Some histologic subtypes almost never exhibit any lymph node metastasis such as the liposarcoma. Other histologic subtypes such as epithelioid sarcoma, synovial sarcoma, malignant fibrohistiocytoma, and embryonal rhabdomyosarcoma more frequently exhibit metastasis to the regional lymph nodes.

## DIAGNOSIS

Prior to planning the treatment to be rendered, a definitive diagnosis must be reached. Superficially located small tumors, e.g., 2 to 3 cm in diameter, may be totally excised (excisional biopsy) for a complete pathologic evaluation and then treatment. In most cases, however, one is dealing with larger masses, often deeply situated, which require prior diagnostic evaluation before surgical treatment is undertaken. The most common diagnostic method is that of a core needle biopsy such as Tru-Cut, which allows determination of not only the general diagnosis of soft tissue sarcoma but also of the histologic subtype. This is performed under local anesthesia by making a small nick in the skin over the most protuberant area and passing through this small skin incision a Tru-Cut needle several times into the mass in order to have several pieces of tumor for pathologic evaluation. The anatomic position of nearby major blood vessels or nerves should be kept in mind so as to avoid incidental injury to any of these structures. In some cases, the Tru-Cut needle biopsy will not offer sufficient diagnostic material. In these cases, an open biopsy may be indicated. The open biopsy should be performed, keeping in mind the outline of the definitive incision to be employed later should the mass turn out to be a soft tissue sarcoma. In the extremities, the definitive incision is longitudinal due to the anatomic configuration of the extremities and, therefore, the open biopsy should also be longitudinal so that it can be encompassed easily in the definitive excision. In an open biopsy, the incision is carried vertically through the subcutaneous fat and investing fascia down to the surface of the tumor without raising any flaps. The tumor surface is incised and a deep biopsy is obtained. A superficial biopsy may render nondiagnostic material. An adequate biopsy should be obtained to allow for sufficient pathologic material. In some cases, frozen section may be indicated to be certain that diagnostic material has been procured. After good hemostasis is achieved, the open biopsy incision is closed in layers so as to allow for primary healing and avoid extravasation and infiltration of blood along tissue planes or oozing through the incision. Extravasation of blood along these planes may carry tumor cells beyond the boundaries of the planned resection. Oozing through a loosely closed biopsy incision may contaminate the field of the definitive operation. To avoid an ecchymosis, the patient is advised to stay in bed the remainder of the day on which the biopsy was performed. The use of a drain should be avoided after an open biopsy. If a drain

has to be used, its exit point should be placed in the same line as that of the incision so as to be encompassed more easily and removed en bloc with the biopsy incision within the elliptical incision to be used in the definitive operation.

## SURGICAL TREATMENT

Prior to surgical treatment, a metastatic workup should be performed to rule out the presence of distant metastases. Given the propensity of soft tissue sarcomas to metastasize to the lungs, a chest x-ray is required as a minimum to detect any possible distant metastases. For high-grade sarcomas, a CT scan of the chest is also advisable. For retroperitoneal sarcomas, a CT scan of the abdomen and pelvis is necessary not only to assess the extent of the tumor mass but also to evaluate the presence or absence of any intraabdominal metastases. Generally, an en bloc resection of the biopsy tract should be performed with the underlying tumor mass. In most cases, this technique is feasible, with the exception of situations where the biopsy track traverses an intervening free space such as the peritoneal or thoracic cavity. In most cases, however, such as those with extremity sarcomas or sarcomas of the retroperitoneum and chest, the tumor mass abuts against the wall of the trunk and a biopsy is usually taken from this area. The definitive incision is a longitudinal one for the extremities or, for other anatomic areas, one disposed along the long axis of the tumor mass, and is an elliptical incision encompassing the previous biopsy tract. A previous review of the CT or MRI scans should identify for the surgeon the location of the tumor mass and, therefore, provide indications as to how the flaps should be made. For a sarcoma located in the subcutaneous fat or protruding through the fascia into the subcutaneous fat, after the elliptical incision is made the flaps obviously should be thin for a distance well beyond the probable extent of the tumor mass. For sarcomas that are situated deep to the investing fascia, the flaps can be made thick to the fascia level and then dissection superficial to the fascia should be carried out to beyond the probable extent of the tumor mass. For large tumor masses situated deeply within the extremities, such as a muscle compartment in the thigh, it is best not to develop the flaps on the basis of external palpatory findings only because these do not allow for precise identification of the lateral borders of the tumor and one usually ends up with an unnecessarily wide flap. In these cases, it is best to enter through the deep fascia well proximal and distal to the tumor mass and then through the additional appreciation of the deeper palpatory findings one is better able to determine the lateral width of the flaps. Sharp dissection is employed using a scalpel and/or cautery, with the tissues to be divided under tension through traction and countertraction, which is a basic condition for accurate, precise dissection. Blunt dissection is seldom, if ever, indicated because it does not permit an accurate delineation of the plane or course of dissection. Metzenbaum scissors may be used in the case of transparent structures, but in most situations where the tissues are opaque, scalpel or cautery dissection should be performed. When the cautery is used, it is placed at a low setting and with the tissues under tension, the tip of the cautery is applied continuously and lightly in cutting through the tissues layer by layer. This provides more effective use of the cautery for hemostasis and offers a safer technique compared to using the cautery in strokes. At each plane, the incision is carried from end to end, avoiding the trap of getting into a deep "hole" where exposure is limited. Involvement of the major extremity blood vessels is not an indication for amputation if the tumor otherwise is resectable. Survival and local control for patients with major vessel resection is as good as that of patients without vessel involvement.[12] Whenever there is possible involvement of a major vessel, one proceeds to make an elliptical incision around the biopsy tract and exposes the blood vessels well above as well as below the tumor mass and dissects otherwise all the way around the tumor mass so that the remaining structures to be dissected would be the blood vessels themselves (Fig. 20A-1). One then starts dissection of the blood vessels by entering their sheath on the side opposite to the tumor. One thus may determine on the basis of edema or other tissue changes whether indeed the blood vessels have to be sacrificed or not. Usually by entering the sheath

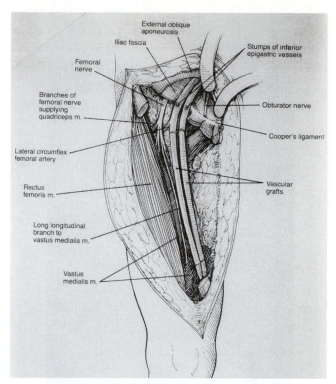

**FIGURE 20A-2.** Operative field following resection of the femoral vessels and repair with vascular grafts due to involvement by a soft tissue sarcoma. *From Karakousis CP: Surgery for soft tissue sarcomas, in Atlas of Surgical Oncology, K. Bland et al (eds). Philadelphia, WB Saunders, 1995, pp 283–400.*

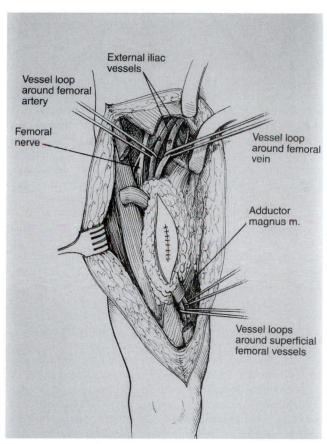

**FIGURE 20A-1.** This drawing illustrates the principle of proximal and distal exposure and control of major blood vessels potentially involved by tumor, and the circumferential mobilization of the specimen from other soft tissues prior to transection of the vessels and removal of the specimen followed by vascular repair. *From Karakousis CP: Surgery for soft tissue sarcomas, in Atlas of Surgical Oncology, K. Bland et al (eds). Philadelphia, WB Saunders, 1995, pp 283–400.*

of the blood vessels and extricating the latter off their sheath and away from the tumor, it becomes possible to preserve them. However, when there is any question of involvement of the blood vessels, there should be no hesitation to sacrifice them and replace them with either an autologous vein or a synthetic graft. Again, before the blood vessels are divided, it is necessary to mobilize the tumor specimen with adjacent normal tissues free all the way around so that the last remaining structure to be divided would be the blood vessels themselves. In this case, the patient is heparinized, the blood vessels are clamped with vascular clamps placed distally and proximally, and the specimen is removed (Fig. 20A-2). Long-term patency with autologous or synthetic grafts is excellent for the major blood vessels. For smaller blood vessels below the knee or elbow, reconstruction may not be necessary because there is sufficient collateral circulation through other arterial branches. In some cases, when the vein distal to the point of involvement is extensively thrombosed, there is no need to replace the thrombosed vein with a graft, and in this case one relies on the existing collateral circulation, which is facilitated, postoperatively with leg elevation and elastic support. Although in most cases of vessel involvement, limb-preserving resection is possible with removal of the involved segment of vessels and reconstruction, this may not be a practical goal in cases where vessel involvement is associated with extensive edema of the lower

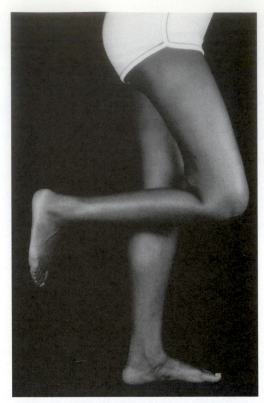

**FIGURE 20A-3.** Functional extremity following resection of the sciatic nerve due to a malignant schwannoma arising from this nerve, en bloc with posterior compartment resection. The patient is able to walk unassisted with the characteristic gait of foot drop.

extremity. One should then discuss frankly the option of amputation with the patient because in these cases there is obviously a significant compromise of the extremity, and the wide surgical resection for the removal of the tumor, necessitates a variable interruption of the lymphatic outflow of the extremity and may result in a worsening of the edema and functional compromise that elevation and elastic support can only partially ameliorate. Involvement of one of the major nerves, including the sciatic nerve, is not in itself an indication for amputation if the tumor can otherwise be resected completely with a satisfactory margin (Fig. 20A-3). In cases of possible nerve involvement, the nerve under consideration is exposed well above and below the tumor mass and the tumor mass is otherwise mobilized; one then enters the sheath of the nerve proximal and distal to the tumor mass and incises the sheath of the nerve on the side away from the tumor so as to extricate the nerve from its sheath, leaving the sheath itself on the surface of the tumor. Again, as one develops the plane between the sheath and the nerve and comes close to the area of the tumor, if there are indications of involvement of the nerve itself, there should be no hesitation to sacrifice this nerve in preference to performing an amputation. Sacrifice of a single nerve of one of the extremities results in an extremity that although compromised, functions significantly better than a prosthesis following an amputation. Limited involvement of an underlying bone may be

dealt with by resecting the tumor mass with the adjacent normal soft tissues and the involved bone segment with a margin above and below the area of the malignancy followed by reconstruction of the bone continuity. Limb-saving resection should be possible in 95% of extremity sarcomas. However, in about 5% of these cases, the tumor mass is so extensive that it is not possible to perform an en bloc resection of tumor mass with surrounding normal tissues through grossly clean planes and leave a viable extremity, as in the case of circumferential involvement of an extremity and involvement of a major joint.

## SURGERY FOR SARCOMAS OF THE TORSO

### CHEST WALL TUMORS

The definitive incision is made according to the longitudinal axis of the tumor mass, whatever its direction might be. In cases where the tumor mass is grossly spherical, then an incision along the course of the ribs over the center of the mass is made, encompassing any previous biopsy tract. Flaps are then developed to beyond the probable extent of the tumor mass on each lateral side and posterior or anterior to the tumor mass at a distance of 5 cm or greater. The involved rib or ribs are divided, starting first anteriorly or posteriorly away from the tumor by removing a segment of the rib(s) certain to be involved, which allows entry into the chest cavity and palpation of the tumor from both its external and internal aspects so as to determine accurately the lateral extent of the dissection and the necessity to remove any additional ribs in order to maintain an adequate margin around the tumor. The intercostal vessels are carefully ligated and divided and involvement of the underlying lung is dealt with by removing the involved portion of the lung by placing a stapling device around the area of the involvement. Chest tubes are employed to drain the thoracic cavity and the defect in the chest wall is repaired with the use of mesh. The mesh is sutured to the edge of the defect with nonabsorbable sutures, passing around the adjacent ribs or musculoaponeurotic layers and the folded edge of the mesh, which is kept taut at its center and free of wrinkles by continuously folding its edge at the periphery to accommodate the curvature of the defect. This provides coverage of the defect in a straight plane, in contrast to the contoured plane of the curvature of the ribs, but this does not seem to create a significant compromise of the functional capacity of the ipsilateral chest cavity in most cases. Whenever a defect is unusually large, one may consider the use of methylmethacrylate with the mesh to contour a plane that would simulate the curvature of the removed ribs. Closure of the remaining layers is performed, or at least the subcutaneous fat and skin over the mesh. In situations where the skin has been removed also, provision for a flap has to be made in order to provide a seal for the chest cavity.

Chest wall tumors involving the upper ribs present a special challenge. They are often extensive and require removal of the first to the fourth ribs from origin to insertion. In these cases, a curving incision along the medial border of the scapula, the axilla, to the anterior chest wall is made. The trapezius muscles posteriorly, latissimus dorsi inferiorly, and the pectoralis major anteriorly are divided. The levator scapulae and rhomboid muscles medial to the vertebral border of the scapula, anteriorly the pectoralis minor and anterolaterally the serratus anterior are divided sufficiently to allow exposure of the upper ribs and mobilization of the axillary vessels and brachial plexus off the chest wall. Branches or tributaries of the axillary vessels in connection with the upper chest wall are ligated and divided. One then should be able to expose the upper surface of the first rib and divide it medially, close to the sternochondral junction and posteriorly, close to the spine. The same is repeated for the second and third ribs or as necessary according to the location of the tumor mass (Fig. 20A-4).

Sarcomas of the lower chest wall at or near the costal margin may also involve the ipsilateral diaphragm and are resected by removing

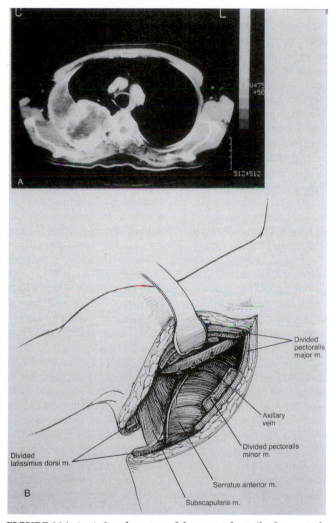

**FIGURE 20A-4.** *A*. Involvement of the upper four ribs from a soft tissue sarcoma on CT scan. *B*. Anterior part of dissection separating the axillary neurovascular bundle from the chest wall. *From Karakousis CP: Surgery for soft tissue sarcomas, in Atlas of Surgical Oncology, K. Bland et al (eds). Philadelphia, WB Saunders, 1995, pp 283–400.*

the lower ribs and corresponding parts of the diaphragm, as well as the upper abdominal wall muscles to a clean surgical margin. Repair of the defect is performed with the use of mesh for the chest and upper abdominal wall, as well as mesh for repair of the diaphragm. The mesh is sutured superiorly on the edges of the defect in the lower chest wall and then, as one reaches the costal margin, another piece of mesh is sutured on the posterior, medial, and lateral edges of the diaphragmatic defect and anteriorly along the imaginary line previously occupied by the costal margin to the first piece of mesh. The first mesh then is held taut and sutured to the edge of the abdominal wall defect. In placing the mesh in any part of the chest or abdominal wall, it is important to keep the mesh taut and then to fold the mesh as the curvature of the defect is encountered so as to prevent wrinkling. For extra security, the mesh is folded and suturing is carried out between the adjacent edge of the defect in the tissues and the folded edge of the mesh. Of course, the extra mesh is trimmed after the mesh has been sutured all the way around.

Sarcomas of the sternum are dealt with by making a longitudinal incision from the lower neck over the middle of the sternum to well below the xiphoid, providing an ellipse around any biopsy tract. Flaps are then developed laterally to well beyond the extent of the edge of the sternum, depending on the precise location and extent of the tumor mass. The ribs are divided lateral to the tumor mass and with a combination of external and internal palpation one is able to carry out the dissection all the way around safely. It is important to remember the location of the internal mammary artery, about one-half inch from the edge of the sternum as it courses along the posterior aspect of the ribs in a longitudinal vertical direction. The medial ends of the clavicles are divided with Gigli's saws (Fig. 20A-5). In the case of resection of the chest wall also involving extensive resection of the skin, myocutaneous flaps may be used, such as that of pectoralis major, latissimus dorsi, rectus abdominis, or transverse rectus abdominis myocutaneous (TRAM) flap.

## SARCOMAS OF THE ABDOMINAL WALL

These tumors may be confined within the abdominal wall or involve the latter by direct extension of an intraperitoneal or retroperitoneal tumor. The resection may be performed preserving one of the layers of the abdominal wall whenever that is feasible and the surgical plane chosen appears free of tumor. However, sarcomas of the abdominal wall often require resection of the entire thickness of the musculature of the abdominal wall and, therefore, require a repair in order to avoid a hernia. A piece of mesh may be used to repair such a defect, as previously described in chest wall defects. However, in repair of abdominal wall defects, extra caution should be exercised because of the situation that exists particularly in the lower quadrants of the abdomen. The loops of bowel there as they gravitate tend to adhere to the mesh and in some instances fistulize. At least in cases of usage of the polypropylene mesh, there is about a 25% incidence of fistula formation due to adherence of loops of bowel to the mesh.[13] This may not be the same for other types of synthetic material; however, it is prudent in choosing a synthetic material to cover the defect in the abdominal wall that may potentially come into direct contact with bowel loops to provide coverage for the inner surface of the synthetic material so as to preclude the possibility

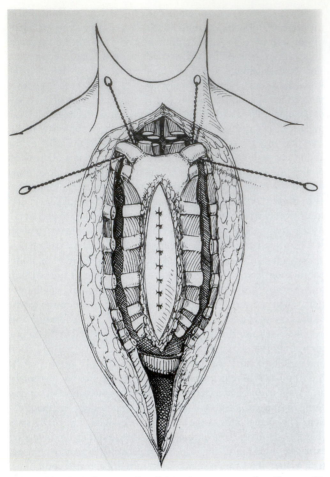

**FIGURE 20A-5.** Sarcoma involving the sternum; the ribs are divided on both sides of the sternum and the medial ends of the clavicles are also divided. *From Karakousis CP: Surgery for soft tissue sarcomas, in Atlas of Surgical Oncology, K. Bland et al (eds). Philadelphia, WB Saunders, 1995, pp 283–400.*

of direct contact with loops of bowel. The greater omentum is the tissue most easily available and suitable for this purpose. It can be elongated to reach to the groin by detaching it from the transverse colon and releasing one of the two corners from which it is hanging, preserving its blood supply through the right gastroepiploic or the short gastric vessels. However, in many instances of cancer surgery of the abdominal cavity and abdominal wall, the omentum has been resected or it needs to be resected due to involvement. In these cases, one may provide coverage for the inner surface of the defect by rotating the contralateral rectus abdominis muscle or simply obtaining a free patch of peritoneum from another site in the abdominal cavity, to suture it to the defect in the peritoneum itself prior to the repair of the fascial defect with the mesh. The last method is, in our experience, the simplest method of dealing with this problem and seems to work well. Such a free patch of peritoneum seems to survive in the low oxygen tension of the peritoneal cavity and prevents dense adhesion formation between the loops of bowel and mesh and subsequent fistulization.[13] After repair of the abdominal wall

defect with the mesh, closed-suction drainage is provided by placing a suction catheter between the mesh and the overlying skin flap. The suction drainage helps to eliminate the lymphatic drainage that tends to accumulate and allows approximation and healing between the subcutaneous fat and the mesh.

## RETROPERITONEAL SARCOMAS

Retroperitoneal sarcomas provide technical challenges to the operating surgeon due to the large size at which they are usually diagnosed and often their inaccessible location.

### SARCOMAS OF THE UPPER QUADRANTS

For sarcomas of the upper quadrants of the abdomen, the patient is placed in a lateral or semilateral position with the affected side up, and a thoracoabdominal incision is used. Depending upon the location of the tumor mass, one may use the 9th, 10th, or 11th intercostal space. The incision starts at the midline and is extended to the costal margin. The thoracoabdominal incision may also be combined with a midline incision, extending from the xiphoid to the umbilicus or below, depending upon the size of the tumor and the need for exposure. Usually the portion of the incision between the costal margin and the midline is made first and is carried through the anterior rectus sheath, rectus abdominis muscle, posterior rectus sheath, and peritoneum. This limited incision from the costal margin to the midline allows entry for at least palpation of the liver and other organs to assess the extent and location of the tumor and the best course the incision should follow between the ribs for optimal exposure, i.e., whether a lower one in the 10th or 11th intercostal space, or a higher one at the 9th or 8th intercostal space. The lower intercostal incisions are supposed to have less morbidity, but all are tolerated well given effective postoperative analgesia. In the thoracic portion of the incision, the pleural cavity is entered. The costal margin is divided and actually, a small segment of the costal margin is removed and then the diaphragm is incised. One then assesses the need for resection of part of the diaphragm if the tumor is adherent to the latter. The diaphragm is divided radially for a few centimeters in order to allow full opening of the incision as the self-retaining chest wall retractors are placed. If the diaphragm is involved, the incision is further carried to circumscribe the area of involvement.

Whenever the diaphragm is not involved, the incision in the diaphragm is extended peripherally as needed for purposes of exposure at a distance of about 3 to 5 cm from the ribs in order to avoid denervation of the central and largest part of the diaphragm from the phrenic nerve. Through the peritoneal aspect of the tumor, any organs that can be separated, such as the hepatic or splenic flexure of the colon, are dissected off if not involved by the tumor mass. The stomach on the left side and the liver on the right side are also separated whenever possible. The parietal peritoneum anterior to the area of involvement is then incised and one enters the retroperitoneal space between the peritoneum and the posterolateral abdominal wall. If the deeper layers of this musculature are involved, then of course one incises the deeper layers of the musculature of

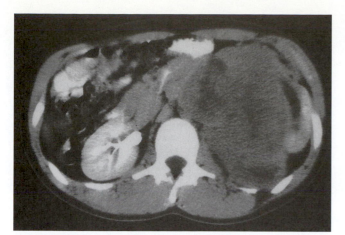

**FIGURE 20A-6.** Left upper quadrant sarcoma.

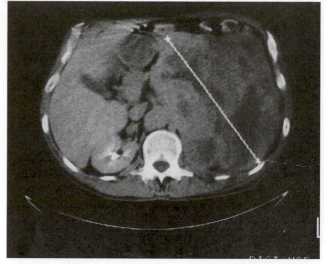

**FIGURE 20A-8.** Left upper quadrant sarcoma. The tumors in Figs. 20A-6, 20A-7, and 20A-8 were removed through a left thoracoabdominal incision in combination with a midline incision.

the abdominal wall in order to obtain a clean plane separating the tumor mass from the more superficial muscle layers, i.e., internal or external oblique. Posteriorly, the quadratus lumborum is separated from the tumor mass, although this muscle can also be resected en bloc with the tumor if necessary. The basic idea is to mobilize the tumor off its bed by freeing all the posterolateral attachments, which should be relatively easy to do, and carry this dissection close to the midline near the aorta on the left side or the inferior vena cava on the right. Following the path of least resistance and the dictates of safe dissection, one then may separate the respective flexure of the colon if not involved, or in case of involvement, the bowel is divided proximally and distally, as well as the relevant section of its mesentery around its area of involvement so as to further mobilize the tumor mass. On the left side, the spleen may have to be resected en bloc with the distal portion of the pancreas (Figs. 20A-6, 20A-7, and 20A-8). In this case, the splenic artery is identified at the superior border of the pancreas in the lesser sac and it is ligated, and

divided. The pancreas is mobilized at its superior and inferior border following mobilization of the spleen by dividing the lienorenal ligament. The splenic vein on the posterior surface of the pancreas is dissected, ligated, and divided. The pancreas is divided medial to the tumor by using a stapler or mattress sutures to control bleeding from its cut surface. On the right side, the right lobe of the liver may have to be resected en bloc with the tumor mass (Figs. 20A-9, 20A-10). In this case, the tumor mass and right lobe of the liver are mobilized posterolaterally by dividing parietal attachments and the right triangular ligament. In the porta hepatis, the right hepatic artery, right branch of the portal vein, and the right hepatic duct are ligated and divided. The trunk of the right branch of the portal vein

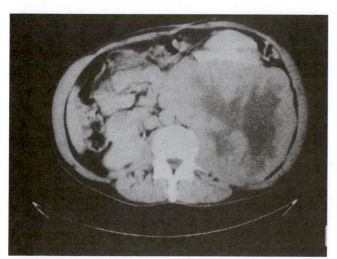

**FIGURE 20A-7.** Left upper quadrant sarcoma displacing the left kidney anteriorly.

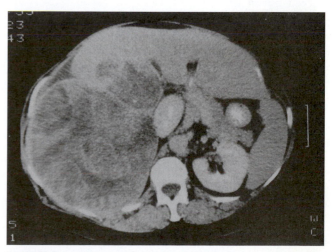

**FIGURE 20A-9.** Tumor mass in the right upper quadrant involving the right lobe of the liver and displacing the right kidney medially.

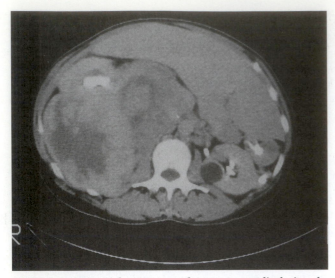

**FIGURE 20A-10.** Right upper quadrant sarcoma displacing the right kidney anteriorly.

is short and it is preferably divided between two tightly placed vascular clamps, the two ends being oversewn with a running vascular suture. The hepatic parenchyma is divided through a plane defined by a line between the gallbladder fossa and hepatic vein confluence anteriorly, and the lateral border of the inferior vena cava posteriorly. Maintaining this plane helps avoid injury to the supply of the left lobe. If a kidney has to be resected, this organ is mobilized posterolaterally from the quadratus lumborum; the ureter is exposed, ligated, and divided inferiorly. The renal artery is ligated and divided posteriorly, and anteriorly the renal vein is identified, ligated, and divided. The proximal stump of the vein is preferably sutured with a running vascular suture (Fig. 20A-11). The essential aspects of an

upper quadrant retroperitoneal sarcoma resection are

1. The use of a thoracoabdominal incision in the lateral position. The thoracoabdominal incision should be combined with a midline incision in most cases for exposure.
2. The mobilization of the tumor off its bed by separating it posterolaterally off the inner layers of the abdominal wall and diaphragm to nearly the midline with en bloc resection of any involved portions of abdominal wall layers or diaphragm. Through the transperitoneal part of the exposure, the tumor mass is separated off adjacent viscera or the involved visceral organs are mobilized en bloc.
3. After the tumor mass is mobilized off its bed, both posterolaterally as well as anteromedially, it can be lifted off its bed and then midline attachments or major blood vessels connecting the tumor mass to the inferior vena cava on the right or the aorta on the left are dealt with.

It is wrong to attempt to resect a retroperitoneal sarcoma of the upper quadrant with the patient in the supine position through a midline incision and to try to define first the resectability of the tumor by attempting to develop a plane between the tumor mass and the adjacent major vascular structures such as the aorta and inferior vena cava. The latter policy is hazardous and apt to lead to abandonment of resection of the tumor mass.

## RETROPERITONEAL SARCOMAS OF THE FLANK

These tumors are dealt with by placing the patient in a lateral position with the affected side up (Figs. 20A-12, 20A-13). A flank incision is made over the center of the mass, the length of which depends on the location of the tumor. This incision is usually joined with a midline incision in a T fashion for the appropriate amount of exposure. Again, retroperitoneal dissection between the tumor mass and the

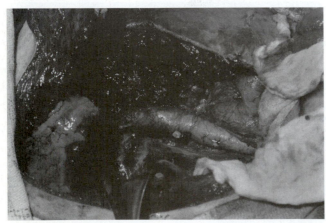

**FIGURE 20A-11.** Operative field following resection of the tumor shown in Fig. 20A-9, which required en bloc resection of the right lobe of the liver and right kidney. The inferior vena cava and divided hepatic parenchyma are clearly shown.

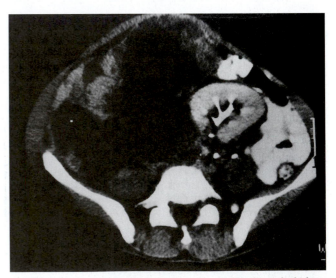

**FIGURE 20A-12.** Right flank sarcoma displacing the right kidney to the left.

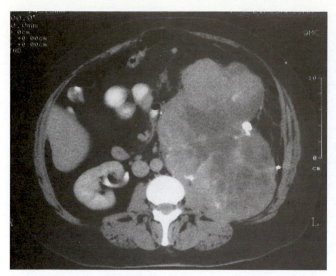

**FIGURE 20A-13.** Left flank sarcoma.

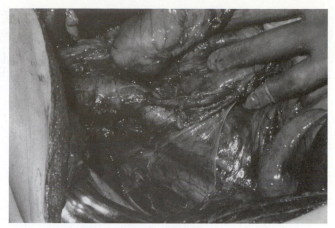

**FIGURE 20A-15.** Operative field following resection of the sarcoma shown in Figs. 20A-12 and 20A-14, en bloc with the right kidney and the infrarenal portion of the inferior vena cava.

posterolateral abdominal wall is carried out mobilizing the tumor mass. On the anteromedial aspect of the tumor mass, any viscera that can be separated are dissected off or, if involved, left on the surface of the tumor mass, in the case of bowel by separating the involved portion from its continuity. Again, resection is carried out in a lateral position, the tumor is mobilized both posterolaterally and anteromedially, and then the plane of dissection and the vascular connections between the tumor mass and the aorta on the left or the inferior vena cava on the right are dealt with (Figs. 20A-14, 20A-15).

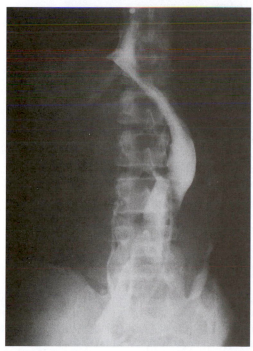

**FIGURE 20A-14.** Right flank sarcoma displacing the inferior vena cava.

Flank sarcomas often require resection of the ipsilateral kidney and the ipsilateral portion of the colon.

## SARCOMAS IN THE EPIGASTRIC REGION AND MESENTERY OF THE BOWEL

Sarcomas in the epigastric region, i.e., in the midline of the upper abdomen, are operated on with the patient in a supine position through a long midline incision. One then proceeds to separate the tumor mass from the adjacent structures (or remove the latter en bloc). Limiting anatomic factors are the superior mesenteric vessels and porta hepatis.

For sarcomas in the mesentery of the bowel, the approach is also through a midline incision with the patient in the supine position and loops of bowel that can be separated from the tumor mass are separated. Then, one identifies the involved loops of bowel and locates the first free loop immediately proximal to the tumor mass and the first free loop immediately distal to the tumor mass. One then incises the peritoneal leaves of the mesentery, proximal and distal to the area of involvement of the mesentery by following visible mesenteric branches down to the base of the mesentery. This will expose the superior mesenteric vein first and then any tributaries to the vein from the involved area of the mesentery are ligated and divided (Fig. 20A-16). Immediately to the left of the superior mesenteric vein and slightly more posteriorly, the superior mesenteric artery is exposed and the branches of the superior mesenteric artery to the involved segment of the mesentery are ligated and divided. Mere palpation of the tumor mass in the mesentery of the small bowel is not sufficient to determine resectability. One needs to expose and dissect the superior mesenteric vessels.[14] This not only will provide a definite answer as to the resectability of the mesenteric tumor, but also will provide the maximum margin toward the root of the mesentery and allow removal of the tumor mass, whenever that is feasible, with full knowledge that the distal uninvolved loops of bowel will continue to have their blood supply. Thus, the dissection is carried out safely with secure and precise knowledge of the

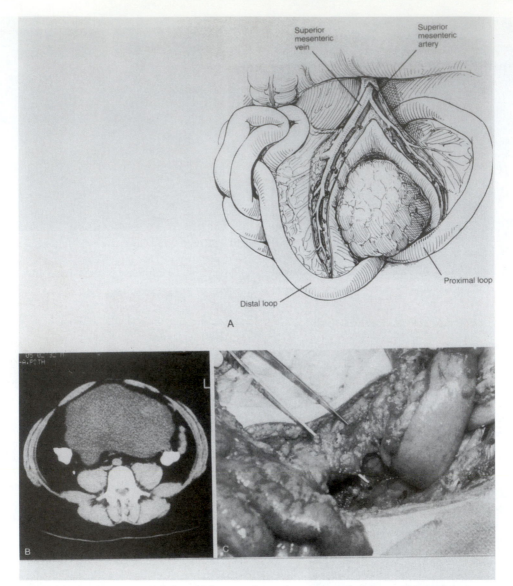

**FIGURE 20A-16.** Sarcoma of the mid-line involving the mesentery of the small bowel shown on CT scan (*B*). Drawing *A* shows the principle of dissection and exposure of the superior mesenteric vessels at the base of the mesentery and ligation of the branches and tributaries from the involved area of mesentery. In *C*, the forceps shows the superior mesenteric vessels surrounded by some adipose tissue supplying the distal uninvolved loops of bowel. *From Karakousis CP: Surgery for soft tissue sarcomas, in* Atlas of Surgical Oncology, *K. Bland et al (eds). Philadelphia, WB Saunders, 1995, pp 283–400.*

loops that have to be sacrificed in removing the specific mesenteric tumor. Blind application of clamps through the mesentery without dissection and identification of the vessels supplying the tumor is discouraged because it may end up with unintended injury of vessels and the need to resect all of the bowel distal to the area of involvement of the mesentery. Of course, if the area of involvement of the mesentery is near the ileocecal area that is not a problem, but for tumors situated near the ligament of Treitz, it is crucial to dissect and expose the superior mesenteric vessels.

## SARCOMAS IN THE LOWER QUADRANTS OF THE ABDOMEN

Masses in these locations, i.e., in the right or left iliac fossa, may be exposed and resected with the patient in a supine position using the abdominoinguinal incision[15] (Fig. 20A-17). The ipsilateral groin is draped in the field and the extremity is covered with a sterile stockinet which makes it possible to relax the femoral nerve and iliofemoral vessels and to dissect them more easily off the area of

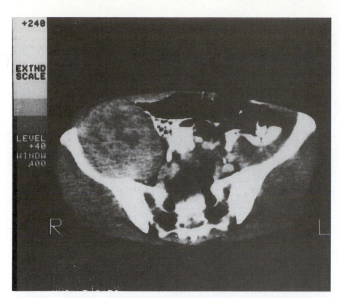

**FIGURE 20A-17.** Sarcoma of the right lower quadrant resected through a right abdominoinguinal incision.

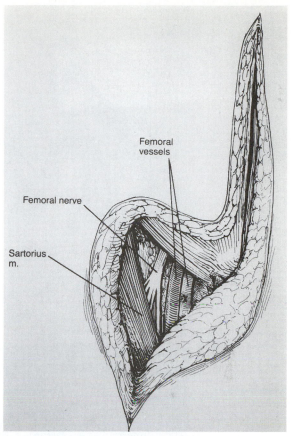

**FIGURE 20A-18.** Drawing illustrates a right abdominoinguinal incision exposing the femoral vessels and nerve. *From Karakousis CP: Surgery for soft tissue sarcomas, in* Atlas of Surgical Oncology, *K. Bland et al (eds). Philadelphia, WB Saunders, 1995, pp 283–400.*

the tumor when the extremity is flexed at the knee and hip joints. The abdominoinguinal incision is made by making a midline incision from the umbilicus or above the umbilicus down to the pubic symphysis. The peritoneal cavity is entered and initial assessment of the extent of the tumor or the existence of any metastasis is determined. Assuming there is no contraindication to resection of the tumor mass, in order to resect it by completing the abdominoinguinal incision, one extends the incision from its lower end at the pubic symphysis to the midinguinal point on the affected side. The incision is further continued from the midinguinal point for about 5 to 10 cm below the inguinal ligament exposing the femoral vessels. The ipsilateral rectus abdominis and sheath are divided near the pubic crest (Fig. 20A-18). The inguinal ligament is divided near the pubic tubercle, and as the abdominal wall is retracted, the inferior epigastric vein and inferior epigastric artery are serially ligated and divided (Fig. 20A-19). The lateral part of the inguinal ligament is detached off the iliac fascia, and this opens up the whole area of the lower quadrant, exposing in continuity the lower abdominal aorta and inferior vena cava and the ipsilateral common iliac, external iliac, and common femoral vessels so as to have full exposure for the manipulation and removal of the tumor mass (Fig. 20A-20). It also becomes possible in this case to resect the vessels if they are involved by having one continuous exposed field. Any attachments of the tumor mass onto the abdominal wall are freed by dissecting through the appropriate plane, removing the peritoneum and any involved muscle layers of the anterior abdominal wall en bloc with the tumor mass. Then the tumor mass is dissected posterolaterally off the iliac bone. The femoral nerve is exposed lateral to the femoral and external iliac arteries. It is located underneath the iliac fascia. After the femoral nerve is exposed at the level of the inguinal ligament, it is dissected in its course between the iliacus and psoas muscles. The nerve, if involved by the tumor, can be sacrificed. In this case, the patients lose the capacity

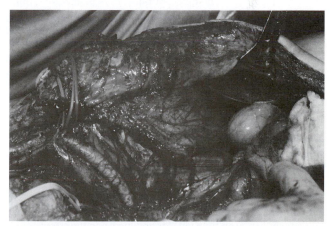

**FIGURE 20A-19.** The tumor shown in Fig. 20A-17 is exposed through a right abdominoinguinal incision. Vessel loops are around the inferior epigastric vein and artery prior to their ligation and division.

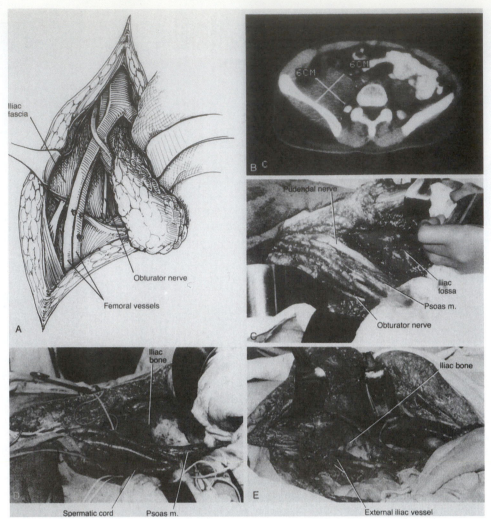

**FIGURE 20A-20.** *A*. The abdominoinguinal incision fully developed exposes the iliofemoral vessels in their continuity. *B*. Right iliac fossa tumor. *C*, *D*, and *E* show operative fields after resection of iliac fossa tumors. *From Karakousis CP: Surgery for soft tissue sarcomas, in* Atlas of Surgical Oncology, *K. Bland et al (eds). Philadelphia, WB Saunders, 1995, pp 283–400.*

for active extension of the knee, but they manage in the first month or two to ambulate by using a walker, crutches, or a cane. They finally manage to passively extend the knee by flexing the hip as they walk, and they are able to walk without any support. In most cases, however, it should be possible to save the nerve if it is not actually invaded by the tumor. The iliacus or psoas muscles can be removed en bloc with the tumor mass. The femoral vessels are distally exposed and vessel loops are passed around the common femoral vessels. Vessel loops are also passed around the origin of the common iliac artery and the common iliac vein. The latter is situated lateral to the artery on the right side and medial to the artery on the left side. The abdominoinguinal incision is indicated for

1. Sarcomas of the lower abdomen that extend from the midline over the iliac vessels to the iliac crest

2. Sarcomas of the iliac fossa
3. Large tumor masses over the external iliac vessels with or without involvement of these vessels
4. Sarcomas involving the lateral wall of the lesser pelvis
5. Those extending to or through the obturator foramen involving the pubic bone and/or the proximal portion of the adductor group of muscles

Rarely, a bilateral abdominoinguinal incision may be required by extending the lower end of the midline incision from the pubic symphysis to both groins, as described before. The repair of this incision is fairly straightforward. The inguinal ligament, if still present, is sutured lateral to the vessels to the iliac fascia when the fascia is available, if not, to the underlying iliacus muscle if available, or finally, to the ligaments of the anterior capsule of the hip joint.

Medial to the vessels, the inguinal ligament is sutured to Cooper's ligament. When making the abdominoinguinal incision, the spermatic cord in the male can be preserved by incising the inguinal floor from inside all the way to the internal inguinal ring and extricating the spermatic cord off the inguinal canal. The spermatic cord after it goes through the deep inguinal ring bifurcates into the internal spermatic vessels coursing superiorly, and the ductus deferens coursing posteromedially. The internal spermatic vessels, if close to the tumor, can be ligated and divided. The viability of the testis is preserved if the internal spermatic vessels are ligated and divided as long as the testis has not been mobilized off its scrotal bed. In cases of resection of the lower abdominal wall, including the inguinal ligament, reconstruction may be performed by using a mesh to replace the missing part of the lower abdominal wall and inguinal ligament. In this case, however, attention should be paid to cover the vessels with the mobilized sartorius or other muscle, so as to avoid direct contact between the mesh and the vessels as the mesh may erode into the artery if in direct contact and cause bleeding from the femoral artery. A preferred method of reconstruction is that of using the contralateral rectus abdominis, which includes the peritoneum, posterior rectus sheath, and the rectus muscle based on the inferior epigastric vessels. The rectus is divided at a sufficiently high level so as to permit its lateral mobilization. The contralateral rectus abdominis will reach the iliac crest easily and therefore can be used to repair the lower part of the abdominal wall and inguinal ligament. Whether the mesh or the mobilized contralateral rectus abdominis, the inferior edge of the tissue used for reconstruction is sutured lateral to the vessels to the iliac fascia, iliacus muscle, or the ligaments of the anterior capsule of the hip joint, depending upon the availability of tissues and medial to the vessels to Cooper's ligament. The rectus abdominis and anterior sheath are, of course, approximated to the pubic crest. Nonabsorbable interrupted sutures are used.

In many cases of sarcomas or other tumors of the lesser pelvis, which adhere to the wall of the lesser pelvis and extend to the obturator foramen, one may not have to use the entire length of the abdominoinguinal incision, but simply use a lateral transverse extension from the lower end at the pubic symphysis to the pubic tubercle. The ipsilateral rectus abdominis and anterior sheath are divided off the pubic crest, and this permits sufficient exposure to dissect a tumor off the external iliac vein, the wall of the lesser pelvis, the internal iliac artery and the obturator foramen. The obturator nerve and vessels can be clearly exposed through this approach. If necessary, the obturator nerve and vessels can be removed en bloc with the tumor mass. There is no noticeable deficit after removal of the obturator nerve, since in the upright position adduction is performed by gravity, and only in the supine position may patients have to help adduct the extremity with their hands, although in some cases, apparently due to innervation of the adductor magnus by the sciatic nerve, younger patients are able to actively adduct their extremity even after removal of the obturator nerve.

## SARCOMAS OF THE MIDLINE OF THE PELVIS

These tumors are dealt with with the patient in a supine position and a midline incision of appropriate length is made. Most pelvic sarcomas can be resected with portions of the adjacent organs as needed,

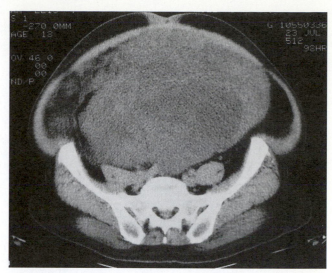

**FIGURE 20A-21.** Midline sarcoma of the upper pelvis that required resection of the right colon and a segment of the right ureter.

e.g., bladder or rectum, and rarely do they require pelvic exenteration. If a significant part of or the entire bladder has to be resected, reconstruction with an ileal loop is performed. If a substantial portion of the ureter on one side has been involved, reconstruction can then be done by using a defunctionalized segment of ileum to which is anastomosed the proximal end of the ureter on the proximal end of the bowel in an end-to-side fashion near the divided edge of the bowel and then the distal end of the bowel is anastomosed directly to the bladder (Figs. 20A-21, 20A-22).

It is inadvisable to anastomose the distal end of the bowel to the distal end of the ureter, if available, because the thick mucus secretions of the intestinal segment used as a conduit may have difficulty going through the distal ureterointestinal anastomosis. It is therefore preferable to perform an end-to-side anastomosis between the distal end of the defunctionalized ileal conduit directly to the bladder by using a two-layer anastomosis with running absorbable sutures for the inner layer, and Lembert silk sutures for the outer layer. This type of reconstruction works very well on a long-term basis and preserves kidney function. Through the midline part of the incision, in order to assess the situation, it is important to incise the peritoneum inferiorly and separate the bladder from the wall of the pelvis. This allows greater exposure and, if necessary, the lower end of the incision can be extended bilaterally to the pubic tubercle on each side by dividing the rectus abdominis and anterior rectus sheath on each side. This allows greater exposure on the inferior aspects of the pelvis and full exposure of the obturator foramen and the lateral wall of the lesser pelvis (Fig. 20A-23).

If the tumor is adherent to the lateral wall of the lesser pelvis, the fascia covering the obturator internus and the obturator internus itself can be resected en bloc with the adjacent tumor mass. Of course, the internal iliac artery needs to be exposed and possibly ligated at its origin, certainly the branch from the internal iliac artery to the bladder, i.e., the superior vesical artery should be ligated and divided, which facilitates exposure without creating any problems

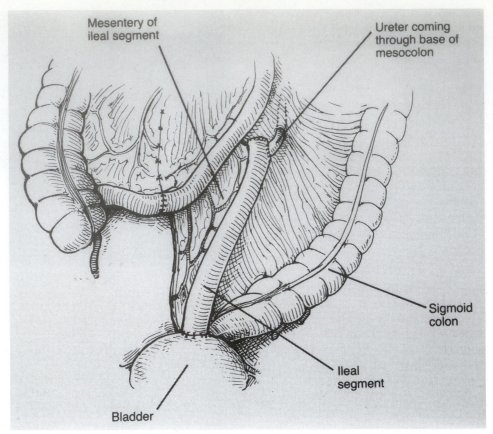

**FIGURE 20A-22.** Drawing illustrating repair of the resected left ureter through a piece of ileum proximally anastomosed to the proximal end of the ureter and distally to the bladder. *From Karakousis CP: Surgery for soft tissue sarcomas, in* Atlas of Surgical Oncology, *K. Bland et al (eds). Philadelphia, WB Saunders, 1995, pp 283–400.*

with the vascularization of the bladder. In some cases, a low anterior resection of the rectosigmoid has to be performed with end-to-end anastomosis which, if one is not secure about it being leakproof, can be protected by a transverse cutaneous loop colostomy.

## SACRAL INVOLVEMENT

Sarcomas involving the anterior or posterior surface of the sacrum can be approached in a lateral position if it is anticipated that extensive dissection of pelvic organs will also be required. Otherwise, the prone position is preferable. A midline incision over the sacrum is performed from the lumbosacral junction to the tip of the coccyx and below. Flaps are then developed to the left and right of the sacrum beyond the palpable extent of the sacrum, and then the origin of the gluteus maximus is divided off the sacrum. Inferiorly, the anococcygeal raphe is divided and the presacral space is entered. The sacrotuberous ligament is then divided. The ischiorectal fossa is explored. The pudendal nerve is identified on the lateral wall of the ischiorectal fossa on the surface of the obturator fascia. The nerve is traced proximally and the sacrospinous ligament is divided. By palpation both from the posterior aspect of the sacrum and the anterior aspect of the sacrum, one can estimate the cephalad extent of the tumor

mass and with neurosurgical rongeurs, one enters the posterior sacral plate above the area of involvement and enters the sacral canal.

Sacral roots can then be identified, and the ones not very close to the tumor can be preserved. The pudendal nerve consists of S2, S3, S4 roots on each side. One should try to preserve as many roots as possible from each side. Apparently, bilateral preservation of S2 roots or at least unilateral preservation of S2, S3 roots and their continuation to the pudendal nerve preserve anal and urinary sphincteric control and the capacity for erection in men. Having identified some of the proximal sacral roots to the pudendal nerve, one may divide the bone transversely with osteotomes through the fused vertebral bodies. One can perform a resection of the coccyx and distal part of the sacrum, i.e., below the S2 vertebra with preservation of sphincter control.[16] If one can divide the sacrum in a straight line across (the highest such transverse line is the one connecting the lower ends of the sacroiliac joints), then one is below the S2 vertebra. Higher divisions of the sacrum are possible but fraught with the risks of sphincter denervation and incomplete tumor resection due to anatomic limitations for wide resection encountered in this area. When the tumor involves a viscus such as the rectum and is situated between the sacrum and the rectal wall, then the patient is placed in a lateral position, a midline abdominal incision is made to mobilize the bowel

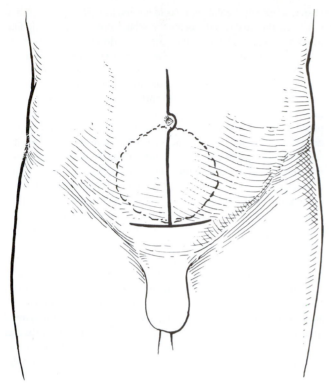

**FIGURE 20A-23.** For low, midline pelvic sarcomas extending close to the obturator foramen, the midline portion of the incision is combined with a transverse extension bilaterally, transecting the rectus abdominis muscle and anterior rectus sheath off the pubic crest bilaterally for greater exposure.

and divide it above its level of involvement, separating the anterior rectal wall off the bladder and prostate in the male or uterus in the female. Through a posterior longitudinal incision over the middle of the sacrum one can then divide the rectum distally through the divided anococcygeal raphe, remove the specimen of sacrum-tumor-rectum, and perform a low end-to-end anastomosis through a posterior approach. In patients where it is not possible to perform a low anastomosis, a complete abdominoperineal resection may be performed in a lateral position by extending the incision over the sacrum and coccyx around the anus and then dissecting between the anterior wall of the rectum, and vagina in the female or prostate in the male.

## SARCOMAS OF THE LOWER EXTREMITY

Sarcomas in the iliac fossa without bone involvement may be resected through an abdominoinguinal incision, as was described in the section on retroperitoneal sarcomas. Whenever there is involvement of the iliac bone, however, the technique of *internal hemipelvectomy* is required.[17] In this operation, the patient is placed in a semilateral position so as to have more exposure of the anterior abdominal wall but also of the buttock. An incision along the iliac crest from the posterior inferior iliac spine along the iliac crest to the anterior superior iliac spine is made. The incision is then extended to the pubic

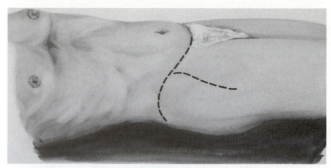

**FIGURE 20A-24.** The incision for an internal hemipelvectomy. The extension of the incision to the greater trochanter is used only in cases of complete internal hemipelvectomy, or resection of some of the gluteal muscles en bloc with the iliac bone.

tubercle over the inguinal ligament (Fig. 20A-24). The retroperitoneal space is entered medial to the iliac crest by dividing the external oblique, internal oblique, and transversus abdominis muscles. The peritoneum is displaced by blunt dissection. Superomedially, the ureter is identified, as are the common iliac and external iliac vessels. The lateral third of the inguinal ligament is detached off the iliac fascia. The inferior epigastric artery and the epigastric vein are ligated and divided at their origin (Fig. 20A-25) and the medial end

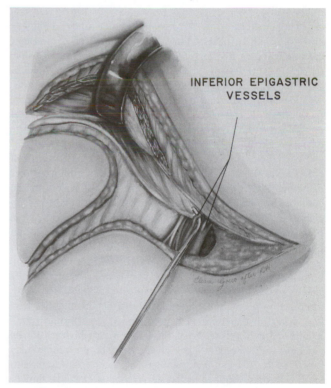

**FIGURE 20A-25.** The retroperitoneal space has been entered and the inferior epigastric vessels are being dissected in order to be ligated and divided. *From Karakousis CP: Internal hemipelvectomy. Surg Gynecol Obstet 158:279, 1984.*

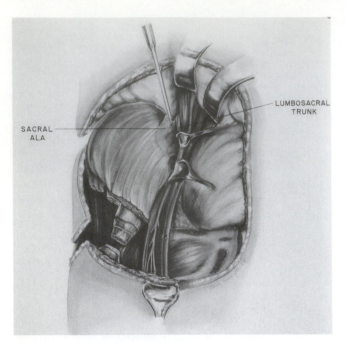

**FIGURE 20A-26.** Drawing illustrating in the case of complete internal hemipelvectomy proximal division through the sacral ala, retracting medially the lumbosacral trunk. *From Karakousis CP: Internal hemipelvectomy. Surg Gynecol Obstet 158:279, 1984.*

of the inguinal ligament is divided off the pubic tubercle. This type of incision suffices for resection of the iliac bone and adjacent musculature when the division of the bone distally is carried just above the acetabulum. Proximally the bone may be divided through the sacroiliac joint or the sacral ala for a safer surgical margin. When dividing the bone through the sacral ala, it is important to remember that the lumbosacral trunk (L4, L5) crosses in front of the sacral ala en route to joining the sacral nerve roots (S1-S3) in order to form the sciatic nerve (Fig. 20A-26).

When the tumor is confined to the bone or it extends medially only into the iliacus muscle and there is no evidence of involvement of the gluteal muscles, on the lateral side of the incision along the iliac crest the gluteal fascia is incised and the gluteal musculature, i.e., the gluteus medius and minimus anteriorly and the gluteus maximus posteriorly, are separated with a periosteal elevator off the iliac bone posterolaterally until the greater sciatic notch is identified. As one approaches the notch, the inferior and superior gluteal arteries or branches of may be encountered and need to be ligated and divided. These provide blood supply to the gluteus maximus and medius-minimus, respectively. On the medial side behind the iliac fascia and, lateral to the common femoral artery, the femoral nerve is identified and it is dissected off the tumor mass whenever possible and preserved. In order to have greater laxity on the femoral nerve as well as the iliac and femoral vessels, it is important to have the lower extremity wrapped with a sterile wrap so it can be flexed at the knee and hip joints, a maneuver which allows for relaxation and better retraction of these structures.

The attachments of quadratus lumborum and the fascia of the latissimus dorsi posteriorly are divided off the iliac crest. The

posterior edge of the iliac bone is identified as well as the sacroiliac joint. On the medial side again the sciatic notch is exposed. The psoas muscle may or may not be preserved depending on the location and extent of the tumor. The iliacus muscle, which usually has to be resected, is divided at the level of the inguinal ligament. The sartorius muscle is divided off its origin as well as the tensor fascia lata. The rectus femoris is divided off its origin from the anterior inferior iliac spine. With blunt dissection the iliac bone is then exposed from the level below the anterior inferior iliac spine to the greater sciatic notch. A Gigli saw is passed around the greater sciatic notch and the bone is divided from the greater sciatic notch to below the anterior inferior iliac spine. This plane of division is just above the acetabulum and leaves about 2 cm of iliac bone at the roof of the acetabulum. The bone is divided proximally through the sacroiliac joint or the sacral ala, maintaining careful orientation as one proceeds to divide the bone with an osteotome (Fig. 20A-27). A Gigli saw is not appropriate for division of the bone proximally.

Whenever part of the gluteal musculature has to be resected due to penetration of the tumor through the lateral plate of the iliac bone into the gluteal muscles, one has to extend the incision from the anterior superior iliac spine to the greater trochanter sufficiently so as to develop a posterolateral flap that leaves the gluteus maximus attached to the flap whenever possible. The gluteus maximus has only a small area of origin from the posterior aspect of the iliac bone and usually can be preserved because most of it originates from the sacral edge.

Whenever the entire innominate bone has to be resected, the incision mentioned above is carried from the posterior-inferior iliac spine along the iliac crest to the anterior-superior iliac spine to the pubic tubercle and then medially all the way to the pubic symphysis. The ipsilateral rectus abdominis and the anterior rectus sheath are divided off the pubic crest and the peritoneum is more extensively

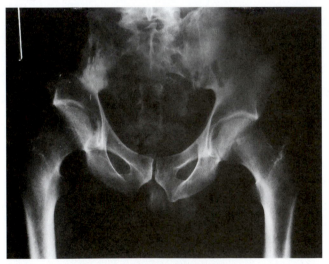

**FIGURE 20A-27.** X-ray of the pelvis following resection of the right iliac bone from above the acetabulum to the sacroiliac joint. The roof of the unsupported acetabulum migrates cephalad and forms a callus with the adjacent sacral ala.

displaced medially. The incision from the anterior superior iliac spine toward the greater trochanter is extended more posteriorly, the fascia lata is incised, and the insertion of the gluteus maximus to the gluteal line of the femur is divided, as well as the insertions of gluteus medius and minimus, piriformis, gemelli, obturator internus and externus, quadratus femoris around the greater trochanter. The sciatic nerve is exposed and dissected all the way to the greater sciatic notch. In these cases, for a complete resection of the innominate bone, the common femoral vessels are mobilized and surrounded in their continuity with the iliac vessels by umbilical tape. The adductor group of muscles is divided off their origin from the pubic bone. The iliacus and psoas muscles are divided below the level of the inguinal ligament, exposing the anterior aspect of the capsule of the hip joint. The capsule of the hip joint is incised and the neck of the femur is exposed. The neck of the tumor is divided with a Gigli saw. The pubic symphysis is divided with a Gigli saw, the sacroiliac joint, or sacral ala with an osteotome, and following the division of the ipsilateral levator ani, sacrotuberous and sacrospinous ligament, the specimen is removed (Fig. 20A-28).

Following removal of the specimen, one can see the sciatic and femoral nerves in this field along with the iliofemoral vessels, which will continue to supply the lower extremity. A pivotal anatomic point in the incision for internal hemipelvectomy is ligation and division of the inferior epigastric vessels, which allows mobility of the iliofemoral vessels. It allows in-continuity exposure of the iliofemoral vessels, sufficient mobility to work around them, and provides excellent exposure so that the resection of the hemipelvis may be performed with clear visualization of the sciatic and femoral nerves. Following complete internal hemipelvectomy with resection of the entire hemipelvis, the ipsilateral lower extremity shortens by about 2 to 3 cm and there is no function in the hip joint, although there is full function in the ankle and knee joints. The patients are forced to use crutches indefinitely through their lifetime, at least the ones who are younger and able to stand using their arms to support themselves. Older patients end up wheelchair-bound. Most people, however, feel grateful for the preservation of the extremity

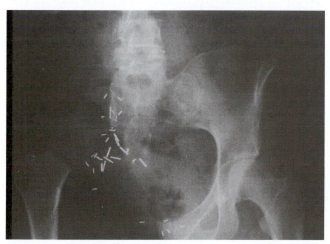

**FIGURE 20A-28.** X-ray of the pelvis following right internal hemipelvectomy.

even if they are not able to use crutches. In cases of a partial internal hemipelvectomy, whenever the iliac bone can be resected with preservation of the acetabulum, the function is vastly superior, although the extremity also shortens about 2 cm because the roof of the acetabulum migrates cephalad and comes to abut against the sacral ala, forming a callus there. Patients with preservation of the acetabulum, although they require the use of a walker and crutches for the first 3 to 6 months, finally graduate to using a cane, and by the end of a year they are able to walk without the use of a cane with a slight tilt in walking, but walking nevertheless fairly freely without any support.

## SARCOMAS IN THE GROIN

These tumors are managed with the patient in a supine position by using the incision for radical groin dissection,[18] which exposes the external iliac vessels for proximal control. In this incision, which is longitudinal over the groin area and may have to be modified according to the location of the tumor, the retroperitoneal space is entered by incising the external oblique aponeurosis, internal oblique, transversus abdominis, and transversalis fascia and by dividing the inguinal ligament lateral to the artery. The inferior epigastric artery and vein are ligated and divided to open up the space, provided the tumor is not that close to the inguinal ligament. If it is close to the inguinal ligament, then, of course, the external oblique, internal oblique, and transversus abdominis muscles are divided above the inguinal ligament, exposing the external iliac vessels above the tumor-involved area and through the continuation of the longitudinal incision in the skin, exposing again the femoral vessels below the area of involvement. The specimen is mobilized all the way around, and then all that is left to decide is whether the vessels can be dissected off the tumor or not. If resection of the vessels is required, the patient is heparinized, vascular clamps are placed proximally and distally, and the vessels are divided. The profunda femoris vessels have to be dealt with, of course, as dictated by the location of the tumor mass. Appropriate vessel reconstruction is performed as necessary.

## SARCOMAS OF THE ANTERIOR COMPARTMENT

In sarcomas of the anterior compartment of the thigh (Fig. 20A-29), a compartment resection may be performed without necessarily removing the entire quadriceps.[19] The fleshy bulge on the medial aspect of the knee is the distal part of the vastus medialis and this is usually out of the way and can be preserved with intact innervation. In sarcomas of the anterior compartment of the thigh, a longitudinal incision is made all the way from the anterior superior iliac spine to near the patella. Flaps are developed. On the medial side, the femoral nerve is dissected lateral to the femoral artery, below the inguinal ligament. At this point, the nerve provides sensory branches to the anteromedial aspect of the skin of the thigh and a motor branch to sartorius. At a deeper plane and a few centimeters below the inguinal ligament, the trunk of the nerve is traced to the point it gives off a leash of nerves, supplying the rectus femoris, vastus intermedius and vastus lateralis, which courses in an

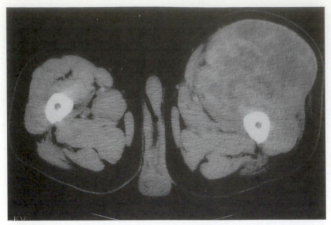

**FIGURE 20A-29.** A CT scan showing soft tissue sarcoma of the left anterior compartment of the thigh.

inferolateral direction under the proximal part of the rectus femoris along with the lateral femoral circumflex branches. There is, however, a long slender branch of the femoral nerve coursing longitudinally on the surface of the vastus medialis, which supplies the vastus medialis at two levels. If this nerve branch can be preserved along with the distal half of the vastus medialis, this is sufficient to provide a very useful extensor capacity for the knee joint (Fig. 20A-30). In addition to controlling the blood supply at the level of the femoral circumflex branches, other blood supply to the quadriceps is from perforator branches from the profunda femoris vessels entering through the posterolateral aspect of the vastus lateralis muscle. Infrequently, when the sarcoma is localized in the inferior medial aspect of the anterior compartment, the vastus lateralis, with intact innervation, may then be preserved. Rarely, the entire quadriceps muscle needs to be resected in order to perform an adequate resection with clean surgical margins. In this case, the extension of the knee joint is lost. The patients require fairly extensive rehabilitation, using a walker initially, then crutches, then a cane, but finally they seem to be able to walk without even a cane, apparently due to passive extension of the knee joint as the hip flexes. Although they walk slowly, they do so fairly well, but occasionally they trip and fall and they walk upstairs step by step. Therefore, it is preferable to preserve part of the quadriceps whenever the location of the tumor permits. Usually the muscle that can be preserved is the distal half of the vastus medialis with intact nervation. This can be done without compromising the adequacy of the resection of the anterior compartment.

## SARCOMAS OF THE MEDIAL COMPARTMENT

These tumors, when large and centrally located, require resection of the entire medial compartment (Fig. 20A-31). The medial compartment consists of pectineus, adductor longus, and gracilis muscles superficially, adductor brevis in the middle, and adductor magnus posteriorly. A longitudinal incision is made over the bulge of the tumor in the medial compartment and then a flap is developed anteriorly to the approximate course of the common and superficial

femoral vessels. By retracting the sartorius, these vessels are exposed. The branches of the profunda femoris vessels (medial femoral circumflex) supplying the adductor group of muscles are ligated and divided at their origin. The continuation of the profunda vessels can usually be preserved. The muscles are divided near the insertion to the linea aspera of the femur all the way to the adductor hiatus, which frees the femoral vessels as they pass through the foramen to become popliteal vessels. The inferior and terminal part of the adductor magnus at the adductor tubercle is divided. Following division of all the adductor muscles at their insertion to the linea aspera, the sciatic nerve is now exposed, dissected out, and preserved on the posterior aspect of adductor magnus. Proximally the adductor muscles are divided off the pubic bone near the origin from this bone. A complete medial compartment resection exposes the common femoral vessels in their continuity with the superficial femoral vessels. It exposes also the profunda vessels, the sciatic nerve posteriorly, and the obturator externus superiorly as the last drapes the obturator foramen en route to its insertion to the femur (Fig. 20A-32). Medial compartment resection can be performed without any appreciable disability as the patient in a standing position adducts the leg with the aid of gravity. Therefore, walking and going up and down stairs is not affected. In a supine position, older patients have difficulty adducting their leg.

## SARCOMAS OF THE BUTTOCK

Sarcomas of the buttock can be resected with the patient in a lateral or prone position. Some authors who described this procedure, which has been called buttockectomy (a more appropriate term is glutectomy), have used an oblique incision along the direction of the fibers of the gluteus maximus. It is preferable, however, to use a longitudinal incision that extends from the iliac crest all the way to the upper femur well below the area of the ischial tuberosity and greater trochanter. This type of incision is much longer than the oblique incision, and it allows for flap development to the edge of the sacrum, permitting the division of the gluteus maximus at its origin from the sacrum and the posterior portion of the iliac bone as well as at its insertion into the femur and the fascia lata. This incision also allows early identification of the sciatic nerve well below the lowermost fibers of the gluteus maximus as the nerve courses lateral to the biceps femoris between the ischial tuberosity and the greater trochanter. By identifying the sciatic nerve in this location, it becomes much safer to proceed with resection of the entire gluteus maximus from its origin to insertion. If the tumor is located somewhat posteriorly, the sacrotuberous ligament is divided near the sacrum and at the ischial tuberosity (removing also a piece of the bone if needed) and removed with the specimen. The posterior femoral cutaneous nerve sensory to the posterior aspect of the skin of the thigh usually has to be sacrificed. As the dissection proceeds superiorly, the inferior gluteal vessels and nerve are ligated and divided at their origin, and a decision is made whether the gluteus medius and minimus should be resected en bloc with the maximus. A resection of the gluteus maximus alone does not substantially impair ambulation. However, resection of all the glutei muscles causes some limping on walking.

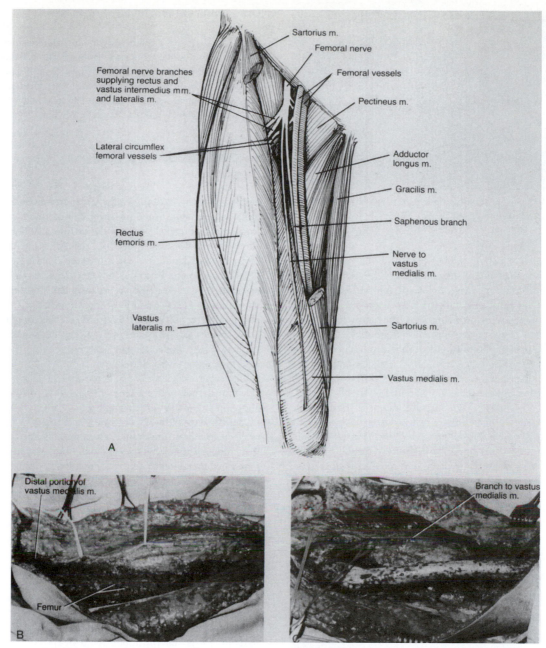

**FIGURE 20A-30.** *A.* Drawing illustrating the nerve supply of the vastus medialis through a long slender branch of femoral nerve. *B* and *C* show operative fields following anterior compartment resection with preservation of the branch to the distal portion of the vastus medialis. *From Karakousis CP: Surgery for soft tissue sarcomas, in* Atlas of Surgical Oncology, *K. Bland et al (eds). Philadelphia, WB Saunders, 1995, pp 283–400.*

## SARCOMAS OF THE POSTERIOR COMPARTMENT OF THE THIGH

For sarcomas of the posterior compartment of the thigh, a longitudinal incision is made starting at the lower border of the gluteus maximus and is continued down to the popliteal fossa with the patient in a prone position. Flaps are then developed around the tumor mass. If the mass is situated somewhat proximally, the fibers of the gluteus maximus are vertically divided at its lower border in order to expose the sciatic nerve superiorly between the ischial tuberosity

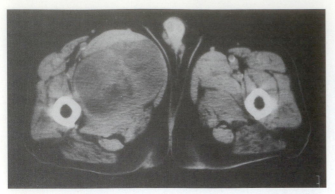

**FIGURE 20A-31.** CT scan showing a soft tissue sarcoma of the medial compartment of the right thigh.

and the greater trochanter. The nerve at this level is lateral to the biceps femoris, but as the latter deviates toward its insertion, the nerve assumes a position between the biceps femoris on the lateral side and semimembranosus on the medial side. The hamstring muscles (biceps, semitendinosus, semimembranosus) are divided off their origin from the ischial tuberosity and also divided inferiorly in the popliteal fossa after the sciatic nerve and its branches into the tibial and common peroneal nerves have been identified and dissected (Fig. 20A-33). The sciatic as the tumor specimen is mobilized is approached from the surface that is free of tumor, the sheath of the nerve is incised, and the nerve trunk extricated from its sheath while the sheath of the nerve is left on the tumor mass (Fig. 20A-34). In some of these tumors, the posterior part of the medial compartment, i.e., adductor magnus, may have to be removed if close to the tumor mass. Inferiorly, the popliteal vessels are recognized as they cross through the adductor hiatus and become common popliteal vessels.

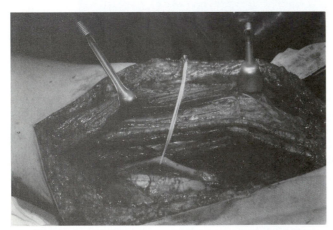

**FIGURE 20A-32.** Operative field following medial compartment resection showing the exposed common and superficial femoral vessels and the sciatic nerve posteriorly retracted with a vessel loop. In this case, it was possible to preserve the profunda femoris vessels.

## SARCOMAS OF THE POPLITEAL FOSSA

In sarcomas of the popliteal fossa, an S-shaped incision may be utilized as in popliteal node dissection.[20] The tibial and common peroneal nerves are dissected, as well as the popliteal vessels. The priority is in dissecting out the nerves that are more superficial, and then the popliteal vessels, which can be resected with the tumor mass, if necessary, and replaced with grafts.

## SARCOMAS BELOW THE KNEE

In sarcomas below the knee, usually wide resection of the sarcoma is performed because compartment resection is associated with functional impairment. In the posterior compartment, the whole gastrocnemius muscle or part of it can be resected. The soleus muscle contributes to the same insertion at the Achilles tendon and, therefore, preserves that flexion capacity of the ankle joint. The posterior tibial vessels and nerve course between the soleus and the deep layer of muscles, i.e., flexor hallucis longus, tibialis posterior, and flexor digitorum longus. The course of the common peroneal nerve is important in resection of the lateral and anterior compartments. This nerve courses along the edge of the biceps femoris and then around the neck of the fibula (deep to peroneus longus origin), enters the anterior compartment, and divides at this point into the superficial and deep peroneal nerves. The anterior tibial vessels enter the anterior compartment between the tibia and fibula through an opening above the interosseous membrane.

Sarcomas near the ankle region and foot can have only local excision in a limb-preserving resection. It is important, however, that complete gross resection of the tumor is performed in order to have a better chance for adjuvant radiation to destroy any potential microscopic residual. In the plantar aspect of the foot, one may resect the skin overlying the tumor as needed, the plantar aponeurosis and the first layer of muscles, placing the skin graft over the second layer of muscles, which preserves the flexion capacity of the toes.

## UPPER EXTREMITY

### SARCOMAS OF THE LOWER NECK.

Sarcomas of the lower neck require dissection around the tumor mass in the manner of wide excision, which may involve resection of the sternocleidomastoid (anteriorly) and the trapezius muscle (posteriorly), the internal jugular vein, the adipose tissue, and nodes down to the surface of the brachial plexus. For sarcomas in the lower part of the neck, it may become necessary to resect the clavicle by dividing this bone medially and laterally and leaving the central portion of the bone on the tumor mass.[21] This improves exposure by also dividing the origin of the pectoralis major at the inferior border of the clavicle and reveals the axillary vessels and brachial plexus at the apex of the axilla. Removal of the clavicle requires the use of a splint postoperatively for a few weeks, although physiotherapy of the upper extremity is carried out during this period as tolerated. Removal of the clavicle does not have any significant long-term functional effects. Removal of the pectoral muscles may be required for sarcomas just below the clavicle in the upper part of the chest near the axillary region.

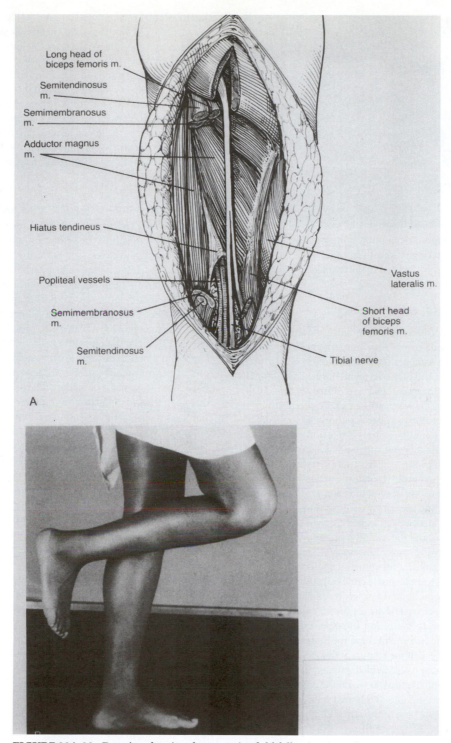

**FIGURE 20A-33.** Drawing showing the operative field following posterior compartment resection. The print shows flexion of the knee in a patient who had the right sciatic nerve resected due to involvement. *From Karakousis CP: Surgery for soft tissue sarcomas, in* Atlas of Surgical Oncology, *K. Bland et al (eds). Philadelphia, WB Saunders, 1995, pp 283–400.*

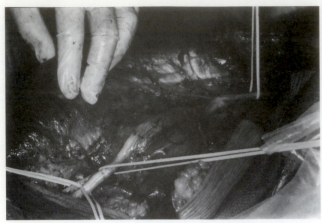

**FIGURE 20A-34.** Intraoperative photograph showing dissection of the sciatic nerve by entering its sheath from the side opposite to the location of the tumor. In the vast majority of cases, the sciatic nerve is preserved.

SARCOMAS INVOLVING THE SCAPULA. For these tumors, partial or complete scapulectomy may be performed depending upon the location of the sarcoma. In order to resect the scapula, an incision from the lower end of the vertebral border of the scapula is carried out to the shoulder joint. Flaps are raised, both medially and laterally. Medially, the trapezius muscle and underneath it the rhomboid muscles and levator scapulae superiorly are divided, inferiorly the relevant portion of latissimus dorsi, and laterally teres major and minor, infraspinatus and supraspinatus muscles are divided near their insertion to the humerus. The serratus anterior is also divided close to the chest wall. The capsule of the shoulder joint is entered and divided. The long head of the triceps is divided off its origin below the glenoid and anteriorly the insertion of subscapularis to the humerus is divided, as well as the origins of biceps brachii and coracobrachialis from, and the insertion of pectoralis minor to, the coracoid process. In most cases, however, one may perform a subtotal or what may be called a functional scapulectomy, removing in essence 95% of the scapula and leaving only the glenoid with an inch or so of the adjacent bone. In other words, one divides the muscles attached to the vertebral border of the scapula and axillary border and then the supraspinatus and infraspinatus just underneath the beginning of the free end of the spine that is divided with a Gigli saw exposing the neck of the scapula at that point. By using a Gigli saw, the neck of the scapula is divided, leaving the glenoid with about 2 cm of adjacent bone attached, as well as the coracoid process. This certainly secures great stability in this area and results in much improved function and better use of the arm with physiotherapy.

SARCOMAS OF THE ARM. Sarcomas of the anterior compartment of the arm require wide excision of the involved muscle or muscles and adjacent normal tissue, keeping in mind the course of the musculocutaneous nerve, which pierces the coracobrachialis and proceeds to enter the space proximally between the biceps and brachialis, supplying both muscles as it courses in an inferolateral direction, emerging on the lateral border of the biceps to become the lateral antebrachial cutaneous nerve (Fig. 20A-35). If the surgeon can preserve one of the two flexors, the flexion ability in the elbow is preserved. If both biceps and brachialis have to be resected, there is a weak flexion ability of the elbow with the forearm in a neutral position between supination and pronation through the action of the brachioradialis, which is supplied by the radial nerve.

In the posterior compartment of the arm, the course of the radial nerve is important as it proceeds in the spiral groove of the humerus emerging between the lateral head of the triceps and brachioradialis laterally and brachialis medially. Usually, wide resection of a portion of the triceps is performed around the sarcoma, preserving the radial nerve.

SARCOMAS OF THE FOREARM AND HAND. In the forearm, it is important to remember that the median nerve passes between the two heads of pronator teres and then proceeds between the superficial and deep layer of flexors. At this point, just below the pronator teres, it gives off the anterior interosseous nerve, which supplies the deep flexors. Resection of the median nerve below this point, if necessary, preserves the flexor capacity of the hand through the deep flexors. The brachial artery above the level of the pronator teres bifurcates into the radial, which proceeds more superficially on the medial side of the brachioradialis and the ulnar artery, which is larger and proceeds under pronator teres in front of the deep flexors of the forearm lateral to the flexor carpi ulnaris and the ulnar nerve. If one of the two major branches of the brachial artery, i.e., the ulnar or radial artery, is too close to the tumor, it can be resected since there is usually a good anastomotic communication at the palmar arch between the two vessels, one of them being adequate to provide circulation to the hand. On the dorsal part of the forearm, the course of the radial nerve in its continuation into the posterior interosseous nerve is important to bear in mind. Again, wide resection is performed in the sense of working around the tumor mass and securing a margin of adjacent normal tissue to the extent the local functional anatomy of the extremity permits. If a muscle has to be resected, adequate margins along this muscle may be provided by removing a sufficient length of the muscle.

In the area of the wrist and hand, local excision is only possible by removing the gross tumor with millimeters of normal tissue around it and relying largely on radiation for control of microscopic disease. This seems to work in most cases. In the distal part of the extremities, local excision followed by adjuvant radiation seems to be more effective than local excision in the upper part of the extremities, perhaps because the planning as well as the delivery of the radiation dose can be more precise and effective in the distal portions of the extremity where the distance between the surgical bed and skin surface the radiation beam has to traverse is a short one without the intervention of bulky tissues in between.

## MAJOR AMPUTATIONS

### HEMIPELVECTOMY

Hemipelvectomy is resection of the hemipelvis and the ipsilateral lower extremity in cases of tumors that cannot be resected with more

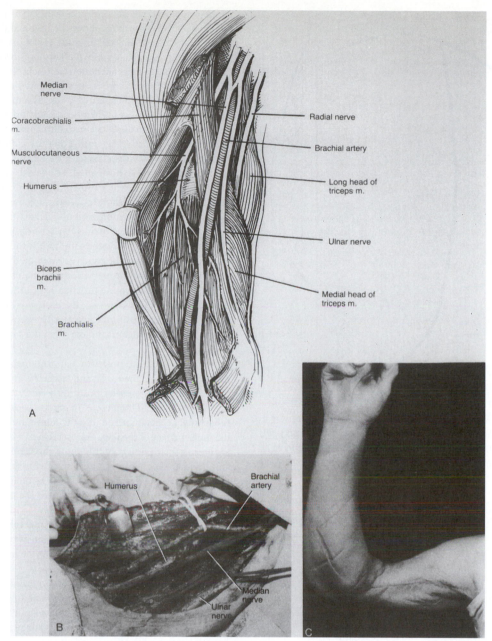

**FIGURE 20A-35.** *A*. Drawing showing anatomy of the anterior compartment of the arm. *B*. Operative field following resection of the anterior compartment sarcoma. *C*. Flexion of the arm through brachioradialis in a patient who had resection of both biceps and brachialis due to recurrent sarcoma after radiation. *From Karakousis CP: Surgery for soft tissue sarcomas, in Atlas of Surgical Oncology, K. Bland et al (eds). Philadelphia, WB Saunders, 1995, pp 283–400.*

conservative procedures. There are two major types of hemipelvectomy, posterior flap hemipelvectomy, which is more common, and anterior flap hemipelvectomy.[22] In posterior flap hemipelvectomy, an incision is made from the posterior inferior iliac spine along the iliac crest to the anterior superior iliac spine and then along the inguinal ligament and pubic crest to the pubic symphysis. The inci-

sion is extended from its posterior end inferiorly toward the greater trochanter and for about 10 cm below the greater trochanter and then transversely across the posterior aspect of the thigh to the medial aspect of the thigh and then vertically up to the pubic tubercle joining the anterior part of incision (Figs. 20A-36, 20A-37). Through the part of the incision along the iliac crest, the external oblique

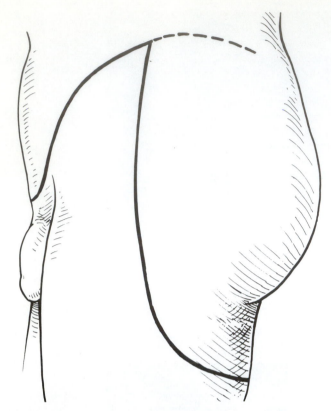

**FIGURE 20A-36.** The anterolateral portion of the incision for a posterior flap hemipelvectomy. *From Karakousis CP: Surgery for soft tissue sarcomas, in* Atlas of Surgical Oncology, *K. Bland et al (eds). Philadelphia, WB Saunders, 1995, pp 283–400.*

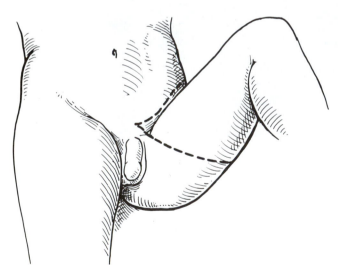

**FIGURE 20A-37.** Medial part of the incision for posterior flap hemipelvectomy. *From Karakousis CP: Surgery for soft tissue sarcomas, in* Atlas of Surgical Oncology, *K. Bland et al (eds). Philadelphia, WB Saunders, 1995, pp 283–400.*

aponeurosis, internal oblique, and transversus abdominis muscles are divided. This continues above the inguinal ligament to the anterior rectus sheath and rectus muscles, which are divided off the pubic crest to the pubic symphysis. This incision opens the inguinal canal, and after the external oblique aponeurosis is divided down to the external inguinal ring, the posterior wall of the inguinal canal is divided. In males the spermatic vessels and vas deferens can be preserved if not involved. The operation is usually extraperitoneal, with the peritoneum dissected medially exposing the ureter, which is also retracted medially. Depending on the location of the tumor, the level of ligation of the vessels is selected, i.e., the common iliac or the external iliac vessels, to be divided. The vessels are divided at the appropriate level above the location of the tumor, and then the iliacus muscle is divided at the same level, exposing medially the greater sciatic notch. The pubic symphysis is divided in the midline with a Gigli saw. The iliac bone is then divided posteriorly, preserving part of the iliac crest with a Gigli saw if the tumor location permits, a procedure known as conservative hemipelvectomy, or through the sacroiliac joint, or if necessary through the sacral ala using an osteotome. If a high division of the bone proximally is anticipated, i.e., through the sacroiliac joint or sacral ala, the patient is better placed in a lateral or semilateral position for posterior exposure. If the iliac bone can be divided through its middle, then the supine position may be satisfactory.

When making the posterior flap, the incision is carried down through the subcutaneous fat and fascia lata and the flap is dissected off the hamstring muscles posteriorly and the adductor group of muscles medially. The gluteus maximus is divided off the gluteal tuberosity, i.e., its insertion into the femur, but it is left attached on the inner surface of the flap. The sciatic nerve is traced all the way to the greater sciatic notch. At this point, the sciatic nerve can be ligated and divided. The femoral nerve is, of course, ligated and divided anteriorly along with the iliac vessels. As the specimen is retracted laterally, the levator ani is divided across the pelvic wall along with sacrotuberous and sacrospinous ligaments, and this permits removal of the specimen. The posterior flap then is folded anteriorly and is sutured to the anterior edge. The fascia lata is sutured to the external oblique aponeurosis. Part of the flap may be trimmed, as necessary. Suction drains are required.

In past descriptions of this operation, the flap necrosis rate of the posterior flap ranged between 60% and 80%. However, in our experience, it has become clear that the viability of the posterior flap is guaranteed if the gluteus maximus is left attached to the flap. The level of ligation of the iliac vessels is not important, since even with ligation of the common iliac vessels, if the gluteus maximus is left attached to the flap, the viability of the flap is secure because the gluteus maximus apparently has sufficient blood supply through its origin from the sacrum other than the main supply through the inferior gluteal vessels. In contrast, with removal of the gluteus maximus, the rate of flap necrosis is significant regardless of the level of ligation of the iliac vessels.[22]

Posterior flap hemipelvectomy is applicable for all sarcomas requiring this high amputation in which the skin of the buttock and gluteus maximus are not involved. Sarcomas of the buttock requiring amputation, however, require what may be called an anterior flap hemipelvectomy. In this operation, the anterior flap is fashioned by extending the incision along the iliac crest from the anterior superior iliac spine vertically on the anterior thigh to just above the patella, then transversely to the medial side of the thigh and then vertically up to the pubic tubercle. The common iliac and external iliac vessels are dissected and mobilized. The inguinal ligament is divided at the anterior superior iliac spine and pubic tubercle. At the distal part of the flap above the knee, the dissection is carried through the subcutaneous fat, fascia lata, and quadriceps femoris, down to the bone. Anteromedially, the sartorius muscle is divided, and under the fascia extending between vastus medialis and adductors, the superficial femoral vessels are identified, ligated, and divided. The quadriceps is dissected off the femur with a periosteal elevator. It is not necessary to dissect vastus medialis or lateralis all the way to the linea aspera. One can cut through the middle of these muscles to the surface of the femur. The superficial femoral vessels are mobilized with the flap. As the dissection proceeds on the surface of the adductor group of muscles, the medial femoral circumflex vessels are ligated and divided as they go into the adductor group of muscles. The rectus femoris is divided off the anterior inferior iliac spine, and this frees up the entire anterior flap (Fig. 20A-38). The anterior flap is composed of a large area of skin from the anterior thigh, subcutaneous fat, and the quadriceps femoris (minus the posterior portions of vastus medialis and lateralis). Its blood supply is based primarily on the lateral circumflex vessels of the profunda, and therefore it is important to preserve the iliac vessels, their continuity to the common femoral vessels, and the lateral circumflex branches of the profunda femoris vessels.

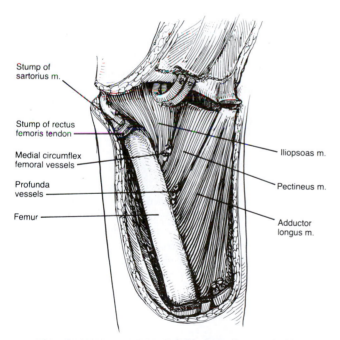

**FIGURE 20A-38.** An anterior flap has been dissected off the anterior surface of the femur (for an anterior flap hemipelvectomy). *From Karakousis CP: Surgery for soft tissue sarcomas, in* Atlas of Surgical Oncology, *K. Bland et al (eds). Philadelphia, WB Saunders, 1995, pp 283–400.*

## HIP DISARTICULATION

In this procedure, an incision is carried out from the anterior superior iliac spine along the inguinal ligament to the pubic tubercle and then around the back of the thigh, creating a posterior flap of sufficient length to be brought over to cover the defect following removal of the extremity. Anteriorly, the dissection is carried out through the subcutaneous fat below the inguinal ligament, and the common femoral vessels are ligated and divided. The femoral nerve is also divided and the adductor group of muscles is divided off their origin from the pubic bone. The sartorius muscles, tensor fascia lata, and rectus femoris are divided near their origin. The insertion of the gluteal muscles (also of piriformis, gemelli, obturators, and quadratus femoris) to the femur is divided. Posteriorly, the flap is composed of skin, subcutaneous fat, fascia lata, and proximally the gluteus maximus. Again, the posterior flap is made sufficiently long so that following removal of the extremity, one may be able to cover the defect. The capsule of the hip joint is entered and the head of the femur disarticulated by dividing the ligamentum teres. This permits removal of the extremity and the rotation of the posterior flap anteriorly to be sutured to the fascia and skin of the anterior portion of the incision.

## FOREQUARTER AMPUTATION

This is a procedure performed with the patient in a lateral or semilateral position for extensive sarcomas near the shoulder joint involving the brachial plexus and vessels. The incision is carried out from the medial end of the clavicle over the lower neck and then over the middle of the scapula to its inferior angle and around the axilla, anteriorly over the pectoral muscles to meet the beginning of the previous incision at the medial end of the clavicle. The pectoralis major and minor are divided. The clavicle is divided by placing a right-angled clamp and then a Gigli saw around the medial end of the clavicle. A piece of the clavicle is removed for exposure. The subclavius muscle and fascia are divided. The subclavian vessels are ligated and divided, as well as the brachial plexus. Posteriorly, the flap is developed to the vertebral border of the scapula, dividing the trapezius, rhomboids, levator scapulae, and around the tip of the scapula the latissimus dorsi, and finally more anteriorly, the insertion of the serratus anterior to the ribs. This permits removal of the upper extremity, and the flaps are then approximated. In case of involvement of the axillary wall, in which case the incision has to be carried well below the area of involvement, there can be a skin defect resulting from this type of incision and, therefore, particularly for a concomitant chest wall resection, it is necessary to provide a flap for coverage.[23] That flap can be created by extending the incision from the medial end of the clavicle along and just below this bone to the anterior border of the deltoid muscle in the shoulder and then along this border to the muscle's insertion and around it along the posterior border of the deltoid to the mid scapula. The skin, subcutaneous fat, and fascia are dissected off the deltoid. This creates a large flap, which is dissected to the lower neck and vertebral border of the scapula. The two ends of the base of this widely based flap (at the medial end of the clavicle and over the scapula) are joined with a curving incision around the axilla, well below the area of any involvement

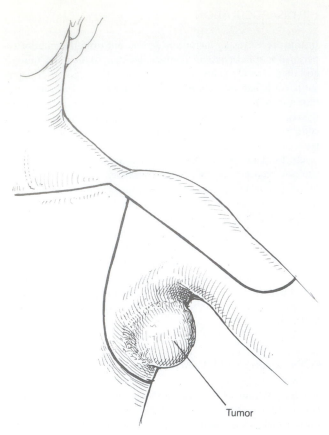

Tumor

**FIGURE 20A-39.** The anterior part of the incision for forequarter amputation in conjunction with a deltoid fasciocutaneous flap. *From Karakousis CP: Surgery for soft tissue sarcomas, in* Atlas of Surgical Oncology, *K. Bland et al (eds). Philadelphia, WB Saunders, 1995, pp 283–400.*

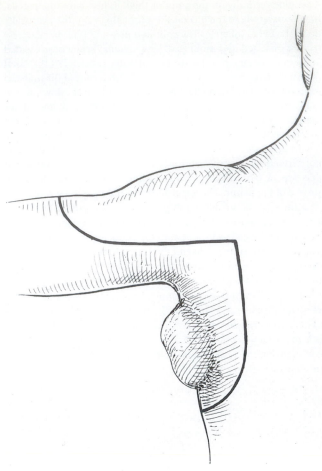

**FIGURE 20A-40.** The posterior part of the incision for forequarter amputation in conjunction with a fasciocutaneous deltoid flap. *From Karakousis CP: Surgery for soft tissue sarcomas, in* Atlas of Surgical Oncology, *K. Bland et al (eds). Philadelphia, WB Saunders, 1995, pp 283–400.*

(Figs. 20A-39, 20A-40). The rest of the operation is described as above, the only difference being the availability of a large flap to cover a skin defect. The procedure of forequarter amputation described above involved early ligation and division of the subclavian vessels and brachial plexus, after the division of the medial end of the clavicle and removal of a 2- to 3-cm portion of this bone. However, dissection around the subclavian vessels can be difficult, particularly in the presence of fibrosis or previous radiation. Even in the absence of these conditions, the limitations of space render the dissection difficult, and as one dissects the subclavian vein with a right-angle clamp, if bleeding is encountered from the posterior surface of the vein, it may be difficult to control. Therefore, in the experience of this author, it is safer and easier to perform the dissection first around the scapula by dividing the muscles around it; dividing the pectoralis major and minor and serratus anterior off its rib attachments; removing a medial segment of the clavicle, and through a posterior approach, ligating and dividing the trunks of the brachial plexus; and as a last stage of the procedure, proceed to control and divide the subclavian vessels. In such a case, even if there is any bleeding around the vessels as the dissection proceeds, a vascular clamp can

be placed around both vessels en bloc with any remaining trunks of the brachial plexus, and the specimen may be removed safely. The deltoid flap is a useful technique in preserving skin that may be used to cover a defect in the axillary area should the need arise because of tumor involvement in the skin of the axilla. This is more important when there is also concomitant resection of ribs, in which case flap coverage is necessary to provide a seal for the thoracic cavity.

## INTEGRATION OF MODALITIES IN SOFT TISSUE SARCOMAS

The high rates of limb preservation and local control in extremity soft tissue sarcomas can be attributed to two factors: (1) The development and refinement of surgical techniques that have made possible complete resection of the tumor and surrounding microscopic extensions with preservation of a well-functioning extremity; (2) the use of adjuvant radiation.

Development of the surgical treatment in various locations in this modern era has been outlined in the section on surgical treatment. There is now abundant evidence that adjuvant radiation helps improve local control, apparently by destroying potential microscopic residue around the tumor site. There are many retrospective studies showing a local recurrence rate in the range of 10% to 20% with resection and adjuvant postoperative radiation,[24–26] which compares favorably with local recurrence rates of 28% to 36%[27,28] after wide excision and 65% to 90%[28,29] after local excision reported in the past when surgical treatment was relied upon exclusively. A randomized study by the National Cancer Institute (NCI) comparing limb-sparing surgery followed by radiation to amputation found a low rate of local recurrence in the limb-sparing group and no difference in survival between the two groups.[30] A prospective randomized study using brachytherapy[31] was performed at Memorial Sloan-Kettering Cancer Center in patients with soft tissue sarcomas, and it was shown that the brachytherapy arm had a local control rate of 90% versus 69% for the surgery-alone group ($p = 0.01$), but in this study there was no improvement in local control of low-grade tumors having a local recurrence rate from 20% to 30%.[6,32,33]

Radiation treatment has been used as a preoperative modality, either alone or in combination with intraarterial infusion of doxorubicin (Adriamycin), which is applicable for extremity locations having a single identifiable artery supplying the area of the tumor.[34] The local control rate in patients with soft tissue sarcoma treated with resection followed by radiation is 80% to 90%. This is true mostly for extremity, neck, and trunk wall locations. For retroperitoneal sarcomas, radiation, although certainly it can be helpful, is not as well established due to limitations in delivering an adequate total dose of radiation because of adjacent viscera that may suffer damage from this treatment if not carefully given. At this point, it is not clear whether preoperative or postoperative radiation has any substantial advantage, although some authors prefer preoperative radiation.[35] The rates of local control appear to be about the same. With preoperative radiation, one has the theoretical advantage of some shrinkage of the tumor and, therefore, potentially an easier resection of a somewhat smaller tumor with limb preservation. The disadvantage of preoperative radiation is that the operation is performed on irradiated tissue with reduced capacities for healing and, therefore, an increased rate of complications. A Canadian prospective randomized study comparing preoperative versus postoperative radiation in the treatment of soft tissue sarcomas terminated prematurely because of a significantly higher rate of wound complications observed in the preoperative radiation group.[36] There is consensus that for low-grade tumors ($\leq 5$ cm) that can be resected with an adequate surgical margin, there is no need for adjuvant radiation.[6] For larger ($> 5$ cm) tumors and all high-grade lesions, the prevailing tendency is to administer adjuvant radiation, either preoperatively or postoperatively.[6] Some groups prefer brachytherapy. The author has used postoperative radiation selectively (in about 20% of patients) whenever it is needed for narrow surgical margins for sarcomas of all grades.[37] The local recurrence rate of sarcomas of all grades that had an adequate resection without radiation was 10%, whereas that of sarcomas with local excision and radiation was 25%.[37] Marginal

resection plus brachytherapy radiation is associated with a local recurrence rate of 30%.[38] Therefore, wide resection alone provides better local control than local excision and radiation. The latter method should be applied to anatomic areas not amenable to wide resection.

Radiation, however, is an effective modality, since the local recurrence rate with local excision alone in the past for these tumors was 65%.[28] A narrow surgical margin is 2 cm or less within the same compartment. Lesser lateral margins may be acceptable in areas covered with a strong aponeurotic layer. What is an adequate surgical margin, however, is of course not known through prospective randomized series, but a minimum of a 2-cm margin and microscopically negative surgical margins are generally desirable before one relies on surgical treatment alone. The surgical treatment is the most important clinical modality in the management of a primary soft tissue sarcoma. It is incumbent upon the surgeon to perform an adequate resection by removing all gross tumor and eliminating microscopic disease around it, or at least minimizing potential microscopic residual disease. A plan to use adjuvant radiation is no excuse for local excision of the tumor with inadequate margins, with the exception of the distal extremities where local excision is done in the interests of limb preservation. In most anatomic areas, adequate margins can be obtained, certainly in most directions around the tumor mass accepting a lesser margin only in the vicinity of critical structures such as major vessels, nerves, or bone. This strategy eliminates local microscopic disease with the gross tumor and certainly tends to minimize potential residual microscopic disease.

In a study of preoperative radiation plus surgery, patients with negative margins had a local control rate of 97%, whereas those with positive margins had a local control rate of 82%.[39]

## MANAGEMENT OF RETROPERITONEAL SARCOMAS

The importance of the surgical treatment is best shown in the management of these tumors. In a collective review, the complete resectability rate was 53%, ranging from 38% to 74% in various centers. In this review, the 5-year survival rate of patients with retroperitoneal sarcomas was 34%, largely because nearly one-half of the patients did not have their tumor resected. The 5-year survival rate, however, for those who had complete resection was 54%, being 74% for grade I tumors, and 24% for grade II and III tumors. The local recurrence rate was 72% at 5 years, and 91% at 10 years of follow-up, pointing to the fact that in the majority of patients with complete resection, it was not possible to obtain a wide margin around the tumor and thus eliminate adjacent microscopic extensions.[40] In the author's series comprising localized retroperitoneal sarcomas, i.e., both primary as well as sarcomas referred with local recurrence, the overall complete resectability rate was 96%, the 5-year survival rate was 63%, and the 10-year survival rate 46%. The 5-year survival rate was 88% for grade I, 52% for grade II, and 45% for grade III tumors ($p = 0.007$). The local recurrence rate was 16% for wide resection and 56% for local excision ($p = 0.001$). The 5- and 10-year survival rates were 72% and 61%, respectively, for the group with wide resection, and 55% and 23%, respectively, for the group with local excision ($p = 0.01$)[41]; there was no imbalance between the two groups regarding the frequency of the various grades. These data demonstrated that complete resection of retroperitoneal sarcoma is a sine qua non for the successful management of the patient and was possible in the vast majority of the patients. With this high resectability rate, the 5-year survival rate of retroperitoneal sarcomas is similar to that of extremity sarcomas. Wide resection in retroperitoneal locations is not only associated with a significantly lower rate of local recurrence but also a significantly higher rate of survival. The local recurrence rate for patients with adjuvant postoperative radiation was 22% and for those without 33%.[41] In retroperitoneal sarcomas local recurrence, in contrast to the situation with extremity sarcomas, has a more ominous prognosis because of the opportunities for local recurrence to further disseminate in the free peritoneal cavity.

## ADJUVANT CHEMOTHERAPY

Nearly half of the patients with soft tissue sarcomas finally succumb to their disease due to distant metastases.[6] The rate of distant metastasis varies according to the grade of the tumor, the size ($\leq 5$ cm or $>5$ cm) and location of the tumor (superficial versus deep to the fascia). The drugs that have been evaluated mostly are various combinations of doxorubicin, dacarbazine, cyclophosphamide, vincristine, actinomycin D, and recently ifosfamide. In a prospective randomized study, there was significant improvement of disease-free survival with adjuvant chemotherapy using the so-called CYVADIC (cyclophosphamide, vincristine, doxorubicin and dacarbazine) combination. The 7-year actuarial survival rate was 56% in the treated group versus 43% for the observation group ($p = 0.007$), but the rate of distant metastases and the overall survival rate between the two groups was not statistically significant.[42] In a study from M.D. Anderson Hospital, there was an advantage in disease-free survival for the treated group, but there was no significant difference in overall survival.[43]

Studies with adjuvant postoperative doxorubicin chemotherapy currently have not shown a survival benefit.[6] In another study from M.D. Anderson Hospital, it was demonstrated that the survival of patients who responded to preoperative therapy was superior to that observed among nonresponding patients.[44] However, it is only a minority of the patients who demonstrate significant response to preoperative chemotherapy; thus, in a prospective trial at Memorial Hospital of 29 patients with primary or recurrent high-grade nonmetastatic soft tissue sarcomas who were treated with two cycles of preoperative chemotherapy, only one patient had a partial response.[45] Furthermore, quantitating the response to chemotherapy in soft tissue sarcomas is difficult.

In conclusion, adjuvant, as well as neoadjuvant chemotherapy in adults with soft tissue sarcomas remains an investigational treatment. The use of the new agent, ifosfamide, which has not been evaluated in past studies, has provided further impetus for combinations of this agent with doxorubicin and possibly other agents in the adjuvant therapy of adult soft tissue sarcomas. In practice, patients with large high-grade sarcomas, because of the poor 5-year survival rate (30% to 45%), often are treated empirically with adjuvant chemotherapy based on a doxorubicin-containing combination.

## RECURRENCE

### LOCAL RECURRENCE

The most common types of recurrence of soft tissue sarcomas are local and hematogenous recurrence. In this author's experience, local recurrence can be resected successfully in the majority (95%) of patients. Of patients with recurrent tumors of an extremity, 90% of them can have limb-preserving resection. The rate of further local recurrence is in the range of about 27% and the 5-year survival for patients with grade I tumors is 100%; grade II, 77%; and Grade III, 45% ($p = 0.0002$). Overall, the 5-year survival rate was 78% for tumors $\leq 5$ cm and 57% for those $>5$ cm ($p = 0.03$).[46] Patients presenting with local recurrence without evidence of distant disease have an excellent chance of long-term survival that equals that of primary soft tissue sarcomas because although patients with local recurrence present greater difficulty for an adequate resection of their recurrence, this is balanced by a lesser biologic aggressiveness because tumors that have a higher biologic aggressiveness in addition to local recurrence will also present with concomitant hematogenous metastases. Therefore, the group of soft tissue sarcoma patients presenting with local recurrence alone is a select group that seems to be biologically less aggressive than the average primary soft tissue sarcoma, and this counterbalances the difficulty of performing an adequate resection in the case of local recurrence.

### DISTANT HEMATOGENOUS METASTASES

Distant hematogenous metastases from soft tissue sarcomas usually appear in the lungs and often concern the lungs only. If the disease in the lungs remains unchecked or progresses, it may cause the demise of the patient from compromise of pulmonary function or it may also spread to other sites. The rather frequent and often exclusive involvement of the lung parenchyma constitutes the biologic basis on which the surgical treatment of lung metastases (pulmonary metastasectomy) has evolved. The 5-year survival rate in many retrospective series ranges from 20% to 30% for patients who undergo metastasectomy.[47] Some of these patients, however, require repeat thoracotomies in order to control recurrences within the lungs. Resection of pulmonary metastases is a standard treatment for patients with soft tissue sarcomas that has spread to the lungs, if there are no other metastatic sites. The 5-year survival rate varies with the completeness of resection, the number of metastatic lesions, and the prior disease-free interval or tumor doubling time. The effect of chemotherapy on survival of these patients is not clear, although the majority of the patients do receive chemotherapy preoperatively or postoperatively. The response rate to combination chemotherapy has varied widely among different series, being most often in the range of about 40%.[6]

In conclusion, early diagnosis and adequate treatment of a primary soft tissue sarcoma is of the utmost importance in the survival of these patients. Wide resection with limb preservation is the surgical treatment of choice and is feasible in most anatomic locations. Adjuvant radiation is an effective adjuvant modality in destroying microscopic residual at the primary site and should be considered, particularly in the presence of narrow surgical margins. Survival depends on the grade, size, and location of the tumor (superficial vs. deep). Patients with local recurrence alone can be salvaged at high rates by thorough resection combined with radiation as necessary, depending upon the surgical margin. Lymph node metastases are infrequent in soft tissue sarcomas, but they should be surgically treated, provided that the rest of the disease can also be resected. If technically feasible, pulmonary metastases, should be resected in order to obtain the best palliation and long-term survival.

# REFERENCES

1. MORTON DL et al: Soft-tissue sarcomas, in *Cancer Medicine*, vol 2, JF Holland et al (eds). Baltimore, Williams & Wilkins, 1997, pp 2559–2589.

2. GREENLEE RT et al: Cancer Statistics 2000. CA Cancer J Clin 50:7, 2000.

3. LI FP, FRAUMENI JF JR: Soft tissue sarcomas, breast cancer and other neoplasms. A familial syndrome? Ann Intern Med 71:747, 1969.

4. STEWART FW, TREVES N: Lymphangiosarcoma in postmastectomy lymphedema. Cancer 1:64, 1948.

5. SORENSEN SA et al: Long-term follow-up of von Recklinghausen neurofibromatosis. N Engl J Med 314:1010, 1986.

6. BRENNAN MF et al: Soft tissue sarcoma, in *Cancer: Principles and Practice of Oncology*, 5th ed, VT DeVita Jr et al (eds). Philadelphia, Lippincott-Raven, 1997, pp 1738–1781.

7. KARAKOUSIS CP, DRISCOLL DL: Treatment and local control of primary extremity soft tissue sarcomas. J Surg Oncol 71:155, 1999.

8. BRENNAN MF: The surgeon as a leader in cancer care: Lessons learned from the study of soft tissue sarcoma. J Am Coll Surg 182:520, 1996.

9. LAWRENCE W JR et al: Adult soft tissue sarcomas. A pattern of care survey of the American College of Surgeons. Ann Surg 205:349, 1987.

10. *AJJC Cancer Staging Manual*, 5th ed, ID Fleming et al (eds). Philadelphia, Lippincott-Raven 1998, pp 139–146.

11. O'BRIAN J, STOUT AP: Malignant fibrous xanthemas. Cancer 17:1445, 1964.

12. KARAKOUSIS CP et al: Major vessel resection during limb-preserving surgery for soft tissue sarcomas. World J Surg 20:345, 1996.

13. KARAKOUSIS CP et al: Use of a mesh for musculoaponeurotic defects of the abdominal wall in cancer surgery and the risk of bowel fistulas. J Am Coll Surg 181:11, 1995.

14. KARAKOUSIS CP et al: Technic of resection of mesenteric tumors. Am J Surg 137:693, 1979.

15. KARAKOUSIS CP: Abdominoinguinal incision in resection of pelvic tumors with lateral fixation. Am J Surg 164:366, 1992.

16. KARAKOUSIS CP: Sacral resection with preservation of continence. Surg Gynecol Obstet 163:270, 1986.

17. KARAKOUSIS CP: Internal hemipelvectomy. Surg Gynecol Obstet 158:279, 1984.

18. KARAKOUSIS CP: Ilioinguinal lymph node dissection. Am J Surg 141:299, 1981.

19. KARAKOUSIS CP et al: Anterior compartment resection of the thigh in soft tissue sarcomas. Eur J Surg Oncol 24:308, 1998.

20. KARAKOUSIS CP: The technique of popliteal lymph node dissection. Surg Gynecol Obstet 151:420, 1980.

21. KARAKOUSIS CP et al: Claviculectomy for the exposure and en bloc resection of adjacent tumors. Am J Surg 164:63, 1992.

22. KARAKOUSIS CP et al: Variants of hemipelvectomy and their complications. Am J Surg 158:404, 1989.

23. VOLPE CM et al: Forequarter amputation with fasciocutaneous deltoid flap reconstruction for malignant tumors of the upper extremity. Ann Surg Oncol 4:298, 1997.

24. SIM FH et al: Soft tissue sarcoma: Mayo Clinic experience. Semin Surg Oncol 4:38, 1988.

25. LINDBERG RD et al: Conservative surgery and postoperative radiotherapy in 300 adults with soft-tissue sarcomas. Cancer 47:2391, 1981.

26. POTTER DA et al: High-grade soft tissue sarcomas of the extremities. Cancer 58:190, 1986.

27. SHIU MH et al: Surgical treatment of 297 soft tissue sarcomas of the lower extremity. Ann Surg 182:597, 1975.

28. ABBAS JS et al: The surgical treatment and outcome of soft-tissue sarcoma. L Arch Surg 116:765, 1981.

29. CADMAN NL et al: Synovial sarcoma. An analysis of 134 tumors. Cancer 18:613, 1965.

30. ROSENBERG SA et al: The treatment of soft-tissue sarcomas of the extremities: Prospective randomized evaluation of (1) limb-sparing surgery plus radiation therapy compared with amputation and (2) the role of adjuvant chemotherapy. Ann Surg 196:305, 1982.

31. BRENNAN MF et al: The role of multimodality therapy in soft-tissue sarcoma. Ann Surg 214:328, 1991.

32. PISTERS PWT et al: A prospective randomized trial of adjuvant brachytherapy in the management of low grade soft tissue sarcomas of the extremity and superficial trunk. J Clin Oncol 12:1150, 1994.

33. PISTERS PWT et al: Long term results of a prospective randomized trial evaluating the role of adjuvant brachytherapy in soft tissue sarcomas. J Clin Oncol 14:859, 1996.

34. EILBER FR et al: Neoadjuvant chemotherapy with radiotherapy in the multidisciplinary management of soft tissue sarcomas of the extremity. Surg Oncol Clin North Am 2:611, 1993.

35. SUIT HD et al: Preoperative, intraoperative, and postoperative radiation in the treatment of primary soft tissue sarcoma. Cancer 55:2659, 1985.

36. O'SULLIVAN B et al: Phase III randomized trial of preoperative versus postoperative radiotherapy in the curative management of extremity soft tissue sarcoma. A Canadian Sarcoma Group and NCI Canadian Clinical Trials Group Study. ASCO Proc 18:2066, 1999.

37. KARAKOUSIS CP et al: Primary soft tissue sarcoma of the extremities in adults. Br J Surg 82:1208, 1995.

38. SHIU MH et al: Brachytherapy and function-saving resection of soft tissue sarcoma arising in the limb. Int J Radiat Oncol Biol Phys 21:1485, 1991.

39. SADOSKI C et al: Preoperative radiation, surgical margins and local control of extremity sarcomas of soft tissue. J Surg Oncol 52:223, 1993.

40. STORM FK, MAHVI DM: Diagnosis and management of retroperitoneal soft-tissue sarcoma. Ann Surg 214:2, 1991.

41. KARAKOUSIS CP et al: Retroperitoneal sarcomas and their management. Arch Surg 130:1104, 1995.

42. BRAMWELL V et al: Adjuvant CYVADIC chemotherapy for adult

soft tissue sarcoma: reduced local recurrence but no improvement in survival: a study of the European Organization for Research and Treatment of Cancer, Soft Tissue and Bone Sarcoma Group. J Clin Oncol 12:1137, 1994.

43. BENJAMIN RS et al: The importance of combination chemotherapy for adjuvant treatment of high-risk patients with soft tissue sarcomas of the extremities, in *Adjuvant Therapy of Cancer*, *V*, SE Salmon (ed). Orlando, Grune & Stratton, 1987, p 735.

44. PEZZI CM et al: Preoperative chemotherapy for soft tissue sarcomas of the extremities. Ann Surg 211:476, 1990.

45. CASPER ES et al: Preoperative and postoperative adjuvant combination chemotherapy for adults with high grade soft tissue sarcoma. Cancer 73:1644, 1994.

46. KARAKOUSIS CP et al: Local recurrence in soft-tissue sarcomas and survival. Ann Surg Oncol 3:255, 1996.

47. VERAZIN GT et al: Resections of lung metastases from soft-tissue sarcomas. A multivariate analysis. Arch Surg 1407, 1992.

# 20B / SARCOMAS OF BONE

*Patrick P. Lin and John H. Healey*

## SARCOMAS OF BONE

### INTRODUCTION

Primary sarcomas of bone are rare. Only 2100 cases occur a year in the United States, which is less than 0.2% of all cases of cancer. Although not nearly as prevalent as lung, breast, prostate, and colon cancer, sarcomas of bone are important because they have provided many lessons for all of oncology. Over the past 30 years, remarkable advances have been made in the diagnosis and treatment of these tumors, and some lesions that were once considered rapidly fatal are now potentially curable. The experience with sarcomas has helped to establish and validate many of the concepts of modern surgical oncology, including principles of wide en bloc surgical excision, adjuvant multiagent chemotherapy, and a multidisciplinary team approach to patient care.

In recent years, there has been a shift away from the surgeon to the medical or pediatric oncologist as the primary coordinator of the patient's care. This has occurred in part as a result of broad changes in health care delivery and managed health care. It is important for the surgeon to remember that he or she is not simply one of many physicians within the system. Surgery remains the primary curative modality for sarcomas, and the overall success of treatment is critically dependent on the success of surgery. Furthermore, the relationship between a surgeon and patient is a very close and special one, and this can enable the surgeon to play an important role as the patient's advocate.

Sarcomas of bone are difficult diseases to treat. The tumors are made up of many different pathologic entities and take on myriad forms. Their occurrence in different parts of the body poses a multitude of surgical challenges, both in terms of resection and reconstruction. These diseases should be treated in major centers and not by the occasional surgical oncologist. Outcome clearly depends on the surgeon's experience. Furthermore, given the rarity of the tumors, collaboration between large centers is crucial for advances to continue to be made. For example, the Children's Cancer Group (CCG) and Pediatric Oncology Group (POG) must pool at least 3 years of cases to answer a therapeutic question striving to improve survival of osteogenic sarcoma or Ewing sarcoma by 15%. Patients treated off protocol at nonparticipating centers compromise the potential to improve the outcome for these diseases.

### CLINICAL MANIFESTATIONS

The presenting symptoms are usually pain and swelling at the affected site. Pain at rest, especially that which awakens a patient at night, is a significant finding that suggests active growth, venous hypertension, or periosteal distension. Conversely, lesions that are found incidentally without symptoms are more likely to be indolent. Often patients ascribe pain to a recent minor injury, and this can mislead the physician. A mechanism of injury that does not adequately explain a pattern of pain should arouse suspicion. A mass may be present, but tumors in the femur and pelvis are easily masked by overlying soft tissues, and the patient may not notice it. A limp may be the result of muscle atrophy, nerve involvement, or pain. Weakness, numbness, and paresthesias may signify impingement on or direct involvement of nerves. Constitutional symptoms such as weight loss, malaise, and fevers may be present, particularly with Ewing sarcoma and malignant fibrous histiocytoma (MFH).

The past medical history and family history can provide valuable information. A number of conditions may predispose the patient to a secondary sarcoma, including previous radiation, Paget's disease, bone infarct, and fibrous dysplasia. Patients with hereditary retinoblastoma have a genetic predisposition to developing sarcomas as a result of a germline mutation in the Rb tumor suppressor gene. Likewise, patients with a germline mutation in the p53 gene may be at risk for multiple cancers, including sarcomas. The pediatric patient with a sarcoma of bone is occasionally the index case for a family with the Li-Fraumeni syndrome. If a patient has a first-degree relative who has had a cancer at a young age (e.g., breast), the syndrome may be present in the family, and affected members may be at risk for multiple primary malignancies.

The physical examination should document areas of swelling, which can be assessed by direct measurement of limb circumference. Areas of tenderness should be carefully noted. When performing range-of-motion tests, the possibility of causing a pathologic fracture through a lesion in the bone must always be kept in mind. Since this may have dire consequences for the patient, it may be prudent to obtain a radiograph prior to completing the examination. A thorough neurologic and vascular examination may reveal focal deficits, which could result from involvement of major nerves or vessels by tumor.

## DIAGNOSIS

The diagnosis of sarcomas of bone is difficult. It is unrealistic to expect a pathologist to make the correct diagnosis with just a small piece of tissue and no other information. For example, chondrosarcoma and chondroblastic osteogenic sarcoma may have areas that appear similar histologically, but the two tumors have markedly different prognosis and treatment. Communication between clinical specialties is vital. In addition to the biopsy specimen, significant findings from the history, physical examination, radiographs, laboratory studies, and other studies should be considered and discussed before a final diagnosis is rendered.

RADIOLOGY. Although the plain radiograph may seem antiquated and unsophisticated, it still remains the single most important radiographic test to obtain for diagnostic purposes. Other imaging modalities, including computed tomography (CT) and magnetic resonance imaging (MRI), cannot easily convey the same information that is present on the plain radiograph, which is far superior in terms of narrowing the differential diagnosis and clinching the final diagnosis.

On a plain radiograph, malignant tumors are characterized by a permeative growth pattern and erosion through the cortex. The borders of the lesion are not well defined and there is usually no sclerotic rim around the lesion. Periosteal reaction in the form of onion-skinning, Codman's triangle, and sunburst formation occurs with rapidly expansile lesions that lift the periosteum off the bone and induce new bone formation. In contrast, a faint, intact rim of cortex around a lesion implies a slower rate of growth that permits cortical bone formation to keep pace with the tumor. The lesion may be purely lytic, or it may have ossified or calcified matrix. Cartilaginous tumors are characterized by "popcorn" calcifications, which differ from the "fluffy" ossification pattern of osteoblastic tumors.

CT scans are excellent for assessing cross-sectional bony detail and are superior to MRI scans in this regard. Benign lesions may expand the intramedullary space and thin the cortex but rarely erode through the cortex. A subtle breach in cortical continuity may not be apparent on plain radiographs but may be readily demonstrated by CT scans.

The quality of MRI scans varies considerably. It is more cost effective for the surgeon to order the particular scan that is needed than to be sent a suboptimal scan. Scans with low-strength magnets and "open" scans give relatively poor resolution. Bilateral scans are rarely indicated and compromise the depiction of the lesion. Certain sequences that are designed for specific purposes, such as evaluation of meniscal tears, are inadequate for tumors. Full-length coronal or sagittal images of the affected bone are necessary to determine the extent of the lesion and presence of skip lesions, but these views are frequently omitted with limited scans.

Different connective tissues have different characteristics on MRI. Bone, calcifications, and dense fibrous tissues appear dark. Normal articular cartilage also appears dark, but the cartilage of tumors has a high water content and is characteristically bright on T2-weighted images. Likewise, myxoid tissue appears intensely bright on T2-weighted images. Fat is bright on T1-weighted images, but becomes dark on short tau inversion recovery (STIR) or fat-saturation type images. Hemorrhage can have different appearances depending on how old the hemorrhage is. Tumors filled with blood, such as telangiectatic osteogenic sarcoma, can show fluid-fluid levels, if sufficient time is allowed during the scan for the red blood cells to settle.

Tumors are typically easier to see on T2-weighted images and usually appear bright on these sequences. However, the tumor is often difficult to distinguish from surrounding edema, which also appears bright on T2-weighted images. The extent of the tumor is actually better represented on T1-weighted images. Fat planes surrounding vessels and nerves are important to note on T1-weighted images, and obliteration of these planes by tumor may indicate invasion of the nerve or vessel. It is also important to pay attention to the lumen of veins, which may harbor tumor. Gadolinium may help in this regard and may also provide enhancement of highly vascularized areas. Dynamic MRI is being investigated to provide information on the metabolic activity and viability of certain areas.

In addition to radiographs of the affected site, the workup of a sarcoma of bone should also include a plain chest x-ray and chest CT since the lung is the most common site of metastasis.

NUCLEAR MEDICINE. A technetium bone scan should be obtained to assess both the primary tumor and screen for distant metastases. The technetium is conjugated to a diphosphonate molecule, which is taken up preferentially at sites of bone formation. The bone scan is not specific for any one disorder, and increased uptake can occur with fracture, infection, and metabolic disorders. Other nuclear medicine scans, such as thallium scans (usually for osteogenic sarcoma) and gallium scans (usually for Ewing sarcoma), have some utility in monitoring the response to chemotherapy as well as screening for distant disease and are used in conjunction with technetium bone scans in some centers.[1–3]

LABORATORY STUDIES. Serum chemistries, a complete blood count, and coagulation profiles should be obtained. Particular attention should be paid to serum calcium level, which may be markedly elevated, and hypoalbuminemia, which can mask hypercalcemia. A high phosphate level in conjunction with hypercalcemia may lead to renal lithiasis as well as calcifications being deposited in soft tissues.

BIOPSY. The gold standard for biopsy is the traditional open biopsy.[4] Although a seemingly simple procedure, great care must be taken in its execution, since technical errors adversely affect chances for limb preservation and cure.[5,6] Sarcomas thrive in connective tissue, including fat, muscle, tendon, and bone, and the risk for seeding these tissues should always be kept in mind. The biopsy is best performed in the operating room under general anesthesia, which allows the patient to be kept under sterile conditions until an adequate sample has been obtained. The frozen section must verify that pathologic tissue of sufficient quality and quantity has been secured. If nondiagnostic material is found initially, more tissue should be taken. Portable x-ray or image intensifier with hard copies can verify that the biopsy was taken from the appropriate site, and this may be important for medicolegal purposes. Strict adherence to sterile technique is necessary, since an infected tumor can result in an unresectable lesion. Care must be taken during the prep when holding the extremity to avoid fracture, which can also result in an unresectable tumor. Exsanguination should be by gravity drainage rather than wrapping with elastic bandages. Antibiotics must be withheld until cultures have been obtained.

The incision should be longitudinal. Transverse incisions are contraindicated since they result in contamination of multiple compartments and fascial planes. The selection of the incision is vital and must be in line with the subsequent incision for the definitive resection. Thus, it has been advised that the biopsy is probably best performed by the surgeon who will perform the definitive resection.[4,7] Skin flaps should not be raised. If a hole must be made in the cortex of a bone, it should be round without corners to reduce chances for postoperative fracture.[8] The dissection during biopsy should be directly through a single muscle compartment. Fascial planes between muscle groups and neurovascular structures should be avoided since everything that is exposed must be considered potentially contaminated with tumor cells. Penetrating retractors may spread tumor cells and should not be used near the tumor.

Hemostasis and wound closure must be meticulous, because hematoma, dehiscence, and infection can spread tumor cells and compromise resectability of the tumor. The hole in the bone should be plugged with Gelfoam, bone wax, methylmethacrylate or some other substance to minimize bleeding from the bone. Direct pressure can be applied to promote clot formation prior to closure. The sutures should penetrate the skin close to the incision since the biopsy incision and suture holes must be completely excised. The use of a drain is controversial. The drain may reduce the chance of a large hematoma forming. However, drains can become clotted and should not be relied upon for hemostasis. The increased risk of infection also argues against the use of a drain. If drains are used, they must be brought out in line with the incision, and the subsequent resection must include the drain tract. Postoperatively, the limb must be protected with some form of immobilization and/or crutches to avoid a pathologic fracture.

Closed percutaneous needle biopsies have been used with varying success, and accuracy ranges from 80% to 98%.[9–14] Tru-cut or core biopsies have had somewhat better accuracy than fine-needle aspirates since core biopsies produce more tissue and are somewhat easier to interpret. Although closed biopsy may seem simpler and quicker than open biopsy, there are several drawbacks. Lesions may be difficult to access if they are calcified, ossified, or covered by cortical bone. The accuracy is highly dependent upon the experience of the pathologist, and one study found that the percentage of correct diagnoses ranged from 87% to 98%, depending on which pathologist interpreted the sample.[11] Multiple needle passes are usually required, and these may not be completely excised at the time of resection. Currently, needle biopsies seem most appropriate when the radiograph alone is diagnostic, and only a small amount of tissue is needed for confirmation. Needle biopsy may become more attractive in the future as molecular diagnostic tests improve.

**OTHER STUDIES.** Patients who are candidates for certain types of chemotherapy may require other tests. For example, patients that receive cardiotoxic agents, such as doxorubicin, should have a baseline ECG and a test for ventricular function such as a MUGA scan.

**TABLE 20B-1.** MUSCULOSKELETAL TUMOR SOCIETY (MSTS) STAGING SYSTEM OF SARCOMAS

| STAGE | GRADE | SITE | METASTASIS |
|-------|-------|------|------------|
| IA | G1 | T1 | M0 |
| IB | G1 | T2 | M0 |
| IIA | G2 | T1 | M0 |
| IIB | G2 | T2 | M0 |
| III | G1 or G2 | T1 or T2 | M1 |

Grade:
G1   Low grade
G2   High grade

Site:
T1   Intracompartmental
T2   Extracompartmental

Metastasis:
M0   No metastasis
M1   Regional or distant metastasis

SOURCE: Enneking WF et al.[15]

## STAGING

The most widely used staging system, which has been adopted by the Musculoskeletal Tumor Society, is based upon grade (G), site of primary tumor (T), and metastasis (M) (Table 20B-1).[15] Nodal involvement is rare and qualifies as a distant metastasis. Grade is either low (G1) or high (G2). Tumors are classified according to whether they are intracompartmental (T1) or extracompartmental (T2). Intracompartmental tumors lie completely within a bone.

The American Joint Committee on Cancer (AJCC) (Table 20B-2) has a very similar staging system for primary malignant bone tumors (excluding myeloma) based on the G, T, N, M concept.[16] Lymph node involvement is separated from distant metastasis in stage IV disease. Four grades are recognized, but grades 1 and 2 (well differentiated and moderately differentiated, respectively) are grouped together, and grades 3 and 4 (poorly differentiated and undifferentiated, respectively) are grouped together.

## SURGICAL TREATMENT

It is vital to have a clear conception of the surgical goals for each patient. These may be divided into oncologic and reconstructive goals. The former should take precedence over the latter since surgical margins should not be compromised for the ease of reconstruction. From an oncologic perspective, surgery may be performed for diagnostic, palliative, adjunctive, or curative intent.[17] When the diagnosis is uncertain, a formal open biopsy is the most prudent course. Exploratory surgery without a clear formulation of goals is strongly discouraged because it is unlikely to be a curative procedure and is likely to result in widespread contamination of tissues.

**TABLE 20B-2. AMERICAN JOINT COMMITTEE ON CANCER (AJCC) STAGING FOR SARCOMAS OF BONE**

| STAGE | GRADE | TUMOR (PRIMARY) | NODES (REGIONAL) | METASTASES (DISTANT) |
|---|---|---|---|---|
| IA | G1–G2 | T1 | N0 | M0 |
| IB | G1–G2 | T2 | N0 | M0 |
| IIA | G3–G4 | T1 | N0 | M0 |
| IIB | G3–G4 | T2 | N0 | M0 |
| III | — | — | — | — |
| IVA | Any | Any | N1 | M0 |
| IVB | Any | Any | Any | M1 |

Grade (G):
G1 Well differentiated
G2 Moderately differentiated
G3 Poorly differentiated
G4 Undifferentiated

Primary tumor (T):
T1 Tumor is confined within cortex
T2 Tumor extends beyond cortex

Regional lymph nodes (N):
N0 No regional lymph node metastases
N1 Regional lymph node metastases

Distant metastases:
M0 None
M1 Distant metastases

SOURCE: Fleming ID et al.[16]

Surgical procedures for removing the tumor have been classified as radical, wide, marginal, or intralesional.[15] A radical resection completely removes all anatomic compartments that are involved by the tumor. A wide excision enters the compartments containing the tumor but leaves a cuff of normal tissue around the tumor. A marginal excision enters the edematous reactive zone around the pseudocapsule without penetrating the tumor. An intralesional excision, as exemplified by curettage, enters the tumor directly. It has been customary to reserve the term *resection* for radical procedures. The term *excision* is generally used for all other procedures. The older term *en bloc resection* is usually synonymous with wide excision, but it has not been defined formally and is somewhat ambiguous. Finally, the concept of "wide margin with contamination" is important because it specifically denotes the situation where a formal wide excision is attempted but the tumor entered. If this is recognized during surgery, it may be possible to excise the area of contamination.

Radical resection and wide excision offer the best chance for cure. The less effective the adjuvant treatment, the greater the need for a wide margin of normal tissue. However, radical resection or wide excision are not necessarily appropriate for all patients. If the goal of surgery is palliative or adjunctive, a marginal or intralesional procedure may be employed in combination with another modality, such as radiation, cryosurgery, or hyperthermia.

**AMPUTATIONS.** Amputations have traditionally been used to treat sarcomas, and it was recognized during the nineteenth century by Samuel Gross and others that cures could sometimes be achieved with amputation alone. However, amputation is not synonymous with radical resection. These procedures may be marginal or intralesional, since it is sometimes impossible to cut through normal uninvolved tissue. This is especially true for massive lesions involving the pelvis and brachial plexus.

The primary indication for amputation is the inability to obtain an adequate margin of normal tissue around the tumor and still retain a useful limb. Certain conditions predispose to amputation, including widespread contamination of soft tissue by previous surgery, fracture, and infection. Another broad indication for amputation is the anticipated loss of vascular and/or nervous supply to the extremity that cannot be adequately restored. Loss of two major nerves in a limb, such as both the sciatic and femoral nerves in the leg, makes amputation advisable. However, loss of only one nerve, even if it is the sciatic nerve, does not automatically mandate amputation. Even without the sciatic nerve, the leg and foot remain sensate to a degree because of the saphenous nerve. An active quadriceps allows ambulation with minimal or even no external support.

An amputation must be regarded as both an ablative and reconstructive procedure. Advances in prosthetics have increased the potential function of amputees. For example, ischial containment sockets have significantly improved the gait of above-knee amputees.[18] Energy-conserving foot-ankle constructs have lowered energy expenditure for most lower-extremity amputees and facilitated return to sports in motivated individuals.[19] In order for patients to achieve their full potential, meticulous technique during surgery and close supervision of rehabilitation is essential.[20–26] Muscle balance by myodesis or myoplasty improves function and prevents debilitating joint contractures, which preclude use of prosthetics. Stretching and range-of-motion exercises are also important to prevent stiffness. Muscle coverage of the end of the bone is desirable, but the amount of soft tissue coverage must be chosen carefully. A tight closure can result in wound breakdown over the stump, whereas excessive soft tissue results in a painful mobile wad that may also break down. A compressive or rigid plaster postoperative dressing and elevation of the limb helps prevent edema, contracture, and wound dehiscence.[27,28] Early prosthetic fitting is beneficial for aerobic conditioning and regaining use of the limb, but immediate prosthetic fitting can be problematic. Shrinkage of the stump results in loss of intimate contact in the socket, which increases shear forces on the skin and predisposes to wound breakdown.[29]

Disadvantages of amputations are well-known and include the psychologic burden of losing a limb and the effect of altered cosmesis on self-image. The expense of maintaining and replacing prosthetic limbs is considerable. Ambulation increases demand on cardiac output and oxygen consumption for lower-extremity amputees.[30] Phantom pain and phantom sensations are common in the early postoperative period, but tend to improve with time. Approximately 10% of patients have severe, intractable pain.[28,31]

**LIMB-PRESERVING SURGERY.** Limb-preserving surgery has become possible for many patients as a result of improvements in surgical technique, reconstructive materials, and adjuvant therapy. The indications for such surgery include not only the technical ability to reconstruct a limb, but more importantly the ability to achieve adequate margins. Previous contamination of tissues by infection, fracture, or inadvisable surgery increase the risk of local recurrence and are relative contraindications. Another important consideration is the rate of complications. Procedures that result in wound dehiscence or infection may interfere with chemotherapy and jeopardize chances for cure.

Reconstructive procedures after limb-sparing procedures usually require large bone grafts, endoprosthetic replacement, or a combination of biologic and artificial materials. At present there is no perfect reconstructive strategy, and there are advantages and disadvantages for any given approach. One of the major problems is durability. As the cure rate for sarcomas improves, a substantial number of patients will live 50 years or more, and thus, the quality of reconstructions must begin to be assessed with regard to long-term outcome.

ALLOGRAFTS. Bulk allografts of bone have been used extensively for major reconstructions (Fig. 20B-1). They are versatile implants, since large bone banks are able to provide bones of essentially all types and sizes. They can be ordered with soft tissue attachments to restore muscle function and provide joint stability. Allografts are fundamentally appealing because they are a biologic reconstruction and provide a scaffold for the potential regeneration of living tissue.

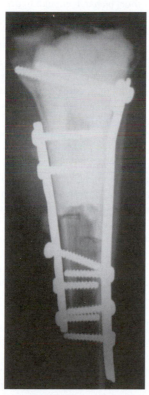

FIGURE 20B-1. An osteoarticular allograft was used to reconstruct the proximal tibia. The allograft was filled with antibiotic (gentamicin) impregnated methylmethacrylate, which may reduce the likelihood of infection and improve fixation.

It is important to note that all normal connective tissues—bones, cartilage, tendons, and ligaments—are alive, and cells continually replenish the matrix to maintain structural integrity of the tissue. With the possible exception of the cartilage in fresh-frozen osteoarticular grafts, allografts are dead. Without some degree of incorporation and regeneration by the host, the grafts will eventually undergo fatigue failure.

The possibility of transmitting infectious agents, particularly viruses, is a concern with allografts. Transmission of the human immunodeficiency virus (HIV) has not occurred with irradiated, freeze-dried grafts, even from an infected donor.[32] It is believed that the virus cannot survive the harsh conditions of graft preparation, which include extensive washing, removal of blood and marrow, defatting with alcohol, and lyophilization. However, fresh allografts and fresh-frozen allografts may potentially transmit the virus. Current methods of sterilization, including radiation to 2 million cGy, freezing, and treatment with ethylene oxide, do not completely destroy HIV particles and, therefore, one is relying primarily upon the screening tests to avoid infection. Two infected donors transmitted HIV to multiple recipients in the 1980s, when screening protocols were not as rigorous as they are today. The risk of HIV infection is currently believed to be extremely low and comparable to the risk of HIV transmission from a unit of blood, which is estimated to be 1:493,000.[33] The risk of infection with other known viral agents is estimated to be 1:641,000 for human T-cell lymphotropic virus-1 (HTLV-1), 1:63,000 for hepatitis B, and 1:103,000 for hepatitis C.[33]

The biomechanical and biologic properties of allografts are affected by the method of processing. Fresh allografts retain the most strength but are also the most immunogenic and consequently may be less likely to be incorporated into the host.[34,35] Freezing in liquid nitrogen reduces immunogenicity with little effect on mechanical strength. Freeze drying increases shelf life and simplifies storage but results in a significant loss (10% to 61%) of bending and torsional strength.[36,37]

The clinical results that have been obtained with allografts vary according to the situation in which they are employed. Intercalary allografts, which replace only part of the diaphysis, have performed the best, and long-term graft survival is between 80% and 100%.[38,39] The worst results have occurred with allograft arthrodesis, and Mankin et al.[38] found that only 40% of the grafts were retained at 10 years. However, the poor results may be related in part to the use of plate fixation for arthrodesis. Resection arthrodesis of the knee with autogenous grafts and a long nail has been reported to have 92% survival of the reconstruction at 10 years.[40] Osteoarticular allografts have had intermediate results. These allografts are frozen fresh in liquid nitrogen. Dimethyl sulfoxide (DMSO) or glycerol solutions are used for cryopreservation of the chondrocytes. Although 40% to 70% of cells survive the experimental freeze-thawing process,[41,42] few survive long-term in animals[43,44] or humans,[45] and one study of specimens retrieved at autopsy found no viable chondrocytes.[46] Degenerative changes occur with time as a result of mechanical wear, subchondral collapse, and possibly immune reaction,[47] but such changes are not always painful. In symptomatic cases, total joint arthroplasty may be able to replace the articular surfaces while retaining the bulk of the allograft.

The major problems with allografts include fracture, nonunion, and infection. The overall rate of fractures is 16% to 19%.[38,48,49]

The occurrence of a fracture is not always a catastrophic event, and up to 75% of allografts can be salvaged by internal fixation and bone grafting. Fractures occur because allograft bone is not live tissue and cannot repair the microfractures that occur with repetitive stress. Over time the allograft becomes revascularized and repopulated with live osteocytes, but this is a very slow process, with less than 20% incorporation at 5 years.[45] Ironically, revascularization may contribute to fractures because it causes resorption and weakening of bone prior to the formation of new live bone. It is prudent not to leave any holes in allograft bone since these defects create a stress riser, provide an avenue for vascular invasion, and stimulate osteoclastic bone resorption.

The incidence of nonunion is difficult to determine because it is anticipated that the healing of the nonviable allograft bone to host bone is much slower than the healing of live native bone to native bone. One large study reported a nonunion rate of 17% but did not define precisely the difference between normal healing, delayed union, and nonunion for allografts.[38] Capanna et al.[50] found that 67% of host-graft junctions were healed at 12 months, but only 2% ultimately failed to unite.[50] Capanna et al.[50] also reported that pulsed electromagnetic fields improved the graft union rate in a randomized trial. Vander Griend et al.[48] reported that 16% of patients had a delayed union or nonunion, but half of these patients healed after bone grafting and other procedures.[48]

A number of factors probably have an impact on the healing process, including periosteal and soft tissue coverage, stressshielding, chemotherapy,[51] and immunologic reactions.[34] Nonunion may also result from technical errors in internal fixation, such as leaving a gap between the ends of bones or failing to achieve a rigid construct.[48] It is notable that in the study by Vander Griend[48] the type of internal fixation did not affect the rate of bone healing, and there was no difference between plate fixation and intramedullary nailing. However, there were more fractures in the group fixed with plates and screws.[48] Recent evidence suggests that the allograft induces resorption by the host and this may contribute to nonunion.

The most serious complication is infection, which occurs in 6% to 13% of patients.[38,52–54] Since the graft is not vascularized, infections are difficult to eradicate, and in most instances necessitate removal of the graft. The rate of infection is especially high for large pelvic allografts.[55] Several measures have been proposed to minimize the risk of infection. Coverage of the graft with well-vascularized muscle and soft tissue is important, particularly in areas such as the proximal tibia where the skin is thin. Injection of antibiotic-impregnated bone cement into the medullary cavity may reduce the rate of infection while at the same time retarding bone resorption.[56] A prolonged period of prophylactic oral antibiotics has been used by many authors, but it is difficult to prove whether this is beneficial or not.

AUTOGENOUS GRAFTS. Autogenous bone grafts avoid problems with immunogenicity and transmission of infectious diseases, but they are not used as extensively as allografts for large skeletal defects. When autogenous bone graft is harvested, a completely separate set of instruments, gowns, and gloves should be used, and the donor site must not be contaminated with tumor cells.

The most common type of autogenous graft is morselized cancellous bone graft from the iliac crest, which is used to stimulate new bone formation and bone healing. In contrast, bulk bone grafts are used to provide structural support, and these are usually harvested from the fibula, iliac crest, and rib. The amount of bone available from these sites is limited, and the graft is often smaller than the skeletal defect. In certain situations, it may be possible to use larger grafts at the risk of seriously weakening the donor bone. For example, the anterior half of the femur and tibia have been used in resection arthrodesis of the knee. In this procedure, a long intramedullary nail extending from the proximal femur to the distal tibia must be inserted and left permanently in place since removal of the nail is associated with a high risk of fracture and collapse.[40,57–59] The rate of infection for large, nonvascularized grafts is substantial and comparable to the rate of infection for allografts.[58]

If the tumor does not significantly compromise the structural integrity of the bone, it may be possible to remove the tumor from the resected bone, sterilize it, and reinsert it into the defect. This approach has not been popular in the United States, partly because of the concern over reimplantation of tumor cells. However, in many parts of the world where large bone banks do not exist and endoprostheses are prohibitively expensive, reinsertion of resected bone has been a major method of reconstruction. Even in advanced countries, the approach has some appeal, since the bone is perfectly matched to the patient both immunologically and structurally. The success of this procedure depends critically upon the method of sterilization, which include autoclaving, prolonged hyperthermia, repetitive freeze-thawing with liquid nitrogen, and massive radiation. The sterilization procedure must be harsh enough to destroy all tumor cells. Unfortunately, this leads to varying degrees of compromise in the quality of the graft. With the possible exception of freeze-thawing in liquid nitrogen,[36] all of these procedures significantly reduce the mechanical strength of bone and inactivate bone-inductive proteins. Nevertheless, reasonable results have been obtained by Harrington et al.[60] when autoclaved grafts were used as part of a composite reconstruction involving both bone graft and endoprosthesis.[60] There were two local recurrences in this series of 42 patients, but the authors maintained that they did not arise from the autoclaved segment.

Vascularized autogenous grafts can be either local pedicular grafts or free grafts, the most versatile being the free fibular graft (Fig. 20B-2). Vascularized grafts have several theoretical advantages as a result of an intact blood supply. It is believed that they are less prone to infection, less susceptible to fatigue damage, more likely to undergo hypertrophy, and more apt to heal promptly than allografts. The limited experience with vascularized grafts after tumor excision is encouraging, but the data suggest that they have not yet fulfilled all previous expectations.[61–66] Although vascularized grafts have been used successfully as a salvage procedure after deep infection, they are not immune from infection themselves, and in the large series from the Mayo Clinic, there was a 16% rate of infection.[64] It has been the impression of many observers that vascularized grafts have the capacity to heal more quickly than allografts, and indeed, vascularized grafts can be used effectively in situations of recalcitrant nonunion. However, the nonunion rate with primary vascularized grafts is 6% to 19% after tumor resection, and this may reflect loss of blood flow to the graft in a certain fraction of cases.[62,64–66] The rate of stress fractures is high, ranging from 8% to 43%, but this is not necessarily catastrophic, and some believe that it may even stimulate hypertrophy of the bone.[62,64,65] Experimentally, vascularized grafts undergo hypertrophy more quickly and to a

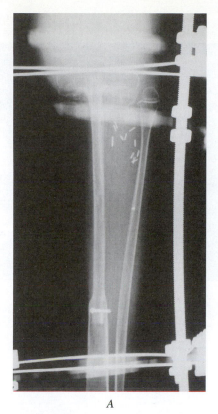
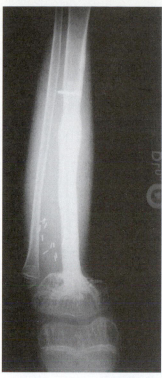

*A*                                              *B*

**FIGURE 20B-2.** A vascularized fibula was used to reconstruct a tibial defect after limb-sparing surgery for Ewing's sarcoma. The growth plate was spared and continues to grow. A thin-wire external fixator was used initially for stabilization. The patient has sustained two fractures, but these have healed, and the graft has hypertrophied.

greater degree than allografts,[67] but clinically, there is great variability in the amount of hypertrophy. One study found hypertrophy in six of seven patients,[65] but in the Mayo Clinic series, hypertrophy occurred in only 37% of patients.[61] Since the grafts are initially weak and prone to fracture, the limb must be protected with a cast, brace, or external fixator for an extended period of time, often 2 years or longer. This may be particularly unpleasant and difficult for cancer patients. Another consideration is that there may be significant donor site morbidity, and patients may experience ankle pain, great toe weakness, peroneal nerve palsy, scarring, and compartment syndrome.

It is likely that the technique of free fibular transfer will continue to improve in the future. Innovative uses, such as combining vascularized fibular grafts with allografts, may prove to be worthwhile and may expand indications for the procedure in the future.[68,69] However, given its present limitations and rate of complications, patients should be carefully selected for this demanding operation.

**ROTATIONPLASTY.** The Van Nes rotationplasty is typically done for a distal femoral lesion in a child less than 10 years old. The procedure involves attachment of the proximal femur to the proximal tibia, which is rotated 180° so that the foot faces backward

(Fig. 20B-3). This effectively converts the ankle joint to a knee joint and changes what would have been a high above-knee amputation (AKA) into a below-knee amputation (BKA). Function is usually quite good, and most patients can use a prosthesis to ambulate without crutches.[70] The procedure allows for continued growth of the limb, which is problematic in young children. An AKA in a young child will result in an extremely short stump when the child reaches maturity. Likewise, an allograft does not continue to grow, and eventually there will be a major leg length discrepancy and incongruity of joint surfaces. Although leg lengthening with distraction osteogenesis can restore some of the lost length,[71] this is a difficult and painful process.

In addition to function, there are many other benefits to rotationplasty. The healing of bone in a rotationplasty is usually prompt, and delayed union occurred in only 2% of patients in one large series.[72] This allows chemotherapy to proceed in a timely manner without interruptions from surgical complications. The reconstruction is durable and less prone to complications of allografts, such as fracture and infection. Finally, there is no phantom pain, and the foot remains fully sensate. Despite these advantages, the operation has not achieved universal acceptance primarily because of the cosmetic appearance of the limb.

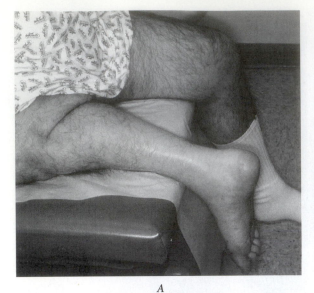

*A*

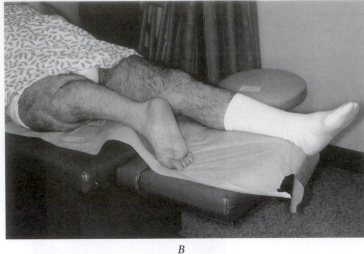

*B*

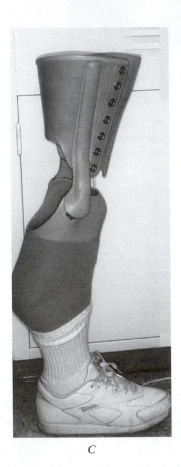

*C*

**FIGURE 20B-3.** Van Nes rotationplasty is usually performed on small children, but it can also be applied to adults with good function, as seen in these photographs. The ankle functions as a knee, and it can extend as well as flex. The orthosis is somewhat different from conventional BKA orthoses. The socket must be larger to accommodate the foot, and the suspension requires a lace-up mechanism.

There are variations of the Van Nes rotationplasty that involve fusion of the distal femur to the pelvis for proximal femoral lesions.[73] This procedure turns the knee into a hip joint and the ankle into a knee joint. The procedure again attempts to convert what would have been a hip disarticulation or hemipelvectomy into a BKA, and utilizes normal native tissue that would have been discarded with a high amputation. The concept of the procedure can also be adapted to the upper extremity. Rather than performing a high above-elbow amputation, the involved segment of the arm can be excised, and the ulna can be fused to the proximal humerus or shoulder. This results in a short arm but retains the hand, which is the most important part of the upper extremity. In all of these procedures, a prerequisite is that the major nerves to the distal limb not be involved with tumor. If only one nerve is involved, consideration may be given to section of the nerve and primary reanastamosis, particularly in a young child, who has greater potential for nerve repair and regeneration.

ENDOPROSTHETIC REPLACEMENT. Although endoprostheses have occasionally been used for intercalary defects in the diaphysis,[74] they are usually employed in situations involving joint reconstruction. The primary advantage to endoprosthetic replacement is immediate skeletal stability and restoration of function. Nonunion is not an issue with endoprostheses, and there is no need to wait for bony healing to occur before patients are permitted to use the limb. This is an important consideration in a patient who may not have very long to live.

Similar to allografts, endoprostheses are prone to a number of complications. Infection occurs in 2% to 9% of patients and usually results in removal of the implant.[75–78] The rate of infection varies for different anatomic sites and is highest for the proximal tibia, where the soft tissue coverage is poorest.[75] Awareness of the problem has led to more aggressive use of muscle flaps and free flaps, which have significantly reduced the rate of infections.[79] Successful reimplantation of a prosthesis is often possible after a deep infection, but this requires thorough surgical debridement, placement of a temporary antibiotic-impregnated cement spacer, and administration of intravenous antibiotics for an extended time. Amputation may be needed to cure refractory infections or those for which treatment would delay resumption of postoperative chemotherapy or jeopardize the patient's life.

In contrast to allografts, fracture of the prosthesis and periprosthetic bone fractures are less common and occur in approximately 5% of patients.[78,79] The major cause of late failure is aseptic loosening, which is a problem unique to endoprostheses (Fig. 20B-4).[77,79–82] The rate of aseptic loosening is related to numerous factors. The location of the implant is important, and the rate of loosening is highest for the proximal tibia, followed by the distal femur, proximal humerus, and finally proximal femur.[79,83] The age of the patient affects prosthetic survival, and younger, more active patients have significantly higher failure rates.[83] The amount of bone resected also affects the rate of loosening. Distal femoral resections that remove greater than 40% of the length of the femur have been found to have a higher rate of failure than resections of less than 40%.[82,84]

Fortunately, there are several factors amenable to design modifications and medical intervention that can reduce the rate of aseptic loosening. The use of less constrained implants has improved longevity of implants. Older, constrained prostheses that allowed motion in only one plane were associated with a high rate of loosening as a result of stress concentration at the stems. The newer rotating hinge prostheses for the knee dissipate forces by allowing motion in multiple planes. Preliminary data seem to indicate that these prostheses have a much lower rate of loosening compared to older single-axis designs.[85]

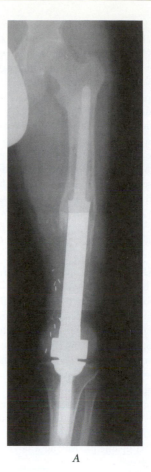
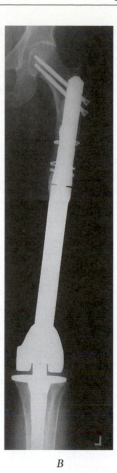

*A*            *B*

**FIGURE 20B-4.** The most common late complication of prosthetic reconstruction is osteolysis and loosening of the implant. *A*. Loosening of a distal femoral prosthesis is manifested by the osteolysis around the stem in the intramedullary canal. The loosening may have been related in part to the fact that the prosthesis had only one axis of rotation. *B*. The prosthesis was revised with a massive, uncemented, rotating hinge knee, with interlocking screws into the femoral head. The rotating hinge relieves stress on the stem and may be less prone to loosening. The prosthesis was stable at 6 years.

In addition to reducing mechanical stress, interruption of the biologic events leading to aseptic loosening is also possible. Aseptic loosening is mediated in part by a reaction of macrophages to particulate debris from polyethylene, metal, and cement. The activated macrophages produce factors that stimulate bone resorption by osteoclasts, which ultimately results in radiographic osteolysis and clinical loosening around the implant. The use of an extramedullary ring of porous ingrowth surfaces has been shown to retard the loosening rate by enhancing fixation with extracortical bone and inducing the formation of a fibrous cuff, which seals the medullary canal from particulate debris.[86,87] There is also some thought to medically halting the process by inhibiting osteoclasts with bisphosphonates such as alendronate. Experimental results in a canine model have shown an arrest of aseptic loosening even after the process has started.[44]

Expandable prostheses have been used primarily for tumors around the knee in adolescent children to maintain growth and prevent leg length discrepancy.[88–92] Although the concept is attractive, there are a number of limitations that dampen the enthusiasm for the procedure. The patients who would benefit most from the device—very young children—are not candidates since their bones are too small to accommodate endoprostheses. The expandable portion of the device is weak in some designs and subject to fracture. The lengthening must be done in small incremental steps to avoid nerve palsy and joint contracture, thus necessitating multiple procedures. The tibial component crosses the tibial growth plate, which further retards growth of the limb. This problem may be diminished by the use of a thin, smooth, sliding tibial stem, but mean growth is still only 76% of normal with this design.[88] Finally, the rate of aseptic loosening and overall rate of failure seems to be higher than the corresponding rates for nonexpandable prostheses.[93]

**COMPOSITE RECONSTRUCTION.** Composite reconstructions utilize a combination of biologic and synthetic materials. Currently, the majority of composite reconstructions involve alloprostheses, which refer to a combination of allografts and endoprostheses (Fig. 20B-5). Since most series on this type of reconstruction are small, there has yet to be demonstrated an overall benefit in comparison to endoprostheses or allografts alone.[38,94] However, there are a number of practical and theoretical considerations that make composite reconstructions appealing and rational.

The main advantage of this approach is that it provides tendinous and other soft tissue attachments to the endoprosthesis. Although tendons can be successfully anchored to endoprostheses, tumor excisions often include tendons and ligaments, leaving a large gap between the muscle and the prosthesis.

Another advantage of composite reconstructions is restoration of bone stock. Although most endoprostheses for the knee survive 5 years, it is likely that the current generation of implants will not outlast a young patient who is cured of disease. At least one, and perhaps many, revisions will have to be performed. If only pure endoprostheses are used and no attempt is made to restore bone stock, there will be progressive bone loss with each revision, making reconstruction increasingly difficult and less likely to succeed.

A potential advantage of alloprostheses is that the rate of aseptic loosening may be lower than with pure endoprostheses. The data on this are too limited at present to draw conclusions. Allograft bone may theoretically reduce some stress on the distal stem, provided that the graft unites to native bone. Moreover, allografts seem more resistant to macrophage-induced osteolysis since they are not vascularized. In the situations where aseptic loosening has been observed, there is usually failure of the allograft, either as a result of resorption of the graft or nonunion at the host-graft junction.[94]

Theoretic disadvantages also exist. Alloprostheses are usually cemented, forgoing the potential enhancement of long-term results by porous ingrowth fixation. Furthermore, operative time is greater than for allografts or prostheses alone, so the risk of infection may increase.

In a sense, all allograft and autograft reconstructions should be considered composite prosthetic reconstructions since the grafts require some form of internal fixation, whether it be screws, plates, nails, or long-stemmed components of endoprostheses. Further-

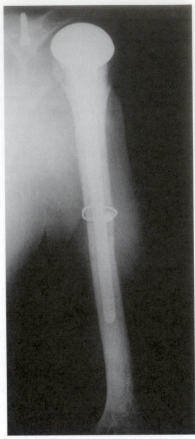

**FIGURE 20B-5.** Composite alloprosthetic reconstruction of the proximal humerus takes advantage of the soft tissues of the allograft to reattach the rotator cuff. The allograft extends halfway down the shaft and joins the native bone at the circumferential cable.

more, the use of endoprostheses after tumor resection often requires some degree of biologic healing, such tendinous attachment, capsular formation, and bony ingrowth, for the device to achieve complete stability and maximal function. In the future, it will be more useful to think in terms of how best to combine biologic and artificial materials in composite reconstructions rather than to dwell upon the old debate over whether pure allografts or endoprostheses are better. The advent of artificially engineered biologic materials and the continued refinement of endoprostheses has opened up many new and exciting possibilities for such composite reconstructions.

**ARTHRODESIS.** Arthrodesis is not often performed now, but it can provide a satisfactory reconstruction. When the procedure is successful, the result is a pain-free, stable limb. Stability is more critical in the lower extremity, which is needed for ambulation, than the upper extremity, where motion is arguably more important. The main drawback to arthrodesis is loss of motion. This can be tolerated surprisingly well in certain joints, such as the hip, but it poses greater functional problems in other joints, such as the elbow, where a large arc of motion is essential.

Arthrodesis after tumor resection is difficult because there is usually a large bony defect. Options for bridging this defect include vascularized grafts, nonvascularized autogenous grafts, allografts, and/or endoprostheses. Although allografts most readily span the gap, they have been associated with a high rate of late fracture and failure when used in this setting, and thus they may not provide a durable reconstruction. Another problem with arthrodesis is that some form of immobilization is required postoperatively until bone union occurs. Large spica casts, such as those used for hip arthrodesis in adults, can create considerable hardship for the patient. As a result, most surgeons now tend to reserve arthrodesis as a salvage procedure, especially after deep infection.

**RESECTION ARTHROPLASTY.** Resection arthroplasty involves simply excising the cartilage and contiguous bones of a joint without reconstructing the joint. The advantage of this approach is the exact opposite of arthrodesis. Patients have motion at the expense of stability and shortening of the limb. Over time, the empty space fills in with fibrous scar tissue, and there is a limited amount of stability. Certain areas are particularly amenable to simple resection without reconstruction of bones or joints, such as the proximal fibula, clavicle, and ribs. However, for most major joints and adjacent bones, resection arthroplasty is not performed often, and function is usually better with a prosthesis or allograft. Resection arthroplasty may be appropriate in certain cases of internal hemipelvectomy where an extensive amount of pelvic and sacral bone is removed (Fig. 20B-6). Endoprosthetic replacement may not be feasible, and reconstruction with massive pelvic allografts may not be efficacious, since they have met with a high rate of infection and fracture.[55] Some patients do regain the ability to ambulate after resection arthoplasty of the hip, albeit with a cane or crutches.

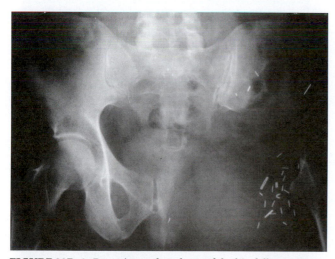

**FIGURE 20B-6.** Resection arthroplasty of the hip following internal hemipelvectomy was selected as the reconstructive option since there was only a small amount of ilium left, which could not easily accommodate a prosthesis or allograft. Comparison of the lesser trochanters reveals approximately 3 cm of shortening.

## ADJUVANT THERAPY

**CHEMOTHERAPY.** Systemic adjuvant therapy in the form of multiagent chemotherapy has been successful for some primary sarcomas of bone and has made a significant improvement in disease-free survival for these tumors. Chemotherapy is now part of the standard treatment of osteogenic sarcoma and Ewing sarcoma. There is encouraging evidence that it may be beneficial for malignant fibrous histiocytoma of bone as well. Unfortunately, other tumors continue to defy attempts at systemic treatment with traditional agents, and it seems likely that these resistant sarcomas will require new cytotoxic or biologic agents for effective systemic treatment.

**RADIATION.** Local adjuvant therapy has traditionally involved radiation treatment. It is widely believed that most sarcomas, apart from Ewing sarcoma, are resistant to radiation, but it should be stressed that resistance is a relative term, and any tissue, normal or neoplastic, becomes sensitive with a sufficiently high dose.

**OTHER FORMS OF LOCAL ADJUVANT THERAPY.** In addition to radiation, many other agents have been tried, including phenol and methylmethacrylate (bone cement), but most of these have not been found to be efficacious.[95,96] One notable exception is liquid nitrogen (cryosurgery), which has been shown to be effective in a number of settings (Fig. 20B-7). It has been used most often in the treatment of aggressive benign bone tumors such as aneurysmal bone cyst and giant cell tumor,[97–100] but has also been used for low-grade chondrosarcoma.[101] Cryosurgery extends the margin of surgical excision by a variable amount in bone, depending on the duration of the freeze, the temperature attained, and the number of cycles of freeze-thawing. Typically a zone of necrosis of 1 to 3 cm is generated in bone, and both normal and neoplastic cells are destroyed. The use of cryosurgery is particularly useful in intralesional procedures. Since many sarcomas are not particularly responsive to chemotherapy or radiation, cryosurgery may be the most effective local adjuvant therapy currently available for these tumors. It is important during cryosurgery to protect normal tissues and to prevent gas embolism by providing a vent for the nitrogen to escape.

## OSTEOGENIC SARCOMA

### INTRODUCTION

Osteogenic sarcoma (osteosarcoma) is the most common of the primary bone sarcomas. Tumor registries indicate that the incidence is 2 to 3 per million people per year, and approximately 600 to 800 cases occur every year in the United States. Males are favored by a ratio of about 3:2. The most commonly affected sites are the distal femur, proximal tibia, and proximal humerus. The peak incidence is in the adolescent years, but a second peak occurs in advanced age.[102]

It is likely that osteogenic sarcoma comprises several distinct disorders with different etiologies and outcomes. Primary, high-grade (so-called conventional) osteogenic sarcoma is the most common type and is characterized by an aggressive, rapidly growing tumor that usually arises in the medullary cavity (Figs. 20B-8, 20B-9). Secondary osteogenic sarcoma develops in the setting of a previous bone

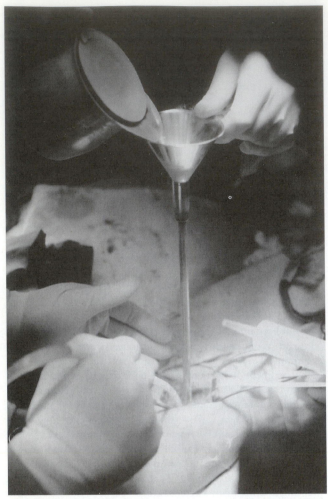

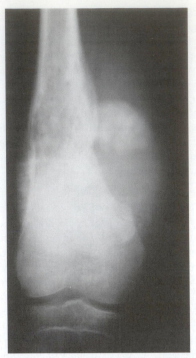

**FIGURE 20B-8.** Osteoblastic osteogenic sarcoma of the distal femur. An osteoblastic lesion in the distal metaphysis of the femur of a skeletally immature person is the classic radiographic presentation of osteogenic sarcoma.

**FIGURE 20B-7.** Intraoperative application of liquid nitrogen is most commonly performed with a funnel and a special insulated vessel to pour the liquid nitrogen. Note the wide exposure with retraction of the skin and soft tissues. Suction of the condensation and vapors is essential for visualization. One assistant has an irrigation bulb ready to irrigate normal tissue that might come in contact with liquid nitrogen.

disorder, such as Paget's disease, bone infarct, fibrous dysplasia, or prior radiation. Secondary osteogenic sarcoma is rare in young patients, but in patients over 60 years of age, it accounts for over half of the cases.[103] These high-grade tumors have a poor prognosis and do not respond well to adjuvant therapy.[104] Primary, low-grade, intramedullary osteogenic sarcoma is a rare variant that is well differentiated and has a low potential for metastasis.[105,106] The tumor can transform into high-grade osteogenic sarcoma, especially after local recurrence. Unlike most low-grade osteogenic sarcomas, it arises from within the medullary canal.

*Parosteal osteogenic sarcoma* is a term used in the past to designate a tumor arising directly adjacent to but distinct from the external surface of a bone. The most common location for the tumor is on the posterior aspect of the distal femur. The majority of tumors

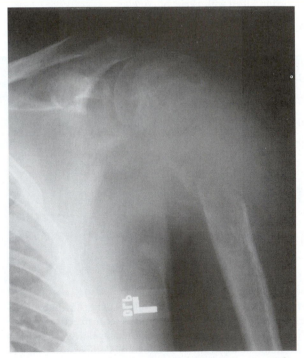

**FIGURE 20B-9.** Telangiectatic osteogenic sarcoma can produce a lytic lesion with little ossification.

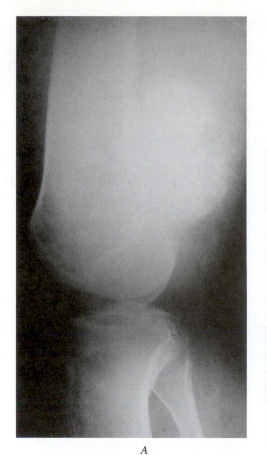
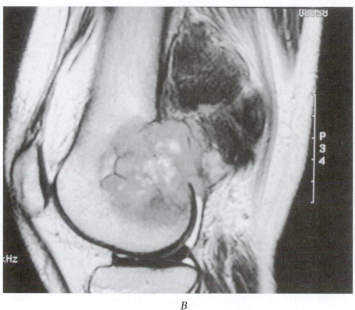

*A*                                                                 *B*

**FIGURE 20B-10.** High-grade juxtacortical osteogenic sarcoma. *A*. Plain radiograph shows a tumor on the posterior aspect of the femur, which is a classic location for juxtacortical osteogenic sarcomas. *B*. MRI demonstrates that the tumors in this location are not always low grade. The lesion has eroded into the medullary canal of the femur and was subsequently proved to be high grade.

are low-grade and have a favorable prognosis, but some are high-grade and metastasize rapidly.[107,108] In addition, invasion of the medullary canal can occur with both low- and high-grade tumors (Fig. 20B-10). The variability in behavior makes the term parosteal osteogenic sarcoma dangerous and unsatisfactory. Since it has historically been associated with well-differentiated lesions amenable to excision only, the unsuspecting physician may render inadequate treatment for the rare high-grade tumor. To avoid any ambiguity, the term *parosteal* should be abandoned in favor of *juxtacortical* or *surface osteogenic sarcoma,* which should be further designated as high or low grade.[107,109,110] Low-grade osteogenic sarcomas of all varieties should not receive chemotherapy.

*Periosteal osteogenic sarcoma* is another variant of osteogenic sarcoma that likewise should be renamed and included in the group of juxtacortical osteogenic sarcomas. Historically, periosteal osteogenic sarcoma referred to a lesion arising from the diaphyseal cortex or periosteum. The distinctive feature of the tumor is a prominent cartilaginous component, which occasionally makes differentiation from chondrosarcoma difficult.[111,112] Most lesions are usually intermediate in grade, and the overall prognosis is better than conventional

high-grade osteogenic sarcoma. However, like parosteal osteogenic sarcomas, these tumors have great variability in behavior. They may be low-grade or high-grade, and they may or may not involve the intramedullary canal. In the past, such variability has led to confusion over proper treatment, and it would therefore seem best to discard the term *periosteal osteogenic sarcoma* in favor of *juxtacortical* or *surface osteogenic sarcoma,* which should be qualified as either high or low grade.

The genetic basis of osteogenic sarcoma is complicated and only beginning to be understood.[113] Unlike Ewing sarcoma, there is no characteristic chromosomal translocation. Complex karyotypes are present in most tumors,[114] and one study found diploid tumors in only 2 out of 9 tumors.[115] Ring chromosomes have been noted in a substantial number of cases of juxtacortical osteogenic sarcoma.[116]

An important observation is that patients with hereditary retinoblastoma are at increased risk of developing osteogenic sarcoma. These patients have a germline mutation in the tumor suppressor Rb gene and have only one copy of a normal, functional Rb gene. A subsequent point mutation in this normal gene is the key genetic event that leads to retinoblastoma in the eye. The same "two-hit hypothesis" presumably applies to the development of osteogenic sarcoma in the extremities. In patients without hereditary retinoblastoma, it has been postulated that inactivation of the Rb gene through different mutational mechanisms may be important to the pathogenesis of osteogenic sarcoma. Indeed, perturbations of the Rb gene have been found in a significant proportion of patients, and one study identified mutations in 8 of 23 tumors.[117] Disruption of Rb-mediated regulation of the cell cycle may occur in as many as 80% of high-grade sarcomas.[118]

Patients with the Li-Fraumeni syndrome also have an increased risk of developing osteogenic sarcoma. These patients have a germline mutation in p53, another tumor suppressor gene. The LiFraumeni syndrome is rare, and analysis of 235 osteogenic sarcoma patients showed that only 3% had germline mutations in p53.[119] However, similar to the Rb gene, inactivation of p53 can occur through different mechanisms, and thus it has been estimated that up to 50% of osteogenic sarcomas may have perturbations of p53.[120–123] One mechanism of inactivation is the amplification of the MDM2 oncogene, which binds to p53 and suppresses its function.[124] The role of p53 in the development of osteogenic sarcoma is supported by experimental work in animals. Knockout mice with deficient p53 have a markedly increased incidence of osteogenic sarcoma.[125,126]

Mutations in Rb and p53 cannot fully explain the pathogenesis of osteogenic sarcoma, since there are tumors and cell lines without mutations of these genes. Genetic perturbations of other tumor suppressor genes, such as p16 and p21, may be important, and a putative tumor suppressor gene is believed to be present on chromosome 3q.[127,128] Dominantly acting oncogenes may also be involved. Osteogenic sarcoma cell lines express a variety of oncogenes, including *ras, met,* (hepatocyte growth factor receptor), and *sis* (platelet-derived growth factor).[129–132] The *myc* oncogene is sporadically amplified in osteogenic sarcoma.[133–135] Expression of the erbB oncogene (epidermal growth factor receptor) was found to be present in 42% of patients,[136] and transforming growth factor β (TGF-β) has been detected in 25 of 25 high-grade osteosarcomas, and the subtypes may have prognostic significance.[137] The v-*fos* oncogene was discovered in murine retroviruses that induced osteogenic sarcomas,[138] and overexpression of the related c-*fos* gene was found by immunohistochemical assay in 61% of human osteogenic sarcomas.[139] Finally, the SV40 virus, which contains SV40 large T antigen, is known to produce osteogenic sarcomas in hamsters and other rodents.[140]

Although the research on oncogenes has provided many tantalizing clues, there is still no clear picture of how osteogenic sarcoma develops. Since the pathogenesis is not completely understood, only limited preventive measures can be recommended at this time. Minimizing exposure to ionizing radiation is a worthy general principle, but the risk of developing osteogenic sarcoma does not rise significantly until the dose exceeds 30 Gy.[103,141] Radiation of benign bone tumors, however, may produce osteogenic sarcoma at markedly increased rates, and this should be done only under exceptional circumstances.[142,143] Patients with familial cancer syndromes such as hereditary retinoblastoma and the Li-Fraumeni syndrome should receive genetic counseling and be followed regularly. Patients with certain abnormalities of bone, such as Paget's disease, previous radiation treatment, fibrous dysplasia, or bone infarct may also benefit from periodic follow-up.

## CLINICAL MANIFESTATIONS

Most patients come to attention because of persistent pain at the affected site. Pathologic fracture is an uncommon but dramatic presentation. A deep, firm, fixed mass may be appreciated by some patients, but swelling may be subtle, especially in areas such as the thigh where there is substantial soft tissue covering the lesion. The tumor may produce relatively mild symptoms that are frequently ascribed to minor injuries, especially in active children.

Examination demonstrates tenderness of the bone directly over the lesion. Measurement of the girth of the limb typically shows an increase in circumference. Warmth, erythema, and occasionally bruits can be appreciated with highly vascular tumors, such as telangiectatic osteogenic sarcoma.

## DIAGNOSIS

On plain radiographs classic high-grade osteogenic sarcoma produces a striking osteoblastic lesion. In children, there are few clinical entities that can mimic this picture, and the diagnosis is strongly suggested by the radiographs. The lesion usually arises in the metaphysis of a long bone and grows outward from the medullary canal. The tumor displays typical features of a malignant lesion, including a permeative growth pattern, poorly defined borders, and erosion through the cortex.

It is important to stress that the radiographic appearance can be quite varied, and the classic features are often absent.[144] Certain histologic subtypes, such as the telangiectatic, and small cell variants, may produce purely lytic lesions in bone with little or no ossified matrix (see Fig. 20B-9). For this reason, lytic lesions of bone should not be diagnosed automatically as "bone cysts." On the contrary, permeative, destructive lesions in children must include osteogenic sarcoma in the differential diagnosis.

CT and MRI scans are not as helpful as plain radiographs in establishing the diagnosis of osteogenic sarcoma, but these studies provide anatomic information that is important for surgical planning. MRI is excellent for imaging lesions in the marrow, which is useful for determining the level of resection, screening for skip lesions, and determining whether there is invasion of the medullary canal by juxtacortical tumors. Penetration of the physeal cartilage and involvement of the epiphysis occurs frequently and is readily demonstrated on MRI but may not be evident on plain radiographs.

## HISTOLOGY

The essential histologic feature of osteogenic sarcoma is the production of osteoid by malignant spindle-shaped cells, which must be directly adjacent to osteoid without any intervening, normal osteoblasts lining the osteoid. However, in addition to the osteoblastic areas, there may be other areas showing varying degrees of cartilage, fibrous tissue, vascular spaces, and sheets of small round cells. The histologic subtypes of primary high-grade osteogenic sarcoma (osteoblastic, chondroblastic, fibroblastic, telangiectatic, and small cell variants) are determined by which type of tissue predominates. The prognostic significance of the different histologic subtypes is uncertain, and there has not been demonstrated a significant difference in survival based upon these subtypes.

In high-grade osteogenic sarcoma, the malignant cells are pleomorphic with large, hyperchromatic nuclei, and mitotic figures are frequent. In contrast, low-grade osteogenic sarcoma is characterized by a paucity of pleomorphic cells and mitotic figures. Although osteoid is present, there are areas of well-differentiated bone, which can make the distinction from heterotopic ossification (myositis ossificans) difficult, especially when the tumor arises in a juxtacortical location. The key to diagnosis is the identification of foci of clearly malignant, neoplastic cells. In addition, heterotopic ossification may demonstrate a zonation phenomenon with more mature, ossified matrix on the periphery, whereas tumors tend to be more immature on the periphery.

The histologic diagnosis of osteogenic sarcoma can be difficult. Fracture callus, especially in the setting of a pathologic fracture through a fibrous tumor, can masquerade as osteogenic sarcoma. The production of osteoid may be minimal in some cases of osteogenic sarcoma, and its presence may be difficult to detect since there are no stains that unequivocally establish its presence. Consequently, telangiectatic osteogenic sarcoma may be mistaken for aneurysmal bone cyst; small cell osteogenic sarcoma may appear to be a round cell tumor such as Ewing's sarcoma; and chondroblastic osteogenic sarcoma may be confused with chondrosarcoma. As currently conceived, osteogenic sarcoma has heterogeneous genetic and morphologic profiles. Osteogenic sarcoma may actually be a constellation of disorders that have similar clinical patterns of disease. Molecular diagnosis and staging promises to subclassify the disease and direct targeted therapy.

## STAGING

The Musculoskeletal Tumor Society staging system, as described above, is the most widely used staging system. This appropriately recognizes stage I lesions as low-grade tumors, which have a much different behavior and prognosis than stage II or III lesions. However, these low-grade tumors are relatively uncommon, and the majority of tumors fall into the category of stage IIb. As a result, the current staging system does not differentiate between subsets of patients that may have markedly different prognosis with current methods of treatment, and more work needs to be done to improve stratification of patients for chemotherapy and other treatment protocols.

A number of factors have been found to have possible prognostic importance besides those currently used for staging. The site of the tumor is important. Axial and pelvic tumors fare worse than tumors of the extremities. This may be related to the difficulty in achieving negative surgical margins. Elevation of alkaline phosphatase level above 400 and lactose dehydrogenase (LDH) level above 400 have both been shown to be independent predictors of an unfavorable outcome.[145–147] Race was found to be important in one study, with blacks having a worse outcome.[145] Secondary osteogenic sarcomas, especially when associated with radiation or Paget's disease, have a worse prognosis. A displaced pathologic fracture through the lesion is associated with decreased survival. Skip lesions, which may represent bone-to-bone metastases, have been associated with a poor prognosis.[148,149] Although one early study reported that 25% of all

patients had skip lesions,[148] other studies indicate that this is an uncommon event, affecting fewer than 5% of patients.[150–155]

Staging studies should include chest x-ray and CT, since the lungs are the most common site of metastasis. A technetium bone scan screens for bony metastases, which are the second most common site of metastasis, as well as skip lesions. Thallium scans are useful for monitoring disease activity, response to chemotherapy, and distant metastases.[156–161] Of the laboratory tests, particular attention should be paid to the alkaline phosphatase and LDH levels.

## TREATMENT

For low-grade osteogenic sarcoma, whether intramedullary or juxtacortical, wide surgical excision alone is the treatment of choice, and the overall survival is estimated to be greater than 90% in studies with at least 5-year follow-up.[105,107,162–165] Intralesional and marginal excisions are inadequate, and local recurrence rates range from 50% to 100% with such treatment.[164,166–168] Adjuvant chemotherapy is not indicated for these patients, but they should have regular, periodic long-term follow-up for systemic and local relapse.

For high-grade osteogenic sarcoma, surgical excision of the primary tumor must be combined with adjuvant chemotherapy. Historical data indicate that survival is less than 20% with amputation alone.[169–171] It is noteworthy that limb-sparing surgery is now possible for the majority of patients as a result of improvements in surgical technique and adjuvant therapy. However, it is still vitally important that an oncologically sound operation be performed. The prognostic factors for local recurrence include both surgical margin and response to chemotherapy. There is a high rate of recurrence with marginal excision, especially in patients with unfavorable responses to chemotherapy.[172] With intralesional procedures, there is an even higher rate of recurrence. The development of a local recurrence bodes poorly for the patient, and the 5-year survival rate is only 11%.[173]

In a combined review of osteogenic sarcoma of the distal femur, Rougraff et al.[174] reported that the rate of local recurrence was 0% for hip disarticulation, 7.8% for transfemoral amputation, and 11% for limb-sparing surgery.[174] The German group reported local recurrence of 2.2% for amputation or rotationplasty in contrast to 11.1% for limb-sparing procedures.[175] The group at the Rizzoli Institute found that local recurrence was 0% for rotationplasty and radical amputation, 8% for wide amputation, and 10% for limb-sparing surgery.[173] Poor responders to chemotherapy who had narrow surgical margins suffered local recurrence in 20% of cases. Taken together, these studies indicate that amputation is more likely to control local disease than limb-sparing surgery. An important question is whether this may affect survival. In the study by Rougraff et al.,[174] there was no statistical difference in overall survival despite the difference in local control. One interpretation of the data is that local recurrence does not affect survival. It is known that microscopic, undetectable pulmonary metastasis is already present in most patients at the time of diagnosis. Patients who do not respond to chemotherapy will die from these metastases, regardless of whether they develop local recurrence. An alternative view is that the power of current studies is not sufficient to detect a small difference in survival. It should be stressed that there is selection bias in determining which patients undergo amputation. There are no randomized surgical trials, and it is likely that the larger, more advanced tumors are treated by amputation. Since overall survival is still the same, the possibility exists that there may be a slight survival advantage for amputation. One study with 46 patients found that survival was 62% for amputation compared to 55% for limb-sparing surgery, but the result was not statistically significant.[176] In the 1980 Cooperative Osteosarcoma Study Group (COSS study), 26% of patients undergoing wide excision developed pulmonary metastases compared to 13% of patients having amputation, but again the difference was not statistically significant.[177] Although not conclusive, these results should encourage the surgeon to exercise caution and restraint. It is important to resist the temptation to extend the indications for limb-sparing surgery to situations where it may not be appropriate.

Surgical excision of metastatic lesions can be beneficial for some patients. Patients that present with metastatic disease have a poor prognosis, with only 11% surviving at 5 years.[178] However, with aggressive treatment, including resection of pulmonary metastases and intensive chemotherapy, survival can be extended for most patients and some patients cured. Bacci et al.[179] reported that 10 of 23 patients were continuously disease free at a mean of 30 months,[179] and Tabone et al.[180] reported a 27% event-free survival rate at 3 years.[180] Complete resection of recurrences seems to be the most important factor for a successful outcome.

Although radiation therapy was commonly used prior to the era of modern chemotherapy, it is no longer part of the standard treatment of primary tumors. Since a high rate of local control has been achieved with limb-sparing surgery alone, the addition of radiation with its attendant complications is not warranted. Osteogenic sarcoma requires high doses of radiation to be effective. At 60 Gy, the response is inconsistent. At doses of 70 to 80 Gy tumoricidal effects become more pronounced, but damage to normal surrounding tissues increases substantially as well.[181-185] Even with high doses of radiation and chemotherapy, it has been found that areas of viable tumor are still present, and thus radiation alone is not suitable as primary treatment for most tumors.[186] However, certain lesions in problematic areas, such as the craniofacial region or spine, may be difficult to excise with wide margins, and radiation may be employed as an adjuvant to surgery or occasionally as primary treatment.[187,188] Adjuvant radiation therapy may also be of benefit in cases of displaced pathologic fracture that are treated with limb-preserving surgery.

## ADJUVANT THERAPY

In most cases of high-grade osteogenic sarcoma, microscopic metastatic disease already exists at the time of diagnosis, and systemic adjuvant chemotherapy is required to eradicate these deposits. Although many advances have been made in the use of chemotherapy, the effectiveness of chemotherapeutic is not such that they could be used without surgery, and the survival rate is less than 25% with chemotherapy alone.[189] From a historical point of view, it is notable that whole lung irradiation is not effective adjuvant therapy for micrometastatic pulmonary disease.[190]

There was initial skepticism and resistance to the idea of adjuvant chemotherapy, and many believed that osteogenic sarcoma was unresponsive to chemotherapy.[191] The response rate to single-agent therapy in various phase II trials was only 0% to 33%.[192] Several randomized studies settled the issue definitively. These had to be terminated prematurely because of the poor survival in the surgery-only arm of the trial.[7,193]

An important principle that is illustrated by osteogenic sarcoma is that chemotherapeutic agents do not have an all-or-none effect. This may have relevance for other cancers and sarcomas that are currently considered to be unresponsive to chemotherapy. When administered with sufficiently high dose intensity and in the right combination, the agents can be effective. Moreover, a positive adjuvant effect can be demonstrated even in patients who do not have an ostensible clinical response to chemotherapy.

A seminal finding by Jaffe in 1972 was that high-dose methotrexate (HDMTX) with leucovorin rescue could result in regression of pulmonary metastases.[194] This observation led to the demonstration that HDMTX could increase survival when used in an adjuvant setting after excision of stage II (nonmetastatic) tumors.[195,196] HDMTX has since been used in most protocols for osteogenic sarcoma and continues to be a major component of current multiagent regimens.

The success of HDMTX-based regimens is critically dependent on a sufficiently high dose of methotrexate.[175,177,197] The term "high dose" has been used loosely in the past, and numerous trials that failed to see a positive effect may have employed insufficient amounts of the medication.[198-200] The range of doses that is considered high dose is 8 to 12 $g/m^2$, but children generally require doses at the high end of the spectrum (12 $g/m^2$).[201,202] Rosen[201] made the important observation that some tumors did not respond with an initial dose of 200 mg/kg (approximately 8 $g/m^2$) of methotrexate but subsequently showed a dramatic complete response when the dose was escalated to 12 $g/m^2$ or more.[201]

Several agents in addition to HDMTX were subsequently found to have efficacy, most notably doxorubicin (Adriamycin)[203,204] and cisplatin.[205-207] Mosende and Rosen[208] reported that the combination of bleomycin, cyclophosphamide, and dactinomycin (BCD) was effective against metastatic disease and employed this combination in institutional and national protocols.[208] Recent sentiment has been to delete these less-active agents in favor of intensification of more active agents.

The results of multiple studies indicate that multiagent adjuvant chemotherapy is superior to single-agent adjuvant therapy. Rosenberg et al.[209] found that HDMTX alone gave only a 38% survival rate at 2 years, and Cortes et al.[204] reported only 39% survival with doxorubicin alone.[204] Most series employing multiagent chemotherapy have reported 5-year disease-free survival rates in the range of 55% to 76%.[145,189,198,210-213]

The T4, 5, 7, 10, and 12 protocols, used previously at Memorial Sloan-Kettering, resulted collectively in a 65% disease-free 5-year survival rate for 279 patients with stage II (nonmetastatic) disease.[145] After 13 years of follow-up there has not been further deterioration of results. This series of protocols was based primarily on HDMTX and doxorubicin, which were used in conjunction with a number of other agents, starting with cyclophosphamide in T4 and T5, then BCD in T7, and finally BCD with cisplatin for poor responders in T10 and T12. It is noteworthy that for the subset of 104 patients aged 21 years or less with a primary tumor in the extremity (i.e., classic osteogenic sarcoma in a young patient), a disease-free survival rate

**TABLE 20B-3.** SELECTED MAJOR SERIES OF ADJUVANT CHEMOTHERAPY IN OSTEOGENIC SARCOMA

| STUDY | YEAR | AGENTS | 5-YR SURVIVAL RATE* | NO. OF PATIENTS | NOTES |
|---|---|---|---|---|---|
| MD Anderson TIOS I, III[189] | 1990 | CDP, HDMTX, Dox, Cy | 57% | 90 | Pre-op intra-arterial CDP |
| Memorial Sloan-Kettering[145] | 1992 | HDMTX, Dox, BCD, CDP | 65% | 279 | Protocols T4, T5, T7, T10, T12 |
| Rizzoli Institute[366] | 1993 | HDMTX, Dox, intra-arterial CDP, [Ifos/etop] | 63% | 164 | Ifos/etop given to poor responders |
| MIOS[193] | 1986 | HDMTX, Dox, BCD, CDP | 66% at 2 yr | 36 | Randomized +/− chemo. |
| COSS80[177] | 1984 | HDMTX, Dox, BCD vs CDP, +/− interferon | 68% at 30 mo. | 116 | No difference: BCD vs. CDP |
| CALGB[203] | 1978 | Dox | 39% | 88 | Single agent |

*Disease-free or continuously disease-free survival.
ABBREVIATIONS: HDMTX = high-dose methotrexate; Dox = doxorubicin; CDP = cis-platin; Cy = cyclophosphamide; BCD = bleomycin, cyclophosphamide, dactinomycin; Ifos/etop = ifosfamide/etoposide.

of 76% at 5 years was achieved, and the survival rate did not diminish significantly at 10 years. The survival rate is worse for older patients, who are more likely to have secondary osteogenic sarcoma in difficult locations such as the pelvis.

Although the protocols used at Memorial Sloan-Kettering were quite successful, the search for more effective combinations of chemotherapy continues, and a summary of some of the major series is shown in Table 20B-3. It is important to note that it is not possible simply to add more drugs to current regimens since this will compromise the dose intensity of the most active agents.[201,214,215] Thus, there have been attempts to substitute certain agents for others. In particular, the efficacy of BCD has been questioned.[216] In the COSS 82 trial, cisplatin was compared with BCD. Although the response to preoperative chemotherapy seemed to favor cisplatin, there was no difference in survival.[213] The following COSS 86 trial achieved a 68% disease-free survival rate with HDMTX, doxorubicin, and cisplatin while eliminating BCD.[212] The results were comparable to the results obtained previously at Memorial Sloan-Kettering.

A large CCG/POG study, which has recently finished accrual, is also based on HDMTX, doxorubicin, and cisplatin. The study includes a double randomization of two agents, ifosfamide and muramyl tripeptide phosphoethanolamine (MTP-PE). High-dose ifosfamide has been found to be active in phase II trials,[217,218] and one group reported a high percentage of good chemotherapeutic responses when it was given preoperatively.[175] MTP-PE is the active agent of BCG and represents a form of biologic therapy. MTP-PE activates monocytes and macrophages and induces them to become tumoricidal. Since it is not a traditional cytotoxic agent and has minimal side effects, it should not compromise the dose intensity of the more conventional chemotherapeutic agents. MTP-PE has been shown to be effective in a randomized, double-blinded study in dogs.[219]

Several aspects of chemotherapy are relevant to surgical treatment and worthy of comment. In most series, chemotherapy for osteogenic sarcoma has included a preoperative, so-called neoadjuvant phase. There are many benefits of preoperative chemotherapy: It immediately treats micrometastatic disease; it provides a safety margin for resection, and may permit potentially less resection of normal tissue if there is a significant response; and it allows time for surgical planning, manufacture of custom prostheses, and procurement of allografts. Nevertheless, in spite of these advantages, a clear survival benefit has not been demonstrated for neoadjuvant therapy.[145]

One of the advantages of preoperative chemotherapy is the ability to assess the histologic response to chemotherapy in the surgical specimen. Various scoring systems exist for determining the histologic response.[216,220] The one currently used at Memorial Sloan-Kettering for histologic response is modified from Huvos' original description and includes four grades: grade I, 0% to 50% necrosis; grade II, 51% to 90% necrosis; grade III, 91% to 99% necrosis; and grade IV, 100% necrosis (Fig. 20B-11).[221,222] Patients with a grade III or IV response to chemotherapy have significantly higher disease-free survival at 5 years than patients with grade I or II response.[145] However, it should be noted that the response to preoperative chemotherapy is highly dependent on which agents are used and the length of neoadjuvant therapy. Single-agent neoadjuvant therapy may result in a poor response for most patients, but subsequent multiagent chemotherapy may result in a higher percentage of survivors.[223] Conversely, a long period of preoperative chemotherapy may result in a high percentage of "good responders," but the rate of survival may be much less.[224]

Conceptually, an attractive idea is to administer different agents postoperatively if a patient does not respond well to the preoperative agents. This "tailoring" of chemotherapy unfortunately has not resulted in improved survival for patients that do not respond well.[145,213] Nevertheless, the idea is still appealing and investigators continue to try to devise therapeutic approaches based upon the response to initial chemotherapy. It should be emphasized that even though certain patients may not show a dramatic response to preoperative chemotherapy, there is still a survival advantage to receiving adjuvant chemotherapy. In the study from Memorial Sloan-Kettering, the patients with a grade I or II (i.e., minimal) chemotherapeutic response still had better survival than historic controls of patients who received surgery only. Moreover, there was not a statistical difference in survival between grade II and grade III chemotherapy response, which reflects the fact that there is a continuum in the responsiveness and effectiveness of chemotherapy. Thus,

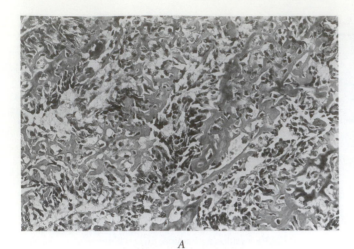

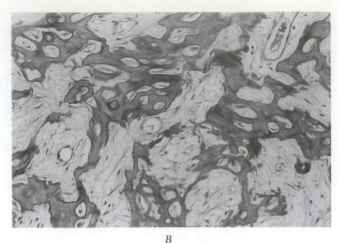

*A*                                                    *B*

**FIGURE 20B-11.** High-grade osteogenic sarcoma. A grade III chemotherapy effect is demonstrated. *A.* Biopsy of the specimen prior to administration of chemotherapy shows pleomorphic, hyperchromatic cells producing abundant osteoid. *B.* After induction chemotherapy and excision of the tumor, widespread necrosis is seen. The marrow is fibrotic with few viable cells. Empty lacunae, or "empty turtle shells," are frequent. Occasional nuclei, representing viable cells, are seen in nuclei (arrow). This photomicrograph demonstrates how chemotherapy could induce massive cell death and yet not affect the extracellular matrix. Thus, it is often observed clinically that the size of a tumor on x-ray or CT scan does not diminish despite an excellent histologic response to chemotherapy.

---

chemotherapy should not be abandoned if there is not a grade III or IV response. On the contrary, the patients with a grade I or II response are precisely the ones who require the most diligence and perseverance in achieving maximum dose intensity. Deviations from protocol and delays in resumption of chemotherapy after surgery were noted to result in decreased survival for these patients.[145]

There was initially some interest in administering chemotherapy intraarterially to deliver high doses to the primary tumor.[207] Although impressive necrosis of the primary tumor was produced, particularly with cisplatin, the rates of local recurrence, disease-free survival, and overall survival have not been shown to be superior to conventional intravenous administration of chemotherapy.[189,212,224–226] This is not surprising, since most deaths from osteogenic sarcoma occur as a result of distant pulmonary metastasis rather than local spread. Since intraarterial chemotherapy is considerably more time-consuming and difficult to give than intravenous chemotherapy, most centers now do not routinely employ this route of drug delivery. However, intraarterial chemotherapy may be valuable in certain cases where the risk of local recurrence is perceived to be high after limb-sparing surgery, such as in the setting of a displaced pathologic fracture. The local therapeutic effects may be further intensified by regional limb perfusion, which permits very high doses to be achieved in the tumor while limiting systemic toxicity. This complex intervention is done in the operating room with the limb under tourniquet. At present, it remains an investigative procedure and is not indicated for most patients.

Future directions for adjuvant therapy include the use of biologic modifiers and other means to increase the therapeutic window for traditional chemotherapeutic agents. Two examples already in use

are granulocyte colony-stimulating factor (GCSF) and granulocyte-macrophage colony-stimulating factor (GMCSF), which are used to treat neutropenia and facilitate dose intensification of cytotoxic agents that are limited by bone marrow suppression. There is also much interest in the development of cardioprotective agents, which may allow greater doses of doxorubicin to be administered. Similarly, isolated lung perfusion may permit extremely high doses of doxorubicin to be achieved in pulmonary metastases while limiting cardiac and systemic toxicity.

Understanding the mechanisms of drug resistance is of paramount importance. The role of the multidrug resistance genes, p-glycoprotein, dihydrofolate reductase amplification, and other processes are being actively investigated. It is important to note that drug resistance may not be limited to proteins within the cell. There may also be problems with delivering drugs to the cell and across the cell membrane. Preliminary experimental work indicates that all of these mechanisms are operative to some degree. A full understanding of drug resistance will be crucial to the development of strategies to enhance the effectiveness of current cytotoxic drugs.

Although dose intensification of chemotherapy is important, equally important in the long run are efforts aimed at reducing dosage. The morbidity and mortality associated with current multi-agent protocols is significant. Stratification of patients must become more sophisticated, and the intensity of chemotherapeutic regimens must be tailored better to the patients' prognosis and expected outcome. It should be remembered that surgery alone cures 15% to 20% of patients and those patients must be identified and spared the ravages of chemotherapy. In addition, the development of biologically based, noncytotoxic therapies will become increasingly important.

MTP-PE is one step in this direction and represents an attempt at immunotherapy. Although previous attempts with interferon and BCG were not successful,[177,227] preliminary data indicate that other agents that augment the immune response, such as interleukin 2 (IL-2), may have some effectiveness.[228] Finally, it is hoped that elucidation of the genetic mutations underlying osteogenic sarcoma will ultimately lead to gene-based therapy that can reverse these changes.[229-231]

## CHONDROSARCOMA

### INTRODUCTION

Chondrosarcoma is the second most common primary bone sarcoma and is half as common as osteosarcoma. Approximately 400 cases occur each year in the United States. All age groups may be affected, but the disease is uncommon in children and may be more aggressive in this population.[232] The peak incidence is in the fourth to sixth decades, and there is a slight male preference. Chondrosarcoma can arise in all bones, but the most common site is the pelvis followed by the proximal femur, proximal humerus, spine, and ribs.[233,234]

The cause of chondrosarcoma is unknown in most instances. Some patients develop chondrosarcoma secondary to multiple osteochondromas (exostoses) or multiple enchondromatosis. Malignant degeneration of an isolated osteochondroma is less common but can occur.[235,236] Malignant degeneration of an isolated enchondroma has been suspected but never clearly proven, since it is difficult to rule out the possibility that the lesion may have started out as a low-grade chondrosarcoma rather than an enchondroma.

The only known preventive measures consist of regular follow-up for patients with multiple exostoses, multiple enchondromas, and other cartilaginous lesions. Sudden growth and increased pain are signs of possible malignant degeneration.

### CLINICAL MANIFESTATIONS

The signs and symptoms may be subtle and persist for a long time before the patient seeks medical attention. Chondrosarcomas tend to grow slowly. In one study the mean duration of symptoms was 33 months.[237] Location in the pelvis or proximal femur may escape notice until the tumor reaches massive proportions. Although pain is often vague and mild, the presence of pain is an important sign since it is one indication that the tumor may be growing and causing pressure within bone. This is especially important in an equivocal lesion that may be difficult to distinguish from enchondroma.

### DIAGNOSIS

The diagnosis of chondrosarcoma can be difficult. Perhaps in no other tumor is the close collaboration between clinical specialties so crucial to making the correct diagnosis. The ultimate test of course is the behavior of the tumor over time. Experience has shown that certain cartilaginous tumors—synovial chondromatosis, enchondromas of the digits—behave as benign tumors, but these lesions may have the exact same histologic appearance as low-grade chon-

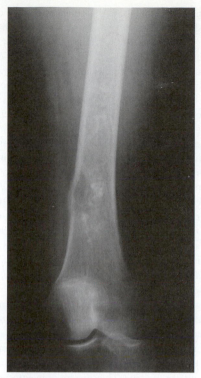

**FIGURE 20B-12.** Chondrosarcoma of the femur. The cartilage in the intramedullary canal is revealed by the small calcifications. Although this appearance is similar to many enchondromas, the small focal area of cortical erosion suggests a more aggressive lesion, and the lytic area adjacent to the erosion raises the possibility of an area of rapid growth and dedifferentiation.

drosarcomas. Therefore, the diagnosis should incorporate not only microscopic findings but other important data, such as the radiographic appearance, location of the tumor, age of the patient, symptoms, and growth over time.

Radiographically, cartilaginous matrix usually produces popcorn or ring calcifications, but not all cartilage becomes calcified (Fig. 20B-12). In fact, it is more important to pay attention to lytic and lucent areas, which may signify a highly cellular, less differentiated, and more aggressive part of the tumor. Enchondromas and low-grade chondrosarcomas tend to remain within bone, but higher-grade lesions produce cortical erosion, which is best demonstrated on CT scans. Unlike normal cartilage, which is dark on MRI scans, the cartilage of tumors, whether benign or malignant, is characteristically bright on T2-weighted images. MRI is better for showing the extent of the lesion than plain radiographs and CT, which may not adequately demonstrate noncalcified portions of the tumor.

### HISTOLOGY

The characteristic feature of all chondrosarcomas is the production of a cartilaginous matrix by malignant cells. Classic chondrosarcoma is a purely cartilaginous lesion, whereas other histologic variants may show differentiation along other lines in certain areas. Chondrosarcoma has traditionally been divided into low, intermediate, and high grades. Low-grade tumors (grade I) are characterized by the presence of double-nucleated chondrocytes in a lacuna, occasional atypical cells with some variation in size and shape, and mild myxoid or cystic changes. Cellular atypia must be interpreted with caution since these changes may be due to fixation artifacts. Chondrocytes normally fill the entire lacuna, but during the process of slide preparation, the cell contracts from the edges of the lacuna, giving the illusion that there is a space between the cell and the cartilage. Some variation in cell size and shape thus occurs with all cartilaginous tissue, and this finding may not necessarily imply pleomorphism. Chondrosarcomas envelop preexisting normal bone trabeculae demonstrating their invasive character. Intermediate-grade lesions (grade II) have noticeably greater cellularity and multiple nuclei or cells in a lacuna, but maintenance of a lobular architecture. Extensive myxoid changes are seen in some intermediate-grade tumors. High-grade lesions (grade III) have greatly increased cellularity with sheetlike areas of malignant cells, loss of lobular architecture, and greater than 2 mitoses per 10 high-power fields.

The recognition of a high-grade tumor is usually not problematic. However, distinguishing a grade I chondrosarcoma from an enchondroma can be extremely difficult and may in fact be impossible with routine histologic methods. The term "grade 1/2" has sometimes been used to describe equivocal lesions, but the notion is nebulous and unsatisfying. The concept of in situ carcinoma may be apt for these low-grade lesions that have a predilection to recur locally but virtually no metastatic potential. Mirra[238] emphasized the inspection of the bony trabeculae as a possible indication of malignancy.[238] A tumor enclosed by trabeculae of normal bone suggests an enchondroma, whereas an infiltrative tumor that engulfs trabeculae of bone is more indicative of a malignant nature.

In addition to classic chondrosarcoma, there are a number of variants of chondrosarcoma. Dedifferentiated chondrosarcoma is a rare high-grade lesion that contains areas that simulate other sarcomas, such as fibrosarcoma, malignant fibrous histiocytoma, and most commonly osteogenic sarcoma. The presence of an osteogenic sarcoma–like area poses a dilemma in classification, since an argument could be made that the tumor is a chondroblastic osteogenic sarcoma. The clinical setting may provide a clue as to the true nature of the tumor. A lesion arising in the distal metaphysis of the femur in a 15-year-old would be more apt to be an osteogenic sarcoma, whereas a pelvic lesion in a 60-year-old would be more likely to be chondrosarcoma. Nevertheless, there is sufficient overlap in histologic and clinical presentation that a distinction can sometimes be difficult to make. The nomenclature is important and not merely an academic exercise since it may define what treatment a patient is eligible for.

Mesenchymal chondrosarcoma is a distinctive variant that has, in addition to classic chondrosarcomatous areas, a small cell component without a clear pattern of differentiation. The small cell portion may mimic Ewing sarcoma or may exhibit a vascular pattern reminiscent of hemangiopericytoma.[239] Often the two areas are present to varying degrees in the same tumor.[240] These tumors may be intermediate or high grade.

Myxoid chondrosarcoma is characterized by abundant myxoid stroma. When it occurs in soft tissue it is associated with a 9;22

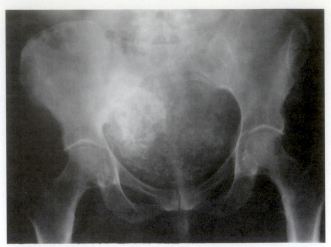

**FIGURE 20B-13.** A massive secondary chondrosarcoma filling the pelvis has arisen from an osteochondroma. The cartilage of the tumor is manifested by the "popcorn" calcifications.

translocation involving the EWS and CHN genes. However, with the possible exception of one case report,[241] the lesions in bone do not carry this translocation and probably represent a different pathologic entity.

Clear cell chondrosarcoma is a rare low-grade tumor distinguished by clear cells with prominent boundaries. Although the appearance may resemble chondroblastoma in areas, clear cell chondrosarcoma is a malignant tumor that has a definite potential for metastasis.

Secondary chondrosarcoma may arise in a variety of settings, most commonly multiple osteochondromas (Fig. 20B-13) or enchondromas (Ollier's disease). Secondary chondrosarcomas pose special problems in diagnosis and treatment. The malignant tumor may be difficult to distinguish from the cartilaginous background, especially since the majority of the chondrosarcomas start out as low-grade lesions. Accelerated growth or an increase in the size of the cartilaginous cap is a worrisome sign, but can occur with pregnancy, lactation, and other normal conditions. It has been stated that if the size of the cap exceeds 1 cm, the tumor is much more likely to be malignant, but this dogma has never been proven.[242]

## STAGING

The three histologic grades of chondrosarcoma pose a problem in terms of staging in the MTS system, which includes only high and low grades. Although AJCC has grouped grade I and II together as low-grade lesions, an argument could be made for considering grade II and III together as high-grade lesions, since these lesions have a significantly greater potential for metastasis. In the series reported by Evans et al.,[243] the rate of metastases was 0%, 10%, and 71% for grade I, II, and III lesions, respectively.[243] Estimates of the risk of metastasis from grade I tumors range from 0% to 9%,[237,244-246] and probably vary according to the criteria used by a particular pathologist to define grade I tumors. Despite the low risk of distant metastasis, the local aggressiveness of grade I tumors should not be underestimated. In one study, patients were three times more likely to die from local progression than distant metastasis.[237]

In addition to histologic grade, there may be other tests to gauge the malignant potential of tumors. Aneuploid tumors have been reported to be associated with a worse prognosis than diploid tumors.[43] The biochemical composition of the cartilaginous matrix also varies with grade, but this has not been successfully used to distinguish benign from low-grade tumors.[247–249] It is expected that additional measures will be found in the future to define better the grade and stage of chondrosarcoma.

## TREATMENT

Some low-grade chondrosarcomas grow slowly. Untreated or undertreated lesions may be compatible with patient survival of many years; hence, survival at 5 years is not the equivalent of cure. Most large series show definite deterioration in survival between 5 to 10 years for all grades, and Springfield[233] has recommended 10 years as the appropriate minimum length of follow-up for comparative studies, as opposed to 5 years for most other tumors. Dedifferentiated chondrosarcoma is an exception, since the disease progresses rapidly and most patients succumb within the first 3 years.

The treatment of chondrosarcoma is critically dependent on surgery. There is no systemic adjuvant therapy that has been proven to be effective, and complete surgical extirpation offers the best chance for cure. It is fairly well established that the treatment of choice for intermediate- and high-grade tumors should be wide excision, since these tumors have a definite potential for metastasis. However, the treatment of grade I chondrosarcoma remains controversial because of the difficulty in distinguishing enchondroma from low-grade chondrosarcoma. A wide excision with the attendant potential loss of normal function seems excessive for what may turn out to be a benign tumor; however, a local, intralesional curettage does not seem adequate for a sarcoma. The results of intralesional curettage has varied between institutions. Ozaki et al.[250] noted that three out of three low-grade tumors treated by local curettage recurred.[250] However, Bauer et al.[244] reported only 9% local recurrence and no metastasis in a group of 23 patients. Similarly, Yasko et al.[251] found a 7.5% local recurrence rate and no metastases at M.D. Anderson. Finally, Marcove[101] reported a 95% success rate with local excision and cryosurgery, but he also noted that during routine rebiopsy that there were viable tumor cells in 4 of 20 specimens, which led to a wider excision. The results of curettage probably depend on many factors, including surgical technique, site of tumor, the use of cryosurgery or other adjuvants, and the exact definition of a grade I tumor at a particular institution. A universal recommendation cannot be made for all tumors and situations. The surgeon should pay attention to all clinical data and should always be aware of the possibility of sampling error in the biopsy specimen. If areas of intermediate- or high-grade tumor are found after an intralesional procedure, a formal wide reexcision is the most prudent course.

Chondrosarcoma is not especially responsive to radiation treatment, but it may be of benefit in difficult surgical areas such as the spine and cranium. In one study high doses of radiation were administered to patients with unresectable tumors or gross residual disease after surgery.[252] Of the 15 patients with sufficient follow-up, six tumors were controlled at least 5 years, four tumors had local control ranging from 1 to 5 years, and five tumors recurred at less than a year. Experimental work with charged particle, proton, and neutron beam radiation has provided some encouraging preliminary data for tumors arising in central areas. These forms of radiation have less scatter and less destruction of surrounding normal tissue than conventional photon beam radiation and may allow very high radiation doses (>70 Gy) to spinal and other sites. Rates of local control, usually with surgical debulking, have ranged from 50% to 78% at 5 years.[253–260]

## ADJUVANT THERAPY

Systemic adjuvant chemotherapy has not had a measurable impact on chondrosarcoma. However, it should be recognized that there are only limited data pertaining to the use of chemotherapy for chondrosarcoma. Frassica et al.[261] reported on a series of dedifferentiated chondrosarcoma and found no effect of chemotherapy, but a variety of protocols were used, and many of the patients already had metastatic disease. In contrast to this study, Huvos et al.[239] found somewhat more encouraging results for patients with mesenchymal chondrosarcoma. Patients received chemotherapy that was similar to the protocols used at Memorial Sloan-Kettering for Ewing's sarcoma or osteogenic sarcoma, depending on whether the histology was primarily small cell or hemangiopericytomatoid, respectively. Of the 11 patients who had preoperative chemotherapy, there were four complete responses, three partial responses, and four nonresponses. However, despite the encouraging histologic responses, disease-free survival for patients with localized disease at presentation was only 50% at short-term follow-up (23 to 49 months).

Several experimental agents have been proposed. $^{35}$S-sulfate is taken up preferentially by chondrocytes, which need sulfate to produce proteoglycans. However, this agent has been associated with granulocytopenia and other severe hematologic disturbances. Other agents that have been considered include retinoic acid and somatostatin, which seem to have some activity in animal studies.[262–267] Unfortunately, there has not yet been a concerted effort to test these and other agents clinically in a rigorous manner.

## EWING SARCOMA

## INTRODUCTION

Ewing sarcoma is a malignant tumor of small round cells arising in bone. The exact nature and origin of the cells has been a matter of much debate.[268,269] Ewing, who is credited with bringing attention to the disorder, preferred to call it "diffuse endothelioma of bone."[270] Others believed it was derived from skeletal mesenchyme.[271] Still others proposed that it was merely a form of metastatic neuroblastoma. As a result of recent cytogenetic and molecular studies, Ewing sarcoma is now thought to be a member of a family of tumors that includes primitive neuroectodermal tumors (PNET), peripheral neuroepithelioma, Askin's tumor of the chest wall, and extraosseous Ewing sarcoma.[269] These tumors probably arise from a neuroectodermal stem cell rather than mesenchymal tissue, but definitive proof is still lacking.

Ewing sarcoma is one-half to one-third as common as osteogenic sarcoma in the United States, but among patients less than 15 years of age, Ewing sarcoma is nearly as common as osteogenic sarcoma.[272] This reflects the fact that Ewing sarcoma has a sharper peak incidence in younger patients than osteogenic sarcoma and is rare beyond the third decade. However, the development of new cytogenetic and molecular diagnostic tools may allow the detection of more cases in the elderly that previously were ascribed to poorly differentiated round cell tumors.

The disease usually affects Caucasians and is distinctly uncommon in blacks and orientals. The male-to-female ratio is approximately 3:2.[273] The pelvis and femur are favored locations, but many other bones may be involved, including the humerus, tibia, and fibula. Primary soft tissue involvement has a predilection for the paravertebral muscles.

The etiology is related to a chromosomal translocation. In over 90% of patients, there is a reciprocal t(11;22)(q24;q12) translocation that results in a fusion of the EWS gene to the FLI-1 gene. In approximately 5% of patients there is a 21;22 translocation that fuses the EWS gene to the ERG gene, and in rare cases the EWS gene may be fused to other genes such as the E1A gene and the ETV1 gene.[274,275] The chimeric proteins function as aberrant transcription factors. It is believed that the fusion proteins activate and/or repress a set of genes and that this results in neoplastic transformation of the cell, but the critical target genes have yet to be identified.

## CLINICAL MANIFESTATIONS

Most patients complain of pain and swelling at the affected site. Growth of the tumor is rapid, and symptoms are typically present for only weeks to months. In most cases, a substantial firm mass is present, and its sudden appearance and enlargement may cause alarm in the patient. The presentation can simulate acute osteomyelitis, and some patients have constitutional symptoms of fevers, malaise, and lethargy. Pathologic fractures can occur.

## DIAGNOSIS

Ewing sarcoma has protean radiographic manifestations and is notorious for its ability to masquerade as other disorders. The most well-known finding—onionskin formation—is not consistently present. Moreover, it is not a unique attribute and can be produced by numerous other diseases, including osteomyelitis, Langerhans cell granuloma, and osteogenic sarcoma. Onionskin formation is one form of reactive periosteal bone formation. Other forms include the sunburst pattern ("hair-on-end" bone) and Codman's triangle. In all of these variations, the new bone is not made by the tumor but by the periosteum, which is elevated off the cortical bone by a rapidly expanding mass. In Codman's triangle, the mass erodes through the central portion of the onionskin laminations, leaving only the tri-

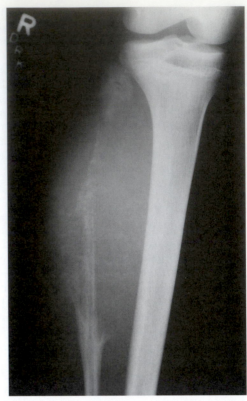

**FIGURE 20B-14.** Ewing's sarcoma is the most common primary malignant tumor of the fibula. Note the radiating spicules of reactive bone and Codman's triangle (arrow), where the periosteum is starting to lift off the bone.

angular ends on the bone. In a sunburst pattern, the central portion is filled in by spicules of new bone radiating outward perpendicular to the shaft (Figs. 20B-14, 20B-15).

Ewing sarcoma usually produces an ill-defined, lytic defect that permeates up and down the medullary canal, giving the bone a moth-eaten appearance. However, in approximately 10% of patients, the tumor may have a predominantly blastic appearance as a result of exuberant reactive bone formation. This can cause it to be confused with osteogenic sarcoma, particularly the small cell variant.[276]

An important clue that suggests the possibility of Ewing sarcoma is the presence of a large soft tissue mass adjacent to the bone. This may be subtle and difficult to appreciate on plain radiographs but becomes apparent with CT or MRI scans. In certain bones such as the pelvis, periosteal reaction is often absent radiographically, and the soft tissue mass becomes more important to making the diagnosis.

Laboratory tests may show leukocytosis with a left shift, and the erythrocyte sedimentation rate may be elevated. These findings, along with the history, examination, and radiographs, can easily deceive the clinician into thinking that the diagnosis is osteomyelitis. The serum lactate dehydrogenase (LDH) level is important to note because it is correlated to the disease burden and has prognostic importance.

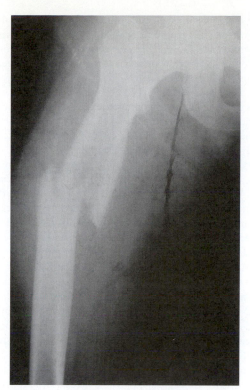

**FIGURE 20B-15.** Ewing's sarcoma of the femur. A pathologic fracture has occurred. Note the onionskin laminations, which represent another type of reactive bone formation.

## HISTOLOGY

The tumor is composed of sheets of small round blue cells with hyperchromatic nuclei. There is scant cytoplasm and little extracellular matrix. The cells are usually glycogen positive. Neural markers are occasionally present, and these can include neuron-specific enolase, CD57, neurofilaments, S100 protein, and Homer-Wright rosettes.[277]

Ewing sarcoma may be morphologically indistinguishable from other small round cell tumors, such as lymphoma of bone and metastatic neuroblastoma. Differentiation from these other entities has been facilitated in recent years by the development of the monoclonal antibodies HBA71 and O13 against Ewing sarcoma.[278] The antibodies recognize the p30/32 MIC2 protein, which was originally described as a cell surface marker of T lymphocytes.[279] The function of the MIC2 protein is not completely understood, but in T cells it is thought to be involved in cell adhesion. Immunohistochemistry with the O13 antibody is positive in most cases of Ewing sarcoma.[280–283] In a large study of 244 cases, the antibody was found to be 91% sensitive.[284] However, the antibody is not 100% specific, and it occasionally cross-reacts with lymphomas and other tumors.[285] This is not surprising since the MIC2 protein has been detected by another antibody 12E7 on most lymphoblastic lymphomas and T-cell acute lymphocytic leukemias.[285] Other tumors that occasionally bind O13 include astrocytomas, neuroectodermal tumors, mesenchymal chondrosarcoma, embryonal rhabdomyosar-

comas, and carcinomas.[280,282] It is notable that neuroblastomas have not been found to react with O13.

The development of reverse transcriptase–polymerase chain reaction (RT-PCR) has also aided the diagnosis of Ewing sarcoma by facilitating the detection of specific chromosomal translocations.[219] RT-PCR is a powerful test, and one study reported 100% sensitivity and specificity in detecting the 11;22 translocation.[286] However, other tumors besides Ewing sarcoma occasionally possess the same translocation, and one study found it in two polyphenotypic tumors and two mixed rhabdomyosarcomas.[287] Thus, like the O13 antibody, RT-PCR cannot be relied upon exclusively to make the diagnosis, and it is still important to consider all of the histologic and clinical data.

## STAGING

The staging system for Ewing sarcoma differs from the system used for most sarcomas of bone. This seems appropriate since the histogenesis of Ewing sarcoma may not be mesenchymally derived and the clinical behavior seems to differ from most sarcomas. Enneking[288] suggested four stages: stage I, solitary intraosseous tumor; stage II, solitary tumor with extraosseous extension; stage III, multicentric skeletal involvement; and stage IV, distant metastases.[288]

The staging system reflects the propensity of Ewing sarcoma to disseminate widely and early in the course of the disease. Lungs and other bones are the usual sites of metastases. A distinctive feature of Ewing sarcoma is its predilection for bone marrow involvement, which is uncommon in other sarcomas.[289] The finding carries a poor prognosis, and Meyers et al.[290] found no survivors when it was present. Bone marrow biopsy should be part of the standard staging studies for Ewing sarcoma.

## TREATMENT

Treatment of the primary tumor consists of radiation therapy, surgery, or a combination of both modalities. Historically, radiation therapy has been used most often. It was recognized by Ewing and others that the tumors are sensitive to radiation. However, survival with radiation treatment alone was less than 10%, reflecting the presence of microscopic disseminated disease at the time of diagnosis. Surgery, which usually involved amputation, produced equally poor results, and consequently, many authors condemned the use of surgery for Ewing sarcoma.[291,292]

Radiation has produced rates of local control ranging from 60% to 90%. There are a number of explanations for the wide variation in results. Techniques of radiation therapy have improved over time. Radiation in older trials may have been hampered by inadequate equipment as well as poor imaging techniques. The advent of CT and MRI has led to more accurate depiction of the tumor and better selection of radiation fields. Yet despite the advances in radiation therapy, a number of recent reports have continued to show disappointing results. A POG study found only 76% local control at 3 years,[293] while a CESS study reported only 77% local control at 5 years.[294] Recurrences have been noted to occur within radiation fields, and autopsies have demonstrated viable malignant cells in irradiated tumors. Tepper et al.[295] found live neoplastic cells in 11 of

28 primary tumors, and Telles et al.[296] found recurrent disease in 13 of 26 tumors.[296] A certain amount of selection bias was inherent in these autopsy studies since only patients who failed treatment were analyzed. Nevertheless, the studies clearly demonstrate that many tumors are not completely eradicated by radiation.

Local recurrence after radiation is associated with a number of factors. The size of the tumor is important. Large tumors (greater than 100 mL volume) are much more likely to harbor a focus of radioresistant cells than small tumors.[294] The location of the tumor is also important. Central and pelvic tumors have much higher rates of local recurrence than distal tumors.[297] This may reflect the difficulty in achieving adequate radiation doses around vital organs.

The response to chemotherapy also affects the likelihood of local recurrence. It was first noted that patients who received chemotherapy had lower overall rates of local recurrence than patients who did not receive chemotherapy.[298,299] Arai et al.[300] subsequently found that patients who responded well to chemotherapy had significantly better local control than patients who responded poorly. In this study, patients who had an objective response to chemotherapy and a tumor less than 8 cm long achieved 90% local control, despite being given a low radiation dose (35 Gy). Patients who had an objective response to chemotherapy and a tumor more than 8 cm long were given a high radiation dose (50 to 60 Gy), but these patients obtained only 52% local control. Finally, patients who failed to show a response to chemotherapy were also given a high dose (50 to 60 Gy), but had only 17% local control.

In addition to improving local control with radiation, effective adjuvant chemotherapy has made limb-sparing surgical excision possible. In fact, surgery may be a superior alternative to radiation treatment. The most cogent argument in favor of surgery is that it can remove a focus of radioresistant and chemoresistant cells that may reside within a large tumor. Another compelling argument is that patients who undergo radiation are at a substantial risk for developing a second primary tumor, particularly osteogenic sarcoma.[301–307] The cumulative risk increases with time and has been estimated to be 8.6% at 20 years, with a mean latency of 7.6 years.[301] Patients who receive a radiation dose of 60 Gy or greater seem to be at greatest risk.[301,308,309]

Many clinicians have objected to surgery on the basis of its being invasive, destructive, and disfiguring. They have preferred radiation because it seems to be noninvasive and limb-preserving. This viewpoint may have had some merit in the past, but it is no longer completely valid. Surgical reconstructive techniques have improved considerably, and function after limb-sparing surgery is significantly better now than in the past. Surgery should no longer be reserved for "expendable" bones, such as the ribs, clavicle, and fibula.[310] With modern surgical techniques, there are few, if any, truly nonexpendable bones, and reconstructive options exist for essentially all anatomic sites. Furthermore, it is worth emphasizing that radiation produces a significant amount of damage to normal tissue and can potentially cause serious functional impairment. Complications of radiation include skin atrophy and breakdown, fibrosis of muscles, contracture of joints, vasculitis, neuropathy, growth plate arrest, limb length inequality, osteonecrosis, and pathologic fractures.[311,312]

Although it is important to compare radiation and surgery with respect to functional outcome, the focus of the current debate should center on oncologic outcome. At present, the published data seem to favor surgery but they are not entirely conclusive. Several studies have shown that surgery produces a higher rate of local control. Bacci et al.[302] found 36% local recurrence with radiation alone compared to 8% local recurrence with either surgery alone or surgery with radiation. Ozaki[313] reported 15% local recurrence with radiation therapy alone compared to 4% local recurrence with surgery alone and 4% with surgery and radiation therapy. The main criticism of these and other studies is that they were not randomized trials, and there may have been a selection bias toward surgical excision of relatively smaller and more distal tumors.

There is only limited data pertaining to large, centrally located tumors, which carry the worst prognosis.[302,314,315] Some have recommended radiation therapy for these sites because it is difficult to obtain negative surgical margins, and the rate of complications is high. However, radiation treatment is also difficult in central locations because of their proximity to vital organs, and these tumors are precisely the ones most likely to recur after radiation.

There is conflicting data on whether surgery may have a positive impact on pelvic tumors. Scully et al.[316] found that there was no difference in survival between radiation therapy and surgery for pelvic tumors.[316] The experience of the Rizzoli Institute was similar, and survival was not improved by the addition of surgery to radiation.[317] In contrast to these findings, several groups have reported more favorable results after surgical treatment of pelvic tumors.[318–321] In the study from Memorial Sloan-Kettering, 9 of 12 patients with pelvic tumors were treated surgically, and there were no local recurrences in these nine tumors.[319] At UCLA, Yang et al.[320] obtained 51% cumulative 5-year survival in patients who had surgical resection compared to 18% survival in patients who did not have surgery.

Some have proposed that a combination of surgery and radiation be used to improve the rate of local control. Data on this subject are limited and confounded by a significant selection bias for patients that receive both radiation and surgery. Often these are the patients with the greatest perceived risk of recurrence—those with positive margins, large tumors, or contamination by previous surgery. This may be the reason that some investigators have not found an advantage to combining surgery with radiation.[313,317] More encouraging results were found by Wunder et al.[322] at Memorial Sloan-Kettering. Among patients who had a complete en bloc resection, the relative risk of local recurrence was 3.9 for patients who did not receive radiation compared to those that did receive radiation. All six patients with local recurrence in this series subsequently died of disease. The results at UCLA also seem to indicate a potential benefit of combined radiation and surgery in selected patients.[320] If indeed there is an increase in both local control and survival, the benefits of combining the two modalities may outweigh the increased risks of complications that would be expected from this aggressive approach. Proposals to conduct randomized trials of radiation versus surgery fail to consider that many patients may benefit from both modalities.

The issue of surgical treatment is further complicated by the choice of margins. Should the margin be outside of the original tumor, outside of the tumor after induction chemotherapy, or outside of the tumor after induction chemotherapy and radiation? Theoretically, it seems most prudent if the margin around the original tumor is chosen, but this requires sacrificing the most tissue. A margin outside of a tumor that has shrunk after induction

**TABLE 20B-4.** SELECTED SERIES OF ADJUVANT CHEMOTHERAPY IN EWING'S SARCOMA

| STUDY | YEAR | AGENTS | 5-YR SURVIVAL RATE* | NO. OF PATIENTS | NOTES |
|---|---|---|---|---|---|
| IESS-1[314] | 1990 | VACA | 60% | 331 | XRT for local control |
| IESS-2[327] | 1990 | VACA | 68% | 214 | High-dose intermittent chemo. better than low-dose continuous |
| CESS81[294] | 1988 | VACA | 55% | 93 | XRT for local control, 23% local relapse |
| Rizzoli Institute[302] | 1989 | VACA | 54% | 144 | Survival only 32% without dactinomycin |
| CCG/POG[333] | 1994 | VACA, Ifos/etop | 69% at 3 yr | 398 | Survival 50% without Ifos/etop |
| Memorial Sloan-Kettering[339] | 1995 | CAV, Ifos/etop | 77% at 2 yr | 36 | Protocol P6: High-dose CAV |
| CESS86[367] | 1991 | VACA VAIA | 62% | 122 | VAIA for high-risk patients |

*Disease-free or continuously disease-free survival.
ABBREVIATIONS: VACA = vincristine, doxorubicin, cyclophosphamide, dactinomycin; CAV = cyclophosphamide, doxorubicin, vincristine; VAIA = vincristine, ifosfamide, cyclophosphamide, dactinomycin; Ifos/etop = ifosfamide/etoposide.

chemotherapy and/or radiation is less optimal but may be chosen to spare important structures such as major nerves.

Pathologic fractures, especially those occurring after radiation, pose another surgical dilemma. In the study by Terek et al.,[323] all femoral lesions treated initially with radiation eventually required surgical treatment, either as a result of recurrence or pathologic fracture that failed to unite.[323] Healing of these postradiation fractures can occur but is often delayed.[324]

It is likely that no single therapeutic strategy will be ideal for all patients. Surgery may theoretically improve the chances for local control, but patients should be carefully selected, and the lesion must be resectable with adequate margins. In patients at high risk of local recurrence, surgery may be combined with radiation, but there may be an increase in wound complications. In the rare, unresectable lesion, radiation alone may be the only choice, but it is possible that after radiation and induction chemotherapy, the lesion may regress and become resectable.

## ADJUVANT THERAPY

The development of chemotherapy for Ewing sarcoma began in the 1960s, when phase II trials in patients with metastatic disease showed promise for cyclophosphamide, actinomycin D, vincristine, and other agents. Successful adjuvant chemotherapy for patients with nonmetastatic disease was reported by Hustu[325] in 1968, who treated five patients with vincristine and cyclophosphamide. It may be more than mere coincidence that the chemotherapy was adapted from protocols for neuroblastoma, and the neurotoxic agent vincristine was used.

The first Intergroup Ewing Sarcoma Study (IESS-1) began accrual of patients in 1973.[326] This involved three major study groups (CCSG, SWOG, and CALBG) and 84 participating institutions. The chemotherapy was based on vincristine, actinomycin D, and cyclophosphamide (VAC), and patients were randomized to three groups: VAC alone, VAC plus doxorubicin (VACA), and VAC plus whole lung irradiation. Radiation was used to treat the primary tumor. The IESS-1 study firmly established the effectiveness of adjuvant chemotherapy. Patients that received VAC plus doxorubicin had a 5-year relapse-free survival of 60%, which was far superior to any historic control. Patients that received only VAC had a survival of only 28%, which demonstrated the effectiveness of doxorubicin. Survival with VAC + whole lung irradiation gave intermediate results with survival of 53%, which was better than VAC alone, but was not as effective as the VACA combination.

In the follow-up IESS-2 trial, intermittent high-dose chemotherapy was shown to be more effective than continuous moderate-dose chemotherapy.[327] Dose intensity, especially that of doxorubicin, was found to be an important factor.[215] A 5-year disease-free survival of 68% was achieved in the intermittent high-dose chemotherapy group, but there was greater cardiotoxicity and one cardiac-related death.[327]

Subsequent trials have corroborated the findings of IESS-1 and confirmed the effectiveness of VACA. The results of selected major trials are shown in Table 20B-4. The CESS 81 study obtained 55% disease-free survival at 69 months,[294] while the Rizzoli group found 54% disease-free survival at 5 years.[302] Hayes et al.[328] used these four agents in a somewhat different protocol and reported 3-year disease-free survival of 82% for tumors less than 8 cm and 64% for tumors greater than 8 cm.[328]

Rosen[319] at Memorial Sloan-Kettering reported a 10-year experience with a series of 67 consecutive patients from 1970 to 1980. The protocols evolved during this period from T2 to T6 to T9. The T2 protocol consisted of VACA, whereas the T6 and T9 protocols employed doxorubicin, cyclophosphamide, high-dose methotrexate, BCD (see osteogenic sarcoma above), and BCNU (T6). Although excellent results were reported, with 79% disease-free survival at 2 years, which was stable to 5 years the interpretation of the study is complicated by the variety of agents and protocols. Many of the early patients received extremely high doses of doxorubicin in the range of 700 to 900 mg/m$^2$, which is beyond the doses allowed under current protocols. In a follow-up study of patients who received T9 and T11 chemotherapy at the same institution, Meyers[290] found 53% event-free survival at 5 years.[290]

This study, however, included patients with metastatic and relapsed disease.

There is currently much interest in the use of ifosfamide and etoposide (VP16), which have been shown to be effective in phase II trials.[329–333] However, addition of these agents to the traditional four-agent VACA regimen may produce only a small increase in survival. A large study from the Rizzoli Institute found only a 4% increase in disease-free survival, which was not statistically significant.[334,335] Preliminary data from a recent large, randomized CCG/POG study of 398 patients showed more encouraging results, and the 5-year event-free survival was increased significantly from 52% to 69%.[333]

In recent years there has been an effort to stratify patients into high-risk versus standard-risk categories. The definition of high risk varies, but usually includes metastatic cases (lung, bone, and/or bone marrow), relapsed cases, and primary tumors in unfavorable locations. The latter category comprises axial and pelvic tumors, but many investigators have also included "proximal" tumors in the humerus and femur. Large tumors have also been included in high-risk categories, with criteria being either larger than 8 cm in greatest dimension or over 100 mL in volume.[328,336]

It seems that if all of the above tumors are considered to be high risk, then only a small percentage of cases would qualify as standard risk. Not all of the high-risk cases are at similarly high risk. The prognosis in axial or pelvic locations is worse than the humerus or femur. Likewise, the prognosis for patients that relapse while on chemotherapy is bleak, whereas the prognosis for patients that present with metastatic disease may be somewhat better.[290,337–339] Cangir et al.,[337] reporting the IESS experience, found that the 5-year survival was 30% for patients that presented with metastases (i.e., patients who did not relapse during treatment).[337] Sandoval[338] similarly found an overall survival of 35% for cases that presented de novo with metastases. The type (location) and timing of metastases appear to be important. Meyers[290] found no survivors in patients with bone marrow involvement or patients that developed metastases while on chemotherapy. These considerations should be kept in mind when reviewing the literature on high-risk cases. The results that pertain to one set of "high-risk" patients may very well not apply to another group.

In contrast to osteogenic sarcoma and other sarcomas, there has not been much success with surgical resection of metastases. Heij[340] reported that all 12 patients who underwent thoracotomy for metastases eventually died of the disease. It is probable that the behavior of Ewing sarcoma differs from osteogenic sarcoma, and Ewing sarcoma has a much greater propensity for widespread microscopic dissemination.

Bone marrow transplant and stem cell rescue have been used for relapsed and high-risk patients.[318,341–343] This approach seems especially applicable to cases of bone marrow metastases, which might respond to bone marrow ablation by total body irradiation and/or high-dose chemotherapy. Total body irradiation has an additional appeal since Ewing sarcoma is radiosensitive. However, it should be recalled that the responses below 30 Gy were unpredictable, and a significant percentage of patients do not respond well to radiation therapy even at high doses.[300]

Cornbleet et al.[344] reported in 1981 on three patients with refractory Ewing sarcoma treated with high-dose melphalan and autolo-gous bone marrow rescue.[344] Two patients had a complete response and survived free of disease for 12 and 13 months, respectively. One patient had a partial response. A more extensive study was performed at the NCI, where patients were treated with VACA, radiation therapy for local control, 8-Gy total body irradiation, and autologous bone marrow rescue.[341] Early results were impressive, with 30 of 31 complete responses, but long-term results were less encouraging. Of the 13 metastatic patients, 9 relapsed and the projected 6-year survival rate was only 10%. The nonmetastatic, high-risk patients fared better, with only 5 of 18 relapsing. Burdach et al.[343] reported more optimistic results in a group of 17 patients with metastatic disease (7 new patients, 10 relapsed patients). Treatment consisted of induction chemotherapy, local treatment, myeloablation with melphalan/etoposide and carboplatin, 12-Gy total body irradiation, and finally bone marrow or stem cell rescue. The 6-year relapse-free survival was 45%.

## MALIGNANT FIBROUS HISTIOCYTOMA OF BONE

Although malignant fibrous histiocytoma (MFH) of bone resembles its soft tissue counterpart histologically, there is evidence to suggest that it is a distinct clinical entity and that the therapeutic approach to the two tumors should be different. The annual incidence is difficult to estimate, but it is likely that fewer than 300 cases occur annually in the United States. As many as 30% of cases arise secondary to another condition, most commonly radiation.[345] Other predisposing conditions include bone infarct, Paget's disease, osteomyelitis, and fibrous dysplasia.[346,347] The disease is most common in the fourth to fifth decades and has a broad age distribution. More men than women are affected. The distal femur, proximal tibia, proximal femur, pelvis, and proximal humerus are the most typical sites.

The clinical presentation is usually one of pain at the affected region. Swelling may or may not be present. In up to a fourth of patients, there may be a pathologic fracture. The clinician should be attuned to the possibility of multifocal disease, which occurred in 16 of 130 patients in one study.[348] This may represent bone-to-bone metastasis or multiple primary tumors.

The radiographic appearance is usually lytic (Fig. 20B-16), but there may be some sclerosis, and rarely a purely sclerotic lesion. The tumor tends to occur in the metaphysis. Periosteal bone formation is usually absent. Underlying bone disease such as radiation osteitis, bone infarcts, and Paget's disease may complicate the radiographic picture.

The tumor is composed of spindle-shaped cells with a fibroblastic, xanthomatous, and/or histiocytic appearance. The cells tend to be arranged in whorled, storiform, or cartwheel patterns. Multinucleated giant cells are present to varying degrees. Numerous histologic subtypes have been described, including myxoid, angiomatoid, hemangiopericytomatoid, fibrous histiocytomatous, and fibrous xanthomatous variants. The prognostic significance of these subtypes is uncertain.

The spindle-shaped cells are probably not true histiocytes despite having phagocytic properties. Instead, they are believed to be derived from primitive mesenchymal cells. Unlike other spindle cell sarcomas, MFH lacks markers of differentiation, such as the

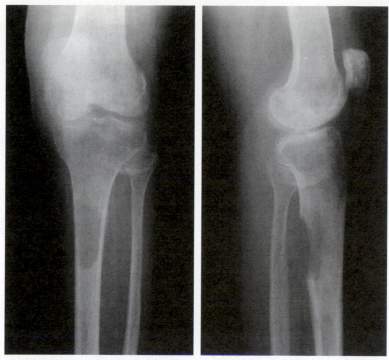

**FIGURE 20B-16.** MFH of the tibia. The AP view demonstrates a lytic lesion without sclerotic borders. The lateral view shows the true aggressive nature of the lesion, as the posterior cortex is completely eroded. A soft-tissue mass can be appreciated.

smooth muscle actin of leiomyosarcoma. The distinction between MFH and fibrosarcoma of bone may be an arbitrary one, since there are no markers that distinguish the two lesions. Well-differentiated fibrosarcoma tends to have more of a "herringbone" pattern of thin, fibroblastic cells. However, pleomorphic, high-grade fibrosarcoma is indistinguishable from high-grade MFH. Prior to the term MFH becoming popular, the tumors were called poorly differentiated fibrosarcoma.

Staging is according to the MTS system. MFH is usually a high-grade lesion,[348] but low-grade lesions do occur. Metastases develop most often in the lungs. The propensity for lymph node metastasis is probably low,[348] but estimates have varied from 0% to 27%.[349–352] The prognosis is better for low-grade lesions, younger patients, and primary MFH as opposed to secondary MFH arising in another lesion.[348] Huvos[345] also found that MFH arising in a field of radiation had a better prognosis than other types of secondary MFH.

The treatment of MFH of bone is still evolving. The experience with MFH is not as extensive as with other sarcomas of bone, and many principles of treatment are based upon the experience with osteogenic sarcoma. Part of the difficulty in comparing various studies is that the histologic definition, particularly the distinction from fibrosarcoma of bone, is somewhat nebulous. Furthermore, most studies have combined primary and secondary MFH of bone, but these may behave differently and have different prognosis.

The treatment of the primary tumor should be wide surgical excision. The results that have been reported with surgery vary widely and may reflect the heterogeneity of the tumors included in the studies. Patients with secondary MFH of bone in the setting of Paget's disease or prior radiation typically have a poor prognosis, and these tumors tend not to respond to adjuvant therapy. Overall, the survival at 5 years with surgery alone is approximately 30%, but estimates range from 6% to 50%. Several authors have noted that the survival of patients diminishes significantly between 5 and 10 years, which suggests that evaluation of patients at early follow-up may not be an accurate reflection of actual cure.[349,350] The role of radiation therapy, either as primary treatment or an adjuvant to surgery, has not been extensively investigated, and there have been only anecdotal reports of tumors responding to radiation.[349–351]

There is some evidence that adjuvant chemotherapy has a beneficial effect. Rosen[353] noted that three of four patients had a complete response when HDMTX was given preoperatively.[353] Weiner et al.[354] similarly reported favorable results with vincristine, HDMTX, and doxorubicin in a small group of patients. Bacci et al.[355] reported survival in 7 of 12 patients treated with surgery and chemotherapy, but only 1 of 18 patients treated with surgery only. In a follow-up study, these authors reported 78% event-free survival at 3 years with a protocol based upon osteogenic sarcoma protocols that included HDMTX, ifosfamide, cisplatin, and doxorubicin.[356] Yokoyama et al.[357] found that five patients with surgery and chemotherapy (HDMTX, doxorubicin, and vincristine) were alive at 5 years, but 10 of 12 patients who were treated with inadequate surgery died in 2 years.[357] Others have also found that in order for adjuvant

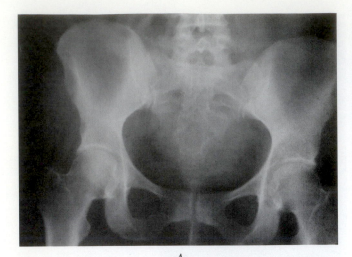
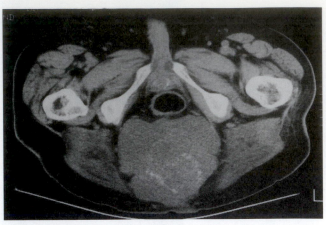

*A*                                        *B*

**FIGURE 20B-17.** Sacral-coccygeal chordoma. *A*. AP pelvis x-ray shows a subtle lytic lesion in the lower sacrum with a sclerotic border. *B*. CT scan shows a much larger and extensive lesion than is appreciated on plain x-ray. Faint calcifications are present.

systemic therapy to work, a formal wide excision is necessary,[349] and this recalls the experience with osteogenic sarcoma.

## CHORDOMA

A chordoma is a malignant tumor derived from remnants of notochordal tissue. These rare lesions make up only 1% of malignant bone tumors. Most chordomas are low-grade, locally aggressive tumors. The potential for metastasis is estimated at approximately 20% to 30% and appears to be higher for tumors of the mobile spine than the sacrum. Because of their central location in sensitive areas, they are more often lethal from uncontrolled local growth than distant metastasis. Rarely, lethal sarcomatous degeneration has been reported, especially after radiation therapy.

The peak age of occurrence is in the sixth decade, and males are favored by a 2:1 ratio. The most common sites are the sacrum, which makes up over half of the cases, followed by the clivus and sphenoocciput. The remaining cases are distributed throughout the spine. It is intriguing that the nucleus pulposus of intervertebral disks, which is derived from notochord, does not seem to develop into chordomas. A possible explanation is that the nucleus pulposus is a normal developmental structure and not a vestigial nest of fetal cells. In contrast, the sacrum and sphenoid often contain residual, unresorbed notochordal tissue.

In the sacral region, the tumors tend to cause only vague discomfort early in the course of the disease, which often results in the tumors attaining a large size before discovery. Bowel changes and obstipation are common. As the tumors progress, they can involve lumbosacral nerve roots and cause incontinence, urinary retention, numbness, and motor weakness. The tumors may also invade the rectum, other vital organs, and major vessels in the pelvis. Rectal examination is critical to identify the mass and to assess the mobility of the rectum over the mass.

In the sphenoid, patients most often complain of headache. Compression of the hypothalamus and pituitary gland can result in endocrine abnormalities, such as diabetes insipidus, polydipsia, and amenorrhea. Impingement on cranial nerves may give rise to visual disturbances, paresthesias, and facial paralysis.

Radiographically, the tumors produce lytic lesions in bone. They are often overlooked since the sacral region and the skull are difficult to interpret on plain x-ray (Fig. 20B-17). CT and MRI usually show intraspinal extension even in the absence of neurologic findings. A large soft tissue mass is typically present in the pelvis. Although usually centrally located, the mass may extend unilaterally along the sciatic nerve or into the piriformis or gluteus maximus.

Histologically, the tumor is composed of large, distinctive "physaliferous" cells, which have a vacuolated, soap-bubbly appearance. Most of the vacuoles are actually extracellular deposits of glycoproteins. Some chondrosarcomas and mucinous adenocarcinomas may have cells that appear similar, and the distinction between these tumors can sometimes be difficult.

Chordomas may be staged according to the MTS system, and most tumors are low-grade extracompartmental lesions (stage IB). The surgeon should pay particularly close attention to areas of local extension, including nerve roots, spinal canal, spinal cord, major vessels, and viscera. Dedifferentiation to a high-grade lesion can occur, especially after radiation treatment, and is uniformly fatal.

The treatment of sacral tumor consists of wide surgical excision, which usually entails complete or partial sacrectomies. These represent some of the most formidable surgical challenges and may be associated with considerable morbidity.[358] Total extirpation of the sacrum has a 10% mortality rate.[359] Exposure is difficult, and wound healing can be problematic with extensile posterior approaches, especially those that involve a T or Y incision. A simultaneous anterior approach is sometimes necessary and can greatly increase exposure, but entrance into the peritoneal cavity should not be done lightly, since this risks widespread dissemination of tumor in the abdomen.

High blood loss is to be expected from engorged epidural veins, which may be difficult to control. Restoration of spinal-pelvic continuity can be quite demanding. Ligation of the internal iliac vessels may be helpful if there is a large soft tissue mass anteriorly. Laparoscopic mobilization of anterior structures is a recently reported technique.[360]

Section of the sacral roots should be performed as necessary. Division of the nerves on only one side usually does not result in incontinence. If both S3 nerve roots are preserved, the patient is expected to be continent. If both S2–S4 nerve roots are sacrificed, the patient is likely to lose voluntary control of the bladder, anal sphincter, and erectile function.[358,359]

Adjuvant chemotherapy has not had a demonstrable effect on these tumors and is not routinely used. The role of adjuvant radiation is more controversial. Since chordomas grow slowly, they are not especially radiosensitive. In order to produce a response, relatively high doses are needed, but this is difficult to achieve near the central nervous system. In the sacral area, blood supply to skin flaps is tenuous and skin slough is a major concern. Samson et al.[358] maintained that adjuvant radiotherapy was beneficial for sacral tumors but could not demonstrate a statistical difference in recurrence in a retrospective analysis. These authors recommended preoperative radiation up to a maximum of 50 Gy when contamination during surgery was likely to occur and an additional 16 Gy postoperatively if contamination did indeed occur.

Charged particle and proton beam radiation have been used experimentally with some success, and 5-year actuarial relapse rates vary from 36% to 55%, with mean doses of 65 to 70 Gy.[259,260] These beams can deliver higher doses to tumors compared to conventional radiation therapy since there is less scatter and involvement of sensitive adjacent tissues. Radiation may be especially useful in cranial and high cervical lesions, where the surgical procedure may be limited to intralesional debulking.[256,257,259,361]

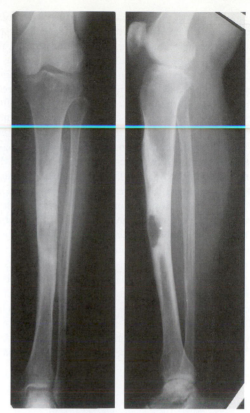

**FIGURE 20B-18.** Adamantinoma. On the AP view, the lesion is seen to extend throughout much of the shaft of the tibia with mixed lytic and sclerotic areas. On the lateral view, a lytic lesion is noted to arise in the anterior cortex of the tibia. This is typical for adamantinomas but unusual for other tumors of bone.

## ADAMANTINOMA

Adamantinomas are rare, distinctive tumors that typically arise in the tibia. Most lesions are low grade and do not metastasize early. The tumors favor men by approximately 3:2, and they are rarely encountered in children. The usual presenting complaint is localized pain.

Radiographically, the appearance can be quite variable. The lesion may be purely lytic or it may have a mixed lytic-sclerotic pattern (Fig. 20B-18). The tumor may be an isolated, discrete lesion, but it may also permeate throughout the entire bone. Some patients have multifocal areas of involvement, and in up to 10% of patients, the fibula is involved simultaneously with the tibia.

Histologically, adamantinomas are characterized by an unusual biphasic appearance, which bears a superficial resemblance to the ameloblasts of the teeth. However, they are not derived from ameloblasts, and the name adamantinoma is thus somewhat a misnomer. The tumor is composed of rows of compact epithelial-like cells with intervening, fibrous, spindle-shaped cells. Staining for keratins may be positive in the epithelial-like cells. The histologic picture, like the radiographic appearance, can be varied and areas of tubular, alveolar, or vascular formation may also be seen. In cases where small foci of osteoid are present, the appearance can resemble osteofibrous dysplasia, and there is controversy over whether there might be a relationship between the two lesions.[362] A review of 30 patients by one author did not demonstrate the presence of osteofibrous dysplasia,[273] but it is possible that in rare cases adamantinoma may arise from osteofibrous dysplasia.

A formal wide excision should be performed, since intralesional procedures result in a high rate of recurrence.[362] Surgical treatment alone is curative for the majority of patients[363,364] The rate of metastasis in one series was 29%, occurring most commonly in the lungs, but half of these were associated with previous intralesional surgery.[362] A more representative estimate may be closer to 10%.[364,365] Prolonged survival after surgical excision of pulmonary metastasis is possible.

## OTHER PRIMARY SARCOMAS OF BONE

Other types of sarcomas can arise primarily in the bone. The histologic appearance of these tumors is similar to their soft tissue counterparts. As primary bone lesions, all of these lesions are quite rare, and metastatic disease from a primary site elsewhere in the body should be considered in the differential diagnosis.

Fibrosarcomas recall the appearance of fibrous connective tissue and contain a variable amount of extracellular collagen. The spindle-shaped fibroblasts tend to form a herringbone pattern. The tumor lacks differentiation along cartilaginous, osseous, myogenic, or vascular lines. Some of these tumors may arguably be considered MFH, especially the more pleomorphic and poorly differentiated lesions, and as a result the incidence of fibrosarcoma is difficult to assess. In Dahlin's[350] review of cases from the Mayo Clinic, fibrosarcoma was considered to be three times as common as MFH, but some of these were subsequently reclassified as MFH. In contrast, in Huvos'[348] review of cases at Memorial Sloan-Kettering, MFH was more common than fibrosarcoma. The distinction may be more than simply a semantic one, since the treatment of fibrosarcoma has traditionally been wide surgical excision alone, whereas there is justification for adjuvant chemotherapy in the case of MFH. It is unknown if chemotherapy will have an impact on fibrosarcoma of bone.

Leiomyosarcoma may bear a superficial resemblance to other spindle cell sarcomas, but it is distinguished by the presence of smooth muscle actin and other markers of smooth muscle differentiation. Like the soft tissue tumor, it is notable for resistance to chemotherapy and radiation. Wide surgical excision offers the best chance for cure.

Hemangioendotheliomas are tumors derived from cells of blood vessels. They are characterized by the presence of vascular spaces surrounded by neoplastic cells. Hemangioendothelioma is notable for a peculiar tendency for multifocal involvement especially of one limb, in up to 30% of patients (Fig. 20B-19). This phenomenon suggests a developmental aberration in the pathogenesis of the tumor. The potential for multiple tumors to arise throughout a limb bud can make treatment decisions difficult and frustrating. Even radical resections cannot guarantee prevention of recurrence. Curiously, multifocal lesions may be less likely to metastasize. Careful staging is needed for the entire limb bud and MRI or PET scan is recommended.

Special mention should be made of the rare "malignant giant cell tumor of bone." Most giant cell tumors of bone are locally aggressive but benign tumors. Malignant giant cell tumors occur in two settings.[273] Most commonly, the tumor is benign initially but becomes malignant after attempted treatment, especially when radiation is used. Less commonly, the tumor is diagnosed de novo as a malignant giant cell tumor. The criteria for such a diagnosis should include, in addition to the presence of malignant spindle cells, the presence of an area of the tumor that appears exactly as a benign giant cell tumor. The treatment for these tumors is wide surgical excision. There is a definite potential for metastases, which occur in a minority of patients, but the overall prognosis is favorable with adequate surgical treatment.

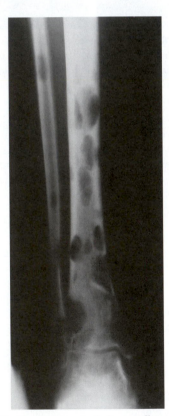

**FIGURE 20B-19.** Hemangioendothelioma of bone with multifocal involvement. Note involvement of both the tibia and fibula.

## SUMMARY

The treatment of osteogenic sarcoma offers a paradigm for spindle cell tumors, whereas the treatment of Ewing sarcoma provides a paradigm for small round cell tumors. The success with these two tumors offers hope for the treatment of other sarcomas of bone that have not yet met with equal success. Cooperative studies between institutions are needed if improvements in care are to be achieved in the treatment of these rare tumors.

## REFERENCES

1. CALUSER CI et al: The value of thallium and three-phase bone scans in the evaluation of bone and soft tissue sarcomas. Eur J Nucl Med 21:1198, 1994.
2. KIRCHNER PT, SIMON MA: Radioisotopic evaluation of skeletal disease. J Bone Joint Surg Am 63:673, 1981.
3. SIMON MA, KIRCHNER PT: Scintigraphic evaluation of primary bone tumors: Comparison of technetium-99m phosphonate and gallium citrate imaging. J Bone Joint Surg Am 62:758, 1980.
4. SIMON MA, FINN HA: Diagnostic strategy for bone and soft-tissue tumors (review). J Bone Joint Surg Am 75:622, 1993.
5. SIMON MA, BIERMANN JS: Biopsy of bone and soft-tissue lesions (Review). Bone Joint Surg Am 75:616, 1993.
6. MANKIN HJ et al: The hazards of the biopsy, revisited. Members of the Musculoskeletal Tumor Society (see comments). J Bone Joint Surg Am 78:656, 1996.
7. EILBER F et al: Adjuvant chemotherapy for osteosarcoma: A randomized prospective trial. J Clin Oncol 5:21, 1987.
8. CLARK CR et al: The effect of biopsy-hole shape and size on bone strength. J Bone Joint Surg Am 59:213, 1977.

9. BALL AB et al: Diagnosis of soft tissue tumours by Tru-cut biopsy. Br J Surg 77:756, 1990.

10. WHITE VA et al: Osteosarcoma and the role of fine-needle aspiration. A study of 51 cases. Cancer 62:1238, 1988.

11. KISSIN MW et al: Value of Tru-cut biopsy in the diagnosis of soft tissue tumours. Br J Surg 73:742, 1986.

12. AKERMAN M et al: Aspiration cytology of soft-tissue tumors. The 10-year experience at an orthopedic oncology center. Acta Orthop Scand 56:407, 1985.

13. DESANTOS LA et al: The value of percutaneous needle biopsy in the management of primary bone tumors. Cancer 43:735, 1979.

14. HAJDU SI, MELAMED MR: Needle biopsy of primary malignant bone tumors. Surg Gynecol Obstet 133:829, 1971.

15. ENNEKING WF et al: A system for the surgical staging of musculoskeletal sarcoma. Clin Orthop Rel Res 153:106, 1980.

16. FLEMING ID et al: AJCC Cancer Staging Manual. Philadelphia, Lippincott, 1997.

17. ENNEKING WF: Surgical procedures, in Musculoskeletal Tumor Surgery. New York, Churchill Livingstone, 1983, pp 89–122.

18. MICHAEL JW: Overview of prosthetic feet (review). Instructional Course Lectures 39:367, 1990.

19. MICHAEL JW: Current concepts in above-knee socket design (review). Instructional Course Lectures 39:373, 1990.

20. MALAWER MM, BAKER A: Amputations for tumor, in Surgery of the Musculoskeletal System, CM Evarts (ed). New York, Churchill Livingstone, 1990, pp 5163–5191.

21. GRAY DW, NG RL: Anatomical aspects of the blood supply to the skin of the posterior calf: Technique of below-knee amputation. Br J Surg 77:662, 1990.

22. HOLLOWAY GA JR, BURGESS EM: Cutaneous blood flow and its relation to healing of below knee amputation. Surg Gynecol Obstet 146:750, 1978.

23. HUMZAH MD, GILBERT PM: Fasciocutaneous blood supply in below-knee amputation (review). J Bone Joint Surg Br 79:441, 1997.

24. BURGESS EM et al: Segmental transcutaneous measurements of $PO_2$ in patients requiring below-the-knee amputation for peripheral vascular insufficiency. J Bone Joint Surg Am 64:378, 1982.

25. BURGESS EM: Wound healing after amputation: Effect of controlled environment treatment. A preliminary study. J Bone Joint Surg Am 60:245, 1978.

26. ROMANO RL, BURGESS EM: Level selection in lower extremity amputations. Clin Orthop Rel Res 74:177, 1971.

27. MOONEY V et al: The below-the-knee amputation for vascular disease. J Bone Joint Surg Am 58:365, 1976.

28. FINSEN V et al: Transcutaneous electrical nerve stimulation after major amputation. J Bone Joint Surg Br 70:109, 1988.

29. PINZUR MS: New concepts in lower-limb amputation and prosthetic management (review). Instructional Course Lectures 39:361, 1990.

30. OTIS JC et al: Energy cost during gait in osteosarcoma patients after resection and knee replacement and after above-the-knee amputation. J Bone Joint Surg Am 67:606, 1985.

31. NIKOLAJSEN L et al: Randomised trial of epidural bupivacaine and morphine in prevention of stump and phantom pain in lower-limb amputation (see comments). Lancet 350:1353, 1997.

32. TOMFORD WW: Transmission of disease through transplantation of musculoskeletal allografts (review). J Bone Joint Surg Am 77:1742, 1995.

33. SCHREIBER GB et al: The risk of transfusion-transmitted viral infections. The Retrovirus Epidemiology Donor Study (see comments). N Engl J Med 334:1685, 1996.

34. STEVENSON S et al: Critical biological determinants of incorporation of non-vascularized cortical bone grafts. Quantification of a complex process and structure. J Bone Joint Surg Am 79:1, 1997.

35. STEVENSON S et al: The fate of cancellous and cortical bone after transplantation of fresh and frozen tissue-antigen-matched and mismatched osteochondral allografts in dogs. J Bone Joint Surg Am 73:1143, 1991.

36. PELKER RR et al: Effects of freezing and freeze-drying on the biomechanical properties of rat bone. J Orthop Res 1:405, 1984.

37. PELKER RR et al: Biomechanical properties of bone allografts. Clin Orthop Rel Res 174:54, 1983.

38. MANKIN HJ et al: Long-term results of allograft replacement in the management of bone tumors. Clin Orthop Rel Res 324:86, 1996.

39. MAKLEY JT: The use of allografts to reconstruct intercalary defects of long bones. Clin Orthop Rel Res 324:58, 1985.

40. WOLF RE et al: Ten year follow-up of resection-arthrodesis of the knee (abstract). 44, 1997.

41. TOMFORD WW et al: Experimental freeze-preservation of chondrocytes. Clin Orthop Rel Res 197:11, 1985.

42. FRIEDLAENDER GE, MANKIN HJ: Bone banking: Current methods and suggested guidelines. Instructional Course Lectures 30:36, 1981.

43. KREICBERGS A et al: Cytological diagnosis of bone tumours. J Bone Joint Surg Br 78:258, 1996.

44. MALININ TI et al: Cryopreservation of articular cartilage. Ultrastructural observations and long-term results of experimental distal femoral transplantation. Clin Orthop Rel Res 303:18, 1994.

45. ENNEKING WF, MINDELL ER: Observations on massive retrieved human allografts. J Bone Joint Surg Am 73:1123, 1991.

46. HEALEY JH et al: Mechanism of failure of allogeneic bone transplants. Surg Forum 34:527, 1985.

47. STEVENSON S: The immune response to osteochondral allografts in dogs. J Bone Joint Surg Am 69:573, 1987.

48. VANDER GRIEND RA: The effect of internal fixation on the healing of large allografts. J Bone Joint Surg Am 76:657, 1994.

49. BERREY BH JR et al: Fractures of allografts. Frequency, treatment, and end-results. J Bone Joint Surg Am 72:825, 1990.

50. CAPANNA R et al: Effect of electromagnetic fields on patients undergoing massive bone graft following bone tumor resection. A double blind study. Clin Orthop Rel Res 306:213, 1994.

51. FRIEDLAENDER GE et al: Effects of chemotherapeutic agents on bone. I. Short-term methotrexate and doxorubicin (adriamycin) treatment in a rat model. J Bone Joint Surg Am 66:602, 1984.

52. LORD CF et al: Infection in bone allografts. Incidence, nature, and treatment. J Bone Joint Surg Am 70:369, 1988.

53. DICK HM, STRAUCH RJ: Infection of massive bone allografts. Clin Orthop Rel Res 306:46, 1994.

54. MNAYMNEH W et al: Massive distal femoral osteoarticular allografts after resection of bone tumors. Clin Orthop Rel Res 303:103, 1994.

55. OZAKI T et al: High complication rates with pelvic allografts. Experience of 22 sarcoma resections. Acta Orthop Scand 67:333, 1996.

56. OZAKI T et al: Intramedullary, antibiotic-loaded cemented, massive allografts for skeletal reconstruction. 26 cases

compared with 19 uncemented allografts. Acta Orthop Scand 68:387, 1997.

57. ENNEKING WF, SHIRLEY PD: Resection-arthrodesis for malignant and potentially malignant lesions about the knee using an intramedullary rod and local bone grafts. J Bone Joint Surg Am 59:223, 1977.

58. CAMPANACCI M, COSTA P: Total resection of distal femur or proximal tibia for bone tumours. Autogenous bone grafts and arthrodesis in twenty-six cases. J Bone Joint Surg Br 61-B:455, 1979.

59. ARROYO JS et al: Arthrodesis of the knee with a modular titanium intramedullary nail. J Bone Joint Surg Am 79:26, 1997.

60. HARRINGTON KD et al: Limb salvage and prosthetic joint reconstruction for low-grade and selected high-grade sarcomas of bone after wide resection and replacement by autoclaved [corrected] autogeneic grafts (published erratum appears in Clin Orthop 216:312, 1987). Clin Orthop Rel Res 211:180, 1986.

61. HSU RWW et al: Free vascularized fibular graft for skeletal defect reconstruction after tumor resection, in Limb Salvage—Major Reconstructions in Oncologic and Nontumoral Conditions, F Langlais, B Tomeno (eds). Berlin, Springer-Verlag, 1991, pp 225–231.

62. MINAMI A et al: Vascularized fibular graft for bone reconstruction of the extremities after tumor resection in limb-saving procedures. Microsurgery 16:56, 1995.

63. MALIZOS KN et al: Free vascularized fibula in traumatic long bone defects and in limb salvaging following tumor resection: Comparative study. Microsurgery 14:368, 1993.

64. HAN CS et al: Vascularized bone transfer. J Bone Joint Surg Am 74:1441, 1992.

65. ABERG M et al: Reconstruction with a free vascularized fibular graft for malignant bone tumor. Acta Orthop Scand 59:430, 1988.

66. MOORE JR et al: Use of free vascularized bone grafts in the treatment of bone tumors. Clin Orthop Rel Res 175:37, 1983.

67. BROWN KL: Limb reconstruction with vascularized fibular grafts after bone tumor resection. Clin Orthop Rel Res 262:64, 1991.

68. OZAKI T et al: Reconstruction of tibia by ipsilateral vascularized fibula and allograft. 12 cases with malignant bone tumors. Acta Orthop Scand 68:298, 1997.

69. CAPANNA R et al: Indications to vascularized fibula transplantation in limb salvage surgery (abstract), in 9th International Symposium of Limb Salvage, JH Healey (ed). New York, ISOLS, 1997, p 123.

70. CAMMISA FP JR et al: The Van Nes tibial rotationplasty. A functionally viable reconstructive procedure in children who have a tumor of the distal end of the femur. J Bone Joint Surg Am 72:1541, 1990.

71. TSUCHIYA H et al: Limb salvage using distraction osteogenesis. A classification of the technique (published erratum appears in J Bone Joint Surg Br 79:693, 1997. J Bone Joint Surg Br 79:403, 1997.

72. GOTTSAUNER-WOLF F et al: Rotationplasty for limb salvage in the treatment of malignant tumors at the knee. A follow-up study of seventy patients. J Bone Joint Surg Am 73:1365, 1991.

73. WINKELMANN WW: Hip rotationplasty for malignant tumors of the proximal part of the femur. J Bone Joint Surg Am 68:362, 1986.

74. ABUDU A et al: The outcome and functional results of diaphyseal endoprostheses after tumour excision. J Bone Joint Surg Br 78:652, 1996.

75. CAPANNA R et al: Modular uncemented prosthetic reconstruc-

tion after resection of tumours of the distal femur. J Bone Joint Surg Br 76:178, 1994.

76. ROBERTS P et al: Prosthetic replacement of the distal femur for primary bone tumours. J Bone Joint Surg Br 73:762, 1991.

77. ECKARDT JJ et al: Endoprosthetic replacement for stage IIB osteosarcoma. Clin Orthop Rel Res 270:202, 1991.

78. UNWIN PS et al: Distal femoral arthroplasty using custom-made prostheses. The first 218 cases. J Arthroplasty 8:259, 1993.

79. HOROWITZ SM et al: Prosthetic and extremity survivorship after limb salvage for sarcoma. How long do the reconstructions last? Clin Orthop Rel Res 293:280, 1993.

80. WARD WG et al: Five to ten year results of custom endoprosthetic replacement for tumors of the distal femur (abstract), in Complications of Limb Salvage: Prevention, Management and Outcome, KLB Brown (ed). Montreal, ISOLS, 1991, pp 483–491.

81. MUSCHLER GF et al: A custom distal femoral prosthesis for reconstruction of large defects following wide excision for sarcoma: Results and prognostic factors. Orthopedics 18:527, 1995.

82. UNWIN PS et al: Aseptic loosening in cemented custom-made prosthetic replacements for bone tumours of the lower limb. J Bone Joint Surg Br 78:5, 1996.

83. CANNON SR: Massive prostheses for malignant bone tumours of the limbs (review). J Bone Joint Surg Br 79:497, 1997.

84. KAWAI A et al: Prosthetic knee replacement after resection of a malignant tumor of the distal part of the femur: Medium to long-term results. J Bone Joint Surg Am 80(5):636, 1998.

85. KAWAI A et al: A rotating-hinge knee replacement for malignant tumors of the femur and tibia. Journal of Arthroplasty 14(2):187, 1999.

86. WARD WG et al: Extramedullary porous coating to prevent diaphyseal osteolysis and radiolucent lines around proximal tibial replacements. A preliminary report. J Bone Joint Surg Am 75:976, 1993.

87. CHAO EY, SIM FH: Modular prosthetic system for segmental bone and joint replacement after tumor resection (review). Orthopedics 8:641, 1985.

88. COOL WP et al: Growth after extendible endoprosthetic replacement of the distal femur. J Bone Joint Surg Br 79:938, 1997.

89. UNWIN PS, WALKER PS: Extendible endoprostheses for the skeletally immature. Clin Orthop Rel Res 322:179, 1996.

90. KENAN S et al: Limb-sparing surgery in skeletally immature patients with osteosarcoma: The use of an expandable prosthesis. Clin Orthop Rel Res 270:223, 1991.

91. FINN HA, SIMON MA: Limb-salvage surgery in the treatment of osteosarcoma in skeletally immature individuals (review) [32 refs]. Clin Orthop Rel Res 262:108, 1991.

92. SCHINDLER OS et al: Stanmore custom-made extendible distal femoral replacements: Clinical experience in children with primary malignant bone tumours. J Bone Joint Surg Br 79:927, 1997.

93. SHANBHAG AS et al: The John Charnley Award. Inhibition of wear debris mediated osteolysis in a canine total hip arthroplasty model. Clin Orthop Rel Res 344:33, 1997.

94. ZEHR RJ et al: Allograft-prosthesis composite versus megaprosthesis in proximal femoral reconstruction. Clin Orthop Rel Res 322:207, 1996.

95. MALAWER MM et al: The effect of cryosurgery and polymethylmethacrylate in dogs with experimental bone defects comparable to tumor defects. Clin Orthop Rel Res 226:299, 1988.

96. YUN YH et al: An investigation of bone necrosis and healing

after cryosurgery, phenol cautery or packing with bone cement of defects in the dog femur. Int Orthop 17:176, 1993.

97. MARCOVE RC et al: The treatment of aneurysmal bone cyst. Clin Orthop Rel Res 311:157, 1995.

98. MALAWER MM, DUNHAM W: Cryosurgery and acrylic cementation as surgical adjuncts in the treatment of aggressive (benign) bone tumors: Analysis of 25 patients below the age of 21 (review). Clin Orthop Rel Res 262:42, 1991.

99. MARCOVE RC: A 17-year review of cryosurgery in the treatment of bone tumors. Clin Orthop Rel Res 163:231, 1982.

100. MARCOVE RC et al: Cryosurgery in the treatment of giant cell tumors of bone: A report of 52 consecutive cases. Clin Orthop Rel Res 134:275, 1978.

101. MARCOVE RC et al: The use of cryosurgery in the treatment of low and medium grade chondrosarcoma: A preliminary report. Clin Orthop Rel Res 147:147, 1977.

102. DORFMAN HD, CZERNIAK B: Bone cancers. Cancer 75(Suppl):203, 1995.

103. HUVOS AG: Osteogenic sarcoma of bones and soft tissues in older persons: A clinicopathologic analysis of 117 patients older than 60 years. Cancer 57:1442, 1986.

104. HEALEY JH, BUSS D: Radiation and pagetic osteogenic sarcomas (Review). Clin Orthop Rel Res 270:128, 1991.

105. CHOONG PF et al: Low grade central osteogenic sarcoma: A long-term followup of 20 patients. Clin Orthop Rel Res 322:198, 1996.

106. KURT AM et al: Low-grade intraosseous osteosarcoma. Cancer 65:1418, 1990.

107. AHUJA SC et al: Juxtacortical (parosteal) osteogenic sarcoma: Histological grading and prognosis. J Bone Joint Surg Am 59:632, 1977.

108. UNNI KK et al: Parosteal osteogenic sarcoma. Cancer 37:2644, 1976.

109. RAYMOND AK: Surface osteosarcoma (review). Clin Orthop Rel Res 270:140, 1991.

110. SCHAJOWICZ F et al: Osteosarcomas arising on the surfaces of long bones. J Bone Joint Surg Am 70:555, 1988.

111. CAMPANACCI M, GIUNTI A: Periosteal osteosarcoma: Review of 41 cases, 22 with long-term follow-up. Italian J Orthop Traumatol 2:23, 1976.

112. SCHAJOWICZ F: Juxtacortical chondrosarcoma. J Bone Joint Surg Br 59-B:473, 1977.

113. POMPETTI F et al: Oncogene alterations in primary, recurrent, and metastatic human bone tumors (review). J Cell Biochem 63:37, 1996.

114. FLETCHER JA et al: Cytogenetic aberrations in osteosarcomas: Nonrandom deletions, rings, and double-minute chromosomes. Cancer Genet Cytogen 77:81, 1994.

115. HOOGERWERF WA et al: Chromosome analysis of nine osteosarcomas. Genes Chromosomes Cancer 9:88, 1994.

116. SZYMANSKA J et al: Ring chromosomes in parosteal osteosarcoma contain sequences from 12q13-15: A combined cytogenetic and comparative genomic hybridization study. Genes Chromosomes Cancer 16:31, 1996.

117. ARAKI N et al: Involvement of the retinoblastoma gene in primary osteosarcomas and other bone and soft-tissue tumors. Clin Orthop Rel Res 270:271, 1991.

118. CANCE WG et al: Altered expression of the retinoblastoma gene product in human sarcomas. N Eng J Med 323:1457, 1990.

119. MCINTYRE JF et al: Germline mutations of the p53 tumor suppressor gene in children with osteosarcoma. J Clin Oncol 12:925, 1994.

120. MILLER CW et al: Frequency and structure of p53 rearrangements in human osteosarcoma. Cancer Res 50:7950, 1990.

121. MASUDA H et al: Rearrangement of the p53 gene in human osteogenic sarcomas. Proc Nat Acad Sci US 84:7716, 1987.

122. MILLER CW et al: Alterations of the p53, Rb and MDM2 genes in osteosarcoma. J Cancer Res Clin Oncol 122:559, 1996.

123. LONARDO F et al: p53 and MDM2 alterations in osteosarcomas: Correlation with clinicopathologic features and proliferative rate. Cancer 79:1541, 1997.

124. LADANYI M et al: MDM2 gene amplification in metastatic osteosarcoma. Cancer Res 53:16, 1993.

125. DONEHOWER LA et al: Mice deficient for p53 are developmentally normal but susceptible to spontaneous tumours. Nature 356:215, 1992.

126. LAVIGUEUR A et al: High incidence of lung, bone, and lymphoid tumors in transgenic mice overexpressing mutant alleles of the p53 oncogene. Mol Cell Biol 9:3982, 1989.

127. YAMAGUCHI T et al: Allelotype analysis in osteosarcomas: Frequent allele loss on 3q, 13q, 17q, and 18q. Cancer Res 52:2419, 1992.

128. KRUZELOCK RP et al: Localization of a novel tumor suppressor locus on human chromosome 3q important in osteosarcoma tumorigenesis. Cancer Res 57:106, 1997.

129. FERRACINI R et al: The Met/HGF receptor is over-expressed in human osteosarcomas and is activated by either a paracrine or an autocrine circuit. Oncogene 10:739, 1995.

130. NARDEUX PC et al: A c-ras-Ki oncogene is activated, amplified and overexpressed in a human osteosarcoma cell line. Biochem Biophys Res Commun 146:395, 1987.

131. HELDIN CH et al: A human osteosarcoma cell line secretes a growth factor structurally related to a homodimer of PDGF A-chains. Nature 319:511, 1986.

132. GRAVES DT et al: Detection of c-sis transcripts and synthesis of PDGF-like proteins by human osteosarcoma cells. Science 226:972, 1984.

133. LADANYI M et al: Sporadic amplification of the MYC gene in human osteosarcomas. Diagn Mol Pathol 2:163, 1993.

134. ISFORT RJ et al: Analysis of oncogenes, tumor suppressor genes, autocrine growth-factor production, and differentiation state of human osteosarcoma cell lines. Mol Carcinogen 14:170, 1995.

135. OZAKI T et al: Alterations of retinoblastoma susceptible gene accompanied by c-myc amplification in human bone and soft tissue tumors. Cell Mol Biol 39:235, 1993.

136. ONDA M et al: ErbB-2 expression is correlated with poor prognosis for patients with osteosarcoma. Cancer 77:71, 1996.

137. KLOEN P et al: Expression of transforming growth factor-beta (TGF-beta) isoforms in osteosarcomas: TGF-beta3 is related to disease progression. Cancer 80:2230, 1997.

138. CURRAN T et al: Viral and cellular fos proteins: A comparative analysis. Cell 36:259, 1984.

139. WU JX et al: The proto-oncogene c-fos is over-expressed in the majority of human osteosarcomas. Oncogene 5:989, 1990.

140. DIAMANDOPOULOS GT, MCLANE MF: Effect of host age, virus dose, and route of inoculation on tumor incidence, latency, and morphology in Syrian hamsters inoculated intravenously with oncogenic DNA simian virus 40. J Nat Cancer Instit 55:479, 1975.

141. HUVOS AG et al: Postradiation osteogenic sarcoma of bone and soft tissues: A clinicopathologic study of 66 patients. Cancer 55:1244, 1985.

142. CAHAN WG et al: Sarcoma arising in irradiated bone: Report of eleven cases, 1948 (classical article). Cancer 82:8, 1998.

143. CAHAN WG: Radiation-induced sarcoma: 50 years later (editorial). Cancer 82:6, 1998.

144. ROSENBERG ZS et al: Osteosarcoma: Subtle, rare, and misleading plain film features. AJR 165:1209, 1995.

145. MEYERS PA et al: Chemotherapy for nonmetastatic osteogenic sarcoma: The Memorial Sloan-Kettering experience (see comments). J Clin Oncol 10:5, 1992.

146. BACCI G et al: Prognostic significance of serum lactate dehydrogenase in patients with osteosarcoma of the extremities. J Chemother 6:204, 1994.

147. BACCI G et al: Prognostic significance of serum alkaline phosphatase measurements in patients with osteosarcoma treated with adjuvant or neoadjuvant chemotherapy. Cancer 71:1224, 1993.

148. WUISMAN P, ENNEKING WF: Prognosis for patients who have osteosarcoma with skip metastasis. J Bone Joint Surg Am 72:60, 1990.

149. MALAWER MM, DUNHAM WK: Skip metastases in osteosarcoma: Recent experience. J Surg Oncol 22:236, 1983.

150. PAN G et al: Osteosarcoma: MR imaging after preoperative chemotherapy. Radiology 174:517, 1990.

151. CAMPANACCI M, LAUS M: Local recurrence after amputation for osteosarcoma. J Bone Joint Surg Br 62-B:201, 1980.

152. deSANTOS LA et al: Computed tomography in the evaluation of osteosarcoma: Experience with 25 cases. AJR 4:535, 1994.

153. LEWIS RJ, LOTZ MJ: Proceedings: Medullary extension of osteosarcoma: Implications for rational therapy. Cancer 33:371, 1974.

154. DAHLIN DC, COVENTRY MB: Osteogenic sarcoma: A study of six hundred cases. J Bone Joint Surg Am 49:101, 1967.

155. ANANI AP et al: Metastatic skipping in the bone marrow (skip metastases) in osteosarcoma: Frequency and clinical implications? Annal Pathologie 7:193, 1987.

156. LIN J et al: Quantitative evaluation of thallium-201 uptake in predicting chemotherapeutic response of osteosarcoma. Eur J Nucl Med 22:553, 1995.

157. ROSEN G et al: Serial thallium-201 scintigraphy in osteosarcoma: Correlation with tumor necrosis after preoperative chemotherapy. Clin Orthop Rel Res 293:302, 1993.

158. NADEL HR: Thallium-201 for oncological imaging in children (review). Semin Nucl Med 23:243, 1993.

159. YEH SD et al: Semiquantitative gallium scintigraphy in patients with osteogenic sarcoma. Clin Nucl Med 9:175, 1984.

160. OHTOMO K et al: Thallium-201 scintigraphy to assess effect of chemotherapy in osteosarcoma. J Nucl Med 37:1444, 1996.

161. MENENDEZ LR et al: Thallium-201 scanning for the evaluation of osteosarcoma and soft-tissue sarcoma: A study of the evaluation and predictability of the histological response to chemotherapy (see comments). J Bone Joint Surg Am 75:526, 1993.

162. SHETH DS et al: Conventional and dedifferentiated parosteal osteosarcoma: Diagnosis, treatment, and outcome. Cancer 78:2136, 1996.

163. OKADA K et al: Parosteal osteosarcoma: A clinicopathological study. J Bone Joint Surg Am 76:366, 1994.

164. RITSCHL P et al: Parosteal osteosarcoma: 2-23-year follow-up of 33 patients. Acta Orthop Scand 62:195, 1991.

165. LUCK JV JR et al: Parosteal osteosarcoma: A treatment-oriented study. Clin Orthop Rel Res 153:92, 1980.

166. BERTONI F et al: Osteosarcoma: Low-grade intraosseous-type osteosarcoma, histologically resembling parosteal osteosarcoma, fibrous dysplasia, and desmoplastic fibroma. Cancer 71:338, 1993.

167. ENNEKING WF et al: The surgical treatment of parosteal osteosarcoma in long bones. J Bone Joint Surg Am 67:125, 1985.

168. CAMPANACCI M et al: Parosteal osteosarcoma. J Bone Joint Surg Br 66:313, 1984.

169. FRIEDMAN MA, CARTER SK: The therapy of osteogenic sarcoma: Current status and thoughts for the future (review). J Surg Oncol 4:482, 1972.

170. McKENNA RJ et al: Osteogenic sarcoma in children. CA 16:26, 1966.

171. MARCOVE RC et al: Osteogenic sarcoma under the age of twenty-one: A review of one hundred and forty-five operative cases. J Bone Joint Surg Am 52:411, 1970.

172. GHERLINZONI F et al: Limb sparing versus amputation in osteosarcoma: Correlation between local control, surgical margins and tumor necrosis: Istituto Rizzoli experience. Ann Oncol 3 (Supp 2):S23, 1992.

173. PICCI P et al: Relationship of chemotherapy-induced necrosis and surgical margins to local recurrence in osteosarcoma (see comments). J Clin Oncol 12:2699, 1994.

174. ROUGRAFF BT et al: Limb salvage compared with amputation for osteosarcoma of the distal end of the femur: A long-term oncological, functional, and quality-of-life study. J Bone Joint Surg Am 76:649, 1994.

175. WINKLER K et al: Treatment of osteosarcoma: Experience of the Cooperative Osteosarcoma Study Group (COSS) (review). Cancer Treat Res 62:269, 1993.

176. GOORIN AM et al: Weekly high-dose methotrexate and doxorubicin for osteosarcoma. The Dana-Farber Cancer Institute/the Children's Hospital—study III. J Clin Oncol 5:1178, 1987.

177. WINKLER K et al: Neoadjuvant chemotherapy for osteogenic sarcoma: Results of a Cooperative German/Austrian study. J Clin Oncol 2:617, 1984.

178. MEYERS PA et al: Osteogenic sarcoma with clinically detectable metastasis at initial presentation. J Clin Oncol 11:449, 1993.

179. BACCI G et al: Osteogenic sarcoma of the extremity with detectable lung metastases at presentation: Results of treatment of 23 patients with chemotherapy followed by simultaneous resection of primary and metastatic lesions. Cancer 79:245, 1997.

180. TABONE MD et al: Osteosarcoma recurrences in pediatric patients previously treated with intensive chemotherapy. J Clin Oncol 12:2614, 1994.

181. LEE ES, MACKENZIE DH: Osteosarcoma: A study of the value of preoperative megavoltage radiotherapy. Br J Surg 51:252, 1964.

182. TEFFT M et al: Radiation in bone sarcomas: A re-evaluation in the era of intensive systemic chemotherapy. Cancer 39 (Suppl):806, 1977.

183. de MOOR NG: Osteosarcoma a review of 72 cases treated by megavoltage radiation therapy, with or without surgery. S African J Surg 13:137, 1975.

184. LEE ES: Osteosarcoma: A reconnaissance (review). Clin Radiol 26:5, 1975.

185. POPPE E et al: Osteosarcoma. Acta Chir Scand 134:549, 1968.

186. ROSEN G et al: Combination chemotherapy and radiation therapy in the treatment of metastatic osteogenic sarcoma. Cancer 35:622, 1975.

187. CHAMBERS RG, MAHONEY WD: Osteogenic sarcoma of the mandible: Current management. Am Surg 36:463, 1970.

188. Martinez A et al: Intra-arterial infusion of radiosensitizer (BUdR) combined with hypofractionated irradiation and chemotherapy for primary treatment of osteogenic sarcoma. Int J Radiat Oncol Biol Phys 11:123, 1985.

189. Hudson M et al: Pediatric osteosarcoma: Therapeutic strategies, results, and prognostic factors derived from a 10-year experience. J Clin Oncol 8:1988, 1990.

190. Rab GT et al: Elective whole lung irradiation in the treatment of osteogenic sarcoma. Cancer 38:939, 1976.

191. Taylor WF et al: Trends and variability in survival from osteosarcoma. Mayo Clin Proc 53:695, 1978.

192. Bode U, Levine AS: The biology and management of osteosarcoma, in Cancer in the Young, AS Levine (ed). New York, Masson Publishing, 1982, pp 575–602.

193. Link MP et al: The effect of adjuvant chemotherapy on relapse-free survival in patients with osteosarcoma of the extremity. N Engl J Med 314:1600, 1986.

194. Jaffe N: Recent advances in the chemotherapy of metastatic osteogenic sarcoma. Cancer 30:1627, 1972.

195. Jaffe N et al: Weekly high-dose methotrexate-citrovorum factor in osteogenic sarcoma: Pre-surgical treatment of primary tumor and of overt pulmonary metastases. Cancer 39:45, 1977.

196. Rosen G et al: Chemotherapy, en bloc resection, and prosthetic bone replacement in the treatment of osteogenic sarcoma. Cancer 37:1, 1976.

197. Bacci G et al: Primary chemotherapy and delayed surgery (neoadjuvant chemotherapy) for osteosarcoma of the extremities: The Istituto Rizzoli Experience in 127 patients treated preoperatively with intravenous methotrexate (high versus moderate doses) and intraarterial cisplatin. Cancer 65:2539, 1990.

198. Bramwell VH et al: A comparison of two short intensive adjuvant chemotherapy regimens in operable osteosarcoma of limbs in children and young adults: The first study of the European Osteosarcoma Intergroup. J Clin Oncol 10:1579, 1992.

199. Edmonson JH et al: A controlled pilot study of high-dose methotrexate as postsurgical adjuvant treatment for primary osteosarcoma. J Clin Oncol 2:152, 1984.

200. French Bone Tumor Study Group: Age and dose of chemotherapy as major prognostic factors in a trial of adjuvant therapy of osteosarcoma combining two alternating drug combinations and early prophylactic lung irradiation. French Bone Tumor Study Group. Cancer 61:1304, 1988.

201. Rosen G et al: Primary osteogenic sarcoma: The rationale for preoperative chemotherapy and delayed surgery. Cancer 43:2163, 1979.

202. Wang YM et al: Age-related pharmacokinetics of high-dose methotrexate in patients with osteosarcoma. Cancer Treat Rep 63:405, 1979.

203. Cortes EP et al: Amputation and adriamycin in primary osteosarcoma. N Engl J Med 291:998, 1974.

204. Cortes EP et al: Amputation and adriamycin in primary osteosarcoma: A 5-year report. Cancer Treat Rep 62:271, 1978.

205. Ochs JJ et al: cis-Dichlorodiammineplatinum (II) in advanced osteogenic sarcoma. Cancer Treat Rep 62:239, 1978.

206. Nitschke R et al: Cis-diamminedichloroplatinum (NSC-119875) in childhood malignancies: A Southwest Oncology Group study. Med Pediatr Oncol 4:127, 1978.

207. Jaffe N et al: Osteosarcoma: Intra-arterial treatment of the primary tumor with cis-diammine-dichloroplatinum II (CDP): Angiographic, pathologic, and pharmacologic studies. Cancer 51:402, 1983.

208. Mosende C et al: Combination chemotherapy with bleomycin, cyclophosphamide and dactinomycin for the treatment of osteogenic sarcoma. Cancer 40:2779, 1977.

209. Rosenberg SA et al: Treatment of osteogenic sarcoma. I. Effect of adjuvant high-dose methotrexate after amputation. Cancer Treat Rep 63:739, 1979.

210. Ettinger LJ et al: Adjuvant adriamycin and cisplatin in newly diagnosed, nonmetastatic osteosarcoma of the extremity. J Clin Oncol 4:353, 1986.

211. Cortes WW et al: Adjuvant chemotherapy in primary treatment of osteogenic sarcoma: A Southwest Oncology Group study. Cancer 36:1598, 1975.

212. Winkler K et al: Effect of intraarterial versus intravenous cisplatin in addition to systemic doxorubicin, high-dose methotrexate, and ifosfamide on histologic tumor response in osteosarcoma (study COSS-86). Cancer 66:1703, 1990.

213. Winkler K et al: Neoadjuvant chemotherapy of osteosarcoma: Results of a randomized cooperative trial (COSS-82) with salvage chemotherapy based on histological tumor response. J Clin Oncol 6:329, 1988.

214. Bacci G et al: The importance of dose-intensity in neoadjuvant chemotherapy of osteosarcoma: A retrospective analysis of high-dose methotrexate, cisplatinum and adriamycin used preoperatively. J Chemother 2:127, 1990.

215. Smith MA et al: Influence of doxorubicin dose intensity on response and outcome for patients with osteogenic sarcoma and Ewing's sarcoma (see comments). J Nat Cancer Instit 83:1460, 1991.

216. Pratt CB et al: Bleomycin, cyclophosphamide, and dactinomycin in metastatic osteosarcoma: Lack of tumor regression in previously treated patients. Cancer Treat Rep 71:421, 1987.

217. Harris MB et al: Treatment of osteosarcoma with ifosfamide: Comparison of response in pediatric patients with recurrent disease versus patients previously untreated: A Pediatric Oncology Group study. Med Pediat Oncol 24:87, 1995.

218. Pratt CB et al: Clinical studies of ifosfamide/mesna at St Jude Children's Research Hospital, 1983–1988. Semin Oncol 16 (Suppl 3):51, 1989.

219. MacEwen EG et al: Therapy for osteosarcoma in dogs with intravenous injection of liposome-encapsulated muramyl tripeptide. J Natl Cancer Instit 81:935, 1989.

220. Picci P et al: Histologic evaluation of necrosis in osteosarcoma induced by chemotherapy: Regional mapping of viable and nonviable tumor. Cancer 56:1515, 1985.

221. Huvos AG et al: Primary osteogenic sarcoma: Pathologic aspects in 20 patients after treatment with chemotherapy en bloc resection, and prosthetic bone replacement. Arch Pathol Lab Med 101:14, 1977.

222. Rosen G et al: Primary osteogenic sarcoma: Eight-year experience with adjuvant chemotherapy. J Cancer Res Clin Oncol 106(Suppl):55, 1983.

223. Solheim OP et al: The treatment of osteosarcoma: Present trends. The Scandinavian Sarcoma Group experience. Ann Oncol 3 (Suppl 2):S7, 1992.

224. Petrilli AS et al: Increased survival, limb preservation, and prognostic factors for osteosarcoma. Cancer 68:733, 1991.

225. Malawer M et al: Impact of two cycles of preoperative chemotherapy with intraarterial cisplatin and intravenous doxorubicin on the choice of surgical procedure for high-grade bone sarcomas of the extremities. Clin Orthop Rel Res 270:214, 1991.

226. Jaffe N et al: Comparison of intra-arterial cis-diamminedichloroplatinum II with high-dose methotrexate and

citrovorum factor rescue in the treatment of primary osteosarcoma. J Clin Oncol 3:1101, 1985.

227. STRANDER H et al: Adjuvant interferon treatment in human osteosarcoma. Cancer Treat Res 62:29, 1993.

228. KHANNA C et al: Interleukin-2 liposome inhalation therapy is safe and effective for dogs with spontaneous pulmonary metastases. Cancer 79:1409, 1997.

229. HANSEN MF: Molecular genetic considerations in osteosarcoma (review). Clin Orthop Rel Res 270:237, 1991.

230. HUANG HJ et al: Suppression of the neoplastic phenotype by replacement of the RB gene in human cancer cells. Science 242:1563, 1988.

231. WOMER RB: The cellular biology of bone tumors. Clin Orthop Rel Res 262:12, 1991.

232. HUVOS AG, MARCOVE RC: Chondrosarcoma in the young: A clinicopathologic analysis of 79 patients younger than 21 years of age. Am J Surg Pathol 11:930, 1987.

233. SPRINGFIELD DS et al: Chondrosarcoma: A review (review). Instruct Course Lect 45:417, 1996.

234. HEALEY JH, LANE JM: Chondrosarcoma. Clin Orthop Rel Res 204:119, 1986.

235. WUISMAN PI et al: Secondary chondrosarcoma in osteochondromas: Medullary extension in 15 of 45 cases. Acta Orthop Scand 68:396, 1997.

236. UNNI KK: Osteochondroma (osteocartilaginous exostosis), in Dahlin's Bone Tumors, Anonymous. Philadelphia, Lippincott-Raven, 1996, pp 11–24.

237. PRITCHARD DJ et al: Chondrosarcoma: A clinicopathologic and statistical analysis. Cancer 45:149, 1980.

238. MIRRA JM: Bone Tumors. Philadelphia, Lea & Febiger; 1989, p 502.

239. HUVOS AG et al: Mesenchymal chondrosarcoma: A clinicopathologic analysis of 35 patients with emphasis on treatment. Cancer 51:1230, 1983.

240. NAKASHIMA Y et al: Mesenchymal chondrosarcoma of bone and soft tissue: A review of 111 cases. Cancer 57:2444, 1986.

241. GILL S et al: Fusion of the EWS gene to a DNA segment from 9q22-31 in a human myxoid chondrosarcoma. Genes Chromos Cancer 12:307, 1995.

242. LICHTENSTEIN L: Bone Tumors, St. Louis, CV Mosby, 1972.

243. EVANS HL et al: Prognostic factors in chondrosarcoma of bone: A clinicopathologic analysis with emphasis on histologic grading. Cancer 40:818, 1977.

244. BAUER HC et al: Low risk of recurrence of enchondroma and low-grade chondrosarcoma in extremities: 80 patients followed for 2-25 years. Acta Orthop Scand 66:283, 1995.

245. GITELIS S et al: Chondrosarcoma of bone: The experience at the Istituto Ortopedico Rizzoli. J Bone Joint Surg Am 63:1248, 1981.

246. LINDBOM A et al: Primary chondrosarcoma of bone. Acta Radiol 55:81, 1961.

247. MILLER DR, MANKIN HJ: A comparison of collagen synthesis by different categories of human chondrosarcoma in organ culture. Clin Orthop Rel Res 168:252, 1982.

248. MANKIN HJ et al: The biology of human chondrosarcoma. II. Variation in chemical composition among types and subtypes of benign and malignant cartilage tumors. J Bone Joint Surg Am 62:176, 1980.

249. MANKIN HJ et al: The biology of human chondrosarcoma. I. Description of the cases, grading, and biochemical analyses. J Bone Joint Surg Am 62:160, 1980.

250. OZAKI T et al: Influence of intralesional surgery on treatment outcome of chondrosarcoma. Cancer 77:1292, 1996.

251. YASKO AW et al: Low-grade chondrosarcoma of the long bones: Late results of curettage versus wide excision (abstract). Proceedings of the 65th Annual Meeting of the American Academy of Orthopaedic Surgeons 141, 1998.

252. HARWOOD AR et al: Radiotherapy of chondrosarcoma of bone. Cancer 45:2769, 1980.

253. SUIT H: Regaud Lecture, Granda 1994: Tumors of the connective and supporting tissues (review). Radiother Oncol 34:93, 1995.

254. HUG EB et al: Locally challenging osteo- and chondrogenic tumors of the axial skeleton: Results of combined proton and photon radiation therapy using three-dimensional treatment planning. Int J Radiat Oncol Biol Phys 31:467, 1995.

255. SUIT HD et al: Increased efficacy of radiation therapy by use of proton beam. Strahlentherapie Onkologie 166:40, 1990.

256. AUSTIN-SEYMOUR M et al: Fractionated proton radiation therapy of chordoma and low-grade chondrosarcoma of the base of the skull. J Neurosurg 70:13, 1989.

257. BERSON AM et al: Charged particle irradiation of chordoma and chondrosarcoma of the base of skull and cervical spine: The Lawrence Berkeley Laboratory experience. Int J Radiat Oncol Biol Phys 15:559, 1988.

258. SUIT HD et al: Definitive radiation therapy for chordoma and chondrosarcoma of base of skull and cervical spine. J Neurosurg 56:377, 1982.

259. CASTRO JR et al: Experience in charged particle irradiation of tumors of the skull base: 1977–1992 (see comments) (review). Int J Radiat Oncol Biol Phys 29:647, 1994.

260. NOWAKOWSKI VA et al: Charged particle radiotherapy of paraspinal tumors. Int J Radiat Oncol Biol Phys 22:295, 1992.

261. FRASSICA FJ et al: Dedifferentiated chondrosarcoma: A report of the clinicopathological features and treatment of seventy-eight cases. J Bone Joint Surg Am 68:1197, 1986.

262. HORTON WE et al: Retinoic acid rapidly reduces cartilage matrix synthesis by altering gene transcription in chondrocytes. Develop Biol 123:508, 1987.

263. REUBI JC: A somatostatin analogue inhibits chondrosarcoma and insulinoma tumour growth. Acta Endocrinol 109:108, 1985.

264. MEROMSKY L, LOTAN R: Modulation by retinoic acid of cellular, surface-exposed, and secreted glycoconjugates in cultured human sarcoma cells. J Nat Cancer Instit 72:203, 1984.

265. ETTLIN R et al: Histological changes during regression induced by retinoic acid in a transplantable rat chondrosarcoma. Virchows Arch 1:1, 1994.

266. THEIN R, LOTAN R: Sensitivity of cultured human osteosarcoma and chondrosarcoma cells to retinoic acid. Cancer Res 42:4771, 1982.

267. SHAPIRO SS et al: Effect of aromatic retinoids on rat chondrosarcoma glycosaminoglycan biosynthesis. Cancer Res 36:3702, 1976.

268. NOGUERA R et al: Dynamic model of differentiation in Ewing's sarcoma cells: Comparative analysis of morphologic, immunocytochemical, and oncogene expression parameters (see comments). Lab Invest 66:143, 1992.

269. RETTIG WJ et al: Ewing's sarcoma: New approaches to histogenesis and molecular plasticity (editorial; comment) Lab Invest 66:133, 1992.

270. EWING J: Diffuse endothelioma of bone. Proc New York Pathol Soc 21:17, 1921.

271. MIRRA JM: Bone Tumors. Philadelphia, Lea & Febiger, 1989.

272. GURNEY JG et al: Trends in cancer incidence among children in the U.S. Cancer 78:532, 1996.

273. HUVOS AG: *Bone Tumors*. Philadelphia, WB Saunders, 1991.

274. URANO F et al: A novel chimera gene between EWS and E1A-F, encoding the adenovirus E1A enhancer-binding protein, in extraosseous Ewing's sarcoma. Biochem Biophys Res Commun 219:608, 1996.

275. JEON IS et al: A variant Ewing's sarcoma translocation (7;22) fuses the EWS gene to the ETS gene ETV1. Oncogene 10:1229, 1995.

276. ZELAZNY A et al: Quantitative analysis of the plain radiographic appearance of Ewing's sarcoma of bone. Invest Radiol 32:59, 1997.

277. FELLINGER EJ et al: Comparison of cell surface antigen HBA71 (p30/32MIC2), neuron-specific enolase, and vimentin in the immunohistochemical analysis of Ewing's sarcoma of bone. Am J Surg Pathol 16:746, 1992.

278. HAMILTON G et al: Characterization of a human endocrine tissue and tumor-associated Ewing's sarcoma antigen. Cancer Res 48:6127, 1988.

279. FELLINGER EJ et al: Biochemical and genetic characterization of the HBA71 Ewing's sarcoma cell surface antigen. Cancer Res 51:336, 1991.

280. FELLINGER EJ et al: Immunohistochemical analysis of Ewing's sarcoma cell surface antigen p30/32MIC2. Am J Pathol 139:317, 1991.

281. LEE CS et al: EWS/FLI-1 fusion transcript detection and MIC2 immunohistochemical staining in the diagnosis of Ewing's sarcoma. Pediatr Pathol Lab Med 16:379, 1996.

282. DEVANEY K et al: MIC2 detection in tumors of bone and adjacent soft tissues. Clin Orthop Rel Res 310:176, 1995.

283. WEIDNER N, TJOE J: Immunohistochemical profile of monoclonal antibody O13: Antibody that recognizes glycoprotein p30/32MIC2 and is useful in diagnosing Ewing's sarcoma and peripheral neuroepithelioma (see comments). Am J Surg Pathol 18:486, 1994.

284. PERLMAN EJ et al: Ewing's sarcoma—Routine diagnostic utilization of MIC2 analysis: A Pediatric Oncology Group/ Children's Cancer Group Intergroup Study. Human Pathol 25:304, 1994.

285. RIOPEL M et al: MIC2 analysis in pediatric lymphomas and leukemias. Human Pathol 25:396, 1994.

286. SCOTLANDI K et al: Immunostaining of the p30/32MIC2 antigen and molecular detection of EWS rearrangements for the diagnosis of Ewing's sarcoma and peripheral neuroectodermal tumor. Human Pathol 27:408, 1996.

287. THORNER P et al: Is the EWS/FLI-1 fusion transcript specific for Ewing sarcoma and peripheral primitive neuroectodermal tumor? A report of four cases showing this transcript in a wider range of tumor types. Am J Pathol 148:1125, 1996.

288. ENNEKING WF: *Musculoskeletal Tumor Surgery*. New York, Churchill Livingstone, 1983, p 1351.

289. OBERLIN O et al: Incidence of bone marrow involvement in Ewing's sarcoma: Value of extensive investigation of the bone marrow. Med Pediatr Oncol 24:343, 1995.

290. MEYERS PA et al: Ewing's sarcoma (ES)/primitive neuroectodermal tumor (PNET) of bone: Histological response (HR) to pre-operative chemotherapy (CT) predicts event free survival (EFS) (Meeting abstract). Proc Annu Meet Am Soc Clin Oncol 14:A1407, 1995.

291. FALK S, ALPERT M: Five-year survival of patients with Ewing's sarcoma. Surg Gynecol Obst 124:319, 1967.

292. BOYER CW JR et al: Ewing's sarcoma: Case against surgery. Cancer 20:1602, 1967.

293. DONALDSON S et al: The Pediatric Oncology Group (POG) experience in Ewing's sarcoma of bone. Med Pediatr Oncol 17:283, 1989.

294. JURGENS H et al: Multidisciplinary treatment of primary Ewing's sarcoma of bone. A 6-year experience of a European Cooperative Trial. Cancer 61:23, 1988.

295. TEPPER J et al: Local control of Ewing's sarcoma of bone with radiotherapy and combination chemotherapy. Cancer 46:1969, 1980.

296. TELLES NC et al: Ewing's sarcoma: An autopsy study. Cancer 41:2321, 1978.

297. RAZEK A et al: Intergroup Ewing's Sarcoma Study: Local control related to radiation dose, volume, and site of primary lesion in Ewing's sarcoma. Cancer 46:516, 1980.

298. CHAN RC et al: Management and results of localized Ewing's sarcoma. Cancer 43:1001, 1979.

299. FERNANDEZ CH et al: Localized Ewing's sarcoma: Treatment and results. Cancer 34:143, 1974.

300. ARAI Y et al: Ewing's sarcoma: Local tumor control and patterns of failure following limited-volume radiation therapy. Int J Radiat Oncol Biol Phys 21:1501, 1991.

301. KUTTESCH JF et al: Second malignancies after Ewing's sarcoma: Radiation dose-dependency of secondary sarcomas. J Clin Oncol 14:2818, 1996.

302. BACCI G et al: Long-term results in 144 localized Ewing's sarcoma patients treated with combined therapy. Cancer 63:1477, 1989.

303. GASPARINI M et al: Long-term outcome of patients with monostotic Ewing's sarcoma treated with combined modality. Med Pediatr Oncol 23:406, 1994.

304. STRONG LC et al: Risk of radiation-related subsequent malignant tumors in survivors of Ewing's sarcoma. J Nat Cancer Instit 62:1401, 1979.

305. SMITH LM et al: Second cancers in long-term survivors of Ewing's sarcoma. Clin Orthop Rel Res 274:275, 1992.

306. NOVAKOVIC B et al: Late effects of therapy in survivors of Ewing's sarcoma family tumors. J Pediatr Hemat/Oncol 19:220, 1997.

307. NICHOLSON HS et al: Late effects of therapy in adult survivors of osteosarcoma and Ewing's sarcoma (see comments). Med Pediatr Oncol 20:6, 1992.

308. HAWKINS MM et al: Radiotherapy, alkylating agents, and risk of bone cancer after childhood cancer. J Nat Cancer Instit 88:270, 1996.

309. TUCKER MA et al: Bone sarcomas linked to radiotherapy and chemotherapy in children. N Engl J Med 317:588, 1987.

310. NEFF JR: Nonmetastatic Ewing's sarcoma of bone: The role of surgical therapy. Clin Orthop Rel Res 204:111, 1986.

311. JENTZSCH K et al: Leg function after radiotherapy for Ewing's sarcoma. Cancer 47:1267, 1981.

312. LEWIS RJ et al: Ewing's sarcoma: Functional effects of radiation therapy. J Bone Joint Surg Am 59:325, 1977.

313. OZAKI T et al: Significance of surgical margin on the prognosis of patients with Ewing's sarcoma: A report from the Cooperative Ewing's Sarcoma Study. Cancer 78:892, 1996.

314. NESBIT ME JR et al: Multimodal therapy for the management of primary, nonmetastatic Ewing's sarcoma of bone: A long-term follow-up of the First Intergroup study. J Clin Oncol 8:1664, 1990.

315. WILKINS RM et al: Ewing's sarcoma of bone: Experience with 140 patients. Cancer 58:2551, 1986.

316. SCULLY SP et al: Role of surgical resection in pelvic Ewing's sarcoma. J Clin Oncol 13:2336, 1995.

317. PICCI P et al: Outcome of patients with non-metastatic Ewing's sarcoma of the pelvis: Results in 65 patients (meeting abstract). Proc Annu Meet Am Soc Clin Oncol 13:A1656, 1994.

318. EVANS RG et al: Multimodal therapy for the management of localized Ewing's sarcoma of pelvic and sacral bones: A report from the second intergroup study. J Clin Oncol 9:1173, 1991.

319. ROSEN G et al: Ewing's sarcoma: Ten-year experience with adjuvant chemotherapy. Cancer 47:2204, 1981.

320. YANG RS et al: Surgical indications for Ewing's sarcoma of the pelvis. Cancer 76:1388, 1995.

321. FRASSICA FJ et al: Ewing sarcoma of the pelvis: Clinicopathological features and treatment. J Bone Joint Surg Am 75:1457, 1993.

322. WUNDER JS et al: The histologic response to chemotherapy as a predictor of oncologic outcome of operative treatment of Ewing sarcoma. J Bone Joint Surg Am 80:1020, 1998.

323. TEREK RM et al: Treatment of femoral Ewing's sarcoma. Cancer 78:70, 1996.

324. SPRINGFIELD DS, PAGLIARULO C: Fractures of long bones previously treated for Ewing's sarcoma. J Bone Joint Surg Am 67:477, 1985.

325. HUSTU HO et al: Treatment of Ewing's sarcoma with concurrent radiotherapy and chemotherapy. J Pediatr 73:249, 1968.

326. NESBIT ME JR et al: Multimodal therapy for the management of primary, nonmetastatic Ewing's sarcoma of bone: An Intergroup Study. Nat Cancer Inst Monogr 56:255, 1981.

327. BURGERT EO JR et al: Multimodal therapy for the management of nonpelvic, localized Ewing's sarcoma of bone: Intergroup study IESS-II (see comments). J Clin Oncol 8:1514, 1990.

328. HAYES FA et al: Therapy for localized Ewing's sarcoma of bone. J Clin Oncol 7:208, 1989.

329. MEYER WH et al: Ifosfamide plus etoposide in newly diagnosed Ewing's sarcoma of bone. J Clin Oncol 10:1737, 1992.

330. JURGENS H et al: High-dose ifosfamide with mesna uroprotection in Ewing's sarcoma. Cancer Chemother Pharmacol 24(suppl 1):S40, 1989.

331. WEXLER LH et al: Ifosfamide and etoposide plus vincristine, doxorubicin, and cyclophosphamide for newly diagnosed Ewing's sarcoma family of tumors. Cancer 78:901, 1996.

332. JURGENS H et al: Ifosfamide in pediatric malignancies (review). Semin Oncol 16(suppl 3):46, 1989.

333. GRIER H et al: Improved outcome in nonmetastatic Ewing's sarcoma (EWS) and PNET of bone with the addition of ifosfamide (I) and etoposide (E) to vincristine (V), Adriamycin (Ad), cyclophosphamide (C), and actinomycin (A): A Children's Cancer Group (CCG) and Pediatric Oncology Group (POG) report (meeting abstract). Proc Annu Meet Am Soc Clin Oncol 13:A1443, 1994.

334. BACCI G et al: No advantages in the addition of ifosfamide and VP-16 to the standard four-drug regimen in the maintenance phase of neoadjuvant chemotherapy of Ewing's sarcoma of bone: Results of two sequential studies. J Chemother 5:247, 1993.

335. BACCI G et al: Neoadjuvant chemotherapy for Ewing's sarcoma of bone: No benefit observed after adding ifosfamide and etoposide to vincristine, actinomycin, cyclophosphamide,

and doxorubicin in the maintenance phase-results of two sequential studies. Cancer 82:1174, 1998.

336. DUNST J et al: Radiation therapy in Ewing's sarcoma: An update of the CESS 86 trial (see comments). Int J Radiat Oncol Biol Phys 32:919, 1995.

337. CANGIR A et al: Ewing's sarcoma metastatic at diagnosis: Results and comparisons of two intergroup Ewing's sarcoma studies. Cancer 66:887, 1990.

338. SANDOVAL C et al: Outcome in 43 children presenting with metastatic Ewing sarcoma: The St. Jude Children's Research Hospital experience, 1962 to 1992. Med Pediatr Oncol 26:180, 1996.

339. KUSHNER BH et al: Very-high-dose short-term chemotherapy for poor-risk peripheral primitive neuroectodermal tumors, including Ewing's sarcoma, in children and young adults. J Clin Oncol 13:2796, 1995.

340. HEIJ HA et al: Prognostic factors in surgery for pulmonary metastases in children. Surgery 115:687, 1994.

341. MISER JS et al: Preliminary results of treatment of Ewing's sarcoma of bone in children and young adults: Six months of intensive combined modality therapy without maintenance. J Clin Oncol 6:484, 1988.

342. BADER JL et al: Intensive combined modality therapy of small round cell and undifferentiated sarcomas in children and young adults: Local control and patterns of failure. Radiother Oncol 16:189, 1989.

343. BURDACH S et al: Myeloablative radiochemotherapy and hematopoietic stem-cell rescue in poor-prognosis Ewing's sarcoma. J Clin Oncol 11:1482, 1993.

344. CORNBLEET MA et al: Treatment of Ewing's sarcoma with high-dose melphalan and autologous bone marrow transplantation. Cancer Treat Rep 65:241, 1981.

345. HUVOS AG et al: Postradiation malignant fibrous histiocytoma of bone: A clinicopathologic study of 20 patients. Am J Surg Pathol 10:9, 1986.

346. MIRRA JM et al: Malignant fibrous histiocytoma and osteosarcoma in association with bone infarcts; report of four cases, two in caisson workers. J Bone Joint Surg Am 56:932, 1974.

347. MCCARTHY EF et al: Malignant fibrous histiocytoma of bone: A study of 35 cases. Human Pathol 10:57, 1979.

348. HUVOS AG et al: The pathology of malignant fibrous histiocytoma of bone: A study of 130 patients. Am J Surg Pathol 9:853, 1985.

349. CAPANNA R et al: Malignant fibrous histiocytoma of bone. The experience at the Rizzoli Institute: Report of 90 cases. Cancer 54:177, 1984.

350. DAHLIN DC et al: Malignant (fibrous) histiocytoma of bone: Fact or fancy? Cancer 39:1508, 1977.

351. SPANIER SS et al: Primary malignant fibrous histiocytoma of bone. Cancer 36:2084, 1975.

352. YUEN WW, SAW D: Malignant fibrous histiocytoma of bone. J Bone Joint Surg Am 67:482, 1985.

353. URBAN C et al: Chemotherapy of malignant fibrous histiocytoma of bone: A report of five cases. Cancer 51:795, 1983.

354. WEINER M et al: Adjuvant chemotherapy of malignant fibrous histiocytoma of bone. Cancer 51:25, 1983.

355. BACCI G et al: Adjuvant chemotherapy for malignant fibrous histiocytoma in the femur and tibia. J Bone Joint Surg Am 67:620, 1985.

356. BACCI G et al: Neoadjuvant chemotherapy for osseous malignant fibrous histiocytoma of the extremity: Results in 18 cases and comparison with 112 contemporary osteosarcoma patients

treated with the same chemotherapy regimen. J Chemother 9:293, 1997.

357. Yokoyama R et al: Prognostic factors of malignant fibrous histiocytoma of bone: A clinical and histopathologic analysis of 34 cases. Cancer 72:1902, 1993.

358. Samson IR et al: Operative treatment of sacrococcygeal chordoma: A review of twenty-one cases. J Bone Joint Surg Am 75;1476, 1993.

359. Stener B, Gunterberg B: High amputation of the sacrum for extirpation of tumors: Principles and technique (published erratum appears in Rev Chir Orthop 73: following 217, 1987). Spine 3:351, 1978.

360. Conlon KC, Boland PJ: Laparoscopically assisted radical sacrococcygectomy: A new operative approach to large sacrococcygeal chordomas. Surg Endosc 11:1118, 1997.

361. Castro JR et al: Charged particle radiotherapy for lesions encircling the brain stem or spinal cord. Int J Radiat Oncol Biol Phys 17:477, 1989.

362. Mao X et al: The FLI-1 and chimeric EWS-FLI-1 oncoproteins display similar DNA binding specificities. J Biol Chem 269:18216, 1994.

363. Gebhardt MC et al: The treatment of adamantinoma of the tibia by wide resection and allograft bone transplantation. J Bone Joint Surg Am 69:1177, 1987.

364. Huvos AG, Marcove RC: Adamantinoma of long bones: A clinicopathological study of fourteen cases with vascular origin suggested. J Bone Joint Surg Am 57:110, 1975.

365. Unni KK et al: Adamantinomas of long bones. Cancer 34:1796, 1974.

366. Bacci G et al: Primary chemotherapy and delayed surgery for nonmetastatic osteosarcoma of the extremities: Results in 164 patients preoperatively treated with high doses of methotrexate followed by cisplatin and doxorubicin. Cancer 72:3227, 1993.

367. Dunst J et al: Radiation therapy as local treatment in Ewing's sarcoma: Results of the Cooperative Ewing's Sarcoma Studies CESS 81 and CESS 86. Cancer 67:2818, 1991.

# CHAPTER 21

# NEOPLASMS OF THE ENDOCRINE SYSTEM

*Jeffrey A. Norton*

## INTRODUCTION

Endocrine cancer includes the thyroid, parathyroid, endocrine pancreas, and the adrenal. Cancer of the endocrine system is uncommon. Since ovary and breast cancers are not included in the heading of endocrine cancer, thyroid cancer is the most common type. There are approximately 12,000 new cases of thyroid cancer each year in the United States. The remaining types are even less common, with an annual incidence of 1 to 6 per million population. The purpose of this chapter is to inform the reader about these rare tumors. Further, we will carefully consider the multiple endocrine neoplasia (MEN) syndromes, several autosomal dominant familial endocrine cancer syndromes that simultaneously affect multiple endocrine glands.

## THYROID CANCER

### EPIDEMIOLOGY

The estimated number of new cases of thyroid cancer each year in the United States is approximately 12,000 with nearly 9000 occurring in women.[1] Thyroid cancer is the most common endocrine malignancy. It accounts for 89% of all endocrine cancers and 59% of deaths from endocrine cancer. The incidence of thyroid cancer is increasing, whereas the death rate is decreasing. Most patients are females between the ages of 25 and 65 years; but thyroid cancer can occur in children and the elderly. For well-differentiated thyroid cancers, age at diagnosis is an important prognostic variable. Older patients have a poorer prognosis. Thyroid cancer can be one of the most indolent tumors and one of the most aggressive.[2] Patients with papillary thyroid cancer are usually cured, although patients with anaplastic thyroid cancer seldom live longer than 6 months.

### RISK FACTORS

Papillary thyroid cancer is associated with neck irradiation.[3] The incidence increases with radiation exposure between 200 and 2000 cGy. Interestingly, radiation-induced papillary thyroid cancer has a similar prognosis to papillary thyroid cancer not associated with radiation. Follicular thyroid cancer is associated with iodine deficiency and goiter. Medullary thyroid cancer (MTC) may occur as part of an autosomal dominant familial endocrine syndrome in patients with multiple endocrine neoplasia (MEN) type 2A or B and familial MTC (see Multiple Endocrine Neoplasia for details).

### PRESENTATION

Most patients with thyroid cancer present with a thyroid nodule that is palpable on physical examination. Thyroid nodules are common; the prevalence is estimated to be between 4% and 7% of the U.S. adult population, or approximately 15 million people. Only about 5% to 10% of these nodules are cancerous. The goal of the evaluation is to select cancerous nodules for surgery and to avoid surgery in benign nodules that are not causing symptoms. Previously, thyroid scan and ultrasound were recommended as part of the workup of most patients with thyroid nodules. Currently, neither is recommended because studies have demonstrated that neither is able to accurately discriminate between benign and malignant disease.[4] It is now clear that the single best test to select patients for surgery is fine-needle aspiration (FNA) for cytology.[5] Results of FNA can be divided into benign, suspicious, or malignant (Fig. 21-1). If a nodule appears benign on FNA, there is only a low probability that the mass is cancerous (<3%). Therefore, in patients with benign FNA results, surgery can be safely avoided. If the FNA results suggest that the nodule is malignant, there is a high probability of malignancy (>95%), so definitive surgery can be planned. FNA can reliably

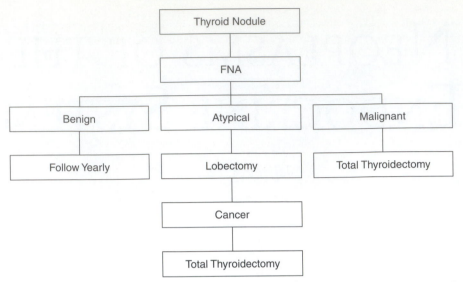

**FIGURE 21-1.** Algorithm for evaluation of the results of fine needle aspiration of a thyroid nodule.

determine papillary thyroid cancer by specific cytologic findings, including Orphan Annie nuclei, nuclear grooves, and psamomma bodies. Similarly, medullary thyroid cancer and anaplastic thyroid cancer can also be readily identified. However, follicular thyroid cancers are problematic on cytology. If the FNA findings indicate atypical follicular cells that are suspicious, but not diagnostic for cancer, thyroid lobectomy is indicated for diagnosis. Lobectomy allows the pathologist to examine the relationship of the nodule to the surrounding thyroid tissue. Follicular thyroid cancer is diagnosed by the detection of capsular or vascular invasion. FNA is the study of choice to evaluate thyroid nodules. It has been shown to save health care dollars, because it accurately selects patients who need surgery from those who do not.

## TYPES OF THYROID CANCER, TREATMENT AND OUTCOME

Neoplasms of the thyroid gland include papillary thyroid cancer (75%), follicular thyroid cancer (15%), medullary thyroid cancer (5%), and anaplastic thyroid cancer (<5%) (Table 21-1). Some patients may have the follicular variant of papillary thyroid cancer or mixed papillary follicular thyroid cancer, which are really subtypes of papillary thyroid cancer and behave like papillary thyroid cancer.

**TABLE 21-1.** INCIDENCE, TYPE, AND SURVIVAL OF THYROID CANCER

| TYPE | INCIDENCE, % | 10-YEAR SURVIVAL |
|------|--------------|------------------|
| Papillary | 75 | 90 |
| Follicular | 15 | 70 |
| Medullary | 5 | 50 |
| Anaplastic | <5 | 0 |

Hurthle cell carcinomas are a subtype of follicular carcinoma and have the same prognosis as follicular cancer. Only approximately 10% to 15% of individuals with well-differentiated thyroid cancer (papillary and follicular) die from it. Nearly twice as many patients die from follicular thyroid cancer as papillary cancer.

For patients with well-differentiated thyroid cancer, a combination of surgery, radioactive iodine therapy, and thyroid suppression therapy is indicated depending on the type and extent of tumor (Fig. 21-2). Total thyroidectomy, radioactive iodine treatment, and thyroxin to suppress thyroid-stimulating hormone (TSH) levels have each been demonstrated to prolong disease-free and overall survival in retrospective studies done by Mazzaferri.[6] For all patients with papillary thyroid cancer, the 1-year survival is approximately 90% (see Table 21-1). Survival is not adversely affected by the presence of lymph node metastases. Old age (>45 to 50 years), tall cell variant of papillary thyroid cancer, extrathyroidal invasion, and distant metastases each portend a poor prognosis and are associated with

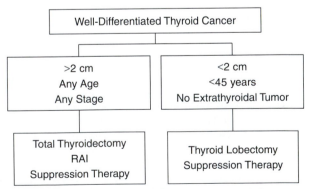

**FIGURE 21-2.** Algorithm for the determination of the management of well-differentiated thyroid cancer according to type and extent of the tumor.

decreased survival. Patients with follicular thyroid cancer have a 10-year survival rate of 70%.[7] Although fewer individuals are diagnosed with follicular thyroid cancer than papillary thyroid cancer, more patients die from follicular thyroid cancer than any type of thyroid malignancy.[2] Therefore, most experts recommend maximum treatment for this diagnosis, which involves total thyroidectomy, radioactive iodine treatment, and thyroid suppression therapy. Further, for patients with well-differentiated thyroid cancer, this treatment allows the use of thyroglobulin levels to detect persistent or recurrent disease.

MTC is associated with a sensitive and specific blood hormone marker, calcitonin.[8] If serum levels of calcitonin are elevated either as basal levels or in response to pentagastrin and calcium, it is diagnostic of MTC. Surgery is the only effective treatment. Total thyroidectomy and central lymph node dissection are recommended because this tumor may be bilateral and it commonly metastasizes early to lymph nodes. Early diagnosis and treatment of individuals from MEN 2 families is almost always curative.[9] However, when MTC spreads to cervical lymph nodes, the long-term survival is 50%. Recently, efforts to aggressively resect lymph node metastases within the neck and mediastinum from individuals with biochemical but not imaging evidence of tumor (hypercalcitonemia) have resulted in complete remission in 30% of patients.

Anaplastic thyroid cancer is best treated nonsurgically with a combination of doxorubicin chemotherapy and hyperfractionated external beam radiation.[10] Surgery is not indicated except for individuals with very small tumors in whom resection may improve local control. Aggressive treatment with low-dose doxorubicin and hyperfractionated radiation therapy appears to improve local control of these tumors. However, patients will still develop metastatic disease and the 2-year survival rate is less than 5%.

## PARATHYROID CANCER

Parathyroid cancer is an uncommon endocrine tumor. Although primary hyperparathyroidism (HPT) is relatively common with an incidence of 3 to 5 per 100,000 population, parathyroid cancer is unusual because it occurs in only 1% of individuals with HPT. Parathyroid cancer most commonly occurs sporadically, but it may occur in families (Table 21-2).[11]

**TABLE 21-2. DIFFERENTIATION OF PARATHYROID CANCER FROM ADENOMA AND HYPERPLASIA**

| TYPE | ETIOLOGY | INCIDENCE, % | CALCIUM, mg/dL | SURGICAL PROCEDURE |
|------|----------|--------------|----------------|--------------------|
| Hyperplasia | Familial | 14 | 11–12 | 3½- or 4-gland excision + transplant |
| Adenoma | Radiation | 85 | 11–12 | Excise adenoma |
| Cancer | Familial | <1 | >14 | Excise gland with ipsilateral thyroid |

Patients with parathyroid cancer have a severe form of HPT. They present with significant hypercalcemia (>14 mg/dL). Symptoms include weakness, bone pain, lethargy, tiredness, kidney stones, and altered mental status. The diagnosis is made by measuring serum levels of total or ionized calcium and intact parathyroid hormone. Serum calcium levels are generally greater than 14 mg/dL and levels of intact parathyroid hormone are markedly elevated. Patients may also have a neck mass or hoarse voice. Physical examination may demonstrate a palpable firm mass in the neck. Indirect laryngoscopy may identify a paramedian immobile vocal cord diagnostic of recurrent laryngeal nerve paralysis. Computed tomography (CT) of the neck and chest is indicated if there is a high suspicion of parathyroid cancer. CT may demonstrate local invasion into surrounding neck structures like the esophagus or strap muscles and/or pulmonary metastases.

At surgery, the diagnosis is made by identification of a firm, immobile whitish-gray mass that is composed of parathyroid cells and is diffusely invasive. Parathyroid cancers are distinguished from adenomas based on findings at surgery. Parathyroid adenomas are usually reddish-brown, soft, and noninvasive, whereas cancers are whitish-gray, firm to rock hard, and locally adherent or diffusely invasive. There are pathologic criteria for parathyroid cancer including frequent mitoses, fibrosis, local invasion, vascular invasion, and nuclear pleomorphism.[12] However, most parathyroid cancers do not meet all the criteria, and the diagnosis may be uncertain unless one is able to detect either lymph node or distant pulmonary metastases. When the diagnosis is suspected, concomitant thyroid lobectomy is performed as well as extensive lymph node dissection. The goal of surgery is to remove all the soft tissue from the affected side while preserving the function of the recurrent laryngeal nerve. If preoperative examination demonstrates vocal cord paralysis, the recurrent laryngeal nerve should be sacrificed with the specimen. Excision of one recurrent laryngeal nerve makes the voice weak and hoarse temporarily, but near complete recovery is anticipated within 6 months.[13] Removal of both recurrent laryngeal nerves if associated with the need for permanent tracheostomy and should be avoided. Parathyroid cancer may be multifocal in the familial setting and total parathyroidectomy may be indicated.[11] Parathyroid cancer may be first identified as a locally recurrent parathyroid tumor[14] or pulmonary metastases.[15] A major issue is control of hypercalcemia. Reexcision of locally recurrent tumors has been effective at controlling serum calcium levels,[14] but removal of distant metastases has not.[15] Medications including diphosphanates may ameliorate hypercalcemia. DTIC (Diethyl-triazeno-indazole-carboxamide) chemotherapy has produced a complete response in one patient with pulmonary metastases.[16]

## ADRENAL CANCER

### ADRENAL CORTICAL CARCINOMA

Adrenal cortical carcinoma is a malignant neoplasm of adrenal cortical cells demonstrating partial or complete histologic and functional differentiation. Adrenal cortical carcinomas are rare and make up between 0.05% and 0.2% of all cancers. This incidence translates to a rate of only 2 per million in the world population. Women develop

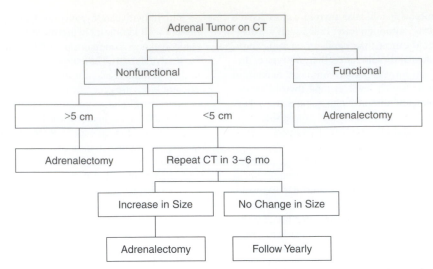

**FIGURE 21-3.** Algorithm for the work-up of adrenal masses (incidenluomas) detected by CT.

functional adrenal cortical carcinomas more commonly than men. However, men develop nonfunctioning malignant adrenal tumors more commonly than women. There is a bimodal occurrence by age, with a peak incidence in those under 5 years of age and a second peak in the fourth and fifth decade. Adrenocortical carcinoma has been described as part of a complex hereditary syndrome including sarcoma and breast and lung cancers.

Adrenal cortical carcinomas are usually greater than 6 cm in size and weigh between 100 and 5000 g.[17] Areas of necrosis and hemorrhage are common. Invasion and metastases also occur. Microscopically the appearance is variable. Cells with big nuclei, hyperchromatism, and enlarged nucleoli are all consistent with malignancy. Nuclear pleomorphism is more common in tumors greater than 500 g. Vascular invasion and large numbers of mitoses are diagnostic of malignancy. Broad desmoplastic bands are associated with cancer.

## SIGNS AND SYMPTOMS OF HYPERCORTISOLISM

Patients with adrenal cortical cancer commonly present with signs and symptoms of hypercortisolism.[18,19] These include weight gain, hirsutism, hypertension, menstrual irregularity, diabetes, truncal obesity, osteoporosis, opportunistic infections, muscle atrophy, and mental changes. The diagnosis is established by measuring a 24-h urinary level of free cortisol or 17-hydroxycorticosteroids.

Adrenal CT can detect normal adrenal glands in most patients. CT can reliably distinguish tumor from normal glands. CT has great sensitivity (>95%); however, it lacks specificity. CT can be used to image the primary tumor plus local and distant metastases. Magnetic resonance imaging (MRI) has similar resolution to CT; however, it is much more expensive so it is not recommended. Adrenal cancers are usually greater than 6 cm in size. In patients with endogenous hypercortisolism, it is necessary to exclude Cushing's disease

(ACTH-secreting pituitary tumor), because most (85%) patients will have this cause.

## INCIDENTALOMA

With the advent of more CT scans, incidentally discovered adrenal masses (incidentaloma) are becoming a common problem for the clinician.[20] The two indications for surgical resection of an incidentaloma are cancer and/or hormonal function. Therefore, the workup of an incidentaloma is designed to make these determinations (Fig. 21-3). Size is the most important determinant of a potentially malignant tumor. Adrenal cortical carcinomas are generally at least 6 cm in diameter. Therefore, surgery is necessary for large adrenal masses (>5 cm). FNA for cytology of an adrenal mass cannot differentiate a benign from a malignant adrenal cortical tumor. Further, FNA may be catastrophic in a patient with an unsuspected pheochromocytoma, so urinary catecholamine levels must be measured prior to a needle biopsy. FNA is indicated for patients with possible metastatic cancer to the adrenal or a diagnosis of lymphoma.

Complete biochemical assessment and blood pressure should be measured in every patient with an incidentally discovered adrenal mass to identify excessive hormonal function. This includes measurement of serum level of potassium, 24-h urinary levels of free cortisol, catecholamines, vanillylmandelic acid (VMA), and metanephrine. If a functional tumor is identified, adrenalectomy is indicated. If the mass in less than 5 cm and nonfunctional, repeat follow-up CT examination in 6 months is indicated to determine if there is any increase in size. If size increases, surgical excision is necessary. If there is no change, it is most likely an adenoma and subsequent CT scans are only necessary yearly.

Adrenocortical carcinoma may also present with signs and symptoms of sex hormone secretion. These signs (virilization in females or feminization in males) are usually detected on physical examination. If sex hormone excess is suspected, blood levels of the appropriate hormone are measured, as are 24-h urinary levels of 17-ketosteroids.[20]

## TREATMENT OF ADRENAL CORTICAL CANCER

The mainstay of treatment of adrenal cortical carcinoma is complete resection of all tumor. In general, surgery is best performed as an open, rather than a laparoscopic procedure. It may be necessary to remove contiguous structures at the time of definitive surgery. It is important to consider that the best time for curative resection is the initial time. The surgeon needs adequate imaging of the extent of tumor that can be achieved by either CT or MRI. Imaging should include the chest to rule out pulmonary metastases. The overall 5-year survival rate of resected adrenal cancer is approximately 22%. If complete resection cannot be achieved, tumor debulking is attempted to decrease the amount of cortisol-secreting tissue and to minimize complications due to tumor mass. If a localized recurrence is detected, it should be removed surgically.[21] Prolonged remissions have been reported following resection of hepatic, pulmonary, and cerebral metastases from adrenal cortical carcinoma.[21] Palliation of bony metastases may be achieved by radiation therapy. Abdominal radiation therapy may be useful in two-thirds of patients with local recurrences not amenable to resection.

Once the patient has recurrent and/or metastatic unresectable adrenal cortical carcinoma, chemotherapy with o,p-DDD (mitotane) is used. Mitotane has been reported to have a 20% response rate.[22,23] Other chemotherapy regimens have been used but are generally ineffective.[24] Partial responses have been reported with doxorubicin and alkylating agents. Cisplatin and etoposide have also been useful. Suramin and gossypol have been tried, but have minimal efficacy.

## PHEOCHROMOCYTOMA

Pheochromocytomas are tumors that arise from chromaffin cells and secrete catecholamines.[17] Chromaffin cells are widespread throughout the body along the sympathetic nerves. Most are found in the adrenal medulla, which explains why the tumors most commonly occur in the adrenal. The rule of 10 applies to pheochromocytoma: 10% malignant, 10% extraadrenal, and 10% bilateral. Extraadrenal pheochromocytomas may arise anywhere, including the organ of Zuckerkandl, carotid body, heart, along the aorta (both thoracic and abdominal), and within the urinary bladder. Extra adrenal pheochromocytomas are more often malignant. Bilateral adrenal pheochromocytomas occur in familial syndromes including MEN 2A and MEN 2B (see section on MEN).[25]

Malignant pheochromocytomas tend to be larger and weigh more than benign tumors. The only absolute criteria for malignancy are the presence of secondary tumors in sites where chromaffin cells are not usually present and visceral metastases. Size of tumor (weight) and amount of necrosis correlate with malignant potential.[17] *ras* gene mutations are seen in pheochromocytomas and other neuroendocrine tumors.[26]

## CLINICAL MANIFESTATIONS AND DIAGNOSIS

Patients with pheochromocytoma present with a range of symptoms from mild hypertension to sudden death. Patients usually describe "spells" of paroxysmal headaches, pallor, palpitations, hypertension, and diaphoresis. In 50%, the hypertension is intermittent, whereas in the others it is sustained.

The diagnosis of pheochromocytoma is based on measuring levels of catecholamines and their metabolites in the urine.[27] The recommended study is a 24-h urine for catecholamines, metanephrine, and VMA. Methods of measuring urinary levels of catecholamine metabolites (VMA and metanephrine) are more sensitive than those for measuring levels of total catecholamines, epinephrine, or norepinephrine.

## LOCALIZATION STUDIES

CT and MRI are the two radiologic (nonnuclear medicine) procedures of choice to localize pheochromocytomas. Both are noninvasive and sensitive, being able to detect tumors approximately 1 cm in diameter. MR may be more specific because of increased signal intensity on different imaging sequences.

Nuclear scanning with labeled metaiodobenzylguanidine (MIBG) is another useful method to image pheochromocytoma.[28,29] The sensitivity of MIBG scanning is 78% in sporadic pheochromocytoma, 91% in malignant pheochromocytoma, and 94% in familial pheochromocytoma. The overall sensitivity is 87%. The specificity is nearly 100%. MIBG scanning is efficacious for the localization of pheochromocytomas, especially those that arise in nonadrenal sites, and those that may be malignant.

## PREOPERATIVE PREPARATION OF PATIENTS WITH PHEOCHROMOCYTOMA

Once the diagnosis is established and the tumor localized, preoperative preparation includes alpha-adrenergic blockade. Patients are started on phenoxybenzamine 10 mg P.O. BID or TID. If tachycardia develops (heart rate >100 beats/min), beta-adrenergic blocking agents (propranolol) are added. Propranolol should never be started prior to phenoxybenzamine. Patients need to be on phenoxybenzamine for at least 7 days prior to surgery. Alpha-blockade restores the circulating plasma volume in these patients and allows safe anesthesia and surgery.

## MALIGNANT PHEOCHROMOCYTOMAS

Malignant pheochromocytomas are thought not to occur in MEN syndromes and are present in approximately 10% of patients. Pathologic analysis may be not be helpful in predicting which tumors are malignant. Malignancy is diagnosed by the presence of distant or recurrent disease in areas without sympathetic nerves. Metastases may not develop until many years after the initial surgery. Incidence of detection of recurrent or metastatic disease during the first 9 years after surgery is 5% per year. Males are more likely to develop metastases. Imaging with [131]I-MIBG is usually able to detect recurrent or metastatic tumor.[28,29] Some recommend yearly [131]I-MIBG scans to detect recurrence in all patients following surgery. Others recommend lifelong follow-up with measurement of blood pressure and urinary levels of catecholamines. The detection of recurrent or metastatic tumor should be based on the same methods as primary tumor. It appears that with careful follow-up the incidence of malignant pheochromocytoma may be significantly greater than 10% and may approach 30% to 50%.

The basic principles in the treatment of malignant pheochromocytoma are to surgically resect localized recurrences or metastases and to treat hypertensive symptoms by catecholamine blockade. Painful bony metastases respond well to radiotherapy. Soft tissue masses may also respond. Standard chemotherapy regimens including streptozotocin, BCNU, and doxorubicin have had limited efficacy. Combination of cyclophosphamide, vincristine, and dacarbazine has had a 60% response rate for metastatic pheochromocytoma, including one complete response.[30] Patients whose tumors are imaged by MIBG are eligible for [131]I-MIBG therapy, which has had a 60% response rate.

Survival data of patients with malignant pheochromocytoma are difficult to obtain because of the rarity and indolence of the tumor. The 5-year survival rate is between 36% and 60%.

## PANCREATIC ISLET CELL TUMORS

Endocrine tumors of the pancreas are classified primarily according to the associated clinical syndrome.[31] Signs and symptoms are due to uncontrolled excessive secretion of hormone. For example, patients with insulinoma have altered mental status, confusion, seizures, and other neuroglycopenic symptoms related to hypoglycemia caused by excessive uncontrolled insulin secretion.[32] Pancreatic endocrine tumors share a number of common features, including similar microscopic appearance, hormonal symptoms, special issues in patients with MEN type 1,[33] and malignant growth affecting survival. Pancreatic endocrine tumors are usually slow-growing, and even patients with extensive tumor may still live for long periods. However, if liver metastases occur, survival will be affected by the malignant nature of the tumor. Effective treatment must address the symptoms associated with the clinical syndrome and the malignant potential of the tumor.

### EPIDEMIOLOGY

Endocrine tumors of the pancreas are rare, having an incidence of less than 10 per million people per year.[31] Insulinomas are the most common islet cell tumors, with a prevalence of approximately 1 per million per year, and gastrinomas are a close second. The remaining islet cell tumors are less common.

Pancreatic neuroendocrine tumors arise from cells that have been termed APUDomas, which means amine precursor uptake and decarboxylation. Islet cell tumors are composed of monotonous sheets of small round cells with uniform nuclei and cytoplasm. Mitotic figures are unusual. Tumors have dense secretory granules. When stained by immunohistochemistry, most pancreatic neuro-

endocrine tumors are positive for more than one hormone. However, in most instances only one peptide is secreted into the circulation.

Because patients with pancreatic islet cell tumors are now living longer, the development of a secondary symptomatic pancreatic hormonal syndrome is becoming increasingly problematic. It occurs more commonly in patients with malignant islet cell tumors. Patients with a long history of malignant gastrinoma may develop signs and symptoms of hypercortisolism secondary to ectopic ACTH secretion. In patients with multiple or metastatic islet cell tumors, it may not be possible to determine which tumor produces the hormone that is responsible for the symptoms and syndrome. Therefore, the surgeon must be aware that excision of a specific tumor may not improve the symptoms of the syndrome.

### PATHOLOGY

In general, microscopic pathologic analysis of pancreatic endocrine tumors has failed to predict the growth pattern of the tumor and is not able to determine whether a tumor is benign or malignant. In addition, there is no correlation between histologic pattern and clinical syndrome. At present, the only clear determination of malignancy is detection of metastases, either in lymph nodes or liver. Microscopic invasion of blood vessels and surrounding pancreas is another indicator of malignancy, but is not as precise as the detection of distant metastatic disease. Because of this, it is unclear exactly what proportion of pancreatic islet cell tumors are malignant. The benign nature of an individual tumor can only be determined by careful long-term follow-up studies. In general, few (<10%) insulinomas are cancerous;[34] 60% of gastrinomas are malignant (lymph node or liver metastases);[35] and the majority (50% to 90%) of all other islet cell tumors are malignant (Table 21-3).

The size of an individual islet cell tumor does not appear to correlate with the severity of the hormonally mediated symptoms. There is, however, a clear correlation between the size of the tumor and the occurrence of malignancy; the larger the tumor, the greater the probability of metastases, especially liver metastases. Insulinomas, like duodenal gastrinomas, are generally small tumors, <2 cm.

**TABLE 21-3.** ISLET CELL TUMOR, MEN-1, DIAGNOSIS, LOCATION, AND MALIGNANT POTENTIAL

| TUMOR | MEN-1, % | DIAGNOSIS | LOCATION | MALIGNANT, % |
|---|---|---|---|---|
| Gastrinoma | 20 | Gastrin, BAO, secretin | Duodenum, pancreas | 60 |
| Insulinoma | 10 | Glucose, insulin | Pancreas | <10 |
| Glucagonoma | rare | Glucagon | Pancreas | 100 |
| Somatostatinoma | rare | Somatostatin | Pancreas, duodenum | 100 |
| VIPoma | rare | VIP | Pancreas, duodenum | 60 |
| PPoma | 100 | PP, mass | Pancreas | 50 |

However, duodenal gastrinomas still have a 60% chance of nodal metastases, while small insulinomas seldom spread. Glucagonomas, somatostatinomas, pancreatic polypeptidomas, and other islet cell tumors are frequently large at the time of detection, >5 cm, and are usually malignant. Most pancreatic endocrine tumors are solitary, encapsulated, and within the pancreas. However, islet cell tumors may also occur in the duodenum and other extrapancreatic locations. Primary gastrinomas have been described within the heart, liver, stomach, and ovary. When metastases occur, they are usually found in peripancreatic lymph nodes (60%) or liver (30%). Late in the course of disease, tumor spreads to lung, bone, and even heart.

Pancreatic endocrine tumors occur in either a nonfamilial (sporadic) form or in a familial form associated with MEN-1 (see section on MEN-1). The exact proportion of patients with pancreatic islet cell tumors who manifest MEN-1 varies in different series from <5% to 25%. The recognition of MEN-1 syndrome is important, because these patients always have multiple pancreatic islet cell tumors. Furthermore, screening of other family members is indicated. Finally, the presence of one hormonal abnormality in MEN-1 patients may affect another. Primary hyperparathyroidism worsens the manifestations of Zöllinger-Ellison syndrome and should be corrected first. Functional islet cell tumors are the second most frequent abnormality in MEN-1, and are present in approximately 80% of individuals. Gastrinomas, insulinomas, glucagonomas, and vasoactive intestinal peptide tumors (VIPomas) occur in decreasing prevalence in MEN-1 patients with gastrinomas in 54% and insulinomas, 20%. In addition to MEN-1, studies suggest that pancreatic islet cell tumors are found more commonly in patients with von Recklinghausen's disease, von Hippel Lindau syndrome, and tuberous sclerosis. In patients with von Recklinghausen's disease, duodenal somatostatinomas and gastrinomas have been reported. In patients with von Hippel Lindau syndrome, 17% of patients had pancreatic endocrine tumors, including both adenomas and carcinomas. However, it is unusual for these tumors to be functional and few have a clinical hormonal syndrome. Patients with tuberous sclerosis have insulinomas and nonfunctional pancreatic islet cell tumors.

## SPECIFIC ISLET CELL TUMORS

Insulinomas occur in the pancreas and are evenly distributed among the head, body, and tail.[34] Glucagonomas also occur within the pancreas (see Table 21-3). In contrast, primary gastrinomas usually occur within the duodenum (50%), and the second most common site is the pancreas (20% to 40%). Further, approximately 80% to 85% of primary gastrinomas are found within the gastrinoma triangle, an area that includes the head of the pancreas and the duodenum.[35] VIPomas are usually in the pancreas, but they may also occur within the duodenum. Somatostatinomas are commonly in the pancreas but may be extrapancreatic. In a recent review of 48 primary somatostatinomas, 56% were in the pancreas and 44% were in the duodenum or jejunum. Similar to glucagonomas, somatostatinomas usually are large, >5 cm, and metastases are present at the time of diagnosis.[31]

Patients with insulinoma or gastrinoma have symptoms of hypoglycemia and ulcer diathesis with or without diarrhea, respectively,

which raise the possibility of an islet cell tumor. The diagnosis is established biochemically based on the results of standardized tests. Insulinoma is diagnosed by a 72-h fast with the development of neuroglycopenic symptoms. Insulinoma is proven by hypoglycemia (glucose <45 mg/DL) and hyperinsulinism (insulin >5 μIU/mL). Close supervision is necessary to exclude factitious hypoglycemia use of medications to falsely decrease blood glucose levels. Gastrinoma or Zöllinger-Ellison syndrome (ZES) is diagnosed by elevated fasting serum levels of gastrin (>100 pg mL) and elevated levels of basal acid output (BAO >15 mEq/h). All antiacid medications should be discontinued during testing because these drugs may falsely elevate serum gastrin levels. Secretin stimulation test is also used to diagnose ZES; 2 IU/kg of secretin is given intravenously and serum levels of gastrin are measured before and after. An increase of 200 pg/mL over basal levels of gastrin is consistent with ZES.

Nonfunctioning pancreatic islet cell tumors are usually large (>5 cm) and symptoms are related to tumor mass. Other less common functioning islet cell tumors such as those associated with acromegaly (GRFoma, or growth hormone–releasing factor), hypercalcemia, or ectopic ACTH production are usually quite large, with liver metastases found at diagnosis.

## RADIOLOGIC IMAGING

Despite the fact that there are numerous studies to image pancreatic islet cell tumors, some patients will have no imageable tumor. CT has been an excellent study for identifying large tumors within the pancreas and liver. It can reliably visualize tumors that are greater than 2 to 3 cm in diameter; however, smaller tumors may be missed. CT is indicated in all patients with suspected islet cell tumors, especially to exclude liver metastases. The results with MRI are similar to CT. It has the advantage that no radiation is used. However, it is much more expensive and is not recommended. Somatostatin receptor scintigraphy (SRS) images islet cell tumors based on the density of somatostatin receptors.[36] It is an excellent study at identifying both primary and metastatic tumors. It has a sensitivity and specificity of approximately 85% to 90%. It is the imaging study of choice for gastrinomas. However, it must be realized that it may fail to identify small tumors within the duodenum. Further, it is not useful for insulinomas, because most tumors are not imaged. Endoscopic ultrasound is best for imaging small pancreatic islet cell tumors within the pancreas like insulinoma. It has a sensitivity and specificity of 85% for pancreatic islet cell tumors. However, it is observer-dependent and not all institutions have had excellent results. Occult insulinomas and gastrinomas can be regionally localized by portal venous sampling for hormone concentration or provocative angiogram. Arteries that perfuse the pancreas are injected with an agent that causes the tumor to secrete hormone, which can be measured in the hepatic vein. Calcium is used to stimulate insulin secretion by insulinoma and secretin is used for gastrinoma. These studies provide correct regional localization in approximately 90% of patients. Secretin angiogram is not recommended for gastrinomas because occult tumors are generally within the gastrinoma triangle, but calcium angiogram may be useful for insulinomas that are uniformly distributed throughout the pancreas.

## TREATMENT

Treatment should be designed to control the signs and symptoms of excessive hormone secretion and the malignant growth and spread of the tumor. The only curative treatment is complete surgical resection of all tumor. Resection of primary gastrinoma has been shown to decrease the probability of liver metastases.[37] Even localized liver metastases can be removed for apparent amelioration of symptoms and prolongation of survival.[38] Since SRS is a total body imaging study, it can be used to exclude unsuspected sites outside the liver.[36]

Medical management of the gastric acid hypersecretion in patients with gastrinoma can usually be achieved with 20 to 40 mg of omeprazole twice a day.[31] The hypoglycemic symptoms of insulinoma are treated by more frequent feedings. Drugs like diazoxide, ictreotide, and verapamil may occasionally be helpful.[34] However, in general, the hypoglycemia of insulinomas is not able to be controlled medically. The symptoms of glucagonoma (rash) and VIPoma (diarrhea) can be controlled with octreotide, the long-acting somatostatin analogue. The malignant tumoral process of islet cell tumors can seldom be controlled with chemotherapy.[39] Approximately 30% to 40% of tumors respond to doxorubicin (Adriamycin), 5-fluorouracil (5-FU), and streptozotocin as single drugs or in combination. Interferon-α has also produced some partial responses. Chemoembolization of liver metastases using interventional radiology techniques and doxorubicin has had a 90% response rate with improvement in symptoms. However, there have been no complete responses, and it doesn't appear to prolong survival. Patients with liver metastases have a 20% 5-year survival.[31] However, because of the indolent nature of the tumor, some patients may live for many years with distant disease despite the inadequacy of treatment.

## CARCINOID TUMORS

Carcinoid tumors are neuroendocrine tumors derived from the diffuse neuroendocrine system.[41] They are composed of monotonous sheets of small round cells with uniform nuclei and cytoplasm. Pathologists cannot differentiate benign from malignant tumors based on histology. Malignancy can only be determined by the detection of metastases either to lymph nodes or distant sites. Carcinoid tumors synthesize numerous bioactive amines and peptides, including neuron-specific enolase (NSE), 5-hydroxytryptamine (serotonin), 5-hydroxytryptophan, synaptophysin, chromogranin A and C, substance P, tachykinins, and hormones like ACTH, calcitonin, and growth hormone–releasing hormone. Carcinoid tumors are fairly common in autopsy series and are present in approximately 21 per million autopsies. Similarly, 1 in 300 appendectomies will have a carcinoid tumor. Carcinoid tumors occur with greater frequency in patients with the MEN-1 syndrome.

Carcinoid tumors generally originate in four sites: bronchus, appendix, rectum, and small intestine (Table 21-4). Carcinoid tumors most commonly occur in the appendix (40%), small intestine (27%), rectum (13%), and bronchus (12%). Carcinoid tumors may also be divided into those of foregut, midgut, and hindgut. Foregut tumors include the bronchus, stomach, and thymus, which most commonly produce peptide hormones like ACTH and calcitonin. These tumors also cause the atypical carcinoid syndrome because

**TABLE 21-4. CARCINOID TUMORS: LOCATION, METASTASES, AND CARCINOID SYNDROME BY LOCATION**

| GUT | SITE | INCIDENCE, % | METASTASES, % | CARCINOID SYNDROME, % |
|---|---|---|---|---|
| Fore | Stomach, | 2 | 22 | 10 |
| | duodenum, | 3 | 20 | 3 |
| | bronchus, | 12 | 50 | 13 |
| | thymus | 2 | 25 | 0 |
| Mid | Jejunum, | 1 | 35 | 9 |
| | ileum, | 23 | 35 | 9 |
| | appendix, | 38 | 2 | <1 |
| | ovary | <1 | 6 | 50 |
| Hind | Rectum | 13 | 3 | 0 |

they secrete 5-hydroxytryptophan and lack the enzyme to convert it to 5-hydroxytryptamine or serotonin. Midgut carcinoid tumors include the appendix and small intestine. These tumors most commonly secrete serotonin, which causes the typical carcinoid syndrome. However, because the liver metabolizes serotonin, signs and symptoms of the carcinoid syndrome are not present without liver metastases and the release of serotonin into the systemic circulation. Hindgut carcinoid tumors occur in the rectum and generally secrete no hormones.

Foregut carcinoid tumors most commonly occur in the bronchus and are a common cause of ectopic ACTH syndrome (Cushing's syndrome). The tumors occur in the major bronchi. They appear like a red cherry on bronchoscopy because of increased vascularity. Biopsy is contraindicated because of the risk of uncontrolled hemorrhage. MRI of the chest is the best method to diagnose bronchial carcinoid tumors because it can distinguish a tumor from hilar vessels. Lobectomy is the surgical procedure of choice because 50% have lymph node metastases. Thymic carcinoid tumors are another potential cause of ectopic ACTH syndrome. These tumors are commonly malignant. CT and MRI are excellent studies to image the extent of disease and make the diagnosis. The tumor appears as a mass within the anterior superior mediastinum and the thymus. Radical thymectomy is the procedure of choice. Care should be taken to avoid injury to one or both phrenic nerves. Stomach carcinoid tumors account for 3 of every 1000 gastric neoplasms. Recent studies suggest that all gastric carcinoid tumors are not similar. Some are associated with chronic hypergastrinemic states like achlorhydria and ZES. These tumors arise from the enterochromaffin-like (ECL) cells, are small, multiple, and seldom malignant (9% overall). These are contrasted to sporadic carcinoid tumors of the stomach, which are large, single, and atypical on histology and are associated with the carcinoid syndrome in 15% to 50% of patients. These tumors cause the syndrome without liver metastases because the bioactive substances can enter the systemic circulation; 55% to 66% of these large gastric carcinoid tumors are malignant based on the detection of nodal or liver metastases.

Midgut carcinoid tumors most commonly occur within the appendix. Most carcinoid tumors occur at the tip of the appendix and are totally removed by an appendectomy. Appendiceal carcinoid tumors are usually smaller than 1 cm in diameter and simple appendectomy is adequate. Tumors between 1 and 2 cm are more worrisome, especially when present at the base of the appendix. These tumors have a 50% chance of lymph node metastases and are best treated by right hemicolectomy. Tumors greater than 2 cm in size have a high probability of nodal spread and are also treated by right hemicolectomy. However, most appendiceal carcinoids are smaller than 1 cm, appear at the tip of the appendix, and only require simple appendectomy. Primary small intestinal carcinoid tumors may be multiple and most occur within the ileum. In fact, 40% are within 2 ft of the ileocecal valve. Unlike appendiceal carcinoid tumors that are usually benign, these tumors are generally malignant. They spread to local lymph nodes and cause a dense fibrotic reaction that distorts the gut and may cause symptoms of small bowel obstruction. This fibrosis may obliterate venous outflow and result in venous mesenteric infarction. The incidence of nodal metastases from ileal carcinoid tumors is dependent on the size of the tumor. If the tumor is less than 1 cm, nodal metastases are present approximately 15% of the time. If the tumor is between 1 and 2 cm, nodal metastases occur 60% to 80% of the time. If the tumor is larger than 2 cm, metastases nearly always occur. Liver metastases also occur, and if present, patients have symptoms of the malignant carcinoid syndrome. Duodenal carcinoid tumors may also occur, but most are asymptomatic and are found on endoscopy as an incidental finding. Duodenal carcinoid tumors less than 1 cm in size are clinically insignificant, whereas approximately one-third of larger tumors spread to lymph nodes. Thus duodenal carcinoid tumors are rarely clinically significant, but it must be considered that gastrinomas and somatostatinomas can appear like a small duodenal carcinoid. Immunoperoxidase staining for various hormones helps to differentiate the various tumors.

In approximately 1 in every 2500 sigmoidoscopies, a hindgut carcinoid tumor will be identified. Rectal carcinoids occur submucosally on the anterior or lateral walls of the rectum between 4 and 13 cm from the dentate line. Approximately 80% of these tumors are less than 1 cm in size and never metastasize. Tumors greater than 2 cm, which are rare, almost always metastasize. These larger tumors are locally invasive and have a large number of mitoses. Either simple resection with negative margins or low anterior resection is the procedure of choice for rectal carcinoid tumors. Abdominoperineal resection is not recommended, because small tumors are seldom malignant and large tumors are usually not cured by surgery. Rectal carcinoid tumors seldom cause the carcinoid syndrome.

## CARCINOID SYNDROME

The carcinoid syndrome is associated with severe flushing attacks. Flushing attacks are characterized by the sudden onset of a deep red color over the upper part of the body, primarily the neck and face, and an unpleasant feeling of warmth, lacrimation, itching, palpitations, and diarrhea. Flushing spells may be precipitated by stress, certain foods like cheese or wine, exercise, and drugs. Attacks are generally brief, lasting 2 to 5 min, and are episodic. Typical flushing attacks are most commonly seen with carcinoid tumors that originate in the midgut and have liver metastases. Diarrhea is also associated with carcinoid syndrome. Ovarian carcinoid tumors also commonly cause the carcinoid syndrome (see Table 21-4). Diarrhea usually occurs with the flushing but it may also occur alone. Typically

the stools are watery with the number of movements ranging from 3 to 30 per day. Patients commonly develop wheezing and airway constriction during an attack. Cardiac manifestations are also part of the carcinoid syndrome. The cardiac disease is typically caused by fibrosis that involves primarily the right side of the heart. Fibrous deposits tend to cause constriction of the tricuspid and pulmonic valve that results in regurgitation. In the atypical carcinoid syndrome, the flushing may be prolonged, lasting several days, more diffuse over the entire body, and may be a constant red or cyanotic color. The atypical rash is frequently provoked by food and may be associated with intense pruritus.

In general, the signs and symptoms of the carcinoid syndrome are caused by serotonin (5-HT) secretion by the tumor. Most patients (>85%) with the carcinoid syndrome have elevated urinary levels of 5-hydroxyindolacetic acid (5-HIAA), the major metabolite of serotonin. The carcinoid syndrome is diagnosed by elevated urinary levels of 5-HIAA. It is also important to remember that foregut carcinoid tumor may produce the atypical carcinoid syndrome. These tumors lack the appropriate decarboxylase enzyme to convert 5-hydroxytryptophan to serotonin (5-hydroxytryptamine). Therefore, in patients with atypical carcinoid syndrome urinary levels of 5-HIAA may be normal but urinary metabolites of tryptophan will be elevated. Further, platelet levels of serotonin will be elevated because platelets have the enzyme to convert 5-hydroxytryptophan to serotonin. However, most patients with carcinoid syndrome have midgut carcinoid tumors with liver metastases and these patients will have elevated urinary levels of 5-HIAA.

## LOCALIZATION STUDIES

Patients with the carcinoid syndrome typically have a mass in the small bowel on CT with cicatrization and narrowing of the bowel with partial obstruction. These patients usually have liver metastases. Tumor is best imaged by somatostatin receptor scintigraphy (SRS), which has approximately a 90% sensitivity and specificity for the tumor. SRS is especially useful because it will also image bone and other distant metastases.

## PROGNOSIS AND TREATMENT

For all patients with the carcinoid syndrome the 5-year survival is approximately 25% (Table 21-5). The prognosis varies with the site of origin and extent of disease. Patients with the carcinoid

**TABLE 21-5. SURVIVAL WITH CARCINOID TUMORS BY SITE AND STAGE**

| SITE | 5-YEAR SURVIVAL, % | | |
| --- | --- | --- | --- |
| | LOCAL | NODAL | DISTANT |
| Appendix | 99 | 99 | 27 |
| Rectum | 92 | 44 | 7 |
| Bronchus | 96 | 71 | 11 |
| Ileum | 75 | 60 | 20 |
| Stomach | 93 | 23 | 0 |

syndrome usually have distant metastases. The most immediate life-threatening complication is the carcinoid crisis that may occur during chemotherapy, surgery, or anesthesia. The crisis only happens in patients with 24-h urinary 5-HIAA levels greater than 200 mg. The crisis initially presents with upper body flush, hypertension, and tachycardia, and subsequently severe hypotension and death may develop. Treatment with intravenous octreotide (long-acting somatostatin analogue) ameliorates the symptoms and signs and can be life-saving.

The manifestations of the carcinoid syndrome should be managed medically. The flush is initially controlled by avoiding precipitating agents, diarrhea by antidiarrheal drugs, wheezing by bronchial dilators, and valvular heart disease by inotropic drugs and diuretics. However, the syndrome may not be completely controlled by these measures and eventually patients become more symptomatic. At this point, patients are treated by the somatostatin analogue octreotide, 100 to 150 μg subcut TID, which markedly improves all symptoms. Patients who are treated chronically with this drug may become refractory to it and require larger and larger doses. Interferon-α has also been used to treat the carcinoid syndrome and may be helpful in some patients.

Carcinoid tumors are best managed surgically. However, in patients with liver or other distant sites of metastasis, surgery is seldom curative. Patients with distant metastases may have symptoms related to a partial small bowel obstruction that warrant surgery. Further, in some reports aggressive surgery to debulk the primary and metastatic tumor is associated with amelioration of symptoms and prolongation of survival. Hepatic metastases may also be treated with chemoembolization, cryotherapy, radiofrequency ablation, and liver transplantation. Each of these procedures may improve symptoms, but none has been shown to prolong survival. Chemotherapy with doxorubicin, 5-FU, and streptozocin has a 30% partial response rate. However, there have been no complete responses and no improvement in survival. Immunotherapy with interferon-α has also decreased tumor size and may improve symptoms. In general, patients with carcinoid tumors live for long periods (see Table 21-5) and treatments are used to provide specific goals like relief of symptoms and prolongation of survival.

## MULTIPLE ENDOCRINE NEOPLASIA

Multiple endocrine neoplasia type 1 (MEN-1) is an inherited endocrine disorder that includes hyperplasia of the parathyroid glands, tumors of the pancreatic islets and anterior pituitary, and occasionally carcinoid tumors and lipomas. It is inherited as an autosomal dominant disorder with variable penetrance. This means that 50% of the offspring will develop the disease, but each may not express all of the components (Table 21-6).

### GENETIC ABNORMALITIES IN MEN-1

The causative gene in MEN-1 has been mapped to the long arm of chromosome 11 (see Table 21-6). The exact gene has been identified and named menin. Menin is a tumor suppressor gene, but its exact function is unknown.[41] Screening for the presence of disease should begin during the second or third decade of life.

**TABLE 21-6. MULTIPLE ENDOCRINE NEOPLASIAS: GENETICS AND CLINICAL SYNDROMES**

| VARIABLE | MEN-1 | MEN-2A | MEN-2B | FMTC |
|---|---|---|---|---|
| Chromosome | 11q12–13 | 10 | 10 | 10 |
| Gene | Menin | RET | RET | RET |
| Autosomal dominant | Yes | Yes | Yes | Yes |
| Phenotype | No | No | Yes | No |
| MTC | No | Yes | Yes | Yes |
| Virulence of MTC | None | ++ | ++++ | + |
| Pheochromocytoma | No | Yes | Yes | No |
| Islet cell tumors | Yes | No | No | No |
| Parathyroid hyperplasia | Yes | Yes | No | No |
| Pituitary tumors | Yes | No | No | No |

Individuals at risk should be questioned and examined for kidney stones, lipomas, hypercortisolism, hypoglycemia, peptic ulcer disease, headaches, acromegaly, and visual field defects. Blood levels of calcium, glucose, prolactin, gastrin, and pancreatic polypeptide are measured.

### PARATHYROID HYPERPLASIA IN MEN-1

Primary hyperparathyroidism (HPT) is the most common endocrine disorder in patients with MEN-1.[42,43] The manifestations are similar to those seen in non–MEN-1 patients with HPT and include asymptomatic hypercalcemia, weakness, fatigue, kidney stones, and bone pain from decreased bone density. The prevalence of HPT in MEN-1 increases with age and is nearly 100% after age 50. The age of onset is 25 years, which is younger than sporadic HPT. Primary hyperparathyroidism is diagnosed by measurement of elevated serum levels of total calcium, ionized calcium, and parathyroid hormone (PTH). The intact PTH assay has seldom given false-positive results and is very specific for HPT. These patients always have parathyroid hyperplasia, but at surgery there can be some asymmetry in size.[43] The operation of choice is either 3½-gland parathyroidectomy or 4-gland parathyroidectomy with forearm transplant. The cervical thymus should also be removed as supernumerary glands can occur and are usually within the thymus.

### PANCREATIC ISLET CELL TUMORS IN MEN-1

MEN-1 patients also develop pancreatic or duodenal neuroendocrine tumors.[31] These tumors may be malignant and there is a correlation between the size of the tumor and the chance of metastases.[44] Pancreatic islet cell tumors may be nonfunctional or produce excessive hormones that cause a characteristic clinical syndrome. The most common functional islet cell tumor in MEN-1 is gastrinoma. Moreover, any islet cell tumor can occur in patients with MEN-1 including gastrinoma, insulinoma, glucagonoma, VIPoma, GRFoma, somatostatinoma, and nonfunctional tumor or pancreatic polypeptide (PPoma).

Surgery is indicated to remove a potentially malignant islet cell tumor and to cure the hormonal effects. At surgery these patients commonly have multiple pancreatic islet cell tumors and also multiple duodenal neuroendocrine tumors.[45] Recent studies indicate that tumors that produce insulin, glucagon, and VIP are more commonly within the pancreas, whereas tumors that secrete gastrin are usually within the duodenum.[46] The goal of surgery is to remove tumor without excessive morbidity and mortality. Surgical resection seldom cures ZES patients,[47] but it reduces the probability of liver metastases.[37]

## PITUITARY TUMORS IN MEN-1

The most common pituitary tumor in MEN-1 is a prolactinoma. Elevated serum levels of prolactin are diagnostic and are used as a screening study. Prolactinomas cause galactorrhea and impotence. Pituitary tumors in MEN-1 may also secrete other hormones including corticotropin (ACTH), growth hormone, and thyroid-stimulating hormone (TSH). These tumors are associated with Cushing's disease, acromegaly, and hyperthyroidism, respectively. Biochemical diagnosis of each is based on recognition of the clinical signs and symptoms. MRI or CT of the sella and visual field examination are ordered for patients suspected to have pituitary tumors. Bitemporal hemianopsia may occur when large tumors compress the optic chiasm. Pituitary adenomas that produce prolactin are usually treated with bromocriptine. Pituitary tumors can also be removed surgically or less commonly treated with irradiation.

## LESS COMMON TUMORS IN MEN-1

Less common tumors that may be associated with MEN-1 include bronchial or thymic carcinoids, intestinal carcinoids, gastric carcinoids, lipomas, benign adenomas of the thyroid gland, benign adrenocortical adenomas, and rarely adrenocortical carcinomas. Carcinoid tumors should be removed surgically when identified. Cortical adenomas of the thyroid gland and benign cortical adenomas of the adrenal cortex usually require no treatment, unless there is evidence of excessive hormonal function. Lipomas are usually large and should be excised when symptomatic. Adrenal cortical carcinomas commonly present with signs and symptoms of hypercortisolism and are identified as a large adrenal tumor on CT (≥6 cm). Surgical resection is the treatment of choice.

## MEN TYPE 2A, 2B, AND FAMILIAL MTC

MEN type 2A (MEN-2A) is an autosomal dominantly inherited endocrine syndrome that is characterized by MTC, adrenal pheochromocytoma(s), and parathyroid hyperplasia[9] (see Table 21-6). MEN type 2B (MEN-2B) is an autosomal dominantly inherited endocrine syndrome that is characterized by MTC, adrenal pheochromocytoma(s), and a characteristic phenotype that includes mucosal neuromas, puffy lips, bony abnormalities, marfanoid habitus, intestinal ganglioneuromas, and corneal nerve hypertrophy.[48] Unlike MEN-2A, parathyroid disease is not associated with MEN-2B. Familial medullary thyroid carcinoma (FMTC) is characterized by an autosomal dominant inheritance of only MTC without any other endocrine abnormalities.[49]

## GENE DEFECT IN MEN-2

The gene for MEN-2A, MEN-2B, and FMTC has been localized to the pericentromeric region of chromosome 10 (see Table 21-6). The responsible gene is a transmembrane protein kinase receptor called RET.[50,51] RET is an oncogene in that mutations enhance cellular growth. The exact mechanism by which RET enhances cellular growth is unknown. Recent studies have detected missense mutations in RET in all individuals with MEN-2A, MEN-2B, and FMTC.[50,51] MEN-2A and FMTC mutations have been identified within the extracellular portion of the molecule, whereas MEN-2B mutations have been identified within the intracellular domain.

## MEDULLARY THYROID CARCINOMA

In patients with MEN-2A, MTC generally appears between the ages of 5 and 25 years prior to development of pheochromocytoma or primary hyperparathyroidism.[9,52,53] Recently, detection of RET mutations in the peripheral white blood cells of patients from kindreds with MEN-2A has been used as a screening procedure to diagnose an affected individual[9,52] (Fig. 21-4). Since 100% of individuals with MEN-2A will develop MTC, total thyroidectomy has been performed when RET mutations are detected.[9] Prior to thyroid surgery, it is important to rule out the presence of a pheochromocytoma by measuring 24-h urine levels of VMA, metanephrines, and total catecholamines.[53] When total thyroidectomy has been performed based solely on genetic testing, either premalignant C-cell hyperplasia or in situ MTC has been identified.[9]

Individuals with MEN-2B have a characteristic phenotype.[48] These patients have prognathism, puffy lips, poor dentition, mucosal neuromas, corneal nerve hypertrophy, and multiple bony abnormalities. The presence of MEN-2B can be ascertained by the observation of corneal nerve hypertrophy on slit light examination. Patients with MEN-2B usually have locally advanced medullary thyroid carcinoma at presentation.[48] These patients are seldom cured by thyroidectomy and usually die of the MTC.

Individuals with FMTC have the best prognosis.[49] In these patients, the MTC occurs at an older age and patients seldom die from medullary thyroid cancer. Thus, in the three different familial settings, although the same oncogene is affected, the virulence of the MTC is different. The most virulent form is MEN-2B, the intermediate form is MEN-2A, and the least virulent is FMTC. Total thyroidectomy is indicated for the familial types of MTC because each involves both lobes of the gland.

## PHEOCHROMOCYTOMA IN MEN-2A AND MEN-2B

Individuals with either MEN-2A or MEN-2B may develop bilateral benign intraadrenal pheochromocytomas.[53] The diagnosis of pheochromocytoma is made by detection of elevated 24-h urinary levels of VMA, metanephrines, or total catecholamines. Urinary metanephrines are the single best diagnostic study. Imaging studies can identify which adrenal gland is involved. CT, MR, and MIBG scan each have utility. Both MR and CT can image pheochromocytomas as small as 1 cm. There is controversy as to the extent of adrenalectomy in patients with MEN-2. Some recommend bilateral

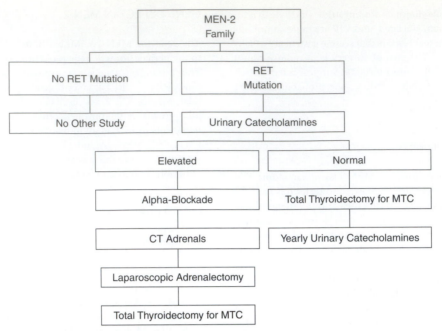

**FIGURE 21-4.** Algorithm for the diagnosis and treatment of MEN-2A.

adrenalectomy for all individuals with biochemical evidence of pheochromocytoma, because studies have shown that 70% are bilateral and sudden death can be caused by an untreated pheochromocytoma. Others remove only the adrenal gland in which a tumor is seen. If an unilateral adrenalectomy is performed, careful follow-up is warranted because some patients may develop another tumor in the contralateral gland. Recent studies have demonstrated that laparoscopic adrenalectomy is the method of choice to remove these tumors. Resection should be performed after the patient has been prepared preoperatively with α-adrenergic blocking drugs like phenoxybenzamine. Adrenal surgery should be performed prior to thyroidectomy (see Fig. 21-4).

### PARATHYROID DISEASE IN MEN-2A

Patients with MEN-2A may also develop symptomatic primary hyperparathyroidism. The diagnosis is ascertained by measurement of elevated serum levels of calcium and parathyroid hormone. HPT is caused by multiple gland disease or parathyroid hyperplasia (see Table 21-6). The proper surgical treatment is either 3½-gland parathyroidectomy or 4-gland parathyroidectomy with transplant.

### GASTROINTESTINAL MANIFESTATIONS OF MEN-2A OR MEN-2B

Some individuals with MEN-2A may also have Hirschsprung's disease. Recent evidence suggests that Hirschsprung's disease is also associated with RET mutations; however, these mutations are inactivating for RET. Individuals with MEN-2B commonly complain of severe constipation, and megacolon or diverticulosis has been described. MEN-2B patients are known to have abnormal gut motility secondary to intestinal ganglioneuromatosis. Constipation should be treated as symptoms arise. As the MTC becomes metastatic, patients may develop severe secretory diarrhea. Medullary thyroid carcinoma can secrete a wide variety of peptide hormones that cause diarrhea. Octreotide has been used to inhibit the diarrhea in this setting.

## REFERENCES

1. SILVERBERG E et al: Cancer statistics. CA 40:9, 1990.
2. ROBBINS J et al: Thyroid cancer: A lethal endocrine neoplasm. Ann Intern Med 115:133, 1991.
3. SCHNEIDER AB et al: Radiation-induced tumors of the head and neck following childhood irradiation. Medicine 64:1, 1985.
4. BRANDER A et al: Thyroid gland: U.S. screening in an adult population. Radiology 181:683, 1991.
5. GHARIB H, GOELLNER JR: Fine needle aspiration biopsy of the thyroid: An appraisal. Ann Intern Med 118:282, 1993.
6. MAZZAFERRI EL et al: Papillary thyroid carcinoma: The impact of therapy in 576 patients. Medicine 56:171, 1977.
7. BRENNAN MD et al: Follicular thyroid cancer treated at the Mayo Clinic 1946–1970: Initial manifestations, pathology findings, therapy and outcome. Mayo Clin Proc 66:11, 1991.
8. VAN HEERDEN JA et al: Long term course of patients with persistent hypercalcitoninemia after apparent curative primary surgery for medullary thyroid cancer. Ann Surg 212:395, 1990.
9. WELLS SA JR et al: Predictive testing and prophylactic thyroidectomy in patients at risk for multiple endocrine neoplasia type-2a. Ann Surg 220:237, 1994.
10. KIM JH, LEEPER RD: Treatment of anaplastic giant and spindle cell carcinoma of the thyroid gland with combination adriamycin and radiation therapy: A new approach. Cancer 52:954, 1983.

11. STREETEN EA et al: Studies in a kindred with parathyroid carcinoma. J Clin Endocrinol Metab 75:362, 1992.

12. SCHANTZ A, CASTLEMAN B: Parathyroid carcinoma, a study of 70 cases. Cancer 31:6600, 1973.

13. PATOW C et al: Vocal cord paralysis and reoperative parathyroidectomy: A prospective study. Ann Surg 203:282, 1986.

14. FRAKER DL et al: Locally recurrent parathyroid neoplasms as a cause for persistent or recurrent hyperparathyroidism. Ann Surg 213:58, 1991.

15. FLYE MW, BRENNAN MF: Surgical resection of metastatic parathyroid carcinoma. Ann Surg 193:425, 1981.

16. CALANDRA DB et al: Parathyroid carcinoma. Biochemical and pathological response to DTIC. Surgery 96:1162, 1984.

17. PAGE DL et al: Tumors of the adrenal, in *Atlas of Tumor Pathology*. AFIP, Washington DC, 1986.

18. KASPERLIK-ZALUSKA AA et al: Adrenal carcinoma. A clinical study and treatment results of 52 patients. Cancer 75:2587, 1995.

19. LUTON JP et al: Clinical features of adrenocortical carcinoma, prognostic factors and the effect of mitotane therapy. N Engl J Med 322:1195, 1990.

20. ROSS NS, ARON DC: Hormonal evaluation of the patient with an incidentally discovered adrenal mass. N Engl J Med 323:1401, 1990.

21. JENSEN JC et al: Recurrent or metastatic disease in select patients with adrenocortical carcinoma. Arch Surg 126:457, 1991.

22. DECKER RA et al: ECOG mitotane and adriamycin in patients with ACC. Surgery 110:1006, 1991.

23. HAAK HR et al: Mitotane therapy of adrenocortical carcinoma. N Engl J Med 322:758, 1990.

24. POMMIER R, BRENNA MF: An 11 year experience with adrenocortical cancer. Surgery 112:1963, 1992.

25. LAIRMORE TC et al: Management of pheochromocytomas in patients with multiple endocrine neoplasia type 2 syndromes. Ann Surg 217:595, 1993.

26. MOLEY JF et al: Low frequency of ras gene mutations in neuroblastomas, pheochromocytomas and medullary thyroid cancers. Cancer Res 51:1596, 1991.

27. DUNCAN MW et al: Measurement of norepinephrine and 3,4-dihydroxyphenylglycol in urine and plasma for the diagnosis of pheochromocytoma. N Engl J Med 319:136, 1988.

28. SHAPIRO B et al: Iodine-131 metaiodobenzylguanidine for the locating of suspected pheochromocytoma: Experience in 400 cases. J Nucl Med 26:576, 1985.

29. KREMPF M et al: Use of $^{131}$I m iodobenzylguanidine in the treatment of malignant pheochromocytoma. J Clin Endocrinol Metab 72:455, 1991.

30. AVERBUCH SD et al: Malignant pheochromocytoma: Effective treatment with a combination of cyclophosphamide, vincristine and dacarbazine. Ann Intern Med 109:267, 1988.

31. NORTON JA: Neuroendocrine tumors of the pancreas and duodenum. Curr Prob Surg 31:77, 1994.

32. DOHERTY GM et al: Results of a prospective strategy to diagnose, localize and resect insulinomas. Surgery 110:989, 1991.

33. NAKAMURA Y et al: Localization of the genetic defect in multiple endocrine neoplasia type 1 within a small region of chromosome 11. Am J Hum Genet 44:751, 1989.

34. SERVICE FJ et al: Functioning insulinoma—incidence, recurrence, and long-term survival of patients: A 60-year study. Mayo Clin Proc 66:711, 1991.

35. NORTON JA et al: Curative resection in Zollinger-Ellison syndrome: Results of a 10 year prospective study. Ann Surg 215:8, 1992.

36. LAMBERTS SW et al: Somatostatin receptor imaging in the localization of endocrine tumors. N Engl J Med 323:1246, 1990.

37. FRAKER DL et al: Surgery in Zollinger-Ellison syndrome alters the natural history of gastrinoma. Ann Surg 220:320, 1994.

38. NORTON JA et al: Aggressive resection of metastatic disease in selected patients with malignant gastrinoma. Ann Surg 203:352, 1986.

39. MODLIN IM et al: Management of unresectable malignant endocrine tumors of the pancreas. Surg Gynecol Obstet 176:507, 1993.

40. JENSEN RT, NORTON JA: Carcinoid tumors and the carcinoid syndrome, in *Cancer Principles and Practice of Oncology*, 5th ed, VT DeVita Jr et al (eds). Philadelphia, Lippincott-Raven, 1997, pp 1704–1723.

41. CHANDRASEKHARAPPA SC et al: Positional cloning of the gene for multiple endocrine neoplasia type 1. Science 276:404, 1997.

42. FRIEDMAN E et al: Multiple endocrine neoplasia type 1 pathology, pathophysiology, molecular genetics and differential diagnosis, in *The Parathyroids*, JP Eilezikian et al (eds). New York, Raven Press, 1994, pp 647–680.

43. METZ DC et al: Multiple endocrine neoplasia type 1 clinical features and management, in *The Parathyroids*, JP Bilezikian et al (eds). New York, Raven Press, 1994, pp 591–646.

44. WEBER HC et al: Determinant of metastatic rate and survival in patients with Zollinger-Ellison syndrome: A prospective long-term study. Gastroenterology 108:1637, 1995.

45. VELDHUID JD et al: Surgical vs. medical management of multiple endocrine neoplasia type 1. J Clin Endocrinol Metab 82:357, 1997.

46. PIPELEERS-MARICHAL M et al: Gastrinomas in the duodenums of patients with multiple endocrine neoplasia type 1 and the Zollinger-Ellison syndrome. N Engl J Med 322:723, 1990.

47. MACFARLAND MP et al: Prospective study of surgical resection of duodenal and pancreatic gastrinomas in multiple endocrine neoplasia type 1. Surgery 118:973, 1995.

48. NORTON JA et al: Multiple endocrine neoplasia type 2-B: The most aggressive form of medullary thyroid carcinoma. Surg Clin North Am 59:109, 1979.

49. FARNDON JR et al: Familial medullary thyroid carcinoma without associated endocrinopathies: A distinct clinical entity. Br J Surg 73:278, 1986.

50. MULLIGAN LM et al: Specific mutations of the RET protooncogene are related to the disease phenotype in MEN-2A and FMTC. Nature Genet 6:70, 1994.

51. SANTORO M et al: Activation of RET as a dominant transforming gene by germline mutations of MEN-2A and MEN-2B. Science 267:381, 1995.

52. LIPS CJM et al: Clinical screening as compared with DNA analysis in families with multiple endocrine neoplasia type 2A. N Engl J Med 331:828, 1994.

53. HOWE J et al: Prevalence of pheochromocytoma and hyperparathyroidism in multiple endocrine neoplasia type 2A: Results of long-term follow-up. Surgery 114:1070, 1993.

# CHAPTER 22

# BENIGN AND MALIGNANT MESOTHELIOMA

*Sunil Singhal and Larry R. Kaiser*

## INTRODUCTION

Mesotheliomas are neoplasms of the serosal membranes of the body cavities; 80% of mesotheliomas originate in the pleural space. Other sites of tumor growth include the peritoneum, pericardium, tunica vaginalis testis, and ovarian epithelium. Pleural mesotheliomas occur ten times more frequently than peritoneal mesotheliomas.

Mesotheliomas can be classified into three general categories: diffuse malignant, localized benign, and localized malignant mesotheliomas. Diffuse mesotheliomas account for 90% of these tumors. They are of special interest because of their increasing frequency, dismal prognosis, and medicolegal issues related to asbestos exposure. Localized mesotheliomas usually are benign and these lesions are more correctly labeled as solitary benign fibrous tumors, since they likely are not of mesothelial cell origin. However, 10% of localized-mesotheliomas may be malignant.[1]

Of all tumors seen in the pleura, 95% are metastatic, not primary, but the most common primary tumor of the pleural cavity is mesothelioma. This chapter details the etiology, pathology, and pathophysiology of malignant mesothelioma and considers the clinical aspects of presentation, diagnostic studies, and therapeutic modalities.

## DIFFUSE MALIGNANT MESOTHELIOMA

### ETIOLOGY

**BACKGROUND.** Asbestos inhalation is an established cause of malignant mesotheliomas; 80% of cases are estimated to be caused by asbestos. Hundreds of cohort studies and case reports have been reported about the connection between asbestos and pleural malignancies. Together, these epidemiologic studies have analyzed over 50,000 male and female asbestos-related workers and come to the same conclusion: asbestos unequivocally causes mesotheliomas.

**HISTORY.** The earliest recorded use of asbestos dates back to the fifth century B.C. in Greece where the material was used as wicks in gold lamps for the goddess Athena. Theophrastus noted that the wick would remain well after the oil was burned off. Asbestos, the Greek word for "unquenchable," predicted the persistence this fiber would come to have in human tissues.[2] Benjamin Franklin gave an asbestos purse to the Englishman Sir Han Sloane and Charlemagne dazzled his dinner guests by throwing his asbestos tablecloth into the fireplace to clean it.

Not until centuries later during the 1850s did asbestos production dramatically rise. Large deposits of asbestos were rediscovered and developed in South Africa (crocidolite asbestos) and Canada (chrystolite asbestos). Uses as diverse as packaging and insulating material were employed. During the two world wars, the full potential of asbestos began to be realized. By 1947, the journal *Asbestos* listed hundreds of possible uses for this natural material. Asbestos was commercially useful because it was extremely resistant to heat and combustion, inexpensive, and had high tensile strength. Asbestos was used in electrical and heat insulation, woven and molded brake linings, textiles, sheet packaging, shingles, paper, fireproofing, and floor tiles.

By the turn of the century, the association between pulmonary diseases and asbestos exposure was beginning to be elucidated; however, the specter of tuberculosis and respiratory infections precluded physicians from making the etiologic connection. Not until the 1960s, in a classic report by J.C. Wagner, was the causal relationship accepted.[3] He described 33 patients with histologically proven pleural mesotheliomas in an asbestos mining community in the northwest province of South Africa. Over the ensuing decade, numerous case reports, cohort studies, and experimental evidence would strengthen Wagner's claim.

In the United States, however, asbestos was not accepted as a cause of pleural malignancies until 1964.[4] In the 1970s the Occupational Safety and Health Administration (OSHA) established 5 fibers per cubic millimeter as acceptable exposure, which still exposed workers to 4 million fibers a day. Subsequently, in 1976, the standard exposure level was reduced to 2 fibers per cubic millimeter; the current level of exposure is set at 0.2 fibers per cubic millimeter. Excess exposure legally mandates respirators, shower and changing facilities, and protective clothing.[5]

The U.S. Environmental Protection Agency estimates that over 700,000 buildings contain asbestos material. Recently, they ordered inspection of all public and commercial buildings which is estimated to cost over $50 billion. Up until 1972, asbestos was sprayed in thousands of schools and other public buildings. Based on conditions, the estimates for the cost of removal of the asbestos in these buildings approximate $100 to $150 billion.[6]

CHARACTERISTICS OF ASBESTOS. Asbestos is a naturally occurring fiber that has two major structural forms: serpentines (chrystolite) and amphiboles (crocidolite, amosite, tremolite, anthopyllite, actinolite) (Fig. 22-1). Serpentines are curly, pilable, short fibers. Amphiboles are long (>4 $\mu$m length), thin (<0.25 $\mu$m diameter), silica-rich fibers. Chrystolite, crocidolite, and amosite fibers are the most important fiber types because they are used commercially, whereas the others are natural contaminants. Numerous studies have demonstrated that there is variable carcinogenicity among the different asbestos types. Crocidolite fibers are associated with the highest risk of mesotheliomas because of their fiber dimensions, unique physical and chemical properties, and inability of the immune system to clear them from tissues.

Animal studies have demonstrated that mesothelioma can be induced by virtually any insoluble mineral. By altering the fiber

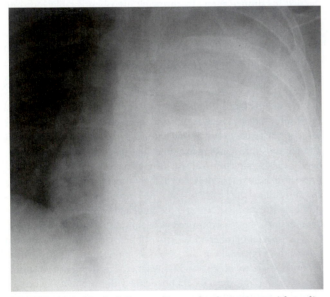

**FIGURE 22-1.** Typical chest radiograph of a patient with malignant mesothelioma presenting with increasing shortness of breath and chest pain demonstrating a large pleural effusion. Cytologic examination of the fluid often is unreliable.

dimensions of other materials such as fiberglass, it has been demonstrated that these are as potent as crocidolite asbestos fibers of similar length. Fibers that are sufficiently small, particularly a diameter less than 0.25 $\mu$m and length greater than 4 to 8 $\mu$m, have an increased risk of carcinogenicity.[7] A length to diameter ratio of 10:1 is associated with increased carcinogenesis.[5] Therefore, long, needlelike crocidolites are claimed to be more mutagenic.

For the most part, carcinogenicity is independent of the biochemical consistency of the fibers and depends mainly on the fiber dimensions. However, some increased risk of cancer is noted with fibers of asbestos compared to fibers of identical size of glass wool and rock wool.[8] Therefore, there must be some additional uncharacterized risk associated with asbestos itself. Furthermore, comparable fibers of erionite, another rare naturally occurring mineral, are even more potent than asbestos in inducing tumors.[9] Cations within the crystal lattice contribute to the toxicity of mineral fibers. Magnesium ($Mg^{2+}$) on the surface of chrystolite asbestos is important to the cytotoxicity and carcinogenicity in experimental animals.[10] The iron ($Fe^{2+}$ and $Fe^{3+}$) content of amphibole fibers is important because when catalyzed by the Fenton reaction, it generates highly toxic and potentially mutagenic reactive oxygen species.

The "amphibole hypothesis" argues that crocidolite fibers are responsible for causing mesotheliomas because they are found in the pulmonary tissues at autopsy, whereas chrystolite fibers are not. Chrystolite fibers are broken down in lung parenchyma and are thought to be cleared from tissues, whereas amphibole fibers are retained longer and cleared less by the immune system.[8] Crocidolite fibers are greater than 10 $\mu$m, so they can be retained longer because they cannot be ingested by macrophages (12 $\mu$m diameter). Also, crocidolite fibers have chemical modification of the surface of their fibers that protect them from digestion. Crocidolite fibers have been demonstrated to be associated with an increased risk of mesothelioma. Debate continues, however, as to the carcinogenicity of chrystolite fibers that account for 95% of all asbestos used worldwide, and, thus, it is economically important to determine its biologic effects. Many authors suggest chrystolite is either mildly mutagenic or not at all carcinogenic. Instead, they argue almost all natural sources of chrystolite are usually mixed with other amphiboles, particularly tremolite. It is these contaminating asbestos fibers, they argue, that cause the increased incidence of neoplasms.[11] Others argue that chrystolite fibers are independently carcinogenic.[6,12,13] Likely, there exists a gradient from crocidolite through amosite to chrystolite asbestos fibers in the potential likelihood to cause mesotheliomas.

The cumulative dose of asbestos is of greater importance than the period of exposure. There is overwhelming evidence of a dose-response relationship of asbestos fibers in lung tissue. Increased severity of exposure and increasing length of exposure are associated with increased death rate due to mesothelioma.[11,14–16] Even intense, localized occupational exposures to asbestos can have effects decades after exposure has ended. Asbestos workers with heavy exposure have a higher risk of developing peritoneal mesothelioma, whereas those exposed for relatively brief periods are at higher risks of developing pleural disease. However, there is a significant percentage of patients with mesotheliomas who have little apparent asbestos exposure yet still develop mesotheliomas. It is possible they have had significant submicroscopic environmental exposure. Also, there is a group of patients who have a significantly large exposure to asbestos who remain tumor free. Therefore, a qualitative dose-response relationship is hard to demonstrate. Another problem in trying to quantitate asbestos exposure and mesothelioma incidence is that reliable information regarding the actual level of asbestos dust in the air cannot be found prior to the late 1960s.

Instead of a direct linear relationship between dose and tumorigenicity, it is suggested that different individuals have different thresholds of susceptibility. Familial clustering of malignant mesothelioma supports the hypothesis that individual threshold is variable and may be predicted genetically. For practical purposes, though, increasing dose can be assumed to have increasing cancer risk.

## EPIDEMIOLOGY

Pleural mesotheliomas occur with a five times greater incidence in men than in women. This reflects the increased work-related exposure of men to asbestos. Incidence rates rise steadily with age and are approximately tenfold higher in men between 60 and 64 than among those between 30 and 34. The disease usually presents in the sixth or seventh decade of life, although it has been seen in individuals ranging in age from 4 years to over 90. There is also significant geographic variation of the incidence of mesothelioma with sections of New England, Philadelphia, Seattle, San Francisco, and Hawaii (all locations of large shipbuilding and asbestos use in World War II) with fivefold higher rates of mesothelioma than other regions of the country.[17,18]

In the past, it has been difficult to estimate how many people died of mesothelioma because physicians were reluctant to diagnose serosal-based tumors and rarely coded them separately from other pulmonary carcinomas. Death certificates rarely can be counted on to determine mesothelioma as a cause of death.[11,19] The incidence of mesothelioma was estimated at 2.7 per million people in 1972 and has been trending upward (Fig. 22-2). More accurate statistics

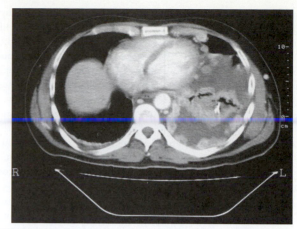

**FIGURE 22-3.** CT scan demonstrating pleural thickening and nodularity consistent with malignant mesothelioma.

now suggest that mesothelioma currently accounts for 20 deaths per million male population in industrialized nations. There are approximately 4000 new cases each year in the United States alone.[20] Various epidemiologic estimates based on data from the Surveillance, Epidemiology, and End Results (SEER) program suggest the peak of 3000 to 4000 new cases a year should be reached at the turn of the century and decline over the next 40 years (Fig. 22-3),[21–23] 75,000 new cases are expected to occur over the next 20 years. The current trend in female mesothelioma incidence is flat at 3 cases per million women. In the third world, mesothelioma incidence rates are predicted to continue to rise indefinitely because of poor regulation of asbestos mining and widespread industrial and household utilization of asbestos.

All urban dwellers are exposed to some asbestos in the environment. As high as 97% to 100% of people from cities demonstrate asbestos exposure on autopsy. Quantitative methods and isolation of ferruginous (asbestos) bodies, the hallmark of asbestos exposure, can be demonstrated in 90% to 100% of the general population.[24] However, the highest death rates occur among workers exposed to asbestos. Death rates vary among different workers depending on the type of asbestos to which they are exposed, degree of exposure, and length of exposure. Those working directly with asbestos are more likely to receive high enough concentrations to cause significant accumulations in their pulmonary parenchyma. The risk of any cancer death in the United States is currently 18%; in asbestos workers, this rises to 50%.[5] Of all cancers that occur, 3% are related to occupational asbestos exposure. The highest death rates tend to occur among asbestos manufacturers and insulation workers. Some cohorts of asbestos insulation workers have shown a greater than 300-fold increased incidence in malignant mesothelioma compared to the general population. From World War II through the 1960s, asbestos was the main material used in insulating pipes and decks of naval vessels and commercial ships. In some studies, as high as 11% of shipyard and dockyard workers present with malignant mesotheliomas.[17,25] Utilizing 7000 pathologists throughout the United States and Canada to study various professions, asbestos-related insulation producers were found to have a 46-fold increased risk of mesotheliomas.[11] In one cohort of railroad machinists, there

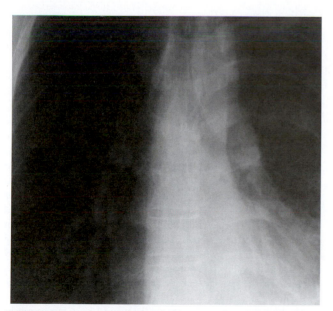

**FIGURE 22-2.** Chest radiograph demonstrating left pleural effusion and the nodularity characteristic of mesothelioma.

were 88.1 pleural mesotheliomas per 1000 deaths.[26] Other groups at increased risk of asbestos exposure in the past included textile manufacturers, miners, gas mask manufacturers, and cigarette filter manufacturers.[12] Currently, asbestos is used in cement, ceiling and floor tiles, and automobile brake linings. Of the United States supply of asbestos, 90% comes from Canadian chrystolite asbestos deposits.

Families of asbestos workers are also at an increased risk of mesotheliomas. Asbestos fibers may be brought home on hair and clothing. Estimates of 1% to 7% of children in these families risk household contamination and developing pulmonary malignancies.[25] The most important risk factor in females developing malignant mesothelioma is a family member that works in an asbestos-related occupation.

Epidemiologic studies have concluded that there is an average 35- to 40-year latency period from asbestos exposure to clinical presentation. There is little risk before 20 years from onset of exposure. Thereafter, it rises by nearly 100-fold over the ensuing 30 years.[27,28] At least 96% have a latency period greater than 20 years.[29,30] There is little known about this so-called latency period. Some postulate that repetitious injury to the DNA of mesothelial cells genetically alters them. This also suggests that multiple neoplastic transformations are necessary. The steep rise in malignant mesothelioma that began in the 1940s is reflected by the parallel rise in the asbestos industry starting in 1910.[11] Therefore, people exposed in the 1970s will not start presenting until the turn of the century, at the earliest. Eight million people are estimated to have been exposed to asbestos by the mid-1970s. Smoking is an established risk factor in the development of primary bronchogenic carcinoma, but epidemiologic studies have failed to show any association between tobacco and mesothelioma development. However, there is significant danger in asbestos-exposed smokers. The increased risk of developing lung cancer in smokers with asbestos exposure is 90-fold, higher than either smoking or asbestos exposure alone. Animal experiments and epidemiologic studies have confirmed this synergistic effect of asbestos exposure and cigarette smoking.

Asbestos exposure also is linked to an increased risk of a number of other pulmonary diseases. Besides malignant mesothelioma and lung carcinoma in smokers, these include asbestosis and benign changes to the pleura (pleural effusions, fibrosis, and plaques). Asbestosis (pulmonary fibrosis) generally requires higher doses of asbestos than mesotheliomas. The severity of asbestosis does not seem to influence the incidence of mesothelioma. Asbestos is also associated with lymphoid system dyscrasias, leukemias, and lymphomas. Asbestos workers also have been shown to have increased risk of cancers of the gastrointestinal tract, larynx, kidney, pancreas, ovary, and eyes.

## OTHER ETIOLOGIES

There is a wide variation in individuals developing malignant mesothelioma attributable to asbestos. Even with a thorough history and review with family members, 20% of patients are unable to recount prior asbestos exposure. Some other etiologies that have been associated with malignant mesothelioma including zeolite and other organic fibers, thorium dioxide, prior iatrogenic radiation exposure, and chronic inflammation. Regardless of these different etiologies,

the natural history and prognosis for non-asbestos–related malignancies are equally dismal.

In southern Turkey, in a circumscribed volcanic area of central Cappadocia, the mortality rate is as high as 40% from pleural mesothelioma. Many villagers live in cavelike dwellings where the natural rock is rich in erionite, a specific fibrous zeolite mineral. In Louisiana and other parts of the globe, there have been case reports of other organic fibers from materials such as sugar cane causing malignant mesothelioma.[11]

Another significant etiologic factor for mesothelioma is radiation for other primary malignancies. There have been case reports of individuals developing malignant mesotheliomas years after radiation for testicular seminoma, cervical cancer, breast cancer, and Hodgkin's disease.[31–33] In contrast to asbestos-induced malignant mesothelioma, postirradiation malignant mesothelioma has a shorter latency period of 19.5 years, equal probability in men and females, and younger average age of 45 years.[34,35]

There are reports of malignant mesothelioma arising after thorium dioxide (radiographic contrast dye) use.[36] Chronic inflammation has been a proposed risk factor to pleural malignancies. Previous lung disease, recurrent lung infections, recurrent pleural effusions, and recurrent spontaneous pneumothoraces have been associated with higher incidences of pleural mesotheliomas. Repeated studies of intrapleural injections of SV-40 virus induces mesothelioma in up to 100% of animals.[37–39]

The issue of genetic susceptibility is currently being investigated but is difficult to discern from shared household exposure.[40,41] One study has suggested a high association of HLA-B27 antigens in those with malignant mesotheliomas.[42] In a Finnish study, patients with malignant mesotheliomas were found to have decreased expression of the glutathione-S-transferase M1 (GSTM1) gene. This gene is important in detoxification of several carcinogens, including polycyclic aromatic hydrocarbons.[43,44]

## PATHOPHYSIOLOGY

Asbestos fibers enter the airway by inhalation and tend to deposit in the right lung. This reflects the anatomic variation of a more vertical right mainstem bronchus and the increased surface area of the right pleural cavity. Asbestos fibers are transported through the airways along their long axis according to the principles of laminar flow. Therefore, the depth of penetration of the fibers into the respiratory system correlates with fiber diameter, not fiber length. Inhaled particles tend to preferentially deposit at airway bifurcations through impaction, sedimentation, interception, and by Brownian motion for particles under 1 $\mu$m.[8,45] Thin rigid amphibole fibers deposit preferentially near the pleural surface, usually in the lower one-third of the lungs. The curly, pliable chrystolite fibers deposit more centrally.[46,47] Two peaks of clearance have been observed from the lower respiratory tracts of animal models: one at 11 h and the second at 29 days. Two-thirds of the daily dose is eliminated by coughing and swallowing, only to appear in the feces. This has been postulated to be a possible mechanism for the development of peritoneal mesothelioma.

The fibers can eventually settle in the pleural space by two mechanisms: direct penetration or migration from lung parenchyma.

Those fibers longer than 8 μm are inhaled and retained at the mesothelial lining and subserosal connective tissue. Other inhaled fibers that deposit in the lung parenchyma are capable of migrating to the pleura.[48] The lymphatic flow from the pleural space goes exclusively through the parietal pleura, and this would probably lead tumor cells to implant here. For this reason there is more involvement of the parietal pleura early on in disease. These fibers remain trapped because the openings of the lymphatic channels draining these spaces are 8 to 12 μm in diameter.[47] Fibrous plaques develop on the parietal pleura lining the intercostal region. The location of these fibrous plaques corresponds to the sites of the lymphatic clearance from the pleural space. Early lesions and malignant mesothelioma arise at these sites of lymphatic clearance.[49]

It should be noted that although smoking is not directly associated with mesotheliomas, it appears to affect tumorigenesis by various means. First, it impairs clearance of asbestos and second, inhaled tobacco smoke may make it easier for asbestos fibers to penetrate through bronchial walls. Finally, smoking causes increased alveolar macrophage–induced reactive oxygen species.[50]

**MESOTHELIAL CELL DAMAGE.** Debate continues as to whether asbestos is directly carcinogenic to mesothelial cells. Asbestos is not directly electrophilic like other carcinogens, nor does it form adducts with DNA.[51] Asbestos has not been shown to directly cause base substitutions or frameshift mutations in bacterial-mutation assays. Of the 23 agents designated as Group 1 human carcinogens by the International Agency for Research on Cancer, only asbestos and conjugated estrogens were not mutagenic. Carcinogens, as described throughout this textbook, usually evoke a multistep process that involves an initiation phase and promoter phase. There is uncertainty as to whether this multistage model is applicable to asbestos-related oncogenesis, or if it is, whether it is involved in the initiation phase.[50]

Asbestos fibers less than 5 μm are encapsulated by a portion of the plasma membrane and engulfed by mesothelial cells. Rieder[52] speculates that the surface of asbestos fibers is positively charged and shows a high affinity for polar proteins. These fibers have a tendency to be coated with tubulin and microtubule-associated proteins that can interact along the surface that the kinetochores of chromosomes can move. They undergo translocation to the perinuclear region by cytoplasmic microtubule-dependent saltatory transport.[51,53] There they mechanically interfere with mitotic spindle formation and chromosomal movement.[54] Interestingly, ten times the concentration of asbestos is necessary to cause the same level of toxicity in bronchial epithelial cells as in mesothelial cells.[9] What makes mesothelial cells unique to the effects of asbestos? In culture, rapidly dividing mesothelial cells lack keratin filaments, whereas other types of epithelia often contain a cage of keratin filaments surrounding the interphase and mitotic nucleus. This keratin cage may prevent asbestos fibers from invading the forming spindle.[52]

**CHROMOSOMAL ALTERATIONS.** Malignant mesothelioma is associated with complex and heterogeneous cytogenetic changes with no specific aberrations common to all tumor samples. Asbestos fibers induce numerical chromosomal changes: aneuploidy in diploid cells and polyploidy in tetraploid cells. Structural chromosomal alterations are also induced, but only at low levels.[9,55]

Chromosomal loss or deletions can result in the loss of a normal allele of a tumor suppressor gene. Specific nonrandom chromosomal alterations have been observed in human and animal mesothelioma cell lines, particularly in chromosomes 1, 2, 3, 4, 5, 6, 7, 9, 11, 17, and 22.[9,52,56]

Alterations in chromosome 1 have been detected in as many as 60% to 100% of mesothelioma cell lines.[57,58] A gene important for cellular senescence is thought to be lost, causing cellular immortalization. Chromosome 3 often loses the region between 3p14 and 3p25.[59] Polysomy of chromosome 7 has been seen frequently in human mesothelioma lines. Chromosome 7 is the site of the protooncogene HER-1, which encodes the epidermal growth factor. Arguably, the most common chromosomal abnormality in malignant mesothelioma is monosomy 22, correlated with mutations in neurofibromatosis (NF2) tumor suppressor genes.[60]

**ONCOGENE/TUMOR SUPPRESSOR GENES ACTIVATED.** Cytogenetic changes in oncogenes and tumor suppressor genes have been reported in many mesotheliomas. However, it is possible that these changes are overestimated due to extensive inferences from results obtained with established mesothelioma cell lines rather than primary tumors.[61] Various groups have reported variable results about gene loss or activation. Some claim alteration of p53 on chromosome 17p in up to 25% to 50% of mesothelioma cell lines, whereas others find no significant contribution of p53 to tumor pathogenesis.[62–66] Amplification of N-*myc*, c-*myc*, H-*ras*, K-*ras*, Rb gene, V-*fos*, and HER 2/neu have not been detected.[37,64] The presence of Wilms' tumor suppressor gene mutations on chromosome 11 in human mesotheliomas raises the possibility that alterations in this gene or binding of the WT1 gene product to the p53 tumor suppressor may predispose to mesothelial carcinogenesis.[67,68]

## CLINICAL PRESENTATION

### HISTORY

The typical patient with malignant pleural mesothelioma presents in his early 60s.[69] Children of asbestos workers may present under 50 years of age, reflecting the 30-year latency period. The two most important pieces of medical history to obtain are history of asbestos exposure and tobacco use. A comprehensive history must focus on the period 20 to 40 years before and should include the occupations of family members living with the patient at the time. Even a complete history may fail to establish the exposure history in 20% to 30% of patients.[5]

Patients who present with malignant mesothelioma often are in surprisingly good general health. There is an average 3-month delay before patients seek medical attention, but this period may be considerably longer. The most common presenting symptoms are dyspnea (60% to 70%) and insidious onset of chest pain (50% to 70%).[70] At later stages, patients will begin experiencing weight loss (25% to 30%), cough (27%), fever (33%), weakness (33%), and anorexia (10%) (Table 22-1). Other symptoms noted at presentation have included stridor, nausea, headache, and perceived tachycardia. Five percent of patients will present with complaints of acute onset of

**TABLE 22-1.** BUTCHART CLASSIFICATION OF STAGING

I.      Tumor confined within the "capsule" of the parietal pleura, i.e., involving only ipsilateral pleura, lung, pericardium, and diaphragm.

II.     Tumor invading chest wall or involving mediastinal structures, e.g., esophagus, heart, opposite pleura. Lymph node involvement within the chest.

III.    Tumor penetrating diaphragm to involve peritoneum: involvement of opposite pleura. Lymph node involvement outside the chest.

IV.     Distant blood-borne metastases.

excruciating chest pain and dyspnea. Emergency evaluation will reveal a hemothorax or spontaneous pneumothorax.[69,71] Ten percent of patients will be referred due to asymptomatic abnormalities on routine chest roentgenogram.[70] Rarely will the patient present with nonspecific constitutional symptoms or evidence of metastatic disease.

The symptoms of malignant mesothelioma result from the effects of the tumor in the pleural cavity: the enlarging mass, invasion of adjacent structures, and production of fluid by mesothelial cells (Fig. 22-4). By the time the patient presents, the tumor has often become bulky and there may be a large pleural effusion. Pain and shortness of breath are the two most common symptoms. A dry cough may be elicited when the patient is asked to breathe deeply. Weight loss may be a common finding.

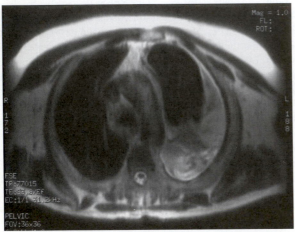

*A*

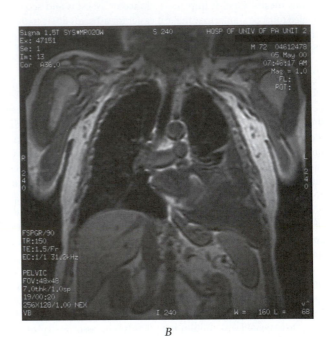

*B*

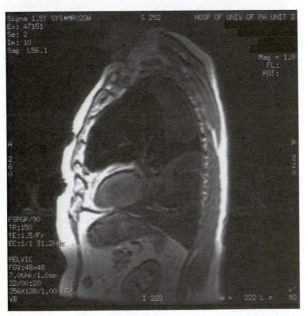

*C*

**FIGURE 22-4.** *A.* An axial reconstruction from a magnetic imaging scan (MRI) demonstrating malignant mesothelioma. *B.* Likewise, the coronal MRI reconstruction aids in detecting penetration through the hemidiaphragm. *C.* Sagittal MRI reconstruction that also aids in assessing penetration through the hemidiaphragm.

The character of the chest pain varies from a heavy feeling to a dull aching sensation in the posterolateral chest to a severe pain that frequently radiates to the upper abdomen, shoulder, and arms. Although the pain may be pleuritic in nature, it is more commonly unrelated to respiratory or other chest wall movements. Almost all patients with mesothelioma present with a pleural effusion, but the occasional patient may have bulky tumor with no fluid present.

## PHYSICAL EXAMINATION

The most common (80%) physical examination findings usually are secondary to the pleural effusion or pleural mass: decreased ipsilateral chest wall movement, dullness to percussion over involved lung fields, and decreased intensity of breath sounds. The right side is more commonly affected, and bilateral involvement at presentation is rare.[72] If the tumor has eroded through the chest wall, focal tenderness or a palpable mass may be felt. In later disease, there may be signs of compression or invasion of the mediastinal structures such as superior vena cava compression or involvement of the phrenic nerve and cervical lymph nodes, but these are unusual manifestations.[70] Signs of weight loss are common, although signs of extrathoracic involvement are uncommon at presentation, occurring in fewer than 10% of patients.[73]

## DIAGNOSTIC APPROACH

### DIFFERENTIAL DIAGNOSIS

When a patient presents to the surgeon with the clinical presentation above, he or she has usually been referred for evaluation of pleural thickening or an effusion noticed on radiographic studies. In addition to primary or metastatic pleural malignancy, a pleural effusion could be secondary to congestive heart failure, cirrhosis, pneumonia, empyema, or benign asbestos pleurisy.

Ninety-five percent of pleural neoplasms are metastatic. The most common primary neoplasms that metastasize to the pleura and cause malignant effusions are lung cancer (36%), breast cancer (25%), ovarian cancer (5%), and gastric cancer (2%).[74] The similarities between metastatic adenocarcinoma and mesothelioma may be so striking that the term pseudomesotheliomatous adenocarcinoma is sometimes used. Pseudomesotheliomatous tumors resemble malignant mesothelioma both clinically and in gross appearance. Prognosis is poor and treatment difficult.[75] Lymphomas account for another 10% of metastatic pleural tumors.

It is reasonable to consider that a pleural effusion could be a manifestation of a reactive process that occurs in the pleural space, either reactive mesothelial proliferation or reactive fibrosis. Reactive processes can arise from a number of benign growths and inflammatory processes. These often mimic desmoplastic variants of malignant mesothelioma. Desmoplastic malignant mesotheliomas are especially hard to characterize accurately because large portions of the tumor are composed of bland-appearing fibrous tissue.[76]

## LABORATORY STUDIES

There are no specific diagnostic tests, short of obtaining tissue, that characterize malignant mesothelioma. The most common finding is thrombocytosis ($>400,000/mm^3$) noted in 60% to 90% of patients.[77] Approximately 15% of patients have platelet counts over $1,000,000/mm^3$. Occasionally, patients will develop anemia of chronic disease.[72] Elevated sedimentation rate ($>100$ mm/h) is noted early in disease, but is nonspecific.[69] There have been occasional reports of hypercalcemia, nephrotic syndrome, and hemolytic anemia.[70]

## IMAGING STUDIES

Pancoast[78] described the first radiographic changes associated with asbestos 80 years ago. In order to differentiate tuberculosis from dust inhalation, he described increased thickness of the prominent linear shadows that uniquely extended from the hilum to the base. Since then, computed tomography, magnetic resonance imaging, and most recently positron emission tomography (PET) have changed the diagnosis and staging of malignant mesothelioma. Radiologic diagnosis of pleural mesothelioma requires a high degree of clinical suspicion. The major pathologic features of mesothelioma are well demonstrated by conventional chest radiography and computed tomography, yet the features are not specific to this tumor. Computed tomography, however, demonstrates the findings in greater detail.[79]

The most common radiologic presentation (40% to 95%) is a large, unilateral pleural effusion (Fig. 22-5). Only 10% of patients present with bilateral effusions.[74] The effusion may be quite large with near complete opacification of the hemithorax. Fluid may be loculated, surrounded by areas of thickened or nodular pleura, and thus there may only be a small amount of free-flowing pleural fluid. Aspiration of the fluid may reveal the underlying tumor radiographically, particularly if a pneumothorax is produced at the same time. The production of a pneumothorax may sometimes be used as a diagnostic aid. A shadow that persists after removal of the fluid is highly suggestive of an underlying tumor. Mediastinal shift is a variable finding, both before and after aspiration of the effusion. Shift may occur, either toward the affected side (suggesting invasion and fixation of tissue by tumor) or to the contralateral side ("tension effusion," a relatively late manifestation).[80]

Asbestos-caused pleural disease should be part of the differential diagnosis in a patient with a pleural effusion and history resembling malignant mesothelioma. Asbestos pleurisy occurs in 3% to 5% of asbestos workers and is usually recurrent and bilateral. Also associated with chest pain, 33% of the effusions secondary to asbestos pleurisy are bloody. The other common radiographic finding with malignant pleural mesothelioma is diffuse, circumferential pleural thickening (60% to 100%), usually associated with plaques and effusions. Neoplastic growth usually is unilateral at presentation, with two-thirds located on the right side.[70] This may reflect the larger surface area of the right pleural cavity as well as the anatomic distinction of the more vertical right bronchial tree. Pleural thickening commonly extends along pleural spaces into the fissures and medially to involve the mediastinal pleural reflection. The interlobar fissure

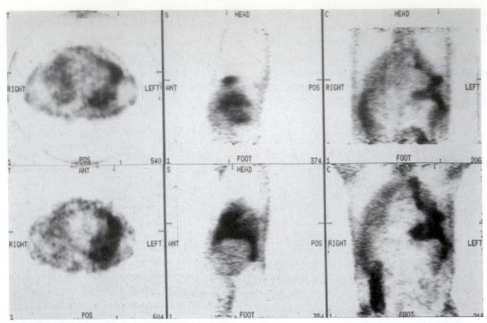

**FIGURE 22-5.** Positron emission tomogram (PET) demonstrating visualization of mesothelioma and progression of the disease.

becomes markedly thickened due to a combination of fibrosis, tumor, and associated fluid. A thick rind of neoplasm results in restriction and over time causes a decrease in size of the hemithorax, a common finding in patients with mesothelioma. The lower hemithorax tends to be more affected by the tumor than the upper, a phenomenon termed *gravitational metastasis*.[80] Additionally, the mediastinum frequently becomes fixed by the rigid rind of disease. The nodular densities can become large and a mass lesion will predominate with only minimal pleural thickening. Pleural plaques are the most common manifestation of prior asbestos exposure.[81] These are focal areas of fibrosis believed to occur when the asbestos fibers that have not undergone phagocytosis flow out of the lungs via the lymphatics into the surrounding pleura and soft tissues, where they

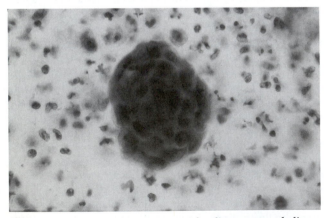

**FIGURE 22-6.** Cytologic appearance of malignant mesothelioma.

elicit a submesothelial reaction. They are usually thin (3 to 5 mm), discrete, irregular, and separate and, therefore, usually there is no confusion with a malignant process. They develop predominantly in the parietal pleura, although they may form in the visceral pleura in the fissures. They are bilateral and often symmetric, forming adjacent to rigid structures, most commonly next to the fifth and eighth ribs or tendinous insertions of the diaphragm.[80] They usually spare the lung apices and costophrenic sulcus and are more commonly seen along the posterior reflection of the pleura.[82] However, pleural plaques of asbestosis can extend and coalesce into diffuse pleural thickening. Eighty-five percent of plaques show some calcification at autopsy, although this is not often seen on plain chest films.[81] CT detects almost all cases of pleural plaques, whereas plain films miss over 10%.[79] It should be noted that whenever calcifications are seen on CT, the possibility of osteoid differentiation in neoplastic cells must be considered. There have been several reports describing densely calcified pleural masses on CT that on necropsy were later diagnosed as osteosarcomatous changes within pleural mesotheliomas.[83-85]

Up to one-third of patients with mesothelioma have evidence of pleural or parenchymal asbestosis (pulmonary fibrosis).[86] The severity of asbestosis does not seem to correlate with the incidence of mesothelioma. Asbestosis presents as an interstitial infiltrate characterized by irregular linear densities, septal lines, and parenchymal bands. Often there are fine nodular opacities, honeycombing, and a "ground-glass" appearance.[87]

Lung nodules may be present in up to 50% of patients and are usually seen as multiple discrete tumor masses. They are often greater than 5 cm in size when first detected. These nodular masses represent either parenchymal extension from pleural-based masses that have become surrounded by lung parenchyma or more uncommonly metastatic disease. Although intraparenchymal extension has little diagnostic significance, metastases portend a poor outcome.[79] Diffuse pulmonary parenchymal metastasis in a miliary pattern is occasionally seen at the time of presentation of pleural mesothelioma.[88,89] Lung nodules must be differentiated from rounded atelectasis, a finding caused by localized fibrous thickening of the pleura with lung folded around it, with associated curving vessels and bronchi, producing a cochlealike appearance.[90] Radiologic features that can differentiate between rounded atelectasis and mesothelioma are blurring of the border by entering vessels causing a tail or comet sign, chronic pleural thickening near the mass, and a stable appearance on serial films.

Involvement of the chest wall with rib destruction is not uncommon (up to 20% of patients) and can be best demonstrated by CT scan.[86] Degrees of involvement include "roof tiling" deformities due to periosteal reaction or complete destruction of ribs usually along the axillary line. There are a variety of other findings that may be seen on radiologic examination of the thorax. Up to 30% of patients present with radiologic evidence of hilar or mediastinal lymph node involvement. Other findings include pericardial infiltration or transdiaphragmatic invasion.

### CHEST ROENTGENOGRAMS.

On the plain chest radiograph, a large pleural effusion, pleural thickening, and nodularity with decreased volume of the involved hemithorax is sufficiently classic to permit a consideration of the diagnosis of mesothelioma. In many cases, there is blunting of the costophrenic angle. The tumor may flatten the dome of the thorax. A composite picture of a lowered shoulder, elevated hemidiaphragm, contracted intercostal spaces, and scoliosis is often seen. Ribs may be eroded. Only 20% of patients with pleural mesothelioma demonstrate characteristic signs of asbestosis—a low diaphragm, interstitial fibrosis, or pleural plaques.[5] Lateral and oblique films are extremely helpful in radiographic screening for pleural plaques. Close to 20% to 40% of plaques not otherwise seen by posteroanterior (PA) views are seen on other angles.[81]

### COMPUTED TOMOGRAPHY.

CT scan is the most accurate noninvasive method for assessing the stage and progression of mesothelioma.[91,92] The prime importance of CT lies in its ability to define the extent of disease and it also may be useful in assessing response to treatment and in longitudinal follow-up. It is also used to look for metastatic disease in the contralateral hemithorax or peritoneal cavity, and is particularly helpful in assessing the mediastinal lymph nodes.

A CT scan may aid in differentiating benign from malignant pleural thickening. The most common finding on CT scans with malignant mesothelioma is unilateral thickening with irregular pleuropulmonary contours.[93] There is a spectrum of appearances of malignant mesothelioma on CT scans: focal nodular masses or lesions, pleural effusions, diffuse pleural thickening extending circumferentially around the hemithorax, spread of the tumor within the ipsilateral or contralateral parenchyma, through the ribs, into the mediastinum, or across the diaphragm, or distant hematogenous spread.[80,94,95]

### MAGNETIC RESONANCE IMAGING.

MRI adds significantly to our ability to image malignant mesothelioma. The differ-

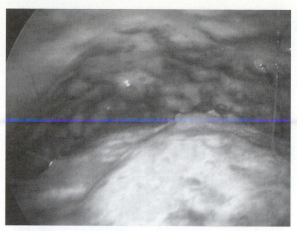

**FIGURE 22-7.** The appearance of malignant mesothelioma at the time of a videothoracoscopic biopsy. (See also Plate 33.)

ential signal intensity allows pleural mesothelioma infiltration and pleural fluid to be seen as a high-intensity signal on T2-weighted images.[74] The major advantage of MRI is the ability to image in the coronal and sagittal planes, which is especially useful in determining whether the disease extends through the diaphragm and into the peritoneal cavity, a distinction that is extremely important for a patient being considered for operative intervention (Fig. 22-7). The extent of the tumor within the chest, particularly the mediastinal pleura, and the mass effect of the tumor are very well demonstrated on the coronal MR images.[96]

### POSITRON EMISSION TOMOGRAPHY.

As opposed to other imaging modalities, PET is a metabolic scan that relies on a positron-emitting isotope (fluorodeoxyglucose, FDG) that is metabolized at a differential rate between tumor cells and normal cells. The FDG is phosphorylated to FDG-6-PO$_4$ that is not further degraded and trapped within the tumor cell. PET may have advantages over other imaging studies in differentiating benign from malignant pleural thickening, assessing extent of tumor involvement, and locating optimal sites for thoracoscopic biopsy. PET may also be more useful in assessing progression or regression of disease following therapy (Fig. 22-8).

### INVASIVE DIAGNOSTIC STUDIES.

Since no imaging study is absolutely specific for the diagnosis of mesothelioma, pleural fluid cytology or a specimen of pleura must be obtained. Techniques applicable for the diagnosis of pleural malignancy include thoracentesis, pleural needle biopsy, thoracoscopy, and open pleural biopsy. In order to balance optimal diagnostic sensitivity with minimal invasiveness, it is reasonable to start with thoracentesis to look for malignant cells. This procedure often is combined with pleural needle biopsy, although this procedure (closed-needle biopsy) is becoming a lost art. Even if sufficient material is obtained, it may be difficult to differentiate malignant mesothelioma from benign reactive mesothelial proliferation. Thoracentesis and needle biopsy each are associated with 40% to 60% accuracy, but combined they may yield an accuracy of 90%. With the advent of video thoracoscopy, it has become more

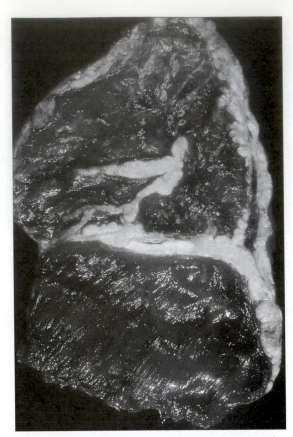

**FIGURE 22-8.** Surgical specimen following extrapleural pneumonectomy showing mesothelioma encasing the lung and involving the major fissure.

common for patients to undergo this procedure in order to obtain sufficient diagnostic material.

The main problem with the less invasive diagnostic techniques is the size of the sample. Malignant pleural mesotheliomas vary in differentiation, cell type, and histologic pattern from one anatomic region to another; therefore, thorough sampling is often needed. The size of tumor specimens influences the diagnosis. More biphasic mesotheliomas are diagnosed with larger (thoracotomy, autopsy) than smaller (thorascopy, closed needle) biopsy techniques.[97] Sarcomatoid mesotheliomas account for 20% of the tumors regardless of the method the tissue is obtained, indicating the increased incidence of the biphasic variant is due to the epithelial type. Thus, one may assume that a specimen demonstrating sarcomatoid histology is probably sarcomatoid; however, a biopsy that is epithelial may have sarcomatoid features elsewhere in the tumor, a distinction important with regard to prognosis.[97,98]

The most worrisome complication of invasive biopsy techniques, whether thoracentesis, needle biopsy, or thoracoscopy, is seeding of the needle tract, chest tube drain, trocar site, or incision with malignant cells; 10% to 50% of patients develop seeding of the chest wall that grows into a painful site of tumor invasion.[72,99,100] Boutin[101] routinely waits 10 to 12 days to allow the incision to heal and then gives a dose of radiotherapy directed at the biopsy site on the chest wall.[101]

**THORACENTESIS.** Up to 80% of patients with mesothelioma present with a pleural effusion and almost all will develop an effusion at some point in the course of their disease.[70,102] Whenever an effusion is suggestive of a malignancy, a thoracentesis should be performed to obtain cells for cytologic evaluation. Epithelioid malignant mesothelioma presents more frequently with pleural effusion than sarcomatoid variants (Fig. 22-6).

Mesothelial cells synthesize collagen, laminin, elastin, and proteoglycans, including hyaluronic acid into the pleural space. In malignant mesothelioma, the fluid is frequently serosanguinous, but approximately 50% of effusions are bloody. Fluid chemistry is usually exudative (protein >30 g/L). Pleural fluid has a lactose dehydrogenase (LDH) concentration 36 to 600 IU and a glucose concentration of 21 to 155 mg/dL (which is inversely correlated with the number of malignant cells present).[69] Some studies have demonstrated pleural effusions with a low pH (<7.30) are a poor prognostic indicator of survival.[103] Hyaluronic acid (HA) level is consistently elevated in patients with malignant mesothelioma. HA level is 70% to 90% sensitive for malignant mesotheliomas, but up to 20% of nonmalignant inflammatory effusions also have elevations of equal level. Other neoplasms retain near normal values. Some authors report hyaluronic acid levels greater than 0.8 mg/mL are diagnostic for malignant mesothelioma, but this level alone is not sufficient for diagnosis.[104–106]

Fluid cytology has value in diagnosing malignant mesotheliomas with 30% to 70% accuracy and false-negative results likely coming from sampling error and not an error in interpretation.[102] When looking at fluid cytology, the most important finding indicative of malignant mesothelioma is numerous cell aggregates of varying size. Clumps composed of 5 to 200 or more cells are frequently irregular with protruding edges. They may also be frondlike and appear to be papillary fragments (Fig. 22-9). Metastatic adenocarcinoma, on the other hand, has rounded, smooth-appearing cell aggregates. Reactive mesothelial processes also have cellular aggregates of smaller, less complex size. Other cytologic features suggestive of mesothelioma include a characteristic cytoplasm with cell enlargement, specialized cell borders, multinucleation, cell-to-cell apposition, and a uniform cell population.[107] Routine cytogenetic analysis of chromosomal aberrations in these samples is unhelpful in making the diagnosis of malignancy.[102]

**FINE-NEEDLE ASPIRATION.** With closed-needle biopsy, malignant mesothelioma is often hard to distinguish from reactive mesothelial proliferation mainly because of the small size of the sample. In diffuse pleural thickening there may only be small, localized foci of malignant cells admixed with fibrous tissue. Some clinicians prefer to use an Abrams or Cope needle in the presence of pleural fluid, whereas others recommend a cutting needle in an attempt to obtain adequate pleural tissue for histopathologic examination.[70] The use of mechanically operated biopsy instruments has improved the ease and speed of biopsy while producing high-quality specimens without shear artifacts.[108] The most common complications of this procedure are pneumothorax, focal pulmonary hemorrhage, and local seeding of the tumor.

To improve diagnostic accuracy, ultrasound and CT scan may be used to guide fine-needle aspiration. Approximately an 80% diagnostic accuracy can be achieved in the first two attempts utilizing these imaging modalities to direct the needle.[108,109]

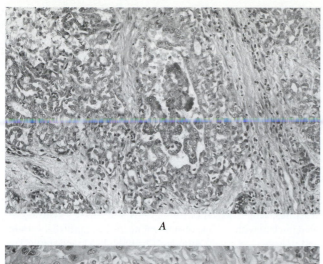

*A*

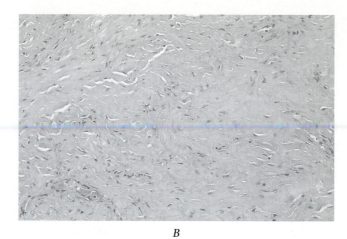

*B*

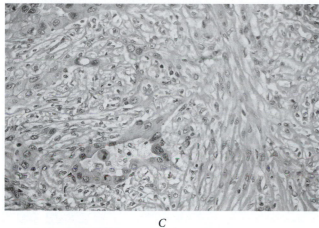

*C*

**FIGURE 22-9.** *A.* Photomicrograph of the epithelial subtype of malignant mesothelioma. *B.* The sarcomatous subtype of mesothelioma. *C.* Biphasic malignant mesothelioma.

**VIDEOTHORACOSCOPY.** Videothoracoscopy, with a 90% to 100% diagnostic sensitivity and specificity, is the best and most expeditious way to obtain a prompt diagnosis. It permits complete visualization of the pleural cavity and the opportunity for thorough sampling of various sites. It also allows the surgeon to more accurately stage the disease.[110,111] The procedure can be performed under local or general anesthesia.[112–114] The appearance varies from diffuse pleural thickening to multiple tiny nodules on either the parietal pleura, visceral pleura or both (Fig. 22-10).[100,113] Complications of thoracoscopy usually are minor and the procedure is associated with almost no mortality (<0.02%). The patient typically leaves the hospital the day following the procedure unless pleurodesis has been carried out, which may prompt a longer stay with an indwelling chest tube. Thoracoscopy may not be possible if the pleural space is obliterated completely by tumor and adhesions.

**DIAGNOSTIC THORACOTOMY.** If repeated attempts to obtain diagnostic material have failed, more tissue may be needed, or if the pleural space is obliterated, a thoracotomy may be the only alternative. However, open biopsy should be avoided whenever possible because of the attendant morbidity. There is a significantly increased tendency for malignant mesothelioma to track through the incision site. The procedure should be kept simple. No attempt should be made to carry out an extensive procedure, and often simply opening the intercostal space (dividing the intercostal muscle) down to the thickened pleura allows a piece of pleura to be removed.

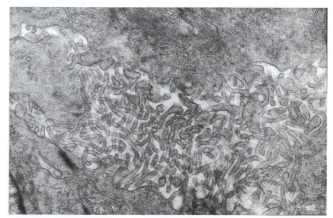

**FIGURE 22-10.** Electron micrograph of malignant mesothelioma demonstrating the characteristic microvilli.

## PATHOLOGY

### GROSS

Grossly, early malignant mesothelioma appears as many small nodules on the pleural surface, both visceral and parietal, although very early only the parietal pleural surface may be involved. Progression of the tumor results in coalescence of the nodules to form plaques that merge to form a sheet of tumor. In later stages, malignant mesotheliomas appear with diffuse involvement of the visceral and parietal pleura with involvement of the fissures and obliteration of the pleural space. This white, hard tumor spreads over the entire lung, encasing it with tumor up to several centimeters thick (Fig. 22-11). Areas of necrosis and hemorrhage are often seen. The neoplasm may invade the chest wall and mediastinum and may spread to the opposite pleural cavity or the peritoneal cavity. Pleural effusions and ascites are a common finding.

### MICROSCOPIC

Malignant mesotheliomas present in three different histologic variations: epithelial (50%), sarcomatous or fibrous (20%), and biphasic or mixed (30%) type. Histologic variants of malignant mesothelioma are thought to originate from the same precursor cell at various points of differentiation and maturity.[115] Primitive subserosal mesothelial cells start out as precursors to sarcomatoid variants. Sarcomatous cells maintain the potential to differentiate into the epithelial form. The epithelial form is thought to be the end stage, completely differentiated mesothelial cell. Sarcomatous variants therefore demonstrate more mitotic activity and reflect a more primitive status. The epithelial subtype has a better prognosis than the sarcomatoid subtype.[98,116] Other rare variations of mesotheliomas such as desmoplastic and lymphohistiocytoid mesotheliomas have been reported.

Of pleural mesotheliomas, 50% are epithelioid. The cells tend to be cuboidal or polyhedral in appearance, forming sheets, papillary structures, acinar spaces, or lining clefts. They have a centrally located nucleus with a single prominent nucleolus. Epithelial variants tend to have moderately abundant eosinophilic cytoplasm.[117] This variant uniquely has a constant nuclear-to-cytoplasm ratio with variable cell size.[118,119] Anaplasia, atypical mitotic figures, and pleomorphism are uncommon among these tumor cells. Epithelial malignant mesotheliomas are arranged in a combination of different patterns: papillary (small, irregular cystic spaces are lined by tumor cells and filled by papillary projections with cores of connective tissue and

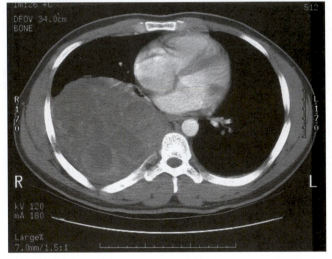

*B*

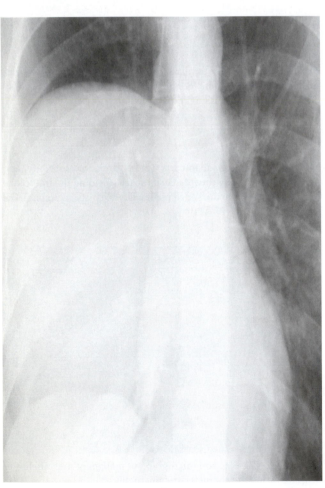

*A*

**FIGURE 22-11.** *A.* Chest radiograph demonstrating a giant solitary benign fibrous tumor. *B.* CT scan of a giant solitary benign fibrous tumor. These usually arise from the visceral pleural surface and are connected by a narrow pedicle.

a covering of tumor cells), tubular (well-formed glandular spaces), and tubulopapillary.[120] Longer survival time is associated with tubulopapillary subtypes compared to nonglandular solid types.[98] The most important differential in the examination of this variant is metastatic adenocarcinoma. Adenocarcinomas tend to have high nuclear-to-cytoplasm ratios. As epithelial mesotheliomas become increasingly anaplastic, they can become impossible to distinguish from adenocarcinomas with the light microscope.

Sarcomatous (fibrous or spindle cell) mesotheliomas account for 20% of pleural mesotheliomas, and probably a higher percentage in younger patients.[69] The cells tend to be elongated with high mitotic activity. The spindlelike cells are surrounded by a collagen matrix. Unlike epithelioid variants, sarcomatous tumors can show different patterns that are nonspecific and overlap with soft tissue tumors arising in the chest wall. These sarcomas include fibrosarcoma, liposarcoma, malignant fibrous histiocytoma, rhabdomyosarcoma, malignant schwannoma, and extraosseous osteosarcoma.[84,118]

Biphasic mesotheliomas demonstrate sheets of mesothelioma cells with a mixture of epithelial and sarcomatous characteristics. The transition from one to another can be gradual or abrupt. Metastasis can be from one type or the other or both.

Desmoplastic mesothelioma is an unusual variant that appears like individual neoplastic cells widely separated by thick bands of hyalinized collagen, often arranged in intertwining bundles or whorls in a storiform pattern. Desmoplastic variants have a rapid clinical course with early metastasis to liver, lung, and bone.[121,122] Desmoplastic variants are easily confused with reactive fibrotic processes. In comparing the two, desmoplastic mesotheliomas tend to be avascular, have increased cellularity, randomly arranged collagen bundles, areas of bland necrosis, and infiltration into adjacent tissues.

Lymphohistiocytoid mesothelioma is a variant of predominantly sarcomatoid histology and may look like non-Hodgkin's lymphoma. There is intense lymphocytic infiltration with scattered histiocytoid-appearing mesothelial cells among sporadic mesothelial cells with sinous villous processes and intracytoplasmic neolumina lined by microvilli. Nuclei appear rounded to oval with finely divided chromatin and small to prominent nucleoli.[123]

In patients with malignant mesothelioma regardless of the histologic type, two forms of asbestos fibers are seen microscopically in the lung: uncoated fibers and asbestos bodies. The ratio of uncoated fibers to asbestos bodies falls anywhere from 5 to 10,000:1. Uncoated fibers usually require electron microscopy to be visualized. Polarized light is of limited value because these thin fibers are only weakly birefringent. Asbestos bodies or ferruginous bodies, the hallmark of asbestos exposure, are transparent fibers of 10- to 300-μm length coated with protein and iron compounds. A histologic stain for iron is useful in demonstrating asbestos bodies in tissues.[124,125] Ferruginous bodies may be seen in the sputum but cannot be readily associated with asbestos exposure since many people with known asbestos exposure do not have them. Malignant mesothelioma patients have asbestos body counts intermediate between those of the general population and those with asbestosis.[126]

## SPECIAL STUDIES

Accurate pathologic diagnosis cannot be accomplished in a vacuum, but depends on close interaction between the surgeon and

the pathologist. Once the tissue specimen has been obtained, it is the work of the pathologist to distinguish among a diverse number of pleural diseases. Techniques beyond light microscopy available to the pathologist include histochemistry, immunohistochemistry, and electron microscopy. The main differential diagnosis in specimens of pleura falls into four groups:

1. Reactive mesothelial proliferation and adenocarcinoma versus epithelial type of mesothelioma
2. Fibrosarcomas versus sarcomatous variants of mesothelioma
3. Fibrosing pleuritis versus desmoplastic variant of mesothelioma
4. Lymphomas versus lymphohistiocytoid variants[76]

An experienced pathologist is key to differentiating malignant mesothelioma from metastatic pleural disease. There should be no hesitation on the part of the pathologist to send slides out for a second opinion from a pathologist experienced in the diagnosis of mesothelioma.

HISTOCHEMISTRY. Although histochemical findings may supplement the gross and microscopic features in the diagnosis of mesothelioma, they are not in themselves reliable independent diagnostic criteria.[126] Mesothelial cells synthesize collagen, laminin, elastin, and proteoglycans, particularly hyaluronic acid (HA). Mesotheliomas tend to produce HA, whereas metastatic adenocarcinoma synthesizes neutral mucin. Histochemistry is often of limited value with mucopolysaccharides because they are water-soluble and tend to bind to aqueous fixatives. Alternatively, electrophoresis is extremely reliable, but is not generally diagnostically available. Histochemical staining has moderate specificity and sensitivity; 50% of epithelial mesotheliomas have undetectable levels of HA.[117] Of nonmalignant inflammatory processes in the pleural space, 25% also stain positive for HA. However, there is significant quantitative difference of HA between malignant mesotheliomas and other lung adenocarcinomas.[127]

HA can be readily stained with alcian blue or colloidal iron stains. Alcian blue–positive material that is entirely removed by hyaluronidase reaction supports a diagnosis of malignant mesothelioma, whereas staining unaffected by enzymatic degradation suggests adenocarcinoma. Adenocarcinomas can be stained with periodic acid-Schiff (PAS) to demonstrate cytoplasmic vacuoles containing neutral mucin. The PAS stain is used before and after diastase digestion. Diastase-positive neutral mucopolysaccharide staining is extremely suggestive of adenocarcinoma. Although histochemical stains for mucins are useful in distinguishing between epithelial mesothelioma and adenocarcinoma, they are not helpful in separating sarcomatous mesotheliomas from other spindle cell tumors.

IMMUNOHISTOCHEMISTRY. Immunohistochemical studies are an exciting area of diagnosis of malignant mesotheliomas. Immunoglobulins are designed to target particular proteins unique to a cell line. In diagnosing malignant mesotheliomas, immunoglobulins to intermediate filaments, CEA, WT-1, B72.3, Leu M1, and SC are used. Formalin-fixed and paraffin-imbedded tissue blocks can be immunoperoxidase-stained for these techniques.

A wide range of intermediate filaments (IFs) are expressed by mesenchymal cells. Neoplasms often express the same pattern of IFs as their tissue of origin. Therefore, immunoglobulins specific to cytoskeletal elements can be used to differentiate cell types. Staining for IFs is not specific for neoplastic mesothelial proliferations versus reactive mesothelial growth. Quiescent submesothelial cells express only vimentin. As they differentiate into surface mesothelial cells, they acquire low-molecular-weight cytokeratins and begin to decrease vimentin expression. Fully differentiated surface mesothelial cells express both high- and low-molecular-weight cytokeratins without vimentin.[128,129] Staining for IFs is indicated in differentiating sarcomatous mesotheliomas (cytokeratin-positive) from soft tissue sarcomas (cytokeratin-negative).[98,117,130]

Carcinoembryonic antigen (CEA), an oncofetal protein abundant in neoplasms of endodermal origin, is most useful for distinguishing mesothelial cells from adenocarcinoma.[131] Anywhere from 70% to 100% of adenocarcinomas will stain positive for CEA, whereas mesothelial cells rarely are positive for CEA.[132,133]

One marker that may be particularly valuable in the diagnosis of mesothelioma is the Wilms' tumor 1 (WT-1) gene product. WT-1 is a tumor suppressor gene that is restricted primarily to mesenchymally derived tissue and therefore appears to be selectively expressed in tumors of mesodermal origin, such as mesothelioma.[67,134]

Many other major antigens are being explored for immunohistochemical staining, including monoclonal antibodies to B73.3, SC, and Leu M1.[135,136] The monoclonal antibody Leu M1 is a myelomonocytic marker expressed by the neoplastic cells of Hodgkin's disease that stains positive for metastatic adenocarcinoma and negative for malignant mesothelioma in the majority of patients. B72.3 is a monoclonal antibody to TAG-72, a common antigen in breast adenocarcinoma that also binds lung adenocarcinomas but is negative in most mesotheliomas. SC (secretory component) is an antigenically distinct portion of secretory immunoglobulin A positive for mesotheliomas that is found in external secretion and in a variety of normal epithelial cells and their neoplasms.

ELECTRON MICROSCOPY. With electron microscopy, the ultrastructural characteristics of the microvilli, intracellular junctions, tonofilaments, basal lamina, and intracellular lumens may be examined. The presence of microvilli is key to the diagnosis of mesothelioma. Length-to-diameter (L/D) ratio is used as a primary means to separate mesothelial cells from other cells. Epithelial malignant mesothelioma has a L/D ratio twice as large as metastatic adenocarcinoma and an average L/D ratio greater than 11, whereas adenocarcinoma has an average L/D ratio less than 6. They possess long, wavy-appearing surface microvilli that project into the cavity.[137,138] Desmosomes are well-developed but tight junctions are poorly formed and are incomplete. Normal mesothelial cells have a complex cytoskeletal network of IFs. IFs are organized into tonofibrillar bundles in a perinuclear distribution.[139] Numerous pinocytic vesicles are associated with the basal layer with large collections of intracytoplasmic glycogen. Mesotheliomas have limited cytoplasmic organelles, decreased rough endoplasmic reticulum, and an absence of secretory granules.[140] In contrast, adenocarcinomas have decreased numbers of IFs, short microvilli, numerous lamellar bodies, and mucous granules.

DIFFERENTIAL DIAGNOSIS. Histochemistry best differentiates metastatic adenocarcinoma from epithelioid mesotheliomas. Mucicarmine and PAS with diastase are the two most frequently used stains in excluding the diagnosis of adenocarcinoma. HA staining rarely is used in clinical practice. To distinguish between reactive mesothelial proliferation and epithelioid mesotheliomas is more difficult. Since reactive mesothelial proliferation and epithelial malignant mesotheliomas both involve mesothelial cells, histochemistry and immunohistochemistry are not as helpful. It has been found that mesothelial cells express epithelial membrane antigen (EMA) strongly, whereas reactive mesothelial cells are negative or weakly staining. It also has been thought that silver staining for nuclear organizer regions may help to make a distinction between benign and malignant mesothelioma, with more organizer regions being present in the malignant cells.[133,141,142]

Immunohistochemical staining for intermediate filaments best distinguishes fibrosarcomas from sarcomatoid mesotheliomas. To distinguish reactive fibrosis from desmoplastic variants of mesothelioma remains a pathologic dilemma. Attempts at histiochemical and immunohistochemical techniques have provided no single useful means of differentiation.[133,143]

## STAGING AND PROGNOSIS

Staging of malignant mesothelioma is important to assess prognosis and to guide treatment. Unfortunately, in the past and even now there has been no widely accepted staging system. Most of the proposed systems for staging are based on stage I–IV classifications or tumor, node, metastasis (TNM) staging. The most commonly used system in the past was that of Butchart, put forth in 1976[144] (Table 22-2). Because of the lack of a single agreed-upon staging system, it has been difficult to interpret clinical trials because these trials have lacked uniform descriptors to classify treatment and mortality rates. In the past, the fundamental problem with staging malignant mesothelioma was twofold. Due to the long latency period of the disease, we did not have the knowledge to describe its natural history. Secondly, we lacked adequate techniques to define the extent of mesothelioma radiographically because of the unique platelike growth pattern exhibited by the tumor.[91]

In order to improve the staging, The International Mesothelioma Interest Group met during the Seventh World Conference of the International Association for the Study of Lung Cancer. The meeting included many of the originators of the previous proposed staging systems. The staging system proposed by this group was based on the analysis of emerging information about the impact of tumor and nodal status on survival. It incorporates very specific TNM descriptors based on emerging information about the natural history of the disease[145] (Table 22-3).

The new staging system is better at delineating early disease—particularly at recognizing the improved survival of T1, N0 disease. T1 is separated into T1a and T1b. The key feature between these two is involvement of the visceral pleura, which in many cases is assessed thoracoscopically. Tumor tends to arise in the parietal and diaphragmatic pleura and later advances to the visceral pleura. Patients usually have a free pleural space and present with a large pleural effusion. T1 disease may be amenable to resection by pleurectomy with decortication.[145] Another key aspect is distinction between T1b and T2. T2 defines disease that extends into the pulmonary parenchyma; thus tumor cannot be resected without taking part of the underlying

**TABLE 22-2. INTERNATIONAL MESOTHELIOMA INTEREST GROUP STAGING**

| | |
|---|---|
| T1 | T1a tumor limited to the ipsilateral parietal pleura, including mediastinal and diaphragmatic pleura. No involvement of the visceral pleura. |
| | T1b tumor involving the ipsilateral parietal pleura, including mediastinal and diaphragmatic pleura. Scattered foci of tumor also involving the visceral pleura. |
| T2 | Tumor involving each of the ipsilateral pleural surfaces (parietal, mediastinal, diaphragmatic, and visceral pleura) with at least one of the following features: |
| | • Involvement of diaphragmatic muscle. |
| | • Confluent visceral pleural tumor (including the fissures) or extension of tumor from visceral pleura into the underlying pulmonary parenchyma. |
| T3 | Describes locally advanced but potentially resectable tumor. Tumor involving all of the ipsilateral pleural surfaces (parietal, mediastinal, diaphragmatic, and visceral pleura) with at least one of the following features: |
| | • Involvement of the endothoracic fascia. |
| | • Extension into the mediastinal fat. |
| | • Solitary, completely resectable focus of tumor extending into the soft tissues of the chest wall. |
| | • Nontransmural involvement of the pericardium. |
| T4 | Describes locally advanced technically unresectable tumor. Tumor involving all of the ipsilateral pleural surfaces (parietal, mediastinal, diaphragmatic, and visceral) with at least one of the following features: |
| | • Diffuse extension or multifocal masses of tumor in the chest wall with or without associated rib destruction. |
| | • Direct transdiaphragmatic extension of tumor to the peritoneum. |
| | • Direct extension of tumor to the contralateral pleura. |
| | • Direct extension of tumor to one or more mediastinal organs. |
| | • Direct extension of tumor into the spine. |
| | • Tumor extending through to the internal surface of the pericardium with or without a pericardial effusion; or tumor involving the myocardium. |

N—Lymph nodes

| | |
|---|---|
| NX | Regional lymph nodes cannot be assessed. |
| N0 | No regional lymph node metastases. |
| N1 | Metastases in the ipsilateral bronchopulmonary or hilar lymph nodes. |
| N2 | Metastases in the subcarinal or the ipsilateral mediastinal lymph nodes, including the ipsilateral internal mammary nodes. |
| N3 | Metastases in the contralateral mediastinal, contralateral internal mammary, ipsilateral, or contralateral supraclavicular lymph nodes. |

M—Metastases

| | |
|---|---|
| MX | Presence of distant metastases cannot be assessed. |
| M0 | No distant metastasis. |
| M1 | Distant metastasis present. |
| T4 | Tumor extends to any of the following: Contralateral pleura or lung by direct extension, peritoneum or intra-abdominal organs by direct extension, cervical tissues. |

Supraclavicular, or scalene lymph nodes

M—Metastases

| | |
|---|---|
| MX | Presence of distant metastases cannot be assessed. |
| M0 | No (known) distant metastasis. |
| M1 | Distant metastasis present. |

| STAGE: | DESCRIPTION: |
|---|---|
| Stage I | |
| 1a | T1aN0M0 |
| 1b | T1bN0M0 |
| Stage II | T2N0M0 |
| Stage III | Any T3M0 |
| | Any N1M0 |
| | Any N2M0 |
| Stage IV | Any T4 |
| | Any N3 |
| | Any M1 |

**TABLE 22-3.** SUGARBAKER STAGING SYSTEM FOR MESOTHELIOMA

| STAGE NO. | DEFINITION |
| --- | --- |
| I | Disease confined to within capsule of the parietal pleura; ipsilateral pleura, lung, pericardium, diaphragm, or chest-wall disease limited to previous biopsy sites. |
| II | All of stage I with positive intrathoracic (N1 or N2) lymph nodes. |
| III | Local extension of disease into chest wall or mediastinum; heart, or through diaphragm, peritoneum; with or without extrathoracic or contralateral (N3) lymph node involvement. |
| IV | Distant metastatic disease. |

**TABLE 22-4.** PLEURECTOMY WITH OR WITHOUT DECORTICATION

| YEAR | AUTHOR | N | MEDIAN SUR (MO) | 2-YR SUR % | BIBLIOGRAPHY REFERENCE |
| --- | --- | --- | --- | --- | --- |
| 1997 | Pass | 39 | 14.5 | | Pass[97] |
| 1996 | Rusch | 51 | 18.3 | 40 | Rusch[96] |
| 1994 | Allen | 56 | 9 | 8.9 | Allen[94] |
| 1991 | Brancatisano | 45 | 16 | 21 | Brancatisano[91] |
| 1990 | Harvey | 9 | 11.9 | 0 | Harvey[90] |
| 1989 | Ruffie | 63 | 9.8 | | Ruffie[89] |
| 1989 | Achatzy | 46 | 10 | 11 | Achatzy[89] |
| 1988 | Faber | 33 | 10 | 12 | Faber[88] |
| 1986 | DaValle | 23 | 11.2 | | DaValle[86] |
| 1984 | Law | 28 | 20 | 32 | Law[84] |
| 1982 | Brenner | 69 | 15 | | Brenner[82] |
| 1982 | Chahinian | 30 | 13 | 27 | Chahinian[82] |
| 1976 | Wanebo | 33 | 16.1 | | Wanebo[76] |
| | Totals | 515 | 13.4 | | |

parenchyma. Usually the diaphragm is involved and an extrapleural pneumonectomy may be required. T3 disease describes a locally advanced tumor that usually precludes an extrapleural pneumonectomy. By this stage, the tumor involves the entire ipsilateral pleural space and usually extends into the endothoracic fascia, chest wall, and mediastinal fat, and involves structures that are not resectable. T4 disease designates a locally advanced tumor that clearly involves the ipsilateral pleural surfaces, with at least one or the other structure directly invaded.

This staging system is based primarily on surgical and pathologic findings that may be at least partly assessed by CT. At present, CT remains the best noninvasive staging technique but usually is supplemented by MRI to assess transdiaphragmatic extension. Up to 85% accuracy in staging can be achieved by CT as validated by findings at thoracotomy or autopsy.[92] Neither CT nor MRI can always distinguish among T1a, T1b, or T2 because these techniques cannot differentiate parietal from visceral involvement. However, CT can evaluate the presence of a significant pleural effusion (T1 disease) and usually can differentiate it from extension of the tumor through the visceral pleura to involve the lung parenchyma (T2 disease).[146] CT frequently can distinguish T3 from T4 disease by defining involvement of soft tissues of the chest wall and pericardium. However, little information is available about nodal involvement assessed by CT. Two factors account for this: involved nodes may not be enlarged and large portions of the hilum and mediastinum are often obscured by bulky tumor. With any imaging modality used to stage this disease, the tendency is to understage the true extent of malignant pleural mesothelioma.[146]

Even with this new international classification for which there is significant consensus, difficulties remain in assigning the correct stage to individual patients.[147] The sensitivity of CT scanning is poor in detecting early stages of invasion into the chest wall, mediastinum, and diaphragm.[148] Ideally, complete assessment would include thoracoscopy for pleural extent and mediastinoscopy for suspicious lymph nodes. Laparoscopy has been demonstrated to be safe and accurate for detecting transdiaphragmatic tumor extension over and above the capability of the CT scan or MRI. In fact, laparoscopy should probably be performed routinely prior to a contemplated extrapleural pneumonectomy to assure that resection is justified. Both the presence of transdiaphragmatic extension or diffuse peritoneal involvement can be accurately assessed with laparoscopy.

Sugarbaker and colleagues[149] have recently proposed a revised staging classification based on findings established in a large series of extrapleural pneumonectomies (Table 22-4). They have made major advances in our knowledge of prognostic indicators and have been able to identify a subgroup of patients who do extremely well. This staging system takes into account lymph node involvement (whether intrapleural or extrapleural) and a number of features related to findings at the time of operation. Patients with pure epithelial histology, lack of nodal involvement, and negative resection margins can be expected to be long-term survivors.

## PROGNOSIS

The overall prognosis of malignant mesothelioma is poor. As the tumor progresses, dyspnea on exertion is followed by shortness of breath at rest. The tumor encases the lung and obliterates the pleural space. Significant ventilation-perfusion mismatching occurs as deoxygenated blood is shunted into lung trapped by tumor and effusions. This leads to hypoxemia that is refractory to supplemental oxygen.

Symptoms begin to develop secondary to tumor invasion of thoracic structures.[69] Compression of the esophagus leads to dysphagia, which results in rapid weight loss and death. Infiltration of the vertebral column causes cord compression and paraplegia. Invasion of the sympathetic and thoracic nerves can cause recurrent laryngeal nerve paralysis, brachial plexopathy, Horner's syndrome, and Pancoast syndrome.[150] Involvement of the great vessels of the mediastinum can cause superior vena cava syndrome. Growth into the epicardium leads to right-sided heart failure and arrhythmias, causing death in 10% of patients.[5] Any biopsy, trocar, or chest tube sites may be seeded with tumor and may be sites of significant chest pain.

Metastasis is an end-stage complication of malignant mesothelioma but is rarely the cause of death. Of patients at necropsy, 20% to 80% have evidence of hematogenous spread.[50,151] Sarcomatous variants of malignant mesothelioma resemble sarcomas clinically in that they are more commonly associated with extrathoracic metastasis, little or no effusions, and shorter survival times. Epithelial variants behave more like carcinomas in that they are associated with local invasion causing large pleural effusions, contralateral pleural involvement, ascites, and metastasis to regional lymph nodes.[152,153] In a review of 143 autopsies, Henderson reported that intrathoracic spread occurs most commonly to the pericardium and contralateral pleura and lung. Transdiaphragmatic spread and hilar, mediastinal, retroperitoneal, and cervical lymph node metastasis are other common locations of invasion. The most common sites of distant metastasis are liver (25%), bone (16%), adrenal gland (14%), and kidney (13%).[50,154] Hilar and mediastinal lymph node involvement is present in approximately 50% of patients, however, extrathoracic lymph node involvement is particularly uncommon (<1%).[74,155] Brain metastases are rare, but have been reported.[75,156–159]

Most patients die of complications related to local disease. Progressive tumor bulk compromises pulmonary function and chest wall invasion requires high doses of narcotics to control pain. Death often occurs from respiratory failure, pulmonary infections, and small bowel obstruction secondary to peritoneal involvement.

In a review of 11 studies encompassing 560 patients receiving supportive care or treatment, median survival was 8.6 months.[77] It is difficult to interpret exact mean survival because some reports measure survival from diagnosis, whereas others measure survival from the development of symptoms. As well, the natural history of the disease can be variable, with the occasional long-term survivor despite no treatment. The range of survival ranges from 1 month to greater than 10 years.[160]

In a retrospective analysis of 131 patients at Memorial Sloan-Kettering Cancer Center, survival was reported using the new staging system based on clinical stage from the International Mesothelioma Interest Group.[145] Stage I disease had a 35-month median survival, whereas stage II disease had a 16-month survival, stage III 11.5 months survival, and stage IV, 5.9 months median survival.[145] Prior studies based survival analysis on Butchart's staging criteria, which are far less precise in the prognostic characteristics. Six different studies, including over 500 patients staged by Butchart's system, found median survival for stage I to be 11 to 17 months; stage II, 8 to 17 months; stage III, 1 to 9 months; and stage IV, 0 to 4 months.[144,161–164]

Multiple prognostic indicators have been proposed to correlate with survival. The most common variables influencing survival based on the largest studies to date include epithelioid histology, stage I disease by Butchart's staging system, and age under 60.[77,162] Epithelioid histology has consistently been found to be a prognostic indicator of survival, associated with a 10- to 17-month survival time compared to the sarcomatous variant where survival is in the 4- to 7-month range.[98,100,165] Many authors diverge on whether sarcomatous or biphasic histology is the worst prognostic indicator.[98,116] Survival rate in older patients is significantly worse than in younger patients. Other important prognostic indicators associated with longer survival include good performance status, absence of weight loss,

absence of chest pain, and an interval greater than 6 months from the onset of symptoms and presentation.[98,116] Absence of chest pain likely reflects limited disease with minimal pleural involvement. Although some authors suggest females survive longer, this may merely reflect that females are more likely to have an epithelioid histology. Fever of unknown origin and clotting abnormalities (including thrombocytosis) are poor prognostic signs.[166]

## THERAPEUTIC APPROACH

### CHEMOTHERAPY

Chemotherapy has proven to have limited efficacy in malignant mesothelioma. Over the past 45 years, scores of controlled studies, case reports, and retrospective analyses have compared single-drug and combination therapies. Most of these have been small, single-institution trials of single agents or combination regimens. In some reports, mesotheliomas have been included in phase II studies of sarcoma therapy. Several authors have reviewed the literature extensively in recent years.[167,168]

Consistently, the maximal response rate seen with any single agent has been 20%. Average response rates vary from 9% to 12%. Various combinations have not significantly improved his figure. The most promising drugs against mesotheliomas have included doxorubicin, epirubicin, cyclophosphamide, and mitomycin.

In many of these clinical trials, problems exist in assessing the efficacy of treatment since they utilize variable criteria to define response. Because of the unique characteristics of this diffuse malignancy, response is difficult to quantify and the usual WHO criteria for partial resonse rarely are used. Many studies use development or resolution of pleural effusion or other subjective criteria to assess efficacy, factors that are not accurate predictors of mesothelioma outcome. Second, the patient population included in these studies is heterogeneous, because some investigators are selectively choosing patients who likely will do well while others are lax in describing their inclusion criteria. Third, there are only a handful of studies with large cohorts of patients since mesothelioma is a rare disease. Many studies base results on less than 15 patients, making it difficult to draw conclusions on response rates. With better staging criteria and a critical mass of clinicians with an interest in treating this disease, we are likely to be able to better assess outcome of therapy, an important consideration in new drug development. Furthermore, over the past decade a number of chemotherapeutic agents have entered phase I and II clinical trials.[169–178]

Anthracyclines have shown the greatest promise among chemotherapeutic agents. Doxorubicin, the most extensively studied agent, has a partial response rate in the range of 10% to 40%, with the average usually quoted at 20%.[167,173,179–182] Cisplatin, another anthracycline, appears to be more effective in combination with other drugs. Carboplatin, a cisplatin analog, has been shown to have some activity against mesothelioma when used as a single agent, and it has the advantage of being less nephrotoxic and better tolerated than cisplatin.[148,174–176,183,184] Currently, the chemotherapy regimen of choice is carboplatin combined with paclitaxel.

Plant derivatives as a group have shown poor responses against mesotheliomas. A number of trials have shown vincristine and vinblastine to be inactive against mesothelioma. Isolated reports of partial response to paclitaxel as a single agent have appeared; however, there is a high association of cardiac arrythmias and painful peripheral neuropathy.[185-187] Alkylating agents such as ifosfamide, mesna, cyclophosphamide, and mitomycin have been studied in over 400 patients in numerous studies. One of the most promising alkylators is mitomycin. In a single phase II trial, 21% of patients were found to have some degree of response; however, this was associated with significant pulmonary toxicity. Ifosfamide and cyclophosphamide have demonstrated only minimal activity against pleural mesotheliomas.[163,188] Other promising antimetabolites include methotrexate and fluorouracil. Methotrexate was found to have an overall response rate ranging from 35% to 45% in several small studies, possibly one of the leading treatment options for mesothelioma. Fluorouracil at best shows a 15% response rate over many studies.[167,173,179]

A large number of combination drug trials have tried to improve on the 20% accepted response rate for doxorubicin. Combination regimens have not resulted in a significant improvement in survival. There have been over 20 different multidrug trials since 1978, the majority combining anthracyclines (doxorubicin) with alkylating agents (cyclophosphamide, mitomycin, ifosfamide) or platinum agents (cisplatin, carboplatin).[166,167,170,185,189-197] The Cancer and Leukemia Group B (CALGB) has conducted four phase II and phase III mesothelioma studies since 1985, with no notable improvement over single-agent therapy.[170,175] One of the most promising trials compared doxorubicin and cisplatin, but objective response rates were similar (9% versus 12%, respectively).[170] The combination of doxorubicin, cisplatin, bleomycin, and mitomycin has produced response rates of 44% in one study; however, this has not been repeated.[167]

Intracavitary chemotherapy that theoretically achieves high local concentrations of drug has been tried in patients with early-stage disease. In advanced disease the pleural space often is obliterated, thus making intracavitary therapy not feasible. Agents that have been evaluated by the intracavitary route include cisplatin, cytosine arabinoside, doxorubicin, and mitomycin C.[198-201]

## RADIATION THERAPY

External beam radiation therapy, when used as a single modality, is ineffective. There is modest regression of gross disease in many studies: however, no study has shown any prolongation of survival when patients were treated with radiation as primary treatment.[202]

There are a number of reasons why pleural tumors are not conducive to radiation therapy. There is a large volume of tissue included in treatment that can be damaged, including the heart, lungs, liver, and esophagus. More than 5000 cGY is needed over the course of treatment to achieve adequate palliation in most cases, and the target beam must include the pleural surface, diaphragm, and mediastinum. The field borders include the first rib superiorly, the diaphragmatic reflection of pleura inferiorly (12th thoracic vertebral body), the full width of the mediastinum, and the ipsilateral margin of the bony rib cage. CT scans can help delineate sites of gross disease.[203]

Many new techniques have been designed to protect the pulmonary parenchyma from significant radiation damage that is likely to occur with the large-volume field. Combined photon and electron beams use large, opposed anterior and posterior external beam ports with central lung blocking. The pleural areas underneath the blocks are treated with electron beams of appropriate energy (10 to 15 MeV). Tissue compensators can help improve dose distribution. Off-axis beam rotation technique radiates a maximal area of the pleural space to a high dose while shielding the underlying lung. However, even with these complex techniques, up to one-third of the lung can still be damaged.[148,203] With fractions of 180 to 200 cGy given five times a week, the dose to the esophagus can be limited to 4500 to 5000 cGy, the whole lung to 2000 cGy, the liver to 3000 cGy, and 50% of the heart to 4000 cGy.[203] The major role of radiation therapy in mesothelioma is an adjunct following surgical resection. Demarcation of the sites of residual gross tumor with surgical clips at thoracotomy helps plan accurate, high-dose external radiation. Radiation therapy also plays a role in palliative treatment, specifically for the management of pain and subcutaneous lesions at incision sites.

## SURGERY

Two surgical operations are important in the management of diffuse malignant mesothelioma: pleurectomy with or without decortication and extrapleural pneumonectomy (EPP). One of the earliest attempts to resect a mesothelioma was in 1922 in Germany by Eiselsberg, when an "endothelioma of the pleura" was removed from a 46-year-old man. He recommended radical surgery, but removed only the fourth through eighth ribs and a portion of the lung. An EPP was done as early as 1949 by Mason and endorsed by others beginning in 1959.[205]

At most 20% to 30% of all patients with malignant mesothelioma are surgical candidates.[206] The indications for surgical management are threefold. First, thoracotomy for biopsy may be necessary if other invasive diagnostic techniques have failed. Second, attempts at cure may be attempted with early, potentially resectable disease. Third, if cure is unattainable, surgical palliation may be considered, because pleurectomy is the most definitive, albeit most invasive, procedure for effecting pleurodesis. However, it is accompanied by significant morbidity.

Often, whether the tumor is resectable or not is determined at surgery. A tumor of any size may be completely resectable depending mainly on whether it is confined to one hemithorax, has not extended through the hemidiaphragm or the epicardium, and does not invade the chest wall.[207] The CT and MRI criteria for resectability include.

1. Preserved extrapleural planes
2. Normal CT attenuation values and MR signal intensity characteristics of structures adjacent to the tumor
3. Absence of extrapleural soft tissue masses
4. A smooth diaphragmatic surface on sagittal and coronal images

Patz concluded that the most reliable indicator of resectability was a clear plane between the inferior surface of the diaphragm and adjacent abdominal organs and a smooth inferior diaphragmatic contour. Patients with distant metastases are not surgical candidates. Criteria for unresectability as determined by CT or MRI include tumor encasement of the diaphragm, invasion of the extrapleural soft tissues or fat, infiltration or displacement or separation of ribs by tumor, and bone destruction.[207] Although there are numerous reports involving over 800 patients, it is difficult to assess the effect of surgical resection because of the diversity of the procedures.[205,208,209]

PERIOPERATIVE MANAGEMENT. Patients should be evaluated with regard to their fitness to undergo a major chest operation that likely will involve pneumonectomy. The patient's overall health and nutritional status should be considered. The cardiac status should be routinely evaluated by electrocardiogram as well as echocardiogram, and any history of heart disease should be pursued. Any significant ventricular dysfunction rules the patient out of surgical consideration. Obviously any patient with a history of a myocardial infarct within the past 3 months or who has an arrhythmia requiring medication should not be considered for extrapleural pneumonectomy.[77] Operation tends to be indicated in younger patients and EPP should probably be limited to patients under 70, with a few exceptions.

Furthermore, pulmonary function test results should ensure adequate pulmonary reserve following pneumonectomy. Many potential candidates may have borderline flows that preclude operation. The degree of pulmonary dysfunction correlates with the degree of costophrenic angle involvement, width and length of pleural fibrosis, and presence of either circumscribed plaque or diffuse pleural thickening.[77] Forced expiratory volume ($FEV_1$) should be greater than 2 L/s or greater than 70% of predicted. If less, a ventilation-perfusion scan should be performed to assess the contribution of the involved lung. Relative contraindications include $FEV_1 < 1$ L/s, $Pao_2 < 55$ mmHg, or $Pco_2 > 45$ mmHg.

PROCEDURES. Parietal pleurectomy involves stripping the pleura from the apex of the hemithorax to the diaphragm. Extrapleural dissection of the parietal pleura is facilitated by removing a rib after a generous posterolateral thoracotomy. All of the chest wall pleura can be removed, but the diaphragmatic pleura and mediastinal pleura cannot be completely resected. This procedure is feasible if there is a patent pleural space and minimal involvement of the visceral pleura. If the space is obliterated by the fusion of the visceral and parietal pleura, pleurectomy and decortication would be necessary, a difficult procedure when tumor is involved, as opposed to infection, where a fibrous peel is present. This procedure requires that a decortication plane be established between the peel (tumor and/or fibrosis) and the visceral pleura. Since the tumor likely involves the visceral pleura, the chance of being able to establish a clean decortication plane is small, and significant damage of the underlying lung parenchyma with resultant bleeding and air leak is likely to result. Usually EPP is required when there is significant involvement of the visceral pleura. Two large intercostal catheters are used to drain blood and to manage peripheral air leaks. Large air leaks may prevent full expansion of the lung, as will incomplete decortication. A residual space increases the likelihood of prolonged air leak and empyema. Operative mortality rate should be less than 2%. Various studies using this approach have reported median survival ranging from 9 to 18 months (Table 22-5).

Complications reported following this procedure include air leaks, hemorrhage, and infection. The most common complication (10%) is prolonged air leak (>7 days). Other postoperative complications include pneumonia, and occasionally empyema. Vocal cord

## TABLE 22-5. EXTRAPLEURAL PNEUMONECTOMY

| YEAR | AUTHOR | N | MEDIAN SUR (MO) | 2-YR SUR % | BIBLIOGRAPHY REFERENCES |
|---|---|---|---|---|---|
| 1997 | Pass | 39 | 9.4 | | Pass[97] |
| 1996 | Sugarbaker | 120 | 21 | 45 | Sugarbaker[96] |
| 1996 | Rusch | 50 | 9.9 | | Rusch[96] |
| 1994 | Allen | 40 | 13.3 | 22.5 | Allen[94]; Faber[94] |
| 1990 | Geroulenos | 18 | 20 | | Geroulenos[90] |
| 1990 | Harvey | 7 | 5.4 | 28.5 | Harvey[90] |
| 1989 | Ruffie | 23 | 9.3 | 17 | Ruffie[89] |
| 1988 | Faber | 33 | 13.5 | 24 | Faber[88] |
| 1986 | DaValle | | 17.8 | 24 | DaValle[86] |
| 1982 | Chahinian | 6 | 18 | 33 | Chahinian[82] |
| 1978 | DeLaria | 11 | | 18 | DeLaria[78] |
| 1976 | Butchart | 29 | 4.5 | 10.3 | Butchart[76] |
| | Totals | 376 | 12.9 | | |

paralysis because of recurrent laryngeal nerve injury has also been noted.[77,210,211]

EPP is a radical procedure that includes en bloc removal of the parietal pleura, lung, pericardium, and ipsilateral hemidiaphragm. It is designed to remove all gross disease, but it must be recognized that some disease likely remains because of the nature of this diffuse tumor. It is necessary to include the pericardium not only to ensure removal of as much tumor as possible but also to facilitate control of the pulmonary vessels.[77] This procedure is indicated for stage I disease, that is, technically resectable tumors that are encapsulated by the parietal pleura.[77] A number of authors have reported series of EPP with median survival ranging from 4 to 21 months. Since this procedure is associated with high morbidity and mortality rates, it is best carried out on carefully selected patients by a surgeon experienced in the performance of the procedure and the management of these patients postoperatively. Details of the operative procedure are available elsewhere.[212]

Prior to opening the chest, we advocate the performance of a diagnostic laparoscopy to assess transdiaphragmatic extension or peritoneal spread.[213] Either of these situations would preclude EPP. EPP is carried out through a generous posterolateral thoracotomy incision that extends down toward the diaphragm. To facilitate entry into the extrapleural plane, the sixth rib is removed and extrapleural dissection is begun extending inferiorly toward the diaphragm and superiorly toward the apex. Care must be taken to avoid the brachiocephalic vessels. The dissection extends around the apex toward the mediastinal pleura. The pericardium is incised, leaving the phrenic nerve intact if possible, and the pericardial dissection is carried around the inferior pulmonary vein and across the inferior raphe until the posterior pericardium is entered. The inferior vena cava must be identified and the pleura dissected off this structure. Care must be taken to avoid damage to the esophagus when dissecting posteriorly. The hemidiaphragm is incised down to the peritoneum, which is preserved if possible. If necessary, the peritoneum is taken as well, but often the muscular diaphragm may be dissected away from the peritoneum. Again, care must be taken when incising the diaphragm over the inferior vena cava. The pulmonary artery is encircled, as are the superior and inferior pulmonary veins. We divide these structures using staplers. The bronchus is dissected as far proximal as is feasible and is closed with a stapler and divided. The bronchial closure is buttressed with a flap of pericardial fat or pericardium.

Once the lung is removed, the pericardium is closed with a fenestrated patch of either bovine pericardium or polytetrafluoroethylene (PTFE). The hemidiaphragm likewise is reconstructed with a PTFE patch to prevent migration of abdominal viscera. We place a chest tube attached to a balanced drainage system; the tube is removed within 24 h.

Mortality rate following extrapleural pneumonectomy should not exceed 5% to 10%, and ideally should be 5% or less. This procedure often has been associated with a mortality of 20%, which is unacceptable and points out the requirement that EPP should only be performed in centers where at least 10 of these procedures are done per year. Patient selection is also key in minimizing mortality statistics, as is vigilant postoperative care. Patients over the age of 70 rarely are candidates for this operation.

The most common complication following EPP is supraventricular arrhythmias requiring medical treatment, which occur in up to 25% to 40% of patients.[214] A small number of patients develop bronchopleural fistulas, especially with right-sided extrapleural pneumonectomies.[77] Other complications include empyema, vocal cord paralysis, chylothorax, arrhythmia, myocardial infarct, congestive heart failure, gastrointestinal complications, and respiratory insufficiency. In some patients there is a tendency for the operated hemithorax to fill rapidly, causing hemodynamic compromise. This must be promptly recognized and the chest drained in order to restore hemodynamics. If not recognized, this may be a fatal complication. Patients should be transfused as necessary.

Butchart and associates[144] reported on 29 patients in one of the first series of extrapleural pneumonectomies. Although median survival was approximately 4 months and perioperative mortality hovered around 30%, three major lessons came out of this study. First, there were two long-term survivors. Secondly, the histology of the tumor was analyzed, and a correlation with epithelial histology as a positive prognosis was established. And finally, the Butchart staging system was presented.[140]

Allen and Faber[215–217] have twice reported on their experience at the Rush-Presbyterian-St. Luke's Medical Center. In their series, 40 patients underwent EPP and 56 patients had pleurectomy/decortication with lung preservation. Most patients were treated additionally with adjuvant chemotherapy or radiotherapy. They reported similar operative mortality rates, 7.5% for extrapleural pneumonectomies and 5.4% for pleurectomies. Although the extrapleural pneumonectomy group had a 13.3-month median survival and 22.5% two-year survival, pleurectomy patients had a 9.0-month median survival and a 8.9% 2-year survival. However, this trend did not reach statistical significance.

A third major series was reported by the Lung Cancer Study Group (LCSG).[218] From 1985 to 1988, 83 patients were entered into the study. The first mesothelioma trial, LCSG 851, defined the patient population seen by the LCSG, and the feasibility of performing surgical resection by extrapleural pneumonectomy in a multiinstitutional setting. Only 20 of the 83 patients (24%) underwent extrapleural pneumonectomy. Patients who were not extrapleural pneumonectomy candidates had a more limited operation with or without adjuvant therapy or had nonsurgical management. Of these 20 patients,

3 (15%) died postoperatively. The recurrence-free survival time was significantly longer for the patients undergoing extrapleural pneumonectomy than for the other two groups ($p = 0.03$), but there was no difference in overall survival among the three groups. This experience prompted the LCSG to explore combining a potentially less morbid operation, pleurectomy/decortication, with adjuvant therapy. The results of another LCSG trial (LCSG 861) and of a small single-institution pilot study demonstrated the feasibility of intrapleural cisplatin-based chemotherapy, and led to the development of LCSG 882, which combined pleurectomy/decortication with postoperative intrapleural and subsequent systemic cisplatin-based chemotherapy.[219]

A 1996 report from Memorial Sloan-Kettering Cancer Center described 131 thoracotomies, resulting in 101 resections, 72 of which were complete. Extrapleural pneumonectomy was done in 50 patients and pleurectomy/decortication in 51. Local recurrence occurred mainly after pleurectomy/decortication and distant metastases developed after extrapleural pneumonectomy. Median survival was 9.9 months and 18.7 months for extrapleural pneumonectomy and pleurectomy, respectively.[220,221]

Most recently, Sugarbaker and colleagues[149] reported the results following extrapleural pneumonectomy in 183 patients and noted the importance of resection margins, cell type, and extrapleural lymph node status.[149] All of these patients were enrolled in a protocol that involved trimodality therapy including operation and postoperative chemotherapy and radiation therapy. The perioperative mortality was an astonishing 3.8% and the morbidity was 50%. The most common complications included pulmonary morbidity; infection, including sepsis; and gastrointestinal problems. Complications related to technical problems were noted in 12 patients, with 9 patients returning to the operating room for reexploration for bleeding or suspected tamponade. Ten patients had vocal cord paralysis. Median survival for the series was 19 months with 2- and 5-year survival of 38% and 15%, respectively. Epithelial cell type, negative resection margins, and lack of extrapleural lymph node involvement all were associated with prolonged survival. In 31 patients where all three of these variables were present, there was a 68% 2-year survival rate, a 46% 5-year survival rate, and a median survival time of 51 months, indicating that all is not hopeless with this disease.

## ADJUVANT THERAPY

Single-modality treatment, whether chemotherapy, radiation, or surgery, is seen to be of limited value in treating mesothelioma. Adjuvant therapy and combined modalities are being utilized to work synergistically to improve efficacy and there is reason for optimism.[222–224]

Bimodal and trimodal treatment plans have been tried: chemotherapy with radiation, surgery with chemotherapy, surgery with radiation, and all three combined modalities. Rare studies of chemotherapy with radiation therapy have met with only limited success.[225–227]

For over a decade at the Dana Farber Cancer Institute, trimodality treatment combining extrapleural pneumonectomy with sequential postoperative chemotherapy (doxorubicin at 60 mg/m$^2$, cyclophosphamide at 600 mg/m$^2$, cisplatin at 70 mg/m$^2$) for four to six cycles, and then up to 5500 cGy adjuvant radiotherapy to the postoperative hemithorax has been used. Overall median survival of 44 Butchart stage I patients improved to 16 months. The most common site of failure was the ipsilateral hemithorax.[228–231] As noted above, Sugarbaker et al.[149] recently updated this experience and reported on results in 183 patients treated with the trimodality regime. Overall perioperative mortality was 3.8% and the median survival was 19 months, with 15% of patients alive at 5 years. They defined several variables that are associated with prolonged survival. It is probably safe to conclude from their data that patients with sarcomatoid histology should probably not be offered extrapleural pneumonectomy. Likewise, if there is obvious mediastinal lymph node involvement, a nonoperative approach likely is the procedure of choice.

A similar approach has been tried in Germany on 93 patients.[232] Aggressive surgical management in selected patients is followed by doxorubicin, vindesine, and cyclophosphamide. A group of these patients who demonstrated partial remission received 4500 to 6000 cGy using rotating tangential technique. Median survival was 13 months. In a series of 26 patients, Alberts[163] reported only a 10.9-month median survival time after maximal pleural cytoreduction, 4500 cGy postoperative radiation therapy, and doxorubicin, cyclophosphamide, and procarbazine administration.

In the past, operation was combined with brachytherapy.[233,234] This approach is of historical interest only, at present. After debulking by partial pleurectomy, gross residual tumor was treated with $^{125}$I, $^{192}$Ir, or $^{32}$P radioactive colloids, which delivers 3000 cGy over 3 days within 1 cm of the site of implantation. This is then followed by external radiation to 4500 cGy over 4.5 weeks; 41 patients received external beam irradiation after pleurectomy and decortication, and 54 patients with gross residual disease received an implant and external beam therapy. Median survival time for the entire group was 12.6 months, with a 2-year survival rate of 35%. Those with pure epithelial histology who did not require an implant had a median survival of 22.5 months and a 2-year survival of 41%. The majority of the complications were secondary to the radiotherapy—pneumonitis, pulmonary fibrosis, esophagitis, and pericardial effusion.

Pleurectomy/decortication has also been combined with intracavitary chemotherapy and at times postoperative systemic chemotherapy. Intrapleural chemotherapy has variable toxicity depending on the patient, the most notable being acute renal insufficiency. Rusch combined intrapleural chemotherapy with cisplatin and cytosine arabinoside following pleurectomy and decortication and systemic cisplatin chemotherapy. In a subsequent phase II trial, pleurectomy and decortication were followed by immediate postoperative intrapleural cisplatin and mitomycin. Two cycles of systemic cisplatin and mitomycin were given starting 4 to 6 weeks postoperatively. Of the 36 patients entered on study, 28 had pleurectomy/decortication and intrapleural chemotherapy. The median survival was 17 months and locoregional disease was the most common site of relapse.[218,220,221] Other investigators have reported series of intrapleural cisplatin and mitomycin after pleurectomy followed by systemic chemotherapy. Median survival ranges from 13 to 17 months.[198,236] Some authors claim that this approach has a role for palliation and occasional long-term disease-free survival. Others have felt that it is inadequate and produces significant toxicity.[199]

Chemoimmunotherapy is also being studied as an alternative form of therapy. A number of investigators have tried using various combinations of chemotherapy (doxorubicin, mitomycin, cisplatin) with immunomodulators (α-IFN). No significant difference in survival or relapse rates have been noticed in comparison to single modalities; however, further trials need to be evaluated.[190,237–239]

## IMMUNOTHERAPY

Like the majority of human malignancies, mesothelioma is frequently resistant to multiple effector mechanisms. This phenomenon appears to represent active immune evasion or deviation mediated in part by mesothelioma-derived cytokines. Also, multiple mesothelioma-derived cytokines appear to be involved at several levels of tumorigenesis. Recent research has focused on how proliferation-related and other tumorigenic cytokine-mediated processes may be inhibited by some of the agents, which are already partially successful against mesotheliomas.[240] Attempts have been made to utilize systemic administration of interferon (IFN) α, β, γ, interleukin 2, and lymphokine-activated killer cells.

IFN-α has consistently been shown to inhibit the cellular proliferation of mesothelioma and has demonstrated additive or synergistic growth when combined with other chemotherapeutic agents. However, IFN-α has produced only a 12% response rate in some of the most promising studies.[241–244]

IFN-β is unlikely to be useful because it is associated with significant toxic side effects. The Southwest Oncology Study Group noted no response at all to 6 weeks of IFN-β treatment after evaluating 14 patients.[245,246]

IFN-γ is a lymphokine produced by T lymphocytes in response to specific antigenic or mitogenic stimuli. Transient partial responses have been noted in early mesothelioma, but no response is seen with later disease.[247] Intrapleural delivery of IFN-γ also has been studied, since this cytokine shares the antiproliferative effects of other interferons, and in addition is a potent activator of macrophage cytotoxicity against tumor cell lines. In a study of 89 patients over 46 months, overall partial response of 15% to 20% was seen in early disease with good tolerance of IFN. Eight patients had histologically confirmed complete remissions and nine had partial responses with greater than 50% reduction in tumor volume. Overall, patients with stage I disease had a response rate of 45%. IFN-γ was found to have limited efficacy in Butchart stage I disease, especially if the tumor was confined to the parietal and diaphragmatic pleura.[100,248]

Human mesothelial cells grown in tissue culture have been shown to be susceptible to lysis by lymphokine-activated killer cells, an effect enhanced by IL-2. Intrapleural administration of IL-2 has been associated with good tolerance, moderate toxicity, and 90% initial response rate.[148] Administration of IL-2 in patients with malignant mesothelioma, either alone or in combination with autologous IL-2–activated killer cells, has been evaluated by several groups. IL-2 shows some promise.[247,249] Intrapleural recombinant IL-2 has been infused with little to no improved efficacy over other modalities.[250,251] The median survival time of the largest intrapleural IL-2 study ($n = 15$) was 21 months for half the patients that responded to treatment.

## EMERGING MODALITIES

As discussed, regardless of the modality used, conventional forms of treatment for malignant mesothelioma have proven disappointing. Only 20% of tumors can be approached surgically, chemotherapy has limited results, and the neoplasm appears to be radioresistant. Immunotherapy and gene therapy offer new approaches to treatment. Other modalities for treatment include photodynamic therapy, immunoconjugate therapy, and chemohyperthermia.[252]

**GENE THERAPY.** Because of the propensity for mesothelioma to remain localized to the hemithorax, it is an ideal target for regional gene therapy. After demonstrating preclinical efficacy, our group embarked on a clinical trial of regional gene therapy via instillation of an adenoviral vector containing a so-called suicide gene, thymidine kinase, into the involved pleural space.[253–255] This approach relies on the conversion of systemically administered ganciclovir to a toxic triphosphate moiety that kills the tumor cells that are expressing the novel genes. A "bystander effect" allows the response to be spread within the tumor.

Twenty-six patients were treated in the initial phase I clinical trial. Patients with all stages of disease were eligible for participation. The treatment proved to be safe with a maximal tolerated dose (MTD) not reached. The most significant toxicity was a self-limited fever just after adenoviral vector administration. Gene transfer was consistently seen at the higher dose levels. A few radiographic responses were seen. A second trial with an improved vector is under way. There are a number of ways to optimize gene delivery and the potential efficacy of this approach that holds great promise for the treatment of localized malignancies such as mesothelioma.

**PHOTODYNAMIC THERAPY.** PDT is based on administering light-sensitive porphyrin molecules followed by direct intracavitary PDT aimed at destroying the porphyrin-containing tumor cells. Photosensitive molecules injected intrapleurally are taken up preferentially by malignant cells. When 630-nm light is used to activate the molecule, it generates free radicals to selectively lyse neoplastic cells.[256] Moderate success has been achieved in good-risk patients with low tumor burden.[257–259] Attempts as a surgical adjuvant show limited results, with a series of early reports suggesting a high rate of esophagopleural fistulas and esophageal perforations mainly due to poor monitoring of light delivery.[260–262]

A phase II trial of surgery and PDT has been evaluated in 54 patients to determine the optimal light dose. Patients with isolated hemithorax pleural malignancy (mesothelioma or lung adenocarcinoma) were prospectively entered into the trial in groups of three to receive light doses between 15 to 35 $J/cm^2$ 2 days after delivering the porphyrin molecules. Another arm of the trial delivered light doses between 30 to 32.5 $J/cm^2$ after a day. The MTD was determined to be 30 $J/cm^2$ 1 day after receiving the sensitizer molecule.[259] Further trials are being conducted to determine survival curves.

Friedberg and Hahn [personal communication] currently are conducting a trial using PDT following maximal tumor debulking. Light delivery is measured in real time using multiple strategically placed light sensors. Thus far the approach has proven to be safe and not associated with any of the light-related toxicity seen in previous trials.

**IMMUNOCONJUGATE THERAPY.** Immunoconjugate therapy makes use of monoclonal antibodies with specificity of tumors, usually conjugated to a toxin or radioactive particle. Clinical trials have been slow in appearing because of absence of mesothelial-specific target cells.[263] Chemohyperthermia combines intracavitary chemotherapy with intracavitary hyperthermia. Although proven to be safe, no survival advantage has been demonstrated yet.[264,265]

**PALLIATIVE MANAGEMENT.** Palliative treatment often is the only help the thoracic surgeon can offer to the patient with mesothelioma. The two major symptoms addressed are pain and shortness of breath. Once a pleural effusion has developed, it is persistent and recurs rapidly after simple drainage. Several liters of fluid may be removed in a matter of weeks. Diuretics do not prevent reaccumulation. With repeated drainage, thickening of the pleura begins to occur, leading to difficulty in aspiration because of development of rigid-walled loculations in the pleura. Ultrasound or CT guidance may be required at this stage to access these sites. Repeat thoracentesis is not definitive therapy for symptomatic pleural effusion.

Complete drainage and full reexpansion of the lung are necessary before any of the common intrapleural agents can be expected to effect pleurodesis. Full reexpansion is often difficult to achieve in mesothelioma because the thick rind of tumor on the surface of the lung prevents it from expanding sufficiently to create apposition with the chest wall. Pleurectomy with decortication may be required if the patient is well enough to undergo the procedure.[148] Talc is considered more effective than bleomycin or tetracycline in promoting pleural adhesions.[266]

If a chest tube can be placed, a sclerosing agent, usually talc slurry, is instilled if the lung expands enough to create pleural apposition. It may be preferable to proceed with videothoracoscopy, drainage of the effusion, and immediate insufflation of dry talc as a sclerosant.[77,267] Another option involves placement of a pleuroperitoneal shunt, especially in the situation where the lung is unable to completely reexpand.

A number of modalities exist to manage pain in patients with malignant mesothelioma. Radiation therapy has been successful in palliating the pain from tumor involvement of the chest wall. Radiation in moderate doses of 4000 to 5000 cGy has been shown to relieve symptoms of pain, superior vena cava obstruction, dyspnea, and dysphagia in up to two-thirds of patients.[202,203]

Narcotics usually are needed in late-stage disease to control the pain associated with malignant mesothelioma invasion of the chest wall. Transdermal delivery of a narcotic is effective in many cases. At other times, chronic epidural narcotic administration may be necessary and can be achieved with an implanted catheter.[77]

## PERITONEAL MESOTHELIOMA

Although both pleural and peritoneal mesotheliomas are related to asbestos exposure, there are significant differences between the two. Pleural mesotheliomas occur in a ratio of 10:1 relative to peritoneal mesotheliomas.[268] Patients with peritoneal mesotheliomas consistently are younger than those with pleural tumors, tending to be in their late 40s or early 50s. This reflects the fact that a higher cumulative dose of asbestos is necessary to develop peritoneal mesotheliomas.

Asbestos fibers enter the body through inhalation. By ciliary clearance, the fibers are brought out of the respiratory tract into the oropharynx and swallowed. Up to 75% of inhaled fibers eventually are found in the feces. Some of the fibers come in contact with the gastrointestinal epithelium. There is ample opportunity for penetration of the gut wall in the middle and lower portions of the small intestines, as well as some opportunity to enter the cecum due to stasis. From there they are absorbed into the circulation and lymphatics. Once in the splanchnic circulation, asbestos fibers can settle in the mesothelial lining of parenchymal organs and epithelium of the biliary and urinary tracts.[269] There have been various reports of peritoneal mesotheliomas developing after Thorotrast contamination during cholangiography and during routine use for angiography, even 50 years later.[270]

## PATHOLOGY

Similar to pleural mesotheliomas, malignant peritoneal mesotheliomas can have epithelioid, sarcomatous, or biphasic variants. Histochemical, immunohistochemical, and electron microscopic findings are similar to pleural mesotheliomas.[271] Epithelioid histology greatly predominates (80% to 90%) and presents with diffuse omental thickening and multiple nodular plaques in the mesentery.[272] Ascites is a common feature. Sarcomatoid variants more often are well-defined masses in the mesentery and omentum.[273,274] Various other lesions, specifically metastatic adenocarcinoma, may be confused with epithelioid peritoneal mesothelioma. Fibrosarcomas, leiomyosarcomas, and malignant fibrous histiocytomas can be confused with sarcomatous variants.

Other histologic variations unique to peritoneal mesotheliomas are papillary serous, well-differentiated papillary, and multicyctic mesotheliomas and various mixes of these types. Well-differentiated papillary mesotheliomas are considered of low-grade malignant potential and are associated with long-term survival. Often on presentation this variant is confused with peritoneal carcinomatosis. It is important to distinguish this from epithelioid subtypes because of the differences in epidemiology, clinical behavior, treatment, and prognosis.[275,276] The cystic or multicystic mesotheliomas lie between borderline benign to malignant potential. Cystic mesotheliomas usually occur in females (90% of patients) with a mean age of 38 years. It shows a natural affinity for pelvic surfaces.

## CLINICAL PRESENTATION

The most common presenting symptoms are abdominal pain, increasing abdominal girth secondary to ascites, and weight loss. Unfortunately, these nonspecific symptoms delay diagnosis unless an asbestos history is elicited early and the physician's suspicion is aroused. Rarely at presentation does a patient have a palpable abdominal mass. The tumor usually is confined to the peritoneal cavity. Malaise, fever, weakness, and constipation are occasionally present. The abdominal pain usually is progressive and migratory in nature and unchanging with movement or food. The pain is nonfocal and variable, described as anything from constant epigastric to burning hypogastric pain. Rarely does the patient have significant constipa-

tion or obstipation because intestinal obstruction is a late complication.

The physical examination often is normal at presentation; the ascites can be difficult to detect and the fluid can obscure the detection of masses.

## DIAGNOSIS

The diagnosis of peritoneal mesothelioma usually is made late, most commonly at laparotomy or autopsy. This is due to a lack of specific early symptoms and nonspecific screening studies. Peritoneal mesothelioma is included in a long differential diagnosis of other abdominal pathologies including adenocarcinoma, carcinomatosis, sarcoma, lymphoma, small bowel obstruction, inguinal hernia, lymphomas, localized peritoneal processes, inflammatory or granulomatous bowel disease, progressive systemic sclerosis, intestinal carcinoid tumor, mesenteritis, endometriosis, pseudomyxoma peritonei, and postirradiation enteritis.[277–280] The most important disease to rule out is adenocarcinoma, particularly from the ovaries or remnants from the Müllerian ducts.[281] If at surgical exploration enlarged, cystic, or solid ovaries with irregular surfaces are found, the most likely diagnosis is that of surface epithelium–derived adenocarcinoma.

Similar to malignant pleural mesothelioma, thrombocytosis is a common accompaniment and is a poor prognostic indicator. Clotting abnormalities including hemolytic anemia and disseminated intravascular coagulation (DIC) may occur. Patients have been noted to have hypergammaglobulinemia, and there have been reports of ectopic hormone production and recurrent hypoglycemic episodes due to the production of an insulinlike substance. Hyponatremia and hyperkalemia due to ectopic ADH or ACTH also have been observed.[278]

Peritoneal mesotheliomas present with a wide spectrum of radiographic appearances.[274] Imaging studies should be limited to the chest and abdomen because distant metastases rarely occur with malignant peritoneal mesothelioma. CT evaluation is the most important to assess chest and pelvic involvement.

One-half of all chest roentgenograms will reveal pleural plaques in cases of peritoneal mesothelioma, whereas only 25% of pleural mesothelioma patients have these plaques.[282] This reflects the fact that peritoneal mesothelioma requires a much higher exposure to asbestos. There is a wide variety of findings on abdominal roentgenograms, anywhere from normal to diffuse involvement. There may be some thickening of bowel lining. Extrinsic masses may reveal displacement of bowel loops and bowel obstruction. Rarely are abdominal calcifications noted.[279] Barium contrast studies can reveal compression and dislocation of bowel loops by extrinsic masses. Also, mesenteric retraction, segmental stenosis, and signs of intestinal obstruction can be observed. Rarely is there intraluminal involvement.[283]

Contrast-enhanced CT should always be used to evaluate the gastrointestinal, biliary, and urinary tracts. Classic findings on CT scan include ascites (75% to 90%), mesenteric thickening (75%), pleural involvement (57%), peritoneal studding, and hemorrhage within the tumor mass.[269] CT can also reveal local invasion of bowel and pancreas, liver metastases, and visceral involvement. Peritoneal thickening is most commonly seen on the parietal peritoneum around the liver and spleen and in the flanks. Mesenteric involvement can be present in numerous patterns: stratified, fishbone, stellate, and pleated. All of the mesenteric reflections can be involved, including the small bowels, cecum, and colon. Sheetlike masses with entrapped fat indicate massive peritoneal infiltration.[279] Poor prognostic indicators include bone destruction and retroperitoneal lymph node involvement.

Finally, ultrasound is commonly used to visualize abdominal pathology, specifically to differentiate masses from ascitic fluid. The most dramatic finding is thickening of the omentum, described as an omental cake. It characteristically surrounds the bowels and is continuous with the abdominal wall.[279]

Definitive diagnosis of peritoneal mesothelioma is rarely confirmed until some invasive diagnostic study, usually laparoscopy or laparotomy, is performed. Up to 90% of patients have ascites, so paracentesis can be attempted. Peritoneal fluid from malignant ascites is often viscous in nature. Similar to pleural malignant effusions, it may be high in hyaluronidase. Cytologic analysis rarely establishes the diagnosis. As with pleural biopsies, one must be concerned about seeding the biopsy site with malignant cells. Laparoscopy is a very effective technique to visualize the abdominal cavity. It permits the surgeon to examine the anterior surface and lateral parietal peritoneum, the pelvic peritoneum, the surface of the intestine, and anterior surface of the liver.[269] Definitive diagnosis may require laparotomy, depending upon extent of disease, but with current laparoscopic techniques this should rarely be necessary. Open biopsy allows the surgeon to inspect the abdomen for sites of tumor nodules, extension into the bowels and ovaries, and transdiaphragmatic extension, but laparoscopy may provide the same information in the hands of an experienced operator.

## STAGING AND PROGNOSIS

Too few cases of malignant peritoneal mesothelioma have been scrutinized to devise a staging system. The overall prognosis is poor, although some suggest that patients with malignant peritoneal mesothelioma survive longer than those with pleural mesotheliomas.[284] Median survival of untreated patients is 4 to 12 months. Complications related to the disease include esophageal achalasia, dysphagia, secondary amyloidosis, and dermatomyositis. One of the most difficult management issues in these patients is control of their clotting abnormalities: DIC, thrombosis, thrombophlebitis, and Coombs-positive hemolytic anemia.

Metastasis is a rare complication of peritoneal malignant mesothelioma.[278] The tumor is more likely to spread regionally to the pleural cavities than to metastasize. At autopsy, 75% of occurrences are limited to the abdomen. The most common sites of metastasis are abdominal organs and lymph nodes. Extrathoracic sites of metastasis include the lung, pleura, and pericardium.

Death tends to occur as a result of local intraabdominal disease. As the tumor enlarges, it continues to seed the peritoneal surfaces. As these nodules enlarge, they coalesce. This causes intestinal adhesions, nodularity, and infiltration of the omentum. The most accumulation of tumor tends to occur in the lower abdomen, the leaves of mesentery, pelvis, and beneath the right hemidiaphragm. This suggests that the tumor cells are distributed via gravity and peritoneal fluid.[269,284] Intestinal peristalsis may prevent tumor cells from adhering to the visceral peritoneal surfaces. Eventually, as the tumor encases the abdomen, it begins to coat the liver, spleen, and small bowel surface. Rarely does the tumor actually penetrate through the liver capsule or retroperitoneal structures. Also, peritoneal mesotheliomas rarely pass through the diaphragm, whereas pleural mesotheliomas are known to commonly transgress the diaphragm. Finally, patients do eventually die from small bowel obstruction, malnutrition, and weight loss.

The most favorable prognostic indicator, similar to pleural mesotheliomas, is epithelioid histology. Most peritoneal mesotheliomas are epithelioid, suggesting why patients may have a longer survival period than those with pleural mesotheliomas. Other favorable indicators are age under 50, 0-1 performance status, and no prior surgery or diagnostic complications.[284]

## THERAPY

Due to the limited number of patients that develop peritoneal mesothelioma, clinical trials have been sparse. Unlike pleural mesotheliomas, there is some suggestion that chemotherapy has a significant effect on long-term outcome. Therefore, if no acute symptoms of small bowel obstruction are present, intraperitoneal or systemic chemotherapy should be started. During this time, the patient can be evaluated for distant metastases and surgery.[284]

Surgery rarely is an option with peritoneal mesothelioma. Although the tumor is usually confined to the abdominal cavity, there is extensive intracavitary involvement. Surgery has not been demonstrated to enhance survival. The only indications for surgery include biopsy or palliation of obstruction or relief of ascites.

Development of ascites is often rapid. Relief can be accomplished with peritoneovenous shunting or repeated paracentesis.[280] The use of peritoneovenous shunting of intractable malignant ascites is controversial. In most patients, it can improve appetite, ambulation, and strength. However, shunts have also been associated with extensive metastatic dissemination to both lungs, pulmonary edema, sepsis, bowel perforation, and tumor embolization.[285] Surgical resection may be considered in patients with low-malignant-potential histologies such as well-differentiated papillary or cystic variants. Some authors suggest that debulking can prolong survival because of the slow natural history of these variants.

Chemotherapy has had some success in the management of peritoneal mesothelioma. Most trials have involved intracavitary administration. Two concepts have been proposed: (1) Extensive cryoreduction of the tumor prior to intraperitoneal chemotherapy is necessary, and (2) peritoneal chemotherapy must be administered before wound healing and abdominal adhesions prevent uniform distribution.[284]

Intraperitoneal chemotherapy is used to enhance local delivery. However, due to the large surface area of the bowel, penetration through the peritoneum in high concentrations is unlikely. Intraperitoneal chemohyperthermia has been used to enhance the cytotoxicity of anticancerous drugs such as mitomycin C.[286] There is a suggestion of some response to doxorubicin and cyclophosphamide, but favorable response to intraperitoneal chemotherapy does not necessarily translate to improved survival in many of these cases.[280]

Combination chemotherapy and multimodal regimens containing doxorubicin have been used to treat malignant peritoneal mesothelioma. In one series by Antman,[287] 18 patients received doxorubicin, 7 received additional surgery, and 6 received radiotherapy. One complete response and four partial responses were observed, ranging from 6 to 36 months. Significant clotting abnormalities, including DIC, massive thrombosis, fatal pulmonary emboli, Coombs-positive hemolytic anemia, and phlebitis, occurred in 22% of patients.

Alternatively, tumor debulking used prior to intraperitoneal chemotherapy may contribute to improved survival. Intraperitoneal cisplatin has been given to patients following surgical debulking. Median survival time was extended to 19 to 22 months.[288,289] Radiotherapy has also been used as an adjunctive measure. External beam radiation of the whole abdomen has had a limited role due to the poor tolerance by abdominal viscera. Intracavitary placement of radioactive colloids has had some limited success. The radioisotopes are thought to distribute poorly though due to gravity and adhesions.

Finally, trimodality therapy including surgical debulking, external beam radiation, and intraperitoneal chemotherapy has been utilized. Reports from the Dana Farber Cancer Institute suggest that aggressive multimodal treatment provides the best outcome survival ranging from 9 to 34 months in a small series of patients.[290,291] Unfortunately, aggressive management of these patients often is associated with high morbidity.

## PERICARDIAL MESOTHELIOMA

Primary pericardial tumors are extremely rare. Mesotheliomas are the most common primary pericardial tumor. Pericardial mesotheliomas are a diagnostic and therapeutic dilemma. The male:female ratio is 2:1, with a wide range of ages. One-half of the cases occur between the fifth and seventh decade.[292] The initial signs and symptoms are nonspecific. Pericardial mesotheliomas may present with a picture of constrictive pericarditis, systemic lupus erythematosus, or rheumatic heart disease. Most patients have pleuritic chest pain and evidence of cardiac tamponade.[293,294]

The gross appearance may be of a localized mass that is solid, cystic, or angiomatous, or of diffuse nodules. Complete encasement of the heart is rare. The tumor may penetrate the myocardium and invade the conducting tissue or coronary arteries or compress the great vessels.[294] There is one report of a presentation with intracardiac invasion to the atrium resembling cardiac myxoma.[295]

Chest roentgenograms may reveal an enlarged cardiac silhouette. Occasionally there is an associated pleural effusion, mediastinal widening, or the appearance of an anterior mediastinal mass. Echocardiography, especially transesophageal echo, may be useful in differentiating tumor from fluid. The most common findings on transcutaneous echocardiography are pericardial effusions, tamponade, thickened pericardium, mitral valve abnormalities, and pericardial masses.[292,296] Two-thirds of reported cases are associated with hemorrhagic pericardial effusions; however, cytologic analysis is negative in more than 75% of patients.[293,297] CT and MRI can be used to clearly depict the location and anatomic extent of a pericardial mass.[298–301]

Pericardial mesothelioma is a highly lethal disease. Mean survival is 3.5 months from time of presentation.[292] Local spread is common, but extrathoracic metastases are rare. The tumor commonly is diagnosed at a late stage and often results in pericardial constriction caused by tumor expansion or associated serous or hemorrhagic pericardial effusion.[294] No data have demonstrated prolonged survival from surgical intervention. Thoracotomy is probably necessary to make a definitive pathologic diagnosis. Complete tumor resection usually is impossible; therefore, operations mostly are limited to relieving obstruction. Systemic chemotherapy or radiotherapy has not demonstrated any effect. Local intrapericardial space injection of chemotherapeutics or sclerosing agents have been tried.[302]

## TUNICA VAGINALIS TESTIS MESOTHELIOMA

Tumors arising from the tunica vaginalis testis also are extremely rare. Tumors present in a wide age range of patients with an even distribution throughout the second to eighth decade.[303] Most patients present with a hydrocele or paratesticular mass. Grossly, the tumor presents as multiple, firm papillary nodules studding a hydrocele sac, often associated with a mass infiltrating the spermatic cord or adjacent testis.[303] Müllerian-type tumors, carcinomas of the rete testes, adenomatoid tumors, and metastatic carcinomas need to be differentiated from testis mesotheliomas.[303,304]

Malignant mesothelioma of the tunica vaginalis testis has an aggressive natural history with the potential for late recurrence or metastasis of even well-differentiated histologies. There is a need for early, aggressive surgical management.[303] Hemiscrotectomy or radical orchiectomy should be performed whenever possible. Patients should receive adjunctive inguinal or retroperitoneal lymph node dissection, radiation, or both.[305,306] In order for patients to obtain long-term survival, complete removal of the tumor must occur.

## LOCALIZED BENIGN MESOTHELIOMA

Localized benign mesotheliomas, now called solitary benign fibrous tumors, are believed to arise from submesothelial fibroblasts, not mesothelial cells; thus these tumors are not mesotheliomas and the term should not be used.[307] They can arise from the pleura, peritoneum, and tunica vaginalis testis.[308–310] Occasionally these tumors have arisen from the liver, adrenal, and atrioventricular node. Solitary fibrous tumors are not associated with asbestos exposure and they can arise in any age group, although peak incidence is in the fourth to sixth decade.[311] In stark contrast to malignant mesotheliomas, these tumors tend to occur in a 2:1 ratio of women to men.[1]

Grossly, they are well-circumscribed, encapsulated, and attached to the mesothelial surface of organs by a thin strip of tissue on a stalk that contains hypertrophic arteries and veins. Occasionally, there is calcification, hemorrhage, or central necrosis.[312] Approximately 80% of solitary fibrous tumors of the pleura originate on the visceral surface of the pleura.[309] There is a great deal of variation in size, ranging from subcentimeter nodules to large 30-cm-diameter masses.[308,310] Some authors report fibrous tumors involving the entire pleural cavity and hemithorax.[1]

Histologically, these neoplasms are composed of bland spindle-shaped cells with a wide range of cellular density and variability in vascularity.[313,314] They are fibrocellular or sarcomatous in character. Occasionally, there is a component of epithelial-like cells in a papillary pattern.[311] There is minimal nuclear pleomorphism and absent mitoses. Ultrastructural analysis reveals both fibroblasts and mesothelial cells.[309] In the peritoneum, benign cystic-appearing mesotheliomas have also arisen.

Solitary benign fibrous tumors often are asymptomatic and found unexpectedly on routine roentgenograms. Other patients may present due to symptoms from enlarging masses, metabolic abnormalities, and paraneoplastic syndromes. Large pleural tumors can give rise to pain and a wide spectrum of symptoms such as progressive dyspnea, atelectasis, pneumonia, and superior vena cava syndrome.[311] Benign cystic mesotheliomas of the peritoneum can present with abdominal pain, distention, early satiety, and other symptoms of mass compression.[315]

Electrolyte and neoplastic syndromes have been noted in benign fibrous tumors, especially with larger lesions. These patients may present with manifestations of hypoglycemia secondary to tumor production of insulinlike growth factor. They also may develop hyponatremia due to neoplastic SIADH production.[150] In benign pleural tumors, extrathoracic symptoms of pulmonary hypertrophic osteoarthropathy and digital clubbing can be seen in up to one-fourth of patients. The affected long bones show periosteal proliferation and new bone formation. Relief of the symptoms can be obtained following tumor resection.

Most solitary benign fibrous tumors should be surgically removed. Plain radiographs, CT, or MRI are all viable options to visualize and delineate the extent of tumor before resection.[316] If resected before extensive intrathoracic or intraabdominal growth, solitary fibrous tumors often are cured.[308,309,317] The best indicator of a good prognosis is the presence of a pedicle supporting the tumor. Local recurrences have occurred as long as 17 years after surgery.[312]

## LOCALIZED MALIGNANT MESOTHELIOMA

Localized malignant mesotheliomas are the rarest of the three categories of mesotheliomas (diffuse malignant, localized benign, localized malignant). Only one out of every six localized mesotheliomas is malignant.[318] They have been known to arise in the pleural and peritoneal space.[319,320] Grossly, these tumors resemble solitary benign fibrous tumors.[320] Histologically, immunohistochemically, and ultrastructurally, they are identical to diffuse epithelioid and biphasic malignant mesotheliomas. These patients rarely survive more than 2 years.[318] When resected, these tumors can appear to be benign; however, they often recur quickly. Recurrences are often characterized by multiple nodules rather than a diffuse rind, typical of malignant mesotheliomas.[320] Occasionally with meticulous resection, cure has been obtained.

## CONCLUSION

Mesothelial malignancies are rare neoplasms, especially when compared to bronchogenic carcinoma. However, the relationship to asbestos has caused these lesions to attract an increased amount of attention. Malignant mesothelioma up to now has defied all attempts

at therapy and continues to carry a poor prognosis. However, recent information suggests that with appropriate therapy a subset of patients with diffuse disease may be long-term survivors. Better staging systems should allow for more precise tailoring of therapy and more accurate information regarding prognosis. These lesions also lend themselves to novel therapies because of their intracavitary location.

## REFERENCES

1. ROBINSON LA, REILLY RB: Localized pleural mesothelioma: The clinical spectrum. Chest 106:1611, 1994.
2. LEE DH, SELIKOFF IJ: Historical background to the asbestos problem. Environ Res 18:300, 1979.
3. WAGNER JC: Epidemiology of diffuse mesothelial tumors: evidence of an association front in South Africa and the United Kingdom. Ann NY Acad Sci 132:575, 1965.
4. ENTERLINE PE: Changing attitudes and opinions regarding asbestos and cancer 1934–1965 (see comments). Am J Ind Med 20:685, 1991.
5. ANTMAN KH: Natural history and epidemiology of malignant mesothelioma. Chest 103(Suppl 4):373S, 1993.
6. HUNCHAREK M: Asbestos and cancer: Epidemiological and public health controversies. Cancer Invest 12:214, 1994.
7. CHURG A et al: Lung asbestos content in chrysotile workers with mesothelioma. Am Rev Respir Dis 130:1042, 1984.
8. LIPPMANN M: Deposition and retention of inhaled fibres: Effects on incidence of lung cancer and mesothelioma. Occup Environ Med 51:793, 1994.
9. WALKER C et al: Possible cellular and molecular mechanisms for asbestos carcinogenicity (see comments). Am J Ind Med 21:253, 1992.
10. CHURG A: Deposition and clearance of chrysotile asbestos. Ann Occup Hyg 38:625, 424, 1994.
11. MCDONALD JC, MCDONALD AD: The epidemiology of mesothelioma in historical context. Eur Respir J 9:1932, 1996.
12. SMITH AH, WRIGHT CC: Chrysotile asbestos is the main cause of pleural mesothelioma. Am J Ind Med 30:252, 1996.
13. POTT F: Asbestos use and carcinogenicity in Germany and a comparison with animal studies. Ann Occup Hyg 38:589, 420, 1994.
14. LIDDELL FD et al: The 1891–1920 birth cohort of Quebec chrysotile miners and millers: Development from 1904 and mortality to 1992 (see comments). Ann Occup Hyg 41:13, 1997.
15. CRAIGHEAD JE: Current pathogenetic concepts of diffuse malignant mesothelioma. Hum Pathol 18:544, 1987.
16. DAVIS JM et al: Mesothelioma dose response following intraperitoneal injection of mineral fibres. Int J Exp Pathol 72:263, 1991.
17. ROSS D, MCDONALD JC: Occupational and geographical factors in the epidemiology of malignant mesothelioma. Monaldi Arc Chest Dis 50:459, 1995.
18. CONNELLY RR et al: Demographic patterns for mesothelioma in the United States. J Nat Cancer Inst 78:1053, 1987.
19. SELIKOFF IJ: Death certificates in epidemiological studies, including occupational hazards: Inaccuracies in occupational categories. Am J Ind Med 22:493, 1992.
20. SPIRTAS R et al: Recent trends in mesothelioma incidence in the United States. Am J Ind Med 9:397, 1986.
21. PRICE B: Analysis of current trends in United States mesothelioma incidence. Am J Epidemiol 145:211, 1997.

22. Peto J et al: Continuing increase in mesothelioma mortality in Britain (see comments). Lancet 345:535, 1995.

23. Walker AM et al: Projections of asbestos-related disease 1980–2009. J Occup Med 25:409, 1983.

24. King JA, Wong SW: Autopsy evaluation of asbestos exposure: Retrospective study of 135 cases with quantitation of ferruginous bodies in digested lung tissue. South Med J 89:380, 1996.

25. Kilburn KH et al: Asbestos disease in family contacts of shipyard workers. Am J Public Health 75:615, 1985.

26. Mancuso TF: Relative risk of mesothelioma among railroad machinists exposed to chrysotile (published erratum appears in Am J Ind Med 15:125, 1989); (see comments). Am J Ind Med 13:639, 1988.

27. Mossman BT et al: Mechanisms of carcinogenesis and clinical features of asbestos-associated cancer. Cancer Invest 14:466, 1996.

28. Nicholson WJ, Raffn E: Recent data on cancer due to asbestos in the USA and Denmark. Med Lav 86:393, 1995.

29. Lanphear BP, Bunchen CR: Latent period for malignant mesothelioma of occupational origin. J Occup Med 34:718, 1992.

30. Selikoff IJ et al: Latency of asbestos disease among insulation workers in the United States and Canada. Cancer 46:2736, 1980.

31. Weissmann LB et al: Malignant mesothelioma following treatment for Hodgkin's disease. J Clin Oncol 14:2098, 1998.

32. Shannon VR et al: Malignant pleural mesothelioma after radiation therapy for breast cancer: A report of two additional patients. Cancer 76:437, 1995.

33. Hofmann J et al: Malignant mesothelioma following radiation therapy. Am J Med 97:379, 1994.

34. Pappo AS et al: Post-irradiation malignant mesothelioma (letter). Cancer 79:192, 1997.

35. Cavazza A et al: Post-irradiation malignant mesothelioma. Cancer 77:1379, 1996.

36. Ishikawa Y et al: Lack of apparent excess of malignant mesothelioma but increased overall malignancies of peritoneal cavity in Japanese autopsies with Thorotrast injection into blood vessels. J Cancer Res Clin Oncol 121:567, 1995.

37. Pass HI et al: Evidence for and implications of SV40-like sequences in human mesotheliomas. Imp Adv Oncol 89, 1996.

38. Carbone M et al: Simian virus 40-like DNA sequences in human pleural mesothelioma. Oncogene 9:1781, 1994.

39. Cicala C et al: SV40 induces mesotheliomas in hamsters. Am J Pathol 142:1524, 1993.

40. Huncharek M: Genetic factors in the aetiology of malignant mesothelioma. Eur J Cancer 31A:1741, 1995.

41. Martensson G et al: Malignant mesothelioma in two pairs of siblings: Is there a hereditary predisposing factor? Eur J Respir Dis 65:179, 1984.

42. Merchant JA et al: The HL-A system in asbestos workers. Br Med J 1:189, 1975.

43. Segers K et al: Glutathione S-transferase expression in malignant mesothelioma and non-neoplastic mesothelium: An immunohistochemical study. J Cancer Res Clin Oncol 122:619, 1996.

44. Hirvonen A et al: Glutathione S-transferase and N-acetyltransferase genotypes and asbestos-associated pulmonary disorders. J Nat Cancer Instit 88:1853, 1996.

45. Rom WN et al: Cellular and molecular basis of the asbestos-related diseases (see comments). Am Rev Respir Dis 143:408, 1991.

46. Gibbs AR et al: Fibre distribution in the lungs and pleura of subjects with asbestos related diffuse pleural fibrosis. Br J Ind Med 48:762, 1991.

47. Craighead JE: The epidemiology and pathogenesis of malignant mesothelioma. Chest 96(suppl 1):92S, 1989.

48. Viallat JR et al: Pleural migration of chrysotile fibers after intratracheal injection in rats. Arch Environ Health 41:282, 1986.

49. Boutin C et al: Black spots concentrate oncogenic asbestos fibers in the parietal pleura: Thoracoscopic and mineralogic study. Am J Respir Crit Care Med 153:444, 1996.

50. Henderson DW et al: *Malignant Mesothelioma.* New York, Hemisphere Publishing, 1992.

51. Barrett JC et al: Multiple mechanisms for the carcinogenic effects of asbestos and other mineral fibers. Environ Health Perspect 81:81, 1989.

52. Rieder CL et al: Some possible routes for asbestos-induced aneuploidy during mitosis in vertebrate cells, in *Cellular and Molecular Aspects of Fiber Carcinogenesis*, C Harris et al (eds). Cold Spring Harbor Laboratory Press, Cold Spring Harbor, NY, 1991, pp 1–26.

53. Cole RW et al: Crocidolite asbestos fibers undergo size-dependent microtubule-mediated transport after endocytosis in vertebrate lung epithelial cells. Cancer Res 51:4942, 1991.

54. Gerwin BI: Asbestos and the mesothelial cell: A molecular trail to mitogenic stimuli and suppressor gene suspects. Am J Respir Cell Mol Biol 11:507, 1994.

55. Bouts MJ et al: Cytogenetic analysis of malignant mesothelioma. Cancer Genet Cytogenet 47:1, 1990.

56. Pass HI, Mew DJ: In vitro and in vivo studies of mesothelioma. J Cell Biochem 24(suppl):142, 1996.

57. Lee WC et al: Loss of heterozygosity analysis defines a critical region in chromosome 1p2: Commonly deleted in human malignant mesothelioma. Cancer Res 56:4297, 1996.

58. Pass HI: Malignant pleural mesothelioma: The thoracic surgeon and gene therapy (editorial; comment). Ann Thorac Surg 57:1383, 1994.

59. Taguchi T et al: Recurrent deletions of specific chromosomal sites in 1p, 3p, 6q, and 9p in human malignant mesothelioma (published erratum appears in Cancer Res 53:5063, 1993). Cancer Res 53:4349, 1993.

60. Kleymenova EV et al: Characterization of the rat neurofibromatosis 2 gene and its involvement in asbestos-induced mesothelioma. Mol Carcinogen 18:54, 1997.

61. Bielefeldt-Ohmann H et al: Molecular pathobiology and immunology of malignant mesothelioma. J Pathol 178:369, 1996.

62. Mor O et al: Absence of p53 mutations in malignant mesotheliomas. Am J Respir Cell Mol Biol 16:9, 1997.

63. Cote RJ et al: Genetic alterations of the p53 gene are a feature of malignant mesotheliomas (published erratum appears in Cancer Res 1:6399, 1991). Cancer Res 51:5410, 1991.

64. Metcalf RA et al: p53 and Kirsten-ras mutations in human mesothelioma cell lines. Cancer Res 52:2610, 1992.

65. Kafiri G et al: p53 Expression is common in malignant mesothelioma. Histopathology 21:331, 1992.

66. Battifora H: p53 Immunohistochemistry: A word of caution (editorial; comment). Human Pathol 25:435, 1994.

67. Amin KM et al: Wilms' tumor 1 susceptibility (WT1) gene products are selectively expressed in malignant mesothelioma. Am J Pathol 146:344, 1995.

68. Langerak AW et al: Expression of the Wilms' tumor gene WT1 in human malignant mesothelioma cell lines and

relationship to platelet-derived growth factor A and insulin-like growth factor 2 expression. Genes Chromosomes Cancer 12:87, 1995.

69. ANTMAN KH: Clinical presentation and natural history of benign and malignant mesothelioma. Semin Oncol 8:313, 1981.

70. MUSK AW, CHRISTMAS TI: The clinical diagnosis of malignant mesothelioma, in *Malignant Mesothelioma,* DW Henderson et al (eds). Hemisphere Publishing, New York, pp 253–258, 1992.

71. WU H et al: Lepidic intrapulmonary growth of malignant mesothelioma presenting as recurrent hydropneumothorax. Human Pathol 27:989, 1996.

72. DIMITROV NV, MCMAHON S: Presentation, diagnostic methods, staging, and natural history of malignant mesothelioma, in *Asbestos-Related Malignancy,* K Antman, J Aisner (eds), Grune & Stratton, Orlando, pp 225–238, 1987.

73. CHAILLEUX E et al: Prognostic factors in diffuse malignant pleural mesothelioma: A study of 167 patients. Chest 93:159, 1988.

74. MILLER BH et al: From the archives of the AFIP. Malignant pleural mesothelioma: Radiologic-pathologic correlation. Radiographics 16:613, 1996.

75. FALCONIERI G et al: Intracranial metastases from malignant pleural mesothelioma: Report of three autopsy cases and review of the literature. Arch Pathol Lab Med 115:591, 1991.

76. COLBY TV: Malignancies in the lung and pleura mimicking benign processes. Semin Diag Pathol 12:30, 1995.

77. PASS HI, POGREBNIAK HW: Malignant pleural mesothelioma. Curr Prob Surg 30:921, 1993.

78. PANCOAST HK et al: A roentgenologic study of the effects of dust inhalation upon the lungs. Trans Assoc Am Physic 32:97, 1917.

79. RABINOWITZ JG et al: A comparative study of mesothelioma and asbestosis using computed tomography and conventional chest radiography. Radiology 144:453, 1982.

80. LANGLOIS SLP, HENDERSON DW: Radiological investigation of mesothelioma, in *Malignant Mesothelioma,* DW Henderson et al (ed). New York, Hemisphere Publishing, 1992, pp 259–277.

81. MILLER WT JR et al: Asbestos-related chest diseases: Plain radiographic findings. Semin Roentgenol 27:102, 1992.

82. SOLOMON A et al: Calcified plaques on mediastinal pleural reflections associated with asbestos exposure: Four case reports. Am J Ind Med 6:53, 1984.

83. RAIZON A et al: Calcification as a sign of sarcomatous degeneration of malignant pleural mesotheliomas: A new CT finding. J Comput Assist Tomog 20:42, 1996.

84. ANDRION A et al: Sarcomatous tumor of the chest wall with osteochondroid differentiation: Evidence of mesothelial origin. Am J Surg Pathol 13:707, 1989.

85. YOUSEM SA, HOCHHOLZER L: Malignant mesotheliomas with osseous and cartilaginous differentiation. Arch Pathol Lab Med 111:62, 1987.

86. SOLOMON A: The radiology of asbestosis and related neoplasms, in *Asbestos-Related Malignancy,* K Antman, J Aisner (eds). Orlando, Grune & Stratton, 1987, pp 239–262.

87. GAMSU G et al: Computed tomography in the diagnosis of asbestos-related thoracic disease. J Thorac Imag 4:61, 1989.

88. OHISHI N et al: Extensive pulmonary metastases in malignant pleural mesothelioma: A rare clinical and radiographic presentation. Chest 110:296, 1996.

89. HUNCHAREK M: Miliary mesothelioma (see comments). Chest 106:605, 1994.

90. LIBSHITZ HI: Malignant pleural mesothelioma and rounded atelectasis (letter). AJR 162:1000, 1994.

91. TAMMILEHTO L et al: Evaluation of the clinical TNM staging system for malignant pleural mesothelioma: An assessment in 88 patients. Lung Cancer 12:25, 1995.

92. MAASILTA P et al: Radiographic chest assessment of lung injury following hemithorax irradiation for pleural mesothelioma. Eur Respir J 4:76, 1991.

93. SAHIN AA et al: Malignant pleural mesothelioma caused by environmental exposure to asbestos or erionite in rural Turkey: CT findings in 84 patients. AJR 161:533, 1993.

94. KAWASHIMA A, LIBSHITZ HI: Malignant pleural mesothelioma: CT manifestations in 50 cases. AJR 155:965, 1990.

95. LEUNG AN et al: CT in differential diagnosis of diffuse pleural disease. AJR 154:487, 1990.

96. LORIGAN JG, LIBSHITZ HI: MR imaging of malignant pleural mesothelioma. J Comp Assist Tom 13:617, 1989.

97. VAN GELDER T et al: The influence of the diagnostic technique on the histopathological diagnosis in malignant mesothelioma. Virchows Arch (Pathol Anat Histopath) 418:315, 1991.

98. JOHANSSON L, LINDEN CJ: Aspects of histopathologic subtype as a prognostic factor in 85 pleural mesotheliomas. Chest 109:109, 1996.

99. LOW EM et al: Prevention of tumour seeding following thoracoscopy in mesothelioma by prophylactic radiotherapy. Clin Oncol 7:317, 1995.

100. BOUTIN C et al: Intrapleural treatment with recombinant gamma-interferon in early stage malignant pleural mesothelioma. Cancer 74:2460, 1994.

101. BOUTIN C et al: Prevention of malignant seeding after invasive diagnostic procedures in patients with pleural mesothelioma: A randomized trial of local radiotherapy (see comments). Chest 108:754, 1995.

102. RENSHAW AA et al: The role of cytologic evaluation of pleural fluid in the diagnosis of malignant mesothelioma. Chest 111:106, 1997.

103. GOTTEHRER A et al: Pleural fluid analysis in malignant mesothelioma: Prognostic implications. Chest 100:1003, 1991.

104. MARTENSSON G et al: The sensitivity of hyaluronan analysis of pleural fluid from patients with malignant mesothelioma and a comparison of different methods. Cancer 73:1406, 1994.

105. HILLERDAL G et al: Hyaluronan in pleural effusions and in serum. Cancer 67:2410, 1991.

106. PETTERSSON T et al: Concentration of hyaluronic acid in pleural fluid as a diagnostic aid for malignant mesothelioma. Chest 94:1037, 1988.

107. ROBERTS GH, CAMPBELL GM: Exfoliative cytology of diffuse mesothelioma. J Clin Pathol 25:577, 1972.

108. SCOTT EM et al: Diffuse pleural thickening: Percutaneous CT-guided cutting needle biopsy. Radiology 194:867, 1995.

109. METINTAS M et al: CT-guided pleural needle biopsy in the diagnosis of malignant mesothelioma. J Comp Assist Tom 19:370, 1995.

110. KOHMAN LJ: Thoracoscopy for the evaluation and treatment of pleural space disease. Chest Surg Clin N Am 4:467, 1994.

111. LODDENKEMPER R, BOUTIN C: Thoracoscopy: Present diagnostic and therapeutic indications. Eur Respir J 6:1544, 1993.

112. ROBINSON GR, GLEESON K: Diagnostic flexible fiberoptic pleuroscopy in suspected malignant pleural effusion (see comments). Chest 107:424, 1995.

113. COLT HG: Thoracoscopic management of malignant pleural effusions. Clin Chest Med 16:505, 1995.

114. BOUTIN C, REY F: Thoracoscopy in pleural malignant mesothelioma: A prospective study of 188 consecutive patients. Part 1: Diagnosis. Cancer 72:389, 1993.

115. KLIMA M, BOSSART MI: Sarcomatous type of malignant mesothelioma. Ultrastruct Pathol 4:349, 1983.

116. VAN GELDER J et al: Prognostic factors and survival in malignant pleural mesothelioma. Eur Respir J 7:1035, 1994.

117. ROGGLI VL: Quantitative and analytical studies in the diagnosis of mesothelioma. Semin Diagn Pathol 9:162, 1992.

118. YOUSEM SA, HOCHHOLZER L: Unusual thoracic manifestations of epithelioid hemangioendothelioma. Arch Pathol Lab Med 111:459, 1987.

119. KAWAI T et al: Glycosaminoglycans in malignant diffuse mesothelioma. Cancer 56:567, 1985.

120. CORRIN B, ADDIS BJ: Histopathology of the pleura. Respiration 57:160, 1990.

121. MACHIN T et al: Bony metastases in desmoplastic pleural mesothelioma. Thorax 43:155, 1988.

122. CANTIN R et al: Desmoplastic diffuse mesothelioma. Am J Surg Pathol 6:215, 1982.

123. HENDERSON DW et al: Lymphohistiocytoid mesothelioma: A rare lymphomatoid variant of predominantly sarcomatoid mesothelioma. Ultrastruct Pathol 12:367, 1988.

124. CRAIGHEAD JE et al: The pathology of asbestos-associated diseases of the lungs and pleural cavities: Diagnostic criteria and proposed grading schema. Report of the Pneumoconiosis Committee of the College of American Pathologists and the National Institute for Occupational Safety and Health. Arch Pathol Lab Med 106:544, 1982.

125. ASHCROFT T: Epidemiological and quantitative relationships between mesothelioma and asbestos on Tyneside. J Clin Pathol 26:832, 1973.

126. ROGGLI VL et al: Pathology of human mesothelioma: Etiologic and diagnostic considerations. Pathol Annu 22:91, 1987.

127. CHIU B et al: Analysis of hyaluronic acid in the diagnosis of malignant mesothelioma. Cancer 54:2195, 1984.

128. BOLEN JW et al: Reactive and neoplastic serosal tissue: A light-microscopic, ultrastructural, and immunocytochemical study. Am J Surg Pathol 10:34, 1986.

129. BLOBEL GA et al: The intermediate filament cytoskeleton of malignant mesotheliomas and its diagnostic significance. Am J Pathol 121:235, 1985.

130. AL-IZZI M et al: Pleural mesothelioma of connective tissue type, localized fibrous tumour of the pleura, and reactive submesothelial hyperplasia. An immunohistochemical comparison. J Pathol 158:41, 1989.

131. ORDONEZ NG: The immunohistochemical diagnosis of mesothelioma: Differentiation of mesothelioma and lung adenocarcinoma. Am J Surg Pathol 13:276, 1989.

132. DEJMEK A: Methods to improve the diagnostic accuracy of malignant mesothelioma. Respir Med 90:191, 1996.

133. MCCAUGHEY WT et al: Diagnosis of diffuse malignant mesothelioma: Experience of a US/Canadian Mesothelioma Panel. Mod Pathol 4:342, 1991.

134. KUMAR-SINGH S et al: WT1 mutation in malignant mesothelioma and WT1 immunoreactivity in relation to p53 and growth factor expression, cell-type transition, and prognosis. J Pathol 181:67, 1997.

135. GUZMAN J et al: Immunocytology in malignant pleural mesothelioma: Expression of tumor markers and distribution of lymphocyte subsets. Chest 95:590, 1989.

136. SINGH G et al: Immunodiagnosis of mesothelioma: Use of antimesothelial cell serum in an indirect immunofluorescence assay. Cancer 43:2286, 1979.

137. DARDICK I et al: Diffuse epithelial mesothelioma: A review of the ultrastructural spectrum. Ultrastruct Pathol 1:503, 1987.

138. WARHOL MJ et al: Malignant mesothelioma: Ultrastructural distinction from adenocarcinoma. Am J Surg Pathol 6:307, 1982.

139. COLEMAN M et al: The ultrastructural pathology of malignant pleural mesothelioma. Pathol Annu 24:303, 1989.

140. DAVID JM: Ultrastructure of human mesotheliomas. J Nat Cancer Inst 52:1715, 1974.

141. HAMMAR SP et al: Mucin-positive epithelial mesotheliomas: A histochemical, immunohistochemical, and ultrastructural comparison with mucin-producing pulmonary adenocarcinomas. Ultrastruct Pathol 20:293, 1996.

142. BOGERS J et al: Stereological evaluation of malignant mesothelioma versus benign pleural hyperplasia. Pathol Res Pract 192:10, 1996.

143. CAGLE PT et al: Immunohistochemical differentiation of sarcomatoid mesotheliomas from other spindle cell neoplasms. Am J Clin Pathol 92:566, 1989.

144. BUTCHART EG et al: Pleuropneumonectomy in the management of diffuse malignant mesothelioma of the pleura: Experience with 29 patients. Thorax 31:15, 1976.

145. RUSCH VW, VENKATRAMAN E: The importance of surgical staging in the treatment of malignant pleural mesothelioma. J Thorac Cardiovasc Surg 111:815, discussion 825, 1996.

146. PATZ EF et al: The proposed new international TNM staging system for malignant pleural mesothelioma: Application to imaging. AJR 166:323, 1996.

147. JETT JR: Malignant pleural mesothelioma: A proposed new staging system (editorial; comment). Chest 108:895, 1995.

148. MORENO DE LA SANTA P, BUTCHART EG: Therapeutic options in malignant mesothelioma. Curr Op Oncol 7:134, 1995.

149. SUGARBAKER DJ et al: Resection margins, extrapleural nodal status, and cell type determine postoperative long-term survival in trimodality therapy of malignant pleural mesothelioma: Results in 183 patients. J Thorac Cardiovasc Surg 117:54, 1999.

150. WARREN W: The clinical manifestations and diagnosis of mesothelioma, in *Mesothelioma Diagnosis and Management*, CF Kittle (ed). Chicago, Year Book Medical Publishers, 1987, pp 31–36.

151. ROGGLI VL et al: Pathology of human mesothelioma: Etiologic and diagnostic considerations (review). Pathol Annu 22 (Pt. 2):91, 1987.

152. HUNCHAREK M, MUSCAT J: Metastases in diffuse pleural mesothelioma: Influence of histological type. Thorax 42:897, 1987.

153. LAW MR et al: Malignant mesothelioma of the pleura: Relation between histological type and clinical behaviour. Thorax 37:810, 1982.

154. KING JA et al: Mesothelioma: A study of 22 gases. South Med J 90:199, 1997.

155. HUNCHAREK M, SMITH K: Extrathoracic lymph node metastases in malignant pleural mesothelioma (letter). Chest 93:443, 1988.

156. KITAI R et al: Brain metastasis from malignant mesothelioma: Case report (review). Neurol Med Chir (Tokyo) 35:172, 1995.

157. WRONSKI M, BURT M: Cerebral metastases in pleural mesothelioma: Case report and review of the literature. J Neurooncol 17:21, 1993.

158. HUNCHAREK M, MUSCAT J: Cerebral metastases in pleural mesothelioma (letter; comment). Am J Clin Oncol 13:180, 1990.

159. HARRISON RN: Sarcomatous pleural mesothelioma and cerebral

metastases: Case report and a review of eight cases. Eur J Respir Dis 65:185, 1984.

160. Mark EJ, Shin DH: Diffuse malignant mesothelioma of the pleura: A clinicopathological study of six patients with a prolonged symptom-free interval or extended survival after biopsy and a review of the literature of long-term survival. Virchows Arch [Pathol Anat] 422:445, 1993.

161. Boutin C et al: Thoracoscopy in pleural malignant mesothelioma: A prospective study of 188 consecutive patients. Part 2: Prognosis and staging. Cancer 72:394, 1993.

162. Antman K: Malignant mesothelioma: Prognostic variables in a registry of 180 patients, the Dana-Farber Cancer Institute and Brigham and Women's Hospital experience over two decades, 1965–1985. J Clin Oncol 6:147, 1988.

163. Alberts AS et al: Malignant pleural mesothelioma: A disease unaffected by current therapeutic maneuvers. J Clin Oncol 6:527, 1988.

164. Brenner J et al: Malignant mesothelioma of the pleura: Review of 123 patients. Cancer 49:2431, 1982.

165. Fusco V et al: Malignant pleural mesothelioma: Multivariate analysis of prognostic factors on 113 patients. Anticancer Res 13:683, 1993.

166. Antman K et al: An intergroup phase III randomized study of doxorubicin and dacarbazine with or without ifosfamide and mesna in advanced soft tissue and bone sarcomas. J Clin Oncol 11:1276, 1993.

167. Ong ST, Vogelzang NJ: Chemotherapy in malignant pleural mesothelioma: A review. J Clin Oncol 14:1007, 1996.

168. Krarup-Hansen A, Hansen HH: Chemotherapy in malignant mesothelioma: A review. Cancer Chemother Pharmacol 28:319, 1991.

169. Vogelzang NJ et al: Trimetrexate in malignant mesothelioma: A cancer and leukemia group B phase II study. J Clin Oncol 12:1436, 1994.

170. Chahinian AP et al: Randomized phase II trial of cisplatin with mitomycin or doxorubicin for malignant mesothelioma by the Cancer and Leukemia Group B. J Clin Oncol 11:1559, 1993.

171. Mattson K et al: Multimodality treatment programs for malignant pleural mesothelioma using high-dose hemithorax irradiation. Int J Radia Oncol Biol Phys 24:643, 1992.

172. Zidar BL et al: A phase II evaluation of ifosfamide and mesna in unresectable diffuse malignant mesothelioma. A Southwest Oncology Group study. Cancer 70:2547, 1992.

173. Solheim OP et al: High-dose methotrexate in the treatment of malignant mesothelioma of the pleura: A phase II study. Br J Cancer 65:956, 1992.

174. Raghavan D et al: Phase II trial of carboplatin in the management of malignant mesothelioma. J Clin Oncol 8:151, 1990.

175. Vogelzang NJ et al: Carboplatin in malignant mesothelioma: A phase II study of the cancer and leukemia group B. Cancer Chemother Pharmacol 27:239, 1990.

176. Mbidde EK et al: Phase II trial of carboplatin (JM8) in treatment of patients with malignant mesothelioma. Cancer Chemother Pharmacol 18:284, 1986.

177. Krarup-Hansen A: Phase II trials of malignant mesothelioma: A commentary and update (comment). Lung Cancer 11:305, 1994.

178. Krarup-Hansen A: Studies concerning high dose ifosfamide to patients suffering from malignant mesothelioma (letter). Lung Cancer 16:101, 1996.

179. Harvey VJ et al: Chemotherapy of diffuse malignant mesothelioma: Phase II trials of single agent 5-fluorouracil and Adriamycin. Cancer 54:961, 1984.

180. Vogelzang NJ et al: Malignant mesothelioma: The University of Minnesota experience. Cancer 53:377, 1984.

181. Lerner HJ et al: Malignant mesothelioma: The Eastern Cooperative Oncology Group (ECOG) experience. Cancer 52:1981, 1983.

182. Rossof AH: Treatment II: Chemotherapy in the management of malignant mesothelioma, in Mesothelioma: Diagnosis and Management, CF Kittle (ed). Chicago, Year Book Medical Publishers, 1987, pp 73–78.

183. Planting AS et al: Phase II study of a short course of weekly high-dose cisplatin combined with long-term oral etoposide in pleural mesothelioma. Ann Oncol 6:613, 1995.

184. Zidar BL et al: A phase II evaluation of cisplatin in unresectable diffuse malignant mesothelioma: A Southwest Oncology Group Study. Invest New Drugs 6:223, 1988.

185. Palackdharry CS: Phase I trial of dose-escalated paclitaxel and carboplatin in combination with ifosfamide and filgrastim: Preliminary results. Semin Oncol 23:78, 1996.

186. van Meerbeeck J et al: Paclitaxel for malignant pleural mesothelioma: A phase II study of the EORTC Lung Cancer Cooperative Group. Br J Cancer 74:961, 1996.

187. Martensson G, Sorenson S: A phase II study of vincristine in malignant mesothelioma: A negative report. Cancer Chemother Pharmacol 24:133, 1989.

188. Magri MD et al: Treatment of malignant mesothelioma with epirubicin and ifosfamide: A phase II cooperative study. Ann Oncol 3:237, 1992.

189. Hunt KJ et al: Treatment of malignant mesothelioma with methotrexate and vinblastine, with or without platinum chemotherapy. Chest 109:1239, 1996.

190. Hasturk S et al: Combined chemotherapy in pleurectomized malignant pleural mesothelioma patients. J Chemother 8:159, 1996.

191. Anand A et al: Prospective study of combination chemotherapy with cyclophosphamide, doxorubicin, and cisplatin for unresectable or metastatic malignant pleural mesothelioma (letter; comment). Cancer 77:1959, 1996.

192. Shin DM et al: Prospective study of combination chemotherapy with cyclophosphamide, doxorubicin, and cisplatin for unresectable or metastatic malignant pleural mesothelioma (see comments). Cancer 76:2230, 1995.

193. Dirix LY et al: A phase II trial of dose-escalated doxorubicin and ifosfamide/mesna in patients with malignant mesothelioma. Ann Oncol 5:653, 1994.

194. Tsavaris N et al: Combination chemotherapy with cisplatin-vinblastine in malignant mesothelioma (see comments). Lung Cancer 11:299, 1994.

195. Gridelli C et al: Mitomycin C and vindesine: An ineffective combination chemotherapy in the treatment of malignant pleural mesothelioma. Tumori 78:380, 1992.

196. Ardizzoni A et al: Activity of doxorubicin and cisplatin combination chemotherapy in patients with diffuse malignant pleural mesothelioma: An Italian Lung Cancer Task Force (FONICAP) Phase II study. Cancer 67:2984, 1991.

197. Chahinian AP et al: Experimental and clinical activity of mitomycin C and cis-diamminedichloro in malignant mesothelioma. Cancer Res 44:1688, 1984.

198. Colleoni M et al: Surgery followed by intracavitary plus systemic chemotherapy in malignant pleural mesothelioma. Tumori 82:53, 1996.

199. SAUTER ER et al: Optimal management of malignant mesothelioma after subtotal pleurectomy: Revisiting the role of intrapleural chemotherapy and postoperative radiation. J Surg Oncol 60:100, 1995.

200. FIGLIN R et al: Intrapleural chemotherapy without pleurodesis for malignant pleural effusions: LCSG Trial 861. Chest 106:3635S, 1994.

201. LERZA R et al: High doses of intrapleural cisplatin in a case of malignant pleural mesothelioma: Clinical observations and pharmacokinetic analyses. Cancer 73:79, 1994.

202. DAVIS SR et al: Radiotherapy in the treatment of malignant mesothelioma of the pleura, with special reference to its use in palliation. Australasian Radiol 38:212, 1994.

203. REDDY S: Treatment III: Radiation in the therapy of malignant mesothelioma, in Mesothelioma: Diagnosis and Management, CF Kittle (ed). Chicago, Year Book Medical Publishers, 1987, pp 79–86.

204. MATTSON K et al: Epirubicin in malignant mesothelioma: A phase II study of the European Organization for Research and Treatment of Cancer Lung Cancer Cooperative Group. J Clin Oncol 10:824, 1992.

205. KITTLE CF: Treatment I: The surgical treatment of mesothelioma, in Mesothelioma: Diagnosis and Management, CF Kittle (ed). Chicago, Year Book Medical Publishers, 1987, pp 61–72.

206. VOGELZANG NJ: Malignant mesothelioma: Diagnostic and management strategies for 1992 (review). Semin Oncol 19:64, 1992.

207. PATZ EF JR et al: Malignant pleural mesothelioma: Value of CT and MR imaging in predicting resectability. AJR 159:961, 1992.

208. PASS HI et al: Surgically debulked malignant pleural mesothelioma. Results and prognostic factors. Ann Surg Oncol 4:215, 1997.

209. AISNER J: Therapeutic approach to malignant mesothelioma. Chest 96:95S, 1989.

210. AISNER J: Current approach to malignant mesothelioma of the pleura. Chest 107:332S, 1995.

211. BRANCATISANO RP et al: Pleurectomy for mesothelioma (see comments). Med J Aust 154:455, 460, 1991.

212. SUGARBAKER DJ et al: Extrapleural pneumonectomy in the treatment of malignant pleural mesothelioma. Ann Thorac Surg 54:941, 1992.

213. CONLON KC et al: Laparoscopy: An important tool in the staging of malignant pleural mesothelioma. Ann Surg Oncol 3:489, 1996.

214. HARPOLE DH et al: Prospective analysis of pneumonectomy: Risk factors for major morbidity and cardiac dysrhythmias. Ann Thorac Surg 61:977, 1996.

215. FABER LP: 1986: Extrapleural pneumonectomy for diffuse, malignant mesothelioma. Updated in 1994. Ann Thorac Surg 58:1782, 1994.

216. ALLEN KB et al: Malignant pleural mesothelioma: Extrapleural pneumonectomy and pleurectomy. Chest Surg Clin North Am 4:113, 1994.

217. FABER LP: Surgical treatment of asbestos-related disease of the chest. Surg Clin North Am 68:525, 1988.

218. RUSCH VW et al: The role of extrapleural pneumonectomy in malignant pleural mesothelioma: A Lung Cancer Study Group trial (see comments). J Thorac Cardiovasc Surg 102:1, 1991a.

219. RUSCH VW et al: Intrapleural cisplatin and cytarabine in the management of mallignant pleural effusions: A Lung Cancer Study Group trial. J Clin Oncol 9:313, 1991b.

220. RUSCH VW: Clinical features and current treatment of diffuse malignant pleural mesothelioma. Lung Cancer 12:S127, 1995.

221. RUSCH VW: Pleurectomy/decortication and adjuvant therapy for malignant mesothelioma. Chest 103:382S, 1993.

222. HUNCHAREK M et al: Treatment and survival in diffuse malignant pleural mesothelioma: A study of 83 cases from the Massachusetts General Hospital. Anticancer Res 16:1265, 1996.

223. SUGARBAKER DJ, NORBERTO JJ: Multimodality management of malignant pleural mesothelioma (review). Chest 113:61S, 1998.

224. KELLER SM: Adjuvant therapy for malignant pleural mesothelioma. Chest Surg Clin North Am 4:127, 1994.

225. LINDEN CJ et al: Effect of hemithorax irradiation alone or combined with doxorubicin and cyclophosphamide in 47 pleural mesotheliomas: A nonrandomized phase II study. Eur Respir J 9:2565, 1996.

226. SINOFF C et al: Combined doxorubicin and radiation therapy in malignant pleural mesothelioma. Cancer Treat Rep 66:1605, 1982.

227. CHAHINIAN AP et al: Diffuse malignant mesothelioma: Prospective evaluation of 69 patients. Ann Int Med 96:746, 1982.

228. SUGARBAKER DJ et al: Extrapleural pneumonectomy, chemotherapy, and radiotherapy in the treatment of diffuse malignant pleural mesothelioma (see comments). J Thorac Cardiovasc Surg 102:10, discussion 14, 1991.

229. BALDINI EH et al: Patterns of failure after trimodality therapy for malignant pleural mesothelioma. Ann Thorac Surg 63:334, 1997.

230. SUGARBAKER DJ et al: Mesothelioma and radical multimodality therapy: Who benefits? Chest 107:345S, 1995.

231. SUGARBAKER DJ et al: Node status has prognostic significance in the multimodality therapy of diffuse, malignant mesothelioma. J Clin Oncol 11:1172, 1993.

232. CALAVREZOS A et al: Malignant mesothelioma of the pleura: A prospective therapeutic study of 132 patients from 1981–1985. Klin Wochenschrift 66:607, 1988.

233. HILARIS BS et al: Pleurectomy and intraoperative brachytherapy and postoperative radiation in the treatment of malignant pleural mesothelioma. Int J Radiat Oncol Biol Phys 10:325, 1984.

234. MARTINI N et al: Pleural mesothelioma. Ann Thorac Surg 43:113, 1987.

235. RUSCH VW: A proposed new international TNM staging system for malignant pleural mesothelioma: From the International Mesothelioma Interest Group (see comments). Chest 108:1122, 1995.

236. LEE JD et al: Intrapleural chemotherapy for patients with incompletely resected malignant mesothelioma: The UCLA experience. J Surg Oncol 60:262, 1995.

237. SOULIE P et al: Combined systemic chemoimmunotherapy in advanced diffuse malignant mesothelioma: Report of a phase I-II study of weekly cisplatin/interferon alfa-2a. J Clin Oncol 14:878, 1996.

238. PASS HW et al: A phase II trial investigating primary immunochemotherapy for malignant pleural mesothelioma and the feasibility of adjuvant immunochemotherapy after maximal cytoreduction. Ann Surg Oncol 2:214, 1995.

239. UPHAM JW et al: Interferon alpha and doxorubicin in malignant mesothelioma: A phase II study. Aust NZ J Med 23:683, 1993.

240. FITZPATRICK DR et al: The role of growth factors and cytokines in the tumorigenesis and immunobiology of malignant mesothelioma. Am J Respir Cell Mol Biol 12:455, 1995.

241. BIELEFELDT-OHMANN H et al: Interleukin-6 involvement in mesothelioma pathobiology: Inhibition by interferon alpha immunotherapy. Cancer Immunol Immunother 40:241, 1995.

242. BIELEFELDT-OHMANN H et al: Potential for interferon-alpha-based therapy in mesothelioma: Assessment in a murine model. J Interferon Cytokine Res 15:213, 1995.

243. ARDIZZONI A et al: Recombinant interferon alpha-2b in the treatment of diffuse malignant pleural mesothelioma. Am J Clin Oncol 17:80, 1994.

244. CHRISTMAS TI et al: Effect of interferon-alpha 2a on malignant mesothelioma. J Interferon Res 13:9, 1993.

245. VON HOFF DD et al: Phase II evaluation of recombinant interferon-beta (IFN-beta ser) in patients with diffuse mesothelioma: A Southwest Oncology Group study. J Interferon Res 10:531, 1990.

246. ROSSO R et al: Intrapleural natural beta interferon in the treatment of malignant pleural effusions. Oncology 45:253, 1988.

247. FITZPATRICK DR et al: Potential for cytokine therapy of malignant mesothelioma. Cancer Treat Rev 21:273, 1995.

248. BOUTIN C et al: Activity of intrapleural recombinant gamma-interferon in malignant mesothelioma. Cancer 67:2033, 1991.

249. BOWMAN RV et al: Capacity of tumor necrosis factor to augment lymphocyte-mediated tumor cells of malignant mesothelioma. Clin Immunol Immunopathol 58:80, 1991.

250. ASTOUL P et al: Intrapleural recombinant Il-2 in passive immunotherapy for malignant pleural effusion. Chest 103:209, 1993.

251. GOEY SH et al: Intrapleural administration of interleukin 2 in pleural mesothelioma: A phase I-II study. Br J Cancer 72:1283, 1995.

252. UPHAM JW et al: Malignant mesothelioma: New insights into tumour biology and immunology as a basis for new treatment approaches. Thorax 50:887, 1995.

253. SMYTHE WR et al: Use of recombinant adenovirus to transfer the herpes simplex virus thymidine (HSVtk) gene to thoracic neoplasms: An effective in vitro drug sensitization. Cancer Res 54:2055, 1994.

254. SMYTHE WR et al: Treatment of experimental human mesothelioma using adenovirus transfer of herpes simplex thymidine kinase gene. Ann Surg 222:78, 1995.

255. STERMAN DH et al: Adenovirus-mediated herpes simplex thymidine kinase/ganciclovir gene therapy in patients with localized malignancy: Results of a phase I clinical trial of malignant mesothelioma. Hum Gene Ther 1, 9:1083, 1998.

256. HENDERSON BW, DOUGHERTY TJ: *Photodynamic Therapy: Basic Principles and Clinical Applications.* New York, M Dekker, 1992.

257. KOREN H et al: Hypericin in phototherapy. J Photochem Photobiol 36:113, 1996.

258. RIS HB et al: Intraoperative photodynamic therapy with *m*-tetrahydroxyphenylchlorin for chest malignancies. Lasers Surg Med 18:39, 1996.

259. PASS HI, DONINGTON JS: Use of photodynamic therapy for the management of pleural malignancies. Semin Surg Oncol 11:360, 1995.

260. TAKITA H et al: Operation and intracavitary photodynamic therapy for malignant pleural mesothelioma: A phase II study. Ann Thorac Surg 58:995, 1994.

261. TEMECK BK, PASS HI: Esophagopleural fistula: A complication of photodynamic therapy. South Med J 88:271, 1995.

262. LUKETICH JD et al: Bronchoesophagopleural fistula after photodynamic therapy for malignant mesothelioma. Ann Thorac Surg 62:283, 1996.

263. GRIFFIN TW et al: Antitumor activity of intraperitoneal immunotoxins in a nude mouse model of human malignant mesothelioma. Cancer Res 47:4266, 1987.

264. CARRY PY et al: A new device for the treatment of pleural malignancies: Intrapleural chemohyperthermia preliminary report. Oncology 50:348, 1993.

265. COULON L et al: Cytokine production during intraperitoneal chemohyperthermia. Oncology 50:371, 1993.

266. HARTMAN DL et al: Comparison of insufflated talc under thoracoscopic guidance with standard tetracycline and bleomycin pleurodesis for control of malignant pleural effusions. J Thorac Cardiovasc Surg 105:743; discussion 747, 1993.

267. VIALLAT JR et al: Thoracoscopic talc poudrage pleurodesis for malignant effusions: A review of 360 cases. Chest 110:1387, 1996.

268. HILLERDAL G: Malignant mesothelioma 1982: Review of 4710 published cases. Br J Dis Chest 77:321, 1983.

269. ANTMAN K, AISNER J: *Asbestos-Related Malignancy.* Orlando, Grune & Stratton, 1987.

270. STEY C et al: Malignant peritoneal mesothelioma after Thorotrast exposure. Am J Clin Oncol 18:313, 1995.

271. EYDEN BP et al: Malignant epithelial mesothelioma of the peritoneum: Observations on a problem case. Ultrastruct Pathol 20:337, 1996.

272. KANNERSTEIN M, CHURG J: Peritoneal mesothelioma. Hum Pathol 8:283, 1977.

273. KASS ME: Pathology of peritoneal mesothelioma. Cancer Treat Res 81:213, 1996.

274. ROS PR et al: Peritoneal mesothelioma: Radiologic appearances correlated with histology. Acta Radiol 32:355, 1991.

275. HOEKMAN K et al: Well-differentiated papillary mesothelioma of the peritoneum: A separate entity. Eur J Cancer 32A:255, 1996.

276. ANTMAN KH et al: Early peritoneal mesothelioma: A treatable malignancy. Lancet 2:977, 1985.

277. ANDRION A et al: Malignant peritoneal mesothelioma in a 17-year-old boy with evidence of previous exposure to chrysotile and tremolite asbestos. Hum Pathol 25:617, 1994.

278. BRENNER J et al: Malignant peritoneal mesothelioma: Review of 25 patients. Am J Gastroenterol 75:311, 1981.

279. RAPTOPOULOS V: Peritoneal mesothelioma. Crit Rev Diagn Imaging 24:293, 1985.

280. PLAUS WJ: Peritoneal mesothelioma. Arch Surg 123:763, 1988.

281. BOLLINGER DJ et al: Peritoneal malignant mesothelioma versus serous papillary adenocarcinoma: A histochemical and immunohistochemical comparison. Am J Surg Pathol 13:659, 1989.

282. REUTER K et al: Diagnosis of peritoneal mesothelioma: Computed tomography, sonography, and fine-needle aspiration biopsy. AJR 140:1189, 1983.

283. COZZI G et al: Double contrast barium enema combined with non-invasive imaging in peritoneal mesothelioma. Acta Radiol 30:21, 1989.

284. AVERBACH AM, SUGARBAKER PH: Peritoneal mesothelioma: Treatment approach based on natural history. Cancer Treat Res 81:193, 1996.

285. NERVINO HE, GEBHARDT FC: Peritoneovenous shunt for intractable malignant ascites: A single case report of metastatic

peritoneal mesothelioma implanted via LeVeen shunt. Cancer 54:2231, 1984.

286. PANTEIX G et al: Study of the pharmacokinetics of mitomycin C in humans during intraperitoneal chemohyperthermia with special mention of the concentration in local tissues. Oncology 50:366, 1993.

287. ANTMAN KH et al: Peritoneal mesothelioma: Natural history and response to chemotherapy. J Clin Oncol 1:386, 1983.

288. LANGER CJ et al: Intraperitoneal cisplatin and etoposide in peritoneal mesothelioma: Favorable outcome with a multimodality approach. Cancer Chemother Pharmacol 32:204, 1993.

289. MARKMAN M, KELSEN D: Efficacy of cisplatin-based intraperitoneal chemotherapy as treatment of malignant peritoneal mesothelioma. J Cancer Res Clin Oncol 118:547, 1992.

290. LEDERMAN GS et al: Long-term survival in peritoneal mesothelioma: The role of radiotherapy and combined modality treatment. Cancer 59:1882, 1987.

291. ANTMAN KM, CORSON JM: Benign and malignant pleural mesothelioma. Clin Chest Med 6:127, 1985.

292. THOMASON R et al: Primary malignant mesothelioma of the pericardium: Case report and literature review (see comments). Texas Heart Inst J 21:170, 1994.

293. HOLLINS J et al: Primary pericardial mesothelioma: Diagnostic and therapeutic challenges in management. South Med J 81:537, 1988.

294. LLEWELLYN MJ et al: Pericardial constriction caused by primary mesothelioma. Br Heart J 57:54, 1987.

295. LIN TS et al: Pericardial mesothelioma with intracardiac invasion into the right atrium. Cardiology 85:357, 1994.

296. AGATSTON AS et al: Echocardiographic findings in primary pericardial mesothelioma. Am Heart J 111:986, 1986.

297. YILLING FP et al: Pericardial mesothelioma. Chest 81:520, 1982.

298. KAMINAGA T et al: Magnetic resonance imaging of pericardial malignant mesothelioma. Magn Res Imaging 11:1057, 1993.

299. STEIN M et al: Magnetic resonance imaging findings in primary pericardial mesothelioma. Israel J Med Sci 31:192, 1995.

300. VOGEL HJ et al: Mesothelioma of the pericardium: CT and MR findings. J Comp Assist Tom 13:543, 1989.

301. GOSSINGER HD et al: Magnetic resonance imaging findings in a patient with pericardial mesothelioma. Am Heart J 115:1321, 1988.

302. SHEPHERD FA et al: Medical management of malignant pericardial effusion by tetracycline sclerosis. Am J Cardiol 60:1161, 1987.

303. JONES MA et al: Malignant mesothelioma of the tunica vaginalis: A clinicopathologic analysis of 11 cases with review of the literature. American Journal of Surg Pathol 19:815, 1995.

304. MOCH H et al: A new case of malignant mesothelioma of the tunica vaginalis testis: Immunohistochemistry in comparison with an adenomatoid tumor of the testis. Pathol Res Prac 190:400, discussion 404, 1994.

305. LOPEZ JI et al: Combined therapy in a case of malignant mesothelioma of the tunica vaginalis testis. Scand J Urol Nephrol 29:361, 1995.

306. TJANDRA BS et al: Papillary mesothelioma of the albuginea testis. Urology 43:118, 1994.

307. DERVAN PA et al: Solitary (localized) fibrous mesothelioma: Evidence against mesothelial cell. Histopathology 10:867, 1986.

308. GOLDBLUM J, HART WR: Localized and diffuse mesotheliomas of the genital tract and peritoneum in women: A clinicopathologic study of nineteen true mesothelial neoplasms, other than adenomatoid tumors, multicystic mesotheliomas, and localized fibrous tumors. Am J Surg Pathol 19:1124, 1995.

309. BRISELLI M et al: Solitary fibrous tumors of the pleura: Eight new cases and review of 360 cases in the literature. Cancer 47:2678, 1981.

310. DALTON WT et al: Localized primary tumors of the pleura: An analysis of 40 cases. Cancer 44:1465, 1979.

311. SHABANAH FH, SAYEGH SF: Solitary (localized) pleural mesothelioma: Report of two cases and review of the literature. Chest 60:558, 1971.

312. OKIKE N et al: Localized mesothelioma of the pleura: Benign and malignant variants. J Thorac Cardiovasc Surg 75:363, 1978.

313. HAMMAR SP: The pathology of benign and malignant pleural disease. Chest Surg Clin North Am 4:405, 1994.

314. WANEBO HJ et al: Pleural mesothelioma. Cancer 38:2481, 1976.

315. POLLACK CV JR, JORDEN RC: Benign cystic mesothelioma presenting as acute abdominal pain in a young woman. J Emerg Med 9:21, 1991.

316. HARRIS GN et al: Benign fibrous mesothelioma of the pleura: MR imaging findings. AJR 165:1143, 1995.

317. KAMPSCHOER PH et al: Benign abdominal multicystic mesothelioma. Acta Obstet Gynecol Scand 71:555, 1992.

318. OBERS VJ et al: Primary malignant pleural tumors (mesotheliomas) presenting as localized masses: Fine needle aspiration cytologic findings, clinical and radiologic features and review of the literature. Acta Cytol 32:567, 1988.

319. GOURTSOYIANNIS N et al: Solitary malignant mesothelioma of the small intestine: Radiological appearances. Abdom Imaging 21:258, 1996.

320. CROTTY TB et al: Localized malignant mesothelioma: A clinicopathologic and flow cytometric study. Am J Surg Pathol 18:357, 1994.

# CHAPTER 23

# SURGICAL ONCOLOGY IN THE MANAGEMENT OF LYMPHOMAS

*Omaida C. Velazquez and Linda S. Callans*

## INTRODUCTION

Lymphomas are tumors of the immune system and include Hodgkin's disease and non-Hodgkin's lymphoma. Non-Hodgkin's lymphomas are mainly derived from lymphocytes (lymphocytic lymphoma), but there are variants, and very rarely tumors arise from histiocytes. Lymphomas occur within lymph nodes or in the lymphoid tissue of specific organs such as the gastrointestinal tract, thyroid, breast, pancreas, lung, or skin (Table 23-1). About 90% of cases of Hodgkin's disease arise in lymph nodes, whereas only 10% have an extranodal origin. Extranodal involvement is more common in non-Hodgkin's lymphomas, with up to 35% arising in an extranodal site and approximately 65% originating within lymph nodes.

The surgeon's role in the management of lymphomas is manifold. For example, surgeons perform lymph node biopsy to establish the diagnosis, assist in the precise staging of the disease, obtain adequate long-term venous access for systemic chemotherapy, and treat complications that occur either during the original presentation of the disease or as a consequence of the treatment. The surgeon may play a more central role for lymphomas that are confined to a single extranodal organ. Although attempted curative surgery has traditionally been the therapy of choice for gastric and other localized gastrointestinal lymphomas, the role of surgery as the primary mode of therapy has become and remains somewhat controversial.

This chapter will present a broad overview of the various types of lymphoma and review the epidemiology, clinical presentation, diagnosis, etiology, histopathology, and staging of lymphoma. Most importantly, this chapter will discuss the role of surgery in the management of lymphomas with a focus on gastrointestinal lymphomas.

## SYSTEMIC LYMPHOMA

### HODGKIN'S DISEASE

**CLINICAL PRESENTATION.** Hodgkin's disease is relatively rare, with a slight male preponderance and a bimodal age distribution curve. This age curve peaks in the late 20s, declines by the mid-40s and increases again after age 45. Most patients with Hodgkin's disease present with asymptomatic lymphadenopathy in the cervical area (Table 23-2). Physical examination can identify other sites of peripheral adenopathy as well as the presence of hepatosplenomegaly. Laboratory evaluation should include routine hematology studies and liver function tests, and bone marrow evaluation should be performed. CT scans of the chest, abdomen, and pelvis are essential for staging and some advocate lymphangiography to further assess retroperitoneal lymph nodes. Constitutional or "B" symptoms such as fever, night sweats, and weight loss indicate widespread disease and unfavorable prognosis.

**DIAGNOSIS.** The diagnosis of Hodgkin's disease is usually established by lymph node biopsy. The largest and most centrally placed lymph node should be selected for excision. When a matted

## TABLE 23-1. SITES OF EXTRANODAL LYMPHOMA

|  | % NON-HODGKIN'S LYMPHOMAS |
| --- | --- |
| Gastrointestinal tract (100%) | 5 |
|   Stomach (50–60%) |  |
|   Small bowel (30%) |  |
|   Colon (6%) |  |
|   Esophagus (1%) |  |
| Waldeyer's ring | Unavailable |
| Skin | Unavailable |
| Thyroid | 2–3 |
| CNS | <2 |
| Pancreas | 1–2 |
| Breast | 1 |
| Lung | <1 |
| Spleen only | <1 |

cluster of nodes is present, either a central node from the group should be excised or a generous incisional biopsy should be performed. Lymph nodes from the lower cervical or axillary regions provide the best results for histologic examination since lymph nodes from other areas such as inguinal, parotid, or submandibular regions often show changes from previous inflammatory processes. If only mediastinal or paraaortic nodes are present, tissue can be obtained via mediastinoscopy, video thoracoscopy, or thoracotomy; less commonly, laparoscopy or laparotomy may be required, depending on the location of the nodal disease. Excised lymph nodes should be sent fresh to pathology for appropriate workup when lymphoma is suspected, since antibodies used for subtyping require fresh cell preparations or frozen sections.

Histologically, Hodgkin's disease is characterized by the presence of Reed-Sternberg multinucleated giant cells. Different histologic subtypes of Hodgkin's disease can be seen (Table 23-3) and these have been associated with varied prognoses. It is now questioned whether the lymphocyte predominance (nodular) type is a true form of Hodgkin's disease since its course is so indolent. In general, prognosis worsens from the classic lymphocyte predominance (diffuse) type to the lymphocyte depletion form of Hodgkin's disease, as listed in Table 23-3, although overall stage of disease is a more important prognostic factor than histologic subtype.

STAGING. Although laparotomy is seldom required for obtaining tissue diagnosis, staging laparotomy is indicated for selected patients with Hodgkin's disease since treatment and prognosis are determined by the stage of disease.[1] Hodgkin's disease tends to

## TABLE 23-2. LOCATION OF PALPABLE LYMPH NODES IN PATIENTS WITH HODGKIN'S DISEASE

| LYMPH NODE BASIN | PATIENTS, % |
| --- | --- |
| Cervical | 65–80 |
| Axillary | 10–15 |
| Inguinal | 6–12 |

## TABLE 23-3. HISTOLOGIC SUBTYPES OF HODGKIN'S DISEASE

- Lymphocyte predominance, nodular
- Lymphocyte predominance, diffuse (or lymphocyte-rich classic disease)
- Nodular sclerosis
- Mixed cellularity
- Lymphocyte depletion

metastasize initially in a predictable, nonrandom pattern via lymphatic channels to contiguous lymph node groups and organs. This predictable mode of spread provides the rationale for staging laparotomy and the basis for radiation treatment to adjacent lymph node areas in patients with apparently localized disease.

Stage is related to the anatomic distribution of disease and the presence or absence of constitutional symptoms as reflected in the Ann Arbor Classification outlined in Table 23-4. Clinically, stage is determined by history, physical exam, initial diagnostic biopsy, and imaging studies. Pathologic stage is more accurate and includes histologic data from the liver, spleen, retroperitoneal and intraabdominal lymph nodes, and bone marrow aspirate and biopsy. Assignment of stage using clinical criteria alone is frequently inaccurate, with a 20% to 25% rate of upstaging and a 10% to 15% downstaging following laparotomy, with a total alteration in stage after laparotomy of 30% to 40%.[1]

Staging laparotomy is not applicable to all patients with Hodgkin's disease and is performed only when results may change treatment plans. Patients with B symptoms, felt to have disseminated disease, and those with advanced stage disease (IIIB, IV) are treated with combination chemotherapy and do not benefit from staging laparotomy. Staging laparotomy, however, is indicated for patients with low-clinical-stage Hodgkin's disease (IA, IIA, IIIA) in whom the results may have a major influence on therapeutic management. Staging laparotomy involves a systematic exploration of the abdomen including splenectomy, core and wedge liver biopsies,

## TABLE 23-4. STAGING OF LYMPHOMA (ANN ARBOR CLASSIFICATION)

- Stage I     Single lymph node chain
  - IE   Single extranodal site or organ
- Stage II   ≥2 lymph node chains, same side of diaphragm
  - IIE  Localized extranodal involvement
- Stage III  Nodal involvement both sides of diaphragm
  - IIIE  With extranodal site or organ
  - IIIS  Splenic disease
- Stage IV  Diffuse disease with multiple extranodal sites or a single extranodal site with distant nodal involvement

Designation for constitutional symptoms:
- A  No symptoms
- B  Fever, night sweats, weight loss (>10% in 6 months)

and selective excision of abdominal and retroperitoneal lymph nodes based on CT, lymphangiography, and intraoperative findings. Staging laparoscopy is an attractive alternative to formal laparotomy for surgeons facile with laparoscopy, but is unproven as an effective staging procedure and has not gained wide acceptance. Oophoropexy is advised in the premenopausal woman in whom radiation therapy to the pelvic nodes is likely to be part of the treatment. Ancillary procedures like appendectomy or cholecystectomy are not recommended. Staging laparotomy carries an operative mortality rate of less than 0.5% and a low morbidity that includes wound infection, pneumonia, subphrenic abscess (1%), and early postoperative small bowel obstruction (1% to 2%). However, the risk of developing postsplenectomy sepsis in patients with Hodgkin's disease is significant, and pneumococcal vaccine should be given to all patients preoperatively. The meningococcal vaccine should be considered in young patients at risk.

**TREATMENT.** The information from pathology obtained at staging laparotomy guides treatment recommendations for either radiation alone (stages IA and IIA) or radiation plus chemotherapy (Stage IIIA). For stages IA and IIA, treatment with radiation only results in 91% and 82% survival respectively, with no advantage being shown with the addition of chemotherapy. For stage IIIA, however, the addition of chemotherapy to radiation improves survival from 65% to 92%.

## NON-HODGKIN'S LYMPHOMA

Non-Hodgkin's lymphomas (NHLs) represent a diverse group of malignancies of the lymphoreticular tissue, and various classification schemes have been employed, including the Kiel, Lukes-Collins, and Rappaport systems (Table 23-5).[2] The National Cancer Institute attempted to simplify these classification schemes in 1982 when it developed a Working Formulation of Non-Hodgkin's Lymphoma for clinical usage. Table 23-5 lists the various types of NHL in the working formulation and compares the various classification schemes.

**CLINICAL PRESENTATION.** NHL has a more variable clinical course and natural history than Hodgkin's disease. The median age at presentation for patients with NHL is 50 years, and there is no gender predilection. Unlike Hodgkin's disease, only two-thirds of patients with NHL are initially asymptomatic. Patients with NHL commonly present with peripheral adenopathy, hepatomegaly, splenomegaly, abdominal mass, and mediastinal adenopathy. NHL occurs in extranodal sites in 20% to 35% of patients. Constitutional (B) symptoms are common at presentation and NHL is often disseminated at the time of diagnosis. The pattern of spread is unpredictable, with disease spreading to distant nodal and extranodal sites through the bloodstream. Consequently, more patients are found to have leukemic features than in the setting of Hodgkin's disease.

**DIAGNOSIS.** The pathologic classifications of NHL are based on light and electron microscopic morphology, immunohistochemical studies, and selected cell surface antigen markers. With the refinements in flow cytometry techniques, lymphoma can sometimes be diagnosed and subtyped using fine-needle aspiration cytology, but surgical excisional biopsy of an involved lymph node remains the gold standard for diagnosis. It is of paramount importance that the pathologist obtain fresh tissue for evaluation of possible lymphoma. Most antibodies used to stain the cell surface markers are only biologically functional against proteins in their native configuration, requiring either fresh cells in suspension or frozen tissue preparations; they cannot be used on paraffin sections.

The different types of lymphomas are distinguished by immunohistochemistry and/or flow cytometry using a panel of monoclonal antibodies to determine the cell line of origin (e.g., B- or T-cell lymphoma; see Table 23-6).[3] Other commonly used molecular biology studies include Southern blot analysis that can distinguish poorly differentiated carcinoma from lymphoma and confirm the subtype of lymphoma by determining clonality and identifying chromosomal rearrangements and amplifications. Various histologic subtypes of lymphoma have been associated with chromosomal rearrangements, some of which involve a cellular protooncogene at, or near, the chromosomal breakpoint (Table 23-7).

**STAGING AND TREATMENT.** Most NHLs are monoclonal B-cell lymphomas. Patients under the age of 35 and over 65 years of age have a higher incidence of diffuse and, therefore, unfavorable histology. Similar to Hodgkin's disease, therapy options are based not only on the histopathologic type but also on the stage as outlined in Table 23-4. Treatment consists primarily of combination chemotherapy with radiation if the disease is localized. Since most NHL are disseminated at the time of presentation, staging laparotomy is seldom required. However, there may be selected rare individuals that present with limited disease in whom staging laparotomy may influence the selection of therapy. Occasional patients with NHL and symptomatic splenomegaly with physiologic hypersplenism may benefit from splenectomy.

## PRIMARY GASTROINTESTINAL LYMPHOMAS

### INTRODUCTION

Although the gastrointestinal (GI) tract is the most common site of extranodal lymphomas, GI lymphomas are uncommon, representing 5% of all NHLs and less than 5% of all primary GI malignancies. They are localized in the stomach in 50% to 60% of patients, in the jejunum and ileum in about 30%, and in the large intestine in about 6% (see Table 23-1).

About 80% of primary GI lymphomas are of B-cell origin, almost all of which are of the non-Hodgkin's variety. Since the classification schemes for GI lymphomas were traditionally adapted from those for nodal lymphomas (see Table 23-5)[2] and several different schemes have been used, controversy exists regarding the influence of histologic type on prognosis, the preferred treatment, and overall outcome in response to different therapy. Furthermore, a significant proportion of GI lymphomas follow a different clinical course from their nodal counterparts despite a similar histology. Thus, Isaacson[4,5] developed a new concept of GI lymphomas based on the observation that the histology of low-grade B-cell GI lymphomas

**TABLE 23-5.** COMPARISON OF CLASSIFICATION SCHEMES FOR NHL

| WORKING FORMULATION | KIEL | LUKES-COLLINS | RAPPAPORT |
|---|---|---|---|
| **LOW GRADE** | | | |
| A. Malignant lymphoma, small lymphocytic (SL) | Lymphocytic, CLL lymphoplasmacytic/ lymphoplasmacytoid | Small lymphocytic and plasmacytoid lymphocytic | Lymphocytic, well-differentiated |
| B. Malignant lymphoma, follicular, predominantly small cleaved and large cell (FSC) | Centroblastic-centrocytic (small), follicular | Small cleaved FCC, follicular or follicular and diffuse | Nodular, poorly differentiated lymphocytic |
| C. Malignant lymphoma, follicular, mixed small cleaved and large cell (FM) | Centroblastic-centrocytic (small), follicular | Small cleaved FCC, follicular large cleaved FCC, follicular | Nodular, mixed lymphocytic-histiocytic |
| **INTERMEDIATE GRADE** | | | |
| D. Malignant lymphoma, follicular, predominantly large cell (FL) | Centroblastic-centrocytic (large), follicular | Large cleaved and/or noncleaved FCC, follicular | Nodular histiocytic |
| E. Malignant melanoma, diffuse small cleaved cell (DSC) | Centrocytic, small | Small cleaved FCC, diffuse | Diffuse lymphocytic, poorly differentiated |
| F. Malignant lymphoma, diffuse, mixed small and large cell (DM) | Centroblastic-centrocytic, diffuse; lymphoplasma-cytoid, polymorphic diffuse | Small cleaved, large cleaved, or large noncleaved FCC | Diffuse mixed lymphocytic-histiocytic |
| G. Malignant lymphoma, diffuse, large cell (DL) | Centroblastic-centrocytic, (large), diffuse; centrocytic (large); centroblastic, diffuse | Large cleaved or noncleaved FCC (diffuse) | Diffuse histiocytic |
| **HIGH-GRADE** | | | |
| H. Malignant lymphoma, large cell, immunoblastic (IBL) | Immunoblastic and T-zone lymphoma | Immunoblastic sarcoma, T- or B-cell type | Diffuse histiocytic |
| I. Malignant lymphoma, lymphoblastic (LBL) | Lymphoblastic convoluted, or unclassified | Convoluted T-cell | Lymphoblastic convoluted/ nonconvoluted |
| J. Malignant lymphoma, small noncleaved cell (SNC) | Lymphoblastic, Burkitt's type and other B-lymphoblastic | Small noncleaved FCC | Undifferentiated, Burkitt's and non-Burkitt's |
| **MISCELLANEOUS** | | | |
| Composite | Extramedullary plasmacytoma | | |
| Mycosis fungoides | Unclassifiable | | |
| Histiocytic | Other | | |

SOURCE: From Parikh AA et al: Gastric lymphoma, in *Management of Upper Gastrointestinal Cancer*, JM Daly et al (eds). Philadelphia, WB Saunders, 1999, p 162.

was similar to that of mucosa-associated lymphoid tissue (MALT), and closely simulated that of the Peyer's patches rather than lymph nodes (Table 23-8).[2] Approximately 40% of gastric lymphomas and 20% of intestinal lymphomas are of the MALT type.

Various studies have shown stage of disease and whether the patient underwent curative surgical resection to be important and independent variables impacting the survival of patients with primary GI lymphomas. In general, low tumor burden suggested by localized tumor mass less than 10 cm, normal serum lactose de-

hydrogenase (LDH) and $\beta_2$-microglobulin levels predict a better response to treatment and a better outcome. Aneuploidy and elevated p53 protein expression are associated with significantly reduced survival, whereas tumor size, grade, and S-phase fraction are not independent prognostic factors.

The preferred treatment for early-stage GI lymphomas continues to be controversial. Some authors advocate an aggressive surgical approach, whereas others recommend primary chemotherapy plus radiotherapy, especially for the treatment of gastric lymphoma. The

## TABLE 23-6. SELECTED MONOCLONAL ANTIBODIES OF INTEREST IN THE STUDY OF LYMPHOID NEOPLASIA

| ANTIGEN CD | ANTIBODIES, COMMON NAME | SPECTRUM OF REACTIVITY |
|---|---|---|
| CD1 | T6, Leu6 | Thymocyte/Langerhans |
| CD2 | T11, Leu5 | Pan T |
| CD3 | T3, Leu4, polyclonal anti-CD3* | Pan T |
| CD4 | T4, Leu3 | T "helper" (MHC II) |
| CD5 | OKT1, Leu1 | Pan T, B subset |
| CD6 | T12, TU33 | Pan T, B subset |
| CD7 | Leu9, TU14, 3A1 | Pan T, early B, early myeloid |
| CD8 | T8, OKT8, Leu2 | T suppressor (MHC I-reactive) |
| CD9 | J2, BA2 | T, B, myeloid |
| CD10 | CALLA, J5 | Pre-B, pre-T, GC |
| CD13 | MY7 | Myeloid, monocyte |
| CD14 | MY4 | Monocyte |
| CD15 | Leu-M1* | Myeloid, monocyte |
| CD19 | B4 | Pan B (not plasma cell) |
| CD20 | B1, L 26* | Pan B (not B-precursor, plasma cell) |
| CD21 | B2 | MZ and GC-B, FDC |
| CD22 | Leu14 | Pan B |
| CD23 | Blast 2 | MZ and GC-B, FDC |
| CD25 | TAC; IL2 receptor | Activated T, B |
| CD30 | Ki-1, Ber H2* | Activated T, B |
| CD33 | MY9 | Myeloid |
| CD43 | Leu 22 (L60)*, MT1* | Pan T, B subset, monocyte |
| CD45 | LCA* | Pan-leukocyte |
| CD45RO | UCHL 1* | Subset T, rare B, monocytes |
| CD45RA | MB1*, 4KB5* | Pan B, rare T |
| Leu 8 | Human Mel 14 analogue | Homing receptor; subset T, subset B |
| | bF1* | T-cell receptor |
| | Tdt | B + T precursors, cortical thymocyte |
| | HLA-DR (MHC class II) | B cells, activated T cells |

*Can be used on paraffin sections.
ABBREVIATIONS: CALLA = common acute lymphoblastic leukemia antigen, CD = cluster designation, FDC = follicular dendritic cells, GC = germinal center, IL2 = interleukin-2, LCA = leukocyte common antigen, MHC = major histocompatibility complex, MZ = mantle zone, PB = peripheral blood, PC = plasma cell, RS = Reed-Sternberg, Tdt = terminal deoxynucleotidyl transferase.
SOURCE: Harris NL: The pathology of lymphomas: A practical approach to diagnosis and classification. Surg Oncol Clin North Am 2:171, 1993.

## TABLE 23-7. CHROMOSOMAL AND ONCOGENE CHANGES IN LYMPHOMA

| HISTOLOGIC SUBTYPE OF LYMPHOMA | CHROMOSOMAL REARRANGEMENT | INVOLVED ONCOGENE |
|---|---|---|
| Burkitt's lymphoma (90%) | t(8;14)(q24;q32) | myc |
| | or t(8;22)(q24;q11) | myc |
| | or t(2;9)(p11;q24) | myc |
| Follicular lymphomas (80–85%) and some GI lymphomas | t(14;18)(q32;q21) | bcl-2 |
| Diffuse intermediately differentiated lymphomas (50%) | t(11;14)(q13;q32) | bcl-1 |
| Diffuse large cell lymphoma | t(3;22)(q27;q11) | |
| Ki-1 + anaplastic large cell lymphoma | t(2;5)(p23;p35) | |

following sections will focus on the clinical presentation, diagnosis and staging, etiology, treatment and outcome of the different sites of primary GI lymphomas.

## PRIMARY GASTRIC LYMPHOMA

The stomach is the site of over 50% of all GI lymphomas and represents the most common organ involved in extranodal lymphoma (see Table 23-1). Lymphoma constitutes an increasing proportion of all gastric neoplasms, accounting for approximately 5% of all

## TABLE 23-8. A CLASSIFICATION SCHEME OF PRIMARY GASTROINTESTINAL LYMPHOMAS

- B cell (80%)
    MALT type
    Low grade
    High grade (with or without a low-grade component)
  Immunoproliferative small-intestinal disease (IPSID)
    Low grade
    High grade (with or without a low-grade component)
  Mantle cell or malignant lymphoma centrocytic (lymphomatous polyposis)
  Burkitt-like
  Other (types that correspond to peripheral lymph node variants)
- T cell (20%)
    Enteropathy-associated T-cell lymphoma (EATL)
    Other types unassociated with enteropathy

SOURCE: Adapted from Parikh AA et al: Gastric lymphoma, in *Management of Upper Gastrointestinal Cancer*, JM Daly et al (eds). Philadelphia, WB Saunders, 1999, p 163.

**TABLE 23-9.** SIGNS AND SYMPTOMS
OF GASTRIC LYMPHOMA

| SYMPTOM/SIGN | FREQUENCY, % |
|---|---|
| Epigastric pain | 70–80 |
| Weight loss | 35–55 |
| Nausea, vomiting | 20–40 |
| Anorexia | 10–40 |
| Mass | 20–25 |
| Bleeding | 20–25 |
| Perforation | 1–2 |

malignant gastric tumors. The diagnosis of primary gastric lymphoma is made when initial symptoms are gastric in origin and when the stomach is found to be either exclusively or predominantly involved with the tumor.

CLINICAL PRESENTATION. Gastric lymphoma is uncommon in children and young adults, with the peak incidence in the sixth and seventh decades. Symptoms are strikingly similar and difficult to differentiate from gastric adenocarcinoma (Table 23-9).[2] The most common presenting symptoms include epigastric pain, weight loss, nausea, and vomiting. Although occult bleeding and anemia are observed in more than half of the patients, gross bleeding is an unusual presentation.

DIAGNOSIS AND STAGING. The study of choice to establish the diagnosis of gastric lymphoma is upper endoscopy with biopsy. Occasionally endoscopic biopsy may be nondiagnostic due to the submucosal growth pattern of lymphoma without ulceration of the overlying mucosa, and full-thickness wedge biopsy may be required. Evaluation should include physical examination and CT scans of the chest, abdomen, and pelvis in search of distant lymphadenopathy and other extranodal sites of disease. Other diagnostic modalities might include lymphangiography, bone marrow biopsy, and biopsy of any enlarged peripheral lymph node. Endoscopic ultrasonography may be useful in detecting regional lymphadenopathy and determining when tumors involve the full thickness of the gastric wall. Staging is based on preoperative studies, intraoperative findings, and pathologic examination. Most authors use a modification of the Ann Arbor staging system for gastric lymphoma depicted in Table 23-10.

**TABLE 23-10.** MODIFIED ANN ARBOR STAGING
SYSTEM FOR GASTRIC LYMPHOMA

| |  | | |
|---|---|---|---|
| • | Stage | IE | Disease confined to the stomach |
| • | Stage | IIE1 | Stomach with perigastric node involvement |
| | | IIE2 | Stomach with regional nonadjacent node involvement |
| • | Stage | IIIE | Nodal involvement both sides of diaphragm, or other localized extralymphatic ± splenic disease |
| • | Stage | IV | Diffuse disease |

**TABLE 23-11.** STAGING SYSTEM FOR PRIMARY
GASTRIC LYMPHOMA ACCORDING TO THE TNM
SYSTEM

T—Primary tumor
| | |
|---|---|
| T1: | Lymphoma confined to the mucosa |
| T2: | Involving the mucosa, submucosa, muscularis propria and extending into but not through the serosa |
| T3: | Penetrating through the serosa with or without involving contiguous structures |
| TX: | Degree of penetration undetermined |

N—Regional lymph nodes
| | |
|---|---|
| N0: | No involvement of nodes |
| N1: | Involvement of perigastric nodes |
| NX: | Nodal involvement undetermined |

M—Distant metastasis
| | |
|---|---|
| M0: | No distant metastasis |
| M1: | Evidence of distant metastasis including nodes beyond the regional area |

| | |
|---|---|
| Stage 1: | No involvement of regional lymph nodes or distant metastasis |
| A: | T1, N-, M0 |
| B: | T2, N0, M0 |
| C: | T3, N0, M0 |
| Stage 2–3: | No involvement of regional lymph nodes T1–3, N1, M0 |
| Stage 4: | Metastatic disease T1–3, N0–1, M1 |

SOURCE: Parikh AA et al: Gastric lymphoma, in *Management of Upper Gastrointestinal Cancer*, JM Daly et al (eds). Philadelphia, WB Saunders, 1999, p 171.

Some authors, however, prefer to use the tumor-node-metastasis (TNM) staging system (Table 23-11).[2]

ETIOLOGY. The etiology is still unknown, but many gastric lymphomas are now thought to arise from MALT that accumulates in the submucosa secondary to chronic inflammation. Evidence suggests that chronic inflammation caused by exogenous agents or antigens results in the pathologic stimulation of lymphoid tissue. *Helicobacter pylori* has been identified in the majority of patients with gastric lymphoma and treatment of *H. pylori* infection results in regression of cases of low-grade gastric lymphomas (MALToma).[6–10] In a subset of gastric MALTomas, homozygous p16 deletions are acquired and may contribute to the transformation from a low-grade to a high-grade malignancy.[11] As in many nodal lymphomas, the chromosomal translocation [t(14:18)] placing the *bcl*-2 protooncogene adjacent to the immunoglobulin heavy chain locus (see Table 23-7) has been identified in some GI lymphomas[12] and variations in *bcl*-2 and p53 expression may correlate with progression from low- to high-grade lesions.

TREATMENT AND OUTCOME. As a result of the data regarding *H. pylori* infection and gastric lymphomas, some authors

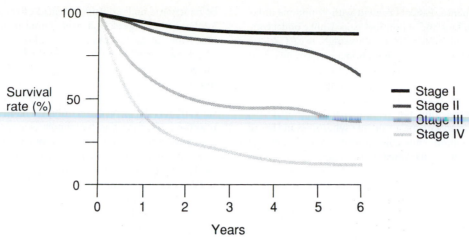

**FIGURE 23-1.** Survival of gastric lymphoma by stage. (*From* Surgery: Scientific Principles and Practice, *LJ Greenfield et al* (eds). *Philadelphia, Lippincott-Raven, 1997, p 803.*)

advocate that antibiotics become the first line of therapy for low-grade gastric MALToma, which has a particularly indolent course. It must be remembered, however, that only low-grade MALTomas have consistently responded to antibiotic therapy, and antibiotics should be considered a part of an armamentarium of treatment in addition to the more traditional modalities such as surgery, radiation, and chemotherapy.

Most centers advocate a multimodality approach to the treatment of primary gastric lymphomas. Gastric resection has traditionally been considered the first step in the therapeutic strategy, since gastrectomy provided more accurate histology and staging, provided cure in cases of localized tumor, and eliminated the risk of life-threatening complications of systemic treatment such as hemorrhage or perforation. Overall 5-year survival rate following surgical resection for early-stage gastric lymphoma ranges from 33% to 84%, with higher cure rates achieved for localized (stage IE and IIE1) disease. Many retrospective studies have shown a significant improvement in 5-year survival rate with curative resection (60% to 75%) compared with noncurative resection (30% to 35%), even when postoperative radiation and chemotherapy are added to palliative surgery.[13–18] Although all gross disease should be resected, extended resection (to include distal esophagectomy, for example) is generally not indicated, and postoperative radiation is effective if margins are microscopically involved. The abdomen can also be explored for nonregional disease at the time of surgery and disseminated disease documented by biopsy if identified.

More recently there has been a trend toward primary radiation and chemotherapy based on the radiosensitivity of the tumor, a better understanding of MALT in the pathogenesis of the disease, and an appreciation of the morbidity associated with gastric resection and postgastrectomy syndromes. Studies comparing surgery with primary radiation have shown similar results, and there are data suggesting that primary radiation can achieve cure rates as high as 85% for stage IE disease.[19–23] Moreover, the complication rates associated with cytolytic therapy are probably not as high as once believed. A broad range of perforation rate has been reported in

the literature ranging from 4% to 43%. The perforation rate, however, probably more closely approximates 5% in most patients with primary gastric lymphomas treated with cytolytic agents alone, although the risk may well be higher for tumors involving the full thickness of the gastric wall.

Survival for gastric lymphoma is closely related to the stage of the disease at the time of diagnosis (Fig. 23-1). In a limited number of cases (stage IE), surgery may be curative without the need for further therapy. Patients with stage IIE disease, however, benefit from postoperative radiation to the gastrectomy bed to improve local and regional control. In addition, these patients have a greater than 30% chance of recurrence outside the treatment field after undergoing attempted curative resection, and most studies show improvement in survival when systemic chemotherapy is given in addition to surgery or primary radiotherapy.[24] Overall 5-year survival rates for primary gastric lymphomas range from 50% to 70%. Patients with early-stage gastric lymphoma (IE and IIE) have survival rates in excess of 70%, whereas those with advanced disease (stage IIIE and IVE) have overall 5-year survival rates of about 20%.

## PRIMARY SMALL-BOWEL LYMPHOMA

Small-bowel lymphomas arise from the lymphoid tissue within the wall of the small intestine and, therefore, predominantly involve the ileum, which has the greatest concentration of gut lymphoid tissue in the Peyer's patches. Almost all of the primary small-bowel lymphomas are non-Hodgkin, B-cell lymphomas, although rare cases of T-cell lymphomas occur either sporadically or as a complication of celiac disease. Most small-intestinal lymphomas are of intermediate to high grade and show large cell or immunoblastic features with a diffuse, rather than nodular, growth pattern.

**CLINICAL PRESENTATION.** Small-intestinal lymphomas occur most frequently during the fifth or sixth decade and have a slight male predominance. Patients present with symptoms of fatigue, malaise, weight loss, and abdominal pain. Unlike nodal lymphomas, constitutional symptoms of fever and night sweats are rare and suggest either diffuse intestinal lymphoma or a complication of the lymphoma such as perforation. Approximately one-third of undiagnosed patients present with an acute complication, including perforation, obstruction, intussusception, or hemorrhage that requires operative intervention. On the other hand, intestinal lymphomas may be associated with malabsorptive syndromes and have a more insidious presentation. Thus, clinical deterioration in a patient with previously controlled celiac disease may suggest the diagnosis of lymphoma.

DIAGNOSIS. The physical exam is generally not specific, although later in the disease many patients may have a palpable abdominal mass. In early disease, the diagnosis is usually first suspected by noting either submucosal nodules, mucosal ulcerations, or diffuse thickened mucosal folds on GI contrast studies.[25] These tumors are multifocal in 15% of patients. Abdominal CT scan can show diffuse thickening of the bowel wall or abdominal mass as well as retroperitoneal lymph node enlargement. Chest CT scans and bone marrow evaluation are important for staging the disease. Laparotomy with a small-bowel biopsy may be indicated to establish the diagnosis of lymphoma and resection of limited disease should be considered as discussed below.

ETIOLOGY. Many medical conditions have been associated with an increased risk of intestinal lymphoma, including celiac sprue; Crohn's disease; dermatitis; rheumatoid arthritis; Wegener's granulomatosis; systemic lupus erythematosus; and immunodeficiency syndromes such as AIDS, X-linked agammaglobulinemia and Wiscott-Aldrich syndrome. There is also an increased incidence seen in patients with states of prolonged or profound immunosuppression such as with transplantation or chemotherapy. An infectious etiology is also suspected in the immunoproliferative disease of the small intestine (IPSID, also known as Mediterranean lymphoma) and other primary GI lymphomas. *Giardia lamblia* is frequently identified in patients with IPSID, and Epstein-Barr-virus (EBV) has been implicated in other settings. Enteropathy-associated T-cell lymphomas may be disorders of an abnormal response to gluten, and a gluten-free diet can markedly reduce the risk for lymphoma in patients with celiac sprue.

TREATMENT AND OUTCOME. Most patients require surgery. As mentioned, about one-third of patients present in the acute setting with obstruction or perforation and require urgent intervention. Other goals of surgical intervention include establishing the diagnosis, staging, and resection for cure in the setting of localized disease. Although the series are small and the studies are retrospective, the available data support the role of curative surgical resection for small-bowel lymphoma, showing improved survival over biopsy or palliative resection followed by adjuvant chemoradiation. Many authors also advocate a role for debulking to minimize the incidence of treatment complications and decrease tumor burden to be treated, thereby enhancing response and outcome, but there are little data to support this approach either way. Intraoperative staging should include a liver biopsy and biopsy of periaortic or mesenteric nodes outside the field of resection. If the tumor is localized, the surgical treatment should involve resection with en bloc lymphadenectomy to allow histologic assessment of nodes for lymphoma involvement. Clips should be placed as radiomarkers for postoperative radiotherapy, especially if there is gross residual disease or suspicion of positive surgical margins.

Most centers advise adjuvant chemotherapy for patients with stage IE and IIE primary small-bowel lymphoma after "curative" resection, assuming that lymphoma is a systemic disease that requires systemic therapy. A regimen of combination chemotherapy with radiotherapy is usually advised for patients that undergo surgical debulking only, or those with diffuse advanced disease (stage IIIE or IVE), and may significantly affect survival depending on the type of lymphoma. Patients with primary small- and large-bowel lymphomas frequently present with advanced disease at diagnosis and their prognosis is generally worse than similar patients with gastric lymphoma. As a group, patients with small-bowel lymphomas do poorly, with 5-year survival rates ranging from 20% to 40%. Those with extensive intraabdominal or disseminated disease rarely survive 1 year after diagnosis. On the other hand, patients with limited disease that can be fully resected may have survival rates as high as 80% in some studies.

## IMMUNOPROLIFERATIVE SMALL-INTESTINAL DISEASE

Immunoproliferative small intestinal disease (IPSID), also known as Mediterranean lymphoma, is a variant of primary small-bowel lymphoma, most commonly seen throughout the Mediterranean basin and Middle East and in lower socioeconomic populations in underdeveloped countries. It is characterized by diffuse involvement of the entire small intestine, and therefore is not amenable to surgical treatment. IPSID may have an infectious etiology, since rare cases of resolution with early antibiotic treatment have been reported. Often, *G. lamblia* can be isolated from these individuals. IPSID has also been named α-chain or heavy-chain disease because of the predominance of the α heavy-chain protein in the serum. There is early mucosal infiltration with benign-appearing plasma cells that then progresses to malignant large cell immunoblastic lymphoma with diffuse nodal involvement.

IPSID affects young adults and has a male predominance. Patients present with weight loss, intestinal cramps, diarrhea, steatorrhea, and clubbing of the fingers. Barium studies of the small bowel are abnormal, with a nodular, polypoid pattern seen on the upper GI with small-bowel follow through. Diagnosis can usually be established by endoscopic biopsy of the distal duodenum or proximal jejunum. The clinical course is that of progressive exacerbations and remissions leading to death from malnutrition or progression to disseminated lymphoma. Treatment is with a combination of antibiotics, chemotherapy, and total abdominal radiation but prognosis is dismal.

## PRIMARY LARGE-BOWEL LYMPHOMA

Colorectal lymphomas are rare, accounting for about 6% of GI lymphomas and less than 0.5% of all colorectal malignancies. Both non-Hodgkin's and Hodgkin's lymphomas of the large bowel have been reported. Generally, disease is disseminated at the time of diagnosis, but an occasional patient will have focal disease limited to the colon. Patients typically present with crampy abdominal pain, anorexia, weight loss, melena or frank bleeding, change in bowel habits, and obstruction. The diagnosis is suspected on barium enema that can show a pattern of cobblestoning, mucosal ulcerations, and thickened folds. Colonoscopic biopsy can usually provide tissue for definitive diagnosis though occasionally surgery is required for diagnosis.

Colorectal lymphoma is generally highly responsive to combination chemotherapy and radiation and surgery is not considered a primary mode of therapy. Surgical resection may be considered in rare instances when the clinical evaluation reveals a focal site of disease in the large bowel. However, for most cases of localized low-grade colorectal lymphomas, radiation therapy alone continues to be the first line of therapy and combination chemoradiation is advised for intermediate- and high-grade colorectal lymphomas. Thus, the role of surgery is limited for colorectal lymphomas.

## PRIMARY ESOPHAGEAL LYMPHOMA

The esophagus is the least commonly involved organ of the GI tract, accounting for only 1% of the primary GI lymphomas. Most commonly, the esophagus is involved by lymphoma secondarily due to cervical and mediastinal lymph node invasion or from contiguous spread from gastric lymphoma. The primary form of esophageal lymphoma arises in the esophageal wall itself and is mostly seen in male patients with Hodgkin's disease. Rare cases of primary non-Hodgkin's lymphoma of the esophagus have also been reported. Esophageal lymphoma may be suggested by double-contrast esophagography and the diagnosis established by histology from tissue obtained by endoscopy with biopsy. Since therapy is primary radiation and chemotherapy, it is critical that the correct diagnosis of esophageal lymphoma be established to avoid unnecessary esophagectomy.

## REFERENCES

1. HUANG PP, URIST M: Evaluation of abdominal Hodgkin's disease. Surg Oncol Clin North Am 2:207, 1993.
2. PARIKH AA et al: Gastric lymphoma, in *Management of Upper Gastrointestinal Cancer*, JM Daly et al (eds). Philadelphia, WB Saunders, 1999, pp. 160–180.
3. HARRIS NL: The pathology of lymphomas: A practical approach to diagnosis and classification. Surg Oncol Clin North Am 2:171, 1993.
4. ISAACSON PG et al: Classifying primary gut lymphomas. Lancet 12:1148, 1988.
5. ISAACSON PG, SPENCER J, WRIGHT DH: Recent developments in our understanding of gastric lymphomas. Am J Surg Pathol 20(Suppl 1):S1, 1996.
6. WOTHERSPOON AC et al: Regression of primary low-grade B-cell gastric lymphoma of mucosa-associated lymphoid tissue type after eradication of *Helicobacter pylori*. Lancet 342:575, 1993.
7. BAYERDORFFER E et al: Regression of primary gastric lymphoma of mucosa-associated lymphoid tissue type after cure of *Helicobacter pylori* infection. Lancet 345:1591, 1995.
8. WEBER DM et al: Regression of gastric lymphoma of mucosa-associated lymphoid tissue with antibiotic therapy for *Helicobacter pylori*. Gastroenterology 107:1835, 1994.
9. ROGGERO E et al: Eradication of *Helicobacter pylori* infection in primary low-grade gastric lymphoma of mucosa-associated lymphoid tissue. Ann Intern Med 122:267, 1995.
10. PARSONNET J et al: *Helicobacter pylori* infection and gastric lymphoma. N Engl J Med 330:1267, 1994.
11. NEUMEISTER P et al: Deletions analysis of the p16 tumor suppressor gene in gastrointestinal mucosa-associated lymphoid tissue lymphomas. Gastroenterology 112:1871, 1997.
12. SHEPHARD NA et al: 14:18 translocation in primary intestinal lymphoma: a detection by polymerase chain reaction in routinely processed tissue. Histopathology 18:415, 1991.
13. ROSEN CB et al: Is an aggressive surgical approach to the patient with gastric lymphoma warranted? Ann Surg 205:634, 1987.
14. GOSPODAROWICZ MK et al: Outcome analysis of localized gastrointestinal lymphoma treated with surgery and postoperative irradiation. Int J Radiat Oncol Biol Phys 19:1357, 1990.
15. BOZZETTI F et al: Role of surgery in patients with primary non-Hodgkin's lymphoma of the stomach: An old problem revisited. Br J Surg 80:1101, 1993.
16. LAW MM et al: Role of surgery in the management of primary lymphoma of the gastrointestinal tract. J Surg Oncol 61:199, 1996.
17. LIN KM et al: Advantage of surgery and adjuvant chemotherapy in the treatment of primary gastrointestinal lymphoma. J Surg Oncol 64:237, 1997.
18. DONOHUE JH, HABERMANN TM: The management of gastric lymphoma. Surg Oncol Clin North Am 2:213, 1993.
19. BURGERS JMV et al: Treatment results of primary stage I and II non-Hodgkin's lymphoma of the stomach. Radiother Oncol 11:319, 1988.
20. SCHUTZE WP, HALPERN NB: Gastric lymphoma. Surg Gynecol Obstet 172:33, 1991.
21. BEN YOSEF R, HOPPE RT: Treatment of early-stage gastric lymphoma. J Surg Oncol 57:78, 1994.
22. KOCH P et al: Primary lymphoma of the stomach: Three-year results of a prospective multi-center study. The German Multi-centers Study Group on GI-NHL. Ann Oncol 8(Suppl 1):85, 1997.
23. KOCHER M et al: Radiotherapy for treatment of localized gastrointestinal non-Hodgkin's lymphoma. Radiother Oncol 42:37, 1997.
24. AMER MH, EL-AKKAD S: Gastrointestinal lymphoma in adults: Clinical features and management of 300 cases. Gastroenterology 106:846, 1994.
25. LEVINE MS et al: Non-Hodgkin's lymphoma of the gastrointestinal tract: Radiographic findings. AJR 168:165, 1997.

# CHAPTER 24

# METASTATIC CANCER

## 24A / BRAIN METASTASES

*Rajesh K. Bindal, Ajay K. Bindal, and Raymond Sawaya*

## INTRODUCTION

Brain metastasis is the most common type of intracranial tumor. The annual incidence of brain metastases is estimated at over 100,000.[1] This may be rising with the increasing incidence of cancer, improved survival of patients with metastatic disease, and use of chemotherapy, which does not penetrate the blood-brain barrier.[2] In contrast, the annual incidence of primary brain tumors is estimated at 17,000.[3] Overall, 20% to 25% of patients dying of cancer have brain metastasis at autopsy.[4] The incidence of brain metastasis varies dramatically based on the type of primary tumor. By far, the most common primary tumors in patients with brain metastasis are lung, breast, melanoma, renal cell, and colon cancers, listed in declining order. Brain metastasis from other types of cancer, such as sarcoma,[5] or ovarian,[6] prostate,[7] and bladder carcinoma[8,9] is less common.

Approximately one-third of patients with lung cancer have brain metastases at autopsy.[4,10] This incidence is higher with small cell carcinomas and adenocarcinoma of lung. Lung cancer metastasizes to the brain relatively early in its clinical course, with the median interval from initial diagnosis of cancer to diagnosis of brain metastasis being only 6 months.[11] Between 20% and 30% of patients dying of breast cancer have brain metastases,[12,13] there being a median interval of 2 to 3 years from initial diagnosis to development of brain metastasis.[14,15] This interval is similar to that observed for melanoma; however, half of the patients dying from melanoma have brain metastases.[16] The incidence of brain metastasis with renal cell carcinoma is 10% to 11%,[4,17] whereas that for colon cancer is 6% to 11%.[4,18]

## CLINICAL SIGNS AND SYMPTOMS

Up to two-thirds of all brain metastases are symptomatic at some time during the patient's life.[19,20] Clinical evidence in terms of neuro-logic signs and symptoms is the first indicator of brain metastasis in most patients. The signs and symptoms of metastatic tumors are very similar to signs and symptoms of other expanding intracranial mass lesions.[21,22] These symptoms have two main etiologies—increased intracranial pressure (ICP) and focal irritation or destruction of neurons.

Increased ICP can be caused by direct mass effect of the tumor, by edematous expansion of surrounding white matter, by obstructive hydrocephalus, or, most commonly, by a combination of these effects. Except in pediatric patients, the skull is a rigid container of fixed volume. Therefore, any increase in intracranial volume via edema or expanding tumor mass must be compensated for in some manner. Initially, the volume of blood in vessels and cerebrospinal fluid (CSF) in ventricles and cisterns is reduced, while ICP is kept constant. However, when this compensatory mechanism is exhausted, ICP rises. Cerebellar lesions often increase ICP by compressing the aqueduct of Sylvius and fourth ventricle, resulting in obstructive hydrocephalus. Symptoms of increased ICP include headache, nausea, vomiting, confusion, and lethargy. These signs and symptoms rarely have any localizing value. Increased ICP can also cause herniation of brain tissue into adjacent compartments, damaging both the herniating tissue and the tissue transgressed. This can give rise to false localizing signs as specific areas of the brain distant to the tumor site are affected.

Focal irritation or destruction of surrounding brain tissue can result from direct compression of neurons, effects of peritumoral edema, or hemorrhage. These events often result in focal signs and symptoms that have very important localizing value, including hemiparesis, visual field defects, aphasia, focal seizures, and ataxia.

The most common symptoms are headache, focal weakness, and mental and behavioral disturbances. Symptoms of brain metastases generally follow a gradual onset. However, acute onset may occur and is often precipitated by hemorrhage into the tumor.[23] Chorio-carcinoma and melanoma have the greatest propensity to present as hemorrhagic metastatic lesions. Up to 80% of brain metastases from melanoma have radiographic evidence of hemorrhage, although bleeding is often clinically silent. Macroscopic evidence of hemorrhage is found at autopsy in 60% of metastases from germ cell tumors, 30% of those from melanoma, 5% of those from lung cancer, and in 1% of breast metastases. In three-fourths of these patients, the hemorrhage may be symptomatic. Acute strokelike onset of symptoms can occur in 43% of these patients.[23]

## RADIOGRAPHIC APPEARANCE

Contrast-enhanced magnetic resonance imaging (MRI) is the single best tool for radiographic evaluation of patients with suspected brain metastasis (Fig. 24A-1).[24] It has been proved by numerous studies to be more sensitive and specific than any other imaging technique in determining presence or absence, location, and number of metastases. Both T1- and T2-weighted images play a role in detecting metastases. Multiplicity, marked vasogenic edema, and mass effect are considered the hallmark of brain metastases. Lesions tend to be spheroid and peripherally located. They often appear at the gray-white matter junction and in vascular border zones.[25] On T1 imaging, metastases appear as loci of increased signal intensity. Larger tumors often appear to have peripheral enhancement with a nonenhancing core, representing central necrosis. Peritumoral edema on T1 appears as a region of decreased signal intensity. In T2 images, tumors often have decreased intensity, whereas edema appears with increased intensity. Presence and extent of edema is far better appreciated on T2 than on T1 images. The contrast agent used with MRI is gadolinium diethylenetriaminepentaacetic acid (GA-DTPA). Use of contrast makes MRI imaging more sensitive, and often lesions that are not evident on nonenhanced scans appear with the use of contrast.

## DIFFERENTIAL DIAGNOSIS

In patients with known systemic cancer, the appearance of clinical symptoms and a radiographically evident lesion consistent with brain metastasis is virtually diagnostic. It has been reported that 89% to 93% of patients with a history of cancer who present with a single supratentorial lesion have brain metastasis.[26,27] Patients with multiple lesions are even more likely to have metastatic disease.

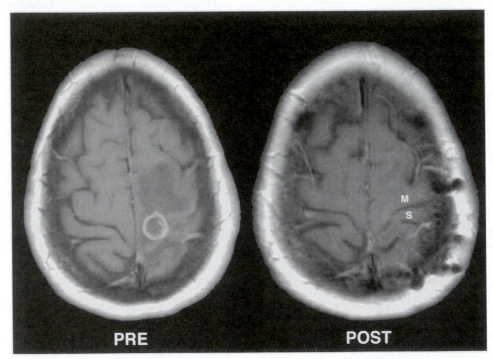

**FIGURE 24A-1.** Preoperative (PRE) and postoperative (POST) T1-weighted MR images with gadolinium contrast enhancement of a single metastatic non–small cell lung carcinoma in the left frontoparietal region with surrounding edema in a patient with severe headaches and weakness in the right foot and leg. The lesion was adjacent to motor (M) and sensory (S) cortices and required transgression of eloquent brain for resection. At the time of discharge on the fifth postoperative day, the patient was ambulating without a walker and had only mild leg weakness, and by the one-month follow-up visit, she was symptom free. (*From Lang FF, Wildrick DM, and Sawaya R. Cancer Control, March/April 1998, with permission.*)

Even so, the physician must always be aware of other disease states that can present in a similar manner, such as a primary brain tumor or a cerebrovascular disorder.

Many patients present with clinical and radiographic signs consistent with brain metastasis but without a previous history of cancer. Such patients with multiple intracranial lesions should be strongly suspected of having metastases. Patients with a single brain lesion and no history of cancer are much less likely to have metastasis, but the possibility must be considered. One study indicated that 15% of such patients had an eventual histologic diagnosis of brain metastasis.[27] Searching for a primary cancer site or for other sites of metastasis is very important. A number of tests should be performed. The patient's medical history and physical exam are extremely important. Chest radiographs, preferably both x-rays and CT scans, must also be performed.[28] These can be used to find lung primaries or metastases, both of which are very common in patients with brain metastasis. Bronchoscopy can be used to confirm diagnosis in these patients. Abdominal CT is useful in visualizing colon or kidney primaries and liver metastases. A stool guaiac test, sputum cytology study, and intravenous pyelogram can also prove helpful. A biopsy is, of course, the very best test for diagnosis.

Patients presenting with brain metastases as the first sign of cancer are found to have lung primaries most of the time. Breast primaries are relatively rare in these patients, probably due to the relative ease of early detection of the primary lesion.

## THERAPEUTIC DECISION MAKING

The major treatment modalities for brain metastases are steroids, whole brain radiation therapy (WBRT), surgery, and radiosurgery. Chemotherapy has not been proved to be of much value except in selected patients with germ cell tumors or small cell lung cancer. Brain metastases are often surrounded by an impressive amount of vasogenic edema relative to the size of the lesion, which results in increased mass effect. Steroids serve to reduce this edema, thereby reducing associated symptoms. In older series, median survival in untreated patients was 1 month and was increased to 2 months by treating patients with steroids alone.[29,30]

### WHOLE BRAIN RADIATION THERAPY

A large percentage of patients with brain metastasis have widespread, uncontrolled systemic cancer. In these patients brain metastasis is not likely to be a substantial survival-limiting factor, and the goal of treatment in these patients is palliation. WBRT is the treatment of choice in this setting, giving symptomatic response rates of 70% to 93%, depending on the individual symptoms.[22,31–33] Radioresistant tumors such as renal cell carcinoma and melanoma appear to respond less well, whereas radiosensitive tumors such as small cell lung cancer respond better.[34–36] Median survival after WBRT is only 3 to 6 months.[19,31,37] Many investigators have examined the optimal dose for WBRT. The use of 30 Gy in 10 fractions has become standard practice at many institutions. Despite numerous studies, there is limited evidence that use of higher radiation doses results in

improved palliation or survival.[31,32,38–40] Unfortunately, palliation from WBRT is only temporary, and it has been shown that metastases will begin to enlarge at a median of 21 weeks after treatment.[26] In a study of patients with a controlled or absent primary tumor, a Karnofsky Performance Scale (KPS) score of 70 to 100, no evidence of metastasis elsewhere, and an age of less than 60 years, the median survival with WBRT alone was only 7.4 months.[41] This group represented the most favorable subset of 87 patients from a group of 700. Thus, WBRT is only indicated for patients not expected to survive for a prolonged period with respect to their systemic disease.

## CHEMOTHERAPY

The results of chemotherapy for brain metastases are generally poor. Treatments have very low overall response rates,[42] and several explanations have been proposed for this phenomenon. Perhaps most importantly, the types of tumors that most often metastasize to the brain are generally not chemosensitive. Additionally, brain metastases often develop after failure of first-line chemotherapeutic agents. Thirdly, the blood-brain barrier may play a role.[43] Chemotherapy may be beneficial in patients with small cell lung cancer, choriocarcinoma, germ cell tumors, and perhaps breast cancer.[44] In patients with primary tumors of other types, chemotherapy has little, if any, role to play in metastasis management.

## SURGICAL DECISION MAKING

A certain percentage of patients will develop brain metastasis in the setting of absent, limited, or controlled systemic disease. Up to 50% of patients with lung cancer[45] and 32% to 65% of patients with breast cancer[14,15,46] are in this category. In these patients, the brain metastasis is likely to be a survival-limiting factor. In this setting, aggressive local control of the brain metastasis via surgery can be expected to result in improved survival and quality of life.

In evaluating a patient for surgery, the number of brain metastases is important. The number of brain metastases varies according to the histology of the primary tumor. Overall, at autopsy, 65% to 85% of patients have multiple lesions.[47,48] On CT scan, 50% to 56% of patients have multiple lesions.[49,50] Melanoma is most likely to present with multiple lesions, followed by lung and breast primaries.[49] Colon cancer presents with multiple lesions 50% of the time, whereas brain metastases from renal cell carcinoma are usually single.[51,52] The overall incidence of multiple lesions seen on MRI has not been quantified but is likely to fall somewhere between the observed autopsy and CT scan data as patients demonstrating a single lesion on CT may be found to have multiple lesions on MRI.[24] Historically, patients with multiple brain metastases have been considered surgical candidates only in rare instances. However, recent data suggest that patients with a limited number of brain metastases in whom all lesions can be removed may benefit from surgery.[53] Thus patients with up to three lesions, or rarely, four, may be considered surgical candidates if all lesions are surgically accessible.

Surgical accessibility has already been referred to and is an important consideration. A lesion is considered accessible if it can be resected with an acceptable risk of morbidity. The definition is therefore dependent on the definition of acceptable risk. Small lesions deep within the brain and lesions in the motor cortex, speech center, internal capsule, thalamus, basal ganglia, and the brainstem are generally considered unresectable. However, with modern surgical techniques such as intraoperative ultrasonography, stereotactic guidance, cortical mapping, and image-guided surgery, some lesions that had previously been considered unresectable can now be safely removed.[54,55] In addition, in rare instances even a lesion in the brainstem may be removed using techniques such as the laser.[56] Thus, each lesion must be carefully evaluated to determine accessibility.

## SURGERY FOR SINGLE BRAIN METASTASES

*RANDOMIZED TRIALS.* In a landmark study, Patchell and colleagues[26] firmly established the role of surgery in the treatment of brain metastasis. In a controlled, randomized trial they compared surgery followed by WBRT to needle biopsy followed by WBRT in patients with a known history of cancer and a KPS score of 70 or higher. Six patients (11%) were found to have nonmetastatic disease, including primary brain tumors and abscesses, and were excluded from the trial. It is interesting to note that 30 of the 48 patients in this trial had either an unresected primary tumor or disseminated metastases at the time of their randomization. Patients in the surgical arm had a longer median survival (40 weeks vs. 15 weeks) and a longer functionally independent survival (38 weeks vs. 8 weeks) than with radiation alone. In addition, recurrence at the site of the original metastasis was lower with surgery (20% vs. 52%). When the length of time to death from neurologic causes was compared, patients in the surgical arm again had a longer survival (median 62 weeks vs. 26 weeks). Thirty-day mortality in both arms was 4%. Thirty-day morbidity rates in the surgical and radiation treatment arms were 8% and 17%, respectively. From this trial, it was definitely proved that surgery with WBRT was superior to WBRT alone in selected patients with a single brain metastasis.

A second controlled, randomized trial from Europe has corroborated these findings.[57] In this trial, survival in the surgical group was 10 months vs. 6 months for the group treated with WBRT alone. Progressive extracranial disease and age over 60 years were negative prognostic indicators. Patients with active extracranial disease had a median survival of 5 months in each arm of the trial. The authors concluded that surgery was indicated for patients with a single lesion in the face of stable systemic disease, especially if they were less than 60 years of age.

A third controlled, randomized trial appears to present a different picture.[58] In this comparison of surgery to WBRT, surgically treated patients survived 5.6 months relative to 6.3 months with WBRT alone, which was not statistically significant. The results of this trial differed dramatically from those of the two previous retrospective studies in that a much shorter survival time was reported for the surgically treated patients, and the reasons for this are discussed below. One explanation for these differences is the inclusion of significant numbers of patients with very poor health in the study by Mintz et al.[58] In this trial, 45% of patients had extracranial metastases, compared to 37.5% in Patchell's trial and 31.7% in the European study. Moreover, unlike the other trials, no exclusion was made for highly advanced systemic disease. Also, 21% of patients had KPS

scores of 50 or 60, indicating that they were incapable of independent living and were in poor condition.

Overall, these trials appear to support the role of surgery in the treatment of brain metastasis. Patient selection is very important. Only patients whose health is not severely compromised would be likely to benefit from surgical resection. In these patients, surgery appears to improve the length and quality of life.

*SURVIVAL AND PROGNOSTIC FACTORS.* Recent studies indicate that the median survival after resection of a brain metastasis is 11 to 16 months, depending on various prognostic factors.[53,59–62] Larger series in the literature have also consistently demonstrated a 5-year survival rate of 10% to 15%. By far the most important prognostic factors are extent of systemic disease and neurologic performance status. In addition, location of tumor and age play a role in postoperative survival. Other possible factors that have not been definitively proved to affect survival include time to development of brain metastasis, tumor histology, and failure of prior WBRT.

The importance of extent of systemic disease and neurologic performance status in predicting postoperative survival has been repeatedly demonstrated. In a study of 125 patients with a single brain metastasis from tumors of various histologies, the median survival of patients with systemic disease was 6 months, whereas that for patients without systemic disease was 22 months, with a greater than 25% 5-year survival.[62] Survival was also stratified according to the neurologic status of patients. Survival was 22 months for patients with no (or minimal) neurologic deficits, 10 months with a moderate deficit, and 6 months with a severe deficit.[62] A special subset of patients may be those having a single brain metastasis and a lung primary that are both resectable, as well as no other evidence of disease. The prognosis for this subset of patients is relatively good. In one study, 4-year survival was 56%, whereas in another, 5-year survival was 45%.[63,64]

Location of the tumor is important in that patients with infratentorial lesions tend to have a poorer survival than those with supratentorial tumors. In a large series, patients with supratentorial lesions survived 12 months compared to 7 months for patients with infratentorial lesions.[65] This finding has been supported by multivariate data analysis.[63,66] Patients with infratentorial lesions have a much higher incidence of developing carcinomatous meningitis after surgery, which is an ominous event. It has been found that 30% to 38% of patients with cerebellar metastases develop a meningeal relapse after surgery, whereas only 4.7% of those with supratentorial tumors do so.[67,68] This may be one factor resulting in the poorer overall survival in these patients.

Age has been shown to be a prognostic indicator in multiple studies, including two randomized trials.[26,57] In the study by Noordijk et al.,[57] patients over 60 years old who were treated with surgery survived 6 months compared to 19 months for younger patients. Multivariate analysis in retrospective studies also supports the prognostic value of age.[69]

Time to development of brain metastasis may also be a prognostic indicator. Multivariate analysis in some studies has indicated that development of brain metastasis soon after diagnosis of cancer may be an independent negative prognostic indicator. In the randomized trial of Patchell et al.,[26] a longer time between diagnosis of the primary cancer and the brain metastasis was shown by multivariate analysis to be a significant prognostic indicator of increased survival. In a study of patients with lung cancer, those with a brain metastasis diagnosed synchronously with the lung primary survived a median of 9.2 months relative to 13 months for patients diagnosed metachronously.[65] However, when multivariate analysis was used to correct for differences in other prognostic factors, time of onset of brain metastasis no longer had any influence on survival. Results from other studies are similarly mixed.

There is minimal information in the literature suggesting the role of primary tumor histology in survival of brain metastasis patients. Very few studies on tumors of varying histologic types have found significant differences in survival relative to tumor histology. In one study of 229 patients who were operated upon largely in the 1970s, lung, gastrointestinal, and genitourinary primaries were associated with longer survival according to multivariate analysis.[66] Yet, in the presence of many recent advances in oncology, the relevance of these data in the modern era is unclear. From an examination of many studies on survival after resection of brain metastases, it does appear that patients with renal primaries may have a superior prognosis, whereas those with melanoma may have a poorer prognosis;[1] however, this is far from definite.

Some data suggest that male gender is associated with a poorer outcome among brain metastasis patients. In studies from the Mayo Clinic and Memorial Sloan-Kettering Cancer Center, multivariate analysis indicated that male gender was an independent negative prognostic indicator.[65,69] The reasons for this are unclear, and additional confirmation of these findings is necessary.

*COMPLICATIONS OF SURGERY.* Brain metastases tend to be located subcortically, at the junction between the gray and white matter, and tend to be well demarcated from surrounding, healthy brain. It is mainly these characteristics that account for the low morbidity and mortality of surgery for brain metastases relative to that for other brain tumors. In recent large series, operative morbidity rate is estimated at 5% or less and 30-day mortality rate is close to 3%.[1] The complication rates are dependent on factors such as tumor location. Lesions in eloquent cortex such as the motor strip will have a higher incidence of morbidity whereas lesions in the posterior fossa may also be associated with increased 30-day mortality. Use of tools such as stereotactic localization and cortical mapping can be helpful in reducing morbidity.[54] Published studies uniformly indicate that the majority of patients will improve neurologically after surgery. Postoperative hospital stays are short, with one study reporting that patients were discharged at a median of 3 days after surgery.[53]

*POSTOPERATIVE WBRT.* The use of postoperative WBRT is standard at most institutions, and a number of studies have examined its efficacy. The first such study, from the Mayo Clinic, examined a series of 85 patients operated on between 1972 and 1982.[69] In this study, patients receiving postoperative WBRT had a 21% rate of tumor recurrence in the brain relative to 85% for those not receiving WBRT. Patients receiving WBRT also had a significantly improved survival. This study has been frequently cited as proof of the efficacy of WBRT, and the 85% relapse figure in patients not receiving WBRT has been widely quoted. Unfortunately, the data from this study may not be applicable to patients currently being treated. Given the years in which patients were treated, it is clear that some patients did not receive an optimal CT scan prior to surgery. In the absence of such imaging, many patients with multiple metastases may have been thought to have only a single lesion at the time of surgery. Certainly, these patients would be more likely to have rapid enlargement of their previously undiagnosed lesions without WBRT. The 85% relapse figure given here[69] is much higher than that reported in any other study.

Five additional studies of this type have been published,[67,70–73] including four that are more recent[67,70,72,73] than that of Smalley et al.,[69] and all of which showed a decrease in recurrence rates with WBRT. Only one of these studies, on patients with melanoma, showed an increased survival with WBRT;[73] however, multivariate analysis was not performed, making it impossible to know whether or not this survival advantage was simply due to a difference in prognostic factors.

There have been numerous reports of neurotoxicity from WBRT, including radiation necrosis and dementia.[67,74–79] In one report, 11% of 1-year survivors developed dementia attributable to WBRT, whereas in the other study, 50% of 2-year survivors were so affected.[62,67] Many of the patients in these studies were treated with doses greater than the 30 Gy in 10 fractions that is currently widely used. However, even in patients receiving 30 Gy in 10 fractions, patients were found to develop leukoencephalopathy not attributable to other causes.[78] Few data have been published on detailed neuropsychologic testing in long-term survivors who underwent WBRT, but the available reports suggest that these patients do develop deterioration.

Although only a minority of patients with brain metastasis will survive in the longer term, toxicity in this subgroup is very important because these survivors represent the greatest beneficiaries of surgery and the greatest incentive for aggressive treatment. In summary, the preponderance of evidence indicates that WBRT probably decreases recurrence rates in the brain and is associated with a definite but unquantified toxicity. A survival benefit with WBRT in the modern neurosurgical practice has not been proved. Despite this, it is considered standard treatment at most institutions. Further studies are required to settle this controversial issue.

## SURGERY FOR MULTIPLE BRAIN METASTASES. 
Historically, patients with multiple brain metastases have not been considered surgical candidates except in rare instances. This was despite the fact that no study had ever carefully examined the role of surgery in such patients. Eventually, however, isolated reports of patients with multiple brain metastases treated with surgery began to appear in the literature.

We recently examined the role of surgery in the treatment of patients with multiple brain metastases at The University of Texas M. D. Anderson Cancer Center.[53] We evaluated 56 patients who underwent resection for multiple brain metastases, 30 of whom had one or more lesions left unresected (Group A) and 26 of whom had all lesions resected (Group B). Twenty-six other patients with a single metastasis who underwent resection (Group C) were selected to match Group B by type of primary tumor, time from first diagnosis of cancer to diagnosis of brain metastases, and presence or absence of systemic cancer at the time of surgery. Statistical analysis indicated that Groups A and B were also homogenous for these prognostic indicators. Median survival duration was 6 months for Group A,

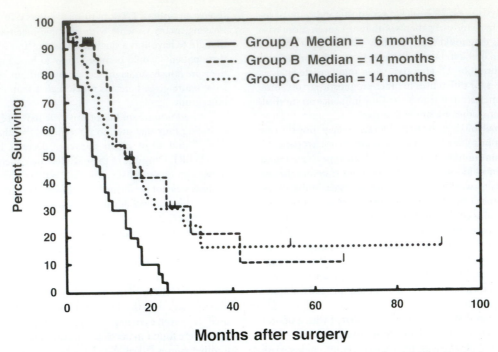

**FIGURE 24A-2.** Survival in patients with multiple brain metastases treated surgically. Group A, patients with multiple metastases in whom one or more lesions were left unresected; group B, patients with multiple metastases in whom all the lesions were resected; group C, patients with solitary, completely resected metastases. (*From Bindal RK, Sawaya R, Leavens MF, and Lee JJ, Journal of Neurosurgery 79:210–216; 1993, with permission.*)

14 months for Group B, and 14 months for Group C. There was a statistically significant difference in survival between Groups A and B ($p = 0.003$) and Groups A and C ($p = 0.012$) but not between groups B and C (Fig. 24A-2). Recurrence of brain metastasis occurred in 31% of patients in Group B and in 35% of patients in Group C. Symptoms improved after surgery in 65% of patients in Group A, 83% of patients in Group B, and 84% of patients in Group C. Groups A, B, and C had complication rates of 8%, 9%, and 8%, respectively, per craniotomy and 30-day mortality rates of 3%, 4%, and 0%, respectively. We conclude that surgical removal of all lesions in selected patients with multiple brain metastases results in significantly increased survival and gives a prognosis similar to that of patients undergoing surgery for a single metastasis.

Recent studies from Memorial Sloan-Kettering Cancer Center have reported similar results. In a study of patients with lung cancer, the presence of multiple brain metastases was not a negative prognostic indicator as assessed by multivariate analysis.[65] In a study of 670 patients with varied tumor histologies, 49 of whom had multiple lesions, multivariate analysis again failed to demonstrate multiple brain metastases to be a negative prognostic factor, as patients with single lesions survived 9.2 months compared to 9 months for those with multiple lesions.[59]

A study from the University of Colorado appears to present a different conclusion.[80] Forty-six patients undergoing surgery for brain metastases were evaluated. Of these, 28 had a single lesion whereas 18 had two or more metastases. The authors found that patients with multiple metastases had a median survival of 5 months compared

with 12 months for patients with a single lesion, a difference that was significant by univariate analysis; however, only one of the patients with multiple lesions underwent excision of all lesions. This patient survived for 46 months following surgery. The 5-month median survival for those patients who did not have all known lesions removed is very consistent with the 6-month survival that we had previously reported for such patients. Thus, although this paper at first glance seems to contradict the previously mentioned studies, the data actually corroborate our conclusion that patients with multiple lesions who do not have all lesions removed have a poorer prognosis.

From these studies, it appears that surgery for multiple brain metastases is warranted in selected cases, especially if all known brain metastases can be removed. Complication rates are low, and multiple craniotomies are well tolerated in achieving the goal of complete resection. Survival appears to be similar to that of patients with a single brain metastasis, and a significant percentage of patients can enjoy prolonged survival. However, there are still only a limited number of studies of this controversial issue, and further research is needed to more clearly define the role of surgery for these patients.

## RECURRENCE AFTER SURGERY

Unfortunately, 31% to 51% of surgically treated patients will develop recurrence of brain metastases.[26,53,62] Treatment options for such patients are limited. Many have already received WBRT, and the results of retreatment with this modality are mixed. Chemotherapy, as previously discussed, generally gives poor results.

We recently studied a group of 44 patients with metastatic recurrence in order to determine the characteristics of such lesions.[81] The median time from initial surgery to recurrence was 6 months. Recurrence was local in 20 patients, distant in 18, and both local and distant in 6 patients. Twenty-nine patients (66%) had a single lesion at the time of diagnosis of recurrence, 8 (18%) had two lesions, 3 (7%) had three, and 4 (9%) had four or more lesions. Thirty patients had known systemic disease at the time of recurrence. Median survival for all patients after recurrence was 8.7 months. A total of 29 (66%) patients, including 3 with multiple lesions, underwent reoperation. Of the 15 patients not undergoing surgery, 10 received chemotherapy. Median survival for patients receiving reoperation was 11 months compared to 3 months for those without reoperation. Patients undergoing reoperation were more likely to have local recurrence, a single metastasis, or a better KPS score, and were less likely to have systemic disease. Multivariate analysis was performed to correct for these differences in the patient population, and reoperation was still found to be a positive independent prognostic factor.

Another study evaluated 109 patients with recurrent brain metastases from non–small cell lung cancer.[82] The median time to recurrence for these patients was 5 months. In 48.5% of patients recurrence was only local, in 13.5% it was both local and distant, in 30% there were one or more distant recurrences, and 8% developed meningeal carcinomatosis. Of 109 patients, 28.5% appeared to develop multiple lesions at recurrence; 32 patients (30%) underwent reoperation and will be discussed later. The survival after recurrence for patients not undergoing reoperation was not stated. In the entire group of 109 patients, reoperation, histology of adenocarcinoma, complete resection of the primary tumor, and female sex were found to be positive independent prognostic indicators.

The literature indicates that the majority of patients developing recurrence have only a single lesion. A significant percentage of such patients may be treated with reoperation. Reoperation has a positive independent influence on survival, and survival is very poor for patients who are not candidates for reoperation.

## REIRRADIATION FOR RECURRENCE

The role of reirradiation for recurrent metastatic brain lesions is controversial. A small number of studies in the literature have examined this issue.[83–86] Results of reirradiation are mixed. Median survival after reirradiation was limited, ranging from 1.8 to 4 months. Response rates varied from 27% to 75%, and the duration of response for patients who improved was short, with a median of 2.7 months, in a recent study by Wong et al.[86] Presence of extracranial metastasis of the primary cancer was found to be a negative prognostic indicator as assessed by multivariate analysis; however, even patients without extracranial disease had a 12-month survival rate of 14% and negligible long-term survival. Toxicity of treatment was low in all studies, probably due to the short survival observed following reirradiation. Thus, although reirradiation remains a treatment option, results are limited.

## REOPERATION FOR RECURRENCE

A study by Sundaresan et al.[87] in 1988 examined the role of reoperation for brain metastases in 21 patients. Radiation necrosis was found in three patients. Thirteen patients improved neurologically after surgery, whereas one patient developed a new deficit. There was no surgical mortality. Two patients developed wound-related complications resulting in loss of the bone flap, and one patient developed a CSF leak and infection. Overall, median survival after reoperation was 9 months.

In a recent study, we evaluated the results of reoperation for brain metastasis at the M.D. Anderson Cancer Center in 48 patients.[88] Systemic disease was present at the time of reoperation in 23 (47.9%) patients. Thirty-three (75.0%) of the 44 symptomatic patients improved after reoperation. There was no operative mortality and 30-day morbidity rate was low (6.3%). The median hospital stay after surgery was 5 days. In this study survival after reoperation was 11.5 months, and the 5-year survival rate was 17%. Multivariate analysis was performed to determine which variables correlated with survival. This analysis revealed that the status of systemic disease, KPS score, time to recurrence, age, and the type of primary tumor significantly influenced survival.

In our study at the M.D. Anderson Cancer Center, a model was developed to predict patients' survival using the five factors determined to be prognostic by multivariate analysis. In this system, a patient was first assigned a score by adding together all of his or her negative prognostic indicators, as presented in Table 24A-1. This score was then converted to a grade (Table 24A-2). For example, a 65-year-old man who presented with a recurrent brain metastasis from lung cancer, who underwent initial craniotomy 9 months ago, who had no evidence of systemic disease, and had a KPS score of 70 was assigned a score of 2 and therefore had grade II disease; 9 patients were classified as grade I, 19 as grade II, 14 as grade III, and 6 as grade IV. Survival correlated significantly with patient grade.

**TABLE 24A-1.** CALCULATION OF SCORE FOR PATIENT GRADE DETERMINATION

| FACTOR EVALUATED | SCORE |
|---|---|
| Status of Systemic Disease | |
|     Present | 1 |
|     Absent | 0 |
| Pre-reoperative Karnofsky Performance Scale Score | |
|     ≤70 | 1 |
|     >70 | 0 |
| Time to Recurrence | |
|     <4 mos | 1 |
|     ≥4 mos | 0 |
| Age | |
|     ≥40 yrs | 1 |
|     <40 yrs | 0 |
| Type of Primary Tumor | |
|     Melanoma or breast cancer | 1 |
|     Lung or other cancer | 0 |

SOURCE: Bindal RK et al: J Neurosurg 83:600, 1995, with permission.

**TABLE 24A-2. SCORE TO GRADE CONVERSION**

| SCORE | GRADE |
| --- | --- |
| 0–1 | I |
| 2 | II |
| 3 | III |
| 4–5 | IV |

Median survival for patients in grade I was not reached. Patients in grades II, III, and IV survived a median of 13.4, 6.8, and 3.4 months, respectively. Patients in grade I had a 5-year survival rate of 57%. Patients in grade II had 3- and 5-year survival rates of 23% and 11%, respectively. Patients in grades III and IV had 1-year survival rates of 17% and 0%, respectively.

Another study from the Memorial Sloan-Kettering Cancer Center is consistent with our results.[82] In this study, 32 patients with non–small cell lung cancer underwent reoperation for recurrent brain metastases. Within this group, 84.4% of patients had a single brain metastasis. Median survival in these patients from the time of reoperation was 10 months. Of these 32 patients, 8 underwent a second reoperation and survived an additional 10.5 months. Reirradiation did not increase survival. Multivariate analysis of the entire group of 109 patients with recurrent brain metastasis upon whom this study was based revealed that reoperation was an independent factor associated with increased survival.

These studies indicate that reoperation plays a role in managing recurrent brain metastasis, especially in patients assigned a low grade according to our model.[88] Reoperation is well tolerated and appears to prolong life. Given the limited treatment options for patients with metastatic recurrence in the brain, reoperation must be strongly considered in selected cases.

## ROLE OF RADIOSURGERY

Stereotactic radiosurgery is a relatively new modality increasingly being used to treat brain metastases. The term refers to the use of small, well-collimated beams of ionizing radiation to ablate intracranial lesions. All stereotactic systems have the ability to: (1) accurately locate and immobilize an intracranial target in three-dimensional space, (2) produce sharply collimated beams of radiation with a steep dose gradient at the beam edge, and (3) target the beam accurately, minimizing radiation exposure to surrounding brain tissue. The radiation dose is usually delivered in a single fraction. Hypofractionation has a more lethal effect on tissue than is possible by delivery of the same dose of radiation in many fractions. The use of numerous beams of radiation converging on the target site results in a high dose of radiation delivery to the tumor site. This dose falls off rapidly away from the target in a ratio dependent upon the size of the target. With a small target, surrounding brain tissue receives a lower radiation dose than with a large target.

The main advantage of stereotactic radiosurgery with regard to brain metastases lies primarily in its ability to treat lesions that are not amenable to surgical resection and secondarily, in its noninvasive nature with fewer attendant risks and a shorter hospital stay. Brain metastases are particularly well suited for treatment by stereotactic radiosurgery because (1) they are often spherical and show enhancing margins on MRI or CT; (2) they are generally small (<3 cm) when first detected; (3) they tend to displace normal brain tissue circumferentially, reducing its chance of being damaged; and (4) brain metastases tend to be well demarcated and minimally invasive. Even so, due to the developing nature of radiosurgery, lesions that would otherwise be surgically resected are rarely treated by this modality. Recurrent brain metastases and lesions located in unreachable regions of the brain are the ones that are often selected for radiosurgical procedures.

## RESULTS OF TREATMENT WITH RADIOSURGERY

Numerous studies have evaluated the results of radiosurgery for brain metastases. Overall survival results range from 6 to 13 months.[89–96] Reported local control rates range from 82% to 95%. A number of factors have been found to affect survival and local control after radiosurgery. Factors affecting survival here are similar to factors affecting survival after surgery. Several studies have demonstrated that extent of extracranial disease and Karnofsky performance status are very important survival factors.[89,91,94] Patients with three or more lesions appear to have a poorer prognosis.[91,94] A longer interval from initial diagnosis of cancer to diagnosis of brain metastasis is favorable. The presence of a radioresistant tumor histology does not appear to be a negative factor in local control.[93] Although it is felt that the best responses are obtained if WBRT is given concurrently with radiosurgery,[93] recent publications suggest that acceptable results may be achievable with radiosurgery alone, leaving WBRT in reserve for treatment of possible recurrence.[97,98] Radiation necrosis develops in up to 16% of patients.[94]

Some studies have shown that radiosurgery is effective in treating brain metastases and appears to be superior to WBRT alone. Some authors have even suggested that radiosurgery is effective enough to replace surgery as the treatment of choice in patients with a limited number of lesions and controlled systemic disease,[96] but this is controversial.

## SURGERY VERSUS RADIOSURGERY FOR BRAIN METASTASES

We recently performed a study comparing these two treatment modalities for brain metastases.[99] We prospectively followed 31 patients treated by radiosurgery and 62 patients treated by surgery who were retrospectively matched. Patients were matched with respect to the following criteria: histology of primary tumor, extent of systemic disease, preoperative KPS score, time to brain metastasis, number of brain metastases, and patient age and sex. For patients treated by radiosurgery, the median size of the treated lesion was 1.96 cm$^3$, and the median dose was 20 Gy. The median survival was 7.5 months for patients treated by radiosurgery and 16.4 months for those treated by surgery; this difference was statistically significant by both univariate ($p = 0.0018$) and multivariate ($p = 0.0009$) analyses (Fig. 24A-3). The difference in survival was due to a higher rate of mortality from brain metastasis in the radiosurgery group

## Overall Survival

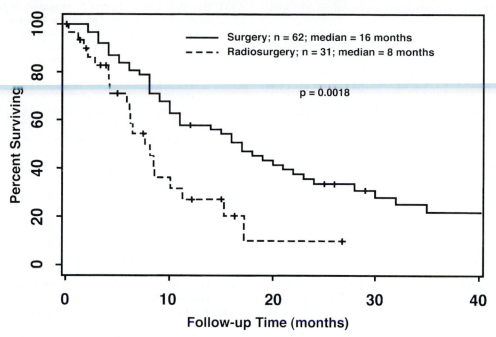

**FIGURE 24A-3.** Graph comparing survival periods in patients treated surgically and radiosurgically. Radiosurgically treated patients had a shorter overall survival period according to both univariate and multivariate analyses. (*From Bindal AK, Bindal RK, Hess KR, Shiu A, Hassenbusch SJ, Shi WM, and Sawaya R. Journal of Neurosurgery 84:748–754; 1996, with permission.*)

than in the surgery group ($p < 0.0001$) and not due to a difference in the rate of death from systemic disease ($p = 0.28$). Log-rank analysis showed that this higher mortality rate in the radiosurgery group was due to a greater progression rate of the radiosurgically treated lesions ($p = 0.0001$) and not due to the development of new brain metastases ($p = 0.75$).

From this study, we concluded that surgery is superior to radiosurgery in the treatment of brain metastases. Patients who undergo surgical treatment survive longer and have better local tumor control. Our data suggest that the indications for radiosurgery are limited to surgically inaccessible metastatic tumors or patients in poor medical condition. Surgery should remain the treatment of choice whenever possible. However, as radiosurgery is a noninvasive treatment, it can be used to treat patients who are not surgical candidates either because of advanced systemic disease or poor medical condition. Radiosurgery is more effective at local control than WBRT and therefore may be used as an adjunct to, or even in lieu of, WBRT for patients in poor medical condition. Thus, radiosurgery remains an important tool in treatment of brain metastases.

## CONCLUSION

Brain metastasis is a deadly disease and portends a very poor overall prognosis. Most patients have widespread disseminated disease. The goal of treatment in such patients is palliation, and surgery very

rarely plays a role. Yet, in a significant subset of patients, an aggressive surgical approach can extend survival, reduce symptoms, and improve quality of life. Combined modality treatment with surgery, fractionated radiation, and radiosurgery can prevent a significant number of patients from dying from their brain metastases and can improve the prognosis of this dismal disease.

## REFERENCES

1. SAWAYA R, BINDAL RK: Metastatic brain tumors, in *Brain Tumors. An Encyclopedic Approach,* Kaye AH, Laws ER (eds). Edinburgh, Churchill Livingstone, 1995, pp 923–946.
2. POSNER JB, CHERNIK NL: Intracranial metastases from systemic cancer. Adv Neurol 19:579, 1978.
3. WALKER AE, ROBINS M, WEINFELD FD: Epidemiology of brain tumors: The national survey of intracranial neoplasms. Neurology 35:219, 1985.
4. TAKAKURA K et al: *Metastatic Tumors of the Nervous System.* New York, Igaku-Shoin, 1982, 346 pp.
5. BINDAL RK et al: Sarcoma metastatic to the brain: Results of surgical treatment. Neurosurgery 35:185, 1994; discussion, pp 190–191.
6. STEIN M et al: Involvement of the central nervous system by ovarian carcinoma. Cancer 58:2066, 1986.
7. CASTALDO JE et al: Intracranial metastases due to prostatic carcinoma. Cancer 52:1739, 1983.

8. Anderson RS et al: Brain metastases from transitional cell carcinoma of urinary bladder. Urology 39:17, 1992.

9. Bloch JL et al: Brain metastases from transitional cell carcinoma. J Urol 137:97, 1987.

10. Galluzzi S, Panye P: Brain metastases from primary bronchial carcinoma: A statistical study of 741 necropsies. Cancer 10:408, 1956.

11. Sorensen JB et al: Brain metastases in adenocarcinoma of the lung: Frequency, risk groups, and prognosis. J Clin Oncol 6:1474, 1988.

12. Lee Y: Breast carcinoma: Pattern of metastases at autopsy. J Surg Oncol 23:175, 1983.

13. Tsukada Y et al: Central nervous system metastasis from breast carcinoma. Cancer 52:2349, 1983.

14. Boogerd W et al: Brain metastases in breast cancer; natural history, prognostic factors and outcome. J Neurooncol 15:165, 1993.

15. Dethy S et al: History of brain and epidural metastases from breast cancer in relation with the disease evolution outside the central nervous system. Eur Neurol 35:38, 1995.

16. Patel J et al: Metastatic pattern of malignant melanoma: A study of 216 autopsy cases. Am J Surg 135:807, 1978.

17. Weiss L et al: Metastatic patterns of renal carcinoma: An analysis of 687 necropsies. J Cancer Res Clin Oncol 114:605, 1988.

18. Weiss L et al: Haematogenous metastatic patterns in colonic carcinoma: An analysis of 1541 necropsies. J Pathol 150:195, 1986.

19. Cairncross JG et al: Radiation therapy for brain metastases. Ann Neurol 7:529, 1980.

20. Hirsch FR et al: Intracranial metastases in small cell carcinoma of the lung: Correlation of clinical and autopsy findings. Cancer 50:2433, 1982.

21. Cairncross JG, Posner JB: The management of brain metastases, in Oncology of the Nervous System, Walker MD (ed). Boston, Martinus Nijhof, 1983, pp 341–377.

22. Posner JB: Diagnosis and treatment of metastases to the brain. Clin Bull 4:47, 1974.

23. Graus F et al: Cerebrovascular complications in patients with cancer. Medicine 64:16, 1985.

24. Sze G et al: Detection of brain metastases: Comparison of contrast-enhanced MR with unenhanced MR and enhanced CT. Am J Neuroradiol 11:785, 1990.

25. Hwang TL et al: Predilection of brain metastasis in gray and white matter junction and vascular border zones. Cancer 77:1551, 1996.

26. Patchell RA et al: A randomized trial of surgery in the treatment of single metastases to the brain. N Engl J Med 322:494, 1990.

27. Voorhies RM et al: The single supratentorial lesion. An evaluation of preoperative diagnostic tests. J Neurosurg 53:364, 1980.

28. Latief KH et al: Search for a primary lung neoplasm in patients with brain metastasis: Is the chest radiograph sufficient? AJR 168:1339, 1997.

29. Markesbery WR et al: Treatment for patients with cerebral metastases. Arch Neurol 35:754, 1978.

30. Ruderman N, Hall T: Use of glucocorticoids in the palliative treatment of metastatic brain tumors. Cancer 18:298, 1965.

31. Borgelt B et al: The palliation of brain metastases: Final results of the first two studies by the Radiation Therapy Oncology Group. Int J Radiat Oncol Biol Phys 6:1, 1980.

32. Hoskin PJ et al: The influence of extent and local management on the outcome of radiotherapy for brain metastases. Int J Radiat Oncol Biol Phys 19:111, 1990.

33. Sheline GE, Brady LW: Radiation therapy for brain metastases. J Neurooncol 4:219, 1987.

34. Giannone L et al: Favorable prognosis of brain metastases in small cell lung cancer. Ann Intern Med 106:386, 1987.

35. Retsas S, Gershuny AR: Central nervous system involvement in malignant melanoma. Cancer 61:1926, 1988.

36. Wronski M et al: External radiation of brain metastases from renal carcinoma: A retrospective study of 119 patients from the M. D. Anderson Cancer Center. Int J Radiat Oncol Biol Phys 37:753, 1997.

37. Patchell RA: Brain metastases. Neurol Clin 9:817, 1991.

38. Gelber RD et al: Equivalence of radiation schedules for the palliative treatment of brain metastases in patients with favorable prognosis. Cancer 48:1749, 1981.

39. Hendrickson F: The optimum schedule for palliative radiotherapy for metastatic brain cancer. Int J Radiat Oncol Biol Phys 2:165, 1977.

40. Shehata WM et al: Rapid fractionation technique and re-treatment of cerebral metastases by irradiation. Cancer 34:257, 1974.

41. Diener-West M et al: Identification of an optimal subgroup for treatment evaluation of patients with brain metastases using RTOG study 7916. Int J Radiat Oncol Biol Phys 16:669, 1989.

42. Greig NH: Chemotherapy of brain metastases: Current status. Cancer Treat Rev 11:157, 1984.

43. Buckner JC: The role of chemotherapy in the treatment of patients with brain metastases from solid tumors. Cancer Metastasis Rev 10:335, 1991.

44. Lee JS et al: Primary chemotherapy of brain metastasis in small-cell lung cancer. J Clin Oncol 7:916, 1989.

45. Patchell RA et al: Single brain metastases: Surgery plus radiation or radiation alone. Neurology 36:447, 1986.

46. DiStefano A et al: The natural history of breast cancer patients with brain metastases. Cancer 44:1913, 1979.

47. Ask-Upmark E: Metastatic tumors of the brain and their localization. Acta Med Scand 154:1, 1956.

48. Chason J et al: Metastatic carcinoma in the central nervous system and dorsal root ganglia. Cancer 16:781, 1963.

49. Delattre JY et al: Distribution of brain metastases. Arch Neurol 45:741, 1988.

50. Swift PS et al: CT characteristics of patients with brain metastases treated in RTOG study 79-16. Int J Radiat Oncol Biol Phys 25:209, 1993.

51. Cascino TL et al: Brain metastases from colon cancer. J Neurooncol 1:203, 1983.

52. Decker DA et al: Brain metastases in patients with renal cell carcinoma: Prognosis and treatment. J Clin Oncol 2:169, 1984.

53. Bindal RK et al: Surgical treatment of multiple brain metastases. J Neurosurg 79:210, 1993.

54. Kelly PJ et al: Results of computed tomography-based computer-assisted stereotactic resection of metastatic intracranial tumors. Neurosurgery 22:7, 1988.

55. Pillay P et al: Minimally invasive brain surgery. Ann Acad Med Singapore 22:459, 1993.

56. Tobler WD et al: Successful laser-assisted excision of a metastatic midbrain tumor. Neurosurgery 18:795, 1986.

57. Noordijk EM et al: The choice of treatment of single brain metastasis should be based on extracranial tumor activity and age. Int J Radiat Oncol Biol Phys 29:711, 1994.

58. Mintz AH et al: A randomized trial to assess the efficacy of surgery in addition to radiotherapy in patients with a single cerebral metastasis. Cancer 78:1470, 1996.

59. ARBIT E et al: Surgical resection of brain metastasis in 670 patients: The Memorial Sloan-Kettering Cancer Center experience, 1972–1992. J Neurosurg 80:386A, 1994.

60. FERRARA M et al: Surgical treatment of 100 single brain metastases. Analysis of the results. J Neurosurg Sci 34:303, 1990.

61. NUSSBAUM ES et al: Brain metastases. Histology, multiplicity, surgery, and survival. Cancer 78:1781, 1996.

62. SUNDARESAN N, GALICICH JH: Surgical treatment of brain metastases. Clinical and computerized tomography evaluation of the results of treatment. Cancer 55:1382, 1985.

63. CATINELLA FP et al: Surgical treatment of primary lung cancer and solitary intracranial metastasis. Chest 95:972, 1989.

64. HANKINS JR et al: Surgical management of lung cancer with solitary cerebral metastasis. Ann Thorac Surg 46:24, 1988.

65. WRONSKI M et al: Survival after surgical treatment of brain metastases from lung cancer: A follow-up study of 231 patients treated between 1976 and 1991. J Neurosurg 83:605, 1995.

66. SMALLEY SR et al: Resection for solitary brain metastasis. Role of adjuvant radiation and prognostic variables in 229 patients. J Neurosurg 77:531, 1992.

67. DeANGELIS LM et al: The role of postoperative radiotherapy after resection of single brain metastases. Neurosurgery 24:798, 1989.

68. KITAOKA K et al: Follow-up study on metastatic cerebellar tumor surgery—characteristic problems of surgical treatment. Neurol Med Chir (Tokyo) 30:591, 1990.

69. SMALLEY SR et al: Adjuvant radiation therapy after surgical resection of solitary brain metastasis: Association with pattern of failure and survival. Int J Radiat Oncol Biol Phys 13:1611, 1987.

70. ARMSTRONG JG et al: Postoperative radiation for lung cancer metastatic to the brain. J Clin Oncol 12:2340, 1994.

71. DOSORETZ DE et al: Management of solitary metastasis to the brain: The role of elective brain irradiation following complete surgical resection. Int J Radiat Oncol Biol Phys 6:1727, 1980.

72. HAGEN NA et al: The role of radiation therapy following resection of single brain metastasis from melanoma. Neurology 40:158, 1990.

73. SKIBBER JM et al: Cranial irradiation after surgical excision of brain metastases in melanoma patients. Ann Surg Oncol 3:118, 1996.

74. ASAI A et al: Subacute brain atrophy after radiation therapy for malignant brain tumor. Cancer 63:1962, 1989.

75. DeANGELIS LM et al: Radiation-induced dementia in patients cured of brain metastases. Neurology 39:789, 1989.

76. JOHNSON BE et al: Neurologic, computed cranial tomographic, and magnetic resonance imaging abnormalities in patients with small-cell lung cancer: Further follow-up of 6- to 13-year survivors. J Clin Oncol 8:48, 1990.

77. LAUKKANEN E et al: The role of prophylactic brain irradiation in limited stage small cell lung cancer: Clinical, neuropsychologic, and CT sequelae. Int J Radiat Oncol Biol Phys 14:1109, 1988.

78. LEE Y et al: Treatment-related white matter changes in cancer patients. Cancer 57:1473, 1986.

79. SUNDARESAN N et al: Radiation necrosis after treatment of solitary intracranial metastases. Neurosurgery 8:329, 1981.

80. HAZUKA MB et al: Multiple brain metastases are associated with poor survival in patients treated with surgery and radiotherapy. J Clin Oncol 11:369, 1993.

81. BINDAL R et al: Recurrent brain metastasis. *American Association of Neurological Surgeons 65th Annual Meeting,* Denver, Colorado, 1997.

82. ARBIT E et al: The treatment of patients with recurrent brain metastases. A retrospective analysis of 109 patients with non-small cell lung cancer. Cancer 76:765, 1995.

83. COOPER JS et al: Cerebral metastases: Value of reirradiation in selected patients. Radiology 174:883, 1990.

84. HAZUKA MB, KINZIE JJ: Brain metastases: Results and effects of re-irradiation. Int J Radiat Oncol Biol Phys 15:433, 1988.

85. KURUP P et al: Results of re-irradiation for cerebral metastases. Cancer 46:2587, 1980.

86. WONG WW et al: Analysis of outcome in patients reirradiated for brain metastases. Int J Radiat Oncol Biol Phys 34:585, 1996.

87. SUNDARESAN N et al: Reoperation for brain metastases. J Clin Oncol 6:1625, 1988.

88. BINDAL RK et al: Reoperation for recurrent metastatic brain tumors. J Neurosurg 83:600, 1995.

89. AUCHTER RM et al: A multiinstitutional outcome and prognostic factor analysis of radiosurgery for resectable single brain metastasis. Int J Radiat Oncol Biol Phys 35:27, 1996.

90. BINDAL RK et al: Survival after radiosurgery for brain metastasis: Regarding Buatti et al. IJROBP 32(4):1161–1166; 1995 [letter; comment]. Int J Radiat Oncol Biol Phys 36:523, 1996.

91. BRENEMAN JC et al: Stereotactic radiosurgery for the treatment of brain metastases. Results of a single institution series. Cancer 79:551, 1997.

92. ENGENHART R et al: Long-term follow-up for brain metastases treated by percutaneous stereotactic single high-dose irradiation. Cancer 71:1353, 1993.

93. FLICKINGER JC et al: A multi-institutional experience with stereotactic radiosurgery for solitary brain metastasis. Int J Radiat Oncol Biol Phys 28:797, 1994.

94. JOSEPH J et al: Linear accelerator-based stereotaxic radiosurgery for brain metastases: The influence of number of lesions on survival. J Clin Oncol 14:1085, 1996.

95. LOEFFLER JS, ALEXANDER EI: Radiosurgery for the treatment of intracranial metastases, in *Stereotactic Radiosurgery.* Alexander EI et al (eds.). New York, McGraw-Hill, 1993, pp 197–206.

96. MEHTA MP et al: Defining the role of radiosurgery in the management of brain metastases. Int J Radiat Oncol Biol Phys 24:619, 1992.

97. SHIAU CY et al: Radiosurgery for brain metastases: Relationship of dose and pattern of enhancement to local control. Int J Radiat Oncol Biol Phys 37:375, 1997.

98. SHIRATO H et al: Stereotactic irradiation without whole-brain irradiation for single brain metastasis. Int J Radiat Oncol Biol Phys 37:385, 1997.

99. BINDAL AK et al: Surgery versus radiosurgery in the treatment of brain metastasis. J Neurosurg 84:748, 1996.

# 24B / PULMONARY METASTASES

*Hiroshi Takita*

## INTRODUCTION

Malignant tumors usually spread either by the lymphatic or the hematogenous route. Lymphatic metastases tend initially to involve regional lymph nodes. Hematogenous metastases usually involve the lungs. Gastrointestinal tumors, however, are an exception, since the first site of hematogenous metastasis is often the liver.[1] Ordinarily, cancer does not disseminate all over the body from the primary site. Tumors often remain at the first site of metastasis such as the lungs or liver for a period of time. Then as time elapses, they will metastasize by systemic circulation to the generalized area of the body.[1] Lungs and liver are rich in capillary vessels. This is especially true for the lungs, since almost the entire volume of circulating blood must go through their capillary vessels for gas exchange. Therefore, lungs and liver might be considered filters of the circulating blood. It is also known that a 50- to 100-fold concentration of white blood cells occurs in the lung capillaries as compared to other parts of the body.[2] Consequently, it may be viewed that lungs are the largest defense organ in the body. Harmful particles in the circulation are trapped in the lung capillaries and may be destroyed by a high concentration of the white blood cells in situ. It may also be stated that lung metastasis is a manifestation of the body's defense mechanism in preventing further tumor dissemination. Control of lung metastasis before the tumor can escape once again into the systemic circulation is a difficult task but a worthwhile goal. Unlike the oil filter of a car, which is easily and completely replaced when harmful particles accumulate, the lungs are usually irreplaceable. Therefore, the surgeon must painstakingly remove these harmful particles (metastases) while preserving normal lung.

## CLINICAL MANIFESTATION

### SIGNS AND SYMPTOMS

Fewer than 50% of those with metastatic pulmonary tumors complain of symptoms such as cough, hemoptysis, chest pain, dyspnea, fever, and pulmonary osteoarthropathy.[3] Generally the lung metastases are radiologically found in the periphery of the lung and present as fairly discrete round lesions. When patients present with respiratory symptoms of hemoptysis, endobronchial metastasis may be found by bronchoscopy. The incidence of endobronchial metastasis (compared to peripheral lung metastasis) of 4% has been reported.[4] Endobronchial metastasis from breast, colon or rectum, kidney, uterus, and melanoma has been reported in the literature.[5]

## DIAGNOSIS

Lung metastasis is usually diagnosed by chest x-ray for patients presenting with symptoms of endobronchial metastasis. Patients with tumors that are known to have a high incidence of lung metastasis such as sarcoma, melanoma, and germ cell tumor may be followed by periodic CT scans.[6] Magnetic resonance imagining (MRI) is at present not recommended for routine use for the staging or follow-up of patients with metastatic lung disease because it is expensive and because relatively long exposure time induces motion artifacts.

## TUMOR DOUBLING TIME

Some metastatic tumors grow very rapidly, and one can easily observe them grow in a matter of a few weeks. Others remain stationary for many months. It is a conventional thought that patients with rapidly growing tumors have a worse prognosis than those with slower-growing tumors. A quantitative measure of the growth rate of metastatic lung lesions, tumor doubling time (TDT), was first introduced by Collins et al. in 1956.[7] They reviewed serial chest x-rays of patients with metastatic lung lesions and found that most of the tumors grew at a constant rate. By plotting the diameter of a metastatic lung lesion in two or more time intervals on a graph paper with logarithm of the cube root, it is possible to measure the rate of growth in terms of TDT (Fig. 24B-1). Subsequently, Spratt and Spratt reported on the statistical correlation between measured growth rates, TDT, and the duration of the survival of patients, in 1964.[8] According to the size and rate of growth (TDT) of the metastatic tumor, they could predict the length of the survival of each patient expressed in the number of the doubling times (Fig. 24B-2).[8] Joseph and others[9] studied metastatic lung lesions of 113 patients and reported good correlation between the TDT and the interval between resection of the primary lesion and the discovery of pulmonary metastasis (disease free interval = DFI). When patients were categorized by TDT of less than 20 days, TDT of 21 to 40 days, and TDT over 40 days, their respective 12-month survival rates were 11%, 45%, and 86%. TDT thus was found to correlate with the survival of the patients.[9]

## Graph for Estimation of Tumor Doubling Time

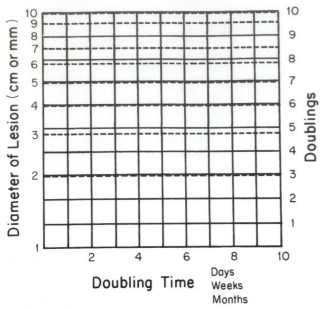

**FIGURE 24B-1.** The scale on the vertical axis on the left side is made of the logarithm of the cube root. The scale on the vertical axis on the right side is made of the cube root of 2 and the lines are drawn equidistant: An increase in the diameter of a tumor by the cube root of 2 indicates doubling of the volume of the tumor.

How to estimate the tumor doubling time (TDT): Choose a set of chest x-rays from a patient with lung lesion(s) taken at a certain time interval (days, weeks, or months). Plot the diameter of the tumor from the first x-ray in the graph on the left side (using the logarithmic scale). Then plot the diameter of the tumor from the second x-ray in the graph at the appropriate time interval (days, weeks, or months). Connect the two dots with a straight line, and read the time interval where the diagonal line crosses two adjacent equidistant lines (doubling scale = vertical axis on the right side). That time interval is the TDT.

## INDICATIONS FOR SURGERY

The following criteria are generally accepted for patients to be considered for surgical intervention[10]:

1. Controlled or controllable primary disease
2. Absence of extrapulmonary metastasis
3. Good operative risk
4. Lack of alternative therapy

Although the above conditions appear reasonable, the efficacy of the surgical therapy of metastatic lung lesions has not been proven by any prospective randomized studies. Historically, in 1939 in the United States, the first metastasectomy for solitary lung metastasis

from a renal cell carcinoma was performed. The patient survived for 23 years.[11] Marcove et al.[12] reported that there were no 5-year survivors among patients diagnosed with osteogenic sarcoma presenting with lung metastasis and no surgical treatment. These past reports are frequently cited for advocating surgical therapy.

## SURGICAL APPROACH

For the surgical procedure on the lung, posterolateral thoracotomy has been the standard approach. In the case of metastasectomy for bilateral lung lesions, either stage bilateral thoracotomies or mediansternotomy are usually utilized.[13] The advantages of the mediansternotomy are that it requires only one incision to reach both lungs and that it is reportedly less painful compared to the lateral thoracotomy. However, the mediansternotomy has the serious drawback of having limited accessibility to the posterior aspect of the lungs as well as the posterior mediastinum. Transsternal bilateral thoracotomy (clamshell incision) was reintroduced in the 1980s for thoracic organ transplantation. For this approach, both fourth intercostal spaces are entered and the sternum is transected at the same level. With this approach, the exposure of the lungs is excellent. The drawback of the clamshell incision is that the patient experiences severe postoperative pain. In one report, 7 of 10 patients required prolonged intubation due to postoperative pain.[14] In order to control the postoperative pain, institution of epidural anesthesia is essential.[15] Recently, the author's option for approach to both lungs has been simultaneous bilateral thoracotomies. However, availability of epidural anesthesia is important for smooth postoperative recovery. Recently the concept of minimally invasive surgical procedures has become popular. The feasibility of using video-assisted thoracic surgery (VATS) technology in metastasectomy was studied by a prospective clinical trial of 18 patients.[16] It was found that in 10 patients (56%), thoracoscopy failed to detect all the metastatic lung lesions to be removed. The investigators concluded that VATS might only be indicated for biopsy diagnosis of suspected metastatic lesions. Moreover, there have been reports of tumor implantation of the chest wall at the surgical scars after thoracoscopic resection of a metastatic tumor.[17] The purpose of the metastasectomy should be to remove completely all of the identified lesions yet try to preserve as much lung as possible. Intraoperatively, when the chest cavity is entered, it is carefully inspected and palpated after the lung is made atelectatic by use of a double-lumen endotracheal tube. For local resection staplers may be used; however, the use of needle tip cautery to cut out each metastatic lesion with a minimum margin of surrounding lung can be a useful technique for the removal of multiple lung lesions (Fig. 24B-3).[18] There have also been reports of using the laser for local excision of metastatic lesions.[19]

## RESULTS

The overall 5-year survival of patients who have undergone metastasectomy has been reported to be approximately 30%.[10] The postoperative survival results have been analyzed according to factors that may influence the overall outcome of patients. From the analysis, one may be able to better define the candidates for the metastasectomy.

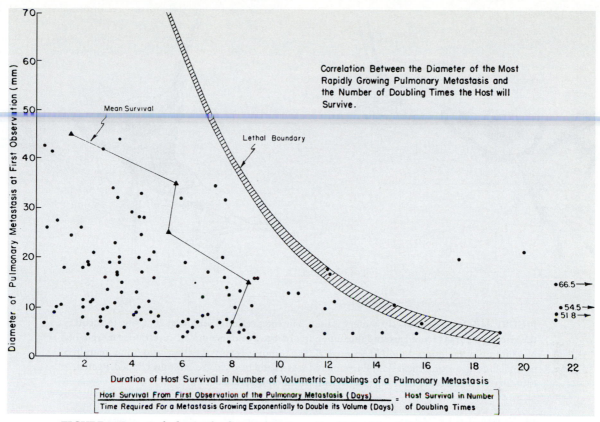

**FIGURE 24B-2.** Each dot in the figure plots the ratio obtained by dividing the TDT (days) of a pulmonary metastasis into the host survival (days) from the time the pulmonary metastases was first observed against the diameter of the metastasis at first observation. For example, a patient presenting with a lung metastasis 2 cm in diameter has a 95% chance of dying within 10.8 doubling times. (*From Spratt and Spratt: Rates of growth of pulmonary metastases and host survival. Ann Surg 159:161–171, 1964, with permission.*)

Prognostic factors are type of tumor, size, number of metastatic lesions, unilateral versus bilateral lesions, TDT, and DFI. As previously mentioned, if one assumes that the rate of growth of lung metastasis is constant, one may be able to replace TDT and DFI. Estimation of TDT requires at least one set of x-rays taken at a certain time interval before preoperative evaluation. Presently, the health care system in the United States is not centralized. Therefore, serial x-ray films for each patient are not available in one place. Consequently, it is difficult to measure TDT in most patients. It is this author's opinion that this is the reason why analysis of the TDT is missing from most of the recently published literature in the United States.

Because the natural history of each tumor is different, it may be logical to discuss the surgical management of metastatic lung tumor according to the type of primary tumor.

## SOFT TISSUE SARCOMA (TABLE 24B-1)

The overall 5-year survival rate following metastasectomy is reported to be 22% to 38%. The survival results are correlated to the DFI, TDT,

histologic grade, number of lesions found or removed, and complete resection.[20–25] Chemotherapy for soft tissue sarcoma produces response rates of up to 25%. In a retrospective study, 77 patients were found to have lung metastasis. Metastasectomy was performed in 34 patients, and 7 patients survived 4 years (21%). Chemotherapy was given to 43 patients, with 13 patients responding. Four of the responders survived 4 years (30%).[26] The authors suggest that the therapeutic benefit of effective chemotherapy may be as good as the results of the surgical therapy. It is expected that future publications on the treatment of lung metastasis from soft tissue sarcoma will describe the combined-modality approach in a prospective study design.[22]

## RENAL CELL CARCINOMA (TABLE 24B-2)

The overall 5-year survival rate of the metastasectomy has been reported to be 35.9% to 55%. The DFI, number of lesions, and complete resection of the lesion(s) correlated with better survival.[27–30]

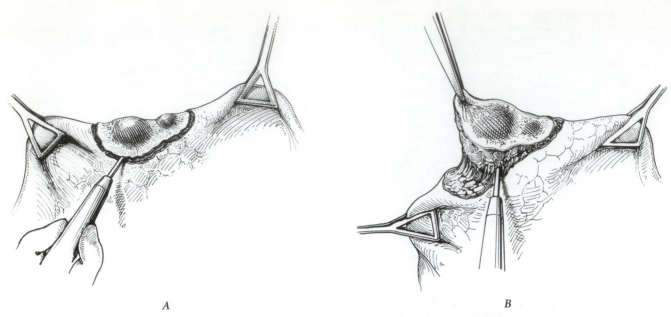

*A*                      *B*

**FIGURE 24B-3.** *A.* A needle tip cautery is used. The coagulation is set low at 20. Using the cautery, the visceral pleura is scored around the tumor. In order to avoid incomplete resection, a margin of 3 to 5 mm from the lesion should be secured. *B.* The tumor is removed with a 3- to 5-mm margin of normal lung all around the lesion. Encountered vessels and bronchi are carefully clipped, ligated, or cauterized. The defect of the lung is sewn with continuous suture of 3-0.

## COLORECTAL CARCINOMA (TABLE 24B-3)

The overall survival rate has been reported to be 24% to 43%.[31–35] Most of the investigators reported correlation between fewer lesions and complete resection to better survival. Ducreux et al.[35] reported normal carcinoembryonic antigen (CEA) level to be a good prognostic indicator. It is of interest that DFI was not found to be a significant factor in most of the reported series.

## MELANOMA (TABLE 24B-4)

The 5-year survival rate has been reported to be 14% to 25%.[36–39] Solitary metastasis and complete resection were good prognostic indicators. Generally, TDT and DFI did not influence the outcome. It is this author's opinion that melanoma may be an exception to the rule of the constant growth rate of the metastatic tumors to the lung. Metastatic melanomas may stay dormant for a long period of time, and unknown factors such as hormonal or immunologic influences may trigger a sudden rapid growth of the tumors.

## HEAD AND NECK TUMORS (TABLE 24B-5)

Five-year survival rates of 29% to 43% have been reported. Mazer et al.[40] stated that metastasis from a laryngeal primary had better survival rates when compared to other organ sites. The presence of mediastinal node metastasis was a poor prognostic indicator. Finley et al.[41] reported a solitary lesion and DFI over 2 years to be good indicators for favorable outcome. There was approximately 20% chance of finding a primary lung cancer when patients with previous history of head and neck cancer were found to have radiologically detected lung lesions.[42]

**TABLE 24B-1.** SURGICAL THERAPY OF LUNG METASTASIS FROM SOFT-TISSUE SARCOMA

| AUTHORS | NO. OF PATIENTS | 5-YR SURVIVAL RATE | SIGNIFICANT FACTORS FOR SURVIVAL |
|---|---|---|---|
| Putnam et al.[20] NCI, 1984 | 63 | 18 mo (median) | TDT, DFI, no. of lesions |
| Casson et al.[21] MDA, 1992 | 58 | 25.8% | TDT, no. of lesions, histologic grade |
| Verazin et al.[22] RPCI, 1992 | 78 | 22% | DFI, complete resection |
| Gadd et al.[23] MSK, 1993 | 65 | 23% (3 yr) | Histologic type, complete resection |
| Ueda et al.[24] Japan, 1993 | 23 | 24.8% | Histologic type, complete resection |
| Vangeel et al.[25] EORTC, 1996 | 255 | 38% | DFI, no. of lesions, histologic grade, complete resection |

ABBREVIATIONS: NCI: National Cancer Institute, MDA: MD Anderson, RPCI: Roswell Park Cancer Institute, MSK: Memorial Sloan Kettering, Japan: Osaka University, EROTC: European Organization for Research and Treatment of Cancer.

**TABLE 24B-2.** SURGICAL THERAPY OF LUNG METASTASIS FROM RENAL CELL CARCINOMA

| AUTHORS | NO. OF PATIENTS | 5-YR SURVIVAL RATE | SIGNIFICANT FACTORS FOR SURVIVAL |
|---|---|---|---|
| Pogrebniak et al.[27] NCI, 1992 | 23 | 43 mo (median) | Complete resection |
| Cerfolio et al.[28] Mayo Clinic, 1994 | 96 (48 = solitary, 48 = multiple) | 35.9% 45.6% 27%   p < .05 | DFI Solitary lesion |
| Fourquier et al.[29] France,* 1997 | 50 | 44% | Complete resection |
| Hoshi, et al.[30] Japan,† 1997 | 17 | 55% | No. of lesions |

* France: Marie Lannelongue Hospital.
† Japan: Tohoku University.

## BREAST CARCINOMA

Isolated pulmonary metastasis from breast carcinoma is uncommon. At the Mayo Clinic, 60 out of 13,502 breast cancer patients (0.4%) were found to have an isolated pulmonary metastasis. More typical in lung metastasis from breast carcinoma is the lymphangitic spread, which is a nonsurgical condition.[43] When patients with a previous history of breast carcinoma presented with discrete lung lesion(s), Casey et al.[44] reported that 52% of them were found to be primary carcinoma of the lung, and 43% were found to have metastatic breast carcinoma. After metastasectomy, a 5-year survival rate of 36% to 50% has been reported.[43–46] Solitary metastasis, DFI over 12 months, and positive estrogen receptor (ER) have been reported to be significant prognostic indicators.[43–46] McDonald et al.[43] reported that there was no difference in the survival between those with complete resection and incomplete resection. This may be explained by availability of effective nonsurgical

therapies such as hormones or chemotherapy.[43] It is this author's opinion that due to the recent development of more effective non-surgical therapy, fewer patients with lung metastasis from breast carcinoma have been considered for surgery. Thoracotomy is advised for patients with a previous history of breast carcinoma who present with a single lesion, because this may turn out to be another primary tumor.[42]

## PROSTATE CANCER

It is known that the majority of lung metastases in prostate cancer are lymphangitic and are not amenable to surgery. It was reported that solitary lung metastasis for prostatic carcinoma was seen in 11 of a total of 1290 patients.[47] In his 30 years at a cancer center, the author recalls one patient with solitary lung metastasis from prostate cancer. This patient underwent a metastasectomy but did not survive long thereafter.

## GYNECOLOGIC CANCERS

CERVIX. Of 817 patients, 50 (6%) in one series were found to have lung metastasis, but only 9 of these patients had a solitary

**TABLE 24B-3.** SURGICAL THERAPY OF LUNG METASTASIS FROM COLORECTAL CARCINOMA

| AUTHORS | NO. OF PATIENTS | 5-YR SURVIVAL RATE | SIGNIFICANT FACTORS FOR SURVIVAL |
|---|---|---|---|
| Sauter et al.[31] Ochsner clinic, 1990 | 18 (solitary = 12; multiple = 6) | 47% 19% | No. of lesions |
| Mori et al.[32] Japan,* 1991 | 35 | 38% | Solitary, size |
| McCormack et al.[33] MSK, 1992 | 144 | 40% | Complete resection |
| VanHalteren et al.[34] Netherlands,† 1995 | 38 | 43% | No. of lesions |
| Ducreux et al.[35] France,‡ 1996 | 86 | 24% | No. of lesions, complete resection, normal CEA |

* Japan = Kyushu University.
† Netherlands = Netherlands Cancer Institute.
‡ France = Institute Mutualiste Montsouris and Gustave Roussy Inst.

**TABLE 24B-4.** SURGICAL THERAPY OF LUNG METASTASIS FROM MELANOMA

| AUTHORS | NO. OF PATIENTS | 5-YR SURVIVAL RATE | SIGNIFICANT FACTORS FOR SURVIVAL |
|---|---|---|---|
| Pogrebniak et al.[36] NCI, 1988 | 49 | 13 mo (median) | Solitary |
| Wong et al.[37] UCLA, 1988 | 47 | 25% | Complete resection |
| Gorenstein et al.[38] MDA, 1991 | 56 | 25% | Lung metastasis as the first site |
| Karakousis et al.[39] RPCI, 1994 | 39 | 14% | Solitary |

**TABLE 24B-5.** SURGICAL THERAPY OF LUNG METASTASIS FROM HEAD AND NECK CANCER

| AUTHORS | NO. OF PATIENTS | 5-YR SURVIVAL RATE | SIGNIFICANT FACTORS FOR SURVIVAL | PRIMARY LUNG CANCER FOUND |
|---|---|---|---|---|
| Mazer et al.[40] MSK, 1988 | 44 | 43% | Nodal status of the primary, mediastinal metastasis | 15% |
| Finley et al.[41] RPCI, 1992 | 24 | 29% | Solitary lesion, DFI | 16% |
| Rendina et al.[42] Italy,* 1986 | 11 | — | Mostly solitary, laryngeal carcinoma | 27% |

* Italy = University of Rome.

lesion.[48] If there is no evidence of disease elsewhere, metastasectomy may possibly be recommended particularly for those patients with solitary lesions.

UTERINE CANCER. In a large series of 1665 patients, 18 (1.8%) were found to have solitary metastasis. Ten patients underwent surgery, and the median survival was 25.6%. Eight patients were treated with hormones and the median survival was 53 months.[49] There was a report from Massachusetts General Hospital of 17 patients with gynecologic tumors who underwent metastasectomy. For 9 patients with a solitary metastasis, the median survival was 64 months. There were no 5 year survivors among 8 patients with multiple metastases.[50]

## OSTEOGENIC SARCOMA (TABLE 24B-6)

Overall 5-year survival rate of 40% to 53% has been reported. Recent progress in therapy of osteogenic sarcoma is the development of the combined-modality approach in which patients are given intensive perioperative chemotherapy.[51–54] When lung metastasis is discovered after completing the initial treatment, there is no consensus of opinion on the treatment plan. Some patients receive surgery only, but some are treated also with perioperative chemotherapy.

Favorable outcome of metastasectomy was related to completeness of resection and number of lesions removed.[51–54]

## TESTICULAR TUMORS

Since the introduction of effective chemotherapy regimens in the 1970s, the surgical therapy is adjunctive therapy to chemotherapy.[55] Patients with radiologically persistent or newly developed lung or mediastinal lesions following completion of chemotherapy are candidates for surgical intervention.[56] Besides intrathoracic lesions, presence of persistent retroperitoneal adenopathy or supraclavicular adenopathy can be surgically treated by staged or simultaneous operations. Surgery is usually not advised if the levels of tumor markers such as α-fetoprotein and human chorionic gonadotropin are elevated.[57] Residual intrathoracic tumors may be low-grade neoplasms such as mature teratoma, but complete resection is required to prevent local recurrence.

## FUTURE DIRECTION IN MANAGEMENT OF LUNG METASTASIS

The combined-modality approach of perioperative chemotherapy and/or immunotherapy will probably be used in prospectively

**TABLE 24B-6.** SURGICAL THERAPY OF LUNG METASTASIS FROM OSTEOGENIC SARCOMA

| AUTHORS | NUMBER OF PATIENTS | | | 5-YR SURVIVAL RATE | SIGNIFICANT FACTORS FOR SURVIVAL |
|---|---|---|---|---|---|
| | INITIALLY TREATED | LUNG METASTASIS | RESECTED | | |
| Putnam et al.[51] NCI, 1983 | 80 | 43 | 39 | 40% | DFI, complete resection, no. of lesions |
| Goorin et al.[52] Boston,* 1984 | 93 | 32 | 26 | 40% | Complete resection, no. of lesions |
| Tabone et al.[53] France,† 1994 | 137 | | 20 | 40% (3 yr) | Complete resection |
| Ward et al.[54] UCLA, 1994 | 111 | | 36 | 53% | Complete resection, effective chemotherapy |

* Boston = Dana Farber Institute.
† France = Gustave Roussy Institute.

designed clinical trials. There have been reports of preclinical and clinical studies of regional infusion chemotherapy. When more effective chemotherapeutic or biologic agents are available such approach may produce interesting results.[58]

## REFERENCES

1. VIADANA E et al: Cascade spread of blood-borne metastases in solid and non-solid cancers of humans, in *Pulmonary Metastasis,* Weiss L, Gilbert HA (eds). Boston, GK Hall, 1978, pp 142–167.

2. ERMERT L et al: Computer-assisted morphometry of the intracapillary leukocyte pool in the rabbit lung. Cell Tissue Res 271:469, 1993.

3. CHOKSI LB et al: The surgical management of solitary pulmonary metastases. Surg Gynecol Obstet 134:479, 1972.

4. SCHULTZ V et al: Invasive-bioptic diagnosis of pulmonary metastases. Contrib Oncol 30:42, 1988.

5. HRUBAN RH, MARSH BR: Endobronchial metastasis. J Thorac Cardiovasc Surg 106:537, 1993.

6. PASS HI et al: Detection of pulmonary metastases in patients with osteogenic and soft tissue sarcomas: The superiority of CT scans compared with conventional linear tomograms using dynamic analysis. J Clin Oncol 3:1261, 1985.

7. COLLINS VP et al: Observations on growth rates of human tumors. AJR 76:988, 1956.

8. SPRATT JS, SPRATT TL: Rate of growth of pulmonary metastases and host survival. Ann Surg 159:161, 1964.

9. JOSEPH WL et al: Prognostic significance of tumor doubling time in evaluating operability in pulmonary metastatic disease. J Thorac Cardiovasc Surg 61:23, 1971.

10. McCORMACK P, MARTINI N: The changing role of surgery for pulmonary metastases. Ann Thorac Surg 23:139, 1979.

11. BARNEY JD, CHURCHILL EJ: Adenocarcinoma of the kidney with metastasis to the lung. J Urol 42:269, 1939.

12. MARCOVE RC et al: Osteogenic sarcoma under the age of twenty-one: A review of one hundred and forty five operative cases. J Bone Joint Surg 52-A: 411, 1970.

13. JOHNSTON MR: Median sternotomy for resection of pulmonary metastasis. J Thorac Cardiovasc Surg 85:516, 1983.

14. SHIMIZU N et al: Transsternal thoracotomy for bilateral pulmonary metastasis. J Surg Oncol 50:105, 1995.

15. REEVES JG et al: Anesthesia and supportive care for cardiothoracic surgery, in *Surgery of the Chest,* 6th ed, Sabiston DC Jr, Spencer FC (eds). Philadelphia, WB Saunders, 1995, pp 117–152.

16. McCORMACK PM et al: Role of video-assisted thoracic surgery in the treatment of pulmonary metastases: Results of a prospective trial. Ann Thorac Surg 62:213, 1996.

17. WALSH GL, NESBITT JC: Tumor implants after thoracoscopic resection of a metastatic sarcoma. Ann Thorac Surg 59:215, 1995.

18. TAKITA H: Surgery for cancer of the lung, in *Atlas of Surgical Oncology,* Bland KI et al (eds). Philadelphia, WB Saunders, 1995, pp 259–282.

19. SALTZMAN DA et al: Aggressive metastasectomy for pulmonic sarcomatous metastases: A follow-up study. Am J Surg 166:543, 1993.

20. PUTNAM JB Jr et al: Analysis of prognostic factors in patients undergoing resection of pulmonary metastases from soft tissue sarcomas. J Thorac Cardiovasc Surg 87:260, 1984.

21. CASSON AG et al: Five-year survival after pulmonary metastasectomy for adult soft tissue sarcoma. Cancer 69:662, 1992.

22. VERAZIN GT et al: Resection of lung metastases from soft tissue sarcomas: A multivariate analysis. Arch Surg 127:1407, 1992.

23. GADD MA et al: Development and treatment of pulmonary metastases in adult patients with extremity soft tissue sarcoma. Ann Surg 218:705, 1993.

24. UEDA T et al: Aggressive pulmonary metastasectomy for soft tissue sarcoma. Cancer 72:1919, 1993.

25. VANGEEL AN et al: Surgical treatment of lung metastases: The European Organization for Research and Treatment of Cancer—Soft Tissue and Bone Sarcoma Group study of 255 Patients. Cancer 77:675, 1996.

26. MENTZER SJ et al: Selected benefit of Thoracotomy and Chemotherapy for sarcoma metastatic to the lung. J Surg Oncol 53:54, 1993.

27. POGREBNIAK HW et al: Renal cell carcinoma: Resection of solitary and multiple metastases. Ann Thorac Surg 54:33, 1992.

28. CERFOLIO RJ et al: Pulmonary resection of metastatic renal cell carcinoma. Ann Thorac Surg 57:339, 1994.

29. FOURQUIER P et al: Lung Metastases of renal cell carcinoma: Results of surgical resection. Eur J Cardiothorac Surg 11:17, 1997.

30. HOSHI S et al: Study on the surgical treatment for pulmonary metastasis from renal cell carcinoma. Nippon Hinyokika Gakkai Zasshi 88:46, 1997.

31. SAUTER ER et al: Improved survival after pulmonary resection of metastatic colorectal carcinoma. J Surg Oncol 43:135, 1990.

32. MORI M et al: Surgical resection of pulmonary metastases from colorectal adenocarcinoma: special reference to repeat pulmonary resections. Arch Surg 126:1297, 1991.

33. McCORMACK PM et al: Lung resection for colorectal metastases: 10 year results. Arch Surg 127:1403, 1992.

34. VAN HALTEREN HK et al: Pulmonary resection for metastases of colorectal origin. Chest 107:1526, 1995.

35. DUCREUX GP et al: Surgery for lung metastases from colorectal cancer: Analysis of prognostic factors. J Clin Oncol 14:2047, 1996.

36. POGREBNIAK HW et al: Resection of pulmonary metastases from malignant melanoma: Results of a 16-year experience. Ann Thorac Surg 46:20, 1988.

37. WONG JH et al: Surgical resection for metastatic melanoma to the lung. Arch Surg 123:1091, 1988.

38. GORENSTEIN LA et al: Improved survival after resection of pulmonary metastases from malignant melanoma. Ann Thorac Surg 52:204, 1991.

39. KARAKOUSIS CP et al: Metastasectomy in malignant melanoma. Surgery 115:295, 1994.

40. MAZER TM et al: Resection of pulmonary metastases from squamous carcinoma of the head and neck. Am J Surg 156:238, 1988.

41. FINLEY RK et al: Results of surgical resection of pulmonary metastases of squamous cell carcinoma of the head and neck. Am J Surg 164:594, 1992.

42. RENDINA EA et al: Pulmonary resection for metastatic laryngeal carcinoma. J Thorac Cardiovasc Surg 92:114, 1986.

43. McDONALD ML et al: Pulmonary resection for metastatic breast cancer. Ann Thorac Surg 58:1599, 1994.

44. CASEY JJ et al: The solitary pulmonary nodule in the patient with breast cancer. Surgery 96:801, 1984.

45. LANZA LA et al: Long-term survival after resection of pulmonary metastases from carcinoma of the breast. Ann Thorac Surg 54:244, 1992.

46. STAREN ED et al: Pulmonary resection for metastatic breast cancer. Arch Surg 127:1282, 1992.

47. Fobozzi SJ et al: Pulmonary metastases from prostate cancer. Cancer 75:2706, 1995.

48. Imachi M et al: Pulmonary metastasis from carcinoma of the uterine cervix. Gynecol Oncol 33:189, 1989.

49. Bouros D et al: Natural history of patients with pulmonary metastases from uterine cancer. Cancer 78:441, 1996.

50. Fuller AF et al: Pulmonary resection for metastases from gynecologic cancers: Massachusetts General Hospital Experience. Gynecol Oncol 22:174, 1985.

51. Putnam JB Jr et al: Survival following aggressive resection of pulmonary metastases from osteogenic sarcoma: Analysis of prognostic factors. Ann Thorac Surg 36:516, 1983.

52. Goorin AM et al: Prognostic significance of complete surgical resection of pulmonary metastases in patients with osteogenic sarcoma: Analysis of 32 patients. J Clin Oncol 2:425, 1984.

53. Tabone MD et al: Osteosarcoma recurrence in pediatric patients previously treated with intensive chemotherapy. J Clin Oncol 12:2614, 1994.

54. Ward WG et al: Pulmonary metastases of stage IIB extremity osteosarcoma and subsequent pulmonary metastases. J Clin Oncol 12:1849, 1994.

55. Merrin C et al: Combination radical surgery and multiple sequential chemotherapy for the treatment of advanced carcinoma of the testis. Cancer 37:20, 1976.

56. Anyanwu E et al: Pulmonary metastasectomy as secondary treatment for testicular tumors. Ann Thorac Surg 57:1222,1994.

57. Bosl GJ et al: Cancer of the testis, in Cancer, Principle and Practice of Oncology, 5th ed, Devita VT Jr et al (eds). Philadelphia, Lippincott-Raven, 1997, pp 1397–1425.

58. Pass HI et al: Isolated perfusion with tumor necrosis factor for pulmonary metastases. Ann Thorac Surg 61:1609, 1996.

# 24C / HEPATIC METASTASES

*David E. Rivadeneira and John M. Daly*

## INTRODUCTION

The liver is the second most common site of metastatic disease, exceeded only by the lymph nodes, and is reported to occur in 25% to 40% of all cancer patients succumbing to their disease.[1] Recent advances in imaging techniques, anesthetic management, better knowledge of liver anatomy, improved results of operative resection, regional anticancer therapies, and tumor immunology have established measurable benefits for some highly selected patients with metastatic disease to the liver. This disease process represents a challenging and often difficult clinical decision process for surgeons, and, therefore, it is imperative for surgeons to become familiar with current therapies available for these patients.

Metastatic colorectal cancer remains the major metastatic disease process in which liver-specific treatment is performed. Colorectal cancer develops in more than 140,000 patients annually and is the third leading cause of cancer deaths in both men and women in the United States with more than 55,000 deaths per year.[2] Hepatic metastases are present in 15% to 25% of patients at the time of diagnosis (synchronous) of colorectal cancer and another 25% to 50% will develop liver metastases within 3 years following resection of the primary tumor (metachronous).[3,4]

## NATURAL HISTORY OF METASTATIC COLORECTAL CANCER TO LIVER

In order to attempt any therapeutic intervention in patients with colorectal liver metastases, one must first understand the natural history of the disease. The median survival of untreated patients with liver metastases from colorectal cancer is usually less than 2 years, and reports indicate less than 1 year when extensive hepatic metastases are present.

Survival is related to extent of tumor burden in the liver. Several series have reported the natural history of patients with metastatic disease to the liver (Table 24C-1). Wood et al.,[5] in a retrospective analysis of 113 patients with untreated colorectal liver metastasis, demonstrated a 6% 1-year survival rate in patients with extensive liver spread compared to 27% in those with disease limited to a segment or lobe, and 60% in patients with a solitary lesion. There were no 5-year survivors in the unresected group of patients. Although these data indicate that solitary lesions or unilobar disease appear to have a better prognosis, the 5-year survival rate for untreated colorectal hepatic metastases, irrespective of the degree of liver involvement, was consistently less than 3% for most studies and survival beyond 5 years is rare.

## RESECTION OF COLORECTAL LIVER METASTASES

The dismal outcome of patients with untreated colorectal liver metastases has served as a yardstick to assess and compare other therapies. The benefit of surgical resection has been addressed by several retrospective, case-controlled studies. Wilson and Adson[6] reported survival rates in 60 patients that underwent resection compared to 60 patients with biopsy only and no resection. Both patient groups were matched with respect to age, sex, and size and number of metastatic lesions. The authors reported no 5-year survivors in the biopsy-only group, compared to a 25% survival rate in the resection group. More recent series have demonstrated a slightly higher 5-year survival rate after liver resection for metastatic colorectal metastases (Table 24C-2).

Scheele et al.[7] compared 183 patients who had resection of liver metastasis to 62 patients that did not have resection but were deemed resectable. Once again, there were no 5-year survivors in the unresected group compared to an actuarial 5-year survival rate of 38% in the resected group. In a large multi-institutional study of 859 patients undergoing hepatic resection for colorectal metastases, a 33% 5-year survival rate was reported. Therefore, during the last 15 to 20 years, hepatic resection has become the widely accepted treatment of choice in selected patients with liver metastases, with numerous large series reporting a postresection 5-year survival rate in the range of 25% to 40%. These findings render a prospective study of surgical resection versus no treatment extremely difficult due to the issue of potentially withholding significant benefit and possible cure for a subgroup of patients. Under these circumstances, with many centers reporting a less than 5% operative mortality rate with major liver resections, surgery is the mainstay therapy for potentially resectable liver metastases from colorectal primaries.

## PREDICTIVE FACTORS

There is little disagreement regarding the benefit of hepatic resection for selected patients. Determining the subset of patients that may benefit from resection remains an important decision.

**TABLE 24C-1.** NATURAL HISTORY OF LIVER METASTASES FROM COLORECTAL CANCER

| REFERENCE | NO. OF PATIENTS | METASTATIC BURDEN | MEDIAN SURVIVAL TIME, MO. | SURVIVAL RATE (%) | | |
|---|---|---|---|---|---|---|
| | | | | 1 YR | 3 YR | 5 YR |
| Wood et al.[5] | 113 | Unilobar and bilobar | 6.6[†] | 15 | 3 | 1 |
| Wanebo et al.[10] | 18 | Unilobar | 19 | 72 | 17 | 0 |
| Bengmark & Hafstrom[3] | 40 | Unilobar and bilobar | 5.7[†] | * | 0 | 0 |
| Bengtsson et al.[82] | 25 | Unilobar and bilobar | 4.5[†] | 12 | 0 | 0 |
| Scheele et al.[7] | 62 | Unilobar and bilobar | 14 | * | * | * |

\* Data not available.
† Represents mean survival time.

The extent of metastatic disease is of paramount importance in evaluating each patient. Concomitant extrahepatic metastases, including positive celiac or periportal lymph nodes is usually considered a contraindication to surgical resection. Inability to resect all gross disease with at least 1 cm of clear margin or if the extent of resection is incompatible with life are generally considered absolute contraindications (Table 24C-3).

Multivariate analysis of various prognostic factors allows for potential identification of patients that will benefit the most from surgery and those in which a procedure may be avoided. Several large studies[8–13] have identified factors with prognostic significance, which include the disease-free interval from primary tumor excision to appearance of metastases, number and size of liver metastases, stage of the primary colorectal carcinoma, elevated preoperative serum carcinoembryonic antigen (CEA) levels, the presence of extrahepatic disease, and involvement of the margin of resection (Table 24C-4).

An association between primary tumor stage and survival has been demonstrated in several studies.[8,9,14] The involvement of lymph nodes with the primary tumor (Duke's C) is associated with a poorer outcome compared to negative nodal status (Duke's B). A multiinstitutional, retrospective study by Hughes et al.[14] reported 47% and 23% 5-year survival rates for patients with node-negative and node-

positive primary colorectal tumors, respectively. However, this association should not preclude liver resection in those patients with node-positive primary tumors.

Although tumor size has not been shown conclusively to affect survival, there appears to be a well-established association with the number of liver metastases. Several reports demonstrated a reduced 5-year survival rate for patients with three or more lesions. A retrospective analysis of 244 patients undergoing curative hepatic resection for colorectal carcinoma showed that number of metastases (three or more lesions) was one of three statistically significant prognosticators. The other two factors were elevated preoperative serum CEA levels and surgical margin.[12]

Additional studies have shown that the presence of satellite nodules, that is, lesions less than 1 cm diameter within 1 cm of the major metastatic deposit, is a poor prognostic sign. Scheele et al.[7] reported 5-year survival rates of 17% and 45% in patients with and without satellite lesions, respectively. In another study an 11% 5-year survival rate was demonstrated in patients with satellite lesions compared to 30% for patients with a solitary lesion.[15]

The pathologic margin of resection is clearly an important prognostic factor for patients undergoing liver resection for colorectal carcinoma. As demonstrated by the Gastrointestinal Study Group (GITSG),[16] noncurative (positive margin) resection provides no benefit to asymptomatic patients, since unresectable and noncurative resection groups had similar survival rates of 17 and 21 months, respectively. Cady et al.[12] showed that surgical margin was the only

**TABLE 24C-2.** RESULTS OF HEPATIC RESECTION FOR METASTATIC COLORECTAL CANCER

| REFERENCE | YEAR | NO. OF PATIENTS | 5-YR SURVIVAL RATE, % |
|---|---|---|---|
| Cady et al.[12] | 1998 | 244 | 30 |
| Elias et al.[44] | 1998 | 136 | 28 |
| Fong et al.[8] | 1997 | 456 | 38 |
| Jamison et al.[13] | 1997 | 280 | 27 |
| Scheele et al.[83] | 1996 | 376 | 39 |
| Gozzetti et al.[45] | 1994 | 108 | 28 |
| Gayowski et al.[29] | 1994 | 204 | 32 |
| Rosen et al.[15] | 1992 | 280 | 25 |
| Nordlinger et al.[9]* | 1992 | 1818 | 26 |
| Doci et al.[28] | 1991 | 100 | 30 |
| Hughes et al.[84]* | 1988 | 859 | 33 |

\* Represents multi-institutional collected series.

**TABLE 24C-3.** ABSOLUTE CONTRAINDICATIONS TO RESECTION OF COLORECTAL LIVER METASTASES

Inability to resect all gross metastases (R0 resection) with at least 1 cm of margin.
*Exceptions:* Symptomatic palliation in patients with neuroendocrine tumors.

Extrahepatic metastases.
*Exceptions:* Patients with local recurrence, direct invasion of adjacent structures, such as the diaphragm, and in a subset of patients with pulmonary metastases.

Lymph node metastases to liver hilum.

**TABLE 24C-4.** FACTORS AFFECTING SURVIVAL AFTER RESECTION OF LIVER METASTASES

| REFERENCE | NO. OF PATIENTS | NO. OF METASTASES | SIZE OF METASTASES | RESECTION MARGIN | EXTRA HEPATIC DISEASE | PRE-OP CEA LEVEL |
|---|---|---|---|---|---|---|
| Fong et al.[8] | 456 | ‡ | ‡ | ‡ | ‡ | ‡ |
| Nordlinger et al.[9]* | 1818 | ‡ | ‡ | ‡ | ‡ | ‡ |
| Wanebo et al.[10] | 74 | ‡ | § | † | † | § |
| Hughes et al.[84]* | 859 | † | ‡ | § | § | † |
| Elias et al.[44] | 269 | § | † | ‡ | § | † |
| Cady et al.[12] | 244 | ‡ | § | ‡ | † | ‡ |
| Jamison et al.[13] | 280 | § | § | § | ‡ | § |

\* Represents multi-institutional collected series.
† Data not available.
‡ Represents significant factor affecting survival.
§ Represents not a significant factor affecting survival.

technical variable that had a statistically significant impact on survival. This study showed 30% of the selected patients undergoing curative hepatic resection with an adequate surgical margin of 1 cm or more were disease-free at 5 years, in comparison to 10% for patients with a positive margin.

Another possible predictor of adverse outcome has been extremely elevated preoperative serum CEA levels.[8,9,12,17] In a retrospective study of 456 patients undergoing liver resection for colorectal metastases at the Memorial Sloan-Kettering Cancer Center, Fong et al.[8] demonstrated that a circulating CEA level greater than 200 ng/mL was associated with a significantly worse outcome than patients with less than 200 ng/mL. Similar findings have been demonstrated by several others in which there were no long-term disease-free survivors in patients with CEA levels greater than 200 ng/mL.[9,12] Although extremely elevated CEA levels appear to be a prognostic indicator, the degree of elevation should not be an absolute contraindication to resection.

Approximately 15% to 25% of patients undergoing laparotomy for resection of the primary colorectal carcinoma will demonstrate synchronous liver metastases.[3,4] These patients often pose a difficult decision-making problem in regard to the timing and extent of resection. Although simultaneous large-bowel and liver resections have been performed with acceptable results, no survival advantage has been demonstrated versus delayed hepatic resection. Therefore, most surgeons recommend delaying the liver resection for 6 to 8 weeks after the primary resection. This time period allows for an extensive diagnostic evaluation for additional metastatic lesions.

As mentioned before, the presence of extrahepatic metastatic disease is usually a contraindication to liver resection. An exception to the no resection rule for patients with extrahepatic metastases may be a particular subset of highly selected patients with limited, resectable pulmonary and hepatic metastases.

The lung represents the next most likely site, after the liver, of metastatic disease. It is estimated that pulmonary metastases will develop in 10% of patients with colorectal carcinoma at some time in the course of their disease.[18] From studies of resectable pulmonary-only metastases isolated to the lungs, a 5-year survival rate of 20% to 43% and a probability of 10-year survival of 20% have been demonstrated.[19–22] These encouraging results have led some inves-

tigators to aggressive resection of metastatic disease isolated to the lung and liver. Gough et al.[23] described the Mayo Clinic experience with nine patients who underwent surgery for liver and lung colorectal metastases and reported a median survival time of 27 months after completion of surgery.

A retrospective series of 33 patients that underwent pulmonary and hepatic resections for colorectal metastases showed a median survival of 25 months. In addition, they demonstrated that patients with synchronous hepatic and pulmonary metastases had a worse prognosis than those with metachronous metastases.[24]

Murata et al.[25] reported on 17 patients who underwent resection of pulmonary metastases after resection of hepatic metastases with a median survival time of 31 months. In addition, the authors reported 10 patients who underwent simultaneous pulmonary and hepatic resections for metastatic disease with a median survival time of 24 months. They showed that the time of appearance of hepatic or pulmonary metastases and the distribution of pulmonary lesions were independently significant prognostic factors influencing survival. Patients with metachronous hepatic or pulmonary lesions or unilateral pulmonary metastases had a longer survival.

Regnard and colleagues[26] reported a retrospective study of patients undergoing pulmonary resection following hepatic resection for colorectal metastatic disease. In 43 patients studied there were no reported operative deaths and a median survival of 19 months was observed. The authors also noted that both elevated prethoracotomy serum CEA levels and an increased number of pulmonary resections were significant poor prognostic indicators. The interval time between hepatic and pulmonary resections for metastatic disease was shown to be a borderline significant prognostic factor, particularly when the interval was more than 36 months.

It is clear that only a highly selected group of patients with combined hepatic and pulmonary metastases from colorectal cancer should be considered for surgical resection.

Based on current information, specific criteria for selection of appropriate surgical candidates include patients with adequate pulmonary function, the absence of poor clinical prognostic factors, and no additional distant metastases. Poor candidates include patients with synchronous lesions, a short latency period, high CEA levels, and those with more than four lesions and a low probability of complete resection.

**TABLE 24C-5. STAGING SYSTEM LIVER METASTASES**[29]

| STAGE I | mT1 | N0 | M0 |
|---|---|---|---|
| Stage II | mT2 | N0 | M0 |
| Stage III | mT3 | N0 | M0 |
| Stage IVa | mT4 | N0 | M0 |
| Stage IVb | Any mT | N1 | M0, M1 |
| | | N0, N1 | M1 |

mT1 = Solitary ≤2 cm.
mT2 = Solitary >2 cm, or multiple ≤2 cm unilobar.
mT3 = Multiple >2 cm, unilobar.
mT4 = Invasion of major branch of portal or hepatic veins or bile duct, and/or bilobar.
N1 = Positive abdominal lymph node.
M1 = Extrahepatic metastases or direct invasion to adjacent organs.

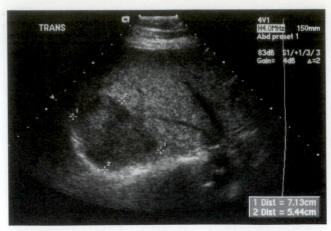

**FIGURE 24C-1.** Transabdominal ultrasound. Large colorectal metastases in segments 7 and 8.

It is evident that the extent of metastatic liver involvement is crucial to patient survival and therefore accurate staging of disease is essential to successful surgical intervention. There is no single universally accepted staging system for colorectal liver metastases, although several have been proposed.[27–29] Gayowski et al.[29] have proposed a staging system that is a modification from the International Union Against Cancer (UICC) and The American Joint Committee on Cancer (AJCC) recommendations for primary liver tumors. This system classifies patients in stages I to IV according to number and size of metastatic tumors, extent of distribution, and the presence or absence of extrahepatic disease (Table 24C-5).

## PREOPERATIVE EVALUATION

The preoperative diagnostic evaluation must address the primary tumor site, the extent of hepatic involvement, and the extent of extrahepatic metastatic disease.

Most patients found to have metastatic disease to the liver from a colorectal primary are asymptomatic. Those patients that present with abdominal pain, anorexia, and a feeling of fullness are usually advanced in their disease. Hepatomegaly, jaundice, or ascites are extremely poor late signs and indicate massive replacement of liver with tumor.

Laboratory tests may provide an indication of metastatic liver involvement. Levels of serum alkaline phosphatase, γ-glutamyl transferase, lactate dehydrogenase (LDH), and serum CEA levels have been reported to be elevated in patients with liver metastases. The best initial laboratory test to indicate liver involvement is serum alkaline phosphatase and γ-glutamyl transferase, with a reported 90% sensitivity and 93% specificity.[30] Several reports have shown that serum CEA levels are elevated in patients with colorectal liver metastases.[12,30–32] Sugerbaker[32] has reported that serum CEA are elevated in 80% to 90% of patients with hepatic metastases.

Careful preoperative selection of patients using imaging modalities is crucial to avoid unnecessary surgical explorations. Routine testing includes bidirectional chest radiographs, abdominal and pelvic dynamic computed tomography (CT) with detailed examination of the liver, and intraoperative ultrasonography. Additional studies may include CT arterial portography (CTAP), magnetic resonance imaging (MRI), and positron emission tomography (PET) scans.

Transabdominal ultrasound has a limited use as a preoperative imaging modality in patients with suspected liver metastases. It is extremely user-dependent and difficult to perform in obese patients and those with ascites. Its use is predominantly in patients with large lesions and to differentiate cystic from solid (Fig. 24C-1). In addition, transabdominal ultrasound with the addition of doppler modality may be used in patients with questionable arterial and venous flow dynamics.

The use of CT has advanced our ability to detect hepatic lesions in patients with colorectal metastases. The reported sensitivity of contrast-enhanced incremental CT for detecting hepatic lesions ranges from 38% to 84%, with most studies reporting a sensitivity between 60% and 75%.[33–36] The sensitivity of incremental CT for lesions less than 1 cm in diameter declines dramatically to rates of 0% to 56%.[37] The relatively low sensitivity of IV contrast-enhanced incremental CT for detecting hepatic tumors has led to the development of other contrast-enhanced techniques, such as CT arterial portography (CTAP). The rationale for CTAP is based on the principle that the arterial blood supply to hepatic tumors is provided mainly by the hepatic artery, not by the portal system. Therefore, contrast material infused to the liver through the vein, bypassing the systemic circulation, will identify tumors as hypodense lesions, whereas increased attenuation indicates normal liver (Fig. 24C-2). Reported sensitivities for detection of hepatic neoplasms range from 78% to 94% and have made it the gold standard for preoperative imaging before hepatic tumor resection.[34,38] Major limitations include a high false-positive rate, which is reported to occur in 13% to 15% of patients, and complications from invasive arterial instrumentation.

Several reports indicate that contrast-enhanced helical or dynamic CT scans may be superior or equal to results from CTAP. Kuszyk et al.[39] demonstrated an overall sensitivity of 81% in 21

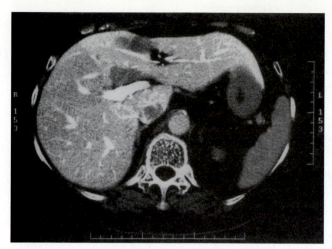

**FIGURE 24C-2.** Computer tomography with arterial portography (CTAP). Low attenuation mass in segment 6 and 8.

patients with hepatic tumors undergoing portal vein phase contrast-enhanced helical CT. The authors reported a false-positive rate of 4% in this study. In addition they demonstrate a substantial cost savings with helical CT. They report the cost of a contrast-enhanced liver CT at their institution is approximately $600 compared to $4600 for the CTAP, not including the cost associated with hospitalization for one day or the management of complications associated with arterial canalization. Therefore, initial studies demonstrate contrast-enhanced helical CT scans provide adequate sensitivity with a lower false-positive rate at eight times less expense than CTAP (Fig. 24C-3). Additional prospective studies are needed to fully appreciate these differences.

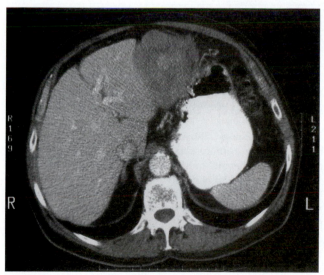

**FIGURE 24C-3.** Spiral CT. Large colorectal metastases to the left hepatic lobe.

The use of routine chest CT for the detection of extrahepatic disease appears to be unwarranted. Povoski and colleagues[40] examined 100 patients with known colorectal hepatic metastases undergoing chest CT after a normal chest radiograph. They reported 11 patients with positive chest CT findings, of which 4 patients had malignant disease (3 metastatic colorectal cancers and one primary lung cancer). This translates into a positive yield of 4% and a positive predictive value of 36% for chest CT. Therefore, chest CT only minimally improved detection of malignant lesions of the lung over conventional chest radiograph and should not be used routinely as a screening modality in patients referred with potentially resectable hepatic colorectal metastases. A chest CT and further investigations are needed if a chest x-ray is abnormal, as demonstrated in the treatment algorithm (Fig. 24C-4).

More recent radiologic modalities employed for the evaluation of disease extent include positron emission tomography (PET). PET scan is a noninvasive imaging technique allowing direct evaluation of cellular glucose metabolism using $^{18}$F-labeled fluorodeoxyglucose (FDG) as a tracer. The principle of this imaging technique is based on malignant cells possessing a relatively low level of glucose-6-phosphatase, which leads to accumulation and trapping of FDG intracellularly, allowing for visualization of increased uptake compared to normal cells (Fig. 24C-5).

Reports have suggested greater sensitivity of PET over conventional imaging in detecting occult hepatic and extrahepatic disease.[41,42] Delbeke et al.[43] reported a prospective blinded comparison of 110 patients undergoing PET scan evaluation after documented 1-cm or larger hepatic lesions as determined by CT scan. They demonstrated that 66 of 66 patients (100%) with metastatic tumors in the liver, either from colorectal carcinomas or sarcoma primaries, had increased accumulation of FDG in tumor areas compared to normal surrounding tissue.

The use of FDG PET appears particularly useful in identifying metastases in patients with recurrent colorectal carcinoma with elevated plasma CEA levels and normal or equivocal CT scans. In a metaanalysis of 378 patients from seven studies, the PET scan has led to a 27% detection of unsuspected metastases and change in management in 37% of patients.[43] Although promising, PET remains a less available and more expensive radiologic modality in the detection of colorectal metastases to the liver. In addition, its capability to identify lesions smaller than 1 cm remains unanswered. Therefore the use of PET must be thought of as investigational at this time.

The preoperative diagnostic evaluation must be followed up with a thorough intraoperative assessment. Intraoperative ultrasound has led to improvements in determining the resectability of liver tumors, and conservation of liver tissue during resection. After inspection and palpation, the use of intraoperative ultrasound is used to systematically scan the liver. It allows for safer resections and needle biopsies by delineating better anatomic structures. In addition to the detection of occult metastases it provides an assessment of freezing tissue planes during cryoablation (discussed later in this chapter).

Occult metastases can be identified in approximately 10% to 15% of patients who are evaluated with intraoperative sonography.[36] Intraoperative ultrasonography provides a significantly higher sensitivity than preoperative transabdominal ultrasonography, CT,

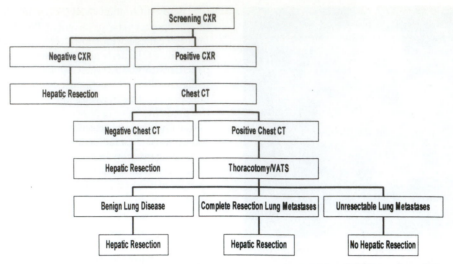

**FIGURE 24C-4.** Treatment algorithm for treatment of chest CT in patients evaluated for hepatic colorectal metastases. (Reproduced with permission from Povosky SP et al: Role of chest CT in patients with negative x-rays referred for hepatic colorectal metastases. Ann Surg Oncol 5:9–15, 1998.)

or surgical exploration with manual palpation in detecting liver metastases from colorectal primaries.[34,36,38] Several studies addressing the sensitivity of the more common radiologic techniques for detection of metastatic liver involvement are listed in Table 24C-6.

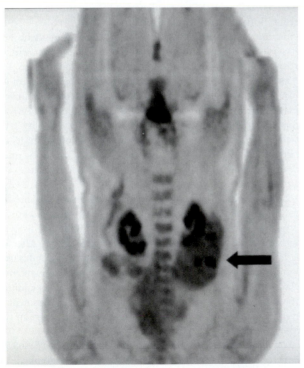

**FIGURE 24C-5.** Positron emission tomography (PET). Multiple colorectal metastases in the liver (arrow).

**TABLE 24C-6.** SENSITIVITIES OF COMMONLY USED IMAGING TECHNIQUES IN DETECTING LIVER METASTASES

| REFERENCE | TUS, % | CT, % | CTAP, % | MRI, % | IOUS, % |
|---|---|---|---|---|---|
| Moran et al.[38] | 56 | * | 95 | * | 98 |
| Hagspiel et al.[35] | 39 | 50 | * | 56 | 80 |
| Soyer et al.[34] | 67 | 72 | 89 | * | 96 |
| Nelson et al.[85] | * | 66 | 85 | 64 | * |
| Yamaguchi et al.[37] | 58 | 56 | 86 | * | * |
| Charnley et al.[36] | 35 | 70 | * | * | 92 |

* Data not available.
ABBREVIATIONS: TUS = transabdominal ultrasound; CT = computed tomography; CTAP = CT arterial portography; MRI = magnetic resonance image; IOUS = intraoperative US.

## PERIOPERATIVE MORBIDITY AND MORTALITY

Advances in radiologic assessment of liver anatomy, resection techniques, and anesthetic care and monitoring have translated into decreasing perioperative morbidity and mortality rates.

The morbidity and mortality rates from several large series in patients undergoing hepatic resection for colorectal metastases are included in Table 24C-7. In a series of 456 consecutive hepatic resections, Fong et al.[8] reported an overall perioperative mortality rate of less than 3% with a median hospital stay of 12 days. Patients who underwent a lobectomy or greater resection had a statistically significant longer hospital stay (13 days) and a higher 30-day mortality rate (4.6%) compared to patients undergoing less than a lobectomy (11 days and 0.5% mortality respectively).

Cady et al.[12] reported a 3.6% perioperative mortality rate in 244 patients undergoing hepatic resections. These included seven

**TABLE 24C-7.** PERIOPERATIVE MORTALITY AND MORBIDITY RATES OF LIVER RESECTION FOR COLORECTAL METASTASES

| REFERENCE | YEAR | PERIOD | NO. OF PATIENTS | MORTALITY RATE | MORBIDITY RATE |
|---|---|---|---|---|---|
| Elias et al.[44] | 1998 | 1984–1996 | 136 | 1.5% | — |
| Cady et al.[12] | 1998 | 1988–1996 | 244 | 3.6% | 7.3% |
| Fong et al.[8] | 1997 | 1985–1991 | 456 | 2.8% | 24% |
| Scheele et al.[83] | 1996 | 1960–1993 | 471 | 4.5% | 16% |
| | | 1990–1993 | 155 | 2.6% | 7% |
| Wanebo et al.[10] | 1996 | 1978–1994 | 74 | 7%* | 38% |
| Rees et al.[46] | 1996 | 1986–1995 | 150 | 0.7% | 23% |
| Gozzetti et al.[45] | 1994 | 1981–1991 | 108 | 0.9% | 21.4% |
| Steele et al.[16] | 1991 | 1984–1988 | 150 | 2.7% | 13% |

* Sixty-day mortality rate.

deaths after lobectomy, two deaths after segmentectomy, and no deaths after extended resections. The majority of deaths occur from perioperative hemorrhage, infection, or hepatic failure. Although significant hemorrhage is rare, occurring in 1% to 3% of patients, it does constitute a major cause of mortality. The reported complication rates range from 10% to 30% in most series.[8,12,44–46] They include complications common to all large abdominal operations including cardiovascular, pulmonary, and infectious processes. Pulmonary complications, which are more frequent, are secondary to the large abdominal incision and formation of sympathetic postoperative pleural effusions. Symptomatic pleural effusions necessitating drainage occur in 5% to 10% of patients and pneumonia occurs in 5% to 22% of postoperative patients.

Complications specific to hepatic resection include liver failure, biliary fistula, and perihepatic abscess. Hepatic failure develops in patients in whom the remaining liver tissue is insufficient to sustain life. This occurs in a reported 3% to 8% of patients undergoing major resections. Bile leak and biliary fistula occur in 2% to 5%, and perihepatic abscesses occur in 2% to 10% of patients.

## REPEAT HEPATIC RESECTION FOR RECURRENT COLORECTAL METASTASES

The main cause of death after liver resection for colorectal metastases is tumor recurrence. From 55% to 80% of patients undergoing liver resections for colorectal metastases will develop tumor recurrence, of which 20% to 40% will have subsequent isolated liver involvement.[9,47] Performing a repeat liver resection in this group of patients has been described in several larges studies, with 5-year survival rates comparable to patients undergoing initial resection (Table 24C-8). Pinson et al.[47] reviewed the results of 10 patients undergoing repeat hepatic resections for colorectal metastases and reported a mean interval of 17 months between the first and second hepatic operation. Increasing plasma CEA levels were the predominant finding in most patients diagnosed with recurrent tumor. They reported no operative mortality but an exceptionally high 60% complication rate, including three transient bile leaks, bile duct stenosis, subphrenic abscess, and transient hepatic failure. Survival was demonstrated in 100% at 1 year and 88% at 2 years. Disease-free survival at 1 and 3 years was 60% and 45%, respectively. In addition, the authors reported the cumulative findings of 15 published series on 134 patients undergoing repeat hepatic surgery for colorectal metastases. In this metaanalysis an actuarial survival of 91% at 1 year, 69% at 2 years, 55% at 3 years, 45% at 4 years, and 40% at 5 years was reported.

In a retrospective analysis of 202 patients undergoing liver resection for metastatic colorectal cancer over a 12-year period, repeat liver resections were done on 23 patients. There was a postoperative morbidity rate of 22% and no operative mortality. The 5-year actuarial survival rate after repeat resection was 32%, with a median length of survival of 40 months. These results are similar to the survival data obtained after first hepatic resection by the same group

**TABLE 24C-8.** SURVIVAL AFTER HEPATIC RE-RESECTION FOR RECURRENT COLORECTAL LIVER METASTASES

| REFERENCE | YEAR | NO. OF PATIENTS | 5-YR SURVIVAL RATE, % | MEDIAN SURVIVAL RATE, MO |
|---|---|---|---|---|
| Kin et al.[86] | 1998 | 15 | 21.2 | 16 |
| Chu et al.[87] | 1997 | 10 | 23 | 16 |
| Tuttle et al.[48] | 1997 | 23 | 32 | 40 |
| Wanebo et al.[10]* | 1996 | 536 | — | 24† |
| Fernandez-Trigo et al.[49]* | 1996 | 170 | 32 | 34 |
| Scheele et al.[83] | 1996 | 26 | 57 | 60 |
| Fong et al.[8] | 1994 | 25 | 0 | 30 |

* Represents collected series.
† Mean survival time.

**TABLE 24C-9.** RANDOMIZED STUDIES OF HAI VERSUS SYSTEMIC CHEMOTHERAPY FOR HEPATIC METASTASES

| | | HAI | | | SYSTEMIC | |
| REFERENCE | NO. OF PATIENTS | DRUG | RESPONSE, % | SURVIVAL RATE % (1-YR/2-YR) | DRUG | RESPONSE, % |
| --- | --- | --- | --- | --- | --- | --- |
| Kemeny et al.[60] | 162 | FUDR | 52 | 60/25 | FUDR | 20 |
| Chang et al.[53] | 143 | FUDR | 42 | 85/44 | FUDR | 10 |
| Rougier et al.[55] | 163 | FUDR | 49 | 61/22 | 5FU | 14 |
| Hohn et al.[54] | 64 | FUDR | 62 | 60/30 | FUDR | 17 |

of surgeons during the same time period.[48] Comparable results have been reported by the Repeat Hepatic Metastases Registry with a 32% 5-year actuarial survival rate after repeat resection of 170 patients from 20 institutions worldwide.[49] Neither of these two large reported series identified any significant prognostic indicators in predicting long-term survival in patients who underwent complete resection.

Although mortality and morbidity data in patients with repeat hepatic resections indicate it to be a safe procedure and survival rates are comparable to patients undergoing an initial resection, it must be emphasized that all studies to date are retrospective and contain highly selected patient populations. Patient selection criteria for repeat hepatic resection should be the same as for the initial resection: satisfactory medical condition, absence of extrahepatic disease, and the ability to obtain a negative margin. Therefore, repeat hepatic resection appears to be a safe and potentially effective treatment for a select group of patients with recurrent colorectal metastases.

## INTRAARTERIAL CHEMOTHERAPY

Since the liver is the most common site for tumor recurrence after liver resection for colorectal metastases, and is the sole site in up to 40% of patients, regional hepatic chemotherapy represents an attractive mode of adjuvant therapy. The most investigated form of providing regional hepatic chemotherapy has been with hepatic artery infusion. The purpose of hepatic arterial infusion is to achieve higher drug delivery directly to the area of tumor involvement without systemic side effects. Breedis and Young[50] initially described that hepatic tumors exceeding 1 cm in diameter derive their blood supply from the hepatic artery, in contrast to the normal hepatic parenchyma, which is supplied predominantly by the portal circulation. Therefore, this difference in blood supply is the rationale for delivering chemotherapy directly into the hepatic artery.

The ideal chemotherapeutic agent for regional infusion would be a drug that is largely extracted by the liver during the first pass and, therefore, produce lower systemic drug concentrations and toxicity. The most common chemotherapeutic agents used in intraarterial infusion have been the antimetabolites 5-flurouracil (5-FU) and its derivative 5-flurodeoxyuridine (FUDR). Both compounds inhibit thymidilate synthase, the enzyme responsible for the rate-limiting step in the production of thymidine, an essential substrate for DNA synthesis. These agents are suitable for intraarterial infusion due to their high hepatic drug extraction (80% to 90%) and short plasma half-lives. Ensminger and Gyves[51] reported a fourfold higher

concentration of FUDR after hepatic arterial injection compared to systemic administration.

The role of hepatic arterial infusion therapy on long-term survival in patients with hepatic metastases continues to be controversial. The use of hepatic arterial infusion has been relegated to the patient with unresectable colorectal liver metastases. Several prospective randomized trials (Table 24C-9) have been conducted to address and compare the efficacy of hepatic arterial infusion versus systemic chemotherapy.[52–55]

A randomized study comparing hepatic arterial infusion with systemic FUDR infusion reported by Kemeny et al.[52] demonstrated a statistically significant difference in the response rate between groups. A response was defined as a greater than 50% reduction in measurable disease. This study reported a 52% response rate in patients receiving hepatic arterial infusion compared to 20% with systemic therapy. However, there was no significant difference in median survival between hepatic artery infusion and systemic groups, 17 and 12 months, respectively. A criticism of this study was that a significant (60%) number of systemic infusion patients crossed over and received intrahepatic therapy. Although the crossover design makes survival data difficult to interpret, other studies have demonstrated similar results.

A study from the Northern California Oncology Group (NCOG) reported a 42% partial response rate in patients receiving intrahepatic infusion of FUDR compared to 10% with systemic FUDR infusion. No survival benefit was demonstrated, with median durations of 16 months for both groups.[54]

Martin et al.[56] described the Mayo Clinic experience in a study that randomized 74 patients to either intrahepatic infusion of FUDR or systemic FU infusion. They reported a response rate of 48% and 21%, respectively. Although there were no crossover patients in this study, no survival benefit was demonstrated.

Intraarterial therapy with multiple chemotherapeutic agents has been used to treat patients with unresectable colorectal liver metastases. Protocols including a combination of FUDR, BCNU, and mitomycin C have been used with reported response rates of 70%, but a major side effect from this regimen was increased regional and systemic toxicity.[57]

Prior to pump placement, a celiac and superior mesenteric artery arteriogram is often performed to delineate the highly variable arterial anatomy of the liver and confirm the patency of the portal vein. Daly et al.[58] have reported the variability of the arterial anatomy of the liver in a review of 100 celiac and superior mesenteric artery angiograms (Fig. 24C-6). At operation, a thorough examination of

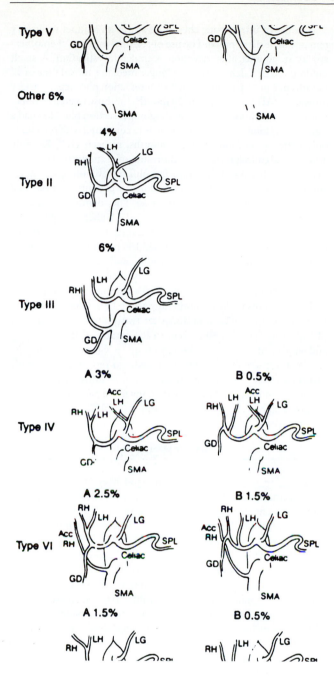

**FIGURE 24C-6.** Hepatic arterial anatomy. (Reproduced with permission from Soballe PW, Daly JM: Hepatic metastases, in *Maingot's Abdominal Operations*, ed 10, MJ Zinner et al (eds). Norwalk, CT, Appleton & Lange, 1997, pp 1591–1602.)

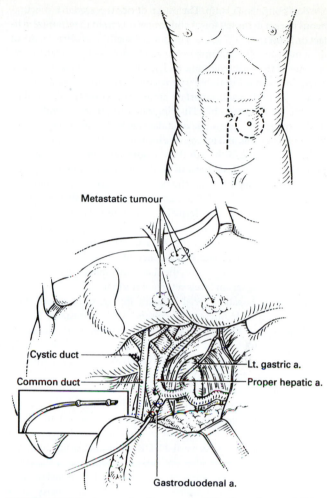

**FIGURE 24C-7.** Anatomic placement of the hepatic arterial infusion pump. The catheter tip is placed into the gastroduodenal artery with the right gastric artery ligated. Note that a cholecystectomy is performed. (Reproduced with permission from Kemeny NE, Sigurdson ER: Intra-arterial chemotherapy for liver tumors, in *Blumgart's Surgery of the Liver and Biliary Tract.* New York, Churchill Livingstone, 1982, p 1482.)

the abdomen is performed to determine the extent of hepatic disease and the presence of any extrahepatic extension. The hepatic artery catheter is usually introduced with the catheter tip placed into the gastroduodenal artery as shown in Fig. 24C-7. The hepatic artery itself is not cannulated due to the risk of vessel thrombosis. Special attention must be taken to identify and ligate small collateral branches from the hepatic artery to the stomach, pancreas, and duodenum. This will prevent inadvertent perfusion and subsequent severe chemoinduced ulcer formation and pancreatitis. In addition, the gallbladder is removed because studies have indicated an increased rate (up to 33%) of chemoinduced cholecystitis. Adequate perfusion to the liver is confirmed at the end of the procedure by infusing fluorescein and visualizing fluorescent liver parenchyma with a Wood's ultraviolet lamp. The pump device is placed in a subcutaneous pocket in the left lower abdominal quadrant to minimize artifact on subsequent CT scans. The device usually holds 30 to 50 mL of drug in a specialized chamber that can be accessed percutaneously.

One of the most common and severe complications of hepatic artery infusion is hepatobiliary toxicity. This is manifested initially as serum elevations of aspartate aminotransferase (AST), alkaline phosphatase, and bilirubin. Histologically, the process resembles biliary sclerosis, with gross bile duct damage and small-artery intimal fibrous thickening, and in its severe form may resemble primary sclerosing cholangitis. Although there is some evidence of hepatocyte necrosis and cholestasis, most of the damage is a combined ischemic and inflammatory effect on the bile duct system. The etiology of biliary toxicity may result from its blood supply. Similar to hepatic tumors, the biliary system derives its blood supply from the hepatic artery and therefore is more susceptible to toxicity. It is therefore imperative for close monitoring of the liver function tests in all patients receiving intraarterial hepatic chemotherapy. When elevations of liver function tests do occur, the chemotherapeutic agent must be withdrawn until serum levels return to normal.

The use of hepatic arterial infusion appears to be a valid therapy in patients with unresectable colorectal liver metastases. Several randomized prospective trials demonstrated a significant tumor response rate compared to systemic therapy. The issue of survival benefit is still unclear because most trials have a significant number of crossover patients.

The addition of biomodulating agents that would increase the effect of drug delivered and reduce complications has been investigated. Adding agents such as folinic acid (leucovorin) and dexamethasone to the FUDR regimen significantly decreased the hepatoxicity of hepatic arterial FUDR while increasing response rates in previously untreated patients. Leucovorin, a reduced folate, is thought to potentiate the inhibition of thymidylate synthase by increasing the active metabolite of 5-FU, flurodeoxyridine monophosphate (FdUMP). The addition of dexamethasone, with its well-known anti-inflammatory effects, decreased biliary toxicity, as determined by resolution of liver function abnormalities in patients receiving FUDR and leucovorin. Kemeny at al.[59] in a prospective double-blinded randomized study of intrahepatic FUDR with dexamethasone versus FUDR alone reported a significant response rate of 71% for the FUDR plus dexamethasone group compared to 40% in the FUDR alone patients. In addition increased survival and decreased hepatotoxicity favored the FUDR plus dexamethasone group, although this did not reach statistical significance, as demonstrated in Table 24C-10.

**TABLE 24C-10. RANDOMIZED TRIAL OF HAI OF FUDR VERSUS FUDR PLUS DEXAMETHASONE (DEX)[59]**

|  | FUDR (n = 25) | FUDR + DEX (n = 24) | P |
|---|---|---|---|
| Response, % | 40 | 71 | 0.03 |
| Bilirubin >3 mg/dL | 30% | 9% | 0.07 |
| Survival, mo | 15 | 19 | 0.06 |

The use of intrahepatic chemotherapy as an adjunct to surgery remains to be determined. The use of regional infusion chemotherapy as an adjunct after resection is under investigation. A small randomized trial demonstrated a longer median survival time of 37 months in 5 of 11 patients treated with resection plus hepatic artery infusion (HAI) compared with 28 months for those treated by resection only. In addition, patients undergoing resection plus HAI had a significantly longer median time to failure compared with resection-only patients, 30 months and 9 months, respectively.[60] Recently Kemeny and colleagues reported the results of a randomized prospective study of hepatic arterial infusion plus intravenous chemotherapy versus systemic chemotherapy alone in patients with resected hepatic metastasis from colorectal cancer. They demonstrated a significantly lower rate of hepatic relapse and a higher rate of survival at two years in patients treated with combined therapy than systemic therapy alone. The study compromised 156 patients randomized to hepatic arterial infusion with floxuridine and dexamethasone plus intravenous fluorouracil versus similar systemic therapy alone. The median survival was 72.2 months in the combined-therapy group and 59.3 months in the monotherapy group (p = 0.03), with a median follow-up of 62.7 months. After two years the survival free of hepatic relapse was 90 percent in the combined-therapy group and 60 percent in the monotherapy group (p < 0.001). Given these results it appears that patients that undergo resection for hepatic metastases may benefit from hepatic arterial infusion plus intravenous chemotherapy. Studies with many more patients are needed to show a significant increase in overall survival.[60a]

## CRYOTHERAPY

Cryoablation is a process in which rapid freeze-thaw treatments cause intracellular ice crystal formation with subsequent cellular membrane damage and death. This is a relatively new modality in the treatment of colorectal hepatic metastasis. Destruction of tumor cells with cryoablation has been demonstrated in various organs, such as the rectum,[61] breast,[62] skin,[63] lung,[64] prostate,[63] pancreas,[63] brain,[65] and liver. However, until recently the inability to properly monitor the freezing process and to treat deep lesions had limited wide clinical application of this modality. Two recent advances in cryotechnology have made cryoablation of hepatic lesions more feasible. These include vacuum-insulated cryoprobes of many different diameters that allow for controlled freezing of deeply located lesions, and intraoperative ultrasound that allows for accurate cryoprobe placement and careful monitoring of the extent of tissue freezing.

Although some advocate the use of cryotherapy as an alternative to liver resection in patients with isolated liver tumors, there have been no prospective randomized trials addressing this issue. Most groups report the use of cryotherapy in patients with colorectal liver metastases that are deemed unresectable because of the extent and/or location of the malignant lesions. These include patients with multiple bilobar lesions that cannot be resected and in patients with disease proximal to major intrahepatic vessels. Gage et al.[61] demonstrated that large blood vessels are more resistant to freezing in cryotherapy than their surrounding tissue. This resistance is attributed to the heat sink effect of flowing blood in the vessel. Therefore, cryotherapy may well be ideal in those patients with tumors adjacent to major vessels such as the portal vein, inferior vena cava, and the hepatic veins. However, some have argued that tumors immediately adjacent to large vessels may not reach adequate freezing levels due to this same heat sink effect and advocate temporary hepatic inflow occlusion in these instances.

In addition, cryotherapy may play a role in patients with positive or "close" margins after hepatic resection. Several series suggest that tumor margin recurrence may be decreased following traditional resection by cryoablation of the resection edge.[66] Furthermore, cryotherapy may be of benefit for those patients who are technically resectable but are medically unfit for a major surgical resection due to confounding medical comorbidities. It may also be beneficial for those with low hepatic reserves, such as the severely cirrhotic patient with a hepatic tumor.

The introduction of intraoperative real-time ultrasonography has allowed for the detection and assessment of additional disease and is an accurate method of monitoring the extent of tissue freezing and accurate cryoprobe placement. Cryoprobe sizes range from 3 to 9 mm in diameter. Larger cryoprobes with diameters of 5 to 9 mm allow for freezing targets of more than 6 cm in diameter and are most frequently used in hepatic cryotherapy. Applying a flat or spike cryoprobe directly to the lesion can treat lesions that are small and superficial. For intraparenchymal lesions a modified Seldinger-type technique is used. An echogenic needle and j-wire are inserted into the center of the lesion and a dilator and cannula are placed over the wire into the tumor. When the wire and dilator position are confirmed with real-time ultrasonography, the wire and dilator are removed and the cryoprobe is inserted through the cannula into the tumor. The use of ultrasonography is essential to allow visualization of the most direct path to the target and avoidance of major vascular structures. Liquid nitrogen is allowed to flow through the center of the cryoprobe and is vented along its lateral edges. The tumor is frozen with a margin of at least 1 cm of surrounding liver tissue. The final appearance of the target is a dense hypoechoic (black) area with a hyperechoic (white) rim, representing complete reflection of the ultrasound waves at the solidification interface between frozen and unfrozen tissue.

Once the determined amount of tissue is frozen, the liquid nitrogen is removed and the frozen tissue is allowed to either passively thaw with the cryoprobe left in place or actively thawed with warmed nitrogen gas through the cryoprobe. After several minutes the cryoprobe is slowly removed and the remaining tract is packed with hemostatic agents such as Gelfoam or Surgicel to minimize bleeding.

Several reports indicate that repeated freeze-thaw cycles are more efficient in killing tumor cells than a single freeze-thaw cycle. It has been demonstrated that repeated freezing of liver tissue shows increased signs of cell damage. Stewart et al.[67] demonstrated that double freeze-thaw cycles in hepatic cryotherapy patients resulted in greater hepatocellular injury as measured by the serum aspartate aminotransferase (AST) level on the first postoperative day. Although advantages to multiple freeze-thaw cycles may exist, they do not come without possible additional complications. Cozzi et al.[68] reported increased thrombocytopenia, which correlated with the increased hepatocellular damage in the early postoperative period, in patients following multiple freeze-thaw cycles. Therefore, one should be aware of possible increased bleeding complications with patients undergoing multiple freeze-thaw cycles.

Many of the major complications of cryotherapy are similar to those seen in hepatic resections and include hemorrhage, pleural effusion, biloma, and perihepatic abscesses. Complications that are more specific to cryotherapy include significant hypothermia, cracking or fragmentation of the parenchyma, increases in circulating hepatic transaminase levels, thrombocytopenia, myoglobinuria, acute renal failure, and cryoshock with severe disseminated intravascular coagulopathy (DIC). Significant hypothermia can occur in patients undergoing cryotherapy, and therefore intravenous fluids and blood products should be warmed prior to administration.

Thermal stress occurring during the rapid freezing and thawing process may cause the liver to fragment or "crack." Although fragmentation of tissue is common after cryoablation, it is usually easily controlled and is rarely associated with massive hemorrhage. In a reported series of 63 patients undergoing cryotherapy, 5 patients (8%) developed fragmentation of the frozen parenchyma with 2 patients (3%) developing massive bleeding.[69]

Myoglobinuria has been reported in several large series.[66,70,71] It usually occurs after the thawing process and resolves by day 3 or 4. Although the mechanism is unclear, it may represent an important component in patients that develop acute tubular necrosis and renal impairment.

The most feared complication of hepatic cryotherapy is the development of DIC. This refractory coagulopathy may be associated with multiple organ failure and is termed *cryoshock*. The etiology for this coagulopathy is unclear, but thought to be mediated by large amounts of circulating products released by necrotizing liver tissue.

Mortality rates in patients undergoing hepatic cryotherapy have ranged from 1% to 8%.[66,70,72,73] Seifert et al.[71] reported, in a recent metaanalysis of 20 published series of hepatic cryotherapy in patients with colorectal liver metastases, 14 postoperative deaths in 869 patients treated, resulting in an overall 1.6% mortality rate. The most common cause for mortality was acute myocardial infarction followed by DIC and multiorgan failure—cryoshock, pulmonary embolus, respiratory failure, cerebrovascular accident, complicated hepatic abscess, and postoperative hemorrhage from coagulopathy. Mortality and morbidity rates from recent published series are listed in Table 24C-11.

The efficacy of cryotherapy in the treatment of colorectal liver metastasis continues to be investigated. Although most series indicate encouraging results, survival and recurrence rates are difficult to interpret due to the limited follow-up time, small sample size, and lack of appropriate controls. Ravikumar et al.,[73] in a study of 18 patients treated by cryotherapy with a median follow-up of 24 months, projected a 5-year survival rate and a 5-year disease-free survival rate of 78% and 39%, respectively. Based on these results, the authors advocated cryotherapy as an alternative to traditional hepatic resection. However, this study is based on a relatively small number of patients and may be confounded by selection bias. The author treated only patients with one to three lesions, and therefore it is difficult to evaluate the true efficacy of cryoablation based on this report. Similarly, Morris et al.[66] noted 3-year survival rates comparable to those after surgical resection in cases where plasma CEA levels returned to normal after cryoablation.

The reported median survival rates of more than 2 years in most cryotherapy series and the possibility of long-term disease-free survival compares well to the median survival times of 13 to 16

**TABLE 24C-11.** MORBIDITY AND MORTALITY RATES WITH HEPATIC CRYOTHERAPY

|  | NO. OF PATIENTS | MORTALITY RATE | HEMORRHAGE RATE | COAGULOPATHY RATE | PLEURAL EFFUSION RATE | BILE FISTULA RATE |
|---|---|---|---|---|---|---|
| Morris et al.[66] | 110 | 2% | 9% | * | 4% | 8% |
| Sharif et al.[72] | 39 | 0% | 3% | 3% | * | 0% |
| Weaver et al.[88] | 140 | 4% | 7% | 1% | 5% | 4% |
| Onik et al.[70] | 86 | 3% | 1% | * | * | 1% |
| Ravikumar et al.[73] | 32 | 0% | 0% | * | * | 0% |
| Seifert et al.[71]† | 869 | 1.6% | 4% | 3.8% | 6% | 3% |

* No data available.
† Represents meta-analysis.

months in patients treated with hepatic artery chemotherapy. The percentage of patients alive and disease-free with a median follow-up time of 14 to 26 months has been reported to be from 20% to 51%.

The use of minimally invasive techniques has allowed laparoscopic cryoablation of hepatic metastases. Cuschieri et al.[74] reported a total laparoscopic or laparoscopic-assisted approach to cryoablation in 10 out of 22 patients with colorectal liver metastases. The

authors reported no significant perioperative morbidity related to the laparoscopic approach. In a retrospective study of 12 patients undergoing laparoscopic cryoablation, the authors reported a mean of 2.7 lesions treated with an average lesion size of 3.3 cm. In addition they reported a remarkable postoperative course with 11 out of 12 patients tolerating a regular diet and ambulating within 24 h and a mean time to discharge of 3.5 days.[75] The laparoscopic approach is demonstrated in Fig. 24C-8. To fully determine the outcome and

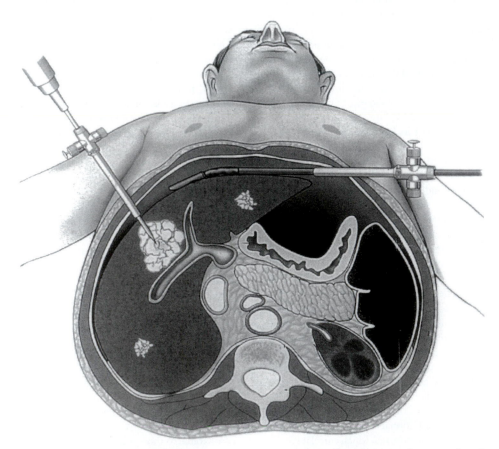

**FIGURE 24C-8.** Laparoscopic hepatic cryosurgery. Ultrasound and cryoprobes are placed through conventional laparoscopic ports. (Reproduced with permission from Henifold BT: Laparoscopic cryoablation of hepatic metastases. Semin Surg Oncol 15:196, 1998.)

potential in decreasing postoperative morbidity in patients receiving aggressive treatment for inoperable hepatic metastases, additional studies are needed to further identify patient selection criteria for laparoscopic cryoablation.

The use of hepatic cryotherapy appears to be well established, with acceptable morbidity in treating patients with unresectable colorectal hepatic metastases. Its role as a substitute for surgical resection has not been substantiated. Future prospective randomized trials are needed to address this issue.

## TREATMENT OF HEPATIC METASTASES FROM NONCOLORECTAL PRIMARIES

The surgical management of hepatic metastases from noncolorectal tumors is less well defined. The literature provides a preponderance of accumulated uncontrolled evidence in a heterogeneous population suggesting benefit of hepatic resection in a carefully selected group of patients. Elias et al.[76] reported a 5-year survival rate of 36% in a prospective analysis of 147 patients undergoing hepatic resections for noncolorectal liver metastases. These results are comparable to the 5-year survival rate of 34% demonstrated in 270 patients submitted to hepatic resections for colorectal primaries from the same institution. There was no difference observed in survival when synchronous and metachronous lesions were compared, or when patients with more or fewer than three liver metastases were compared. Five-year survival rates according to the primary were 20% for breast cancers; 74% for neuroendocrine tumors; 46% for testicular tumors; 18% for sarcomas; and slightly less than 20% for gastric carcinomas, melanomas, and gallbladder adenocarcinomas. Similar results have been reported by Harrison and colleagues,[77] who demonstrated a 37% 5-year survival rate in a series of 96 patients undergoing resections for noncolorectal, nonneuroendocrine hepatic metastases. This appears to be a slightly higher 5-year survival rate compared to the French experience, but may be due to differences in the primary tumor types, with more sarcomas and fewer breast cancers.

Based on these observations, it would appear that a benefit from resection may occur in patients with certain types of primary tumors. The best results are from neuroendocrine, nonseminomatous testicular tumors, Wilm's tumors or adenocarcinomas of the kidney, and sarcomas. Hepatic neuroendocrine metastases pose a unique management decision process due to their biologic behavior. These tumors are usually thought of as having low malignant potential, and although they may present with extensive metastatic liver disease, an indolent course with a long-term natural history is characteristic of neuroendocrine tumors.

Numerous studies have addressed the issue of hepatic resections, either with the intent of cure or for palliation of symptoms for neuroendocrine metastases. Most of these studies indicate that a select group of patients may benefit from hepatic resection. Que et al.[78] reported a 73% 4-year survival rate after resection of hepatic metastases in patients with neuroendocrine tumors. A prospective nonrandomized study by Carty et al.[79] reported in a group of 25 patients with unresectable islet cell tumors a 60% and 28% 2-year and 5-year survival, respectively. In patients that underwent complete resection

of metastatic tumor, there was a demonstrable increase in survival at 2 years to 87% and 79% at 5 years. A prospective nonrandomized study by Frilling et al.[80] also demonstrated potential benefit in hepatic resections in a select group of patients with metastatic neuroendocrine tumors. They reported that close to 14% of patients referred for liver resection with metastatic neuroendocrine disease underwent curative resections. All of these patients were disease-free 2 years after their resection.

Another select group of patients that may benefit from hepatic resections from metastatic disease are those with soft tissue sarcomas to the liver. Jaques et al.[81] reviewed 65 patients with hepatic metastases from soft tissue sarcoma primaries. They identified that the primary site influences the pattern of metastases, with the majority of hepatic metastases from viscera and retroperitoneal leiomyosarcomas, and almost none from extremity or trunk primary sites. Hepatic resection for metastatic soft tissue sarcoma was performed in 14 patients. Three patients underwent wedge resection, ten patients underwent lobar or segmental resection, and one patient had an incomplete resection. The median survival in the resected group was 30 months, and there were no 5-year survivors after hepatic resection. Although the median survival from time of resection of hepatic metastases is similar for colorectal and sarcoma primary tumors (30 months), the 5-year survival rate is clearly not. However, when all patients in the literature undergoing hepatic resection for metastatic soft tissue sarcoma are considered, a 5-year survival occurred in 5 of 48, or 11% of patients.

The use of hepatic resection for patients with noncolorectal metastases appears to benefit a very select group, such as those with neuroendocrine, renal, and testicular tumors. The indications and contraindications have not been fully explored. Before contemplating hepatic resection these patients should be carefully evaluated for possible extrahepatic disease and considered only if all disease can be resected. An exception to this may be a patient with symptomatic neuroendocrine metastatic disease, in which decreasing tumor burden may alleviate symptoms.

## REFERENCES

1. Schwartz S: Liver, in *Principles of Surgery,* 7th ed, Schwartz S et al (eds). New York, McGraw-Hill, 1999.
2. Parker S et al: Cancer statistics, 1997. CA Cancer J Clin 47:5, 1997.
3. Bengmark S, Hafstrom L: The natural history of primary and secondary malignant tumors of the liver: I. The prognosis for patients with hepatic metastases from colonic and rectal carcinoma by laparotomy. Cancer 23:198, 1969.
4. Bozzetti F et al: Patterns of failure following surgical resection of colorectal cancer liver metastases. Rationale for a multimodal approach. Ann Surg 205:264, 1987.
5. Wood C et al: A retrospective study of the natural history of patients with liver metastases from colorectal cancer. Clin Oncol 2:285, 1976.
6. Wilson S, Adson M: Surgical treatment of hepatic metastases from colorectal cancers. Arch Surg 111:330, 1984.
7. Scheele J et al: Indicators of prognosis after hepatic resection for colorectal secondaries. Surgery 110:13, 1991.
8. Fong Y et al: Resection is safe and effective for hepatic colorectal

metastases: An analysis of 456 consecutive cases. J Clin Oncol 15:938, 1997.

9. NORDLINGER B et al: Surgical resection of hepatic metastases: Multicentric retrospective study by the French Association of Surgery, in *Treatment of Hepatic Metastases of Colorectal Cancer*, Nordlinger B, Jaeck D (eds). Paris, Springer-Verlag, 1992, pp 129–161.

10. WANEBO H et al: Patient selection for hepatic resection of colorectal metastases. Arch Surg 131:322, 1996.

11. HUGHES K et al: Resection of the liver for colorectal carcinoma metastases: A multi-institutional study of patterns of recurrence. Surgery 100:278, 1986.

12. CADY B et al: Surgical margin in hepatic resection for colorectal metastasis. Ann Surg 227:566, 1998.

13. JAMISON R et al: Hepatic resection for metastatic colorectal cancer results in cure for some patients. Arch Surg 132:505, 1997.

14. HUGHES K et al: Resection of the liver for colorectal carcinoma metastases: A multi-institutional study of indications for resection. Surgery 103:278, 1988.

15. ROSEN C et al: Perioperative blood transfusion and determinants of survival after liver resection for metastatic colorectal carcinoma. Ann Surg 216:493, 1992.

16. STEELE G et al: A prospective evaluation of hepatic resection for colorectal carcinoma metastases to the liver: Gastrointestinal tumor study group protocol 6584. J Clin Oncol 9:1105, 1991.

17. BAKALAKOS E et al: Is carcino-embryonic antigen useful in the follow-up management of patients with colorectal liver metastases. Am J Surg 177:2, 1999.

18. PHIL E et al: Lung recurrence after curative surgery for colorectal cancer. Dis Colon Rectum 30:417, 1987.

19. GIRARD P et al: Surgery for lung metastases from colorectal cancer: Analysis of prognostic factors. J Clin Oncol 14:2047, 1996.

20. MCAFEE M et al: Colorectal lung metastases: Results of surgical excision. Ann Thorac Surg 53:780, 1992.

21. MCCORMACK P, ATTIYEH F: Resected pulmonary metastases from colorectal cancer. Dis Colon Rectum 22:553, 1979.

22. ROBINSON B et al: Is resection of pulmonary and hepatic metastases warranted in patients with colorectal cancer? J Thorac Cardiovasc Surg 117:66, 1999.

23. GOUGH D et al: Resection for hepatic and pulmonary metastases in patients with colorectal cancer. Br J Surg 81:94, 1994.

24. MINNARD E et al: Surgical resection for hepatic and pulmonary colorectal metastases. Surg Oncol 15:552, 1998.

25. MURATA S et al: Resection of both hepatic and pulmonary metastases in patients with colorectal carcinoma. Cancer 83:1086, 1998.

26. REGNARD J et al: Surgical treatment of hepatic and pulmonary metastases from colorectal cancers. Ann Thorac Surg 66:214, 1998.

27. FORTNER J et al: Multivariate analysis of a personal series of 247 consecutive patients with liver metastases from colorectal cancer. I. Treatment by hepatic resection. Ann Surg 199:306, 1984.

28. DOCI R et al: One hundred patients with hepatic metastases from colorectal cancer treated by resection: Analysis of prognostic determinants. Br J Surg 78:797, 1991.

29. GAYOWSKI T et al: Experience in hepatic resection for metastatic colorectal cancer-analysis of clinical and pathological risk factors. Surgery 116:703, 1994.

30. BEUERS U: Hepatic malignancies—Clinical features and laboratory test. Diag Oncol 1:359, 1991.

31. KEMENY N et al: A prospective analysis of laboratory test and imaging studies to detect hepatic lesions. Ann Surg 195:163, 1982.

32. SUGARBAKER P: Surgical decision making for large bowel cancer metastatic to the liver. Radiology 174:621, 1990.

33. SOYER P et al: Preoperative assessment of resectability of hepatic metastases from colonic carcinoma: CT portography vs sonogram and dynamic CT. AJR 159:741, 1992.

34. SOYER P et al: Detection of liver metastases from colorectal cancer: Comparison of intraoperative US and CT during arterial portography. Radiology 183:541, 1992.

35. HAGSPIEL K et al: Detection of liver metastases: Comparison of superparamagnetic iron oxide enhanced and unenhanced MR imaging at 1.5 T with dynamic CT, intraoperative US and percutaneous US. Radiology 196:471, 1995.

36. CHARNLEY R et al: Detection of colorectal liver metastases using intraoperative ultrasonography. Br J Surg 78:45, 1991.

37. YAMAGUCHI A et al: Detection by CT during arterial portography of colorectal cancer metastases to liver. Dis Colon Rectum 34:37, 1991.

38. MORAN B et al: Computed tomographic portography in preoperative imaging of hepatic neoplasms. Br J Surg 82:669, 1995.

39. KUSZYK B et al: Portal-phase contrast-enhanced helical CT for the detection of malignant hepatic tumors: Sensitivity based on comparison with intraoperative and pathologic findings. AJR 166:91, 1996.

40. POVOSKI S et al: Role of chest CT in patients with negative chest x-rays referred for hepatic colorectal metastases. Ann Surg Oncol 5:9, 1998.

41. VITOLA J et al: Positron emission tomography to stage suspected metastatic colorectal carcinoma to the liver. Am J Surg 171:21, 1996.

42. LAI D et al: The role of whole-body positron emission tomography with 18F-fluorodeoxyglucose in identifying operable colorectal cancer metastases to the liver. Arch Surg 131:703, 1996.

43. DELBEKE D et al: Evaluation of benign vs malignant hepatic lesions with positron emission tomography. Arch Surg 133:510, 1998.

44. ELIAS D et al: Results of 136 curative hepatectomies with a safety margin of less than 10 mm for colorectal metastases. J Surg Oncol 69:88, 1998.

45. GOZZETTI G et al: Undici anni di esperienza nella terapia chirurgica delle metastasi epatiche da tumori colo-rettali. Chirurg Ital 46:30, 1994.

46. REES M et al: One hundred and fifty hepatic resections—The evolution of techniques toward bloodless surgery. Br J Surg 83:1526, 1996.

47. PINSON C et al: Repeat hepatic surgery for colorectal cancer metastasis to the liver. Ann Surg 223:765, 1996.

48. TUTTLE T et al: Repeat hepatic resection as effective treatment for recurrent colorectal liver metastases. J Surg Oncol 4:125, 1997.

49. FERNANDEZ-TRIGO V et al: Repeat liver resections from colorectal metastasis. Surgery 117:296, 1995.

50. BREEDIS C, YOUNG G: The blood supply of neoplasms in the liver. Am J Pathol 30:969, 1954.

51. ENSMINGER W et al: A clinical-pharmacological evaluation of hepatic arterial infusions of 5-fluoro-2'-deoxyuridine and 5-fluorouracil. Cancer Res 38:3784, 1978.

52. KEMENY N et al: Intrahepatic or systemic infusion of fluorodeoxyuridine in patients with liver metastases from colorectal carcinoma—A randomized trial. Ann Intern Med 107:459, 1987.

53. CHANG A et al: A prospective randomized trial of regional versus systemic continuous 5-fluorodeoxyuridine chemotherapy in the treatment of colorectal liver metastases. Ann Surg 206:685, 1987.

54. HOHN D et al: A randomized trial of continuous intravenous versus hepatic intra-arterial floxuridine in patients with colorectal cancer metastatic to the liver: The Northern California Oncology Group Trial. J Clin Oncol 7:1646, 1989.

55. ROUGIER P et al: Hepatic arterial infusion of floxuridine in patients with liver metastases from colorectal carcinoma: Long term results of a prospective randomized trial. J Clin Oncol 10:1112, 1992.

56. MARTIN J et al: Intra-arterial floxuridine vs systemic fluorouracil for hepatic metastases from colorectal cancer. A randomized trial. Arch Surg 125:1022, 1990.

57. KEMENY N et al: Randomized trial of hepatic artery FUDR, mitomycin and BCNU versus FUDR alone: Effective salvage therapy for liver metastases of colorectal cancer. J Clin Oncol 11, 1993.

58. DALY J et al: Long-term hepatic arterial infusion chemotherapy. Arch Surg 119:936, 1986.

59. KEMENY N et al: Phase II study of hepatic arterial floxuridine, leucovorin, and dexamethasone for unresectable liver colorectal carcinoma. J Clin Oncol 12:2288, 1994.

60. KEMENY N et al: Results of a prospective randomized trial of continuous regional chemotherapy and hepatic resection as treatment of hepatic metastases from colorectal primaries. Cancer 57:492, 1986.

60a. KEMENY N et al: Randomized trial of hepatic arterial floxoridine, mitomycin, and carmustine versus floxoridine alone in previously treated patients with liver metastases from colorectal cancer. J Clin Oncol 11:330, 1993.

61. GAGE A: Cryotherapy for inoperable rectal cancer. Dis Colon Rectum 11:36, 1968.

62. RAND R et al: Cryolumpectomy for carcinoma of the breast. Surg Gynecol Obstet 165:392, 1987.

63. GILL W et al: Cryosurgery for neoplasia. Br J Surg 57:494, 1970.

64. UHLSCHMID G et al: Cryosurgery of pulmonary metastases. Cryobiology 16:171, 1979.

65. COOPER I: Cryogenic surgery. A new method of destruction or extirpation of benign or malignant tissues. N Engl J Med 268:743, 1993.

66. MORRIS D et al: Cryoablation of hepatic malignancy: An evaluation of tumour marker data and survival in 110 patients. GI Cancer 1:247, 1996.

67. STEWART G et al: Hepatic cryotherapy: Double-freeze cycles achieve greater hepatocellular injury in man. Cryobiology 32:215, 1995.

68. COZZI P et al: Thrombocytopenia after hepatic cryotherapy for colorectal metastases: Correlates with hepatocellular injury. World J Surg 18:774, 1994.

69. KANE R: Ulrasound-guided hepatic cryosurgery for tumor ablation. Semin Intervention Radiol 10:132, 1993.

70. ONIK G et al: Cryosurgery for liver cancer. Semin Surg Oncol 9:309, 1993.

71. SEIFERT J et al: A collective review of the world literature on hepatic cryotherapy. J R Coll Surg Edinb 43:141, 1998.

72. SHARIF M et al: Cryoablation of unresectable malignant liver tumors. Am J Surg 171:27, 1996.

73. RAVIKUMAR T et al: A 5-year study of cryosurgery in the treatment of liver tumors. Arch Surg 126:1520, 1991.

74. CUSCHIERI A et al: Hepatic cryotherapy for liver tumors: Development and clinical evaluation of a high-frequency insulated multineedle probe system for open and laparoscopic use. Surg Endosc 9:483, 1995.

75. HENIFORD B et al: Laparoscopic cryoablation of hepatic metastases. Semin Surg Oncol 15:194, 1998.

76. ELIAS D et al: Resection of liver metastases from noncolorectal primary: Indications and results based on 147 monocentric patients. J Am Coll Surg 187:487, 1998.

77. HARRISON L et al: Hepatic resection for noncolorectal, nonneuroendocrine metastases: A fifteen-year experience with ninety-six patients. Surgery 121:625, 1997.

78. QUE F et al: Hepatic resection for metastatic neuroendocrine carcinomas. Am J Surg 169:36, 1995.

79. CARTY S et al: Prospective study of aggressive resection of metastatic pancreatic endocrine tumors. Surgery 112:1024, 1992.

80. FRILLING A et al: Treatment of liver metastases in patients with neuroendocrine tumors. Langenbeck's Arch Surg 383:62, 1998.

81. JAQUES D et al: Hepatic metastases from soft-tissue sarcoma. Ann Surg 221:392, 1995.

82. BENGTSSON G et al: Natural history of patients with untreated liver metastases from colorectal cancer. Am J Surg 141:586, 1981.

83. SCHEELE J et al: Chirurgische resektion kolorektaler lebermetastasen: Gold-standard fur solitare and resektable herde. Swiss Surg Suppl 4:4, 1996.

84. HUGHES K et al: Resection of the liver for colorectal carcinoma metastases: A multi-institutional study of long term survivors. Dis Colon Rectum 31:1, 1988.

85. NELSON R et al: Hepatic tumors—Comparison of CT during arterial portography, delayed CT, and MR imaging for preoperative evaluation. Radiology 172:27, 1989.

86. KIN T et al: Repeat hepatectomy for recurrent colorectal metastases. World J Surg 22:1087, 1998.

87. CHU Q et al: Repeat hepatic resection for recurrent colorectal cancer. World J Surg 21:292, 1997.

88. WEAVER M et al: Hepatic cryosurgery in treating colorectal metastases. Cancer 76:210, 1995.

# 24D / MANAGEMENT OF PERITONEAL SURFACE MALIGNANCY: APPENDIX CANCER AND PSEUDOMYXOMA PERITONEI, COLON CANCER, GASTRIC CANCER, ABDOMINOPELVIC SARCOMA, AND PRIMARY PERITONEAL MALIGNANCY

*Paul H. Sugarbaker*

## INTRODUCTION

As surgical oncology evolved in the midst of a technological revolution in patient care, this discipline expanded from the resection of primary tumor to include the surgical management of metastatic disease. For gastrointestinal cancer, the earliest success with this new concept was with complete resection of locally recurrent colon and rectal cancer.[1,2] Then the resection of liver metastases from the same disease was shown to be of benefit to a selected group of patients.[3] Extension of the concept of complete eradication of metastatic disease to bring about long-term survival to patients with peritoneal surface malignancy has been pioneered by our group.[4] The clinical pathways for treatment of a wide variety of abdominal and pelvic malignancies that disseminate to peritoneal surfaces has grown out of extensive experience with appendiceal cancer. Appendiceal cancer is the paradigm for successful treatment of peritoneal carcinomatosis.[5] This review presents the background, the standardized treatments currently in use, and the results of treatment of peritoneal surface malignancy. The selection factors leading to long-term survival with acceptable morbidity and mortality will be a central focus for this work. The peritoneal surface malignancies to be discussed include appendix cancer and pseudomyxoma peritonei, colon cancer with peritoneal carcinomatosis, gastric cancer with peritoneal carcinomatosis, abdominopelvic sarcoma with sarcomatosis, and primary peritoneal surface malignancy including peritoneal mesothelioma, papillary serous cancer, and primary peritoneal adenocarcinoma. A discussion regarding the palliation of debilitating ascites is included.

## PRINCIPLES OF MANAGEMENT

The successful treatment of peritoneal surface malignancy requires a combined approach that utilizes peritonectomy procedures and perioperative intraperitoneal chemotherapy. In addition, knowledgeable patient selection is mandatory. The visceral and parietal peritonectomy procedures that one must utilize in an attempt to resect all visible evidence of disease are illustrated below. Complete cytoreduction is essential for treatment of peritoneal surface malignancy to result in long-term survival. One to six peritonectomy procedures may be required.[6] Their utilization depends on the distribution and extent of invasion of the malignancy disseminated within the peritoneal space.

## PERITONECTOMY PROCEDURES

If a surgeon elects to manage patients with peritoneal surface malignancy, additional knowledge concerning cancer dissemination on peritoneal surfaces and numerous refinements of his or her technical skills are required. The surgeon must be proficient in dissection using lasermode electrosurgery.

### RATIONALE FOR PERITONECTOMY PROCEDURES.
Peritonectomy procedures are necessary if one is to successfully treat peritoneal surface malignancies with curative intent. Peritonectomy procedures are used in the areas of visible cancer progression in an attempt to leave the patient with only microscopic residual disease. Small tumor nodules are removed using electroevaporation. Involvement of visceral peritoneum frequently requires resection of a portion of the stomach, small intestine, or colorectum.

### LOCATIONS OF PERITONEAL SURFACE MALIGNANCY.
Peritoneal surface malignancy tends to involve the visceral peritoneum in greatest volume at three definite sites. These are sites where the bowel is anchored to the retroperitoneum and peristalsis results in less motion of the visceral peritoneal surface. The rectosigmoid colon, as it comes up out of the pelvis, is a nonmobile portion

of the bowel. Also, it is a dependent site; and therefore, it frequently requires resection. Usually a complete pelvic peritonectomy involves stripping of the abdominal sidewalls, the peritoneum overlying the bladder, the cul-de-sac, and the rectosigmoid colon. The ileocecal valve is another area where there is limited mobility. Resection of the terminal ileum and a small portion of the right colon is often necessary. A final site often requiring resection is the antrum of the stomach. The antrum of the stomach is fixed to the retroperitoneum at the pylorus. Tumor coming into the foramen of Winslow accumulates in the subpyloric space and may cause intestinal obstruction as a result of gastric outlet obstruction. Occasionally, tumor in the lesser omentum will cause a confluence of disease on the lesser curvature. This may require total gastrectomy because of encasement of the vascular supply to the stomach.

*LASERMODE ELECTROSURGERY.* In order to adequately perform cytoreductive surgery, the surgeon must use lasermode electrosurgery. Peritonectomies and visceral resections using the traditional scissor and knife dissection will unnecessarily disseminate a large number of tumor cells within the abdomen. Also, clean peritoneal surfaces devoid of cancer cells are less likely to occur with sharp dissection or with electrosurgical dissection. Lasermode electrosurgery leaves a margin of heat necrosis that is devoid of viable malignant cells. Not only does electroevaporation of tumor and normal tissue at the margins of resection minimize the likelihood of persistent disease, but also it minimizes blood loss. In the absence of lasermode electrosurgery, profuse bleeding from stripped peritoneal surfaces may occur during the intraperitoneal wash with chemotherapy.

*CONVERSION OF PERITONEAL SURFACE TO INVASIVE MALIGNANCY BY SURGERY.* Finally, extensive cytoreductions in the absence of perioperative intraperitoneal chemotherapy may actually harm patients in the long run rather than help them. Extensive removal of peritoneal surfaces without intraperitoneal chemotherapy will allow tumor cells to become implanted within a deeper layer of the abdomen and pelvis. This may contribute to obstruction of vital structures such as the ureter or common duct. Also, deep involvement of the pelvic sidewall and tissues along vascular structures will occur. If a surgeon attempts to treat peritoneal surface malignancy, he or she must become thoroughly familiar with the techniques of intraoperative chemotherapy, early postoperative chemotherapy, and induction intraperitoneal chemotherapy. Complete cytoreduction combined with aggressive perioperative intraperitoneal chemotherapy and proper patient selection are the three essential requirements of treatment for peritoneal surface malignancy.

POSITION AND INCISION (FIG. 24D-1). The patient is supine with the gluteal fold advanced to the end of the operating table to allow full access to the perineum during the surgical procedure. This lithotomy position is achieved with the legs extended in St. Mark's leg holders (AMSCO, Erie, PA). The weight of the legs must be directed to the soles of the feet by positioning the footrests so that minimal weight is on the calf muscle. Myonecrosis within the gastrocnemius muscle may occur unless the legs are protected properly. All surfaces of the St. Mark's stirrups are protected by foam padding. The legs are surrounded by alternating-pressure boots

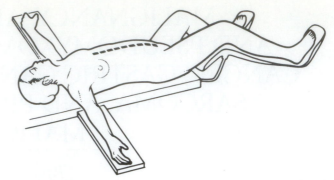

**FIGURE 24D-1.** Modified lithotomy position and maximal midline incision for cytoreductive surgery.

(SCB Compression Boots, Kendall Co., Boston, MA). These should be operative before the start of anesthesia for maximal protection against venothrombosis. A heating/cooling blanket is placed over the chest and arms of the patient (Bair Hugger Upper Body Cover, Augustine Medical, Eden Prairie, MN 55344) and also beneath the torso (Cincinnati Sub-Zero, Cincinnati, OH).

Abdominal skin preparation is from midchest to midthigh. The external genitalia are prepared in the male and a vaginal preparation is used in females. The Foley catheter is placed in position. A Silastic 18-gauge nasogastric sump tube is placed within the stomach (Argyle Salem Sump Tube, Sherwood Medical, St. Louis, MO).

ABDOMINAL EXPOSURE, GREATER OMENTECTOMY, AND SPLENECTOMY (FIG. 24D-2). The abdomen is opened through a midline incision from xiphoid to pubis. Generous

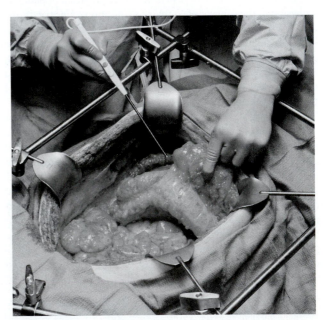

**FIGURE 24D-2.** Abdominal exposure using a self-retaining retractor, complete greater omentectomy and splenectomy. (See also Plate 34.)

abdominal exposure is achieved through the use of a Thompson Self-Retaining Retractor (Thompson Surgical Instruments, Inc., Traverse City, MI). The standard tool used to dissect tumor on peritoneal surfaces from the normal tissues is a 3-mm ball-tipped electrosurgical handpiece (Valleylab, Boulder, CO). The ball-tipped instrument is placed at the interface of tumor and normal tissues. The focal point for further dissection is placed on strong traction. The electrosurgical generator is used on pure cut at high voltage. The 3-mm ball-tipped electrode is used cautiously for tumor removal on tubular structures, especially the ureters, small bowel, and colon. Dissection of parietal peritoneal surfaces presents less risk for heat necrosis and fistula formation.

Using ball-tipped electrosurgery on pure cut creates a large volume of plume because of the electroevaporation (carbonization) of tissue. To maintain visualization of the operative field and to preserve a smoke-free atmosphere, a smoke filtration unit is used (Stackhouse Inc., El Segunda, CA). The vacuum tip is maintained 2 to 3 in (5 to 7.5 cm) from the field of dissection whenever electrosurgery is in use.

To free the midabdomen of a large volume of tumor, the greater omentectomy-splenectomy is performed. The greater omentum is elevated and then separated from the transverse colon using electrosurgery. This dissection continues beneath the peritoneum that covers the transverse mesocolon so as to expose the pancreas. The gastroepiploic vessels on the greater curvature of the stomach are clamped, ligated, and divided. Also, the short gastric vessels are transected. The mound of tumor that covers the spleen is identified. With traction on the spleen, the peritoneum anterior to the pancreas is stripped from the gland using electrosurgery. This freely exposes the splenic artery and vein at the tail of the pancreas. These vessels are ligated in continuity and proximally suture-ligated. This allows the greater curvature of the stomach to be reflected to the right from the pylorus to the gastroesophageal junction.

### PERITONEAL STRIPPING FROM BENEATH THE LEFT HEMIDIAPHRAGM (FIG. 24D-3).
To begin peritonectomy of the left upper quadrant, the peritoneum at the edge of the abdominal

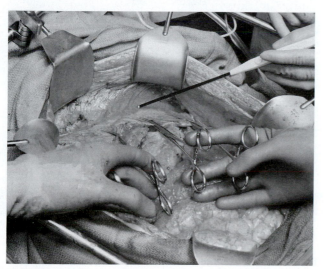

**FIGURE 24D-3.** Peritoneal stripping from the left diaphragm. (See also Plate 35.)

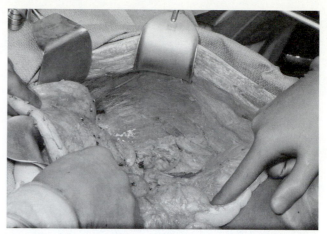

**FIGURE 24D-4.** Left subphrenic peritonectomy completed. (See also Plate 36.)

incision is stripped off the posterior rectus sheath. This allows strong traction to be exerted on the tumor specimen throughout the left upper quadrant and separation of surface tumor from all normal tissue in the left upper quadrant to the diaphragmatic muscle, the left adrenal gland, and the superior half of perirenal fat. The splenic flexure of the colon is severed from the left abdominal gutter and moved medially by dividing the peritoneum along Toldt's line. The dissection beneath diaphragm muscle must be performed with ball-tipped electrosurgery, not by blunt dissection. Numerous blood vessels between the diaphragm muscle and its peritoneal surface must be electrocoagulated before their transection or unnecessary bleeding will occur as the divided blood vessel retracts into the muscle of the diaphragm. Tissues are transected using ball-tipped electrosurgery on pure cut, with all blood vessels electrocoagulated before their division.

### LEFT SUBPHRENIC PERITONECTOMY COMPLETED (FIG. 24D-4).
When the left upper quadrant peritonectomy is completed, the stomach may be reflected medially. Numerous branches of the gastroepiploic arteries that have been ligated are evident. The left adrenal gland, pancreas, and left Gerota's fascia are visualized completely, as is the anterior peritoneal surface of the transverse mesocolon. The surgeon must avoid the left gastric artery and coronary vein to preserve the sole remaining vascular supply to the stomach.

### PERITONEAL STRIPPING FROM BENEATH THE RIGHT HEMIDIAPHRAGM (FIG. 24D-5).
Peritoneum is stripped from the right posterior rectus sheath to begin the peritonectomy in the right upper quadrant of the abdomen. Strong traction on the specimen is used to elevate the hemidiaphragm into the operative field. Again, ball-tipped electrosurgery on pure cut is used to dissect at the interface of tumor and normal tissue. Coagulation current is used to divide the blood vessels as they are encountered and before they bleed.

The stripping of tumor from the undersurface of the diaphragm continues until the bare area of the liver is encountered. At that point, tumor on the superior surface of the liver is electroevaporated

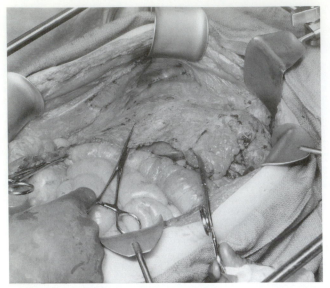

**FIGURE 24D-5.** Peritoneal stripping of the undersurface of the right hemidiaphragm. (See also Plate 37.)

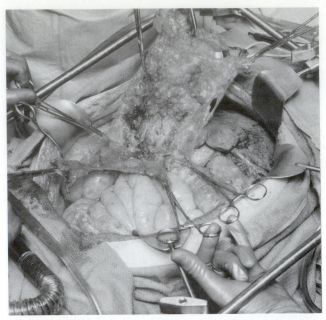

**FIGURE 24D-6.** Stripping of tumor from beneath the right hemidiaphragm, from the right subhepatic space and from the surface of the liver. (See also Plate 38.)

until the liver surface is cleared. With ball-tipped electrosurgical dissection, a thick layer of tumor may be lifted off the dome of the liver by moving beneath Glisson's capsule. Isolated patches of tumor on the liver surface are electroevaporated with the distal 2 cm of the ball tip bent and stripped of insulation ("hockey stick" configuration). Ball-tipped electrosurgery is also used to extirpate tumor from attachments of the falciform ligament and round ligament.

### STRIPPING OF TUMOR FROM BENEATH THE RIGHT HEMIDIAPHRAGM, FROM RIGHT SUBHEPATIC SPACE, AND FROM THE SURFACE OF THE LIVER (FIG. 24D-6).

Tumor from beneath the right hemidiaphragm, from the right subhepatic space, and from the surface of the liver forms an envelope as it is removed en bloc. The dissection is greatly facilitated if the tumor specimen can be maintained intact. The dissection continues laterally on the right to encounter the perirenal fat covering the right kidney. Also, the right adrenal gland is visualized and carefully avoided as tumor is stripped from the right subhepatic space. Care is taken not to traumatize the vena cava or to disrupt the caudate lobe veins that pass between the vena cava and segment 1 of the liver.

### COMPLETED RIGHT SUBPHRENIC PERITONECTOMY (FIG. 24D-7).

With strong upward traction on the right costal margin by the self-retaining retractor and medial displacement of the right liver, one can visualize the completed right subphrenic peritonectomy. The anterior branches of the phrenic artery and vein on the hemidiaphragm are seen and have been preserved. The right hepatic vein and the vena cava below have been exposed. The right subhepatic space, including the right adrenal gland and perirenal fat covering the right kidney, constitutes the base of the dissection.

Frequently, tumor is densely adherent to the tendinous central portion of the left or right hemidiaphragm. If this occurs, the tissue infiltrated by tumor must be resected. This usually requires an elliptical excision of a portion of the hemidiaphragm on either the right or the left. The defect in the diaphragm is closed with interrupted sutures after the intraoperative chemotherapy is completed.

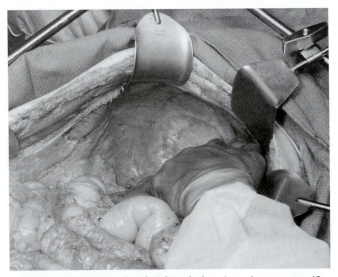

**FIGURE 24D-7.** Completed right subphrenic peritonectomy. (See also Plate 39.)

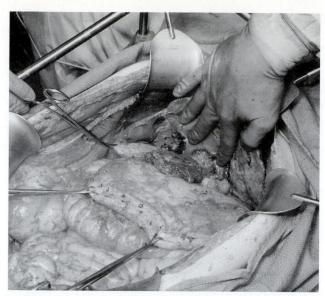

**FIGURE 24D-8.** Lesser omentectomy and cholecystectomy with stripping of the porta hepatis. (See also Plate 40.)

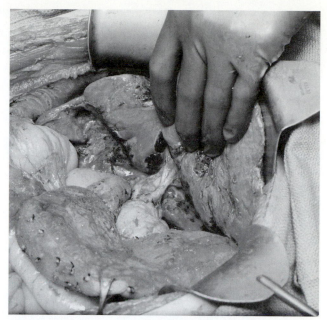

**FIGURE 24D-9.** Stripping of the omental bursa. (See also Plate 41.)

## LESSER OMENTECTOMY AND CHOLECYSTECTOMY WITH STRIPPING OF THE PORTA HEPATIS (FIG. 24D-8).

The gallbladder is removed in a routine fashion from its fundus toward the cystic artery and cystic duct. These structures are ligated and divided. The right lateral portion of the hepatoduodenal ligament that covers the porta hepatis is characteristically heavily layered with tumor. Using strong traction, the cancerous tissue that coats the porta hepatis is bluntly stripped from the base of the gallbladder bed toward the duodenum. The right gastric artery going to the lesser omental arcade is preserved. To continue resection of the lesser omentum, one dissects through the gastrohepatic fissure that divides liver segments 2, 3, and 4 from segment 1. Ball-tipped electrosurgery is used to electroevaporate tumor from the anterior surface of the left caudate process. Care is taken not to traumatize the anterior surface of the caudate process, for this can result in excessive and needless blood loss. The segmental blood supply to the caudate lobe is located on the anterior surface of this segment of the liver, and hemorrhage may occur with only superficial trauma. Also, a replaced left hepatic artery may arise from the left gastric artery and cross through the hepatogastric fissure.

## STRIPPING OF THE OMENTAL BURSA (FIG. 24D-9).

As one clears the left part of liver segment 1 of tumor, the vena cava is visualized directly beneath. To begin to strip the omental bursa, strong traction is maintained on the tumor and ball-tipped electrosurgery is used to divide the fibrous tissue between liver segment 1 and the vena cava. The phrenoesophageal ligament is incised so that peritoneum can be stripped away from the crus of the right hemidiaphragm. The common hepatic artery and the left gastric artery are skeletonized and lymph nodes in this region avoided. The cephalad and caudad branching of the left gastric artery and the coronary vein are identified and avoided. Dissection of lesser omental fat by compressing tissue between the thumb and index finger helps identify the major branches of the left gastric artery. Omental fat not involved by tumor is preserved to ensure adequate blood supply to the stomach. At least two major branches of the left gastric artery to the lesser curvature of the stomach are required to provide blood supply to the stomach. The surgeon dissects in a clockwise direction along the lesser curvature of the stomach, attempting to preserve the arcade. Care is taken to preserve as much omental fat as possible; only tumor tissue is removed. One attempts to spare the anterior vagus nerve going toward the antrum of the stomach.

Sometimes, a pyloroplasty or gastrojejunostomy must be performed if the vagus nerve is divided. As a result of the anterior vagotomy and in the absence of a gastric drainage procedure, gastric stasis may occur.

## COMPLETE PELVIC PERITONECTOMY (FIG. 24D-10).

The tumor-bearing peritoneum is stripped from the posterior surface of the lower abdominal incision, exposing the rectus muscle. The muscular surface of the bladder is seen, as ball-tipped electrosurgery strips peritoneum and preperitoneal fat from this structure. The urachus must be divided and is then elevated on a clamp as the leading point for this dissection. In the female, the round ligaments are divided as they enter the internal inguinal ring.

The peritoneal incision around the pelvis is completed by dividing the peritoneum along the pelvic brim. The right and left ureters are identified and preserved. In women, the right and left ovarian veins are ligated at the level of the lower pole of the kidney and divided. A linear stapler is used to divide the sigmoid colon just above the limits of the pelvic tumor. The vascular supply of the distal portion of the bowel is traced back to its origin on the aorta. The inferior

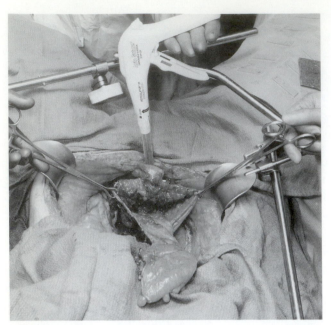

**FIGURE 24D-10.** Complete pelvic peritonectomy. (See also Plate 42.)

mesenteric artery is suture-ligated and divided. This allows one to pack all the viscera, including the proximal sigmoid colon, in the upper abdomen.

### RESECTION OF RECTOSIGMOID COLON AND CUL-DE-SAC OF DOUGLAS (FIG. 24D-11). Ball-tipped electrosurgery is used to dissect at the limits of the mesorectum. The surgeon works in a centripetal fashion. Extraperitoneal ligation of the uterine arteries is performed just above the ureter and close to the base of the

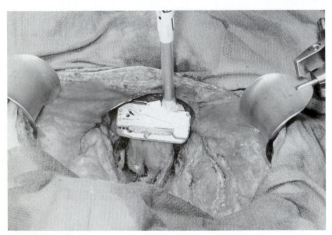

**FIGURE 24D-11.** Resection of rectosigmoid colon and cul-de-sac of Douglas. (See also Plate 43.)

bladder. In women, the bladder is moved gently off the cervix and the vagina is entered. The vaginal cuff anterior and posterior to the cervix is transected using ball-tipped electrosurgery, and the rectovaginal septum is entered. Ball-tipped electrosurgery is used to divide the perirectal fat beneath the peritoneal reflection. This ensures that all tumors that occupy the cul-de-sac are removed intact with the specimen. The rectal musculature is skeletonized using ball-tipped electrosurgery. A roticulator stapler (Autosuture, Norwalk, CT) is used to close off the rectal stump and the rectum is sharply divided above the stapler with scissors.

### VAGINAL CLOSURE AND LOW COLORECTAL ANASTO-MOSIS (FIG. 24D-12). One of the few suture repairs performed prior to the intraoperative chemotherapy is the closure of the vaginal cuff. If one fails to close the vaginal cuff, chemotherapy-containing fluid will leak from the vagina. The circular stapled colorectal anastomosis occurs after intraoperative chemotherapy. A circular stapling device is passed into the rectum, and the trochar penetrates the staple line. A monofilament suture placed in a purse-string fashion is used to secure the staple anvil in the proximal sigmoid colon. The body of the circular stapler and anvil are mated, and the stapler is activated to complete the low colorectal anastomosis (Intraluminal Stapler 33, Ethicon, Sommerville, NJ).

### LEFT COLON MOBILIZATION FOR A TENSION-FREE LOW COLORECTAL ANASTOMOSIS (FIG. 24D-13). A requirement for a complication-free low colorectal anastomosis is absence of tension on the staple line. Adequate mobilization of the entire left colon is needed, and several steps may be required to accomplish this. The inferior mesenteric artery is ligated on the aorta, and then its individual branches are resected as they arise from this vascular trunk. This is the Y-to-V transition that keeps the intermediate arcade intact. The inferior mesenteric vein is divided as it courses around the duodenum. The mesentery of the transverse colon and splenic flexure are completely elevated from the perirenal fat surrounding the left kidney. Taking care to avoid the left ureter, the surgeon divides the left colon mesentery from all its attachments. These maneuvers allow the junction of the sigmoid and descending colon to reach to the low rectum or anus for a tension-free anastomosis. Redundant descending colon should fall into the hollow of the sacrum.

To assess the stapled colorectal anastomosis, the proximal and distal tissue rings are examined for completeness. Air is insufflated into the rectum with a water-filled pelvis to check for an airtight circle of staples. Two hands should easily pass beneath the sigmoid colon to ensure there is no tension on the stapled anastomosis. A rectal examination is done to check for staple-line bleeding at the anastomosis.

### ANTRECTOMY AND GASTRIC RECONSTRUCTION (FIG. 24D-14). The gastric antrum, along with other intraabdominal structures that have restricted peristalsis, may be surrounded so densely by tumor that resection rather than peritoneal stripping is required for complete tumor removal. The right gastric artery is divided and the first portion of the duodenum is separated from the pancreas. A stapler (Ethicon PLC75, Cincinnati, OH) is used to close off and transect the duodenum just below the last visible

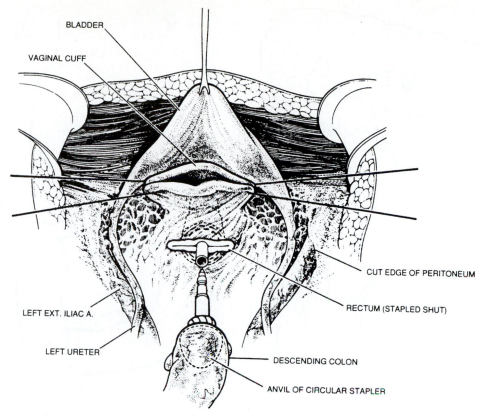

BLADDER

VAGINAL CUFF

CUT EDGE OF PERITONEUM

RECTUM (STAPLED SHUT)

LEFT EXT. ILIAC A.

LEFT URETER

DESCENDING COLON

ANVIL OF CIRCULAR STAPLER

**FIGURE 24D-12.** Vaginal closure and low colorectal anastomosis.

evidence of tumor. Similarly, a stapler (Ethicon TA90, Cincinnati, OH) divides the stomach proximally above the tumor. The duodenal and gastric staple lines are inverted with interrupted sutures after intraoperative chemotherapy has been completed. A side-to-side gastrojejunostomy is performed after the intraoperative chemotherapy is complete.

### TOTAL GASTRECTOMY WITH STAGED RECONSTRUCTION (FIG. 24D-15).

In approximately 10% of patients with pseudomyxoma peritonei, a total gastrectomy will be needed to clear the left upper quadrant of mucinous tumor. In most instances, this indicates that the tumor is a more aggressive type, usually called pseudomyxoma/carcinoma hybrid. Alternatively, the patient may have had many prior surgical procedures with prior extensive dissection in the left upper quadrant.

To perform the gastrectomy, the esophagus is closed off with a linear stapler (Ethicon TA30, Cincinnati, OH) and then transected. The left gastric artery is ligated and suture-ligated. Final attachments of the stomach to the superior portion of the head of the pancreas are divided using ball-tipped electrosurgery. Great care is taken to not damage the anterior surface of the pancreas. To reconstruct the gastrointestinal tract after gastrectomy that is part of a complete cytoreduction, a duodenal exclusion operation is performed. This protects the esophagojejunal anastomosis. Approximately 20 cm below the ligament of Treitz, a portion of jejunum is transected

with a linear stapler and brought in a retrocolic fashion up to the esophagus. The esophageal staple line is removed and a purse-string suture is used to secure the anvil of a circular stapler in the distal esophagus (Ethicon ILS29, Cincinnati, OH). The staple line closing the proximal jejunum is removed and the stapler is passed approximately 5 cm into the jejunum and then out through the jejunal wall. It is mated with the anvil within the esophagus, and the staple line is completed. The proximal jejunum is stapled off, and then the staple line inverted with interrupted sutures. This reconstruction is performed after the intraoperative chemotherapy is complete. The portion of jejunum proximal to the linear staple line is now brought out in the left upper quadrant as an end ostomy in order to divert all bile and digestive enzymes from the gastrointestinal tract. This diverting jejunostomy is closed between 6 and 9 months postoperatively as part of a second-look procedure.

### TUBES AND DRAINS REQUIRED FOR INTRAOPERATIVE AND EARLY POSTOPERATIVE INTRAPERITONEAL CHEMOTHERAPY (FIG. 24D-16).

Four closed-suction drains are placed in the dependent portions of the abdomen. This includes one in the right subhepatic space, one in the left subdiaphragmatic space, and two in the pelvis. A Tenckhoff catheter (Quinton curled peritoneal catheter, Quinton, Inc., Seattle, WA) is placed through the abdominal wall and positioned within the abdomen at the site that is thought

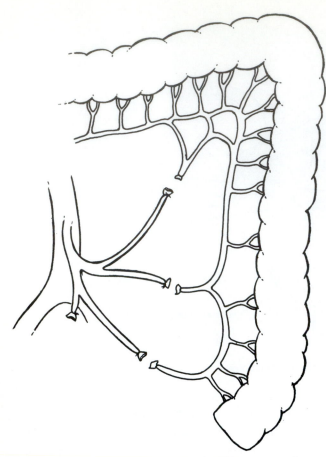

**FIGURE 24D-13.** Left colon mobilization for a low colorectal anastomosis.

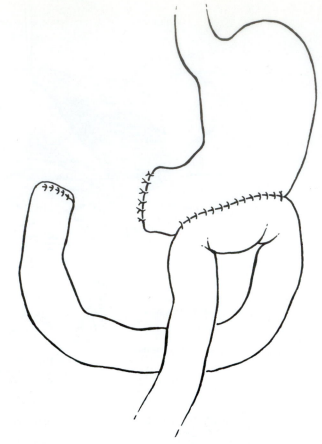

**FIGURE 24D-14.** Antrectomy and gastric reconstruction.

to be the area of greatest risk for recurrence. All transabdominal drains and tubes are secured to the skin in a watertight fashion with a purse-string suture. Temperature probes are placed at the inflow (Tenckhoff catheter) and at a remote site. They are removed after the intraoperative chemotherapy is completed. Right-angle thoracostomy tubes (Deknatel, Floral Park, NY) are inserted on both the right and left sides to prevent abdominal fluid from accumulating in the chest as a result of the subphrenic peritonectomy.

## INTRAPERITONEAL CHEMOTHERAPY

CONCEPTUAL CHANGES WITH INTRAPERITONEAL CHEMOTHERAPY. Changes in the use of chemotherapy in patients with peritoneal carcinomatosis, peritoneal sarcomatosis, and peritoneal mesothelioma have occurred and shown favorable results of treatment. A change in *route* of drug administration has occurred. Chemotherapy is given intraperitoneally, or by combined intraperitoneal and intravenous routes. In this new strategy, intravenous chemotherapy alone is rarely indicated. Also, a change in *timing* has occurred in that chemotherapy begins in the operating

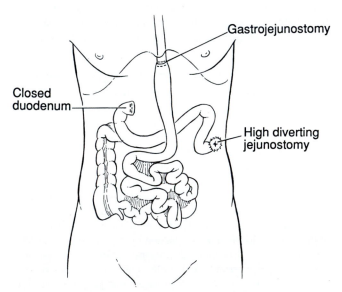

**FIGURE 24D-15.** Total gastrectomy with staged reconstruction.

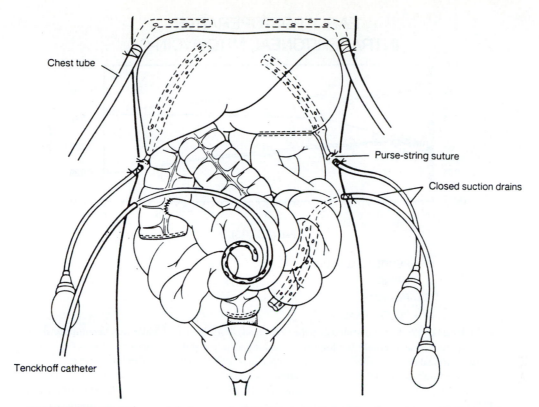

**FIGURE 24D-16.** Tubes and drains required for intraoperative and early postoperative intraperitoneal chemotherapy.

room and may be continued for the first five postoperative days. Third, a change in *selection* criteria for treatment of cancer has occurred, with the nonaggressive peritoneal surface malignancies likely to benefit from this approach. The lesion size of peritoneal implants is of crucial importance. Only patients with small intraperitoneal tumor nodules that have a limited distribution within the abdomen and pelvis are likely to show prolonged benefit. Meticulous cytoreductive surgery is necessary prior to the intraperitoneal chemotherapy instillation. Aggressive treatment strategies for an advanced and invasive intraperitoneal malignancy will not produce long-term benefits, and is often the cause of excessive morbidity or mortality. The initiation of treatments for peritoneal surface malignancy must occur as early as is possible in the natural history of these diseases in order to achieve the greatest benefits. The greatest change that now needs to occur with peritoneal surface malignancy is a change in oncologists' attitudes toward these diseases. They may be cured with early application of combined treatments.

BACKGROUND.  Most cancers that occur within the abdomen or pelvis will disseminate by three different routes. These are hematogenous metastases, lymphatic metastases, and spread through the peritoneal space to surfaces within the abdomen and pelvis. In a substantial number of patients with abdominal or pelvic malignancy, surgical treatment failure is isolated to the resection site or to peritoneal surfaces. This leads to a hypothesis that suggests that the elimination of peritoneal surface spread may have an impact on the survival of these cancer patients, and that a leading cause of death and suffering in patients with these malignancies is progression of peritoneal surface disease. Prior to the use of cytoreductive surgery and intraperitoneal chemotherapy these conditions were uniformly fatal, eventually resulting in intestinal obstruction. Occasionally patients with low-grade malignancies such as pseudomyxoma peritonei survived for several years, but all end-results reportings have shown fatal outcomes.

Current technology for the administration of intraperitoneal chemotherapy demands that it be used as an integral part of the surgical procedure. "Surgically directed chemotherapy" involves several crucial technological modifications of chemotherapy administration. First, an intraperitoneal rather than an intravenous route for chemotherapy is used. The intraperitoneal route, when properly utilized, will allow uniform distribution of a high concentration of anticancer therapy at the site of the malignancy. This is achieved by the surgeon intraoperatively manipulating the intestinal contents to uniformly distribute the chemotherapy. In the early postoperative period, the patient's position is repeatedly changed to assist gravity in maintaining an optimal chemotherapy distribution.

Secondly, the chemotherapy administration is timed so that all of the malignancy, except for microscopic residual disease, will have

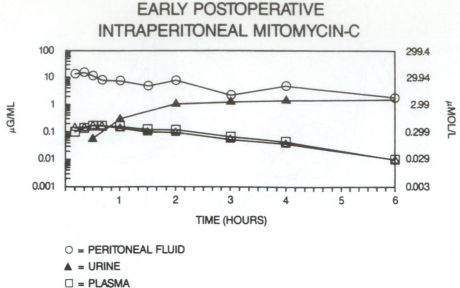

**FIGURE 24D-17.** When instilled into the peritoneal cavity, large molecular weight compounds are sequestered at that site for long time periods. The physiologic barrier to the release of intraperitoneal drugs is called "the peritoneal plasma barrier." In this experiment, 15 mg of mitomycin C was infused into the cavity as rapidly as possible. Intraperitoneal, intravenous, portal venous and urine mitomycin C concentrations were determined by HPLC assay. (From Sugarbaker PH et al: Rationale for early postoperative intraperitoneal chemotherapy [EPIC] in patients with advanced gastrointestinal cancer. Cancer Res 50:5790–5794, 1990 [with permission]).

been removed prior to the chemotherapy treatments. This means that the limited penetration of chemotherapy into tissues, which is approximately 1 mm, will be adequate to eradicate all tumor cells. Also, the chemotherapy will be used prior to the construction of any anastomosis. This means that suture line recurrences should also be eliminated. Finally, since all adhesions have been taken down, there will be no surfaces in the abdomen or pelvis excluded by scar tissue from contact with chemotherapy solutions.

From all theoretical considerations, cytoreductive surgery and intraperitoneal chemotherapy must be used as early in the natural history of the cancer as is possible. No longer can the clinician wait for the patient with peritoneal carcinomatosis to become symptomatic to begin treatments. Protocols to prevent iatrogenic peritoneal surface spread that may occur as a result of the resection of a primary gastrointestinal malignancy must be considered. The treatment of patients with an invasive malignancy that has a wide distribution of a large mass of cancer will not produce long-term benefits. As oncologists accept that peritoneal surface malignancy can be cured, they will initiate aggressive treatments in a timely fashion.

**PERITONEAL-PLASMA BARRIER.** Intraperitoneal chemotherapy gives high response rates within the abdomen because the "peritoneal plasma barrier" provides dose-intensive therapy.[7] Figure 24D-17 shows that large-molecular-weight substances, such

as mitomycin C, are confined to the abdominal cavity for long time periods.[8] This means that the exposure of peritoneal surfaces to pharmacologically active molecules can be increased considerably by giving the drugs via the intraperitoneal route rather than the intravenous route.

For the chemotherapy agents used to treat peritoneal carcinomatosis or peritoneal sarcomatosis, the area-under-the-curve ratios of intraperitoneal to intravenous exposure are favorable. Table 24D-1 presents the area under the curve (intraperitoneal/

**TABLE 24D-1.** AREA UNDER THE CURVE (CONCENTRATION OF DRUG TIMES THE DURATION OF EXPOSURE) RATIOS OF PERITONEAL SURFACE EXPOSURE TO SYSTEMIC EXPOSURE FOR DRUGS USED TO TREAT INTRAABDOMINAL CANCER

| DRUG | MOLECULAR WEIGHT | AREA UNDER THE CURVE RATIO |
|---|---|---|
| 5-Fluorouracil | 130 | 250 |
| Mitomycin C | 334 | 75 |
| Doxorubicin | 544 | 500 |
| Cisplatin | 300 | 20 |
| Taxol | 808 | 1000 |
| Gemcitabine | 263 | 50 |

intravenous) for the drugs in routine clinical use in patients with peritoneal seeding. In our studies, these include 5-fluorouracil, mitomycin C, doxorubicin, cisplatin, taxol, and gemcitabine.

One should not assume that the intraperitoneal administration of chemotherapy eliminates their systemic toxicities. Although the drugs are sequestered within the peritoneal space, they eventually are cleared into the systemic circulation. For this reason, the safe doses of most drugs instilled into the peritoneal cavity are identical to the intravenous dose. The exceptions are drugs with hepatic metabolism such as 5-fluorouracil and gemcitabine. An increased dose of approximately 50% is usually possible with 5-fluorouracil. The dose for a 5-day course of intravenous 5-fluorouracil is approximately 500 mg/m$^2$; for intraperitoneal 5-fluorouracil, the dose is 750 mg/m$^2$ per day. This considerable (50%) increase in the dose of 5-fluorouracil is of great advantage in treating peritoneal carcinomatosis.

**TUMOR CELL ENTRAPMENT.** Sugarbaker and colleagues have advanced the "tumor cell entrapment" hypothesis to explain the rapid progression of peritoneal surface malignancy in patients who undergo treatment using surgery alone.[8] This theory relates the high incidence and rapid progression of peritoneal surface implantation to:

Free intraperitoneal tumor emboli as a result of serosal penetration by cancer

Leakage of malignant cells from transected lymphatics

Dissemination of malignant cells directly from the cancer specimen as a result of surgical trauma and backflow of venous blood

Fibrin entrapment of intraabdominal tumor emboli on traumatized peritoneal surfaces

Progression of these entrapped tumor cells through growth factors involved in the wound-healing process

This phenomenon may cause a high incidence of surgical treatment failure in patients treated for primary gastrointestinal cancer. Also, the reimplantation of malignant cells into peritonectomized surfaces in a reoperative setting must be expected unless intraperitoneal chemotherapy is used.

Chemotherapy employed in the perioperative period not only directly destroys tumor cells, but also eliminates viable platelets, white blood cells, and monocytes from the perioneal cavity. This diminishes the promotion of tumor growth associated with the wound-healing process. Consequently, the results from use of intraperitoneal chemotherapy show a reduction in local recurrence and peritoneal surface recurrence in patients with intraabdominal cancer. Removal of the leukocytes and monocytes also decreases the ability of the abdomen to resist an infectious process. For this reason, strict aseptic technique is imperative when administering the chemotherapy or handling abdominal tubes and drains.

In order to interrupt this widespread implantation of tumor cells on abdominal and pelvic surfaces, the abdominal cavity is flooded with chemotherapy in a large volume of fluid during the operation (heated intraoperative intraperitoneal chemotherapy) and in the postoperative period (early postoperative intraperitoneal chemotherapy).

**PRIOR LIMITED BENEFITS WITH INTRAPERITONEAL CHEMOTHERAPY.** The use of intraperitoneal chemotherapy in the past has met with limited success and acceptance by oncologists. There have been three major impediments to greater success. Intracavitary instillation allows very limited penetration of drug into tumor nodules. Only the outermost layer (approximately 1 mm) of a cancer nodule is penetrated by the chemotherapy. This means that only minute tumor nodules can be definitely treated. In most trials, oncologists have attempted to treat established disease, and this selection of patients has caused disappointment with intraperitoneal drug use. Microscopic residual disease is the ideal target for intraperitoneal chemotherapy protocols.

A second cause for limited success with intraperitoneal chemotherapy is a nonuniform drug distribution. A majority of patients treated by drug instillation into the abdomen or pelvis have had prior surgery, which invariably causes scarring between peritoneal surfaces. The adhesions create multiple barriers to the free access of fluid. Although the instillation of a large volume of fluid will partially overcome the problems created by adhesions, frequently large surface areas will have no access to chemotherapy. Limited access from adhesions is impossible to predict and may increase with repeated instillations of chemotherapy.

Nonuniform drug distribution after surgery may result from fibrin entrapment. Surgery causes fibrin deposits on surfaces that have been traumatized by the cancer resection. Free intraperitoneal cancer cells become trapped within the fibrin. The fibrin is infiltrated by platelets, neutrophils, and monocytes as part of the wound-healing process. As collagen is laid down, the tumor cells are entrapped within scar tissue. The scar tissue is dense and poorly penetrated by intraperitoneal chemotherapy.

Nonuniform drug distribution may be caused by gravity. Intraperitoneal fluid does not uniformly distribute itself to anterior and posterior peritoneal surfaces. Gravity pulls the fluid to dependent portions of the abdomen and pelvis—especially the pelvis, paracolic gutters, and the right retrohepatic space. Unless the patient actively pursues frequent changes in position, the surfaces between bowel loops and the anterior abdominal wall will remain relatively untreated.

A final obstacle to success with the administration of intraperitoneal chemotherapy encountered in the past is the *difficulty and dangers of long-term peritoneal access*. There has been no catheter or technical solution to the requirement for reliable repeated access to the peritoneal space. Repeated instillations of large volumes of chemotherapy solution cause great inconvenience and can result in a large number of serious complications. Whether the oncologist chooses repeated paracentesis or an indwelling catheter, complications such as pain upon instillation, bowel perforation, instillation into soft tissues, or inability to infuse or drain occur repeatedly. At this time, prolonged peritoneal access is a technical challenge without a known solution.

The problems with prolonged peritoneal access have led some surgical oncologists to adopt what has been referred to as the "big bang" approach. All visible abdominal or pelvic cancer should be completely extirpated by surgery. Then in the operating room, a high dose of heated chemotherapy is delivered to eradicate tiny tumor nodules and microscopic cancer cells that remain. This means that all abdominal and pelvic components of the cancer, including

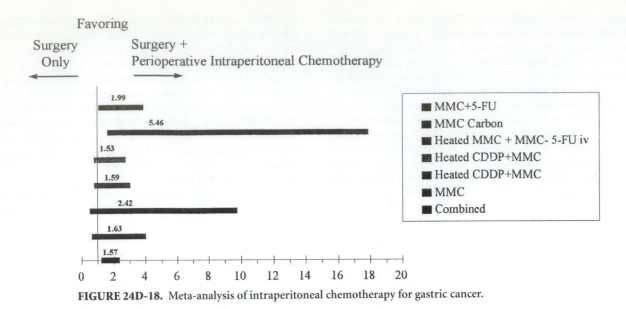

**FIGURE 24D-18.** Meta-analysis of intraperitoneal chemotherapy for gastric cancer.

persistent peritoneal surface malignancy, are eliminated. Systemic components of the disease now become the responsibility of the medical oncologist.

## CLINICAL EVIDENCE THAT CYTOREDUCTIVE SURGERY AND INTRAPERITONEAL CHEMOTHERAPY IS OF BENEFIT TO PATIENTS WITH PERITONEAL SURFACE MALIGNANCY.

Treatments for peritoneal carcinomatosis and sarcomatosis have been shown to provide prolonged survival with some patients alive at 5 years and considered cured. The strategy for treating these patients has always involved three essential components. The first essential component is a complete cytoreduction, utilizing peritonectomy procedures with an attempt to remove all visible tumor. Assuming that microscopic residual disease will eventuate in recurrence in all these patients, the second essential component involves perioperative intraperitoneal chemotherapy. It is becoming increasingly clear that proper patient selection is the third essential component of these treatment strategies. Although no one questions the essential need for complete cytoreduction and for accurate patient selection, many oncologists are not convinced that the intraperitoneal chemotherapy is of benefit to prevent recurrence of peritoneal surface disease. There are data from prospective trials and from clinical observations that suggest that intraperitoneal chemotherapy can reduce or eliminate the recurrence of peritoneal carcinomatosis after surgery.

The first data come from prospective clinical trials. Sugarbaker and coworkers[9] conducted a trial in patients with poor-prognosis colon cancer.[9] Intravenous 5-fluorouracil was randomized against intraperitoneal 5-fluorouracil. Each cycle of treatment was given for 5 days, and the treatments were repeated on a monthly basis for 1 year. Patients who recurred were explored, and the status of their disease was assessed during the surgery. A statistically significant decrease in the incidence of peritoneal carcinomatosis occurred in patients who had received intraperitoneal 5-fluorouracil ( $p = 0.003$ ). In this small group of poor-prognosis patients, there was no improvement in survival but there was a great reduction in the incidence of recurrence of peritoneal carcinomatosis in the patients receiving intraperitoneal 5-fluorouracil.

Several prospective randomized studies in peritoneal carcinomatosis from gastric cancer have been reported. The metaanalysis of eight trials is shown in Fig. 24D-18. In all but one of these trials the intraperitoneal chemotherapy was given in the perioperative period. There was an improved survival in the seven trials utilizing perioperative intraperitoneal chemotherapy.[10] In the study by Yu et al.,[11] perioperative intraperitoneal mitomycin C and 5-fluorouracil were used for the first 5 days following gastrectomy. An analysis by the Cox proportional hazards model showed that the risk of recurrence was nearly twice as great in patients who had surgery alone as compared to those patients who had surgery plus perioperative chemotherapy. In patients with stage III disease, the odds ratio was 4 in favor of the intraperitoneal chemotherapy. In patients who had positive lymph nodes, the odds ratio was 8. These data strongly suggest that microscopic residual disease can be eliminated by adjuvant perioperative intraperitoneal chemotherapy.

Data provided by Gough and coworkers[12] at the Mayo Clinic in patients with pseudomyxoma peritonei show that intraperitoneal chemotherapy is effective in this patient population. In their report on 56 patients, the only long-term survivors were those who had both surgery and intraperitoneal chemotherapy. Patients who had only repeated surgeries had a median survival of 3 years, and only 5% of these patients were alive at the end of 5 years.

The patterns of recurrence in patients treated with intraperitoneal chemotherapy show marked differences in the incidence of recurrence in the abdomen as compared to other anatomic sites. Zoetmulder and colleagues[13] showed that diaphragm perforation in patients with pseudomyxoma peritonei that occurred at the time of cytoreduction was associated with disease progression within the pleural space in 10 of 11 patients. Disease control within the abdomen where intraperitoneal chemotherapy was used occurred in these patients. Small-volume disease that entered the chest through a diaphragm perforation without intraperitoneal chemotherapy resulted in progression. A much larger residual disease found in the abdomen was controlled with perioperative intraperitoneal chemotherapy. Likewise, if drain tracts are used in patients with known peritoneal carcinomatosis, they will become involved by disease. Drain tracts in patients undergoing cytoreductive surgery with intraperitoneal chemotherapy seldom, if ever, develop abdominal wall recurrence. Likewise, the abdominal incision is frequently involved if surgery only is used to treat peritoneal carcinomatosis or sarcomatosis. If the surgery is combined with intraperitoneal chemotherapy, disease within the abdominal incision is not seen. This is also true in ovarian cancer patients with vaginal cuff recurrence. If the vaginal cuff is closed without intraperitoneal chemotherapy, ovarian cancer is inoculated into this anatomic site. If intraperitoneal chemotherapy is used after an ovarian cancer cytoreduction, no recurrence within the vaginal cuff has been observed.

A final site for disease occurrence is the laparoscopy ports after laparoscopy in patients with suspect peritoneal carcinomatosis. Almost invariably, the laparoscopy ports become involved by cancer because disease is disseminated by the puncture sites through the abdominal wall.[14] There is a very definite correlation of the pattern of failure in patients receiving early postoperative intraperitoneal chemotherapy with dye studies that show nonuniform distribution of intraperitoneal chemotherapy in a closed abdomen. Zoetmulder and Sugarbaker[13] found that recurrence in patients with pseudomyxoma peritonei was most likely to occur within the abdominal incision, within colorectal or gastrojejunal suture lines, and at the base of the small-bowel mesentery. In patients given early postoperative intraperitoneal chemotherapy, the closure of the abdominal incision and suture lines prevents adequate chemotherapy access at these sites. Another area for frequent recurrence was the anterior surface of the stomach. Dye studies have shown that the left lobe of the liver almost invariably becomes adherent to the anterior surface of the stomach in patients treated with a closed intraperitoneal chemotherapy technique. Also, dye studies have demonstrated poor chemotherapy access to the base of the small-bowel mesentery. These data strongly suggest that pseudomyxoma peritonei recurs where there is imperfect exposure to the intraperitoneal chemotherapy. Other sites that have been noted to have a high incidence of recurrence after use of intraperitoneal chemotherapy are the inverted appendiceal stump and umbilical fissure.

Elias and coworkers (personal communication) reported an interesting pattern of recurrence in those patients who were treated using a peritoneal expander to deliver intraperitoneal chemotherapy. They reported a high incidence of recurrent disease where the peritoneal expander contacted the peritoneal surface at the edges of the abdominal incision. Cancer cells were pressed into the peritoneal surface at this site and were prevented from coming into contact with the chemotherapy and heated fluid.

Finally, it should be mentioned that surgery has been used for many decades in an attempt to treat patients with recurrent intraabdominal cancer. The fact that surgery alone has been unsuccessful is well established. Patients with peritoneal seeding have never experienced long-term survival by surgery alone. Data presented in this review clearly show that there is a high salvage rate in properly selected patients who are treated with cytoreductive surgery combined with adequate intraperitoneal chemotherapy. These data taken together strongly suggest that intraperitoneal chemotherapy is

an essential component of treatment protocols for peritoneal surface malignancies.

## PATIENT SELECTION FOR TREATMENT

The greatest impediment to lasting benefits from intraperitoneal chemotherapy should be attributed to improper patient selection. A great number of patients with advanced intraabdominal disease have been treated with minimal benefit. Even with extensive cytoreductive surgery and aggressive intraperitoneal chemotherapy, the patient is not likely to have a lasting benefit. Rapid recurrence of intraperitoneal cancer combined with progression of lymph nodal or systemic disease, are likely to interfere with long-term survival in these patients. Patients that benefit must have minimal residual disease isolated to peritoneal surfaces that have access to chemotherapy so that complete eradication of disease can occur. Partial responses are not of great benefit in peritoneal surface malignancies. Complete and durable responses are the reasonable goal. In the natural history of this disease, the time of the initiation of treatment has a great bearing on the benefits achieved. Asymptomatic patients with small volume peritoneal surface malignancy must be selected for intraperitoneal chemotherapy protocols.

### CLINICAL ASSESSMENTS OF PERITONEAL SURFACE MALIGNANCY.

In the past, peritoneal carcinomatosis was considered to be a fatal disease process. The only assessment used was either carcinomatosis present with a presumed fatal outcome or carcinomatosis absent with curative treatment options available. Currently, there are four important clinical assessments of peritoneal surface malignancy that need to be used to select patients who will benefit from treatment protocols.

1. The histopathology to assess the invasive character of the malignancy
2. The preoperative CT scan of abdomen and pelvis
3. The peritoneal cancer index
4. The completeness of cytoreduction score

### HISTOPATHOLOGY TO ASSESS INVASIVE CHARACTER.

The biologic aggressiveness of a peritoneal surface malignancy will have profound influence on its treatment options. Noninvasive tumors may have extensive spread on peritoneal surfaces and yet be completely resectable by peritonectomy procedures. Also, these noninvasive malignancies are extremely unlikely to metastasize by lymphatics to lymph nodes and by the blood to liver and other systemic sites. Therefore, protocols for cytoreductive surgery and intraperitoneal chemotherapy may have a curative intent in patients with a large mass of widely disseminated pseudomyxoma peritonei and peritoneal mesothelioma.[15] Also, some low-grade sarcomas may be aggressively treated with cure as a goal using cytoreductive surgery and intraperitoneal chemotherapy despite extensive disease progression. Pathology review and an assessment of the invasive or nonaggressive nature of a malignancy is essential to treatment planning.

### PREOPERATIVE CT SCAN.

The preoperative CT scan of chest, abdomen, and pelvis may be of great value in planning treatments for peritoneal surface malignancy. Systemic metastases can be clinically excluded and pleural surface spread ruled out. Unfortunately, the CT scan should be regarded as an inaccurate test by which to quantitate intestinal type of peritoneal carcinomatosis from adenocarcinoma. The malignant tissue progresses on the peritoneal surfaces and its shape conforms to the normal contours of the abdominopelvic structures. This is quite different from the metastatic process in the liver or lung, which progresses as three-dimensional tumor nodules and can be accurately assessed by CT.[16]

However, the CT scan has been of great help in locating and quantitating *mucinous* adenocarcinoma within the peritoneal cavity.[17] These tumors produce copious colloid material that is readily distinguished by shape and by density from normal structures. Using two distinctive radiologic criteria, those patients with resectable mucinous peritoneal carcinomatosis can be selected from those with nonresectable malignancy. This keeps patients who are unlikely to benefit from reoperative surgery from undergoing cytoreductive surgical procedures. The two radiologic criteria found to be most useful are: (1) Segmental obstruction of small bowel and (2) presence of tumor nodules greater than 5 cm in diameter on small-bowel surfaces or directly adjacent to small-bowel mesentery.

These criteria reflect radiologically the biology of the mucinous adenocarcinoma. Obstructed segments of bowel signal an invasive character of malignancy on small-bowel surfaces that would be unlikely to be completely cytoreduced. Mucinous cancer on small bowel or small-bowel mesentery indicates that the mucinous cancer is no longer redistributed. This means that small-bowel surfaces or small-bowel mesentery will have residual disease after cytoreduction, because these surfaces are impossible to peritonectomize (Fig. 24D-19 and Fig. 24D-20). The CT is also of great help in the

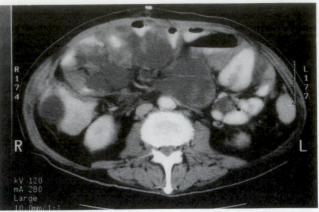

**FIGURE 24D-20.** Patient with intermediate grade mucinous adenocarcinoma who has recurred after extensive prior cytoreductive surgery. Small bowel loops are slightly distended, contain small volumes of air, and its mesenteric surface is coated with mucinous tumor nodules. This patient has less than 5% likelihood of a complete cytoreduction.

identification of nodules of recurrent sarcoma and sarcomatosis. The recurrences on peritoneal surfaces are nodular and the result of fibrin entrapment of traumatically disseminated sarcoma cells. In a CT scan with maximal filling of bowel with oral contrast, even small 1-cm nodular sarcoma recurrences are imaged.

**PERITONEAL CANCER INDEX.** The third assessment of peritoneal surface malignancy is the peritoneal cancer index (PCI). This is a clinical integration of both peritoneal implant size and distribution of peritoneal surface malignancy (Fig. 24D-21). It should be used in the decision-making process as the abdomen is explored. To arrive at a score, the size of intraperitoneal nodules must be assessed. The lesion size or LS score should be used. An LS-0 score means that no malignant deposits are visualized. An LS-1 score signifies tumor nodules less than 0.5 cm are present. The number of nodules is not scored, only the size of the largest nodules. An LS-2 score signifies tumor nodules between 0.5 and 5.0 cm are present. LS-3 signifies tumor nodules greater than 5.0 cm in any dimension are present. If there is a confluence of tumor, the lesion size is scored as 3.

In order to assess the distribution of peritoneal surface disease, the abdominopelvic regions are utilized. For each of these 13 regions, a lesion size score is determined. The summation of the lesion size score in each of the 13 abdominopelvic regions is the PCI for that patient. A maximal score is 39 (13 × 3).

The PCI has been validated to date in three separate situations. First, Steller and colleagues[18] used it successfully to quantitate intraperitoneal tumor in a murine peritoneal carcinomatosis model. Gomez and coworkers[19] showed that the PCI could be used to predict long-term survival in patients with peritoneal carcinomatosis from colon cancer having a second cytoreduction. Berthet and coworkers[20] showed that the PCI predicted benefits for treatment of peritoneal sarcomatosis from recurrent visceral or parietal sarcoma.

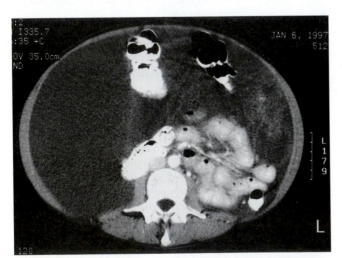

**FIGURE 24D-19.** Patient with adenomucinosis of appendiceal origin (pseudomyxoma peritonei syndrome) who had a complete cytoreduction and remains disease free 2 years postoperatively. The mucinous tumor is very extensive, but the small bowel loops are of normal caliber and are not distended by air. Also, the small bowel has become "compartmentalized" by the mucinous tumor. The small bowel surfaces and small bowel mesentery remain tumor free.

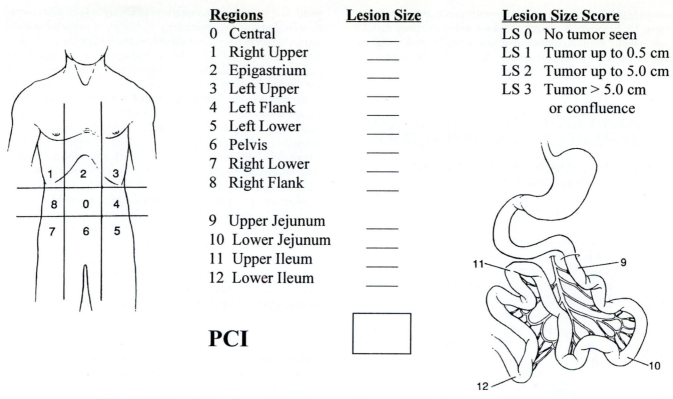

| **Regions** | **Lesion Size** | **Lesion Size Score** |
|---|---|---|
| 0  Central | ____ | LS 0   No tumor seen |
| 1  Right Upper | ____ | LS 1   Tumor up to 0.5 cm |
| 2  Epigastrium | ____ | LS 2   Tumor up to 5.0 cm |
| 3  Left Upper | ____ | LS 3   Tumor > 5.0 cm |
| 4  Left Flank | ____ | or confluence |
| 5  Left Lower | ____ | |
| 6  Pelvis | ____ | |
| 7  Right Lower | ____ | |
| 8  Right Flank | ____ | |
| | | |
| 9   Upper Jejunum | ____ | |
| 10  Lower Jejunum | ____ | |
| 11  Upper Ileum | ____ | |
| 12  Lower Ileum | ____ | |

**PCI**

**FIGURE 24D-21.** Peritoneal cancer index is a composite score of lesion size 0 to 3 in abdominopelvic regions 0–12.

In both clinical studies, the patients with a favorable prognosis had a score of less than 12.

There are some caveats in the use of the PCI. First, noninvasive malignancy on peritoneal surfaces may be completely cytoreduced. Diseases such as pseudomxyoma peritonei and peritoneal mesothelioma are in this category. With these "benign tumors," the status of the abdomen and pelvis after cytoreduction may have no relationship to its status at the time of abdominal exploration. In other words, even though the surgeons may find an abdomen with a PCI of 39, it can be converted to an index of 0 by cytoreduction. In these diseases, the prognosis will only be related to the condition of the abdomen after the cytoreduction (completeness of cytoreduction score).

A second caveat for the PCI is invasive cancer at crucial anatomic sites. For example, invasive cancer not cleanly resected on the common bile duct will cause a poor prognosis despite a low PCI. Invasion of the base of the bladder or unresectable disease on a pelvic side wall may, by itself, result in residual invasive cancer after cytoreduction and imply a poor prognosis. Also, unresectable cancer at numerous sites on the small bowel may by itself confer a poor prognosis. In other words, invasive cancer at crucial anatomic sites may function as systemic disease in assessing prognosis with invasive cancer. Since long-term survival can only occur in patients with a complete cytoreduction, residual disease at anatomically crucial sites may override a favorable score with the PCI.

**COMPLETENESS OF CYTOREDUCTION SCORE.** The final assessment to be used to assess prognosis with peritoneal surface malignancy is the completeness of cytoreduction (CC) score. This information is of less value to the surgeon in planning treatments than the PCI. The CC score is not available until after the cytoreduction is complete, rather than as the abdomen is being explored. If during exploration it becomes obvious that cytoreduction will not be complete, the surgeon may decide that a palliative debulking that will provide symptomatic relief is appropriate and discontinue plans for an aggressive cytoreduction with intraperitoneal chemotherapy. In both noninvasive and invasive peritoneal surface malignancy, the CC score is a major prognostic indicator. It has been shown to function with accuracy in pseudomyxoma peritonei, colon cancer with peritoneal carcinomatosis, and sarcomatosis.[15,20,21]

The size of peritoneal implants used to determine the CC score may vary with the primary site of the peritoneal carcinomatosis. More chemotherapy-responsive malignancies, such as ovarian cancer, may be eradicated even though larger-sized tumor nodules remain after cytoreduction. For gastrointestinal cancer the CC score has been defined as follows: A CC-0 score indicates that no peritoneal seeding was exposed during the complete exploration. A CC-1 score indicates that tumor nodules persisting after cytoreduction are less than 2.5 mm. This is a nodule size thought to be penetrable by intracavity chemotherapy and would, therefore, be designated a complete cytoreduction. A CC-2 score indicates tumor nodules between 2.5 mm and 2.5 cm. A CC-3 score indicates tumor nodules greater than 2.5 cm or a confluence of unresectable tumor nodules at any site within the abdomen or pelvis. CC-2 and CC-3 cytoreduction are considered incomplete.

## CURRENT METHODOLOGY FOR DELIVERY OF INTRAPERITONEAL CHEMOTHERAPY

### HEATED INTRAOPERATIVE INTRAPERITONEAL CHEMOTHERAPY ADMINISTRATION

In the operating room, heated intraoperative intraperitoneal chemotherapy is used. Heat is part of the optimizing process and is used to bring as much dose intensity to the abdominal and pelvic surfaces as is possible. Hyperthermia with intraperitoneal chemotherapy has several advantages. First, heat by itself has more toxicity for cancerous tissue than for normal tissue. This predominant effect on cancer increases as the vascularity of the malignancy decreases. Second, hyperthermia increases the penetration of chemotherapy into tissues. As tissues soften in response to heat, the elevated interstitial pressure of a tumor mass may decrease and allow improved drug penetration. Third, and probably most important, heat increases the cytotoxicity of selected chemotherapy agents. This synergism occurs only at the interface of heat and body tissue at the peritoneal surface. The rationale for using heated chemotherapy as a surgically directed modality in the operating room is presented in Table 24D-2.

After the cancer resection is complete, the Tenckhoff catheter and closed-suction drains are placed through the abdominal wall and made watertight with a purse-string suture at the skin. Temperature probes are secured to the skin edge. Using a long-running #2 monofilament suture, the skin edges are secured to the self-retaining retractor. A plastic sheet is incorporated into these sutures to create a covering for the abdominal cavity. A slit in the plastic cover is made to allow the surgeon's double-gloved hand access to the abdomen and pelvis (Fig. 24D-22). During the 90 min of perfusion, all the anatomic structures within the peritoneal cavity are uniformly exposed to heat and to chemotherapy. The surgeon gently but continuously manipulates all viscera to keep adherence of peritoneal surfaces to a minimum. If bleeding or some other event occurs, the chemotherapy solution is suctioned into the reservoir so that full visualization of the abdomen and pelvis is achieved. Roller pumps force the chemotherapy solution into the abdomen through the Tenckhoff catheter and pulls it out through the drains. A heat exchanger keeps the fluid being infused at 44° to 46°C so that the intraperitoneal fluid is maintained at 42° to 43°C. The apparatus used for the administration of heated intraoperative intraperitoneal chemotherapy is diagrammed in Fig. 24D-23. The smoke evacuator is used to pull air from beneath the plastic cover through activated charcoal, preventing contamination of air in the operating room by chemotherapy aerosols.

After the intraoperative perfusion is complete, the abdomen is suctioned dry of fluid. The abdomen is then reopened, retractors repositioned, and reconstructive surgery is performed. It should be reemphasized that no suture lines are constructed until after the chemotherapy perfusion is complete. One exception to this rule is closure of the vaginal cuff to prevent intraperitoneal chemotherapy leakage. The standardized orders for heated intraoperative intraperitoneal chemotherapy are given in Table 24D-3.

## TABLE 24D-2. RATIONALE FOR THE USE OF HEATED INTRAOPERATIVE INTRAPERITONEAL CHEMOTHERAPY

Heat increases drug penetration into tissue.

Heat increases the cytotoxicity of selected chemotherapy agents.

Heat has an antitumor effect by itself.

Intraoperative chemotherapy allows manual distribution of drug and heat uniformly to all surfaces of the abdomen and pelvis.

Renal toxicities of chemotherapy given in the operation room can be avoided by careful monitoring of urine output during chemotherapy perfusion.

The time that elapses during the heated perfusion allows a normalization of many parameters (temperature, blood clotting, hemodynamic, etc.).

## TABLE 24D-3. STANDARDIZED ORDERS FOR HEATED INTRAOPERATIVE INTRAPERITONEAL CHEMOTHERAPY

### MITOMYCIN ORDERS

1. For adenocarcinoma from appendiceal, colonic, rectal, gastric, and pancreatic cancer; add mitomycin_____mg to 2 L of 1.5% peritoneal dialysis solution.
2. Dose of mitomycin for males, 12.5 mg/m²; for females, 10 mg/m².
3. Use a 33% dose reduction for heavy prior chemotherapy, marginal renal function, age greater than 60, extensive intraoperative trauma to small bowel surfaces, or prior radiotherapy.
4. Send 1 L of 1.5% peritoneal dialysis solution to test the perfusion circuit.
5. Send 1 L of 1.5% peritoneal dialysis solution for immediate postoperative lavage.
6. Send the above to operating room_____at_____o'clock.

### CISPLATIN AND DOXORUBICIN ORDERS

1. For sarcoma, ovarian cancer, and mesothelioma; add cisplatin_____mg to 2 L of 1.5% peritoneal dialysis solution. The dose of cisplatin is 50 mg/m².
2. Add doxorubicin_____mg to the same 2 L of 1.5% peritoneal dialysis solution. The dose of doxorubicin is 15 mg/m².
3. Use a 33% dose reduction for heavy prior chemotherapy, marginal renal function, age greater than 60, extensive intraoperative trauma to small bowel surfaces, or prior radiotherapy.
4. Send 1 L of 1.5% peritoneal dialysis solution to test the perfusion circuit.
5. Send 1 L of 1.5% peritoneal dialysis solution for immediate postoperative lavage.
6. Send the above to operating room_____at_____o'clock.

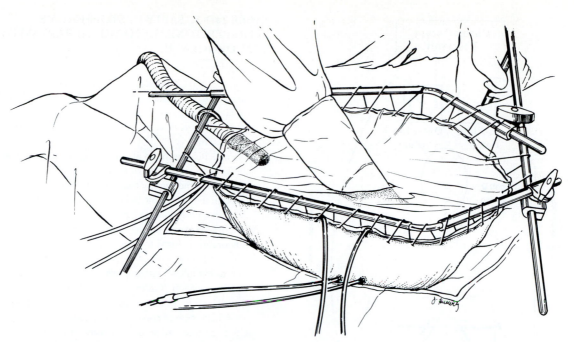

**FIGURE 24D-22.** Coliseum technique for heated intraoperative intraperitoneal chemotherapy. Surgical manipulation of the abdominal contents after complete resection of cancer assures uniform distribution of heat and chemotherapy.

**MITOMYCIN C.** Mitomycin C is used intraoperatively to treat appendiceal, colonic, and gastric cancer.

**CISPLATIN AND DOXORUBICIN.** Doxorubicin and cisplatin together are used to treat sarcomatosis and peritoneal mesothelioma. Also, papillary serous cancer and primary peritoneal adenocarcinoma are treated with the doxorubicin and cisplatin regimen.

### IMMEDIATE POSTOPERATIVE ABDOMINAL LAVAGE

In patients who are to receive early postoperative intraperitoneal 5-fluorouracil, the catheters for drug instillation and abdominal drainage must be kept clear of blood clots and tissue debris. To accomplish this, an abdominal lavage is begun in the operating room. This lavage utilizes the tubes inserted for heated intraoperative intraperitoneal chemotherapy. Large volumes of fluid are rapidly infused and then drained from the abdomen after a short dwell time. The standardized orders for immediate postoperative abdominal lavage are given in Table 24D-4. All intraabdominal catheters are withdrawn before the patient is discharged from the hospital.

### EARLY POSTOPERATIVE INTRAPERITONEAL 5-FLUOROURACIL

The standardized orders for early postoperative intraperitoneal 5-fluorouracil are presented in Table 24D-5. After the patient sta-

bilizes postoperatively, and after the drainage from the immediate postoperative abdominal lavage is no longer blood-stained, the 5-fluorouracil instillation occurs. The patients treated are those with adenocarcinoma from appendiceal, colonic, and gastric primaries. Patients with pseudomyxoma peritonei are not treated with 5-fluorouracil because the intraoperative heated mitomycin is usually sufficient. In some patients who have extensive small-bowel trauma from lysis of adhesions, the early postoperative 5-fluorouracil is withheld for fear of fistula formation.[22,23] These patients are usually recommended for a second-look surgery.

### TABLE 24D-4. IMMEDIATE POSTOPERATIVE ABDOMINAL LAVAGE

**DAY OF OPERATION**

1. Run in 1000 mL 1.5% dextrose peritoneal dialysis solution as rapidly as possible. Warm to body temperature prior to instillation. Clamp all abdominal drains during infusion.
2. No dwell time.
3. Drain as rapidly as possible through the Tenckhoff catheter and abdominal drains.
4. Repeat irrigations q 1 h for 4 h, the q 4 h until returns are clear; then q 8 h until chemotherapy begins.
5. Change dressing at Tenckhoff catheter and abdominal drain skin sites using sterile technique once daily and prn.
6. Standardized precautions must be used for all body fluids from this patient.

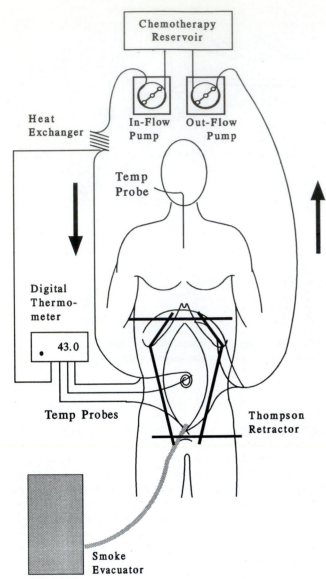

**FIGURE 24D-23.** Circuit for heated intraoperative intraperitoneal chemotherapy perfusion. All plastic tubes are positioned in a standardized fashion except the Tenckhoff catheter for the heated intraoperative perfusion. It is placed at the anatomic site at which the surgeon thinks there is the greatest likelihood of recurrence. This allows for regional dose intensity of the heated chemotherapy.

## INDUCTION TREATMENT WITH INTRAVENOUS MITOMYCIN C AND INTRAPERITONEAL 5-FLUOROURACIL

Patients should be carefully selected to receive induction intraperitoneal chemotherapy. Intestinal adhesions are the most frequent contraindication to its use. Usually, induction intraperitoneal chemotherapy is not recommended in patients with extensive prior surgery. The treatment is directed at the small-bowel surfaces and is

**TABLE 24D-5.** EARLY POSTOPERATIVE INTRAPERITONEAL CHEMOTHERAPY WITH 5-FLUOROURACIL

POSTOPERATIVE DAYS 1–5
1.  Add to____mL 1.5% dextrose peritoneal dialysis solution:
    (a)____mg 5-fluorouracil (650 mg/m², maximal dose 1300 mg)
    (b) 50 mEq sodium bicarbonate
2.  Intraperitoneal fluid volume: 1 L for patients <2.0 m², 1.5 L for >2.0 m².
3.  Drain all fluid from the abdominal cavity prior to instillation, then clamp abdominal drains.
4.  Run the chemotherapy solution into the abdominal cavity through the Tenckhoff catheter as rapidly as possible. Dwell for 23 h and drain for 1 h prior to next instillation.
5.  Use gravity to maximize intraperitoneal distribution of the 5-fluorouracil. Instill the chemotherapy with the patient in a full right lateral position. After ½ h, direct the patient to turn to the full left lateral position. Change position right to left every ½ h. If tolerated, use 10 degrees of Trendelenburg position. Continue turning for the first 6 h after instillation of chemotherapy solution.
6.  Continue to drain abdominal cavity after final dwell until Tenckhoff catheter is removed.
7.  Use 33% dose reduction for heavy prior chemotherapy, age greater than 60, or prior radiotherapy.

designed to eradicate large numbers of minute peritoneal implants. If this goal can be accomplished with the induction intraperitoneal chemotherapy, then the cytoreduction will be greatly facilitated. Parietal peritoneal surfaces, stomach surfaces and the large bowel can usually be completely cytoreduced. Small-bowel surfaces are the most common site for residual disease that prevents the CC-0 or CC-1 cytoreduction. Table 24D-6 presents the standardized orders for induction chemotherapy for adenocarcinoma.

## REOPERATIVE SURGERY PLUS ADDITIONAL INTRAPERITONEAL CHEMOTHERAPY

As the clinical data regarding treatment of peritoneal surface malignancy becomes available, the need for additional operative procedures and additional cycles of intraperitoneal chemotherapy become clear. This seems most evident, at this point in time, with the tumors that do not have a tumor marker by which to monitor for recurrent disease. Peritoneal carcinomatosis from colon cancer is now routinely managed with a second-look surgery at 6 to 9 months. Also, primary peritoneal surface malignancy, especially mesothelioma, has a scheduled second-look surgery at 6 to 9 months.

At the second-look surgery, the abdomen is widely opened and all of the peritoneal surfaces are visualized with a complete take-down of all adhesions. Additional cytoreduction is performed, and additional visceral resections may be required. If a CC-1 cytoreduction can again be achieved, then heated intraoperative intraperitoneal chemotherapy is used. If the patient has adenocarcinoma, then early postoperative intraperitoneal 5-fluorouracil is recommended. If it

**TABLE 24D-6.** INDUCTION INTRAPERITONEAL 5-FLUOROURACIL AND INTRAVENOUS MITOMYCIN CHEMOTHERAPY

CYCLE NO._____

1. CBC, platelets, complete blood chemistries, and appropriate tumor marker prior to treatment; CBC and platelets 10 days after initiation of treatments.
2. 5-Fluorouracil ____mg (750 mg/m², maximum dose 1500 mg) and 50 mEq sodium bicarbonate in 1000 mL 1.5% dextrose peritoneal dialysis solution via intraperitoneal catheter q day × 5 days. Last dose____. Dwell for 23 h, drain for 1 h. Continue with next administration even if no drainage obtained.
3. On Day 3 (Date _____): 500 mL lactated Ringer's solution intravenously over 2 h prior to mitomycin infusion. Mitomycin ____mg (10 mg/m² in women and 12.5 mg/m² in men) in 200 mL 5% dextrose and water intravenously over 2 h.
4. Follow routine procedure for peripheral extravasation of a vesicant if extravasation should occur.
5. Compazine 25 mg per rectum q 4 h prn for nausea. OUTPATIENT ONLY: May dose × 4 for use at home.
6. Percocet 1 tablet PO q 3 h prn for pain. OUTPATIENT ONLY: May dose × 4 for use at home.
7. Routine vital signs.
8. Out of bed at lib.
9. Diet: Regular as tolerated.
10. Daily dressing change to intraperitoneal catheter skin exit site.
11. Use 33% dose reduction for age greater than 60 or prior radiotherapy.

appears from the reoperation that the initial heated chemotherapy and early postoperative chemotherapy treatments were successful for the most part, then the same regimen will be employed again. If there is a "chemotherapy failure" and recurrent disease is seen in areas that have been previously peritonectomized, then a chemotherapy change would be initiated.

## ONCOLOGIC EMERGENCY

As a primary gastrointestinal cancer is resected, intraperitoneal dissemination of cancer cells may sometimes occur. Of course, if a perfusionist is available to administer heated intraoperative intraperitoneal, then this would be the preferred treatment. However, in many instances a perfusion system may not be available, or it may in an emergency situation thought to be unsafe. Resections of gastrointestinal cancers may occur in which there is "intraoperative tumor spill." In these patients treatments to eliminate small volumes of microscopic residual disease are advisable. Other clinical situations that would call for the emergency use of intraoperative intraperitoneal chemotherapy would be the presence of a small volume of localized cancer seeding that would be resected as part of the removal of the primary tumor. Another indication would be

a perforated intraabdominal malignancy when that perforation is through the cancer itself. Positive peritoneal cytology would also be considered an indication for the oncologic emergency.

In this treatment, the abdominal wall is elevated on a self-retaining retractor and a plastic sheet incorporated into the skin sutures. Drains that are placed for fluid removal postoperatively are used to introduce the 3 L of normothermic chemotherapy. Blood warmers are generally used to bring the fluid up to body temperature. For 1 h, the surgeon manipulates all of the peritoneal surfaces by rubbing the peritoneal surfaces that are at greatest risk for the adherence of cancer cells. The doses of drug are the same as for heated intraoperative intraperitoneal chemotherapy (see Table 24D-3). After the peritoneal surfaces are treated, then suture lines are constructed and the abdomen is closed. A majority of these patients will be recommended for a second-look surgery at 6 to 9 months.

## CLINICAL RESULTS OF TREATMENT

### RELIABLE RELIEF OF DEBILITATING ASCITES

Patients with a large volume of malignant ascites are frequently encountered as a cancerous process moves toward its terminal phase. This may be caused by breast cancer, gastric cancer, mucinous malignancies of the colon or appendix, and primary peritoneal surface cancers. Intraperitoneal chemotherapy is uniformly successful in eliminating the debilitating ascites.[24,25] Success usually requires two or three instillations of a systemic dose of appropriate chemotherapy into the abdomen. Frequently combinations of both systemic and intraperitoneal chemotherapy are selected (see Table 24D-6). Also, Link and colleagues[26] used mitoxantrone in this clinical situation.

It is important to inform patients that intraperitoneal chemotherapy as treatment for malignant ascites is for symptomatic relief and should not be considered curative. The mass of solid tumor seen by CT scan will remain unchanged or will progress during treatment. Only the ascites will disappear. The mechanism of action of intraperitoneal chemotherapy on large-volume malignant ascites is destruction of surface cancer. This causes a layer of fibrosis over all malignant deposits and also on normal parietal and visceral peritoneal surfaces. This fibrotic layer of tissue prevents formation of both normal peritoneal fluid and malignant fluids. The fluid that had previously accumulated in the abdomen is directed by the layer of fibrosis into the circulation. After three or four intraperitoneal chemotherapy treatments, the abdominal space may transiently cease to exist as peritoneal surfaces adhere together.

**TECHNIQUE FOR CHEMOTHERAPY INSTILLATION FOR TREATMENT OF ASCITES.** The technique used for repeated instillation of intraperitoneal chemotherapy to palliate malignant ascites is crucial for success. First paracentesis using a temporary all-purpose drain should provide access to the peritoneal space. A long-term indwelling (Tenckhoff) catheter should not be used to provide access because of the high incidence of infection with a foreign body located within a large volume of intraabdominal fluid over a long time period. Also an intraperitoneal subcutaneous port should not be used because of difficulties it creates with drainage of intraperitoneal fluid. Repeated paracentesis is safe if CT or ultrasound is used to select the site on the abdominal wall for puncture. When the ascites is gone or greatly diminished, the paracentesis becomes more dangerous. Of course, if the malignant ascites is greatly reduced then these treatments are discontinued.

### SCHEDULE AND DOSE OF INTRAPERITONEAL CHEMOTHERAPY FOR TREATMENT OF ASCITES.

The all-purpose drain is kept in place for 5 days. Each day the ascites fluid is drained as completely as possible. Multiple changes in the patient's position may facilitate drainage. Then the intraperitoneal chemotherapy solution is instilled for a 23-h dwell. Our first choice of drugs is a combination of cisplatin (15 mg/m$^2$ per day) and doxorubicin (3 mg/m$^2$ per day) instilled as rapidly as possible. As soon as the chemotherapy solution has been instilled, the patient is instructed to turn from front to back and from side to side every half hour. Alternatively, mitoxantrone can be used at 3 mg/m$^2$ per day for 5 days in a row. The cycle of treatments is repeated at 3-week intervals. In a few patients, persistent ascites may require a surgical procedure (debulking) in order to separate adherent bowel loops, remove bulk disease, and allow the use of a single cycle of heated intraoperative intraperitoneal chemotherapy. During the debulking, only large masses of tumor are removed. This generally includes the greater and lesser omentum and pedunculated tumor masses. No attempt at a complete cytoreduction is made. The patient is treated for 90 min with heat, doxorubicin, and cisplatin. The responses achieved in patients that are debulked and then given chemotherapy may be more lasting than in patients given chemotherapy only.

### TREATMENT OF MUCINOUS ASCITES.

One caveat must be mentioned regarding the management of debilitating ascites. If the intraperitoneal fluid is mucinous, it cannot be drained through a tube. Relief of mucinous ascites can only be achieved by laparotomy and manual removal of mucinous tumor. Usually a greater omentectomy is performed as part of the debulking. Liposuction apparatus may greatly facilitate the complete evacuation of the viscous material. If the tumor mass can be reduced to a low level, then intraoperative and early postoperative intraperitoneal chemotherapy may slow the reaccumulation of mucinous tumor.

## CLINICAL RESULTS OF TREATMENT

### APPENDIX CANCER AND PSEUDOMYXOMA PERITONEI

The paradigm for treatment of peritoneal carcinomatosis is appendiceal malignancy. The experience with approximately 350 patients treated over a 15-year time span is presented in this manuscript. The clinical pathway currently utilized for appendix malignancy with peritoneal dissemination is shown in Fig. 24D-24. The survival of all patients is approximately 50% (Fig. 24D-25).

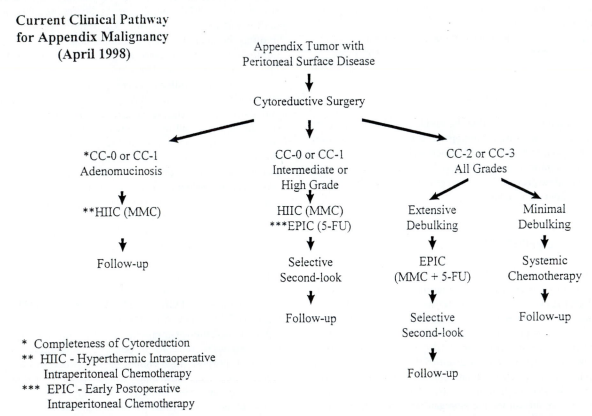

**FIGURE 24D-24.** Clinical pathway in current use for appendiceal malignancy with peritoneal dissemination.

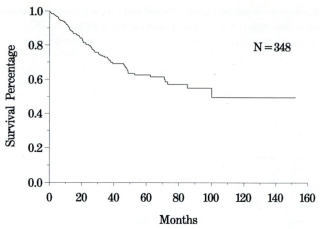

**FIGURE 24D-25.** Survival of 348 patients with established peritoneal surface malignancy from a perforated appendiceal malignancy. Patients were treated by cytoreductive surgery and intraperitoneal chemotherapy.

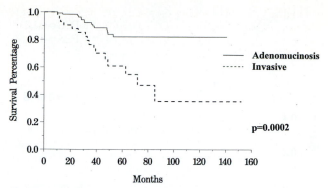

**FIGURE 24D-26.** Survival of appendiceal malignancy with established peritoneal surface disease by histologic appearance.

### APPENDICEAL MALIGNANCY AS A PARADIGM.

The concepts gained from treating peritoneal surface malignancy from an appendiceal primary tumor can be translated to other gastrointestinal cancers. There are unique clinical features of the appendiceal malignancies that have facilitated the rapid progress documented with this tumor. Spread from appendiceal tumors usually occurs in the absence of lymph node and liver metastases. The primary tumor occurs within a tiny lumen. Even small tumors early in the natural history of the disease will cause appendiceal obstruction and cause appendiceal perforation. This results in a release of tumor cells into the free peritoneal cavity. The seeding of the abdomen occurs in almost every patient before lymph node metastases or liver metastases has occurred. Second, there is a wide spectrum of invasion that these tumors exhibit. The ones that are minimally invasive can be totally resected using peritonectomy procedures to achieve a CC-1 cytoreduction. Third, the majority of these tumors are mucinous. The texture of the implants allows greater penetration by chemotherapy than with solid tumors. Finally, the malignancy disseminates so that all of its components are within the regional chemotherapy field. If the intraperitoneal chemotherapy is successful in eradicating the residual tumor on peritoneal surfaces, the patient will be a long-term survivor. If disease persists after chemotherapy, the peritoneal malignancy will recur. In these patients the response achieved by the intraperitoneal chemotherapy determines the outcome; assuming, of course, that a CC-1 cytoreduction was possible.

The treatment strategies used included peritonectomy procedures combined with perioperative intraperitoneal chemotherapy with mitomycin C and 5-fluorouracil. Survival was significantly correlated with the invasive character of the mucinous tumor (Fig. 24D-26), the completeness of cytoreduction (Fig. 24D-27), and the prior surgical score (Fig. 24D-28). In contrast to most studies with gastrointestinal cancer patients, lymph node involvement was not a determinate prognostic factor in patients with peritoneal

dissemination of malignancy if intraperitoneal chemotherapy was used.

Although approximately 50% of patients with carcinomatosis from appendiceal malignancy survive long term with treatment, patients with an adenocarcinoid carcinomatosis from the appendix do not experience prolonged benefit from these aggressive treatments. Neither mitomycin C plus 5-fluorouracil nor cisplatin plus doxorubicin have been effective (Fig. 24D-29).

### COLON CANCER PERITONEAL CARCINOMATOSIS

To date, approximately 100 patients have been treated who have peritoneal carcinomatosis from colon cancer. The clinical pathway currently utilized to treat peritoneal carcinomatosis from colon cancer is shown in Fig. 24D-30. The survival of all patients treated is

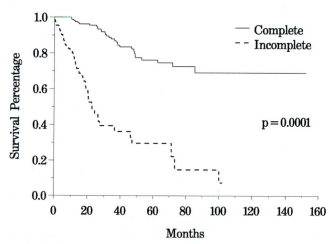

**FIGURE 24D-27.** Survival of appendiceal malignancy with established peritoneal surface disease by completeness of cytoreduction.

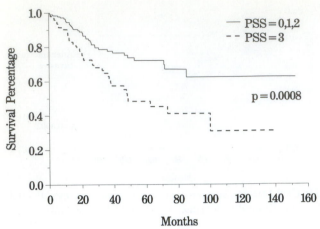

**FIGURE 24D-28.** Survival of appendiceal malignancy with established peritoneal surface disease by the extent of prior surgical interventions. If the prior surgical score is 3 (PSS-3), at least 5 of the 9 abdominopelvic regions (AR 0–8) had been previously dissected without the use of intraoperative or early postoperative intraperitoneal chemotherapy. For the PSS-2, 2 to 5 abdominopelvic regions had been dissected. For PSS-1, only one region had been dissected. These patients had exploratory surgery but no major organ or tissue dissection. For PSS-0, patients had biopsy only. Patients with prior survival score showing little or moderate dissection are compared to patients who had a prior attempt at a complete cytoreduction without perioperative intraperitoneal chemotherapy.

shown in Fig. 24D-31. In this disease, the preoperative lesion size was a significant determinant of prognosis (Fig. 24D-32).

The PCI should provide a score valuable in selecting patients for treatment. In patients who had a complete cytoreduction, there

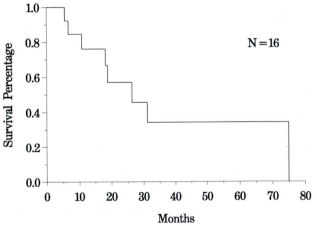

**FIGURE 24D-29.** Survival of appendiceal adenocarcinoid patients with established peritoneal carcinomatosis.

was marked improvement in survival; patients with residual disease show the expected short survival expected with peritoneal carcinomatosis from colon cancer (Fig. 24D-33). These data suggest an early aggressive approach to peritoneal surface spread of adenocarcinoma of the colon in selected patients. Patients with positive lymph nodes at the time of resection of the primary cancer have a reduced prognosis but approximately 15% may enjoy prolonged survival (Fig. 24D-34).

## SARCOMATOSIS

The clinical pathway currently utilized for patients with recurrent abdominopelvic sarcoma is shown in Fig. 24D-35. Berthet and colleagues[20] have reviewed their experience with cytoreductive surgery and intraperitoneal chemotherapy for treatment of selected patients with sarcomatosis. The survival of 43 patients with recurrent abdominopelvic sarcoma is shown in Fig. 24D-36. If the PCI at the time of abdominal exploration was less than 13, there was a 75% 5-year survival. In those who had a PCI of 13 or more, the 5-year survival was only 13% (Fig. 24D-37). The completeness of cytoreduction was also statistically significant for an improved prognosis. Twenty-seven patients with a complete cytoreduction had a 5-year survival of 39%. Sixteen patients with a CC-2 or CC-3 resection had a survival of 14% (Fig. 24D-38).

## PERITONEAL SEEDING FROM GASTRIC CANCER

Extensive studies with peritoneal seeding from gastric cancer have been conducted in Japan. Prior reports from western series are not available. Survival rates for patients in Japan with heated intraoperative intraperitoneal chemotherapy at time of gastrectomy vary from 10% to 43%.[27,28] The clinical pathway currently utilized for gastric cancer is shown in Fig. 24D-39. Our results with resectable stage IV disease in 13 patients who received intraperitoneal chemotherapy are shown in Fig. 24D-40.

## PRIMARY PERITONEAL SURFACE MALIGNANCY

A confusing and poorly understood group of tumors that have been successfully treated with peritonectomy and perioperative intraperitoneal chemotherapy are the primary peritoneal surface malignancies. A clinical pathway currently utilized to treat peritoneal mesothelioma, papillary serous adenocarcinoma, and primary peritoneal adenocarcinoma is shown in Fig. 24D-41. Currently, all patients are being treated with heated intraoperative cisplatin and doxorubicin. A second-look procedure with initiation of these same treatments is performed in 6 to 9 months. As with appendiceal adenocarcinoma, the survival rate was heavily dependent upon the invasive character of the tumor and the completeness of cytoreduction. The median length of survival in a group of 44 patients with primary peritoneal tumors was 18 months (Fig. 24D-42). Further experience with this group of patients is necessary.

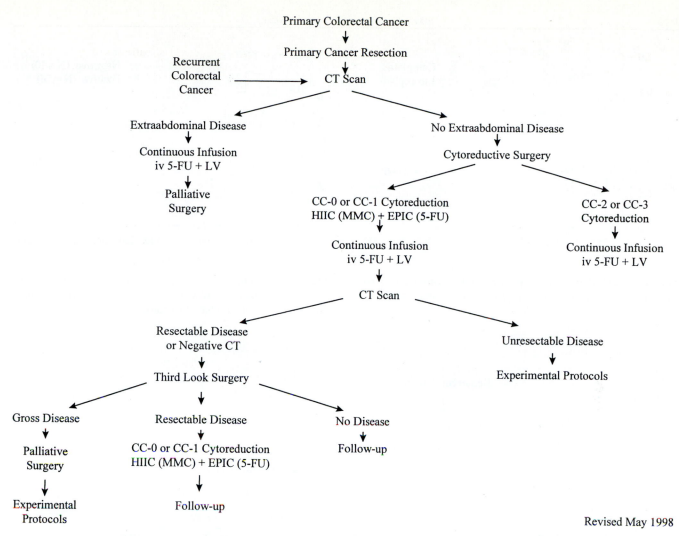

**FIGURE 24D-30.** Clinical pathway currently utilized to treat peritoneal carcinomatosis from colon cancer.

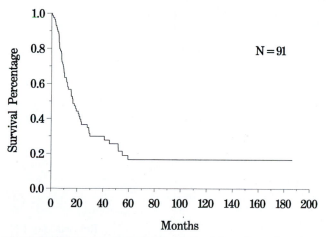

**FIGURE 24D-31.** Survival of all patients with peritoneal carcinomatosis from colon cancer.

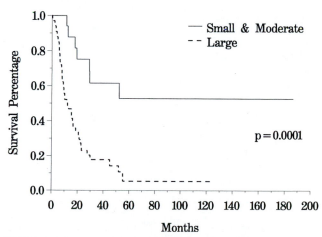

**FIGURE 24D-32.** Survival of patients with peritoneal carcinomatosis from colon cancer by preoperative lesion size.

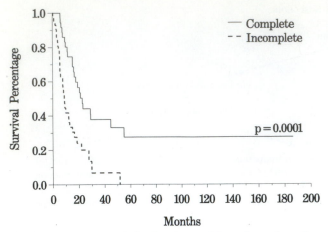

**FIGURE 24D-33.** Survival of patients with peritoneal carcinomatosis from colon cancer by completeness of cytoreduction.

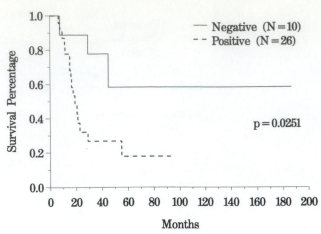

**FIGURE 24D-34.** Survival of patients with peritoneal carcinomatosis from colon cancer with a complete cytoreduction by presence vs absence of lymph node metastases.

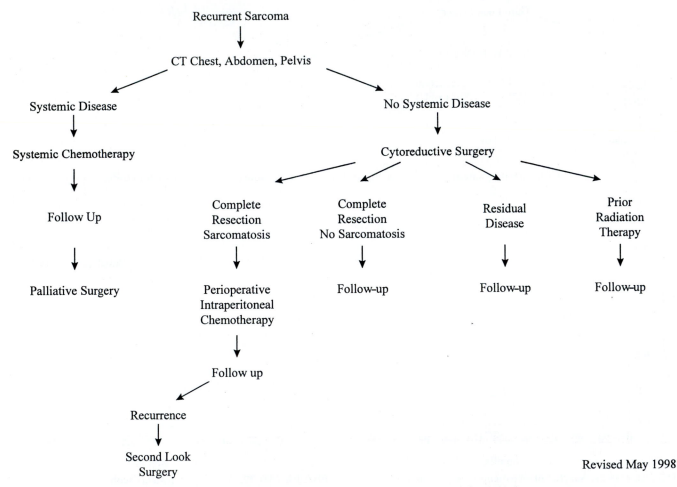

Revised May 1998

**FIGURE 24D-35.** Clinical pathway currently utilized to treat recurrent abdominopelvic sarcoma.

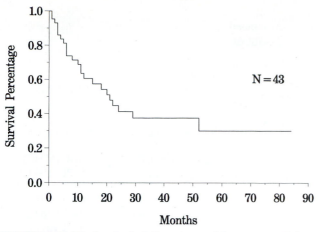

**FIGURE 24D-36.** Survival of 43 patients with recurrent abdominopelvic sarcoma.

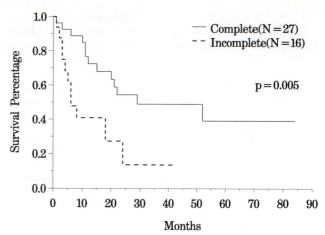

**FIGURE 24D-38.** Survival of patients with recurrent abdominopelvic sarcoma by completeness of cytoreduction.

## RECURRENT AND OBSTRUCTING GASTROINTESTINAL CANCER

Averbach and colleagues[29] looked at their experience with an extremely problematic group of patients. These are patients who developed intestinal obstruction after prior treatment for a gastrointestinal malignancy. With aggressive treatments using a second-look surgery, peritonectomy procedures, and intraperitoneal chemotherapy, a complete cytoreduction resulted in a 5-year survival in 60% of the patients, and an incomplete resection resulted in no 5-year survivals. The patients with appendiceal malignancy had a greatly improved survival as compared to those with colon cancer or other diagnoses. A free interval of greater than 2 years between primary malignancy and the onset of obstruction also correlated favorably with prolonged survival. Only patients with intraperitoneal chemotherapy used in conjunction with cytoreductive surgery were shown to have prolonged survival.

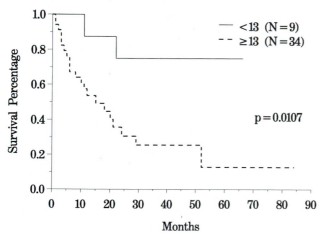

**FIGURE 24D-37.** Survival of patients with recurrent abdominopelvic sarcoma by prior surgical score.

## MORBIDITY AND MORTALITY RATES OF PHASE II STUDIES

The morbidity and mortality rates in 170 consecutive patients who had cytoreductive surgery and heated intraoperative intraperitoneal chemotherapy for peritoneal carcinomatosis have been reported.[30] In these patients, there were three treatment related deaths (1.8%). Peripancreatitis (7.1%) and fistula (4.7%) were the most common major complications. There were 25.3% of patients with grade III or IV complications.

## ALTERNATIVE APPROACHES

Peritoneal carcinomatosis has been treated in the past with systemic chemotherapy. No long-term survivors have been described in the literature. Palliative surgery can give temporary relief of intestinal obstruction. These efforts have always been categorized as low-value surgery because long-term survival was rarely achieved. Other therapies that would include intraperitoneal immunotherapy, intraperitoneal isotopes, and intraperitoneal labeled monoclonal antibody have not shown reproducible beneficial results. In summary, alternative approaches to cytoreductive surgery and intraperitoneal chemotherapy for peritoneal carcinomatosis have not been reported.

## PATIENT CARE CONSIDERATIONS

The major detrimental side effect of combined cytoreductive surgery and intraperitoneal chemotherapy is prolonged ileus. Patients may have a nasogastric tube in place with large volumes of secretions being aspirated for 2 to 4 weeks postoperatively. The length of time required for nasogastric suctioning is dependent upon the extent of the peritonectomy procedures and the extent of prior abdominal adhesions that required lysis.

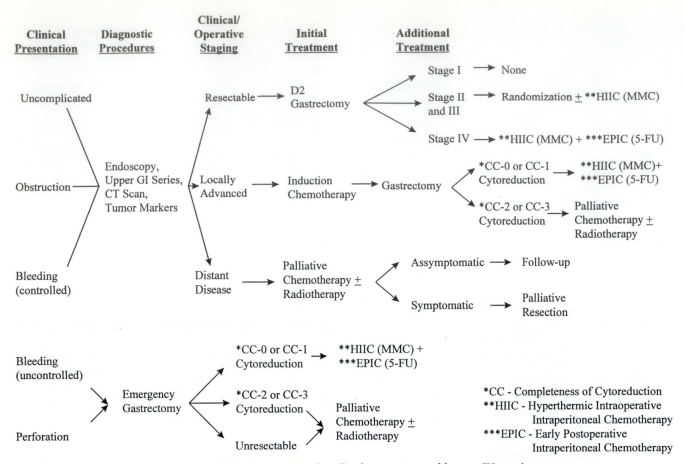

**FIGURE 24D-39.** Clinical pathway currently utilized to treat resectable stage IV gastric cancer.

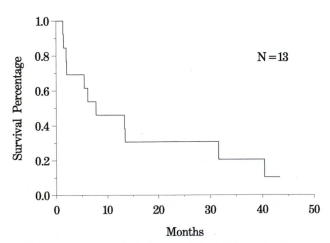

**FIGURE 24D-40.** Survival of resected stage IV gastric cancer patients also receiving perioperative chemotherapy.

The most life-threatening postoperative complication is the fistula. These are almost always sidewall perforations of the small bowel, but colon and stomach perforations have occurred. Patients need to be made aware of the possibility of a fistula before cytoreductive surgery and intraperitoneal chemotherapy are contemplated. As mentioned above, the anastomotic leak rate is low.

Following these treatments, the patient is maintained on parenteral feeding for 2 to 4 weeks. Approximately 20% of patients, especially those who have had extensive prior surgery or who have a short bowel, will need parenteral feeding for several weeks after they leave the hospital.

## ETHICAL CONSIDERATIONS IN CLINICAL STUDIES WITH PERITONEAL SURFACE MALIGNANCY

The sequence of events that should accompany a new program in peritoneal surface malignancy has not yet been defined. The requirements for formal institutional review board approval will vary from one institution to another. Guidelines for an evolution of treatment strategies that allow for reliable clinical research may occur as follows.

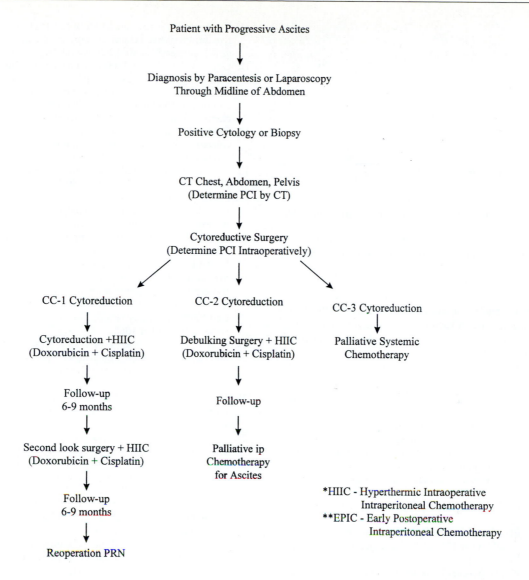

**FIGURE 24D-41.** Clinical pathway currently utilized to treat primary peritoneal surface malignancy, peritoneal mesothelioma, papillary serous cancer, and primary peritoneal adenocarcinoma.

Without exception, adjuvant intraperitoneal chemotherapy studies in patients with primary gastrointestinal cancer must be randomized and require review by a research board. An exception to the need for randomization is resected pancreatic cancer. Also, when a group first attempts to initiate treatment plans with intraperitoneal chemotherapy, the learning curve associated with a new technology is best approached by a startup protocol approved by an institutional review board. This forces the group to standardize the methods and familiarize themselves with the experience of others. Selection criteria to treat patients with a reasonable likelihood of benefit must be evident. An omnibus protocol is suggested that allows aggressive cytoreduction and perioperative intraperitoneal chemotherapy in patients with no systemic dissemination and small-volume peritoneal seeding from recurrent colorectal cancer, resected primary gastric cancer, and resected primary or recurrent abdominopelvic sarcoma. This omnibus protocol should be utilized on a limited time period to treat 10 to 20 patients.

Formal protocols should not be required for the treatment of debilitating ascites. Also, the long-term survival of patients with established peritoneal surface malignancy that has a small volume and limited distribution has been established. After completing the startup protocols, phase II clinical studies on this group of patients by an oncologic team that has demonstrated experience should proceed without the need for further institutional review board approval. The

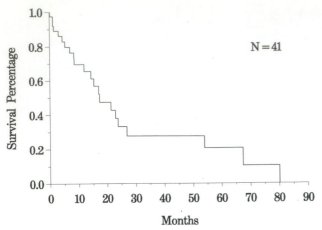

**FIGURE 24D-42.** Survival of 41 patients with primary peritoneal surface malignancy.

peritoneal surface spread of most gastrointestinal cancers that have a low PCI and that after surgery have a completeness of cytoreduction score of 0 or 1 should be routinely treated according to standardized intraperitoneal chemotherapy protocols.

## REFERENCES

1. GUNDERSON LL, SOSIN H: Areas of failure found at reoperation (second or symptomatic look) following "curative surgery" for adenocarcinoma of the rectum: Clinicopathologic correlation and implications for adjuvant therapy. Cancer 34:1278, 1974.
2. SUGARBAKER PH: Surgical management of locally recurrent and metastatic colorectal cancer, in *Atlas of Surgical Oncology*, CP Karakousis et al (eds). Philadelphia, Saunders, 1995, pp 671–692.
3. SUGARBAKER PH, HUGHES KA: Surgery for colorectal metastasis to liver, in *Colorectal Cancer*, H Wanebo (ed). St. Louis, Mosby-Year Book, 1993, pp 405–413.
4. SUGARBAKER PH: *Peritoneal Carcinomatosis: Principles of Management.* Boston, Kluwer, 1996.
5. SUGARBAKER PH: Peritoneal carcinomatosis from appendiceal cancer: A paradigm for treatment of abdomino-pelvic dissemination of gastrointestinal malignancy. Acta Chir Austr 28:4, 1996.
6. SUGARBAKER PH: Peritonectomy procedures, in *Peritoneal Carcinomatosis: Principles of Management*, PH Sugarbaker (ed). Boston, Kluwer, 1996, pp 235–262.
7. JACQUET P et al: Peritoneal carcinomatosis from intraabdominal malignancy: Natural history and new prospects for management. Acta Belg Chir 94:191, 1994.
8. SUGARBAKER PH et al: Rationale for early postoperative intraperitoneal chemotherapy (EPIC) in patients with advanced gastrointestinal cancer. Cancer Res 50:5790, 1990.
9. SUGARBAKER PH et al: Prospective randomized trial of intravenous versus intraperitoneal 5-fluorouracil in patients with advanced primary colon or rectal cancer. Surgery 98:414, 1985.
10. SUGARBAKER PH, YONEMURA Y: Clinical Pathway for the Management of Resectable Gastric Cancer with Peritoneal Seeding: Best Palliation with a Ray of Hope for Cure. Oncology 58:96, 2000.
11. YU W et al: Prospective randomized trial of early postoperative intraperitoneal chemotherapy as an adjuvant for resectable gastric cancer. Ann Surg 223:347, 1998.
12. GOUGH DB et al: Pseudomyxoma peritonei: Long-term survival with an aggressive regional approach. Ann Surg 219:112, 1994.
13. ZOETMULDER FAN, SUGARBAKER PH: Patterns of failure after complete cytoreduction and early postoperative intraperitoneal chemotherapy. Eur J CA 32A(10):1727, 1996.
14. JACQUET P, SUGARBAKER PH: Wound recurrence after laparoscopic colectomy for cancer: New rationale for intraoperative intraperitoneal chemotherapy. Surg Endosc 10:295, 1996.
15. SUGARBAKER PH et al: Management of pseudomyxoma peritonei of appendiceal origin. Adv Surg 30:233, 1997.
16. ARCHER A: Radiology of peritoneal carcinomatosis, in *Peritoneal Carcinomatosis: Principles of Management*, PH Sugarbaker (ed). Boston, Kluwer, 1996, pp 263–288.
17. JACQUET P et al: Abdominal computed tomographic scan in the selection of patients with mucinous peritoneal carcinomatosis for cytoreductive surgery. J Am Coll Surg 181:530, 1995.
18. STELLER EP: Comparison of four scoring methods for an intraperitoneal immunotherapy model. Enhancement and Abrogation: Modifications of Host Immune Influence IL-2 and LAK Cell Immunotherapy (Ph.D. Thesis). Erasmus University Rotterdam, November 1988.
19. GOMEZ PORTILLA A et al: Second-look surgery after cytoreductive and intraperitoneal chemotherapy for peritoneal carcinomatosis from colorectal cancer: Analysis of prognostic features. World J Surg 23:23, 1999.
20. BERTHET B et al: Quantitative methodologies for selection of patients with recurrent abdominopelvic sarcoma for treatment. Eur J Cancer 35:413, 1999.
21. SUGARBAKER PH et al: Peritoneal carcinomatosis from adenocarcinoma of the colon. World J Surg 20:585, 1996.
22. MURIO EJ, SUGARBAKER PH: Gastrointestinal fistula following cytoreductive procedures for peritoneal carcinomatosis: Incidence and outcome. J Exp Clin Cancer Res 12:153, 1993.
23. FERNANDEZ-TRIO V, SUGARBAKER PH: Diagnosis and management of postoperative gastrointestinal fistulas: A kinetic analysis. J Exp Clin Cancer Res 13:233, 1994.
24. GILLY FN et al: Intraperitoneal chemo-hyperthermic (CHIP): A new therapy in the treatment of the peritoneal seedings. Int Surg 76:164, 1991.
25. FUJIMOTO S et al: Intraperitoneal hyperthermic perfusion combined with surgery effective for gastric cancer patients with peritoneal seeding. Ann Surg 208:36, 1988.
26. LINK K et al: Intraperitoneal regional chemotherapy (IPRC) with mitoxantrone, in *Peritoneal Carcinomatosis: Drugs and Disease*, PH Sugarbaker (ed). Boston, Kluwer, 1996, pp 31–40.
27. YONEMURA Y et al: Effects of intraoperative chemohyperthermia in patients with gastric cancer with peritoneal dissemination. Surgery 119:437, 1996.
28. FUJIMOTO S et al: Positive results of combined therapy of surgery and intraperitoneal hyperthermia perfusion for far-advanced gastric cancer. Ann Surg 212:592, 1990.
29. AVERBACH AM, SUGARBAKER PH: Recurrent intraabdominal cancer with intestinal obstruction. Int Surg 80:141, 1995.
30. STEPHENS AD, SUGARBAKER PH: Morbidity and mortality of cytoreductive surgery and hyperthermic intraoperative intraperitoneal chemotherapy with mitomycin C using the coliseum technique. In H Bismuth et al. (eds): *8th World Congress of the International Gastro-Surgical Club.* Bologna, Italy, Monduzzi Editore, 1998, pp 893–897.

# 24E / MANAGEMENT OF MALIGNANT PLEURAL AND PERICARDIAL EFFUSIONS AND MALIGNANT ASCITES

*Harvey I. Pass and Barbara Temeck*

## MALIGNANT PLEURAL EFFUSION

### INTRODUCTION

A pleural effusion may be a presenting sign of a neoplasm or a development later in the course of the disease. Diagnostic workup is essential to distinguish more probable malignant from benign causes for determination of appropriate therapy. The major histologies that cause malignant pleural effusions are lung cancer, breast cancer, and lymphoma. Malignant pleural effusions have been reported to occur in half of the patients with metastatic breast cancer,[1] about one-quarter of the patients with lung cancer[2] and a third of patients with lymphoma.[3] In lung cancer, adenocarcinoma is the most frequent cell type due to its peripheral nature. These histologies account for 73% of malignant pleural effusions, with the remainder including gastrointestinal and genitourinary tract cancers, melanoma, mesothelioma, sarcoma, thyroid cancer, and leukemia. The primary lesion is unknown in about 15% of patients. In malignancy, survival is related to the specific cancer causing the malignant pleural effusion. Although survival rate is usually poor, survival can be prolonged in patients with breast cancer. Relief of a patient's symptoms can usually be achieved with local therapy and thus avoidance of systemic toxicity.

### ANATOMY AND PHYSIOLOGY

The pleural space is the 10 to 20 $\mu$m between the single layers of mesothelial cells comprising the visceral and parietal pleura. The systemic circulation via the intercostals supplies the parietal pleura with drainage into the intercostal and bronchial veins. The bronchial circulation supplies the visceral pleura with drainage into pulmonary veins.[2] Lymphatics from the parietal pleura and from below the diaphragm drain into intercostal and mediastinal nodes, whereas lymphatics from the visceral pleura flow along the interlobar septae. Lymph enters into the right lymphatic trunk or thoracic duct. Formerly it had been considered that up to 10 L of protein-free fluid passed through the pleural space over 24 h, which was rapidly cleared and resulted in a few millimeters of fluid in the pleural space.[4] Flow

as calculated by Starling's law should be from parietal to visceral pleural capillaries due to the difference in hydrostatic and colloid osmotic pressures.[5] This concept has been modified and ascribed to the parietal pleura the major role in the movement of pleural fluid.[6] Stomata, 2 to 12 $\mu$m, form openings between mesothelial cells and permit exit of pleural fluid, cells, and protein from the pleural space. Direct communication occurs from stomata to lymphatic channels. The process involves the formation of only 100 to 200 mL of fluid per 24 h and involves concentration of the protein that is thus taken up by the lymphatics.[7] The protein content of the fluid in the pleural space is about 1.5 g/100 mL.[8] The lymphatic drainage that accommodates the pleura fluid has a reserve up to 500 mL and the equal entry and exit of fluid allow no accumulation of fluid.

Changes in hydrostatic pressure, colloid osmotic pressure, capillary permeability, and lymphatic drainage can lead to the development of a pleural effusion.[4,9,10] Factors implicated in the development of malignant pleural effusion are interference with lymphatic drainage and increased capillary permeability. Blockage of lymphatic drainage occurs through pleural implants, lymph node metastases, or lymphangitic spread. There is no direct correlation between the extent of metastatic pleural involvement and the development of pleural effusion.[11] Pleural implants can change capillary permeability by production of vasomotor peptides. Physiologic disturbances can occur from free-floating cells in the pleural space. In lung cancer, malignant pleural effusions can be caused by pulmonary artery invasion and embolization of tumor cells to the visceral pleura with subsequent spread to the pleural space. Peripheral cancers such as adenocarcinoma of the lung produce direct seeding of the pleural space. In breast cancer malignant pleural effusion can result from extension of the tumor from the chest wall or seeding into the systemic circulation such as by liver metastasis into the inferior vena cava.[12]

It is important to distinguish effusions that do not arise from direct malignant involvement of the pleura. Cardiac and pericardial disease as well as the superior vena cava syndrome alter hydrostatic pressure and can lead to pleural effusion. Other etiologies are decreased colloid osmotic pressure by hypoalbuminemia, impaired lymphatic drainage by radiation or fibrosis, increased capillary permeability by inflammatory reaction to therapy or as a result of a complicating pneumonia, increased negative pleural pressure by atelectasis of the lung and communication of diaphragmatic lymphatic channels, which can result in concomitant pleural effusion and malignant ascites. In patients with malignancy, concurrent conditions such as cirrhosis, pulmonary embolism, and infection must be identified in order to make therapeutic decisions.

## CLINICAL MANIFESTATION

A malignant pleural effusion will present with symptoms in 77% of patients and is the initial presentation in 50% to 90% of patients with primary or metastatic pleural malignancy.[13,14] The time course over which the fluid develops rather than the amount of fluid correlates to the severity of symptom.[15] Atelectasis results in dyspnea and nonproductive cough. Chest pain is present in more than 50% of patients and may be pleuritic from inflammation of the parietal pleura. Ipsilateral shoulder pain occurs from involvement of the diaphragmatic parietal pleura. A sense of heaviness in the chest can be experienced. Physical examination can indicate dyspnea and difficulty in breathing. With small pleural effusions dullness to percussion occurs in the lowermost part of the thorax unless the fluid is eliminated. Respiratory excursions of the thorax are normal in small effusions and vocal fremitus and breath sounds are transmitted poorly to the stethoscope. Large pleural effusions produce dullness to percussion. Alveoli above compressed area of lung may distend resulting in hyperresonance of the lung immediately above the fluid. Loud bronchial breathing from compressed lung may also be auscultated through the fluid. Vocal fremitus is absent. The chest wall may demonstrate restricted expansion and intercostal fullness with undetectable movement of the diaphragm. The thorax may deviate to the unaffected side. Patients can lose weight and appear chronically ill. Other findings include evidence of ascites, pericardial disease, lymphadenopathy, and nonmalignant disease. In malignant chylothorax, loss of protein can lead to cachexia and edema with fluid losses up to 2500 mL over 24 h and resulting hemodynamic compromise.

## DIAGNOSIS (TABLE 24E-1)

**RADIOLOGIC ASSESSMENT.** Initial assessment of pleural fluid by chest radiograph on upright posteroanterior and lateral films presents a ground glass appearance with blunting of the costophrenic angle, concave meniscus, density over the diaphragm and pleural space, capping of the apex, and delineation of interlobar fissures (pseudotumor). In one-third of patients bilateral effusions are evident on presentation; 175 mL of fluid can be seen on an upright chest film and will cause blunting of the costophrenic angle.[16] The posterior angle should be carefully examined as well because it is much deeper and may be below the level of the lateral angle. Old films may confirm that the blunting is a new finding. A lateral film can detect 100 mL of fluid; decubitus films can distinguish free versus loculated fluid and be helpful in planning therapeutic intervention.[16] Lateral decubitus films can assist in distinguishing subpulmonic effusions, which are the most common problem to mimic diaphragmatic elevation. The posteroanterior film suggests subpulmonic effusion when

**TABLE 24E-1. DIAGNOSTIC MODALITIES FOR MALIGNANT PLEURAL EFFUSION**

| HISTORY AND PHYSICAL EXAMINATION | |
| --- | --- |
| Radiologic assessment | Chest radiography, CT, MRI, ultrasound |
| Fluid analysis | Hematology, chemistry, tumor markers, enzymes |
| Cytology | Thoracentesis, thoracoscopy, thoracotomy |
| Histology | Percutaneous closed pleural biopsy, open pleural biopsy via thoracoscopy or thoracotomy |

the dome of the diaphragm appears to be the costophrenic angle with an abrupt dropoff and the lateral view demonstrates a posterior meniscus. In the absence of costophrenic blunting, increased separation between the diaphragmatic surface of the lung and the gastric bubble on upright chest film support the diagnosis of a left subpulmonic effusion.[17]

In large pleural effusions (>1500 mL) opacification of the hemithorax can cause mediastinal shift to the contralateral side. Differential diagnosis involves atelectasis, producing a shift toward the same side with increased retrosternal clear space on the lateral chest film. When the mediastinum is fixed, it may not occur. Additional findings on chest radiograph refer to specific disease processes such as primary lung and metastatic tumors, congestive heart failure, pulmonary embolism, connective tissue disorders, infectious diseases, and intraabdominal processes (e.g., subphrenic abscess).

Computerized tomography (CT) can define small effusions and loculated areas of fluid. It is possible to distinguish pleural fluid collections from solid pleural lesions on the basis of attenuation values. Pleural effusions usually have a density of 20 Housefield units with solid lesions having higher values.[18] However, this is controversial and attenuation values do not distinguish among different causes of pleural fluid. CT is most helpful after drainage of a pleural effusion and permits assessment of the chest wall, pleura, and lungs. High-resolution CT techniques can demonstrate the anatomy of the interface better than conventional CT. CT following contrast injection can differentiate pleural thickening from pleural fluid. Ultrasound is another method to study pleural fluid and distinguish it from pleural thickening.

**PLEURAL FLUID ANALYSIS.** Malignant pleural effusions are clinically described as grossly bloody; however, this applies to only 30% to 60% of the cases. In addition, not all bloody effusions are malignant. However, a bloody effusion is the single strongest positive predictive element of malignancy.[19] Clotting of aspirated fluid within several minutes and a nonuniform color during the procedure point toward a traumatic thoracentesis. Red blood cell counts can range from 10,000 per cubic millimeter in half of the patients to 100,000 per cubic millimeter.[20] Of malignant effusions, 50% to 85% have been reported to be oxidative with diagnostic (but not absolute) characteristics of a pleural protein/serum protein ratio

>0.5, pleural lactic dehydrogenase (LDH)/serum LDH ratio >0.6 or a pleural fluid LDH level of 200 international units.[21,22] Other less specific criteria are protein content over 3 g per 100 mL, pH below 7.30, and specific gravity above 1.016. Error in diagnosis can occur in 10% of patients if fluid is absorbed, leaving an excess of protein in longstanding transudates, making them appear to be exudates.[21] Amylase level can be elevated in the pleural fluid of patients with adenocarcinoma of the lung and/or ovary.[23] The patients with a large tumor burden, low glucose level (less than 60 mg/dL) and pH under 7.3 may signal poor response to therapy and short survival.

**CHYLOTHORAX.** Neoplastic causes of chylothorax are related to thoracic and abdominal malignancies, most frequently lymphoma, lymphosarcoma, and bronchogenic carcinoma. The thoracic duct ruptures due to direct tumor invasion or obstruction by tumor emboli. The milky sterile alkaline fluid contains fat globules that stain with Sudan III. Specific gravity ranges from 1.012 to 1.025, cell count indicates a red cell range of 50 to 600 per cubic millimeter and lymphocyte range of 400 to 7,000 per cubic millimeter. Total fat is 4 to 5 g/dL, cholesterol/triglyceride ratio less than 1, total protein 2 to 6 g/dL, albumin 1 to 4 g/dL, glucose 50 to 100 g/dL, and electrolyte levels similar to those in plasma.

**CYTOLOGY.** Cytologic diagnosis of malignant pleural fluid has been reported to yield a diagnosis of malignancy in 50% of the first aspirate, 65% of the second, and 70% of the third, with the removal of old degenerated cells contributing to the result.[1,24,25] The true positive rate is 42% to 96% of patients with known neoplasm and the false-positive rate is 0% to 3%. Sample size should be at least 250 mL and sent immediately to the laboratory. Location of the effusion, the extent and histology of the disease, and the mode of processing the specimen can influence results. Techniques for processing specimens include wet mounts stained with toluidine blue, smear fixed in 95% alcohol- or air-dried, cytocentrifuged preparations. All cell blocks should be prepared for paraffin embedding and sectioning. Additional techniques involve immunochemistry using monoclonal antibodies, polyclonal antisera to epithelial membrane antigen or carcinoembryonic antigen (CEA), and immunoperoxidase staining. Reaction occurs in 50% of cancer cells to anti-CEA heteroantisera[26] and 54% to polyclonal antisera with no reaction with benign effusions. Of effusions related to adenocarcinoma of the lung, breast, and ovary, 100% are recognized by the IgG-1 antibody B72.3 and there is 95% recognition when including poorly differentiated squamous cell lung cancer and metastatic adenocarcinoma from other sites.[27,28] HMFG-2, AUA-1, Mbr and Mov2 are other monoclonal antibodies that demonstrate reactivity with malignant cells.[29] Cytochemical staining with phosphatase, naphthylacetate esterase, and periodic acid–Schiff and sheep erythrocyte rosetting can identify malignant lymphocytes.

Tissue culture of pleural fluid has been used to identify malignant cells.[30] Cytogenetic studies incorporate cytologic and chromosomal analysis and improve on the result of either technique alone.[19] Correct diagnosis of malignant pleural effusion abnormalities using cytogenetics has been reported in the range of 65% to 91%.[31] In a study of lymphoma and leukemia, cytogenetic abnormalities occurred more frequently than positive cytology.[31] Cytogenetic abnormalities have not been demonstrated in benign effusions.[32] Be-

cause of the time and expense involved, these cytogenetic studies are warranted only when repeat cytologic examinations are negative and the probability of malignancy is considered high.

**BIOCHEMICAL AND OTHER APPROACHES TO ANALYSIS.** In pleural effusions related to adenocarcinoma, pleural fluid CEA levels of 720 ng/mL have a 91% sensitivity and 92% specificity.[19] Of patients with pleural metastases from adenocarcinoma of the lung, 90% have CEA levels greater than 10 ng/mL. Other tumor markers or enzymes that have been investigated are creatinine kinase BB, galactosyl transferase, and adenosine deaminase.[33–35] These tests are expensive, time consuming, and lack sensitivity and specificity for malignancy. Malignant pleural effusions have also been identified on bone scans as the technetium radioactive agent can accumulate in the pleural space.[36]

## DIAGNOSTIC PROCEDURES

Thoracentesis is the standard method to make a cytologic diagnosis of malignant pleural effusion. The procedure can be done under CT or sonographic guidance if more precise fluid localization is required. Prior to the procedure, the patient's clotting function and platelet count should be checked.

Although the evidence of complications is low, the clinician must be prepared to deal with bradycardia due to the "pleural shock" response from crossing the parietal pleura by a needle, bleeding, and pneumothorax. Oxygen therapy and narcotics should be readily available to alleviate dyspnea or pain related to the procedure. Reexpansion pulmonary edema may be avoided by limiting the volume of aspirated fluid to 1500 mL, since large effusions will warrant more definitive methods of treatment.[37,38] Failure to obtain a diagnosis by thoracentesis can be followed by a closed percutaneous pleural biopsy with cytology[24,25,39,40] and CT can facilitate the procedure. A positive diagnosis with pleural biopsy is in the range of 40% to 69% that improves to 81% to 90% when added to cytology. It is important to perform the pleural biospsy prior to thoracentesis. The complications associated with pleural biopsy are similar to thoracentesis. However, implantation of cancer cells occurs in 4.1% of patients.

For the remaining 15% to 20% of patients who remain without a diagnosis, video-assisted thoracoscopy (VATS) should be performed. With high sensitivity and specificity, VATS has positive results in 93% to 96% of malignant pleural effusions.[41,42] The surgeon is able to access the intrapleural pathology and do specific biopsies. Therapy may be given concurrently, such as pleurectomy and sclerosis, or postoperatively via a chest tube inserted at the time of VATS. With multiple adhesions, thoracoscopy may not be feasible, making it necessary to proceed to thoracoscopy and open pleural biopsies for diagnostic and therapeutic purposes. Despite all procedures, a diagnosis is not possible in all patients. In patients who have had a nondiagnostic thoracoscopy, their effusion presented no additional problem in 61% and a benign or malignant disease was evident in 39% within 6 years.[43] Bronchoscopy is warranted prior to thoracoscopy or if there is a pulmonary lesion associated with a pleural effusion, ipsilateral volume loss, or no contralateral shift with a large pleural effusion.[44]

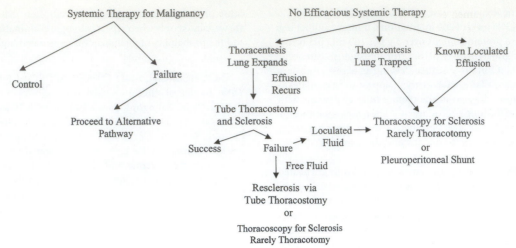

**FIGURE 24E-1.** Algorithm for the treatment of malignant pleural effusion.

## TREATMENT (ALGORITHM IN FIG. 24E-1)

Asymptomatic patients with extensive systemic disease may not need immediate treatment. The condition of the patient, the tumor histology, and extent of the disease must be considered in formulating management. The goal of therapy should be palliation of symptoms and improvement in the quality of life. Malignant pleural effusions in histologies such as breast, lymphoma, small cell lung, and testicular carcinoma can be treated by systemic therapy. Initial thoracentesis can demonstrate the capability of the lung to expand upon removal of fluid and provide immediate relief of symptoms, anticipating effective systemic therapy. Without satisfactory systemic therapy, thoracentesis should not be relied upon to control malignant pleural effusions in solid tumors because the mean time to recurrence is 4.2 days with a 97% recurrence in 30 days. Pneumothorax, empyema, bleeding, and loculation of fluid can complicate the procedure. In addition, chemical sclerotherapy without effective drainage of fluid is less effective than tube thoracostomy because of dilution of the sclerosant by undrained pleural fluid. High recurrence rates, 60% to 100%, also have been reported with tube thoracostomy alone.[45]

Tube thoracostomy with pleurodesis offers the most effective method to prevent the reaccumulation of a malignant pleural effusion. Thorough drainage of the pleural space and a parietal pleura in complete contact with the visceral pleura of a fully expanded lung with a sclerosant distributed around all pleural surfaces is important particularly for creating a chemical pleuritis. The mechanism of action for instilled agents includes chemical pleuritis, cytoreduction, and immunostimulation.

Chest tube placement should be done through an incision in the anterior axillary line and positioned to allow for dependent drainage along the diaphragm. Underwater seal drainage to continuous negative suction at 15 to 20 cm $H_2O$ should be done to allow for maximal lung reexpansion. Complete evacuation of the fluid must be accomplished and a large volume should be drained initially 1,000 mL at a time with intermittent subsequent clamping to prevent ipsilat-

eral pulmonary edema. Sclerotherapy should be administered when chest radiograph has demonstrated resolution of pleural fluid with lung reexpansion and preferably when chest tube drainage is less than 150 for 24 h. Premedication of the patient with narcotic analgesia is essential prior to the procedure; 15 to 25 mL of 1% to 2% lidocaine may be added to the sclerosant for local anesthetic effect. Sclerotherapy is given with the chest tube clamped and the patient rotated every 15 min into various positions to facilitate distribution. However, a study done with tetracycline indicated that movement of the patient did not influence the distribution of the agent.[46] After 4 h of clamping, suction is reestablished on the chest tube and maintained continuously or used only for the first 24 h and discontinued with conversion to only underwater seal drainage. It may be important to leave the chest tube in place for several days for adequate adhesion formation. In general, a 28 or 32 French chest tube is used; however, smaller catheters (7 to 24 French) have been placed under CT or sonographic guidance into loculated areas, and have been used effectively.[47] Such an approach improves patients' comfort and quality of life and may be amenable to outpatient management. Decision to remove the chest tube is based upon full expansion of the lung and drainage less than 150 mL per 24 h. Suture closure of the chest tube site prevents external drainage and sucking chest wound. A chest radiograph should be done after 24 h to document a stable result. Specific agents that have been administered intrapleurally include tetracycline,[48–53] doxycycline,[54–56] minocycline,[57] talc,[58–66] quinacrine,[67–71] methylprednisolone,[72] bleomycin,[53,73,74] cisplatin and cytarabine,[75] doxorubicin with or without LC9018,[76–78] etoposide,[79] OK-432,[80,81] mitomycin,[80] nitrogen mustard,[45,82,83] mitoxantrone,[84,85] radioisotopes,[86] *Corynebacterium parvum*,[87–92] interferons,[93–95] or interleukin 2.[96–98] Most agents are usually given by tube thoracostomy, although one can also perform direct thoracentesis followed by an intracavitary approach. In certain patients, such as those treated with talc poudrage or insufflation, thoracoscopy is generally used. Thoracoscopic technique involves two approaches. The procedure can be done with local anesthesia and intravenous sedation in a nonintubated patient or with general anesthesia and double-lumen endotracheal intubation. Adhesions can be divided under direct vision and loculated effusions drained. Decortication, pleurectomy, and pleural abrasion can also be performed by open thoracotomy, with 85% to 100% of patients experiencing control of malignant effusions. Most recently, talc slurry has been used, which does not require thoracoscopy. The associated morbidity of open thoracotomy is 23% and mortality 9% to 18%, making careful selection of symptomatic patients with trapped lung warranted.[14–45]

When pleural effusions do not respond to initial tube thoracostomy and sclerosis, or they recur, a repeat procedure with the same or different agent may be tried. Factors that require a different approach are trapped lung, loculated fluid, extensive disease, and large volumes of drainage. Thoracoscopy can be helpful; alternatively, patients may be treated with a pleuroperitoneal shunt.[99–101] The Denver shunt (Denver Biometrics, Evergreen, CO), which is most often used, allows the pleural fluid to drain to the peritoneum via a unidirectionally valved chamber that requires manual compression. Palliation of symptoms has been reported to be good in several series with an 8.6-month median duration of function.[99–101] Occlusion of the shunt can occur, and some patients may develop symptomatic ascites.

Often, treatment modalities include radiation therapy (1.4 to 2.3 Gy) combined with chemotherapy for pleural effusions caused by lymphoma. In small cell lung cancer, 80% of the effusions will respond to chemotherapy. An initial thoracentesis will relieve symptoms prior to therapy. A chest tube and sclerosis is reserved for failure of chemotherapy and radiation. In contrast, malignant pleural effusions in non–small cell lung cancer usually require sclerosis for control. However, patients in whom the effusion is not related to tumor spread, and therefore with negative findings for malignancy, may be candidates for resection and adjuvant therapy. These patients have an effusion on the basis of atelectasis, mediastinal nodal involvement, or postobstructive pneumonia. Another clinical indication involves patients with lung cancer recognized at thoracotomy to have intrapleural-disseminated disease and effusion. A study done in 12 patients demonstrated 100% control of effusion by resection of the primary lesion and intrapleural perfusion hyperthermic chemotherapy.[102] After resection the pleural space was irrigated for 2 h with 43° saline solution containing cisplatin using specially devised extracorporeal circuits. Mean survival time was 20 months.

For patients with chylothorax, tube thoracostomy and parenteral nutritional support need to be initiated immediately. Clear liquids and medium-chain triglycerides should only be considered for oral intake. Operative procedures are performed by thoracotomy or preferably by thoracoscopy. Administration of liquid fat as cream or olive oil via a nasogastric tube 2 h prior to operation can help in visualization of the leak and can be removed through the nasogastric tube at the end of the operation. Intraoperative techniques include suture closure of the point of leakage, ligation above and below the leak, ligation of the thoracic duct at the diaphragm with oversewing of the mediastinal pleura and mass ligation of tissue between the aorta and azygous vein when the duct cannot be visualized, pleurectomy, and pleurodesis. A pleuroperitoneal stent can be used in patients who are either refractory or not candidates for the above therapies.

## PROGNOSIS

For patients with malignant pleural effusions, the prognosis is usually poor. Survival time is months for patients with cancer of the lung, ovary, and gastrointestinal tract. The best survival is seen in patients with breast cancer who respond to chemotherapy. Intermediate survival length is seen in patients with lymphoma and testicular cancer. It is essential to establish the ability of the lung to reexpand in order to decide on management, with the goal of palliation of symptoms and improvement of the quality of life. The experience of the clinician must be relied upon. Prospective randomized trials are warranted to evaluate available methods and advance therapeutic knowledge.

## MALIGNANT PERICARDIAL EFFUSION

### INTRODUCTION

In patients with disseminated malignancy the development of a malignant pericardial effusion is common. In clinical and autopsy series the incidence is 5% to 53% depending on histology. Combined cardiac and pericardial metastases occur in 22%, pericardial alone occur in 45%, and myocardial alone occur in 32% of autopsy cases. Primary lesions are most often lung (33%), breast (25%), Hodgkin's and non-Hodgkin's lymphoma (15%), leukemia, melanoma, gastrointestinal tract, and sarcoma.[103,104] Not all patients having malignancy within the pericardium develop a pericardial effusion. In up to one-half of patients with malignancy and a pericardial effusion, the etiology of the effusion is related to radiation therapy, chemotherapy, or infection.[105–107]

### ANATOMY AND PHYSIOLOGY

The normal flow of lymph is from the subendocardium through the myocardium to the subepicardium to the lymphatic trunk that follows the coronary arteries to the root of the aorta. Drainage proceeds to the cardiac node between the superior vena cava and brachiocephalic artery or via the paratracheal nodes to the cardiac node. Ultimate drainage is to the mediastinal lymph nodes. Much less important is the lymphatic plexus of the pericardium whose flow is to the paraaortic node and subsequently to the thoracic duct or paratracheal lymph nodes.[108,109] With metastatic disease to the mediastinal lymph nodes, retrograde lymph flow occurs due to disturbances in the hydrostatic and osmotic pressures and capillary filtration. This is considered the most important mechanism of cardiac metastases with a lesser role played by hematogenous spread and direct tumor invasion.[108]

The normal pericardial space contains a small amount of fluid and the pressure is similar to intrapleural negative pressure. A compliant pericardium can accommodate a slow accumulation of fluid with delay in onset of symptoms and/or hemodynamic instability. Rapid accumulation of fluid or loss of pericardial compliance altered by radiation, inflammation, or tumor implants can result in early development of symptoms and hemodynamic compromise.[110]

## CLINICAL MANIFESTATION

The spectrum of symptoms for malignant pericardial effusion ranges from none to cardiogenic shock, depending on the rate of accumulation and the compliance of the pericardium. Patients experience dyspnea, cough, chest pain, orthopnea, palpitations, malaise, syncope, and dysphagia. With cardiac tamponade, patients develop confusion, anxiety, diaphoresis, facial plethora, and cyanosis. They may attempt to sit up and lean forward to gain relief of symptoms. Loss of consciousness may occur. Examination may reveal tachycardia, jugular venous distention, rales, pericardial friction rub, arrhythmia, cyanosis, hepatosplenomegaly, ascites, peripheral edema, hypertension, and cool extremities. Beck's triad may develop, which is characterized by high venous pressure, low arterial pressure, and distant heart sounds. Pulsus paradoxus reflects an inspiratory decrease in arterial pressure exceeding 10 mm Hg while the respiratory venous pressure remains steady or increases (Kussmaul's sign). The exaggerated waxing and waning in the pulse volume can be palpated or demonstrated by sphygmomanometer and reflects impedance to left ventricular filling by an inspiratory increase in right ventricular filling. Pulsus paradoxus may be missed when there is left ventricular dysfunction, localized right atrial tamponade, positive-pressure breathing, atrial septal defect, severe aortic regurgitation, and pulmonary arterial obstruction. Ultimately, cardiogenic shock, arrest, and death can occur.

## DIAGNOSIS (TABLE 24E-3)

At least 250 mL of pericardial fluid is necessary to produce cardiomegaly on chest radiograph, which has a water bottle appearance. Pleural effusions are present in one-half of the patients. There may be prominence of the epicardial fat pad and loss of the usual contour of the pericardial reflection. Because of its availability and portability echocardiography (ECHO) has become the diagnostic method

## TABLE 24E-2. DIAGNOSTIC MODALITIES FOR MALIGNANT PERICARDIAL EFFUSION

### HISTORY AND PHYSICAL EXAMINATION

| | |
|---|---|
| Cardiac assessment | Electrocardiogram, right heart catheterization |
| Radiologic assessment | Chest radiography, CT, MRI, echocardiogram (two-dimensional) transesophageal, Doppler ultrasound |
| Fluid analysis | Hematology, chemistry, tumor markers, enzymes |
| Cytology | Pericardiocentesis, subxiphoid pericardial window, pericardioscopy, thoracoscopy, thoracotomy |
| Histology | Open pericardial biopsy vs. subxiphoid pericardial window, pericardioscopy, thoracoscopy, thoracotomy |

of choice.[111] Two-dimensional ECHO, transesophageal ECHO, and Doppler ultrasound can delineate location and loculation of pericardial fluid and the pressure of retropericardial masses.[111,112] However, there have been reports of the failure of ECHO to distinguish loculated pericardial effusion, pericardial cysts, diaphragmatic hernias, and pericardial tumors.[111] ECHO has a limited field of view, is dependent upon the operator, and does not define tissue characterization. CT and MRI provide more specific anatomic detail. CT is widely available and can be used to assist in fluid aspiration and biopsy of the pericardium. Calcification of the pericardium is better detected on CT than MRI. In chylopericardium, lymphangiography combined with CT can be helpful in evaluation of the thoracic duct and communications between the pericardium and lymphatic system. Radionuclide imaging techniques may also be helpful for diagnosis of chylopericardium.[113] Although spiral and ultrafast CT scan can provide better-quality images than standard CT with some information as to pericardial and myocardial function, MRI is superior in minimizing blurring of the pericardium and heart. The three-dimensional morphology of the pericardium and its involvement by adjacent disease processes is well depicted on MRI, which should complement ECHO to answer clinical questions. MRI can detect small pericardial effusions and loculated effusions not evident on ECHO. Some tissue characterization can be achieved on MRI. Dynamic MRI (live MRI) can provide information on ventricular function. MRI can show compression or collapse of the right side of the heart chambers during ventricular diastole that is a finding that indicates cardiac tamponade.[114,115]

When symptomatic, 90% of the patients have abnormalities including (in order of decreasing frequency) nonspecific ST segment–T wave changes, low QRS voltage, sinus tachycardia, atrial fibrillation and flutter, premature ventricular contractions, and heart block. Although ECHO can indicate cardiac tamponade by diastolic collapse of the right atrium and right ventricle, Doppler flow velocity abnormalities and overdistention of the inferior vena cava, clinical and hemodynamic assessments are also essential in making a diagnosis, particularly in early tamponade. Hemodynamic parameters are measured by catheterization of the right side of the heart and refer to decrease in cardiac output, elevation of right atrial pressure with loss of diastolic "y" descent, and equalization of diastolic pressure.

For determination of the etiology of a pericardial effusion, pericardiocentesis is the first diagnostic modality. In malignancy the yield is 45% to 87%.[116–118] Hemorrhagic fluid is suggestive but not diagnostic of malignant pericardial effusion. Fluid should also be sent for cell count, protein, glucose, amylase, triglyceride, and bacteriologic studies. In patients with ovarian cancer, measurement of CA 125 levels in the serum and pericardial fluid is of diagnostic and prognostic value.[119] Chylopericardium can occur with lymphoma and other mediastinal neoplasms, as well as mediastinal irradiation. The fluid demonstrates high triglyceride and protein content, a predominance of lymphocytes and fat globules by Sudan III staining. Up to 40% of the symptomatic effusions in patients with a primary malignancy will have other etiologies including radiation, drug-related, uremia, infections, and idiopathic.[120] Open pericardial biopsy is most commonly performed through the subxiphoid route and pericardioscopy can improve diagnostic yield.[121] Other approaches are subcostal video-assisted thoracoscopy and limited

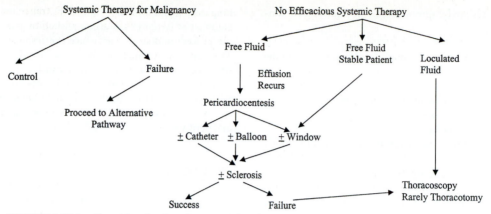

**FIGURE 24E-2.** Algorithm for the treatment of malignant pericardial effusion.

anterior thoracotomy. Results are in the 31% to 55% range for pericardial biopsy.[122,123]

## TREATMENT (ALGORITHM IN FIG. 24E-2)

Patients in cardiac tamponade require emergency pericardiocentesis and may benefit from the administration of volume. Pericardiocentesis is also used initially in the nonacute setting. Without additional therapy the reported recurrence rate is 66% to 100%.[124,125] Pericardiocentesis is performed via the subxiphoid or left parasternal approach. Compared to the blind or electrocardiographically guided technique, the use of ECHO or fluoroscopy decreases the complication rate that is also related to the location and size of the fluid. Two-dimensional ECHO allows a dyspneic patient to sit upright as pericardiocentesis is being performed. When pericardiocentesis is done with right heart catheterization, hemodynamic parameters should be obtained before and after the procedure.[126–128]

Percutaneously placed pericardial catheters are another method of treating malignant pericardial effusions. The catheter should remain in place until draining less than 75 mL per 24 h. Review of the literature indicates that this may require 4.8 days.[129] Prophylactic antibiotics will decrease the occurrence of infection. This approach can work in up to 75% of the patients but has usually been supplemented by systemic therapy or sclerosant agents.[126,128–130] Sclerosing agents can be administered through the pericardial catheter while systemic therapy is given concurrently. The largest clinical experience is with tetracycline. With a dose range of 500 to 1000 mg reported over 1 to 8 consecutive days, responses of 75% to 100% are seen. Associated complications are pain, fever, arrhythmia, and catheter plugging. Doxycycline, now available instead of parenteral tetracycline, is administered as a 500-mg dose and is associated with fever and pain. Lidocaine mixed with this sclerosant can decrease the incidence of pain. Patients should also be premedicated with a narcotic analgesic prior to the procedure if pain is anticipated.

Chemotherapeutic drugs, including bleomycin, 60 mg (range 5 to 60 mg), are used for instillation. A response rate up to 100% has been reported with bleomycin. Fever frequently occurs with bleomycin sclerosis. Other agents in this category with respective response rates are cisplatin (4 of 8 patients), mitoxantrone (9 of 12 patients), nitrogen mustard (9 of 9 patients), thiotepa (3 of 4 patients), 5-fluorouracil (3 of 3 patients), teniposide (2 of 3 patients), quinacrine hydrochloride (2 of 2 patients), and vinblastine (1 of 1 patients).[108,131–143] Concurrent therapy is also given to some of these patients. A different type of agent is OK-432, lyophilized powder of *Streptococcus pyogenes* A3, which is both penicillin- and heat-treated. Responses were seen in 6 of 10 patients.[144] In contrast to the previous agents that may act through an inflammatory reaction induced by the sclerosant or an antitumor effect, OK-432 can stimulate cell-mediated immunity as well as produce cytotoxicity of malignant cells. These patients experienced fever (60%), pain (50%), arrhythmia (30%), and hypotension (20%). Talc, 10 g in 50 mL of saline, may be considered for refractory cases, but the risk of late constrictive pericarditis is not known. The use of radionuclides has been limited and has involved chromic phosphate P32 (23/32 responders), a radioactive iodine added to a tumor-related monoclonal antibody[110] I-HMFG2 (4/4 responders) and gold Au-198 (0/1 responders).[145–149] In general, instillation therapy should allow the agent to remain in contact with the pericardial space for a period of time, after which the pericardium is drained to allow adherence of the visceral and parietal pericardial surfaces. Drainage should continue until less than 75 mL for 24 h, and may require repeated instillation therapy to be accomplished.

As is evident from the above numbers, the experience with pericardial sclerotherapy is limited compared to the use in malignant pleural effusions. Definitive conclusions as to efficiency are not possible because of the small numbers of patients treated with most of the agents. The procedure may be considered particularly appropriate in patients who undergo placement of a pericardial catheter for cardiac tamponade or who are poor surgical candidates.

Another percutaneous approach is balloon pericardiotomy. Following a subxiphoid pericardiocentesis, a balloon is passed over a guidewire and dilated to create a window between the pericardium and pleural spaces. Resolution of pericardial effusions occurred in 87% to 96% of patients.[150,151] The most frequently seen complication is pleural effusion requiring thoracentesis or chest tube drainage reported in up to 18% followed by fever (13%) and small pneumothorax (4%).

Surgical procedures can be appropriate in the following circumstances:

1. Limited chemotherapeutic and radiation options to control the effusion
2. Undiagnosed effusion
3. Medical condition of the patient able to tolerate the procedure
4. Failure of other palliative measures
5. Reasonable expectation of survival
6. Constriction by radiation or neoplasm and satisfactory prognosis

Hemodynamic stabilization of the patient prior to a surgical procedure may be necessary via a pericardiocentesis or pericardial catheter. However, in a stable patient the distention of the pericardial sac may assist with the procedure, particularly with subxiphoid pericardiectomy or the pericardial window approach, the most commonly performed operations. The procedure can be done under local anesthesia or converted to general anesthesia as permitted hemodynamically. The mortality rate of 8% is usually related to the underlying cancer and demonstrates the importance of patient selection.[122–124,152–156] Success is dependent upon the inflammatory fusion of the epicardium to pericardium and is promoted by maintenance of the pericardial tube until drainage is less than 75 mL for 24 h over a period of usually 2 to 8 days. Effusions have been controlled in 93% of reported cases.

In malignant pericardial effusion the role of pericardioscopy as an adjunct for diagnostic and therapeutic purposes to pericardiocentesis, balloon pericardiotomy, and subxiphoid pericardiotomy remains to be defined.[157,158] A loculated or recurrent effusion can be dealt with through the thoracoscopic or thoracotomy approaches. Radiation-induced effusions also tend to have a higher recurrence rate after the subxiphoid approach. Thoracoscopy is performed through the left chest and can be used instead of a left anterior thoracotomy for pericardial drainage. The port site for the video camera is placed high at about the third intercostal space since the distended pericardium may crowd the chest. The second and third ports should be placed anterior and posterior to the pericardial sac. A lateral pericardiotomy can be performed by a left anterior thoracotomy to create a pleuropericardial window by excision of a large segment of anterior pericardium to provide intrapleural communication. The low recurrence rate of 15% must be weighed against the requirement for thoracotomy and general anesthesia.[159] A more extensive pericardiectomy can be done through a left anterolateral thoracotomy, bilateral anterior thoracotomy with transection of the body of the sternum or median sternotomy with a mortality of 13% to 19%. Such a procedure is helpful when there is an element of constrictive pericarditis. Inadequate pericardial resection leads to a recurrence rate of 17%.[160–162] In debilitated patients with a loculated or recurrent malignant pericardial effusion a pericardioperitoneal shunt may be palliative. In chylopericardium with or without chylothorax the thoracic duct may need to be ligated in addition to a pericardial procedure.

## NONSURGICAL THERAPEUTIC MODALITIES

Chemotherapy has been used to treat malignant pericardial effusions in patients with lymphoma, leukemia, breast cancer, small cell lung cancer, and testicular cancer. In 75% of the patients immediate relief of symptoms is accomplished by pericardiocentesis, but the procedure does not influence the response to chemotherapy. The results with radiation therapy by histology are 93% for lymphoma or leukemia, 71% for breast cancer, and 45% for other solid tumors.[134,139,163–167] Initial pericardiocentesis is similarly performed prior to radiation therapy that is then delivered in doses of 2 to 3 Gy over a 2- to 3-week period. Potential complications are myocarditis and pericarditis.[108,143,165,167–169]

## PROGNOSIS

The histology and extent of the malignant disease influence survival of patients with malignant pericardial effusion. After intervention mean survival with lung cancer is 3.5 months, breast cancer 9.3 to 18.5 months, and lymphoma 10 months, and other cancers less than 6 months.[163,169,170] The goal of therapy should be to palliate symptoms, return the patient to good functional status expeditiously, and prevention of recurrence.

## MALIGNANT ASCITES

### INTRODUCTION

Ascites is the result of malignancy in 10% of patients. The most common malignancy associated with ascites is ovarian cancer, and it accounts for 30% to 50% of the cases. Other common cancers are uterine, breast, gastric, colon, pancreatic, lung, and lymphoma. Including ovarian cancer, these histologies make up 80% of cases, and for the remainder, the malignancy may not be identified.[171,172] Treatment is aimed at relief of symptoms and may improve survival although prognosis is usually poor. The patient's medical condition, histology, and extent of disease must be considered to achieve palliation while minimizing the morbidity of therapy.

### PATHOPHYSIOLOGY

Normally there is movement of fluid in and out of the peritoneal cavity. A small amount of transudative fluid, about 50 mL, with a protein content of 20% to 25% of plasma is present because resorption of fluid exceeds production. The movement of fluid is predominantly through the diaphragmatic lymphatics rather than omental, peritoneal lymphatics, and the thoracic duct. Several factors are responsible for the development of malignant ascites. Tumor obstructs the lymphatic flow that reduces the outflow of fluid and precedes the onset of ascites. Later in ascites the increased peritoneal cavity hydrostatic pressure produces increased fluid absorption. Due to the increased production of fluid by visceral capillaries along the involved and uninvolved peritoneal surfaces in cases of malignancy, fluid can move into the peritoneal cavity at a rate that can be more than 10 times normal, which exceeds the flow of fluid out.[173–175] The capillaries occur in the lining of the peritoneum or are new vessels of the tumor circulation and are influenced by a hormonal factor secreted by the tumor and similar to endothelial growth factor.[173,176,177] Another factor contributing to malignant ascites is increased capillary permeability to albumin resulting in an exudative fluid with a protein level that is 85% of plasma level.[173] In a liver involved by metastatic disease, hepatic venous obstruction can result in increased hepatic venous pressure with the elevation of hepatic sinusoidal pressure and fluid transudation into the peritoneal cavity.[178] The protein concentration of hepatic lymph is high because of the increased permeability of the sinusoidal bed. Increased hepatic fluid formation also leads to ascites. Alterations in renal perfusion from decreased effective plasma volume will subsequently lead to secretion of renin. Water retention and ascites are the outcome of sodium conservation by the kidneys through the renin-angiotensin-aldosterone mechanism. Patients with malignant ascites and extensive hepatic metastases may respond to the aldosterone antagonist spironolactone.[179,180] Malignancy can also cause chylous ascites, and when present in the adult population, has resulted from a malignancy in 88% of adults with the condition. Chylous ascites is much less frequent in pediatric patients. There is extensive obstruction of lymphatic and lymphaticovenous collaterals within the abdomen including the retroperitoneal lymphatics.[181,182]

## CLINICAL MANIFESTATIONS

In half of the patients ascites is the first manifestation of malignant disease.[183] Abdominal distention causes discomfort or pain, anorexia, nausea, and emesis. Patients experience malaise, dyspnea, ankle edema, and change in weight, either loss or gain. With at least 500 mL of fluid, signs of ascites include: (1) bulging flanks in the supine position by the weight of fluid, (2) tympany on top of the abdominal curve as a result of gas-filled intestines floating to the surface of the fluid, (3) a fluid wave percussed by the left hand with tapping of the flank with the right hand (an assistant presses downward on the midline of the abdomen to block mesenteric fat), (4) shifting dullness with changes of position of the patient. Sensitivity of the findings varies from 60% to 80% and specificity 65% to 90%.[184] The *puddle* sign can detect as little as 120 mL of fluid. The patient lies prone for 5 min, then assumes the knee-chest position, which allows the fluid to go to the most dependent area. The examiner flicks near the flank with a finger while moving the stethoscope diaphragm further away. The intensity of the sound is loudest at the end of the puddle even though the distance has increased. The difference in sound transmission disappears when the patient sits up.

## DIAGNOSIS (TABLE 24E-3)

A careful history and physical examination is performed. Complete blood count and liver function tests are ordered. Carcinoembryonic antigen (CEA) level can be elevated in malignant and nonmalignant conditions and is most often used to indicate relapse in colorectal cancer. Carbohydrate antigen (CA) 125 is a nonspecific marker for ovarian cancer since it is elevated in other cancers such as pancreatic, lung, colorectal, breast, and in patients without malignancy. Tumor markers do not diagnose ascites as malignant but can help to define histology of the primary tumor. Ultrasonography is the most commonly used radiologic technique and a fluid volume of 100 mL can be detected. Computerized tomography (CT) and especially magnetic resonance imaging (MRI) can provide details about

### TABLE 24E-3. DIAGNOSTIC MODALITIES FOR MALIGNANT ASCITES

HISTORY AND PHYSICAL EXAMINATION

| | |
|---|---|
| Radiologic assessment | CT abdomen and plevis, MRI, ultrasound |
| Fluid analysis | Hematology, chemistry, tumor markers, enzymes |
| Cytology | Paracentesis with/without CT, ultrasound, laparoscopy |
| Histology | Biopsy under CT, ultrasound or laparoscopy |

the fluid in relation to intraabdominal organs. All three techniques demonstrate hepatic metastases. CT and transvaginal ultrasound are useful in ovarian cancer and CT in pancreatic cancer. Percutaneous cytologic and histologic procedures of abnormalities can be done under CT and ultrasonography guidance. Information on the primary tumor can be obtained from chest radiography, and barium studies complement the endoscopic procedures and mammography.

Abdominal paracentesis should be diagnostic and therapeutic and establishes the time to reaccumulation. The procedure should be done with intravenous hydration of the patient or liberal oral fluid intake to prevent orthostatic hypotension from rapid shifts of fluid from the intravascular compartment. The patient should be asked to void prior to the paracentesis to avoid injuring the urinary bladder. Fluid is sent for cell count with differential, protein, lactic dehydrogenase, cholesterol, amylase, glucose, pH, cytology, and microbiologic studies. Studies of the fluid for fibronectin, sialic acid, proteases, and antiproteases, if available, may be helpful. Nonmalignant etiologies as congestive heart failure, cirrhosis, infection, pancreatic disease, myxedema, and complication of chemotherapy and radiation therapy must be eliminated. Elevated protein level in ascites as compared to serum (ratio >0.4) and increased lactic dehydrogenase ratio of ascites to serum of >1.0 suggest neoplasm.[183,185] In the absence of infection, a cell count of greater than 10,000 red blood cells per microliter and more than 1000 white cells per microliter will favor malignancy. Malignant fluid is often blood or serosanguinous. Chylous fluid is milky white. The lipid content is greater than in the plasma, and protein content exceeds more than half that of the plasma. Fat is seen microscopically, with the ratio of neutral fat to total lipid higher than that of plasma.

Cytology for malignant ascites is 60% sensitive and 100% specific.[183,186–188] The cytology will be negative even in the presence of hepatic metastases, hepatocellular carcinoma, or chylous ascites unless there is associated peritoneal carcinomatosis.[188] Laparoscopy with biopsy will yield a diagnosis in 85% to 95% of patients, and it is important to securely close all trocar sites to prevent leakage. Seeding of tumor at trocar sites can occur.[189]

## TREATMENT (ALGORITHM IN FIG. 24E-3)

Dietary salt restriction is ineffective in malignant ascites, but spironolactone in doses of 100 to 450 mg per day has been reported to

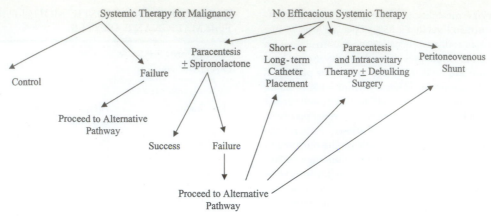

**FIGURE 24E-3.** Algorithm for the treatment of malignant ascites.

control malignant ascites. The effect may be temporary and progressively increasing doses of furosemide may be added to the regimen. The doses of diuretics should be adjusted accordingly so that the patients will lose no more than 1 kg per day so as not to deplete the intravascular volume and cause electrolyte abnormalities.[180,190–192]

The standard method of treatment for malignant ascites is paracentesis. Up to 10 L of fluid can be removed without a hemodynamic problem if the patient is given intravenous albumin replacement. Ultrasonography should be used during the procedure for loculated ascites, extensive solid disease, or suspected adhesions. Associated risks are hypotension, hypoproteinemia, electrolyte abnormalities, bowel perforation, peritonitis, pulmonary embolus, and death.[193] Paracentesis can be accomplished with immediate removal of the catheter or alternatively leaving it in place to drain the fluid over 1 to 3 days. Catheters such as the Tenckoff catheter (Davol, Cranston, RI) can be permanently placed to palliate intractable ascites but it creates the risk of bacterial growth and sepsis in the peritoneum.[194]

## SYSTEMIC CHEMOTHERAPY

Chemotherapy is particularly beneficial to patients with ovarian cancer or lymphoma. Even with malignant ascites, patients with stage I or stage IA ovarian cancer who undergo surgical treatment and chemotherapy have 5-year survival rates of almost 50%. In more advanced stages of ovarian cancer, median survival of 44 months can be seen with agents such as cisplatin and taxol. Overall resolution or marked diminution of malignant ascites is seen in 46% of ovarian cancers and 11% of lymphomas.[195,196]

## INTRACAVITARY THERAPY

Direct treatment into the peritoneal cavity has been performed with several modalities that include chemotherapy, phototherapy, radiocolloids, and immunotherapy. Photodynamic therapy (PDT) was investigated in a phase I study in which 39 patients with disseminated intraperitoneal tumors underwent debulking surgery and light-delivery PDT. The maximal tolerated dose of PDT performed 48 h after intravenous administration of 2.5 mg of dihematoporphyrin ether (Photofrin, QLT Phototherapeutics, Inc., Vancouver British Columbia, Canada) was 3.75 J/cm$^2$ of 514-nm green light to the entire peritoneal surface with boosts of 5 to 7 J/cm$^2$ of 630-nm red light to sites of gross disease encountered at surgery. Nine patients were alive and free of disease 3 to 27 months after treatment, 9 patients died from progressive disease, and 21 patients were reported alive with progressive tumor. Assessment and efficacy will require a phase II or III study using the maximally tolerated dose of PDT.[197]

Phase I and II trials have been performed with chemotherapy in malignant ascites. There are no completed randomized studies comparing intraperitoneal chemotherapy with systemic therapy. With intracavitary chemotherapy, a large volume of fluid is important for instillation of the agents so that adequate distribution of the agents can occur.[198] High concentrations can be present in the peritoneal cavity with low systemic concentration. Systemic side effects may be decreased, but interstitial adhesions can result from the procedure. The procedure has been used in peritoneal carcinomatosis and malignant ascites from ovarian and gastrointestinal carcinomatosis. Agents that have been instilled include nitrogen mustard, cisplatin, etoposide, mitomycin, thiotepa, methotrexate, bleomycin, mitoxantrone, 5-fluorouracil, and doxorubicin.[60,73,199–209] In phase II studies, complete response rates of 45% to 50% have been noted with ovarian cancer. Determination of survival advantage awaits randomized trials. Reports have varied from control of malignant ascites in 50% of patients by intracavitary cisplatin or bleomycin to phase II studies in which 82% to 90% of patients with malignant ascites had resolution of the ascites from gastric or colorectal cancer after debulking surgery and continuous hyperthermic peritoneal perfusion (CHPP) with mitomycin C or mitomycin C and cisplatin.[210–213] Radiocolloids have been used in intracavitary therapy and have been relegated to historical interest.[214,215]

Biologic response modifiers including *Corynebacterium parvum*, OK-432, interferon, and IL-2 have been explored for intracavitary treatment of ascites.[93,216–222] Response rates vary from 29% to 45%, and can be accompanied by the usual flulike syndrome and hematologic/hemodynamic toxicity of this therapy. Newer therapies include the use of antimucin antibody 2G3,[105] and the use of matrix metalloproteinase inhibitors.[223–227]

## PERITONEOVENOUS SHUNTING

Peritoneovenous shunting can be accomplished with the LeVeen (Becton-Dickenson and Leveen, Rutherford, NJ) or Denver (Johnson & Johnson, Evergreen, CO) shunts. The latter has a unidirectional valve that allows flushing of the shunt but has not demonstrated functional superiority.[228] Flow is from the peritoneum to the central circulation due to the pressure differential. Peritoneovenous shunting is appropriate for patients who are refractory to therapies for the underlying malignancy. The shunt should not be used when there is loculated ascites, infection, bloody ascites, or protein content greater that 50 g/L, jaundice with a bilirubin level greater than 10 mg%, pseudomyxoma peritonei, or coagulopathy. Relief of malignant ascites will occur in 64% to 77% of patients.[229,230] A complication rate as high as 25% has been reported due to shunt occlusion, heart failure, coagulapathy, tumor dissemination, thrombosis of the superior vena cava, pulmonary embolus, intestinal obstruction, sepsis, and death.[231,232] All patients with a functioning shunt have a degree of coagulopathy measured by serum parameters such as fibrinogen degradation products.[233,234] Ten to forty percent of patients may have shunt occlusion, which can be treated with flushing with a thrombolytic agent or replacement.[235,236] Diuretics are administered to help with excretion of fluid and to avoid heart failure. Reports of tumor dissemination have not substantiated a problem with hematogenous spread or considered to have impacted on survival.[237,238]

## RADICAL SURGERY

Radical surgery has involved extensive debulking surgery with early postoperative intraperitoneal chemotherapy and in some cases abdominal radiation for carcinomatosis. Survival of greater than 3 years for colorectal and gastric cancer has been reported. Phase III studies with larger numbers of patients obviously are required.[202,239,240]

## PROGNOSIS

The average prognosis with malignant ascites is 20 weeks from the time of diagnosis. Results for individual histologies will vary such as 30 to 35 weeks for ovarian cancer, 12 to 20 weeks for gastrointestinal cancer, and 58 to 78 weeks for lymphoma.[183,214,215,223] In women, it is important to thoroughly investigate for an ovarian primary since therapeutic options can provide effective palliation. When the histology is not identified, the prognosis ranges from 7.5 days to 3 months.[214,240] Malignant chylous ascites portends a grave prognosis. Histology of the tumor, if known, is of major importance in planning therapy. Presently available therapies need to be investigated in prospective randomized studies, and the focus of treatment need to be on palliation of symptoms with minimal morbidity.

## REFERENCES

1. HAWHEER FH, YARBRO JW: Diagnosis and treatment of malignant pleural effusions. Semin Oncol 12:54, 1985.
2. SAHN SA: Pleural effusions in lung cancer. Clin Chest Med 14:189, 1993.
3. BRUNEAU R, RUBIN P: The management of pleural effusion and chylotory in lymphoma. Radiology 85:1085, 1965.
4. BLACK LF: The pleural space and pleural fluid. Mayo Clin Proc 47:493, 1972.
5. KINASEWITZ GT, FISHMAN AP: Influence of alterations in Starling forces on visceral pleural fluid movement. J Appl Physiol 51:671, 1981.
6. HENSCHKE C et al: The pathogenesis, radiologic evaluation, and therapy of pleural effusions. Radiol Clin North Am 27:1241, 1989.
7. BROADDUS C, STAUB N: Pleural liquid and protein turnover in health and disease. Semin Respir Med 9:7, 1987.
8. AGOSTONI E: Mechanics of the pleural space. Physiol Rev 52:57, 1972.
9. LEFF A et al: Pleural effusion from malignancy. Ann Intern Med 88:532, 1978.
10. MEYER PL: Metastatic carcinoma of the pleura. Thorax 21:437, 1966.
11. SAHN SA: Malignant pleural effusions. Clin Chest Med 6:113, 1998.
12. FENTIMEN I et al: Pleural effusion in breast cancer: A review of 105 cases. Cancer 4:2087, 1981.
13. CHERNOW B, SAHN SA: Carcinomatous involvement of the pleura: an analysis of 96 cases. Am J Med 67:695, 1977.
14. MARTINI N et al: Indications for pleurectomy in malignant effusion. Cancer 35:734, 1975.
15. ZEHNER LC, HOUGSTRATEN B: Malignant effusions and their management. Semin Oncol Nurs 1:259, 1985.
16. WOODRING JH: Recognition of pleural effusion on supine radiographs: How much fluid is required. Am J Roentgenol 142:59, 1984.
17. PETERSON JA: Recognition of intrapulmonary pleural effusions. Radiology 74:34, 1960.
18. FLOWER CDR, WILLIAMS MP: The pleural space, in *CT Review*, JES Husband (ed). London, Churchill Livingstone, 1989, pp 23–32.
19. DHILLON DP, SPIRO SG: Pleural disease: malignant pleural effusion. Br J Hosp Med 23:506, 1983.
20. PETERSON T, RISKA H: Diagnostic value of total and differential leukocyte counts in pleural effusion. Acta Med Scand 210:129, 1981.
21. LIGHT RW: Pleural effusion. Med Clin N Am 61:1339, 1977.
22. CARR DT: Diagnostic studies of pleural fluid. Surg Clin North Am 53:801, 1973.
23. KRENER MR et al: High amylase levels in neoplasm related pleural effusion. Ann Intern Med 110:567, 1989.
24. SALYER WR et al: Efficiency of pleural needle biopsy and pleural fluid cytopathology in the diagnosis of malignant neoplasm involving the pleura. Chest 67:536, 1975.
25. PRAKASH UBS, REIMAN HM: Comparison of needle biopsy with cytologic analysis for evaluation of pleural effusion: Analysis of 414 cases. Mayo Clin Proc 60:158–164, 1985.
26. ESTABAN JM et al: Immunocytochemical profile of benign and carcinomatous effusions: A practical approach to difficult diagnosis. Am J Clin Pathol 94:608, 1990.

27. Martin SE et al: Identification of adenocarcinoma in cytologic preparation of effusion using monoclonal antibody B72.3. Am J Clin Pathol 86:10, 1986.

28. Johnston WW et al: Use of a monoclonal antibody (B72.3) as an immunological adjunct to diagnosis of adenocarcinoma in tumor effusions. Cancer Res 45:1894, 1985.

29. Mottolese M et al: Use of selected combination of monoclonal antibodies to tumor associated antigens in the diagnosis of neoplastic effusions of unknown origin. Eur J Clin Oncol 24:1277, 1988.

30. Monif GRG et al: Living cytology: A new diagnostic technique for malignant pleural effusion. Chest 69:626, 1976.

31. Dewald G et al: Usefulness of chromosome examination in the diagnosis of malignant pleural effusion. N Engl J Med 295:1494, 1976.

32. Fraisse J et al: Diagnosis of malignancy by cytogenic means in effusion. Clin Genet 14:288, 1978.

33. Silverman LM et al: Creatinine kinase BB: A new tumor-associated marker. Clin Chem 25:1432, 1979.

34. Kim VD et al: Galactosyltransferase variant in pleural effusion. Clin Chem 28:1133, 1982.

35. Petersson T et al: Adenosine deaminase in the diagnosis of pleural effusions. Acta Med Scand 215:299, 1984.

36. Goldstein HA, Gefte WB: Detection of unsuspected malignant pleural effusion by bone scan. AJR 10:556, 1983.

37. Mahfood S et al: Reexpansion pulmonary edema. Ann Thorac Surg 45:340, 1988.

38. Trachiotis GD et al: Reexpansion pulmonary edema. Ann Thorac Surg 63:1205, 1992.

39. Sarma PR, Moore MR: Approach to the management of pleural effusion in malignancy. South Med J 71:133, 1978.

40. Winkelman M, Pfitzer P: Blind pleural biopsy in combination with cytology of pleural effusion. Acta Cytol 25:373, 1981.

41. Daniel TM: Diagnostic Thoracoscopy for pleural disease. Ann Thorac Surg 56:639, 1993.

42. Colt HG: Thoracoscopic management of malignant pleural effusions. Clin in Chest Med 16:505, 1995.

43. Ryan J et al: The outcome of patients with pleural effusion of indeterminate cause at thoracotomy. Mayo Clin Proc 56:145, 1981.

44. Feinsilver SH et al: Fiberoptic bronchoscopy and pleural effusion of unknown origin. Chest 90:516, 1986.

45. Anderson CB et al: The treatment of malignant pleural effusions. Cancer 33:916, 1974.

46. Lorch DG et al: Effect of patient positioning on distribution of tetracycline in the pleural space during pleurodesis. Chest 93:527, 1988.

47. Morrison MC et al: Sclerotherapy of malignant pleural effusion through sonographically placed small-bore catheters. AJR 158:41, 1992.

48. Wallach HW: Intrapleural tetracycline for malignant pleural effusions. Chest 68:510, 1975.

49. Zaloznik AJ et al: Intrapleural tetracycline in malignant pleural effusions. Cancer 51:752, 1983.

50. Gravelyn TR et al: Tetracycline pleurodesis for malignant pleural effusions. Cancer 59:1973, 1987.

51. Landvater L et al: Malignant pleural effusions treated by tetracycline sclerotherapy. Chest 93:1196, 1988.

52. Sherman S et al: Clinical experience with tetracycline pleurodesis of malignant pleural effusions. South Med J 80:716, 1987.

53. Ruckdeschel JC et al: Tetracycline therapy for malignant pleural effusions. Chest 100:1528, 1991.

54. Muir JF et al: Use of intrapleural doxycycline via lavage-drainage in recurrent effusions of neoplastic origin (French). Revue des Maladies Respiratoires 4:29, 1987.

55. Kitzmura S et al: Intrapleural deoxycycline for control of malignant pleural effusions. Curr Ther Res 30:515, 1981.

56. Mansson T: Treatment of malignant pleural effusions with deoxycycline. Scand J Infect Dis 53:29, 1988.

57. Hatta T et al: Effect of intrapleural administration of minocycline on postoperative air leakage and malignant pleural effusions. Kyobu Gelca 43:283, 1990.

58. Adler RH, Sayek I: Treatment of malignant pleural effusion: A method using tube thoracostomy and talc. Ann Thorac Surg 22:8, 1976.

59. Daniel TM et al: Thoracoscopy and talc poudrage for pneumothoraces and effusions. Ann Thorac Surg 50:186, 1990.

60. Cohen RG et al: Talc pleurodesis: Talc slurry versus thoracoscopic talc insufflation in a porcine model (see comments) Ann Thorac Surg 62:1000; discussion 1003, 1996.

61. Webb WR et al: Iodized talc pleurodesis for the treatment of pleural effusions. J Thorac Cardiovasc Surg 103:881; discussion 885, 1992.

62. Pearson FG: Talc poudrage for malignant pleural effusion. J Thorac Cardiovasc Surg 51:732, 1966.

63. Kennedy L, Sahn SA: Talc pleurodesis for the treatment of pneumothorax and pleural effusion (see comments). Chest 106:1215, 1994.

64. Aelony Y et al: Thoracoscopic talc poudrage pleurodesis for chronic recurrent pleural effusions. Ann Intern Med 115:778, 1991.

65. Rinaldo JE et al: Adult respiratory distress syndrome following intrapleural instillation of talc. J Thorac Cardiovasc Surg 85:523, 1983.

66. Factor SM: Granulomatous pneumonitis: A result of intrapleural instillation of quinacrine and talcum powder. Arch Pathol 99:499, 1975.

67. Taylor SA et al: Quinacrine in the management of malignant pleural effusion. Br J Surg 64:52, 1977.

68. Borda I: Convulsions following intrapleural administration of quinacrine hydrochloride. JAMA 201:1049, 1967.

69. Borja ER, Pugh RP: Single-dose quinacrine (atabrine) and thoracostomy in the control of pleural effusions in patients with neoplastic diseases. Cancer 31:899, 1973.

70. Stiksa G: Treatment of recurrent pleural effusion by pleurodesis with quinacrine: Comparison between instillation by repeated thoracenteses and by tube drainage. Scand J Respir Dis 60:197, 1979.

71. Hickman JA: Treatment of neoplastic pleural effusions with local instillations of quinacrine (mepacrine) hydrochloride. Thorax 25:226, 1970.

72. Bartal AH: Clinical and flow cytometry characteristics of malignant pleural effusions in patients after intracavitary administration of methylprednisolone acetate. Cancer 67:3136, 1991.

73. Ostrowski MJ: An assessment of the long-term results of controlling the reaccumulation of malignant effusions using intracavity bleomycin. Cancer 57:721, 1986.

74. Bitran JD et al: Intracavitary bleomycin for the control of malignant effusions. J Surg Oncol 16:273, 1981.

75. Figlin R et al: Intrapleural chemotherapy without pleurodesis for malignant pleural effusions: LCSG Trial 861. Chest 106:363S, 1994.

76. Ike O: Treatment of malignant pleural effusions with

doxorubicin hydrochloride-containing poly (L-lactic acid) microspheres. Chest 99:911, 1991.

77. MASUNO T: A comparative trial of LC9018 plus doxorubicin and doxorubicin alone for the treatment of malignant pleural effusion secondary to lung cancer. Cancer 68:1495, 1991.

78. DESAI SD: Intracavitary doxorubicin in malignant effusions. Lancet 1:872, 1979.

79. HOLOYE PY et al: Intrapleural etoposide for malignant effusion. Cancer Chemother Pharmacol 26:147, 1990.

80. LUH KT: Comparison of OK-432 and mitomycin C pleurodesis for malignant pleural effusion caused by lung cancer: A randomized trial. Cancer 69:674, 1992.

81. UCHIDA A: Intrapleural administration of OK432 in cancer patients: Augmentation of autologous tumor killing activity of tumor-associated large granular lymphocytes. Cancer Immunol Immunother 18:5, 1984.

82. KEFFORD RF: Intracavitary adriamycin nitrogen mustard and tetracycline in the control of malignant effusions: A randomized study. Med J Aust 2:447, 1980.

83. GREENWALD DW: Management of malignant pleural effusion. J Surg Oncol 10:361, 1978.

84. TORSTEN U: Local therapy of malignant pleural effusion with mitoxantrone. Anticancer Drugs 3:17, 1992.

85. GROTH G: Intrapleural palliative treatment of malignant pleural effusions with mitoxantrone versus placebo (pleural tube alone). Ann Oncol 2:213, 1991.

86. IZBICKI R: Pleural effusion in cancer patients: A prospective randomized study of pleural drainage with the addition of radioactive phosphorous to the pleural space vs. pleural drainage alone. Cancer 36:1511, 1975.

87. OSTROWSKI MJ: A randomized trial of intracavitary bleomycin and Corynebacterium parvum in the control of malignant pleural effusions. Radiother Oncol 14:19, 1989.

88. LEAHY BC: Treatment of malignant pleural effusions with intrapleural Corynebacterium parvum or tetracycline. Eur J Respir Dis 66:50, 1985.

89. HILLERDAL G: Corynebacterium parvum in malignant pleural effusion: A randomized prospective study. Eur J Respir Dis 69:204, 1986.

90. ROSSI GA: Symptomatic treatment of recurrent malignant pleural effusions with intrapleurally administered Corynebacterium parvum: Clinical response is not associated with evidence of enhancement of local cellular-mediated immunity. Am Rev Respir Dis 135:885, 1987.

91. FELLETTI R: Intrapleural Corynebacterium parvum for malignant pleural effusions. Thorax 38:22, 1983.

92. MCLEOD DT: Further experience of Corynebacterium parvum in malignant pleural effusion. Thorax 40:515, 1985.

93. GEBBIA V: Intracavitary beta-interferon for the management of pleural and/or abdominal effusions in patients with advanced cancer refractory to chemotherapy. In Vivo 5:579, 1991.

94. DAVIS M: A phase I-II study of recombinant intrapleural alpha interferon in malignant pleural effusions. Am J Clin Oncol 15:328, 1992.

95. GOLDMAN CA: Interferon instillation for malignant pleural effusions. Ann Oncol 4:141, 1993.

96. VIALLAT JR: Intrapleural immunotherapy with escalating doses of interleukin-2 in metastatic pleural effusions. Cancer 71:4067, 1993.

97. ASTOUL P: Intrapleural recombinant IL-2 in passive immunotherapy for malignant pleural effusion. Chest 103:209, 1993.

98. YASUMOTO K: Intrapleural application of recombinant interleukin-2 in patients with malignant pleurisy due to lung cancer: A multi-institutional cooperative study. Biotherapy 3:345, 1991.

99. LITTLE AG: Pleuroperitoneal shunting for malignant pleural effusions. Cancer 58:2740, 1986.

100. WEESE JL: Pleural peritoneal shunts for the treatment of malignant pleural effusions. Surg Gynecol Obstet 154:391, 1982.

101. REICH H: Pleuroperitoneal shunt for malignant pleural effusions: A one-year experience. Semin Surg Oncol 9:160, 1993.

102. MATSUZAKI Y: Intrapleural perfusion hyperthermo-chemotherapy for malignant pleural dissemination and effusion. Ann Thorac Surg 59:127, 1995.

103. HARRER WV: Carcinoma of the larynx with cardiac metastases. Arch Otolaryngol 91:382, 1970.

104. ADENLE AD: Clinical and pathologic features of metastatic neoplasms of the pericardium. Chest 81:166, 1982.

105. BUCKMAN R: Intraperitoneal therapy of malignant ascites associated with carcinoma of ovary and breast using radioiodinated monoclonal antibody 2G3. Gynecol Oncol 47:102, 1992.

106. POSNER MR: Pericardial disease in patients with cancer: The differentiation of malignant from idiopathic and radiation-induced pericarditis. Am J Med 71:407, 1981.

107. APPLEFELD MM: The late appearance of chronic pericardial disease in patients treated by radiotherapy for Hodgkin's disease. Ann Intern Med 94:338, 1981.

108. FRASER RS: Cardiac tamponade as a presentation of extracardiac malignancy. Cancer 45:1697, 1980.

109. MILLER AJ: The study of the lymphatics of the heart: an overview. Microcirc Endothelium Lymphatics 2:349, 1985.

110. REDDY PS: Spectrum of hemodynamic changes in cardiac tamponade. Am J Cardiol 66:1487, 1990.

111. GILLAM LD: Hydrodynamic compression of the right atrium: A new echocardiographic sign of cardiac tamponade. Circulation 68:294, 1983.

112. SEWARD JB: Transesophageal echocardiography: Technique, anatomic correlations, implementation, and clinical application. Mayo Clin Proc 63:649, 1988.

113. SAVRAN SV: Idiopathic chylopericardium: 131-I-triolein scan for noninvasive diagnosis. Ann Intern Med 82:663, 1975.

114. MONCADA R: Diagnostic role of computed tomography in pericardial heart disease: Congenital defects, thickening, neoplasms, and effusions. Am Heart J 103:263, 1982.

115. WHITE CS: MR evaluation of the pericardium. Top Magn Reson Imaging 7:258, 1995.

116. WIENER HG: The diagnostic value of pericardial cytology: An analysis of 95 cases. Acta Cytol 35:149, 1991.

117. ZIPF REJ: The role of cytology in the evaluation of pericardial effusions. Chest 62:593, 1972.

118. KING DT: The use of cytology to evaluate pericardial effusions. Ann Clin Lab Sci 9:18, 1979.

119. SEO T: Usefulness of serum CA125 measurement for monitoring pericardial effusion. Jpn Circ J 57:489, 1993.

120. HANCOCK EW: Pericardial disease: Differential diagnosis and management. Hosp Pract (Off Ed) 18:101, 1983.

121. MILLAIRE A: Malignant pericardial effusions: Usefulness of pericardioscopy. Am Heart J 124:1030, 1992.

122. CAMPBELL PT: Subxiphoid pericardiotomy in the diagnosis and management of large pericardial effusions associated with malignancy. Chest 101:938, 1992.

123. MILLS SA: Subxiphoid pericardial window for pericardial effusive disease. J Cardiovasc Surg (Torino) 30:768, 1989.

124. GHOSH SC: Clinical experience with subxyphoid pericardial decompression. Int Surg 70:5, 1985.

125. LAHAM RJ: Pericardial effusion in patients with cancer: Outcome with contemporary management strategies. Heart 75:67, 1996.

126. WONG B. The risk of pericardiocentesis. Am J Cardiol 44:1110, 1979.

127. GUBERMAN BA: Cardiac tamponade in medical patients. Circulation 64:633, 1981.

128. CALLAHAN JA: Two-dimensional echocardiographically guided pericardiocentesis: Experience in 117 consecutive patients. Am J Cardiol 55:476, 1985.

129. PATEL AK: Catheter drainage of the pericardium: Practical method to maintain long-term patency. Chest 92:1018, 1987.

130. KOPECKY SL et al: Percutaneous pericardial catheter drainage: report of 42 consecutive cases. Am J Cardiol 58:633, 1986.

131. VAITKUS PT: Treatment of malignant pericardial effusion. JAMA 272:59, 1994.

132. SHEPHERD FA: Medical management of malignant pericardial effusion by tetracycline sclerosis. Am J Cardiol 60:1161, 1987.

133. DAVIS S: Intrapericardial tetracycline sclerosis in the treatment of malignant pericardial effusion: An analysis of thirty-three cases. J Clin Oncol 2:631, 1984.

134. MAHER ER: Intrapericardial installation of bleomycin in malignant pericardial effusion. Am Heart J 111:613, 1986.

135. WEI JY: Recurrent cardiac tamponade and large pericardial effusions: management with an indwelling pericardial catheter. Am J Cardiol 42:281, 1978.

136. van BELLE SJ: Treatment of malignant pericardial tamponade with sclerosis induced by instillation of bleomycin. Int J Cardiol 16:155, 1987.

137. van der GAAST A: Intrapericardial instillation of bleomycin in the management of malignant pericardial effusion. Eur J Cancer Clin Oncol 25:1505, 1989.

138. CORMICAN MC: Intrapericardial bleomycin for the management of cardiac tamponade secondary to malignant pericardial effusion. Br Heart J 63:61, 1990.

139. BINDI M: Intracavitary cisplatin in malignant cardiac tamponade. Tumori 73:163, 1987.

140. FIORENTINO MV: Intrapericardial instillation of platin in malignant pericardial effusion. Cancer 62:1904, 1988.

141. MARKMAN M: Intrapericardial instillation of cisplatin in a patient with a large malignant effusion. Cancer Drug Deliv 2:49, 1985.

142. FIGOLI F: Pharmacokinetics of VM 26 given intrapericardially or intravenously in patients with malignant pericardial effusion. Cancer Chemother Pharmacol 20:239, 1987.

143. SMITH FE: Conservative management of malignant pericardial effusion. Cancer 33:47, 1974.

144. IMAMURA T: Intrapericardial OK-432 instillation for the management of malignant pericardial effusion. Cancer 68:259, 1991.

145. O'BRYAN RM: Critical analysis of the control of malignant effusions with radioisotopes. Henry Ford Hosp Med J 16:3, 1968.

146. MARTINI N: Intrapericardial installation of radioactive chromic phosphate in malignant effusion. AJR Am J Roentgenol 128:639, 1977.

147. SPRENGELMEYER JT: Phosphorus-32-colloidal chromic phosphate: Treatment of choice for malignant pericardial effusion. J Nucl Med 31:2034, 1990.

148. COURTENAY-LUCK NS: Targeting of monoclonal antibodies to tumours. Curr Opin Immunol 2:880, 1989.

149. PECTASIDES D: Antibody-guided irradiation of malignant pleural and pericardial effusions. Br J Cancer 53:727, 1986.

150. PALACIOS IF: Percutaneous balloon pericardial window for patients with malignant pericardial effusion and tamponade. Cathet Cardiovasc Diagn 22:244, 1991.

151. ZISKIND AA: Percutaneous balloon pericardiotomy for the treatment of cardiac tamponade and large pericardial effusions: Description of technique and report of the first 50 cases. J Am Coll Cardiol 21:1, 1993.

152. MILLER JI: Pericardiectomy: Current indications, concepts, and results in a university center. Ann Thorac Surg 34:40, 1982.

153. HANKINS JR: Pericardial window for malignant pericardial effusion. Ann Thorac Surg 30:465, 1980.

154. OSUCH JR: Emergency subxiphoid pericardial decompression for malignant pericardial effusion. Am Surg 51:298, 1985.

155. LITTLE AG: Operation for diagnosis and treatment of pericardial effusions. Surgery 96:738, 1984.

156. SUGIMOTO JT: Pericardial window: Mechanisms of efficacy. Ann Thorac Surg 50:442, 1990.

157. KONDOS GT: Flexible fiberoptic pericardioscopy for the diagnosis of pericardial disease. J Am Coll Cardiol 7:432, 1986.

158. LITTLE AG: Pericardioscopy as adjunct to pericardial window. Chest 89:53, 1986.

159. HILL GJ: Pleural pericardial window for palliation of cardiac tamponade due to cancer. Cancer 26:81, 1970.

160. LIEPMAN MK: Surgical management of pericardial tamponade as a presenting manifestation of acute leukemia. J Surg Oncol 17:183, 1981.

161. APPELQVIST P: Emergency pericardiotomy as primary diagnostic and therapeutic procedure in malignant pericardial tamponade. Report of three cases and review of the literature. J Surg Oncol 21:18, 1982.

162. PIEHLER JM: Surgical management of effusive pericardial disease: Influence of extent of pericardial resection on clinical course. J Thorac Cardiovasc Surg 90:506, 1985.

163. WOLL PJ: Pericardial effusion complicating breast cancer. J R Soc Med 80:490, 1987.

164. PRIMROSE WR: Malignant pericardial effusion managed with vinblastine. Clin Oncol 9:67, 1983.

165. NELSON BE: Malignant pericardial effusion from squamous cell cancer of the cervix. J Surg Oncol 52:203, 1993.

166. SHINDE SR: Cardiac tamponade as the only initial feature of malignancy: A case report and review of the literature. J Surg Oncol 32:96, 1986.

167. SULKES A: Pericardial effusion as first evidence of malignancy in bronchogenic carcinoma. J Surg Oncol 20:71, 1982.

168. CHAM WC: Radiation therapy of cardiac and pericardial metastases. Radiology 114:701, 1975.

169. TERRY LNJ: Pericardial and myocardial involvement by lymphomas and leukemias: The role of radiotherapy. Cancer 25:1003, 1970.

170. CELERMAJER DS: Pericardiocentesis for symptomatic malignant pericardial effusion: A study of 36 patients. Med J Aust 154:19, 1991.

171. RUNYON BA: Care of patients with ascites. N Engl J Med 330:337, 1994.

172. MONTE SA: Positive effusion cytology as the initial presentation of malignancy. Acta Cytol 31:448, 1987.

173. NAGY JA: Pathogenesis of ascites tumor growth: Angiogenesis, vascular remodeling, and stroma formation in the peritoneal lining. Cancer Res 55:376, 1995.

174. FELDMAN GB: Lymphatic drainage of the peritoneal cavity and its significance in ovarian cancer. Am J Obstet Gynecol 119:991, 1974.

175. BRONSKILL MJ: A quantitative measurement of peritoneal drainage in malignant ascites. Cancer 40:2375, 1977.

176. SENGER DR: Tumor cells secrete a vascular permeability factor that promotes accumulation of ascites fluid. Science 219:983, 1983.

177. YEO KT: Vascular permeability factor (vascular endothelial growth factor) in guinea pig and human tumor and inflammatory effusions. Cancer Res 53:2912, 1993.

178. ZINK J: Intraperitoneal pressure in formation and reabsorption of ascites in cats. Am J Physiol 233:H185, 1977.

179. BOSCH J: Hepatic hemodynamics and the renin-angiotensin-aldosterone system in cirrhosis. Gastroenterology 78:92, 1980.

180. POCKROS PJ: Mobilization of malignant ascites with diuretics is dependent on ascitic fluid characteristics. Gastroenterology 103:1302, 1992.

181. PRESS OW: Evaluation and management of chylous ascites. Ann Intern Med 96:358, 1982.

182. UNGER SW: Chylous ascites in infants and children. Surgery 93:455, 1983.

183. GARRISON RN: Malignant ascites. Clinical and experimental observations. Ann Surg 203:644, 1986.

184. WILLIAMS JWJ: Does this patient have ascites? How to divine fluid in the abdomen. JAMA 267:2645, 1992.

185. GREENE LS: Distinguishing between malignant and cirrhotic ascites by computerized step-wise discriminant functional analysis of its biochemistry. Am J Gastroenterol 70:448, 1978.

186. COLLI A: Diagnostic accuracy of sialic acid in the diagnosis of malignant ascites. Cancer 63:912, 1989.

187. CASTALDO G: Total discrimination of peritoneal malignant ascites from cirrhosis- and hepatocarcinoma-associated ascites by assays of ascitic cholesterol and lactate dehydrogenase. Clin Chem 40:478, 1994.

188. RUNYON BA: Ascitic fluid analysis in malignancy-related ascites. Hepatology 8:1104, 1988.

189. WEXNER SD: Port site metastases after laparoscopic colorectal surgery for cure of malignancy. Br J Surg 82:295, 1995.

190. GREENWAY B: Control of malignant ascites with spironolactone. Br J Surg 69:441, 1982.

191. PEREZ-AYUSO RM: Randomized comparative study of efficacy of furosemide versus spironolactone in nonazotemic cirrhosis with ascites: Relationship between the diuretic response and the activity of the renin-aldosterone system. Gastroenterology 84:961, 1983.

192. RAZIS DV: Diuretics in malignant effusions and edemas of generalized cancer. J Med 7:449, 1976.

193. LIFSHITZ S: Ascites, pathophysiology and control measures. Int J Radiat Oncol Biol Phys 8:1423, 1982.

194. LOMAS DA: Palliation of malignant ascites with a Tenckhoff catheter. Thorax 44:828, 1989.

195. RICHARDSON GS: Common epithelial cancer of the ovary (2). N Engl J Med 312:474, 1985.

196. MALIK I: Clinical features and management of malignant ascites. JPMA J Pak Med Assoc 41:38, 1991.

197. DELANEY TF: Phase I study of debulking surgery and photodynamic therapy for disseminated intraperitoneal tumors. Int J Radiat Oncol Biol Phys 25:445, 1993.

198. ROSENSHEIN N: The effect of volume on the distribution of substances instilled into the peritoneal cavity. Gynecol Oncol 6:106, 1978.

199. CASPER ES: Ip cisplatin in patients with malignant ascites: Pharmacokinetic evaluation and comparison with the iv route. Cancer Treat Rep 67:235, 1983.

200. OZOLS RF: Phase I and pharmacological studies of adriamycin administered intraperitoneally to patients with ovarian cancer. Cancer Res 42:4265, 1982.

201. MARKMAN M: Intraperitoneal therapy of ovarian cancer. Semin Oncol 25:356, 1998.

202. SUGARBAKER PH: Rationale for integrating early postoperative intraperitoneal chemotherapy into the surgical treatment of gastrointestinal cancer. Semin Oncol 16:83, 1989.

203. JONES AL: A pilot study of intraperitoneal cisplatin in the management of gastric cancer. Ann Oncol 5:123, 1994.

204. SCHILSKY RL: Phase I clinical and pharmacologic study of intraperitoneal cisplatin and fluorouracil in patients with advanced intraabdominal cancer. J Clin Oncol 8:2054, 1990.

205. BITRAN JD: Intraperitoneal bleomycin: Pharmacokinetics and results of a phase II trial. Cancer 56:2420, 1985.

206. PICCART MJ: Intraperitoneal chemotherapy: Technical experience at five institutions. Semin Oncol 12:90, 1985.

207. HOWELL SB: Intraperitoneal chemotherapy: The use of concurrent systemic neutralizing agents. Semin Oncol 12:17, 1985.

208. OZOLS RF: Phase II trial of 5-FU administered Ip to patients with refractory ovarian cancer. Cancer Treat Rep 68:1229, 1984.

209. ALBERTS DEPARTMENT OF SURGERY: Phase I clinical and pharmacokinetic study of mitoxantrone given to patients by intraperitoneal administration. Cancer Res 48:5874, 1988.

210. GILLY FN: Intra-Peritoneal Chemo-Hyperthermia (CHIP): A new therapy in the treatment of the peritoneal seedings. Preliminary report. Int Surg 76:164, 1991.

211. YAMAGUCHI A: Intraperitoneal hyperthermic treatment for peritoneal dissemination of colorectal cancers. Dis Colon Rectum 35:964, 1992.

212. ALEXANDER HR: Treatment of peritoneal carcinomatosis by continuous hyperthermic peritoneal perfusion with cisplatin. Cancer Treat Res 81:41, 1996.

213. BARTLETT DL: A phase I trial of continuous hyperthermic peritoneal perfusion with tumor necrosis factor and cisplatin in the treatment of peritoneal carcinomatosis. Cancer 83:1251, 1998.

214. ARIEL IM: Intracavitary administration of radioactive isotopes in the control of effusions due to cancer: Results in 267 patients. Cancer 19:1096, 1966.

215. JACKSON GL: Intracavitary chromic phosphate (32P) colloidal suspension therapy. Cancer 48:2596, 1981.

216. TORISU M: New approach to management of malignant ascites with a streptococcal preparation, OK-432. I. Improvement of host immunity and prolongation of survival. Surgery 93:357, 1983.

217. KITSUKI H: Induction of inflammatory cytokines in effusion cavity by OK-432 injection therapy for patients with malignant effusion: Role of interferon-gamma in enhancement of surface expression of ICAM-1 on tumor cells in vivo. Clin Immunol Immunopathol 78:283, 1996.

218. KATO H: Treatment of malignant ascites and pleurisy by a streptococcal preparation OK-432 with fresh frozen plasma: A mechanism of polymorphonuclear leukocyte (PMN) accumulation. Int J Immunopharmacol 11:117, 1989.

219. BEZWODA WR: Intraperitoneal recombinant interferon-alpha 2b for recurrent malignant ascites due to ovarian cancer. Cancer 64:1029, 1989.
220. RAMBALDI A: Intraperitoneal administration of interferon beta in ovarian cancer patients. Cancer 56:294, 1985.
221. WELANDER CE: Interferon in the treatment of ovarian cancer. Semin Oncol 15:26, 1988.
222. D'ACQUISTO R: A phase I trial of intraperitoneal recombinant gamma-interferon in advanced ovarian carcinoma. J Clin Oncol 6:689, 1988.
223. PARSONS SL: Malignant ascites. Br J Surg 83:6, 1996.
224. D'ERRICO A: Augmentation of type IV collagenase, laminin receptor, and Ki67 proliferation antigen associated with human colon, gastric, and breast carcinoma progression. Mod Pathol 4:239, 1991.
225. ZUCKER SM: (r) 92,000 type IV collagenase is increased in plasma of patients with colon cancer and breast cancer. Cancer Res 53:140, 1993.
226. DECLERCK YA: Inhibition of invasion and metastasis in cells transfected with an inhibitor of metalloproteinases. Cancer Res 52:701, 1992.
227. WATSON SA: Inhibition of organ invasion by the matrix metalloproteinase inhibitor batimastat (BB-94) in two human colon carcinoma metastasis models. Cancer Res 55:3629, 1995.
228. FULENWIDER JT: LeVeen vs Denver peritoneovenous shunts for intractable ascites of cirrhosis: A randomized, prospective trial. Arch Surg 121:351, 1986.
229. LEVEEN HH: Peritoneo-venous shunting for ascites. Ann Surg 180:580, 1974.
230. LEVEEN HH: Further experience with peritoneo-venous shunt for ascites. Ann Surg 184:574, 1976.
231. GREIG PD: Complications after peritoneovenous shunting for ascites. Am J Surg 139:125, 1980.
232. HELZBERG JH: Peritoneovenous shunts in malignant ascites. Dig Dis Sci 30:1104, 1985.
233. EDNEY JA: Peritoneovenous shunts palliate malignant ascites. Am J Surg 158:598, 1989.
234. RAGNI MV: Ascites-induced Le Veen shunt coagulopathy. Ann Surg 198:91, 1983.
235. LUND RH: Complications of Denver peritoneovenous shunting. Arch Surg 117:924, 1982.
236. LEVEEN HH: Peritoneovenous shunt occlusion: Etiology, diagnosis, therapy. Ann Surg 200:212, 1984.
237. TARIN D: Absence of metastatic sequelae during long-term treatment of malignant ascites by peritoneo-venous shunting: A clinico-pathological report. Invasion Metastasis 4:1, 1984.
238. TARIN D: Mechanisms of human tumor metastasis studied in patients with peritoneovenous shunts. Cancer Res 44:3584, 1984.
239. SUGARBAKER PH: Intraperitoneal chemotherapy and cytoreductive surgery for the prevention and treatment of peritoneal carcinomatosis and sarcomatosis. Semin Surg Oncol 14:254, 1988.
240. RINGENBERG QS: Malignant ascites of unknown origin. Cancer 64:753, 1989.

# INDEX

Abdominal tumors
abdominal wall sarcomas, 989–990
intraperitoneal chemotherapy for,
171–176
general considerations in, 171–173
hyperthermic perfusion in, 173–174,
173f, 174f
postoperative treatment in, 174–175,
174f
results of, 175–176, 175f, 176f
technique in, 174, 174f, 175f
recurrence sites of, 173t
Achalasia, esophageal carcinoma and, 611
Actinic cell carcinoma, of parotid gland,
532
Actinic cheilitis, 487–488
Actinic keratosis, 486–488
clinical manifestations of, 487, 487f
general considerations for, 486–487
histology of, 487, 487f
treatment of, 487–488, 488f
Adamantinoma, 1043, 1043f
Adenoassociated virus, 185
Adenocarcinoma
anal, 749
of bladder, 778
endometrial, 888, 888t
of esophagus
epidemiology of, 610
prevalence and incidence of, 609
of gynecologic system, 363
metastasis frequency in, 131t
of parotid gland, 532–533
of prostate, 817
renal, metastasis of, 279–281, 280f
of small intestine, 688–689, 689t
of stomach, 623–632
diagnosis of, 626
molecular biology of, 625
multimodal therapy for, 630–632

pathological findings and staging of,
624–625, 625t, 634t
risk factors of, 624
surgical planning for, 626–628, 626t,
627f
surgical technique for, 628–630,
628f–633f
in vaginal cancer, 871, 872, 872f
treatment of, 877
Adenoid cystic carcinoma
of lung, 558–559
of parotid gland, 533
Adenoma
adrenal, 325
carcinoma tumor development
sequence in, 418, 418f
of gallbladder, 345
hepatic, 342, 659–661
clinical manifestation of, 659–660
diagnosis of, 660
histology of, 660
prevalence of, 659
treatment of, 660–661
of small intestine, 688
Adenomatous polyposis gene, 698
Adenovirus, 185
Adjuvant therapy
for bone sarcomas, 1025, 1026f
for chondrosarcoma, 1035
for colon cancer, 713–715
chemotherapy, 713–714
immunotherapy, 714–715
radiation, 715
for Ewing's sarcoma, 1039–1040, 1039t
for melanoma, malignant, 516
for mesothelioma, 1088–1090
gene therapy, 1089–1090
immunoconjugate therapy, 1090
immunotherapy, 1089
palliative management, 1090

photodynamic therapy, 1090
for oral cavity cancer, 525
for osteogenic sarcoma, 1030–1033,
1032f
for ovarian cancer borderline tumors,
939
for pancreas neoplasms, 650–654, 652t,
655f
for parotid gland tumors, 535
for penile cancer, 804
for pulmonary metastases, 563–564
for rectal cancer, 736–738
for soft tissue sarcomas, 1012
for solid tumors, systemic, 151–152
surgery and, 126–128, 127t
Adnexal mass, in ovarian cancer, 917–918,
918f, 919f
Adrenal neoplasms, 1057–1060
adrenal cortical, 1057–1060
hypercortisolism in, 1058
incidentaloma, 1058–1059
signs and symptoms of, 1058
treatment of, 1059
nuclear imaging techniques for,
262–263, 264f–266f
pathology and staging of, 325
pheochromocytoma, 1059–1060
pathology and staging of, 325–326
Aerodigestive cancer, alcohol on, 57
Aflatoxins, 61, 665
Age
on breast cancer, 951
on prostate cancer, 813
Age standardization, 4
AJCC staging system
for bladder cancer, 780t
for bone sarcomas, 1017, 1018t
for breast cancer, 302t, 954, 955t
clinical features of, 704
for colorectal tumors, 340t, 703t

AJCC staging system (cont.)
   for larynx cancer, 307t
   for lymphomas, 368t
   for ovarian tumors, 360t
   for penile cancer, 792–794, 794t
   for testicular tumors, 355t, 356t, 843t
   for vaginal cancer, 873, 873t
   for vulvar cancer, 860, 860t
ALA (5-aminolevulinic acid)
   in cellular injury mechanism, 464–465
   on normal tissue, 465
   in PDT application timing, 465–466
   in protoporphyrin IX synthesis,
      463–464, 463f
Alcohol, 57–59
   on aerodigestive cancer, 57
   on breast cancer, 57–58, 953
   on colorectal cancer, 58–59, 698, 725
   on endometrial cancer, 58
   on esophageal carcinoma, 610
   liver cirrhosis from, 665
   on oropharyngeal cancer risk, 520t, 525
   on prostate cancer, 58
Alimentary tract. See also Gastrointestinal
      tumors
   tumor biomarkers for, 124t
Alkylating chemotherapy agents, 152
Allografts, for bone sarcomas, 1019–1020,
      1019f
Alveolar rhabdomyosarcoma, 384
Aminoglutethimide, 153t
5-Aminolevulinic acid (ALA). See ALA
      (5-aminolevulinic acid)
Ampullary tumors, pathology and staging
      for, 347, 347f
Amputation. See also specific procedures,
      e.g., Mastectomy
   forequarter, 1009–1010, 1010f
   hemipelvectomy, 1006–1009, 1008f,
      1009f
   hip disarticulation, 1006–1009, 1008f,
      1009f
   for sarcomas, 988, 1018
     bone, 1018
Anal cancer, 745–750
   epidermoid tumors in, 745–747
     clinical presentation, 747
     cocarcinogens, 746
     etiology and pathogenesis, 745–746
     histologic types, 746
     investigation, 747
     patterns of spread, 746–747
     premalignant lesions, 746
     staging, 747
   introduction to, 745
   rare, 749–750, 751f
   treatment of, 747–749

chemoirradiation therapy, 748
   current, 748
   historical, 747–748
   radiation-alone therapy, 748
   surgery, 748–749
Anal sphincter resections, 733–735
Androgen receptor blocker, for prostate
      cancer, 834
Anesthesia
   cardiac risk assessment for, 132–133
   in cryosurgery, 439
   for laparoscopy, 389–390
Angiofibroma, 305, 305f
Angiofollicular hyperplasia
   of lymph node, 334
   of mediastinum, 604f, 605
Angiogenesis
   antiangiogenesis agents for, 37
   in metastasis, 110–114
     angiogenic and antiangiogenic
       regulation in, 111–114, 112f,
       113f
     microenvironment regulation of, 114
Angiosarcoma, 985
   of lung, 561
Anoreceptive intercourse, 745
Anterior compartment, sarcomas of,
      1001–1002, 1002f, 1003f
Anthracyclines, 152, 154
   for mesothelioma, 1085
Antiangiogenesis agents, 37
Antiestrogens, 154–155
Antigens, common, 205t
Antioxidants, 36
   dietary, 52–54
Antrectomy, and gastric reconstruction,
      1154–1155, 1156f
Apoptosis, in chemotherapy, 147–148
Appendix cancer, 1168, 1168f–1170f
Arachidonic acid modulators, 37–38
Arginine, 476
Argon, 432
Arm sarcomas, 1006, 1007f
Arsenic, 488
Arthrodesis, 1024–1025
Asbestos, mesothelioma and
   asbestos fibers in, 1070–1071
   background and history in, 1069–1070
   epidemiology of, 1071–1072, 1071f
   pathophysiology of, 1072–1073
Ascites, malignant, 1167–1168, 1184–1187
   chemotherapy for, systemic, 1186
   clinical manifestations of, 1185
   diagnosis of, 1185, 1185t
   intracavity therapy for, 1186–1187
   introduction to, 1184
   laparoscopy and, 390

   pathophysiology of, 1184–1185
   prognosis for, 1187
   surgery for, radical, 1187
   treatment of, 1185–1186, 1186f
ASGE colon surveillance, 422t
Astrocytic tumors, 310–312, 313f–315f
Autogenous grafts, 1020–1021, 1021f
Automated flow cytometry, 291–292
Autopsies, 288
Axillary node dissection, 515

Bacille Calmette-Guérin vaccine
      (BCG), 513
Barium enema, 706
Barium swallow, 611
Barrett's esophagus, 610
Bartholin's carcinoma, 857, 858
   treatment of, 869
Basal cell carcinoma, 494–498
   clinical manifestations of, 494–495,
      495f, 496f
   cryosurgery for, 438–439
   diagnosis of, 495
   etiology and pathogenesis of, 494
   histology of, 296, 296t, 496, 496f, 497f
   modes of spread of, 494
   staging of, 496
   treatment of, 497–498, 497f
   in vulvar cancer, 857, 858
     treatment of, 869
Basal cell nevus syndrome, 420t
Base displacement, 25
Base excision repair, of DNA, 28–29, 28f,
      29t
Benign prostatic hyperplasia, 351
Benzo[a]pyrene (BP), 20, 22–23
Benzoporphyrins, 463
Beta-carotene, 52–53
Bicalutamide, 153t
Bile duct tumors, endoscopy for,
      422–425
   diagnosis and, 422–424, 423f
   therapy and, 424–425, 424t, 425t
Biliary neoplasms, extrahepatic,
      673–682
   benign, 681–682
   conclusions for, 682
   distal, 679–681
     chemotherapy for, 681
     epidemiology of, 679–680
     palliation for, 680–681
     presentation of, 680
     radiotherapy for, 681
     surgical resection of, 680
   introduction to, 673
   nuclear imaging techniques for,
      248–250

gallbladder cancer, 248–249, 249f
large bowel neoplasms, 250, 251f
small intestine neoplasms, 249–250, 250f
proximal, 673–679
chemotherapy for, 679
epidemiology of, 673–674
evaluation of, 674, 675f
history of, 673
palliative therapy for, 679
presentation of, 674
radiotherapy for, 679
surgical therapy for, 674–676
operative conduct in, 676–679, 679f
patient selection in, 675–676, 676f, 678f
results of, 674–675, 677t
Biliary tree inflammation, 344
Biologic diversity, of neoplasms, 103–105, 104f
Biologic response modifiers, 156
Biology, molecular, 191–212. See also Molecular biology
Biomarkers
genetic, 207–209, 207t, 209t
for immunology, 210–211
for ovarian cancer, 916–917, 924t
serum, 64, 123, 124t
Biopsy, 220–221
of bone sarcomas, 1016–1017
of breast, 953–954
fine-needle aspiration, 220
for cytology, 288–289, 289f
of hepatic tumors
benign, 341–342
malignant, 343–344, 344f
of mediastinum neoplasms, 576
for mesothelioma, 1078
of pancreatic neoplasms, 346
for pathologic diagnosis and staging, 125–126
of salivary gland masses, 534
of soft tissue tumors, 369–370
of thyroid neoplasms, 322–324, 322f–324f, 1056, 1056f
of hepatic tumors, 341
of lung and pleura, 334, 334t
of lymph node, 366
of mediastinum neoplasms, 327–328, 576
of sarcomas, 986
sentinel node, for malignant melanoma, 510–512, 511f, 512t, 513f
Bladder cancer, 769–789
clinical manifestations of, 771–772, 771t

diagnosis of, 772–776
endoscopic findings in, 775–776, 777f
history and physical in, 772
laboratory findings in, 772–773
radiographic findings in, 773–775
chest radiograph, 775
CT, 774, 775f, 776f
intravenous pyelogram, 773, 774f, 775f
MRI, 774
nuclear bone scan, 774, 775f
ultrasound, 773–774
etiology of, 769–771, 770f, 770t
follow-up and frequency for, 787–788, 788t, 789t
histology of, 776–779
cell types, 776–778, 777f, 778t
prognostic factors in, 778–779, 779t
incidence of, 6f, 7f, 769
laparoscopy for, 404
nuclear imaging techniques for, 252–253, 253f
preventive measures for, 771
staging of, 779–781, 779t–780t, 780f, 781t
summary of, 788–789
survival rates of, 8f
tobacco on, 20–21
treatment of, 781–787
metastatic disease, 787, 787t
muscle-invasive disease, 783–787, 784f, 785t, 786t
superficial disease, 782
high-risk, 782–783, 783t
Bleomycin, 153t
Body size, on cancer, 48
Bone and joint tumors
biomarkers for, 124t
cryosurgery for, 449–450
lymphoma, 282–284, 283f
pathology and staging of, 373–379
benign, 377–379, 379f
biopsy in, 374–375
clinical assessment in, 373–374, 374t, 375f, 375t
malignant, 375–377, 376f–377f
sarcomas, 1015–1044
adamantinoma, 1043, 1043f
adjuvant therapy for, 1025, 1026f
chondrosarcoma, 1033–1035
adjuvant therapy for, 1035
clinical manifestations of, 1033
diagnosis of, 1033, 1033f
histology of, 1033–1034, 1034f
introduction to, 1033

staging of, 1034–1035
treatment of, 1035
chordoma, 1042–1043, 1042f
clinical manifestations of, 1015
diagnosis of, 1016–1017
Ewing's, 1035–1040
adjuvant therapy for, 1039–1040, 1039t
clinical manifestations of, 1036
diagnosis of, 1036, 1036f, 1037f
histology of, 1037
introduction to, 1035–1036
staging of, 1037
treatment of, 1037–1039
fibrosarcoma, 1044
giant cell tumor, 1044
hemangioendothelioma, 1044, 1044f
introduction to, 1015
leiomyosarcoma, 1044
malignant fibrous histiocytoma, 1040–1042
histology and presentation of, 1040–1041, 1042f
treatment of, 1041–1042
nuclear imaging techniques for, 260–261, 262f
osteogenic, 1025–1033
adjuvant therapy for, 1030–1033, 1032f
clinical manifestations of, 1028
diagnosis of, 1028
histology of, 1028–1029
introduction to, 1025–1028, 1026f, 1027f
staging of, 1029
treatment of, 1029–1030
staging of, 1017, 1017t
summary for, 1044
surgical treatment for
allografts, 1019–1020, 1019f
amputations in, 1018
arthrodesis, 1024–1025
autogenous grafts, 1020–1021, 1021f
composite reconstruction, 1024, 1024f
endoprosthetic replacement, 1023–1024, 1023f
limb-preserving surgery, 1018–1019
resection arthroplasty, 1025, 1025f
rotationplasty, 1021–1023, 1022f
Bone scan
for breast cancer, 259
for prostate carcinoma, 254
Bowel mesentery, sarcomas of, 993–994, 994f

Bowen's disease, 488–489, 488f, 489f
  histology of, 792, 793f
Brain cancer
  cryosurgery for, 440–441
  histologic classification of, 310
  incidence of, 7f
  metastatic, 1113–1121
    clinical signs and symptoms,
      1113–1114, 1114f
    differential diagnosis for, 1114–1115
    introduction to, 1113
    radiosurgery role in, 1120–1121,
      1121f
    recurrence of
      after surgery, 1118–1119
      reirradiation for, 1119
      reoperation for, 1119–1120, 1119t,
        1120t
    therapeutic decision making for,
      1115–1118
      chemotherapy in, 1115
      for multiple metastases,
        1117–1118, 1118f
      postoperative WBRT in, 1117
      randomized trials in, 1116
      surgical complications in, 1117
      survival and prognostic factors in,
        1116–1117
      whole brain radiation in, 1115,
        1117
  survival rates for, 8f
BRCA2 gene, 912–913, 912t, 951–952,
  952t
Breast cancer, 951–976
  alcohol on, 57–58, 953
  biomarkers for
    genetic, 209
    serum, 124t
  chemotherapy for, 969–971
    controversies in, 969t
    locally advanced, 970–971
    ovarian ablation and, 970
    tamoxifen in, 969–970
  conclusions for, 976
  diagnosis of, 953–954, 954f, 956f
  dietary fiber on, 51–52
  fat and caloric intake on, 46–47
  fat type on, 47–48
  follow-up for, 971–973, 973t
    contralateral, 972–973, 973t
    recurrent, 973
  fruits and vegetables on, 49
  genetic basis of, 204t
  grains on, whole, 50
  incidence rate of, United States, 6–7,
    6f, 7f
  invasive, 962, 963t

lactation and, 975
laser therapy for, 460–461
in males, 975
mastectomy for, 957–959
  axillary dissection in, 959
  Langer's lines in, 957, 957f
  Orr incision in, 958, 958f
  skin-sparing, 958–959
  Stewart incision in, 958, 958f
noninvasive, 959–962
  ductal carcinoma in situ, 959–962
    histology of, 960
    surgery only for, 961, 961t
    surgery with radiation for,
      960–961, 960t
    Van Nuys prognostic index for,
      961, 962t
  lobular carcinoma in situ, 959
  nuclear imaging techniques for,
    256–260, 257t
    lymphoscintigraphy and sentinel
      node detection in, 257–260,
      258f
    palliative therapies in, 260
occult, with axillary metastases, 974,
  974t
Paget's disease of nipple in, 975
pathology and staging for, 281–282,
  282f, 298–301, 299f
  AJCC system in, 302t, 955t
  diagnostic sampling in, 299
  microscopy in, 300, 300f
  pathologic evaluation of, 299
  reporting in, 300–302, 300t
  risk assessment in, 301, 301f
  special tissue allocations in, 299–300
p53 gene in, 209, 956
phyllodes tumor in, 974–975
physical activity and body type on, 48
pregnancy and, 975
prognostic factors for, 954–957
pulmonary metastases of, 1129
risk factors for, 951–953, 952t, 953t
staging of, 954, 955t
survival rate for, 8f, 971, 972f
treatment of, early, 963–969
  axillary dissection in, 966–967
  CMF therapy in, 967, 967t
  mastectomy vs. breast conservation
    with radiation, 963–964, 964t
  Milan trials for, 964–965, 965t
  radiation efficacy in, 965–966, 966t
  sentinel lymph node in, 967–969,
    968t
  T1 lesions in, 969, 969t
  tumor characteristics in, 966
treatment of, metastatic, 973–974

Bronchial carcinoids, 557–558
Bronchoscopy, 613
Burkitt's lymphoma, herpes viruses and,
  95–96
Buschke Lowenstein tumors, 749
Buttockectomy, 1002
Buttocks, sarcomas of, 1002

CA 125
  in fallopian tube cancer, 897
  in ovarian carcinoma, 401, 913–914,
    916–917, 919f
Cachexia
  etiology of, 473–475
  introduction to, 473–475
  nutritional support for
    efficacy of, 476–477
    methods of, 475–476
  summary of, 477
Caffeic acid phenethyl ester (CAPE), 36
Calcium, dietary, 54
Caloric intake, on cancer, 46–48
Camptothecin, 156
Cancer. See also specific types,
    e.g., Melanoma
  chemoprevention of, 35–38, 36t
    antiangiogenesis agents in, 37
    antioxidants in, 36
    arachidonic acid modulators in,
      37–38
    cell proliferation decrease in, 37
    detoxifying enzymes modifiers of,
      35–36
    differentiation agents in, 36
    DNA integrity in, 36
    growth factor blockade in, 37
    human trials in, 38
  metastasis of, 101–116
    (See also Metastases)
  multistage model of, 17–18, 18f
  clonal origin of, 18–19, 19f
Carbon dioxide
  in cryosurgery, 432
  in port site metastasis, 390
Carboplatin, 153t, 155
  for mesothelioma, 1085
Carcinoembryonic antigen (CEA)
  in bladder cancer, 773
  in colon cancer, 706–707, 713, 715
  in nuclear imaging techniques,
    250–251
Carcinogenesis
  chemoprevention of, 35–38, 36t, 62–66,
    63t (See also Chemoprevention)
  genetic basis of, 198–203, 198f
    DNA mismatch repair genes, 201,
      203f

familial cancer syndromes, 201–203, 204t
oncogenes in, 199, 200f, 201t
proto–oncogenes in, 199, 200f, 201t
tumor suppressor genes in, 199–201, 202f
multistage mechanisms of, 15–39
clonal origin of cancer model in, 18–19, 19f
DNA damage and mutation induction in, 20–27
carcinogens in, metabolic activation and detoxification of, 22–23, 23f
DNA damage in, 25–27, 26t
endogenous factors of, 23–25, 24f
exogenous factors of, 20–22, 21t
DNA repair mechanisms in, 27–33, 27t
base excision repair in, 28–29, 28f, 29t
cell cycle checkpoint pathways in, 33
direct damage reversal in, 27–28, 27f
double-strand break repair in, 32–33, 32f
mismatch repair in, 30–32, 31f
nucleotide excision repair in, 29–30, 30f
genetic vs. epigenetic factors in, 19–20
historical perspective in, 15–17, 16t
multistage cancer model in, 17–18, 18f
nutrition and, 44–68 (See also Nutrition)
physical agents in, 78–87 (See also Physical agents)
Carcinogens, dietary, 59–62, 60t
food preparation and processing on, 60t, 61–62
mycotoxins, 61
naturally occurring, 59–61, 60t
Carcinoid tumor(s)
of colon, 716
of endocrine system, 1062–1064
carcinoid syndrome in, 1063, 1063t
introduction to, 1062–1063, 1062t
localization studies for, 1063
prognosis and treatment of, 1063–1064, 1063t
of lung, 557–558
pathology and staging for, 336, 337f
of small intestine, 690–691
of stomach, 634–635

Carcinosarcomas, in ovarian epithelial tumors, 922
Cardiac risk, laparoscopy assessment of, 132–133
Cardiopulmonary bypass technique, for renal cell carcinoma, 761–762, 761f
Carotenoids, 56
chemoprevention trials for, 65–66
Case-control study, 10
Castleman's disease, 557
of mediastinum, 604f, 605
pathology and staging for, 334
Castration, 833
Caucasians, carcinoma in, 484t
Caustic strictures, esophageal carcinoma and, 611
Cavitron ultrasonic surgical aspirator (CUSA), 461–462
CEA (carcinoembryonic antigen). See Carcinoembryonic antigen
Cell proliferation, chemoprevention and, 37
Cellulitis, 804
Central nervous system cancer. See also specific types, e.g., Brain cancer
incidence of, 7f
survival rates of, 8f
Cervical cancer, 883–888
carcinoma, 361–362
clinical manifestation of, 884–886
cryosurgery for, 450–451
evaluation of, 886, 886f
genetic markers of, 207t
incidence of, 7f, 883
laparoscopy for, 403, 403t
leiomyomas, 361, 362f
microinvasive, 884, 885t
nuclear imaging techniques for, 255, 256f
pathogenesis and risk factors for, 883–884, 884
pathology and staging in, 361–362, 362f
pulmonary metastases of, 1129–1130
screening and early detection of, 884
staging of, 885t
survival rates of, 8f
treatment of, 886–888
invasive, 886–888, 887f
recurrent, 888
Cervical intraepithelial neoplasia, cryosurgery for, 450–451
Cervical lymph nodes
dissection for, 536–539 (See also under Neck cancers)
oral cavity cancer and, 524–525

Chemoembolization, 227–228
imaging after, 229
Chemoirradiation therapy. See Chemoradiation therapy
Chemoprevention, 35–38, 36t
antiangiogenesis agents in, 37
antioxidants in, 36
arachidonic acid modulators in, 37–38
bladder cancer, 771
cell proliferation decrease in, 37
detoxifying enzymes modifiers of, 35–36
differentiation agents in, 36
DNA integrity in, 36
growth factor blockade in, 37
human trials in, 38
research in, 62–66
biomarkers, 64
chemoprevention trials, 65–66
dietary modification trials, 65
preclinical and early phase clinical testing, 63–64, 63t
Chemoradiation therapy
for anal cancer, 748
for cervical cancer, 886–888
for esophageal carcinoma, 618–620, 619t
for pancreatic neoplasms, 650–656, 652t, 655f
Chemotherapy
apoptosis from, 147–148
for ascites, malignant, 1186
for bone sarcoma, 1025
for brain cancer, metastatic, 1115
for breast cancer, 969–971
controversies in, 969t
locally advanced, 970–971
ovarian ablation and, 970
tamoxifen in, 969–970
for cervical cancer, 886–887
for colon cancer, 713–714
for endocrine neoplasms, 154–155
for esophagus carcinoma, 618
extrahepatic biliary tract
distal, 681
proximal, 679
for fallopian tube cancer, 900, 900t
for gestational trophoblastic tumors, 906–908, 907t, 908t
hemofiltration and, 171
for hepatic metastases, 269–270, 269f, 1140–1142, 1141f, 1142t
for Hodgkin's lymphoma, 598
for hypopharynx cancer, 530–521
for larynx cancer, 530
for lung neoplasms, stage I primary, 549

Chemotherapy *(cont.)*
  for malignant fibrous histiocytoma,
    1041–1042
  for melanoma, 516
  for mesothelioma, 1085–1086
  for nasopharynx cancer, 527
  for nonseminomas, 594, 847–848
  nutritional support for, 477
  for osteogenic sarcoma, 1030–1033,
    1032f
  for ovarian cancer
    intraperitoneal, 937, 937t
    primary, 931–932
    salvage, 935
  for parotid gland tumors, 535
  for penile cancer, 794–795
  for peritoneal malignancies, 171–176,
    1156–1167
    background for, 1157–1158
    benefits of, prior, 1159–1160
    clinical evidence for, 1160–1161,
      1160f
    delivery of, 1164–1167
      heated intraoperative, 1164–1165,
        1164t, 1165f, 1166f
      induction with 5–FU and
        mitomycin C, 1166, 1167t
      oncologic emergency in, 1167
      postoperative abdominal lavage,
        immediate, 1165, 1165t
      postoperative 5–FU, early, 1165,
        1166t
      with reoperative surgery,
        1166–1167
    general considerations in, 171–173
    hyperthermic perfusion in, 173–174,
      173f, 174f
    patient selection for, 1161–1164
      cancer index in, 1162–1163, 1163f
      clinical assessment in, 1161
      CT scan in, 1161–1162, 1162f
      cytoreduction score in, 1163–1164
      histopathology in, 1161
      peritoneal-plasma barrier in,
        1158–1159, 1158f, 1158t
    postoperative treatment in, 174–175,
      174f
    results of, 175–176, 175f, 176f
    technique in, 174, 174f, 175f
    tumor cell entrapment in, 1159
  pharmacokinetics of
    regional, 160–161
    systemic, 148–149, 149t
  for seminomas, 593, 844
  for solid tumors, regional, 159–176
    hemofiltration and, 171
    history of, 159–160

    intraarterial, 161–162, 162f
    intraperitoneal, 171–176
      general considerations in, 171–173
      hyperthermic perfusion in,
        173–174, 173f, 174f
      postoperative treatment in,
        174–175, 174f
      results of, 175–176, 175f, 176f
      technique in, 174, 174f, 175f
    introduction, 159
    limb perfusion in, isolated, 165–168,
      165f–168f, 167t
    locoregional infusion and perfusion
      in, 170–171, 170f, 171f
    locoregional perfusion in, with ECC,
      162–165, 163f, 164f
      general considerations for,
        162–163
      hyperthermia enhancement of,
        163–164
      hypoxia enhancement of, 164–165
    pelvic perfusion in, isolated,
      168–170, 169f
    pharmacokinetics of, 160–161
  for solid tumors, systemic, 147–157
    agents of, 152–156, 153t–154t
      alkylating, 152
      anthracyclines and DNA
        intercalators, 152, 154
      biologic response modifiers, 156
      endocrine, 154–155
      folate antagonists, 155
      platinum compounds, 155
      purine and pyrimidine
        antimetabolites, 155
      taxanes, 155–156
      topoisomerase I inhibitors, 156
      topoisomerase II inhibitors, 156
      vica alkaloids, 156
    biology of, 147–148
    drug evaluation in, 157
    drug resistance mechanisms in, 150,
      150t
    drug resistance models in, 148
    history of, 147
    introduction to, 147
    models for, 148
    pharmacokinetics of, 148–149, 149t
    strategies of, 150–152
      adjuvant, 151–152
      combination, 150
      high-dose, 152
      multimodality, 150–151, 151t
      neoadjuvant, 152
      primary, 150, 151t
    toxicity of, 149–150
  for stomach neoplasms, 630–631

for testicular cancer, 844, 847–848
  for uterine cancer, 892
Chest radiograph. *See* Chest X-ray
Chest wall tumors
  in pediatric patients, 380
  sarcomas, 988–989, 989f, 990f
Chest X-ray
  for bladder cancer, 706
  for colon cancer, 706
Chlorins, 462
Cholangiocarcinoma, 344
  nuclear imaging techniques for,
    248–249, 249f
Cholangioscopy, 423–424
Cholecystectomy, 1153, 1153f
Cholecystojejunostomy, laparoscopy for,
  395–398, 395f–399f
Chondrosarcoma, 377, 377f, 1033–1035
  adjuvant therapy for, 1035
  clinical manifestations of, 1033
  diagnosis of, 1033, 1033f
  histology of, 1033–1034, 1034f
  introduction to, 1033
  staging of, 1034–1035
  treatment of, 1035
Chordoma, 605, 1042–1043, 1042f
Choriocarcinoma, gestational, 905
Chromosomal instability, 33
Cigarettes. *See* Tobacco
Circumcision, 791
Cisplatin, 153t, 155
  for esophageal cancer, 618, 620
  for mesothelioma, 1085
  for ovarian cancer, 932
  for seminoma, 844
Clear-cell tumors, ovarian epithelial, 922
Clonal origin, of cancer model, 18–19, 19f
Coal tar, 15
Cockayne's syndrome, 29, 30
Colon cancer, 697–718
  adjuvant therapy for, 713–715
    chemotherapy, 713–714
    immunotherapy, 714–715
    radiation, 715
  ASGE surveillance of, 422t
  diagnosis, screening and evaluation of,
    704–707
    asymptomatic patients, 704, 705t
    colonoscopy in, 706
    high-risk patients, 705–706
    imaging in, 706
    laboratory studies in, 706–707
    symptomatic patients, 704
  epidemiology of, 697–698
  etiology and pathogenesis of, 698–701
    adenoma-carcinoma sequence in,
      698

genetic predisposition in, 700–701
inflammatory bowel disease, 701
nonsteroidal anti-inflammatory
drugs (NSAIDs), 701
pathways in, 698–700
chromosomal instability, 700
estrogen receptor, 700
mutator pathway, 698–700
suppressor pathway, 698, 699f
previous colorectal cancer, 701
introduction to, 697
malignant lesions in, other, 716–718
carcinoid, 716
lymphoma, 716–717
sarcoma, 717
squamous cell carcinoma, 717–718
pathology of, 701–703
modes of spread, 701–702
staging, 702–703, 703t
results for, 715
surveillance of, 715, 716f
treatment of, 707–713
curative resection, 707–709, 708f
hemorrhage from, 710
laparoscopic colectomy, 709
malignant polyps, 707
metastatic disease, 711–713
liver, 711–713
liver and lung, 713
lung, 713
obstructing, 709–710
oophorectomy, 710–711
perforated, 710
recurrent disease, 711
resection
en bloc, 710
palliative, 711
synchronous colorectal neoplasms,
711
Colonoscopy, 421
for colon cancer, 706
Colorectal anastomosis, 1154, 1155f
Colorectal cancer
alcohol on, 58–59
biomarkers for
genetic, 207t, 209–210
serum, 124t
classification of, 417t
cryosurgery for, 447–448
dietary fiber on, 51
endoscopy for, 416–422
diagnosis and, 416–417, 417f
screening and, 421–422, 422t
therapy and, 417–421, 417t, 418f,
419f, 420t–421t
fat and caloric intake on, 47
fat type on, 47–48

fruits and vegetables on, 49
genetic basis of, 204t
grains on, whole, 50
hepatic metastasis from, 1133–1144
(See also under Hepatobiliary
neoplasms)
host and tumor interactions in,
106–108
imaging of, 225–227
incidence of, 6f, 7f
interventional radiology for, 227–229
laparoscopy for, 400
laser therapy for, 459–460
NSAIDs on, 37–38
peritoneal carcinomatosis in,
1169–1170, 1171f, 1172f
physical activity and body type on, 48
pulmonary metastases of, 1128, 1129t
survival rates of, 8f
tumor angiogenesis and, 110–111, 111f
Combination modalities. See also
Chemoradiation
radiation therapy and, 143–144
surgical therapy and, 126–128, 127t
COMPARE algorithm, 157
Composite reconstruction, for bone
sarcomas, 1024, 1024f
Computed tomography (CT), 224
for bladder cancer, 774, 775f, 776f
for bone sarcomas, 1016
for colon cancer, 706
for esophageal carcinoma staging, 612
for hemangioma, 662–663, 663f
for hepatic adenoma, 660
for hepatic metastases, 1136–1137,
1137f
for hepatocellular carcinoma, 666–667,
666f
for kidney and ureter cancer, 252
for lung neoplasms, 245
for mesothelioma, 1076–1077
for pancreatic tumors, 247
for rectal cancer, 728–729, 728f, 729f
for renal cell carcinoma, 754
for testicular cancer, 842–843
Contraceptives, oral, hepatic adenomas
and, 659, 661
Correlation, 9–10
Cowden's disease, 420t
genetic basis of, 204t
Cox-2 inhibition, 37
Crohn's disease, 701
Cronkite-Canada syndrome, 420t
Cryoablation, for hepatocellular
carcinoma, 668–669
Cryoprobe, 434–435, 434f, 435f
Cryosurgery, 429–452

for bone tumors, 449–450
for brain tumors, 440–441
clinical application of, 430t, 438
cryogenic injury in, 431–432
equipment for, 432–433
apparatus in, 432–433
cryogenic agents in, 432, 432t
for eye tumors, 440
future directions in, 452
for hepatic metastases, 1142–1144,
1143f, 1144t
history of, 429–431
beginning of, 429–430
modern era in, 430–431, 430t
for larynx cancer, 443
for liver tumors, 443–446
postoperative care in, 445
results in, 445–446, 446f
selection criteria in, 444
technique in, 444–445
for melanoma, 440
for miscellaneous sites, 451–452
for oral cancer, 441–442
for pancreatic cancer, 447–448
for pharynx cancer, 443
for prostate cancer, 448–449
for rectal cancer, 447–448
for skin cancer, 438–440, 486
actinic keratosis, 487–488
vs. other therapy, 440
results in, 439–440
selection criteria in, 439
technique in, 439
technique of, 433–437
cryogen selection in, 433
cryonecrosis border zone in, 436,
437f
cryoprobe technique in, 434–435,
434f, 435f
freeze-thaw cycles in, 435–436, 436f
monitoring in, 436–437, 438f
thermocouples in, 437
ultrasound in, 437, 438f
spray and pour technique in, 435
technique selection in, 433–434
for tracheobronchial tumors, 443
for uterine tumors, 450–451
wound healing in, 431–432
Cryptorchidism, 839
Cushing's syndrome, 325
Cutaneous neoplasm
biopsy of, 221
metastasis frequency in, 131t
Cyclooxygenase, colon cancer and, 700
Cyclophosphamide, 152, 153t
on bladder cancer, 770
Cylindroma, 558–559

Cystectomy, 783–787, 784f, 785t, 786t
Cystoscopy, 775–776, 777f
Cysts, mediastinal, 333–334
Cytogenetics, 293, 293f
Cytokines
    cachexia and, 474
    gene transfer strategies of, 182f
    immunosuppression by, 210–211
Cytology, 288–289, 289f, 290f
Cytoreductive surgery, 130
    for ovarian cancer, 928–931, 929t, 930f,
        936

Dacarbazine, 153t
Delbruck-Luria model, 148
Delivery systems, in gene therapy, 184–186
    non-viral vectors, 186
    viral vectors, 184–185, 185t
DES (diethylstilbestrol)
    for testicular cancer, 833–834
    vaginal cancer and, 870
Detoxifying enzymes, 35–36
Diabetes mellitus, 134
Diagnosis and staging, 217–385. See also
        specific cancers, e.g., Vulvar
        cancer
    imaging techniques in, non-nuclear,
        223–232
        computed tomography (CT), 224
        future trends in, 230–232
        for human colon carcinoma, 225,
            226f, 227f
            interventional radiology in,
                227–229
            strategies in, 226–227
        interventional radiology and,
            227–229
            chemoembolization of liver in,
                227–228
            percutaneous ethanol injection in,
                228
            percutaneous tumor ablation in,
                228–229
            post-interventional imaging in,
                229–230, 230f–232f
        introduction to, 223
        for liver tumor, 224–225
            interventional radiology in,
                227–229
        magnetic resonance imaging (MRI),
            224
        ultrasound, 223–224
    imaging techniques in, nuclear,
        235–271
        of biliary neoplasms, extrahepatic,
            248–250
            gallbladder cancer, 248–249, 249f

large bowel neoplasms, 250, 251f
        small intestine neoplasms,
            249–250, 250f
    of bladder carcinoma, 252–253, 253f
    of bone sarcomas, 260–261, 262f
    of breast cancer
        lymphoscintigraphy and sentinel
            node detection in, 257–260,
            258f
        palliative therapies in, 260
    for cardiac risk factor assessment, 271
    CEA level in, 250–251
    of cervix cancer, 255, 256f
    of colorectal cancer, 250–251, 251f,
        252f
    of endocrine neoplasms, 261–263,
        263f, 264f
    of endometrium cancer, 255
    of esophageal cancer, 247
    future of, 271
    of gestational trophoblastic disease,
        255
    of head and neck cancers, 242–245
        parathyroid, 244–245
        thyroid cancer, 242–244, 242f–244f
    introduction to, 235
    of kidney and ureter cancer, 251–252
    of lung neoplasms, 245–246
    of lymphoma, 265–268
    of mediastinal tumors, 246–247, 246f
    of mesothelioma, 263–265
    of metastatic cancer, 268–271
        brain, 268–269
        liver, 268f, 269, 270, 270f
        peritoneal, 270
        pleural effusions, 245–246
    methodologies in, 235–239
        detection systems in, 236–239,
            237t, 239f
        instruments in, 236t
        molecular imaging in, 235, 238f
        nuclear medicine therapy in,
            235–236
        radioisotopes in, 236t
        radiopharmaceuticals in, 237t
    of ovarian cancer, 255–256
    of pancreatic tumors, 247–248, 248f,
        249f
    of penis carcinoma, 253
    of prostate carcinoma, 254–255
    radiolabeled antibodies in, 256
    of skin neoplasms, 239–242, 241f
    of soft tissue sarcoma, 260
    of stomach cancer, 247
    of testis cancer, 255
    of uterine sarcoma, 255
    of vulval and vaginal neoplasms, 255

pathology in, 279–385 (See also
            Pathology)
    for renal cell carcinoma, 754
    of solid tumors, surgical techniques for,
        217–221
        biopsy in, 220–221
        curative surgery principles in,
            219–220
        history and physical examination in,
            218–219
        role of, 217–218, 218f
Diet. See also Nutrition
    on breast cancer, 952–953
    on colon cancer, 697–698
    fat and caloric intake in, 46–48
    on prostate cancer, 815
    on rectum cancer, 725
    as risk factor, 11, 21, 35
Dietary modification trials, 65
Diethylstilbestrol (DES)
    for testicular cancer, 833–834
    vaginal cancer and, 870
Differentiation agents, 36
Diffuse large B-cell lymphoma,
        mediastinal, 330
Difluoromethylornithine (DFMO), 37
Digital rectal exam, 819t, 822
Dimethylbenzanthrene (DMBA), 15, 16f
DNA
    damage to and mutation induction in,
        20–27
        carcinogens in, metabolic activation
            and detoxification of, 22–23, 23f
        DNA damage in, 25–27, 26t
        endogenous factors of, 23–25, 24f
        exogenous factors of, 20–22, 21t
        molecular biology and, 191–212 (See
            also Molecular biology)
        in pathology techniques, 207–208, 207t
        repair mechanisms of, 27–33, 27t
            base excision repair in, 28–29, 28f,
                29t
            cell cycle checkpoint pathways in, 33
            chemoprevention and, 36
            direct damage reversal in, 27–28, 27f
            double-strand break repair in, 32–33,
                32f
            mismatch repair in, 30–32, 31f, 201,
                203f
            nucleotide excision repair in, 29–30,
                30f
        UV light on, 483–484
DNA intercalator chemotherapy agents,
        152, 154
DNA ploidy analysis, 773
Docetaxel, 153t, 155–156
Doege-Potter syndrome, 573, 582, 602

Double-strand break repair, 32–33, 32f
Doubling time
    of pulmonary metastases, 1125–1126,
        1126f, 1127f
    of testicular cancer, 840
Doxorubicin, 153t
    for soft tissue sarcomas, 1012
Drug resistance
    genes in, 184
    mechanisms of, 150, 150t
    models in, 148
Drug-sensitivity genes, 183–184, 183f
Ductal carcinoma in situ, 959–962
    histology of, 960
    surgery only for, 961, 961t
    surgery with radiation for, 960–961,
        960t
    Van Nuys prognostic index for, 961,
        962t
Duke's stage D disease, 106–107, 112f,
    113f
Dumbbell-shaped tumor, 582
Dura, metastatic carcinoma of, 320f

Ear cancer, 308, 308f
Effusions. *See* specific types, e.g., Pleural
    effusion
Elderly patient, laparoscopy assessment
    of, 135
Elective lymph node dissection (ELND),
    for melanoma, malignant,
    508–510, 539
Electromagnetic irradiation, 79
Embryonal (medulloblastoma) tumors,
    312t, 314, 317f, 318f
En bloc resection
    for colon cancer, 710
    for esophageal carcinoma, 614–615,
        616f, 617f
Endochondromas, 378
Endocrine neoplasms, 1055–1066
    adrenal, 1057–1060
        adrenal cortical, 1057–1060
            hypercortisolism in, 1058
            incidentaloma, 1058–1059
            signs and symptoms of, 1058
            treatment of, 1059
        pathology and staging of, 325
        pheochromocytoma, 1059–1060
        pathology and staging of, 325–326
    biomarkers for, 124t
    carcinoid
        carcinoid syndrome in, 1063, 1063t
        introduction to, 1062–1063, 1062t
        localization studies for, 1063
        prognosis and treatment of,
            1063–1064, 1063t

chemotherapy agents for, 154–155
immunohistochemical stains for, 326,
    326f
introduction to, 1055
laparoscopy assessment of, 134
of mediastinum, 600–602
    parathyroid, 600–601, 600f
    thyroid, 601–602, 602t
multiple endocrine neoplasia, 204t,
    1064–1066
    type 1, 1064–1065, 1064t
    type 2 and familial, 1065–1066, 1066f
nuclear imaging techniques for,
    261–263, 263f, 264f
pancreatic, 1060–1062, 1060t
    epidemiology of, 1060
    gastrinoma in, 1061–1062
    insulinomas in, 1061–1062
    pathology of, 1060–1061, 1060t
parathyroid, 1057, 1057t
    of mediastinum, 600–601, 600f
    pathology and staging of, 324–325,
        325f
pathology and staging of, 322–326
thyroid, 1055–1057
    clinical presentation of, 1055–1056,
        1056f
    epidemiology of, 1055
    pathology and staging of, 322–324
        fine-needle aspiration biopsy of,
            322–324, 322f–324f
        nodule of, 322
    risk factors for, 1055
    treatment and outcomes of,
        1056–1057, 1056f, 1056t
    types of, 1056, 1056t
Endometrial carcinoma
    alcohol on, 58
    diagnosis and evaluation of, 889–990
    laparoscopy for, 403
    nuclear imaging techniques for, 255
    in ovarian cancer, 921–922, 921f
    pathology and staging in, 361–362
    risk factors for, 888, 888t
Endometriosis, 363
Endoprosthetic replacement, 1023–1024,
    1023f
Endoscopic retrograde
    cholangiopancreatography
    (ERCP), 422–423
Endoscopic ultrasound (EUS)
    for colorectal tumors, 417, 417f
    for esophageal tumors, 411–413
    for gastric tumors, 416
    for pancreatic and biliary cancer,
        423–424
Endoscopy, 411–425

for bile duct and pancreas tumors,
    422–425
    diagnosis and, 422–424, 423f
    therapy and, 424–425, 424t, 425t
biopsy with, 220
for bladder cancer, 775–776, 777f
for colorectal tumors, 416–422
    diagnosis and, 416–417, 417f
    screening and, 421–422, 422t
    therapy and, 417–421, 417t, 418f,
        419f, 420t–421t
for esophageal tumors, 411–414
    diagnosis and, 411–413, 412f, 413f
    screening and, 414
    therapy and, 413–414
for gastric tumors, 414–416
    diagnosis and, 414–416, 415f, 416f
    screening and, 416
    therapy and, 416
introduction to, 411
Enteral feeding, 475–476
Enzyme detoxifiers, 35–36
Ependymomas, 313–314, 316f
Epidemiology, of cancer, 3–98
    demographics and geographic
        distribution in, 3–14
    analytic epidemiology in, 9–10
    descriptive epidemiology in, 4–9
        general considerations in, 4–5
        incidence rates in, United States,
            6–8, 6f, 7f
        international variations in, 8–9, 9f
        mortality rates in, United States,
            5–6, 5f, 6f
        survival rates in, 8, 8f
    historical aspects in, 3–4
    introduction to, 3
    patterns of care research in, 13
    risk factors and, 10–13
        diet, 11, 21, 35
        genetics, 12–13
        hormones, 11
        medicines and medical
            procedures, 12
        occupation, 11, 16t, 20
        pollution, 11–12
        reproductive variables, 11
        sexual behavior, 11
        sunlight, 12
        tobacco, 10–11, 15, 20–21, 23
            (*See also* Tobacco)
        viruses, 12
    summary of, 13–14
    etiology and, 15–98 (*See also* Etiology)
Epidermal growth factor receptor, 107,
    108
Epidermodysplasia verruciformis, 485

Epidermoid carcinoma, 491–494
  in anal cancer, 745–747
    clinical presentation of, 747
    cocarcinogens, 746
    etiology and pathogenesis, 745–746
    histologic types, 746
    investigation, 747
    patterns of spread, 746–747
    premalignant lesions, 746
    staging, 747
  clinical manifestations of, 492–493,
      492f, 493t
  diagnosis of, 493
  etiology of, 491
  histology of, 493, 493f
  metastasis frequency in, 131t
  modes of spread of, 491–492
  of parotid gland, 533
  pathogenesis of, 491
  staging of, 493
  treatment of, 493–494
Epigastric sarcomas, 993
Epithelial tumors
  of gynecologic system
    in ovarian cancer, 920–922
      biomarkers for, 916
      carcinosarcomas, 922
      clear-cell, 922
      endometroid, 921–922, 921f
      mucinous, 921, 921f
      other, 922
      serous, 920–921, 920f, 921f
      transitional-cell, 922
    pathology and staging in, 357, 357t,
        358f, 358t
      microscopic appearance of,
          358–359, 358f, 359f, 360t
  of nervous system, with glial
      differentiation, 310–314
    astrocytic, 310–312, 313f–315f
    embryonal (medulloblastoma), 312t,
        314, 317f, 318f
    ependymomas, 313–314, 316f
    meningothelial, 314–316, 319f
    oligodendrogliomas, 312–313
Epstein-Barr virus
  herpes viruses and, 95, 95t, 96f
  in lymphoproliferative disorders,
      368–369
  nasopharynx cancer and, 525–526
Erythroplasia of Queyrat, 489, 489f
  histology of, 792, 793f
Esophageal carcinoma, 609–620
  clinical presentation of, 611
  diagnosis of, 611–612
  endoscopy for, 411–414
    diagnosis and, 411–413, 412f, 413f

  screening and, 414
  therapy and, 413–414
epidemiology of, 610
  adenocarcinoma, 610
  squamous cell, 610
laparoscopy for, 394, 394t
laser therapy for, 458–459
lymphoma, 1111
nuclear imaging techniques for, 247
premalignant lesions of, 610–611
  achalasia, 611
  Barrett's esophagus, 610
  caustic strictures, 611
  chronic esophagitis, 611
  Plummer-Vincent syndrome, 611
  tylosis, 611
prevalence and incidence of, 609–610
  adenocarcinoma, 609–610
  squamous cell, 609
staging of, 612–613, 612t
treatment of, 611–620
  chemoradiation in
    preoperative, 618–620, 619t
    primary, 620
  chemotherapy in, preoperative, 618
  radiation therapy in, 617–618, 618t
  surgical therapy in, 613–617
    en bloc resection, 614–615, 616f,
        617f
    three-field lymphadenectomy,
        615–617
    transhiatal esophagectomy, 614
    transthoracic esophagectomy,
        614
Esophagitis, chronic, 611
Esophagoscopy, 611–612
Estramustine, 153t
Estrogen, 154–155
  receptor gene for, 700
Etiology, of cancer
  multistage carcinogenesis mechanisms
      in, 15–39
    cancer chemoprevention in, 35–38,
        36t
      antiangiogenesis agents in, 37
      antioxidants in, 36
      arachidonic acid modulators in,
          37–38
      cell proliferation decrease in, 37
      detoxifying enzymes modifiers of,
          35–36
      differentiation agents in, 36
      DNA integrity in, 36
      growth factor blockade in, 37
      human trials in, 38
    clonal origin of cancer model in,
        18–19, 19f

DNA damage and mutation
    induction in, 20–27
  carcinogens in, metabolic
      activation and, 22–23, 23f
  DNA damage in, 25–27, 26t
  endogenous factors of, 23–25, 24f
  exogenous factors of, 20–22, 21t
DNA repair mechanisms in, 27–33,
    27t
  base excision repair in, 28–29, 28f,
      29t
  cell cycle checkpoint pathways in,
      33
  direct damage reversal in, 27–28,
      27f
  double-strand break repair in,
      32–33, 32f
  mismatch repair in, 30–32, 31f
  nucleotide excision repair in,
      29–30, 30f
future directions in, 38–39
genetic vs. epigenetic factors in,
    19–20
historical perspective in, 15–17, 16t
molecular epidemiology in, 38
multistage cancer model in, 17–18,
    18f
signal transduction and gene
    expression in, 33–35, 34f, 34t
nutrition-related carcinogenesis in,
    44–68
alcohol on, 57–59
  aerodigestive cancer, 57
  breast cancer, 57–58
  colorectal cancer, 58–59
  endometrial cancer, 58
  prostate cancer, 58
body size on, 48
caloric intake on, 46–48
chemoprevention research in, 62–66
  biomarkers, 64
  chemoprevention trials, 65–66
  dietary modification trials, 65
  preclinical and early phase clinical
      testing, 63–64, 63t
dietary carcinogens on, 59–62, 60t
  food preparation and processing
      on, 60t, 61–62
  mycotoxins, 61
  naturally occurring, 59–61, 60t
dietary fiber on, 50–52
fat intake on, 46–48
grains on, whole, 50
historical overview of, 44–46
introduction to, 44
micronutrients on, 52–54
  calcium, 54

folate, 54
   selenium, 53–54
   vitamin A and β-carotene, 52–53
   vitamin C, 53
   vitamin E, 53
  physical activity on, 48
  phytochemicals on, 54–57, 55t
   carotenoids, 56
   general considerations in, 54
   green tea polyphenols, 56–57
   indoles, 57
   isothiocyanates, 57
   organosulfur compounds, 56
   phytoestrogens, 56
  summary of, 68
  trends and directions for, 66–68
  vegetables and fruits on, 48–50
physical agent carcinogenesis in, 78–87
  future trends in, 82–86, 85t
  historical overview of, 78–81
   electromagnetic, 79
   ionizing irradiation, 80–81
   thermal, 78–79
   ultraviolet, 79–80
  introduction to, 78
  ionizing irradiation in, molecular
    mechanism of, 81–82, 83f, 84f,
    84t, 86
  summary of, 86–87
viral carcinogenesis in, 92–98, 93t
  hepatitis viruses, 94–95
  herpes viruses, 95–98
   Burkitt's lymphoma, 95–96
   Epstein-Barr virus, 95, 95t, 96f
   Hodgkin's disease, 96
   human herpes virus 8, 97–98
   lymphoproliferative disease, 96–97
   nasopharyngeal carcinoma, 96
   x-linked lymphoproliferation, 97,
    97t
  historical overview of, 92
  human T-cell leukemia virus
    type 1, 98
  introduction to, 92
  Papovaviridae, 92–94
   papillomaviruses, 92–93, 94f
   polyomaviruses, 93–94
Etoposide, 153t, 156
Ewing's sarcoma, 1035–1040
  adjuvant therapy for, 1039–1040, 1039t
  clinical manifestations of, 1036
  diagnosis of, 1036, 1036f, 1037f
  *vs.* fracture callus, 378
  genetic markers of, 207t
  histology of, 1037
  introduction to, 1035–1036
  pathology of, 376, 376f, 377f

staging of, 1037
  treatment of, 1037–1039
Eye tumors, 440

Fallopian tube carcinoma, 897–900
  clinical manifestations of, 897, 898t
  diagnosis of, 897–898
  histology of, 898, 898f, 898t, 899t
  introduction to, 897
  ovarian cancer and, 942
  pathology and staging of, 361, 898–899,
    899t
  patterns of spread, 899–900, 899t
  treatment of, 900, 900t
Familial adenomatous polyposis (FAP),
    420t, 421, 700
  genetic basis of, 204t
Familial cancer
  genetic markers for, 207t
  ovarian, 911
  prostate, 814–815, 814t
  syndromes in, 201–203, 204t
Fats, 46–48
Fertility drugs, 911–912
Fiber, dietary, 50–52
Fibroblasts, 108–109
Fibrohistiocytic lesions, 985–986
  histology of, 371, 372f
Fibroma(s)
  angiofibroma, 305, 305f
  infantile myofibromatosis, 384f
  of mediastinum, 602
  neurofibromas, 321–322, 321f, 322f
   of mediastinum, 583–585
   of small intestine, 688
  neurofibromatosis, 420t
   genetic basis of, 204t
   neurofibromas and, mediastinal, 584
  ovarian, 924–925
Fibrosarcoma, 985, 1044
Fibrosing mediastinitis, 334
Fibrous lesions, histology of, 370–371,
    371f, 372f
Fibrous mesothelioma, 338
Fibrous polyps, of lung, 557
Finasteride, 37
Fine-needle aspiration biopsy, 220
  for cytology, 288–289, 289f
  of hepatic tumors, malignant, 343–344,
    344f
  for mediastinum neoplasms, 576
  for mesothelioma, 1078
  of pancreatic neoplasms, 346
  for pathologic diagnosis and staging,
    125–126
  for salivary gland masses, 534
  of soft tissue tumors, 369–370

of thyroid neoplasms, 322–324,
    322f–324f
Flank sarcomas, 992–993, 992f, 993f
5–Fluorouracil (5–FU), 153t
  for bile duct cancer, 681
  for colon cancer, 713–714
  for esophageal cancer, 618, 620
  for pancreatic cancer, 654–655
  for peritoneal malignancies, 1165, 1166,
    1166t, 1167t
  for skin cancers, 486
   actinic keratosis, 488
   Bowen's disease, 489
   erythroplasia of Queyrat, 489
Flutamide, 153t
Focal nodular hyperplasia, 340–343, 344f
  hepatic, 661–662, 661f
Folate, 54
  antagonists of, 155
Food preparation and processing, 60t,
    61–62
Forearm sarcomas, 1006
Fracture callus, *vs.* Ewing's sarcoma, 378
Freeze-thaw cycles, 435–436, 436f
Freon, 432
Fruits, 48–50
5–FU. *See* Fluorouracil (5–FU)

Gallbladder tumor(s). *See also* Biliary
    neoplasms, extrahepatic
  bile duct, endoscopy for, 422–425
   diagnosis and, 422–424, 423f
   therapy and, 424–425, 424t, 425t
  nuclear imaging techniques for,
    248–249, 249f
  pathology and staging for, 340–344
   gallbladder and biliary tree
    inflammation in, 344
   gallbladder and extrahepatic bile
    ducts, 345
Gangliocytic paragangliomas, of small
    intestine, 688
Ganglioneuroblastoma, 585, 589f
Ganglioneuromas, 585, 586f, 587f
  of small intestine, 688
Gardner's syndrome, 420t
Gastrectomy, total, 1155, 1156f
Gastric transection, in
    pancreaticoduodenectomy, 645
Gastric tumors. *See* Gastrointestinal
    tumors; Stomach neoplasm(s)
Gastrinoma, 1061–1062
Gastrointestinal tumors. *See also* specific
    types, e.g., Stomach
    neoplasm(s)
  biomarkers for, 124t
  clinical outcomes for, 1173

Gastrointestinal tumors *(cont.)*
  laparoscopy for, 393–400
    esophageal, 394, 394t
    gastric, 394, 394t
    pancreatic, 394–398, 395f–398f
  pathology and staging for, 338–340,
    340t, 341f–343f
  stromal, 340, 343f
Gastrojejunostomy, 650
Gemcitabine, 153t
  for ovarian cancer, 935
  for pancreatic cancer, 656
Gene conversion, 32
Gene expression
  analysis of
    mRNA, 197
    protein, 198
  signal transduction and, 33–35, 34f, 34t
Gene therapy
  for mesothelioma, 1089–1090
  surgical oncology and, 181–187
    cell type-specific regulatory elements
      in, 186–187
    delivery systems in, 184–186
      non-viral vectors, 186
      viral vectors, 184–185, 185t
    expression control in, 186, 186f
    future directions in, 187
    introduction to, 181
    present status in, 187
    strategies in, 181–184, 182t
      drug-resistance genes, 184
      drug-sensitivity genes, 183–184,
        183f
      immunotherapy by gene transfer,
        182–183, 182f
      oncogene inactivation, 181–182
      tumor suppressor gene defect
        correction, 181–182
Genetics
  adenomatous polyposis gene in, 698
  on breast cancer, 951–952, 952t
  cancer markers and, 207–208, 207t
  on colon cancer, 700–701
  estrogen receptor gene in, 700
  on Ewing's sarcoma, 1036
  on MEN-2, 1065
  on osteogenic sarcoma, 1027
  on ovarian cancer, 912–913, 912t
  on rectal cancer, 726
  as risk factor, 12–13
Genistein, 37
Genitourinary carcinoma. *See also* specific
    types, e.g., Bladder cancer
  laparoscopy for, 400–407
    bladder, 404
    cervical, 403, 403t

endometrial, 403
    ovarian, 400–403, 401f, 402f
    pelvic lymphadenectomy in,
      405–407, 405f–407f
    prostate, 404–405, 404t
    renal, 404
Germ cell neoplasms, 589–594
  classification of, 590t
  general considerations for, 589–591
  nonseminomatous tumors, 593–594,
    593f
  nuclear imaging of, 247
  ovarian, 361, 361f, 912, 914, 922–924,
    940–941, 940t
    biomarkers for, 916–917, 924t
    classification of, 922–923, 922t
    dermoid cyst, 923
    dysgerminoma, 923, 923f
    markers of, 924t
    other, 924
    primitive, 923
    teratoma, immature, 923
    yolk sac, 923, 923f
  pathology and staging of, 591t
    mediastinal, 331–332, 332f
    ovarian, 361, 361f
  in pediatric patients, 382, 383f
  seminomas, 593, 593f, 841
  teratomatous lesion of, 591–593, 592f
  testicular, 353–354, 353f, 354f, 355t,
    356t
Germ line gene therapy, for
    radioprotection, 86
Gerota's fascia, 755–756, 756f
Gestational choriocarcinoma, 905
Gestational trophoblastic tumors,
    903–908, 906t
  clinical manifestations of, 903, 904t
  diagnosis of, 903–904
  introduction to, 903
  nuclear imaging techniques for, 255
  pathology of, 904–906, 904f, 905f, 905t
  staging of, 906, 906t
  therapy for, metastatic
    high risk, poor prognosis, 907–908,
      907t, 908t
    low risk, good prognosis, 907
  therapy for, nonmetastatic, 906, 907t
  treatment of, 905
    surgery in, 908
Giant cell tumor, of bone, 377–378, 378f,
    1044
Giant lymph node hyperplasia, of
    mediastinum, 604f, 605
Glutamine, 475
Glutectomy, 1002
Glycosylases, 29, 29t

Goserelin, 153t
Grafts
  allografts, 1019–1020, 1019f
  autogenous, 1020–1021, 1021f
Grains, whole, 50
Granulomatous lymphadenitis, 334
Granulomatous prostatitis, 350–351,
    350f
Granulosa cell tumor, ovarian, 924, 924f
Green tea polyphenols, 56–57
Groin node dissection, for melanoma,
    malignant, 514–515, 514f, 515f
Groin sarcomas, 1001
Gross examination, in pathology, 285,
    285f
Growth factors
  blockade of, 37
  in metastasis, 105–106
Growth hormone, 476
Gynecologic neoplasms. *See also* specific
    types, e.g., Cervical cancer
  pathology and staging for, 354–363
    adenocarcinoma, 363
    endometriosis, 363
    endometrium and cervix carcinoma,
      361–362
    endosalpingiosis, 363
    epithelial tumors, 357, 357t, 358f,
      358t
      microscopic appearance of,
        358–359, 358f, 359f, 360t
    fallopian tubes, 361
    female peritoneum, 363
    germ cell tumors, 361, 361f
    ovary, benign cysts of, 356–357, 356f
    ovary, neoplasms of, 357, 360t
    pulmonary metastases of, 1129–1130
    sex cord-stromal tumors, 359–361
    uterine corpus and cervix, 361, 362f
    vagina and vulva, 362–363

Hamartoma
  of lung, 556–557, 556t
  of small intestine, 687
  of thymus, 576
Hand sarcomas, 1006
Head and neck tumors. *See also* Head
    cancers; Neck cancers
  in pediatric patients, 379–380, 379f,
    380f
  pulmonary metastases of, 1128, 1130t
Head cancers, 519–539
  biomarkers for, 124t
  dissection for, 536–539
    cervical lymph node metastasis, 537
    cutaneous melanoma, 539
    lymphatic anatomy in, 536–537, 536f

metastatic SCC with occult primary tumor, 539
neck dissections in, 536f, 537
nodal metastasis patterns in, 538, 538t, 539t
salivary gland carcinoma, 539
tracheoesophageal (level IV) lymph nodes, 539
fruits and vegetables on, 49
grains on, whole, 50
introduction to, 519, 520t
larynx and hypopharynx, 527–531 (*See also* Larynx)
nasopharynx, 525–527 (*See also* Nasopharynx)
oral cavity, 303–304, 303f, 304f, 519–525 (*See also* Oral cavity)
salivary glands, 531–536 (*See also* Salivary gland tumors)
*Helicobacter pylori,* 17
gastric lymphomas and, 340, 341f, 369f, 634
Hemangioendothelioma, 1044, 1044f
Hemangiomas
hepatic, 662–663, 663f
of small intestine, 688
Hemangiopericytoma, 561, 985
Hematologic malignancies, genetic markers for, 207t
Hematolymphoid system oncology, pathology and staging in, 364–369
clinical manifestation of, 365, 365t
general considerations in, 363–365, 364f
immunodeficiency, 367–369
surgical intervention requirement in, 365–367, 366f–368f, 367t, 368t
Hematoporphyrin, 462
Hematuria, 771–772, 771t
Hemipelvectomy, 999–1001, 999f–1001f
Hemofiltration, chemotherapy and, 171
Hepatic. *See* Hepatobiliary neoplasms
Hepaticojejunostomy, 649–650
Hepatitis virus, 94–95
hepatocellular carcinoma and, 665
Hepatobiliary neoplasms, 659–682
extrahepatic biliary tract, 673–682
benign, 681–682
conclusions for, 682
introduction to, 673
extrahepatic biliary tract, distal, 679–681
chemotherapy for, 681
epidemiology of, 679–680
palliation for, 680–681
presentation of, 680

radiotherapy for, 681
surgical resection of, 680
extrahepatic biliary tract, proximal, 673–679
chemotherapy for, 679
epidemiology of, 673–674
evaluation of, 674, 675f
history of, 673
palliative therapy for, 679
presentation of, 674
radiotherapy for, 679
surgical therapy for, 674–679
operative conduct in, 676–679, 679f
patient selection in, 675–676, 676f, 678f
results of, 674–675, 677t
laparoscopy for, 398–400
metastatic hepatic, 1133–1145
from colorectal cancer, 711–713, 1133, 1134t
repeat, 1138t, 1139–1140
resection of, 1133, 1134t
cryotherapy for, 1142–1144, 1143t, 1144f
intraarterial chemotherapy for, 1140–1142, 1140t, 1141f, 1142t
introduction to, 1133
from noncolorectal primaries, 1145
perioperative morbidity and mortality in, 1138–1139, 1139t
predictive factors for, 1133–1136, 1134t–1136t
preoperative evaluation of, 1136–1138, 1136f–1138f, 1138t
primary hepatic, 659–670, 660t
biomarkers for, 124t
chemoembolization of, 227–228
imaging after, 229
cryosurgery for, 443–446
postoperative care in, 445
results in, 445–446, 446f
selection criteria in, 444
technique in, 444–445
imaging of, 224–225
pathology and staging for, 340–344
benign, 340–343, 344f
malignant, 343–344, 344f, 345f
primary hepatic, benign, 659–663
focal nodular hyperplasia, 661–662, 661f
hemangiomas, 662–663, 663f
hepatic adenoma, 659–661
clinical manifestation of, 659–660
diagnosis of, 660
histology of, 660
prevalence of, 659
treatment of, 660–661

infantile hemangioendothelioma, 663
nodular regenerative hyperplasia, 662
pathology and staging for, 340–343, 344f
solid tumors, 663–664, 664f
primary hepatic, malignant, 664–670, 664t
hepatocellular carcinoma, 664–670
clinical manifestation of, 665–666
diagnosis of, 666–667, 666f, 667f
etiology of, 664–665, 664t, 665t
histology of, 667
prevalence of, 664
staging of, 667, 668f
therapeutic option summary for, 669–670
treatment of, 667–668
intrahepatic cholangiocarcinoma, 670
mesenchymal tumor, 670
pathology and staging for, 343–344, 344f, 345f
Hepatoblastoma, 344
Hepatocellular carcinoma, 664–670
clinical manifestation of, 665–666
diagnosis of, 666–667, 666f, 667f
etiology of, 664–665, 664t, 665t
histology of, 667
prevalence of, 664
staging of, 667, 668f
therapeutic option summary for, 669–670
treatment of, 667–668
Herpes viruses, 95–98
Burkitt's lymphoma, 95–96
Epstein-Barr virus, 95, 95t, 96f
Hodgkin's disease, 96
human herpes virus 8, 97–98
lymphoproliferative disease, 96–97
nasopharyngeal carcinoma, 96
x-linked lymphoproliferation, 97, 97t
HER-2/neu, 209, 211–212
Heterocyclic aromatic amines, 61–62
Heterotopic tissue, in small intestine, 687
Heterozygosity loss, 194–195, 196f
Histiocytoma, malignant fibrous, 561
Hodgkin's lymphoma, 598, 599t, 1103–1105
clinical presentation of, 1103, 1104t
diagnosis of, 1103–1104, 1104t
herpes virus and, 96
laparoscopy for, 391–393, 393f
pathology and staging of, 330, 1104–1105, 1104t
treatment of, 1105
Homologous recombination, 31–32

Homovanillic acid, from mediastinum neurogenic tumors, 582
Hormones. *See also* Endocrine neoplasms
in chemoprevention, 35, 37
mediastinal neoplasms on, 573, 575t
for prostate cancer, 833–834
on prostate cancer, 815
as risk factor, 11
Hospital-based registries, 4
Host and tumor interactions, 105–114
organ-derived growth factors in, 105–106
organ-specific growth regulation in, 106–108
organ-specific phenotype modulation in, 108–110
tissue-specific repairs factors in, 106
tumor angiogenesis in, 110–114
angiogenic and antiangiogenic regulation in, 111–114, 112f, 113f
microenvironment regulation of, 114
HPD/photofrin, 462
Human colon carcinoma (HCC). *See* Colon cancer; Colorectal cancer
Human herpes virus 8, 97–98
Human immunodeficiency virus (HIV), allografts and, 1019
Human papillomavirus, 92–93, 94f
anal cancer and, 746, 749
in cervical cancer, 883–884, 884t
in head and neck cancer, 519
nonmelanoma skin cancer and, 485
in penile cancer, 791, 792
in vaginal cancer, 870
in vulvar cancer, 853–854, 854t
Human T-cell leukemia virus type 1, 98
Hydatidiform mole, 904, 904f, 905f, 905t
Hydroxyl radicals, 24
Hypermetabolism, cachexia and, 474
Hyperparathyroidism, 324–325, 325f
parathyroid tumors and, 600
Hyperthermic isolation limb perfusion (HILP), 513
Hypopharynx cancer, 305, 530–531. *See also* Larynx cancer
Hysterectomy, 886–887, 890–891, 892

Ifosfamide, 153t
for Ewing's sarcoma, 1040
for soft tissue sarcomas, 1012
Iliac fossa sarcomas, 999–1001, 999f–1001f
Imaging techniques. *See also* specific types, e.g., Computed tomography (CT)

for diagnosis and staging, 223–232
computed tomography (CT), 224
future trends in, 230–232
for human colon carcinoma, 225, 226f, 227f
interventional radiology in, 227–229
strategies in, 226–227
interventional radiology and, 227–229
chemoembolization of liver in, 227–228
percutaneous ethanol injection in, 228
percutaneous tumor ablation in, 228–229
post-interventional imaging in, 229–230, 230f–232f
introduction to, 223
for liver tumor, 224–225
interventional radiology in, 227–229
magnetic resonance imaging (MRI), 224
ultrasound, 223–224
nuclear, 235–271 (*See also* Nuclear imaging)
Immunoconjugate therapy, for mesothelioma, 1090
Immunodeficiency, in hematolymphoid system oncology, 367–369
Immunohistochemistry, 205–206, 205t, 206f
endocrine neoplasms stains in, 326, 326f
immunostains in, 290, 291f, 292f
Immunology, biomarkers for, 210–211
Immunoscintigraphy, 131–132
Immunostains, 290, 291f, 292f
Immunosuppression, UV light exposure on, 485
Immunotherapy
for colon cancer, 714–715
by gene transfer, 182–183, 182f
for mesothelioma, 1089
In-transit lesions, in melanoma, 512
Incidence rate. *See* Epidemiology
Indoles, 57
Infantile hemangioendothelioma, 663
Infantile myofibromatosis, 384f
Infection, surgical, 134–135, 134t
Inflammatory bowel disease, 701
Inguinal adenopathy, 799–800
Inguinal metastases, 749
Inguinal nodes, urethral cancer and, 809–810
Insulin-glucagon ratio, cachexia and, 475

Insulinomas, 1061–1062
Interferon, 153t, 156
for mesothelioma, 1089
on metastatic carcinoma cells, 109–110, 111, 114
for skin cancer, 486, 494, 498
Interleukin 2, 153t, 156
for melanoma, 517
for mesothelioma, 1089
Interleukin 8, 114
Interleukin 10, 211
Interstitial laser hyperthermia, 460
Intervention trial, 10
Intraepithelial neoplasia
cervical, cryosurgery for, 450–451
from HPV, 749
prostatic, 351–352, 351f, 352f
vaginal, 871
vulvar, 861–862
Intratubular germ cell neoplasia, 353–354, 353f, 354f, 355t
Intravenous pyelogram, 773, 774f, 775f
Invasion and metastasis, 101–116. *See also* Metastases
Invasive sepsis, laparoscopy in, 134–135, 134t
Ionizing irradiation, 80–82, 83f, 84f, 84t, 86
Irradiation, 79–86. *See also* Radiation therapy
electromagnetic, 79–87
ionizing irradiation, 80–82, 83f, 84f, 84t, 86–87
thermal, 78–79
ultraviolet, 79–80
Isolated limb perfusion, 165–168, 165f–168f, 167t
Isothiocyanates, 57
Itinotecan, 153t

Jackson staging system, for penile carcinoma, 792, 792t
Jejunostomy, laparoscopy for, 395–398, 395f–399f
Jugulotympanic paraganglioma, 308, 308f
Juvenile fibrous tumor, 383, 383f, 384f
Juvenile polyposis syndrome, 421t

K-*ras*, pancreatic neoplasms and, 637–638
Keratoacanthoma, 489–491
clinical manifestations of, 490, 490f
diagnosis of, 490
general considerations for, 489–490
histology of, 296, 296t, 490–491, 490f
treatment of, 491
Keratopalmar keratosis, 611
Kidney. *See also* Renal
benign tumors of, 348, 348f

Knee sarcomas, 1004
Kocher maneuver, in
 pancreaticoduodenectomy,
 643–644, 644f
Krukenberg tumor, 925

Lactation, breast cancer during, 975
Langerhan's cell histiocytosis, 378–379
Laparoscopy, 389–407
 for anal sphincter resection, 735
 for colectomy, 709
 for gastrointestinal tumors, 393–400
  colorectal, 400
  esophageal, 394, 394t
  gastric, 394, 394t
  hepatic, 398–400
  pancreatic, 394–398, 395f–399f,
   642–643
 general approach to, 389–391
  port site metastasis and, 390–391,
   404
  technique for, 390
  ultrasound in, 391
 for genitourinary carcinoma, 400–407
  bladder, 404
  cervical, 403, 403t
  endometrial, 403
  ovarian, 400–403, 401f, 402f
  pelvic lymphadenectomy in,
   405–407, 405f–407f
  prostate, 404–405, 404t
  renal, 404
 for hepatocellular carcinoma, 667
 introduction to, 389
 for lymphoma, 391–393, 393f
 for ovarian adnexal mass, 918
 surgical oncology and, 132–135
  cardiac risk assessment in, 132–133
  elderly patient in, 135
  endocrine disorders in, 134
  invasive sepsis in, 134–135, 134t
  pulmonary risk assessment in,
   133–134
Laparotomy
 cryosurgery and, of liver, 444
 vs. laparoscopy, 132
Large bowel neoplasms. See also Anal
  cancer; Colon cancer;
  Colorectal cancer; Rectal cancer
 lymphoma of, 1110–1111
 nuclear imaging techniques for, 250,
  251f
Large cell non-Hodgkin's lymphoma,
  599–600
Larynx cancer, 527–530
 clinical presentation of, 529, 529f
 cryosurgery for, 443

general considerations in, 527
historical review of, 527–529, 528t
pathology and staging for, 305–306,
 307t
treatment of, 529–530
Laser ablation. See Laser therapy
Laser-induced fluorescence spectroscopy
 (IF), 459–460
Laser therapy
 for breast cancer, 460–461
 for colorectal cancer, 459–460
 for esophageal cancer, 458–459
 interstitial laser hyperthermia in, 460
 laser theory in, 457
 for penile cancer, 795
 for skin cancer
  actinic keratosis, 488
  Bowen's disease, 489
  erythroplasia of Queyrat, 489
 surgical lasers in, 457–458, 458t
 for tracheobronchial tumors, 443
Leiomyomas
 of cervix, 361, 362f
 of lung, 557
 of mediastinum, 602–603
 of small intestine, 249–250, 688
 of stomach, 416f
 of uterus, cryosurgery for, 451
Leiomyosarcomas, 1044
 features of, 985
 of mediastinum, 602–603
 of prostate, 353
 of small intestine, 250, 250f
 in vaginal cancer, 871, 872
 of vulva, 869
Leukemia
 human T-cell virus type 1, 98
 survival rates of, 8f
Leuprolide, 154t
Li-Fraumeni syndrome, 1028
Ligament of Treitz, 645–646, 646f
Limb-preserving surgery
 for bone sarcomas, 1018–1019
 sarcomas and, 127
Linxian Trials, 65
Lipid metabolism, cachexia and, 474
Lipomas
 histology of, 371, 373f
 of lung, 557
 of mediastinum, 602
 of small intestine, 688
Liposarcomas, 985
Liposome-mediated transfection, 186
Liver neoplasms. See Hepatobiliary
 neoplasms
Liver transplantation, 668
Lobular carcinoma in situ, 959

Locoregional perfusion, 162–165, 163f,
 164f
 general considerations for, 162–163
 hyperthermia enhancement of, 163–164
 hypoxia enhancement of, 164–165
 infusion and, 170–171, 170f, 171f
Lower extremities, sarcomas of, 999–1004
 anterior compartment, 1001–1002,
  1002f, 1003f
 below knee, 1004
 buttocks, 1002
 groin, 1001
 iliac fossa, 999–1001, 999f–1001f
 medial compartment, 1002, 1004f
 popliteal fossa, 1004
 posterior compartment, 1003–1004,
  1005f, 1006f
Lung neoplasms, 545–565. See also
  Pulmonary
 biomarkers for, 124t
 fruits and vegetables on, 49
 grains on, whole, 50
 incidence of, 6f, 7f
 metastatic, 561–565, 1125–1131
  adjuvant therapy for, 563–564
  clinical manifestation of, 1125
  clinical presentation of, 561–562
  conclusions for, 564–565, 565t
  diagnosis of, 1125
  future management directions for,
   1130–1131
  historical review of, 561
  introduction to, 1125
  other considerations for, 564
  pretreatment workup for, 562, 562t
  results in, 1126–1130
   breast carcinoma, 1129
   colorectal carcinoma, 713, 1128,
    1129t
   gynecologic cancers, 1129–1130
   head and neck tumors, 1128, 1130t
   melanoma, 1128, 1129t
   osteogenic sarcoma, 1130, 1130t
   prostate cancer, 1129
   renal cell carcinoma, 1127, 1129t
   soft tissue sarcoma, 1127, 1128t
   testicular tumors, 1130
  surgical approach to, 564, 1126, 1128f
  surgical indications for, 1126
  treatment of, 562–563
  tumor doubling time in, 1125–1126,
   1126f, 1127f
 nuclear imaging techniques for,
  245–246
 pathology and staging for, 334–338
  carcinoid tumor, 336, 337f
  carcinoma, 334–336, 335f, 336f

Lung neoplasms (*cont.*)
    lung masses, 334
    metastatic neoplasms, 337
    pleurae, 337–338, 339f
    tumor, benign, 337
    tumor biopsy, 334, 334t
   primary, 545–556, 546f, 546t, 547t
    occult carcinomas, 545–547
    small cell, 556
    solitary synchronous resectable
      metastases, 556
    stage I, 547–549
      chemotherapy for, 549
      radiation therapy for, 548–549
      resection for, 547–548, 548f
      vitamin A and retinoids for, 548
    stage IIIA, 552–555
      N1-3N2MO tumors, 552–555,
        552f–554f, 553t–555t
      T3N1MO tumors, 555
    stage IIIB, 555–556
      T1N1 and T2N1 tumors, 549–550,
        549f
      T3NOMO tumors, 550–552
        superior sulcus tumors, 551
        tumors in proximity to carina, 551
        tumors invading chest wall,
          550–551, 550t
        tumors invading mediastinum,
          551–552
   primary, less common, 556–561
    adenoid cystic carcinoma, 558–559
    benign tumors, 556–557, 556t
    carcinoid tumors, 557–558
    lymphomas, 560t, 561
    mucoepidermoid carcinoma,
      559–560
    sarcomas, 560–561, 560t
   survival rates of, 8f
Luteinizing hormone-releasing hormone,
    834
Lymph node
   biopsy of, 221, 366
   dissection of
    cervical, 536–539
      cervical lymph node metastasis,
        537
      cutaneous melanoma, 539
      lymphatic anatomy in, 536–537,
        536f
      metastatic SCC with occult
        primary tumor, 539
      neck dissections in, 536f, 537
      nodal metastasis patterns in, 538,
        538t, 539t
      salivary gland carcinoma, 539
      tracheoesophageal (level IV)

      lymph nodes, 539
    elective (ELND), for melanoma,
      malignant, 508–510, 539
    for melanoma, malignant, 513–516
      axillary, 515
      groin, 514–515, 514f, 515f
      neck, 516
      popliteal, 515–516
    in penile cancer, 800–804, 800f–804f
    in testicular cancer, 844–850 (*See also*
      *under* Testicular cancer)
   inguinal, in vulvar cancer, 862, 863f
   in ovarian cancer, 927–928, 928f, 931
Lymphadenectomy
   inguinofemoral, 862–863, 863f
   pelvic, laparoscopy for, 405–407,
     405f–407f
   three-field, for esophageal carcinoma,
     615–617
Lymphadenitis, granulomatous, 334
Lymphoblastic lymphoma, 330–331, 331f
Lymphoblastic non-Hodgkin's
    lymphoma, 598–599
Lymphocytoma, of lung, 557, 561
Lymphomas, 1103–1111
   AJCC staging system for, 368t
   bone, pathology of, 282–284, 283f
   in colon cancer, 716–717
   diffuse large B-cell, 330
   esophageal, 1111
   Hodgkin's, 1103–1105
    clinical presentation of, 1103, 1104t
    diagnosis of, 1103–1104, 1104t
    staging of, 330, 1104–1105, 1104t
    treatment of, 1105
   immunoproliferative small-intestinal,
     1110
   incidence of, 7f
   introduction to, 1103, 1105–1107, 1107t
   laparoscopy for, 391–393, 393f
   of large bowel, 716–717, 1110–1111
   of lung, 560–561, 560t
   lymphoblastic, 330–331, 331f
   mantle cell, 368f
   of mediastinum, 594–600
    characteristics of, 597t
    general considerations in, 594–598,
      595f, 596f, 597t
    Hodgkin's, 598, 599t
    non-Hodgkin's, 598–600
    large cell, 599–600
    lymphoblastic, 598–599
   of nasopharynx, 305
   non-Hodgkin's, 1105, 1106t
   nuclear imaging techniques for,
     265–268
   *vs.* parotid gland masses, 533

   of small intestine, 691–693, 692t,
     1109–1110
   of stomach, 632–634, 633t, 634t,
     1107–1109
    clinical presentation of, 1108, 1108t
    diagnosis and staging of, 1108, 1108t
    etiology of, 1108
    treatment and outcome of,
      1108–1109, 1109f
   survival rates of, 8f
   systemic, 1103–1105
    Hodgkin's disease, 1103–1105
    non-Hodgkin's, 1105, 1106t
   working formulation of 1982
    classification of, 367t
Lymphoproliferative disease, herpes virus
    and, 96–97, 97t
Lymphoscintigraphy
   for breast cancer, sentinel node
     detection in, 257–260, 257t, 258f
   in sentinel node biopsy, 511–512
   for skin neoplasms, 239–242, 241f
Lynch syndrome, 31

m-THPC, 462–463
Magnetic resonance imaging (MRI), 224
   for bladder cancer, 774
   for bone sarcomas, 1016
   for head and neck cancers, 242
   for hepatic adenoma, 660
   for hepatocellular carcinoma, 667, 667f
   for mesothelioma, 1077, 1077f
   for pancreatic tumors, 247
   for prostate carcinoma, 254
   for rectal cancer, 731, 731f
   for renal cell carcinoma, 754–755
Male reproductive system cancers. *See also*
    specific types, e.g., Testicular
    cancer
   pathology and staging for, 350–354
    benign prostatic hyperplasia, 351
    intratubular germ cell neoplasia,
      353–354, 353f, 354f, 355t
    prostate and seminal vesicles,
      350–351, 350f
    prostatic intraepithelial neoplasia,
      351–352, 351f, 352f
    radical prostatectomy, 352–353
    testes and paratesticular structures,
      353
Malignant fibrous histiocytoma,
    1040–1042
   histology and presentation of,
     1040–1041, 1042f
   treatment of, 1041–1042
Malnutrition, 473–475. *See also* Nutrition,
    and cancer

Mammography, 953–954, 954f
Mandible, oral cancer on, 522–524, 522f, 523f
Mandibulectomy, 524, 524f
Mantle cell lymphoma, 368f
Masaoka staging, of thymomas, 579–580, 579t, 580t
Mastectomy, 957–959
  axillary dissection in, 959
  Langer's lines in, 957, 957f
  for locally advanced cancer, 971
  Orr incision in, 958, 958f
  skin-sparing, 958–959
  Stewart incision in, 958, 958f
Medial compartment sarcomas, 1002, 1004f
Mediastinum, neoplasms of, 571–605
  anatomic landmarks in, 571, 572f, 572t, 573t
  Castleman's disease, 604f, 605
  chordoma, 605
  classification of, 572t
  endocrine, 600–602
    parathyroid, 600–601, 600f
    thyroid, 601–602, 602t
  germ cell, 589–594
    classification of, 590t
    general considerations for, 589–591
    nonseminomatous tumors, 593–594, 593f
    seminomas, 593, 593f
    staging of, 591t
    teratomatous lesion of, 591–593, 592f
  historical aspects of, 571, 572t
  incidence of, 571–572, 573f, 574t, 575t
  lung primary T3N0M0 tumors, 551–552
  lymphomas, 594–600
    characteristics of, 597t
    general considerations in, 594–598, 595f, 596f, 597t
    Hodgkin's, 598, 599t
    non-Hodgkin's, 598–600
      large cell, 599–600
      lymphoblastic, 598–599
  mesenchymal, 602–605, 603t
    of blood vessel and lymphatic origin, 603–605, 603f
    of soft tissue, 602–603
  neurogenic, 581–589
    general considerations in, 581–583, 581t, 582f
    of nerve sheath origin, 583–585, 583f, 584f
    from sympathetic ganglia, 585, 586f–589f, 587t
  nuclear imaging of, 246–247, 246f

  pathology and staging for, 326–334
    anatomical definition in, 326
    anatomical distribution in, 327, 327t, 328t
    biopsy for, 327–328
    clinicopathologic features in, 328–334
      Castleman's disease, 334
      cysts, 333–334
      diffuse large B-cell lymphoma, 330
      fibrosing mediastinitis, 334
      germ cell tumors, 331–332, 332f
      granulomatous lymphadenitis, 334
      Hodgkin's lymphoma, 330
      lymphoblastic lymphoma, 330–331, 331f
      neurogenic tumors, 332–333, 333f
      thymoma, 328–330, 329f
    primary, 602
    radiologic evaluation of, 573–575
    signs and symptoms of, 572–573, 575t
    thymic, 576–581, 577t
      hamartomatous lesions, 576
      thymic epithelial, 577–581, 578f, 579f, 579t, 580t
        myasthenia gravis and thymectomy in, 580
        thymic carcinoma in, 580–581
        thymomas, 577–580, 578f, 579f, 579t, 580t
      thymolipoma, 576
    tissue-obtaining techniques for, 575–576
Medical history, 218–219
Medicines, as risk factor, 12
Medulloblastoma, 312t, 314, 317f, 318f
Megestrol acetate, 154t
Melanoma, malignant, 505–517
  of anus, 750, 751f
  biomarkers for, 207t, 210
  clinical manifestation of, 506, 506f, 506t
  cryosurgery for, 440
  diagnosis of, 506–507
  etiology of, 79, 505, 506t
  genetic basis of, 204t
  immunohistochemistry of, 206, 206f
  incidence of, 6f, 7f, 505
    United States, 7, 7f
  of limb, perfusion for, 168t
  pathology of, 507, 507f, 509t
  PCR testing for, 208
  preventive measures for, 505
  prognostic factors of, 509t
  pulmonary metastases of, 1128, 1129t
  staging of, 297–298, 298t, 507–508, 508t
  treatment of, 508–517
    of head and neck, 539

    locoregional recurrence, 512–516
      adjuvant therapy in, 516
      in-transit metastases in, 512–513
      local recurrence in, 512–513
    locoregional recurrence, node dissection in, 513–516
      axillary, 515
      groin, 514–515, 514f, 515f
      neck, 516
      popliteal, 515–516
    stage IV, 516–517, 516f
    stages I and II, 508–512
    stages I and II, primary site, 505
    stages I and II, regional nodes, 508–512
      elective dissection, 508–510, 510t
      sentinel node biopsy, 510–512, 511f, 512t, 513f
    stages I and II, sentinel node biopsy, 511f, 512t, 513f
  in vaginal cancer, 871, 872
    prognostic factors for, 874
    treatment of, 877–878
  in vulvar cancer, 856–857, 858, 860f, 861
    treatment of, 868–869
Meningioma, 314–316, 319f
Meningothelial tumors, 314–316, 319f
Merkel cell cancer, 241
Mesenchymal tumors
  in mediastinum, 602–605, 603t
    of blood vessel and lymphatic origin, 603–605, 603f
    of soft tissue, 602–603
  of small intestine, 688
Mesoblastic nephroma, 381–382
Mesothelioma, 1069–1094
  clinical presentation of, 1073–1075
    history in, 1073–1075, 1074f
    physical examination in, 1075
  conclusions for, 1094
  diagnostic approach to, 1075–1078
    differential diagnosis in, 1075
    imaging studies in, 1075–1078
      chest roentgenograms, 1076
      CT scan, 1076–1077
      fine-needle aspiration, 1078
      general considerations in, 1075–1076, 1075f, 1076f
      invasive diagnostic studies, 1077–1078
      MRI, 1077, 1077f
      positron emission tomography, 1077, 1077f
      thoracentesis, 1078, 1079f
      thoracotomy, 1078
      videothoracoscopy, 1078, 1079f

Mesothelioma *(cont.)*
   laboratory studies in, 1075
   diffuse malignant, 1069–1073
      epidemiology of, 1071–1072, 1071f
      etiology of, 1069–1071
         asbestos characteristics in,
            1070–1071
         background in, 1069–1070
         non-asbestos factors in, 1072
      pathophysiology of, 1072–1073
   introduction to, 1069
   localized benign, 1093–1094
   localized malignant, 1094
   nuclear imaging techniques for,
      263–265
   pathology of, 338, 1078–1082
      differential diagnosis in, 1082
      electron microscopy in, 1082
      gross, 1078–1079, 1080f
      histochemistry in, 1081
      immunohistochemistry in,
         1081–1082
      microscopic, 1079–1081
   pericardial, 1093
   peritoneal, 1090–1093
      clinical presentation of, 1091
      diagnosis of, 1091–1092
      pathology of, 1090–1091
      staging and prognosis of, 1092
      therapy for, 1093
   prognosis for, 1084–1085
   staging for, 1082–1084, 1083t, 1084t
   therapeutic approach for, 1085–1090
      adjuvant therapy, 1088–1090
         gene therapy, 1089–1090
         immunoconjugate therapy, 1090
         immunotherapy, 1089
         palliative management, 1090
         photodynamic therapy, 1090
      chemotherapy, 1085–1086
      radiation therapy, 1086
      surgery, 1086–1088
         perioperative management in,
            1086–1087
         procedures in, 1087–1088, 1087t
   tunica vaginalis testis, 1093
Meta-analysis, 10, 67
Metastases, 101–116
   biologic diversity of neoplasms in,
      103–105, 104f
   brain, 1113–1121
      clinical signs and symptoms,
         1113–1114, 1114f
      differential diagnosis for, 1114–1115
      introduction to, 1113
      radiosurgery role in, 1120–1121,
         1121f

      recurrence of
         after surgery, 1118–1119
         reirradiation for, 1119
         reoperation for, 1119–1120, 1119t,
            1120t
      therapeutic decision making for,
         1115–1118
         chemotherapy in, 1115
         for multiple metastases,
            1117–1118, 1118f
         postoperative WBRT in, 1117
         randomized trials in, 1116
         surgical complications in, 1117
         survival and prognostic factors in,
            1116–1117
         whole brain radiation in, 1115
   of colon cancer, 711–713
      liver, 711–713
      liver and lung, 713
      lung, 713
   conclusions for, 115–116
   from endocrine carcinoid tumors,
      1062–1064, 1062t, 1063t
   frequency of, 131t
   genes in, multiparametric studies of,
      114–115, 115f
   from gestational trophoblastic tumors,
      903, 904t
   of head and neck cancers, cervical
      lymph node, 537–538, 538t,
      539t
   hepatic, 1133–1145
      from colorectal cancer, 1133, 1134t
         repeat resection of, 1138t,
            1139–1140
         resection of, 1133, 1134t
      cryotherapy for, 1142–1144, 1143t,
         1144f
      intraarterial chemotherapy for,
         1140–1142, 1140t, 1141f, 1142t
      introduction to, 1133
      from noncolorectal primaries, 1145
      perioperative morbidity and
         mortality in, 1138–1139, 1139t
      predictive factors for, 1133–1136,
         1134t–1136t
      preoperative evaluation of,
         1136–1138, 1136f–1138f, 1138t
   host and tumor interactions in,
      105–114
      organ-derived growth factors in,
         105–106
      organ-specific growth regulation in,
         106–108
      organ-specific phenotype
         modulation, 108–110
      tissue-specific repairs factors in, 106

      tumor angiogenesis in, 110–114
         angiogenic and antiangiogenic
            regulation in, 111–114, 112f,
            113f
         microenvironment regulation of,
            114
   inguinal, 749
   introduction to, 101
   at laparoscopy port site, 390–391, 404
   nuclear imaging techniques for,
      268–271
      brain, 268–269
      hepatic arterial chemotherapy in,
         269–270, 269f
      liver
         nonresectable, 270, 270f
         staging of, 268f, 269
      peritoneal, 270
      pleural effusions, 245–246
   pathogenesis of, 101–103, 102f
   of prostate cancer, 824, 824f
   pulmonary, 1125–1131
      clinical manifestation of, 1125
      diagnosis of, 1125
      future management directions for,
         1130–1131
      introduction to, 1125
      results in, 1126–1130
         breast carcinoma, 1129
         colorectal carcinoma, 1128, 1129t
         gynecologic cancers, 1129–1130
         head and neck tumors, 1128, 1130t
         melanoma, 1128, 1129t
         osteogenic sarcoma, 1130, 1130t
         prostate cancer, 1129
         renal cell carcinoma, 1127, 1129t
         soft tissue sarcoma, 1127, 1128t
         testicular tumors, 1130
      surgical approach to, 1126, 1128f
      surgical indications for, 1126
      tumor doubling time in, 1125–1126,
         1126f, 1127f
   of renal adenocarcinoma, pathology of,
      279–281, 280f
   of salivary gland tumors, 539
   from soft tissue sarcoma, 1012–1013
   surgical oncology and, 130, 130t
Methotrexate, 154t, 155
   for gestational trophoblastic tumors,
      906, 907t
   for malignant fibrous histiocytoma,
      1041
   for osteogenic sarcoma, 1030–1031
MIBG, in endocrine neoplasm, 261–262
Micronutrients, 52–54
   calcium, 54
   folate, 54

selenium, 53–54
vitamin A and β-carotene, 52–53
vitamin C, 53
vitamin E, 53
Microsatellite instability, 31, 33, 194–195, 196f
Microscopy, conventional, 285, 286f
Mismatch repair, of DNA, 30–32, 31f
Mitomycin, 154t
Mitoxantrone, 154t
Mohs' micrographic surgery
for penile cancer, 795
for skin cancer, 486
squamous cell, 493
for skin neoplasms, 294
Molecular biology, 191–212
antitumor agent sensitivity and, 211–212, 211t
gene expression analysis in
mRNA, 197
protein, 198
gene isolation and analysis in, 193
genetic basis of cancer and, 198–203, 198f
DNA mismatch repair genes, 201, 203f
familial cancer syndromes, 201–203, 204t
oncogenes in, 199, 200f, 201t
proto-oncogenes in, 199, 200f, 201t
tumor suppressor genes in, 199–201, 202f
introduction to, 191
molecular pathology in, 203–208
DNA-based techniques for, 207–208, 207t
immunohistochemistry of, 205–206, 205t, 206f
Northern blotting in, 197–198, 197f
overview of, 191–193, 192f, 193f
prognostic indicators in, 208–211, 209t
breast cancer, 209
colorectal cancer, 209–210
immunologic, 210–211
melanoma, 210
Southern blotting in, 193–197, 194f
heterozygosity loss in, 194–195, 196f
microsatellite instability in, 194–195, 196f
mutation detection in, 195–197
polymerase chain reaction in, 195, 196f
Molecular probes, 293
Moles, vs. melanoma, 506t
Monomorphic adenoma, of parotid gland, 532
Mortality data, 4–5. See also Epidemiology

mRNA, analysis of, 197
Mucinous tumors
of breast, 962
ovarian epithelial, 921, 921f
Mucoepidermoid carcinoma
of lung, 559–560
of parotid gland, 532
Mucosa-associated lymphoid tissue (MALT), gastric lymphoma and, 634
Muir-Torre syndrome, 490
Multinodular fibrolamellar carcinoma, of liver, 345f
Multiple endocrine neoplasia (MEN), 204t, 347, 1064–1066
type 1, 1064–1065, 1064t
type 2 and familial, 1065–1066, 1066f
Multiple-gated acquisition (MUGA) scan, 132
Muscle-invasive disease
follow-up for, 788, 788t, 789t
treatment of, 783–787, 784f, 785t, 786t
Mutation
induction of, DNA damage and, 20–27
carcinogens in, 22–23, 23f
DNA damage in, 25–27, 26t
endogenous factors of, 23–25, 24f
exogenous factors of, 20–22, 21t
Southern blotting detection of, 195–197
Mutator phenotype, 19–20
Myasthenia gravis, thymectomy and, 580
Mycotoxins, 61
Myeloma
biomarkers for, 124t
pathology of, 375–376
Myxopapillary ependymoma, 314

Nasoenteric feeding, 475–476
Nasopharynx cancer, 525–527
clinical presentation of, 526, 526f
demographics of, 525–526
herpes virus and, 96
pathology and staging of, 305, 305f
prognostic factors of, 527
radiographic evaluation of, 526
staging of, 526, 526t
treatment of, 527
Neck cancers
biomarkers for, 124t
dissection for, 536–539
cervical lymph node metastasis, 537
cutaneous melanoma, 539
lymphatic anatomy in, 536–537, 536f
metastatic SCC with occult primary tumor, 539
neck dissections in, 536f, 537

nodal metastasis patterns in, 538, 538t, 539t
salivary gland carcinoma, 539
tracheoesophageal (level IV) lymph nodes, 539
fruits and vegetables on, 49
grains on, whole, 50
introduction to, 519, 520t
larynx and hypopharynx, 527–531
nasopharynx, 525–527 (See also Nasopharynx)
nuclear imaging techniques in, 242–245
parathyroid, 244–245
thyroid cancer, 242–244, 242f–244f
oral cavity, 519–525 (See also Oral cavity)
salivary gland tumors, 531–536 (See also Salivary gland tumors)
sarcomas, 1004
Neck node dissection
in melanoma, malignant, 516
in oral cavity cancer, 524–525
Neoplasms. See also specific types, e.g., Lung
biologic diversity of, 103–105, 104f
Nephrectomy
laparoscopy for, 404
for renal cell carcinoma
partial, 756–760, 757f–759f
radical, 755–756, 756f–757f
Nephroureterectomy, 764, 764f
Nerve sheath, tumors of
in mediastinum, 583–585, 583f, 584f
pathology and staging of, 321–322, 321f, 322f
Nervous system cancers. See also specific types, e.g., Brain cancer
neural tumors, histology of, 371–373, 374f
pathology and staging of, 309–322
anatomical description in, 309
brain, histologic classification of, 310, 312t
metastatic neoplasia, 318, 320f
nerve sheath tumors, 321–322, 321f, 322f
neuroepithelial tumors, with glial differentiation, 310–314
astrocytic, 310–312, 313f–315f
embryonal (medulloblastoma), 312t, 314, 317f, 318f
ependymomas, 313–314, 316f
meningothelial, 314–316, 319f
oligodendrogliomas, 312–313
pituitary gland, 319–320
primary tumors

Nervous system cancers (cont.)
    brain, histologic classification of, 310
    intraoperative diagnosis of, 309–310, 311t
    staging of, 310
    topographic classification of, 310
Neurilemmomas, of mediastinum, 583–585, 583f, 584f
Neuroblastoma, 585, 587f, 587t, 588f
    nuclear imaging techniques for, 262, 264f
    in pediatric patients, 381f, 382
Neuroepithelial tumors, pathology and staging of, 310–314
    astrocytic, 310–312, 313f–315f
    embryonal (medulloblastoma), 312t, 314, 317f, 318f
    ependymomas, 313–314, 316f
    meningothelial, 314–316, 319f
    oligodendrogliomas, 312–313
Neurofibromas, 321–322, 321f, 322f
    of mediastinum, 583–585
    of small intestine, 688
Neurofibromatosis, 420t
    genetic basis of, 204t
    neurofibromas and, mediastinal, 584
Neurofibrosarcomas, 985
    features of, 985
    genetic markers for, 207t
Neurogenic tumors. See also specific types, e.g., Neuroblastoma
    mediastinal, 332–333, 333f
Nilutamide, 154t
Nitrosamines
    on DNA, 24–25
    on esophageal carcinoma, 610
    nasopharynx cancer and, 525
    on pancreatic neoplasms, 637
N-Nitroso compounds, 62
Nitrous oxide, 432
Node. See Lymph node
Nodular regenerative hyperplasia, hepatic, 662
Non-Hodgkin's lymphomas, 598–600, 1105, 1106t
    genetic markers of, 207t
    laparoscopy for, 391–393, 393f
    large cell, 599–600
    lymphoblastic, 598–599
Nonsteroidal antiinflammatory drugs (NSAIDs)
    on arachidonic acid metabolism, 37–38
    on colon cancer, 701
Nonseminomatous tumors, 593–594, 593f
Northern blotting, 197–198, 197f
Norton-Simon hypothesis, 148

Nose cancer, 306–308, 306f
Nuclear imaging, 235–271
    of biliary neoplasms, extrahepatic, 248–250
        gallbladder cancer, 248–249, 249f
        large bowel neoplasms, 250, 251f
        small intestine neoplasms, 249–250, 250f
    for bladder cancer, 774, 775f
    of bladder carcinoma, 252–253, 253f
    of bone sarcomas, 260–261, 262f
    of breast cancer
        lymphoscintigraphy and sentinel node detection in, 257–260, 258f
        palliative therapies in, 260
    for cardiac risk factor assessment, 271
    CEA level in, 250–251
    of cervix cancer, 255, 256f
    of colorectal cancer, 250–251, 251f, 252f
    of endocrine neoplasms, 261–263, 263f, 264f
    of endometrium cancer, 255
    of esophageal cancer, 247
    future of, 271
    of gestational trophoblastic disease, 255
    of head and neck cancers, 242–245
        parathyroid, 244–245
        thyroid cancer, 242–244, 242f–244f
    introduction to, 235
    of kidney and ureter cancer, 251–252
    of lung neoplasms, 245–246
    of lymphoma, 265–268
    of mediastinal tumors, 246–247, 246f
    of mesothelioma, 263–265
    of metastatic cancer, 268–271
        brain, 268–269
        liver
            nonresectable, 270, 270f
            staging of, 268f, 269
        peritoneal, 270
        pleural effusions, 245–246
    methodologies in, 235–239
        detection systems in, 236–239, 237t, 239f
        instruments in, 236t
        molecular imaging in, 235, 238f
        nuclear medicine therapy in, 235–236
        radioisotopes in, 236t
        radiopharmaceuticals in, 237t
    of ovarian cancer, 255–256
    of pancreatic tumors, 247–248, 248f, 249f
    for penile cancer, 253
    of penis carcinoma, 253
    of prostate carcinoma, 254–255
    radiolabeled antibodies in, 256

    of skin neoplasms, 239–242, 241f
    of soft tissue sarcoma, 260
    of stomach cancer, 247
    of testis cancer, 255
    of uterine sarcoma, 255
    of vulval and vaginal neoplasms, 255
Nucleotide excision repair, 29–30, 30f
Nutrition, and cancer, 44–68, 473–477
    alcohol on, 57–59
        aerodigestive cancer, 57
        breast cancer, 57–58
        colorectal cancer, 58–59
        endometrial cancer, 58
        prostate cancer, 58
    body size on, 48
    cachexia etiology in, 473–475
    caloric intake on, 46–48
    chemoprevention research in, 62–66
        biomarkers, 64
        chemoprevention trials, 65–66
        dietary modification trials, 65
        preclinical and early phase clinical testing, 63–64, 63t
    dietary carcinogens on, 59–62, 60t
        food preparation and processing on, 60t, 61–62
        mycotoxins, 61
        naturally occurring, 59–61, 60t
    dietary fiber on, 50–52
    fat intake on, 46–48
    grains on, whole, 50
    historical overview of, 44–46
    introduction to, 44, 473
    micronutrients on, 52–54
        calcium, 54
        folate, 54
        selenium, 53–54
        vitamin A and β-carotene, 52–53
        vitamin C, 53
        vitamin E, 53
    nutritional support in
        clinical efficacy of, 476–477
        methods of, 475–476
    physical activity on, 48
    phytochemicals on, 54–57, 55t
        carotenoids, 56
        general considerations in, 54
        green tea polyphenols, 56–57
        indoles, 57
        isothiocyanates, 57
        organosulfur compounds, 56
        phytoestrogens, 56
    summary of, 68, 477
    trends and directions for, 66–68
    vegetables and fruits on, 48–50

Obstetric system, 354–363. *See also* Gynecologic neoplasms

Occupation
  on bladder cancer, 769
  as risk factor, 11, 16t, 20

Oligodendrogliomas, 312–313

Oltipraz, 36

Omega-3 fatty acids, 475, 476

Omental bursa stripping, 1153, 1153f

Omentectomy
  greater, 1150–1151, 1150f
  lesser, 1153, 1153f
  in ovarian cancer, 930, 930f

Oncogenes, 16, 199, 200f, 201t
  inactivation of, 181–183
  in mesothelioma, 1073
  in pancreatic cancer, 637–638, 638t
  viral, on tumor suppressor genes, 94t

Oncology, surgical, 123–135. *See also* Surgical oncology

Oophorectomy
  in colon cancer, 710–711
  laparoscopy for, 401–403, 401f, 420f

Opsoclonus-polymyclonus syndrome, 582

Oral cavity cancer, 519–525
  adjuvant radiation therapy for, 525
  cervical lymph nodes in, 524–525
  clinical aspects of, 520–522, 521f, 522f
  cryosurgery for, 441–442
  general considerations in, 519–520, 520t
  management of, 522–524, 523t, 524f
  pathology and staging for, 303–304, 303f, 304f
  second primary tumors and, 525
  staging of, 523t
  surgical approach for, 524f
  survival rates of, 8f

Oral contraceptives, 659, 661

Orchiectomy, 833

Organosulfur compounds, 56

Oropharynx cancer, 304–305

*Orpisthorchis viverrini*, 17

Osteogenic sarcomas, 1025–1033
  adjuvant therapy for, 1030–1033, 1032f
  clinical manifestations of, 1028
  diagnosis of, 1028
  histology of, 1028–1029
  introduction to, 1025–1028, 1026f, 1027f
  pulmonary metastases of, 1130, 1130t
  staging of, 1029
  treatment of, 1029–1030

Osteomyelitis, 378

Osteosarcoma, 1015–1025. *See also* Bone and joint tumors

Ovarian cancer, 911–942

adnexal mass management in, 917–918, 918f, 919f
biomarkers for, 124t, 916–917, 924t
borderline tumors in, 938–940
  adjuvant therapy for, 939
  epidemiology of, 938
  prognostic factors for, 938
  pseudomyxoma peritonei in, 939–940
  recurrent disease in, 939
  surgical treatment of, 938–939
in children and adolescents, 942
clinical presentation of, 914
epidemiology of, 911–912
fallopian tube cancer in, 942
genetics on, 912–913, 912t
germ cell tumors in, 940–941, 940t
  pathology of, 922–924
incidence of, 7f
laparoscopy for, 400–403, 401f, 402f
management algorithm for, 926f
nuclear imaging techniques for, 255–256
pathology of, 357, 360t, 918–926, 926f
  cell types in, 918–920, 919f
  epithelial tumors, 920–922
    carcinosarcomas, 922
    clear-cell, 922
    endometroid, 921–922, 921f
    mucinous, 921, 921f
    other, 922
    serous, 920–921, 920f, 921f
    transitional-cell, 922
  germ cell tumors, 922–924
    classification of, 922–923, 922t
    dermoid cyst, 923
    dysgerminoma, 923, 923f
    markers of, 924t
    other, 924
    primitive, 923
    teratoma, immature, 923
    yolk sac, 923, 923f
  metastatic, 925–926, 926f
  sarcomas, 925
  sex cord-stromal tumors, 924–925
pattern of spread, 914–915
peritoneal carcinoma in, primary, 941–942
prognostic factors for, 915–916
screening and prevention of, 913–914
sex cord-stromal tumors in, 941
  pathology of, 924–925
staging of, 357, 360t, 915, 915t
survival rates of, 8f
treatment principles for, 926
  chemotherapy in
    intraperitoneal, 937, 937t
    primary, 931–932
    salvage, 935
  cytoreduction in, secondary, 936
  follow-up after primary treatment in, 934–935
  inadequately staged patient in, 937
  radiation therapy in, 936–937
  reproductive conservation in, 937
  surgery in, disease management and, 926–931
    advanced stage, 928–931, 929t, 930f
    early stage, 927–928, 927t, 928f, 928t
    preoperative evaluation, 926–927
  surgery in, palliative, 936
  surgery in, second-look, 932–934
    findings of, 933–934, 933t, 934t
    outline of, 932–933
    patient management and, 934, 935f
    patient selection for, 933
    secondary debulking in, 934

Ovarian sex cord tumor with annular tubules (SCTAT), 925

Ovary, benign cysts of, 356–357, 356f

*p*53 gene, 26
  angiogenic and antiangiogenic factors and, 111, 114
  in breast cancer, 209, 956
  in gene therapy, 181–182
  in osteogenic sarcoma, 1028
  pancreatic neoplasms and, 638

Paclitaxel, 154t, 155–156
  for mesothelioma, 1085
  for ovarian cancer, 932

Paget's disease
  in breast cancer, 975
  in vulvar cancer, 857, 858f
    treatment of, 861–862

Pancreatic neoplasms, 637–656, 1060–1062, 1060t
  adjuvant treatment for, 650–654, 652t, 655f
  angiography for, 642–643
  biomarkers for, 124t
  clinical manifestations of, 638–639
  clinical staging of, 639–641, 639t, 640t, 641f–643f
  cryosurgery for, 447–448
  CT-resectable disease in, 641
  CT-unresectable disease in, 641
  endoscopy for, 422–425
    diagnosis and, 422–424, 423f
    therapy and, 424–425, 424t, 425t
  epidemiology of, 1060

Pancreatic neoplasms (cont.)
gastrinoma in, 1061–1062
general considerations in, 637–638, 638t
incidence of, 7f
insulinomas in, 1061–1062
laparoscopy for, 394–398, 395f–399f, 642–643
locally advanced, treatment for, 654–656
management algorithm for, 641, 642f
MEN-1 and, 1064–1065
metastatic and recurrent, treatment of, 656
nuclear imaging techniques for, 247–248, 248f, 249f
pancreaticoduodenectomy for, 643–646, 644f
gastric transection in, 645
infrapancreatic SMV exposure in, 643, 644f
Kocher maneuver in, 643–644, 644f
ligament of Treitz dissection in, 645–646, 646f
portal dissection in, 645, 645f
retroperitoneal dissection in, 646, 646f–648f
SMV resection and reconstruction in, 646–647, 649f–651f
specimen evaluation from, 647–649, 647t, 652f, 653f
pancreaticojejunostomy, 649, 655f
pathology and staging for, 340–347, 1060–1061, 1060t
ampullary tumors, 347, 347f
pancreatic neoplasms, 345f, 346–347, 347f
Whipple specimen in, 347
pretreatment diagnostic evaluation of, 639–641, 639t, 640t, 641f–643f
pylorus preservation in, 650
survival rates of, 8f
Pancreaticojejunostomy, 649, 655f
Pancreatitis, pancreatic neoplasms and, 637
Pancreatoscopy, 423–424
Pap smear, 884
Papillary carcinoma, of thyroid, 323–324, 323f
Papillary cystadenoma, of parotid gland, 532
Papillomas, of lung, 557
Papovaviridae viruses, 92–94
papillomaviruses, 92–93, 94f
polyomaviruses, 93–94
Paraganglioma, 308, 308f
Paranasal sinuses, 306–308, 306f

Parathyroid tumors, 1057, 1057t
of mediastinum, 600–601, 600f
MEN-1 and, 1064
MEN-2A and, 1064t, 1066
nuclear imaging techniques for, 244–245
Parotid gland tumors, 531–535
adjuvant therapy for, 535
benign tumors of, 531–532, 532f
clinical aspects of, 533–534, 534f
malignant tumors of, 532–533
mixed, 533
prognostic factors of, 535
surgical approach for, 534–535
Parotidectomy, 534–535
Pathology and staging, in surgical oncology, 279–385. See also specific cancers, e.g., Breast cancer
of bone and joint tumors, 373–379
benign, 377–379, 379f
biopsy in, 374–375
clinical assessment in, 373–374, 374t, 375f, 375t
malignant, 375–377, 376f–377f
of breast, 298–301, 299f
AJCC system in, 302t
diagnostic sampling in, 299
microscopy in, 300, 300f
pathologic evaluation of, 299
reporting in, 300–302, 300t
risk assessment in, 301, 301f
special tissue allocations in, 299–300
case examples in, 279–284
bone lymphoma, primary malignant, 282–284, 283f
breast carcinoma, 281–282, 282f
metastatic renal adenocarcinoma, 279–281, 280f
endocrine, 322–326
adrenal, 325
adrenal adenoma, 325
immunohistochemical stains for, 326, 326f
parathyroid, 324–325, 325f
pheochromocytoma, 325–326
thyroid, 322–324
fine-needle aspiration biopsy of, 322–324, 322f–324f
nodule of, 322
of gastrointestinal tract, 338–340, 340t, 341f–343f
of head and neck, 301–309
ear and temporal bone, 308, 308f
frozen sections in, 301
hypopharynx, 305
introduction to, 301

larynx, 305–306, 307t
nasopharynx, 305, 305f
nose and paranasal sinuses, 306–308, 306f
oral cavity, 303–304, 303f, 304f
oropharynx, 304–305
premalignant lesions in, 301–303
resection margins in, 301
salivary glands, 308–309, 309t
of hematolymphoid system, 364–369
clinical manifestation of, 365, 365t
general considerations in, 363–365, 364f
immunodeficiency, 367–369
surgical intervention requirement in, 365–367, 366f–368f, 367t, 368t
of liver, biliary tract, and pancreas, 340–347
ampullary tumors, 347, 347f
gallbladder and biliary tree inflammation in, 344
gallbladder and extrahepatic bile ducts, 345
hepatic tumors, benign, 340–343, 344f
hepatic tumors, malignant, 343–344, 344f, 345f
pancreatic neoplasms, 345f, 346–347, 347f
Whipple specimen in, 347
of lung and pleura, 334–338
carcinoid tumor, 336, 337f
carcinoma, 334–336, 335f, 336f
lung masses, 334
metastatic neoplasms, 337
pleurae, 337–338
tumor, benign, 337
tumor biopsy, 334, 334t
of male reproductive system, 350–354
benign prostatic hyperplasia, 351
intratubular germ cell neoplasia, 353–354, 353f, 354f, 355t
prostate and seminal vesicles, 350–351, 350f
prostatic intraepithelial neoplasia, 351–352, 351f, 352f
radical prostatectomy, 352–353
testes and paratesticular structures, 353
mediastinal, 326–334
anatomical definition in, 326
anatomical distribution in, 327, 327t, 328t
biopsy for, 327–328
clinicopathologic features in, 328–334

Castleman's disease, 334
cysts, 333–334
diffuse large B-cell lymphoma, 330
fibrosing mediastinitis, 334
germ cell tumors, 331–332, 332f
granulomatous lymphadenitis, 334
Hodgkin's lymphoma, 330
lymphoblastic lymphoma,
    330–331, 331f
neurogenic tumors, 332–333, 333f
thymoma, 328–330, 329f
of nervous system, 309–322
    anatomical description in, 309
    brain, histologic classification of,
        310, 312t
    metastatic neoplasia, 318, 320f
    nerve sheath tumors, 321–322, 321f,
        322f
    neuroepithelial tumors, 310–314
        astrocytic, 310–312, 313f–315f
        embryonal (medulloblastoma),
            312t, 314, 317f, 318f
        ependymomas, 313–314, 316f
        meningothelial, 314–316, 319f
        oligodendrogliomas, 312–313
    pituitary gland, 319–320
    primary tumors, intraoperative
        diagnosis of, 309–310, 311t
    staging of, 310
    topographic classification of, 310
of obstetric and gynecologic system,
    354–363
    adenocarcinoma, 363
    endometriosis, 363
    endometrium and cervix carcinoma,
        361–362
    endosalpingiosis, 363
    epithelial tumors, 357, 357t, 358f,
        358t
        microscopic appearance of,
            358–359, 358f, 359f, 360t
    fallopian tubes, 361
    female peritoneum, 363
    germ cell tumors, 361, 361f
    ovary
        benign cysts of, 356–357, 356f
        neoplasms of, 357, 360t
    sex cord-stromal tumors, 359–361
    uterine corpus and cervix, 361, 362f
    vagina and vulva, 362–363
pathology principles for, 284–293
    automated flow cytometry, 291–292
    autopsies, 288
    cytogenetics, 293, 293f
    cytology, 288–289, 289f, 290f
    gross examination, 285, 285f
    immunostains, 290, 291f, 292f

intraoperative methods, 285–288,
    287f, 288f
microscopy, 285, 286f
molecular probes, 293
stains, conventional special, 289–290
of pediatric patients, 379–385
    chest wall tumors, 380
    germ cell neoplasms, 382, 383f
    head and neck masses, 379–380,
        379f, 380f
    neuroblastoma, 381f, 382
    renal neoplasms, 380–382, 381f
    soft tissue neoplasms, 382–385, 383f,
        384f
practice recommendations in, 284
of skin lesions, 293–298
    cutaneous malignancies in, 295–298,
        296f, 297f, 298t
    cutaneous tumors in, 295, 295f
    Mohs' micrographic surgery in, 294
    surgical approach to, 294
of soft tissue tumors, 369–373
    definition of, 369
    evaluation and diagnosis in, 369–370
    histologic classification in, 370–373
        fibrohistiocytic lesions, 371, 372f
        fibrous lesions, 370–371, 371f, 372f
        lipomatous tumors, 371, 373f
        neural tumors, 371–373, 374f
        round cell sarcomas, 373
        smooth muscle tumors, 373
    pathobiology in, 369
    reporting in, 370
    specimens in, 370
surgeon and pathologist in, 279
of urologic system, 348–350
    kidney tumors
        benign, 348, 348f
        malignant, 348–349, 349f
    renal masses, 348
    urothelial tumors, 349–350, 350f
Whipple specimen in, 347
PCR. See Polymerase chain reaction
Pediatric patients, pathology and staging
    for, 379–385
    chest wall tumors, 380
    germ cell neoplasms, 382, 383f
    head and neck masses, 379–380, 379f,
        380f
    neuroblastoma, 381f, 382
    renal neoplasms, 380–382, 381f
    soft tissue neoplasms, 382–385, 383f,
        384f
Pelvic lymphadenectomy
    laparoscopy for, 405–407, 405f–407f
    for penile cancer, 803
Pelvic peritonectomy, 1153–1154, 1154f

Pelvis sarcoma, 997–998, 997f–999f
Penectomy
    partial, 795, 796f, 797f
    total, 795–799, 797f–799f
Penile cancer, 791–805. See also Urethral
    cancer
    clinical manifestations of, 791–792
    diagnosis of, 792
    etiology and incidence of, 791
    histology of, 792, 793f
    nuclear imaging techniques for, 253
    staging of, 792–794, 792t, 794t
    treatment of, 794–805
        adjuvant modalities in, 804
        general considerations in, 794
        locally advanced lesions, 795–799
            follow-up, 799
            penectomy, partial, 795, 796f,
                797f
            penectomy, total, 795–799,
                797f–799f
        low tumor burden, 794–795
        regional disease, 799–804
            anatomic considerations in, 800f,
                801
            ilioinguinal lymph node dissection
                in, 801–804, 801f–806f
            inguinal adenopathy in, 799–800
            inguinal lymph node dissection in,
                801, 801f
            node dissection in, 800–801, 800f
        therapeutic options summary in,
            805, 807f
Percutaneous acetic acid injection, for
    hepatocellular carcinoma, 669
Percutaneous biopsy, 220
Percutaneous ethanol injection, 228
    for hepatocellular carcinoma, 669
Percutaneous tumor ablation, 228–229
Pericardial effusions, malignant,
    1181–1184
    anatomy and physiology in, 1181
    clinical manifestation of, 1182
    diagnosis of, 1182–1183, 1182t
    introduction to, 1181
    nonsurgical therapeutic modalities for,
        1184
    prognosis for, 1184
    treatment of, 1183–1184, 1183f
Peritoneal malignancies, 1149–1176
    chemotherapy for, intraperitoneal,
        1156–1167
        background in, 1157–1158
        benefits of, prior, 1159–1160
        clinical evidence for, 1160–1161,
            1160f
        delivery of, 1164–1167

Peritoneal malignancies (cont.)
　heated intraoperative, 1164–1165,
　　1164t, 1165f, 1166f
　induction with 5–FU and
　　mitomycin C, 1166, 1167t
　oncologic emergency in, 1167
　postoperative 5–FU, early, 1165,
　　1166t
　postoperative abdominal lavage,
　　immediate, 1165, 1165t
　with reoperative surgery,
　　1166–1167
　patient selection for, 1161–1164
　　cancer index in, 1162–1163, 1163f
　　clinical assessment in, 1161
　　CT scan in, 1161–1162, 1162f
　　cytoreduction score in, 1163–1164
　　histopathology in, 1161
　　peritoneal-plasma barrier in,
　　　1158–1159, 1158f, 1158t
　　tumor cell entrapment in, 1159
　clinical results in, 1167–1174
　　alternative approaches, 1173
　　appendix cancer, 1168,
　　　1168f–1170f
　　ascites, 1167–1168
　　colon cancer peritoneal
　　　carcinomatosis, 1169–1170,
　　　1171f, 1172f
　　gastrointestinal cancer, 1173
　　patient care considerations,
　　　1173–1174
　　peritoneal seeding from gastric
　　　cancer, 1170, 1174f
　　phase II studies, 1173
　　primary peritoneal malignancy,
　　　1170, 1175f, 1176f
　　sarcomatosis, 1170, 1172f, 1173f
　ethical considerations in, 1174–1176
　introduction to, 1149
　in ovarian cancer, 941–942
　peritonectomy procedures in,
　　1149–1156
　　abdominal exposure, 1150–1151,
　　　1150f
　　antrectomy and gastric
　　　reconstruction, 1154–1155,
　　　1156f
　　chemotherapy tubes and drains,
　　　1155–1156, 1157f
　　cholecystectomy, 1153, 1153f
　　colon mobilization, left, 1154, 1156f
　　gastrectomy, total, 1155, 1156f
　　omental bursa stripping, 1153, 1153f
　　omentectomy, greater, 1150–1151,
　　　1150f
　　omentectomy, lesser, 1153, 1153f

　　pelvic peritonectomy, 1153–1154,
　　　1154f
　　peritoneal stripping
　　　from beneath left hemidiaphragm,
　　　　1151, 1151f
　　　from beneath right
　　　　hemidiaphragm, 1151–1152,
　　　　1152f
　　position and incision, 1150, 1150f
　　rationale for, 1149–1150
　　rectosigmoid colon resection, 1154,
　　　1154f
　　splenectomy, 1150–1151, 1150f
　　subphrenic peritonectomy, left, 1151,
　　　1151f
　　subphrenic peritonectomy, right,
　　　1152, 1152f
　　tumor stripping, from beneath right
　　　hemidiaphragm, 1152, 1152f
　　vaginal closure and low colorectal
　　　anastomosis, 1154, 1155f
Peritoneum, female, 363
Peutz-Jeghers syndrome, 420t
Pharmacokinetics, of chemotherapy
　　agents
　regional, 160–161
　systemic, 148–149, 149t
Pharynx cancer
　cryosurgery for, 443
　incidence of, 7f
　survival rates of, 8f
Phenacetin, 770
Pheochromocytoma, 262, 263f,
　　1059–1060
　multiple endocrine neoplasia and,
　　1065–1066, 1066f
　pathology and staging of, 325–326
Photoactivation, 464
Photodynamic therapy, 462–467
　application timing in, 465–466
　cellular injury mechanism and, 464–465
　current state of, 466–467
　limitations of, 466
　for mesothelioma, 1090
　on normal tissue, 465
　photoactivation in, 464
　photosensitizer toxicity in, 466
　for skin cancer, 486
　tumor detection and, 466
　in tumor localization, 464
Photosensitization, 462–464
　endogenous, 463–464, 463f
　exogenous, 462–463
　tumor localization and, 464
Phthalocyanines, 463
Physical activity, 48
Physical agents, carcinogenesis and, 78–87

　future trends in, 82–86, 85t
　historical overview of, 78–81
　　electromagnetic, 79
　　ionizing irradiation, 80–81
　　thermal, 78–79
　　ultraviolet, 79–80
　introduction to, 78
　ionizing irradiation in, molecular
　　mechanism of, 81–82, 83f, 84f,
　　84t, 86
　summary of, 86–87
Physical examination, 218–219
Phytochemicals, 54–57, 55t
　carotenoids, 56
　general considerations in, 54
　green tea polyphenols, 56–57
　indoles, 57
　isothiocyanates, 57
　organosulfur compounds, 56
　phytoestrogens, 56
Phytoestrogens, 56
Pituitary tumors, 1065
Placental site trophoblastic tumor, 905
Plasmacytoma, of lung, 561
Platinum compounds, 155
Pleomorphic adenoma, of parotid gland,
　　532
Pleurae cancer, 337–338, 339f7
Pleural effusions, malignant,
　　1177–1181
　anatomy and physiology in,
　　1177–1178
　clinical manifestation of, 1178
　diagnosis of, 1178–1179, 1178t
　　biochemical analysis in, 1179
　　chylothorax in, 1179
　　cytology in, 1179
　　fluid analysis in, 1178–1179
　　radiologic assessment in, 1178
　diagnostic procedures in, 1179
　introduction to, 1177
　prognosis for, 1181
　treatment of, 1180–1181, 1180f
Plexiform neurofibroma, 322f
Plummer-Vincent syndrome, esophageal
　　carcinoma and, 611
Pollution, 11–12
Polycyclic aromatic hydrocarbons (PAHs),
　　20, 62
　activation of, 22
Polymerase chain reaction (PCR)
　for melanoma, 208
　in PSA testing, 821
　in Southern blotting, 195, 196f
Polyp Prevention Trial, 65
Polyphenols, 56–57
Polyposis syndromes, 420t–421t

Polyps
  in colon cancer, 707
  of stomach, 623
Popliteal fossa sarcoma, 1004
Popliteal node dissection, 515–516
Population-based cancer registries, 4
Port site metastasis, laparoscopy and, 390–391, 404
Portal dissection, in pancreaticoduodenectomy, 645, 645f
Positron emission tomography (PET)
  for breast cancer, 259
  for colorectal cancer, 250–251, 251f, 252f
  for endocrine neoplasms, 262–264, 264f
  for esophageal cancer, 247
  for head and neck cancers, 242
  for hepatic adenoma, 660
  for hepatic metastases, 1137–1138
  for large bowel neoplasms, 250, 251f
  for lung neoplasms, 245–246
  for mesothelioma, 1077, 1077f
  for ovarian cancer, 255–256
  for pancreatic tumors, 247
  on patient management, 125t
  for prostate carcinoma, 254
  for rectal cancer, 732
  for small intestine neoplasms, 250, 250f
  for stomach cancer, 247
  for testis cancer, 255
Posterior compartment sarcoma, 1003–1004, 1005f, 1006f
Prednisone, 154t
Pregnancy
  breast cancer during, 975
  on ovarian cancer risk, 911
  partial molar, 904, 905f
Primitive neuroectodermal tumor, 383–385
Prostate cancer, 813–836
  advanced, 834–835
  alcohol on, 58
  biomarkers for
    genetic, 207t
    serum, 124t
  cryosurgery for, 448–449
  diagnosis of, 818–822
    prostate-specific antigen, 818–822, 818f, 819f, 819t
      age-specific PSA level, 819–820, 820t
      free and total PSA, 820, 821f, 821t, 823t
      hypersensitive measurement in, 820–821
      PCR techniques, 821

PSA density, 819
PSA velocity, 819, 819f
recurrent disease and, 820
summary for, 822
  epidemiology of, 813–816
    age in, 813
    detection methods in, 813, 814t
    dietary factors in, 815
    family history in, 814–815, 814t
    hormones in, 815
    race in, 814
    summary for, 815–816
    United States, 6–7, 6f, 7f
    vasectomy in, 815
    vitamins in, 815
  fat and caloric intake on, 47
  fat type on, 48
  fruits and vegetables on, 49–50
  grains on, whole, 50
  histology of, 816–818
    grading, cytologic, and nuclear features, 816, 817f
    other carcinomas, 817–818
    precursor lesions, 816, 816f
    summary for, 818
    surgical specimens, 816–817
    tumor volume, 816, 817f
  hormonal therapy for, 833–834
  hormone refractory disease in, 835–836, 836t
  introduction to, 813–836
  laparoscopy for, 404–405, 404t
  management of, 825
  nuclear imaging techniques for, 254–255
  observation of, 825–830
    general considerations in, 825–826
    preoperative preparation in, 827
    prostatectomy in
      perineal, 830, 831f
      radical, 826–827, 827f, 830, 832f
    PSA and DRE detection in, 826
    surgical procedure in, 827–830, 828f–831f
  pathology and staging for, 350–351, 350f, 823–824, 823t, 824f
  physical activity and body type on, 48
  pulmonary metastases of, 1129
  radiotherapy for, 830–833
    advanced stage of, 832–833, 835
    after prostatectomy, 833
    evaluation of, 832
    general considerations in, 830–832
    hormonal therapy with, 832
    salvage prostatectomy after, 833
  transrectal ultrasound for, 822–823, 822f, 823f

Prostate-specific antigen (PSA), 813, 814f, 818–822, 818f, 819f, 819t
  age-specific PSA level, 819–820, 820t
  free and total PSA, 820, 821f, 821t, 823t
  hypersensitive measurement in, 820–821
  PCR techniques, 821
  PSA density, 819
  PSA velocity, 819, 819f
  recurrent disease and, 820
  summary for, 822
Prostatectomy, 352–353
  perineal, 830, 831f
  radical, 826–827, 827f, 830, 832f
  radiotherapy and, 833
Prostatic intraepithelial neoplasia, 351–352, 351f, 352f
Prostatitis, granulomatous, 350–351, 350f
Protein kinase C, 34
Proto-oncogenes, 199, 200f, 201t
Proton beam therapy, 142
Protoporphyrin IX, 463–464, 463f
PSA testing. See Prostate-specific antigen (PSA)
Pseudomyxoma peritonei, 939–940
Pseudotumors, of lung, 557
Pulmonary blastoma, 561
Pulmonary metastases, 561–565, 1125–1131. See also Lung neoplasms
  adjuvant therapy for, 563–564
  clinical presentation of, 561–562, 1125
  conclusions for, 564–565, 565t
  diagnosis of, 1125
  future management directions for, 1130–1131
  historical review of, 561
  introduction to, 1125
  other considerations for, 564
  pretreatment workup for, 562, 562t
  results in, 1126–1130
    breast carcinoma, 1129
    colorectal carcinoma, 1128, 1129t
    gynecologic cancers, 1129–1130
    head and neck tumors, 1128, 1130t
    melanoma, 1128, 1129t
    osteogenic sarcoma, 1130, 1130t
    prostate cancer, 1129
    renal cell carcinoma, 1127, 1129t
    soft tissue sarcoma, 1127, 1128t
    testicular tumors, 1130
  surgical approach to, 564, 1126, 1128f
  surgical indications for, 1126
  treatment of, 562–563
  tumor doubling time in, 1125–1126, 1126f, 1127f

Pulmonary risk, laparoscopy assessment of, 133–134
Pulsatility index, of ovarian adnexal masses, 917
Purine antimetabolites, 155
Purpurins, 462
Pyelogram, intravenous, 773, 774f, 775f
Pyrimidine antimetabolites, 155

Race
    on carcinoma, 484t
    on prostate cancer, 814
Radiation exposure
    on bladder cancer, 770
    on breast cancer, 953
Radiation therapy, 137–144
    for adenoid cystic carcinoma, 559
    biology of, 137–141, 139f–141f
    for bladder cancer, 783–784
    for bone sarcoma, 1025
    for breast cancer, 960–961, 960t, 965–966, 966t
    for cervical cancer, 886–888
    clinical results of, 137, 138t
    for colon cancer, 715
    combined modality therapy with, 143–144
    for esophageal carcinoma, 617–618, 618t
    for Ewing's sarcoma, 1037–1039
    for extrahepatic biliary tract
        distal, 681
        proximal, 679
    for fallopian tube cancer, 900
    for Hodgkin's lymphoma, 598
    for hypopharynx cancer, 530–531
    for larynx cancer, 529–530
    for lung neoplasms, 548–549
    for mesothelioma, 1086
    nutritional support for, 477
    for pancreatic neoplasms, 650–654, 652t, 655f
    for parotid gland tumors, 535
    for penile cancer, 795
    for prostate cancer, 830–833
        advanced stage of, 832–833, 835
        after prostatectomy, 833
        evaluation of, 832
        general considerations in, 830–832
        hormonal therapy with, 832
        salvage prostatectomy after, 833
    for seminomas, 593
    for soft tissue sarcomas, 1011
    for stomach neoplasms, 631–632
    treatment methods of, 141–143, 142f–144f

for uterine cancer, 891
for vaginal cancer, 875–877
Radicality, 219–220
Radiofrequency ablation, for hepatocellular carcinoma, 669
Radioimmunodetection, for rectal cancer, 731
Radioiodine scans, 243–244, 243f, 244f
Radiology
    for bone sarcomas, 1016, 1028
    for chondrosarcoma, 1033, 1033f
    for Ewing's sarcoma, 1036, 1036f
    interventional, 227–229
        chemoembolization of liver in, 227–228
        percutaneous ethanol injection in, 228
        percutaneous tumor ablation in, 228–229
        post-interventional imaging in, 229–230, 230f–232f
    for renal cell carcinoma, 754–755
Radon, 21–22
Reactive oxygen species (ROS), 23–24
    antioxidant micronutrients on, 52
Recklinghausen's disease, 584
Rectal cancer, 725–739. See also Colorectal cancer
    diagnosis of, 727, 727f
    epidemiology of, 725–726
        United States, 6f, 7, 7f
    imaging techniques for, 728–732
        CT, 728–729, 728f, 729f
        endorectal ultrasound, 729–731, 730f, 731t
        MRI, 731, 731f
        PET, 732
        radioimmunodetection, 731
    incidence of, 7f
    pathologic staging and prognosis for, 726–727
    survival rates of, 8f
    treatment of, 732–739
        adjuvant therapy, 736–738
        locally recurrent, 738–739
        surgery in, 732–736
            abdominoperineal resection, 733
            general considerations for, 732–733, 732f
            local excision, 735–736
            sphincter-saving resections, 733–735
Rectosigmoid colon resection, 1154, 1154f
Renal. See Kidney; Renal cancer
Renal cancer. See also Renal cell carcinoma
    adenocarcinoma metastasis, 279–281, 280f

genetic markers for, 207t
incidence of, 7f
laparoscopy for, 404
nuclear imaging for, 251–252
pathology and staging for, 348–350, 349f
    kidney tumors, benign, 348, 348f
    kidney tumors, malignant, 348–349, 349f
    renal masses, 348
    urothelial tumors, 349–350, 350f
in pediatric patients, 380–382, 381f
survival rates of, 8f
transitional cell carcinoma, 762–766
    diagnosis of, 763
    etiology of, 762
    management of, 763–764
    nephroureterectomy for, 764, 764f
    pathology and grade of, 762–763
    staging of, 763
    surgery for, conservative, 765–766, 765f
    ureterectomy for, distal, 764–765, 765f
Renal cell carcinoma, 348–349, 349f, 753–762. See also Renal cancer
    clinical presentation of, 753
    cytogenetics of, 753–754
    histopathology of, 753–754
    pulmonary metastases of, 1127, 1129t
    radiographic imaging of, 754–755
    staging of, 754
    surgical treatment of, 755
        general considerations in, 755
        nephrectomy
            partial, 755–756, 756f–757f
            radical, 755–756, 756f–757f
        with vena cava involvement, 760–762, 760f
            cardiopulmonary bypass in, 761–762, 761f
            contraindications for, 762
            general considerations for, 760–761
            venous bypass in, 761, 762f
Reproductive variables, as risk factor, 11
Resection arthroplasty, for bone sarcomas, 1025, 1025f
Retinoblastoma
    genetic markers for, 204t, 207t
    osteogenic sarcoma and, 1027–1028
Retinoids
    as differentiation agents, 36
    for lung neoplasms, stage I, 548
    for skin cancer, 486, 498
Reverse transcriptase PCR, 197–198, 197f
Revised European American Lymphoma (REAL) system, 598

Rhabdomyoma, of mediastinum, 603
Rhabdomyosarcoma, 383–385, 384f
    features of, 985
Risk factor(s), 10–13
    diet, 11
    genetics, 12–13
    hormones, 11
    medicines and medical procedures, 12
    occupation, 11
    pollution, 11–12
    reproductive variables, 11
    sexual behavior, 11
    sunlight, 12
    tobacco, 10–11
    viruses, 12
Rotationplasty, 1021–1023, 1022f
Round cell sarcomas, histology of, 373

Sacrococcygeal teratoma, 383, 383f
Sacrum sarcoma, 998–999
Salivary gland tumors, 531–536
    metastasis of, 539
    parotid gland, 531–535
        adjuvant therapy for, 535
        benign tumors of, 531–532, 532f
        clinical aspects of, 533–534, 534f
        malignant mixed tumors of, 533
        malignant tumors of, 532–533
        prognostic factors of, 535
        surgical approach for, 534–535
    pathology and staging for, 308–309,
        309t
    submandibular gland neoplasms,
        535–536
Sarcoma botryoides, 872, 873f
Sarcomas
    of bone, 1015–1044 (See also under
        Bone and joint tumors)
    chemotherapy for, intraarterial, 162,
        162f
    in colon cancer, 717
    isolated limb perfusion for, 165–168,
        165f–168f, 167t
    limb amputation and, 127
    of lung, 560–561, 560t
    metastasis frequency in, 131t
    of small intestine, 689–690
    of soft tissue, 983–1013 (See also Soft
        tissue sarcomas)
    uterine, 892
    in vaginal cancer, treatment of, 877
    in vulvar cancer, 857, 858
        treatment of, 869
Sarcomatosis, peritoneal malignancies
        and, 1170, 1172f, 1173f
Satellitosis, in melanoma, 512
Scapula sarcomas, 1006

Schwannoma, 321–322, 321f, 322f
    of mediastinum, 583–585, 583f, 584f
    of small intestine, 688
Sciatic nerve sarcoma, 988f
Sclerosing hemangiomas, 557
Selenium, 53–54
Seminal vesicles, 350–351, 350f
Seminomas, 593, 593f
    histology of, 841
Sentinel lymph node
    biopsy of
        lymphoscintigraphy in, 240–241
        for melanoma, malignant, 297–298,
            510–512, 511f, 512t, 513f
        in breast cancer, 967–969, 968t
        lymphoscintigraphy detection,
            257–260, 257t, 258f
Sepsis, laparoscopy in, 134–135, 134t
Serous tumors, ovarian epithelial,
        920–921, 920f, 921f
Sertoli-Leydig tumor, 359–361, 925
Serum tumor markers, 123, 124t
Sex cord-stromal tumors
    biomarkers for, 917
    in ovarian cancer, 941
    pathology and staging in, 359–361
Sexual behavior
    anoreceptive intercourse, 745
    penile reconstruction for, 799
    as risk factor, 11
Sigmoidoscopy, 421
Signal transduction, 17
    tumor promoters and, 33–35, 34f, 34t
Single-strand conformational
        polymorphism (SSCP), 196–197
Sinonasal polyps, 306, 306f
Skin color, 485
Skin neoplasms, 483–498
    basal cell carcinoma, 494–498
        clinical manifestations of, 494–495,
            495f, 496f
        diagnosis of, 495
        etiology and pathogenesis of, 494
        histology of, 496, 496f, 497f
        modes of spread of, 494
        staging of, 496
        treatment of, 497–498, 497f
    cryosurgery for, 438–440
        vs. other therapy, 440
        results in, 439–440
        selection criteria in, 439
        technique in, 439
    etiology of, 483–485
        external factors in, 12, 21, 79,
            483–485
        host factors in, 485
    incidence and epidemiology of, 483

    introduction to, 483
    lymphoscintigraphy for, 239–242, 241f
    melanoma, malignant, 505–517 (See
        also Melanoma)
    pathology and staging for, 293–298
        cutaneous malignancies in, 295–298,
            296f, 297f, 298t
        cutaneous tumors in, 295, 295f
        Mohs micrographic surgery in, 294
        surgical approach to, 294
    precancerous lesions and carcinoma in
        situ, 486–491
        actinic keratosis, 486–488
            clinical manifestations of, 487,
                487f
            general considerations for,
                486–487
            histology of, 487, 487f
            treatment of, 487–488, 488f
        Bowen's disease, 488–489, 488f, 489f
        erythroplasia of Queyrat, 489, 489f
        introduction to, 486
        keratoacanthoma, 489–491
            clinical manifestations of, 490,
                490f
            diagnosis of, 490
            general considerations for,
                489–490
            histology of, 490–491, 490f
            treatment of, 491
        squamous cell (epidermoid
            carcinoma), 491–494
            clinical manifestations of, 492–493,
                492f, 493t
            diagnosis of, 493
            etiology of, 491
            histology of, 493, 493f
            modes of spread of, 491–492
            pathogenesis of, 491
            staging of, 493
            treatment of, 493–494
        treatment methods for, 485–486,
            485t
Skipper-Schabel model, 148
Small cell carcinoma
    of lung, 556
    of parotid gland, 533
Small intestine neoplasms, 685–693
    anatomy in, 685–686
    benign, 687–688
    diagnosis of, 687
    epidemiology of, 686, 686t
    etiology of, 686–687, 686t
    introduction to, 685
    malignant, 688–693
        adenocarcinoma, 688–689, 689t
        carcinoid tumor, 690–691

Small intestine neoplasmas *(cont.)*
  lymphoma, 691–693, 692t,
      1109–1110
    immunoproliferative, 1110
  sarcoma, 689–690
  nuclear imaging techniques for,
      249–250, 250f
Smoking. *See* Tobacco
Smooth muscle tumors, 373
Soft tissue sarcomas, 983–1014. *See also*
      Soft tissue tumors
  chemotherapy for, adjuvant, 1012
  diagnosis of, 986
  histologic subtypes of, 985–986
  incidence of, 983
  modality integration for, 1009–1010
  nuclear imaging techniques for, 260
  pathological classification of, 983, 984t
  presentation and initial workup of, 984
  prognostic factors for, 984
  pulmonary metastases of, 1127, 1128t
  recurrence of, 1012–1013
  retroperitoneal, 1011–1012
  sites of, 984, 984t
  staging of, 984–985, 985t
  surgical treatment of
    abdominal wall, 989–990
    amputation in, 988, 1006–1010
      forequarter, 1009–1010, 1010f
      hemipelvectomy, 1006–1009,
          1008f, 1009f
      hip disarticulation, 1006–1009,
          1008f, 1009f
    bowel mesentery, 993–994, 994f
    chest wall, 988–989, 989f, 990f
    epigastric region, 993
    flank, 992–993, 992f, 993f
    general considerations in, 986–988,
        987f
    lower extremities, 999–1004,
        999–1006
      anterior compartment,
          1001–1002, 1002f, 1003f
      below knee, 1004
      buttocks, 1002
      groin, 1001
      iliac fossa, 999–1001, 999f–1001f
      medial compartment, 1002, 1004f
      popliteal fossa, 1004
      posterior compartment,
          1003–1004, 1005f, 1006f
    lower quadrants, 994–997, 994f–996f
    pelvis, midline, 997–998, 997f–999f
    sacrum, 998–999
    sciatic nerve, 988f
    upper extremities, 1004–1006
      arm, 1006, 1007f

  forearm, 1006
  hand, 1006
  lower neck, 1004
  scapula, 1006
  upper quadrants, 990–992, 991f, 992f
  in vaginal cancer, 871
Soft tissue tumors. *See also* Soft tissue
      sarcomas
  pathology and staging of, 369–373
    definition of, 369
    evaluation and diagnosis in, 369–370
    histologic classification in, 370–373
      fibrohistiocytic lesions, 371, 372f
      fibrous lesions, 370–371, 371f, 372f
      lipomatous tumors, 371, 373f
      neural tumors, 371–373, 374f
      round cell sarcomas, 373
      smooth muscle tumors, 373
    pathobiology in, 369
    reporting in, 370
    specimens in, 370
  in pediatric patients, 382–385, 383f,
      384f
Solution effects, 431
Southern blotting, 193–197, 194f
  heterozygosity loss in, 194–195, 196f
  microsatellite instability in, 194–195,
      196f
  mutation detection in, 195–197
  polymerase chain reaction in, 195, 196f
Soy, 37
Spinal cord compression, 833
Spindle pole body checkpoint, 33
Splenectomy, 1150–1151, 1150f
  in hematolymphoid disorders, 365
  laparoscopic, 391–393, 392f–393f
  in ovarian cancer, 931
Splenomegaly, 366f
Squamous cell carcinoma, 491–494
  in bladder cancer, 778
  clinical manifestations of, 492–493,
      492f, 493t
  in colon cancer, 717–718
  cryosurgery for, 438–439
  diagnosis of, 493
  of ear, 308
  of esophagus
    epidemiology of, 610
    prevalence and incidence of, 609
  etiology of, 491
  histology of, 296, 297t, 493, 493f
  of hypopharynx, 305
  of larynx, 306
  of maxillary sinus, 308
  metastasis frequency in, 131t
  modes of spread of, 491–492
  of mouth, 304

  of oropharynx, 304–305
  pathogenesis of, 491
  of penis, 792, 793f
  staging of, 493
  treatment of, 493–494
  in vaginal cancer, 871
    prognostic factors for, 874
  in vulvar cancer, 856, 858, 861–869
    distant metastatic, 868
    recurrent, 868
    T1, 862–863, 863f
    T2, 863–866
      additional treatment, 866
      conservative treatment, 863–864
      inguinofemoral lymphadectomy,
          864–866, 864f, 865f
      radical vulvectomy, 864–866, 864f,
          865f
      surgical defect closure, 866, 867f,
          868f
    T3 and T4, 866–868
Squamous papillomas, of larynx, 305–306
Staging. *See* Diagnosis and staging;
      specific cancers, e.g., Testicular
      cancer
Stains
  conventional special, 289–290
  for endocrine neoplasms, 326, 326f
  immunostains in, 290, 291f, 292f
Steroid cell tumors, ovarian, 925
Stomach neoplasm(s), 623–635
  adenocarcinoma in, 623–632
    diagnosis of, 626
    molecular biology of, 625
    multimodal therapy for, 630–632
    pathological findings and staging of,
        624–625, 625t, 634t
    risk factors of, 624
    surgical planning for, 626–628, 626t,
        627f
    surgical technique for, 628–630,
        628f–633f
  biomarkers for, 124t
  carcinoid tumors in, 634–635
  endoscopy for
    diagnosis, 414–416, 415f, 416f
    screening, 416
    therapy, 416
  gastric lymphoma, 1107–1109
    clinical presentation of, 1108, 1108t
    diagnosis and staging of, 1108, 1108t
    etiology of, 1108
    treatment and outcome of,
        1108–1109, 1109f
  incidence of, 7f
  introduction to, 623
  laparoscopy for, 394, 394t

lymphoma in, 632–634, 633t, 634t
mesenchymal tumors in, 634
metastatic tumors in, 635
nuclear imaging techniques for, 247
peritoneal seeding from, 1170, 1174f
polyps in, 623
survival rates of, 8f
Stop-flow technique, 170–171, 170f, 171f
Stromal cells, 109
Subependymomas, 314
Submandibular gland neoplasms, 535–536
Sugar tumors, 557
Sun-reactive skin typing system, 485
Sunburn, 483–485
Sunlight, 12, 21, 483–485
Superior mesenteric artery, pancreatic
        neoplasms and, 639–641, 640f
Superior mesenteric vein, in
        pancreaticoduodenectomy,
        646–647, 649f–651f
Surgical malignancies, gene therapy for,
        181–187. See also under Surgical
        oncology
Surgical oncology, 123–135. See also under
        specific sites, e.g., Lung
    cryosurgery and, 438
    diagnosis and staging in (See also
            Diagnosis and staging)
        of solid tumor, 217–221
            biopsy in, 220–221
            curative surgery principles in,
                219–220
            history and physical examination
                in, 218–219
            role of, 217–218, 218f
    future of, 131–132
    gene therapy for, 181–187
        cell type-specific regulatory elements
            in, 186–187
        delivery systems in, 184–186
            non-viral vectors, 186
            viral vectors, 184–185, 185t
        expression control in, 186, 186f
        future directions in, 187
        introduction to, 181
        present status in, 187
        strategies in, 181–184, 182t
            drug-resistance genes, 184
            drug-sensitivity genes, 183–184,
                183f
            immunotherapy by gene transfer,
                182–183, 182f
            oncogene inactivation, 181–182
            tumor suppressor gene defect
                correction, 181–182
    laparoscopy and, diagnostic,
            132–135

cardiac risk assessment in, 132–133
    elderly patient in, 135
    endocrine disorders in, 134
    invasive sepsis in, 134–135,
        134t
    pulmonary risk assessment in,
        133–134
for lymphoma management,
        1103–1111
for lymphoma management,
        introduction to, 1103
for lymphoma management, primary
        gastrointestinal, 1105–1111
    esophageal, 1111
    gastric, 1107–1109
        clinical presentation of, 1108,
            1108t
        diagnosis and staging of, 1108,
            1108t
        etiology of, 1108
        treatment and outcome of,
            1108–1109, 1109f
    immunoproliferative
        small-intestinal, 1110
    introduction to, 1105–1107, 1107t
    large bowel, 1110–1111
    small-bowel, 1109–1110
for lymphoma management, systemic,
        1103–1105
    Hodgkin's disease, 1103–1105
        clinical presentation of, 1103,
            1104t
        diagnosis of, 1103–1104, 1104t
        staging of, 1104–1105, 1104t
        treatment of, 1105
    non-Hodgkin's, 1105, 1106t
pathology and staging in, 125–126,
        279–385 (See also Pathology
        and staging)
preoperative assessment in, 123–125,
        124t, 125f, 125t
surgical therapy in, 126–130, 131t
    combination modalities and,
        126–128, 127t
    cytoreductive, 130
    local vs. systemic cancer and,
        129–130
    for metastatic disease, 130, 130t
    palliative, 130
    primary, 126
    tumor resection principles in, 128,
        129t
Survival rates. See also Epidemiology of
        cancer, 8, 8f
Sympathetic ganglia tumors, 585,
        586f–589f, 587t
Synovial sarcoma, 985

Tamoxifen, 154t
    for breast cancer, 969–970
    on breast cancer, 35, 37
Taxanes, 155–156
T-cell leukemia virus type 1, 98
Temporal bone cancer, 308, 308f
Teniposide, 156
Teratomas
    of germ cell, 591–593, 592f
    pathology of, 382
Testicular cancer, 839–850
    biomarkers for, 124t
    clinical manifestations of, 839
    diagnosis of, 839–840
    etiology of, 839
    histology of, 841
    introduction to, 839
    nonseminoma in, 844–850
        bulky retroperitoneal disease,
            848–849
        RPLND following chemotherapy in,
            849, 850f
        RPLND modifications for, 849–850
        stage I, 845–847
            RPLND for, 845–846, 845f, 846f
            RPLND for, modified-template,
                846–847, 847f
        stage II, 847, 848f
            chemotherapy for, 847–848,
                848f
        widely metastatic, 849
    nuclear imaging techniques for,
            255
    orchiectomy for, radical inguinal, 840,
            841, 841f, 842f
    pathology and staging for, 353,
            841–843, 842t, 843t
    preoperative evaluation of, 840
    pulmonary metastases of, 1130
    seminoma in, 843–844
        low-stage, 843
        stage II, 843–844
        stage III, 843–844
        treatment of, 843, 844f
    summary of, 850
Texaphyrins, 463
Thecomas, ovarian, 924–925
Thermal burns, 78–79
Thermocouples, 437
Thiotepa, 154t
Thoracentesis, for mesothelioma, 1078,
        1079f
Thoracotomy
    for mesothelioma, 1078
    skin incision for, 582f
Three-field lymphadenectomy, for
        esophageal carcinoma, 615–617

Thymic neoplasms, 576–581, 577t
  hamartomatous lesions, 576
  nuclear imaging of, 246–247, 246f
  thymic epithelial, 577–581, 578f, 579f, 579t, 580t
    myasthenia gravis and thymectomy in, 580
    thymic carcinoma in, 580–581
    thymomas, 577–580, 578f, 579f, 579t, 580t
  thymolipoma, 576
Thymolipoma, 576
Thymoma, pathology and staging for, 328–330, 329f
Thymomas, 577–580, 578f, 579f, 579t, 580t
Thyroid cancer, 1055–1057
  biomarkers for, 124t
  clinical presentation of, 1055–1056, 1056f
  epidemiology of, 1055
  of mediastinum, 601–602, 602t
  multiple endocrine neoplasia and, 1065
  nuclear imaging techniques for, 242–244, 242f–244f
  pathology and staging of, 322–324
    fine-needle aspiration biopsy of, 322–324, 322f–324f
    nodule of, 322
  risk factors for, 1055
  treatment and outcomes of, 1056–1057, 1056f, 1056t
  types of, 1056, 1056t
Tissue inhibitors of metalloproteinases (TIMPs), 109
Tobacco
  β-carotene trials and, 66
  on bladder cancer, 770, 770t
  on colon cancer, 698
  on esophageal carcinoma, 610
  on lung cancer, 545
  on oropharyngeal cancer, 519, 520, 525
  on pancreatic neoplasms, 637
  as risk factor, 10–11, 15, 20–21, 23
  on urinary bladder cancer, 20–21
Tongue cancer. See also Oral cavity cancer
  cryosurgery for, 442
Tonsils, 304–305
Topoisomerase inhibitors, 156
Topotecan, 154t
  for ovarian cancer, 935
Toxicity, of chemotherapy agents, 149–150
Tracheobronchial tumors
  cryosurgery for, 443
  laser therapy for, 443
Transcatheter arterial chemoembolization (TACE), 669

Transforming growth factor beta 2, 105–106
  immunosuppression and, 210–211
Transhiatal esophagectomy, 614
Transitional cell carcinoma, 762–766
  diagnosis of, 763
  etiology of, 762
  management of, 763–764
  nephroureterectomy for, 764, 764f
  ovarian epithelial, 922
  pathology and grade of, 762–763
  pharmaceutic agents and, 770
  of prostate, 817–818
  staging of, 763
  surgery for, conservative, 765–766, 765f
  ureterectomy for, distal, 764–765, 765f
Transrectal ultrasound, 822–823, 822f, 823f
Transthoracic esophagectomy, 614
Transurethral prostatic resection (TURP), 351
Trophoblastic tumors, biomarkers for, 124t
Tumor(s). See also Carcinogenesis; specific types, e.g., Lung neoplasms
  angiogenesis of, 110–114, 112f, 113f
    angiogenic and antiangiogenic regulation in, 111–114, 111f, 113f
    microenvironment regulation of, 114
  biomarkers for
    genetic, 207–209, 207t, 209t
    melanoma, 210
    ovarian cancer, 916–917
    serum, 123, 124t
  chemotherapy for
    regional, 159–176 (See also under Chemotherapy)
    systemic, 147–157 (See also under Chemotherapy)
  localization of, photosensitization and, 464
  surgical techniques for (See also Surgical oncology)
  resection of, 128, 129t
  solid, diagnosis and staging in, 217–221
    biopsy in, 220–221
    curative surgery principles in, 219–220
    history and physical examination in, 218–219
    role of, 217–218, 218f
Tumor-associated globulin (TAG), 131
Tumor cell heterogeneity, 19–20
Tumor growth factor-b, 37

Tumor necrosis factor (TNF), cachexia and, 474–475
Tumor promoters, 17–18, 18f
  signal transduction and, 33–35, 34f, 34t
Tumor suppressor genes
  defect correction for, 181–183
  in mesothelioma, 1073
  molecular biology of, 199–201, 202f
  in pancreatic cancer, 637–638, 638t
  viral oncogenes on, 94t
Turcot syndrome, 420t
Tylosis, esophageal carcinoma and, 611

Ulcerative colitis, 701
Ultrasound, 223–224
  for bladder cancer, 773–774
  in cryosurgery, 437, 438f
  endorectal, for rectal cancer, 729–731, 730f, 731t
  endoscopic
    for colorectal tumors, 417, 417f
    for esophageal tumors, 411–413
      staging of, 612–613
    for gastric cancer, 416
    for pancreatic and biliary cancer, 423–424
  for extrahepatic biliary tract, proximal, 674, 675f
  for focal nodular hyperplasia, 661f
  for hepatic metastases, 1136, 1136f
  for kidney and ureter cancer, 251–252
  in laparoscopy, 391
  for ovarian adnexal mass, 917, 918f, 919f
  for prostate cancer, 822–823, 822f, 823f
Ultraviolet light, 12, 21, 79–80, 483–485
Upper extremities, sarcomas of, 1004–1006
  arm, 1006, 1007f
  forearm, 1006
  hand, 1006
  lower neck, 1004
  scapula, 1006
Ureter cancer
  nuclear imaging for, 251–252
  transitional cell carcinoma, 762–766
    diagnosis of, 763
    etiology of, 762
    management of, 763–764
    nephroureterectomy for, 764, 764f
    pathology and grade of, 762–763
    staging of, 763
    surgery for, conservative, 765–766, 765f
    ureterectomy for, distal, 764–765, 765f
Ureterectomy, 764–765, 765f

Urethral cancer, 805–810. *See also* Penile cancer
  anatomy and histology of, 805
  presentation, diagnosis, and staging of, 805–806, 808t
  treatment of, 807–810
    female, 807–809, 810
    male, 809–810
Urinalysis, for bladder cancer, 772–773
Urinary bladder. *See* Bladder
Urologic system neoplasms, 753–766.
        *See also* Bladder cancer; Renal cancer; Ureter cancer; specific types, e.g., Renal cell carcinoma
Urothelial tumors
  etiology of, 762
  pathology and staging for, 349–350, 350f
Uterine cancer, 888–892
  clinical manifestations of, 888–889, 889f
  cryosurgery for, 450–451
  diagnosis and evaluation of, 889–890
  incidence of, 6f, 7f, 888
  nuclear imaging techniques for, 255
  pathology and staging in, 361, 362f
  pulmonary metastases of, 1130
  risk factors for, 888, 888t
  staging of, 890, 890t
  survival rates of, 8f
  treatment of, 890–892
    uterine sarcoma, 892

Vaccine, Bacille Calmette-Guérin (BCG), 513
Vaccinia virus, 185
Vaginal cancer, 869–878
  anatomy in, 870, 871f
  clinical presentation of, 871–872, 872f, 873f
  epidemiology of, 870
  follow-up and survival for, 878
  histology of, 871
  introduction to, 869–870
  natural history in, 871
  nuclear imaging techniques for, 255
  pathology and staging of, 362–363, 873–874, 873t, 874t
  patterns of spread in, 871
  prognostic factors in, 874
  summary of, 878
  treatment of, 874–878
    nonsquamous cell, 877–878

  preinvasive disease, 874, 875f
  squamous cell, 875–877
    complications in, 876
    recurrent, 876–877
    stage I, 875–876
    stage II, 876
    stage III, 876
Vaginal closure, 1154, 1155f
Vaginal intraepithelial neoplasia (VAIN), 871
Vanillylmandelic acid, 582
Vascular endothelial cell growth factor (VEGF), 11, 110, 114
Vasectomy, 815
Vegetables, 48–50
Vegetarian diet, 52
Venous bypass technique, for renal cell carcinoma, 761, 762f
Verrucous carcinoma, 304, 304f
  histology of, 792, 793f
  in locally advanced penile cancer, 795
Vica alkaloids, 156
Videothoracoscopy, 1078, 1079f
Vinblastine, 154t, 156
Vincristine, 154t, 156
Vinorelbine, 154t, 156
Viruses, 92–98, 93t
  in head and neck cancer, 519
  hepatitis, 94–95
  herpes, 95–98
    Burkitt's lymphoma, 95–96
    Epstein-Barr virus, 95, 95t, 96f
    Hodgkin's disease, 96
    human herpes virus 8, 97–98
    lymphoproliferative disease, 96–97
    nasopharyngeal carcinoma, 96
    x-linked lymphoproliferation, 97, 97t
  historical overview of, 92
  human immunodeficiency virus (HIV), 1019
  human T-cell leukemia virus type 1, 98
  introduction to, 92
  Papovaviridae, 92–94
    papillomaviruses, 92–93, 94f
    polyomaviruses, 93–94
  as risk factor, 12
Vitamin A, 52–53
  for lung neoplasms, 548
  on prostate cancer, 815
Vitamin C, 53
Vitamin D, on prostate cancer, 815
Vitamin E, 53
von Hippel-Lindau disease, 204t

Vulvar cancer, 853–869
  anatomy in, 854–855, 854f, 855f
  clinical presentation of, 857–858, 857f–860f
  diagnosis in, 858–859
  epidemiology of, 853–854, 854t
  follow-up and survival in, 869
  histology in, 856–857
  introduction to, 853
  natural history in, 855–856, 856t
  nuclear imaging techniques for, 255
  pathology and staging of, 362–363, 859–860, 860t, 861t
  patterns of spread in, 855–856, 856t
  prognostic factors for, 860–861
  summary of, 869
  treatment of, 861–869
  treatment of, nonsquamous cell carcinoma, 868–869
  treatment of, preinvasive disease, 861–862
  treatment of, squamous cell carcinoma
    distant metastatic, 868
    recurrent, 868
    T1, 862–863, 863f
    T2, 863–866
      additional treatment, 866
      conservative treatment, 863–864
      inguinofemoral lymphadectomy, 864–866, 864f, 865f
      radical vulvectomy, 864–866, 864f, 865f
      surgical defect closure, 866, 867f, 868f
    T3 and T4, 866–868
Vulvar intraepithelial neoplasia, 861–862

Warthin's tumor, 532
Western blotting, 198
Whipple specimen, 347
Wilm's tumor, 204t
  pathology of, 380–381, 381f
Women's Health Initiative, 65
Women's Health Study, 65
World Health Organization, on bladder tumor classification, 778t

X-linked lymphoproliferation, herpes virus and, 97, 97t
X-rays. *See* Radiology